Associate Editors

GENETIC PRINCIPLES AND HEREDITARY DISEASES

ALEXANDER G. BEARN, M.D.

Professor and Chairman, Department of Medicine, Cornell University Medical College

ENDOCRINE AND METABOLIC DISEASES

NICHOLAS P. CHRISTY, M.D.

Professor of Medicine, Columbia University College of Physicians and Surgeons
at the Roosevelt Hospital

HEMATOLOGIC AND HEMATOPOIETIC DISEASES

RALPH L. NACHMAN, M.D.

Professor of Medicine and Chief of the Division of Hematology,
Cornell University Medical College

DISORDERS OF THE NERVOUS SYSTEM AND BEHAVIOR

FRED PLUM, M.D.

Ann Parrish Titzell Professor and Chairman, Department of Neurology,
Cornell University Medical College

DISEASES OF THE DIGESTIVE SYSTEM

MARVIN H. SLEISENGER, M.D.

Professor and Vice Chairman, Department of Medicine, University of California,
San Francisco

Fourteenth Edition

TEXTBOOK OF MEDICINE VOLUME II

Edited by

PAUL B. BEESON, M.D.

Distinguished Physician, United States Veterans Administration,
University of Washington School of Medicine;
Formerly Nuffield Professor of Clinical Medicine, University of Oxford

WALSH McDERMOTT, M.D.

Professor of Public Affairs in Medicine, Cornell University Medical College;
Attending Physician, The New York Hospital; Special Advisor to the
President, Robert Wood Johnson Foundation

W. B. SAUNDERS COMPANY · Philadelphia · London · Toronto

W. B. Saunders Company: West Washington Square
Philadelphia, PA 19105

12 Dyott Street
London WC1A 1DB

833 Oxford Street
Toronto, Ontario M8Z 5T9, Canada

Library of Congress Cataloging in Publication Data

Main entry under title:

Textbook of medicine.

First–13th editions by R. L. Cecil.

Includes index.

1. Internal medicine.   I. Beeson, Paul B.   II. McDermott,
Walsh, 1909–   III. Cecil, Russell La Fayette, 1881–1965.
Textbook of medicine. [DNLM: 1. Medicine. WB100 T354]

RC46.C4 1975   616   74–4553

ISBN 0–7216–1660–7

Listed here are the latest translated editions of this book, together with
the language of the translation and the publisher:

Portuguese (13th Edition)–Editoria Guanabara Koogan,
                          Rio de Janeiro, Brazil
Serbo-Croat (11th Edition)–Medicinska Knjiga, Belgrade, Yugoslavia
Spanish (13th Edition)–Nueva Editorial Interamericana S.A., de C.V.,
                       Mexico

Textbook of Medicine

Single Vol: ISBN 0-7216-1660-7
Vol I: ISBN 0-7216-1661-5
Vol II: ISBN 0-7216-1662-3

Last digit is the print number: 9   8   7   6   5   4   3   2

Contents

VOLUME I

PART VII. GRANULOMATOUS DISEASES OF UNPROVED ETIOLOGY

PART VIII. MICROBIAL DISEASES

SECTION ONE. VIRAL DISEASES, 182

Viral (and Filter-Passing Microbial) Infections of the Respiratory Tract, 184

PART X.   DISORDERS OF THE NERVOUS SYSTEM AND BEHAVIOR

PART XI. RESPIRATORY DISEASE

SECTION ONE. STRUCTURE AND FUNCTION, 808

SECTION TWO. THE DIAPHRAGM, *J. B. L. Howell,* 816

SECTION THREE. THE CHEST WALL, *J. B. L. Howell,* 817

SECTION FOUR. AIRWAY OBSTRUCTION, 821

Generalized Airway Obstruction: Chronic Obstructive Lung Disease, 821

VOLUME II

PART XII. CARDIOVASCULAR DISEASES

PART XIV.   DISEASES OF THE DIGESTIVE SYSTEM

SECTION ELEVEN. DISEASES OF THE LIVER, *Graham H. Jeffries,* 1324

PART XV. DISEASES OF NUTRITION

PART XVI. HEMATOLOGIC AND HEMATOPOIETIC DISEASES

SECTION ONE.   THE ANEMIAS, 1399

SECTION TWO.   HEMOLYTIC DISORDERS, 1434

PART XVII. DISEASES OF METABOLISM

PART XVIII. DISEASES OF THE ENDOCRINE SYSTEM

PART XX. CERTAIN CUTANEOUS DISEASES WITH SIGNIFICANT SYSTEMIC MANIFESTATIONS

PART XXI. MISCELLANEOUS HEREDITARY DISORDERS AFFECTING MULTIPLE ORGAN SYSTEMS

PART XXII. NORMAL LABORATORY VALUES OF CLINICAL IMPORTANCE

SUMMARY OF CONTENTS

TEXTBOOK
OF
MEDICINE

Part XII
CARDIOVASCULAR DISEASES

541. HEART FAILURE

Alfred P. Fishman

The heart is part of an elaborate circulatory apparatus that is designed to serve two major functions: (1) in the usual course of events, to provide the tissues with sufficient blood (carrying oxygen, substrates, and nutrients) for their metabolic needs, both at rest and during activity; and (2) as a temporary expedient, to reapportion the cardiac output according to the physiologic priorities of the moment, e.g., muscular exercise, heat loss, digestion. The same regulatory mechanisms that satisfy physiologic priorities in health also serve to protect vital organs, e.g., the heart and brain, when cardiac output is seriously compromised.

As a pump, the heart is remarkable not only for its capacity to adjust rapidly to metabolic need and to varying loads, but also for its durability. Unfortunately, it is also vulnerable to a wide array of congenital, metabolic, inflammatory, and degenerative disorders that affect its muscular walls, its linings, its valves, and particularly its nutrient vessels, i.e., the coronary arteries. Some cardiac disorders, such as arteriosclerosis of the small coronary arteries, progress slowly and insidiously, and their disease takes a lifetime to become clinically evident. Others, such as bacterial infection of the aortic valve, are often dramatic in onset and catastrophic in their consequences.

In general, signs and symptoms of heart disease are of two different kinds: those referable to the heart itself, such as pain and palpitation, and others that are extracardiac and originate in congested circulatory beds and hypoperfused organs. Considered out of context, each extracardiac manifestation may be disappointingly nonspecific. For example, breathlessness is a common symptom that is shared by disorders of the heart, the lungs, and the brain. Nonetheless, when breathlessness develops in a patient with left heart disease in association with other evidence of congested and edematous lungs, and grows worse when the patient lies flat, there is little question that the patient is suffering from left heart failure.

Subsequent chapters in Part XII will deal with individual cardiac disorders. The present chapter will be concerned with heart failure, a final common pathway for many of the diverse etiologies and pathogenic mechanisms that will be discussed subsequently.

GENERAL ASPECTS

Heart failure may be considered in clinical, physiologic, or biochemical terms. In the clinic, "heart failure" refers to a distinctive constellation of symptoms and physical signs that has emerged in a patient with an underlying cardiac disorder. The hemodynamic counterpart at that time is an inability of the heart to match its output to the metabolic needs of the body (determined as O_2 consumption) even though filling pressures of the heart are adequate. The biochemical equivalent is not as certain as the hemodynamic, but appears to involve defective conversion by the heart muscle of chemical energy to mechanical work.

By convention, the designation "heart failure" is used as a synonym for myocardial failure. Consequently, heart failure is concerned with a myocardium that is performing inadequately because of either overload or intrinsic disorder. This stipulation automatically excludes syndromes in which the seat of the difficulty is in abnormalities of the heart valves or pericardium or excessive heart rates—each of which can compromise the circulation even though the cardiac muscle is normal.

Disproportion between hemodynamic load and myocardial capacity to cope with it initiates the sequence that culminates in heart failure. In general, the heart tolerates volume overloads better than pressure overloads. For example, *volume* overload of the left ventricle produced by aortic insufficiency may exist for years without causing distress; in contrast, *pressure* overload from aortic stenosis generally elicits signs and symptoms of heart failure much earlier. Sustained overloads are also accommodated better than acute overloads. Thus chronic mitral regurgitation caused by rheumatic heart disease may last for years without signs of heart failure, whereas the acute mitral regurgitation produced by a ruptured chorda tendinea is apt to precipitate a disastrous syndrome of heart failure.

The myocardium responds differently to volume and pressure loads. Volume overloads generally elicit dilatation followed by hypertrophy; conversely, pressure overloads characteristically elicit hypertrophy until late in the natural history when dilatation supervenes. Primary myocardial disease generally elicits both dilatation and hypertrophy.

Categories of Heart Failure

In the clinic, the type of heart failure is generally identified by its durations (acute or chronic), initiating mechanisms, the ventricle that is primarily affected, the characteristic clinical syndrome, and the underlying physiologic derangements.

Acute vs. Chronic Heart Failure. The manifestations of heart failure usually begin insidiously, blurring at the outset with those of the underlying cardiac disorder and continuing gradually into a chronic state. However, the syndrome may also begin acutely, as after myocardial infarction. Between these extremes of acute and chronic heart failure are many instances of subclinical heart failure in which a successful cardiotonic program, coupled with self-restriction of activity by the patient, minimizes signs and symptoms even though cardiac performance remains seriously compromised. On the other hand, it is not uncommon for the course of chronic heart failure that is nicely controlled to be punctuated by bouts of acute heart failure that stem either from lapses in therapy or from progression of the underlying heart disease.

Both acute and chronic heart failure elicit compensatory adjustments. These include increase in peripheral vascular resistance, redistribution of blood flow, and increase in erythropoietic activity. But the adaptive mechanisms differ strikingly in type, degree, and intensity, and even in direction. For example, *acute* distention of the left atrium generally promotes a sodium-poor diuresis, whereas *chronic* distention of the left atrium elicits salt and water retention. This distinction between acute and chronic heart failure must be borne in mind when attempting to relate observations on experimental heart failure in animals to the clinical syndrome of chronic heart failure in man, because experimental heart failure is generally acute in onset, is fulminating in course, and is generally ended abruptly by the death of the animal.

Initiating Mechanisms. Each initiating mechanism generally imposes its own distinctive stamp upon the clinical syndrome. Thus rheumatic heart disease leads to a different constellation of symptoms and signs from that of hypertensive heart disease; in turn, both have a different natural history from cor pulmonale. Indeed, even a single etiology, arteriosclerosis, may have distinctly different consequences; progressive narrowing and gradual occlusion of *peripheral* branches of the coronary arteries may be so covert that the characteristic shortness of breath and undue fatigue of left ventricular failure may be misinterpreted as evidence of the general physical decline of advancing age. Conversely, abrupt closure of a major coronary artery, as a consequence of thrombosis superimposed on an arteriosclerotic plaque, may elicit massive myocardial necrosis, followed by extensive myocardial scarring and unremitting heart failure.

Left vs. Right Heart Failure. With rare exception, one ventricle fails before the other. Because of the prevalence of cardiac disorders which overload or damage the left ventricle, e.g., coronary arteriosclerosis and hypertension, heart failure usually begins with the left ventricle. Breathlessness, the key clinical expression of pulmonary congestion and edema, is the most common initial complaint. Conversely, when the right ventricle fails, systemic venous congestion and peripheral edema generally predominate. Left ventricular failure is the most common cause of right ventricular failure, and breathlessness often improves as right ventricular output falls and pulmonary congestion diminishes.

The mechanism by which left ventricular failure causes the right ventricle to fail is not entirely clear, although pulmonary (venous and arterial) hypertension from the failing left ventricle and the continuity of heart muscle around both ventricles are undoubtedly involved. In contrast to the accepted sequence of left ventricular failure followed by right ventricular failure, it is still debated whether isolated right ventricular failure inevitably elicits left ventricular failure. The latter association is difficult to prove because of the frequent coexistence of independent and unrelated left ventricular disease in patients with right ventricular failure.

The combination of combined left and right ventricular failure, in which evidences of systemic and pulmonary venous hypertension predominate, is traditionally referred to as "congestive heart failure." This is a colloquialism that conveys the image of severe physical incapacity, breathlessness, distended neck veins, hepatic engorgement, and troublesome peripheral edema. But it

also highlights clinical features that can be measured at the bedside: a high venous pressure, a prolonged circulation time, and a diminished vital capacity, all of which improve as the patient gets better.

Backward vs. Forward Heart Failure. Somewhat reminiscent of the fable about the blind men and the elephant is the vintage controversy about "backward" versus "forward" heart failure. "Backward failure" calls attention to the damming up of blood in the veins proximal to the failing ventricle and attributes to this venous congestion a critical role in the evolution of the syndrome of heart failure; "forward failure" assigns the same pivotal role to a decrease in cardiac output and underfilling of the arterial tree. In reality this distinction is meaningless, because it is inevitable in a closed circuit that the inability of the heart to sustain its output (forward failure) and the pooling of blood on the venous inflow side (backward failure) must go hand in hand.

Low vs. High Output Failure. Cardiac catheterization in man has made it possible to sort myocardial failure according to the level of the cardiac output. This practice has served at least three purposes: (1) to separate, on clinical and physiologic grounds, a type of myocardial failure ("high output failure") in which the circulation remains vigorous and the extremities remain warm despite venous congestion, edema, and a lower cardiac output than existed prior to the heart failure; (2) to emphasize that the level of the cardiac output and the circulatory adjustments during myocardial failure are, to large extent, a consequence of the cardiac output that existed prior to heart failure; and (3) to relate etiology and clinical evidences of heart failure to the state of the circulation: the more common causes of heart failure – arteriosclerosis, hypertension, myocardial disease, valvular disease, and pericardial disease – tend to be low output states; less common causes, such as hyperthyroidism, Paget's disease, anemia, beriberi, arteriovenous fistula, tend to be high output states. But the hemodynamic hallmark of cardiac failure remains the same regardless of the level of cardiac output at rest: an inability of the heart to increase its output (or stroke volume or stroke work) as end-diastolic volume (as well as pressure) is increased (see Frank-Starling Principle, below).

The separation into "high" and "low" output failure is concerned with the clinical manifestations, rather than the causes, of myocardial failure. But it is also a hemodynamic frame of reference to which the anatomist and the biochemist can relate the myocardial origins of heart failure. For example, "high output" failure probably has different biochemical bases from "low output" failure. Nor are all types of "low output" or "high output" failure apt to have the same biochemical origins. For example, it is unlikely that the "high output" failure of a peripheral arteriovenous fistula has the same anatomic or biochemical beginnings and evolution as the "high output" failure of severe anemia or malnutrition.

Congestive Failure vs. Congested State. Overfilling of both venous circulations, without myocardial failure, is the hallmark of the "congested state." It may be induced by rapid infusions; it may also occur in the course of "hyperkinetic" circulatory states as diverse as severe anemia and peripheral arteriovenous fistula. Similar but less dramatic venous congestion may also complicate Paget's disease or beriberi. In each of these situations, venous hypertension may arise from a combination of an expanded venous volume and heightened venomotor tone, rather than from heart failure.

It is true that persistence of a "hyperkinetic" congested state may, in time, cause the heart muscle to fail from overwork. The onset of myocardial failure may then be difficult to detect on clinical grounds, because the hyperkinetic circulation persists and the congestion may be only slightly increased during myocardial failure. Accordingly, the transition from the congested state to congestive heart failure may be difficult to detect on clinical grounds alone. But when heart failure does supervene, cardiac catheterization will disclose an inadequate increase in cardiac output during exercise as well as a considerable increase in cardiac output after digitalis. Fortunately, identification of the transition from a "congested state" to "congestive heart failure" is of greater theoretical than practical importance, because therapeutic measures, such as the administration of diuretics and the replacement of particular nutrients, e.g., thiamin in beriberi, are effective in both situations. However, digitalis will exert an important therapeutic effect once the myocardium has failed, whereas it is clinically useless when administered to a heart that is coping well with an overfilled circulation.

Subcellular Bases for Contraction

With each beat, the heart develops force and expends energy. Electrical activity at the cell surface activates the contractile machinery. Connecting the electrical activity at the surface and the contractile machinery within the muscle cell is the sarcoplasmic reticulum which plays a critical role in the release and uptake of calcium during contraction and relaxation.

For the development of the contractile force, heart muscle depends on interactions among contractile proteins, the hypothetical "elastic components" with which they are connected in series, and the constraining bounds within which the contractile elements function. The contractile proteins are contained within sarcomeres, repeating units that comprise the individual muscle fibers (myofibrils). Within the sarcomere, the contractile proteins are arranged in two orderly groups of myofilaments, one consisting of myosin, the other predominantly of actin. Holding the contractile apparatus at bay are two modulator proteins, troponin and tropomyosin. Delivery of calcium to troponin from the sarcoplasmic reticulum and sarcolemma sets the contractile process into motion.

To account for changes in the length of heart muscle during contraction and relaxation, the sliding filament hypothesis of Huxley is generally invoked: during contraction, the thin actin filaments slide past the thicker myosin filaments to shorten the sarcomere; the entire muscle cell follows suit. Conversely, during relaxation, the sarcomeres and the muscle cell resume their initial lengths as the original actin-myosin relationships are restored. Nearby mitochondria generate energy for the contractile machinery by oxidative phosphorylation of free fatty acids and glucose supplied by the circulation.

The tension that is developed in cardiac muscle during contraction depends on actin-myosin relationships. Projecting from the myosin filaments are cross-bridges. Before activation, these bridges are not attached to actin filaments. Upon activation, the cross-bridges on the myosin filaments lock into receptor sites on the actin filaments, thereby developing the force that leads to contraction. As the muscle shortens, the cross-bridges disengage and slide along the actin filament, like a pawl on a ratchet, to engage other sites. Depending on the number of cross-bridges that are interlocked at the same time, different tensions will be developed.

In addition to these subcellular elements that are directly involved in the contractile process, there appears to be a subcellular beta sympathomimetic system that can enhance the inotropic state. Although an increase in intracellular calcium is involved, the precise mechanism is unclear.

Evidence exists that for the sarcomere, as for the whole heart (see Frank-Starling Principle), the tension developed during contraction is directly related to its initial length. This correspondence implies that, for the whole heart, stretching increases the ability of its individual contractile elements to develop force. Also, since stretching does not affect the rate of interaction of active sites, elongation of cardiac muscle fibers before contraction should not affect the velocity of the subsequent contraction. These considerations underlie many current notions about cardiac contractility. But it is still unclear whether the ultrastructural-physiologic correlations are real or simply models for eliciting a new kind of reflection about an exceedingly complicated problem.

PATHOPHYSIOLOGIC INTERPLAY

Each ventricle functions as a separate muscular pump supplied by its own booster pump (atrium). The two ventricles empty in unison, simultaneously dispatching their respective contents: the right ventricle sending blood to the lungs for arterialization, the left ventricle sending arterialized blood to the rest of the body for metabolic purposes. In the normal heart, at least 50 per cent of the end-diastolic volume is ejected with each beat. Much of the ejection force is the result of the inherent properties (fiber-length and inotropism) of the myocardium. But a wide range of adaptability to the ever-changing metabolic needs of daily life is provided by a superimposed series of extrinsic neurohumoral adjustments which, in daily life, modify and obscure the intrinsic inherent properties of the heart muscle.

Each ventricle, as with any man-made machine, is endowed with a finite capacity for stress, strain, and repair. The two ventricles also have somewhat different designs in keeping with their different long-range functions as pumps. The rate of obsolescence of each ventricle depends on the wear and tear to which it is subjected, its supply of nutriments and substrates, and its continuing state of good health. Before birth, both ventricles are taxed equally, because they bear the same pressure loads. After birth, as pulmonary arterial pressure falls, the right ventricular burden decreases and its walls thin. Consequently, other influences remaining equal, the durability of right ventricular performance is destined from birth to exceed that of the left ventricle. The brighter prospects of the right ventricle for longevity in performance are intensified by the greater vulnerability of the left side of the heart to disease and to disorders in its blood supply.

Chronic Compensatory Mechanisms

Two principal mechanisms mark the progression from normal myocardial performance to myocardial failure: hypertrophy and dilatation.

Hypertrophy.   An increase in the muscle mass of a ventricle takes time to develop. It involves increased protein synthesis in response to mechanical overload or dilatation. The common denominator for these two mechanisms may be the Laplace relationship (Fig. 1) which indicates that an increase in wall tension (stress) follows an increase in pressure or radius. Early in hypertrophy, muscle mass and capillary vessels increase proportionately and the contractile properties of the myocardium are preserved. But later, the inotropic behavior becomes abnormal and the capacity of the myocardium to synthesize adrenergic transmitter decreases. Indeed, once hypertrophy begins, the myocardium has been eased on to the road to failure.

In the depressed inotropic state associated with hypertrophy, circulatory function is maintained for a long while by the combination of the increase in muscle mass, the Frank-Starling mechanism (Fig. 2), and augmented sympathetic stimulation. But as the myocardial inotropic state continues to deteriorate, perhaps after intrinsic catecholamine stores have been depleted, circulatory compensation can no longer be maintained. Resting cardiac output then falls and filling pressures increase, leading to the clinical and hemodynamic manifestations of overt congestive heart failure.

Dilatation. Progressive and persistent dilatation marks the transition between ventricular hypertrophy and failure. For a long while, dilatation may serve as a compensatory mechanism, increasing the contractile force of the heart by way of the Frank-Starling relationship. But dilatation gradually becomes inadequate to maintain stroke output.

Several different mechanisms seem to be involved in the ultimate inability of the dilated heart to maintain its output: (1) slippage and rearrangement of sarcomeres during progressive dilatation; as a result, they neither produce a coordinated contraction nor are properly stretched to enhance contractility as the heart dilates further; (2) high wall tension in accord with the law of Laplace (Fig. 1); as the volume of the ventricle increases so that its wall tension for a given pressure in the ventricular cavity during contraction is greater than normal, the myocardial oxygen consumption increases accordingly; (3) protracted maintenance of high wall tension during contraction; in contrast to the normal heart, in which the wall tension decreases in the course of systole, wall tension remains high in the dilated heart; (4) high energy requirements coupled with an inefficient conversion of chemical to mechanical energy; despite the decrease in stroke output, the dilated heart does more internal work and has a higher myocardial oxygen consumption than does the normal heart. Because of these limitations, chronic enlargement is an inefficient and ill-fated mechanism for achieving sustained improvement in cardiac performance.

Assessment of Cardiac Performance

With respect to evaluating cardiac performance, the heart may be regarded from three points of view: as a pump; as a muscle; and as a component of the circulation. Hemodynamic measurements are used to characterize its behavior as a pump: cardiac output, stroke output, stroke work, stroke power, ventricular end-diastolic pressure, ejection fraction, and ventricular end-diastolic volume. To ascertain its behavior as a muscle, principles of muscle mechanics are applied. Its adequacy as a component of the circulation is reflected in the derangements that result from the low cardiac output, the redistribution of blood flow among tissues and organs, organ hypoperfusion, and venous congestion.

Heart as a Pump: Hemodynamics

By the time the heart fails, a variety of mechanisms are operating to bolster its flagging performance. In contrast to the inappropriately low cardiac output, the blood pressure generally remains normal or even increases.

Cardiac Output. At each level of activity, in health and disease, a complicated interplay automatically adjusts the extent of shortening of myocardial fibers and, consequently, the stroke volume and the cardiac output. Four principal determinants set the stroke volume: preload (end-diastolic volume), afterload (impedance to ventricular emptying during systole), the inotropic characteristics of the heart, and the coordinated pattern of contraction. A fifth determinant, the heart rate, sets the cardiac output (stroke volume times heart rate). For practical purposes, three of these five principal determinants of cardiac output—preload, afterload, heart rate—are quantifiable. The fourth, the pattern of contraction, can be evaluated qualitatively. But the fifth, inotropic state, remains difficult to determine except when distortions are so gross that they can be detected at the bedside or visualized by fluoroscopy.

Relationships among these determinants are not fixed; they play greater or lesser roles, depending on the state of the heart. Thus when the inherent contractility (inotropic state) is impaired, stroke output and cardiac output may be maintained by ventricular dilatation (Frank-Starling mechanism). This flexible arrangement limits the value of cardiac output as a measure of cardiac contractility (inotropic state) to situations in which preload, afterload, and heart rate can be held constant. Unfortunately, this degree of control of loading conditions and heart rate is easier to achieve in the experimental laboratory than in clinical situations.

Indicator-dilution techniques are now widely used for the bedside determination of cardiac output. The normal range in adults at rest is between 2.5 and 3.6 liters per minute per square meter. A decrease in cardiac output at rest represents a late stage in abnormal cardiac performance. Failure to increase cardiac output during exercise occurs much earlier. Thus in normal subjects exercising in a supine position, the increase in cardiac output

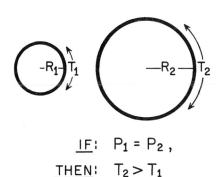

IF: $P_1 = P_2$,

THEN: $T_2 > T_1$

Figure 1. An illustration of the Laplace equation ($T = P \times R$). The mean tension in the wall of the heart during systole (T) is directly proportional to the product of the mean radius (R) and the mean transmural pressure (P) that the wall is supporting. Dilatation of the heart ($R_2 > R_1$) at the same pressure ($P_1 = P_2$) is associated with an increase in wall tension ($T_2 > T_1$).

exceeds 600 ml per minute for each 100 ml increase in oxygen consumption. Lower values indicate abnormal cardiac performance. In heart failure, the arteriovenous difference for oxygen is abnormally wide, resulting almost entirely from the low oxygen content of venous blood returning to the heart rather than from impaired oxygenation in the lungs.

During exercise, heart rate and cardiac output increase as linear functions of oxygen consumption. This is true during both supine and upright exercise, but for any level of exercise the cardiac output is appreciably lower in the upright position. These increases in cardiac output are accomplished principally by acceleration of the heart rate rather than by increase in the stroke volume. In heart failure, cardiac output is even more dependent on heart rate, both at rest and during exercise.

Ventricular End-Diastolic Pressure. Inadequate ventricular emptying during systole leads to an increase in the residual volume of blood in the ventricle after systole, and thereby to an increase in end-diastolic ventricular volume. Since end-diastolic ventricular volumes are difficult to measure, end-diastolic ventricular pressures are generally substituted, thereby taking advantage of the predictable relationship between diastolic pressure and volume in the ventricle as long as the compliance of the ventricular wall remains normal. Accordingly, if ventricular compliance can be assumed to be normal, an end-diastolic pressure in the *left* ventricle greater than 12 mm Hg is a sign of depressed myocardial function; correspondingly, a value greater than 10 mm Hg in the *right* ventricle is abnormal. It is rather simple to estimate the right ventricular end-diastolic pressure by measuring the central venous pressure; the left ventricular end-diastolic pressure is more difficult to estimate because of its inaccessibility. However, in the absence of mitral obstruction or of an increase in pulmonary vascular resistance, pulmonary arterial diastolic pressure may be used to obtain an estimate of left ventricular end-diastolic pressure. Similar information can be obtained from a pulmonary wedge pressure.

Frank-Starling Principle. The Frank-Starling principle describes the force of contraction, generally measured as the work done by the ventricle per beat, as a function of ventricular end-diastolic volume. The end-diastolic volume (initial fiber length) depends in large measure upon the venous return. According to the Frank-Starling relationship, ventricular function curves may be determined by successively increasing venous return, thereby increasing the volume of blood in the ventricle at the end of diastole and the subsequent stroke output (Fig. 2).

The shape and position of the ventricular function curve are modified by autonomic nervous activity. Figure 2 illustrates the displacement of the curve produced by sympathetic nervous activity or the administration of norepinephrine. It also illustrates the effects of heart failure in displacing the curve. It is noteworthy that the failing heart operates on a lower curve instead of slipping over the hump of a single curve onto a descending limb; digitalis relocates the position of the curve toward normal. Although a descending limb has been described in experimental heart failure and occasionally in human subjects with diffuse myocardial disease who have been subjected to physical stress, ventricular function curves in man generally do not show a descending limb.

In the normal heart, the Frank-Starling mechanism operates chiefly to match the stroke outputs of the two ventricles. But in heart failure this mechanism plays an important role in sustaining the cardiac output.

Ejection Fraction. Normally the ratio of stroke volume to left ventricular end-diastolic volume (determined angiographically) ranges from 0.56 to 0.78. A reduced ejection fraction suggests a decrease in myocardial performance.

Systolic Time Intervals. Simultaneous recording of the electrocardiogram, phonocardiogram, and carotid arterial pulse allows indirect bedside appraisal of cardiac function. By this combination of recordings, total electromechanical systole is subdivided into left ventricular ejection time and the pre-ejection period. In patients with abnormalities of myocardial contractility—even before overt congestive heart failure—pre-ejection time usually lengthens, whereas ejection time shortens (the normal ratio of pre-ejection time to left ventricular ejection time is 0.35 ± 0.04 SD). This noninvasive technique is most useful in chronic coronary artery disease, arterial hypertension, and the cardiomyopathies. It does not distinguish between inotropic state and other mechanical determinants of contractility, particularly loading of the ventricle. Disturbances in conduction, valvular disease, and other unanticipated disorders may invalidate the determinations.

Heart as a Muscle

The contractile performance of the heart depends on two essential components: fiber length (Frank-Starling mechanism) and the inherent contractility (inotropic state) of the muscle.

Contractility. Increase in sympathetic nervous activity provides the major inotropic effect for the normal heart (in conjunction with increase in heart rate and venous tone). In contrast to the Frank-Starling mechanism, the increase in force and velocity of contraction is accomplished without corresponding increase in fiber length (end-diastolic ventricular volume).

Inotropic State. Clinicians would welcome an objective index of myocardial contractility in which the inotropic state (intrinsic contractility of the muscle) could be measured independent of change in the length of

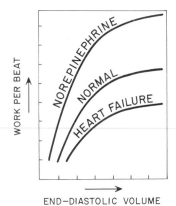

Figure 2. Hypothetical Frank-Starling relationships for different states of myocardial contractility. Enhanced contractility, as after sympathetic nervous stimulation or the administration of norepinephrine, moves the normal curve toward one in which more stroke work is done at lower filling pressures. In heart failure, as contractility is progressively impaired and the heart continues to dilate, the relationship is displaced to a lower curve instead of slipping along a single curve on to a descending limb.

myocardial fibers (Frank-Starling relationship). This would be useful in three different ways: (1) to examine the effects on the myocardium of an acute intervention, such as the administration of digitalis, (2) to determine consecutive changes in the inotropic state of the myocardium in the same individual during the evolution of heart failure and in response to treatment; and (3) to compare the inotropic state in different individuals.

Unfortunately, distinction between the effects of fiber length and of intrinsic contractility is difficult to accomplish for the heart. The main obstacle stems from the strong influence of mechanical loading conditions on hemodynamic measurements. Thus a change in either the preload (length of ventricular fibers at end-diastole) or the afterload (force developed in ventricular muscle during systole) can modify ventricular performance greatly without affecting its intrinsic inotropic state. Another complication is the inability of conventional hemodynamic measurements to take heart size into account so that comparisons of contractility in hearts of different size are generally unreliable.

Because changes in mechanical loading conditions confuse determinations of inotropic state, attempts are being made (1) to make these determinations under constant conditions of mechanical loading (constant diastolic volume, aortic pressure) and heart rate, (2) to devise methods for determining inotropic state that are insensitive to loading conditions, or (3) to interpret hemodynamic values in terms of a change in inotropic state when loading conditions can be adequately discounted. But when determinants of mechanical performance other than inotropic state cannot be discounted – which is usually the case – more independent indices of contractility have been sought, particularly the rate of rise in ventricular pressure in the pre-ejection phase of ventricular contraction and force-velocity relationships.

Rate of Increase in Intraventricular Pressure (dp/dt). Several indices of dp/dt are being used. In practice, dp/dt is determined electronically as the first derivative of the ventricular pressure. For comparative purposes, measurements are generally made at some preselected point(s) in the cardiac cycle, e.g., at 40 mm Hg. Often the value for dp/dt is further standardized by reference to some common denominator; e.g., peak dp/dt may be divided by total pressure instead of being used as dp/dt, per se. At present, application in man of the dp/dt determinations is handicapped by the need for extraordinarily high fidelity recording systems and by the difficulty in reproducing loading conditions. Although it holds considerable promise for comparisons of contractile performance in a single patient before and after intervention, it has little prospect for comparing different hearts. Attempts to obtain a related kind of information by using an end-catheter velocity gauge to determine the rate at which blood is ejected into the aorta are promising but are still in their infancy.

As in the case of pressure, the rate of development of wall tension is also decidedly abnormal in heart failure. Moreover, in contrast to the normal heart in which wall tension decreases during systole, wall tension in heart failure remains high throughout systole so that both the velocity and the degree of shortening are abnormal.

Velocity of Contraction. The use of the velocity of contraction as a measure of contractility involves the force-velocity relationship originally developed by A. V. Hill for skeletal muscle. According to this relationship, the velocity of shortening in skeletal muscle is inversely related to the magnitude of the tension that the muscle develops, i.e., the greater the load that the muscle is obliged to lift during contraction, the slower its speed of shortening. In skeletal muscle, this relationship is a hyperbolic one, the intercept on the velocity axis being called V_{max} (velocity at zero force), whereas the intercept on the force axis (force at zero velocity) is called P_0.

Applying this relationship to the myocardium (Fig. 3), the position of the force-velocity curve would be affected both by a change in end-diastolic fiber length (initial stretch or preload) and by a change in inherent inotropic activity. But the effects would be different. Thus a change in the degree of initial stretch of the heart muscle, and presumably in the number of active sites at which the chemical reactions of contraction can occur, would modify the total force that the muscle develops; in Figure 3, this change would shift the horizontal, but not the vertical, intercept (P_0). In contrast, a change in inotropic activity by cardiotonic agents, on the one hand, or myocardial failure, on the other, would be expected not only to affect the horizontal intercept (total force) but also to displace the force-velocity curve with respect to the vertical axis (rate of force-generating processes). Indeed, the original observations on skeletal muscle even suggested that an ideal measure of contractility might be obtained by extrapolating the force-velocity relationships to the vertical axis (V_{max}), thereby determining the maximal velocity of shortening that would exist at zero load. Although it is acknowledged that P_0 is length dependent, the claim has been made that for heart muscle V_{max} is independent of length. Unfortunately, the latter claim has not been substantiated; consequently, V_{max} does not automatically distinguish between effects of Frank-Starling relationship and changes in inotropic state.

It should be stressed that the assessment of force-velocity relations in the human heart is still empirical and in its infancy. Serious reservations have been expressed about the relevance of the ultrastructural model, which depicts contractile elements in series with elastic elements, to heart muscle. At present, the assessment of force-velocity relations is a technical feat which involves a combination of cineangiography, high fidelity

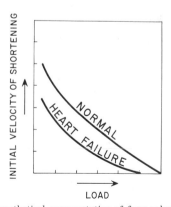

Figure 3. Hypothetical representation of force-velocity changes in heart failure. Under special conditions of loading, the position of the force-velocity curve is determined by the inotropic state of the myocardium. The force-velocity relationship shifts as shown during heart failure, decreasing both the velocity of shortening at any given load and the maximal developed tension. V_{max}, which may be obtained by extrapolation to the vertical axis, is not shown, because the interpretation of this extrapolation is uncertain. (Modified from Braunwald, E., Ross, J., Jr., and Sonnenblick, E. H.: Mechanisms of Contraction of the Normal and Failing Heart. Boston, Little, Brown & Company, 1968.)

recording of ventricular pressures, and an assumed geometric model of the ventricular cavity as a basis for relating wall stress to the velocity and extent of shortening. But these practical limitations should not obscure the conceptual values of the new approaches to contractility. Moreover, even though direct determinations of force-velocity relationships have yet to be made on the human heart in failure, there is little reason to doubt that in the human heart, as in the isolated papillary muscle, myocardial failure will prove to be associated with a decrease in both the force and the velocity of myocardial contraction.

Finally, although the experimental techniques described in this chapter for determination of inotropic state are invasive, elaborate, and expensive, they not only promise fresh insights into myocardial contractility but may also pave the way for noninvasive, bedside techniques by providing reliable standards of reference and calibration as well as a bank of useful empirical information about myocardial performance.

Relaxation and Distensibility. Although most studies of ventricular performance during heart failure have centered around the contraction phase, the course of the relaxation phase (diastole) influences the pattern of the subsequent cardiac contraction. The filling of the ventricle during diastole depends not only on the time available but also on the pattern of relaxation. Relaxation consists of two components: an active one, which promotes relaxation by way of intrinsic mechanisms; and a passive one, arising from extension of the fibers by the inflowing blood. Incomplete relaxation would be expected not only to increase the filling pressure of the heart but also to dissipate energy. In the normal heart, the active and passive components appear to work synergistically to minimize losses in chemical energy. But in heart failure the viscous and elastic properties of the heart muscle seem to change so that there is a diminished resistance to filling (decreased "impedance") and an increased extent of ventricular expansion on filling (increased "compliance"). Thus not only the velocity and duration of relaxation but also changes in the physical properties of the muscle seem involved in heart failure.

Energetics. The heart does work and expends energy during contraction. The principal determinants of myocardial oxygen consumption are the tension developed in the ventricular wall during systole (a function of systolic pressure and ventricular volume), the heart rate, and the inotropic state (contractility) of the ventricular muscle; of less importance is the stroke volume. Myocardial wall tension is described by the Laplace relation which relates pressure, radius, and wall thickness.

For its contraction, the heart depends on the conversion of the chemical energy of oxidizable substrates into the mechanical energy of muscular contraction. ATP participates in this process as the principal store of energy released by oxidation; its breakdown by myosin ATPase is the principal way by which chemical energy is transformed into mechanical energy. ATP resynthesis in the myocardium is accomplished chiefly through oxidative phosphorylation. The rate of ATP breakdown and the quantity of energy used by the myocardium depend chiefly on the tension that is developed in the myocardial fibers rather than on the degree of shortening or the work done; this developed tension causes the ventricular walls to contract and the blood to be ejected. From a biochemical point of view, the muscle of a ventricle has failed when its generation of free energy, or its utiliza-

tion of that energy in the process of contraction, is insufficient for the circulatory load which it has to handle.

Unfortunately, the biochemical basis for heart failure is not yet settled. But it is now clear that there are no consistent defects in energy metabolism or in protein synthesis. The investigative focus at present is on excitation-coupling and the role of calcium in the contractile process.

Heart as Component of Circulation

As the overburdened ventricle fails, it elicits venous hypertension and slowed circulation, and sets into motion peripheral mechanisms to sustain blood pressure and cardiac output.

Venous Hypertension. With the onset of failure, the ventricle fails to empty properly during systole so that the volume of blood left in the ventricle after contraction increases, i.e., ejection fraction decreases. An increase in diastolic pressure in the ventricles and in the atrium and veins that lead to the ventricle accompanies the increase in ventricular volume. Several other elements contribute to the venous hypertension: (1) heightened venomotor tone; (2) expansion of the blood volume as a consequence of sodium retention by the kidney; and, on occasion, (3) regurgitation of blood from ventricle to atrium as the atrioventricular valve becomes incompetent either from ventricular dilatation of from improper closure during an arrhythmia.

Slowed Circulation. The circulation time depends on the cardiac output and the volume of blood interposed between the sites of sampling and injection. Should either ventricle fail, the time for a tracer substance to pass from the site of intravenous injection to the site of detection will be prolonged. For example, in left heart failure, the arm-to-tongue circulation time, measured by using Decholin as a tracer, will be prolonged beyond the normal limits of 10 to 15 seconds; delay of the tracer in traversing the pulmonary circulation and dilated left heart, as well as excessive dilution of the tracer by the enlarged intervening blood volume, contributes to the delay. Similarly, the arm-to-breath circulation time measured after the intravenous injection of ether will be prolonged in right heart failure. By relating the circulation times to the central venous pressure, it may be possible to establish at the bedside which ventricle has failed. For example, in left heart failure, central venous pressure and ether circulation time will be normal, whereas Decholin time will be prolonged.

Peripheral Mechanisms to Sustain Cardiac Output and Blood Pressure. In order to sustain the cardiac output, to apportion it selectively, and to maintain the systemic arterial blood pressure, a variety of peripheral mechanisms are activated.

Autonomic Nervous System. Normally, a four- or fivefold increase in oxygen consumption elicits a doubling of the cardiac output. When the increase in cardiac output cannot keep pace with the level of activity, distribution of blood flow is altered to defend vital areas, e.g., brain and heart. The autonomic nervous system is deeply involved in this rearrangement of the circulation. It also contributes to activation of the mechanisms for retaining sodium and water.

Peripheral vasoconstriction and tachycardia are the hallmarks of the usual forms of heart failure. Paradoxically, despite a generalized increase in sympathetic nervous activity, norepinephrine stores in the heart muscle are depleted because of defective local synthesis. Consequently, the failing heart, denied local adrenergic support for its inotropic and chronotropic responses, is obliged to rely on norepinephrine delivered to it by the blood from the adrenal medulla and the peripheral vasculature. Pharmacologic agents, such as guanethidine, which further deplete the heart of its catecholamines, aggravate heart failure. In many respects, the performance of the human heart that has failed resembles that of both the "denervated" heart and the isolated heart-lung preparation that Starling used. The role that the parasympathetic nervous system plays in heart failure is ill defined, but evidence does exist to indicate that its contribution to the control of heart rate and baroreceptor activity is impaired.

PERIPHERAL VASOCONSTRICTION. Peripheral arteriolar and venoconstriction, mediated by heightened sympathetic nervous activity, are essential compensatory mechanisms in heart failure. The extent to which accumulation of sodium and water in the arteriolar wall contributes to increased arteriolar resistance is as yet unclear. Selective arteriolar vasoconstriction helps not only to sustain the blood pressure but also to preserve function in critical organs. The pattern of selective vasoconstriction, in turn, influences the cardiac output by determining the total peripheral resistance to cardiac emptying.

Selective venoconstriction promotes venous return by transfer of returning blood to the central veins. Although peripheral venoconstriction may contribute importantly to the increase in central venous pressure, the major determinant is myocardial incompetence in coping with the venous return.

REDISTRIBUTION. In order to maintain oxygen delivery to vital organs (brain and myocardium) during heart failure, blood flow is diverted by heightened sympathetic nervous activity from skin, kidneys, splanchnic viscera, and muscle. At first the redistribution of blood flow among organs occurs during activity or stress, i.e., as cardiac output fails to increase appropriately for the increment in metabolism; later it operates also at rest. The mechanism for diversion is the balance between sympathetic innervation and local metabolism: the circulations to skin, kidney, splanchnic organs, and skeletal muscle are richly innervated, and these viscera have low metabolic rates; sympathetic nervous vasoconstriction easily overrides local metabolites. In contrast, the circulations to brain and myocardium are poor in alpha-adrenergic receptors; these organs, with high oxygen consumption, produce ample metabolic dilators to counterbalance heightened sympathetic activity.

In the normal subject during exercise, as need for heat dissipation increases, cutaneous hyperemia develops. In contrast, the patient in heart failure fails to develop cutaneous hyperemia despite increasing need for heat dissipation. The net effect is that the patient in heart failure, suffering from a low cardiac output during exercise, preserves blood pressure and blood flow to vital organs by paying the penalty of impaired heat loss as well as inadequate blood flow to exercising muscles.

VALSALVA MANEUVER. An abnormal response to the Valsalva maneuver, in which intrathoracic pressure is maintained at approximately 40 mm Hg for 10 to 12 seconds, is a useful test for left heart failure. The autonomic nervous system, operating in conjunction with the expanded volume of blood in the left side of the heart and pulmonary venous system, contributes to the abnormal response. During strain, the normal subject manifests a characteristic decrease in blood pressure and pulse pressure and increase in heart rate; when straining stops, the blood pressure, pulse pressure, and bradycardia "overshoot." In contrast, the patient in left heart failure demonstrates a "square wave response" of blood pressure: at the start of straining, blood pressure increases abruptly, stays high during the maneuver, and drops precipitously to baseline after the maneuver, without overshoot. Throughout the procedure there is little or no change in pulse pressure and no tachycardia. The lack of reflex changes stems from the failure of stroke output or arterial pulse pressure to change during the straining phase, so that no reflex changes are elicited in peripheral vessels.

Salt and Water Retention. As the patient slips into heart failure, the reduction in cardiac output is associated with a decrease in renal blood flow and glomerular filtration rate, and with a redistribution of blood flow within the kidneys. These hemodynamic changes undoubtedly contribute to the sodium and water retention of heart failure, but in different ways and to different degrees according to the stage of heart failure. Early in heart failure, when filtration rate is decreased, much of the sodium retention is attributable to the decrease in the filtered load of sodium presented to the tubules for reabsorption. Later on, humoral factors, predominantly hyperaldosteronism and a group of extra-adrenal, sodium-retaining influences ("factor III") predominate.

There is little doubt that disturbed hemodynamics are importantly involved in the release of the humoral factors. Thus a large role is currently envisaged for diminished baroreceptor stimulation in the renal afferent arterioles or a decrease in the sodium load passing the macula densa, or both, in activating the renin-angiotensin-aldosterone mechanism. In addition, baroreceptor effects arising in the distended left atrium or underfilled arterial tree may affect renal hemodynamics and the renin-angiotensin-aldosterone system. Other reflexes engaged in the intense sympathetic activity of heart failure may also be involved. Clearly, the hemodynamic-neurohumoral interplay that results in sodium and water retention is complex and incompletely understood. On the other hand, awareness of the important role of hyperaldosteronism in the genesis of sodium and water retention has provided new approaches to the therapy of heart failure using aldosterone antagonists.

Not only urine but also sweat and saliva are sodium poor. But the underlying mechanisms are different. Antidiuretic hormone is not directly involved in the genesis of the edema of heart failure.

The expansion of the circulating blood volume contributes to sustaining the cardiac output and the perfusion of vital organs. Rarely is the expansion in blood volume marked, usually ranging from 10 to 20 per cent in moderately severe heart failure to 30 to 50 per cent in severe, refractory heart failure. But even modest expansion helps to augment the ventricular end-diastolic volume, thereby improving ventricular performance by way of the Frank-Starling principle. Unfortunately, the high end-diastolic volume and pressures promote the formation of edema by raising capillary pressures in the circulation behind the failing ventricle. At a time when circulation blood volume may be increased by 20 per cent, the extravascular fluid volume may have doubled.

CLINICAL MANIFESTATIONS OF HEART FAILURE

The signs and symptoms of heart failure depend on the ventricle that has failed and the duration of the failure. The clinical syndrome of left ventricular failure is dominated by *symptoms* of pulmonary congestion and edema. In contrast, right ventricular failure is dominated by *signs* of systemic venous congestion and peripheral edema. Fatigue and weakness are common in both types of heart failure.

Left Ventricular Failure

Symptoms

Complaints of respiratory discomfort or distress dominate the symptoms of left ventricular failure. They vary with position, stress, and activity. They are often associated with physical signs of disturbances in the lungs or in respiratory control mechanisms.

Dyspnea. Like pain or anxiety, dyspnea is subjective and difficult to quantify. Because breathing is ordinarily automatic and effortless except after strenuous exertion, the complaint of breathlessness may signify anything from awareness to distress. Dyspnea during modest exertion is usually the first symptom of left heart failure. Usually dyspnea is associated with increased rate of breathing (tachypnea).

The physiologic basis for the sensation of dyspnea remains unclear. Both lungs and the chest muscles may contribute. Thus interstitial edema in the vicinity of the pulmonary capillaries stimulates juxtacapillary receptors ("J-receptors"), thereby reflexly setting a pattern of rapid, shallow breathing; associated with this abnormal pattern is an increase in the work and oxygen cost of moving the stiff lungs. However, this increased amount of work on the lungs is done in the face of diminished blood flow to the respiratory muscles, a consequence of the diminished cardiac output and redistribution of blood flow. Consequently, the disproportion between work done by the respiratory muscles and the supply of blood delivered to them may contribute to fatigue of the respiratory muscles and to the sensation of dyspnea. Sensory elements within the respiratory muscles may also contribute to respiratory discomfort by registering the disproportion between the inordinate amount of energy that is being spent by muscles and the amount of ventilation that they produce.

Although precise mechanisms for dyspnea remain uncertain, its occurrence in left heart failure clearly depends on the increase in the blood and water content of the lungs at the expense of the air volume. Ventilation increases as the air volume is progressively encroached upon, and, as the minute ventilation approaches the maximal ventilatory capacity, the likelihood of dyspnea increases.

Orthopnea. Progressive, and often urgent, dyspnea that occurs soon after lying flat is designated as orthopnea; it is relieved by sitting up. The physiologic basis for orthopnea is the augmented venous return from the lower extremities and splanchnic bed to the lungs that results from redistribution of gravitational forces in the supine position and the reabsorption of diurnal edema. In the patient with heart disease, orthopnea is reliable evidence of left ventricular failure. In contrast, the dyspnea of chronic lung disease or musculoskeletal disorders is rarely aggravated by lying flat.

The patient learns to avoid respiratory distress at night by supporting head and thorax by two or more pillows. In severe heart failure, orthopnea may force the patient to sleep upright in a chair rather than in bed. In some patients with extensive coronary artery disease and left ventricular failure, orthopnea occurs only in the left lateral position; the mechanism for this is unclear.

Cough and expectoration are common in left heart failure, presumably a consequence of reflexes from the congested lungs and bronchi. The patient may also manifest an orthopneic cough which has the same significance as orthopnea, and is presumably the consequence of venous congestion and edema of the tracheobronchial walls. In some patients, precordial distress may substitute for breathlessness in the supine position. This "nocturnal angina" is also somehow related to the mobilization of water from the tissues to the circulation when the patient goes to bed.

Paroxysmal Nocturnal Dyspnea. A bout of urgent respiratory distress, verging on suffocation, may rouse the patient unexpectedly from sleep and cause him to seek relief desperately, either by sitting up or by rushing to the open window to breathe "fresh air." Respiration may be labored and wheezing, hence the designation "cardiac asthma." The episodes represent intolerable aggravation of pulmonary congestion and edema during sleep in the supine position. A combination of dulling of the respiratory center to sensory input from the lungs during sleep and increase in venous return to the lungs makes it possible for pulmonary venous congestion and edema to accumulate to the point of precipitating the frightening episode of breathlessness.

Acute Pulmonary Edema. In an acute episode of left ventricular failure, such as that which follows myocardial infarction, the inability of the left ventricular myocardium to handle the blood that the competent right ventricle is delivering to it may result in an abrupt increase in pulmonary venous and capillary pressure, followed by flooding of the interstitial spaces and alveoli. If the edema is confined to the interstitial spaces of the lungs, an increase in respiratory frequency because of stiff lungs would be expected to produce alveolar hyperventilation and respiratory alkalosis; conversely, once free fluid enters the terminal bronchioles and mounts the respiratory tree, respiratory acidosis may occur because of imbalances between alveolar ventilation and alveolar blood flow (ventilation-perfusion inhomogeneities).

Pulmonary edema may begin with a cough, with wheezing, or with breathlessness. Often there is a sense of oppression in the chest. At first, except for the abnormal breathing pattern and the evidences of heart disease, there may be few physical signs. In time, as free fluid enters the distal airways, rales become audible, most marked in the dependent parts of the lungs, but extending upward as the attack worsens. In a severe attack, the patient is pale, sweating, cyanotic, obviously gasping for breath, and usually producing frothy sputum which may be blood tinged.

Hemoptysis. Rusty sputum, laden with heart failure cells (alveolar macrophages containing hemosiderin), occurs frequently in severe left heart failure. Frankly bloody sputum is generally a sign of pulmonary infarction. In severe pulmonary edema caused by left ventricular failure, the frothy fluid that pours from the bronchial tree is often pink, i.e., blood tinged, owing to the escape of red cells into the alveoli from the congested minute vessels of the lungs.

Cheyne-Stokes Respiration. Some patients with severe heart failure display periodic breathing characterized by alternate periods of apnea and hyperventilation. Cyclic changes in arterial blood gas tensions accompany this waxing and waning of the ventilation: during apnea, the arterial Po_2 reaches its peak, whereas the arterial Pco_2 reaches its nadir. At the same time, alveolar gas tensions are exactly opposite: the alveolar Po_2 reaches its peak during hyperpnea; the alveolar Pco_2 reaches its nadir during hyperpnea. This discrepancy between arterial and alveolar gas tensions has been attributed to the fact that changes in arterial blood gases *cause* the swings in ventilation, whereas the changes in alveolar gas tension are the *consequences* of the changes in ventilation. The critical role of the arterial blood gases stems from the prolonged circulation time between the lungs and the respiratory centers in the brain. This slowing of the circulation exposes the central respiratory control mechanisms to arterial blood that differs in gaseous composition from that in pulmonary venous blood. In essence, because of slowing of the circulation, negative feedback is delayed. As expected, the longer the circulation time, the longer the cycles of hyperventilation and apnea. The neurologic and cerebrovascular changes of old age predispose to Cheyne-Stokes breathing.

Physical Signs

In addition to being breathless, the patient is generally pale, a bit dusky, and sweaty. His handshake is cold because of peripheral vasoconstriction. The heart rate is rapid and the pulse pressure is narrow, with a modest increase in diastolic blood pressure. If only the left ventricle has failed, the neck veins are not distended.

The Heart. Enlargement of the heart is usually evident to inspection and palpation of the apical impulse and is confirmed by roentgenologic and radiographic examination. Angina pectoris is not a manifestation of heart failure, nor is palpitation common unless overzealous administration of digitalis and diuretics has occasioned digitalis toxicity. As the left ventricle fails and pulmonary venous pressure increases, pulmonary arterial pressure also increases, and the heart sound attributable to pulmonary valve closure increases in intensity. Also, as the left ventricle dilates, the mitral valve leaflets fail to appose properly, resulting in mild mitral incompetence.

Gallop Rhythm. The advent of a third heart sound during diastole in an adult with heart disease signifies the advent of heart failure. The fixed sequence of the two normal sounds and the abnormal third sound, in conjunction with an increase in heart rate, is responsible for the characteristic cadence of a gallop rhythm. The third heart sound ("S-3 gallop") occurs early in diastole during the state of rapid ventricular filling. This ventricular gallop presumably originates in the vibrations of the ventricular walls as the rapidly inflowing blood is abruptly arrested; this extra sound, normal in young children and in young adults, is generally a reliable sign of ventricular failure in the middle-aged or elderly patient with heart disease.

A gallop rhythm may also originate in the atrial contribution to ventricular filling. This atrial or "S-4 gallop" is not unique for heart failure, because it may reflect diminished ventricular compliance resulting from hypertrophy or ischemia rather than myocardial failure. If a patient with a fourth heart sound develops heart failure, a third sound appears to cause a quadruple rhythm. If the heart rate is rapid or the P-R interval is prolonged, the atrial and ventricular gallop sounds summate ("summation gallop"). In the candidate for heart failure, summation gallop has the same implication as other diastolic gallop rhythms, particularly if it persists as the heart is slowed.

Pulsus Alternans. In patients with heart disease, particularly if the cause is hypertension, cardiomyopathy, or coronary arteriosclerosis, the appearance of alternating strong and weak beats, even though the fundamental rhythm remains regular, heralds the onset of heart failure. This pulsus alternans may be detected by palpation or by sphygmomanometry. It often follows an extrasystole. Rarely is this mechanical alternans associated with electrical alternans. The mechanism for pulsus alternans has been attributed to alternations in fiber length (ventricular end-diastolic volume) or to alternating increase and decrease in the number of contractile units, or to both.

The Lungs. A characteristic consequence of interstitial edema and pulmonary venous congestion is tachypnea. As left heart failure progresses, interstitial edema is succeeded by alveolar edema and fluid in the terminal bronchioles, particularly at the lung bases. Accordingly, bilateral basal rales are common in moderate failure of the left ventricle.

Electrocardiogram

Abnormalities in the electrocardiogram arise from the underlying cardiac disorder and from therapeutic agents, e.g., digitalis and diuretics, rather than from heart failure, per se.

Radiologic Aspects

The x-ray can be exceedingly helpful in the diagnosis of left ventricular failure. Typically, the cardiac silhouette is enlarged, often assuming telltale configurations that are determined by the underlying disorder. In contrast to the normal, in which pulmonary *arteries* are prominent in the lower lung fields, pulmonary vasculature is prominent at the apices, reflecting pulmonary *venous* hypertension and redistribution of blood flow because of edema and fibrosis at the bases. Enlarged hilar shadows accompany the prominent pulmonary veins in the upper lung fields.

Prominent septal lines, particularly near the costophrenic angles (Kerley's lines), indicate the presence of interstitial edema. The advent of alveolar edema is signaled by a generalized clouding of the lung fields. Pleural effusion may occasionally occur in left heart failure, but is much more apt to occur in biventricular heart failure. Evidence of interstitial and alveolar edema often lessens or disappears when right ventricular failure supervenes. However, hydrothorax generally persists. A widened shadow of the superior vena cava may provide reliable evidence of right ventricular failure and systemic venous congestion.

Pulmonary Function Tests

Traditionally, the course of overt failure of the left ventricle, particularly the response to treatment, has been followed by consecutive determinations of vital capacity. This is an insensitive measure, usually associated with decrease in compliance and occasionally with increase in airway resistance. Recently it has been shown that earlier in the course of pulmonary edema—presumably when the excess fluid is still confined to the interstitial space around alveoli and terminal airways (less than 2 mm in diameter)—expiratory flow rates at *low lung volumes* are reduced and peripheral airways tend to close prematurely during expiration, trapping gas within the lungs and disturbing the distribution of alveolar gas with respect to pulmonary capillary blood. This has led to a variety of tests (e.g., "closing volumes") which are designed to detect premature closure and resultant maldistribution of air—presumably by interstitial edema—long before compliance falls and total resistance of airways increases. During recovery there is usually a delay before expiratory flow rates and closing volumes return to normal, even though left atrial pressure is again within normal limits. The basis for the persistent abnormalities is presumably the gradual removal of interstitial edema from the vicinity of the small airways and blood vessels.

Associated with the high closing volume is evidence of ventilation-perfusion abnormalities manifested by widening of the alveolar-arterial ΔP_{O_2} and a decrease in arterial P_{O_2} caused by "venous admixture." Nonetheless, arterial oxygen saturation is generally near normal unless independent lung disease is present. Along with the decrease in arterial P_{O_2} is a widening of the arterial venous difference in O_2 content owing to the increased extraction of oxygen in the tissues. Arterial CO_2 tension remains normal or low unless free fluid enters the terminal airways in the course of pulmonary edema. Abnormally high values for CO_2 tension indicate that considerable free fluid has made its way into the airways.

Right Ventricular Failure

Clinical Manifestations

Isolated failure of the right ventricle is uncommon, generally a consequence of cor pulmonale secondary to intrinsic lung disease. More often, right ventricular failure is a sequel to left ventricular failure. In right ventricular failure, neck veins are distended and fill from below; the engorged liver may be tender to gentle pressure, and compression causes a surge of blood into the neck veins (hepatojugular reflux). In time, when both ventricles have failed, evidence of right ventricular failure may dominate the scene; but continuing dyspnea and rales attest to the persistence of left ventricular failure, and the continuing low cardiac output is manifested by signs of increased sympathetic nervous activity and of organ hypoperfusion.

Weakness may be marked and is occasionally associated with anorexia, weight loss, and malnutrition ("cardiac cachexia"). Not only severe heart failure, but also digitalis, diuretics, and electrolyte disturbances are generally involved in the genesis of this cachectic state.

Cyanosis. Bluish discoloration of the skin and mucous membranes is designated as cyanosis. It is due to an abnormal concentration of reduced hemoglobin (more than 5 grams per 100 ml) in the subpapillary venous plexus of the skin. In right heart failure, the congested venules, containing blood from which considerable oxygen has been extracted because of the slow flow, account for the cyanosis. In left heart failure, cyanosis is usually caused

by a complication, e.g., pneumonia, unless overt pulmonary edema is present.

Abnormal Heart and Lungs. Although the breathlessness of the left ventricular failure may be somewhat relieved by right heart failure, usually some dyspnea persists along with tachypnea and basal rales. Severe right heart failure (and dilatation) may produce tricuspid valvular insufficiency, thereby contributing to systemic venous engorgement. The murmur of tricuspid insufficiency is distinguished from that of mitral insufficiency by its location (lower left border of sternum) and by its tendency to increase during inspiration. Hydrothorax, generally unilateral, is more common than in isolated left ventricular failure.

Systemic Venous Congestion. Distention of systemic veins is a hallmark of right heart failure. Several different mechanisms contribute to its genesis: (1) the inability of the failing right ventricle to cope adequately with the venous return; (2) the increase in the quantity of blood contained in the large systemic veins; and (3) increased venomotor tone, resulting from heightened sympathetic nervous activity. The increase in systemic venous pressure underlies the hepatomegaly, splenomegaly, and peripheral edema that characterize right heart failure. Less apparent are the congestion and edema of the gastrointestinal tract that the systemic venous hypertension produces.

Pressure in the superficial jugular vein is a useful index of right atrial pressure and, with experience, may be reliably estimated from the height of the fluid column distending the cervical vein. Normally, the cervical veins are flat in the erect position, whereas in right heart failure they are prominent and distended, usually with a level that pulsates. Functional tricuspid insufficiency, complicating dilatation of the right heart, distorts the normal venous pulse by increasing its v wave. Usually superficial venous distention precedes the onset of hepatomegaly and peripheral edema. Occasionally, compression of the abdomen over the liver (hepatojugular reflux) is necessary to display the increased blood volume in the venous system.

Liver. The liver is usually enlarged and palpable in right heart failure, often in association with mild abdominal discomfort, and generally somewhat tender to compression. In severe right heart failure, particularly if the onset is acute, constraint of the swollen liver by its tight capsule may cause right upper quadrant pain. Tricuspid insufficiency accompanying right ventricular dilatation may cause synchronous pulsations in neck veins and liver. Splenomegaly is uncommon except in prolonged congestion of the liver. Rarely is the enlarged spleen tender from congestion per se.

Early in hepatic congestion, sensitive liver function tests, such as the handling of Bromsulphalein, are apt to be abnormal, and modest increases in the concentrations of cellular enzymes in serum, such as glutamic oxaloacetic transaminase (SGOT) increases in serum bilirubin, are not uncommon. The hyperbilirubinemia consists of a combination of quick- and slow-reacting bilirubin, presumably a consequence of decreased oxygen delivery to the liver arising from hypoperfusion and venous hypertension. But jaundice is uncommon unless hepatic congestion is associated with longstanding pulmonary congestion and, often, with pulmonary infarction.

If cardiac output is severely curtailed and liver congestion is marked and protracted, hypoglycemia may occur, presumably owing to depletion of glycogen stores in the liver and increased formation of lactic acid from glucose because of hypoxia. During physical activity, hepatic blood flow in heart failure decreases further, resulting in a marked decrease in aldosterone breakdown, thereby furthering sodium retention.

Repeated bouts of right heart failure elicit atrophy and necrosis of liver cells in the vicinity of the central veins and stimulate extensive fibrosis ("cardiac cirrhosis"). Many months of reduced hepatic blood flow and high venous pressures are required for this reaction, which may result in a shrunken, fibrotic liver difficult to distinguish from posthepatitic cirrhosis. Hepatic coma is a rare, preterminal complication of severe hepatic congestion and fibrosis.

Extracellular Fluid Compartments. In normal subjects, the fluid compartments of the body are held remarkably constant as the result of an automatic interplay among *intake* (governed by thirst and appetite), *transcellular exchanges* of fluid and electrolytes (governed by passive and active mechanisms), and *excretion* (regulated mainly by the kidneys). In heart failure, this automatic balance tends to be upset mainly because of inordinate retention of salt and water by the kidneys. The result is an isosmotic expansion of the extracellular fluid in which the circulating blood volume shares. It is conceivable that early in heart failure the conservation of salt and water may serve a useful purpose by expanding the blood volume either to sustain venous return to the failing heart or to relieve the arterial baroreceptors from undue stimulation as the cardiac output fails. But this teleologic explanation does not apply when the myocardium can no longer respond to increased filling pressures and volumes, and the retention of salt and water only aggravates congestion and edema.

The distribution of the excess extracellular fluid varies from patient to patient. In the patient who is up and about, edema accumulates in the feet and ankles under the influence of gravity; in the bedridden patient, the fluid shifts to the sacral region. Low tissue pressure, as around the back of the ankle, predisposes to localization. The level of colloid osmotic pressure and the integrity of the lymphatic system also influence the distribution of the excess fluid.

Subcutaneous Edema. Dependent edema, manifested as swelling of feet or ankles, developing gradually during the day and subsiding by morning, is a characteristic feature of right heart failure. Invariably, it is anteceded by systemic venous congestion, but after diuresis subcutaneous edema may linger even though systemic venous hypertension has been relieved by the reduction in venous blood volume. Usually a gain in weight precedes clinical evidence of edema. If edema is allowed to persist, complications such as low-grade cellulitis may occur. The combination of edema and slowed venous flow predisposes to thrombosis and to pulmonary embolism. The massive pitting edema of the lower extremities that was commonly seen before the advent of potent diuretics is now rarely encountered except in instances of gross neglect.

Hydrothorax. It is so uncommon for hydrothorax to complicate isolated failure of the right ventricle, that the association of pleural effusion and cor pulmonale should lead to search for an independent mechanism for the pleural effusion, e.g., pulmonary infarction. On the other hand, as indicated previously, it is quite common in combined heart failure (right and left). The pathogenesis of hydrothorax involves impaired removal of water from the pleural space because of high venous pressures in both the pulmonary and systemic circulations, thereby not only compromising transcapillary exchange of water in the pleura but also impeding lymphatic drainage. Hydrothorax contributes to dyspnea not only by encroaching on the air volume but also reflexly, probably by stimuli from lungs and chest wall. Pulmonary infarction may cause pleural effusion in two ways: by direct contiguity of the infarcted area of the lung and the pleural space, or by aggravation of heart failure.

Ascites. Clinically evident excess of free fluid in the abdominal cavity is designated as ascites. It is a late manifestation of right heart failure, generally associated with marked systemic venous hypertension, severe peripheral edema, and hydrothorax. It occurs most frequently in patients with tricuspid valvular disease (or with constrictive pericarditis). Portal and hepatic venous hypertension, coupled with high pressure in the systemic veins draining the peritoneum, seem to be involved in the etiology of ascites; but retention of salt and water is a fundamental prerequisite for ascites to occur. Usually ascites is first noticed by the patient as a gradual increase in abdominal girth. But in severe right heart failure, it may cause anorexia, abdominal discomfort, or pain.

Pericardial Effusion. In severe and persistent heart failure, abnormal quantities of transudate may accumulate in the pericardial sac. Rarely does fluid accumulate to the level of tamponade.

Anasarca. Massive right heart failure may cause excess fluid to accumulate everywhere in the body, most conspicuously in subcutaneous tissues and abdominal and thoracic cavities. Because of the influence of gravity, face and arms are spared until preterminally.

Gastrointestinal Tract. The bowel wall shares in the systemic venous congestion and edema. These changes rarely interfere with absorption of drugs or foods unless heart failure is extreme. In severe congestive heart failure, anorexia, nausea, and vomiting may occur from reflex, central, or local causes. Occasionally, when right heart failure is severe, a protein-losing enteropathy may develop.

Brain. Neurasthenia, headache, and insomnia are common in heart failure. Usually these manifestations are attributed to a combination of a modest diminution of cerebral blood flow and triggering mechanisms, e.g., dyspnea contributing to insomnia. Cerebral manifestations are more frequent when the reduction in cerebral blood flow is superimposed on antecedent cerebrovascular disease, e.g., arteriosclerosis, or personality disorder. Severe heart failure is often associated with irritability, restlessness, and difficulty in fixing attention, particularly in older persons. Preterminally, stupor and coma may develop. The possibility exists that central nervous abnormalities may be enhanced by the delivery to the brain of abnormal products elaborated by remote organs (liver, endocrines, gastrointestinal tract) that suffer deranged metabolism during heart failure as a result of congestion and hypoperfusion.

Kidney. Oliguria occurs in both right and left heart failure but is much more striking in the latter. As the heart improves, urinary output increases. The urine is poor in sodium but has a high specific gravity (1.020 to 1.030). Azotemia is common but generally moderate except when intrinsic renal disease is present or after vigorous diuresis. The combination of azotemia and high specific gravity is distinctive for heart failure (and dehydration) and contrasts with the low specific gravity of intrinsic renal disease. Proteinuria is common but rarely severe—usually less than 1 gram per day. A variety of casts accompany the proteinuria. Renal function, as determined by clearance techniques, is only slightly depressed except in severe right heart failure of long standing.

Other Manifestations.   In severe congestive heart failure, the accumulation of edema may obscure the gradual loss of tissue mass. Often this tissue wasting is associated with *weakness*. In extreme instances, *cachexia* may develop. At this late stage, the patient is usually suffering from anorexia, gastrointestinal upsets, anemia, and electrolyte upsets. Part of the picture undoubtedly stems from organ hypoperfusion and congestion, but often a large contribution has been made by overvigorous use of diuretics and digitalis.

Anxiety.   It is not surprising that patients with organic heart disease become anxious. Indeed, anxiety is a regular feature by the time the heart fails. But not always is it an easy matter to distinguish between cardiac complaints as manifestations of anxiety or of the cardiac disorder. Part of the difficulty stems from the nonspecific nature of complaints, such as breathlessness, especially if the patient does have organic heart disease. The difficulty is compounded if the patient misinterprets or exaggerates his symptoms unconsciously. For example, the severely anxious patient may hyperventilate to the point of alkalosis, producing the characteristic lightheadedness, cold hands, and tingling fingers of hypocapnia, reduced cerebral blood flow, and peripheral vasoconstriction, thereby reinforcing his view of the organic nature of his breathlessness. Palpitation is also commonly misinterpreted by the patient suffering from anxiety as a telltale sign of organic heart disease.

The standard approach for the physician is the separate assessment of the organic versus the psychosomatic aspects of the heart disease. Particularly helpful in this regard are excessive or inconsistent complaints for the extent of the cardiac disease. Not infrequently, hemodynamic measurements may be required to settle the role of organic heart disease in producing the clinical symptoms.

CLINICAL MANAGEMENT

General Measures

The aim of treatment in heart failure is to arrest and reverse the pathogenic sequence that led to the clinical signs and symptoms. The response to treatment of the more common types of heart failure, i.e., hypertensive and arteriosclerotic, is often dramatic. But each relapse marks another milestone on the road to refractory heart failure, not only by signaling progressive deterioration of the myocardium, but also because intensified and protracted treatment enhances the prospect for eliciting the toxic manifestations of the therapeutic agents.

Increasing Cardiac Output.   In most forms of chronic heart failure, the cardiac output can be made to increase by decreasing the cardiac load, by improving myocardial contractility, or by a combination of the two. In the patient with severe bradycardia associated with heart failure, acceleration of the heart rate by cardiac pacing may cure heart failure that would otherwise be refractory. Conversely, severe tachycardia must be arrested if filling times of the ventricles are too greatly curtailed by the abbreviated diastole.

Decreasing the Work of the Heart.   The excess load on the heart may be in the form of pressure, e.g., arterial hypertension, or volume, e.g., the physiologic expansion of the blood volume in late pregnancy. Lightening the load is prerequisite for a successful cardiotonic program. In recent years, serious attention has been paid to decreasing the pressure load during heart failure by administering vasodilator agents. But rarely is specific antihypertensive therapy necessary unless hypertension antedated the heart failure and persists after heart failure is relieved. If hypertension led to heart failure, small doses of ganglionic blocking agents may be helpful.

Rest is an effective way to decrease the cardiac burden in conventional types of heart failure. Rest must be both physical and mental; after recovery from an acute bout of heart failure, a new life style of lessened activity may be required as part of the cardiotonic program. Reassurance is essential, because anxiety automatically augments metabolic activity and induces peripheral arterial constriction. Should reassurance prove inadequate, sedatives or tranquilizers (such as chloral hydrate, 0.5 to 1.0 gram, phenobarbital, 15 to 30 mg, or diazepam, 2 to 10 mg, taken orally three times per day and at bedtime) may be needed to promote mental ease, particularly as the patient improves and grows restless. Narcotics are rarely needed in heart failure unless pulmonary edema has generated intolerable anxiety. Excessive sedation, to the point of immobilizing the patient, enhances the risk of venous thrombosis and embolism, particularly in the elderly.

In left heart failure, the sitting or semisitting position, either in bed or in a chair, usually relieves tachypnea and dyspnea. Oxygen by nasal catheter (4 to 6 liters per minute) also seems to make the patient more comfortable even though hypoxemia is generally mild in heart failure. Finally, mental rest is impossible if urinary retention and constipation are unattended.

It is remarkable how often the proper use of rest as the initial step in treatment will promote a vigorous diuresis, slow the heart rate, and relieve dyspnea, thereby allowing a more leisurely use of other cardiotonic agents, such as digitalis and diuretics. On the other hand, if metabolic demands remain high, as during undetected thyrotoxicosis or fever, heart failure may prove refractory to the conventional cardiotonic program until the thyroid overactivity is curtailed.

Acute Pulmonary Edema

Treatment of the acute pulmonary edema of left ventricular failure is begun with the patient in the sitting position, thereby draining the upper portions of his lungs of excess fluid. Meperidine, 50 mg, or morphine, 10 to 15 mg, is administered intravenously for restlessness or dyspnea. These agents seem to act primarily by relieving anxiety and agitation. Morphine is the traditional agent, but distressing side effects, such as nausea, vomiting, and urinary retention, have detracted from its popularity. Dramatic and immediate relief may be accomplished by reducing venous return to the right heart; this may be done by one or two small phlebotomies (250 ml of blood), by rotating tourniquets (releasing one at a time for five minutes every half hour), or by intermittent positive pressure breathing which raises pleural pressure, thereby impeding venous return. A rapid-acting diuretic, ethacrynic acid or furosemide, is administered intravenously. Even though arterial oxygenation may be near normal, high concentrations of humidified oxygen, 50 to 100 per cent, are frequently used empirically to relieve dyspnea, restlessness, and confusion. Severe hypotension is a contraindication to phlebotomy and to assisted ventilation.

Digitalis (digoxin or lanatoside C, 1.0 mg) may be administered intravenously if the patient has had none during the preceding two weeks. However, the urgency for intravenous injection of digitalis has decreased considerably since the advent of potent, rapid-acting diuretics. An exception to this generalization is the attack of pulmonary edema precipitated by a bout of tachycardia which can be slowed by digitalis, e.g., paroxysmal atrial fibrillation. In this instance, digitalis relieves the heart failure primarily because of its effect on slowing atrioventricular conduction, and consequently the ventricular rate, rather than because of its inotropic effect on the heart. In ectopic tachycardias, it may be necessary to resort to DC electroshock in order to restore normal heart action and tolerable heart rates.

Face to face with a patient in pulmonary edema, the physician often feels compelled to apply a battery of strenuous measures in rapid succession or simultaneously. Especially for patients in poor condition, this treatment may be worse than the disorder which is usually self-limited once the upright position has been assumed, mental rest accomplished, and a potent diuretic administered. As soon as the crisis is over, a more conventional cardiotonic program is begun, and a search is made for the cause of the left heart failure as well as for the mechanism that precipitated the episode.

The role of left heart failure in producing high-altitude pulmonary edema is not clear. Prompt recovery usually follows bed rest, descent to lower altitude, and the administration of oxygen.

Inotropic Agents: Digitalis

Although immediate therapeutic agents for coping with the acute episode of heart failure may not include digitalis, once the crisis is over, lasting improvement almost invariably requires the use of digitalis glycosides. Unfortunately, establishing the proper dose of digitalis is not always straightforward, because optimal doses vary somewhat from patient to patient and with associated clinical disorders. Moreover, unless standard brands of predictable potency are prescribed, tablets may vary considerably in effectiveness. Finally, the concomitant administration of other, apparently unrelated, medications may lead to drug interactions which interfere with the effects of the digitalis.

Drug Interactions. Multiplicity of drugs is the rule in modern therapy. Some drugs are deliberately prescribed in combinations, either to reinforce a desirable therapeutic effect or to avoid an untoward side effect. A familiar example of this practice is the combination of digitalis, a potassium-losing diuretic, and potassium supplements for the treatment of heart failure; the dosage of each is individualized to achieve maximal inotropic effect on the heart and to relieve circulatory congestion. But other drugs, such as sleeping pills and anticoagulants that are administered concomitantly for subsidiary or unrelated purposes, may interact and decrease the effectiveness of the cardiotonic program.

There are several ways by which one therapeutic agent can influence the effects of another. Among these are (1) chemical interaction (cholestyramine, a cholesterol-lowering, ion-exchange resin, impedes absorption of digitoxin [and, to a much lesser extent, of digoxin] by binding in the intestine); (2) competition for binding sites on plasma proteins (digitoxin and ethacrynic acid compete for albumin); (3) induction of drug-metabolizing enzymes (phenobarbital and phenylbutazone enhance the metabolism of digitoxin by hepatic microsomal enzymes); and (4) enhanced excretion (polar metabolites of digitoxin are eliminated more rapidly in urine and bile than is digitoxin per se). In conventional dosages, few of these interactions seem to be clinically significant even though cholestyramine has been advocated in treating digitoxin intoxication. But they do introduce an element of unpredictability into standard therapeutic programs, and they do urge caution whenever medications are either added to or deleted from a stable therapeutic regimen.

Related to the concept of drug interaction is the broader concept of drug-biologic interaction which determines how drugs act. This broader concept includes reactions between the pharmacologic agent and some biologic aspect of the living subject. For example, digitalis effects depend heavily on ion fluxes at ultrastructural membranes; changes in ionic composition and behavior are known to modify the clinical influence of digitalis. Or the physiologic state of the patient may shape the response: acidosis blunts the effectiveness of norepinephrine; the administration of a conventional dose of a ganglionic blocking agent, when sympathetic vasomotor tone is high because of vigorous diuresis and depletion of blood volume, may precipitate circulatory collapse.

The concept of drug-biologic interaction is complicated by individual variability in responsiveness to drugs. Part of this variability is undoubtedly inherited; part is immunologic; most remains to be explained.

Digitalis: General Aspects. Digitalis improves the contractility of the failing myocardium regardless of the type of heart failure, the rate, or the rhythm. After digitalis has been given in effective doses and myocardial contractility has increased, the heart shrinks in size, cardiac output increases, end-diastolic volume and pressure decrease, venous pressure normalizes, and evidences of peripheral vasoconstriction, circulatory congestion, and organ hypoperfusion disappear. In the reordering of the circulation that follows relief of congestive heart failure, blood that had been sequestered in the splanchnic venous bed is redirected to the systemic veins by appropriate adjustments in vascular tone, thereby helping to sustain the improved cardiac output.

Molecular Bases. Although the full picture of how the digitalis glycosides improve cardiac contractility is not yet clear, they do seem to act by altering surface and intracellular (sarcoplasmic reticulum and mitochondria) membranes so that they release calcium ions more readily. Another manifestation of a change in cellular membrane characteristics caused by the glycosides is inhibition of the Na^+-K^+-ATPase activity. However, it is unsettled whether this interference with ATPase, as well as the associated decrease of sodium pumping into the cell, is directly related to the inotropic effect of the glycosides.

Effect on Inotropic State. In low output heart failure, digitalis increases the cardiac output and restores the end-diastolic pressure in the left ventricle to normal.

This is a consequence of increased myocardial contractility. A similar effect on contractility occurs in the normal myocardium, but the cardiac output does not increase because of a direct vasoconstricting effect of digitalis on the peripheral resistance vessels. But in low output heart failure in which sympathetic nervous activity is consistently high, restoration of the cardiac output by digitalis reflexly diminishes sympathetic tone, thereby overriding the direct vasoconstricting effects of digitalis on the vessels. These distinctions underscore the unique property of digitalis glycosides as inotropic agents because of their ability to improve myocardial contractility in heart failure without simultaneously eliciting antagonistic effects, such as peripheral vasoconstriction (or tachycardia).

Myocardial Oxygen Consumption. The increase in the strength of contraction produced by the digitalis glycosides increases the oxygen consumption of the myocardium in the normal heart. But this tendency is neutralized in the failing heart which responds to glycosides by shrinking in volume, thereby reducing wall tension and its associated oxygen consumption. Accordingly, the increase in contractility produced in the dilated failing heart is generally accomplished with no increase in myocardial oxygen consumption.

Catecholamine Depletion. Although reduction in cardiac catecholamines is a feature of chronic heart failure, this depletion leaves unaffected the positive inotropic effects of the digitalis glycosides.

Coronary Circulation. In the normal unanesthetized animal, ouabain elicits coronary vasoconstriction. Unfortunately, nothing is known about the behavior of the coronary circulation in response to digitalis during heart failure.

Systemic Circulation. Digitalis elicits an increase in cardiac output, thereby reducing the reflex vasoconstriction of the low output state. But because of the direct constrictor action of cardiac glycosides on vascular smooth muscle, there is apt to be a brief period of increase in systemic arterial pressure, particularly if large doses of cardiac glycosides are administered intravenously.

Choice of Digitalis Preparation. Five digitalis preparations are in common use today in the United States: digitalis leaf, digoxin, digitoxin, deslanoside (Cedilanid-D), and ouabain. Their basic pharmacologic actions on the heart and their toxic-therapeutic ratios are quite similar. But they do differ considerably with respect to the rate and degree of absorption from the intestine and both the onset and duration of action.

Digoxin and digitoxin have replaced digitalis leaf for chronic oral administration; ouabain and deslanoside, as well as digoxin, are administered intravenously. Digitoxin is not as satisfactory an intravenous agent, because it is relatively slow in reaching its peak effect. Digitalis leaf is gradually disappearing from use, because it varies in potency, requires bioassay for standardization, and has no therapeutic advantage over digitoxin which is its principal constituent.

Traditional practice in digitalization has relied on a preliminary loading phase to achieve a therapeutic level, followed by maintenance dosage to sustain a balance between intake and elimination. Accordingly, the preset loading dose is administered over a period of one to three days (Table 1), providing enough digitalis to load body stores and to compensate for daily elimination. Unless a desperate situation—such as a life-threatening cardiac arrhythmia—calls for acute digitalization, slow digitalization is preferable. Indeed, if there is no hurry, continued administration of the maintenance dose, without a loading dose, has proved to be a practical way to achieve digitalization.

Dosages listed in Table 1 are intended to indicate orders of magnitude rather than precise schedules. Dosage is determined individually according to the nature and severity of the heart disease, the clinical setting, the use of other drugs such as potassium-losing diuretics, and continued observation of the patient's response.

Oral Preparations. Digoxin and digitoxin have replaced digitalis leaf for chronic oral administration.

DIGOXIN. The maintenance dosage of digoxin is determined by a balance between renal excretion, dose, and absorption. Ordinarily, between 75 and 90 per cent of an oral dose is absorbed. Digoxin is lipid soluble and absorbed from the small intestine by diffusion. Some variation in absorption may occur, depending on the solubility of digoxin molecules in the intestinal fluids. Variability in absorption may also result from different preparations of digoxin. Consequently, once a digoxin preparation from one manufacturer has proved effective, changes should be avoided.

Digoxin is excreted primarily by the kidney, and most of the drug appears unchanged in the urine. When fully digitalized, the concentration of digoxin in serum is approximately 1 per cent or less of total body stores of digoxin. If renal function is normal, approximately one

TABLE 1. Administration of Common Cardiac Glycosides

| Preparation | Digitalization | | | Cardiotonic Effects | | Blood Levels | |
	Loading Dose* (mg/24 hrs)	Initial Dose† (mg)	Maintenance Dose (mg)	Onset of Activity (min)	Peak Effect (hrs)	Steady State Therapeutic Level¶ (mg/ml)	Half-Life (hrs)
Digoxin (oral)	2.5	1.0	0.25	60–120	1–3	1.5	36
Digitoxin (oral)	1.2	0.75‡	0.1	30–120	4–6	17	96–144
Deslanoside (IV)	1.6	0.8§	—	10–30	1–2	—	33
Ouabain (IV)	0.25	0.25§	—	3–10	0.5–2	0.5	21
(These values are examples to illustrate orders of magnitude.)							

*Total quantity to be administered in 24 hours for therapeutic effect.
†Assuming no prior digitalis during previous two weeks.
‡The same dose may be administered intravenously if urgent digitalization is required.
§When feasible, switch to oral maintenance doses of digoxin or digitoxin.
¶On conventional maintenance doses.

TABLE 2.   Features of Cardiac Glycoside Preparations in Common Use

Preparation	Source	Usual Route of Administration*	Gastrointestinal Absorption	Protein Binding†	Principal Route of Elimination
Digoxin	*Digitalis lanata*	Oral	75–90%‡	23%‡	Kidneys
Digitoxin	*Digitalis purpurea*	Oral	90–100%	97%	Liver; kidney for metabolites
Deslanoside	*Digitalis lanata*	Intravenous	Erratic	—	Kidneys
Ouabain	*Strophanthus gratus*	Intravenous	Erratic	0	Kidneys

(These values are examples to illustrate orders of magnitude.)

*All can be administered intravenously.
†Affinity for protein (albumin) determines rate of urinary excretion and persistence in body.
‡Varies according to preparation. Different tablets differ in bioavailability of digoxin.

third of the body stores is eliminated per day; the maintenance dose replenishes this daily loss. The half-life of digoxin in serum is approximately the same in normal subjects and in patients with heart failure, averaging one and one half days. However, the half-life is prolonged in renal failure. The serum level of digoxin in renal insufficiency is directly related to the creatinine clearance and inversely to the concentration of urea nitrogen in the blood (BUN). Formulas have been devised to take these relationships into account, recognizing that, in contrast to the normal daily elimination of one third of body stores of digoxin, the anuric patient eliminates about one seventh. Accordingly, the anuric patient will require one half or less of the usual maintenance dose.

Only 5 per cent of digoxin in serum is bound to protein. Its polar structure accounts for the difference between its concentration and that of digitoxin (nonpolar) in the serum (Table 2).

Without an initial loading dose, patients receiving digoxin orally reach a steady state in the serum, reflecting equilibrium between body stores, intake, and elimination in about one week. The steady state level in serum is approximately 1 per cent or less of total body stores of digoxin. Body stores are related to lean body weight, because digoxin does not accumulate in fat or interstitial fluid. In an adult patient, body stores are generally of the order of 0.01 mg per kilogram of body weight. Rarely are body stores required greater than 0.02 mg per kilogram of body weight. Therefore for a 70 kg patient, digitalization usually requires a minimal dose of approximately 0.7 mg. Should this digitalizing dose be exceeded in order to achieve better control of the clinical state, the prospects for toxicity will increase accordingly.

The essential features in using digoxin therapeutically are summarized in Table 1. Because of its short half-life, a single dose per day will cause a wide swing in serum concentration (and in body stores, including the heart) before the next dose is administered. In practice this swing is often unimportant; but, if desirable, its magnitude may be reduced (and therapeutic control improved) by administering one half the daily dose at 12-hour intervals. Many clinicians use digoxin for intravenous as well as oral administration, because its hemodynamic and biologic properties are comparatively well understood, and dosages are relatively easy to adjust.

DIGITOXIN.   This agent is widely used for chronic administration. It differs importantly from digoxin in its metabolism and its slow rate of elimination; the main route of elimination is by metabolism in the liver, only a small fraction being eliminated by the kidney.

Digitoxin is completely absorbed after oral administration so that oral and intravenous dosages are identical. Body stores and digitalizing doses are approximately the same, but maintenance doses are quite different because of different rates of elimination. Approximately 12 per cent of body stores of digitoxin is eliminated per day in patients with normal renal function. The usual body store is estimated to be of the order of 0.8 mg in a 70-kg adult. Therefore the daily maintenance dose is generally 0.1 mg per day (0.12 × 0.8 mg). Because of its slow dissipation and elimination, serum levels of digitoxin vary less from hour to hour than do digoxin levels. But the drug accumulates insidiously so that maintenance doses established at the onset often prove to be toxic in time.

In contrast to digoxin, digitoxin has a strong avidity for albumin so that 97 per cent in plasma is nondialyzable. This combination is a critical factor in limiting glomerular filtration and excretion of digitoxin by the kidneys. After an oral dose of 1.0 mg, 50 per cent of the inotropic effect is reached in one hour; 85 to 100 per cent is achieved in four hours and sustained for the rest of the day. The average half-life is approximately five days. Digitoxin enters into an enterohepatic cycle. Between 30 and 60 per cent of the 1.0 mg dose is eliminated in the feces and urine, the larger fraction generally in the urine. The remainder is metabolized, primarily to digoxin, which is eliminated in the urine. Digoxin is preferable to digitoxin in renal or hepatic insufficiency.

Intravenous Preparations.   As a rule, these are reserved for life-threatening situations. These include acute heart failure complicating a bout of atrial fibrillation with rapid ventricular rate, fulminating pulmonary edema as a complication of left ventricular failure, and the onset of heart failure or a serious arrhythmia during surgery. As a rule, the larger the dose of the glycoside, the more apt it is to create problems, particularly arrhythmias, of its own.

An intravenous bolus of a digitalis preparation may elicit a bout of hypertension, particularly if the dose is large, e.g., 1.0 mg of digoxin. The increase is generally of the order of 20/10, and the effect is generally short lived. But it may suffice to overburden the failing heart and to aggravate the situation until it subsides and is succeeded by the inotropic effect. Hypertension is rarely a problem if the intravenous dose is modest and administered slowly.

OUABAIN.   This is the traditional digitalis preparation for intravenous use. It is a pure crystalline substance that is unsuitable for oral use because of erratic absorption from the gastrointestinal tract. Its latency after intravenous injection is exceedingly brief (less than five minutes); it is rapidly eliminated so that it is not suitable for maintenance of digitalization. The initial intravenous dose is 0.25 to 0.3 mg, administered slowly. An additional 0.15 or 0.3 mg may be repeated after 24 hours.

DESLANOSIDE. This preparation is identical with digoxin except for the addition of a glucose residue. It is gradually replacing ouabain in popularity for intravenous use. Its digitalizing effect appears in 10 to 30 minutes after intravenous injection, reaches peak effect in one to two hours, and regresses in 24 hours. For rapid intravenous digitalization, the full 1.6 mg may be given at once, or, preferably, 0.8 mg may be followed by another 0.8 mg, either in four hours or in divided doses, at two- to four-hour intervals for two to three additional doses. Maintenance of digitalization is preferably done by oral digoxin or digitoxin. But, if necessary, 0.4 mg may be given intravenously or intramuscularly at 8- to 12-hour intervals.

DIGOXIN. For rapid digitalization, 0.5 mg is given initially, followed by 0.25 mg every two to four hours as needed, but taking care to avoid exceeding a total dose of 2 mg in 12 hours. As soon as practical, the oral route is substituted for the intravenous route.

Diagnostic Preparations. ACETYLSTROPHANTHIDIN. This is a partial synthetic which, because of its exceedingly rapid onset of action and dissipation, has been advocated more as a diagnostic test for adequacy of digitalization than as a therapeutic agent for heart failure. In practice, repeated injections of the substance (0.25 mg in 5 ml of glucose and water) are made until toxic or therapeutic effects are observed. Because it is potentially dangerous, other diagnostic tests are being investigated.

Guides to Proper Dosage of Digitalis. A major problem in using digitalis for its inotropic effect is the threat of inducing arrhythmias by virtue of its other effects on the heart (Fig. 4). On the other hand, if rapid atrial fibrillation coexists with heart failure, slowing of the ventricular rate, a consequence of slowed atrioventricular conduction, has proved to be a practical guide to digitalis

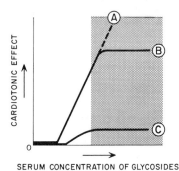

SERUM CONCENTRATION OF GLYCOSIDES

Figure 4. Hypothetical effects on contractility elicited by increasing doses (and serum concentrations) of digitalis. Once the inotropic effect of the digitalis preparation begins, it is unlikely that it will continue indefinitely as in A. Instead, it is likely that beyond a certain point the inotropic effects will taper to a plateau despite increasing serum concentration. When this plateau will occur depends on the capability of the heart to respond; a left ventricle that is suffering its first bout of failure is apt to manifest an excellent inotropic response for small increments in serum concentration before the plateau is reached (B). On the other hand, a spent heart that has suffered multiple myocardial infarctions may only manifest a sluggish inotropic response from the start and plateau early despite enormous increments in serum levels of glycoside (C). The shaded area is intended as a reminder of the increasing likelihood of serious arrhythmias as serum glycoside levels continue to increase.

dosage. Fortunately, slowing of the heart rate when atrial fibrillation coexists with heart failure also provides a rough measure of the inotropic effect (and of serum levels of the glycoside). On the other hand, when heart failure coexists with a normal sinus rhythm, slowing of the heart is a treacherous index of inotropic effect. Digitalis toxicity is common if large doses are administered in the attempt to slow the sinus tachycardia, particularly if a mechanism such as pulmonary emboli, infection, or hyperthyroidism is operating to sustain the rapid heart action.

The clinician now has available several different and effective digitalis preparations. Although none of these have any intrinsic advantage over the others with respect to myocardial contractility, they vary considerably with respect to speed of action, time course of effectiveness, and rates of elimination. Because of the ever-present prospect of digitalis toxicity, before starting to administer digitalis it is important to know whether digitalis, in any form, has been taken during the preceding week or two. Longer may be required if renal failure is present, particularly if digoxin was used. It cannot be overemphasized that the intravenous administration of a bolus of a digitalis preparation to a patient who has recently taken digitalis may precipitate ventricular tachycardia or fibrillation.

Clinical manifestations and the electrocardiogram are the key guides to dosage. As the circulation improves and signs and symptoms of heart failure abate, conventional dosage schedules are tailored to individual needs. The usual changes in the S-T segment and in the T waves produced by digitalis merely indicate that appreciable quantities of digitalis have been taken but provide no measure of dosage or efficacy. On the other hand, digitalis toxicity may first be manifested by electrocardiographic changes of abnormal conduction and of ectopic pacemakers.

Prophylactic. The perennial question of administering digitalis prophylactically, especially before surgical procedures, is again being discussed. This practice requires the administration of a preset dose without conventional criteria for distinguishing between adequacy versus toxicity. Therefore uncertain guidelines for safe administration are coupled with questionable therapeutic benefits. Compounding this uncertainty is the prospect of hypoxia and electrolyte imbalance during surgery. Because of the availability of digitalis preparations that do act rapidly and effectively, there seems to be little basis at present for prophylactic digitalization.

Digitalis Toxicity. Digitalis preparations are among the most dangerous, as well as the most useful, of current medications. The incidence of cardiotoxicity is staggering—of the order of 10 to 20 per cent in hospitalized patients receiving conventional doses of digitalis—and mortality from digitalis cardiotoxicity is estimated to run into the thousands per year.

Several different reasons account for much of this morbidity and mortality. (1) The narrow margin between therapeutic and toxic doses; this predisposes to digitalis toxicity during ordinary use but enhances its prospects when dosages are increased in the attempt to deal with increasing congestive heart failure. (2) The heavy reliance on slowing of heart rate and clearance of circulatory congestion as indices of improved contractility; this practice works well in atrial fibrillation but may be disastrous in normal sinus rhythm. (3) The ease with which changes in the clinical situation can derange stability of control; among the more common upsetting influences are electrolyte disturbances (particularly hypopotassemia), acute myocardial ischemia, upset acid-base balance, hypoxemia, renal impairment, autonomic nervous imbalances, other drugs, and infection. (4) Incomplete understanding by the physician of the distinctions in the clinical pharmacology of the various digitalis preparations; for example, differences in the renal handling of digoxin and digitoxin must be taken into account when choosing the proper glycoside in patients with renal insufficiency.

Recognition. The electrocardiogram is generally the final arbiter of digitalis cardiotoxicity. But three categories of clinical clues direct attention to the electrocardiogram: (1) the appearance of central nervous system evidence of digitalis toxicity, particularly anorexia and aversion to food; (2) a change in the arrhythmia, including unusual slowing or acceleration of the heart rate; and (3) regularization of the heart rate in the patient with atrial fibrillation while taking maintenance doses of digitalis.

Although serum levels are now quite popular as indices of digitalis toxicity, the lack of close correspondence between serum levels of glycosides and moderate cardiotoxicity in individual patients has kept alive interest in other tests to evaluate myocardial sensitivity to digitalis. These include the acetylstrophanthidin tolerance test, which is dangerous and should be reserved for experts. Among the more recent and innocuous is the salivary electrolyte test which relies on increases in the concentration of calcium and potassium in the saliva as an index of digitalis toxicity. This test is as yet empirical, because the mechanism for the increase in the concentration of these electrolytes is unknown. The practical value of this test remains to be established.

Digitalis cardiotoxicity is primarily a matter of arrhythmias. As might be expected from the diverse effects of digitalis on the heart, the arrhythmias are generally nonspecific. However, the coincidence of depressed atrioventricular conduction and stimulation of ectopic pacemakers is virtually unique for digitalis toxicity. This combination accounts for arrhythmias characterized by simultaneous rapid atrial rates and slow ventricular responses, for escape beats, and for nonparoxysmal junctional tachycardia. For example, atrial tachycardia with atrioventricular block, generally precipitated by overzealous administration of potassium-losing diuretics, is characteristic, although not specific, for digitalis toxicity. Even more distinctive is atrioventricular dissociation with junctional rhythm, in which two pacemakers operate independently above and below the intervening area of atrioventricular block. In atrial fibrillation, the advent of serious digitalis toxicity may be signaled by regularization of the ventricular rate because of acceleration of an ectopic focus below a high degree of atrioventricular block.

The usual cause of death in digitalis toxicity is ventricular fibrillation. Rarely does it appear unexpectedly. More often, it is presaged by multifocal premature contractions and runs of ventricular tachycardia. Consequently, premature ventricular beats that appear after digitalis has been started or during maintenance therapy have to be regarded as serious warnings of toxicity, particularly if they are multifocal in origin and if there is bigeminy involving premature beats that are bizarre in appearance. Rarely do ventricular arrhythmias occur

without other evidence of digitalis intake, including the characteristic ST-T deformations, disturbances in atrial ventricular conduction, and atrial arrhythmias.

Treatment. The mainstay for treating digitalis cardiotoxicity is to stop the digitalis and to discontinue diuretics that contributed to hypokalemia. There is no specific antidote. Fortunately, most digitalis-induced arrhythmias are arrested by stopping digitalis. Thus junctional rhythms without excessive ventricular rates or evidence of ventricular irritability are generally treated without specific medication or intervention. But if the arrhythmia is characteristic of ventricular irritability or if it has caused hemodynamic upset in the form of hypotension, heart failure, and pulmonary edema, medical intervention is mandatory.

Potassium is the agent of choice for suppressing digitalis-induced automaticity. But because it slows conduction through the myocardium and specialized conduction tissues, thereby potentiating the depression produced by digitalis, it must be used with extreme caution when atrioventricular block is severe. In the latter case, the introduction of a temporary perivenous cardiac pacemaker may prove useful in tiding the patient over the period needed to eliminate the excess digitalis, particularly if antiarrhythmic drugs are to be used to suppress ectopic atrial or ventricular beats.

If the arrhythmia has produced no crisis, if renal function is adequate, and if there is no hyperkalemia, potassium salts (4 to 6 grams of potassium chloride per day) may be administered orally. On the other hand, if the situation is deteriorating rapidly because of ectopic beats or uncontrollable tachycardia, potassium salts may be administered intravenously. Continuous electrocardiographic monitoring is mandatory during intravenous administration. The combination of continuous monitoring and careful intravenous titration of the arrhythmia is generally safer than is oral administration. The usual preparation for intravenous use contains 40 mEq of potassium in a 500 ml solution of 5 per cent glucose in water; this is administered slowly, e.g., at a rate of 40 mEq per hour. This may be repeated, if necessary, for up to three doses. Hypotension may limit the amount of potassium that can be given by vein. The electrocardiogram is monitored throughout, recognizing that high plasma concentrations of potassium may per se cause death through cardiac depression, arrhythmias, or arrest. The characteristic changes in the EKG are disappearance of the P wave, widening of the QRS complexes, changes in the S-T segments, and tall, peaked T waves.

Antiarrhythmic drugs which decrease ventricular automaticity by slowing diastolic depolarization, such as procainamide, lidocaine, propranolol, and diphenylhydantoin, are effective but must be used cautiously. Procainamide is useful when potassium fails to control the arrhythmia or if potassium is contraindicated because of uremia or hyperkalemia. It also has the advantage of sustained action if digitalis toxicity should persist. But it runs the risk of hypotension, depression of contractility, and producing AV block.

Lidocaine (1 to 2 mg per kilogram in one to two minutes by intravenous injection or as continuous infusion) has been used to control premature ventricular beats and ventricular tachycardia resulting from digitalis. It produces an effect within 45 to 90 seconds which is dissipated within 20 minutes. It has the advantage over procainamide of not causing hypotension. Doses less than 750 mg per hour are rarely associated with significant toxic effects, i.e., neurologic disorders and convulsions.

Diphenylhydantoin has been advocated for the treatment of digitalis-induced arrhythmias because it does not depress atrioventricular conduction. It is administered intravenously at a rate of 5 to 10 mg per kilogram over a 5- to 15-minute period. Propranolol, quinidine, and chelating agents are also being used. Electroconversion by DC shock, which has proved to be remarkably effective in controlling many arrhythmias, is a desperate measure of last resort in digitalis-toxic arrhythmias because of the likelihood of producing uncontrollable paroxysmal ventricular arrhythmias.

Blood Levels. The pharmacologic effectiveness of most drugs depends on concentration at the site of action. Dosage may be a poor guide to this effective concentration because of biologic unpredictability with respect to absorption from the gastrointestinal tract, patterns of distribution throughout the body, and in rates of metabolism and excretion. In general, it is anticipated that concentration of a drug in the blood (serum or plasma) will relate better to therapeutic consequences, including toxicity, than will dosage.

In recent years, as a result of advances in radioimmunoassay technology, determination of serum concentrations of some cardiac glycosides became practical and available as well as reliable, accurate, and specific. The application of these tests to patients taking digitalis preparations (digoxin, digitoxin) has shown that the frequency and severity of toxic effects increase progressively as serum concentrations exceed therapeutic levels.

But some overlap in concentrations does occur, particularly in the zone between toxic and therapeutic levels. Moreover, occasionally there is a complete disparity between serum concentration and clinical consequences. These divergences are not unexpected because of the multiplicity of physiologic, pathologic, and biochemical influences that can modify the response to a given concentration of glycoside in the serum (and at the site of action): e.g., hypokalemia, acid-base disturbances, hypoxemia, interaction with other drugs, hypoproteinemia, acquisition of tolerance. But the exceptions do emphasize that serum concentrations must be interpreted critically in the light of the clinical setting.

Currently, determination of serum concentration of a digitalis glycoside is most useful in patients who are suspected of digitalis toxicity but are unable to provide an accurate account of digitalis dosage. It also has a place in guiding dosage in candidates for digitalis toxicity, e.g., heart failure complicated by renal insufficiency or by violent biochemical and physiologic perturbations, as after cardiac surgery. At the other extreme, determination of serum concentration may indicate that refractory heart failure may simply be a consequence of inadequate dosage.

Digitalis in Acute Myocardial Infarction. As a general rule, digitalis is the drug of choice for myocardial failure. Since some degree of left ventricular failure is characteristic of acute myocardial infarction, it might seem reasonable to afford high priority to digitalis in the therapeutic program. Although this generalization still applies to *severe* heart failure during acute myocardial infarction, particularly if the heart is enlarged, the value of digitalis in less urgent degrees of left ventricular failure during acute myocardial infarction is much less certain.

The dilemma stems from the noninfarcted myocardium. If the noninfarcted ventricle has failed, considerable improvement is to be expected from the inotropic effects of digitalis; conversely, if the noninfarcted ventricle is normal, the inotropic effect will be of little consequence, particularly when compared to the inotropic effects of circulating catecholamines that the acute crisis has promoted. The possibility also exists that, even if digitalis does enhance contractility of the noninfarcted area, the net effect on cardiac performance may not be impressive because of the paradoxical motion of the infarcted area during cardiac contraction.

In addition to these uncertainties concerning enhanced contractility, the threat exists that digitalis may promote ventricular irritability in the peri-infarcted, ischemic zone of the myocardium, thereby predisposing to ectopic foci and uncontrollable ventricular arrhythmias. This likelihood is accentuated by a variety of other concomitant influences that predispose to ventricular arrhythmias: increased sympathetic activity, hypokalemia, and hypoxemia (to which excess sedation may contribute).

These reservations, plus the availability of effective diuretics to clear pulmonary congestion and edema during the first few days of an acute myocardial infarction, encourage extraordinary circumspection in using digitalis during the acute episode. On the other hand, if heart failure persists after the acute crisis—because of either extensive scarring or unremitting hemodynamic overload—digitalis is clearly required because the myocardium has failed globally. Moreover, should atrial fibrillation with a rapid ventricular response complicate acute myocardial infarction early or late in its course, digitalis may be lifesaving. For other supraventricular arrhythmias, which generally require larger doses of digitalis and may even prove refractory, antiarrhythmic agents or electrical conversion are preferable during the phase of increased ventricular irritability.

Other Inotropic Agents: Sympathomimetic Amines. Although fashions in diuretics continue to change, no inotropic agent has as yet been found to compete with digitalis. Substitutes have been sought among the sympathomimetic amines which also stimulate the myocardium but differently from digitalis. The qualifications that have been sought include effectiveness after oral administration, improved contractility in conjunction with peripheral vasodilatation, increased renal excretion of sodium, and a greater increase in coronary blood flow than in myocardial oxygen consumption. Three catecholamines have been singled out for close scrutiny because of their ability to stimulate the heart and to decrease peripheral resistance: epinephrine, isoproterenol, and dopamine. Unfortunately, none of these is on a clinical par with digitalis: all three provoke tachycardia; epinephrine decreases the elimination of sodium by the kidney, whereas isoproterenol usually has no effect on sodium excretion; dopamine has to be given intravenously, acts briefly, and causes undesirable increments in systemic arterial pressure.

Glucagon, a polypeptide hormone produced chiefly by the α cells of the pancreas, attracted considerable attention for a while as a possible adjunct for the patient in refractory heart failure who can tolerate no more digitalis. Like the catecholamines, glucagon presumably exerts its cardiotonic effects by activating adenyl cyclase. It has been given by continuous intravenous infusion (2 to 4 mg per hour for 10 to 13 days) and by injections of large single doses (10 to 25 mg). In these doses, the major side effect was nausea; abnormalities in blood sugar levels were uncommon. Unfortunately, enthusiasm for this agent has begun to wane because of recent evidence that the effects of glucagon on myocardial contractility are far less consistent in chronic heart failure than in the normal heart.

Cardiac Assist Devices.   In some clinics, attempts have been made to gain temporary respite for the heart in acute refractory failure, using devices which share the load for hours to days while the heart recuperates. The most popular methods are (1) venoarterial bypass, which assists the heart by diverting blood from the heart and returning it by a pump to the arterial tree, and (2) counterpulsation, which is synchronized with the heart beat to modify aortic pressure by rhythmically changing either the blood volume in the aorta, using an external pump, or the capacity of the aorta, using an intra-aortic balloon. All methods aim to reduce the external work of the heart, the developed tension, and the myocardial oxygen consumption while improving coronary perfusion. Technical problems have restricted the use of these appliances in man to desperate circumstances (e.g., cardiogenic shock) and for as brief a period as possible. As yet, there are exceedingly few long-term survivors.

Diuretics

Inordinate retention of salt and water, followed by expansion of the plasma and the interstitial tissue compartments of the extracellular fluid volume, is a hallmark of congestive heart failure and is responsible for many of its symptoms. Consequently, elimination of the excess salt and water and contraction of the extravascular fluid volume by diuresis are essential for the successful treatment of heart failure.

"Dry" Weight.   The use of diuretics entails two separate problems: elimination of excess fluid, and the maintenance of edema-free ("dry") weight. In the hospital, where the patient is at rest and salt intake is precisely controlled, low dosages of diuretics may suffice to maintain dry weight. Out of the hospital, where the patient engages in various degrees of exercise, and salt intake is neither readily monitored nor controlled, larger doses may be needed. However, continued use of large doses of diuretics inevitably leads to serious derangements in electrolyte balance, often predisposing to digitalis toxicity by way of hypokalemia. Consequently, once the urgent need for brisk diuresis has passed—as during an episode of acute pulmonary edema—the optimal cardiotonic program relies heavily on digitalis and salt restriction and depends on diuretics as an ancillary measure.

Salt and Water Restriction.   Restriction of sodium intake should be directed not only at sodium chloride per se but also at sodium-containing medications, e.g., antacids. Restriction of water intake is rarely necessary except after the use of potent diuretics which predispose to hyponatremia and water intoxication. In mild heart failure, salt intake is generally restricted to less than 3 grams per day; in severe congestive heart failure, intake of less than 0.5 gram per day is often needed to promote diuresis and to reduce the blood volume and venous pressure. Overzealous sodium restriction in conjunction with potent sodium-losing diuretics, particularly in the elderly or in others with impaired renal function, may lead to weakness, oliguria, and azotemia.

The Sodium Control System.   The major diuretics increase the rate of sodium excretion by the renal tubule. As indicated previously, the tubule is the end organ of an elaborate control system that is influenced by hemodynamic and neurohumoral mechanisms. For some mysterious reason, the control system seems to be reset in heart failure so that an expanded extracellular fluid volume, usually a stimulus to diuresis, coexists with antidiuresis. Nonetheless, despite this reset, it is possible to modify the handling of sodium by intervening at several different sites in the control system.

The diuretics that will be considered interfere with the control system by modifying the reabsorption of sodium, with its accompanying anions and water, by the end organ, the renal tubule (Fig. 5). Five distinct categories of diuretics are in common use (Table 3). Each affects tubular reabsorption somewhat differently, and each produces its own characteristic abnormalities in electrolyte pattern, hydration, and acid-base balance. These abnormalities represent the pharmacologic consequences of effective drug action. When carried to extremes, or when effects interact, they are responsible for the toxicity of these different diuretics.

Thiazides.   Because of their effectiveness by mouth, their reliability, and their relative freedom from toxicity if administered circumspectly, the benzothiadiazine drugs are usually the diuretics of choice in cardiac edema. The prototypes of this group are chlorothiazide and hydrochlorothiazide (Table 4). *Acute* administration promotes the urinary excretion of sodium, chloride, and potassium without consistent change in urinary pH or bicarbonate excretion. The predominant diuretic effect (natriuresis and chloruresis) has been localized to inhibi-

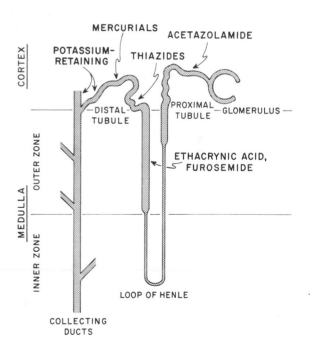

Figure 5. Schematic representation of a nephron, indicating predominant sites of action of the five groups of diuretics. Carbonic anhydrase inhibitors exert predominant effects on the proximal tubule. The potassium-retaining diuretics affect the distal nephron. The major diuretic effect of the thiazides is at a site of urine dilution in the cortical portion of the ascending limb of the loop of Henle. Ethacrynic acid, furosemide, and the organomercurials act chiefly on the loop of Henle, affecting both the diluting and concentrating segments to achieve potent diuretic effects.

TABLE 3.   Diuretic Agents in Heart Failure

Type of Diuretic	Effect on Kidney		Effect on Electrolytes		Toxic Manifestations	Special Features
	Principal Site of Action	Mechanism	In Urine	In Blood		
Thiazides (chloruretic sulfonamides)	Ascending limb of loop of Henle; distal tubule	Interference with dilution of urine	Increased excretion of Na, Cl, K	Hypochloremic alkalosis; hypokalemia	Nausea; vomiting; skin rashes; hyperuricemia; hypercalcemia; hyperglycemia; azotemia	Loss of effectiveness and hypokalemia are common on continued administration
Ethacrynic acid*	Ascending limb of loop of Henle; distal tubule; probably proximal tubule	Interference with dilution and concentration of urine	Increased excretion of Na, Cl, HCO_3, K, H	Hypochloremic alkalosis; hypokalemia; hyponatremia	Hypotension; contraction alkalosis; hyperuricemia; hypercalcemia; azotemia; hyperglycemia; hearing loss	Causes renal vasodilatation; effective in renal insufficiency; systemic acidosis or alkalosis; potent diuresis often followed by rebound
Organomercurials	Proximal and/or distal tubule	Decrease of isosmotic reabsorption	Increased excretion of Na, Cl, H	Hypochloremic alkalosis	Mercury intoxication; sudden death (after IV injection); occasional agranulocytosis	Inactivated by hypochloremic alkalosis; hazardous in oliguria
Potassium-sparing†	Distal tubule	Aldosterone antagonism for Na-K exchange	Decreased excretion of K and H; slight increase in Na, Cl, HCO_3	Hyperkalemia	Generally nontoxic; GI upset; gynecomastia; rare agranulocytosis	Synergistic with thiazides and ethacrynic acid; avoid in renal insufficiency and in hyperkalemia
Carbonic anhydrase inhibitors	Proximal tubule	Inhibition of enzyme involved in acidification of urine	Increased excretion of Na, K, HCO_3; decrease in H	Hyperchloremic acidosis; hypokalemia	Generally nontoxic; mild GI and mental upsets; occasional sulfonamide idiosyncrasy	Not very potent and loses effectiveness in a few days

*Furosemide (Lasix), a nonthiazide sulfonamide, has practically the same indications and effects despite its different chemical structure.
†Spironolactone (Aldactone) operates as a competitive inhibitor of endogenous aldosterone; triamterene and amiloride are noncompetitive inhibitors and produce the characteristic effects on the urine even though aldosterone is absent.

TABLE 4.   Administration of Diuretics

	Example	Relevant Chemical Structure	Preferred Route of Administration	Usual Range of Daily Dosage	Suggested Pattern of Administration
Thiazides	Chlorothiazide (Diuril)	Benzothiadiazine derivative	Oral	500 mg × 2–4	Standard type of diuretic to start treatment; few days on, few days off to avoid refractoriness and serious electrolyte disturbances
Ethacrynic acid*	Ethacrynic acid (Edecrin)	Ketone derivative of aryloxyacetic acid	Oral or IV*	50 mg × 2–3	Reserve for serious or refractory edema
Organomercurials	Meralluride (mercuhydrin)	Theophylline plus organic mercurial	IM	2 ml	Adjunct diuretic or for moderately rapid response in hospital
Potassium sparing†	Triamterene (Dyrenium)	Pteridine derivative	Oral	200 mg	Continuous administration in conjunction with more potent potassium-losing diuretics; do not use with potassium supplements
Carbonic anhydrase inhibitors	Acetazolamide (Diamox)	Sulfanilamide derivative	Oral	250 mg × 4–6	Episodic as booster diuretic; useful before injection of organomercurial for chloride-retaining effect

*Furosemide and ethacrynic acid may be given intravenously as well as by mouth. For ordinary use, however, furosemide is administered as a single oral dose in the morning. In an urgent situation (pulmonary edema), furosemide, as well as ethacrynic acid, may be administered intravenously (50 mg). Intravenous administration should not be administered at less than six-hour intervals.

†Spironolactone (Aldactone), 75 to 100 mg per day, is commonly used as a potassium-sparing diuretic. In refractory heart failure doses of 100 to 600 mg per day have proved helpful.

tion of sodium absorption at a diluting site in the distal nephron (Fig. 5). Although there is also a carbonic anhydrase-inhibiting effect, it is generally insignificant until large daily doses are reached (of the order of 2000 mg per day). Kaliuresis depends on an increase in the quantity of sodium delivered to the distal nephron. Intravenous administration of chlorothiazide is uricosuric, whereas chronic administration results in hyperuricemia. The mechanisms responsible for the paradoxical uric acid effects are still unclear.

Hypokalemia is particularly apt to arise after intensive diuresis with thiazides or after prolonged thiazide therapy. Supplementary doses of potassium may then be required. Several generalizations have proved useful as practical guides to therapy. Acute hypokalemia that is modest in degree is managed by diet; if diet fails to correct the hypokalemia, supplementary doses of potassium may be required. Potassium chloride is generally the agent of choice for oral supplementation, because hypochloremic metabolic alkalosis usually accompanies diuretic-induced hypokalemia. For severe hypokalemia, intravenous infusions are used. To prevent hypokalemia during chronic administration of potassium-losing diuretics, aldosterone inhibitors are useful.

Certain precautions merit attention in applying these guides to therapy. Potassium salts administered orally in any form cause gastric irritation. This side effect is generally tolerable, especially in the hospital, where potassium chloride can be safely given in liquid form after meals. Prolonged administration of potassium salts, particularly if enteric coated, is particularly hazardous because of the high incidence of intestinal ulceration, perforation, and peritonitis, often followed by intestinal stenosis and obstruction. No matter how administered, excessive doses of potassium are apt to lead to hyperkalemia. This likelihood is enhanced in older persons who often have slight renal impairment, especially if an aldosterone inhibitor is given concomitantly.

Ethacrynic Acid and Furosemide.   These are the most potent natriuretic agents currently available. Both are organic acids but otherwise are quite different chemically. Furosemide is a sulfonamide–anthranilic acid derivative related to the thiazide diuretics, whereas ethacrynic acid is a ketone derivative of aryloxyacetic acid (Table 4). Like the thiazides, they are effective orally and are rapid acting. They exert powerful diuretic effects by inhibiting both the renal diluting and concentrating mechanisms in the ascending limb of the loop of Henle (Fig. 5). Ethacrynic acid is without appreciable effect on carbonic anhydrase, whereas furosemide does elicit modest anti-carbonic anhydrase activity.

Ethacrynic acid, administered orally, exerts its effects in 30 minutes and continues to act for six to eight hours; administered intravenously, it acts within a few minutes, reaching its peak activity in one hour. Both agents elicit a marked increase in urine flow containing large quantities of sodium and chloride (of the order of 20 to 30 per cent of the filtered load). Kaliuresis is consistent and appreciable. In conventional doses, neither drug consistently increases bicarbonate secretion or modifies urine pH. But chronic administration of ethacrynic acid promotes hydrogen loss in a bicarbonate-free urine, i.e., produces metabolic alkalosis.

A cardinal virtue of these agents (in contrast with thiazides and carbonic anhydrase inhibitors) is their lack of effect on filtration rate or renal plasma flow unless sodium depletion occurs. This lack of direct hemodynamic effect is fortunate, because a decrease in filtration rate interferes with their action; conversely, increase in filtration rate, as by intravenous administration of mannitol or albumin, enhances their effects. At peak effect, both agents decrease renal vascular resistance.

Ethacrynic acid and furosemide remain effective despite gross electrolyte disturbances and hypoalbuminemia. If pushed, either may cause hyponatremia, volume depletion, fall in blood pressure, fall in urine volume, azotemia, and water retention. Because of the upsets in the electrolyte concentrations which they induce, other diuretics are preferred for maintenance treatment. They are most valuable in three situations: in acute pulmonary edema (25 to 50 mg intravenously), in severe or refractory heart failure, or when renal function is impaired (because they increase renal blood flow). Both agents produce "contraction alkalosis," i.e., an increase in plasma bicarbonate consequent to the decrease in extracellular fluid volume that follows excretion of a large volume of bicarbonate-poor urine. The metabolic alkalosis that follows hydrogen depletion and "contraction" predisposes to alveolar hypoventilation through its depressant effects on respiratory control mechanisms.

Organomercurial Diuretics. Until the advent of potent oral diuretics, the organomercurials, generally a combination of an organic mercurial and theophylline, were the diuretic agents of choice in heart failure. Now they are generally reserved for parenteral administration in hospital. After administration of a maximally effective dose intravenously, large (and approximately equal) amounts of sodium and chloride are eliminated in the urine. The normal subject is apt to eliminate 10 per cent of the filtered load, whereas the individual that has been primed to the stage of hyperchloremic acidosis by prior administration of ammonium chloride may eliminate up to 20 per cent of the filtered load. Bicarbonate excretion does not increase, and urinary acidity persists during the diuresis. The effect on potassium excretion is variable and generally small, depending on prior rates of excretion. Generally they tend to decrease potassium.

Like ethacrynic acid and furosemide, the organomercurials exert an important inhibitory effect on sodium reabsorption in the loop of Henle, impairing both the diluting and concentrating mechanisms. In Figure 5, the organomercurials are shown as acting predominantly on the distal tubule, beyond the predominant sites of action of the thiazides, ethacrynic acid, and furosemide. However, these distinctions are far from absolute. Theophylline-containing mercurials usually elicit transient increases in filtration rate, but this effect is generally neutralized by volume concentration if diuresis is effective.

The organomercurials are almost invariably administered intramuscularly. After intramuscular injection, the onset of action is in one to two hours, reaching a peak in six hours, and lasting for 12 to 24 hours. Early in treatment, a brisk diuresis and natriuresis occur. But with continued use, refractoriness may result, generally for one of two reasons: (1) the onset of a hypochloremic hypokalemic alkalosis (with fairly normal sodium levels); responsiveness may then be restored by administering ammonium chloride; or (2) the advent of a low-salt syndrome in which sodium as well as chloride levels in the serum are severely depressed; this state responds to water restriction.

Aldosterone Antagonists. A characteristic feature of chronic heart failure is high circulating levels of renin and aldosterone. Aldosterone, either by providing energy for active transport or by increasing permeability, enhances the movement of sodium through the distal tubular cell, from lumen to interstitium. Water follows passively. In addition to promoting sodium reabsorption, aldosterone also increases potassium excretion by a mechanism that is not entirely clear but is more than an ion-exchange mechanism. In heart failure the hyperaldosteronism causes continuing sodium retention, whereas potassium excretion remains normal, i.e., no hypokalemia. Aldosterone antagonists interfere with these actions, causing potassium retention and sodium excretion.

Three agents are available: spironolactone, triamterene, and amiloride (MK-870). Spironolactone is most popular; amiloride is not yet available for general use. Although all three act by competing for receptor sites in the distal tubule, the intimate mechanisms involved in electrolyte secretion may be quite different. The major site of action of spironolactone is in the distal tubule, in the region of the aldosterone-stimulated secretion of hydrogen and potassium. It is a specific competitive inhibitor of aldosterone and has no action if aldosterone is absent. It promotes natriuresis, water loss, and potassium retention by depressing aldosterone-dependent sodium-potassium exchange in the distal tubule. It is only effective in the presence of high levels of mineralocorticoid activity; it is devoid of effect after adrenalectomy. Conversely, triamterene (Table 4) and amiloride are noncompetitive inhibitors that inhibit potassium and hydrogen ion excretion even if aldosterone is absent. Their mechanism of action is unclear. Although these natriuretic agents are far less potent than the thiazides, ethacrynic acid, furosemides, and the organomercurials, they have the extraordinary advantage for prolonged use of continuing effectiveness, minor electrolyte derangements, and the virtual absence of toxicity as long as hyperkalemia is avoided. These agents are unique in that they are given without interruption, because, in contrast to the thiazides, ethacrynic acid, and furosemide, they do not lose effectiveness in a few days nor do they cause violent electrolyte upheavals.

Spironolactone is expensive but effective. Oral doses, ranging from 50 to 600 mg per day, are well tolerated for months. A few days may elapse before its action becomes apparent. It is currently being used primarily to potentiate the effects of the more powerful diuretics, particularly if potassium depletion is a serious consideration.

Carbonic Anhydrase Inhibitors. These agents are effective by mouth. They elicit an increase in excretion of bicarbonate, sodium, and potassium and an increase in urine pH. The most striking increments are in bicarbonate and potassium. By interfering with carbonic anhydrase activity in the kidney, they inhibit hydrogen ion secretion primarily in the proximal and distal portions of the nephron, exerting lesser effects on the loop of Henle, i.e., little effect on urinary diluting or concentrating mechanisms.

The prototype of this group is acetazolamide (Table 4). It is a weak diuretic and loses its effectiveness as hyperchloremic metabolic acidosis develops because of diminished hydrogen ion excretion (usually in 48 hours). Like ammonium chloride, this class of diuretics is particularly valuable in patients with high serum bicarbonate, as occurs in cor pulmonale or metabolic alkalosis. They are valuable in preparing for a mercurial diuresis because of the hyperchloremic acidosis that they produce. This group also enhances natriuresis produced by thiazides, ethacrynic acid, and furosemide. A contraindication for its use is severe acidosis, as from renal failure or hepatic insufficiency.

Special Diuretics. This is a miscellaneous group of agents that are used with extreme caution and under special conditions. For example, osmotic diuretics such as mannitol and albumin, which expand the circulating blood volume, have the potential for increasing the renal blood flow and for blocking the reabsorption of sodium and water at the proximal tubule. However, in heart failure they entail the risk of circulatory overload and pulmonary edema.

Combinations. There are two main reasons for introducing a combination of diuretics into a cardiotonic program: to avoid serious electrolyte upsets that are bound to occur if the powerful primary diuretics are administered without pause, in large dosage, for long periods; and to stimulate diuresis when the prevailing cardiotonic program no longer suffices to prevent edema. In either case, the net diuretic effect of the combination will be determined by a wide variety of influences: the respective sites of action on the renal tubule of each agent, the extent of competitive inhibition at common receptor sites, the dose-response curves of the individual drugs, strategic timing of the administration of one agent with respect to the other, and the acid-base and electrolyte balances at the time that the agents are given.

A currently popular duo of diuretics is a potassium-sparing agent (triamterene or spironolactone) that is taken daily and a thiazide that is taken intermittently (e.g., for four days of each week). In time, the thiazide may be succeeded by ethacrynic acid or ethacrynic acid may be given sporadically as needed to sustain the edema-free state. On occasion, particularly in the hospital, a mercurial diuretic (after prior acidification) may prove helpful in overcoming a resistant state of edema. In contrast to the foregoing, other combinations hold little promise for success. Thus the combined use of acetazolamide and a mercurial diuretic is not apt to be exceedingly effective, because, by preventing acidification of the urine, the carbonic anhydrase inhibitor is apt to block, rather than to enhance, the diuretic effect of the mercurial.

The same general principles govern the use of combinations of diuretics in the treatment of refractory edema. This troublesome state is now relatively uncommon because of the advent of powerful primary diuretics, particularly furosemide and ethacrynic acid, coupled with a better understanding of the sites of action of the auxiliary diuretics. On the other hand, refractory edema may again become tractable by reversing electrolyte and acid-base imbalances that have been produced by unremitting administration of the primary diuretics for long periods. As a working principle, resistance to diuresis is overcome by deliberate selection of agents that act on different parts of the tubule. This approach presupposes that digitalis dosage is optimal. On occasion, aminophylline, by its inotropic effect, may reinforce the diuretic action of a thiazide or ethacrynic acid. Clearly, many opportunities exist for the physician to devise original sequences and combinations of diuretics. However, a restraining influence is imposed by the complicated interplay that is to be expected, not only between the diuretic agents per se, but also within the broad context of a deranged internal environment that generally is a feature of the state of refractory edema.

Refractory Edema. This is a state of edema that resists conventional cardiotonic and diuretic measures. Before embarking on an endless train of drug combinations, the patient should be carefully re-evaluated for either a complication or an underlying disorder that has been overlooked: a surgically correctable disorder, such as mitral stenosis or constrictive pericarditis; a medical disorder, including hyperthyroidism, anemia, pulmonary emboli, bacterial endocarditis, persistent infection, and arrhythmias; inappropriate or excessive diuretic therapy that elicits serious disturbances in blood volume and electrolyte composition, digitalis toxicity, and water intoxication; physical overactivity; excessive salt intake and renal disease; sodium-containing medicaments, such as antacids, or agents such as reserpine, propranolol, and guanethidine which depress the myocardium to the point of failure.

Complications. A variety of disturbances may complicate effective diuretic therapy. These include hypotension and vascular collapse from rapid, massive diuresis; sodium depletion, usually the consequence of prolonged and effective diuretic therapy in conjunction with excessive water intake; hypokalemia from uninterrupted use of diuretics, predisposing to digitalis toxicity; hyperkalemia from injudicious administration of aldosterone antagonists and potassium supplements; metabolic alkalosis, either from a massive excretion of a bicarbonate-poor urine or from a combination of increased hydrogen ion excretion in the urine and alveolar hypoventilation as produced by ethacrynic acid or potassium depletion; and hyperuricemia after prolonged administration of small doses of the thiazides, ethacrynic acid, and furosemide, which share an inhibiting effect on uric acid excretion. In predisposed individuals, the hyperuricemia of prolonged diuretic therapy may precipitate an episode of gout. The thiazides, and occasionally furosemide, may precipitate diabetes which is rarely severe.

General Comments. In treating heart failure, rarely is there a desperate need to restore everything to normal at once by vigorous diuresis. The temptation to restore the patient immediately to dry weight and to free him of breathlessness and congestion must be tempered by the penalty of dehydration and severe electrolyte disturbances. The more leisurely the diuretic therapy, the more durable and tolerable the relief.

The ability of these potent diuretics to elicit dramatic diuresis has led to their abuse. Thus without direct inotropic effect on the heart, a single injection of ethacrynic acid can effect a decrease in blood volume, a decrease in intracardiac filling pressures, an increase in cardiac output, and clear edema. But ethacrynic acid is rarely advisable as the mainstay of therapy unless edema is refractory and less drastic measures have proved ineffective. Only when coupled with a full cardiotonic program can judicious control of heart failure be maintained, particularly if the underlying heart disease is progressive and severe complications of diuretic therapy are to be avoided.

Cherniack, N. S., and Longobardo, G. S.: Cheyne-Stokes breathing. *In* Physiology in Medicine. N. Engl. J. Med., 288:952, 1973.

Dollery, C. T., George, C. F., and Orme, M. L'E.: Drug interaction in cardiovascular disease. Prog. Cardiology, 1:31, 1972.

Fishman, A. P.: Pulmonary edema. The water-exchanging function of the lung. Circulation, 46:390, 1972.

Fishman, A. P., and Richards, D. W. (eds.): Circulation of the Blood. Men and Ideas. New York. Oxford University Press, 1964.

Goldberg, M.: The renal physiology of diuretics. *In* Berliner, R. W., and Orloff, J. (eds.): Handbook of Physiology—Renal Physiology. Washington. American Physiological Society, 1973.

Lee, K. S., and Klaus, W.: The subcellular basis for the mechanism of inotropic action of cardiac glycosides. Pharmacol. Rev., 23:193, 1971.

Marshall, R. J., and Shepherd, J. T.: Cardiac Function in Health and Disease. Philadelphia. W. B. Saunders Company, 1968.

Mason, D. T., Zelis, R., and Wikman-Coffelt, J. (eds.): Symposium on congestive heart failure. Am. J. Cardiol., 32:395, 1973.

Noble, M. I. M.: Problems concerning the application of concepts of muscle mechanics to the determination of the contractile state of the heart. Circulation, 45:252, 1972.

Ross, J., Jr., and Peterson, K. L. (editorial): On the assessment of cardiac inotropic state. Circulation, 47:435, 1973.

Smith, T. W., and Haber, E.: Digitalis. N. Engl. J. Med., 289:945, 1010, 1063, 1125, 1973.

·542. SHOCK

Alfred P. Fishman

GENERAL FEATURES

Circulatory shock ("shock") is a life-threatening state in which vital processes are profoundly depressed because of inadequate organ blood flow. Often the interval between the onset of shock and death is less than 48 hours. The circulatory inadequacy may stem from a large decrease in cardiac output, in venous return to the heart, or in peripheral vascular resistance. Of these three potential mechanisms, a considerable decrease in venous return, as after massive hemorrhage, is most common. Not uncommon is acute enfeeblement of the left ventricle after extensive myocardial infarction. Rarely does shock *begin* with massive peripheral vasodilation. On the other hand, peripheral vasodilation invariably complicates prolonged circulatory inadequacy and often is responsible for the fatal outcome.

A diverse assortment of initiating mechanisms (Table 5) can set into motion the sequence culminating in shock. Since each mechanism registers its own distinct imprint on the final picture, the clinical manifestations of shock can vary greatly. But certain features occur quite regularly, particularly if shock is advanced or progressing: arterial hypotension (see below); a decrease in cardiac output sufficient to elicit signs of organ hypoperfusion; metabolic acidosis; and a need for therapeutic intervention to sustain cerebral, cardiac, or renal function at levels compatible with life.

The longer shock lasts, the worse the prognosis. In time, a stage of refractory shock may be reached in which the peripheral circulation continues to dilate despite intense sympathetic nervous activity and vigorous therapy; at the same time, cardiac output falls progressively because of inadequate venous return and inadequate blood flow to the myocardium. The nature of refractory shock is still unsettled, particularly with respect to the role of toxins in producing the fatal outcome. Many toxic factors have been proposed. Most of these are held to arise in splanchnic organs (liver, spleen, pancreas, intestine), from which they are distributed throughout the body by blood and lymph, exerting their principal noxious effects on heart, lungs, microcirculation, and reticuloendothelial system.

Organ Hypoperfusion. The common denominator in shock is cellular dysfunction and death from organ hypoperfusion. This "cellular hypoperfusion" compromises the delivery of metabolic nutriments, substrates, and oxygen to cells and allows metabolic end products to accumulate, thereby deranging intracellular and extracellular environments, disturbing energy pathways, and disordering cellular function. The decrease in blood flow does not affect all organs and tissues equally: first deprived are the nonvital tissues of the gastrointestinal tract, muscle, connective tissue, and skin; only later do the kidneys, liver, heart, lungs, and brain become ischemic. One clinical manifestation of organ hypoperfusion is the lower skin temperature than rectal temperature, caused by cutaneous vasoconstriction; another is oliguria, reflecting diminished renal blood flow.

Arterial Hypotension. A decrease in arterial blood pressure used to be considered a sine qua non for the clinical diagnosis of shock. This stricture no longer applies, because blood pressure in shock may vary considerably, depending on initiating mechanism, severity of shock, duration, and complications. Early in traumatic or hemorrhagic shock, if anxiety is high and pain is intense, blood pressure may be high because of an outpouring of catecholamines into the circulation. This is a treacherous phase, for the hypertension is apt to be fleeting and followed by a precipitous drop in blood pressure. Oppositely, blood pressure inevitably falls to hypotensive levels before death. Between these two extremes are areas of critical clinical importance. A modest decrease in arterial blood pressure, of the order of 10 to 20 mm Hg, quite common at the start of shock, generally represents success of compensatory mechanisms, at least transiently, in stabilizing the circulation; frank arterial hypotension (systolic blood pressure less than 80 mm Hg) signals that shock is progressing and that compensatory mechanisms are proving inadequate. From the point of view of therapy, a more favorable prognosis is to be anticipated from early recognition and intervention than from relying on definite hypotension as the indication for therapy.

The significance of hypotension in shock depends largely on the concomitant state of vasomotor activity. Clinically the assessment of vasomotor activity is generally quite simple: low blood pressure in conjunction with warm hands and good urine flow indicates vasodilation and good cardiac output; hypotension, cold hands, and oliguria represent intense vasoconstriction. Interpretation of these findings in terms of prognosis may vary according to etiology, duration, and severity of the shock. Warm hands may occur early in septic shock when opportunity for successful treatment is at its peak. Later on in septic shock, warm hands may reflect paralysis of

TABLE 5.   Categories of Shock

Type	Etiology
Medical:	
1. Hypovolemic shock: decrease in blood volume by loss of blood, plasma or extracellular fluid	Hemorrhage, burns, vomiting, diarrhea, metabolic acidosis, Addisonian crisis, heat exhaustion
2. Septic shock	Bacteremia, endotoxemia
3. Cardiogenic shock	Myocardial infarction
4. Shock from inadequate cardiac filling	Severe tachycardia
Surgical:	
1. Shock from inadequate cardiac filling	Pericardial tamponade, tension pneumothorax
2. Shock from acute cardiac defects	Ruptured valve cusp or chorda, perforated ventricular septum
3. Shock from mechanical obstruction in central circulation	Massive pulmonary embolus, ball-valve thrombus of mitral valve

arterioles and opening of arteriovenous shunts in the skin before death. Conversely, persistence of warm hands and good urine flow in cardiogenic shock after acute myocardial infarction raises the prospects for reversibility.

When peripheral vasoconstriction is intense, the sphygmomanometer may give artificially low values in shock because of the low cardiac output and the narrow pulse pressure. Consequently, many clinics use arterial cannulation to follow the course of the blood pressure during shock. The cannula affords the additional advantage of providing blood samples for the determination of arterial oxygen tension and pH.

Individual Clinical Syndromes. The diverse etiologic agents in shock are sorted in Table 5 according to medical versus surgical management. Only those amenable to medical management will be considered in this chapter. Moreover, this chapter will not deal with states of circulatory inadequacy that mark the end of chronic cardiac disability, such as prolonged heart failure or myocarditis, in which the spent myocardium is no longer capable of improving its performance.

HYPOVOLEMIC SHOCK

Depletion of the blood volume by hemorrhage, trauma, or burns may produce shock. At least 1 liter of blood must be withdrawn from a healthy man before signs of shock appear; these disappear if the blood is returned at once. Trauma to skeletal muscles may also cause shock as blood escapes into the muscles. Extensive burns produce shock because of loss of plasma from the denuded surface. Despite these individual differences, the net effect is hypovolemia. Prompt restoration of the blood volume after hemorrhage restores the circulation to normal. However, extensive burns or trauma to muscle are generally more difficult to manage because the effects of depleted blood volume are complicated by the products of local infection and dead tissue.

The blood volume may be depleted by ways other than direct loss of blood or plasma from the bloodstream. The same end result may be produced by vomiting, diarrhea, intestinal obstruction, diabetic acidosis, and Addison's disease, all of which cause severe loss of water and electrolytes.

The patient who has just experienced a massive hemorrhage is restless and agitated, dimly aware that he is the victim of a calamity but not quite clear about its nature. Organ hypoperfusion is evident in the pallor, oliguria, and disordered cerebration. He asks for water but becomes nauseated after a few sips. The pulse is rapid and thready. The arterial blood pressure is low, and the pulse pressure is narrow. In essence, he is manifesting the consequences of a decrease in cardiac output, heightened sympathetic nervous activity, and redistribution of blood flow.

Pathophysiology. The clinical syndrome is a consequence of an acute decrease in venous return → low cardiac output → arterial hypotension → baroreceptor stimulation → sympathetic nervous activation (including release of epinephrine and norepinephrine) → nonuniform organ perfusion.

The microcirculation of the skin and viscera contains alpha receptors and responds therefore to the increase in circulating catecholamines by vasoconstricting. In turn, the viscera that are poorly endowed with alpha receptors, i.e., brain, heart, and muscle, receive a disproportionately large fraction of the cardiac output. Moreover,

since heart and muscle contain beta receptors that are also stimulated by the circulating catecholamines, the heart exhibits inotropic and chronotropic effects in conjunction with arteriolar and venular dilatation. The cerebral circulation, which has neither alpha nor beta receptors, does not vasoconstrict.

As a result of the low cardiac output and nonuniform vasoconstriction, blood flow slows in the affected vascular beds and formed elements in the blood tend to clump. Cells become damaged and die, releasing lactic acid and enzymes, such as lactic dehydrogenase and glutamic oxaloacetic transaminase, into the blood; coagulation mechanisms are disturbed. If hypoperfusion persists, irreversible metabolic changes in the cells may preclude restoration. Consequently, early treatment of shock is mandatory.

For comparable decrements in cardiac output, the patient in shock is almost invariably worse off than the patient in chronic left ventricular failure. In large measure this clinical discrepancy stems from the acuity of onset and the initiating mechanisms. Thus the same hemodynamic abnormality may operate differently in the two states: the high atrial pressure of *chronic* ventricular failure is characteristically associated with antidiuresis, whereas *acute* elevation of left atrial pressure elicits a diuresis. The left atrial receptors involved in these responses are currently under intensive study. Another important modifying influence is expansion of the blood volume during chronic heart failure as a consequence of salt and water retention by the kidneys; this compensation is lacking in shock.

Peripheral Vascular Resistance. Because of generalized arteriolar constriction, peripheral vascular resistance is generally high in hypovolemic shock. Calculations of peripheral vascular resistance, expressed as the ratio of drop in blood pressure across the systemic circulation to the cardiac output, are commonly advocated as guides to therapy in hypovolemic shock. Usually the ratio is increased, a consequence of heightened sympathetic nervous activity and of increase in circulating catecholamines. But rarely does this calculation provide a more reliable guide to treatment than do the clinical appearance of the patient, the warmth of the skin, the level of blood pressure, the rate and fullness of the pulse, and the urine output. Moreover, because of the nonuniform effects of heightened sympathetic activity, such calculations often tend to obscure the complicated and heterogeneous engagement of the different systemic vascular beds in the different types of shock.

Oxygen Delivery. In addition to the slowed circulation, which impairs oxygen delivery to tissues, disturbances in acid-base balance upset erythrocyte metabolism, including that of the organic phosphate, 2,3-diphosphoglyceric acid (2,3-DPG), thereby increasing the affinity of hemoglobin for oxygen and hindering oxygen delivery to the tissues.

The Heart. In shock that is simply due to an acute decrease in venous return, the heart is rarely seriously affected unless hypotension persists at levels that are insufficient to sustain coronary arterial blood flow, i.e., less than 70 to 80 mm Hg. Toxins from splanchnic viscera may also contribute to depressed contractility when hypotension is prolonged. One potentially toxic substance has been designated "myocardial depressant factor." It is a peptide which is released from the pancreas during hypotension from any cause. During splanchnic hypoperfusion consequent to systemic hypotension, splanchnic tissues release lysosomal hydrolases which not only exert a negative inotropic action on the heart but also sensitize the myocardium to the myocardial depressant factor from the pancreas.

Shock Lung. Early in shock, unless the tracheobronchial tree or chest is abnormal, the lungs generally pose no clinical problem: alveolar ventilation is usually high, and even though there may be some imbalance in alveolar ventilation-perfusion relationships, arterial hypoxemia and hypocapnia are slight and generally insignificant. But as shock continues and grows worse, pulmonary performance deteriorates. Arterial hypoxemia then becomes more marked, principally because of continued blood flow through airless lungs. This situation may be aggravated by narcotics and sedatives which depress alveolar ventilation, by inspissated bronchial secretions which block ventilation in perfused parts of the lungs, by oxygen toxicity which damages the alveolar-capillary membrane, and by overtransfusion which causes pulmonary edema.

Entirely different from this *progressive* deterioration in pulmonary performance in the course of refractory shock is the entity of "shock lung" (or "wet lung" or "Da Nang lung") which has been applied to the syndrome of respiratory failure that interrupts recovery from circulatory collapse. The typical sequence of shock lung was popularized during the Vietnam war: a soldier who experiences severe *nonthoracic* injury, blood loss, and hypotension during combat; successful resuscitation, using tourniquets, transfusions, and opiates on the battlefield; prompt evacuation to a sophisticated medical facility for more deliberate management and recovery; and then, a few days later, the unexpected interruption of convalescence by progressive respiratory distress and failure.

Only a few who reached the hospital in Da Nang developed shock lung. But in them, the clinical syndrome was unmistakable; interruption of convalescence by the insidious onset (over days) of rapid shallow breathing, breathlessness, and productive cough; somewhat later, rales and wheezes; finally, refractory cyanosis. Paralleling this clinical sequence, x-ray examinations showed enlarging interstitial and alveolar infiltrates that continued to extend and to coalesce until the entire lung was enveloped in a diffuse haze. Enriched oxygen mixtures and assisted ventilation became less and less effective in achieving tolerable levels of oxygenation. Finally, death occurred from respiratory insufficiency, often complicated by circulatory collapse. At autopsy the morbid anatomy was stereotyped; vascular congestion, interstitial and alveolar edema, and focal atelectasis ("congestive atelectasis"). Other anatomic changes were common but not quite as consistent: hemorrhage in the interstitial spaces and alveoli, vascular thrombi, fat emboli, fibrin deposits, and hyaline membranes.

The physiologic picture of shock lung observed in Vietnam held no surprises: its features were reduced compliance and arterial hypoxemia. In part, the reduced compliance reflected stiffening of the lungs by congestive atelectasis; the extent to which loss of surfactant contributed was, and still is, enigmatic. The progressive arterial hypoxemia (without hypercapnia) was shown to represent increasing "venous admixture," evidence of continuing blood flow through parts of the lungs which were functionless in gas exchange.

Unfortunately, many of the links that relate injury and resuscitation on the battlefield to respiratory insufficiency during convalescence are missing. Those that

have been proposed include damage to hypoperfused areas of the lungs during the hypotensive episode, endotoxinemia, fat emboli, release of injurious fatty acids and proteolytic agents, discharge of leukocyte lysosomes in the pulmonary capillaries, and disseminated intravascular coagulation or microemboli. There is also the haunting prospect that therapeutic measures which are lifesaving on the battlefield may be involved in the subsequent respiratory distress during convalescence. Thus overzealous administration of liquids immediately after injury, particularly of crystalloid solutions, predisposes to pulmonary congestion and edema. Also, if bank blood was administered, thrombi may have embolized the lungs, thereby contributing to congestive atelectasis. Even the hospital provides opportunity for inflicting lung damage by way of injudicious administration of enriched oxygen mixtures and oversedation. Once the syndrome is full blown, distinctions between cause and effect tend to become blurred as self-perpetuating mechanisms become operative.

The designation "shock lung" has carried over from Vietnam to civilian life and has been applied indiscriminately to a wide variety of adult respiratory distress syndromes. Favoring this practice is the stereotyped "congestive atelectasis" found at autopsy. However, the high mortality from "shock lung" has stimulated re-evaluation of the civilian disorders in the hope of elucidating unique etiologies and pathogenetic mechanisms at which specific therapeutic measures may be directed.

The Liver. Blood flow through the liver increases early in shock but decreases later on. Accompanying the decrease in hepatic blood flow is a sequestration of blood in the splanchnic venous bed. As hepatic blood flow decreases, the effectiveness of the liver in detoxification and in performing its metabolic activities decreases. Consequently, organic acids accumulate in the blood. The metabolic acidosis is associated with hyperglycemia and hyperkalemia and the release of toxic products from splanchnic viscera.

The Kidneys. Oliguria (less than 25 ml per hour) and anuria are common, particularly if systemic arterial hypotension is marked; prerenal azotemia may also be prominent. As the circulation is restored and blood pressure increases, urinary output improves and the azotemia disappears. But if severe hypotension and renal vasoconstriction have persisted for hours, particularly in patients who have abnormal pigments from hemolysis or muscle trauma in the blood, irreversible injury to the kidneys may occur from tubular necrosis.

SEPTIC SHOCK

Septic shock is a state of circulatory collapse associated with toxicity that results from the spread of bacteria and/or their products throughout the body from a focus of infection. A wide range of microbial organisms can elicit septic shock. Chief among these are the common gram-positive and gram-negative pathogens. But even relatively avirulent microorganisms can produce the syndrome of circulatory collapse if sufficient numbers enter the bloodstream for dissemination. Before the days of antimicrobial drugs, gram-positive organisms, including the Staphylococcus, Streptococcus, Pneumococcus, and *Clostridium perfringens* (septic abortion), were common invaders of the bloodstream; the shock then seemed to originate in the primary infection rather than in the bacteremia. But in recent years, gram-negative organisms have emerged as the principal basis for shock associated with sepsis. All gram-negative bacteria—Escherichia, Klebsiella, Pseudomonas, Proteus, Bacteroides—contain a complex lipopolysaccharide, called endotoxin, in their cell walls. In contrast with gram-positive shock, bloodstream invasion by endotoxin seems to elicit the shock.

Endotoxin Shock. Endotoxin shock is a subset of septic shock. It is a complication of a gram-negative infection associated with the death of the bacteria and the consequent release of endotoxin from their walls. Some investigators believe that the action of endotoxin is primarily via an immune response involving complement. Within the bloodstream endotoxin combines with complement of leukocytes, and activates latent systems, to produce a variety of agents, including sympathomimetic amines (epinephrine, norepinephrine, histamine), that derange the control of circulation. Other vasoactive substances, including kinins, are also present, as well as enzymes released from cellular lysosomes. In addition, there are serious aberrations in the coagulation mechanism, resulting in intravascular coagulation with the consumption of fibrinogen and the production of hemorrhage.

The most common organisms involved in endotoxin shock reside in the human intestinal tract. In the elderly male, endotoxin shock usually follows urethral instrumentation for prostatism. In many adults, it is associated with infections of the urinary tract, gastrointestinal tract (including peritonitis), or biliary tree; often endotoxin shock follows trauma and manipulation (including surgery) of these areas.

Clinical Manifestations. Since septic shock is a complication of bloodstream invasion from a focus, the clinical manifestations reflect both the underlying disorder and the sepsis. The patient is cold, pale, often cyanotic, and oliguric; hypotension is the rule, but it is usually not as marked as after hemorrhage, trauma, or burns. The death rate from endotoxin shock is high, and most patients die if pulmonary complications, particularly "shock lung," appear.

Pathophysiology. Both the associated disorder and the endotoxinemia contribute to the cardiovascular and pulmonary disorders. The endotoxin molecule has no direct depressant effect on the myocardium. Arterial blood pressure is generally near normal, but different mechanisms may be operative: high or normal cardiac output associated with a decrease in peripheral vascular resistance or low cardiac output associated with an increase in peripheral vascular resistance. Hemodynamic combinations may vary with time, but predominant vasodilatation generally supervenes.

The vasodilatation of septic shock has been attributed to fever, bacterial toxins, and the generation of vasodilator substances (including histamine and kinins) and metabolic end products evoked by endotoxin. But despite extensive peripheral vasodilation, these patients also manifest organ hypoperfusion and heightened sympathetic nervous activity: cold fingertips indicate activation of alpha-adrenergic sensitive beds; oliguria suggests that renal blood flow has decreased even though the cardiac output may be high. Catecholamines, released into the circulation in response to stress, not only contribute to local vasoconstriction but also exert direct inotropic effects on the heart.

Lactic acidosis is common, partly attributable to organ hypoperfusion. Its presence should be suspected when a considerable decrease in serum bicarbonate concentration is accompanied by an increase in unmeasured anions ("anion gap"). An increasing anion gap is a bad prognostic sign that signals need for a prompt reappraisal of therapy. In contrast to the metabolic acidosis of hemorrhagic shock, early endotoxin shock is often associated with a high pH and evidence of a mixed respiratory alkalosis and metabolic acidosis. As shock persists and the lungs become involved in the picture of "shock lung," venous admixture increases because of ventilation-perfusion inhomogeneities. Intravascular coagulation may produce the syndrome of disseminated coagulation, afibrinogenemia, and hemorrhage. The coup de grâce in septic shock may be delivered by a generalized Shwartzman phenomenon (intravascular coagulation, deposition of fibrin in glomeruli, and bilateral renal cortical necrosis).

CARDIOGENIC SHOCK

Cardiogenic shock refers to a combination of heart failure and shock that follows extensive myocardial infarction (more than 40 per cent of left ventricular muscle). Evidence of shock, particularly of organ hypoperfusion and hypotension, predominates over that of left ventricular failure. Approximately 15 per cent of patients hospitalized for acute myocardial infarction develop cardiogenic shock. Mortality from cardiogenic shock is high, averaging about 80 per cent in different coronary care units.

Clinical Manifestations. The full-blown picture is characteristic. A patient who has suffered a recent myocardial infarction develops signs of a falling cardiac output, peripheral vasoconstriction, and organ hypoperfusion. Mentation is disturbed; the patient is restless; the skin becomes cold and clammy, and beads of perspiration appear on the head and neck. A persistent tachycardia develops in association with weak peripheral (femoral) pulses. Auscultatory blood pressure (including pulse pressure) decreases.

Of great importance is the urine output. As long as it remains high, the patient may recover without therapy. Conversely, if oliguria appears and progresses in conjunction with evidence of peripheral vasoconstriction, therapy to restore the circulation is mandatory. Delay in starting treatment may be crucial, because the syndrome may cascade precipitously, within hours, from premonitory signs to death.

At the outset, the lungs are often free of rales, because pulmonary edema is confined to the interstitial spaces. However, the increase in respiratory frequency produced by the stiff lungs will elicit respiratory alkalosis. If shock progresses, hypocapnia will become associated with a low pH as metabolic acidosis supervenes. Oxygenation of arterial blood is generally well maintained at the outset but may be compromised in time as venous admixture increases. Consequently, an arterial cannula is valuable in early cardiogenic shock not only for monitoring blood pressure but also for serial sampling to detect the advent of metabolic acidosis and of impaired arterialization.

Occasionally, generalized vasodilation ("warm-handed shock") may dominate the course of cardiogenic shock, usually without apparent reason. The arterial blood pressure decreases, the cardiac output is normal or nearly normal, and the renal blood flow and urine volume remain within the normal range; there is no evidence of organ hypoperfusion. There is neither acidosis nor an increase in the "anion gap" or in lactic acid in blood. The prognosis is generally better than in those patients who manifest hypotension and intense vasoconstriction after myocardial infarction.

Mechanisms other than massive myocardial damage may elicit a shocklike syndrome after acute myocardial infarction: arrhythmias (bradycardia or tachycardia); long-lasting effects of pharmacologic agents, such as propranolol, administered before the episode of infarction; rupture of a necrotic area (papillary muscle, septum, or free wall). Each of these influences requires individual consideration and attention.

Pathophysiology. Cardiogenic shock in the course of acute myocardial infarction is characterized by left ventricular failure, low cardiac output, and arterial hypotension. The damaged left ventricular wall, high left atrial pressure, pulmonary venous congestion, and pulmonary edema initiate one set of reflexes that modify the circulation through remote organs, including kidney and muscles. A different set of reflexes results from the decrease in cardiac output and in filling of the arterial tree. Consequently, it is not surprising that hemodynamic patterns may range from intense peripheral vasoconstriction, as usually occurs in hemorrhagic shock, to mixtures of vasoconstriction and vasodilatation, as may occur in septic shock. But despite these variations, the consistent feature is organ hypoperfusion signaled by oliguria, pale skin, and disturbed mentation. That the kidney can still respond by vasodilating can be shown by a brisk diuretic response to furosemide administered intravenously.

Because of the limited capacity of the cerebral and coronary beds for autoregulation, their blood flow depends largely on the aortic pressure. With respect to cardiogenic shock this dependence is critical, because a decrease in coronary arterial blood pressure entails the prospect of extending the myocardial infarct and of compromising further the performance of the residual viable muscle. Consequently, persistent hypotension enhances the prospects for irreversible cardiac damage and unremitting cardiogenic shock.

That indirect methods for determining arterial blood pressure are unreliable in patients with decreasing cardiac output and peripheral vasoconstriction has been amply demonstrated in cardiogenic shock. Therefore intra-arterial pressure should be monitored directly in patients with early signs of cardiogenic shock. A suitable pressure transducer and a recording or monitoring device are essential for the bedside monitoring. If this electronic system is not available, the physician bases his assessment of arterial pressure on the strength of the femoral pulses and on his indirect assessment of the adequacy of coronary and cerebral perfusion.

SHOCK FROM INADEQUATE FILLING

Excessively rapid heart rates sharply curtail diastolic filling, thereby decreasing cardiac output. In many respects, the clinical picture resembles that of acute pericardial tamponade or acute tension pneumothorax which restrict filling of the heart by mechanical obstruction to venous inflow rather than by excessive heart rate. Success in treatment depends on controlling the arrhythmia.

OTHER HYPOTENSIVE STATES

Acute Disorders

These disorders include the syndromes of vasomotor paralysis and syncope. They differ from shock in etiology, duration, clinical course, and prognosis.

Vasomotor Paralysis. This syndrome represents paralysis of arterioles and is usually manageable. The clinical picture is diametrically opposite to that of hypovolemic shock in which sympathetic vasomotor tone is high. On the other hand, it does share some features of the picture of peripheral vasodilation that occurs frequently in septic shock and occasionally in cardiogenic shock.

The prototype of this syndrome is the massive vasodilatation and circulatory collapse induced by a severe blow to an unguarded abdomen (e.g., a blow to the solar plexus). The same effect can be elicited by spinal anesthesia or by giving vasodilator agents during hypovolemia or anaphylaxis. The onset of hypotension is often precipitous, and proper treatment usually arrests the disorder in minutes.

Treatment of vasodilated hypotension begins with volume expansion, on the assumption that the *effective,* rather than the *actual,* circulating blood volume has been reduced by vasodilatation. But should volume expansion fail to provide prompt relief, vasoconstrictors, such as levarterenol or metaraminol, are in order.

Syncope. A precipitous decrease in systemic arterial blood pressure may produce a transient loss of consciousness, or syncope. The drop in blood pressure may be due to an abrupt decrease in cardiac output or to sudden vasodilatation. The syncope stems from inadequate delivery of oxygen and glucose to the brain as a consequence of the decrease in cerebral blood flow that accompanies the drop in blood pressure.

Syncope is distinguished from shock by the loss of consciousness, by its brief duration, and by its prompt reversal once the initiating mechanism is removed. Any episode of severe hypotension that lasts for more than a few seconds can elicit syncope (see Ch. 353). The most familiar example is the common episode of fainting.

The common faint (vasovagal or vasodepressor syncope) stems from a sudden and precipitous fall in peripheral resistance, probably involving both arterioles and veins, unaccompanied by the increase in cardiac output that usually follows peripheral vasodilatation. The usual setting is one of intense emotional stress, often when the discomfort or anxiety is relieved. Thus it occurs in blood donors after only small quantities of blood have been withdrawn, in subjects with indwelling arterial needles who experience gnawing, dull pain at the puncture site, and in anxious subjects who realize suddenly that they are not about to be harmed. The upright subject feels light-headed, becomes pale, breaks into a cold sweat, complains of nausea, and abruptly passes out. The heart rate slows, and arterial pressure falls precipitously. The cardiac output shows only a slight decrease or remains unchanged from the precollapse level. Vasodilatation is marked in skeletal muscles, but the compensatory increase in heart rate and cardiac output fails to materialize because of intense parasympathetic discharge. The syndrome usually ends abruptly when the subject lies or falls down. Smelling salts usually help. Atropine is rarely needed.

Chronic Disorders

Two states of arterial hypotension, one benign and the other incapacitating, also pertain to the function of the autonomic nervous system in regulating the circulation.

Chronic Arterial Hypotension. Many persons maintain a blood pressure of 90 systolic and 60 diastolic for a lifetime without dire results. Indeed, systemic hypotension predisposes to longevity. They differ from the hypotensive patient in shock in that the low blood pressure is not associated with evidences of intensified sympathetic nervous activity or organ hypoperfusion.

Orthostatic Hypotension. In normal individuals, an elaborate system of cardiovascular reflexes prevents pooling of blood in the periphery when the upright posture is assumed. Central to these mechanisms is the carotid sinus reflex which constricts arterioles and venules and increases heart rate and myocardial contractility. Mechanical pumping by leg muscles and release of neurohumoral substances (catecholamines, renin, and angiotensin) are also involved in maintaining the blood pressure.

Disturbances in the autonomic nervous system (see Ch. 377) that interfere with the cardiovascular reflexes may elicit postural hypotension and syncope. Thus orthostatic hypotension generally represents a chronic inadequacy of the sympathetic nervous contribution to the control of the circulation.

TREATMENT

Mortality from hypovolemic types of shock has decreased dramatically because of prompt administration of blood, plasma, plasma substitutes, and saline solutions. But mortality from septic and cardiogenic shock remains at 70 per cent or higher. Consequently, it is much more difficult to be categorical about managing cardiogenic and septic shock than hypovolemic shock.

Five separate components enter into the planning of therapeutic regimens: initiating mechanisms, duration of shock, level of autonomic nervous activity, state of the peripheral circulation, and performance of the myocardium. The importance of each of these components varies according to the nature of the shock. For example, effective treatment of septic shock is impossible without control of bacterial infection. Also, prolonged shock of any cause is apt to be associated with depressed myocardial contractility and a refractory peripheral circulation even though sympathetic nervous activity is intense.

The crux of any program for treating shock is early detection and prompt intervention. An essential determinant of prognosis is the health of the patient before the onset of shock. A patient who has an underlying debilitating disease or has been receiving anticancer medications may be incapable of recovering from the episode that precipitated shock.

General Measures

Among the general measures that may promote recovery are several simple maneuvers: (1) proper positioning, generally supine in hypovolemic and endotoxin shock and partially upright in cardiogenic shock; (2) judicious relief of pain and restlessness, using morphine (15 mg) or meperidine (100 mg) administered intravenously, while avoiding excess analgesia and narcosis that predispose to arterial hypotension; (3) withholding food, allowing sips of water for thirst, in order to minimize the prospects of vomiting and aspiration; (4) adequate oxygenation accomplished as simply as possible, e.g., oxygen by nasal catheter; and (5) prevention of acidosis, e.g., by restoring circulating blood volume and blood pressure and, if necessary, by administering sodium bicarbonate intravenously, in order to maintain peripheral vascular responsiveness to endogenous and exogenous catecholamines.

Once incipient shock is recognized, a central venous catheter is introduced for the administration of fluid and medications, for blood sampling, and for measuring right atrial pressure. Should shock materialize, steps are immediately taken for intensive treatment. Blood is withdrawn for typing and cross-matching. The electrocardiogram is monitored for early detection of arrhythmias. If the patient is oliguric or anuric, a urinary catheter is placed for reliable determinations of urine flow. A cannula introduced into a peripheral artery will provide not only serial determinations of blood pressure but also blood samples for Po_2 and pH. From the outset, attention is paid to adequate ventilation. If arterial Po_2 falls below 60 to 70 mm Hg, tracheal intubation and assisted ventilation are required to maintain tolerable levels of oxygenation.

Once these general measures — volume replacement and provisions for monitoring — have been instituted, a decision has to be reached concerning priorities: continued transfusions to replenish the decreased circulating blood volume; use of autonomic agents to change the calibers of systemic blood vessels; or cardiotonic agents, such as digitalis, to improve cardiac performance.

Replenishment of the Circulating Blood Volume. In shock associated with hypovolemia, intravenous administration of fluids is clearly the first line of treatment. If blood has been lost, it should be replaced. The aim is to restore arterial blood pressure to tolerable levels rather than to original levels, e.g., systolic pressure of 90 to 100 mm Hg rather than 120 or 130 mm Hg. Crystalloid solutions, such as isotonic saline or glucose, may serve as temporary expedients while matching blood is obtained. More lasting support for the circulation is provided by macromolecular agents, particularly the dextrans of low viscosity and molecular weight (about 40,000), which remain longer in the circulation. Care is taken when blood substitutes are administered to avoid excess hemodilution. Except in states of hypofibrinogenemia and bleeding dyscrasias, low molecular weight dextran is remarkably free of side effects. It is usually administered intravenously as a 6 per cent solution, either in physiologic saline or glucose solution. Five hundred milliliters generally expands the blood volume by an average of approximately 1200 to 1800 ml; the effect is over in a few hours because of its loss via the kidneys unless an additional slow infusion is administered. If oliguria persists during the infusion, the plasma volume may be overexpanded, and pulmonary edema may be precipitated. Colloidal solutions of albumin (25 grams in 100 ml of 0.9 per cent saline) are as effective but much less available. Albumin is preferable to plasma because it does not entail the risk of hepatitis.

The therapeutic goal in the administration of fluids is the re-establishment of an adequate circulating volume and a near-normal distribution of blood flow among organs and tissues without severely upsetting the electrolyte balance. If treatment has to be prolonged, different sequences and combinations of fluids are generally needed, depending on whether the problem is to maintain electrolyte balance, to provide energy, or to combat acidosis. Assuming the judicious selection of fluids, the key clinical guides for administration of adequate amounts of fluid intravenously are clearing of the sensorium, improved circulation to the skin, restoration of the arterial blood pressure, slowing of the heart rate, and increase in urine flow. Unfortunately, consecutive determinations of blood volume have proved to have little practical value as guides to fluid replacement because of the changing natures of most kinds of shock and the inevitable delays that are involved between the times of sampling, the analysis, and the final reporting.

The clinical state of intense peripheral vasoconstriction and organ hypoperfusion, manifested by the cold, clammy skin, thready pulse, and oliguria, clearly calls for intravenous fluids. Arterial blood pressure, governed by an elaborate baroregulatory apparatus, is a complicated guide to fluid replacement. Indeed, overzealous attempts to restore arterial blood pressure to preshock levels are responsible for many attacks of frank pulmonary edema, especially if the left ventricle has been damaged previously.

Currently, central venous pressure is the popular guide to fluid replacement. Its determination involves the measurement of blood pressure in a large intrathoracic vein close to the heart. Normally, this value is of the order of −2 to +5 cm of water. Unfortunately, like the arterial blood pressure, the value may be difficult to interpret, because central venous pressure is a function not only of blood volume but also of venous tone, of the competence and distensibility of the right ventricle, of heart rate, and of intrathoracic pressure. The interpretation of central venous pressure as a guide to fluid administration is even more complicated when vasopressors are being administered, because they raise venous pressure by local effects on venous walls. The greatest value of central venous pressure is in hypovolemic shock in which the myocardium generally performs well. Conversely, it is potentially misleading in cardiogenic shock in which the competent right ventricle responds to an increase in venous return by flooding the lungs with blood that the damaged left ventricle cannot handle.

In hypovolemic and septic shock, the central venous pressure is used as follows: fluids are administered intravenously in an attempt to increase the arterial blood pressure and the urine output without driving the central venous pressure to abnormally high levels (to more than 10 to 15 cm of water). A modest increase in central venous pressure, e.g., to 15 cm of water, may prove necessary during intravenous infusions in order to sustain the cardiac output, particularly if shock is protracted. But should the central venous pressure start mounting abruptly, a state of overtransfusion has been reached and the right ventricle is assumed to have failed.

In cardiogenic shock in which the competence of the left heart is in question, the pulmonary arterial diastolic pressure may be used as an approximate index of left ventricular end-diastolic pressure and as a more meaningful guide for the intravenous administration of fluids than is the central venous pressure.

Autonomic Agents. Endogenous catecholamine levels in the blood are generally high throughout the course of shock, often continuing to increase as shock grows refractory. Moreover, a wide variety of sympathomimetic amines are currently being used to supplement endogenous levels when shock either has failed to respond

to administration of fluids or has reached the stage where fluid overload is in prospect. By exerting their effects on alpha or beta receptors, their actions are excitatory, inhibitory, or a combination of the two. Alpha-excitatory drugs, such as methoxamine (Vasoxyl) cause vasoconstriction; beta-excitatory drugs, such as isoproterenol (Isuprel), relax vascular smooth muscle while exerting positive inotropic, chronotropic, and dromotropic effects on the myocardium. Norepinephrine (levarterenol) exerts both alpha and beta effects and is particularly useful in producing vasoconstriction in conjunction with inotropic and chronotropic effects on the myocardium. Metaraminol can serve the same purpose if the stores of catecholamines in myocardium and vascular smooth muscle are not depleted; it has the advantage over norepinephrine of avoiding local injury and necrosis should leakage occur from a misdirected needle at the site of infusion.

Opinions vary concerning the proper use of vasoactive agents in managing shock. In general, vasoconstrictors constitute first-line drugs that are used in early forms of shock if response to volume expansion is delayed or inadequate. Vasodilators, on the other hand, are generally reserved for shock that is refractory to fluids and in which vasoconstriction is intense. When central venous pressure is high, vasodilators (e.g., phentolamine, isoproterenol) usually increase cardiac output and renal blood flow, raise blood pressure, promote diuresis, and relieve peripheral vasoconstriction. Unless central venous pressure is high, vasodilators are apt to promote deterioration in the clinical state. Resort to vasodilators underscores the common experience that excessively high levels of circulating catecholamines may impede recovery. Consequently, fluids remain the mainstay of therapy for shock, and when vasopressors are given, doses are kept as small as possible.

Despite divergent views and incomplete data, it is possible to distill a few general principles for the use of autonomic agents in treating the common types of shock in which sympathetic activity is high: (1) Vasoconstrictive and inotropic agents, such as norepinephrine, are most likely to be effective if the blood volume is normal or somewhat expanded. (2) Since increasing the level of arterial blood pressure by vasoconstrictors generally increases flow to the brain and heart at the expense of flow to other organs, such as the kidneys, the use of any one of these agents should be as brief and in as small a dose as possible. (3) Acidosis, a regular concomitant of severe shock, lessens the effectiveness of vasoconstrictive agents such as norepinephrine, leading to larger doses and increasing side effects. (4) Vasodilators seem to be in order when volume expansion and intense peripheral vasoconstriction have proved ineffective. (5) Prolonged and severe oliguria that has resisted both volume expansion and the administration of vasoconstrictors during shock may respond to diuretic agents that elicit renal vasodilation, such as furosemide, thereby helping to prevent serious renal injury. (6) Massive doses of adrenocortical steroids, such as hydrocortisone, may be useful in states of bacteremic shock and merit trial in other instances of refractory shock; they have a mandatory role in preventing shock in those patients on maintenance doses of steroids for systemic illness, e.g., rheumatoid arthritis, who are about to be subjected to the stress of anesthesia or surgery.

Oxygen Therapy. It has been noted above that patients in shock are candidates for a wide variety of pulmonary disorders, including atelectasis, pneumonia, and pulmonary edema; the prospects for these grave complications to occur increase as shock persists. Early in shock, when abnormalities in pulmonary performance are generally mild, administration of oxygen by nasal catheter generally suffices. But should shock be severe and protracted, patients may require tracheal intubation and assisted ventilation to relieve labored breathing and to improve alveolar ventilation. Since the use of mechanical respirators to improve gas exchange entails the risk of aggravating shock by impeding venous return, particularly if blood volume is depleted, assisted ventilation in shock should be undertaken only by experts.

Cardiotonic Agents. Even though the normal myocardium may suffer somewhat in early shock from being hypoperfused, rarely is it sufficiently compromised to require the support of digitalis. More justifiable is the administration of digitalis in protracted shock if the heart has previously been damaged by disease or by aging. Even then, extraordinary care is required in digitalization because of the potentiating effects of acidosis, hypoxia, and electrolyte disturbances in severe shock on the production of ventricular arrhythmias and conduction disturbances by digitalis.

In cardiogenic shock, digitalization is apt to be helpful only if evidence can be accrued that the noninfarcted part of the ventricle has failed. Digitalis therapy is then undertaken cautiously, while monitoring the electrocardiogram carefully for arrhythmias.

Intravascular Coagulation. Defects in coagulation are common in shock, but bleeding is uncommon. Despite the tendency to intravascular aggregation and clotting disorders, none of these seem to require anticoagulant therapy. Improvement in the circulation suffices to correct these deficiencies.

Specific Measures

Special attention should be called to certain therapeutic measures that are used in septic and cardiogenic shock.

Septic Shock. Elimination of the cause of sepsis is of cardinal importance in treating septic shock. Intensive treatment on several fronts must be started as soon as the diagnosis is made. While the blood pressure is being sustained by intravenous infusions—usually plasma, dextran, crystalloids, or blood if the hematocrit is low—and possibly by pharmacologic agents, it is critical to administer the proper antimicrobials as soon as blood cultures have been taken. Since most cases of septic shock in a general hospital are due to gram-negative bacilli, it is reasonable to institute antimicrobial therapy with Escherichia, Klebsiella, Pseudomonas, and Enterobacteriaceae in mind, e.g., with an aminoglycoside (gentamicin or kanamycin) and a cephalosporin (cephalothin).

If there is a likelihood of a complicating bacteremia with penicillinase-producing staphylococci, nafcillin or oxacillin should be added.

This regimen can be modified after the results of blood cultures are known, e.g., by adding clindamycin if a gastrointestinal strain of bacteroides is identified or carbenicillin if pseudomonas infection and severe neutropenia coexist (see Ch. 214).

Often the patient relapses after a brief period of response to intravenous fluids. This is presumably due to continuing intravascular stagnation and extravascular fluid loss. Massive doses of glucocorticosteroids (e.g.,

hydrocortisone, 50 to 150 mg) have been proved helpful, particularly if used early in septic shock. Presumably, the corticosteroids correct the defects produced by endotoxin: restore the normal microcirculation by vasodilation, stabilize cell walls to prevent release of vasoactive and proteolytic substances, and decrease adhesiveness of blood cells and platelets. Other vasodilating agents (e.g., phenoxybenzamine) are currently under trial, but there is no great optimism about their therapeutic prospects.

Cardiogenic Shock. Patterns for treating cardiogenic shock after myocardial infarction have been set by coronary intensive care units in which extensive monitoring of blood pressures and of the electrocardiogram are routine. The patient is positioned semiupright, a compromise between the need for cerebral blood flow and the threat of pulmonary edema. The ideal way to support the blood pressure in cardiogenic shock is to increase the cardiac output and to decrease the peripheral resistance. Patients in cardiogenic shock who have only a modest increase in left ventricular pressure often improve after cautious expansion of the circulating blood volume or cautious administration of inotropic agents. Since fluid overload is particularly undesirable after myocardial infarction, failure to restore blood pressure to tolerable levels by volume expansion is generally followed by the administration of vasopressor agents.

In cardiogenic shock the use of inotropic agents, chiefly isoproterenol and levarterenol, is done cautiously, realizing that although the increase in blood pressure does increase coronary blood flow, it does so at the cost of increasing cardiac work and oxygen demand. Hopefully the increased coronary flow will offset the increased work. Unfortunately, this goal is often elusive, and myocardial anoxia may be intensified, leading to extension of the myocardial damage that originally caused the shock. Rarely does isoproterenol have any advantage over levarterenol as the initial catecholamine in cardiogenic shock; not only may it fail to raise the blood pressure if the direct inotropic effects on the heart are neutralized by peripheral vasodilation, but it is also likely to evoke troublesome arrhythmias. Dopamine has staunch advocates because of its vasodilating effects on the kidney, but it is generally reserved as an alternative for levarterenol or isoproterenol. New vasoactive and inotropic agents continue to be tried. But at the moment it seems that cautious administration of levarterenol holds the brightest prospect for restoring the blood pressure unless the patient is already maximally vasoconstricted; isoproterenol is then generally tried. As prerequisites for administering catecholamines, hypoxemia should be corrected and arterial pH should be restored to normal. Disturbances in cardiac rhythm should be handled promptly, with care taken to avoid interventions and drugs that depress myocardial function.

Medical therapy in cardiogenic shock is directed toward maintaining coronary blood flow and preventing extension of the myocardial infarct. Should medical measures prove ineffective, mechanical circulatory assistance is currently being tried in some medical centers. The widest experience has been gained with the intraaortic balloon pump which requires little surgery and offers circulatory assistance by way of counterpulsation. The limited long-term survival rate after balloon-pumping alone has encouraged the use of coronary revascularization procedures, particularly aortic–coronary artery bypass grafts, to restore myocardial blood flow on an emergency basis. These surgical procedures are complicated, requiring preoperative coronary angiography and left ventriculography while the heart is being assisted mechanically. The role of surgical measures in cardiogenic shock remains to be established.

Fishman, A. P.: Shock lung. A distinctive non-entity. Circulation, 47:921, 1973.
Forscher, B. K., Lillehei, R. C., and Stubbs, S. S.: Shock in Low- and High-Flow States. Amsterdam, Excerpta Medica, 1972.
Guyton, A. C., and Jones, C. E.: Central venous pressure: Physiological significance and clinical implications. Am. Heart J., 86:431, 1973.
Hershey, S. G., Del Guercio, L. R. M., and McConn, R. (eds.): Septic Shock in Man. Boston, Little, Brown & Company, 1971.
Lefer, A. M.: Blood-borne humoral factors in the pathophysiology of circulatory shock. Circ. Res., 32:129, 1973.
Lluch, S., Moguilevsky, H. C., Pietra, G., Shaffer, A. B., Hirsch, L. J., and Fishman, A. P.: A reproducible model of cardiogenic shock in the dog. Circulation, 39:205, 1969.
Swan, H. J. C.: Power failure of the heart in acute myocardial infarction. In Likoff, W., Segal, B. L., and Insull, W., Jr. (eds.): Arteriosclerosis and Coronary Heart Disease. New York, Grune & Stratton, 1973.

THROMBOEMBOLIC DISEASES

Sol Sherry

543. INTRODUCTION

Thrombosis is the formation from the constituents of the blood of a solid mass or plug in the heart or blood vessels. The thrombus which forms may be dislodged in whole or in part to another vascular site; when this occurs the thrombus or its fragment is referred to as an embolus. Collectively the states associated with such thrombi or emboli are referred to as the thromboembolic diseases or disorders, and when viewed together they represent a leading cause of serious illness and death in the Western world; furthermore, their importance is likely to grow with increasing longevity. This chapter is concerned with only one form of the thromboembolic disorders, i.e., peripheral venous thrombosis and its major complication, pulmonary artery embolism. The thromboembolic disorders involving the heart, brain, systemic arteries, and selected veins, e.g., hepatic, portal, and renal, are considered elsewhere in the text.

Alterations in blood flow, damage to the vessel wall, and changes in the coagulability of the blood have been stressed as the major factors responsible for thrombus formation in vivo. To these we need add the formed elements (notably the platelets) and fibrinolysis. The interplay among these factors, whose importance varies with the circumstances, controls the initiation and the dynamics of thrombus growth. *In the arterial system*, a vascular lesion is generally accepted as the most frequent primary cause of an acute thrombotic event, and the latter is viewed as an exaggeration of the normal hemostatic response to vascular injury. Thrombi originate adjacent to lesions in arterial walls, and each is composed primarily of a large white head containing platelets and some fibrin; a variable amount of fresh clot then extends from this white head. It is postulated that platelets adhere to the exposed microfibrils and collagen fibers at the site of vascular injury, e.g., fissured or ul-

cerated atheromatous plaque. After adherence and in response to a continuing stimulus, platelets release certain constituents like ADP (adenosine diphosphate) which stimulate platelet aggregation and the formation of a platelet mass. Subsequently, there is activation of the clotting mechanism; this results in formation of fibrin within the the platelet head (so as to stabilize it) and the superimposition of a fresh clot.

The pathogenesis of *venous thrombosis* is less well understood, except when there is direct injury or infection of the vein wall which leads to a thrombus much like that in an artery. However, in most instances, thrombus formation takes place in the absence of a demonstrable vascular lesion, because the venous intima, unlike the arterial, is much less exposed to injury from high fluid pressure or atherosclerosis. Furthermore, in contrast to the arterial, the venous thrombus is composed primarily of a red, gel-like mass similar to a test tube blood clot; a white platelet head is either inconspicuous or absent. Most venous thrombi are postulated to be initiated through local activation of the clotting mechanism with the insular accumulation of thrombin. The latter then triggers both fibrin formation and platelet aggregation and accounts for the successive layers of fibrin coagulum and platelets (lines of Zahn) commonly observed histologically in growing venous thrombi. Local activation of the clotting mechanism is believed to arise as a consequence of two considerations: (1) the presence in the general circulation of activated enzymatic components of the clotting reactions consequent to recent or ongoing tissue damage, trauma, or necrosis and possibly in association with impaired inhibitory or clearing mechanisms; and (2) stasis, which serves to sustain the action of the activated enzymatic clotting factors, as in the animal model developed by Wessler. In this model, immediately after the systemic injection of early activated components of the clotting mechanism (either in purified form or as serum), isolation of a venous segment by ligatures or clamps, so as to effect stasis, results in rapid formation of a thrombus in situ; thrombosis is not seen in the freely flowing circulation and is markedly delayed in the isolated venous segment of control animals.

Venous thromboembolism is a frequent, important, and challenging clinical problem and a particularly frustrating one, because in most instances it can be prevented. In the United States it is estimated that 250,000 cases of deep vein thrombosis are diagnosed yearly, but this is only a fraction of the total because most are silent. Pulmonary embolism, the main complication of thrombosis in the deep veins of the lower extremity, is currently estimated to cause 50,000 deaths yearly; furthermore, the morbidity and mortality of other diseases are significantly influenced when a pulmonary embolism occurs.

544. THROMBOPHLEBITIS AND PHLEBOTHROMBOSIS

The presence of a thrombus in a vein is referred to clinically as thrombophlebitis or phlebothrombosis. Adherence to the vein wall incites an inflammatory reaction with local symptoms, and because of the associated phlebitis the process is referred to as thrombophlebitis. When the thrombus is poorly adherent and extends primarily into the free-flowing circulation, local symptoms of phlebitis may be minimal or absent, and the process may be referred to as phlebothrombosis. Since the two states are, for the most part, identical and subject to the same complications, little virtue attaches to such a clinical differentiation; hereafter only the term thrombophlebitis will be used.

Etiology, Risk Factors, Pathogenesis, and Prevalence. Mutliple causes probably initiate venous thrombosis. Injury to the vessel wall by mechanical trauma, infection, chemical irritants, or the process of thromboangiitis obliterans is responsible for some cases, particularly the superficial variety.

In most instances, stasis with slowing of blood flow and venous distention appears to be the major predisposing factor, e.g., in the venous thrombi which frequently complicate the use of constricting garments, and in such clinical conditions or states as the hyperviscosity syndromes (including polycythemia vera), severe obesity, varicose veins, postoperative and postpartum states, trauma (particularly when extensive or involving fractures of the pelvis or femur), acute myocardial infarction, heart failure, hemiplegia, debility, and cachexia. Long periods of cramped sitting, e.g., in travel or watching television, or in fact any state involving partial or complete immobilization, particularly in the older age group, because of the loss of the normal pumping action of the leg muscles, is subject to an increased incidence of venous thrombosis. The risk of stasis-mediated as well as other forms of venous thrombosis is increased when there has been a previous episode of thrombophlebitis or pulmonary embolism.

Alterations in blood components have received much attention, but a "hypercoagulable state," i.e., one predisposing to thrombus formation, has defied simple description. Rather, it is recognized that many disorders of the blood may be associated with predisposition to venous thrombosis. These include thrombocythemia as well as certain thrombocytopathies, particularly those involving shortened survival and increased platelet functional activities (adhesion, aggregation, and coagulant properties), dysfibrinogenemias, accelerated thromboplastin generation, constitutionally elevated levels of plasma factors V and VIII, heightened antifibrinolytic activity, and decreased antithrombin III activity.

Finally, many other clinical conditions are associated with an increased incidence of thrombophlebitis, but the responsible factors have not been adequately elucidated. These include ulcerative colitis, malignancies of all types (possibly more so of the pancreas), homocystinuria, and prolonged administration of large doses of estrogens or estrogen-containing oral contraceptive agents. The presence of a "migratory thrombophlebitis" should cause suspicion of an underlying malignancy, collagen disease, thromboangiitis obliterans, or polycythemia vera. When thrombosis occurs without evidence of a known predisposing factor or associated clinical condition, the term *idiopathic* thrombophlebitis may be used.

Thrombosis in veins occurs most commonly in the deep and superficial veins of the lower extremities. Deep leg vein thrombi usually begin in the soleal arcade of the calf muscles where they may resolve, organize, extend, or trigger additional thrombi at independent sites. As long as the thrombus remains limited to the soleal veins, no significant clinical problem is posed. However, once extension into the major deep vessels of the leg occurs, or additional thrombi appear at other sites in the major deep veins, the patient is at significant risk for one or more complications (circulatory obstruction, valve damage, pulmonary embolism). When extension occurs from the soleal vessels, the thrombus extends proximally into larger vessels, frequently progressing to involve the popliteal, superficial femoral, common femoral, and iliac veins. More rarely the inferior vena cava is also affected. Thrombi originating in the major deep veins usually begin at the base of valve pockets and then extend either up along the vein wall or into the flowing circulation, or they may completely obstruct the entire vascular lumen. When the latter occurs, retrograde thrombosis as well as continued proximal growth is likely.

Next in frequency to thrombi in the deep leg veins are thrombi in the pelvic venous network, the right cardiac chambers, and the veins of the upper extremities. However, thrombi may occur in any veins (retinal, cerebral, renal, hepatic, portal, mesenteric) and contribute significantly to disease of the organ system involved.

Until recently, data on the incidence and frequency of leg vein thrombi were inadequate, because most of these are inapparent clinically. In studies in which leg vein dissections were carried out post mortem, the incidence was shown to be very high, varying from 27 to 80 per cent, depending on the nature of the series and the extent of the dissection; in most, the incidence ranged from 44 to 65 per cent. This incidence did not appear to depend on sex or clinical diagnosis, for the likelihood of thrombosis was similar in patients dying of medical, surgical, and traumatic causes. The most important factors influencing the frequency of leg vein thrombosis appeared to be the duration of bed rest and advancing age, although other factors undoubtedly contributed to those incidence figures.

With the advent of the ^{125}I labeled fibrinogen leg-scanning technique, important epidemiologic and prevalence data are being obtained on leg vein thrombi appearing during life and in nonfatal situations. For example, in Kakkar's study of 469 consecutive patients aged 40 or over, undergoing elective surgery, 28 per cent developed deep vein thrombosis; older patients undergoing major operations had an incidence of over 50 per cent. Half the thrombi developed within the first 24 hours postoperatively, and the remainder occurred three to seven days after surgery; in one third of the patients, the thrombi were bilateral. The incidence in other conditions was as follows: fractured hips, 75 per cent of pertrochanteric and 34 per cent of subcapital femoral neck fractures; retropubic prostatectomy, 50 per cent; acute myocardial infarction, 38 per cent; stroke, 60 per cent in the hemiplegic lower extremity; gynecologic patients over 30 years of age and undergoing major abdominal or vaginal surgery, 18 per cent; and obstetric patients during the puerperium, 4 per cent. Probably the highest risk is in patients undergoing reconstructive or total hip replacement.

In over 90 per cent of the patients undergoing thrombosis, leg vein thrombi appear first in the veins of the calf; one fifth of these soleal thrombi extend proximally into the major deep vessels of the leg and thigh; of the latter, half embolize. In acute myocardial infarction, in which the over-all incidence of leg vein thrombosis is approximately 30 per cent, 6 per cent of patients may be expected to develop thrombi in the major deep vessels of the leg or thigh, and in 3 per cent the illness will be complicated by an acute pulmonary embolism; the risk of leg vein thrombosis, extension, and embolization, however, is doubled in patients in the older age group who develop shock or congestive heart failure with their infarction.

Clinical Manifestations and Diagnosis. Thrombophlebitis occurs suddenly or gradually. Superficial thrombophlebitis is not difficult to diagnose, because the thrombosed vessel can usually be felt beneath the skin as a tender cord, and the lesion may be accompanied by a surrounding area of localized inflammation. With more extensive use of the venous route both for therapy and drug abuse, the incidence of this form of thrombophlebitis has increased sharply. Although usually benign, a significant number of patients may become infected, e.g., after the use of contaminated equipment or when intravenous catheters have been left in situ for periods of more than 48 hours, and this may lead to a serious septic state.

Deep vein thrombophlebitis is much more difficult to diagnose, because it may or may not be accompanied by local (pain and tenderness) and systemic (fever) symptoms; these occur in only 20 to 30 per cent of patients. In the absence of local findings, the diagnosis should be suspected when there is a "doughy" feeling or an unexplained increase in the circumference of the limb and the presence of *Homans' sign* (pain in the calf and/or popliteal space on dorsiflexion of the foot). The *sphygmomanometer cuff pain test of Lowenberg* may also prove useful, particularly when carried out during ambulation. A blood pressure cuff around the involved part of the extremity is slowly inflated to 200 mm Hg and then deflated. During inflation, discomfort is normally experienced at or above 160 mm Hg. In venous obstructive disease, discomfort or tenderness is evident at a lower level (60 to 150 mm Hg). The test may often be positive when other symptoms and signs are absent, but it is not sufficiently specific to be considered diagnostic. The most useful noninvasive diagnostic techniques are the *augmented Doppler ultrasound examination* and *electrical impedance phlebography* with a thigh cuff. However, these tests are positive only when the major deep veins are obstructed; they do not detect thrombi limited to the soleal veins. *Venography* is the most specific for diagnostic purposes, but it has limitations; it is expensive, may require a cut-down, and cannot be interpreted properly unless all the deep veins, including the soleal vessels, are filled adequately; there is also the possibility (still unresolved) that the large amounts of dye used in the procedure will aggravate an underlying thrombophlebitis.

Unless the patient has local complaints, the signs of venous thrombosis are often overlooked until the occurrence of pulmonary embolism calls attention to the limbs. Therefore special attention should be paid to the possibility of venous thrombi in all patients who are predisposed, and frequent observations should be made in older patients immobilized for any period of time.

Local tenderness in the calf and pain on forced dorsiflexion of the foot should suggest involvement of the deeper branches of the popliteal vein. Edema and mottled cyanosis will be present when the superficial femoral vein is affected; these findings are absent when adequate collateral channels exist. When the disease extends to involve the common femoral and iliac veins, edema and cyanosis of the leg may develop rapidly, often with diminished pulsation of the femoral artery. When associated perivenous inflammation and pelvic lymphatic involvement accompany thrombosis of the iliac vein, the swelling can be massive and result in a "milk leg" or *phlegmasia alba dolens.* In a particularly serious form of deep vein thrombosis called *phlegmasia cerulea dolens,* cyanosis and swelling of the extremity are associated with a disappearance of the arterial pulses; the leg becomes cold; gangrene appears imminent and may follow. This is associated with massive venous occlusion involving the deep, superficial, and intercommunicating veins so that there is almost total outflow obstruction; the rapid rise in tissue pressure compromises the arterial inflow and produces the picture of combined arterial and venous occlusive disease.

Damage to the venous valves resulting from an extensive episode or repeated attacks of deep vein thrombophlebitis may cause venous stasis and insufficiency; this leads to chronic edema, fibrosis, pigmentation, and trophic ulceration in the limb. The eventual deformity in this *postphlebitic syndrome* may be extreme and disabling. However, the most frequent and serious complication of thrombophlebitis is pulmonary embolism, a subject discussed in Ch. 545.

Prophylaxis. Stasis should be eliminated whenever possible, particularly in the older patient. This includes the wearing of elastic or supportive hose in the presence of varicose veins; avoidance of long periods of cramped sitting and of constricting garments about the abdomen and lower extremities; and the use of appropriate measures during periods of immobilization or illness or after surgery, trauma, or fracture. The value of elastic hose during periods of immobilization is very limited, as are foot and leg exercises, even when carried out frequently and in the elevated position. More effective are physical devices which ensure repeated calf muscle contraction or intermittent pulsation of the leg veins. Early but active ambulation is to be encouraged after illness, surgery, or trauma. Whether the elimination of contaminants by filtering parenteral fluids during their administration will reduce the risk of thrombophlebitis is being evaluated.

Iatrogenic thrombophlebitis can be minimized by avoiding prolonged use of intravenous catheters or administration of hypertonic or chemically irritating solutions.

Prophylactic therapy with anticoagulants is to be considered in high risk groups, i.e., those most likely to develop venous thrombi and pulmonary embolism. Included in this category are patients over the age of 50 who will be bedridden or immobilized for long periods of time as a result of extensive fractures, particularly of the femur, or other forms of trauma, debilitating disease, cardiac failure, myocardial infarction, or surgery, particularly hip arthroplasty. The pharmacologic basis for the use of anticoagulation in the prevention of venous thrombotic disease is sound, and its effectiveness in reducing thromboembolic complications after fractured hips or extensive trauma, during the postoperative state, and after acute myocardial infarction has been established in several series of observations. When indicated, anticoagulant therapy should be instituted immediately; it can be carried out solely with *oral agents (coumarin or indandione compounds),* for although these agents take several days to induce an appropriate antithrombotic state, the danger period for pulmonary embolism usually begins somewhat later. Anticoagulation should be continued until full mobilization is completed, because the risk of thrombosis remains as long as stasis exists. Such anticoagulation is not a contraindication to surgery or other procedures. Surgery can be performed without much danger either before or shortly after the institution of anticoagulant treatment, because hemostasis is not impaired for several days; later, in the more chronically anticoagulated patient, surgery can be undertaken after reduction of the level of anticoagulation with careful attention to wound hemostasis. Nevertheless, despite its proved value, physicians have been reluctant to use such prophylactic anticoagulant therapy except in cases of recurrent thrombophlebitis or pulmonary embolism; cited are the hazard of bleeding and the difficulties in maintaining adequate anticoagulation in older patients. Some of these difficulties can be avoided by elimination of a loading dose and recognition of the various factors which influence drug responsiveness (see below).

Infusion of *dextran* 40 or 75 (500 to 1000 ml on day of surgery, 500 ml daily for next five days) can also be used to prevent postoperative thrombophlebitis, presumably by increasing blood flow and preventing surface interactions. However, although effective, it provides little advantage over anticoagulants, because it also enhances the risk of bleeding and is tolerated poorly in individuals with impaired cardiac reserve.

The most promising development in the prevention of deep vein thrombi in immobilized patients is administration of small doses of *heparin,* i.e., 5000 units twice a day subcutaneously into the abdominal wall during periods of high risk. This regimen maintains circulating heparin blood levels at a fraction of that ordinarily achieved with conventional therapeutic doses as used in the treatment of established thrombosis (see below), and does not significantly affect the Lee-White clotting time and activated partial thromboplastin time; nor does it enhance the risk of bleeding. However, there is sufficient circulating heparin to activate enough heparin cofactor (antithrombin III) to block the action of earlier activated enzymes of the clotting reaction (notably Xa and IXa). In several trials, prophylactic therapy with low dose heparin has strikingly reduced the incidence of venous thrombosis occurring postoperatively (except after femoral fractures and hip arthroplasty) and after acute myocardial infarction as measured by ^{125}I labeled fibrinogen scanning. Should trials currently underway also reveal a significant reduction in pulmonary embolism, this mode of prophylaxis is likely to receive widespread acceptance.

The use of *platelet function inhibitors,* e.g., *aspirin, dipyridamole,* and *sulfinpyrazone,* for the prevention of deep vein thrombosis remains unclear; however, sulfinpyrazone (600 to 800 mg daily) has been found useful in reducing the incidence of arteriovenous shunt thrombosis in patients undergoing chronic renal dialysis, and in decreasing the frequency of attacks in patients with recurrent thrombophlebitis who are refractory to coumarin therapy. When sulfinpyrazone is used with coumarin, the dose of the latter should be lowered because of occupation by sulfinpyrazone of coumarin-binding sites.

Treatment. *General Measures.* Acute superficial thrombophlebitis is most often self-limited, unless infected, and usually responds promptly to analgesics, bed rest, warm moist packs, and elevation of the affected limb. Pulmonary embolism is a rare complication unless there is also involvement of the deep venous system. Antimicrobial drugs are not indicated except in septic phlebitis, in which the choice of agent depends on the organism responsible for the infection.

Acute deep vein thrombophlebitis must be managed more aggressively because of the tendency of these thrombi to extend, embolize, and produce serious venous obstruction and damage to venous valves (a postphlebitic insufficiency syndrome occurs in about 5 per cent of those with an ascending thrombophlebitis). In addition to the local measures described above, the objectives of treatment are to prevent further disease and, if indicated, to remove the obstructing thrombus.

Anticoagulants. Currently the principal therapeutic agents for the prevention of further extension and embolization are the anticoagulants, and with their use alone most cases can be managed successfully and without complication. In the absence of contraindications (bleeding diathesis, hemorrhagic lesion, malignant hypertension, known allergy to heparin) anticoagulation should be instituted immediately with heparin, for it is the most effective of the agents available and induces an immediate antithrombotic state.

Heparin can be administered intravenously or by the intramuscular and subcutaneous routes. Based on control of antithrombotic effects, the intravenous route is most often recommended, particularly for the first several days of therapy. Because of local pain and frequent hematomas, intramuscular injections are the least desirable. Even with the intravenous route, dosages and regimens vary. Continuous intravenous infusions of heparin, although requiring special care in administration, are becoming the preferred mode of therapy; control of dosage is easier and, more important, evidence is accumulating that bleeding complications can be reduced significantly. A suggested procedure is to begin with a loading dose of 75 IU per pound of body weight, followed by a sustaining infusion of 10 IU per pound per hour through an indwelling plastic catheter placed above the antecubital fossa. Subsequent dosage is adjusted to maintain the activated partial thromboplastin time at twice normal (range $1^{1}/_{2}$ to $2^{1}/_{2}$); with Lee-White clotting times, the range is 2 to $2^{1}/_{2}$ times normal). If the intermittent injection technique is employed, it is suggested that 60,000 IU be given during the first day (e.g., 10,000 units every four hours) and that, beginning on the second day, dosage be regulated by coagulation determinations; one hour before the next injection, the activated partial thromboplastin time or Lee-White clotting time should be at the level recommended above for sustaining infusions.

Once the dose requirement has been established, the clotting time may be checked once daily at an appropriate time to exclude possible increase or decrease in the anticoagulant effect and to allow for variations in heparin requirement during the course of therapy. Not infrequently, patients in whom thrombosis is occurring require more heparin in the first 24 to 48 hours of treatment than several days after the institution of therapy. Heparin therapy is recommended for periods of seven to ten days before relying solely on oral anticoagulation with coumarin drugs; this will ensure the most potent antithrombotic state and allow the underlying thrombus to become firmly fixed to the vessel wall.

"Burning fingers" and an occasional allergic reaction may be seen with heparin (osteoporosis and alopecia are additional adverse effects associated with long-term administration), but the primary risk in heparin therapy is bleeding. In one series it was as high as 50 per cent in women over the age of 60; usually the incidence is of the order of 5 to 8 per cent. This risk can be reduced by better control of the anticoagulant state, eliminating aspirin and aspirin-containing compounds, and avoiding intramuscular injections and invasive procedures. When significant bleeding occurs, heparin in the circulation can be immediately neutralized with protamine sulfate; the latter reacts with heparin stoichiometrically and on a milligram per milligram basis. Protamine is administered slowly intravenously after dilution in physiologic saline in an amount equivalent to half the last dose of heparin but not in excess of 100 mg. For this calculation 100 units of heparin can be taken to represent 1 mg.

Oral anticoagulation with *coumarin* (or, less popularly, *indandione*) compounds should be instituted several days before the discontinuation of heparin therapy. It should be continued for six weeks to six months, unless the phlebitis is associated with immobilization, in which case the drug should be continued until full physical activity is resumed. If thrombi recur when anticoagulants are discontinued, the treatment should be resumed, and long-term therapy may be necessary. Patients with known recurrent episodes of phlebitis may require prophylactic anticoagulant therapy extending over years.

The action of coumarin compounds is indirect, i.e., the induction of a hypocoagulable state, in contrast to the action of heparin as an immediate activator of antithrombin III. At present, the aim of therapy is to reduce the level of the prothrombin complex factors (factors II, VII, IX, and X) to approximately 20 per cent of normal and sustain it there. (Antithrombin III levels are increased during coumarin administration and may contribute to the antithrombotic effect.) This is achieved by regulating dosage so as to prolong the one-stage prothrombin time test to one and a half to two times the control time by the Quick test. Levels of two and a half times or greater are associated with an increased incidence of bleeding, and levels of less than one and a half times the control may not be effective.

There is little difference in the onset of effect or smoothness of control among the various coumarin derivatives, and vitamin K_1 is equally effective in counteracting their action. Because factor VII of the various vitamin K dependent factors (II, VII, IX, and X) has the shortest half-life, it is depressed most quickly by coumarin therapy. However, the rapid depression of factor VII does not provide good antithrombotic protection but does enhance the risk of bleeding. Accordingly, previous regimens involving the use of a loading dose are being employed less frequently. A suggested regimen is to give warfarin, 10 to 15 mg daily, until the desired effect on the prothrombin time is achieved and the dose adjusted to maintain that level. Individualization of dosage is essential, because a variety of drug interactions, other pharmacologic considerations, and metabolic factors influence the sensitivity and response to the coumarin compounds. *Drugs to be avoided during warfarin therapy* include aspirin, phenylbutazone, oxyphenbutazone, and indomethacin, and the following have been shown to potentiate its effect: anabolic steroids, certain antimicrobials (particularly chloramphenicol and those which affect the intestinal bacterial flora), chloral hydrate, clofibrate, disulfiram, ethacrynic acid, glucagon, mefenamic acid, methylphenidate, quinidine, quinine, and sulfinpyrazone. Those agents which inhibit the prothrombinopenic effect of warfarin include barbiturates, corticosteroids, cholestyramine, ethchlorvynol, glutethimide, griseofulvin, haloperidol, meprobamate, and oral contraceptives. Also, older patients, particularly women, are more sensitive to warfarin, as are individuals suffering from febrile illnesses, malnutrition, steatorrhea, and hepatic or pancreatic disease, as well as those in the im-

mediate postoperative state. Increased resistance to warfarin is associated with hyperlipidemia and hyperuricemia. Warfarin also interferes with the metabolism of other drugs; it enhances the action of diphenylhydantoin, chlorpropamide, and tolbutamide.

In patients being switched from heparin to warfarin therapy, a period of overlap is necessary because of the delay in the antithrombotic effect of the coumarin. A suggested procedure is to give warfarin, 10 to 15 mg daily for two to three days, until the desired therapeutic range for the prothrombin time is achieved; then, while continuing maintenance warfarin therapy, heparin dosage is progressively reduced over another three- to four-day period before discontinuation. Since prothrombin times are influenced by the presence of heparin, such assays should be carried out on blood specimens with a normal or near normal activated partial thromboplastin time; for patients on sustaining infusions of heparin, this may require the in vitro addition of protamine.

Bleeding is a significant hazard, with oral anticoagulation occurring in 3 per cent or more of patients on long-term therapy; vitamin K_1 in doses of 5 to 10 mg is usually corrective. Long-term therapy should not be undertaken unless a reliable laboratory is available and the patient's cooperation can be assured. Individuals on such therapy should avoid contact exercise, aspirin, and aspirin-containing compounds, and should be observed carefully even after slight trauma (subdural hematoma in the aged is often an unsuspected complication of coumarin therapy). Invasive procedures, including needle biopsies and spinal taps, are to be avoided unless the prothrombin time is first restored to or near the normal range. Other adverse effects are minimal; probably of most interest is the occasional appearance of skin necrosis and the rare "purple toe syndrome." Contraindications to coumarin therapy are similar to those previously mentioned for heparin and, in addition, pregnancy. Not only has coumarin administration been shown to increase teratogenicity in animals during the first trimester but, unlike heparin, it crosses the placental barrier and can produce fetal hemorrhage. The use of coumarins also should be avoided, when possible, for patients with severe liver disease or advanced renal insufficiency.

Other Antithrombotic Agents. Low molecular weight *dextran* infusions, based on their ability to improve flow rates by expanding plasma volume and to inhibit platelet adherence and aggregation, have been recommended by some as a useful adjunct in the management of acute thrombophlebitis. In contrast to its proved value in prevention, the efficacy of such therapy for thrombophlebitis remains to be established; at present there is little justification to have dextran infusions replace anticoagulant therapy. Also, there is considerable interest in the use of defibrinating agents; the most promising agents in this respect are the highly purified fraction *(Arvin)* obtained from the venom of the Malayan pit viper, and *Defibrase*. It remains to be established whether these agents will have advantages over heparin.

Surgical Therapy. Surgical procedures may be helpful in the management of some cases of thrombophlebitis; *proximal interruption of venous flow* can be employed to prevent embolization, and thrombectomy to relieve obstruction. The surgical procedures of choice to protect adequately against pulmonary embolization from the lower extremities and pelvis are inferior vena caval ligation, plication, or the insertion of an appropriate filter or umbrella. The last-named can be accomplished transvenously and does not require abdominal surgery. Each procedure has its adherents, and all but the first obviate the difficulty of sudden acute fluid sequestration with hypovolemia and impaired venous return, an event which may be tolerated poorly by people with underlying heart disease. Since all these procedures are usually followed by retrograde thrombosis, and consequently carry a significant incidence of distressing sequelae, both immediate and late, and do not permanently protect (large collaterals develop in several months and may provide a new route for embolization), they are not given consideration except in the presence of pulmonary embolism, or when pulmonary embolism has been known to occur in the past and there is a contraindication to the use of anticoagulant therapy.

Thrombectomy, including the use of Fogarty and similar types of catheters, has been employed successfully in the management of occasional cases of phlegmasia cerulea dolens. However, since this procedure is often followed by venous rethrombosis as well as complicating the subsequent use of anticoagulation, it is currently indicated only for those patients in whom acute fluid sequestration and high tissue tension sufficiently jeopardize the arterial circulation as to threaten the survival of the limb.

Thrombolytic Therapy. Clot-dissolving agents ultimately should prove useful as adjuncts in the management of deep vein thrombophlebitis, for they provide the only medical means for directly lysing a thrombus already formed. The most useful agents for thrombolytic therapy are *streptokinase* and *urokinase,* activators of the naturally occurring human fibrinolytic enzyme system. Streptokinase is a secretory product of the hemolytic Streptococcus and can be produced readily in large quantities and relatively inexpensively for therapeutic purposes. Its major disadvantage is its antigenicity; this poses problems in dosage and, more important, in retreatment should thrombosis recur. Urokinase, a normal constituent of human urine, is nonantigenic and simpler to use therapeutically, but more expensive. Although originally prepared from urine, currently it is being processed from the culture medium of fetal kidney tissue cells. Both agents are given intravenously; for thrombophlebitis, a suggested procedure for streptokinase is to give 250,000 units as a loading dose over a 20- to 30-minute period, followed by a sustaining infusion of 100,000 units per hour for 48 to 72 hours; with urokinase, 2000 units per pound of body weight is given as a loading dose, followed by a sustaining infusion of the same amount per hour for 24 to 48 hours. Heparin therapy is instituted at the termination of the fibrinolytic therapy so as to prevent rethrombosis. Although both agents when used in appropriate dosage are capable of lysing large thrombi in the deep leg veins, the intense fibrinolytic state has a propensity to induce bleeding. Consequently, current recommendations are to limit their use to those patients with extensive occlusions of the major deep veins of the extremity or with a rapidly ascending thrombophlebitis or pulmonary embolism. If lower doses of these agents can be shown to be effective and safe when combined with anticoagulants, as now under test, they may prove an important adjunct to the management of all cases of deep vein thrombosis.

Both urokinase and streptokinase are still under evaluation in the United States and neither is as yet commercially available. The only available preparation, human fibrinolysin, is in reality a mixture of steptokinase and human plasmin. At the dosages recommended by the manufacturer, the fibrinolytic activity induced in the patient is extremely variable, and currently little enthusiasm exists for use of this material for thrombolytic purposes.

Follow-up Therapy. When the systemic symptoms and signs of thrombophlebitis have subsided and the involved limb is pain free and nontender, the patient can begin walking with the leg supported by elastic stockings, unless such activity is followed by return of symptoms. After walking has been resumed, the patient should be advised to elevate the extremity above heart level for several half-hour periods a day. Elastic stockings should be worn until measurement of the extremity reveals no accumulation of edema fluid. Early and persistent therapy is important to prevent development of the postphlebitic syndrome. Once the brawny swelling and induration of the postphlebitic limb have occurred, they may be relieved somewhat by long periods of elevation, elastic compressions, vigorous massage, special exercises and mechanical devices, providing that there has been no recent recurrence of phlebitis. Gross deformities, ulcerations, and persistent or repeated infections may ultimately require one or more surgical procedures.

545. PULMONARY EMBOLISM AND INFARCTION

Definition. Pulmonary embolism is the impaction in the pulmonary vascular bed of a previously detached thrombus or foreign matter. Its major complication, pulmonary infarction, is the necrosis of lung parenchyma resulting from interference with blood supply. Since pulmonary embolism is the more common event, is not invariably accompanied by infarction, and has distinguishing features of its own, this chapter will be devoted primarily to pulmonary embolism; however, discussion of pulmonary infarction will be included as indicated.

Etiology. Pulmonary embolism is a complication, not a primary disease; therefore its etiology is considered in terms of the nature and source of the offending embolus. Almost all pulmonary emboli originate as thrombi; on occasion nonthrombotic materials such as amniotic fluid, fat, air, bone marrow, or tumor may embolize to the lung.

Venous thrombi in the deep veins of the lower extremities are the most common source for pulmonary emboli, accounting for 80 to 90 per cent. Another important source for pulmonary embolization is thrombi in the pelvic veins and prostatic plexus. Prostatic vein thrombosis may accompany malignant disease of the prostate but more frequently follows prostatic surgery. In the female, thrombosis in the pelvic veins may follow parturition or surgery; a particularly severe form, with frequent and protacted embolization, may complicate septic abortion. Pulmonary emboli may also arise from the right heart and are seen in association with cardiac failure, atrial fibrillation, myocardial infarction, the primary cardiomyopathies, and bacterial endocarditis (involving the tricuspid or pulmonic valves). Thrombi in the right heart frequently embolize and are said to account for approximately 25 per cent of pulmonary emboli among cardiac patients.

The factors controlling detachment of the whole or part of a venous thrombus into the general circulation are even less well understood than thrombus formation itself; frequently such thrombi will break away without apparent cause. It was formerly believed that embolization occurred more frequently with phlebothrombosis, but evidence to support this concept is lacking, and symptomatic thrombophlebitis is often complicated by embolization. Of more importance are the location of the vessel (embolism is rare from a superficial vein but very frequent from the iliofemoral vein), the presence of a free floating tail, and factors which acutely change pressure relationships in veins or suddenly increase venous blood flow; these include straining at stool, exertion, and ambulation after a long period of immobilization.

Once a thrombus is released into the venous circulation, it is usually carried rapidly through the great veins and right heart into the pulmonary arteries, except under those circumstances in which the embolus is shunted, through a patent foramen ovale or other defect, into the left heart and systemic circulation (*paradoxical embolization*). However, even this latter condition tends to occur most frequently after a bout of pulmonary embolism, for the associated pulmonary hypertension predisposes to paradoxical embolization.

Incidence and Prevalence.　Pulmonary embolism with or without infarction is a common disorder and a most important cause of morbidity and mortality. It is frequently misdiagnosed. Next to pneumonia, it is the most common acute pulmonary lesion seen in hospitalized patients today. Thirty per cent of pulmonary emboli occur in cardiac patients, another 30 per cent occur among medical noncardiac patients (particularly among the aged), and most of the remainder occur postoperatively. Immobilization, venous disease, and prior cardiopulmonary disease are the factors most frequently predisposing to pulmonary embolism. The over-all incidence of pulmonary embolism in general autopsy series ranges from 5 to 14 per cent, but the incidence is considerably higher (25 per cent) in institutions for the care of the aged, and highest (30 to 45 per cent) among cardiac patients. The incidence of pulmonary embolism appears to have increased progressively over the past several decades.

Embolism to the main pulmonary artery or its primary branches so as to occlude acutely the major portion of the circulation through the lungs, although less frequent than embolism of smaller vessels, is the third most common cause of sudden death (5 per cent) among hospitalized patients. It occurs in about 3 per cent of general autopsy series, but with antemortem diagnosis of only one in eight.

Embolism to medium-sized vessels, i.e., lobar and segmental vessels, is observed approximately three to five times more frequently in autopsy series than is embolism of the major vessels; but since the former is commonly not fatal and is often recurrent, the actual incidence of acute episodes is relatively much greater. Furthermore, in contrast to embolism of the major vessels, the presence of medium-sized emboli at autopsy can be considered only incidental in two thirds of the cases; in the other third, the clinical features are such as to suggest some relation to the fatal termination. Pulmonary infarction complicates embolism of medium-sized arteries in less than 25 per cent of cases. In cardiac patients, the incidence of infarction after such embolism is considerably increased; in one autopsy series, more than

90 per cent of the lungs of cardiac patients with emboli were found to have areas of infarction.

Embolism to small-sized vessels, i.e., subsegmental arteries and their branches, probably occurs with great frequency, but the incidence is difficult to assess. As an isolated and focal lesion, such embolization has little clinical significance, for it usually is not large enough to produce a macroinfarction, and in routine autopsies the lesion is likely to be overlooked unless there are associated thrombi in the larger vessels. However, multiple small emboli scattered throughout the lungs are frequently observed in association with thrombotic occlusions of larger vessels; under these circumstances they contribute significantly to the impairment of pulmonary circulation and associated morbidity. Miliary small vessel occlusion is also the major cause of morbidity when nonthrombotic emboli, such as fat, amniotic fluid, air, or nitrogen, are involved.

Pathology.　Pulmonary emboli may be single or multiple and vary in size from microscopic particles to large saddle emboli that completely occlude the pulmonary artery and its major branches. In addition, a large embolus may break up during passage through the heart or upon impaction and not only obstruct a major vessel but further embolize into one or more smaller branches in both lung fields. Also, there is evidence that, subsequent to impaction, emboli may shift or further fragment into previously unobstructed pulmonary vessels.

With occlusion of the main pulmonary artery or of both its primary branches, or when there is extensive involvement of medium-sized vessels so as to cut off the major portion of the pulmonary arterial circulation, there is acute mechanical obstruction to pulmonary blood flow; the pulmonary artery is distended by the presence of both clot and blood, the right ventricle is acutely dilated, the peripheral veins are engorged, and the liver is congested. Acute infarction rarely occurs; either the lung parenchyma is fairly normal or there is moderate atelectasis, usually explained by the loss of surfactant, and edema. Although the low incidence of acute infarction is possibly attributable to the rapidity with which death occurs (90 per cent of the deaths from acute pulmonary embolism occur within the first two hours), other factors are probably responsible for this phenomenon. In 40 per cent of the cases there is evidence of previous embolization and infarction.

Emboli which pass beyond the pulmonary artery and its major branches tend to impact the arteries of the lower lobes, more often the right than the left. Embolism to other lobes is much less frequent; combined, they account for only 25 per cent of cases. The more frequent involvement of the lower lobes is believed to be due to the fact that these areas lie in the more direct stream of the pulmonary arteries.

When *infarction* occurs, it spreads to involve a pleural surface, either peripheral or interlobar. The infarcted area is airless and hemorrhagic; the hemorrhage is both interstitial and alveolar. Because of the associated pleuritis, hypoventilation, and pre-existing disease, there may be surrounding atelectasis and edema as well. Although occlusion of the larger medium vessels, e.g., interlobar arteries, tends to be associated with infarcts of larger size, the relation between size of vessel occlusion and infarction is a poor one; other factors appear to be more critical in determining the presence and size of the infarct. By roentgenography, infarcts are poorly visualized on the first day. Thereafter they usually appear as humped, wedge-shaped, or, less commonly, rounded shadows. When they occur near the bases, considerable diaphragmatic elevation and restriction of motion may be observed. In 30 to 40 per cent of cases, infarcts are associated with a variable amount of *pleural effusion* that may be serous, serosanguineous, or frankly hemorrhagic; usually the specific gravity is in the range of 1.014 to 1.017 (protein, 3 to 3.5 grams per 100 ml) and there is mild to moderate increase in cell content.

Some shadows clear rapidly (two to three days) on roentgenographic examination and have been referred to as "incomplete" infarcts; however, it is likely that this clearing represents reventilation of an atelectatic or congested area occasioned by the embolic occlusion rather than true resolution of an infarct. "Complete" infarcts clear slowly over a two- to three-week period, ending as an area of linear fibrosis.

Mechanisms of Disease, Including Pulmonary Infarction. Emboli lodging in the pulmonary arterial tree acutely reduce the circulation distal to the site of obstruction. Potentially, the effects are fourfold: (1) less blood proceeds through the pulmonary circuit to the left heart and systemic circulation; (2) there is a damming back of blood behind the mechanical obstruction; (3) hemorrhagic necrosis of the ischemic area may occur; and (4) pulmonary function is impaired (pulmonary capillary perfusion and diffusion; later, ventilation may be compromised as well).

Except for the occurrence of infarction, which must be considered as a localized or focal disorder, the average person is believed capable of withstanding considerable obstruction of the pulmonary arterial bed without serious consequences to the vascular dynamics; in normal animals, a 60 to 70 per cent obstruction is usually well tolerated. Nevertheless, exceptions occur, particularly in the presence of underlying heart disease, when less extensive occlusions may elevate pulmonary arterial pressure or significantly reduce pulmonary venous outflow and when pulmonary circulation has been previously impaired by disease or prior embolization.

With a large occlusion of the main pulmonary artery or its primary branches, the effects are acute and primarily mechanical: rapidly rising pulmonary artery pressure, failure of the right ventricle, cyanosis, venous engorgement, and hepatic congestion. The consequences of impaired pulmonary venous return are sharp reduction in left ventricular filling, diminished cardiac output, reduced coronary and cerebral blood flow, hypoxia (also caused by pulmonary blood shunting), dyspnea, pallor, tachycardia, and hypotension, often progressing quickly to shock and death. Sudden dyspnea and retrosternal pain are frequently the most prominent initial complaints; the dyspnea is believed to be due to anoxia, apprehension, and stimulation of Hering-Breuer and other reflexes; the angina is usually attributed to acute coronary insufficiency, but direct stimulation of sensory nerves in the wall of a rapidly distending pulmonary artery may also play a significant role.

The effects of embolization to medium-sized vessels depend on the number, size, and distribution of the emboli and the prior state of the lung and circulation. Several patterns may be observed. (1) There may be no observable effects; a transient episode of dyspnea may be the only clue to its occurrence. (2) The picture may be predominantly one of pulmonary infarction with hemoptysis, pleuritic chest pain, friction rub, and abnormal roentgenographic shadows. Often, however, some elements of this pattern may be absent, notably the hemoptysis or the evidence of pleural involvement. (3) There may be an acute picture similar to, but frequently not as severe as, that seen with embolization of the main pulmonary artery or its primary branches, in which pattern the primary difficulty is one of extensive and sudden compromise of the pulmonary arterial circulation but here by multiple emboli or recurrent embolization; it may or may not be complicated by infarction. (4) There may be a chronic and insidiously developing syndrome of cor pulmonale from progressive pulmonary hypertension that has evolved slowly after repeated episodes of embolization with or without infarction. This is often superimposed and obscured by the presence of other underlying chronic disease.

Controversy exists concerning the factors that acutely compromise the pulmonary circulation when emboli impact in medium-sized or smaller vessels. Some hold that vasoconstriction (pulmonary and perhaps coronary), mediated through reflexes from occluded arterioles or by the local release of serotonin or other vasoactive substances, plays an important role. It seems probable, however, that the continuing effects of most pulmonary emboli are primarily mechanical; when a major segment of the circulation is organically occluded, pulmonary hypertension and decreased venous outflow result. The suggestion has been made, and experimental studies have been cited to support the concept, that idiopathic pulmonary hypertension and pulmonary arteriosclerosis may result from repeated small pulmonary emboli.

The mechanism of pulmonary infarction is poorly understood. It does not result from ligation of pulmonary vessels and is unusual after embolization in animals with normal lungs; however, it does occur with great frequency in the congested, infected, or hypoventilated lung. Currently the best working hypothesis is that when medium-sized embolization occurs, enhancement of the circulation through the bronchial artery collaterals and bronchopulmonary vascular anastomoses distal to the embolus ordinarily serves to sustain the lung. However, in the presence of congestion or other conditions that predispose to local intrapulmonic circulatory stasis, augmentation of the collateral circulation is delayed or its benefits voided, and infarction occurs.

Hemorrhagic necrosis of the lung tissue and the overlying pleural inflammation are responsible for the characteristic clinical features of pulmonary infarction. The former accounts for the hemoptysis, cough, and fever; the latter for the pleural friction rub and pain. Since both lung tissue and the visceral pleura are devoid of sensory nerves, infarcts that do not extend to the outer surface of the lung to involve the parietal pleura do not cause pleural pain. When pain is present, it usually occurs over the ribs in the axillary region, but occasionally it may appear in the abdomen along the costal margin, or, when there is involvement of the parietal diaphragmatic pleura, in the shoulder or neck. The mechanism of the pain has usually been attributed to friction over an inflamed pleura, but an alternative explanation that may better explain its features (accentuation only on inspiration) is tension exerted during inspiration on those sensitized nerve ends of the parietal pleura that are attached to the intercostal muscles.

Clinical Manifestations. The manifestations of *massive pulmonary embolism* (defined for clinical purposes as occlusion of 50 per cent or more of the pulmonary arterial circulation and representing approximately one third to one half of the suspected cases) may include sudden dyspnea; tachypnea; cyanosis; precordial or substernal oppressive pain, occasionally with radiation to shoulders and neck; evidences of right-sided cardiac dilatation and failure; tachycardia; restlessness; anxiety; syncope, occasionally with convulsions; and hypotension.

With massive embolism, death may be sudden or may occur over a period of several hours. In the latter instance, shock with vascular collapse becomes prominent. In an additional 2 to 3 per cent of patients, death may be delayed from one to several days; but when blood pressure spontaneously returns to normal, recovery is likely (unless the course is complicated by recurrence or an underlying disease). The physical signs noted include pulsation in the second left interspace, accentuation of P_2, a pseudo- or pleuropericardial friction rub, systolic or diastolic murmurs in the second left interspace, and interscapular bruit, S_3 or S_4 gallop rhythm, increased cardiac dullness to the right, distended neck veins, increased venous pressure with an hepatojugular reflex, and enlarged liver. Dislodgment of a large obstructing embolus may be associated with the dramatic transient appearance of a "red arterial wave" suddenly passing over a pallid cyanotic face.

Serial *electrocardiograms* reveal transient changes in most patients (85 per cent), but the pattern is extremely variable. The most frequent initial finding is T wave inversion (40 per cent). The electrocardiographic signs of acute cor pulmonale ($S_1Q_3T_3$, complete right bundle branch block, P pulmonale, or right axis deviation) are present in only 25 per cent of patients; left axis deviation is observed more frequently than right axis deviation. Rhythm disturbances (most commonly, premature ventricular beats) are observed in 10 per cent, as is a pseudoinfarction pattern. Patients with prior cardiopulmonary disease have a greater frequency of arrhythmias, conduction disturbances, and QRS changes; patients with extensive embolization demonstrate more QRS, RST, and T wave changes. In general, little change occurs during the first 24 hours, but after five to six days the QRS, primary RST segment, and T wave abnormalities begin to disappear. Roentgenographically, massive pulmonary embolism may result in the appearance of a large pulmonary arterial shadow that terminates abruptly; in some cases the ischemia may produce radiolucency of portions of the lung field (Westermark's sign).

With *submassive embolism,* i.e., occlusion of less than 50 per cent of the pulmonary circulation and usually involving the medium-sized or smaller vessels, the clinical manifestations may vary from a transient episode of dyspnea or the sudden or insidious worsening of an underlying pulmonary or cardiac disease, to the full-blown picture described for massive embolism (submassive embolism in patients with prior embolism or severe underlying cardiopulmonary disease frequently presents with the findings usually attributable to massive embolism); however, when pulmonary infarction occurs, its manifestations may also be superimposed.

The manifestations of *pulmonary infarction* are usually less dramatic. They vary in intensity from silent to those characterized by pleuritic chest pain, hemoptysis, cough, moderate dyspnea, fever, tachycardia, pleural friction rub, areas of dullness or flatness on percussion, and diminished breath sounds, occasionally with tubular breathing and rales. The leukocyte count is usually elevated, the sedimentation rate is accelerated, and, subsequently, the serum bilirubin and serum lactic dehydrogenase levels rise. Roentgenographic examination may show typical humped or wedge-shaped shadows; on occasions the lesions are rounded or indistinguishable from pneumonic infiltrates. At other times, a pleural effusion may be the only clue to an underlying infarct. The average patient with pulmonary infarction runs a moderately febrile course for a few days, which is followed by clearing of roentgenographic and physical signs in one to three weeks.

Diagnosis.   Despite the introduction of such diagnostic aids as pulmonary isotopic and ventilation photoscanning and selective pulmonary angiography, the diagnosis of pulmonary embolism with or without infarction is accurately made in no more than 50 per cent of cases when compared to autopsy findings. Frequently the diagnosis is overlooked because the disorder appears in the guise of congestive heart failure or pneumonia rather than as a distinctive syndrome; furthermore, the cardinal features do not occur with any great regularity. In half the patients subsequently proved to have recurrent infarction, no evidence of phlebitis, pleural pain, pleural friction rub, or hemoptysis is present, and in any one episode the incidence of each of these is less than 20 per cent. Thus in the absence of classic features, the diagnosis must be made on the basis of a high index of suspicion followed by confirmatory laboratory findings.

Pulmonary embolism with or without infarction should be suspected in all cases of chest pain of unknown cause, atypical pleural effusion, or bronchopneumonia. The possibility of this complication should also be considered in any patient who has a proved or suggestive history of a previous episode (present in 25 per cent of cases), in groups at high risk for deep vein thrombosis, and, most carefully, in critically ill patients with congestive heart failure; the incidence among the last-named group approaches 50 per cent and is much higher among those who exhibit unexplained fever or the *triad of tachycardia, digitalis toxicity, and edema unresponsive to diuretic therapy.*

Actually, the presence of one or more of the following symptoms, signs, or laboratory findings should raise the possibility of pulmonary embolism for consideration: sudden or increased dyspnea, tachypnea, cough, or cyanosis; substernal or pleuritic chest pain; hemoptysis; phlebitis; acute right-sided failure or sudden worsening of congestive heart failure; shock; pulmonary consolidation; pleural friction rub; roentgenographic evidence of pulmonary infiltration, elevated diaphragm, large areas of increased radiolucency, or pleural effusion; unexplained arrhythmias or electrocardiographic changes, particularly when the latter is indicative of acute right-heart strain or dilatation; pulmonary function studies indicating an increased ventilatory dead space, i.e., reduction in the mean alveolar carbon dioxide tension in the presence of a normal or nearly normal arterial carbon dioxide tension; or unexplained fever, leukocytosis, elevated erythrocyte sedimentation rate, serum bilirubin, lactic dehydrogenase, and fibrinogen/fibrin split products (normal levels of fibrinogen/fibrin split products and fibrin monomer are rare in pulmonary embolism).

The most reliable *screening procedures* for excluding an acute pulmonary embolism are pulmonary isotopic photoscanning with technetium-labeled microspheres or macroaggregates of human serum albumin, and an arterial Po_2 determination; a negative four-positional (anterior, posterior, and both laterals) lung scan virtually eliminates acute embolism, and it is rare when the arterial Po_2 is 90 mm Hg or above.

Confirmation of the diagnosis can often be achieved through the use of either selective pulmonary angiography or pulmonary isotopic photoscanning; on occasion, both techniques will be necessary. Since selective *pulmonary angiography* provides direct visualization of the vascular tree, it is the more definitive of the two procedures, and is the choice for establishing the diagnosis of pulmonary embolism. However, there are limitations to its usefulness. It is expensive and requires a skilled team; catheterization of the pulmonary artery is associated with some morbidity; the technique does not distinguish between new and old emboli; the subsegmental and smaller vessels are not visualized adequately; and there may be errors in interpretation unless the angiographer is experienced and strict criteria are used.

Pulmonary isotopic photoscanning has the advantages of convenience and lack of significant morbidity, and allows for repeated observation in following the course of the patient. However, unlike pulmonary arteriography, photoscanning does not visualize the pulmonary arterial tree; rather, it is a measure of the distribution of blood flow or pulmonary capillary perfusion, and defects in perfusion may be misinterpreted as to cause, especially in the presence of any underlying pulmonary lesion, e.g., infiltrates, blebs, cysts, emphysema, an acute asthmatic attack, or alterations in perfusion as a result of previous or associated disease. Since the scan is not specific for pulmonary embolism, perfusion defects should be characterized as to whether they are segmental or not and only interpreted as having a high, medium, or low probability of being due to an embolism. Although emphysema may also be responsible for high probability perfusion defects, the differential diagnosis can usually be resolved by a radioactively labeled xenon ventilation scan, because such a scan is unaffected by pulmonary embolism, at least for a period of five days. Pulmonary isotopic photoscanning is most useful for demonstrating and quantitating the perfusion defect of a pulmonary embolism when the chest roentgenogram is normal; it may also be diagnostic by revealing multiple perfusion defects (indicative of multiple pulmonary embolism) when only an isolated infiltrate or lesion is present roentgenographically. Resolution of the perfusion defect after an embolism occurs progressively (50 per cent in two weeks), and this, too, may be useful diagnostically. It is noteworthy that patients with underlying cardiac disease have an impaired resolution rate.

Acute pulmonary embolism may be most readily confused with acute myocardial infarction, pulmonary edema, acute asthma, atelectasis, pericarditis, spontaneous pneumothorax, ball-valve thrombus in the left atrium, dissecting aneurysm, and pulmonary artery thrombosis. The last-named condition occurs rarely as a primary form of obscure cause or as a complication of a partially obstructing embolus, invading tumor, narrowed vascular lumen, or atherosclerotic plaque.

The differential diagnosis of pulmonary infarction includes pneumonia, pleurisy, other forms of pleural effusion, neoplasm, acute upper abdominal conditions, and the various causes of pulmonary hemorrhage. During resolution, an occasional infarct may slough out, leaving a thin-walled cavity which may be confused with an abscess.

To distinguish between an infarct and pneumonia may be difficult, yet this question arises frequently. Findings that are helpful in pointing to the diagnosis of infarct are a history or the presence of one of the preconditions of infarct, e.g., recent surgery, trauma, cardiac disease, previous venous disease, or pulmonary embolism; an extremely rapid appearance of roentgenographic abnormalities from the time of the first respiratory symptom; illness that seems disproportionately mild in relation to the extent of the pulmonary involvement or leukocytosis; and relative lack of cough or lack of preceding respiratory disease.

A spontaneous form of pulmonary infarction occurs in sickle cell disease, in the mixed sickle cell hemoglobinopathies, or in persons with sickle cell trait who are exposed to high altitude.

Treatment. *General Measures.* Supportive treatment for the usual acute embolism should include bed rest, an analgesic or narcotic (preferably meperidine hydrochloride [Demerol]) for pain and apprehension, and oxygen as indicated. The administration of antimicrobial drugs to prevent bacterial disease of the lungs is not indicated unless a septic infarct is suspected. All sudden effort should be avoided, especially straining at stool. Stool softeners and colonic lavages may prove useful. Pleural effusions may require aspiration, particularly if dyspnea is progressive. Digitalization is indicated if cardiac failure appears or worsens, but usually is of little benefit.

In more severe cases, continuous oxygen therapy should be employed, and positive pressure oxygen may prove particularly useful when pulmonary edema is present. Cardiac arrhythmias, which occur in 10 per cent of cases, should be treated appropriately. If shock occurs, fluids and isoproterenol should be given. Intravenous fluids should be monitored by central venous pressure measurements but maintained below 150 mm saline to prevent pulmonary edema. For hypotension, isoproterenol, because of its inotropic effect on the heart, is the agent of choice. It should be given intravenously slowly, usually at a rate of 2 μg per minute to sustain the systolic blood pressure at about 100 mm Hg (preferably at 120 mm Hg in previously hypertensive patients). Aminophylline, 250 to 500 mg (by suppository, intramuscularly, or by slow intravenous administration), may prove useful, particularly when dyspnea is prominent or pulmonary edema is present. Venesection may be dangerous, however, because of impaired left ventricular filling. The value of pulmonary vasodilators, e.g., papaverine, and bronchodilators, e.g., atropine, is still highly controversial.

Anticoagulants. In the absence of contraindications, heparin therapy should be instituted immediately in all patients with pulmonary embolism to lessen the danger of a recurrent and frequently fatal embolic accident (when heparin allergy is present, anticoagulation should be instituted immediately with coumarin compounds). Hemoptysis from pulmonary infarction is not a contraindication to anticoagulant therapy. The regimen for heparin therapy and subsequent oral coumarin anticoagulation is as described under the treatment of thrombophlebitis. Aspirin and aspirin-containing compounds should be avoided because of the increased risk of bleeding. Coumarin therapy is continued for six weeks unless there is a chronic disease, e.g., cardiac failure, that predisposes to repeated venous thrombus formation; under these circumstances anticoagulant therapy should be continued for prolonged periods.

Thrombolytic Agents. When available, these will

provide an important adjunct to the management of the more seriously ill patient with pulmonary embolism. Clinical trials have demonstrated that urokinase and streptokinase lyse pulmonary emboli extensively, reduce the hemodynamic abnormalities, improve pulmonary capillary perfusion, and increase gas exchange. These effects are observed fairly rapidly and are most striking in patients with massive embolism. Regimens as described previously for thrombophlebitis also should reduce significantly the need for surgical embolectomy, particularly when the therapy is combined with temporary cardiac bypass to tide the patient over the most critical period. Whether local perfusion of the agent directly into the pulmonary artery has any advantage over intravenous administration remains to be established. At present, thrombolytic agents are not indicated for the treatment of submassive embolism when stable vital signs are present; in the absence of complications, the patient is destined to recover and there is little need to increase the risk of bleeding. *Arvin*, the defibrinating agent, may also prove to be of benefit in the managment of acute pulmonary embolism, but its advantage over heparin remains to be established.

Surgical Therapy.   Inferior vena caval ligation, plication, or the insertion of a filter or umbrella should be reserved for those patients in whom anticoagulants are contraindicated, must be discontinued, or whose disease for one reason or another cannot be successfully managed with this form of therapy. Since these procedures carry a significant incidence of sequelae, they are not indicated unless there has been massive embolism or there is evidence of recurrent embolization (a minor recurrence is observed in about 10 per cent of patients during the first few days of heparin therapy, and should not be considered as a failure of anticoagulant therapy unless the episode is significant clinically or continues to recur during adequate levels of anticoagulation).

Surgical embolectomy may be lifesaving in critically ill patients. However, this procedure requires cardiac bypass, and because of the condition of the patients, the mortality in patients treated with surgical embolectomy is still very high. At present, the indication for embolectomy is limited to patients with angiographic evidence of massive embolism of the main pulmonary artery or its primary branches and with sustained peripheral hypotension despite the use of appropriate supportive measures. Pulmonary embolectomy may also be considered for patients who have survived a massive embolism but in whom pulmonary hypertension resulting from the presence of an accessible embolus is leading to the development of cor pulmonale.

Prognosis.   The prognosis of pulmonary embolism is difficult to establish because the clinical diagnosis is frequently obscure. Of those who succumb, approximately 90 per cent die immediately or within the first two hours. Another 2 to 3 per cent die of protracted shock during the next 48 hours. Once stable vital signs are established, subsequent mortality approximates 7 per cent and is usually attributable to recurrent embolism or adverse effects on an underlying cardiopulmonary disease. The likelihood of a fatal episode is increased with succeeding embolic attacks and, most important, in the presence of a significant impairment of cardiopulmonary reserve. The greatest hope for the management of this problem is prevention.

Unfortunately, such measures as the use of elastic stockings or bandages, leg exercises for immobilized pa-

tients, and early ambulation postoperatively have not greatly affected the high incidence of pulmonary embolism; nevertheless, the intelligent use of such measures, and particularly of the more recently developed mechanical devices which enhance blood flow, is to be encouraged. In addition, serious consideration should be given to the use of anticoagulants for all patients predisposed to thrombus formation. When used carefully, anticoagulants have significantly reduced the incidence of pulmonary embolism after fracture of the femur and in cases of congestive heart failure. This form of therapy should not be undertaken lightly, because the hazards, in any specific case, may outweigh the benefits to be derived. Low-dose heparin, should it prove successful, will obviate this problem.

Anticoagulation also has an important role to play in the *prevention of arterial embolism.* Coumarin therapy is useful in avoiding systemic embolization from endocardial mural thrombi in the left ventricle, e.g., after acute transmural infarction, and in the left atrium, e.g., in rheumatic mitral disease or during an electrical conversion of an arrhythmia. For acute myocardial infarction, coumarin therapy should be administered to those at high risk for such embolic episodes; the high risk factors include age over 60, previous myocardial infarction, shock, congestive heart failure, and evidence of large transmural infarction as judged by the levels of serum enzymes, fever, leukocytosis, sedimentation rate, and the extent of the electrocardiographic abnormalities. Therapy should be initiated at the onset of the illness and continued for a period of four weeks. Patients with rheumatic mitral disease with a nonseptic embolus (anticoagulants are contraindicated in subacute bacterial endocarditis) should be maintained on long-term anticoagulation or until surgical correction of the lesion. For individuals undergoing electrical conversion of an arrhythmia, coumarin therapy should be initiated two to three weeks prior to attempting reversion to a sinus rhythm in all patients with previous emboli or evidence of mitral stenosis; in other situations the need for anticoagulation should be considered and evaluated on an individual basis.

Coumarin anticoagulation is less effective for the prevention of platelet emboli such as may occur from prosthetic heart valves and in the transient ischemic attack syndrome. Better results are being obtained for the former condition when coumarin anticoagulation is combined with antiplatelet agents, e.g., sulfinpyrazone (800 mg daily) or dipyridamole (400 mg daily). For the transient ischemic attack syndrome, sulfinpyrazone alone appears to be yielding good results (aspirin, 1.2 grams daily, is also under study).

Medical therapy of an acute embolic event with antithrombotic agents is as described under the management of thrombophlebitis and pulmonary embolism.

Anticoagulants in acute myocardial infarction. Results of a cooperative clinical trial. J.A.M.A., 225:724, 1973.

Basu, D., Gallus, A., Hirsh, J., and Cade, J.: A prospective study of the value of monitoring heparin treatment with the activated partial thromboplastin time. N. Engl. J. Med., 287:324, 1972.

Coon, W. W., Willis, P. W., III, and Keller, J. B.: Venous thromboembolism and other venous disease in the Tecumseh Community Health Study. Circulation, 48:239, 1973.

Foster, C. S., Genton, E., Henderson, M., Sherry, S., and Wessler, S. (eds.): The epidemiology of venous thrombosis. Milbank Memorial Fund Quarterly, 50 (1), Part 2:9, 1972.

Gallus, A. S., Hirsh, J., Tuttle, R. J., et al.: Small subcutaneous doses of heparin in prevention of venous thrombosis. N. Engl. J. Med., 288:545, 1973.

Genton, E.: Guidelines for heparin therapy. Ann. Intern. Med., 80:77, 1974.

Hume, M., Sevitt, S., and Thomas, D. P.: Venous Thrombosis and Pulmonary Embolism. Cambridge, Mass., Harvard University Press, 1970.

Kakkar, V. V., Howe, C. T., Flanc, C., and Clarke, M. B.: Natural history of postoperative deep vein thrombosis. Lancet, 2:230, 1969.

Koch-Weser, J., and Sellers, E. M.: Drug interaction with coumarin anticoagulants. N. Engl. J. Med., 285:547, 1971.

McIntyre, K. M., and Sasahara, A. A.: The hemodynamic response to pulmonary embolism in patients without prior cardiopulmonary disease. Am. J. Cardiol., 28:288, 1971.

O'Reilly, R. A., and Aggeler, P. M.: Studies on coumarin anticoagulant drugs. Institution of warfarin therapy without a loading dose. Circulation, 38:169, 1968.

Paraskos, J. A., Adelstein, S. J., Smith, R. E., et al.: Late prognosis of acute pulmonary embolism, N. Engl. J. Med., 289:55, 1973.

Sasahara, A., Hyers, T. M., Cole, C., et al. (eds.): The urokinase pulmonary embolism trial. Circulation, 47 (Supplement II): II-5, 1973.

Stein, M., and Moser, K. M. (eds.): Pulmonary Thromboembolism. Chicago, Year Book Medical Publishers, 1973.

PULMONARY HYPERTENSION

Daniel S. Lukas

546. INTRODUCTION

Morphologically and physiologically, the circulation of the lungs differs from that of all other organs. Although the entire cardiac output passes through the lungs, a mean pressure in the pulmonary artery only one ninth of the pressure in the aorta is needed to sustain this flow. Under a wide variety of physiologic circumstances, simple adjustments of the pulmonary vascular bed minimize increases of pulmonary arterial pressure. Because many diseases of the heart and lungs can seriously compromise this regulatory capacity, pulmonary hypertension is a common clinical phenomenon. In some disorders elevations of pulmonary arterial pressure are acute and episodic, whereas in others the pulmonary hypertension is chronic and progressive.

The mechanisms producing pulmonary arterial hypertension in the major categories of disease are sufficiently different to warrant separate consideration and are best appreciated in the context of the normal structure and function of the pulmonary circulation.

THE NORMAL PULMONARY CIRCULATION

Structure. The pulmonary arterial tree consists of three distinct types of arteries that differ from each other in the composition of their walls and in size. The elastic arteries include the main pulmonary artery, its major branches, and arteries with external diameters greater than 1.0 mm. The muscular pulmonary arteries range in diameter from 0.1 to 1.0 mm. The smallest pulmonary arteries, the arterioles, have diameters less than 0.1 mm. The walls of all three types of arteries are much thinner than those of systemic arteries, and aside from the main pulmonary artery and its branches, these vessels have no strict anatomic counterparts in the systemic vascular bed.

The media of the main pulmonary artery and the elastic arteries contains a small amount of smooth muscle, collagen, and elastic fibers that are short, irregularly branching, and fragmented in appearance. The media of the aorta, in contrast, is 1.5 to more than 2 times thicker, and its elastic fibers are long, unbranching, and distributed in parallel fashion.

The muscular pulmonary arteries are closely apposed to the bronchioles and alveolar ducts. They have a large lumen and a thin wall that is composed of an intima and a thin media of concentrically oriented smooth muscle fibers bounded by internal and external elastic laminae.

The arterioles differ vastly from those of the systemic circuit, because they contain no muscle except at their point of origin. They consist of an endothelium, a single elastic lamina, and a scanty adventitia.

The pulmonary capillaries are the most prominent structural component of the alveolar walls, in which they form an extensive, interlacing network that is separated from the alveolar air by the lining cells of the alveoli and their basement membrane. The total surface of the capillaries that is available for gas exchange in adults has been estimated to comprise 60 to 70 square meters.

The pulmonary venules are thin-walled structures histologically indistinguishable from the arterioles. The structure of the veins is less ordered than that of the muscular arteries. The media, which is not bounded by well-defined elastic laminae, blends indistinguishably with the adventitia, and both contain smooth muscle and fragmented elastic fibers. The main venous trunks acquire a layer of cardiac muscle before they enter the left atrium. The venules and veins, unlike the arteries, do not course with the bronchial tree but are lodged in the septa that separate lobules and segments of the lung.

The bronchial arteries wind in spiral fashion around the bronchi and anastomose extensively with each other in and around the walls of the airways. They also form vasa vasorum in the adventitia of the elastic and larger muscular pulmonary arteries. Evidence that the two arterial systems intercommunicate in the normal lung is inconclusive. The bronchial veins, however, normally form numerous, small anastomotic channels with the pulmonary veins.

It is of considerable significance that the pulmonary arteries in the fetus and newborn differ structurally from those of the adult and do not attain their final form until the sixth to twelfth month of postnatal life. In the newborn, the media of the main pulmonary artery is as thick as that of the aorta and contains numerous, tightly packed, long, elastic fibers that are fairly uniform in thickness and are arranged in parallel fashion as in the aorta. Progressively after birth, the media diminishes in thickness, and the elastic fibers become fragmented, irregularly shaped, randomly distributed, and less densely packed, until they assume the full adult appearance. The muscular pulmonary arteries in the newborn resemble small systemic arteries. Typically, the wall contains a wide media composed of circularly oriented smooth muscle, and its thickness exceeds the diameter of the lumen. Rapid increase in luminal and external diameters and thinning of the media occur during the first sixth months of life. The arterioles at birth are surrounded by dense connective tissue and their lumina are barely patent. Their wall:lumen ratio likewise rapidly diminishes in the first few months of life.

During the early days of the postnatal period, the mean pulmonary arterial pressure is two or more times greater than that of the adult and may be high enough to reverse flow through the ductus arteriosus. The pulmonary arterial pressure declines to normal adult values within the first month, well before the metamorphosis of the pulmonary vasculature has been completed.

Hemodynamics. The average normal pressure in the pulmonary artery at rest is 19/6 mm Hg (systolic/diastolic) with a mean pressure of 11 mm Hg. Normally at rest, the systolic pressure does not exceed 25 mm Hg, and the mean pressure is not greater than 15 mm Hg. Mean pressures in the large pulmonary veins and left atrium are essentially identical, ranging from 3 to 8 mm Hg, with an average of 5 mm Hg. Thus a pressure gradient from the pulmonary artery to the large pulmonary veins of only 6 mm Hg is sufficient to sustain a blood flow in the normal adult at rest of approximately 6.0 liter per minute. These values are eloquent testimony to the low resistance offered to the flow of blood by the thin-walled and capacious pulmonary vessels. Calculated in the conventional manner as the mean pressure gradient divided by flow, the normal pulmonary vascular resistance is 1.0 mm Hg per liter per minute, or 80 dyne sec cm^{-5}, a value only 7 per cent of the normal systemic vascular resistance. The linear distribution of resistance in the pulmonary vascular bed is uncertain, but measurements in dogs indicate that the pulmonary arteries are responsible for approximately half the total resistance, the pulmonary capillaries for 30 per cent, and the veins for 20 per cent.

Several observations testify to the capacity of the pulmonary vascular bed to accommodate increases in blood flow with disproportionately small increases in pressure. During exercise, two- to threefold increases in cardiac output are associated with increments of only 25 to 50 per cent in mean pulmonary arterial pressure, but the pressure doubles when the output rises to four to five times the resting value. Large left-right shunts through an atrial septal defect that commonly triple the pulmonary blood flow are tolerated for many years with no more than slight elevations of pulmonary arterial pressure. After pneumonectomy or occlusion of either main branch of the pulmonary artery by a balloon catheter and in patients with congenital absence of a main branch of the pulmonary artery, the pulmonary arterial pressures remain within the normal range at rest if the perfused lung is normal.

Augmentation of pulmonary blood flow is facilitated and concomitant changes in pressure are minimized by several mechanisms that combine to expand the net cross-sectional area of the pulmonary vessels and thereby decrease the resistance they offer to the flow of blood. One of these mechanisms relates to the effect of changes in intravascular pressures on the caliber of the vessels. It has been demonstrated that increases in pulmonary arterial pressure well within the normal operational range are associated with large decreases in pulmonary vascular resistance and that the resistance declines further with the addition of a 2 to 3 mm Hg rise in left atrial pressure. The vessels are also subjected to the deforming effects of the pressures that surround them. The total pressure that acts on the vascular wall is the transmural pressure, or the difference between the intravascular and perivascular pressures. Some uncertainties exist regarding perivascular pressures in the lungs, but for vessels that are not intrinsic components of the alveolar structure, perivascular pressure is considered to approximate pleural pressure; for intra-alveolar vessels, the alveolar pressure has been regarded as the extravascular pressure. Since the vessels that account for the major fraction of the pulmonary vascular resistance are exposed to the normally negative pleural pressure, their transmural pressures exceed the hydrostatic pressures within them.

During exercise, the more negative pleural pressures generated to augment tidal volume increase the transmural pressure gradients acting on the extra-alveolar vessels, thereby stretching them open further and decreasing their resistance to flow. Pressure changes within the pleura and the lungs can profoundly affect the pulmonary vasculature. For example, when intrapleural and alveolar pressures are greatly increased, as during a Valsalva maneuver, pulmonary vascular transmural pressures fall, some vessels collapse, and the resistance rises markedly.

Primarily because of gravitational effects on regional intravascular pressures, the lungs are not evenly perfused. In the erect position, the height of the blood column from the apices of the lungs to the midpoint of the left atrium is sufficient to reduce pressures within the pulmonary arteries at the apex almost to zero and decrease the transmural pressures of the pulmonary capillaries and veins in these regions to less than zero. Consequently, the vascular bed in the apices is not open, whereas at the bases of the lungs the vessels are subjected to the distending effects of the overlying column of blood and all are patent. These regional differences in vascular resistance produce a progressive decrease in regional blood flow within the lungs from base to apex, and in the upright position blood flow per unit volume of lung is eight times greater at the base than at the apex. At some point below the apices of the lungs, the transmural pressures of the arteries and the arterial limbs of the alveolar capillaries are high enough to maintain patency of the vessels, but the pressure within the venous segment of the capillaries or the venules is less than or just equals the perivascular pressure. The collapsible vascular segments in this region behave like sluices; they are either barely open or closed, and flow of blood through them no longer depends on the pressure gradient between the arterial and venous limbs but varies directly with the pressure difference between the arterial end of the segment and the pressure surrounding the collapsed segment. These hemodynamic conditions have been compared to those of a waterfall.

With increases in pulmonary flow, small changes in intravascular pressures open previously closed or partially collapsed vessels, thus expanding the size of the vascular bed and further lowering resistance to flow. This recruitment of small vessels and capillaries partly explains the increase of pulmonary diffusing capacity that occurs during exercise.

The volume of blood contained by the pulmonary vessels of an average size adult is approximately 400 to 500 ml, 70 to 100 ml of which is in the pulmonary capillaries. Because of its geometric complexity and the probably nonuniform dimensional rearrangements that the pulmonary vascular bed undergoes with changes in volume, the interrelationships among resistance, pressures, flow, and blood volume in the vessels of the lungs are far from simple. It is clear that the distensibility of the pulmonary arterial tree is much greater than that of the systemic arteries, and that this partially accounts for its lower resistance to flow. The large pulmonary veins, however, are less compliant than the major systemic venous segments. Also, the compliance of the small pulmonary vessels is not uniform; the capillaries are less distensible than the arteries and veins. In one study of normal subjects during an exercise that evoked an almost twofold increase in cardiac output, the pulmonary blood volume increased by only 27 per cent, mean pulmonary arterial pressure increased slightly, and pulmonary vascular resistance fell. The pulmonary vasoconstriction produced by hypoxia is associated with a decrease in pulmonary blood volume, despite the increase of pressure in the elastic pulmonary arteries.

The compliance of the pulmonary vessels is finite, and changes in the volume of blood in the lungs do produce changes in vascular pressures. For example, the intense constriction of the systemic vessels that sometimes occurs after injury to the brain *(Cushing reflex)* results in systemic hypertension, displacement of blood from the systemic circuit into the lungs, and marked pulmonary venous and pulmonary arterial hypertension.

Whereas the systemic vessels are closely regulated by the autonomic nervous system and respond to a wide variety of endogenous compounds and drugs, adjustments of the pulmonary vascular bed appear to result almost entirely in response to physical forces. The pulmonary arteries are supplied with autonomic nerves, and there is experimental evidence in animals that the larger pulmonary arteries can be reflexly induced to stiffen, but reflex control of the pulmonary circulation has not been convincingly demonstrated in man. Similarly, many pharmacologic agents considered on the basis of experiments in animals to exert a vasoconstrictor action on the pulmonary arteries (norepinephrine, epinephrine, and serotonin) or a vasodilator effect (bradykinin, isoproterenol, and acetylcholine) have been shown to have either little or no direct action on the normal human pulmonary vascular bed. Because these compounds profoundly affect the systemic circulation and may alter pulmonary mechanics, the changes in pulmonary vascular pressures and resistance that are observed after they are administered are mainly secondary consequences of their actions elsewhere.

Hypoxia. Ample evidence of several types indicates that hypoxia directly constricts the pulmonary bed and elevates the pulmonary vascular resistance by direct action on the muscular pulmonary arteries, which are separated from the inner surface of the small airways by only 0.1 mm. The mechanism of this effect is not completely understood, but there is evidence that the smooth muscle cells of the pulmonary arteries, unlike those of systemic arteries, lose intracellular potassium and gain sodium when exposed to low oxygen tension; consequently, their transmembrane potential falls to levels close to the threshold for discharge, and the frequency of muscular contraction increases. A recent study suggests that prostaglandins E and F synthesized in the lung may mediate the vasoconstriction.

The vasoconstrictor response to hypoxia is greatly potentiated by increases in blood hydrogen ion and is almost abolished by alkalosis. The hypoxic reflex serves a useful local regulatory function by limiting blood flow to underventilated pulmonary segments and thereby restores the regional ventilation-perfusion ratio to normal, but when the hypoxia is generalized, the response is far from beneficial. Inhalation of 12 per cent oxygen at sea level (P_{O_2}: 91 mm Hg) promptly results in twofold increases of pulmonary vascular resistance and pulmonary arterial mean pressure, with no increase in cardiac output or left atrial pressure.

Pulmonary Arterial Pressure at High Altitude. Chronic exposure to the hypoxia of high altitude produces a sustained increase in pulmonary arterial pressure. The average values of pulmonary arterial pressure in natives of Morococho, Peru, which is at 14,900 feet above sea level (P_{O_2}: 80 mm Hg), are 41/15 mm Hg (systolic/diastolic), with a mean pressure of 28 mm Hg at rest and 77/40 (mean: 60 mm Hg) during exercise. Their right ventricles are hypertrophied, and their small pulmonary arteries are thicker and contain increased amounts of smooth muscle, which extends farther down into the smallest vessels than normally. After two years of residing at sea level, the pulmonary arterial pressures of these people fall to normal values at rest but still rise to abnormal values with exercise.

Studies of the pulmonary circulation in residents of Leadville, Colorado (altitude: 10,200 feet; P_{O_2}: 100 mm Hg), have emphasized the considerable individual variation in the reactivity of the pulmonary vasculature to chronic hypoxia. The average mean pulmonary arterial pressure at rest in one group of subjects was increased to 25 mm Hg, but it varied from 10 to 45 mm Hg, and in one 15-year-old woman the pressure rose to 105 mm Hg during exercise. This subject's pressure became normal after she had resided at sea level for 11 months.

The individuality of the response to hypoxia is further emphasized by the occurrence of acute pulmonary edema at high altitudes in susceptible persons who are otherwise normal. The pathogenesis of the pulmonary edema, which responds promptly to inhalation of oxygen, has not been fully elucidated, but it is not due to left ventricular failure, and pulmonary venous constriction has not been proved to be the cause. It occurs at altitudes greater than 9000 feet in persons who have not previously been exposed to altitude as well as in residents at high altitude within 12 to 36 hours after returning from even a brief sojourn at a lower level. Such persons are liable to recurrence of pulmonary edema with each transition from low to high altitude. Studies of susceptible subjects have revealed hyper-reactivity of their pulmonary vessels to hypoxia. Their pulmonary hemodynamics and pulmonary function were normal at sea level, but at 10,000 feet after a day of exposure to the altitude and a period of vigorous activity at higher altitude, despite the maintenance of normal pulmonary wedge pressures and no evidence of pulmonary edema, their pulmonary arterial pressures were two to three times greater than those of normal subjects at the same altitude.

In many disease states affecting the pulmonary circulation, including those not producing alveolar hypoxia, individual variations in pulmonary vascular reactivity are common, and the spectrum of physiologic and structural abnormalities of the pulmonary vessels in each condition is usually wide.

547. PRIMARY PULMONARY HYPERTENSION

Primary pulmonary hypertension is a disease of unknown cause characterized by marked increase in the pulmonary vascular resistance and pulmonary arterial pressure. Despite exhaustive search while the patient is alive, or at autopsy, no evidence can be found of underlying diseases known to produce pulmonary arterial hypertension, such as congenital or acquired heart disease, pulmonary disease, disorders of respiration, and systemic diseases that affect the pulmonary vessels.

Incidence. Primary pulmonary hypertension is uncommon. In one series of 10,000 patients with heart disease, it was found in only 17. Among reported cases, the patients ranged in age from 1 to 68 years, but most were 20 to 40 years old. There were three times as many women as men; most of the women were in their early thirties and had borne children. The disease is known to occur in a familial form. Among the 14 families reported, 22 female members and 12 males were affected. In six families, apparent parent-to-offspring transmission was documented, and in one kindred five members of three generations manifested the disease. The mode of genetic transmission is uncertain. In five families, the mother and either a daughter or a son were affected; in the other family, the father and his son and daughter died of the disease.

Pathology. In all patients, the pulmonary arteries show structural abnormalities characteristic of hypertensive pulmonary vascular disease usually of the most advanced degree (Grades 4 to 6 of Heath and Edwards). The walls of the muscular arteries and arterioles are greatly thickened, and their lumina are markedly narrowed and even obliterated. The smooth muscle in the media of the muscular arteries is hypertrophied and extends well down into the arterioles, which normally do not have a distinct media. In the arterioles and extending back to the smaller muscular pulmonary arteries less than 0.3 mm and occasionally those as large as 0.5 mm, marked cellular proliferation and fibrosis of the intima are seen. In some of the vessels, the intimal proliferation is concentric, shows an onion-layering appearance, and encroaches evenly on the lumen; in others, the masses of protruding fibrous tissue are unevenly distributed and create an eccentric, irregularly shaped lumen. The fibrous tissue contains elastic fibrils and eventually assumes a hyaline appearance.

Although the media attains a thickness equivalent to 30 per cent of the external diameter of the small arteries in some areas, in other areas the media is atrophied and the vessels dilated. Such generalized dilatations of the arterial wall are often found at and downstream from an occluded segment of a small muscular artery or arteriole and upstream from occlusions in the medium-sized arteries.

In addition to the generalized dilatations, localized dilatations that form morphologically complex, saccular structures develop from the walls of the smallest muscular arteries and arterioles. One of these structures, known as a plexiform lesion, is characterized by a thin-walled sac protruding from the wall of the vessel. The sac frequently contains a thrombus, over which an area of cellular intimal tissue has proliferated to form a complex, plexiform pattern. An overlying layer of fibrous tissue is continuous with the intimal proliferative layer of the artery. In other dilatation lesions, groups of thin-walled, cavernous vessels arise from thin-walled branches of muscular arteries, or occluded arteries give rise to veinlike branches that have been misinterpreted as arteriovenous anastomoses. Because of their thin walls, the vessels of dilatation lesions are subject to rupture and are associated with focal collections of hemosiderin-laden macrophages in the pulmonary tissue.

In the most advanced stage of hypertensive pulmonary vascular disease (Grade 6), fibrinoid necrosis occurs in the media of some of the muscular arteries. The necrotic muscle produces an inflammatory reaction consisting of polymorphonuclear leukocytes and some eosinophils that may invade all layers of the vessel. The necrotizing arteritis may destroy the entire vessel or only a segment of it, and thrombi are found in the lumina of some of the affected arteries.

The elastic pulmonary arteries, especially the main trunk and its branches, are greatly dilated, but the walls are thick. The media shows an increase in muscle mass that in the main pulmonary artery causes the thickness of the media to approximate or exceed that of the aortic media. The elastic fibers in the media are fragmented, irregularly shaped, and arranged in a loose network characteristic of the adult pulmonary artery. This configuration of the elastic tissue is evidence that the pulmonary hypertension was acquired rather than present at birth, because in patients with congenital heart diseases that produce pulmonary arterial hypertension from birth, the elastic fibers of the main pulmonary artery retain their fetal form and appear like those in the aorta. The media contains an excess of acid mucopolysaccharides that can accumulate in cystic fashion. A few atheromas are often found in the intima of the main pulmonary arteries; in occasional patients, they are numerous and scattered throughout the intima of all the elastic arteries.

The capillaries, veins, and parenchyma of the lungs are normal.

The right ventricle is extensively hypertrophied and dilated, and the ring of the tricuspid valve is often dilated. The right atrium is also dilated, and in a few patients, the foramen ovale is patent. The systemic arteries are usually free of significant abnormalities, although James has reported the occurrence of fibrous lesions in the intima of the small arteries of the sinus node in patients with primary pulmonary hypertension.

Etiology and Pathogenesis. None of the several theories proposed for the pathogenesis of primary pulmonary hypertension has been verified. Amniotic fluid embolization of the pulmonary arteries has been suggested as a cause because of the preponderance of young women among patients with the disease, some of whom experienced their first symptoms after pregnancy. Congenital defects in the pulmonary arteries, such as medial aplasia or failure of the pulmonary arteries to undergo normal transformation from their fetal form, have been suggested; however, the appearance of the elastic fibers in the media of the main pulmonary artery of patients with primary pulmonary hypertension indicates that the hypertension was not present from birth, as would be expected if the pulmonary arteries maintained their thick-walled, fetal form. The theory of medial aplasia holds that the areas of dilatation and thinning of the media observed in the muscular arteries represent congenital defects of the media and that the intima over these areas is subject to the development of intimal proliferation that then acts as the primary obstructive lesion. This explanation neglects the fact that all patients with primary pulmonary hypertension do not manifest dilatation lesions or defects of the media other than hypertrophy.

The occurrence of Raynaud's disease in some patients with primary pulmonary hypertension has prompted the speculation that the hypertension is due to vasospasm or to involvement of the pulmonary arteries by a systemic disease of a collagen, autoimmune, or allergic variety. Pulmonary vascular lesions and marked pulmonary hypertension are the predominant abnormalities in rare patients with lupus erythematosus, scleroderma, or sarcoidosis, but other stigmata of these diseases are evident during life or at autopsy. Neurogenically or humorally induced spasm of the pulmonary arteries is an attractive possibility, especially because these vessels in a few patients manifest medial hypertrophy with only slight abnormalities of the intima, but the hypothesis lacks support. Alveolar hypoxia, a potent pulmonary vasoconstrictor, is not present in these patients, and there is no history of residence at altitude, although an occasional patient may first experience symptoms during an excursion to a region several thousand feet above sea level.

The possibility that primary pulmonary hypertension is the consequence of multiple pulmonary emboli is most difficult to deny. Recurrent, small emboli to the lungs are often "silent" and can eventually produce marked increase in pulmonary arterial pressure and a clinical and physiologic syndrome identical to that of primary pulmonary hypertension. It is also often difficult to distinguish between the two conditions by examination of the vasculature of the lungs, because the small pulmonary arteries in widespread pulmonary embolization often exhibit the medial hypertrophy and intimal proliferation of hypertensive pulmonary vascular disease, and recanalized, fibrotic emboli in the small arteries can resemble occlusive intimal lesions. Differentiation of the two conditions depends on identification in the embolic disease of intraluminal thrombi, recent or old, throughout the pulmonary arteries, especially in the larger elastic arteries, and absence of dilatation lesions and necrotizing arteritis, which do not occur in the embolic disorder.

The practical difficulty in discriminating between pulmonary hypertension of the primary type and that caused by recurrent pulmonary embolization can be illustrated by the author's experience with 14 patients who after extensive study were considered to have primary pulmonary hypertension. Nine of these came to autopsy, and no cause for the hypertension other than the pulmonary vascular lesions of primary pulmonary hypertension was found in five. All five were women 32 to 33 years of age, except for one who was 44. In the other four patients, multiple thromboemboli were present in the pulmonary arteries. Two of these were men age 37 and 60 years, and two were women, 48 and 53 years of age. This and other reported experiences suggest the likelihood of an embolic cause of unexplained pulmonary hypertension in patients older than 40 years, especially if they are men. These data were collected before the widespread use of oral contraceptives, and it is conceivable that the proportion of young women with thromboembolism among patients with cryptic pulmonary hypertension may be modified in the future.

Whatever the cause, it appears that once pulmonary hypertension is established, the media of the pulmonary arteries reacts by progressive hypertrophy of its smooth muscle mass, probably as a consequence of increased arterial wall tension and work. The intima subsequently responds to the elevated pressure by proliferation, perhaps as the arterioles do in systemic hypertension. Thus each structural response of the pulmonary arterial tree leads to further compromise of its patency, further elevation of pressure, and the eventual development of the highest grades of hypertensive pulmonary vascular disease.

Pathologic Physiology. The cardinal hemodynamic abnormality is marked increase in the pulmonary vascular resistance with no evident physiologic cause. The resistance is usually 12 to 18 times normal and in the range of the systemic vascular resistance, and in an occasional patient it exceeds the systemic resistance. In one series, the average pulmonary arterial systolic pressure was approximately 110 mm Hg and the mean pressure approximately six times normal. During exercise the pulmonary vascular resistance remains fixed, and the pulmonary arterial pressures rise further. At rest and during exercise, the pulmonary wedge and left atrial pressures are normal. In contrast, the right ventricular end-diastolic and right atrial pressures are usually greatly increased. In some patients, the cardiac output is normal at rest, but more often it is only 50 to 60 per cent of normal and fails to increase appropriately with exercise. As the function of the right ventricle declines under its enormous afterload, cardiac output dwindles further, and evidences of tricuspid regurgitation may appear. Because of the small stroke volume, systemic arterial systolic and pulse pressures are frequently low.

The arterial oxyhemoglobin saturation is usually normal at rest and during exercise, but a few patients display mildly (91 to 92 per cent) and rarely substantially diminished (less than 90 per cent) saturation. Slight reduction in arterial carbon dioxide tension reflects the hyperventilation that commonly exists.

Infusion of tolazoline or acetylcholine into the pulmonary artery has been observed to produce slight to moderate decrease of pulmonary vascular resistance and pulmonary arterial pressure in some patients. Inhalation of oxygen has little effect.

Clinical Manifestations. These are the direct result of the physiologic and anatomic disturbances produced by the disease. Dyspnea during exertion, closely intertwined with fatigue and weakness, is a universal symptom. An oppressive substernal sensation and even frank angina are commonly experienced during effort, although this symptom, which is most likely the result of right ventricular ischemia, can occur in some patients in the form of recurrent and exceedingly disturbing episodes at rest. Syncope on exertion is an ominous sign because patients with primary pulmonary hypertension are subject to sudden death. There is evidence that an abrupt fall in cardiac output secondary to acute right ventricular failure or arrhythmia is the essential mechanism producing the syncopal attacks. Rupture of the flimsy walls of localized arterial dilatation lesions probably accounts for the intermittent minor hemoptyses experienced by some patients. An occasional patient may experience hoarseness related to compression of the left recurrent laryngeal nerve by the enlarged left pulmonary artery.

Overt signs of right ventricular failure develop in many patients before death and initially respond to digitalis and diuretics, but within a short period of time become increasingly more difficult to control. Because of the marked and fixed obstruction to flow in the pulmonary vessels and severe impairment of right ventricular function, the cardiac output is not only low but does not increase on demand to meet peripheral needs. Consequently, systemic arterial pressure can fall precipitously and fatally during anesthesia; after vasodepressor drugs, such as barbiturates; with physiologic stresses, such as fever and hemorrhage; and during diagnostic procedures, such as cardiac catheterization and angiocardiography. Because of the enormous obstruction to blood flow in the lungs, resuscitation from cardiopulmonary arrest is usually unsuccessful.

The patient usually appears normally developed and in good nutritional state. Occasionally the nail beds are slightly cyanotic, but the peripheral origin of the cyanosis is demonstrated by its disappearance after rubbing the digits. Clubbing is absent. Its presence should promptly suggest other causes of the pulmonary hypertension. Depending on the state of right ventricular function, the jugular veins may be distended; almost invariably, they show a prominent and sustained atrial contraction wave ("a" wave). If right ventricular failure and dilatation are advanced, the systolic wave of tricuspid regurgitation can also appear. The carotid arterial pulse is usually small.

The heart may be of normal size or considerably enlarged to the left and right. In contrast to the localized and unimpressive apical impulse, the heave associated with vigorous contraction of the hypertrophied right ventricle can be seen and felt along the left sternal border. Especially in patients with thin-walled and long chests, the prominent systolic pulsation of the enlarged main pulmonary can be seen and palpated for several centimeters to the left of the sternal border in the second left intercostal space. In almost every patient, a loud, sharp, pulmonic ejection sound can be heard and often felt. The second sound is usually closely split (0.02 to 0.03 sec), but in some patients the splitting may be wider (0.04 to 0.05 sec) and may vary relatively little during the respiratory cycle. The sound of pulmonic valvular closure is invariably accentuated in intensity, sharp or ringing in quality, and often palpable. Murmurs may be absent, but in many patients a systolic ejection murmur that is rarely harsh is heard in the third left interspace and extends well up along the left sternal border over the pulmonary artery. The diminuendo, medium-high-pitched murmur of pulmonic valvular regurgitation is audible in the third and fourth left interspaces in patients whose main pulmonary artery is very large, and is most easily detected with the patient erect and his chest held in full expiration. Either an atrial gallop sound (fourth sound) or an early diastolic gallop sound (third sound) or both are often heard over the lower right ventricle; increase in their intensity with inspiration signifies that they are generated in the right heart. When both gallop sounds are present, they can create the auditory illusion of a mitral diastolic rumble, an illusion that is enhanced by the early ejection sound, which may be misidentified as the loud closure sound of a stenotic mitral valve. A systolic murmur of tricuspid regurgitation that increases with inspiration may be heard in the fourth and fifth intercostal spaces along the left sternal border; it occasionally radiates well toward the apex if the tricuspid valve has been displaced to the left by a very enlarged right atrium and right ventricle. The usual signs of right ventricular failure and systemic venous congestion may be present.

Early in the course of the disease, the only abnormality in radiograms of the chest is enlargement of the main pulmonary artery and its major branches. Hypertrophy of the right ventricle is first manifested by its encroachment on the retrosternal space in lateral films and by a globular appearance of the heart in the posteroanterior projection. The heart is seldom massively enlarged, but the right ventricle may be sufficiently hypertrophied and dilated to displace the heart posteriorly, thereby creating some difficulty in assessing the size of the left ven-

tricle. The right atrium usually appears rounded in frontal view, and eventually it and the superior vena cava dilate well into the right chest. The lung fields appear normal or slightly avascular, and the normal size of the small pulmonary arteries contrasts sharply with the dilated central arteries, which can attain considerable size. The pulmonary veins and left atrium are normal in size.

The electrocardiogram invariably reveals evidences of right ventricular hypertrophy, usually of the type associated with a systemic arterial systolic pressure in the ventricle. The mean QRS axis is at 90 degrees or more to the right. Lead V_1 shows an R wave of 1.0 to 1.5 mV with a small S wave, and the T waves in leads V_1 and V_2 are inverted. The P waves are tall (greater than 0.25 mV) and peaked in leads II, III, and aV_f; in V_1 the P wave is upright, peaked, narrow, and associated with a long PR segment. Higher grades of right ventricular hypertrophy are reflected by increasing amplitude of the R wave in V_1 and V_2, prominent S waves in the left precordial leads, and depression of the S-T segment and increasingly negative and coved T waves in V_1 and V_2 and even V_3.

Polycythemia occurs in some patients late in the course of the disease despite a normal or only slightly decreased arterial oxyhemoglobin saturation.

Diagnosis. Although the diagnosis of primary pulmonary hypertension can be made on the basis of the clinical, radiographic, and electrocardiographic manifestations, it is very difficult in some patients to be certain on these grounds alone that an underlying lesion of the heart, such as septal defect, cor triatriatum, or silent mitral stenosis, does not exist. It is especially difficult to exclude multiple pulmonary emboli or a systemic disease as the fundamental disorder. Cardiac catheterization should be performed to establish the diagnosis and to demonstrate that a congenital defect or mitral stenosis is not present. In pulmonary angiograms, filling defects or occlusions of the larger elastic pulmonary arteries are certain signs of pulmonary thromboemboli that are not found in primary pulmonary hypertension. Large areas lacking radioactivity in the lung fields in radioisotopic perfusion scans of the lungs constitute further evidence of the presence of embolic obstruction of large pulmonary arteries.

Because death of patients with primary pulmonary hypertension has been reported to occur during cardiac catheterization and angiocardiography, considerable judgment and care must be exercised in performing these studies and determining how extensive they should be. The general state of the patient, the blood pressure, and the electrocardiogram should be meticulously monitored throughout the procedure and for some time afterward. Arrhythmias and frequent ectopic beats should be promptly suppressed; significant falls in blood pressure should be immediately corrected with an infusion of norepinephrine to maintain perfusion of the right ventricular myocardium. Many patients with primary pulmonary hypertension have undergone these essential diagnostic studies without complication.

The appropriate laboratory tests, including skin biopsy to exclude scleroderma and lupus erythematosus, should be performed in all patients with primary pulmonary hypertension, especially those who manifest Raynaud's phenomenon. Sarcoidosis involving the pulmonary arteries almost exclusively and producing pulmonary hypertension is exceedingly rare and has only recently been reported. The author has also observed one such case in which the cause was uncovered only at autopsy. The possibility of reversing the pulmonary hypertension by the administration of corticosteroids should prompt a search for signs of this disease.

Lung biopsy should not be performed because of the great risk. A small pneumothorax in a patient with primary pulmonary hypertension was reported to precipitate an alarming increase in pulmonary arterial pressure and death.

Pulmonary function studies in patients with primary pulmonary hypertension usually reveal no major abnormalities aside from slight arterial hypoxemia and hyperventilation. If the patient does not have a right-left shunt through a patent foramen ovale, substantial hypoxemia at rest or during exercise owing to intrapulmonary arteriovenous shunting greatly increases the probability that thromboemboli are the cause of the pulmonary hypertension.

Treatment. No effective method for producing a sustained decrease in the pulmonary arterial pressure has been found. Chronic treatment with tolazoline or prolonged infusions of this drug or acetylcholine into the pulmonary artery have proved to be ineffective. Nor is there evidence that long-term administration of oxygen decreases the pulmonary arterial pressure or in any way modifies the course of the disease. Transplantation of a single lung is an appealing therapuetic maneuver but is impractical because of the currently short viability of pulmonary homotransplants. Because of the difficulty in excluding recurrent pulmonary emboli and because in situ thrombosis can occur in pulmonary arteries affected by hypertensive pulmonary vascular disease, chronic anticoagulation therapy has been widely advocated. Such therapy should be closely monitored in view of the deleterious consequences of hemorrhage in these patients. The usual cardiac glycosides, diuretic agents, and restriction of sodium intake should be used to control cardiac failure. The patient should not travel to altitudes above sea level.

Prognosis. The patient usually dies during a syncopal spell, or after an acute, short-lived, shock-like episode, or of intractable right heart failure within three to four years after the onset of symptoms. Rarely, dissection of the main pulmonary artery is the lethal event. An occasional patient may survive for 12 or more years, but with progressively disabling dyspnea, angina, and syncope with exertion.

548. OTHER CAUSES OF PULMONARY VASCULAR DISEASE

CONGENITAL HEART DISEASE

These remarks are intended to supplement the discussion of congenital heart disease in Ch. 551 to 555.

Pulmonary arterial hypertension is exceedingly common in patients with congenital defects that produce left-right shunting of blood within the heart or between the great vessels. The hypertension is usually the result of augmentation of pulmonary blood by the left-right shunt, structural abnormalities within the pulmonary arterial tree, or most commonly both. There are distinct differences in the frequency and severity of the pulmonary vascular abnormalities associated with these congenital lesions.

In patients with left-right shunts that traverse the left ventricle, such as those produced by ventricular septal defect, patent ductus arteriosus, aortic septal defect, and ostium atrioventricularis with a large ventricular septal defect, hypertensive pulmonary vascular disease is very frequent. The severity of the arterial lesions varies among patients, depending on the size of the defect, the magnitude of the left-right shunt it is capable of conducting, and individual susceptibility. If the communication is small and produces a pulmonary blood flow that exceeds systemic blood by 50 per cent or less, the pulmonary arteries are usually normal or show minimal changes and the pulmonary vascular resistance and pulmonary arterial pressure are also normal or only slightly elevated.

With larger defects, hypertensive pulmonary vascular disease of the type described in Ch. 547 is almost universally present. Most commonly, the small pulmonary arteries and arterioles simply manifest thickening of their walls owing to hypertrophy of the smooth muscle of the media (Grade 1 hypertensive pulmonary vascular disease, according to the classification of Heath and Edwards), but other obstructive lesions may be superimposed on this basic abnormality to produce increasingly advanced vascular disease. An early additional change is cellular proliferation of the intima of the arteries (Grade 2), which may subsequently undergo fibrosis and fibroelastic organization (Grade 3). The development of generalized and localized dilatations of the arterial wall with the formation of complex vascular structures occurs in Grade 4 disease, and in Grade 5 the dilatations are scattered throughout the lung and associated with hemosiderosis. Necrotizing arteritis occurs in the most severe form of the disease (Grade 6).

The development of the vascular disease is initiated shortly after birth by failure of the pulmonary arteries to undergo normal transformation from their fetal form. Instead of regressing, the increased mass of smooth muscle in the arterial walls persists, hypertrophies, and extends distally into the arterioles. The elastic fibers in the media of the main pulmonary artery and its major branches also fail to develop their adult form. They persist as dense, thick structures in parallel array, closely resembling their appearance in the media of the aorta. This important histologic sign indicates that the pulmonary vascular disease began in the neonatal period; it is not found in patients who acquired their pulmonary hypertension later in life. The size of the communication determines the subsequent development of arterial lesions. Ventricular septal defects larger than 1 sq cm and patent ducti that approximate 1 cm in diameter are usually associated with more advanced grades of pulmonary vascular disease. Progression of the vascular lesions appears to occur early in life, but the most advanced abnormalities are found in patients older than 15 to 20 years. The pulmonary vascular resistance, however, in patients with only moderate pulmonary arterial hypertension (systolic pressure of 50 to 60 mm Hg) does not appear to increase significantly during the course of many years.

Why pulmonary vascular lesions develop in patients with post-tricuspid valvular shunts is uncertain. One possible factor is that these shunts early in life load the left ventricle and consequently produce higher left ventricular diastolic, left atrial, and pulmonary venous pressures than would normally exist, thus from the outset exhausting the distensibility of the pulmonary arteries and subjecting them thereby to higher pressures. Another theory holds that the transmission directly into the pulmonary arteries of part of the kinetic energy that is generated in the left ventricle is the responsible factor.

The height of the pulmonary arterial pressure in patients with ventricular septal defect or patent ductus arteriosus is determined by the pulmonary vascular resistance, the size of the left-right shunt, and consequently the magnitude of the pulmonary blood flow. If the resistance is only slightly increased, large shunts and pulmonary flows as large as twice the systemic blood flow can occur with pulmonary arterial mean pressures three times normal and systolic pressures of 60 to 70 mm Hg. With increasing resistance, the pulmonary arterial pressures rise and the left-right shunt diminishes. Evidence of right-left shunting at first appears only during exercise when pulmonary arterial and right ventricular pressures increase further or under circumstances when the systemic vascular resistance falls. Eventually, the pulmonary arterial systolic pressure attains systemic arterial levels at rest and the right-left shunt becomes larger and more sustained. Despite persistence of bidirectional shunting, the pulmonary blood flow declines to values usually less than normal. As a consequence of the right-left shunt and the diminished pulmonary blood flow, chronic arterial hypoxemia that is accentuated by exertion appears. In patients with patent ductus arteriosus, because the right-left shunt is directed into the descending segment of the aortic arch, the arterial unsaturation is more pronounced or even confined to the lower body and, occasionally, may also appear in the left arm and left side of the head. It is possible that the polycythemia and consequent increase in blood viscosity contribute to the resistance to flow in the pulmonary vessels.

Aside from cyanosis, which is usually accompanied by clubbing of the fingers and toes, the clinical signs and symptoms of patients with marked pulmonary hypertension and right-left shunts are similar to those of patients with primary pulmonary hypertension, but the course is usually considerably longer, and survival to an age of 30 to 40 years occurs frequently. The cyanosis is especially striking when polycythemia is marked. In patent ductus arteriosus with bidirectional shunting, the toes are cyanotic and clubbed, whereas the fingers are not or are much less so. Some signs of the underlying cardiac lesion are often evident. A precordial bulge is usually present. In some patients, the characteristic murmurs are intermittently audible, but in most, the murmurs are greatly modified. A pulmonic ejection sound is almost always present; the sound of pulmonic valvular closure is loud and sharp in quality, and a diastolic murmur of pulmonic regurgitation is frequent. Persistent enlargement of the left ventricle may be manifested by a forceful, diffuse apical thrust. Suggestive evidences of left ventricular enlargement may also be present in radiograms of the heart and in the electrocardiogram, but these and the radiographic signs of increased pulmonary blood flow tend to disappear as the pulmonary vascular disease advances.

In patients with a left-right shunt that does not traverse the left ventricle, structural abnormalities in the pulmonary arteries are slight, and the pulmonary arterial pressure remains normal or only slightly increased until late in the course of the disease. An atrial septal defect of the secundum type is the most common lesion producing such a shunt; other causes are partial or complete anomalous drainage of the pulmonary veins into the right atrium or its main venous trunks. Only in occasional patients with enormous shunts, caused by complete anomalous pulmonary venous drainage or an atrial septal defect of such size that the atria are converted into a common chamber, are pulmonary vascular disease and significant pulmonary hypertension established early in life. In most patients, despite pulmonary blood flows consistently 2.5 to 3 times greater than normal, the pulmonary arterial pressure remains at the upper limits of normal for 20 to 30 years and even longer. Thereafter, however, pulmonary vascular lesions begin to appear and the pulmonary arterial pressure rises. The earliest structural abnormality is fibrosis of the pulmonary veins followed by cellular proliferation of the endothelium of the widely dilated arterioles and small muscular arteries. At this stage, the pulmonary vascular resistance may no longer be less than normal as it must be to maintain a normal pulmonary arterial pressure in the presence of the large blood flow. The resistance is also fixed, and even though its value is within the limits of normal, the persistently augmented flow produces a proportionate increase in pulmonary arterial pressure.

The pulmonary venous pressure remains normal in atrial septal defect until the onset of myocardial failure, manifested by elevation of the diastolic pressures of both ventricles. As a consequence of the increased left ventricular diastolic pressure, the pressures in the left atrium and pulmonary veins rise to three to four times their usual values. A substantial left-right shunt nevertheless persists, and pulmonary arterial systolic pressure commonly attains values of 60 to 70 mm Hg.

Episodes of pulmonary embolization, which are common in patients with atrial septal defect, and progression of the hypertensive pulmonary arterial lesions eventually produce sevenfold or greater increases of pulmonary vascular resistance that throttle the pulmonary flow and promote right-left shunting through the defect.

The classic clinical, radiographic, and electrocardiographic features of atrial septal defect (see Ch. 552) usually persist throughout the patient's course, and provide for ready recognition of the lesion. The diagnosis is less evident in the occasional patient who has developed high-grade pulmonary vascular disease and pulmonary hypertension early in life and shows little evidence of increased pulmonary blood flow and a hypertrophied but not very large right ventricle.

Treatment. The response of the pulmonary arterial pressure to closure of a septal defect or patent ductus arteriosus is governed by the relative roles of the left-right shunt and the pulmonary vascular resistance in elevating the pressure. If the pulmonary vascular resistance is normal preoperatively, the pulmonary arterial pressure declines to normal values postoperatively. When the shunt constitutes 50 per cent or more of the pulmonary blood flow and the resistance is only moderately increased, a substantial decrease can be expected. When the left-right shunt is small and the pulmonary vascular resistance and pressures approximate those in the systemic circuit, and especially if a significant right-left shunt exists, the pressure does not decrease and the risk of death during or shortly after the surgical procedure is great. Decision as to advisability of surgical correction of the lesion should be made on an individual basis after consideration of all physiologic and clinical data. Some have advocated preoperative measurements of the response of the pulmonary arterial pressure and pulmonary vascular resistance to infusion of tolazoline or inhalation of oxygen as a means of identifying a vasospastic component of an increased resistance.

Except in occasional infants with lower grades of hypertensive pulmonary vascular disease, the pulmonary vascular resistance does not usually fall after closure of an atrial or ventricular septal defect, and although the patient may be greatly benefited by the procedure, some degree of pulmonary hypertension persists.

Stenosis of Pulmonary Arterial Branches. Although multiple coarctation-like, congenital stenoses of the large branches of the pulmonary artery produce an increase in pressure only in the pulmonary arterial segments upstream from the stenotic regions, the malformation in some patients raises the systolic pressure in the main pulmonary artery and right ventricle to 70 or 80 mm Hg and can create difficulty in diagnosis. The lesions can occur in isolated form, but they often coexist with supravalvular aortic stenosis or an atrial septal defect. The total obstructive effect is usually slight, and the systolic pulmonary arterial pressure is increased to only 35 to 40 mm Hg at rest. The stenoses generate a continuous murmur or simply a systolic murmur that can be heard over the upper right or left precordial region. The diagnosis is conclusively established by an angiogram of the pulmonary arteries.

PULMONARY EMBOLI

Thrombi, globules of fat, and particulate matter of amniotic fluid can embolize the pulmonary arteries and produce acute pulmonary hypertension. The pathophysiologic basis for the hypertension is described in Ch. 543 to 545. Repeated embolization of the pulmonary arteries by thrombi (see Ch. 543 to 545 and Ch. 547) schistosomal ova (see Ch. 296), tumors, and cotton fibers and foreign matter contained in some drugs illicitly administered by vein cause chronic, progressive pulmonary hypertension by their primary obstructive effects and by the subsequent development of hypertensive pulmonary vascular lesions. In addition, schistosomal ova and particulate foreign matter evoke a granulomatous inflammatory reaction in the intima and walls of the arteries.

Although fragments of several types of cancer can embolize the pulmonary arteries after the tumor has invaded the liver or the inferior vena cava, the propensity of choriocarcinoma (chorioepithelioma) to metastasize in this manner deserves special consideration. Choriocarcinoma may remain undetected for several years after pregnancy, but soon after it originates it can invade the inferior vena cava and repeatedly discharge fragments of tissue into the pulmonary circulation. These embolic episodes may give rise to symptoms and signs of acute pulmonary embolization, or they can be clinically silent. The consequent obstruction of the larger pulmonary arteries can be extensive and give rise to marked pulmonary hypertension before the tumor invades the walls of the pulmonary arteries and appears in the lung fields.

Choriocarcinoma should be suspected in a woman who has had a recent pregnancy or even one a few years previously and has repeated bouts of pulmonary embolization or unexplained pulmonary hypertension. An increased concentration of human chorionic gonadotrophin and the demonstration of multiple occlusions of the pulmonary arteries by angiography confirm the diagnosis. The tumor is exquisitely sensitive to methotrexate, actinomycin D, and 6-mercaptopurine, and complete cure has been achieved in 50 per cent or more of patients by administration of these agents.

COLLAGEN AND MULTIPLE SYSTEM DISEASES

Pulmonary hypertension caused by the pulmonary arterial lesions of scleroderma, lupus erythematosus, and sarcoidosis has been discussed in Ch. 547. The clinical features and diagnosis of these diseases are presented in Ch. 79, 81, and 102, respectively. It is worth emphasizing that the pulmonary hypertension and its secondary effects may rarely be the only clinically apparent manifestations of these disorders. Hemodynamic studies of patients with scleroderma have demonstrated the high frequency of increases in pulmonary vascular resistance and slight pulmonary hypertension without involvement of the pulmonary parenchyma by the disease.

549. LEFT ATRIAL AND PULMONARY VENOUS HYPERTENSION

Elevation of pulmonary venous pressure is the most common cause of pulmonary arterial hypertension. Most frequently, left atrial and pulmonary venous hypertension are the result of dysfunction of the left ventricle characterized by impairment of its contractile state, decrease in its compliance, or both. Even in the absence of clinical signs of left ventricular failure, left ventricular end-diastolic pressure can be elevated, at first only with physical exertion or stress; later, as ventricular function becomes more impaired, it is chronically increased even at rest. Twofold increases in left atrial, pulmonary venous, and pulmonary arterial pressures are common. During episodes of acute left ventricular failure, pressures in the pulmonary veins and capillaries rise to levels exceeding 25 mm Hg.

The state of left atrial function is a significant determinant of the degree of left atrial and pulmonary venous hypertension. A properly timed, vigorous atrial contraction will generate a considerably increased left ventricular end-diastolic pressure without the need for much increase in left atrial pressure during the rest of diastole, but when the pumping function of the left atrium is lost because of atrial arrhythmia or left atrial failure, its pressure throughout diastole becomes greater. Thus for a given level of ventricular end-diastolic pressure, mean pressures in the atrium and the entire pulmonary vascular circuit are higher in the presence of left atrial failure or arrhythmia, such as atrial fibrillation, than in the presence of normal atrial function.

Disorders of the mitral valvular apparatus are another frequent cause of left atrial hypertension. In general, stenosis of the mitral valve and stenosis combined with regurgitation produce more severe degrees of left atrial hypertension than does mitral regurgitation alone. Nevertheless, in certain patients with chronic, marked mitral regurgitation caused by rheumatic valvular disease or rupture of the chordae tendineae, high-grade hypertension can occur in the left atrium, pulmonary veins, and pulmonary artery.

Less common causes of obstruction at the mitral valve are left atrial myxoma and left atrial ball-valve thrombus. A ball-valve thrombus almost invariably occurs with pre-existing mitral stenosis. A myxoma, which is tethered by a stalk attached to the atrial septum in the region of the fossa ovalis, produces left atrial hypertension by obstructing blood flow through the mitral orifice in diastole, but it can also pass through the mitral valve and obstruct left ventricular outflow. Other tumors of the left atrium can obstruct the mitral valve and may also grow into and obstruct the main pulmonary veins.

Cor triatriatum, a congenital anomaly in which an abnormal diaphragm with one or more small perforations partitions the pulmonary venous outflow region from the main left atrial chamber, mimics mitral stenosis in its effects on the pulmonary circulation. However, it is often not associated with a diastolic murmur and can thus escape clinical detection. Although cor triatriatum and left atrial myxoma are rare, their recognition is of great importance because they can be completely corrected by appropriate surgical procedures.

Mediastinal collagenosis with constriction of the extrapulmonary veins and diffuse pulmonary veno-occlusive disease are rare causes of pulmonary venous hypertension. The etiology of the latter disease, which occurs predominantly in women, is unknown. The small and medium sized pulmonary veins are narrowed and occluded by thrombi and fibrous tissue without evidence of inflammation in the venous walls. The clinical picture resembles that of primary pulmonary arterial hypertension; however, because of increased pressure in the pulmonary capillaries, radiographic evidence of pulmonary congestion and edema are present. The disease leads relentlessly to death in a few weeks to five years after the onset of symptoms.

Pulmonary Circulation in Mitral Stenosis

The physiologic and anatomic modifications of the pulmonary circulation induced by various degrees of chronic pulmonary venous hypertension are well illustrated by the extensive observations that have been made in patients with mitral stenosis. When the mitral orifice is only slightly restricted, left atrial pressure and intravascular pressures throughout the pulmonary circuit may be normal when the patient is at rest, but they exceed normal values with exercise or during other states accompanied by augmentation of cardiac output, such as fever, anemia, pregnancy, thyrotoxicosis, and hypermetabolism of other causes. Tachycardia alone, by abbreviating diastole, requires the generation of a higher left atrial pressure to maintain cardiac output through the stenotic valve. At this stage, as in animals with acutely produced mitral stenosis not severe enough to cause pulmonary edema, the modest vascular hypertension dilates the small pulmonary vessels and produces a decrease in their resistance to flow. In these circumstances, the increase in pulmonary arterial pressure is less pronounced than the increase in pulmonary venous and left atrial pressures.

In moderate and severe mitral stenosis with valvular orifice areas less than 1.5 sq cm, left atrial mean pressure at rest is often in the range of 25 to 30 mm Hg and rises with slight exercise to values of 40 to 55 mm Hg,

especially if cardiac output increases substantially. Even if the pulmonary vascular resistance is normal, the pronounced pulmonary venous hypertension causes the mean pressure in the pulmonary artery to exceed normal values by three- to sixfold. In most patients, however, pulmonary vascular resistance is greater than normal, resulting in an increase of pulmonary arterial pressure that is disproportionately greater than that caused by the left atrial hypertension alone.

The range of abnormality of pulmonary vascular resistance in mitral stenosis is wide. In one series of 180 patients, the resistance was two or more times greater than normal in 67 per cent of the patients. In 11 per cent, the resistance and consequently the pulmonary arterial pressure equaled or exceeded systemic arterial values. Patients with such advanced disturbances usually have very severe mitral stenosis and appear also to have a predisposition to advanced alterations in the pulmonary arteries in response to hypertension in the pulmonary veins and arteries that is not shared by other patients whose mitral obstruction and left atrial hypertension are equally pronounced. The clinical features of such patients resemble in many respects those of patients with primary pulmonary hypertension. A mitral diastolic murmur may not be audible, mainly because the cardiac output is greatly diminished as the result of the pulmonary vascular restriction and marked right ventricular dysfunction. Normal sinus rhythm persists in many of them despite the advanced mitral stenosis. Unlike patients with primary pulmonary hypertension, however, they do not experience frequent syncope.

In mitral stenosis, structural lesions are present in all segments of the pulmonary vascular bed. The pulmonary veins are dilated, and their walls are greatly thickened by medial hypertrophy and proliferation of the intima. In some patients, numerous anastomoses develop between the pulmonary and bronchial veins. These anastomotic channels form submucosal varicosites in the bronchi that can rupture and produce brisk hemoptysis when the left atrial pressure rises acutely.

The basic anatomic expression of increased hydrostatic pressure in the pulmonary capillaries is dilatation and engorgement of these vessels with edema of the alveolar walls and leakage of edema fluid into the alveolar spaces. Measurements made by the simultaneous injection of isotopically labeled water and a nondiffusible indicator into the pulmonary artery of patients with mitral stenosis and with pulmonary venous hypertension of other causes have demonstrated expansion of the interstitial pulmonary water volume directly related to the increase in left atrial pressure. At left atrial pressures of 25 to 30 mm Hg, the extravascular water volume is three or more times normal. Increased transport by the lymphatics is reflected by dilatation of these vessels. When the pulmonary capillary pressure exceeds values of 20 mm Hg, which is on the threshold of plasma protein osmotic pressure, the lymphatic vessels and the edematous interlobular septa at the bases of the lungs become sufficiently radiopaque to appear as short lines extending horizontally to the pleura *(Kerley B lines)* in radiograms of the chest.

Rupture of alveolar capillaries and pulmonary venules leads to scattered microhemorrhages and subsequent hemosiderosis. When the edema is of long standing, it promotes the development of interstitial fibrosis in the alveolar walls and the surrounding parenchyma most marked in the bases of the lower lobes and the lower segments of all lobes. These regional differences attest to the gravitational augmentation of capillary pressure and the greater and more persistent edema in the dependent regions of the lungs. In these regions, the alveolar septa are greatly thickened and the pulmonary capillaries are compressed or obliterated. Rarely, the fibrotic regions become ossified and appear as small calcified nodules scattered throughout the lower lung fields.

The small pulmonary arteries manifest the medial hypertrophy, proliferation and fibrosis of the intima, increased wall thickness, and diminished internal diameter characteristic of hypertensive pulmonary vascular disease; however, dilatation lesions and necrotizing arteritis that are the hallmarks of the most advanced grades of pulmonary vascular disease are very rarely found. Also, in contrast to the hypertensive pulmonary vascular disease associated with congenital heart disease and primary pulmonary hypertension, the distribution of the arterial lesions is not uniform throughout the lungs. The arteries in the lower lobes are most affected and show the greatest restriction of their lumina; even in the upper lobes, in which the larger arteries are dilated and the small arteries are relatively spared, the vascular lesions are more prominent in the lower segments. As a consequence of the pattern of distribution of the vascular abnormalities and probably because of the more pronounced interstitial fibrosis in the lower lobes, blood flow is preferentially directed to the upper zones of the lungs and away from the lower zones, resulting in reversal of the normal ratio of perfusion between the two zones. The ratio of upper zone perfusion to lower zone perfusion can be as large as 4:1 in contrast to the normal ratio of 1:8. The degree to which perfusion of the upper zones exceeds that of the lower regions is directly related to the height of the pulmonary venous pressure. The ratio also increases directly with the pulmonary vascular resistance, but when the resistance attains values in the range of the systemic vessels, the ratio decreases toward normal, probably because of more widespread distribution of the vascular abnormalities.

Pulmonary embolization and infarction are exceedingly frequent in mitral stenosis and in one series were found at autopsy in approximately one third of the patients who had manifested moderate to severe pulmonary arterial hypertension during life. These occlusions and their secondary effects on the parenchyma of the lung undoubtedly contribute to the restriction of the pulmonary vascular bed.

The main pulmonary artery and its central branches are dilated, and their intima often contains atherosclerotic plaques. The cross-sectional diameter of these vessels increases directly with the pulmonary arterial pressure. When the internal diameter of the main pulmonary artery is 4.0 cm or more, the murmur of pulmonic regurgitation (Graham Steell murmur) commonly appears.

Some insight into the mechanisms producing the pulmonary arterial hypertension and the relative roles of the various vascular disturbances in the genesis of the increased pulmonary vascular resistance is offered by observations of the hemodynamic changes that occur after successful mitral valvotomy or replacement of the mitral valve by a prosthetic valve with a functionally adequate orifice. In almost all patients whose left atrial pressure is lowered by the surgical procedure, the pulmonary vascular resistance decreases and the decline in pulmonary arterial pressure is consequently even greater than that

of the pulmonary venous pressure. Substantial decreases in pulmonary vascular resistance have been observed as early as two days after surgery and have been attributed to dilatation of muscular pulmonary arteries that had been reflexly induced to constrict by the pulmonary venous hypertension. However, failure of the resistance to fall immediately after the surgical procedure despite the decrease in left atrial pressure has been interpreted as indicating that interstitial and perivascular edema exert a cardinal role in the pathogenesis of the increased resistance and that resolution of the edema lags behind the fall of pulmonary venous pressure. In the ensuing weeks and months, the pulmonary vascular resistance often decreases further; even in patients whose preoperative values exceeded systemic vascular resistance, the arterial pressure and vascular resistance in the lungs can eventually attain values only slightly in excess of normal. The most striking changes occur in patients whose left atrial pressures postoperatively at rest and during exercise are normal or only slightly greater than normal. Evidence is now available that regression of the medial hypertrophy and intimal proliferation in the small pulmonary arteries is responsible for the progressive decline of the vascular resistance, but the way in which the pulmonary venous hypertension initiated the development of the structural abnormalities in the pulmonary arteries remains uncertain.

550. PULMONARY DISEASES AND DISORDERS OF RESPIRATION

Constriction of the pulmonary arteries by hypoxia and destruction or restriction of the pulmonary vascular bed are the two basic mechanisms that operate to increase the pulmonary arterial pressure in diseases of the lungs and disorders of the respiratory system. Primary alveolar hypoventilation is an example of a condition in which the disturbances in gas exchange alone initiate the pulmonary hypertension; but in most diseases of the lungs, anatomic restriction of the pulmonary vessels alone in the early stages of these diseases usually increases pulmonary arterial pressure only slightly because of the enormous reserve capacity of the pulmonary vasculature. By the time that the disease process has obliterated enough of the vessels to produce high-grade pulmonary hypertension, structural damage of the pulmonary parenchyma is sufficiently advanced to result in marked disturbances in gas exchange. In most pulmonary diseases therefore both mechanisms are operative.

Since diseases of the lungs and respiratory system are described in Part XI, only those features of significance in the production of pulmonary hypertension, its consequences, manifestations, and treatment are considered here.

Pathologic Physiology. In *chronic obstructive pulmonary disease,* loss of pulmonary capillaries accompanies the loss of alveoli. Some muscular arteries adjacent to terminal bronchioles may show intimal fibroelastosis of sufficient extent to obliterate their lumina. The media of the muscular arteries is slightly thickened, but these vessels and the arterioles show few of the changes characteristic of hypertensive pulmonary vascular disease.

The loss of pulmonary vessels is tolerated with little or

no increase of pulmonary arterial pressure at rest, although the pressure does rise to abnormal levels when pulmonary blood flow is augmented by exercise. In such patients, defects in distribution of ventilation and perfusion within the lungs and reduction in diffusing capacity exist but are not severe enough to cause hypercapnia and more than slight hypoxemia. With increase in the extent of hypoventilated but perfused pulmonary segments, marked hypoxemia develops and the pulmonary arterial pressure rises in direct proportion to the degree of oxygen unsaturation of systemic arterial blood. The hypercapnia that accompanies more widespread alveolar hypoventilation does not appear to affect the pulmonary arteries directly, and its effect on blood pH is minimized by concomitant increase in plasma bicarbonate concentration. Acidosis, arising as the consequence of sudden increase in carbon dioxide tension or failure of the buffering capacity to keep pace with the hypercapnia, potentiates the pulmonary vasoconstrictor response to the hypoxia and further raises the pulmonary arterial pressure.

The greater afterload to ejection of blood created by the increased pulmonary vascular resistance and pulmonary hypertension is met by hypertrophy of the right ventricle. Since the pulmonary arterial mean pressure at this stage is usually no more than twice normal, the right ventricle does not fail until a bronchopulmonary infection or some other event aggravates the bronchial obstruction and the disturbances in gas exchange and produces marked, generalized alveolar hypoventilation. Under such circumstances, as much 80 per cent of the cardiac output perfuses underventilated alveoli, and the arterial oxyhemoglobin saturation falls to values of 40 to 80 per cent; the arterial carbon dioxide tension rises to 60 or 80 mm Hg, and the arterial pH falls to values as low as 7.20. Renal blood flow and glomerular filtration decrease; the excretion of sodium and water diminishes, and the extracellular volume expands. The consequent increase in blood volume is augmented by hypoxia-induced polycythemia of variable degree. The end-diastolic pressure of the right ventricle increases and raises the pressure in the right atrium and systemic veins. The contractile function of the right ventricular myocardium is progressively depressed, and the right ventricle dilates and fails. Several studies have demonstrated that left ventricular function, if it was previously normal, is not disturbed by these events, and that left atrial and pulmonary venous pressures remain within the range of normal.

The relative pathogenic role of each physiologic disturbance in producing the sudden increase in pulmonary arterial pressure in this complex state has been difficult to assess. Correction of the hypoxemia or the acidosis while the failure persists reduces the pulmonary arterial pressure, but it remains considerably elevated. Phlebotomy does not promptly lower the pulmonary arterial pressure. In some patients, because of infection and hypermetabolism, the cardiac output is higher than in the prefailure period, but in many patients the cardiac output is subnormal.

It is striking that as the manifestations of acute respiratory insufficiency and congestive right ventricular failure resolve with appropriate treatment, the pulmonary arterial pressure gradually falls and, together with the systemic arterial oxyhemoglobin saturation, finally returns to its prefailure values. It is difficult to avoid assigning a cardinal role to hypoxia in the pathogenesis of the marked pulmonary hypertension and the overt cor pulmonale.

During recurrent acute exacerbations of respiratory failure, and occasionally as the result of pulmonary thromboembolism to which these patients are prone, signs of increased pulmonary hypertension and right ventricular failure reappear. Eventually these manifestations and the disturbances in gas exchange do not respond fully to treatment, and the cor pulmonale becomes chronic.

In *fibroproliferative and chronic inflammatory diseases of the lungs,* the pulmonary vascular bed is compromised in many ways. In the diffuse interstitial disorders that affect the alveolar walls, such as *sarcoidosis* and other granulomatous diseases, the *Hamman-Rich syndrome, scleroderma, polymyositis, berylliosis, asbestosis, lymphangitic carcinomatosis, radiation fibrosis,* and *idiopathic pulmonary hemosiderosis,* the alveolar capillaries are compressed or obliterated. In massive pulmonary fibrosis caused by *silicosis* or coal miner's *pneumoconiosis,* the fibrotic nodules develop in proximity to muscular and small elastic arteries, and as they enlarge, they engulf and obliterate these vessels.

In all these disorders, increasing disruption of parenchymal structures and fibrosis cause progressive distortion, obstruction, and obliteration of pulmonary vessels. With the development of pulmonary hypertension, the medial hypertrophy and intimal proliferation of hypertensive pulmonary vascular disease are superimposed.

Early in the course of the pulmonary disease, as for example in the interstitial disorders of the lung, pulmonary hypertension may be only slight at rest despite marked restriction of lung volume, but the pressure usually rises steeply with exercise. Similarly, hypoxemia is only mild at rest, but the arterial oxygen saturation usually falls during exercise. With diminution of pulmonary diffusion capacity, the development of marked maldistribution of alveolar ventilation and perfusion, and increase in the extent of intrapulmonary arteriovenous shunting, oxygenation of arterial blood is progressively impaired, pulmonary arterial pressure rises further, and the right ventricle fails. Episodic exacerbations of failure are often precipitated by respiratory infections as in obstructive pulmonary disease, but reduction of pulmonary arterial pressure with treatment is less impressive, and once right ventricular failure occurs, it usually becomes chronic. The highest grades of chronic pulmonary hypertension secondary to pulmonary disease are found in fibrotic diseases of the lungs.

In bronchiectasis, tuberculosis, and other chronic inflammatory diseases of the lungs, extensive intercommunications can develop between the bronchial and pulmonary arteries; occasionally, the mammary and intercostal arteries participate in the formation of the anastomoses. The bronchial collateral flow through these channels is usually small, but in a rare patient it is large enough to constitute a significant left-right shunt that increases the pulmonary blood flow, further elevates the pulmonary arterial pressure, and taxes the left ventricle.

Alveolar hypoventilation pronounced enough to produce hypoxemia and hypercapnia, secondary constriction and hypertension in the pulmonary arteries, and right ventricular failure is encountered in a group of disorders characterized by a *defective ventilatory apparatus.* The fundamental defect exists in the chest bellows, as in *kyphoscoliosis, marked obesity,* and *neuromuscular diseases* that affect the respiratory muscles, or in the respiratory control centers, as in hypoventilation of central nervous origin *(Ondine's curse)*. The lungs and pulmonary vessels are intrinsically normal except in patients with severe kyphoscoliosis, whose pulmonary vascular bed is restricted by the inordinately small dimensions of the lungs and in whom concomitant bronchiectasis, areas of atelectasis, and bronchopulmonary infections are common.

Regardless of the nature of the basic defect in this group of diseases, alveolar ventilation not only is diminished at rest, but also fails to increase normally with exercise and increased metabolic demand, which consequently accentuates the hypoxemia and hypercapnia. In patients with these disorders, as well as in those with primary lung diseases who have had bouts of hypercapnia, the sensitivity of the chemoreceptors to both carbon dioxide and hypoxemia is progressively impaired, and the loss of ventilatory response to these stimuli enhances the propensity to the development of cor pulmonale. A respiratory infection commonly precipitates the development of marked pulmonary hypertension and right ventricular failure.

Clinical Manifestations and Diagnosis. Pulmonary disease is usually readily identified by the history, the physical findings, and radiograms of the chest, but clues to the presence and severity of pulmonary hypertension may be masked by the pulmonary disease. In some patients, the classic signs of pulmonary hypertension described in Ch. 547 may be present, but in others, especially those with chronic obstructive disease, the cardiac sounds are barely audible or are obscured by adventitious pulmonary sounds, and enlargement of the right ventricle and main pulmonary artery cannot be detected with certainty. Despite considerable pulmonary hypertension, the sound of pulmonic valvular closure may not be audibly accentuated.

The patient with right ventricular failure typically presents a history of a recent respiratory infection followed by exacerbation of his usual respiratory symptoms and progressive dyspnea. He presents the appearance and physical signs of a patient with acute pulmonary insufficiency. Cyanosis is usually marked, especially in the presence of polycythemia, but often it is not impressive despite pronounced decrease in the arterial oxyhemoglobin saturation. If hypercapnia exists, drowsiness and the other central nervous system manifestations of hypercapnia may be evident. The jugular veins are distended and are further engorged by applying pressure over the enlarged, usually tender liver. Edema of the lower extremities may be present. The cardiac rate is rapid, and an early diastolic gallop sound may be audible over the mid-left precordium.

Radiograms usually reveal a prominent main pulmonary artery and enlargement of its main branches; but if the pulmonary hypertension is not marked or has not been sustained for a prolonged period of time, these vessels may appear normal in size. Especially in patients who have manifested chronic cardiac failure, the right ventricle and the right atrium are grossly enlarged. In other patients with obvious failure, the cardiac dimensions seem surprisingly normal, but serial films will often show diminution in the size of the right ventricle and right atrium with recovery from the failure.

The electrocardiographic manifestations of right ventricular hypertrophy are also modified by lung disease; even in patients with considerable pulmonary hypertension and right ventricular hypertrophy, the usual criteria considered diagnostic of hypertrophy and enlargement of the right ventricle are often not present. Large S waves in the precordial leads as far to the left as V_5 or V_6, a small rS or rSR' complex in V_1, negative T waves in the right precordial leads, a vertical or slight rightward displacement of the mean QRS axis in the frontal plane, and peaked P waves in the limb leads (P pulmonale) may be the only signs that the right ventricle is hypertrophied. These electrocardiographic alterations may not be present if the pulmonary arterial pressure is not two or more times greater than normal at rest. Regression of these electrocardiographic features in the course of recovery from an episode of respiratory failure often permits a retrospective appreciation of their significance. Atrial arrhythmias, especially flutter and fibrillation, and ventricular premature contractions are common in patients with acute respiratory insufficiency and cor pulmonale.

The findings of a reduced oxyhemoglobin saturation, diminished oxygen tension and pH and elevated carbon dioxide tension in the arterial blood, increase in plasma bicarbonate, and polycythemia support the diagnosis of pulmonary hypertension caused by pulmonary disease or respiratory disorder. Studies of pulmonary function are useful in defining the disorder, monitoring the effects of treatment, and assessing the probability that cor pulmonale will develop. Primary alveolar hypoventilation of central origin as the cause of pulmonary hypertension and congestive cardiac failure may go undetected without measurements of arterial blood gases and studies of the ventilatory response to carbon dioxide. In some patients with cardiac murmurs or evidence of left ventricular enlargement, the issue of whether the pulmonary hypertension is primarily due to the pulmonary disease or is secondary to an intracardiac lesion or left ventricular dysfunction may sometimes be resolved only by hemodynamic and angiographic studies. Pulmonary disease does not protect the patient from the development of coronary arteriosclerosis or systemic hypertension, which may compromise left ventricular function. The left ventricle may also be directly affected by scleroderma, polymyositis, sarcoidosis, certain forms of muscular dystrophy, and obesity.

Treatment. Treatment must be simultaneously directed at improving the function of both the lungs and the heart. The specific measures to be used are described in Part XI. When cardiac failure appears, a cardiac glycoside and a diuretic, such as hydrochlorothiazide or furosemide, should be administered. Losses of body potassium during diuresis should be replaced, but because of pre-existing disturbances in potassium balance and impairment of renal function, serum potassium should be closely monitored as a guide to such replacement. The hypoxemia, hypercapnia, acidosis, and electrolyte imbalances appear to predispose the heart of patients with cor pulmonale to arrhythmias and to the toxic effects of cardiac glycosides. Daily maintenance doses larger than 0.1 mg of digitoxin or 0.25 mg of digoxin should be used with caution, and manifestations of digitalis intoxication should be watched for. Correction of hypoxemia by inhalation of oxygen in concentrations that do not depress alveolar ventilation is a cardinal feature of therapy during an acute episode of failure, and chronic administration of oxygen may be indicated to control pulmonary hypertension in patients with marked chronic hypoxemia. Because polycythemia enhances the tendency to develop thromboemboli and increases viscosity of the blood and consequently the resistance to its flow, periodic phlebotomy is indicated to maintain the hematocrit at 50 per cent in patients with marked polycythemia.

Prognosis. The development of pulmonary arterial hypertension and right ventricular failure in patients with pulmonary disease is a serious complication, but its prognostic significance depends on the underlying disorder. With appropriate treatment, the patient with chronic obstructive pulmonary disease may survive repeated bouts of cardiac and pulmonary failure over the course of many years. In patients with pulmonary fibrosis, the course after the onset of cardiac failure is variable but generally much shorter.

Bergofsky, E. H., and Holtzman, S.: A study of the mechanisms involved in the pulmonary arterial pressor response to hypoxia. Circulation Res., 20:506, 1967.

Blount, S. G., Jr., and Grover, R. F.: Pulmonary hypertension. *In* Hurst, J. W., and Logue, R. B. (eds.): The Heart. Arteries and Veins. 2nd ed. New York, McGraw-Hill Book Company, 1970, p. 1126.

Enson, Y., Giuntini, C., Lewis, M. L., Morris, T. Q., Ferrer, M. I., and Harvey, R. J.: The influence of hydrogen ion and hypoxia on the pulmonary circulation. J. Clin. Invest., 43:1146, 1964.

Harris, P., and Heath, D.: The Human Pulmonary Circulation. Its Form and Function in Health and Disease. Baltimore, Williams & Wilkins Company, 1962.

Tsagaris, T. J., and Tikoff, G.: Familial primary pulmonary hypertension. Am. Rev. Respir. Dis., 97:127, 1968.

Yu, P. N.: Pulmonary Blood Volume in Health and Disease. Philadelphia, Lea & Febiger, 1969.

CONGENITAL HEART DISEASE

Joseph K. Perloff

551. INTRODUCTION

Definition. *Congenital* is a Latin derivative from "con," together, and "genitus," born. However, the simple implication that congenital heart disease merely means "present at birth" requires qualification. The natural history begins before birth, because most anomalies compatible with six months of intrauterine life permit live offspring at term. A "congenital" anomaly originating in the developing fetus is often considerably modified, at least physiologically, by the dramatic circulatory adjustments at birth; it may then take weeks, months, or even years for the anomaly to evolve into the prototype pattern recognized as the "typical" clinical picture. Both physiologic and structural changes may subsequently continue. The ductus in a premature infant sometimes remains widely patent for months, finally closing spontaneously, leaving the baby with a normal heart. A ventricular septal defect that delivers a large left to right shunt in infancy may gradually develop progressive infundibular pulmonic stenosis, so that years later the physiologic and the clinical picture resembles classic cyanotic Fallot's tetralogy. A congenital bicuspid aortic valve that is functionally normal at birth may take two, three, or more decades to stiffen, calcify, and present as overt aortic stenosis. Accordingly, congenital heart disease should not be viewed narrowly as a static group of anatomic defects present at birth, but instead as a dynamic group of anomalies that originate in fetal life and

change during the course of postnatal natural histories. Certain defects that are not "anatomic" in the gross morphologic sense are considered congenital, such as congenital complete heart block, whereas others that are "anatomic," such as the aortic root disease of Marfan's syndrome are, by convention, generally not dealt with as congenital.

Incidence, Changing Population, and Role of the Internist and Medical Cardiologist. The prevalence of congenital heart disease has little meaning unless certain preconditions are considered. An impression of over-all prevalence can be derived from 1970 population figures when 3,718,000 live births were registered in the United States. An estimated 28,000 infants were born with congenital heart disease, i.e., 0.8 per cent. About half died within the first year, leaving 14,000 survivors. Thus well in excess of 20,000 infants with congenital heart disease are probably born annually in the United States. Both over-all incidence and incidence of specific defects vary according to patient age (neonate, infant, child, adolescent, young adult, older adult) and according to whether figures are derived from living subjects or necropsy material. A further distinction must be made between incidence based upon *natural* history and the incidence modified by *palliative* or *corrective surgery*. It is now possible to perform palliative or corrective surgery on almost all congenital cardiacs, even the most complex. Survival patterns are affected, often profoundly. We are therefore confronted with a changing population of congenital heart disease. Recent decades of intense diagnostic and therapeutic effort have resulted in survival of larger numbers of adolescents, postadolescents, and adults with congenital defects of the heart or circulation. Accordingly, postpediatric congenital heart disease is increasingly represented not only by anomalies with a natural tendency for long survival, but also by those in which palliative or corrective surgery has been successfully employed. Operation not only increases life expectancy in anomalies with a natural tendency for long survival, but may also permit increasing numbers of patients with disorders hitherto fatal in infancy or childhood to reach postadolescence or even adulthood. Intelligent long-term management requires an understanding of both the preoperative anomaly and the effects of surgical repair. *Thus congenital heart disease from the point of view of patient care should be considered not only in terms of age of onset, but also in terms of the age range that potential survival now permits.* Such patients require specialty care, be it by a pediatric cardiologist who extends an interest to older subjects or by a medical cardiologist who has a satisfactory comprehension of congenital cardiac disease. By the same token, it is no more important for the pediatrician to provide primary general pediatric care for the infant or child with congenital heart disease than for the internist to provide primary general medical care for the late teenager and adult with these malformations.

Etiology. Congenital heart disease is etiologically multifactorial, the result of a complex interplay between genetic and environmental factors. These determinants in part include heredity, chromosomal defects, teratogens, prematurity, altitude at birth, sex, and maternal age.

Some tendency exists for congenital heart disease to run in families. There is an increased incidence of defects in the offspring of propositi. Distribution and incidence are difficult to ascertain, because survival into the reproductive age is a necessary requirement for transmission. Atrial septal defect commonly permits adult survival, and can be not only familial but recurrent through a number of generations. Parents who in childhood experienced spontaneous closure of ventricular septal defects may live to adulthood and produce offspring with ventricular septal defects. There is also the prospect that increasing numbers of operated congenital cardiacs will reach childbearing age and produce a higher incidence of offspring with congenital defects of the heart or circulation. About 2 per cent of siblings of propositi have congenital heart disease. If one of a nonidentical twin pair has a congenital cardiac anomaly, the incidence in the co-twin is about the same as for sibs in general, but about 25 per cent of identical twins with congenital heart disease have affected co-twins with a high probability of identical defects.

Certain abnormal chromosome patterns are associated with predictable types of congenital cardiac disease, although chromosomal abnormalities per se are uncommon in the general population of congenital cardiacs. Down's syndrome (trisomy 21) has a high incidence of endocardial cushion defects, and about 50 per cent of patients with complete endocardial cushion defects have trisomy 21. Typical Turner's syndrome (phenotypic female with XO) occurs with coarctation of the aorta; trisomy 18 occurs with right ventricular origin of both great arteries; the Holt-Oran syndrome heightens suspicion of ostium secundum atrial septal defect, and the Ellis–van Creveld syndrome predicts common atrium.

The role of *teratogens* at critical times in fetal development is epitomized by the effects of thalidomide taken by the pregnant mother. Maternal rubella (German measles) during the first trimester increases the risk of offspring with patent ductus arteriosus and stenosis of the pulmonary artery and its branches.

Ventricular septal defect and patent ductus arteriosus are relatively common in *premature infants*. It has been postulated that the expected intrauterine time of ventricular septal closure is not limited to early fetal life but sometimes continues through gestation into the postpartum period. Delayed closure of the ductus arteriosus is more likely to occur in premature infants in whom the duct may remain patent for as long as four to six months after birth. Incompletely developed cholinergic innervation and reduced constrictor response to oxygen of the premature ductus may in part account for this.

The *altitude at birth* is another factor affecting the occurrence of congenital heart disease. Persistence of the ductus arteriosus is six times as frequent in people born at high altitudes as in those born at sea level. Reduced oxygen tension in ambient air at high altitudes may provide inadequate stimulus for ductal constriction even if cholinergic innervation of the ductal wall is well developed.

Parental age has been considered an etiologic factor. There is no evidence that paternal age plays a role, but *maternal age* has been called into question. Late maternal age (immediate premenopausal) seems to increase the risk of Fallot's tetralogy.

Sex distribution has been a point of interest in congenital diseases of the heart and circulation. The bicuspid aortic valve is predominantly a male disease. In fact, aortic valve disease in general has a strong male prevalence. The male-to-female ratio in ventricular septal defect with aortic regurgitation is twice as high as in uncomplicated ventricular septal defect. Aortic atresia is almost exclusively a disease of male infants. On the other hand, patent ductus arteriosus predominates in females (sex ratio of 2 or 3:1). Female predominance in ostium secundum atrial septal defect is estimated to be as high as 3.5:1, and females predominate in partial endocardial cushion defects. Congenital aneurysms of sinuses of Valsalva carry a male-to-female ratio of 4:1. A similar male-to-female ratio occurs in complete transposition of the great arteries, with a range of 2 to 4:1.

Physiologic Adaptation after Birth. The concept has been underscored that congenital heart diseases are not static in time, but change anatomically and functionally during the course of their natural histories. The most spectacular change in this context occurs at birth. A given congenital cardiac defect may exist in harmony with the fetal circulation, but is confronted with dramatic circulatory changes at birth that alter this harmony to widely varying degrees. It is therefore appropriate to examine briefly the principal immediate and delayed circulatory alterations at birth and in the neonatal period. The immediate changes consist of (1) a colossal fall in pulmonary vascular resistance associated with expansion of the lungs; (2) a pronounced rise in systemic vascular resistance associated with elimination of the low resistance placental circulation; (3) a fall in blood flow to the right atrium owing to abolition of umbilical venous return; (4) an abrupt rise — as much as tenfold — in pulmonary blood flow, which is promptly translated into a rise in left atrial volume and pressure; (5) functional closure of the valve of the foramen ovale caused by the rise in left atrial and the fall in right atrial pressure; and (6) constriction of the ductus arteriosus at about 12 hours after birth in response to an increase in systemic arterial Po_2. Several important delayed changes complete the picture. The thick-walled fetal pulmonary arterioles are designed to meet the full force of systemic right ventricular pressure the instant the lungs expand. After this need has been met, the fetal arterioles involute during the first two months of life. As respiration is established at birth, there is a marked rise in alveolar and systemic arterial oxygen tension to which pulmonary arterioles are exquisitely sensitive, setting the stage for dilatation and anatomic involution. A possible effect of bradykinin in this regard should also be mentioned. In addition, the larger pulmonary arteries may also play a role — though much less — in determining the total drop in pressure across the lungs after birth. Maturational changes may affect the neonatal disparity in size between the main and branch pulmonary arteries as well as the angulation at the origins of the right and left branches; both these factors have been held responsible for a physiologic drop in pressure distal to the pulmonary trunk. The third important delayed change relates to the fetal right ventricle, which slowly loses its relative thickness during the first year of life. Adaptive hypertrophy is an expected feature of the fetal right ventricle, which ejects at systemic pressure via the ductus arteriosus. After birth, with the stimulus of right ventricular afterload eliminated, there is a gradual reduction in its thickness relative to septum and left ventricle. The thick neonatal right ventricular wall does not undergo regression; it merely does not increase its thickness as rapidly as the left in the growing infant.

These physiologic adaptations of the normal heart to the events at birth are remarkable in their own right. It is no surprise that congenital defects of the heart or circulation will, to varying degrees, interact with or be modified by adaptations to extrauterine life. A few examples suffice. At one end of the spectrum is the ductus arteriosus, which is a normal part of the fetal circulation. However, when the fetal ductus remains widely patent after birth, the neonatal fall in pulmonary vascular resistance establishes a left to right shunt; pulmonary blood flow increases, and the left ventricle is volume overloaded and may fail under the burden. What was a normal structure in the fetus becomes a potentially hazardous congenital defect after birth. At the other end of the spectrum, aortic atresia is a case in point. This anomaly is characterized by an atretic aortic valve, a rudimentary left ventricular cavity, and a rudimentary or atretic mitral valve. The left atrium has no effective exit, but in the fetus this is not a serious handicap, because flow into the left atrium via the lungs is negligible and right to left flow across the foramen ovale is not vital. Accordingly, survival to term is the rule, because systemic venous blood received by the fetal right heart is pumped into the systemic circulation via the fetal ductus, bypassing the left heart. However, at birth, the lungs expand and pulmonary blood flow suddenly and dramatically increases, abruptly delivering a large volume into a left atrium that has no effective outlet, because forward flow through the left ventricle is totally obstructed by the atretic mitral and/or aortic valves. Temporary survival depends upon decompression of the left atrium via a herniated valve of the foramen ovale. Death follows in short order. An intermediate case in point is large ventricular septal defect which, although abnormal, does not disturb the fetal circulation, because it allows right ventricular blood to enter the aorta in a fashion analogous to the fetal ductus. However, after birth, a fall in pulmonary vascular resistance establishes a left to right shunt which may significantly disturb the postnatal circulation. Subsequently, the pulmonary vascular resistance may rise again and, in a decade or more, reverse the shunt (Eisenmenger's complex).

The principle to be extracted from these examples is clear. The anatomy and physiology of the heart and circulation in congenital heart disease change with the passage of time from the fetus, to the dramatic changes at birth, to further changes in the infant, child, adolescent, and adult survivor. Some of these changes result in neonatal death; others express themselves gradually over weeks, months, years, or decades. A satisfactory comprehension of the clinical manifestations of congenital heart disease requires that these patterns be taken into account.

Diagnosis. Clinical diagnosis of congenital heart disease can represent the epitome of clinical logic. The pathologic anatomy should first be clarified to shed light on the resulting physiologic derangements. The question can then be asked: "What clinical manifestations result from these anatomic and physiologic derangements?" The stage is then set for the clinical diagnosis, which depends upon a synthesis of information derived from the history, the physical signs, the electrocardiogram, the x-ray, and the laboratories (noninvasive and cardiac catheterization). Similarly, the physical diagnosis consists of a synthesis of its own five parts, namely, physical appearance, the arterial pulse, the venous pulse, precordial movements and palpation, and auscultation. Maximal data should be extracted from each clinical source, relating the information from one source to that from another. A simple principle emerges—on the one hand, depth; on the other, synthesis. Each step should advance

our thinking and narrow the diagnostic possibilities. By the end of the clinical appraisal, untenable considerations should have been abandoned, diagnostic *possibilities* retained for due consideration, and high priority *probabilities* brought into sharp focus.

Diagnostic thinking benefits from the devices of anticipation and supposition. Anticipate what the next step holds, and less will be missed. Once tentative conclusions have been drawn from the history, it is useful to pause momentarily and ask, "If these assumptions are correct, what can I expect the physical examination to show? What specific points might I anticipate in the electrocardiogram or x-ray in order to support or refute the conclusions based on the history?" The device of *anticipation* not only helps achieve a synthesis of each step with the next but also serves to heighten interest as the clinical assessment progresses. The device of *supposition* lends itself to the clinical classification of congenital heart disease proposed in Table 1. As clinical information becomes available, it can be directly related to this classification so that orderly thinking begins apace. For example, we can ask, "*Suppose* this were a *congenital* cardiac defect in an *acyanotic* patient with a *left to right shunt;* which if any of the malformations in this category are appropriate to the information thus far at hand?" By simply asking, "Suppose this were so, what is likely to follow?" one is permitted the dual advantages of thoughtful consideration without inflexible commitment.

Diagnostic information is best handled within the framework of an orderly classification (Table 1) which was selected because it is practical and clinical and can be effectively used irrespective of which of the five sources of diagnostic information one is dealing with. The classification is based essentially on the answers to five simple questions: *(1) Is the patient acyanotic or cyanotic? (2) Is pulmonary arterial flow increased or not? (3) Does the malformation originate in the left or right heart? (4) Which is the dominant ventricle? (5) Is pulmonary hypertension present or absent?* It is not even necessary to ask all five questions for each patient. If the answer to question 1 is "acyanotic," only two additional questions need be posed, namely, "Is a shunt absent or present" (i.e., is pulmonary arterial flow increased or not?), and if a shunt is absent, "On what side of the heart does the malformation originate, left or right?" (Table 2). On the other hand, if the answer to question 1 is "cyanotic," three additional questions need be asked. First, "Is pulmonary arterial flow increased or not?" If the answer is "normal" or "decreased," we need ask, "Which is the dominant ventricle?" and "Is pulmonary hypertension present or absent?" (Table 3).

To illustrate, begin with an acyanotic patient (Table 4). If the answer to question 2 is negative (acyanotic without shunt), then we must ask, "Does the malformation originate in the left or right heart?" (Table 2). Now move step by step through the heart in the direction of blood flow (Table 4). If the malformation originates in the right heart, is it at the level of the venae cavae, right atrium, tricuspid valve, right ventricular inflow, right ventricular outflow, pulmonary artery and its branches, or pulmonary arterioles? Similarly, if the malformation originates in the left heart (Table 5), is it at the level of the pulmonary veins, left atrium, mitral valve, left ventricular inflow, left ventricular outflow, aortic root (supravalvular) or thoracic aorta? If the answer to question 2 is that pulmonary arterial blood flow

TABLE 1. A Clinical Classification of Congenital Heart Disease*

General

Innocent or normal murmurs
Congenital complete heart block
Congenitally corrected transposition of the great arteries
Congenital positional anomalies of the heart — the cardiac malpositions

Acyanotic without a Shunt

Malformations originating in the left heart
1. Aortic stenosis
   a. Valvular
   b. Discrete subvalvular
   c. Muscular subvalvular
   d. Supravalvular
2. Coarctation of the aorta
3. Congenital mitral incompetence
   a. Endocardial cushion defect
   b. Congenitally corrected transposition of the great arteries
   c. Primary endocardial fibroelastosis
   d. Anomalous origin of the left coronary artery from the pulmonary artery
   e. Miscellaneous (double orifice mitral valve, congenital perforations, accessory commissures with anomalous chordal insertion, congenitally short or absent chordae, cleft posterior leaflet, Marfan's syndrome, etc.)
4. Primary endocardial fibroelastosis
5. Congenital obstruction to left atrial flow
   a. Cor triatriatum
   b. Mitral stenosis
   c. Pulmonary vein stenosis
6. Congenital aortic incompetence
Malformations originating in the right heart
1. Pulmonic stenosis
   a. Valvular
   b. Infundibular
   c. Supravalvular (stenosis of the pulmonary artery and its branches)
   d. Subinfundibular
2. Idiopathic dilatation of the pulmonary artery
3. Congenital pulmonary valve incompetence
4. Primary pulmonary hypertension
5. Ebstein's anomaly of the tricuspid valve
6. Hypoplastic right ventricle

Acyanotic with a Shunt (Left to Right)

Shunt at atrial level
1. Atrial septal defect (isolated)
   a. Ostium secundum
   b. Ostium primum
   c. Sinus venosus
2. Atrial septal defect with mild pulmonic stenosis
3. Total anomalous pulmonary venous connection with low pulmonary vascular resistance
4. Partial anomalous pulmonary venous connection with intact atrial septum
5. Atrial septal defect with mitral stenosis (Lutembacher's syndrome)
Shunt at ventricular level
1. Ventricular septal defect (isolated)
   a. Infracristal
   b. Supracristal
   c. Muscular
   d. Endocardial cushion location
2. Ventricular septal defect with mild pulmonic stenosis (acyanotic Fallot's tetralogy)
3. Ventricular septal defect with right ventricular origin of both great arteries
4. Ventricular septal defect with congenitally corrected transposition of the great arteries
5. Ventricular septal defect with aortic incompetence
6. Ventricular septal defect with left ventricular to right atrial shunt
7. Ventricular septal defect with complete interruption of the aortic arch

Shunts between aortic root and right heart
1. Coronary arteriovenous fistula
2. Ruptured sinus of Valsalva aneurysm
Shunt at aorticopulmonary level
1. Patent ductus arteriosus
2. Aorticopulmonary septal defect
3. Anomalous origin of the left coronary artery from the pulmonary artery
4. Truncus arteriosus with large pulmonary arteries and low pulmonary vascular resistance
Shunts at more than one level
1. Complete endocardial cushion defect (complete persistent common atrioventricular canal)
2. Ventricular septal defect with patent ductus arteriosus
3. Ventricular septal defect with atrial septal defect

Cyanotic with a Shunt (Right to Left)

Increased pulmonary blood flow
1. Complete transposition of the great arteries
2. The Taussig-Bing anomaly (right ventricular origin of both great arteries with supracristal ventricular septal defect or right ventricular aorta with biventricular pulmonary trunk)
3. Truncus arteriosus with large pulmonary arteries
4. Total anomalous pulmonary venous connection
5. Single ventricle with low pulmonary resistance and no pulmonic stenosis
6. Common atrium
7. Fallot's tetralogy with pulmonary atresia and increased bronchial arterial flow
8. Tricuspid atresia with large ventricular septal defect and no pulmonic stenosis
Normal or decreased pulmonary blood flow
  Dominant left ventricle
   a. Tricuspid atresia
   b. Ebstein's anomaly with right to left interatrial shunt (mechanical dominance)
   c. Pulmonary atresia with intact ventricular septum and diminutive right ventricle
   d. Congenital vena caval to left atrial communication
   e. Single ventricle with pulmonic stenosis and noninversion of the infundibulum
   f. Large pulmonary arteriovenous fistula in infancy
  Dominant right ventricle
  Normal or low pulmonary arterial pressure
   a. Pulmonary stenosis or atresia with ventricular septal defect and right to left shunt (cyanotic Fallot's tetralogy)
   b. Pulmonic stenosis with right to left interatrial shunt
   c. Complete transposition of the great arteries with severe pulmonic stenosis and large ventricular septal defect
   d. Pulmonic stenosis with right ventricular origin of both great arteries
   e. Pulmonic stenosis with single ventricle and inversion of the infundibulum (electrical dominance)
   f. Pulmonary atresia with intact ventricular septum and dilated right ventricle
   g. Truncus arteriosus with hypoplastic or absent pulmonary arteries
  Normal or nearly normal ventricles
   a. Pulmonary arteriovenous fistula
   b. Congenital vena caval to left atrial communication
  Elevated pulmonary arterial pressure (pulmonary hypertension)
1. Ventricular septal defect with reversed shunt (Eisenmenger's complex)
2. Patent ductus arteriosus or aorticopulmonary septal defect with reversed shunt
3. Atrial septal defect with reversed shunt
4. Right ventricular origin of both great arteries with high pulmonary vascular resistance
5. Hypoplastic left heart (aortic atresia, mitral atresia, complete interruption of the aortic arch)
6. Complete transposition of the great arteries with high pulmonary vascular resistance
7. Single ventricle with high pulmonary vascular resistance
8. Total anomalous pulmonary venous connection with pulmonary venous obstruction

---

*Modified from Perloff, J. K.: The Clinical Recognition of Congenital Heart Disease. Philadelphia, W. B. Saunders Company, 1970.

TABLE 2

Acyanotic

Shunt absent or present?

(Left to right)

Malformation originating in the left heart   Malformation originating in the right heart

TABLE 4

Acyanotic without a shunt, malformation originating in the right heart. Start proximally (venae cavae) and end distally (pulmonary arteries):

1. Venae cavae
2. Right atrium
3. Tricuspid valve
4. Right ventricular inflow
5. Right ventricular outflow
6. Pulmonary artery and branches
7. Pulmonary arterioles

is increased, then the shunt by definition is left to right, because cyanosis is absent. We can then methodically consider the origin of the shunt and the chamber or vessel that receives it. Again, move step by step through the heart in the direction of blood flow, i.e., shunts at atrial level, ventricular level, from aortic root to right heart, or from aortic arch to pulmonary artery (Table 6).

Next, consider cyanotic patients (Table 3). If pulmonary arterial blood flow is increased, there are for all practical purposes, a total of eight possibilities, but only the first four are likely (Table 1, cyanotic with a shunt, increased pulmonary blood flow). If pulmonary arterial flow is normal or decreased, and the left ventricle is dominant, there are a total of six possibilities, only two of which are likely, i.e., tricuspid atresia or Ebstein's anomaly of the tricuspid valve (Table 1). If the right ventricle is dominant, question 5 must be asked, "Is pulmonary hypertension present or absent?" If pulmonary hypertension is present (Table 7), again, move step by step through the heart in the direction of blood flow; i.e., is one dealing with a pulmonary hypertensive right to left shunt at atrial, ventricular, or great vessel level? If pulmonary hypertension is absent (Table 8), this necessarily implies obstruction to outflow into the pulmonary bed, i.e., normal or low pulmonary arterial pressure with high right ventricular pressure. In practical terms, the probabilities are two, pulmonic stenosis with right to left shunt at either atrial or ventricular level.

In dealing with the history, physical examination, electrocardiogram, x-ray, and diagnostic laboratories, it is worthwhile briefly to call attention to a few points especially appropriate to congenital heart disease. In the history, questions should include the pregnancy, for example, maternal exposure to teratogens such as rubella in the first trimester, or the altitude at which the patient was born. Maternal age may be important. Details of a

cardiac murmur—the detection of which often heralds the diagnosis of congenital heart disease—should be precise regarding onset and intensity. Was the murmur present at birth (newborn nursery), or was it first detected in early infancy, adolescence, or young adulthood? Was the murmur always readily heard irrespective of patient cooperation (conspicuous murmur), or was it absent at times, difficult to hear, or believed to be unimportant? Was a new murmur even commented upon (ventricular septal defect with subsequent aortic regurgitation)? Cyanosis should similarly be defined precisely according to time of onset, degree, and distribution. A history of squatting in a cyanotic patient is classic information suggesting Fallot's tetralogy. Patterns of growth and development should be established. It is worth recalling that the clinical manifestations of congestive heart failure differ in infants, older children, and adults. Family history of congenital cardiac disease may shed light on the defect in the patient, especially if kinship is close. Susceptibility to lower respiratory infections suggests large left to right shunts. Neck pulsations (arterial or venous) may provide useful clues. A history of infective endocarditis calls attention to a relatively limited number of defects.

Physical appearance should consider the presence of certain *somatic* congenital defects that are associated with specific types of congenital *cardiac* anomalies, such as *mongolism* (endocardial cushion defect), *Turner's syndrome* (coarctation of the aorta), *peculiar facies and dentition* associated with supravalvular aortic stenosis and pulmonary artery stenosis, the *Holt-Oram syndrome* (defects in the atrial septum), the *Ellis–van Creveld syndrome* (common atrium), or trisomy 18 (double outlet right ventricle).

The arterial pulses should be compared in the upper and lower extremities (coarctation of the aorta), but the brachials should also be palpated (cyanotic male infant with absent brachials and present femorals may mean aortic atresia). Right and left arterial pulses should be compared (increased pulse pressure in the right carotid and brachial arteries in supravalvular aortic stenosis). The jugular venous pulse deserves special attention as soon as the patient is old enough to permit such observa-

TABLE 3

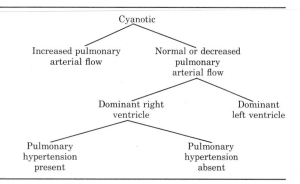

Cyanotic

Increased pulmonary arterial flow   Normal or decreased pulmonary arterial flow

Dominant right ventricle   Dominant left ventricle

Pulmonary hypertension present   Pulmonary hypertension absent

TABLE 5

Acyanotic without a shunt, malformation originating in the left heart. Start proximally (pulmonary veins) and end distally (aorta):

1. Pulmonary veins
2. Left atrium
3. Mitral valve
4. Left ventricular inflow
5. Left ventricular outflow
6. Thoracic aorta

TABLE 6

Acyanotic with a shunt. Where is the left to right communication, i.e., where does it originate and what chamber or vessel receives the shunt? Start proximally and end distally:

1. Atrial level
2. Ventricular level
3. Great vessel level (aortic root, aortic arch)

TABLE 8

Cyanotic with normal or decreased pulmonary arterial flow, dominant right ventricle, and no pulmonary hypertension.

1. Pulmonic stenosis or atresia with right to left shunt at ventricular level.
2. Pulmonic stenosis or atresia with right to left shunt at atrial level.

tion (the short neck of the infant usually makes examination difficult or impossible). Percussion is useful in establishing visceral positions (cardiac and hepatic dullness and gastric tympany) to avoid missing a congenital positional anomaly. Palpation should carefully define each precordial movement according to chamber or vessel of origin, avoiding vague, meaningless terms such as point of maximum impulse. During auscultation, designations such as pulmonary area, aortic area, or mitral area should be avoided, because they assume normal topographical anatomy of the heart, i.e., situs solitus without transposition of the great arteries and without ventricular inversion, assumptions which cannot be made, especially in the context of congenital heart disease. Simple descriptive terms should be used, such as apex, left or right lower, mid or upper sternal border, and the like. Murmurs should be precisely characterized, especially their timing in the cardiac cycle, with systolic murmurs classified as early, mid, late or holosystolic; diastolic murmurs as early diastolic, mid-diastolic or presystolic; and the continuous murmur defined as one that begins in systole and continues without interruption through the second heart sound into all or part of diastole.

The 12-lead surface electrocardiogram should be supplemented by leads V_3R and V_4R, and a vectorcardiogram is often necessary to clarify complex electrocardiograms.

Technically satisfactory plain films of the chest in the posteroanterior, lateral, right and left oblique positions with barium have for all practical purposes replaced cardiac fluoroscopy except for the detection of intracardiac calcium. The noninvasive technique of *echocardiography* is a valuable source of diagnostic information that is available repeatedly and without risk. Cardiac catheterization and angiocardiography should be an extension of clinical judgment, a judgment which should decide not only which patients should be selected for study, but also which type of investigation is most appropriate for a given subject. Accurate diagnosis depends upon synthesis of the broad range of clinical data with results of carefully planned and well-executed laboratory studies.

Scope of These Chapters. Survival in congenital heart disease results from natural selection or from surgical intervention. These chapters will emphasize those defects with a natural tendency to survive beyond the pediatric age group. Such emphasis is appropriate for a text-

book of medicine. It must be stated, however, that congenital cardiac disease is a continuum from birth to adult life and that the only way to understand the patterns of postpediatric survival is to have dealt at some point with the same disorders in the infant and young child. The following categories will be considered: (1) *common* congenital cardiac defects in which postpediatric survival is expected; (2) *uncommon* congenital cardiac defects in which postpediatric survival is expected; (3) *common* congenital cardiac defects in which postpediatric survival is exceptional; and (4) *uncommon* congenital cardiac defects in which postpediatric survival is exceptional. Congenital cardiac anomalies (common or uncommon) in which postpediatric survival is unknown will not be considered. Chief emphasis will be placed on the common or uncommon anomalies with *expected* postpediatric survival. The common or uncommon defects with exceptional postpediatric survival will be touched upon more briefly to provide necessary perspective. It should be borne in mind, however, that as time goes on more and more congenital cardiacs beyond the pediatric age group will be postoperative; this is only as it should be.

552. COMMON CONGENITAL CARDIAC DEFECTS IN WHICH POSTPEDIATRIC SURVIVAL IS EXPECTED

FUNCTIONALLY NORMAL BICUSPID AORTIC VALVE

The frequency of congenitally bicuspid aortic valves — functionally normal, stenotic, and/or incompetent — may approach 2 per cent of the population. If this figure is correct, it would mean that the bicuspid aortic valve is not only the most frequent congenital anomaly of the heart or great vessels, but that the most common congenital cardiac defect in man manifests itself in the *postpediatric population.* The typical bicuspid aortic valve consists of two commissures and two cusps. One cusp, generally the larger, contains a low ridge or raphe ("false commissure"), adjacent to the aortic wall but not reaching the edge of the leaflet. If the free edges of a congenital biscuspid aortic valve are sufficiently redundant to permit unimpeded forward flow (no systolic gradient) yet not redundant enough to cause malapposition in diastole (little or no aortic regurgitation), then the bicuspid aortic valve is said to be "functionally normal." The natural history of such a valve is variable. A bicuspid aortic valve that functions normally at birth may continue to do so throughout life and be found as an incidental necropsy finding in late adult life. However, the same valve may take three unfavorable courses. The first is the tendency to become thickened, fibrotic, calcified, and

TABLE 7

Cyanotic with normal or decreased pulmonary arterial flow, dominant right ventricle, and pulmonary hypertension. Where is the right to left shunt? Start proximally and end distally.

1. Atrial level
2. Ventricular level
3. Great vessel level

stenotic during early or mid-adult life. Second, infective endocarditis may convert a functionally benign lesion into the catastrophic mechanical fault of severe aortic regurgitation. Third, the larger of the two cusps may progressively evert or prolapse, causing progressive aortic regurgitation that ultimately can be severe. It is not yet known what determines which of these courses a given functionally normal congenitally bicuspid valve will take.

Clinical recognition of a functionally normal bicuspid aortic valve can be suspected especially in teenagers and young adults. Innocent systolic murmurs in this age group, except for infraclavicular radiation of the innocent brachiocephalic systolic murmur, are not heard at the right base. Accordingly, a short, somewhat impure Grade I to II midsystolic murmur at the right base in a child, adolescent, or young adult is suspect. If that murmur is introduced by an ejection sound and if careful auscultation detects the soft murmur of aortic regurgitation, the clinical diagnosis reaches a high degree of probability. Physical interventions that increase aortic pressure (squatting, isometric tension with clenched fists) increase the audibility of the soft murmur of aortic regurgitation. Suspicion is always greater in the male, because the congenital bicuspid aortic valve, whether functionally normal or not, is predominantly a male disease. If clinical suspicion is high, an argument can be made for verification by thoracic aortography, because the bicuspid aortic valve is highly susceptible to infective endocarditis and appropriate antimicrobial prophylaxis must be recommended.

CONGENITAL VALVULAR AORTIC STENOSIS

Congenital obstruction to left ventricular outflow can be *valvular, subvalvular,* or *supravalvular.* The most common type is valvular and is usually characterized by narrowing of a bicuspid valve which can be intrinsically stenotic from birth or can become stenotic after progressive thickening and calcification (see above). Unicommissural unicuspid aortic valves are relatively common causes of intrinsically stenotic aortic valves at birth but, like the congenital bicuspid valve, sometimes exhibit delayed obstruction owing to thickening and rigidity.

Congenital valvular aortic stenosis is much more common in males, with a sex ratio approximating 4 or 5:1. If the obstruction is present at birth, the murmur is likely to date from the newborn nursery. On the other hand, the functionally normal congenital bicuspid aortic valve usually goes undetected in infancy or childhood, but may subsequently generate the prominent murmur of aortic stenosis in the second, third, or fourth decade. Angina and effort syncope arouse suspicion of aortic stenosis in acyanotic young patients with a history of dyspnea, fatigue, and either a prominent cardiac murmur dating from infancy or a murmur appearing in the second, third, or fourth decades. Cerebral symptoms can be subtle, consisting of nothing more than mild giddiness or lightheadedness, especially with effort. On the other hand, recurrent syncope is dangerous and heralds sudden death even in childhood or adolescence. Inappropriate sweating sometimes occurs and increases with the advent of cardiac failure. Infective endocarditis is a serious complication of congenital valvular aortic stenosis; all varieties are susceptible. The pulse pressure is

small, and there are a slow rate of rise, a sustained peak, and a gentle collapse when obstruction is severe.

Precordial palpation reveals a left ventricular impulse that varies from normal (mild stenosis) to the strong, sustained heaving movement of the hypertrophied left ventricle with severe obstruction. Presystolic distention of the left ventricle implies increased force of left atrial contraction, and is good evidence in young adults that the obstruction is significant. The thrill of aortic stenosis may be trivial or absent with mild obstruction or with severe obstruction and advanced heart failure. The typical aortic stenotic thrill radiates upward and to the right, is maximal in the second right interspace, and is readily detected in the suprasternal notch and over both carotids. In some patients the thrill is confined to the apex or, if the heart is small, to the lower left sternal edge where the atypical location can be misleading. In addition to the thrill, the sharp impact of an ejection sound can often be palpated at the apex in congenital valvular aortic stenosis.

An ejection sound is a characteristic although not invariable feature of congenital valvular aortic stenosis. The sound is caused by abrupt upward movement of the dome-shaped or truncated stenotic valve and implies good valve motion. In adults calcification may impair valve mobility so that the ejection sound diminishes or vanishes. The aortic stenotic murmur begins after the first sound (or with the ejection sound), rises in a crescendo to a systolic peak, and declines in a decrescendo to end before the aortic component of the second sound. The quality at the right base is harsh, rough, and grunting, especially when loud. Although configuration, length, and loudness do not necessarily relate to the degree of obstruction, the longer and louder the murmur and the later its systolic peak, the greater the likelihood of severe obstruction. However, an unimpressive midsystolic murmur — or none at all — may occur in severe aortic stenosis with advanced heart failure or in adults with increased anteroposterior chest dimensions. The right basal location and radiation of the murmur of valvular aortic stenosis are related to the upward and rightward direction of the high velocity jet within the ascending aorta. The second heart sound should be judged with regard to the intensity of the aortic component and the presence, degree, and type of splitting. In congenital valvular aortic stenosis with mobile valve, the aortic component of the second sound is well preserved even in the presence of significant obstruction. Prominent inspiratory splitting usually (but not invariably) means mild obstruction, because the duration of left ventricular ejection is not prolonged by that standard. *Paradoxical* splitting is a sign of severe obstruction and generally indicates that the duration of left ventricular ejection is appreciably prolonged. However, the majority of patients with aortic stenosis exhibit a second sound that is single or closely split through a wide range of severity.

A soft murmur of aortic regurgitation may be heard with congenital valvular aortic stenosis but is more common with discrete subvalvular aortic stenosis because of cusp distortion (see below). A fourth heart sound in aortic stenosis is the acoustic counterpart of presystolic distention of the left ventricle and is likely to mean appreciable obstruction. However, after age 40, the fourth heart sound is not a reliable sign of severity, because there is an age-related incidence.

Electrocardiographic estimates of severity should be made with caution, because mild valvular aortic stenosis occasionally occurs with left ventricular hypertrophy, and severe obstruction occasionally exists with a normal electrocardiogram. Occasionally sudden death occurs in patients with severe congenital aortic stenosis and normal electrocardiograms. Although these points must be kept in mind, they should not obscure the value of the scalar tracing. The best electrocardiographic index of appreciable obstruction is the combination of both voltage and repolarization criteria for left ventricular hypertrophy, especially in preadolescent patients. In congenital valvular aortic stenosis the x-ray features are poststenotic dilatation of the aorta with a relatively convex, globular left ventricular contour. In adults, aortic calcification is presumptive evidence of valvular obstruction and must be sought with the aid of an image intensifier.

Despite considerable clinical sophistication, cardiac catheterization and angiocardiography are generally required to be precise about the morphologic type and severity of congenital valvular aortic stenosis. If clinical evidence strongly points to mild obstruction, diagnostic intervention may be deferred, the risk of postoperative endocarditis far exceeding the risk and benefits of surgery. When clinical findings point to severe obstruction, diagnostic investigation should precede selection for surgery. If valvular obstruction is severe and the patient is *asymptomatic,* surgical intervention depends in large part on the morphologic type of obstruction. In relatively young patients with mobile congenital bicuspid aortic valves intrinsically stenotic at birth because of commissural fusion, direct repair provides excellent results at low risk. Severe valvular aortic stenosis in the *symptomatic* patient—especially with angina or syncope but without significant congestive heart failure—is appropriately selected for surgical intervention even if this means valve replacement. The more severe the left ventricular dysfunction, the smaller the gradient, the smaller the ejection fraction, the higher the surgical risk, and the poorer the results.

COARCTATION OF THE AORTA

The basic anatomic defect is a localized deformity of the media manifested by a curtain-like infolding that eccentrically narrows the aortic lumen. The zone of coarctation is characteristically located distal to the origin of the left subclavian artery at or just beyond the insertion of the ligamentum arteriosum. Occasionally coarctation is situated at or just proximal to the left subclavian artery so that the orifice of that vessel is in the low pressure zone.

Nearly 25 per cent of patients with coarctation of the aorta have bicuspid aortic valves which may be functionally normal or may take one of the courses described above. The most important noncardiac anomaly is an aneurysm of the circle of Willis which may remain clinically silent or may announce itself by rupture.

Aortic coarctation occurs predominantly in males. After early infancy, these patients are usually asymptomatic when the malformation is first diagnosed. Serious symptoms are relatively uncommon before age 15 years, but it is uncommon for symptoms to be absent beyond age 30. The majority of patients live to adult life, but only a minority reach age 40, and only 10 per cent live beyond age 50. The longest survival was recorded in 1828 by Reynaud in his account of coarctation in a 92-year-old man. Discovery of systemic hypertension provides the initial suspicion unless the brachial and femoral pulses are palpated. A number of minor symptoms such as headache, spontaneous epistaxes, and leg fatigue sometimes occur. The major symptoms are related to four complications: congestive heart failure, rupture of the aorta or dissecting aneurysm, infective endocarditis or endarteritis, and cerebral hemorrhage. The incidence of cardiac failure is highest in early infancy or after the third decade and can develop in adults previously devoid of symptoms related to the malformation. Rupture of the aorta or dissecting aneurysm occurs most frequently in the 20's and 30's. The rupture originates either in the proximal ascending aorta or in a postcoarctation aneurysm. Infective endocarditis or endarteritis occurs most commonly on the peculiarly susceptible bicuspid aortic valve; endarteritis at the site of coarctation occurs less frequently. Cerebral hemorrhage, the fourth major complication, is usually due to rupture of an aneurysm of the circle of Willis. In the pregnant female with coarctation, blood pressure fluctuations are similar in direction to those of uncomplicated pregnancy. The incidence of toxemia is lower in women with coarctation than in pregnant women with other forms of hypertension, intracranial hemorrhage is not more likely to occur, and cardiac failure seldom develops. However, pregnancy does increase the risk of rupture of the aorta, especially at the end of the third trimester. Furthermore, the bacteremia that accompanies labor and delivery can cause endocarditis or endarteritis.

The physique in coarctation is at times especially good, and an athletic appearance of the chest and shoulders contrasts with narrow hips and thin legs. Coarctation of the aorta can sometimes be suspected because of the characteristic physical appearance of *Turner's syndrome,* namely, a female with short stature, webbing of the neck, absent or scanty pubic and axillary hair, wide-set nipples, low hairline, small chin, and wide carrying angle of the arms.

Abnormal differences in upper and lower extremity arterial pulses are the clinical hallmarks of coarctation of the aorta. Diagnostic differences in arm and leg blood pressures should be based upon systolic and not diastolic levels. These pressure differences between arm and leg are exaggerated by exercise, which can therefore be a useful adjunct in confirming mild coarctation. The level of upper extremity blood pressure must be interpreted according to the patient's age. A blood pressure that is normal in an adult may be hypertensive in a child. As patients with coarctation grow older, the systolic pressure rises relatively more than the diastolic, so the pulse pressure increases. Such patients may exhibit conspicuous, forceful carotid and suprasternal pulsations resembling aortic regurgitation, which may coexist. In addition, the subclavian arteries can sometimes be seen pulsating below the clavicles. Collateral vessels are seldom obvious and must be specifically sought by having the patient stand and bend forward with the arms hanging at the sides. The examiner inspects the back, particularly around and between the scapulae, using a tangential light source to expose the subcutaneous collaterals in shadowed relief. The retinal arteries may be tortuous and narrowed, but hypertensive retinopathy is rare.

The right and left brachial arteries should also be simultaneously compared by palpation and blood pressure determination. An absent or relatively small left brachial pulse means that the coarctation is at or just proximal to the left subclavian artery. In aortic stenosis with coarctation, the brachial arterial pulse (and pressure) may be relatively normal rather than hypertensive, whereas the femoral pulses are diminished or absent. Conversely, aortic regurgitation increases the femoral pulse, especially in mild coarctation, so the clinical diagnosis of the combined defects may be overlooked.

Precordial palpation detects a left ventricular impulse that varies from normal to the sustained heaving impulse of ventricular hypertrophy. A dilated ascending aorta can cause a visible and palpable systolic impulse at the right base. Suprasternal thrills are relatively frequent in uncomplicated coarctation, but precordial thrills are seldom present without coexisting aortic stenosis.

An aortic ejection sound increases suspicion of coexisting bicuspid aortic valve, although such sounds may arise in the dilated aortic root. Coarctation of the aorta is associated with systolic, diastolic, or continuous murmurs. Systolic murmurs originate from arterial collaterals, the coarctation itself, and the bicuspid aortic valve. Collateral systolic murmurs are distributed widely over the thorax. There is a tendency for these murmurs to be especially conspicuous along the left sternal border (the left internal mammary artery). Collateral murmurs are crescendo-decrescendo in shape and delayed in onset because of origin in vessels distant from the heart. The coarctation itself is responsible for a localized midline posterior murmur, the level of which is related to the site of coarctation. With mild coarctation, the posterior systolic murmur is relatively short; as the degree of obstruction increases, the murmur gets longer and may extend well into diastole, becoming "continuous." The most common diastolic murmur is aortic regurgitation, a useful sign of coexisting bicuspid aortic valve.

Isolated *right* ventricular hypertrophy is for all practical purposes confined to infants in the first six months with heart failure and reactive pulmonary hypertension. In uncomplicated coarctation, left ventricular hypertrophy is manifested by both voltage and repolarization criteria. However, prominent S-T segment depressions with deeply inverted T waves seldom occur with uncomplicated coarctation and suggest coexisting aortic stenosis.

The x-ray provides considerable information regarding both the diagnosis and the anatomic variations of coarctation of the aorta. Notching of the ribs results from collateral flow through dilated, tortuous, pulsatile *posterior* intercostal arteries. The notches typically appear as irregular, scalloped areas on the undersurfaces of the posterior ribs. The *anterior* ribs are spared because the anterior intercostal arteries do not run in costal grooves. Notching seldom appears before six or seven years. When the coarctation is located *distal* to the left subclavian artery, collateral circulation fails to develop on the left side; *unilateral* notching appears in the *right* posterior ribs. In older children or adults, the lateral x-ray may show *retrosternal* notching caused by dilated tortuous internal mammary arteries. In classic coarctation of the aortic isthmus, the hypertensive ascending aorta is dilated. Aortic dilatation *distal* to the zone of coarctation (poststenotic enlargement) produces a recognizable leftward convexity of the descending thoracic aorta. When this sign is accompanied by the convex shadow of a dilated left subclavian artery, the two convexities form a typical "figure 3" in the frontal projection.

Cardiac catheterization and angiocardiography define the anatomic features of coarctation, including the collateral circulation, but as a rule they are not necessary for a secure clinical diagnosis upon which a therapeutic decision can be based. If there is clinical suspicion of coexisting bicuspid aortic valve, the inclination to perform thoracic aortography is increased, because the diagnosis gives insight into the postoperative natural course and the need for continued prophylaxis for infective endocarditis. The presence of all but mild coarctation warrants consideration for surgical correction. There is still a consensus that optimal age for correction awaits the seventh year. On the other hand, selection of patients for elective repair at earlier ages has progressed, because subsequent recurrence of coarctation has been shown to be negligible when correction is done in early childhood. In fact primary repair in small infants with persistent heart failure is now selectively and successfully accomplished. In older patients, risk of technical complications during surgical correction increases. Irrespective of the quality of the repair, the risk of infective endocarditis on a coexisting bicuspid aortic valve is not diminished, and we do not know whether the risk of intracranial hemorrhage (berry aneurysm) is affected. Although the incidence of heart failure continues to rise during the fourth decade in unoperated coarctation, after age 40 there appears to be an even chance of death from incidental causes. In those surviving to this age, the efficacy of correction becomes debatable. Furthermore, long-term analyses of patients after surgical correction of coarctation of the aorta have revealed a high incidence of premature cardiovascular disease despite adequate surgical repair. Particularly disturbing in this regard are the data on unexplained late postoperative hypertension.

PULMONIC STENOSIS

Congenital obstruction to right ventricular outflow can be valvular, subvalvular, or supravalvular. *Valvular* pulmonic stenosis, the most common variety, is characterized by a conical or dome-shaped valve with a narrow outlet at its apex. Three raphes extend from the small central opening to the wall of the pulmonary artery, although separate leaflets cannot be identified. Rarely, valvular pulmonic stenosis is caused by myxomatous dysplasia of the valve.

The functional consequences of valvular pulmonic stenosis are related to the resistance to right ventricular outflow. Males and females are equally affected. Early discovery of the murmur is the rule, because the anatomic and physiologic conditions necessary for its production are present at birth. Survival into adulthood is relatively common. The tendency for the valve to grow in proportion to body size may in part account for this. However, with advancing age fibrous thickening and even calcification may reduce valve mobility and increase the degree of obstruction.

Familial occurrence is not a feature of the history of ordinary valvular pulmonic stenosis, but a convincing family history may occur with valvular pulmonic stenosis caused by myxomatous dysplasia.

Subjective complaints tend to increase with age, although equivalent degrees of stenosis may handicap one patient in childhood and yet leave another relatively unlimited in the fourth decade. An appreciable number of patients with moderate to severe stenosis are virtually symptom free well into the postpediatric age group. Dyspnea and fatigue are the most common symptoms.

These complaints tend to remain absent as long as the right ventricle can maintain a normal stroke volume at rest and augment its output with effort. Right ventricular failure is the single most common natural cause of death. Patients with valvular pulmonic stenosis sometimes experience giddiness, lightheadedness, or frank syncope, especially with effort. Children as well as adults occasionally have chest pain resembling myocardial ischemia. Some patients with severe pulmonic stenosis may be subjectively aware of giant A waves in the jugular venous pulse, especially during effort or excitement. These patients are susceptible to infective endocarditis.

Infants with isolated typical valvular pulmonic stenosis may appear remarkably healthy, with good fat deposits and chubby round faces. Even older patients may have faces that are wide, full, or even bloated, with highly colored cheeks. Turner's syndrome with small stature, shield chest, and web neck is occasionally associated with valvular pulmonic stenosis. *Myxomatous dysplasia* causing valvular pulmonic stenosis may be associated with slow body growth and abnormal facies (triangular face with hypertelorism, ptosis of the eyelids, and low-set ears).

The jugular venous pulse exhibits an A wave that generally gets progressively larger as the degree of obstruction increases. Exercise and excitement augment these A waves. In addition, powerful right atrial contraction may be associated with presystolic pulsation of the liver. An increase in the height of the V wave occurs with the advent of right ventricular failure and tricuspid regurgitation.

Thrills mirror the location and intensity of accompanying murmurs (see below). In valvular pulmonic stenosis, the thrill is maximal in the second or occasionally third left interspace, radiating upward and toward the left, because the intrapulmonary jet is directed toward the left pulmonary artery. A right ventricular systolic impulse is an important physical sign of pulmonic stenosis and, when absent, the diagnosis should be in doubt. The location of the parasternal right ventricular impulse can sometimes be related to the level of obstruction, because the transmitted systolic movements originate in the high-pressure zone proximal to the stenosis. Presystolic distention of the right ventricle is caused by forceful contraction of the right atrium and is typically accompanied by a large jugular venous A wave.

An ejection sound is a characteristic feature of valvular pulmonic stenosis and serves an important function in identifying this form of obstruction. The pulmonic ejection sound is high pitched, sharp or clicking, and maximal in the second left interspace, often selectively decreasing during inspiration. An ejection sound is not present in valvular pulmonic stenosis caused by myxomatous dysplasia.

The systolic murmur of typical valvular pulmonic stenosis is maximal in the second left interspace, although it may be just as loud in the third. The lower location may be related to secondary subvalvular hypertrophy. The murmur, like the thrill, radiates upward and to the left, and when loud may be heard in the suprasternal notch and at the base of the neck, especially on the left. Loudness per se is not necessarily an index of severity, although as a rule intensity tends to vary directly with the degree of obstruction. However, the magnitude of obstruction is a major determinant of the *duration* of right ventricular ejection which, in turn, determines the *length* of the systolic murmur. A soft, symmetrical murmur, peaking late in systole and extending well beyond aortic closure, is a feature of severe obstruction.

The intensity of the pulmonic component of the second sound varies from normal to inaudible as severity increases. However, the *timing* of the pulmonic component is more important than intensity in assessing the degree of obstruction. A relatively slight increase in expiratory splitting, with normal intensity of the pulmonic component, is evidence of mild stenosis, whereas a marked increase in splitting with a faint or absent pulmonic component is evidence of severe obstruction.

The electrocardiogram commonly shows tall, peaked P waves. The QRS axis in the frontal plane shifts to the right, the degree of right axis deviation tending to vary directly with right ventricular pressure. The severity of pulmonic stenosis corresponds fairly well to the R/S ratios in V_1 and V_6 and to the height of the R wave in V_1. In mild pulmonic stenosis an rSr' pattern in V_1 is sometimes difficult to distinguish from normal. In severe pulmonic stenosis, leads V_1 and V_3R exhibit tall monophasic R waves, and lead V_6 shows an rS pattern. Between these extremes all gradations exist. In severe pulmonic stenosis, deeply inverted T waves that curve upward on the downstroke and that extend beyond V_2 are typical and assume greater significance when accompanied by ST segment depressions. Upright T waves occur with increased right ventricular pressure in young children, and upright T waves in the right precordium are the only electrocardiographic signs of right ventricular hypertension in some children with mild pulmonic stenosis.

The x-ray evaluation of valvular pulmonic stenosis should concentrate on (1) the peripheral (interpulmonary) vascular pattern, (2) the main pulmonary artery and its branches, and (3) the size and contour of the right ventricle and right atrium. The pulmonary vascular pattern is normal even in severe valvular stenosis until the output of the right ventricle falls. Poststenotic dilatation of the pulmonary trunk is characteristic and is often accompanied by conspicuous enlargement of the left branch. Poststenotic dilatation is not a feature of myxomatous dysplasia of the valve. Calcification of the congenitally stenosed pulmonary valve is rare, although examples have been reported. The left anterior oblique view is best for defining the contour of right ventricular enlargement even though a prominent right atrial sweep may be seen in the posteroanterior projection. A conspicuous increase in right heart size is almost always a sign of severity, especially at an early age. Cardiac catheterization and angiocardiography permit definitive diagnosis of the level, morphologic type, and severity of obstruction to right ventricular outflow. However, patients with typical trivial to mild valvular pulmonic stenosis can be identified with such clinical confidence that further diagnostic investigation is generally not required. But in this group, clinical distinction from idiopathic dilatation of the pulmonary trunk may be difficult or impossible.

In typical valvular pulmonic stenosis, surgical repair is probably indicated for all patients with resting gradients of 50 mm Hg or more, although a single determination may be misleading, because gradients vary considerably with cardiac output. The risk of operative repair in typical valvular pulmonic stenosis is low, and technical results are excellent. Postoperative pulmonary regurgitation often occurs, but as a rule it is mild and is a small price to pay. Occasionally, in very severe valvular pulmonic stenosis, secondary hypertrophic subpulmonic stenosis may require infundibular resection. This intervention is relatively uncommon, and its value is still debated; it should not be taken lightly, because right ventriculotomy is necessary.

ATRIAL SEPTAL DEFECT

Atrial defects are designated according to their sites in the septum: (1) in the region of the fossa ovalis (ostium secundum); (2) inferior to the fossa, i.e., between the fossa and the inferior vena cava; (3) in the upper part of the atrial septum (sinus venosus); (4) in the lower part of the septum (ostium primum); and (5) in the position normally occupied by the coronary sinus. The most common variety to be dealt with here is generally referred to as *ostium secundum defect.*

The physiologic consequences of an atrial septal defect depend chiefly upon the magnitude and duration of the shunt and upon the behavior of the pulmonary vascular bed. Two mechanisms have been proposed to explain the left to right shunt. First, in infancy the right and left ventricles have similar distensibility characteristics and hence should have similar end-diastolic volumes. As pulmonary vascular resistance falls in the neonatal period, the right ventricle ejects into a low resistance bed and would be expected to have a larger ejection fraction than the left. During the subsequent diastole the volume received by the right ventricle would increase, and a left to right shunt would therefore be established. Second, as the pulmonary arterioles involute, the relatively thick-walled neonatal right ventricle becomes thinner and offers less resistance to filling than the left. Conditions become appropriate for augmenting flow from left atrium across the defect. This may in part explain the relative infrequency of pulmonary hypertension in young people with atrial septal defect. Pulmonary hypertension is rare in infants and children with uncomplicated atrial septal defects and does not reach its peak incidence of about 14 per cent until early adult life.

In ostium secundum atrial septal defect the female-to-male ratio ranges from 2 to 3.5:1. Family history is important, because these defects not only can be familial, but also may recur through a number of generations.

Atrial septal defects often go unrecognized for years, because symptoms may be trivial or absent and physical signs subtle. The relatively soft pulmonic midsystolic murmur is easily overlooked in restless or crying children and may be mistaken for an innocent murmur in both children and young adults. In apparently healthy normal adults, atrial septal defect is often first suspected because of a routine chest x-ray. Life expectancy is shortened, although adult survival is the rule, and some may live to an advanced age. Survival is more limited in young adults who develop pulmonary hypertension, but even in them the span of life appears to average more than 40 years. It is not rare to find atrial septal defects in patients beyond age 70 years. Death may be unrelated to the defect; but when a relationship exists, cardiac failure is the most common natural cause. Since the natural history of uncomplicated ostium secundum atrial septal defect spans the childbearing age and since the majority of such patients are female, it is important to note that pregnancy is usually well tolerated. After the third or fourth decade, complications generally arise, and practically all patients who survive to the sixth decade are symptomatic. Effort dyspnea and fatigue are most frequent. Older patients with large left to right shunt atrial septal defects may experience not only effort dyspnea but also orthopnea. In the presence of decreased lung compliance caused by longstanding large left to right shunts, the work of breathing is greater in the supine than in the sitting position.

Infective endocarditis is rare in isolated ostium secundum atrial septal defect, a rarity attributed to the absence of jet lesions or turbulence because of low velocity flow across the interatrial communication.

Older patients with ostium secundum atrial septal defects deteriorate chiefly on two accounts. First, degenerative diseases such as coronary artery disease or systemic hypertension cause the left ventricle to become less distensible, so a larger volume of left atrial blood preferentially flows across the defect, adding to the work of an already overloaded right ventricle. The second problem is the advent of atrial arrhythmias—fibrillation, flutter, or paroxysmal atrial tachycardia. After the fourth decade atrial arrhythmias increase in frequency and represent one of the most serious complications.

Physical appearance of adults with ostium secundum atrial septal defect is generally normal, but children often exhibit delicate, frail, or gracile builds, with weight affected more than height. A left precordial bulge is common and is often associated with Harrison's grooves. A distinctive appearance that heightens suspicion of an ostium secundum atrial septal defect is the *Holt-Oram syndrome.* The thumb is hypoplastic, with an accessory phalanx that gives it a "crooked" appearance. Apposition of the thumb with other digits is difficult, and in some cases the thumb is rudimentary or absent.

The jugular venous pulse in ostium secundum atrial septal defect may show A and V waves of equal heights, because the two atria are in communication. Pulmonary hypertension results in an increased force of right atrial contraction and a dominant A wave which may reach giant proportions.

Precordial movement and palpation characteristically detect a right ventricular impulse that is hyperdynamic and relatively brief in duration. This pattern occurs because the left to right shunt distends the right ventricle in diastole, and the chamber then contracts vigorously into a low resistance pulmonary bed. The dilated pulmonary trunk is often palpable in the second left interspace. A systolic thrill in the second left interspace indicates either a very large shunt or coexisting valvular pulmonic stenosis. In the presence of pulmonary hypertension, the right ventricular impulse becomes sustained and less dynamic, and presystolic distention may result from an increased force of right atrial contraction.

The "first heart sound" at the left sternal edge and apex may be split and the *second component* relatively loud. It has been variously proposed that the loud second component originates in the tricuspid valve or represents a pulmonic ejection sound. The location favors the former, although the two mechanisms may coexist. The typical murmur of atrial septal defect results from rapid ejection of a large right ventricular stroke volume into a dilated pulmonary trunk. The murmur is usually Grade 3 or less, maximal in the second left intercostal space, beginning after the first heart sound, crescendo-decrescendo in shape, peaking in early or midsystole, and ending well before both components of the second heart sound. The septal defect itself is, with rare exception, acoustically silent. A murmur exceeding Grade 3 is likely to mean an unusually large shunt or associated valvular pulmonic stenosis. In slightly built patients, widely distributed thoracic systolic murmurs can sometimes be heard in the right chest, axilla, and back because of rapid flow through peripheral pulmonary arteries in low resistance, high-flow atrial septal defects.

A hallmark of atrial septal defect is the behavior of the second heart sound. The aortic and pulmonic components are widely and persistently split and exhibit little or no change in the degree of splitting with respiration or Valsalva's maneuver. The relative loudness of the two components is usually normal, although at times the second component is increased despite little or no pulmonary hypertension. Proximity of the dilated pulmonary trunk to the chest wall and the brisk elastic recoil of the distended pulmonary trunk may account for this.

Two types of diastolic murmurs occur in atrial septal defect with left to right shunt. One is mid-diastolic and is caused by torrential flow across the tricuspid valve, indicating a sizable left to right shunt. The second diastolic murmur is rare and is due to pulmonary regurgitation in the absence of pulmonary hypertension; a very large pulmonary trunk is probably responsible.

Atrial septal defect with pulmonary hypertension exhibits auscultatory signs that differ considerably from the foregoing. The pulmonic midsystolic flow murmur is replaced by a softer, shorter midsystolic murmur caused by ejection of a normal stroke volume into a dilated pulmonary trunk. Tricuspid flow murmurs vanish. Typical pulmonic ejection sounds appear, especially in the second left interspace, and exhibit characteristic respiratory variation in intensity. The pulmonic component of the second heart sound becomes progressively louder, although fixed splitting persists as long as a significant left to right shunt exists. With abolition or reversal of the shunt, the pulmonic component becomes very loud, and the wide fixed split disappears. A *Graham Steell murmur* may develop. The holosystolic murmur of tricuspid regurgitation appears when the pressure load of pulmonary hypertension results in right ventricular failure. Since the right ventricle occupies the apex in atrial septal defect, the tricuspid murmur is heard at that site and mistaken for the murmur of mitral regurgitation.

After the third decade *atrial arrhythmias* increase, with atrial fibrillation the most common, but atrial flutter and paroxysmal atrial tachycardia also occur. When right atrial P waves are present, they generally manifest themselves by peaking in lead II rather than by an increase in amplitude. The QRS duration is usually upper limits of normal with a tendency to increase with age. As QRS duration increases, the pattern resembles complete right bundle branch block, but this rarely develops before the fourth decade. Depolarization is typically clockwise, with q waves in inferior leads and a vertical QRS axis. These electrical directions are important, because they distinguish ostium secundum defects from ostium primum defects in which the axis is directed upward and to the left and depolarization is counterclockwise (see below).

An electrocardiographic sign of atrial septal defect is the rSr′ complex in right precordial leads. This feature is believed to stem from localized hypertrophy of the crista supraventricularis, depolarization of which causes the terminal electrical forces to be directed superiorly, to the right, and anteriorly. These terminal force patterns do not result from interference of electrical impulses through the right bundle branch. In fact, the sequence of ventricular activation is normal, so the term "incomplete right bundle branch block" is inappropriate. With the advent of pulmonary hypertension, the right ventricular free wall thickens and lead V_1 exhibits an increase in the amplitude of the R′ wave together with a gradual decrease in the depth of the S wave.

The *chest x-ray,* especially in postadolescents and adults, is often distinctive. The lung fields show increased pulmonary arterial vascularity that generally extends to the periphery. The combination of a small aorta and a markedly dilated pulmonary trunk with disproportionate enlargement of the right branch can be striking. With the advent of pulmonary hypertension, peripheral pulmonary vascularity is replaced by relatively clear lung fields, the pulmonary trunk and its proximal branches get still larger, and the right branch presents as a huge inverted comma with an abrupt cutoff that makes the contrast between the large central vessels and the clear lung field stand out in bold relief. In an occasional older subject, the main pulmonary artery and its branches dilate aneurysmally and calcify.

Right atrial enlargement is ordinarily seen as a rightward convexity in the posteroanterior projection. Although radiographic signs of left atrial enlargement are occasionally found in adults, this is rarely so in children. Dilatation of the right ventricle is an expected feature, resulting in a convex lifted apex that usually forms an acute angle with the diaphragm. Dilatation of the outflow tract sometimes causes relatively smooth continuity or even a hump-shaped appearance below the enlarged pulmonary trunk. In the left oblique projection the right ventricle casts a rather typical convex anterior shadow.

Although uncomplicated ostium secundum atrial septal defect in the young is among the most easily diagnosed congenital malformations of the heart, the same anomaly may be most misleading in some adults. Mitral stenosis with pulmonary hypertension comes under suspicion because of dyspnea, orthopnea, atrial fibrillation, an increased V wave in the jugular venous pulse, a right ventricular impulse, a loud first heart sound, a delayed pulmonic component of the second sound that is mistaken for an opening snap, a tricuspid flow murmur mistaken for a mitral diastolic murmur, vascular peripheral lung fields believed to represent pulmonary venous congestion, and a cardiac silhouette that exhibits dilatation of the pulmonary trunk and occasionally of both right and left atria. Similarly, mitral regurgitation may be suspected because the holosystolic murmur of tricuspid regurgitation is heard at the apex which is occupied by the right ventricle. A delayed pulmonic component of the second sound followed by a tricuspid flow murmur may be mistaken for the opening snap and the mid-diastolic murmur of coexisting mitral stenosis. In older subjects, coronary artery disease, systemic hypertension, atrial arrhythmias, or inverted left precordial T waves may cloud the issue. A catalogue of these misleading clinical points makes impressive reading, but it is rare to be confronted with all of them at once. However, even when the entire clinical picture is considered, the correct diagnosis may remain uncertain, although clues generally emerge to provide the background for an intelligently planned laboratory study.

Echocardiography has been a major step forward in the noninvasive diagnosis of atrial septal defect, defining not only the expected large right ventricular dimensions but, more important, the paradoxical motion of the interventricular septum. Normally, the interventricular septum moves *away* from the anterior chest wall during systole, behaving as part of the left ventricle. In ostium secundum atrial septal defect (volume overload of the right ventricle), the septum moves *toward* the anterior chest wall in systole, functioning as part of the right ventricle.

Cardiac catheterization is generally employed even in patients in whom the clinical diagnosis is not in doubt. Such an intervention provides precise preoperative quantitative data that set the stage for comparative postoperative assessment. In addition to quantification of the shunt and confirmation of intracardiac pressures, there are a number of other reasons why cardiac catheterization is undertaken. An attempt should be made to separate ostium secundum from sinus venosus atrial septal defects which clinically are usually indistinguishable. Patients with pure ostium secundum atrial septal defects sometimes exhibit mitral leaflet prolapse—especially posterior—analogous to the systolic click—late systolic murmur syndrome. This movement can be detected by left ventricular angiography or echocardiography and need not be accompanied by auscultatory signs. Theoretically, such patients are at risk of infective endocarditis whether the atrial septal defect is repaired or not.

Patients with high flow, low resistance uncomplicated ostium secundum atrial septal defect (pulmonary to systemic flow ratios of at least 2:1) should be electively repaired, optimally in childhood. At this age, surgical risk is minimal, and delay always gives rise to concern over postoperative residua, especially resolution of dilatation and hypertrophy of the right ventricle. There has been some debate regarding surgical correction in older patients (beyond age 40), but current experience has shown that patients in the fifth, sixth, or even seventh decades with relatively low resistance–high flow ostium secundum atrial septal defects benefit from surgical repair which can be undertaken at comparatively low risk. What is still more encouraging is that older patients benefit at an acceptable risk despite the presence of moderate pulmonary hypertension and cardiac failure, provided there is still a sizable left to right shunt. In an occasional patient, irrespective of age, in whom pulmonary resistance has reached or exceeded systemic so that the left to right shunt has been abolished, operative repair is contraindicated.

PATENT DUCTUS ARTERIOSUS

Patent ductus arteriosus represents persistence of the normal fetal vascular channel between the pulmonary artery and the aorta. The pulmonary orifice of the ductus is located immediately to the left of the bifurcation of the pulmonary trunk. The aortic end of the duct usually arises just beyond the origin of the left subclavian artery. A patent ductus is apt to be largest at its aortic insertion, exhibiting the shape of a truncated cone, because the tendency to close begins at the pulmonary arterial end. The ductus arteriosus in full-term infants normally undergoes an initial stage of *functional* closure, followed by a later stage of *anatomic* closure. At the end of a week the ductus is generally no more than probe patent, and by four to eight weeks anatomic closure is usually established.

The physiologic consequences of persistent patency of the ductus arteriosus depend upon the size of the communication and the level of pulmonary vascular resistance. When the ductus is small, the pulmonary arterial pressure remains normal; the left to right shunt and hemodynamic burden are insignificant despite continuous aortic to pulmonary flow across the ductus. When the duct is large, aortic pressure is transmitted directly into the pulmonary trunk, so pulmonary hypertension exists with pressure overload of the right ventricle. Under these circumstances the direction of flow through the ductus depends upon the relative resistances in the pulmonary and systemic beds. If the pulmonary resistance is appreciably lower than systemic, a sizable left to right shunt exists, with volume overload of the left heart together with pressure overload of the right. If the pulmonary resistance is appreciably higher than systemic, left to right flow through the ductus is abolished, leaving a pure right to left shunt and pure pressure overload of the right ventricle. The vast majority of patients with isolated patent ductus arteriosus, literally 95 per cent, have left to right shunts with pulmonary arterial pressures considerably below systemic. Only 5 to 7 per cent have very high pulmonary vascular resistances with exclusive right to left shunts.

For all practical purposes the history in patent ductus arteriosus does not begin at birth, because the diagnosis is not entertained in the newborn nursery. The mother is likely to report that her infant was examined as a newborn and pronounced normal. As the neonatal pulmonary vascular resistance falls, a left to right shunt is established, the ductus murmur emerges, and the diagnosis becomes apparent. Patent ductus arteriosus predominates in females, with a sex ratio as high as 3:1. The female preponderance is even greater in older patients with this anomaly. Family history is important, because patent ductus tends to recur in siblings. The prenatal history also deserves comment, especially regarding maternal rubella in the first trimester. Patent ductus arteriosus (together with pulmonary artery stenosis) is the most common congenital cardiac defect in the offspring of mothers who have had rubella in the first trimester. Birth weight in uncomplicated patent ductus is normal but in the rubella syndrome low birth rate is common, and there is failure to thrive even though the shunt is small and cardiac failure absent. Another interesting point in the history is the *altitude* at which the patient is born. It has been estimated that persistence of the ductus arteriosus is six times as frequent in patients born at high altitudes as in those born at sea level, and there is a tendency for such patients to develop pulmonary hypertension. The physical appearance in patent ductus may be one of underdevelopment, owing to a large shunt, cardiac failure, and recurrent respiratory infections. In addition, maternal rubella results not only in patent ductus and low birth weights, but also in poor growth irrespective of the size of the duct. Differential cyanosis and clubbing occur when pulmonary vascular resistance exceeds systemic so that unoxygenated pulmonary arterial blood flows through the ductus and enters the aorta distal to the left subclavian artery; this unoxygenated blood goes to the lower body so that the toes will be cyanosed and often clubbed.

A wide pulse pressure is an important physical sign of patent ductus with large left to right shunt. Diastolic flow from aortic root into pulmonary artery lowers the aortic diastolic pressure, whereas the large left ventricular stroke volume caused by the left to right shunt results in elevation of aortic systolic pressure.

Precordial impulses are normal with small patent ductus. A moderately large ductus causes isolated volume overload of the left heart; the left ventricular impulse is moderately dynamic, the right ventricular impulse is unimpressive, and a continuous thrill with systolic accentuation is present in the first or second left intercostal space. A large ductus with appreciable left to right shunt results in marked volume overload of the left ventricle with pulmonary hypertension; the left ventricular impulse is hyperdynamic, and a heaving right ventricular impulse appears. If a thrill is present, it is more likely to be systolic. When flow through the ductus is reversed, pulmonary hypertension exists without volume overload of the left ventricle. Palpation detects a right ventricular and pulmonary arterial impulse, a loud pulmonic component of the second sound, but the ductus thrill is absent and a left ventricular impulse is trivial or absent.

Auscultation is virtually diagnostic when the classic murmur of uncomplicated patent ductus arteriosus rises to a peak in latter systole, continues without interruption through the second sound, and then declines in intensity during the course of diastole. High velocity flow through a small duct results in a relatively soft high-frequency continuous murmur. The larger ductus is likely to cause a loud, noisy "machinery" murmur, accentuated in latter systole and punctuated with "eddy" sounds. The ductus murmur is typically loudest in the first or second intercostal space or just beneath the left clavicle. With progressive elevations in pulmonary vascular resistance, the classic murmur is shortened, always beginning with the diastolic portion, and is finally abolished, to be replaced by auscultatory and phonocardiographic signs of pulmonary hypertension per se. Such patients present with a pulmonic ejection sound, a short pulmonic midsystolic murmur, a single or closely split second heart sound, and a loud pulmonic component of the second sound followed by the Graham Steell murmur of pulmonary regurgitation. Under these circumstances the diagnosis of patent ductus arteriosus cannot be made on auscultatory grounds. Differential cyanosis may be the key.

The electrocardiogram can be entirely normal when the ductus is small. Variations from normal depend upon the degree and duration of volume overload of the left heart and pressure overload of the right.

In the x-ray, the ductus can sometimes be seen in the frontal projection as a separate convexity between the aortic knuckle and the pulmonary trunk. In older patients calcium is occasionally identified in the ductus; this should be sought in the frontal, left oblique, and lateral projections. A large left to right shunt *without* appreciable pulmonary hypertension results in varying degrees of pulmonary plethora while the pulmonary trunk and its branches increase in size. The ascending aorta is normal in infants but tends to enlarge in older children or adults. Volume overload of the left heart results in left ventricular dilatation and left atrial enlargement. The increase in left atrial size is usually mild to moderate but can occasionally be marked. Right atrial and right ventricular dilatation develop when pulmonary arterial pressure is elevated in patent ductus with left to right shunt. In infants and young children, a sizable patent ductus arteriosus with left to right shunt and pulmonary hypertension is often associated with congestive heart failure and appreciable cardiomegaly; all four chambers contribute to the cardiac silhouette.

When flow through the ductus is reversed (suprasystemic pulmonary vascular resistance), a different radiologic picture emerges. The left ventricle and the left atrium are normal in size, and the right ventricle is hypertrophied but not conspicuously dilated. The pulmonary trunk and its main branches enlarge, but the ascending aorta tends to be normal, and the peripheral pulmonary vasculature is normal or reduced.

The typical patient with uncomplicated patent ductus in childhood, adolescence, or early adult life can be confidently diagnosed clinically and does not, as a rule, require cardiac catheterization for preoperative confirmation. However, the sick infant with congestive heart failure and large left to right shunt should be investigated preoperatively, not only to confirm the clinical suspicion of patent ductus but also to determine the presence or absence of coexisting anomalies, especially ventricular septal defect. Also requiring diagnostic investigation are those patients (generally postadolescent) with increased pulmonary vascular resistance, in whom the degree of left to right shunt must be firmly established before division of the ductus is recommended.

For all practical purposes typical patent ductus presenting in childhood is uniformly corrected by surgical division. A number of variations in therapeutic judgment are required, however. Since persistent patency of the ductus with *delayed* spontaneous closure is frequent in premature infants, there is a tendency to delay surgery in such patients because of the prospect of spontaneous closure within several months. On the other hand, large patent ductus is a relatively common cause of congestive heart failure in acyanotic infants, and generally requires operative intervention which may take the form of ligation rather than division. After the first year of life most patients with patent ductus are asymptomatic. Division of the ductus in such patients not only carries a low risk but also results in complete anatomic and physiologic correction. The tendency to wait until the child is at least five years old has been modified in most centers so that the disorder in younger children is now corrected. The adult poses a more complex problem. The simplest decisions in the adult group are in patients—generally women—with large left to right shunt, relatively low resistance patent ductus in which the duct is not calcified. These should be surgically divided once the diagnosis is established. Calcification of the patent ductus increases the risk, but, if the shunt is large, operation is still advisable. When pulmonary resistance has exceeded systemic, abolishing the left to right shunt, patients are inoperable. A difficult decision occurs in the occasional adult with a very small patent ductus that is hemodynamically insignificant. The question is a comparison of the risk of infective endocarditis as opposed to the risk of surgery. Each case requires individual judgment. If there has been a previous episode of infective endocarditis and the patient expresses concern regarding recurrence, surgical correction should be advised. If there has been no previous episode of infective endocarditis and the patient is reluctant to undergo thoracotomy, operation should be deferred.

VENTRICULAR SEPTAL DEFECT WITH PULMONIC STENOSIS
(Fallot's Tetralogy)

This combination encompasses a wide anatomic, physiologic, and clinical spectrum. Two elements of the tetralogy are of prime importance, namely, pulmonic stenosis and large ventricular septal defect with right ventricular pressure at systemic levels. Large ventricular septal defect with mild to moderate pulmonic stenosis is looked upon as *acyanotic* Fallot's tetralogy; large ventricular septal defect with severe pulmonic stenosis and right to left shunt as *classic cyanotic Fallot's tetralogy;* and large ventricular septal defect with complete pulmonic stenosis as *Fallot's tetralogy with pulmonary atresia.* It is wise to remain flexible, however, and use appropriate *anatomic* designations instead of, or coupled with, the eponym, to serve the cause of clarity.

In classic cyanotic Fallot's tetralogy, a *large* ventricular septal defect approximates the size of the aortic orifice. The aorta may be entirely left ventricular in origin, or biventricular to varying degrees, but the aortic wall maintains anatomic continuity with the anterior mitral leaflet. Pulmonic stenosis can be located in the pulmonary trunk, pulmonary valve, infundibulum, or subinfundibular zone, although typically the obstruction is infundibular. Pulmonary atresia can be viewed as the ultimate expression of pulmonic stenosis and therefore the most severe form of Fallot's tetralogy. With pulmonary atresia, the pulmonary circulation is supplied chiefly by large bronchial collateral arteries.

The degree of obstruction to right ventricular outflow does not always remain constant but may progress with the passage of time. When life expectancy is prolonged by an anastomotic operation, the patient may develop progressive narrowing of the zone of stenosis until complete closure (atresia). Furthermore, infundibular stenosis can progress sufficiently to reverse the interventricular shunt. Accordingly, a single patient may exhibit a broad spectrum of severity ranging from mild stenosis with large left to right shunt to marked obstruction with reversed shunt.

A number of *additional congenital cardiac malformations* have a tendency to occur in patients with Fallot's tetralogy: (1) right aortic arch, (2) persistent left superior vena cava, (3) hypoplasia, stenosis, or absence of a pulmonary artery, (4) absence of the pulmonary valve, (5) incompetence of the aortic valve, and (6) a coronary arterial anomaly consisting of right coronary arterial origin of the left anterior descending coronary artery.

The *physiologic consequences* depend upon three variables, namely, the degree of pulmonic stenosis, the size of the interventricular communication, and, to a lesser extent, the systemic vascular resistance. These variables can best be understood by beginning with the idea of a large ventricular septal defect upon which increasing degrees of pulmonic stenosis are imposed. When the stenosis is mild, the shunt is entirely left to right, and the condition closely resembles large isolated ventricular septal defect with increased pulmonary blood flow and volume overload of the left heart. As the degree of obstruction increases, the left to right shunt diminishes. When the resistance offered by the obstruction equals systemic resistance, the shunt is balanced. As the stenosis increases still further, a right to left shunt is established, because it becomes easier for the right ventricle to eject into the aorta than into the pulmonary trunk. Since right ventricular blood under these circumstances preferentially enters the aorta, blood flow through the lungs is reduced and the left heart underfilled. When the stenosis is complete (pulmonary atresia), the entire right ventricular output is ejected through the ventricular septal defect into the aorta. No matter how severe the pulmonic stenosis, the right ventricle decompresses into the aorta via the large ventricular septal defect, so right ventricular systolic pressure does not exceed systemic. The magnitude of right ventricular systolic overload is then determined by *aortic* pressure.

The *history in typical Fallot's tetralogy* generally dates from the neonatal period because of detection of a murmur or cyanosis. Arterial unsaturation is usually obvious by three to six months. When an infant is born with very severe pulmonic stenosis or atresia, cyanosis dates from birth, and the murmur is relatively inconspicuous. A history of *squatting for relief of dyspnea* has long been a hallmark of Fallot's tetralogy. In addition, Taussig clearly described the preference for certain other postures, such as the knee-chest position, sitting with the legs drawn underneath, or lying down. A history of right ventricular failure is rare in classic Fallot's tetralogy. The neonatal right ventricle is well equipped to pump at systemic pressures, and is seldom called upon to do more, because the ventricular septal defect permits direct decompression into the aorta. A number of other complications may occur in the natural history, such as recurrent cerebral hypoxia that can lead to brain damage and mental retardation, cerebral venous sinus thromboses, cerebral embolism, or brain abscess. Death from brain abscess is twice as frequent in cyanotic Fallot's tetralogy as in any other form of congenital cardiac disease. Infective endocarditis sometimes occurs on the zone of pulmonic stenosis. There are two chief determinants of long survival: a moderate degree of pulmonic stenosis that permits adequate but not excessive pulmonary blood flow with little or no cyanosis, and pulmonary stenosis that evolves gradually enough to permit the formation of a well developed collateral circulation.

After age four, most cyanotic children with congenital heart disease have Fallot's tetralogy. This malformation is also present in the largest number of *cyanotic adults* with congenital heart disease.

The physical appearance of the majority of patients with either classic cyanotic Fallot's tetralogy or pulmonary atresia reflects small size and physical underdevelopment. When Fallot's tetralogy occurs with little or no cyanosis, the physical appearance is generally normal.

Knowledge of the brachial arterial systolic pressure allows an accurate bedside estimate of the gradient in cyanotic Fallot's tetralogy. Since right ventricular systolic pressure is the same as systemic, the gradient across the zone of stenosis is simply the difference between the brachial arterial systolic pressure and the estimated pulmonary arterial systolic pressure (15 to 25 mm Hg).

The jugular venous pulse in classic cyanotic Fallot's tetralogy is seldom elevated, and the A wave is normal or nearly so, because the right ventricle maintains its neonatal capability of ejecting at systemic pressures without extra help from its atrium.

Precordial movement and palpation in classic Fallot's tetralogy detect a right ventricular systolic impulse that is quiet and usually located inferior to the third left intercostal space because of the stenosed infundibulum. The right ventricle ejects at systemic pressures without an appreciable increase in the vigor of contraction and without dilating. In cyanotic Fallot's tetralogy, especially in the presence of pulmonary atresia, a right aortic arch is relatively frequent, and its pulsation can be detected at the right sternoclavicular junction.

The auscultatory signs mirror the pathologic physiology of cyanotic Fallot's tetralogy. The incidence of aortic ejection sounds varies inversely with the degree of obstruction; the more hypoplastic the pulmonary trunk, the larger the aortic root. The systolic murmur in cyanotic Fallot's tetralogy originates at the zone of stenosis and not across the ventricular septal defect. The murmur tends to be maximal in the third left interspace, because obstruction is usually infundibular. The length and loudness of the murmur (and accompanying thrill) are of considerable importance in estimating the severity of obstruction. A loud, long murmur extending up to the aortic component of the second sound means that an appreciable amount of blood is being ejected into the pulmonary trunk. As resistance at the zone of stenosis rises, there is an increase in the right to left shunt and a reciprocal fall in pulmonary blood flow; the murmur gets shorter and softer. When obstruction is complete (pulmonary atresia), the pulmonic stenotic murmur vanishes altogether and is replaced by a soft midsystolic murmur caused by ejection into the dilated aorta. A continuous murmur is an auscultatory sign of pulmonary atresia because of flow through bronchial collateral circulation. The pulmonic component of the second heart sound is typically inaudible in cyanotic Fallot's tetralogy and pulmonary atresia, but when cyanosis is mild or absent a soft delayed sound can sometimes be detected. When a large ventricular septal defect is associated with mild pulmonic stenosis, the auscultatory signs resemble those of uncomplicated ventricular septal defect, although the murmur tends to have midsystolic accentuation (a combination of the ventricular septal defect and pulmonic stenotic murmurs) and there is likely to be moderately wide splitting of the second heart sound.

The *electrocardiogram* is another useful index of the physiologic spectrum encompassed by ventricular septal defect with pulmonic stenosis. Since the force of right atrial contraction is not appreciably increased, P waves of right atrial enlargement are absent about half the time. The mean QRS axis in the frontal plane is rarely to the right of 150 degrees so that right axis deviation takes the form of a dominant S wave in lead I but dominant R waves in leads II and III. In the precordial leads, a tall monophasic R wave is usually confined to lead V_1 with rS complexes in the remaining chest leads. In the left precordial leads, q waves are conspicuous by their absence in classic cyanotic Fallot's tetralogy, because the left ventricle is underfilled. When the shunt is balanced, right ventricular pressure remains at systemic levels, so the electrocardiogram continues to exhibit right ventricular hypertrophy as described. However, the left heart is no longer underfilled, so left precordial leads exhibit well developed R waves and small q waves. When a large ventricular septal defect appears with mild pulmonic stenosis, the electrocardiogram resembles that of isolated ventricular septal defect with right ventricular hypertension.

The *x-ray* in ventricular septal defect with pulmonic stenosis shows vascular markings that are normal or increased when a large defect exists with a balanced or left to right shunt. More severe obstruction to right ventricular outflow diverts more right ventricular blood into the aorta, so that pulmonary blood flow falls and lung vascularity diminishes. In adults, these oligemic lungs may have an emphysematous appearance. In cyanotic Fallot's tetralogy the pulmonary artery segment is characteristically represented by a *concavity*. The aortic arch size varies inversely with the pulmonary trunk. In pulmonary atresia the aorta receives the entire output from both ventricles, so the rightward sweep and knuckle are especially prominent. A right aortic arch occurs in 20 to 30 per cent of patients with cyanotic Fallot's tetralogy, the incidence increasing with the severity of pulmonic stenosis, so that a right arch is most frequent with pulmonary atresia. In typical cyanotic Fallot's tetralogy the left atrium and left ventricle are normal or small because the left heart is underfilled; the right atrium and right ventricle cope with systemic pressures without dilating, so the cardiac size is normal or nearly so. In pulmonary atresia, however, the cardiac silhouette tends to be larger, especially in older subjects. The configuration of the heart has long been a subject of interest in cyanotic Fallot's tetralogy because of the distinctive boot-shaped appearance caused by a combination of concentric hypertrophy of the right ventricle, an abnormally small left ventricle, a relatively horizontal ventricular septum, and a concave pulmonary artery segment. In Fallot's tetralogy with little or no cyanosis (balanced or bidirectional shunt), the right ventricle remains concentrically hypertrophied, but the left ventricle is not underfilled. The cardiac apex is more likely to be smooth and rounded. When a large ventricular septal defect exists with mild pulmonic stenosis, the x-ray in many ways resembles that of large isolated ventricular septal defect except that the size of the pulmonary trunk may be comparatively small.

The *echocardiogram* serves a useful purpose in identifying continuity between posterior aortic wall and the anterior mitral leaflet, confirming Fallot's tetralogy rather than right ventricular origin of both great arteries. Cardiac catheterization and angiocardiography are important in characterizing the morphology of the right ventricular outflow tract, in identifying the location of the ventricular septal defect, and in ruling out right ventricular origin of both great arteries. Intracardiac repair is technically a lesser problem in the patient with large ventricular septal defect, left ventricular aorta, and acquired pulmonic stenosis, even if the stenosis is severe enough to have reversed the shunt.

Large ventricular septal defect with biventricular aorta and hypoplastic right ventricular outflow tract is far more difficult to repair (classic cyanotic Fallot's tetralogy). Primary intracardiac repair (total correction) is the treatment of choice and can be accomplished even in infancy. Nevertheless, shunt operations (Waterston or Blalock) are appropriately applied in cyanotic symptomatic infants, especially those less than one year old. A previous shunt operation does not materially add to the risk of complete repair. After age five and certainly after age eight, complete repair should be employed, with few exceptions. Similarly, total correction can be undertaken in adults without anticipation of significantly greater operative mortality. Postoperative "complete right bundle branch" is expected after right ventriculotomy. The long-term effects of a patch for relief of outflow obstruction are still to be assessed.

553. UNCOMMON CONGENITAL CARDIAC DEFECTS IN WHICH POSTPEDIATRIC SURVIVAL IS EXPECTED

Situs Inversus. The term "situs inversus" refers to an organ arrangement the reverse of normal (mirror image dextrocardia). Situs inversus is often accidentally discovered on a routine chest x-ray or physical examination, because the malposition is likely to occur with an otherwise normal heart. Such patients experience normal longevity and hence fall into age groups that are susceptible to acquired cardiac disease. Pain of myocardial infarction may be referred to the *right* chest and pain of acute appendicitis to the *left* lower quadrant. Palpation and percussion identify the cardiac apex and stomach on the right and the liver on the left; the left ventricular impulse forms the apex. The heart sounds are louder in the right chest, and splitting of the second sound is detected in the second right intercostal space. The electrocardiogram shows negative P, QRS, and T waves in lead I; the complexes in lead aVR and aVL are the reverse of normal, and right precordial leads resemble those normally recorded from the left chest. The x-rays are the exact mirror image of normal, so that the reader must identify the symbols on the film that designate left and right. The aortic arch and stomach bubble are on the right, together with the cardiac apex.

Dextroversion of the Heart. This term applies when thoracic and abdominal viscera are in normal position but the cardiac *apex* is on the *right* (right thoracic heart). In early fetal life the cardiac apex begins on the side opposite to that which it ultimately occupies. When the apex remains on the right while the aortic arch, left atrium, and stomach are in their normal left-sided positions, the term "dextroversion" is used. Dextroversion of the heart is likely to be detected because of other congenital cardiac anomalies which almost invariably coexist. The most common of these are congenitally corrected transposition of the great arteries (see below), pulmonic stenosis, and ventricular or atrial septal defect. Palpation and percussion identify the cardiac apex and liver on the right with the stomach on the left (normal abdominal situs with right thoracic heart). Heart sounds and murmurs are louder on the right. The electrocardiogram shows upright P waves in lead I, because the atrial situs is normal. Prominent R waves or RS complexes are recorded from the right chest, whereas the left chest leads exhibit small septal q waves and small r waves. The x-ray shows the aortic arch and stomach bubble on the left but the apex on the right; the heart retains its peculiar silhouette whether or not the film is reversed.

Congenital Complete Heart Block. This is a straightforward diagnosis by electrocardiogram. The AV block is likely to be congenital if the slow heart rate existed from infancy (or in utero) and if the QRS configuration exhibits a "supraventricular configuration," i.e., a normal sequence of ventricular excitation. If liberal use were made of the electrocardiogram in infants and children with inappropriately slow heart rates, few cases of congenital heart block would be missed. The conduction defect is generally discovered accidentally in otherwise healthy asymptomatic children, or an alert obstetrician may detect a slow fetal heart rate. The arterial pulse is inappropriately slow for age, the upstroke brisk, the pulse pressure wide, and the rhythm regular. The jugular venous pulse shows intermittent "cannon waves" (right atrial contraction against a closed tricuspid valve), with independent A waves occurring at rates faster than the carotid pulse. The left ventricular impulse is dynamic (large stroke volume). The first heart sound varies in intensity from booming to soft, and there are short midsystolic basal flow murmurs, soft intermittent

fourth heart sounds, and intermittent summation sounds. The x-ray may show mild cardiac enlargement related to increased diastolic filling (slow heart rate). The slow rate, regular rhythm, intermittent cannon waves, and variation in intensity in the first heart sound are a diagnostic combination.

Congenitally Corrected Transposition of the Great Arteries. In this anomaly there is a right to left interchange of the ventricles and their respective AV valves. Right atrial blood flows across an AV valve that is morphologically mitral into a venous ventricle that is morphologically left, and then into the pulmonary trunk. Left atrial blood flows across an AV valve that is morphologically tricuspid into an arterial ventricle that is morphologically right, and then into the aorta. Since the pulmonary trunk springs from an anatomic left ventricle and the aorta from an anatomic right ventricle, the term "transposition of the great arteries" is appropriate. Since right atrial blood finds its way into the pulmonary trunk (across a mitral valve and through an anatomic left ventricle) and since left atrial blood finds its way into the aorta (across an anatomic tricuspid valve and through an anatomic right ventricle), the "transposition" can be considered "congenitally corrected." Hemodynamic consequences of congenitally corrected transposition depend chiefly upon the presence of *associated defects,* the most common of which are (1) incompetence of the left AV valve which is tricuspid and deformed by Ebstein's anomaly (see below), (2) ventricular septal defect, and (3) disturbances in AV conduction. Theoretically, *uncomplicated* congenitally corrected transposition (a rarity) should cause little or no physiologic disturbance. However, even when the malformation is uncomplicated, "spontaneous" failure of the systemic ventricle tends to occur before the fourth decade, although a few patients live longer. The unanswered question is the durability of an anatomic right ventricle as a systemic pump, i.e., whether a right ventricle subjected to systemic work loads will fail for that reason alone.

Idiopathic Dilatation of the Pulmonary Trunk. The malformation is characterized by congenital dilatation of the main pulmonary artery and occasionally its branches in the absence of anatomic or physiologic cause. Patients are asymptomatic, and physical appearance, arterial pulse, and jugular venous pulse are entirely normal. Palpation of the precordium may detect a pulmonary arterial impulse but no right ventricular impulse. Auscultation detects a characteristic pulmonic ejection sound that introduces a soft, short pulmonic midsystolic murmur and generally normal splitting of the second heart sound. The electrocardiogram is normal. The chest x-ray is also normal except for a conspicuous convexity caused by the dilated pulmonary trunk.

Congenital Discrete Subvalvular Aortic Stenosis. Discrete subvalvular aortic stenosis is usually characterized by a circumferential fibrous collar that encircles the left ventricular outflow tract and attaches to both the ventricular septum and the anterior mitral leaflet. The fibrous collar is located so close to the aortic leaflets that they may be mildly incompetent. The arterial pulse is similar to that of valvular aortic stenosis. The systolic thrill is maximal in the first or second right interspace with radiation into the neck. The left ventricular impulse is sustained, and presystolic distention with an accompanying fourth heart sound may be present. *An aortic ejection sound is typically absent.* The midsystolic stenotic *murmur* is rough and noisy, and its location and radiation correspond to the thrill. The sound of aortic valve closure is normal or reduced; a soft early diastolic murmur of aortic regurgitation is relatively common. The electrocardiogram is indistinguishable from other forms of discrete aortic stenosis. In the x-ray, the ascending aorta is usually normal, although slight to moderate dilatation may occur.

Precise characterization of the level and degree of obstruction requires cardiac catheterization and angiocardiography. Echocardiography sometimes detects relatively normal systolic opening of at least two leaflets. Discrete subvalvular aortic stenosis is amenable to direct surgical repair, although it should be remembered that the aortic leaflets are often distorted and that care must be taken not to damage the anterior mitral leaflet to which the subvalvular fibrous collar is attached.

Supravalvular Aortic Stenosis. This malformation is characterized by a segmental hourglass-shaped narrowing immediately above the aortic sinuses. Occasionally there is tubular hypoplasia of the ascending aorta. Associated mental retardation is presumptive evidence that the aortic stenosis is supravalvular. Under these circumstances stenosis of the pulmonary artery and its branches almost always coexists. Physical appearance is sometimes sufficiently typical to permit these diagnoses to be entertained at a glance: small chin, large mouth, malformed teeth, abnormal bite, and retarded growth. The brachial and carotid arterial pulses are sometimes asymmetrical, with the pulse pressure and rate of rise conspicuously greater on the right. The left ventricular impulse is similar to other forms of discrete aortic stenosis. An aortic ejection sound is typically absent, and the midsystolic stenotic murmur tends to be more conspicuous in the first right intercostal space with disproportionate radiation to the right neck. The aortic component of the second sound is normal or soft, and the murmur of aortic regurgitation is rare. The electrocardiogram is similar to those of valvular or discrete subvalvular aortic stenosis. The x-rays are distinguished by one chief feature—not only is poststenotic dilatation of the aorta absent but the ascending aorta is usually undersized. Precise diagnosis of morphology and severity requires cardiac catheterization and angiocardiography. Surgical repair, although possible, is difficult and at times untenable, especially with tubular hypoplasia of the ascending aorta.

Subvalvular Pulmonic Stenosis. The location can be either infundibular or, rarely, subinfundibular. Discrete infundibular stenosis generally results from localized narrowing of the entrance to the outflow tract, beyond which the infundibulum may be somewhat dilated. Subinfundibular stenosis, a rare variety of right ventricular outflow obstruction, may be caused by hypertrophy of either abnormal muscle groups or normal bulbar muscle. Subvalvular pulmonic stenosis is uncommon as an isolated anomaly and is generally associated with ventricular septal defect. Isolated infundibular pulmonic stenosis can be suspected if the right ventricular impulse does not reach the third left interspace, if the murmur and thrill are maximal in the fourth interspace, if an ejection sound is absent, and if the x-ray shows a nondilated pulmonary trunk, a right aortic arch, and a local indentation at the site of the ostium or the infundibulum. Cardiac catheterization and angiocardiography delineate the level of obstruction, its morphologic type, and the degree of severity. It must be borne in mind that surgical

correction requires right ventriculotomy, so operative risk is greater than with valvular pulmonic stenosis.

Supravalvular Pulmonic Stenosis (Stenosis of the Pulmonary Artery and Its Branches). This defect results from narrowing of the pulmonary trunk, its bifurcation, or its primary or peripheral branches; it may be unilateral or bilateral, single or multiple. Stenosis of the pulmonary artery and its branches causes hypertension in the proximal pulmonary trunk, whereas the converse is true with valvular or subvalvular obstruction. Isolated stenosis of the pulmonary artery and its branches exhibits the following features: murmurs, sometimes discovered in early life but sometimes inconspicuous or even absent in infants and young children; an occasional history of maternal rubella with low birth weight, physical and mental underdevelopment, cataracts, and deafness; familial occurrence; occasional hemoptysis from rupture of thin-walled poststenotic aneurysms; or the distinctive appearance associated with supravalvular aortic stenosis (see above). Auscultatory signs include absence of an ejection sound, normal intensity and splitting of the second heart sound, and left basal midsystolic murmurs with peripheral murmurs of nearly equal intensity in the axillae and back. X-rays show little or no dilatation of the pulmonary trunk but may reveal clusters of poststenotic dilatations of intrapulmonary vessels. Cardiac catheterization and angiocardiography establish the severity and define the anatomic pattern and distribution. Stenosis of the pulmonary artery and its branches is not currently amenable to surgical repair except in the occasional patient with isolated obstruction confined to a discrete zone within the pulmonary trunk.

Congenital Pulmonary Valve Regurgitation. Healthy, asymptomatic individuals may be found to have cardiac murmurs and dilatation of the pulmonary trunk on routine chest x-rays. When congenital pulmonary regurgitation accompanies *idiopathic dilatation of the pulmonary trunk,* the clinical features are those of idiopathic dilatation (see above) plus the characteristic diastolic murmur described below. Regurgitation caused by *structural abnormalities of the valve itself* results in the following picture. Palpation detects a right ventricular impulse that becomes progressively more dynamic as the degree of incompetence increases. Systolic expansion of the pulmonary trunk may impart an additional impulse in the second left intercostal space. Auscultation reveals a characteristic diastolic murmur maximal in the second or third left interspace, medium to low in frequency, crescendo-decrescendo in shape, delayed in onset, short in duration, and louder during inspiration. A midsystolic pulmonic flow murmur may be heard; the second sound can be normal or widely split and the pulmonic component soft or inaudible. The electrocardiogram is generally normal or exhibits volume overload of the right ventricle with an rSr' pattern in lead V_1. The x-ray shows moderate dilatation of the pulmonary trunk and occasionally of the right ventricle.

Ebstein's Anomaly of the Tricuspid Valve. Displaced, fused, malformed portions of tricuspid valvular tissue project into the right ventricular cavity. The portion of the right ventricle underlying the adherent tricuspid valvular tissue is thin and functions as a receiving chamber analogous to the right atrium *("atrialized right ventricle").* Abnormal function of the right heart is related to three derangements: the malformed tricuspid valve, the "atrialized" portion of right ventricle, and the reduced capacity of the pumping portion of the right ventricle. Ineffective emptying of the right atrium may result in an appreciable increase in right atrial volume and a right to left shunt through a foramen ovale or an atrial septal defect, although most are acyanotic. Tricuspid regurgitation caused by the malformed leaflets adds to the hemodynamic burden. However, Ebstein's anomaly is compatible with a relatively long and active life, because there is a considerable range of severity. The majority of patients survive into the second, third, or fourth decade, but fewer than 5 per cent live beyond age 50.

Ebstein's anomaly can generally be diagnosed clinically. Bouts of paroxysmal rapid heart action — especially in cyanotic subjects — raise the index of suspicion. A key to the clinical recognition of Ebstein's malformation with right to left shunt is the combination of cyanosis with normal or diminished pulmonary blood flow and a functionally dominant left ventricle (see Table 1). A right ventricular impulse is conspicuously lacking, although the infundibulum may be palpable. A large jugular venous V wave is lacking despite tricuspid regurgitation because of the large size of the right atrium. The murmur of tricuspid regurgitation is either absent or early systolic, because tricuspid regurgitation occurs with normal or low right ventricular systolic pressure. The murmur is usually rough, scratchy, and of medium frequency, tending to be maximal over the region of the displaced tricuspid valve, i.e., further toward the cardiac apex. Third and fourth heart sounds commonly cause triple or quadruple rhythms. Short mid-diastolic or presystolic murmurs occur, especially when the P-R interval is prolonged, which is often the case. Type B Wolff-Parkinson-White electrocardiograms are noteworthy, and, in the context of cyanotic congenital heart disease, are likely to mean Ebstein's anomaly. The electrocardiogram otherwise shows prominent right atrial P waves and generally right bundle branch block but no right ventricular hypertrophy. The chest x-ray may have a relatively characteristic appearance with normal or clear lung fields, small vascular pedicle, and a globular cardiac silhouette caused by rightward convexity of the enlarged right atrium and leftward convexity of the infundibulum.

Congenital Pulmonary Arteriovenous Fistula. This defect is believed to be caused by abnormal development of pulmonary arteries and veins from a common vascular complex. The fistula consists of either one or more relatively large vascular trunks or of a thin aneurysmal sac or a tangle of distended tortuous vascular channels. The arterial supply is derived from one or more abnormal branches of the pulmonary artery. Drainage is almost always through anatomically recognizable dilated pulmonary veins. Such connections are truly *pulmonary* arteriovenous. The physiologic consequences depend chiefly on the amount of unoxygenated blood delivered through the right to left shunt. As a rule the shunt is large enough to result in cyanosis but small enough to cause no significant hemodynamic burden. These fistulas are usually discovered in healthy young adults who are found to have abnormal densities in routine chest x-rays or who exhibit cyanosis or hereditary hemorrhagic telangiectasia. Dyspnea and fatigue are mild even in the presence of conspicuous cyanosis. Intermittent hemoptysis may punctuate the history. Recurrent bleeding also occurs from nose, mouth, or lips from the telangiectasia, and members of the family may have similar complaints.

Cerebral symptoms include dizziness, vertigo, paresthesias, faintness, visual aberrations, speech disturbances, headache, extremity weakness, mental confusion, and convulsions, although the mechanisms are unclear. Physical appearance is characterized by cyanosis and clubbing, together with small ruby patches (telangiectasia) on the face, tongue, lips, skin and nail beds, and nasal or oral mucous membranes. Thoracic auscultation may detect delayed systolic murmurs or occasionally continuous murmurs with systolic accentuation, usually located over the lower lobes or the right middle lobe. The murmurs are generally less than Grade 3 and may get louder with inspiration or Müller's maneuver and softer with expiration or Valsalva's maneuver. The lung fields show densities that may be single or multiple, unilateral or bilateral, and small or large; they are typically located in the lower lobes or right middle lobe. The opacities are homogeneous, rounded or lobulated, fairly well demarcated, and attached to the hilus by bandlike shadows that represent dilated vessels entering and leaving the fistula. The size of a mass tends to decrease with Valsalva's maneuver and increase with Müller's maneuver. In simple terms, pulmonary arteriovenous fistula is a cause of cyanosis with normal ventricles (see Table 1). The combination of cyanosis and telangiectasia with normal electrocardiogram and normal cardiac silhouette is distinctive in its own right, and conclusive when the fistulas cause shadows in the films.

Lutembacher's Syndrome. This syndrome generally consists of a congenital atrial septal defect upon which acquired mitral stenosis is superimposed. A large atrial septal defect has an ameliorating effect upon mitral stenosis, which in turn aggravates the hemodynamic effects of the interatrial communication. Left atrial pressure is relatively low, and symptoms of pulmonary venous congestion are attenuated. Atrial fibrillation is relatively common, and the systemic arterial pulse may be small owing to a decrease in left ventricular stroke volume. The jugular venous pulse may exhibit a prominent A wave in the absence of pulmonary hypertension, because the left atrial pressure is transmitted into the right atrium. The right ventricular impulse tends to be especially dynamic. Auscultation does not readily detect the telltale signs of mitral stenosis which as a rule are incomplete or absent altogether. The pulmonary flow murmur is prominent, because a large right ventricular stroke volume is ejected into a dilated pulmonary trunk. The electrocardiogram shows P waves of combined atrial enlargement, although left atrial P waves need not occur; evidence of right ventricular hypertrophy is common. The x-ray exhibits pulmonary plethora without pulmonary venous congestion; the right atrium and right ventricle are conspicuously dilated, and the pulmonary trunk may reach a remarkable size. Lutembacher's syndrome is more common in females, because this sex predilection exists for both isolated atrial septal defect and isolated mitral stenosis.

Common Atrium. This relatively rare variety of interatrial communication is the result of complete or virtual absence of the atrial septum. The right-sided portion of the common chamber has anatomic features of a *right* atrium and receives both venae cavae and the coronary sinus. The left-sided portion has anatomic features of a left atrium and receives the pulmonary veins. Absence of the septum means that the septum primum is deficient so that elements of the endocardial cushion malformation coexist, especially a cleft anterior mitral leaflet with or without mitral regurgitation. Appearance of the Ellis–van Creveld syndrome heightens suspicion. The clinical picture resembles large atrial septal defect, with the following exceptions: (1) symtpoms begin earlier and are generally more severe; (2) cyanosis exists without sufficient pulmonary hypertension to account for its presence; (3) the physical signs are those of atrial septal defect in which a large left to right shunt persists despite the presence of cyanosis (cyanosis with shunt vascularity; see Table 1); (4) the P wave axis tends to shift leftward, because there is absence of the upper or sinus venosus portion of the atrial septum with absence of a left sinus node), and the QRS shows left axis deviation resembling endocardial cushion defect; and (5) the chest x-ray resembles a large atrial septal defect in which pulmonary arterial blood flow is increased even though cyanosis is present.

Congenital Coronary Arteriovenous Fistula. Here both coronary arteries arise from the aorta, but a fistulous branch of one communicates directly with a cardiac chamber or the pulmonary trunk. The right coronary artery is more frequently involved than the left. However, the *drainage* site is of greater clinical importance than the vessel of origin. Ninety per cent of coronary arterial fistulas drain into the right heart (arteriovenous). Most of these enter the right atrium, coronary sinus, or right ventricle, whereas relatively few enter the pulmonary trunk. Congenital coronary arteriovenous fistula should be considered when an asymptomatic acyanotic child or young adult is found to have an atypically located precordial continuous murmur that is relatively soft and "superficial"; the suspicion is heightened when the murmur does not peak around the second heart sound but instead is louder in either systole or diastole. The precordial location is determined by the chamber or vessel that receives the fistula and not by the vessel of origin. In young patients with small fistulas, an "atypical" continuous murmur is likely to be the only clinical abnormality. Larger flows acting over longer periods of time can result in the following pictures. When the fistula enters the *right atrium* or *coronary sinus*, precordial palpation detects both left and right ventricular impulses; the continuous murmur tends to be louder in systole and maximal along the right sternal border, over the lower sternum, or close to the lower left sternal edge; volume overload of both ventricles may be seen in the electrocardiograms; the x-ray shows increased pulmonary arterial flow. When the communication drains into the body of the *right ventricle,* palpation detects right and left ventricular impulses; the continuous murmur is louder in either systole or diastole and is maximal along the mid- to lower left sternal border or subxiphoid area; volume overload of both ventricles may be seen in the electrocardiogram; the x-rays exhibit increased pulmonary arterial flow. When the pulmonary artery receives the fistula, palpation detects only a left ventricular impulse; the continuous murmur is usually indistinguishable from patent ductus arteriosus in both configuration and location; volume overload of the left ventricle may appear in the electrocardiogram; the x-ray may show increased pulmonary arterial flow.

Congenital Aneurysms of the Sinuses of Valsalva. Sinuses of Valsalva are three small dilatations in the wall of the aorta immediately above the attachments of each aortic cusp. More than 90 per cent of congenital aneurysms originate in the right or noncoronary sinus and project into the right ventricle or right atrium. The typical aneurysm begins as a blind pouch or diverticulum; the entire sinus is not dilated, but instead the aneurysm projects as a finger-like or nipple-like extension with a perforation at its tip. Acute rupture of a large aneurysm creates a dramatic clinical picture; a previously healthy young adult, generally male, develops sudden chest pain, dyspnea and a loud continuous murmur, bounding arterial pulse, and relentless cardiac failure that follows a period of temporary improvement. The arterial pulse resembles that of aortic regurgitation, the jugular venous pulse is elevated, and dynamic biventricular impulses are palpable. The continuous murmur is maximal below the third intercostal space along the right or left sternal border or over the lower sternum. The murmur is usually louder in either systole or diastole and does not peak around the second heart sound as in patent ductus. The electrocardiogram is likely to show biatrial P waves and left ventricular or combined ventricular hypertrophy. The chest x-ray indicates increased pulmonary arterial flow which may be obscured by pulmonary venous congestion, dilatation of both ventricles, and enlargement of the right and occasionally the left atrium. Small perforations sometimes progress slowly and at first go unnoticed. Such patients come to attention because continuous murmurs are detected. Occasionally, unruptured aneurysms are discovered because of accompanying to-and-fro or diastolic murmurs, or because of heart block or myocardial ischemia resulting from coronary arterial compression by the aneurysm.

Cardiac catheterization and angiocardiography are usually definitive. Such studies must be undertaken, because ruptured congenital aneurysms of the sinuses of Valsalva are amenable to complete correction by relatively simple intracardiac repair.

Vena Caval to Left Atrial Connection. Isolated drainage of a vena cava into the left atrium is a rare anomaly, but its presence can be suspected with a high degree of accuracy. The malformation is a form of cyanotic congenital heart disease without right ventricular hypertrophy (see Table 1). Cyanosis dates from early life, but cardiac symptoms are absent or nearly so. A right ventricular impulse is absent, whereas the left ventricle is normal or slightly thrusting. There are no significant murmurs. The electrocardiogram is usually normal but occasionally exhibits left ventricular hypertrophy. The x-ray reveals a normal cardiac silhouette, normal or diminished pulmonary blood flow, and perhaps the shadow of a persistent left superior vena cava.

554. COMMON CONGENITAL CARDIAC DEFECTS IN WHICH POSTPEDIATRIC SURVIVAL IS EXCEPTIONAL

Ventricular Septal Defect. The most common variety of ventricular septal defect lies below and posterior to the crista supraventricularis in the region of the membranous septum. Variations in size of ventricular septal defects deserve special comment. The normal growth of the heart is most rapid in the first two years of life, during which the ventricular septal defect remains about the same in size or enlarges less rapidly than the rest of the heart. Accordingly there is a tendency for the *relative* size of the defect to diminish. This tendency occasionally results in complete spontaneous closure. Ventricular septal defects are seldom seen after the fourth decade, not because patients have succumbed but probably because their communications have spontaneously closed or diminished to the point that they are clinically unrecognizable. The physiologic consequences of isolated ventricular septal defect depend chiefly on the size of the defect and the pulmonary vascular resistance. Both variables may change with time, and the physiologic and clinical manifestations vary accordingly. A small defect causes little or no functional disturbance, because the shunt is negligible and the pressures in the right heart are normal. With moderately large defects, the left to right shunt increases and, up to a point, occurs with little or no elevation in pulmonary arterial pressure. In such patients the physiologic derangements are essentially due to volume overload of the left heart. A large defect (equal to or greater than aortic orifice size) results in equalization of systolic pressures in the two ventricles. The amount of flow into the pulmonary and systemic beds then depends on their relative vascular resistances. Three regulatory mechanisms affect the volume and direction of the interventricular shunt and the level of pulmonary arterial pressure in infants born with large ventricular septal defects: first, the pattern taken by the pulmonary vascular resistance; second, the relative decrease in size that the defect undergoes, especially in the first two years of life; and third, the development of obstruction to right ventricular outflow, i.e., acquired infundibular pulmonic stenosis.

A *small ventricular septal defect* is ordinarily suspected because of a prominent holosystolic parasternal murmur in a patient in whom cardiac evaluation is otherwise normal. The murmur is generally absent at birth but is readily detected at the first well-baby examination. With passage of time, if the size of the defect decreases, the holosystolic murmur becomes softer, shorter, and higher pitched and is usually early systolic prior to complete closure. Similarly, *very small defects* are associated with soft, localized high frequency early systolic murmurs. *Large ventricular septal defects* with appreciable left to right shunts cause congestive heart failure in infancy, with retarded growth and development, recurrent lower respiratory infections, diaphoresis, and malaise. Physical examination reveals an elevated jugular venous pressure, hyperdynamic biventricular impulses, a harsh holosystolic left parasternal murmur accompanied by a thrill, an apical mid-diastolic flow murmur, and normal or wide splitting of the second heart sound with a relatively prominent pulmonic component. The electrocardiogram exhibits biatrial and biventricular hypertrophy with volume overload of the left ventricle. The x-ray shows pulmonary plethora, a large pulmonary trunk, a normal ascending aorta, dilatation of both ventricles, and often dilatation of the left and right atria as well. Spontaneous improvement is related to a reduction in left to right shunt caused by a decrease in the size of the defect, especially in the first year, by an increase in pulmonary vascular resistance, or by acquired infundibular pulmonic stenosis.

In *large ventricular septal defect with reversed shunt (Eisenmenger's complex),* cyanosis ordinarily dates from childhood, although not from birth. Effort dyspnea occurs without left ventricular failure. The jugular venous pulse is usually normal and the precordium quiet, with moderate right ventricular and pulmonary arterial impulses. There are auscultatory signs of pulmonary hypertension but *no murmur of ventricular septal defect.* The electrocardiogram shows right ventricular hypertrophy with little or no evidence of volume overload of the left heart. The x-ray exhibits normal or decreased pulmonary vasculature, a relatively normal cardiac silhouette, moderate dilatation of the pulmonary trunk, and normal aortic arch (see Table 1).

In patients with typical small ventricular septal defects, the clinical diagnosis is so evident and the physiologic consequences are so benign that cardiac catheterization and angiocardiography are not necessary, and such patients should be followed expectantly. They are, however, at risk of infective endocarditis. Patients with *large* ventricular septal defects, especially those with clinical evidence of pulmonary hypertension, should be investigated to determine the presence and degree of the left to right shunt, the pulmonary arterial pressure and vascular resistance, and the angiographic location of the defect or defects.

Large ventricular septal defect with congestive heart failure in infancy is a special problem that will not be dealt with here. Beyond infancy, patients with ventricular septal defects and pulmonary to systemic flow ratios in excess of 1.5 to 1.7:1 should have elective correction. If the pulmonary to systemic flow ratio is less than 1.5:1 because the defect is small, the benign functional consequences do not warrant the risk of operative repair. If a similar flow ratio is the result of *high pulmonary resistance* with *large* ventricular septal defect, operative risk is high and results are poor, because little or no beneficial effect on the pulmonary resistance follows elimination of such a small shunt.

Ventricular Septal Defect with Aortic Regurgitation. Here the murmur of the ventricular defect is usually known from infancy. Between the ages of three and eight years a *new* murmur appears, together with the gradual development of bounding arterial pulses and a dynamic left ventricular impulse. The combined murmurs are *not* continuous but are holosystolic and early diastolic. The electrocardiogram and x-ray may show left ventricular hypertrophy and enlargement out of proportion to what would be expected on the basis of the estimated size of the left to right shunt. As time goes on, the ventricular septal defect may decrease in size and the aortic regurgitation will progressively worsen. Survival to adult life occurs, although cardiac failure eventually develops because of progression of the regurgitation.

Endocardial Cushion Defect. The endocardial cushions of the embryo contribute to the development of the mitral and tricuspid valves and to the growth and convergence of the atrial and ventricular septa. Defects therefore include varying combinations of anomalies in these four contiguous parts of the heart. Three general categories are recognized, namely, complete endocardial cushion defect, partial or incomplete endocardial cushion defect, and transitional forms. In the complete variety, separate atrioventricular valves do not exist as such. There is a common AV valve in a canal formed by an atrial septal defect above and a ventricular septal defect below. The partial or incomplete form is represented by an ostium primum atrial septal defect and a cleft mitral valve. Transitional forms represent intermediates between complete and partial or incomplete endocardial cushion defects. Less commonly, any one of the four component lesions occurs as an isolated anomaly. The physiologic consequences depend upon the presence and degree of the various combinations of the four anatomic components. The following remarks will relate to partial endocardial cushion defects in which postpediatric survival is possible.

An ostium primum atrial septal defect with cleft mitral valve occurs more frequently in females than males. The physical signs resemble those of ostium secundum atrial septal defect except that the left ventricle occupies the apex and is accompanied by the holosystolic murmur of mitral regurgitation. Congestive heart failure may begin in childhood, especially when marked mitral regurgitation exists with a large left to right shunt. Growth and development are poor and lower respiratory infections frequent. If mitral regurgitation is relatively mild and the left to right shunt moderate, symptoms may be delayed for one or two decades. The incompetent left atrioventricular valve is susceptible to infective endocarditis, and mongolism occurs, but not so frequently as with complete endocardial cushion defects. The electrocardiogram is important, because the frontal plane consists of counterclockwise depolarization with left axis deviation, with precordial leads that show the rSr' pattern of expected volume overload of the right ventricle. In persistent ostium primum with cleft but competent mitral valve, this electrocardiogram is the only distinguishing clinical feature from ostium secundum defect.

The most important laboratory study in identifying endocardial cushion defect is a left ventricular angiocardiogram in the frontal projection which shows a characteristic "goose neck" deformity of the outflow tract caused by the cleft anterior mitral cusp and its abnormal chordal arrangements. Surgical repair in partial endocardial cushion defect is limited chiefly by the degree of mitral regurgitation rather than the presence of the atrial septal defect.

Tricuspid Atresia. In this disorder tricuspid valvular tissue cannot be identified. A small imperforate dimple is found on the floor of the right atrium, but no direct pathway exists between right atrium and right ventricle. The only outlet for the right atrium is an interatrial communication which can take the form of a fossa ovale or an atrial septal defect. Variations beyond the mitral valve form the basis of Edwards' anatomic classification from which physiologic inferences can be drawn and clinical expressions of tricuspid atresia understood. According to this classification, tricuspid atresia occurs either with or without transposition of the great arteries and, in each category, with no pulmonic stenosis, with pulmonic stenosis, or with pulmonary atresia. Pulmonary blood flow is the key determinant of longevity. Longevity is greatest when pulmonic stenosis of just the right degree exists so that blood flow to the lungs is favorably regulated. When the great vessels are normally related, the subpulmonic obstruction is generally marked, and most patients die in the first year. Nevertheless, occasional examples of survival have been recorded from the second through the fifth decade, with one exceptional survival to age 57. When the great vessels are *transposed,* coexisting pulmonic stenosis is more likely to permit longer survival. In isolated cases in this category patients have lived into the second, third, and fourth decades, and one died at age 56. The key to the clinical diagnosis of tricuspid atresia is the presence of cyanosis, normal or diminished pulmonary blood flow, and a dominant left ventricle (see Table 1). The electrocardiogram shows right atrial P waves with left axis deviation and adult progression of the QRS in the precordial leads. Definitive diagnosis is achieved by angiocardiography. Palliative surgery is possible through (1) creation of an atrial septal defect in those patients with a foramen ovale, or (2) a shunt operation to improve pulmonary blood flow. More recently, blood from the right atrium has been directed through a conduit to the pulmonary arteries, permitting the right atrium to act as a pumping chamber for the pulmonary circulation.

Complete Transposition of the Great Arteries. According to Elliott and Edwards: "In complete transposition, there are two ventricles. . . . The aorta, with the coronary arteries arising from it, takes origin from the right ventricle, while the pulmonary trunk takes origin exclusively from the left ventricle. Both atrioventricular valves are patent and have the corresponding structure of the right and left sided atrioventricular valves of the normal heart. The connections of the systemic, pulmonary and coronary veins are normal." Survival in complete transposition requires the presence of some means of blood exchange between the pulmonary and systemic circulations which exist in parallel rather than in series, as in hearts with nontransposed great arteries. Connections between the greater and lesser circulations may take the form of interatrial communication, ventricular septal defect, or patent ductus arteriosus. The pathologic physiology of complete transposition of the great arteries depends largely upon three variables: the types of communications that join the pulmonary and systemic circulations, the resistance to flow through the pulmonary bed, and the pressure gradients between the communications that join the greater and lesser circulations. As a general rule, complete transposition of the great arteries is characterized as a congenital cardiac anomaly that exists with cyanosis and increased pulmonary blood flow (see Table 1). Life expectancy is best when the anomaly exists with large ventricular septal defect *and* pulmonic stenosis sufficient to exert a favorable regulation of pulmonary blood flow, so that flow is adequate to prevent serious hypoxia but not great enough to cause left ventricular failure. Even so, the large majority of patients with complete transposition of great arteries die within the first year, often within the first months. Isolated examples of unusual longevity have been recorded into the second, third, or fourth decade; one patient aged 56 years at autopsy was believed to have complete transposition. Definitive diagnosis is by angiocardiography. Two physiologic corrective operations are currently applied. The Mustard operation redirects venous inflows, whereas the Rastelli operation achieves redirection of ventricular outflows.

555. UNCOMMON CONGENITAL CARDIAC DEFECTS IN WHICH POSTPEDIATRIC SURVIVAL IS EXCEPTIONAL

Anomalous origin of the left coronary artery from the pulmonary trunk is characterized by normal origin of the right coronary artery from the aorta and anomalous origin of the left coronary artery (LCA) from the pulmonary trunk. The aberrant left coronary artery is relatively small and thin walled, resembling a venous channel, whereas the right coronary artery is dilated and tortuous, especially in patients who reach adult life. Myocardial ischemia is a serious problem. The ischemic derangement is not due to the fact that only *one* coronary artery originates from the aorta, but is due to direct flow from the right coronary artery to the LCA through intercoronary anastomoses which bypass the capillary bed. Thus the anomalous left coronary artery flows retrograde into the pulmonary artery but does not receive blood from it.

In the natural history of this anomaly, three general patterns emerge: serious symptoms in early infancy with death before one year; early illness followed by improvement so that by childhood symptoms may be absent or nearly so; and absence or virtual absence of early symptoms with survival into adulthood. About 15 or 20 per cent of individuals with anomalous origin of the LCA reach adulthood, but relatively few survive through the fourth decade, although one of the first known patients with this anomaly was a 50-year-old woman. The intercoronary anastomoses often result in a continuous murmur, and the myocardial ischemia results in papillary muscle dysfunction with mitral regurgitation. The electrocardiogram is important, because at a relatively early age deep Q waves appear in leads I and aVL. Definitive diagnosis is by cardiac catheterization and angiocardiography. A left to right shunt from right coronary through intercoronary anastomoses to anomalous LCA into the pulmonary trunk is identified. Selective coronary arteriography (injection into the right coronary) traces this pathway and provides specific anatomic diagnosis. Two surgical interventions have been applied. In infancy, ligation of the anomalous left coronary artery interrupts retrograde flow and improves capillary circulation. In older children or adults, the left subclavian artery or the internal mammary artery or a saphenous vein graft can be directly anastomosed to the left coronary artery, which is then ligated at its origin from the pulmonary artery.

Cor triatriatum is characterized by drainage of the pulmonary veins into an accessory left atrial chamber that lies proximal to the true left atrium. The distal compartment communicates with the mitral valve and contains the left atrial appendage and the fossa ovalis. The fibrous or fibromuscular diaphragm that partitions the left atrium contains one or more openings, the size of which determines the degree of left atrial obstruction. Cor triatriatum is therefore a congenital anomaly that is acyanotic without a shunt, with the malformation originating in the left heart (see Table 1). Severe cor triatriatum is ordinarily detected in infants or young children, but symptoms may not begin until adolescence or adulthood. Patients with mild obstruction may be entirely asymptomatic. The functional consequences are analogous to those of mitral stenosis with elevated pulmonary venous and pulmonary arterial pressures. However, the auscultatory signs of mitral stenosis are lacking, and enlargement of the left atrial appendage is absent, because that structure is in the distal low pressure compartment. It is wise to consider cor triatriatum in postadolescents with clinical signs of obstruction to left atrial flow but without signs of mitral stenosis. The diagnosis is materially assisted by echocardiography that detects normal movements of anterior and posterior mitral leaflets, and by angiocardiography which, with pulmonary arterial injection of contrast material, defines the zone of obstruction as dye opacifies the left heart. Surgical intervention can completely remove the partition and relieve the left atrial obstruction.

Total anomalous pulmonary venous connection (TAPVC) applies to a condition in which all venous blood from both lungs enters the right atrium directly or through one of its tributary veins. The four anomalously connecting pulmonary veins emerge individually from the lungs and either enter the right atrium directly or, more often, unite in the mediastinum to form a confluence which joins the right atrium via (1) the coronary sinus; (2) an anomalous vertical vein or left superior vena cava that connects the left innominate vein to the right superior vena cava; or (3) the right superior vena cava, directly or via the azygos vein. In the right atrium, there is mixing of systemic and pulmonary venous blood, part of which enters the left heart via an atrial septal defect and most of which enters the right ventricle and low-resistance pulmonary bed. Accordingly, TAPVC can be classified as a cyanotic congenital anomaly with increased pulmonary arterial blood flow (see Table 1). The clinical picture in many ways resembles isolated atrial septal defect with large left to right shunt except for cyanosis, which varies from clinically subtle to marked. However, the patient is likely to be male, and symptoms generally begin in early childhood, although some patients reach adult life with surprisingly little disability. The jugular venous pulse may exhibit a large A wave because of pulmonary hypertension. Palpation and auscultation are similar to atrial septal defect with large left to right shunt, but signs of pulmonary hypertension are more likely to coexist. Similarly, the electrocardiogram shows right atrial and right ventricular hypertrophy. The x-ray may resemble atrial septal defect with large left to right shunt, but there is one distinctive picture. When the pulmonary veins communicate with the left innominate vein via a left vertical vein or left superior vena cava, the heart may exhibit a "figure of 8" appearance. The upper part of the figure of 8 is the left vertical vein on the left and the dilated right superior vena cava on the right. The lower part is the cardiac silhouette itself, i.e., dilated right atrium and right ventricle.

Diagnosis is established by cardiac catheterization and angiocardiography; the latter defines the specific connecting pathways. Surgical correction can be achieved, especially when the confluence of pulmonary veins can be anastomosed directly to the left atrium and the vascular channel to the systemic venous bed divided.

Right ventricular origin of both great arteries and "double outlet right ventricle" are synonymous terms for a congenital malformation in which the pulmonary artery arises in its normal position but the aorta arises wholly from the right ventricle. A ventricular septal defect provides the left ventricle with its only outlet. Pulmonic stenosis may or may not coexist. Right ventricular origin of both great arteries can exist with a ventricular septal defect inferior or superior to the crista supraventricularis. In double outlet right ventricle with infracristal ventricular septal defect and no pulmonic stenosis, two steps help in clinical diagnosis. The first step involves recognition of large ventricular septal defect with left to right shunt and pulmonary hypertension. Since both great vessels originate from the right ventricle, pulmonary arterial pressure is by definition systemic. It is a good rule to consider double outlet right ventricle in all patients who present with the picture of large left to right shunt pulmonary hypertensive ventricular septal defect. The second step in the clinical diagnosis consists of the following additional points: (1) a QRS that exhibits left axis deviation and counterclockwise depolarization, and (2) mild to moderate cyanosis with increased pulmonary arterial blood flow in the presence of persistent murmur of ventricular septal defect. It can be seen that the clinical diagnosis depends chiefly on left axis deviation in the presence of a pulmonary hypertensive ventricular septal defect with a large left to right shunt. Favorable adjustments in pulmonary vascular resistance sometimes regulate pulmonary blood flow so that, even though increased, it is not excessive. Under these circumstances longevity is improved; patients occasionally survive into young adulthood, and one underwent successful surgical correction at 53 years of age.

In right ventricular origin of both great vessels with supracristal ventricular septal defect, the defect lies just beneath the pulmonary valve. At times the pulmonary artery straddles the defect. This anomaly, called the *Taussig-Bing complex,* is a diagnostic consideration in patients with increased pulmonary blood flow and cyanosis from birth or early infancy. Radiologic, electrocardiographic, and physical signs of pulmonary hypertension are obligatory. In the presence of patent ductus arteriosus (which often coexists) and high pulmonary vascular resistance, a distinctive type of reversed cyanosis occurs in which the toes are less cyanotic than the fingers, because oxygenated blood from the left ventricle is ejected into the pulmonary trunk and then through the ductus into the descending aorta, whereas unsaturated right ventricular blood is ejected into the aortic root and brachiocephalic vessels. It is a good rule to consider the Taussig-Bing anomaly in patients who appear to have Eisenmenger's complex but in whom cyanosis dates from birth or early infancy.

Right ventricular origin of both great vessels occurs with all grades of pulmonic stenosis (mild to severe to complete, i.e., pulmonary atresia). The ventricular septal defect is usually infracristal if pulmonic stenosis coexists. Double outlet right ventricle with mild to moderate pulmonic stenosis resembles ordinary large ventricular septal defect with equivalent pulmonic stenosis except for three points: (1) the electrocardiogram may exhibit counterclockwise depolarization with left axis deviation; (2) the murmur of ventricular septal defect may persist despite pulmonic stenosis; and (3) there is a tendency for cyanosis to develop in the presence of increased pulmonary blood flow.

Right ventricular origin of both great vessels with severe pulmonic stenosis closely resembles cyanotic Fallot's tetralogy and should be considered whenever the clinical diagnosis of cyanotic Fallot's tetralogy is entertained. Clinical distinction between the two is difficult or impossible, although some points favor double outlet right ventricle: (1) auscultatory evidence of a holosystolic murmur at the lower left sternal edge despite the presence of cyanosis (obligatory left to right shunt through the ventricular septal defect); (2) palpable left ventricular impulse in this context; and (3) electrocardiogram showing small q waves in leads I and aVL and relatively broad slurred S waves in leads I, aVL, and V_{5-6}. The echocardiogram may assist in identifying lack of continuity between the posterior aortic wall and anterior mitral leaflet, because in double outlet right ventricle

there is no continuity between the anterior mitral leaflet and the wall of either great vessel. Definitive diagnosis is angiographic. Corrective surgery is technically feasible, although it is more complex than with closure of isolated large ventricular septal defect or with repair of Fallot's tetralogy.

Truncus arteriosus is a congenital anomaly in which a single great artery leaves the base of the heart through a single semilunar valve. The truncus is situated just above a ventricular septal defect, receives blood from both ventricles, and gives rise to the coronary arteries and to the pulmonary and systemic circulations. No remnant of the second semilunar valve is present. Truncus arteriosus with large pulmonary arteries may occur with cyanosis and pulmonary plethora (see Table 1). Both pulmonary branches may arise from a short main pulmonary artery that emerges from the truncus, or the two pulmonary arterial branches may arise directly from the truncus. Truncus with absent pulmonary arteries is debatable and is physiologically analogous to pulmonary atresia with ventricular septal defect.

The outlook is better when there is an appropriate increase in pulmonary vascular resistance or relatively small pulmonary arteries, either mechanism advantageously controlling pulmonary blood flow and delaying death from cardiac failure. Occasional patients with favorably regulated pulmonary circulations have survived into the third or fourth decade, and one died at the age of 43 years. However, postpediatric survival is rare, especially with truncus arteriosus and large pulmonary arteries.

Definitive diagnosis of truncus arteriosus is by angiocardiography. Physiologic correction is feasible, employing an operation which joins the two pulmonary arteries to the outflow of the right ventricle with an aortic homograft.

Single ventricle refers to a rare congenital anomaly in which there are two atria but only one ventricular chamber that receives both the mitral and tricuspid valves. The usual type is a morphologic left ventricle with a small outlet chamber that represents the infundibular portion of the right ventricle. The infundibulum represents a subdivision of the single left ventricle, not a separate ventricular chamber. The great arteries are almost always transposed. If the infundibulum is situated at the right basal aspect of the heart, this arrangement is called "noninversion"; if the infundibulum is situated at the left basal aspect of the heart (corresponding to its expected location with congenitally corrected transposition), this arrangement is termed "inversion." Pulmonic stenosis may or may not coexist. Single ventricle without pulmonic stenosis occurs with increased pulmonary blood flow, and hence is an anomaly exhibiting cyanosis with pulmonary plethora (see Table 1). In single ventricle with high pulmonary vascular resistance, cyanosis is conspicuous and pulmonary blood flow is normal or diminished (see Table 1). Single ventricle with pulmonic stenosis is an anomaly exhibiting cyanosis with normal or diminished pulmonary blood flow (see Table 1).

This malformation has also been referred to as *cor triloculare biatriatum,* which merely means that there is a three-chambered heart with two atria. Clinical diagnosis is difficult, and definitive diagnosis depends upon cardiac catheterization and angiocardiography. Surgical intervention is palliative, and consists of either banding the pulmonary trunk to limit pulmonary plethora or providing a shunt operation to improve pulmonary blood flow in patients with critical pulmonic stenosis or atresia.

Carter, J. B., Sethi, S., Lee, G. B., and Edwards, J. E.: Prolapse of semilunar cusps as causes of aortic insufficiency. Circulation, 43:922, 1971.

Davis, J. E., Cheitlin, M. D., and Bedynek, J. L.: Sinus venosus atrial septal defect: Analysis of 50 cases. Am. Heart J., 85:177, 1973.

de la Cruz, M. Z., Anselmi, G., Romero, A., and Monroy, G.: A quantitative and qualitative study of the ventricles and great vessels of normal children. Am. Heart J., 60:675, 1960.

Edwards, J. E., Carey, L. S., Neufeld, H. N., and Lester, R. G.: Congenital Heart Disease. Philadelphia, W. B. Saunders Company, 1965.

Feigenbaum, H.: Echocardiography. Philadelphia, Lea & Febiger, 1972.

Gault, J. H., Morrow, A. G., Gay, W. A., and Ross, J., Jr.: Atrial septal defect in patients over age 40 years. Clinical and hemodynamic studies and the effects of operation. Circulation, 37:261, 1968.

Higgins, C. B., and Mulder, D. G.: Tetralogy of Fallot in the adult. Am. J. Cardiol., 29:837, 1972.

Higgins, I. T.: The epidemiology of congenital heart disease. J. Chronic Dis., 18:699, 1965.

Maron, B. J., Humphries, J. O., Rowe, R. D., and Mellits, E. D.: Prognosis of surgically corrected coarctation of the aorta. A 20-year postoperative followup. Circulation, 47:119, 1973.

Nadas, A. S., and Flyer, D. C.: Pediatric Cardiology. 3rd ed. Philadelphia, W. B. Saunders Company, 1972.

Nora, J. J.: Multifactorial inheritance hypothesis for the etiology of congenital heart disease. Circulation, 38:604, 1968.

Perloff, J. K.: Pediatric congenital cardiac becomes a postoperative adult. The changing population of congenital heart disease. Circulation, 47:606, 1973.

Perloff, J. K.: The Clinical Recognition of Congenital Heart Disease. Philadelphia. W. B. Saunders Company, 1970.

Polani, P. E., and Campbell, M.: An aetiological study of congenital heart disease. Ann. Hum. Genet., 19:209, 1955.

Roberts, W. C.: The congenitally bicuspid aortic valve. Am. J. Cardiol., 26:72, 1970.

ACQUIRED VALVULAR HEART DISEASE

John Ross, Jr.

556. INTRODUCTION

Before considering the characteristic features and treatment of each acquired valvular heart lesion, it will be useful to consider broad differences in the physiologic effects of these lesions and to suggest a general diagnostic approach to the patient with valvular heart disease. It will also be worthwhile to discuss the indications for cardiac catheterization, as well as the general considerations that enter into a decision to recommend surgical treatment.

GENERAL PHYSIOLOGIC EFFECTS OF VALVULAR HEART DISEASE

The consequences of stenosis or regurgitation of the heart valves may be considered in relation to their direct effects on the cardiac chamber that must compensate for the valvular lesion by undergoing hypertrophy or dilatation, and their secondary effects on intravascular pressures and blood flow in the aorta, pulmonary vascular bed, and systemic veins. When a semilunar valve of the heart (aortic or pulmonic) is stenotic or regurgitant, or when an atrioventricular valve (mitral or

tricuspid) is regurgitant, the primary burden is placed upon the adjacent *ventricle*. With aortic stenosis and regurgitation, important secondary effects occur in the aortic pressure pulses, and with mitral regurgitation there are major secondary effects on the pulmonary venous bed. When an atrioventricular valve is stenotic, the primary burden is placed on the *atrium,* and secondary effects are prominent on the adjacent venous bed; in tricuspid stenosis, for example, there are right atrial overload and secondary elevation of pressure in the systemic veins. These general consequences of stenotic and regurgitant valvular lesions are summarized in the accompanying figure.

Aortic stenosis places an overload on the left ventricle during systole, a pressure gradient being developed to overcome the obstruction at the aortic valve (see figure). This leads to progressive hypertrophy of the left ventricular wall without an increase in chamber volume. Aortic regurgitation, in contrast, places a volume overload on the left ventricle during diastole. This leads to an augmented forward stroke volume into the aorta which, in turn, causes a substantial increase in the systolic pressure in the aorta and left ventricle, an increase in left ventricular volume, and moderate hypertrophy of the left ventricular wall. An excessive oxygen consumption by the left ventricle occurs in aortic stenosis because of the hypertrophy and increased pressure required to drive blood across the narrowed valve, and myocardial oxygen consumption also is increased to some degree in aortic regurgitation because of the large stroke volume and the increased systolic pressure in the aorta. In addition, there is a low diastolic aortic pressure available for coronary artery perfusion in aortic regurgitation and a low aortic pressure relative to left ventricular pressure in severe aortic stenosis (see figure), which can lead to imbalances between coronary blood flow and myocardial oxygen demands. Angina pectoris is therefore common in both these conditions. Both aortic stenosis and regurgitation, in time, lead to left ventricular myocardial dysfunction.

Mitral regurgitation also places a diastolic volume overload on the left ventricle, but it differs importantly from aortic regurgitation in that the regurgitant leak occurs during ventricular systole and takes place into a relatively low pressure chamber, the left atrium (see figure). The ventricular chamber dilates to allow the increased total stroke volume (forward plus backward flow), but the ventricular systolic pressure is not elevated, wall hypertrophy is only moderate, oxygen demands are not greatly augmented, and coronary artery perfusion pressure is normal. Therefore this lesion, when it develops slowly, tends to be well tolerated, and left ventricular myocardial dysfunction develops late in the course of the disease. Mitral stenosis does not place an overload on the left ventricle; rather, obstruction at the mitral valve overwhelms the capacity of the atrial booster pump to maintain forward blood flow, and progressive elevation of left atrial pressure ensues (see figure).

The secondary effects of these valvular lesions on the arterial and venous beds are many. As mentioned above, the reduced aortic pulse in aortic stenosis and the wide aortic pulse pressure with low diastolic pressure in aortic regurgitation have important effects on coronary artery perfusion. In addition, when valvular lesions are sufficiently severe, or when left ventricular myocardial failure supervenes, the forward cardiac output becomes

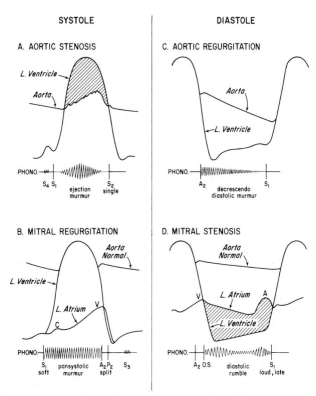

Diagrams of pressure tracings and phonocardiograms in valvular heart disease. The left-hand panels illustrate systole; the right-hand panels, diastole.

A, Pressure tracings in the aorta and left ventricle in aortic stenosis. The shaded area indicates the pressure gradient between left ventricle and aorta. The presystolic (A wave) in the left ventricle is shown, which correlates with the atrial diastolic gallop (S_4) on the phonocardiogram (Phono.). The murmur follows the time course of the pressure gradient during ventricular ejection, and the prolonged left ventricular ejection time results in a single second heart sound (S_2).

B, Pressure tracings in the aorta, left ventricle, and left atrium in mitral regurgitation. (Similar events occur in the right atrium, jugular venous pulse, and right ventricle in tricuspid regurgitation.) A prominent V wave is visible in the left atrium, and the pansystolic murmur on the phonocardiogram persists as long as there is a pressure gradient from left ventricle to left atrium across the leaking mitral valve. The A_2P_2 interval is more widely split than normal because of a shortened left ventricular ejection time in severe mitral regurgitation. The rapid filling wave in the left ventricle and left atrium is illustrated, which is often accompanied by a ventricular diastolic gallop (S_3).

C, Pressure tracings in the aorta and left ventricle in aortic regurgitation. There is a widened arterial pulse pressure with a rapidly falling aortic diastolic pressure. On the phonocardiogram the decrescendo diastolic murmur can be seen to follow the time course of the diminishing diastolic pressure gradient from the aorta to the left ventricle across the leaking aortic valve.

D, Pressure tracings in the aorta, left ventricle, and left atrium in mitral stenosis. (Similar events occur in the right atrium, jugular venous pulse, and right ventricle in tricuspid stenosis.) The left atrial pressure is elevated and the pressure gradient between left atrium and left ventricle during diastole is indicated by the shaded area. The slow fall in left atrial pressure after the V wave (slow Y descent) indicates obstruction to left atrial emptying, and the prominent A wave of left atrial contraction is not transmitted to the ventricle. The dumbbell-shaped diastolic rumble of mitral stenosis in the presence of normal sinus rhythm follows the time course of the pressure gradient, which is greatest early and again late in diastole. It can be seen how an increase or a decrease in the height of the left atrial pressure will move the mitral opening snap (O.S.) closer to or farther from, respectively, the aortic closure sound (A_2); similarly a higher left atrial pressure will result in a later and louder first heart sound (S_1).

reduced, the arterial pulse weakens, and there is reflex systemic vasoconstriction with cool extremities and peripheral cyanosis. Such signs constitute evidence of *"forward" cardiac failure.* The effects of *"backward" cardiac failure* in the presence of left-sided valvular lesions are due to left atrial and pulmonary venous hypertension, and they are reflected in the lungs and the right heart. In mitral stenosis, obstruction to left atrial emptying leads to left atrial hypertension, distention of the pulmonary veins, interstitial edema of the lung, reactive pulmonary arteriolar constriction, and eventually pulmonary arterial hypertension. However, the same sequence of effects can also occur when aortic stenosis becomes extremely severe, or when left ventricular myocardial dysfunction becomes significant in the presence of aortic valve disease or mitral regurgitation. The common denominator under these conditions is marked elevation of the left ventricular diastolic pressure, and late in the course of each of these left-sided valvular lesions left atrial and pulmonary venous hypertension, lung congestion, and pulmonary arterial hypertension can also occur, as in mitral stenosis.

Once severe pulmonary hypertension develops, the resulting pressure overload on the right ventricle may then result in secondary right ventricular failure, tricuspid regurgitation, and right atrial hypertension. This, in turn, leads to congestion of the systemic venous bed and the peripheral tissues (liver, abdomen, and extremities). Tricuspid stenosis alone can produce such effects, the right atrial hypertension being caused by mechanical obstruction at the tricuspid valve.

APPROACH TO THE PATIENT WITH VALVULAR HEART DISEASE

Five basic steps in the evaluation of a patient with acquired valvular heart disease should be taken in a logical sequence: (1) the history, (2) the physical examination, (3) the chest roentgenogram (usually with multiple views and barium swallow), (4) the electrocardiogram, and (5) other special tests (phonocardiogram, echocardiogram, cardiac catheterization). The patient is often seen initially, of course, because of an abnormal finding in one of these areas (cardiac murmur, abnormal electrocardiogram, unusual chest x-ray).

History. The clinical course of patients with each major type of acquired valvular lesion tends to be rather characteristic, and often the findings to be encountered on physical examination can be predicted on the basis of a careful history alone. Thus in mitral stenosis the earliest symptoms are those due to episodic left atrial hypertension and pulmonary congestion, occurring particularly when the heart rate is rapid during exercise, and during intermittent atrial fibrillation or tachycardia. Such symptoms often begin in early adult life, and the dyspnea increases as the mitral valve narrowing progresses and reaches a critical degree. In contrast, patients with aortic stenosis or regurgitation, or mitral regurgitation, tend to develop dyspnea in relation to the duration and severity of the overload on the left ventricle. In acquired isolated aortic stenosis, there is often a long period without symptoms while the stenosis progresses and left ventricular hypertrophy increases; this is followed by a rather abrupt downhill course over four or five years, beginning at age 55 or 60, as the compensatory mechanisms are exhausted. The average downhill course in patients with chronic rheumatic aortic regurgitation tends to be less precipitous than that of aortic stenosis after symptoms begin, taking place over seven or eight years, but it usually begins somewhat earlier in life. On the other hand, in chronic mitral regurgitation the onset of symptoms is gradual and deterioration tends to be slow owing to the relatively favorable loading conditions on the left ventricle, discussed above.

These average clinical courses represent those of patients who experienced rheumatic fever in childhood, or who develop progressive stenosis of a congenitally bicuspid aortic valve. Departures from the typical patterns occur when, for example, coronary artery disease leads to angina pectoris in the presence of mild aortic stenosis, or when mitral regurgitation occurs acutely as a consequence of chordal rupture or papillary muscle dysfunction associated with coronary heart disease. Such deviations from the usual history should arouse the suspicion of a nonrheumatic etiology of valve dysfunction, or of other associated disease.

Physical Examination. In examining the heart, it is well to develop an ordered approach, commencing with careful inspection of the neck veins, palpation of the carotid arteries, and inspection and palpation of the precordium. Palpation of the carotid arteries may be highly useful, for example, in differentiating aortic stenosis caused by valvular obstruction from that caused by hypertrophic subaortic stenosis. Estimation of the jugular venous pressure (which, with practice, can be done reliably within 1 or 2 cm H_2O) and examination of the contour of the jugular venous pulse waves carry great importance, because these veins provide direct clues to events occurring in the right atrium. The jugular veins therefore serve as an "external manometer," and the characteristically slow downslope of the jugular venous pulse (Y descent) associated with tricuspid stenosis (see figure) or the dominant V wave of tricuspid regurgitation, may suggest organic tricuspid valve involvement.

The jugular venous pulse waves often disclose atrial arrhythmias, or provide a clue to the presence of pulmonary hypertension and right ventricular hypertrophy, evidenced by a prominent venous A wave.

Auscultation of the heart is of course the key to an accurate diagnosis in valvular heart disease. An orderly sequence for listening should be developed, each area being examined first for normal or abnormal heart sounds and then for cardiac murmurs. Simultaneous palpation of the carotid artery and observation of the neck veins should be used as aids in the proper timing of the heart sounds and murmurs. By listening first at the aortic area, the aortic component of the second heart sound can be readily identified; the intensity of the pulmonic closure sound and its movement with respiration can then be assessed at the pulmonic area. As one moves down the left sternal border with the diaphragm of the stethoscope, the opening snap of mitral stenosis may be revealed even before the murmur is heard at the apex, or the high-pitched blowing murmur of aortic regurgitation may be audible. The tricuspid and mitral areas should then be examined for the characteristics of the first heart sound. Sometimes a very loud first heart sound alerts the examiner to the possibility of mitral stenosis, whereas mitral regurgitation leads to a reduction in the intensity of the first heart sound at the apex (see figure).

The duration and intensity of the murmurs of valvular heart disease occur with, and tend to follow, the time course of pressure gradients between two adjacent cardiac chambers or between a chamber and its great vessel. Thus the diamond-shaped systolic murmur ("ejection" murmur) of aortic stenosis increases and decreases as the pressure gradient, and the velocity at which blood is forced across the narrowed aortic orifice rises and falls (see figure); this type of murmur does not occur during isovolumetric ventricular contraction and relaxation, and therefore begins well after the first heart sound and ends before the second sound. The decrescendo murmur of aortic regurgitation occurs as the diastolic pressure gradient between the aorta and the left ventricle gradually falls during left ventricular filling (see figure). The holosystolic (pansystolic) murmur of mitral or tricuspid regurgitation begins with the first heart sound and persists as long as active ventricular contraction maintains a positive pressure gradient from the ventricle to the passively filling atrium (see figure). The duration and intensity of the diastolic rumbling murmurs of mitral or tricuspid stenosis closely follow the diastolic pressure gradient across the valve from atrium to ventricle (see figure). Presystolic accentuation of the murmur during the A wave of atrial systole tends to disappear when atrial fibrillation occurs, and if the stenosis is mild the pressure gradient and the murmur may disappear midway during diastole. It also can be seen from the figure why the first heart sound is both late and loud in mitral stenosis, the left ventricle contracting rapidly and forcefully by the time it has built up sufficient pressure to close the mitral valve, and why the interval between the aortic closure sound and the mitral opening snap becomes progressively shorter as left atrial pressure rises.

Finally, it is important that changes in body position and certain other maneuvers become a regular part of the complete physical examination in a patient with valvular heart disease. The murmur of mitral stenosis may not be heard until the patient is placed in the left lateral decubitus position; the same position may be required to move the left ventricle sufficiently close to the chest wall to allow a ventricular diastolic gallop to be appreciated. The diagnosis of mitral stenosis should also not be excluded until a brief period of muscular exercise, or an isometric handgrip, has been performed to accentuate the murmur by increasing the heart rate and cardiac output, thereby augmenting the pressure gradient across the mitral valve. The handgrip maneuver tends to increase aortic pressure as well, and it is useful for augmenting a left ventricular gallop, or for accentuating the murmur of aortic regurgitation. The faint murmur of mild aortic regurgitation may also be detected only when the patient leans forward and breathes out completely. Sometimes the standing position is required to bring out the murmur of hypertrophic subaortic stenosis; the Valsalva maneuver is also useful for accentuating this murmur and for diminishing the murmur of valvular aortic stenosis.

Chest Roentgenogram. As mentioned above, the jugular venous pulse provides a "direct access" route to the right atrium and allows estimation of the right atrial or systemic venous pressure. The pulmonary veins, of course, are inaccessible to physical examination, and therefore the chest roentgenogram is relied upon heavily to aid in detecting left atrial and pulmonary venous hypertension. Often, when there is left atrial hypertension, enlargement of the upper lobe pulmonary veins reflects redistribution of pulmonary blood flow, with reduced perfusion of the lung bases relative to the upper lobes (reversing the normal pattern in the upright posture), and there are signs of interstitial pulmonary edema (such as the Kerley B line) which usually precede the development of pulmonary (intra-alveolar) edema.

Oblique, overpenetrated views of the heart with barium swallow provide valuable information in evaluating valvular heart disease. Left atrial enlargement may be evidenced in the frontal view by a round "double density" or by elevation of the left main-stem bronchus in the frontal view, but it also may be detected only in the right anterior oblique view as a discrete, posterior displacement of the barium-filled esophagus. This view is also useful for identifying right ventricular enlargement in patients suspected of having pulmonary hypertension. The left anterior oblique projection is the most reliable for detecting enlargement of the left ventricle. Other clues to the location of valvular heart lesions include poststenotic dilatation of the aorta in valvular aortic stenosis or calcification in a heart valve. Sometimes the latter is detected only by image intensification fluoroscopy.

The Electrocardiogram. In acquired valvular heart disease, the electrocardiogram should be carefully scrutinized for signs of chamber enlargement. Left atrial enlargement may be the only electrocardiographic sign of isolated mitral stenosis in the patient with sinus rhythm, and this single sign disappears when atrial fibrillation occurs. The presence or absence of left ventricular hypertrophy is of importance in considering the hemodynamic severity of aortic stenosis and in assessing the degree of mitral regurgitation; in the patient with mitral stenosis who has an apical systolic murmur, the presence of left ventricular hypertrophy may indicate that associated mitral regurgitation is of significance. The suspicion of associated coronary heart disease or myocardial disease may be raised by a bundle branch block pattern or by evidence of a previous myocardial infarction. Prominent (septal) Q waves associated with left

ventricular hypertrophy can also occur with hypertrophic subaortic stenosis. Right axis deviation or right ventricular hypertrophy suggests significant pulmonary hypertension. Sometimes the vectorcardiogram is employed to confirm the presence or absence of myocardial infarction or ventricular hypertrophy.

Special Laboratory Tests. Short of cardiac catheterization (discussed below), two other noninvasive tests are highly useful in the precise diagnosis of acquired valvular heart disease: the *phonocardiogram* and the *echocardiogram.*

The *phonocardiogram* is of value particularly for ascertaining the timing of normal and abnormal heart sounds. Recorded with the heart sounds are the indirect carotid pulse wave, which substitutes for the arterial pressure tracing; the indirect jugular venous tracing, which resembles the atrial pressure pulse; and the apex cardiogram, which corresponds roughly to the diastolic left ventricular pressure pulse. For example, a mitral opening snap can be identified by its close relation to the onset of left ventricular filling on the apexcardiogram, and its precise timing in relation to the aortic closure sound can be determined from the carotid pulse wave (see figure). A prolonged left ventricular ejection time and a single second heart sound are often associated with the abnormal carotid pulse wave of severe aortic stenosis (see figure). The phonocardiogram is not particularly useful for detecting soft cardiac murmurs; these are better identified by careful auscultation at various locations and by the several maneuvers described above.

The *echocardiogram* can aid considerably in reaching an accurate clinical diagnosis. Thus the characteristically abnormal pattern of anterior mitral valve leaflet motion can be demonstrated in mitral stenosis, or the fluttering movement of this leaflet associated with a diastolic Austin-Flint murmur can be identified. The echocardiogram may show posterior mitral leaflet prolapse when mitral regurgitation is associated with click-murmur syndrome or with papillary muscle dysfunction. The characteristic anterior movement of the mitral leaflet during systole and echocardiographic identification of septal hypertrophy have simplified the diagnosis of hypertrophic subaortic stenosis. The applications of echocardiography are many, and the technique is finding increasing application in the study of cardiac diseases of all types.

DECISIONS CONSIDERING CARDIAC CATHETERIZATION AND OPERATION

Cardiac catheterization is rarely necessary for the *diagnosis* of valvular heart disease. An accurate diagnosis can usually be accomplished by careful application of the approaches described above, including the use of special noninvasive techniques such as echocardiography when necessary. Therefore cardiac catheterization and angiography are generally reserved until the patient is considered a potential candidate for a corrective operation. Of course there are some occasions when cardiac catheterization is used to make a definitive diagnosis, such as in differentiating angina pectoris caused by aortic stenosis from that resulting from associated coronary atherosclerosis, or in the differential diagnosis of pulmonary hypertension. In the latter situation, it is clearly important not to make a diagnosis of primary pulmonary hypertension until mitral valve obstruction has been carefully excluded by hemodynamic studies.

Prior to considering a surgical procedure, cardiac catheterization is usually undertaken for several purposes: (1) To determine whether the valve lesion (stenosis or regurgitation) is sufficiently severe to make it likely that surgical correction will relieve symptoms. (2) To assess carefully the degree of left ventricular myocardial dysfunction or failure associated with aortic valve lesions and mitral regurgitation. (3) To detect significant associated lesions, such as unexpectedly severe mitral regurgitation or aortic stenosis in a patient with mitral stenosis. (4) To study the coronary circulation, particularly in older subjects or in patients with aortic valve disease in whom symptoms may be due primarily to coronary heart disease rather than the valvular lesion. (5) To assess the relative significance of myocardial and valvular disease in patients with recurrent symptoms after previous cardiac surgery.

Once appropriate information has been assembled concerning the mechanical severity of the valve defect, the degree of involvement of the left ventricular myocardium, the severity of any associated coronary artery disease, and possible complicating illnesses (such as diabetes mellitus, liver disease, anemia, or thyroid disease), a decision concerning the advisability of a cardiac operation can be undertaken. Such a decision must also be based upon knowledge in several other important areas:

1. The risk to the patient's life of the proposed operation versus the risk of medical management alone. Operative risk is related to the nature of the surgical intervention required. Must a valve prosthesis be inserted, or is a commissurotomy possible? Is more than one valve involved? Is there associated coronary artery disease that will require a myocardial revascularization procedure? The patient's age and the presence of associated noncardiac illness also influence the operative risk.

2. The usual natural course of the valve lesion and the long-range outlook after operation. Knowledge of the natural history as well as the likely course after operation is important. For example, once significant symptoms begin in patients with aortic stenosis, the downhill course is usually rapid and the risk of *not* operating outweighs that of the surgical procedure. The average downhill course is somewhat slower after the onset of symptoms in patients with aortic regurgitation, but the degree of secondary left ventricular myocardial dysfunction must be considered, and operation should be undertaken before myocardial disease becomes irreversible. A similar consideration applies in patients with chronic mitral regurgitation, but their more gradual downhill course allows a more leisurely decision concerning the proper time for surgical intervention. The probable finite limitations in the life span of the various valvular prostheses should be taken into account before recommending operation in a young patient who has only moderate limitation of activity.

3. The social setting. This must be considered carefully, for in the final analysis the expected benefits of the operation must be judged in relation to the patient's age, occupational needs, family responsibilities, and expectation of substantially improved longevity and functional capacity.

557. MITRAL STENOSIS

Etiology and Pathology.   Stenosis of the mitral valve in the adult usually develops as a sequel to rheumatic fever;

only rarely is it caused by such malformations as congenital cor triatriatum (see Ch. 555) or left atrial myxoma. It is the most common single valvular lesion to follow acute rheumatic fever, accounting for over half the patients with chronic rheumatic heart disease. About two thirds of the subjects are female.

The rheumatic mitral valve shows fibrosis and thickening of the cusps, with partial fusion of the commissures; in patients with longstanding disease, leaflet fusion may produce restriction of the mitral orifice to as little as 0.5 sq cm. There are thickening and shortening of the chordae tendineae, and there may be heavy calcium deposits in the valve. The left ventricle is generally normal in size and weight unless there is associated mitral regurgitation or disease of the aortic valve, but the left atrium is enlarged and thick walled. Microscopic examination of the myocardium often shows evidence of old rheumatic myocarditis (Aschoff bodies). In the lungs, there is thickening of the muscular walls of the pulmonary arterioles and venules with intimal proliferation, and in the late stages of mitral stenosis there is diffuse hemosiderosis (primarily disintegrated hemoglobin within alveoli), and there may be interstitial fibrosis and pulmonary infarction.

Pathologic Physiology.   The primary physiologic abnormality in mitral stenosis is mechanical obstruction to emptying of the left atrium produced by the narrowed valve orifice. Left ventricular function is usually normal, and therefore the defect in mitral stenosis stands in marked contrast to that of mitral regurgitation, or of aortic valve disease, in each of which a chronic overload is placed in the left ventricle.

When the mitral valve orifice is only mildly reduced, the mean left atrial pressure and filling of the left ventricle remain normal at rest. However, the rate of blood flow across the mitral valve is dependent not only on the orifice area of the valve and the driving pressure gradient (from left atrium to left ventricle), but also on the *time* available for flow across the mitral valve during diastole. With an increase in heart rate, the duration of left ventricular systole shortens only slightly, and tachycardia therefore occurs mainly at the expense of diastolic filling time per minute. Hence patients with mild mitral stenosis generally experience their earliest symptoms only during severe exertion, or with the onset of rapid atrial fibrillation. With exertion, both the normal tachycardia of exercise and the increased cardiac output lead to an increased left atrial pressure, whereas with atrial fibrillation and an uncontrolled ventricular rate the increased rate alone leads to a left atrial pressure elevation because of compromised filling time per minute.

With increased narrowing of the mitral orifice, the mean left atrial pressure becomes somewhat elevated at rest (over 12 mm Hg), but as the mitral orifice is reduced to below 1 sq cm the resting cardiac output can be maintained only at the expense of a markedly elevated left atrial pressure (often in excess of 20 mm Hg), in which the high pressure gradient forces blood across the narrowed orifice at high velocity. In this stage of the disease, the increased left atrial pressure and critically narrowed mitral valve often lead to pulmonary edema. Although pulmonary edema theoretically should occur when the pulmonary venous pressure exceeds about 30 mm Hg, higher levels have occasionally been recorded without its occurrence. This may be related to thickening of the alveolar-capillary membrane, which has been noted in the lungs of patients with mitral stenosis.

As the disease progresses, the elevated pressure in the pulmonary veins leads to pulmonary artery hypertension. When pulmonary hypertension becomes persistent at rest, it reflects two major factors: first, the elevated left atrial pressure is transmitted retrogradely and requires an increased pressure head in the pulmonary artery to drive blood forward; and second, pulmonary arteriolar vasoconstriction occurs. This vasoconstriction is accompanied in time by organic changes, mainly intimal proliferation and medial thickening in the walls of the small pulmonary arteries. At this stage, the pulmonary vascular resistance becomes elevated, which in turn leads to a reduction in the resting cardiac output. This sequence tends to limit any further increase in the left atrial pressure, which may even fall somewhat as the cardiac output becomes diminished. Symptoms of pulmonary venous congestion and pulmonary edema often diminish at this stage. In late mitral stenosis, pulmonary hypertension may become extreme, with the systolic pressure in the pulmonary artery equal to or exceeding that in the systemic arterial bed. Even with less marked elevations in pulmonary arterial pressure, the right ventricular end-diastolic volume and pressure become elevated, and this may lead to functional tricuspid regurgitation. Finally, signs of right ventricular failure appear with peripheral venous congestion.

Clinical Manifestations. *Symptoms and Clinical Course.* After one or more attacks of rheumatic fever in childhood, there is a latent period averaging about 12 years before mitral stenosis becomes clinically manifest, symptoms and signs usually first becoming apparent in young adulthood. There is commonly then a relatively long period (five to eight years) of mild to moderate symptoms as the scarring and obstruction at the valve gradually progress.

The earliest manifestation of mild to moderate mitral stenosis is dyspnea caused primarily by the increased cardiac output and tachycardia of exercise, leading to transient elevation of left atrial pressure, as discussed above. Elevation of the left atrial pressure causes pulmonary venous hypertension, increasing lung stiffness and the work of breathing, and thereby leads to the subjective sensation of dyspnea. As the disease progresses, orthopnea at night commences as a result of redistribution of the peripheral blood volume into the central circulation and of peripheral resorption of fluid caused by the supine posture. Coughing, particularly at night, may also be a troublesome symptom. Dyspnea eventually becomes extreme with minimal activity, and hemoptysis may occur owing to rupture of dilated endobronchial vessels, which appear to form collateral channels between the pulmonary and bronchial venous systems. The hemoptysis, consisting of bright red blood which can accumulate in sufficient quantities to cause atelectasis, usually subsides with bed rest and sedation with opiates; most commonly it occurs in patients who do not have severe elevation of the pulmonary vascular resistance. An increased number of pulmonary infections may occur, perhaps related to the interstitial pulmonary edema present in this stage of the disease, and other factors such as severe emotional stress, sexual activity, and fever with tachycardia may acutely worsen the patient's symptoms.

Significant left atrial enlargement develops as the left atrial hypertension becomes persistent, and atrial premature beats, paroxysmal atrial tachycardia, or atrial fibrillation commonly occur. The sudden onset of atrial fibrillation with rapid ventricular rate may precipitate acute pulmonary edema when the obstruction at the mitral orifice is of sufficient severity. Eventually, sustained atrial fibrillation supervenes, requiring control of the ventricular response with digitalis. Intermittent atrial fibrillation, in particular, may be associated with peripheral embolic phenomena, and the incidence of emboli in patients with chronic atrial fibrillation is substantial. As the left atrium enlarges and stasis occurs, thrombus formation is most frequent within the left atrial appendage, and adherent clots have been found at operation in this location in about 30 per cent of patients. Small emboli may break loose to become lodged in the renal, splenic, or cerebral circulations, and the effects of such emboli, causing a convulsion or perhaps a renal infarction, sometimes provide the initial symptom in a patient with mitral stenosis. Coronary artery embolization with myocardial infarction has also been reported. Sometimes a large embolus to the brain results in serious and permanent sequelae, and saddle embolus in the aorta has been encountered on a number of occasions. Infrequently a thrombus within the left atrium may become sufficiently large to obstruct a pulmonary vein, leading to localized unilateral pulmonary edema, and rarely a pedunculated "ball-valve thrombus" can be formed which mimics the findings of left atrial myxoma (see below).

As mitral stenosis progresses further, the pulmonary vascular resistance rises, tending to limit flow across the pulmonary bed; with the associated diminution of pulmonary venous hypertension, hemoptysis and pulmonary interstitial edema diminish. Thus in patients with longstanding, severe mitral stenosis, dyspnea on exertion and orthopnea often become less prominent, and fatigue now predominates. The development of functional tricuspid regurgitation may result in a further drop in the cardiac output and some reduction in the pulmonary artery pressure. In this stage of the disease weakness and signs of right heart failure become extreme, and abdominal discomfort with hepatomegaly, ascites and peripheral edema dominate the clinical picture. Pulmonary embolus with pulmonary infarction are common late complications.

Physical Findings. The patient (usually a female) with severe mitral stenosis may exhibit peripheral cyanosis and a "mitral facies" (blue-tinged with malar flush), and often there is some degree of emaciation. In such advanced cases, peripheral edema and ascites may also be evident.

The peripheral arterial pulses are typically small, and the blood pressure is normal or low. The jugular venous pulse is initially normal in the presence of moderate mitral stenosis, but as pulmonary hypertension develops, the mean venous pressure is increased and the A wave becomes prominent owing to right ventricular hypertrophy and elevation of the right ventricular end-diastolic pressure. In the presence of atrial fibrillation, there is a dominant V wave in the jugular veins.

In patients with mitral stenosis without pulmonary hypertension, palpation of the precordium may be unremarkable except for the presence of a diastolic thrill localized just inside the left ventricular apex. The apical impulse is otherwise normal, and the heart is not enlarged. In patients with pulmonary hypertension, there is a right ventricular lift in the left parasternal area, and the bulging pulmonary artery segment and pulmonic closure sound may be palpable at the upper left base if the mean pulmonary arterial pressure is in excess of 50 mm Hg.

On auscultation, the first heart sound is generally loud, snapping in quality, and somewhat delayed. These features occur because the left atrial pressure is elevated, and additional time is required for the left ventricle to build up sufficient pressure to close the mitral valve; the rate of change of left ventricular pressure (dP/dt) is rapid by that time, which results in the more forceful than normal mitral valve closure. The aortic closure sound is normal, but a mitral opening snap follows the second sound, the snap being audible at the lower left sternal border and the apex. A general correlation exists between the severity of mitral stenosis and the timing of the opening snap, necessitating careful evaluation of the interval between aortic closure and the opening snap. As the left ventricular pressure declines during the isovolumetric relaxation period after aortic valve closure, eventually it falls below the left atrial pressure and the stenotic mitral valve then snaps open. The higher the left atrial pressure, the closer this event must occur in relation to aortic closure (A_2). This time interval (the so-called A_2-OS interval) tends to be long (0.10 second or more) in patients with mild mitral stenosis and mean left atrial pressures below 15 mm Hg, whereas in patients with severe mitral stenosis and mean left atrial pressures of 20 mm Hg or more, the interval is usually shorter (less than 0.09 second). As might be expected, however, the interval will vary considerably with the heart rate. If the heart rate is below 100 and the interval 0.07 second or less, the mitral stenosis is usually of significant degree.

The opening snap is followed immediately by a low-pitched *diastolic rumble* resulting from turbulent flow across the stenotic mitral orifice. The murmur is usually localized to an area about 2 cm in diameter near or just inside the left ventricular apex in the fourth or fifth left intercostal space, and it is best brought out by positioning the patient in the lateral decubitus position. The mitral rumble is loudest in early diastole; it diminishes somewhat as the pressure gradient between left atrium and left ventricle falls, and, in patients with sinus rhythm, it then becomes loud (presystolic accentuation) as the left atrium contracts to again raise the pressure gradient (see figure in Ch. 556). When the stenosis is mild, the diastolic murmur may not be audible until the patient is placed in the lateral decubitus position *after* performing mild exercise or during a handgrip maneuver, when the cardiac output and heart rate are increased, thereby augmenting the pressure gradient across the valve. In the presence of atrial fibrillation, presystolic accentuation disappears; when the ventricular rate is slow, the murmur may occur only in the early and middle phases of long diastolic periods, because given sufficient time the left atrial and left ventricular pressure will come into equilibrium. In patients with severe mitral stenosis and a very low cardiac output, the murmur may be unusually difficult to appreciate. It is most important therefore to position the patient properly and to listen carefully over a wide area of the left chest for the well localized murmur, as well as to carry out the aforementioned exercise maneuvers. When such precautions are taken, "silent" mitral stenosis will be encountered rarely. Occasionally the murmur is inaudible when massive right ventricular enlargement places the left ventricle far posteriorly from the chest wall.

Individuals with "pure" mitral stenosis have a small fixed orifice, and it is not uncommon to hear a soft systolic murmur at the cardiac apex, which represents a trivial mitral regurgitant leak. When a louder pansystolic murmur at the left ventricular apex is accompanied by a third heart sound, by left ventricular enlargement on physical examination, or by electrocardiographic signs of left ventricular hypertrophy, the associated mitral regurgitation is undoubtedly of significance. In the patient with severe pulmonary hypertension, when a very large right ventricle fills the anterior chest and displaces the left ventricle posteriorly, the murmur of tricuspid regurgitation can mimic that of mitral regurgitation. The systolic murmur of tricuspid regurgitation is ordinarily heard best at the lower left sternal border; it increases with inspiration, and is not heard in the axilla or over the spine posteriorly, features which serve to distinguish it from the murmur of mitral regurgitation. With severe pulmonary hypertension the high-pitched, early diastolic blowing murmur of pulmonic regurgitation (the Graham Steell murmur) may also be audible. This murmur, heard best at the left sternal border, is usually indistinguishable from that of mild aortic regurgitation.

Diagnosis. *Electrocardiogram.* In patients with moderate mitral stenosis and sinus rhythm, the electrocardiogram may show only left atrial enlargement, with a notched and prolonged P wave in the limb leads and an increased negative component of the P wave in lead V_1. When there is atrial fibrillation, patients with rheumatic heart disease tend to show coarse fibrillation waves, presumably owing to the thickened atrial wall and enlarged chamber volume, a finding which contrasts with the fine fibrillatory waves often found in patients with coronary heart disease.

In severe mitral stenosis with pulmonary hypertension, the electrocardiogram often shows right axis deviation, and voltage criteria for right ventricular hypertrophy are sometimes present. Evidence of left ventricular hypertrophy in a patient with mitral stenosis generally indicates accompanying aortic valve disease or significant associated mitral regurgitation.

Roentgenographic Features. Minimal enlargement of the left atrium may be the only radiographic abnormality in patients with moderate mitral stenosis. It may be apparent only with barium swallow, the right anterior oblique view showing best the localized, posterior displacement of the barium-filled esophagus. As the disease progresses, left atrial enlargement becomes distinct, and this chamber is visible as a large round "double density" in the center of the cardiac shadow on the frontal view. The left main-stem bronchus is elevated by the enlarged left atrium (the angle formed by the bronchus with a central, vertical line increasing to more than 45 degrees), and enlargement of the left atrial appendage results in straightening of the left heart border.

As left atrial and pulmonary venous hypertension develop, there is a redistribution of the pulmonary vascularity in the lung fields. Initially, in the upright posture the normal, relative avascularity of the upper lobes is lost, and the pulmonary vascular pattern appears equal in the upper and lower lungs. In later stages of the disease, vascularity in the upper lobe vessels is increased. Redistribution of the pulmonary vascular pattern generally occurs when left atrial pressure exceeds 15 mm Hg, and evidence of interstitial pulmonary edema commonly appears when the mean left atrial pressure at rest exceeds 20 mm Hg. Interstitial edema may be evidenced by *Kerley's B lines,* transverse linear densities about 1 cm in length and located at the lung bases laterally above the diaphragm, representing engorged septal lymphatic vessels. Acute pulmonary edema is reflected by typical butterfly densities in the hilar regions.

As pulmonary hypertension develops, the pulmonary artery segment becomes enlarged, the peripheral pulmonary arteries become dilated, and enlargement of the right ventricle and right atrium is evident. With longstanding pulmonary hypertension a diffuse reticular pattern in the lung fields may result from pulmonary hemosiderosis. Calcification in the mitral valve should be searched for, using image intensification fluoroscopy. The presence of calcification makes it less likely that the valve will prove amenable to valvuloplasty.

Echocardiography. Reflected ultrasound to confirm the presence of mitral stenosis and to estimate its severity has found increasing application. The echo recorded from the mitral leaflets exhibits characteristic features in the presence of significant mitral stenosis, the degree of the abnormality correlating in general with the severity of stenosis. Thickening of the anterior and posterior leaflets can often be identified, and there is a reduced anterior excursion of the leaflet during diastole. Both the anterior and posterior leaflets move forward with diastole as the domed, stenotic valve opens (in a normal valve, the posterior leaflet opens in an opposite direction to the anterior leaflet). Because of the persistent pressure gradient from left atrium to left ventricle, the normal posterior floating motion of the anterior mitral leaflet during mid-diastole does not occur; the leaflet is held open in an anterior position and moves only slowly posteriorly. This posterior motion (the so-called E to F slope) is reduced to less than 12 mm per second with severe mitral stenosis (normally it is 40 mm per second or more).

The detection of characteristic moving echoes from behind the mitral valve can indicate the presence of left atrial myxoma or a ball-valve thrombus.

Pulmonary Function Tests. Patients with longstanding mitral stenosis generally have a reduced pulmonary compliance owing to elevation of the left atrial pressure and interstitial pulmonary edema. The vital capacity, total lung capacity, maximal breathing capacity, and oxygen uptake per unit of ventilation may be reduced, and abnormalities of ventilation-perfusion relations are often seen as well.

Cardiac Catheterization. In the young patient with obvious features of pure mitral stenosis and marked symptoms, cardiac catheterization is not performed in some centers prior to operation. On the other hand, when there is uncertainty about the severity of the stenosis in relation to the level of symptoms, cardiac catheterization should be performed to document objectively the degree of valve narrowing, and to calculate the orifice area. At cardiac catheterization, the typical patient with significant mitral stenosis will exhibit an elevated mean pulmonary artery wedge pressure. If a satisfactory wedge pressure tracing cannot be obtained, transseptal left atrial puncture is often performed. If the patient is in sinus rhythm, the forceful left atrial contraction produces a dominant A wave in the tracing, and there is a slow fall in the pressure after the V wave (reduced rate of the Y descent), reflecting obstruction to left atrial emptying during diastole. The left ventricular end-diastolic pressure is usually normal (below 12 mm Hg). The pressure gradient from left atrium to left ventricle is high early in diastole, falling progressively as left ventricular filling occurs, but the gradient is again increased late in diastole by left atrial contraction (see figure in Ch. 556). In patients with atrial fibrillation, the V wave is dominant and left atrial pressure continues to fall throughout diastole until the onset of ventricular systole.

The *mitral valve orifice area* can be calculated if both the cardiac output and the pressure gradient are known. By the Gorlin formula, the valve orifice area is directly proportional to the flow across the valve per second of diastole and is inversely proportional to the square root of the pressure gradient. In simple terms, this means that if the flow doubles, the pressure gradient will quadruple. Because of this nonlinear relation, measurement of the left atrial or wedge pressure alone can be misleading in assessing the severity of the mitral stenosis. Thus if the cardiac output is unusually high, an elevated left atrial mean pressure may give a false picture of the severity of the stenotic lesion; if it is low, a moderate left atrial pressure elevation may belie the presence of severe stenosis. Also, if the heart rate is abnormally rapid or slow and a shorter or longer diastolic filling time is available, the left atrial mean pressure may not reflect accurately the size of the mitral orifice. The area of the normal mitral valve is about 4 sq cm. Mitral stenosis is generally considered mild when the calculated orifice area is over 1.2 sq cm, moderate when it is between 1.2 and 0.9 sq cm, and severe when it is below 0.8 sq cm. Thus an area of 1.1 sq cm or less is usually considered to represent stenosis of sufficient severity to warrant operation.

Left ventriculography usually shows the left ventricle to contract normally, with a normal end-diastolic volume. It also provides information concerning the degree of thickening and fusion of the chordal attachments of the mitral valve, the pliability of its leaflets, and the degree of associated mitral regurgitation. All these factors, together with the presence or absence of valve calcification, weigh in the decision of whether to perform closed or open mitral valvuloplasty, or whether to recommend replacement of the valve with a prosthesis.

In older patients, selective coronary arteriography is indicated to search for significant coronary vascular disease. Cardiac catheterization will also document the severity of any associated aortic valvular disease; in patients with recurrent systemic emboli, a pulmonary angiogram may verify the presence of a left atrial thrombus.

Differential Diagnosis. Clinical findings of pulmonary hypertension should raise the suspicion of mitral stenosis. *Primary pulmonary hypertension* usually occurs in young females; it is associated with hyperventilation, chest pain, fatigue and dyspnea, and effort syncope, but with a relative paucity of objective physical findings. Whenever this diagnosis is considered, mitral stenosis and left atrial myxoma, treatable causes of left atrial and pulmonary hypertension, should be excluded by measurement of left atrial pressure directly or from an adequate pulmonary arterial wedge pressure. *Pulmonary hypertension caused by severe chronic lung disease* usually presents no diagnostic difficulty; but sometimes patients are given a diagnosis of ordinary bronchial asthma, when in fact their wheezing is due to mitral stenosis with left atrial hypertension ("cardiac asthma").

The murmur of rheumatic mitral stenosis may be mimicked by that resulting from a *left atrial myxoma.* However, with the latter lesion there may be other abnormal diastolic sounds, and the murmur may disappear when the patient's position is altered. In addition, symptoms can vary with changes in body position, syncope may occur, and there is usually an elevated sedimentation rate, anemia, fever, or other evidence of systemic disease. Echocardiography may detect the left atrial myxoma. In the young patient, *congenital cor triatriatum* (a rare malformation consisting of a fibrous partition within the left atrium above the mitral valve) may be considered.

The diastolic rumble which occurs in the presence of severe aortic regurgitation, the *Austin Flint murmur*, may be attributed to organic mitral stenosis. This murmur is typically ushered in by a ventricular diastolic gallop (S_3) rather than an opening snap, and it is loudest in mid-diastole. Amyl nitrite inhalation decreases this murmur by lowering diastolic aortic pressure, but the reflex tachycardia and increased cardiac output increase the murmur of mitral stenosis. Echocardiography is particularly helpful in differentiating the Austin Flint murmur from that of mitral stenosis by detecting a characteristic fluttering motion of the anterior leaflet during diastole as its motion is affected by the regurgitant jet.

In the older patient, *atrial septal defect* is occasionally mistaken for mitral stenosis. In atrial septal defect, the tricuspid closure sound is loud, the widely split second heart may mimic the opening snap of mitral stenosis, and the rumble of excessive flow across the tricuspid valve may be confused with the murmur of mitral stenosis. The murmur of mitral stenosis diminishes with inspiration, in contrast to this murmur and the murmur of tricuspid stenosis, which increase.

Treatment. *Medical Management.* In the patient with mild mitral stenosis and few symptoms, restriction of strenuous activity may result in many years of comfortable existence. If the patient is under 40 years of age, monthly Bicillin injections or oral penicillin (sulfonamides may be used in the allergic patient) are advisable to prevent infection with the beta-hemolytic Streptococcus and recurrence of acute rheumatic fever (see Ch. 191). In addition, antimicrobial drugs in therapeutic doses should be recommended prior to and after dental procedures or surgical manipulations, particularly those on the genitourinary tract, to prevent bacterial endocarditis (see Ch. 192).

In patients with moderate symptoms, limitation of activity should be combined with *sodium restriction* and/or administration of a *diuretic* agent. There is little rationale for the use of digitalis in patients with sinus rhythm, because left ventricular function is normal and this agent has no effect on exercise-induced tachycardia. *When atrial fibrillation occurs* for the first time, one or more attempts at *electrical reversion of the rhythm,* followed by maintenance with oral quinidine, are generally indicated. When mitral stenosis is significant, however, permanent atrial fibrillation will generally supervene in time, despite such therapy. In the presence of chronic atrial fibrillation, *digitalis* should be administered to maintain the ventricular rate at an acceptable level both at rest and during moderate exertion. In patients who are particularly sensitive to digitalis, the addition of a *beta-adrenergic blocking agent* (such as propranolol) in small doses may result in very effective control of the ventricular response. Moreover, during acute stress, such as a pneumonia, patients with atrial fibrillation may develop a rapid ventricular response caused by enhanced atrioventricular conduction con-

sequent to excessive sympathetic nervous discharge; under these circumstances the addition of a beta-adrenergic blocking agent to digitalis may allow effective reduction of the ventricular rate in a safer manner than with high doses of digitalis alone. When the ventricular rate is refractory to digitalis in the absence of acute stress, or when signs of heart failure are out of proportion to the degree of mitral stenosis, hyperthyroidism should be suspected. Obvious signs of thyrotoxicosis may be masked in the presence of cardiac disease; but if such hyperthyroidism is detected and treated, symptoms caused by mild mitral stenosis may disappear.

In patients who have suffered a systemic embolus originating from the left atrium, long-term *anticoagulation* with Coumadin derivatives has been shown to be effective in preventing recurrence. Minor neurologic episodes, or a frank convulsion, often provide the earliest sign of systemic embolization. Emboli also may occur to the legs, or to the mesenteric artery (causing abdominal and bowel necrosis), and prompt surgical treatment with embolectomy is required. If systemic embolization recurs while the patient is on adequate anticoagulant therapy, a mitral valve operation with removal of left atrial clot may be recommended for the patient with somewhat milder mitral stenosis, or with less marked symptoms than are usually required for an elective operation.

When pregnancy occurs in a patient with mitral stenosis, symptoms frequently develop for the first time or intensify. Such symptoms become most severe during the second trimester, when increased cardiac output and blood volume are maximal, and a substantial period of hospital treatment may be required. Generally, such symptoms diminish during the third trimester, and only rarely is a mitral commissurotomy necessary during pregnancy.

Once severe symptoms begin in the patient with tight mitral stenosis (New York Heart Association [N.Y.H.A.] Class III), the average mortality in patients treated medically approaches 30 per cent at five years. In severely limited patients (Class IV), the outlook without operation is extremely poor, less than 20 per cent of patients being alive after five years if data gathered prior to the cardiac surgical era are considered. Surgical treatment has greatly altered this outlook.

Surgical Treatment. In the typical younger patient with symptoms on normal activity (N.Y.H.A. Class II) and findings of pure mitral stenosis, the decision of whether to recommend operation is usually reached by considering the individual in his desired activity setting. In the patient with significant mitral stenosis who has had a complication such as a systemic embolus and who develops symptoms on ordinary exertion, operation is usually recommended. In the older patient in functional Class II who has evidence of mitral valve calcification on x-ray and physical findings suggesting a thickened and immobile mitral leaflet (soft first heart sound and reduced or absent opening snap), or in whom significant associated mitral regurgitation is suspected, a waiting period until symptoms are more severe is justified, because mitral valve replacement with a prosthesis will undoubtedly be necessary. In patients with symptoms on less than normal activity (N.Y.H.A. Class III) or at rest (Class IV), the outlook without surgical treatment is poor and the indication for operation is clear.

The presence of severe pulmonary hypertension was considered at one time to represent a relative contraindication to operation, but more recent studies have indicated that even marked elevations of the pulmonary vascular resistance invariably regress postoperatively. Some reduction in the pulmonary vascular resistance occurs within a few hours postoperatively. In most patients studied by cardiac catheterization six months to one year after operation, the pulmonary artery pressure and pulmonary vascular resistance have returned to normal or near normal levels, provided the left atrial pressure is normal.

Surgical practices differ somewhat as to the type of procedure performed in the patient with mitral stenosis. Closed mitral valvulotomy by opening the valve commissures with the finger, inserted through the left atrial appendage, sometimes combined with the use of a mechanical dilator passed through the left ventricular apex, is still employed by some surgeons without the use of cardiopulmonary bypass (heart-lung machine). In many centers, open mitral commissurotomy is now carried out even in the uncomplicated patient, the left atrium being opened with the patient on cardiopulmonary bypass and the mitral stenosis relieved by blunt and sharp dissection under direct vision. The operative risk of such a mitral valvuloplasty is now about equal to that of cardiopulmonary bypass alone (under 4 per cent). This approach also allows removal of any clot that may be present within the left atrium. If significant mitral regurgitation is produced by the attempted valvuloplasty, it is then possible to proceed readily with replacement of the mitral valve by a ball-valve or other prosthesis.

The late results of valvuloplasty have been poor when there is significant mitral regurgitation, or if there is calcification with severe shortening and thickening of the chordae tendineae and immobilization of the mitral valve leaflets. When the valve exhibits such unfavorable anatomic signs, it is replaced with a prosthetic device. The average operative mortality for valve replacement ranges between 6 and 10 per cent.

After a valvuloplasty, the average patient experiences 8 to 12 years of symptomatic relief, but a second operation is often necessary (usually mitral valve replacement). The late results of mitral valve replacement have been generally favorable, with improved life expectancy and relief of symptoms. Long-term anticoagulation is required for many types of prosthetic devices.

558. MITRAL REGURGITATION

Etiology and Pathology. A wide spectrum of disease processes can result in mitral regurgitation, although rheumatic involvement is by far the most common cause. Rheumatic mitral regurgitation occurs more commonly in males, in contrast to mitral stenosis, and the murmur is commonly heard during or soon after the acute rheumatic episode, again in contrast to the relatively late development of the murmur of mitral stenosis. In chronic rheumatic disease, the left ventricle is generally dilated and the wall thickened, there is left atrial enlargement, and the mitral valve exhibits mild, diffuse scarring of the leaflets associated with some thickening of the chordae tendineae. The finding of associated aortic valve disease favors a rheumatic cause.

Other forms of mitral regurgitation include rupture of one or more chordae tendineae, most commonly resulting from bacterial endocarditis, but also sometimes attributed to rheumatic disease, trauma, or unknown causes. Papillary muscle dysfunction is usually secondary to necrosis or fibrosis of one or both papillary muscles owing to coronary artery disease, mitral regurgitation resulting from poor contraction of the muscles, and systolic eversion of the mitral leaflets. In acute myocardial infarction, rupture of a papillary muscle causes sudden, severe mitral regurgitation (see Ch. 567). Mitral regurgitation caused by ballooning with prolapse of the posterior leaflet during systole, or to abnormally long chordae, the so-called *"floppy valve syndrome,"* sometimes is inherited, and increased acid mucopolysaccharide deposits may be found in the valve. Congenital mitral regurgitation can occur as an isolated condition, but more commonly it accompanies such lesions as ostium primum atrial septal defect or Marfan's syndrome in which the valve may resemble that found in the floppy valve syndrome, but is associated with other stigmata.

Mitral regurgitation also occurs as a secondary phenomenon in patients with idiopathic hypertrophic subaortic stenosis, as discussed subsequently. In primary myocardial disease, mitral regurgitation may be secondary to massive dilatation of the left ventricle and the mitral anulus. Acquired, heavy calcification of the mitral anulus, which typically occurs in elderly women, is sometimes associated with significant mitral regurgitation.

Pathologic Physiology. With insufficiency of the mitral valve of the type found in chronic rheumatic heart disease, regurgitation of blood from the left ventricle into the left atrium commences as soon as the left ventricular pressure during early systole exceeds that in the left atrium, and persists until the left ventricular pressure falls below the left atrial pressure. Therefore the regurgitation is pansystolic, commencing with the first heart sound and often ending with or just after the second heart sound, and at the peak of the atrial V wave. The prominent V wave in the left atrial pressure pulse is due to the normal inflow of blood from the pulmonary veins (when the mitral valve is ordinarily closed) which is augmented by the regurgitant leak.

An important physiologic characteristic of mitral regurgitation relative to the function of the left ventricle is that this lesion provides a relatively low impedance pathway for blood to exit from the left ventricle, pressure in the left atrium being lower than that in the aorta. The pressure in the left ventricle tends to fall more abruptly than normal late in ventricular systole because of the leak, and the average afterload or active tension in the wall of the left ventricle is thereby reduced. This effect favors increased shortening of the myocardial wall because of the inverse relation between force and fiber shortening (and velocity), and the ratio of stroke volume to end-diastolic volume (ejection fraction) may therefore be normal or even high in mitral regurgitation. In addition, although myocardial oxygen consumption is greatly enhanced by lesions which cause increased systolic pressure work or augmented wall tension, it is little affected by the increased volume load imposed by mitral regurgitation. These favorable mechanical loading conditions and the minimal effect of this lesion on oxygen consumption help to explain the prolonged clinical course observed in many patients with chronic mitral regurgitation.

In chronic mitral regurgitation the diastolic volume of the left ventricular chamber becomes increased because of ventricular dilatation and increased muscle mass. The increased diastolic ventricular size allows delivery of a much larger than normal *total* stroke volume during systole (forward stroke volume plus the regurgitant volume), but with a normal extent of shortening of each unit of the enlarged left ventricular circumference. When left ventricular myocardial function is not impaired, the left ventricular end-diastolic pressure is normal or only slightly elevated, and the forward cardiac output is well maintained. Under these conditions, the *mean* left atrial pressure may be minimally elevated, because the exaggerated V wave occurs only briefly during the cardiac cycle. There is no impairment of left atrial emptying into the left ventricle and hence little or no rise in mean left atrial pressure during exercise.

With longstanding, severe mitral regurgitation, left ventricular myocardial contractility is eventually depressed. When this happens, the extent of shortening of the left ventricular wall become reduced, the residual volume in the left ventricle at the end of ejection increases, the ejection fraction falls, and the end-diastolic volume and left ventricular end-diastolic pressure rise. The latter, in turn, leads to elevation of the mean left atrial pressure and subsequently to pulmonary hypertension. Left atrial hypertension also occurs when there is some associated narrowing of the mitral valve. The mechanism of pulmonary hypertension in mitral regurgitation resembles that in mitral stenosis, and in later stages elevations of the pulmonary vascular resistance as severe as those seen with mitral stenosis have been encountered.

The aforementioned description encompasses most patients with chronic rheumatic mitral regurgitation, but there are unusual physiologic manifestations seen late in the course of chronic disease or with acute mitral regurgitation, such as that caused by ruptured chordae tendineae. In the former category is the finding of giant left atrium with low mean left atrial pressure and greatly reduced cardiac output. This syndrome appears to be due to a combination of poor left ventricular function, with reduced forward cardiac output and diminished regurgitant volume, as well as to a capacious and compliant left atrium, which absorbs the regurgitant leak with little change in the pressure. At the other extreme is the situation in sudden, severe mitral regurgitation. In this setting, the left atrium is small, distended, and noncompliant, and the large regurgitant leak produces a giant V wave which can reach 70 to 80 mm Hg (so-called "ventricularization" of the left atrial pressure pulse). Severe pulmonary hypertension and reduced forward cardiac output accompany such marked, acute regurgitation.

Clinical Manifestations. *Symptoms and Clinical Course.* As mentioned earlier, the mean left atrial pressure may not be significantly elevated at rest in patients with mitral regurgitation in whom the left ventricle is compensated, and, unlike mitral stenosis, there is little increase in left atrial pressure during exercise or with tachycardia. Therefore the earliest symptom in mitral regurgitation is often exertional fatigue, which reflects inability to maintain a normal forward cardiac output to supply the exercising skeletal muscles. Mild symptoms of this type may persist for many years without significant dyspnea or pulmonary congestion.

Later in the course of severe chronic mitral regurgitation, with the onset of early left ventricular failure, the ventricular end-diastolic pressure increases, left atrial hypertension develops, and dyspnea on exertion and orthopnea occur. However, paroxysmal nocturnal dyspnea and acute pulmonary edema are distinctly unusual in this condition. With the onset of pulmonary hypertension, right heart failure accompanied by venous distention and peripheral edema may occur. Atrial fibrillation is a common complication, but left atrial thrombi are relatively unusual, and systemic emboli occur much less commonly than with mitral stenosis.

Chronic mitral regurgitation is the best tolerated of the lesions involving the left side of the heart. Frequently, patients remain relatively asymptomatic for 10 or 20 years, even in the presence of severe regurgitation, and it is not uncommon for patients to respond well to medical therapy for an additional 10 years or more before progressive left ventricular failure causes serious progressive difficulty and death. This long clinical course undoubtedly reflects in part the favorable loading conditions of this lesion on the left ventricle, as discussed earlier. It seems likely that a sizable number of patients with only moderate mitral regurgitation never experience serious difficulty and may have a normal life expectancy.

Physical Findings. When mitral regurgitation is severe, the peripheral pulse is sharp and abbreviated, owing to lack of sustained forward stroke volume in the face of the regurgitant leak. The jugular venous pulse is normal unless there is pulmonary hypertension or tricuspid valve disease. Atrial fibrillation is frequently present.

On palpation of the precordium, the left ventricle is enlarged, the apex beat is hyperactive and displaced laterally, and frequently there is a systolic thrill at the apex. In the lateral decubitus position, a rapid outward movement in early diastole (rapid filling wave) may be palpable. If pulmonary hypertension is present, there is a right ventricular lift. When the left atrium is markedly enlarged and the mitral regurgitation is severe, expansion of this chamber during systole may push the right ventricle and pulmonary artery out against the chest wall in the third and fourth left interspaces during late systole, a finding which may be confused with right ventricular enlargement.

The characteristic feature of mitral regurgitation in chronic rheumatic disease is a high-pitched *pansystolic murmur* at the cardiac apex which is transmitted to the left axilla (see figure in Ch. 556). If the lesion is severe, it is accompanied by four other findings: (1) soft first heart sound, (2) loud ventricular diastolic gallop (third heart sound), (3) short early diastolic rumble, which accompanies the rapid inflow of blood to the left ventricle, and (4) wide splitting of the second heart sound caused by early closure of the aortic valve. The last-named finding is caused by shortening of the left ventricular ejection time consequent to the regurgitant leak.

Although the murmur of mitral regurgitation is usually pansystolic, variations may be heard. When mitral regurgitation is due to papillary muscle dysfunction, the murmur begins well after the first heart sound and may have a crescendo-decrescendo quality. These characteristics result from posterior herniation of the mitral leaflet as the papillary muscles fail to contract normally late during ventricular systole. In the *click-murmur syndrome,* late ballooning of the mitral leaflets into the left atrium also occurs, but caused by intrinsic mitral valve disease. In this condition the late systolic murmur may be ushered in by one or more midsystolic clicks. In sudden, severe mitral regurgitation, sinus rhythm is often preserved and there may be a loud fourth heart sound, a most uncommon finding in chronic mitral regurgitation. When a giant left atrial V wave accompanies acute mitral regurgitation, the murmur may occur early in systole; but it is short and terminates before the end of systole, because the left ventricular pressure and massive left atrial V wave equalize near or even before the time of aortic valve closure.

Diagnosis. *Electrocardiogram.* In patients with mild to moderate mitral regurgitation the electrocardiogram may be normal; but with longstanding moderate disease or with severe regurgitation, the electrocardiogram usually shows left ventricular hypertrophy and atrial fibrillation. Typically, there is evidence of a so-called diastolic overload pattern, with upright T waves and voltage criteria for left ventricular hypertrophy. Right ventricular hypertrophy may develop in the late stages of the disease when there is pulmonary hypertension. If sinus rhythm is present, left atrial enlargement may be evident.

In the "click-murmur syndrome" S-T segment and T wave abnormalities may be seen; in the familial form, the QT interval may be prolonged. Evidence of old or recent myocardial infarction may be seen with papillary muscle dysfunction caused by coronary heart disease.

Roentgenographic Features. The left ventricle and left atrium are usually enlarged. Occasionally, the left atrium is of giant size and can extend well into the right chest. The left ventricle is observed to contract vigorously on fluoroscopy, and systolic expansion of the left atrium may be striking. The presence of calcium in the mitral valve suggests some degree of associated mitral stenosis. If left atrial hypertension is marked, the findings in the lung fields resemble those of mitral stenosis.

Echocardiography. The echo from the mitral valve leaflets can be particularly useful in detecting abnormal posterior prolapse of one or both mitral leaflets into the left atrium during systole. This distinctive echocardiographic pattern may allow a definitive diagnosis in the *click-murmur syndrome* or papillary muscle dysfunction.

Cardiac Catheterization. Cardiac catheterization is indicated prior to considering cardiac surgery in order to confirm the presence of severe regurgitation, assess the degree of left ventricular myocardial dysfunction, exclude associated coronary artery disease, and assess the severity of any associated valvular lesions.

The severity of mitral regurgitation can be estimated by cineangiography, with injection of contrast medium into the left ventricle. The backward regurgitation of contrast medium into the left atrium during ventricular systole is readily apparent, and it is also possible to calculate the diastolic volume of the left ventricle, the total stroke volume, and the ejection fraction. If the forward cardiac output and forward stroke volume are calculated by the Fick method, when the regurgitation is severe the regurgitant volume per beat may be well in excess of the forward stroke volume.

An elevated V wave in the left atrium (peak of the V wave over 20 mm Hg) may be detected on the pulmonary artery wedge pressure tracing, or from direct measurement by transseptal puncture, with relatively normal mean left atrial pressure. The increased V wave is followed by a rapid pressure fall (the Y descent) as the ventricle relaxes, the mitral valve opens, and an excessively rapid inflow of blood (forward plus regurgitant volume) crosses the mitral valve in early diastole (see

figure in Ch. 556). Even with pure mitral regurgitation, there is often a pressure gradient across the mitral valve in early diastole, reflecting functional mitral stenosis in the presence of increased flow. A normal, simultaneous rise in left atrial and left ventricular pressures then ensues later in diastole, with no pressure gradient.

With the onset of left ventricular dysfunction, the ventricular end-diastolic pressure increases, the ratio of stroke volume to ventricular end-diastolic volume (ejection fraction) falls to less than 55 per cent, and the forward cardiac output diminishes. At this stage of the disease, pulmonary hypertension of moderate degree is generally present.

Differential Diagnosis. Several conditions may produce a systolic murmur resembling that of mitral regurgitation. The thrill and murmur of *ventricular septal defect* are pansystolic, but their location at the lower left sternal border is characteristic. The murmur of *tricuspid regurgitation* may be heard well to the left of the sternum whenever the right atrium and right ventricle are markedly enlarged, but the prominent V waves in the jugular venous pulse and the characteristic increase in intensity of the murmur with inspiration should help differentiate this lesion from mitral regurgitation.

When the jet of mitral regurgitation caused by a leak through the posterior mitral leaflet strikes the interatrial septum, the murmur is heard well in the aortic area, and it may be confused with the murmur of aortic stenosis. However, the murmur of mitral regurgitation increases when systemic arterial pressure is raised (as with the handgrip maneuver), and it decreases when the systemic arterial pressure is lowered (as with amyl nitrite inhalation), whereas opposite responses tend to occur in aortic stenosis.

The ejection type of murmur associated with *idiopathic hypertrophic subaortic stenosis* may be well heard at the apex, as well as at the left sternal border. The characteristic increase of this murmur with the Valsalva maneuver should provide a point of differentiation.

Treatment. *Medical Management.* In the absence of significant symptoms, the only therapeutic measures necessary are *antimicrobial prophylaxis* against streptococcal infections in the younger patient with a history of rheumatic fever and antimicrobial prophylaxis against bacterial endocarditis with dental or surgical procedures. With the onset of fatigue, dyspnea, or atrial fibrillation, the use of *digitalis* is indicated both to control the ventricular rate and to improve the contractile function of the left ventricle. Frequently, even in patients with severe mitral regurgitation, the use of an oral diuretic and digitalis, together with reduced sodium intake, will serve to maintain the patient in a comfortable status for a number of years.

Surgical Treatment. Surgical treatment is generally indicated when symptoms of severe fatigue or dyspnea occur on less than normal activity (N.Y.H.A. Class III or IV), despite appropriate medical management. Such symptoms generally indicate the onset of significant left ventricular myocardial disease. Obviously, in reaching the decision to recommend operation, the prolonged natural course of this disease should be kept in mind, and the low incidence of serious complications such as acute pulmonary edema, systemic emboli, and sudden death should be considered. Nevertheless, it is desirable to recommend operation prior to the development of irreversible left ventricular myocardial disease, and the persistence of significant symptoms while the patient is maintained on adequate medical therapy is generally considered to presage the onset of this process.

Occasionally, the surgical repair of a ruptured chorda or of a deficient posterior leaflet is possible. Almost always, however, in rheumatic and other forms of mitral regurgitation, replacement of the valve with a prosthesis is necessary. The average operative mortality is 6 to 10 per cent for this procedure, and with most types of valve prostheses, there is need for prolonged anticoagulant therapy. Sudden, severe mitral regurgitation is not well tolerated and generally requires early surgical intervention.

559. AORTIC STENOSIS

Etiology and Pathology. There is evidence that a congenitally bicuspid aortic valve is present in more than one half of adult patients with isolated aortic stenosis, most of the remainder being of rheumatic cause. Although the bicuspid valve is frequently not stenotic in early life, this malformation sets up abnormal stresses within the valve, leading to progressive fibrosis and thickening, with eventual immobility of the leaflets and calcification. This sequence may take many years, and the typical patient presents with findings of significant stenosis in the sixth decade of life. Three quarters of patients with isolated valvular aortic stenosis in adult life are male. The varieties of congenital aortic stenosis as they present in childhood and adolescence are discussed in Ch. 552. When aortic stenosis is due to rheumatic heart disease, the sex distribution is relatively equal, and frequently there is evidence of associated mitral valve involvement. With rheumatic disease, the aortic valve is tricuspid and shows fusion of one or more commissures and scarring and thickening of the leaflets; calcification may also be present. Acquired aortic stenosis may also occur in elderly subjects as a degenerative process without fusion of the commissures, stenosis resulting from heavy deposition of calcium within the valve leaflets. When calcification of the aortic valve is marked, the calcium may extend into the anulus and even into the upper portion of the ventricular septum, leading to involvement of the bundle of His or the left bundle branch.

When aortic stenosis is significant, the left ventricle shows concentric hypertrophy with marked thickening of the left ventricular wall, and there is poststenotic dilatation of the ascending aorta. The left atrium is usually normal unless there has been left ventricular failure.

Pathologic Physiology. The earliest physiologic response to obstruction at the aortic valve, as in acute experimental constriction of the ascending aorta, is to cause an increased left ventricular diastolic volume and pressure and compensatory use of the Frank-Starling mechanism. Consequent to the more forceful contraction, the systolic left ventricular pressure is elevated and a pressure gradient is created across the aortic valve, forcing blood across the narrowed orifice at high velocity. The chronic effect of longstanding systolic pressure overload on the left ventricle is to induce hypertrophy of the ventricular wall, a compensatory process which tends to maintain the force or tension in the wall at relatively normal, without substantial enlargement of the left ventricular cavity. (Wall tension, or stress, is directly related to systolic pressure but inversely proportional to wall thickness, and the increased pressure load is distributed over a larger number of muscle fibers.) The stroke volume is generally well maintained by these mechanisms until very late in the disease. Even when the pressure gradient across the aortic valve is quite large, the compensatory left ventricular hypertrophy, coupled with a forceful left atrial contraction, serves to maintain the cardiac output at normal. This strong left atrial "booster pump" generates a prominent presystolic wave in the pressure tracings, leading to an elevated end-diastolic pressure in the hypertrophied and noncompliant ventricle (often near 20 mm Hg). However, elevation of the end-diastolic pressure by this mechanism does not indicate left ventricular failure, and the mean left atrial pressure is maintained at relatively normal.

It should be recognized that a significant gradient is not produced across the aortic valve until the valve orifice is narrowed substantially, by more than 60 per cent of its normal area. A murmur may be created by turbulent flow in the absence of a pressure gradient; but as the stenosis progresses beyond this critical point, an increasing systolic pressure gradient develops between the left ventricle and aorta.

With the increased heart rate which accompanies muscular exercise, diastole is primarily abbreviated, and therefore more time is available per minute for systolic ejection. Hence the aortic valve gradient does *not* tend to increase during exercise, despite an augmented cardiac output, and the left ventricular end-diastolic pressure and mean left atrial pressure may also remain unchanged. This finding is in marked contrast to the situation in mitral stenosis, when filling occurs during diastole and less time is available for flow during exercise.

The arterial pulse pressure is usually narrow when there is significant aortic stenosis, and an important accompanying effect is a tendency toward reduction of the diastolic aortic pressure. The perfusion pressure available to the coronary circulation is therefore diminished. In addition, the oxygen demands of the left ventricle are increased because of the hypertrophy and the need to maintain an elevated systolic pressure in the ventricle (often well over 200 mm Hg in severe aortic stenosis). Heart rate, as well as pressure development, is an important determinant of myocardial oxygen consumption, and the increased heart rate during exertion, together with a limitation of coronary perfusion pressure, can lead to an imbalance between oxygen supply and demand in the left ventricle. Thus *angina pectoris* is common in aortic stenosis in the absence of coronary artery disease. Transient myocardial ischemia in the hypertrophied heart may also explain, at least in part, the tendency toward *sudden serious arrhythmia* which can lead to sudden death. Likewise, this mechanism, perhaps coupled with transient hypotension caused by momentary inability to maintain cardiac output (such as may occur with sudden assumption of the upright posture), may have a role in the *syncopal attacks* which sometimes mark the clinical course of patients with aortic stenosis.

Longstanding pressure overwork by the hypertrophied left ventricle in aortic stenosis eventually leads to evidence of myocardial disease with inability of the heart muscle to maintain normal basal contractile processes, often associated with some degree of myocardial fibrosis. With the onset of left ventricular dysfunction, the degree of emptying becomes reduced. This, in turn, leads to an increased residual ventricular volume and elevation of the end-diastolic volume, with a further increase in the end-diastolic pressure. Elevation of the left atrial mean pressure then ensues, with the onset of orthopnea and exertional dyspnea through the same mechanisms discussed in Ch. 557. In the late phases of myocardial failure, pulmonary hypertension develops and cardiac output falls.

Clinical Manifestations. *Symptoms and Clinical Course.* Usually there is a latent period of many years, during which aortic stenosis is present and progressing in severity but symptoms are absent. When congenital aortic stenosis is severe, symptoms may occur in childhood, but typically they begin in middle or late life. If there is associated mitral valve disease in patients with rheumatic aortic stenosis, particularly mitral stenosis, the onset of symptoms may be much earlier and may lead to earlier detection of the associated aortic lesion. The three cardinal symptoms of aortic stenosis are (1) angina pectoris, (2) syncope, and (3) symptoms caused by left ventricular failure.

The pathophysiology of *angina pectoris* in aortic stenosis, an imbalance between oxygen supply and demand, is discussed above. It may mimic in every way the exertional chest pain which occurs in patients with coronary artery disease. In the older patient, the *coexistence* of coronary heart disease should be considered. Thus even when the aortic stenosis is moderate, or when stenotic lesions in the coronary vessels are moderate, increased oxygen utilization by the myocardium may lead to angina pectoris. Angina pectoris is often the first symptom in patients with aortic stenosis, and in the young patient it usually indicates severe obstruction to left ventricular ejection.

Syncope is sometimes the initial symptom in patients with aortic stenosis. This may be due to a transient arrhythmia such as atrial or ventricular tachycardia. The tendency of the hypertrophied ventricle to develop transient ischemia undoubtedly makes it more susceptible to ventricular fibrillation or ventricular tachycardia. Other mechanisms for syncope may consist of a transient fall in blood pressure during or immediately after exercise, or upon abruptly assuming the upright posture; such mechanisms are related to transient inability of the left ventricle to maintain a normal forward cardiac output, as discussed earlier, or are perhaps associated with metabolic or reflex peripheral vasodilatation. So-called presyncope may also occur, in which the patient experiences a transient graying out or loss of vision.

One of the major problems in the patient with hemodynamically significant aortic stenosis is the occurrence of *sudden death,* which is occasionally the first sign of the disease. In postmortem studies of patients who have died from aortic stenosis, death was sudden in about 15 per cent. It should be recognized, however, that most of these patients had significant symptoms, and that only 3 to 4 per cent of the patients who die do so without prior symptoms. The mechanism of sudden death is unclear, but it may be due to serious arrhythmia or mechanisms similar to those occurring with syncope.

With longstanding pressure overload, and increasing obstruction at the aortic valve, *left ventricular myocardial dysfunction* eventually develops. The earliest symptom of left ventricular dysfunction is usually orthopnea, caused by elevation of the left atrial mean pressure. Mild dyspnea on exertion may then ensue, which progresses to dyspnea on minimal exertion. In the late stages of aortic stenosis, pulmonary edema or evidence of pulmo-nary hypertension with right ventricular failure and peripheral edema may occur.

The onset of atrial fibrillation in patients with aortic stenosis is uncommon, but when it occurs in the absence of mitral valve disease it is ominous. Usually it indicates an elevated mean left atrial pressure with left atrial distention. Because of the loss of left atrial contribution to ventricular filling, further elevation of the mean left atrial pressure, fall in the cardiac output, and severe cardiac failure may ensue.

The onset of symptoms in a patient with significant aortic stenosis has real importance, because the subsequent course is generally downhill. Although earlier mortality figures based on retrospective clinical analyses of patients with aortic stenosis may be modified somewhat by the advent of modern diuretic, antiarrhythmic, and antimicrobial therapy, the typical course after symptoms begin remains relatively short. Thus the average life expectancy in an adult patient after the onset of congestive heart failure is 18 months to 2 years; after the onset of angina pectoris it is about 5 years; and when syncope begins it is about 6 years, although survivals as long as 18 to 20 years after onset of syncope have been reported. The natural history in the patient with severe stenosis who has few or no symptoms has not been clearly established.

Complications of aortic stenosis include *bacterial endocarditis,* which has been estimated to occur in as many as 25 per cent of patients during their lifetime. Rarely, hemolytic anemia has been seen in patients with severe calcific aortic stenosis, presumably owing to local blood trauma at the valve, and perhaps also to intrinsic red blood cell abnormalities. Systemic emboli have been reported as a result of calcium or fibrin particles breaking loose from the aortic valve.

Physical Findings. The primary findings on physical examination can be related to three features: abnormal ejection of blood into the arterial bed, turbulent flow and prolonged ejection across the stenotic aortic orifice, and left ventricular hypertrophy. Physical findings reflecting all three phenomena can generally be detected in hemodynamically significant aortic valve obstruction; but despite their helpfulness, such signs do not always predict accurately the degree of stenosis in the individual patient.

The patient with aortic stenosis is typically not debilitated or wasted, the cardiac output being well maintained until late in the course of the disease. The mean jugular venous pressure is generally normal, although the A wave may be prominent in patients with hemodynamically significant aortic stenosis, presumably because of septal hypertrophy with decreased right ventricular compliance. The carotid pulse is small, the upstroke is delayed, and a systolic thrill may be felt in the carotid vessels. The blood pressure is usually low-normal, with narrowing of the pulse pressure, but in elderly patients having reduced compliance (increased stiffness) of the aortic wall and arteries it is not unusual to find an elevated *systolic* blood pressure, even in the presence of significant aortic stenosis. However, marked systemic hypertension with a substantial diastolic pressure elevation is not encountered in the presence of severe aortic stenosis.

On palpation of the precordium, there is a systolic thrill at the aortic area, the apex beat is enlarged, and there is a sustained apical impulse. A presystolic atrial impulse may be palpable at the apex in the lateral decubitus position. The first heart sound is usually normal, and the aortic component of the second heart sound is diminished. Often, the second heart sound is single owing to a prolonged left ventricular ejection time; or aortic valve closure may even follow pulmonic valve closure, leading to paradoxical splitting of the second heart sound (decreased splitting during inspiration) (see figure in Ch. 556). The *systolic murmur* of aortic stenosis is crescendo-decrescendo in quality, is loudest at the aortic area, is transmitted to the carotid arteries, and is also audible at the apex. Being ejection in type, the murmur begins well after the first heart sound and ends before the second heart sound. In the presence of severe aortic stenosis, the murmur is long and peaks in mid- or late systole. Frequently there is an atrial diastolic gallop (fourth heart sound), which reflects both reduced compliance of the thickened left ventricular wall and forceful left atrial contraction. This gallop is best heard in the left lateral decubitus position.

When aortic stenosis is mild, there tends to be less delay of the carotid upstroke, the duration of ventricular ejection may be normal, and the second heart sound splits normally with respiration. The systolic murmur tends to be less intense and shorter, peaking early in systole. It should be appreciated, however, that in the late stages of aortic stenosis, when cardiac failure and low cardiac output supervene, the murmur of aortic stenosis may also become markedly diminished in intensity. Under these circumstances, the left ventricle is generally substantially enlarged, and there are symptoms and signs of cardiac failure.

It is not uncommon to hear a soft, early diastolic blowing murmur at the left sternal border caused by mild aortic regurgitation, even in patients with severe aortic stenosis. This small leak occurs because of the small, fixed orifice. The murmur of associated mitral stenosis should be searched for carefully, particularly in female patients with aortic stenosis, because the association of these two obstructive lesions serves to diminish the physical findings of each. When mitral and aortic stenosis coexist, the cardiac output tends to be reduced, the severity of aortic stenosis may be underestimated, and the murmur of mitral stenosis may be difficult to appreciate.

Diagnosis (see table). *Electrocardiogram.* In both children and adults, a normal electrocardiogram is rarely found in the presence of significant aortic stenosis. In children under 10 or 12 years of age, the degree of left ventricular hypertrophy on the electrocardiogram tends to relate to the degree of obstruction, but in adults relatively marked degrees of left ventricular hypertrophy are sometimes seen in mild or moderate obstruction. Typically, the electrocardiogram shows voltage criteria for left ventricular hypertrophy, with associated S-T segment and T wave changes and left atrial enlargement. Occasionally, intraventricular conduction delay or left bundle branch block is seen, particularly late in the course of the disease, and atrial fibrillation is a late and relatively uncommon problem. Complete heart block has been reported in some patients resulting from extension of aortic calcification into the conduction system.

Roentgenographic Features. There may be little or no over-all cardiac enlargement, but when aortic stenosis is significant some degree of left ventricular enlargement is usually discernible, with straightening of the left heart border, downward displacement of the left ventricular apex, and overlapping of the spine by the left ventricular shadow at 60 degrees of rotation in the left anterior oblique view. In the presence of left ventricular failure, the chamber is enlarged and the left atrium is also usually dilated, causing posterior displacement of the barium-filled esophagus. When significant left atrial enlargement is seen, however, it should always raise the suspicion of associated mitral stenosis. Poststenotic dilatation of the ascending aorta is common in the frontal view, and calcification of the aortic valve should be searched for on the plain roentgenogram. However, image intensification fluoroscopy may be necessary for detection of mild valve calcification. In the presence of left ventricular failure, there is evidence of pulmonary venous engorgement and interstitial pulmonary edema.

Cardiac Catheterization. In patients who have symptoms, cardiac catheterization is carried out to determine whether the degree of mechanical obstruction at the aortic valve is sufficient to warrant surgical treatment. It is important to measure both the systolic pressure gradient between left ventricle and aorta (see figure) and the cardiac output at the time of left heart catheterization because of the nonlinear relation between the pressure and flow across the stenotic orifice, the orifice area being directly related to flow and inversely proportional to the square root of the pressure gradient (see Ch. 557). Thus if the cardiac output is reduced by 30 per cent, the pressure gradient will fall by about 50 per cent and the severity of the stenosis will be underestimated if the pressure gradient alone is relied upon. For example, when myocardial failure is responsible for a reduced resting cardiac output, the peak gradient from left ventricle to aorta may be below 50 mm Hg, even in the presence of marked aortic valve narrowing.

When the cardiac output is normal, with relatively mild aortic stenosis the aortic valve orifice area is between 0.75 and 1.5 sq cm in the adult (normal area 2.5 sq cm), and the systolic pressure gradient across the aortic valve is small. When aortic stenosis is moderate, the orifice area is 0.5 to 0.75 sq cm and the peak pressure gradient usually exceeds 50 mm Hg. With very severe or "tight" aortic stenosis, the orifice area is 0.5 sq cm or less, there may be a left ventricular systolic pressure in excess of 250 mm Hg, and transvalvular pressure gradient is often over 100 mm Hg. The right heart pressures are normal, unless there is left ventricular failure which can produce pulmonary hypertension. Simultaneous measurements should be made of the pulmonary artery wedge pressure and the left ventricular pressure to exclude associated mitral stenosis.

It is important that selective left ventricular angiography be carried out to document the functional status of the left ventricle. Such a study will indicate whether or not the left ventricular end-diastolic volume is elevated and the ejection fraction reduced to below 55 per cent, factors which bear on the operative risk in the individual patient. In older patients, it is also important that selective coronary arteriography be performed. Lack of appreciation of significant coronary artery lesions can lead to difficulty during surgical treatment, and coronary revascularization procedures are sometimes carried out at the time of the aortic valve replacement.

Phonocardiography. Recording of heart sounds and the external carotid pulse wave may help in assessing the severity of aortic stenosis by documenting the presence or absence of a single second heart sound, paradoxical splitting, or a prolonged ejection time. A slow rising carotid pulse wave and the characteristics of the ejection murmur can also be documented.

Differential Diagnosis. An ejection murmur at the aortic area and lower left sternal border can be heard in the patient with *idiopathic hypertrophic subaortic stenosis,* although the murmur is generally poorly transmitted to the carotid vessels and has other special features (see Ch. 560). The key differentiating points between this lesion and valvular aortic stenosis are shown in the accompanying table.

In the younger patient who has a murmur suggesting congenital aortic stenosis, other locations for the lesion (supravalvular, subvalvular membrane) should be considered. Occasionally the murmur of papillary muscle dysfunction or ruptured chordae tendineae, caused by mitral regurgitation through the posterior leaflet, can mimic the murmur of aortic stenosis. The mitral regurgitant jet impinges on the interatrial septum, which is directly contiguous to the posterior wall of the aorta, leading to transmission of the murmur to the aortic area; however, this murmur tends to transmit poorly to the carotid arteries; it increases with isometric handgrip and diminishes with amyl nitrite inhalation, whereas the murmur of aortic stenosis will behave in an opposite manner with these two maneuvers.

Treatment. *Medical Management.* The adult patient with findings suggestive of moderate aortic stenosis and no symptoms may be followed carefully, although cardiac catheterization is sometimes done to be certain of the severity of obstruction. In such patients, very strenuous physical exertion, such as competitive athletics, should be prohibited in order to minimize risk of sudden death. Antimicrobial prophylaxis for dental or surgical procedures is advised to prevent the development of bacterial endocarditis. In children or adolescents with con-

genital aortic stenosis who are suspected of having severe obstruction, cardiac catheterization is generally advised even when they are without symptoms.

Early symptoms of orthopnea or mild dyspnea may respond temporarily to digitalis, sodium restriction, and diuresis. However, as soon as significant symptoms appear (angina, syncope, or symptoms of left ventricular failure), the adult patient should usually be sent for cardiac catheterization and coronary arteriography, and consideration should be given to early operation.

Surgical Treatment. In children or young adult patients with congenital aortic stenosis, surgical treatment is generally advocated even in the absence of significant symptoms if the obstruction is severe, because the risk of operation appears to be lower than the risk of sudden death. The bicuspid valve in the young patient is generally favorable for a valvuloplasty, and clinical improvement may be experienced for a number of years.

In the adult patient with symptoms and significant narrowing of the aortic orifice (less than 0.75 sq cm) or peak systolic pressure gradient over 50 mm Hg with normal cardiac output, aortic valve replacement, using a prosthesis or a graft, is carried out, using cardiopulmonary bypass. In patients with severe associated coronary artery disease, saphenous vein bypass grafting may also be performed. If there is associated severe mitral valve disease, double valve replacement is sometimes necessary.

The question whether the adult patient with documented, hemodynamically severe aortic stenosis but with few symptoms should be operated upon is not settled at present. The risk of aortic valve replacement is now between 5 and 10 per cent in many centers, but whether the risk of sudden death in asymptomatic patients over a period of several years approaches this figure is unknown. Therefore older patients are referred for operation if they have significant symptoms.

Differential Diagnosis in Aortic Stenosis

	Valvular Aortic Stenosis	Idiopathic Hypertrophic Subaortic Stenosis
Carotid pulse	Delayed	Rapid and bifid
Systolic murmur, location	Second right ICS, neck and apex	LLSB and apex
Effect of Valsalva maneuver	Murmur decreased	Murmur increased
Aortic closure sound	Soft	Normal
Systolic ejection click	Common when valve not calcified	Rare
Diastolic murmur of aortic regurgitation	Common	Rare
Electrocardiogram	LVH	Marked LVH; deep Q waves (septal in origin); left atrial enlargement
Chest roentgenogram	Normal heart size	Cardiomegaly (left ventricular); left atrial enlargement
Poststenotic dilatation of aorta	Present	Absent
Calcium in aortic valve	Present	Absent

LLSB = Lower left sternal border; ICS = intercostal space; LVH = left ventricular hypertrophy.

560. IDIOPATHIC HYPERTROPHIC SUBAORTIC STENOSIS

Definition. Idiopathic hypertrophic subaortic stenosis (IHSS) is synonymous with the terms muscular subaortic stenosis and hypertrophic obstructive cardiomyopathy. Because all patients with this form of left ventricular hypertrophy do not exhibit hemodynamic obstruction within the left ventricular outflow tract, the more general term asymmetric septal hypertrophy is sometimes used.

Etiology and Pathology. Hypertrophy of the muscular wall of the left ventricle is particularly prominent in the region of the interventricular septum. The septum may be several times as thick as the free wall, and abnormalities in the direction of fibers and in the connections between myofilaments have been demonstrated by electron microscopy in the septal region. In cases in which obstruction is present, the anterior leaflet of the mitral valve is thickened, probably secondary to contact with the hypertrophied septum, and the chordae tendineae may be thickened and elongated. The aortic valve is normal.

An autosomal dominant mode of inheritance has been recognized in some patients with this disease. When echocardiography is used to identify enlargement of the interventricular septum in individuals without other physical findings, it has been claimed that in the great majority of instances this pattern of inheritance can be documented in the relatives of patients who have evident disease.

Pathologic Physiology. Although hypertrophy of the left ventricular wall is most marked in the region of the interventricular septum, hypertrophy also is present elsewhere in the ventricle, and reduced ventricular compliance leads to increased resistance to ventricular filling from the left atrium. The left ventricular end-diastolic pressure is usually elevated in patients with or without obstruction. There is a prominent atrial contraction wave, and the mean left atrial pressure may be somewhat elevated.

The hallmark is variable obstruction to left ventricular ejection below the aortic valve, in the ventricular outflow tract. There is a pressure gradient between the body of the left ventricle and the outflow tract, and the obstruction has been shown to result from abnormal forward movement of the anterior mitral valve leaflet during systole. This leaflet forms the posterior wall of the ventricular outflow tract; when the leading edge of the anterior mitral leaflet meets the hypertrophied septum during ejection, obstruction is produced. This malposition of the anterior mitral valve leaflet probably results largely from lateral displacement of the papillary muscles by the enlarged interventricular septum, and the abnormal position produces some mitral regurgitation as well.

Because of the dynamic nature of the obstruction, the pressure gradient tends to develop progressively during the course of each cardiac systole. There is no obstruction initially, leading to the sharp, early arterial upstroke, but the arterial pulse falls rapidly as the obstruction develops. The pressure gradient may also be variable over time, and can be altered by a variety of interventions. Influences which alter left ventricular volume, systemic arterial pressure (which affects the distending pressure in the outflow tract during systole), or the force of muscular contraction change the caliber of the muscular outflow tract and affect the degree of obstruction. For example, the Valsalva maneuver or assumption of the upright posture produces a decrease in venous return, a fall in arterial pressure, and reflex tachycardia, all of which reduce ventricular volume and outflow tract size. The associated reflex increase in contractility further augments the degree of obstruction with these maneuvers, and the pressure gradient across the outflow tract increases.

Clinical Manifestations. *Symptoms and Clinical Course.* Patients may be detected because of a long-standing heart murmur, sometimes first noted in childhood. In patients with severe left ventricular hypertrophy and outflow tract obstruction, the chief symptoms resemble those of valvular aortic stenosis: angina pectoris (which may be atypical in character), syncope, and manifestations of left ventricular failure. Angina pectoris results from an imbalance between oxygen supply and demand in the hypertrophied ventricle (see Ch. 559) and is usually exertional in nature. However, patients with this disease may experience prolonged, severe chest pain mimicking that of myocardial infarction, undoubtedly related to increased oxygen demand consequent to the elevated left ventricular systolic pressure and marked ventricular hypertrophy. Symptoms caused by

pulmonary congestion and low cardiac output may occur, in part related to the reduced left ventricular compliance and impaired left atrial emptying which characterize this disease, as well as to severe obstruction. However, all these symptoms, including sudden death, also occur in patients without significant obstruction. The clinical picture in such patients can resemble that of a generalized cardiomyopathy.

The course tends to be variable, particularly in patients with mild to moderate symptoms, and periods of spontaneous improvement may be noted. With severe obstruction the disease may be progressive, death usually being due to congestive heart failure. Tachyarrhythmias and atrial fibrillation are poorly tolerated complications, and may lead to severe hypotension. Bacterial endocarditis, once considered rare, has recently been reported in between 5 and 10 per cent of cases.

Physical Findings. The jugular venous pulse generally exhibits a prominent A wave, owing to reduced right ventricular compliance. The carotid pulse is sharp, and when a gradient is present across the outflow tract, the pulse is bisferious with a secondary tidal wave. The left ventricular apex is displaced laterally, in the lateral decubitus position a presystolic apical impulse can usually be felt, and sometimes there is a double impulse during systole as well. With significant obstruction, a systolic thrill may be felt at the lower left sternal border.

On auscultation, there is a low-pitched systolic ejection murmur at the lower left sternal border, which is also heard at the apex but transmits poorly to the base and is not transmitted to the carotid arteries or the left axilla. Sometimes there is a separate pansystolic murmur at the cardiac apex associated with mitral regurgitation. If a murmur is absent in an individual without obstruction at rest, it may be induced by the Valsalva maneuver. If the murmur is present, it can be markedly augmented during the Valsalva maneuver, and it is greatly diminished or disappears after release of the Valsalva maneuver. The murmur of hypertrophic subaortic stenosis may also be increased by having the patient suddenly assume the upright posture, and it may be abolished by squatting.

Diagnosis (see table in Ch. 559). *Electrocardiogram.* A normal electrocardiogram is very rare in the presence of this disorder. Usually there is evidence of left ventricular hypertrophy, which is often striking, with secondary S-T segment and T wave changes. Left atrial enlargement is common. In addition, the hypertrophied septum frequently leads to enlarged initial QRS forces, and prominent "septal" Q waves may be seen in leads II, III, AVF, AVL, or the precordial leads. These changes often resemble those of previous myocardial infarction. There also may be prominent R waves in the limb or right precordial leads. In about 10 per cent of patients, there is a short P-R interval and a partial delta wave, suggestive of a variant of the Wolff-Parkinson-White syndrome. An intraventricular conduction delay is sometimes seen, and left bundle branch block occurs occasionally.

Roentgenographic Features. The plain chest roentgenogram shows left ventricular enlargement, often with a bulge along the lateral wall of the left ventricle in the frontal view, and left atrial enlargement is frequent. The aorta is small, and there is no poststenotic dilatation. There is no calcification in the aortic valve.

Phonocardiogram. When obstruction is present, the indirect carotid pulse wave shows a characteristic sharp upstroke followed by a tidal wave. The murmur is of the ejection type, beginning after the first heart sound and ending before the second sound, and varying intensity of the murmur with provocations can be documented by the phonocardiogram.

Echocardiogram. Ultrasound provides the most useful noninvasive method for diagnosis. In patients with obstruction, the tracing shows an abnormal systolic anterior movement of the mitral valve leaflet. In addition, there is disproportionate thickness in the region of the interventricular septum, as compared to the posterior free wall.

Cardiac Catheterization. The characteristic finding in hypertrophic subaortic stenosis is a pressure gradient within the outflow tract of the left ventricle, the pressure being high in the left ventricular chamber and reduced in the outflow tract, with no pressure gradient across the aortic valve. It is important to measure the elevated systolic pressure in the *inflow tract* of the left ventricle just in front of the mitral valve, because when the catheter is entrapped in the apex, artifactually high ventricular systolic pressures may be measured. Usually the left ventricular end-diastolic pressure is elevated to 20 mm Hg or more owing to a large presystolic wave in the left ventricle, reflecting a large A wave in the left atrium.

If there is no pressure gradient across the outflow tract at rest, or if the gradient is small, it may be increased by having the patient perform a Valsalva maneuver. This decreases venous return, augments heart rate, and increases left ventricular contractility, all of which serve to narrow the outflow tract further and enhance the gradient. In fixed, valvular aortic stenosis the pressure gradient diminishes during the Valsalva maneuver. In addition, an infusion of isoproterenol or administration of amyl nitrite may bring out the pressure gradient, although these agents also will increase the gradient in valvular aortic stenosis.

The pressure gradient tends to diminish markedly during the systemic arterial pressure overshoot after the release of the Valsalva maneuver in hypertrophic subaortic stenosis, and the pressure gradient may be greatly reduced or abolished by infusion of a pressor agent such as methoxamine, or by administration of propranolol. All these maneuvers tend to increase left ventricular volume and reduce contractility and heart rate, thereby widening the outflow tract and decreasing the obstruction.

A characteristic sign, which helps differentiate this lesion from valvular aortic stenosis, is the alteration of pulse pressure in the beat after a ventricular extrasystole. In hypertrophic subaortic stenosis, the systemic arterial *pulse pressure decreases* during this beat, the increased force of contraction produced by postextrasystolic potentiation leading to a narrower outflow tract, increased obstruction, and fall in stroke volume. In valvular aortic stenosis, however, the stroke volume increases and the pulse pressure is augmented. Although 25 to 30 per cent of patients exhibit a small pressure gradient across the right ventricular outflow tract caused by septal bulging, in a few patients a subvalvular pressure gradient may be quite marked on the right side.

Left ventricular angiography shows characteristic findings. There is enormous hypertrophy of the interventricular septum, often with marked distortion of the shape of the left ventricular cavity, and with lateral tilt-ing of the papillary muscles. During systole, the mitral valve can be visualized as it is held forward in an abnormal position, obstructing the left ventricular outflow tract. Mitral regurgitation, usually moderate, occurs beneath this displaced leaflet and is best seen in the oblique or lateral view.

Differential Diagnosis. The murmur of hypertrophic subaortic stenosis may be confused with that of valvular aortic stenosis, but a number of differences in the physical examination, x-ray, and electrocardiogram clarify the diagnosis (see table in Ch. 559).

The systolic murmur is also frequently mistaken for that of mitral regurgitation alone, or of papillary muscle dysfunction. The Valsalva maneuver may be useful in differentiating these murmurs, and the echocardiogram will show characteristically different movements of the anterior mitral valve leaflet. The occurrence of angina pectoris and Q waves in the electrocardiogram sometimes causes a mistaken diagnosis of coronary heart disease.

Treatment. *Medical Treatment.* Beta-adrenergic blocking agents, such as propranolol, have been shown to acutely reduce the pressure gradient at cardiac catheterization in patients with hypertrophic subaortic stenosis. Chronic oral administration of these agents may relieve angina pectoris, and they appear to be particularly effective in patients with latent obstruction. Propranolol also tends to slow the heart rate and improve ventricular filling, and syncope may be relieved. Digitalis and nitroglycerin tend to increase the obstruction; they should be used with caution or avoided.

Atrial fibrillation is poorly tolerated by patients with hypertrophic subaortic stenosis because of loss of the atrial contribution to ventricular filling, and the noncompliant left ventricle then requires an elevated mean left atrial pressure to maintain an adequate diastolic ventricular volume. In addition, if the ventricular response is rapid in atrial fibrillation (or if atrial tachyarrhythmias occur), the hypertrophied left ventricle relaxes poorly and hypotension with pulmonary congestion may result. Therefore such arrhythmias should be promptly terminated by appropriate drugs or electrical reversion.

If the patient with hypertrophic subaortic stenosis becomes hypotensive, the use of isoproterenol will increase the obstruction and generally worsen the patient's condition. Therefore drugs of choice are peripheral vasoconstrictor agents, such as methoxamine or phenylephrine.

Surgical Treatment. Operation is usually reserved for patients with severe symptoms and marked outflow tract obstruction. The most widely used surgical procedure consists of resecting a portion of the hypertrophied left ventricular outflow tract, the septum being approached through the aorta and aortic valve. In some centers, simple myotomy with division of the fibers of the outflow tract has also resulted in relief of the obstruction. These operations have generally been successful, often producing complete or nearly complete relief of the left ventricular pressure gradient, but operative mortality has ranged between 10 and 20 per cent. Replacement of the mitral valve with a prosthesis in order to remove the posterior component of the obstruction (the anterior mitral valve leaflet) has been used with some success, but the complications associated with insertion of a prosthetic device limit the application of this approach.

561. AORTIC REGURGITATION

Etiology and Pathology. Aortic regurgitation is usually the result of rheumatic fever, but it has been described as a complication of an increasing number of systemic diseases (see below). A careful history may be of substantial help in ascertaining etiology. In chronic aortic regurgitation of rheumatic etiology, the aortic valve leaflets are scarred, thickened, and retracted and do not close during diastole. With longstanding disease, marked dilatation of the ascending aorta and the aortic anulus may add further to the insufficiency. Combined aortic stenosis and regurgitation are most frequently associated with rheumatic disease, but can also be seen in the late stages of a congenitally bicuspid valve. Aortic regurgitation may be associated with the most marked enlargement and hypertrophy of the left ventricle encountered in valvular heart disease. Approximately 70 per cent of patients with predominant aortic regurgitation are male.

Isolated congenital aortic regurgitation has rarely been reported as a consequence of a bicuspid aortic valve, but congenital aortic regurgitation can occur as a complication of discrete subvalvular stenosis which produces secondary thickening and insufficiency of the aortic leaflets. In younger children, ventricular septal defect may be complicated by prolapse of an aortic valve leaflet, thereby causing aortic regurgitation.

Acquired aortic regurgitation occurs in association with the following conditions: (1) *Syphilis,* which causes scarring and degeneration of the media and intima of the ascending aorta, resulting in part from disease of the vasa vasorum. There can be an aneurysm in the ascending aorta and dilatation of the aortic anulus, with thickening of the aortic leaflets, as well as narrowing of the coronary ostia caused by syphilitic involvement of the aortic intima. (2) *Ankylosing spondylitis,* in which associated medial disease of the aorta results in significant aortic regurgitation. (3) *Rheumatoid arthritis;* degeneration of the aortic valve leaflets and the ascending aorta have been described. (4) *Marfan's syndrome,* in which loss of elastic tissue and connective tissue degenerative changes can lead to marked dilatation of the aorta and aortic anulus with severe aortic regurgitation. (5) *Hurler's syndrome,* or mucopolysaccharidosis, which may be accompanied by significant aortic regurgitation. (6) *Severe systemic hypertension,* which can be associated with aortic dilatation and relative aortic insufficiency; other complications associated with hypertension, such as ascending aortic aneurysm or dissecting aneurysm, may also cause aortic regurgitation. (7) *Bacterial endocarditis,* which usually occurs on a deformed valve, and can lead to rapid progression of aortic regurgitation or to fenestration of the leaflets.

Pathologic Physiology. The physiologic defect in aortic regurgitation is retrograde leakage of blood from the aorta into the left ventricle during diastole. This results in low diastolic aortic pressure and increase in the end-diastolic volume of the left ventricle. The amount of blood ejected during systole is abnormally large, because it consists of the normal stroke volume plus blood regurgitated during the previous diastolic period. In severe aortic regurgitation the amount of blood regurgitated per beat may equal or even exceed the forward stroke volume. The initial compensation to this volume overload on the left ventricle is by the Frank-Starling mechanism (increased end-diastolic volume), and in mild aortic regurgitation there is increased systolic emptying as well, with little chronic dilatation of the ventricle. As regurgitation becomes more severe, the left ventricle slowly dilates, and new sarcomeres are laid down both in parallel and in series in the left ventricular wall during the process of dilatation and hypertrophy. This compensatory mechanism allows the enlarged left ventricle to deliver a greater stroke volume, but with normal shortening of each unit of the enlarged circumference.

The pathophysiology of aortic regurgitation somewhat resembles the volume overload of mitral regurgitation, but there are two important differences. (1) The increased forward stroke volume is delivered into a high impedance system (the aorta), and because the total forward stroke volume is increased, the left ventricular and aortic systolic pressures are elevated (sometimes to 160 mm Hg or higher). This, together with the increased size of the left ventricular chamber, leads to pressure as well as volume overloading and a somewhat elevated myocardial oxygen consumption. (2) The lowered diastolic aortic pressure tends to impair coronary artery perfusion. Normally the coronary blood flow occurs during diastole; with the reduced diastolic pressure which accompanies aortic regurgitation, coronary blood flow may become inadequate either during exercise or when heart rate and hence the diastolic pressure become very low, as during sleep. The increased myocardial oxygen consumption coupled with relative underperfusion of the coronary bed may lead to an imbalance between oxygen supply and demand. Thus unlike patients with mitral regurgitation, patients with severe aortic regurgitation commonly develop *angina pectoris* in the absence of coronary artery disease.

With adequate left ventricular myocardial contractility the ejection fraction of the left ventricle (ratio of stroke volume to end-diastolic volume) is maintained at normal (over 55 per cent), the forward cardiac output is normal, and left ventricular end-diastolic pressure may remain nearly normal despite ventricular dilatation. However, because longstanding overload leads to myocardial damage and depression of contractility, the extent of wall shortening during ejection tends to diminish, the residual volume in the left ventricle rises, and the end-diastolic pressure in the left ventricle becomes elevated. Indeed, in the late stages of severe aortic regurgitation the diastolic pressure in the aorta and that in the left ventricle may reach equilibration near the end of diastole, leading to an abbreviation of the murmur. Occasionally, "preclosure" of the mitral valve even occurs, leading to a dissociation between the rising left ventricular diastolic pressure and the left atrial pressure, which remains at a lower level. This situation may occur in sudden severe aortic regurgitation, such as with bacterial endocarditis, when sufficient time has not elapsed for ventricular dilatation and hypertrophy to occur. Such mitral valve preclosure may be audible as a snapping sound in mid- to late diastole.

In the late stages of aortic regurgitation the cardiac output decreases, and the left ventricular end-diastolic pressure becomes further elevated because of myocardial failure. The mean left atrial pressure then rises, leading to decreased pulmonary compliance and interstitial edema, and acute pulmonary edema occasionally occurs.

Clinical Manifestations. *Symptoms and Clinical Course.* The typical patient with rheumatic aortic regurgitation has experienced acute rheumatic fever in childhood, and a period of about ten years then follows during which the severity of the regurgitant lesion progresses. Marked aortic regurgitation may become apparent by age 18 or 20, and there often follows a period of compensation during which the patient is asymptomatic, despite the presence of severe regurgitation. Occasionally during this stage of the disease, palpitations caused by transient atrial arrhythmias, headache caused by the high systolic blood pressure during exercise, or subjective sensations resulting from cardiac hyperactivity may be noted. Studies in children followed for many years after developing severe aortic regurgitation indicate that even after 20 years about 25 per cent of the individuals with this lesion remained asymptomatic. However, the average duration of the latent or asymptomatic period in severe aortic regurgitation is about ten years.

The earliest symptoms are usually due to the onset of left ventricular dysfunction or to coronary insufficiency. Mild dyspnea on exertion is noted as a result of elevation of the left ventricular end-diastolic and mean left atrial pressures during exercise. The length of time between onset of this symptom and death of the patient averages seven to ten years, although it should be recognized that many of these data were derived before the advent of modern diuretic therapy and rheumatic fever prophylaxis. Angina pectoris usually begins somewhat later, postdating the onset of dypsnea by two to three years. It may occur during exertion, and may or may not respond to nitroglycerin. Angina pectoris can also be atypical and occur at rest or at night, presumably caused by low heart rate which can lead to very low diastolic aortic pressure and inadequate coronary perfusion during long diastolic periods. The onset of severe nocturnal angina associated with profuse sweating, particularly in young patients, can portend a poor prognosis.

Once left ventricular decompensation begins, patients with severe aortic regurgitation usually tolerate infections poorly. They may experience severe congestive heart failure, and they are also at some risk of unexpected death. There are no clear-cut figures on the incidence of sudden death in patients with severe aortic regurgitation; although not as common as in aortic stenosis, it is by no means rare and probably results from sudden ventricular arrhythmia. In the late stages of severe aortic regurgitation, orthopnea and paroxysmal nocturnal dyspnea occur, and eventually symptoms and signs of right ventricular failure may supervene.

The natural history in the other forms of aortic regurgitation depends largely on the rapidity with which the lesion develops and on its severity. Patients with aortic regurgitation caused by syphilis may exhibit a course resembling that of rheumatic disease, although it usually begins later in life. With acute regurgitation such as that in bacterial endocarditis, there is insufficient time for chronic compensation to occur, and the clinical course may be fulminating. Under these circumstances, severe intractable left ventricular failure may develop.

Physical Findings. The diastolic pressure determined by sphygmomanometry correlates generally with the severity of the regurgitant leak, although in some patients there is severe regurgitation with diastolic pressure as high as 60 mm Hg. A diastolic sound over the artery is usually audible down to 0 mm Hg when regurgitation is severe, but the level at which the diastolic sound muffles corresponds reasonably well to the directly measured aortic pressure at the end of diastole, deter-

mined by a needle within the artery. The systolic arterial pressure is elevated. Characteristic clinical features caused by the large stroke volume and rapid runoff of blood from the aorta consist of *head bobbing* (a nodding motion of the head with each systole, which may be visible from a considerable distance), *visible pulsations of the carotid arteries,* a *Corrigan or water-hammer pulse* (sharp upstroke with collapsing quality), *Quincke's sign* (on light compression of the fingernail, alternate blushing and blanching are visible in the nailbed with each cardiac cycle), *pistol shot sounds* on auscultation with a stethoscope over the femoral arteries, and *Duroziez' murmur* (a to-and-fro bruit over the femoral artery, using slight compression with stethoscope diaphragm). Palpation of the carotid arteries may reveal a bisferious or bifid pulse, particularly if there is some associated aortic stenosis.

On palpation of the precordium, a diastolic thrill may be felt at the lower left sternal border, and a systolic thrill is palpable at the aortic area, the jugular notch, and the carotid arteries. The left ventricle is enlarged, the apex is displaced laterally, and the apex beat is hyperkinetic with marked retraction during systole.

The first heart sound may be normal or slightly reduced; the aortic component of the second heart sound is diminished or inaudible in the presence of severe regurgitation. Frequently, a loud third heart sound is audible at the apex, and there may also be a fourth heart sound. The most characteristic feature of the lesion is a decrescendo, blowing *diastolic murmur* at the left sternal border in the third and fourth intercostal spaces (see figure in Ch. 556). In the presence of mild aortic regurgitation, this murmur is high pitched, soft, and heard only in early diastole; it may be appreciated only with the patient in an upright position, leaning forward, and with held expiration. With a more severe regurgitant leak, the murmur may have a somewhat rougher quality and may last throughout diastole. Late in the course of severe aortic regurgitation, or with acute aortic regurgitation, the diastolic murmur may be shortened by equilibration of aortic pressure with markedly elevated left ventricular end-diastolic pressure before the end of diastole; occasionally, a snapping sound caused by mitral valve "preclosure" is audible (see above). In patients in whom the aortic regurgitation is due primarily to aneurysmal dilatation of the ascending aorta or to enlargement of the aortic anulus, as in Marfan's syndrome, the diastolic murmur may be loudest to the *right* of the sternum, thereby providing a clue to the cause.

Invariably, when aortic regurgitation is severe, there is a systolic ejection murmur at the aortic area which is transmitted to the jugular notch and carotid arteries. This may be very loud even in the presence of pure aortic regurgitation, reflecting the extremely large stroke volume delivered across a deformed aortic valve, but usually there is little or no pressure gradient from left ventricle to aorta during systole. Frequently in the presence of severe aortic regurgitation, an *Austin Flint diastolic rumble* is audible at the apex. Although true mitral stenosis may accompany aortic regurgitation of rheumatic origin, the Austin Flint rumble is characterized by its onset with a third heart sound; it is loudest in mid-diastole and often exhibits some presystolic accentuation. The Austin Flint murmur is probably due not only to interference with opening of the anterior mitral leaflet by the regurgitant jet, but also to a more rapid rise in the left ventricular than the left atrial diastolic pressure. The effect is to prevent full opening of the normal mitral leaflets during diastole, leading to turbulent flow across the mitral orifice (see Ch. 557, Differential Diagnosis).

Sometimes, in the late stages of aortic regurgitation when left ventricular dilatation and failure are present, a holosystolic murmur of relative mitral regurgitation may be audible at the cardiac apex. Signs of pulmonary hypertension and right ventricular enlargement may also be encountered in the late stages of the disease.

Diagnosis. *Electrocardiogram.* The electrocardiogram usually shows left ventricular hypertrophy, sometimes of marked degree, with associated S-T segment and T wave changes. Left atrial enlargement may also be present, particularly when the left ventricular end-diastolic pressure becomes elevated. When myocardial disease develops, left axis deviation, intraventricular conduction defects, or left bundle branch block may occur. Atrial fibrillation is a late and relatively uncommon complication.

Roentgenographic Features. The major findings are enlargement of the left ventricle and aorta with vigorous pulsations of the ascending aorta on fluoroscopy. The left ventricular enlargement is characterized by a downward and lateral displacement of the left ventricular apex, the left ventricle being particularly prominent and overlying the spine in the left anterior oblique view. With severe aortic regurgitation, left atrial enlargement may be apparent on the right anterior oblique view with barium in the esophagus. When aortic regurgitation is associated with aortic root disease, the ascending aorta may be markedly dilated or aneurysmal, although sometimes the major dilatation takes place posteriorly and may not be visible on the plain chest film. Occasionally, calcium is seen in the aortic valve, and calcification in the ascending aortic wall is characteristic of syphilitic involvement.

Echocardiography. By the use of ultrasound, calculation of the diameter of the aortic root and of left ventricular chamber size may be feasible. In addition, in the presence of an Austin Flint rumble there is a characteristic fluttering motion of the anterior mitral leaflet during diastole caused by the impinging aortic regurgitant jet. This finding, together with absence of mitral valve thickening and normal excursion of the posterior leaflet, provides evidence against organic mitral stenosis.

Cardiac Catheterization. It is generally desirable to perform cardiac catheterization prior to undertaking cardiac surgery in order to characterize the status of left ventricular myocardial function and to exclude associated lesions. Supravalvular injection of contrast medium into the aortic root often provides adequate radiographic visualization of the left ventricle and the anatomy of the ascending aorta, and also allows assessment of the severity of the aortic regurgitation. The systolic, left ventricular, and aortic pressures are moderately elevated; there may be a slight systolic pressure gradient across the aortic valve and a low diastolic aortic pressure (see figure in Ch. 556); a normal or moderately elevated left ventricular end-diastolic pressure (less than 20 mm Hg) is encountered when left ventricular myocardial function is maintained, and the forward cardiac output is normal. There may be an early diastolic gradient across the mitral valve from the pulmonary artery wedge or left atrial pressure tracing to the left ventricle; this is probably related to the rapid early rise of left ventricular diastolic pressure and impaired opening

motion of the anterior mitral leaflet consequent to the aortic regurgitation. Simultaneous recordings of this nature should exclude the presence of associated organic mitral stenosis, in which there is usually a pressure gradient throughout diastole. In longstanding aortic regurgitation there is elevation of the calculated left ventricular end-diastolic volume (in excess of 90 ml per square meter), with or without an elevation of the left ventricular end-diastolic pressure.

A reduced ejection fraction, an impaired forward cardiac output, and marked elevation of the left ventricular end-diastolic pressure all indicate depressed left ventricular myocardial function, which may increase the operative risk. Under these conditions, the left ventricular and aortic diastolic pressures may become equal late in diastole at a pressure of 35 to 40 mm Hg, or even higher. It is under the latter circumstances that early closure of the mitral valve can occur (see above), leading to a higher pressure in the left ventricle than in the left atrium in the last portion of diastole. Finally, selective coronary arteriography should be carried out in older patients to search for significant coronary artery disease.

Differential Diagnosis. When mild aortic regurgitation is associated with mitral valve disease, the aortic pulse pressure may be normal and the early diastolic blowing murmur may be confused with that of pulmonic regurgitation (Graham Steell murmur). If severe mitral valve disease with pulmonary hypertension is present, it may not be possible to make this differentiation on physical examination; but when aortography is performed, such a murmur has been shown to be due most commonly to aortic regurgitation. Handgrip, which increases aortic pressure, augments the murmur of aortic regurgitation but usually does not affect that of pulmonic regurgitation.

Treatment. *Medical Management.* In marked aortic regurgitation, some restriction of physical exertion is advisable to reduce the likelihood of sudden arrhythmia. In the younger patient with a history of rheumatic fever, prophylaxis against streptococcal infection is indicated, and the use of antimicrobial drugs to prevent bacterial endocarditis during and after dental or surgical procedures is important at all ages. Patients with syphilitic aortic regurgitation should receive a full course of treatment with penicillin.

In the patient with angina pectoris, nitroglycerin is not always effective, but it may be worth a cautious trial; it should be recalled, however, that nitroglycerin causes peripheral arterial vasodilatation and may lower the aortic diastolic pressure even further. With the onset of dyspnea or orthopnea (symptoms of early left ventricular failure), the use of digitalis, sodium restriction, and diuretics when necessary can result in substantial improvement, and consideration for operation can sometimes be postponed.

Surgical Treatment. Once signs of left ventricular failure become significant, the course of the disease tends to be downhill. Although the natural course is not as abrupt as that in aortic stenosis, the life expectancy averages only about seven years after onset of significant symptoms. When dyspnea or angina becomes troublesome on less than ordinary activity (N.Y.H.A. Class III) despite optimal medical management, surgical treatment should clearly be considered.

An additional factor in selecting the appropriate time for operation is the finding that in some patients, despite hemodynamic improvement after aortic valve replacement, left ventricular dilatation and myocardial dysfunction may persist. Therefore it is desirable that surgical treatment be undertaken prior to the onset of such irreversible left ventricular disease. It may be hoped that improved noninvasive methods eventually allow detection of this potential problem before permanent changes occur.

Sudden, severe aortic regurgitation is poorly tolerated, and the average life expectancy is short. Therefore surgical treatment should usually be undertaken promptly.

In the great majority of patients, replacement of the diseased aortic valve with a prosthesis is necessary. In some patients with marked dilatation of the aortic root and aneurysm formation, aortic valve replacement is combined with replacement of a portion of the ascending aorta.

562. TRICUSPID VALVE DISEASE

TRICUSPID STENOSIS

Tricuspid stenosis is rare as an isolated lesion. Almost always it accompanies rheumatic involvement of other cardiac valves, and it is of clinical significance in only about 5 per cent of patients with rheumatic heart disease. Seventy to 80 per cent of patients with tricuspid stenosis are female, and most often they have accompanying disease of both the mitral and aortic valves. *Rare causes* of tricuspid stenosis include *carcinoid heart disease, endomyocardial fibroelastosis, congenital malformations,* and obstruction from a *right atrial myxoma.*

The primary abnormality in tricuspid stenosis, like that in mitral stenosis, is mechanical obstruction to atrial emptying. This results in an elevated right atrial pressure and a pressure gradient across the tricuspid valve during diastole. It is important to measure simultaneous pressures in the right atrium and right ventricle at cardiac catheterization, because signs of peripheral venous congestion may occur with substantially lower pressure gradients (less than 10 mm Hg; often only 3 or 4 mm Hg) than are observed with mitral stenosis. Generally, the cardiac index is reduced substantially.

Tricuspid stenosis should be suspected particularly in the patient who has signs of multivalve disease and severe right-sided venous congestion but no evidence of marked pulmonary hypertension. The patient may also be relatively free of signs and symptoms of pulmonary venous congestion, despite the presence of mitral valve stenosis. This feature may be due to a limiting effect of this lesion on the cardiac output (a protective effect of the tricuspid stenosis) which may prevent sudden augmentation of blood flow into the pulmonary vascular bed. Such an effect would help explain the unusually prolonged clinical course seen in some patients with tricuspid stenosis.

On physical examination, the mean jugular venous pressure is elevated, and in patients with sinus rhythm there is a very sharp, prominent A wave which reflects right atrial contraction against the stenotic valve. There is a characteristic slow fall in the jugular V wave (delayed Y descent), caused by the obstruction to right atrial emptying and the resulting slow fall in right atrial pressure during diastole (see figure in Ch. 556).

On palpation of the precordium, the right ventricle is not enlarged, and a diastolic thrill may be palpable at the lower left sternal border. The diastolic murmur of tricuspid stenosis will often be missed unless specifically searched for at that location. It resembles that of mitral stenosis, having a low-pitched rumbling quality often beginning with a tricuspid valve opening snap (somewhat later than a mitral opening snap), and an early diastolic decrescendo murmur is followed by presystolic accentuation if sinus rhythm is present. A characteristic feature in differentiating the murmur from that of mitral stenosis is augmentation in the intensity of the tricuspid rumble during *inspiration,* or during the *Müller maneuver* (attempted inspiration against a closed glottis). This augmentation is due to the transitory increase in right atrial filling and tricuspid valve flow, which results from the negative intrathoracic pressure. Both these maneuvers diminish the murmur of mitral stenosis. There may be an associated abnormal increase in the venous pressure during such inspiration in tricuspid stenosis. When atrial fibrillation is present, the murmur is even more difficult to detect, because it may occur only in early diastole and can be confused with the murmur of pulmonic regurgitation.

The electrocardiogram, if sinus rhythm is present, exhibits peaked P waves in leads II and V_1, evidence of right atrial enlargement, but atrial fibrillation is often present. There is no evidence of right ventricular hypertrophy. On the chest roentgenogram, in addition to the findings caused by associated valvular lesions, there is enlargement of the right atrium.

Surgical treatment is not indicated for mild tricuspid stenosis, but if it is severe or if the patient must undergo operation for a mitral valve lesion, surgical treatment may be undertaken. The tricuspid valve is usually not favorable for valvuloplasty, and most often a tricuspid valve prosthesis is inserted. Sometimes the tricuspid stenosis is not detected prior to a mitral valve operation, and is recognized only when unexpected signs of right-sided congestion develop postoperatively.

TRICUSPID REGURGITATION

Tricuspid regurgitation, like tricuspid stenosis, is usually associated with rheumatic disease of other cardiac valves, particularly the mitral. It may occur as an organic lesion, usually combined with some degree of tricuspid stenosis, or more commonly it is a functional lesion secondary to right ventricular dilatation with severe pulmonary hypertension. Such functional tricuspid regurgitation usually occurs late in the course of mitral valve disease. Other forms of severe pulmonary hypertension, such as the Eisenmenger reaction in congenital heart disease or pulmonary hypertension caused by chronic lung disease, can also cause functional tricuspid regurgitation. Rheumatic involvement of the tricuspid valve can result in tricuspid regurgitation when the right ventricular systolic pressure is normal, although most frequently such organic lesions are of a mixed variety, with both stenosis and regurgitation. Isolated tricuspid regurgitation can occur congenitally (as in Ebstein's malformation), and progressive tricuspid regurgitation caused by traumatic damage to the valve has been reported after crush injuries of the chest. The normal tricuspid valve can serve as a focus for bacterial endocarditis, particularly in drug addicts.

Tricuspid regurgitation constitutes a leakage of blood retrograde into the right atrium during right ventricular systole, which places an augmented volume load on the right ventricle. The pathophysiology resembles that of mitral regurgitation but involves the right heart. In mild tricuspid regurgitation, when the right ventricular end-diastolic pressure is not elevated, the right atrial mean pressure is normal and the V wave may not be particularly prominent. As the right ventricular and mean right atrial pressures rise in the presence of more severe regurgitation, the V wave becomes increased. If the right ventricle fails, the right ventricular diastolic and mean right atrial pressures rise, and the V wave becomes markedly enlarged.

Examination in severe tricuspid regurgitation may show the V wave in the jugular venous pulse high in the neck, with the patient in the upright position. Sometimes the height of the venous pressure may be difficult to discern, because the mean pressure may exceed 20 cm of water, and the top of the column may not be visible even in the sitting position. Systolic hepatic pulsations may be present, and there may be marked hepatomegaly, ascites, and peripheral edema. In tricuspid regurgitation secondary to severe pulmonary hypertension, there is a palpable pulmonary artery segment in the second left interspace, and a markedly accentuated pulmonic closure sound is evident. With severe tricuspid regurgitation, there is a thrill over the lower left sternal border and lower sternum, and an enlarged right ventricle is palpable along the left sternal edge and in the subxiphoid region. A pansystolic murmur is heard near the lower left sternal border and lower sternum, transmitted to the right sternal edge or the subxiphoid region. An early diastolic rumble caused by increased blood across the tricuspid valve flow may be audible; when there is organic involvement of the tricuspid valve by rheumatic disease, a longer diastolic murmur caused by associated tricuspid stenosis may be present. A characteristic feature of the murmur of tricuspid regurgitation is its augmentation during inspiration *(Carvallo's sign),* and the murmur can also be increased by the Müller maneuver (see Tricuspid Stenosis, above). These maneuvers lead to decreased intensity of a mitral regurgitant murmur.

There is electrocardiographic evidence of right ventricular hypertrophy, and atrial fibrillation is usually present in severe tricuspid regurgitation. Enlargement of both the right atrium and the right ventricle is evident on the chest roentgenogram.

The *treatment* of tricuspid regurgitation, if moderate and secondary to severe pulmonary hypertension, is conservative. Generally, the patient will respond to medical measures aimed at the left-sided valvular disease (sodium restriction, diuresis, digitalis). When aortic or mitral valve surgery is undertaken, such functional tricuspid regurgitation generally disappears gradually after relief of the left-sided lesion, as the pulmonary hypertension regresses. Occasionally, plication of the tricuspid valve anulus is done in patients with functional tricuspid regurgitation who are undergoing operation on other cardiac valves. If the functional tricuspid regurgitation is very severe, or if organic disease of the tricuspid valve is present in the absence of severe pulmonary hypertension, replacement with a prosthesis is necessary.

563. PULMONIC VALVE DISEASE

PULMONIC REGURGITATION

Regurgitation at the pulmonic valve most commonly accompanies severe pulmonary hypertension caused by left-sided valvular heart disease. The murmur is high pitched, decrescendo in quality, and best heard at the lower left sternal border. It may be indistinguishable from the murmur of mild aortic regurgitation; however, it should be noted that by far the most common cause of such a murmur in the patient with rheumatic valvular heart disease is aortic regurgitation. Isolated congenital pulmonic regurgitation with a normal pulmonary arterial pressure occurs rarely, and in this situation the murmur occurs later in diastole, is lower in pitch, and may be confused with the murmur of tricuspid stenosis. Pulmonic regurgitation with a normal pulmonary artery pressure can also occur in association with bacterial endocarditis on a normal pulmonic valve, particularly in drug users. Occasionally, if antimicrobial therapy is unsuccessful in this condition, excision of the pulmonic valve has been used to eradicate the source of infection, and this procedure does not appear to result in serious hemodynamic difficulties.

PULMONIC STENOSIS

Pulmonic stenosis usually occurs as a congenital malformation and is discussed in Ch. 552. Occasionally, acquired subpulmonic stenosis occurs in association with hypertrophic subaortic stenosis, owing to bulging of the interventricular septum into the right ventricular chamber. Rarely an intrapericardial tumor can compress the main pulmonary artery or right ventricular outflow tract, resulting in a pressure gradient between the right ventricle and the pulmonary artery.

Braunwald, E., Lambrew, C. T., Rockoff, S. D., Ross, J., Jr., and Morrow, A. G.: Idiopathic hypertrophic subaortic stenosis. I. A description of the disease based upon an analysis of 64 patients. Circulation, 30:Suppl.4:213, 1964.

Cohen, L. S., Gault, J. H., and Ross, J., Jr.: Mitral regurgitation. *In* Barondess, J. A. (ed.): Diagnostic Approaches to Presenting Syndromes. Baltimore, Williams & Wilkins Company, 1971, p. 1.

Dexter, L., and Werko, L. (eds.): Evaluation of Results of Cardiac Surgery. American Heart Association Monograph, No. 22, New York, 1968; also: Circulation 37 and 38 (Suppl. V), V-1, 1968.

Hancock, E. W., and Fleming, R. R.: Aortic stenosis. Quart. J. Med., 29:209, 1960.

Kirklin, J. W., and Karp, R. B.: Surgical treatment of acquired valvular heart disease. *In* Hurst, J. W. (ed.): The Heart. 3rd ed. New York, McGraw-Hill Publishing Company, 1974, p. 971.

Pluth, J. R., and McGoon, D. C.: Current status of heart valve replacement. Mod. Concepts Cardiovasc. Dis., 43:65, 1974.

Rees, R. J., Epstein, E. J., Criley, J. M., and Ross, R. S.: Haemodynamic effects of severe aortic regurgitation. Br. Heart J., 26:412, 1964.

Ross, J., Jr., Braunwald, E., Gault, J. H., Mason, D. T., and Morrow, A. G.: On the mechanism of the intraventricular pressure gradient in idiopathic hypertrophic subaortic stenosis. Circulation, 34:558, 1966.

Salazar, E., and Levine, H. D.: Rheumatic tricuspid regurgitation, the clinical spectrum. Am. J. Med., 33:111, 1962.

Sanders, C. A., Harthorne, J. W., De Sanctis, R. S., and Austen, W. G.: Tricuspid stenosis: A difficult diagnosis in the presence of atrial fibrillation. Circulation, 33:26, 1966.

Segal, J., Harvey, W. P., and Hufnagle, C.: A clinical study of one hundred cases of severe aortic insufficiency. Am. J. Med., 21:200, 1956.

Wood, P.: An appreciation of mitral stenosis. Parts I and II. Br. Med. J., 1:1051, 1113, 1954.

564. ARTERIAL HYPERTENSION

W. S. Peart

Definition. A statement that a given arterial pressure is above normal requires a knowledge of the range of normality. For a true definition of a raised arterial pressure, such as is used in epidemiologic studies, a rise above the mean of a population studied under standard conditions is usually used. It is easy to say that an arterial pressure of 120 systolic, 80 diastolic in mm of mercury is normal from the age of 15 years on and that an arterial pressure of 250 systolic, 150 diastolic in mm of mercury is abnormal at any age. The intermediate ranges are decided somewhat arbitrarily. In clinical practice this is of little help. It is wise when there is some doubt not to state either that hypertension exists or that it does not exist, but to substitute observation over a period of time to make sure that casual arterial pressure readings are consistently on the higher side of what is usually encountered in a completely normal subject. Again, it must be realized that single readings taken with a sphygmomanometer under varying circumstances may not reflect the usual arterial pressure in a given person. Measurements taken with automatic apparatus over 24-hour periods have shown considerable lability of pressure in many persons. This does not mean that high casual pressures may not be harmful, but in an individual case it must not be readily assumed that they are, because in these days of intensive therapy and investigation a great deal depends on this decision.

There are thus the two approaches: epidemiologic, which may have to depend upon isolated single readings of large populations that give information only about the range of casual readings, and the clinical approach, in which other factors have to be taken into account. It seems quite clear that most manifestations of disease in patients with raised arterial pressure are the consequences of, or are made worse by, the presence of raised pressure. This applies, for example, to the incidence of atheroma and other vascular disease. There is no doubt either that the higher the arterial pressure, whether systolic or diastolic, the higher the morbidity and mortality, and there is a distinct quantitative relation between these factors in many population studies. The fact that some patients withstand high arterial pressures without showing very many significant changes in their vascular systems compared with other patients with lower pressures and more serious vascular diseases does not invalidate this thesis. One individual's blood vessels may be of better quality than another's.

Some patients have mainly a rise in systolic arterial pressure. This particularly applies to the elderly, in whom such figures as 200 systolic, 90 diastolic in mm of mercury are not uncommon. It is likely that this mainly systolic hypertension represents increasing rigidity of the aorta and main vessels with less effect on the arterioles. There are all gradations from rise of the diastolic pressure with a relatively small rise in the systolic pressure to rise in the systolic pressure with a relatively smaller rise in the diastolic pressure. Too much has been made of the greater importance of diastolic hypertension in morbidity. It is highly likely that rise in the mean pressure is of greatest importance whatever way it is produced.

Measurement of Arterial Pressure. The ordinary sphyg-momanometric method of measuring has been shown to be subject to considerable error. This has emerged in epidemiologic studies of distribution of arterial pressure and must be taken into account clinically, particularly in following the results of treatment. Quite apart from the influence of arm circumference, so that those with fat upper arms have higher recorded pressures than those with thin arms for the same true direct intra-arterial measurements, observer error creeps in. Many observers show conspicuous digit preference in measuring the arterial pressure, and this can make 10 mm of mercury difference in one reading. It should now be agreed that the diastolic pressure is the point at which the Korotkoff sounds become muffled and not where they disappear. To reduce observer bias, an essential goal in epidemiologic or drug treatment studies, automatic or concealed measurement instruments have been introduced. The importance of observer bias cannot be overemphasized; it is best brought out when the examining doctor, after an initial reading which he considers too high, makes the patient recumbent for a variable period so that the pressure then falls below some cutoff point which he regards as normal. This maneuver is often used when a great deal depends on the measurement, such as an insurance policy or a job. It is self-deception and not in the best interests of the patient.

Causes of Hypertension. In most cases of hypertension (high arterial pressure) it is impossible at present to establish a cause. These cases, probably about two thirds of all those seen, are called "essential" or "idiopathic" hypertension. Fortunately, inroads are continually being made into this majority as greater knowledge accrues about disorders known to cause raised arterial pressure. These may be classified as follows:

I. Nonrenal causes
  A. Adrenal cortical overactivity
    1. Cushing's syndrome: Overproduction of hydrocortisone and corticosterone
    2. Conn's syndrome: Overproduction of aldosterone
    3. Pseudohermaphroditism: Overproduction of androgenic steroids
    4. Deoxycorticosterone production due to enzyme defect
  B. Adrenal medullary overactivity
    1. Pheochromocytoma: Overproduction of epinephrine, norepinephrine, and occasionally other amines such as hydroxytyramine
  C. Pregnancy
    Although pregnancy exacerbates the effects of underlying renal disease, the arterial pressure may be raised without any obvious renal disease as part of the "toxemia of pregnancy" syndrome.
  D. Coarctation of the aorta
    Although the coarctation has to take place above the level of the renal arteries for hypertension to exist, no conclusive evidence of renal involvement has yet been provided.
  E. Miscellaneous
    1. Ovarian tumors of varying histologic type: Overproduction of various steroid hormones similar to those in Cushing's syndrome is sometimes seen.
    2. Porphyria during acute attacks
    3. Lead poisoning during acute phase
    4. Raised intracranial pressure, more usually of acute onset, as with subarachnoid hemorrhage
    5. Administration of monoamine oxidase inhibitors followed by cheese ingestion
    6. Licorice, usually used for peptic ulcer treatment
    7. Contraceptive pill
II. Renal causes
  Practically all renal diseases known have been associated with hypertension. Important examples are:
  A. Acute and chronic glomerulonephritis
  B. Pyelonephritis
  C. Diabetic kidney
  D. Polyarteritis nodosa
  E. Polycystic disease
  F. Hemangiopericytoma (renin-producing tumor)

The probable link is interference with blood supply to the kidney, best exemplified by renal artery stenosis due to atheroma, extrinsic bands, or fibromuscular disease.

Incidence and Prevalence. In a given population group there is no comprehensive information about the distribution of causes. Attempts have been made to define this in selected groups of the population. It has been found, for example, by population study in both Wales and Jamaica, that there is a similar incidence of symptomless bacilluria in some subjects with hypertension, but whether cause or effect is uncertain. It is not known how many patients have atheromatous renal artery stenosis or fibromuscular hyperplasia of the renal arteries, or even chronic glomerulonephritis. To completely exclude a renal cause of hypertension requires considerable investigation in depth, including pyelography, arteriography, and renal biopsy, and even with such aids the presence of occult pyelonephritis as a scattered disease of the kidney may be missed. It still seems likely, however, that the bulk of cases picked up in epidemiologic surveys will have no known cause at present with the most intensive of our investigations. The prevalence varies widely in different parts of the world and among various races. For example, blacks in Georgia have a very high incidence of hypertension, as do coastal dwellers in northern Japan. The black population in various parts of Africa may also have a high incidence of hypertension, and although environmental factors, especially dietary ones like salt as in Japan, have been incriminated, the evidence is weak and incomplete. In some areas hypertension is very uncommon, as in many isolated island communities (for example, the Gilbert Islands), and studies of such groups moving to "civilized" environments show a rise of pressure.

Epidemiology. Much effort has been devoted to the epidemiology. Most of the studies depend upon casual arterial pressures taken under reasonably standard conditions, and the results show certain definite features. In general, arterial pressure in urban communities rises with age. The tendency is less marked or nonexistent in some communities, for example, the Gilbert Islands and northern Kenya, and does not seem to be associated with obvious disease but rather with body build and calorie intake. The rise applies to both the systolic and diastolic pressures in both males and females, although the rise in females is greater from the age of 30 to 40 years. This difference in the female has been noted in widely separated populations in different parts of the world. There is a quantitative likeness in the arterial pressure of blood relatives. Despite the common occurrence of hypertension in certain families, over-all there is no evidence of a common dominant genetic inheritance but rather of multiple factors. Environment as well as genetic inheritance has a common role in families. For example, the husbands of multiparous women in a study in South Wales had a lower than average arterial pressure, as did their wives. Unexpected correlations of this sort emerge in epidemiologic studies. Another is the higher incidence of hypertension among the relatives of subjects with hypertension and pyelonephritis. Nevertheless, identical twins may develop severe hypertension at about the same age even though they have spent their lives apart.

Pathology. Certain changes are common to all forms of hypertension and may properly be regarded as due solely to the level of arterial pressure. Other changes are peculiar to each cause of high arterial pressure, and they will be considered separately. In nearly all diseases associated with hypertension, the malignant phase may follow, so that a complicated picture resulting from the presence of the disease and the effects of malignant hypertension may be seen. Despite occasional suggestions to the contrary, the best evidence points to the malignant phase (necrotizing or accelerated phase) of hypertension as being mainly related to the absolute height of the mean pressure or the rate of rise of the mean pressure. Efforts to segregate malignant hypertension as a peculiar disease in its own right have been unrewarding, and the fact that some patients have all the evidence of malignant hypertension at mean pressures lower than other patients who have been withstanding higher pressures for many years does not disprove this general thesis. In any study of a large number of patients, those with malignant hypertension have a higher arterial pressure than those without. The manifestations of malignant hypertension in pathologic terms are acute vascular changes with fibrinoid necrosis in arterioles. The brunt of the damage is borne by vessels in the kidney, pancreas, mesentery, adrenal, and retina. It is rarely seen in voluntary muscle, and no cause can be suggested for this type of distribution. Since the kidney is always involved in all forms of hypertension, it is often difficult to be sure of the difference between primary change causing the hypertension and secondary damage because of the hypertension. It is reasonably certain that there is a primary disease in the kidney when the changes are most clearly seen in the glomeruli, as in glomerulonephritis, disseminated lupus erythematosus, amyloidosis, and diabetes. The glomerular changes with interference of blood flow lead to tubular atrophy, and in those cases in which the blood pressure is elevated, the most common changes are initially hypertrophy of the muscular wall of the afferent arteriole; next, hyalinization; and finally, in the malignant phase, intimal hyperplasia of the onion skin variety, which occurs also in slightly larger arteries, as well as the definitive fibrinoid arteriolar necrosis. All the elements of the blood, including cells, may be demonstrated in these lesions. Since this may resemble a vasculitis, the suggestion that it is part of an immunologic disorder has been made, but this is unlikely because the lesions heal readily with reduction of pressure. The occurrence of microangiopathic hemolytic anemia, with reduction of all formed elements in the blood, and the occurrence of platelets and fibrin on the damaged arterioles, with the potentiality of rapid decrease in renal function, are similarly reversible by rapid reduction of arterial pressure. In the larger arteries within the kidney, from the interlobar to the arcuates, hypertension causes intimal thickening, replication of the internal elastic lamina, and fibrosis with atheromatous deposits, sometimes in a very uniform manner but often as a nodular process. It is thought that this change, when it occurs in the apparently normal kidney, may be responsible for perpetuation of hypertension when the opposite abnormal kidney, the seat of pyelonephritis or involved by renal artery stenosis, is removed. The signs of ischemic change are best seen when the main renal artery is stenosed. The kidney volume shrinks; the glomeruli are crowded but generally appear normal; the juxtaglomerular apparatus in the afferent arteriole and the cells surrounding close to the macula densa of the distal convoluted tubule hypertrophy, sometimes grossly, and become hypergranulated, whereas the tubules between the glomeruli are atrophic and the interstitium may be expanded or fibrotic. The opposite kidney may show all the signs of hypertensive change previously described. The effects of acute narrowing of the arteriolar lumen on the performance of the relevant organs are seen, so that, in the case of the kidney, diminution of function with proteinuria, microscopic hematuria, and even frank hematuria occur. In the retina, exudation and hemorrhage caused by small infarcts, and papilledema associated with a raised intracranial pressure, which is of uncertain origin, are the main features. When this process occurs in the brain, various disturbances result, according to the part of the brain affected; fits and unconsciousness are not rare and are given the clumsy name of hypertensive encephalopathy. Arteriolar spasms may underlie some of these attacks as opposed to cerebral edema, previously implicated, and full recovery may occur. Because the impact may be apparently greater in some organs than in others, it is possible to find fibrinoid necroses in renal biopsies without any characteristic change in the retina. The converse is perhaps less common. In most untreated cases this disorder runs its course to death within two years of diagnosis. The features it shares with all other hypertensive manifestations are those due to the increased load put upon the heart and the blood vessels in different territories. A main finding is the increased incidence of atheroma, both experimentally and pathologically. The increased pressure leads to hypertrophy of the left ventricle and a tendency to angina pectoris and myocardial infarction. The increased load on the left heart leads to raised pulmonary venous pressure, pulmonary edema, raised pulmonary artery pressure, and congestive cardiac failure. The increased pressure in the vessels to the brain leads to a high incidence of strokes caused by cerebral hemorrhage, thrombosis, and subarachnoid hemorrhage. The site of these is probably the arterial microaneurysms originally described by Charcot. Vascular damage in the kidney leads to renal failure. It must be emphasized again that all these manifestations may be linked quantitatively with the level of arterial pressure. There is no doubt that in such conditions of acute onset as acute glomerulonephritis and eclampsia, the manifestations of malignant hypertension, particularly in the brain and retina, may appear at lower pressures and may seem more florid in the presence of renal failure. The latter, however, is not essential to the appearances, for example, of multiple cotton wool exudates and hemorrhages. It is likely that the rate of rise of pressure at least in part governs the severity of the signs.

The Mechanisms of Hypertension. *Circulatory Pattern.* The major factors controlling the arterial pressure are the cardiac output and the total peripheral resistance. If the cardiac output rises, the arterial pressure will rise unless there is a corresponding drop in the peripheral resistance. Most peripheral resistance occurs in the arterioles and is governed by contraction of their muscular walls. A given level of arterial pressure depends on the interplay between these two major factors and, in order to describe the pattern of the circulation, it is necessary to be able to say what the peripheral resistance is and in which part of the body the major changes are occurring. Although it has been claimed that changes in cardiac output are responsible for rises in pressure and may even ultimately lead to persistent high arterial pressure, the evidence for this is weak. In most cases of high arterial pressure, either experimental or in man, the one uniform feature is a raised peripheral resistance. The cardiac output in most cases of established hypertension in man is within normal limits. Theoretically, it might be thought that to know the particular pattern of peripheral resistance could give important clues to the cause of high arterial pressure. In only one form of high arterial pressure is there a very distinctive pattern, and this is pheochromocytoma. Epinephrine and norepinephrine, the amines most commonly released by these tumors, are particularly potent as vasoconstrictors in the skin. Measurements of skin blood flow show very low levels in such patients, unlike other causes of high arterial pressures. Removal of the tumor is followed by a rise in skin flow. If there were a wide variety of different agents raising the arterial pressure by increasing the peripheral resistance in various territories, certain characteristic patterns might emerge. However, in either renal hypertension or hypertension of unknown origin, the pattern is strikingly the same, so that the distribution of resistance is much the same from patient to patient. Admittedly, simultaneous measurements of flow in different parts of the body have not been done. Certain organs show the increased resistance most, the kidney and splanchnic area in particular. The general impression is, however, of a widely distributed increase of peripheral resistance in every tissue and organ of the body except the voluntary muscles.

Increased Cardiac Output. There are a few situations in which increased cardiac output seems to play an important role in raising the arterial pressure: renal failure, toxemia of pregnancy, and acute glomerulonephritis. Most studies have been made of patients with renal failure; these patients are particularly susceptible to fluid load, and the arterial pressure may rise abruptly when the patients are overloaded with water.

Cause of Rise in the Peripheral Resistance. This is uncertain in most cases of hypertension except those associated with high plasma levels of norepinephrine and epinephrine or renin and angiotensin, as in pheochromocytoma or hemangiopericytoma of the kidney. Hypertension itself causes changes in peripheral resistance in the sense that at a high arterial pressure the vessels contract, whereas lowering the arterial pressure causes decreased contraction. This is presumably a direct effect of pressure on the smooth muscle of the arteriolar wall, leading not only to contraction but also to hypertrophy, as was first shown by Folkow and his colleagues (1958). At one extreme, Borst (1963) has claimed that the sequence may be retention of salt and water caused by a renal fault, rise in the cardiac output, rise in arterial pressure to enable the kidney to excrete the salt and water, and secondary contraction of peripheral arterioles, leading to further rise in arterial pressure. Others believe that there is a primary cause for a rise in peripheral resistance, leading inevitably to a rise in arterial pressure. Guyton has emphasized the importance of correlating the many factors, including blood volume, cardiac output, peripheral resistance, the nervous system, and hormonal influences in terms of homeostatic mechanisms. The following major fields require deeper discussion.

Hypertension Associated with Retention of Water and Salt, with or without the Action of Adrenocortical Steroids. The best example, mentioned before, is of the patient with renal failure who tolerates fluid load badly and who is incapable of adjusting cardiac output and peripheral resistance so as to maintain his arterial pressure at normal levels. Removing body fluid by dialysis and lowering the salt intake will control this high arterial pressure in most instances. Even here another renal factor is revealed by the further lowering of arterial pressure brought about in this type of patient by total nephrectomy prior to renal transplantation. In some patients it is the only way in which the arterial pressure may be controlled, and these patients have some of the highest levels of renin activity, angiotensin, and aldosterone yet observed, which is of obvious importance. It was in animals that the condition of "renoprival hypertension" was described, but from closer studies made recently it seems that the hypertension that develops without kidneys is most likely to be due to increased sensitivity to salt and water overload with a rise in cardiac output. One of the experimental links of hypertension with salt and water metabolism is the observation that salt feeding in the rat leads to hypertension and also to renal damage, particularly if deoxycorticosterone (DOCA) is administered subcutaneously. Dahl and his colleagues have shown that there are salt-sensitive and salt-insensitive strains of rats, so that the possibility exists of a genetic factor acting in conjunction with an environmental one to produce high arterial pressure. The high incidence of hypertension and cerebral hemorrhage in northern Japan may be related, because there is a high salt intake in that area, but the exact mechanism is uncertain. In Cushing's syndrome with excess secretion of cortisol from hyperplastic adrenals, hypertension may be very severe and is associated with sodium and water retention as well as increased potassium excretion. The condition may be cured by removal of the suprarenals. It is still not certain whether there are other adrenal steroids capable of raising the arterial pressure, although since every patient with severe Cushing's syndrome does not have hypertension, it is at least suggestive.

Renal Hypertension. That the kidney is directly and primarily responsible for some cases of raised arterial pressure is shown by the successful cure of hypertension by unilateral nephrectomy when one of the two kidneys is diseased. Among the many renal diseases known to be associated with curable hypertension, pyelonephritis, tuberculosis, carcinoma, and, perhaps most important, obstruction to the main renal artery by atheroma or fibromuscular hyperplasia need to be mentioned. The link seems to be interference with blood supply to the kidney. Similar arguments can be applied to bilateral disease. Recent work has made much clearer the way in which the kidney raises the arterial pressure, and this includes experimental hypertension produced by a clip on the renal artery, first successfully accomplished by Goldblatt and his colleagues (1934).

Following are some of the major ways in which the kidney may be associated with elevation of the arterial pressure.

Failure to Excrete or Destroy an Extrarenal Pressor Substance. This has been partly touched on in the discussion of renoprival hypertension, in which the emphasis was on extracellular fluid volume sensitivity, but certain experimental observations suggest that some metabolic function of the kidney might be important apart from its effect on extracellular fluid volume. The hypotensive effect of introducing a normal kidney into the circulation of an animal with hypertension caused by a renal clip and the way in which a kidney with normal blood supply yet deprived of excretory function by a ureteric tie prevents the rise in pressure caused by a clip on the opposite renal artery point to this suggestion. The

ready reversal of renal stenosis hypertension both in man and in animals by removal of the obstruction, even with hypertension of long duration, argues against a very potent extrarenal pressor system.

Failure to Produce a Vasodilator. The hypothesis that the kidney has its main effect on the arterial pressure by providing a vasodilator to keep the arterial pressure down and that hypertension may be due to a failure of vasodilator production has received much recent study. Various extracts, particularly of the medulla of the kidney, have appeared to lower the arterial pressure on injection into animals. Some of these substances are prostaglandins, mainly of the E series, and they have been shown to appear in renal venous blood when the circulation to the kidney is reduced. It is uncertain whether they play a part in general hemodynamic changes in any form of renal hypertension, and the same uncertainty surrounds a possible local role in the renal circulation, particularly of the medulla.

Increased Response of a Normal Pressor Mechanism. An obvious candidate for this role is the sympathetic nervous system and its higher neural centers. If the kidney produced some substance that increased the over-all activity of the sympathetic system, this might be reflected in high arterial pressure. The main substance which has been shown to stimulate the vasomotor centers in the brain as well as facilitate the action of the sympathetic nervous system peripherally is angiotensin. Studies of norepinephrine metabolism have advanced considerably, and it is now possible to get a better estimate of the degree of activity of the sympathetic nervous system since it was discovered that not only norepinephrine but also dopamine beta hydroxylase is released into the circulation as a result of sympathetic activity. The latter substance, unlike norepinephrine, may not be taken up again after discharge, and therefore its plasma level, taken in conjunction with that of norepinephrine, may reflect sympathetic activity. Higher levels of both substances have been reported in hypertension.

Another way in which an increased response in the body could occur would be for the arterioles to respond more markedly than usual to a normal stimulus. For example, if the degree of contraction produced by a given dose of norepinephrine were markedly increased, then a state of high arterial pressure might follow. In hypertension, renal or otherwise, the degree of response to norepinephrine and angiotensin is not easy to quantitate in terms of the familiar log dose-response curve in comparison with a normal situation, so that the apparent decreased response in severe hypertension may be caused by the responses being tested at the top of the curve; although there is no positive evidence of this, the possibility has not been excluded.

Decreased Response of Baroreceptors. The view has been proposed that the fault in hypertension may lie in the baroreceptors and that by an alteration in their response the arterial pressure is allowed to rise to a higher level. Both in man and in animals it has been shown that the baroreceptor can be affected so as to permit a rise of pressure, and changes in stretch of the aortic wall at the root and arch produced experimentally have been associated with such a rise. It is clear that the baroreceptor mechanism in the carotid sinus is easily modified and seems to respond only to change or rate of change in pressure, so the depressor mechanism rapidly becomes reset at higher levels of arterial pressure and operates again only when the arterial pressure is even further elevated. There is need for much greater knowledge of baroreceptors, both central and peripheral in man, and merely to consider the carotid sinus is inadequate.

Renin-Angiotensin System. The development of better methods of measuring renin activity and angiotensin in plasma, especially by sensitive and specific radioimmunoassay methods, makes it possible to assign a role in various physiologic and pathologic situations, especially related to hypertension.

ANATOMY. Renin is stored in granules in the modified smooth muscle cells of the afferent arteriolar wall to the glomerulus, contiguous with the macula densa of the ascending limb of the loop of Henle (Goormaghtigh apparatus).

RELEASE OF RENIN. There are beta receptors within the kidney, stimulation of which governs renin release. Catecholamines, e.g., isoproterenol, epinephrine, and norepinephrine, which stimulate these receptors, liberate renin, whereas stimulation of alpha receptors seems to inhibit release, as does the use of beta blockers like propranolol. It may be that the sympathetic nerve endings close to the juxtaglomerular apparatus may act through the beta receptor. The way in which diuretics like furosemide release renin is not clear, but it is thought that altered sodium concentration in the urine may act as a stimulus, perhaps through the macula densa. In the normal animal or man, renin is released readily by changing from the supine to the erect posture and by sodium deprivation or blood volume depletion; it seems to be released readily by stimuli leading to autoregulation of renal blood flow. The quickest inhibitor of renin release is angiotensin itself, and longer-term effects are brought about by mineralocorticoid excess, e.g., of aldosterone. The way in which the latter inhibition occurs is unclear.

FUNCTIONING OF THE SYSTEM. Renin is probably released in a protein-bound form which reacts with substrate to produce first the decapeptide angiotensin I, which is mainly converted to the pressor octapeptide angiotensin II by cleavage of the two C-terminal amino acids in passage through the lung as well as other sites. Both peptides are readily cleared from the circulation by various tissues and readily destroyed by peptidases.

ACTIONS OF ANGIOTENSIN. Although angiotensin I has some actions of its own, the operation of the system mainly depends on angiotensin II. This peptide is the most potent direct smooth muscle vasoconstrictor known. It also raises the arterial pressure by a direct action on vasomotor centers in the brain, especially the hindbrain, and is known to facilitate sympathetic ganglionic transmission as well as the final sympathetic nerve ending effect. In some species it will liberate epinephrine from the adrenal medulla. The effect of vasoconstriction varies in different organs, but in the kidney, since it tends to reduce renal blood flow, it acts as an antidiuretic agent. Its other major action is in stimulating production of aldosterone from the adrenal cortex, and in different physiologic and pathologic situations it acts as a major but not unique stimulus.

ROLE IN HYPERTENSION. The first point to establish is that the actions of angiotensin are much influenced by electrolyte and water balance. For this reason it is possible to have very high levels of renin and angiotensin in the circulation of subjects with quite normal arterial pressure, as, for example, in cirrhosis of the liver with ascites, in Addison's disease, or in women taking contraceptive pills. Conversely, it may well be true that without too much elevation of the level, an expansion of intravascular volume and sodium retention markedly increases arterial pressure. Simple estimation of renin activity and angiotensin does not allow very precise definition of their action.

HIGH RENIN GROUP. In both human and experimental hypertension it has become clear that when the renin and angiotensin levels are high, reduction will usually lead to a fall of pressure. Good examples are bilateral nephrectomy in patients with terminal renal failure in whom intensive hemodialysis has failed to lower the pressure; the inhibition of renin release by beta-blocking drugs, e.g., propranolol, in malignant hypertension; and the reduction of arterial pressure in experimental renal clip hypertension by competitive angiotensin analogues (sarcosyl-1-alanine-8-octapeptide) or high titer angiotensin II antibodies.

LOW RENIN GROUP. Soon after the discovery by Conn (1961) of primary hyperaldosteronism caused by small tumors of the zona glomerulosa in the adrenal cortex, removal of which cured the hypertension and returned the high plasma and total body sodium, low plasma and body potassium, and high plasma aldosterone and secretion rate to normal, it was discovered that these patients had very low plasma renin activity and angiotensin levels which were difficult to elevate by any of the usual stimuli but which responded to spironolactone, an aldosterone antagonist. There followed the discovery that as many as 20 per cent of patients with hypertension had low plasma renin values. Most of these patients do not have excess mineralocorticoid; but in addition to increased aldosterone, some may have increased deoxycorticosterone or some other steroid, e.g., 18-hydroxydeoxycorticosterone, but the evidence is less convincing. Many of these patients have unexplained hyperplasia of the zona glomerulosa. The elaborate methods needed to distinguish patients with definite tumors from the others indicate some of the difficulties, but definition of the tumor by venography or by radioisotope scanning techniques shows that anatomy still has a place. Surgery is useless unless the patient has been shown to have a convincing drop of arterial pressure after administration of spironolactone in a dose of 300 mg daily for one month.

HYPERTENSION IN PREGNANCY. In patients in whom the arterial pressure rises without subsequently proved underlying renal disease, plasma renin and angiotensin levels tend to fall rather than rise, and although aldosterone production rises in pregnancy, there is also a fall with the development of hypertension.

RENIN-PRODUCING TUMOR (HEMANGIOPERICYTOMA). After the first description by Robertson and his colleagues (1967) of a patient with high arterial pressure, low plasma potassium, high aldosterone levels, and a small tumor on the outside of the renal cortex with a high content of renin, several other such patients have been reported. Such patients represent the clearest examples of the effects of overproduction of renin, because they are cured by removal of the tumor.

Clinical Manifestations. The symptoms and signs are usually secondary to effects on blood vessels in the various organs and tissues or to the increased load borne by the heart.

Cerebral. *Headache* is common, and the early morning occipital headache with stiffness of the neck, sometimes awakening the patient from sleep, commonly associated with vomiting attended by relief, is almost diagnostic of hypertension. Many patients have headache only on Saturday or Sunday mornings when they sleep later. The mechanism of this typical headache is uncertain. It is not closely related to the level of arterial pressure, and many patients with severe hypertension never experience it, but it is uncommon at diastolic pressures less than 120 in millimeters of mercury. It is most likely to be related to changes in cerebrospinal fluid pressure, as in patients with cerebral tumors. Various other forms of headache are associated, but are not diagnostic of hypertension. *Giddiness* short of true vertigo is a common complaint. Although disturbances in the balancing mechanisms are suggested by this, no direct evidence can be offered. *Personality changes* are not uncommon with the severe forms of hypertension and are presumably secondary to vascular damage. Some of these can be reversed by lowering the arterial pressure effectively; for example, ill-defined symptoms of anxiety may disappear. With extreme vascular disease, of course, *fits*, including jacksonian epilepsy, *minor strokes*, and *cerebral deterioration*, all occur. The experimental demonstration that the blood vessels in the brain may contract vigorously in response to high arterial pressure must obviously be related to these manifestations collected under the term *hypertensive encephalopathy*, quite apart from any more permanent vascular change induced by hypertension.

Thoracic. *Angina pectoris* is common and that it is linked to the high pressure and not necessarily to pure narrowing of coronary arteries is demonstrated by its alleviation on lowering the arterial pressure by drugs. An early symptom is *shortness of breath* on effort. This presumably is due to a change in the physical properties of the lung, leading to the sensation of dyspnea. This is often ascribed to left ventricular failure but perhaps more accurately should be attributed to a rise in left atrial pressure and consequently in pulmonary venous pressure. This process may occur acutely at night when the patient has been recumbent and asleep for, usually, about two hours. The typical attack of *cardiac asthma* ensues in which the patient has to sit up, gasping for breath. He dangles his legs over the edge of the bed and may get up and sit by an open window until his breathing is restored to normal. In extreme cases, frank pulmonary edema occurs and may be recognized by the coughing up of pink, frothy sputum. Listening over the chest reveals crackling sounds of all degrees from fine to coarse, depending on the degree of edema, and even wheezing noises may be produced, leading occasionally to confusion with so-called bronchial asthma. Acute lowering of the pressure by drugs alleviates these attacks dramatically. A surprising and unexplained feature is the fact that when the patient resumes his slumbers, he is very rarely reawakened by a second attack.

Because of the increased tendency to vascular disease, *myocardial infarction* may be superimposed on angina or may occur without warning. This may in some patients lead to a permanent cure of the hypertension, presumably because of reduced cardiac output. After a period in which there has been shortness of breath on effort and cardiac asthma, right-sided heart failure may follow, with improvement in the shortness of breath and cardiac asthma but with the other consequences of congestive cardiac failure. Some patients who have had few or no previous symptoms present for the first time in *congestive cardiac failure*. No convincing explanation has been offered for this, but perhaps the response of the pulmonary vasculature in some patients is different, so that the symptoms of left heart failure are minimized until the load on the right heart produces its own failure.

Vascular. The peripheral arteries may be observed to be either occluded in part or conspicuously tortuous. In this respect, a curly right carotid is common, as are tortuous brachial and radial arteries. The heart may show obvious hypertrophy of the left ventricle with an apex outside the midclavicular line, forcefully lifting the ribs above it. Auscultation of the heart typically reveals a presystolic triple rhythm heard usually best between the apex and the sternum. This disappears with successful treatment of the hypertension. The second sound in the right second space is loud and may have a distinctly twangy quality. Otherwise, in the absence of secondary cardiac disease, the sounds are unremarkable.

A rare observation is the presence of *pulsus alternans*, occasionally appreciated by variation in the strength of alternate beats at the wrist. Pulsus alternans may be observed more easily on taking the arterial pressure with a sphygmomanometer; the apparent rate of the pulse doubles as the pressure is slowly decreased. This again may be abolished by lowering the arterial pressure. The presence of failure of all types may be readily recognized from the rales in the lungs or the raised venous pressure, edema, hepatic enlargement, and congestive failure.

Bleeding from unexpected sites occurs in the higher ranges of arterial pressure. Nosebleeds, in the absence of uremia, and hemospermia are not rare.

In addition to the vascular disease already mentioned, involvement of the blood vessels to the legs is perhaps most commonly indicated by the complaint of *intermittent claudication*. This feature may, in fact, be made worse when the arterial pressure is lowered, since the usual cause is a block in the arteries somewhere between the external iliac and the popliteal.

A rare cause of *absent or delayed femoral pulses* is coarctation of the aorta. Although this is often diagnosed in childhood, it may present in young adults. It is fairly easily recognized clinically by the pulse changes. The collateral vessels are clearly seen and felt around the posterior scapular margin and the intercostal spaces, particularly on the back. In the other main vessels, the most striking occurrence is dissecting aneurysm through the media, which is practically always associated with hypertension in the older age group. Aneurysmal dilatation of other vessels and the rupture of berry aneurysms within the skull indicate other types of strain imposed on the vascular system.

Ocular. Patients commonly present with *vascular manifestations in the eye*, and bilateral or unilateral blurring of vision or scotoma is common. In the malignant phase, the changes include papilledema, in which characteristically the swelling is in the retina around the disc and encroaches on the edge, eventually involving the whole; a small, circumscribed so-called "hard" exudate, often arranged like grains of salt, between the disc and the macula; the "cotton-wool" exudate commonly associated with acute rise of arterial pressure as in acute glomerulonephritis and eclampsia, but especially florid in uremia; the typical macular fan or star figure of white lines of exudate between the nerve fibers leading from the macula; and hemorrhages, both linear and round. Papilledema is occasionally unilateral without hemorrhages or exudates, and, conversely, hemorrhages and exudates of all varieties may occur without papilledema; yet all are associated with this accelerated phase. Less severe changes are tortuosity in the arteries and nipping of the veins so that they are distended distally from crossings. Actual white sheathing of the arteries from the disc may be seen, as well as variations in caliber. Spontaneous variations in caliber have been reported in severe hypertension, but this must be an extremely rare observation. One of the most common retinal changes is segmental venous thrombosis, usually starting in the vessels on the temporal side of the retina and clearly occurring at a point of arteriovenous crossing. Central venous obstruction is another similar manifestation. Less common are central retinal arterial obstruction and, perhaps surprisingly, segmental arterial obstruction.

Renal.   The symptom resulting purely from hypertension and not related to the underlying renal disorder is increased *nocturnal frequency.* This may be an early manifestation of hypertension, usually occurring when the diastolic pressure is 120 in mm of mercury or more, and it may be alleviated by lowering the arterial pressure by any means. In severe hypertension of recent onset, diuresis may be extreme and associated with increased water, sodium, and potassium loss, leading to thirst, weakness, and cramps. Longstanding hypertension with vascular damage to the kidneys leads to all the secondary consequences of renal failure and ultimately to uremia.

Special Investigations.   *Urine.*   The presence of protein in the urine is a most important sign in hypertension. It may indicate the presence of the malignant phase, congestive cardiac failure, or a primary renal disease causing hypertension. When proteinuria is associated with glycosuria and ketones, a diabetic kidney, as in the Kimmelstiel-Wilson syndrome, may be present. Alternatively, glycosuria with very little proteinuria may raise the suspicion of a pheochromocytoma with associated hyperglycemia. Examining the centrifuged deposit may reveal the red cells and red cell casts typical of acute glomerulonephritis, polyarteritis nodosa, or the malignant phase of hypertension. Pus cells and motile bacteria characterize urinary infection and point to pyelonephritis. Greater precision is given to the diagnosis of chronic pyelonephritis with sterile urine by quantitative demonstration of the increased rate of cellular excretion, particularly when further stimulated by intravenous injections of prednisolone.

If proteinuria persists, it may be impossible to decide the underlying renal disease without percutaneous renal biopsy and light or electron microscopy. The presence of chronic glomerulonephritis, lupus erythematosus, and other renal diseases causing hypertension may readily be shown by this procedure. It is of much less help in the absence of proteinuria.

One other striking feature of the urine in hypertension is persistent alkalinity in the presence of potassium deficiency, which is most important because it points to hyperaldosteronism. The presence of an inappropriately high potassium excretion for the level of plasma potassium is further evidence of hyperaldosteronism. Estimation of the catecholamine content of the urine, including the free amines epinephrine and norepinephrine, together with measurements of their metabolic products, vanillylmandelic acid and the metanephrines, adds precision to the diagnosis of pheochromocytoma. A simple test of renal function is failure to raise the specific gravity above 1.010 or the osmolality above 500 mOsm per liter after overnight water deprivation.

Blood.   The level of blood urea gives only a rough indication of renal performance, because it is much influenced by dietary protein, and a better estimation, particularly in following the results of treatment, is that of creatinine clearance, which is still probably the most reliable and easily repeated of the tests of renal function. Electrolyte patterns have become of very great importance and are essential to the investigation of any case of hypertension. A low potassium and high bicarbonate point to hyperaldosteronism, and if associated with a higher than normal sodium level, they are strongly suggestive. The most common cause, however, of low plasma potassium and raised bicarbonate is previous administration of a thiazide or similar diuretic. With a suspicion of hyperaldosteronism, either primary or secondary, the use of radioactive isotopes to measure total exchangeable sodium which is high and potassium which is low, is often helpful. Measurement of plasma and urinary levels of aldosterone by radioimmunoassay has provided a practical procedure in suspected cases, although the posture of the patient and the sodium balance when the blood or urine is collected require careful standardization to avoid misleading results. Failure to suppress aldosterone production by DOCA administration points to autonomy either of the tumor or of the zona glomerulosa itself. Epinephrine and norepinephrine in the blood can now be measured either by a double isotope technique, which is laborious, or more readily by radioimmunoassay, but the diagnosis of pheochromocytoma is best made upon urinary excretion of catecholamine derivatives. Plasma renin activity and angiotensin levels will be considered later.

Feces.   The sodium and potassium content in the stools reflects the function of the colonic wall which is under the influence of mineralocorticoids like aldosterone. Increased aldosterone activity promotes sodium reabsorption and potassium excretion, altering the sodium-to-potassium ratio. A real advance was the finding that the electrical potential between the skin and the colonic wall is influenced by mineralocorticoid action, and that with increasing sodium reabsorption the difference increases (Edmonds and Godfrey, 1970). This can be used in a quantitative manner as a simple clinical procedure to indicate the action of aldosterone, especially when combined with changes induced by the aldosterone antagonist spironolactone.

Chest Roentgenogram.   In the roentgenogram of the chest, signs purely related to the hypertension and not to its cause are increased size of the heart, particularly the left ventricle, and increased vascularity of the lung fields caused by pulmonary venous congestion, often with edema, shown initially by small horizontal lines in the costophrenic angles ("B" lines) before the typical hilar butterfly shadows develop. The heart may not appear obviously enlarged according to ordinary roentgenologic criteria, even though enlargement is clinically obvious by the thrust of the left ventricle. Special signs occur in coarctation of the aorta, in which the notching of the lower margin of the rib by the collateral intercostal arteries is diagnostic.

Electrocardiogram.   Even with well marked hypertension, the electrocardiogram may show no definite changes, but probably the most reliable evidence of left ventricular hypertrophy is high voltage in the precordial leads. Left axis deviation is common, and depression of the S-T segments and T wave inversion over the lateral chest leads are usually present in a well established case of severe hypertension. This is often termed "left ventricular strain pattern," but it is uncertain whether this is on an ischemic basis, particularly as it may merge with the changes of ischemia resulting from coronary artery disease.

Intravenous Pyelography. Using this technique, it is possible to pick out those patients with a nonfunctioning kidney and those in whom the clubbed calices and the irregular outline of the scarred kidney point to pyelonephritis. Dilatation of the pelvicaliceal system points to the need to look for obstruction in the urinary tract, because, particularly when associated with infection, this type of obstruction from the urethra upward can be a cause of hypertension. Naturally stone or calcification in the kidney can be seen and may be relevant to the hypertension. It is worth examining the pelvic films carefully for evidence of iliac arterial calcification. On pyelography the delayed appearance on one side of a small volume system in rapid sequence films taken at 1-minute intervals up to 5 minutes, together with increased contrast of dye in the later films up to 20 or 30 minutes, is typical of renal artery obstruction, especially when associated with a smaller kidney. Retrograde ureteric pyelography is used only when obstruction is either apparent or suspected and caliceal anatomy is indistinct. The use of high dose intravenous pyelography has reduced the frequency and need for retrograde examination. The size and shape of the kidney may be better appreciated by the use of tomography, which, when combined with intravenous pyelography, will not only give better indication of these factors, but may also show tumors in the renal areas.

Arteriography. In the search for renal causes of hypertension, arteriography is used only when surgical intervention is intended should an appropriate renal disorder be discovered. The clearest pictures are given by selective catheterization of each renal artery, with a final aortogram to pick up multiple arteries, one of which may be stenosed. Small scars or poor cortical filling can be seen by this technique as well as major blocks in the main renal arteries. Cysts show as avascular round filling defects, and tumors, such as hypernephromas, as areas of increased and irregular vascularity. Renin-producing tumors (hemangiopericytoma) are shown on the outer edge of the cortex and appear as filling defects. Pheochromocytomas can be demonstrated as round or ovoid vascular blush areas by using aortography under the protection of epinephrine-blocking drugs (phentolamine).

Venography. The adrenal veins may be catheterized selectively, the right with difficulty from the wall of the cava, and the left via the renal vein. The anatomy of the gland can be shown by retrograde dye injection, and tumors may be demonstrated. This technique is also used for collecting blood from the renal vein for assay of renin and the adrenal vein for assay of corticosteroids.

Renography. Most information is gained by comparing the curves of radioactivity obtained from the two kidneys simultaneously after the administration of ^{131}I hippuran. This gives quantitative information about individual renal function which is extremely useful in relation to vascular and parenchymal disease as well as obstructions in the urinary tract. Combined with scanning techniques, either instantaneous using a gamma camera, or slowly using a scintillation scanner, information about both function and morphology can be gained. Development of technetium-labeled compounds enables the gamma camera to be used for external tests of individual renal function by steadily improving methods.

Divided Renal Function Studies. Divided renal function tests, in which the urine is collected through separate ureteric catheters and the composition is compared, are the ultimate tests of renal function, despite their technical difficulties, but are being superseded by improvements in radioisotope renography. For example, in stenosis of the main renal artery, water reabsorption increases markedly, leading to increased concentration but reduced clearance of such filtered substances as creatinine, inulin, and para-aminohippuric acid (PAH). The sodium concentration in contrast drops markedly. In parenchymal disease, as for example pyelonephritis, the water reabsorption is reduced and the concentration, as well as the clearance, of inulin, creatinine, and PAH drops, and the sodium concentration may be higher than or no different from that on the normal side. As a preliminary to surgery of the kidneys, such tests are essential.

Essential (Idiopathic) Hypertension. Hypertension for which no recognizable cause can be found is called essential or idiopathic. It should be emphasized that even if a known cause appears to exist—for example, renal disease—an etiologic relationship has not been established conclusively. Frequently the removal of an apparently diseased kidney is not followed by a fall in arterial pressure. (In some cases, secondary damage in the vascular system or opposite kidney may account for this.)

A great deal of controversy has gone on over the role of inheritance in hypertension. The most reasonable position on the basis of data now available seems to be that many factors, predominantly environmental but also inherited, lead to similar arterial pressures in members of certain families. In some families there is perhaps a stronger inherited tendency than in others; for example, twins have been described who developed malignant hypertension at about the same age while in different environments. The tendency to develop high arterial pressure certainly seems to be present at an early age and long before high arterial pressure itself is present. This is shown by the effects of pregnancy. In some women a high arterial pressure may occur for which no cause can be discovered; the arterial pressure may drop after pregnancy and may rise again later in life. They usually come from families with a history of high arterial pressure.

No consistent factor in hypertension of unknown origin has yet emerged that tells us anything about mechanism apart from these few clues.

Prognosis and Treatment. The outlook for a patient with high arterial pressure may in general be quantitatively related to the level of arterial pressure. The higher the pressure, the lower the survival rate over any period. This has been shown repeatedly in population studies. In an attempt to differentiate the outlook for various patients with hypertension, the terms *benign* and *malignant hypertension* have been used; the latter is also called the *accelerated* or *necrotizing phase* to describe both the rapidity of the course and the fibrinoid arteriolar necroses that define the histologic condition. The term "benign" should be abandoned, because it is a poor description for a condition that leads to death by stroke, myocardial infarct, and renal failure. It is easier from the epidemiologic viewpoint in describing large populations to give a quantitative prognosis, but in the individual patient seen for the first time the wise clinician takes account of all the variable factors discussed previously that may influence a particular value measured on the sphygmomanometer. This analysis, of course, influences his decision about whether the patient needs treatment or not.

There is no doubt in malignant hypertension that, unless the arterial pressure is successfully lowered, the patient will be dead usually within two years. It has been shown many times that it is possible to prolong life well over ten years by successful medical or surgical treatment of this phase of hypertension. Now that controlled trials of treatment in less severe grades of hypertension have been carried out, it is clear that improvement in outlook is conferred by successful treatment. In these cases, the prognosis depends on many factors, such as the presence of obvious vascular disease in major organs and the level of arterial pressure in relation to age. Although malignant hypertension may arise abruptly in a patient with previously normal pressure, it commonly supervenes after many years of moderately severe hypertension and seems clearly related to a rise over some months. Adequate treatment keeps this sort of patient out of this dangerous situation. The treatment depends in part on whether a potentially curable cause has been found. The curable causes of hypertension include pheochromocytoma, Cushing's syndrome, Conn's syndrome, renin-producing tumor, coarctation of the aorta, unilateral renal disease, and, occasionally, bilateral renal disease caused by surgically correctable renal artery stenosis. By "cure" in these cases is meant that the arterial pressure is returned to a completely normal level after operation.

Philosophy of Investigation and Treatment. *The first decision* a physician has to make is whether the arterial pressure as measured is too high for the individual, considering both the circumstances of the measurement and any of the other factors that can influence a single arterial pressure reading. *Time is on the side of the physician,* and repeated measurements under similar conditions, weeks or months apart, are often necessary to determine this point in the absence of any obvious signs of the effects of hypertension. It is also good to take the pressure three times in succession at one visit, because it is striking in many patients that the second and third pressures are lower when the stimulus of the initial cuff tightening has worn off. Measurements made over 24 hours by portable apparatus have shown how variable a pressure may be and how it may only be elevated when being measured by the physician. The next decision to be made after deciding that the arterial pressure is too high is given by the answer to the question, *"Am I seeking a cure or merely alleviation?"* Clearly in a young person with severe hypertension and no evidence of vascular disease, a cure is always sought. In a patient of 65 years with evidence of vascular disease of considerable degree, the answer may well be alleviation. In the first place this means that all the investigations that are currently available will be used to obtain a diagnosis, whereas in the second, one will be content with a few investigations useful in the management but concentrating on treatment by drugs. This is a good rule for other conditions than hypertension. The next important therapeutic rule is to make sure that the *symptoms complained of are caused by hypertension* and that the treatment by drugs

is not going to cause more trouble than the underlying condition. Too many elderly patients in their seventies with pressures of 190 systolic, 90 diastolic in mm of mercury are treated with potent hypotensive drugs for symptoms of giddiness caused by positional changes or for headaches as a manifestation of anxiety or depression that have nothing to do with hypertension, and are made much worse. Age needs no additional therapeutic hazards, and when treatment is indicated the arterial pressure should be brought down gently.

With severe hypertension it is unusual to be able to control the pressure by one major drug alone. A diuretic is needed in at least two thirds of the cases.

There is no particular "best" drug for the treatment of high arterial pressure. One of the mysteries of high arterial pressure is the way in which some patients respond well to one drug, some to another, without any other obvious difference between the patients. It is best to become accustomed to the actions and side effects of a small variety of drugs and to use them on all the patients who need treatment, exploiting each one to the full or to the limit of side effects before adding the adjunct or shifting to a new major drug. In the higher range of drug dose in which side effects accrue, multiple therapy is to be encouraged and not sneered at. Some patients do better, for example, on alpha-methyldopa plus guanethidine plus chlorothiazide than on either of the main drugs alone. There is now emerging the possibility of selecting more appropriate drugs for particular patients from studies of plasma renin levels. Some patients with high levels respond to inhibitors of renin release like propranolol, whereas some in the low renin group respond best to an aldosterone antagonist like spironolactone, or even to a thiazide.

Curable Hypertension. Once the rarities such as pheochromocytoma, coarctation of the aorta, Cushing's syndrome, and renin-producing tumors have been considered, two less rare conditions are of great interest because of the problems posed.

RENAL ARTERY STENOSIS. Once clearly diagnosed, prediction as to success of either nephrectomy or reconstructive arterial surgery depends upon other factors. It is best to be under 40 years with fibromuscular hyperplasia of one renal artery on the left side and a high peripheral plasma renin activity or angiotensin level with a higher concentration of renin in venous blood from the affected kidney than from the other side, and with a PAH clearance on the normal side that is well above 200 ml per minute. This enables the surgeon to bring down the splenic artery distal to the stenosis with the knowledge that if the blood flow can be restored satisfactorily, the arterial pressure will be lowered and not maintained, for example, by disease in the opposite kidney. The plasma renin activity is useful in conjunction with clear evidence of ischemia determined by pyelography, renography, and divided renal function studies. By contrast, it is bad to be over 40 years with an atheromatous block and other evidence of atheromatous vascular disease elsewhere as, for example, in the coronary arteries, and an absence of the criteria noted above.

CONN'S SYNDROME. Although initially primary hyperaldosteronism associated with a single tumor of the suprarenal cortex was believed to be easily identified by the presence of hypokalemia, moderate hypertension, raised plasma aldosterone or aldosterone secretion, and a suppressed plasma renin activity, it has now become clear that there are patients with all these criteria who have bilateral hyperplasia of the suprarenal cortex and whose hypertension is not cured by adrenalectomy. It is not even true that all patients with undoubted tumors of the zona glomerulosa have their arterial pressure brought down to normal levels after removal, even though evidence of hyperaldosteronism may disappear. As with most other conditions causing hypertension, there is a variable percentage of patients whose arterial pressure either does not fall at all or does not completely return to normal after operation (for example, pheochromocytoma); presumably secondary changes maintain the hypertension. In general the criteria of curable hypertension associated with an aldosterone adenoma are suppressed plasma renin level which fails to rise in the upright posture on a low sodium diet and injections of furosemide; high aldosterone plasma level resistant to lowering by DOCA administration; increased colonic potential difference reversed by spironolactone; low plasma potassium (less than 3.4 mEq per liter) and total body potassium; and plasma sodium usually above 142 mEq per liter with increased total body sodium. Anatomic demonstration of the tumor by venography, isotope localization with external scanning, or high aldosterone-to-cortisol ratios in adrenal venous blood complete the arduous diagnostic path.

Medical Treatment. From the results in large series of patients medically treated for hypertension, there is no doubt that morbidity and mortality are both reduced so long as the arterial pressure has been consistently lowered. Symptoms and signs both improve, as shown, for example, by the early relief of angina and the diminution in cardiac size roentgenographically. The occurrence of a cerebrovascular stroke in hypertension is an indication for lowering the pressure in order to lessen the risk of further stroke, because it is clear that a major reduction in mortality rate in treated hypertension is due to stroke prevention. Only occasionally in the older age group when the pressure has been reduced too quickly do signs of reduction of cerebral blood flow occur. Similarly, the presence of renal damage with hypertension is usually an indication for lowering the pressure to minimize further deterioration. The creatinine clearance may drop for a short time on lowering the arterial pressure but usually rises again, often to higher levels than at the outset if successful treatment is maintained. This temporary drop must not be used as an argument for lessening the vigor of treatment, and this is also true of intermittent claudication in which the condition will often improve.

The *drugs used in treatment* have known major actions as well as a number of others that are not altogether well defined. It is fair to say that very few of the drugs in current or in past use have had their action of lowering the arterial pressure completely explained. Various types of drugs are used, as follows:

Ganglion Blockers. The best example of these is hexamethonium. The basic chemical structure of this drug has been altered in various ways to produce substances of more desirable properties that are capable of predictable absorption by mouth and predictable duration of action. Acting on parasympathetic and sympathetic ganglia, these agents produce a widespread blockade, leading to changes in peripheral resistance and in venous tone, so that part of their action, seen best with the patient in the standing position, is due to venous pooling and diminished cardiac output. Most of these drugs will lower the arterial pressure in many patients, particularly in the standing or sitting position. The major undesirable side effects are dryness of the mouth, paralysis of ocular accommodation, constipation, and impotence.

Pempidine tartrate may be used in a dose of 5 mg three times a day, which may be increased by 5 mg on each dose. This is probably the best of this type of drug for oral use. It should not be used in patients with distinct uremia (blood urea nitrogen over 50 mg per 100 ml), because paralytic ileus is a real risk. This drug, because of its quick onset of action and relatively short duration, is best given three times daily. The paralysis of ocular accommodation may be overcome by the use of pilocarpine hydrochloride 0.5 per cent eye drops. There is now very little place for this type of drug except as an adjunct in a very severe and resistant hypertensive patient.

Sympathetic Blockers. These have largely replaced the ganglion blockers, and either deplete or interfere with catecholamine metabolism at nerve endings or centrally. A prototype is *guanethidine*, which is concentrated in the postganglionic sympathetic fibers and interferes with the release of norepinephrine from the nerve endings. It also clearly has central effects, shown by the sleepiness and depression produced in some patients. Like the ganglion blockers, these agents produce a fall in pressure, mainly with the patient in the standing position, and, because of the sympathetic blockade, a distinct slowing in heart rate is seen. The major side effects are tiredness, peculiar muscular achings affecting the thighs and upper arms, shortness of breath, giddiness and postural hypotension on exercise owing to failure of vasoconstriction, diarrhea, and occasional impotence after failure of ejaculation.

Guanethidine sulfate in a starting dose of 10 to 25 mg daily is recommended. The full effects of the drug take a few days to become apparent, so that increases of dose (5 mg) should not be made more frequently than about every four or five days. Since it has a prolonged action, it need only be given once daily.

Bethanidine is like guanethidine in its actions but is quicker in onset and shorter in duration of action and has the merit of not causing diarrhea. The initial dose is 10 mg three times daily.

Debrisoquine sulfate has few central effects psychologically, does not cause diarrhea, and has a prolonged action. The starting dose is 10 mg twice daily.

Reserpine (various extracts of *Rauwolfia serpentina*) depletes nerve endings and organ stores of norepinephrine and epinephrine. It can be useful as long as a dose of 0.5 mg daily is not exceeded; beyond this amount, its major side effect of depression, even to suicide, becomes common. It is best used in a dose of 0.25 mg daily in conjunction with a thiazide diuretic, and even then the physician must remember that depression may slowly occur after several apparently trouble-free months; this can be reversed by removing the drug.

Alpha-methyldopa, among its other actions, serves as a competitive substrate for dopa decarboxylase on the route of production of norepinephrine via dopamine. It has marked central effects with tiredness and depression. Patients commonly seem to escape from its effects after some months of treatment. The starting dose is 250 mg either twice or three times daily, with a warning to the patients that they will feel extremely sleepy for the first few days, but that this usually wears off. The dose may be increased slowly as with guanethidine; because of its sedative action, it is well to begin by increasing the night dose. Occasional cases of jaundice and hemolytic anemia have been reported. In higher doses, especially if renal or brain damage is present, a state like akinetic parkinsonism may occur.

Propranolol hydrochloride is different from the aforementioned group in that it is mainly a beta blocker and acts not only on blood vessels, but also on the heart. It perhaps lowers the supine pressure relatively more than the other group of drugs and, apart from its beneficial effect in angina pectoris, it may provoke cardiac failure in those patients with a poor myocardium. The starting dose is 40 mg twice daily for one week, increasing to 80 mg twice daily, and so on. Its main interest now lies in its use in the high renin group of hypertensive patients, and some of these patients are very responsive when the renin levels are effectively suppressed. Another important side effect is shortness of breath on effort or asthma; it should never be used when this is present, and it should be remembered that the wheeziness may take some time to become troublesome.

Pargyline hydrochloride is a monoamine oxidase inhibitor, has a marked central effect, and is often useful in the depressed patient with hypertension. Like all other drugs of this type, it is dangerous if the patient is not warned about taking cheese, yeast and beef extracts, and heavy red wine, all of which may provoke severe hypertension and cerebral hemorrhage. Nevertheless some patients do well.

Adjuvant Drugs. Various drugs are used mainly as adjuvants to these main lines of treatment. They include hydralazine hydrochloride (starting dose 20 mg three times daily), whose mode of action is obscure, and phenoxybenzamine hydrochloride (starting dose 10 mg three times daily), which antagonizes the action of norepinephrine or epinephrine on the vessel wall but is surprisingly ineffective by itself.

Diuretics. In any case of severe hypertension, one of the previously described drugs is usually used in conjunction with a diuretic. The addition of a diuretic increases the hypotensive action and may make possible the use of a smaller dose of the major drug. The most commonly used are the thiazide derivatives, and there is nothing to choose between any of them. For example, chlorothiazide, 0.5 gram daily, is an adequate adjuvant, but has largely been replaced by smaller dose derivatives. The maximal adjuvant action is between two and four times the basic dose. Most doctors give potassium supplements because of the fear of potassium depletion. In general this is quite unnecessary, and a plasma potassium of 3 mEq per liter is not usually associated with any symptoms. Symptomatic hypokalemia in a patient on thiazides needs investigation for possible hyperaldosteronism. The initial mode of action is probably by sodium depletion and reduction in plasma volume, but action still continues when the plasma volume and sodium have been repleted, probably by diminished peripheral resistance. If it is nevertheless wished to give potassium, combined tablets should not be given, because small gut ulceration and stricture occur. Slow-release tablets of potassium chloride are safer. The thiazides may also occasionally precipitate diabetes mellitus, and more commonly gout and light-sensitive rashes. Although it was initially thought that only mild cases of hypertension would respond to a thiazide, experience has shown that quite severe cases may often respond to a thiazide alone; and if there is no particular urgency, then it is worth using, for example, 25 mg of hydrochlorothiazide twice daily. The full effect may take three to six weeks to be demonstrated but is undoubted. Furosemide in a dose of 40 to 80 mg daily is often used instead of a thiazide, but the very rapid diuresis may prove inconvenient.

Spironolactone. Although this can also be used as an adjuvant, it has a place of its own quite apart from its use in lowering the arterial pressure of patients with definite Conn's syndrome. In a dose of 25 mg twice daily, it can be introduced and the dose increased. It must be taken after meals, because otherwise it may cause nausea; it is contraindicated in peptic ulcer which it may cause to bleed. In some males it causes gynecomastia; in fewer females, interference with the menstrual cycle occurs, presumably because of its estrogenic effects. In the presence of renal failure, it should be used cautiously because of the elevation of plasma potassium it causes. Given together with a thiazide, it can provide smooth, well controlled, and symptomless control of hypertension. Suitable treatment is hydrochlorothiazide, 25 mg, spironolactone, 25 mg, each twice daily, or a combination tablet of spironolactone, 25 mg, and hydroflumethiazide, 25 mg, twice daily. Unless there is urgency, this is an excellent approach to the treatment of even severe hypertension. The combination which may well replace this treatment is that of a thiazide with amiloride. The latter is a potent, potassium-sparing diuretic which antagonizes potassium loss by a thiazide; together they can be very effective.

Treatment of Acute Pulmonary Edema and Hypertensive Encephalopathy. Two situations in hypertension demand emergency treatment in which it is essential to bring the arterial pressure down as rapidly as possible. The first is pulmonary edema caused by left ventricular failure, and the second is the state of fits and unconsciousness called hypertensive encephalopathy. In the first, if the patient is overloaded with fluids as in acute glomerulonephritis, the best form of treatment is to reduce the extracellular fluid volume, either by bleeding or by dialysis, although even with quite marked degrees of renal failure, the intravenous injection of furosemide, 40 to 400 mg, usually provides a rapid and dramatic diuresis without notable toxicity. It is always worth trying first, especially when there is doubt about the patient's fluid balance. If there is no obvious fluid overload, the dyspnea may be relieved by use of pentolinium tartrate in a dose starting at 1.5 mg intramuscularly and increasing until the pressure is brought down. The patient should, if possible, be sitting up for this procedure. Good results have been obtained with other drugs such as reserpine (5 mg intramuscularly), alphamethyldopa as an intravenous injection (50 mg per ml, total 250 mg), guanethidine sulfate as an intramuscular injection (25 mg), and sodium nitroprusside by continuous intravenous infusion (25 to 400 μg per minute); in a particular patient it may be necessary to try various of these in sequence. Relief of symptoms can be speedy. It is dangerous to use guanethidine sulfate intravenously, because the release of norepinephrine raises the arterial pressure even higher. Diazoxide (300 mg intravenously) given as a rapid injection produces flushing, nausea, and occasionally vomiting; nevertheless it can usually prompt a fall in arterial pressure within 15 minutes which may last 12 to 24 hours before a further injection is needed. Its mode of action is unknown. If given over a long period, it may cause hyperglycemia and frank diabetes, and even occasional pancreatitis. It is best in fulminating hypertension, but given by the oral route (starting dose, 40 mg three times daily) it has been very effective in patients with hypertension complicating renal impairment when the commonly used remedies have failed. Long-term treatment demands vigilance for the development of diabetes.

Typical Drug Dosages. Pempidine, 5 to 20 mg three times daily; guanethidine, 10 to 100 mg daily; bethanidine, 10 to 30 mg three times daily; debrisoquine, 10 to 80 mg twice daily; reserpine, 0.25 to 0.5 mg daily; alphamethyldopa, 250 mg twice daily to 750 mg three times daily; propranolol, 40 to 160 mg two to three times daily; pargyline, 10 to 25 mg twice daily. To each of these drugs in moderate to severe hypertension, hydrochlorothiazide, 25 to 50 mg or equivalent thiazide is added daily.

Combined therapy in severe resistant hypertension: e.g., alpha-methyldopa, 250 mg three times daily, guanethidine, 25 mg daily, and hydrochlorothiazide, 25 mg daily. Debrisoquine, 20 mg twice daily, propranolol, 40 to 80 mg twice daily, and hydrochlorothiazide, 25 to 50 mg daily. Aldomet, 250 mg twice daily, propranolol, 40 to 80 mg twice daily, and hydrochlorothiazide, 25 to 50 mg daily. It is possible to replace hydrochlorothiazide with another diuretic such as Lasix, 40 to 80 mg daily, or spironolactone, 25 to 50 mg daily. Although combination treatment reduces side effects of each of the main drugs, some combinations have particular although occasional complications. The most important to recognize are dreaming and hallucinations, as well as muscle ache even to the point of severe pain, on combinations of the guanethidine group with propranolol.

Conclusion. Finally, the main aim of treatment is that the patient should live a more comfortable life than before treatment. The patient with diarrhea, impotence, tiredness, and a normal arterial pressure is not a therapeutic triumph. To treat hypertensive subjects requires patience, perseverance, optimism, and a belief that the drugs can be manipulated in most cases to lower the arterial pressure while keeping the patient comfortable.

Aldosterone in Clinical Medicine. Copyright by Searle & Company, San Juan, Puerto Rico. New York, Medcom, Inc., 1972.

Britton, K. E., and Brown, N. J. G.: Clinical Renography. London, Lloyd-Luke (Medical Books) Ltd., 1971.

Conn, J. W.: Aldosteronism and hypertension: Primary aldosteronism versus hypertensive disease with secondary aldosteronism. Arch. Intern. Med., 107:813, 1961.

Gross, F. (ed.): Antihypertensive Therapy, Principles and Practice. Proceedings of the Symposium held in Siena, Italy, June 28 to July 3, 1965, sponsored by CIBA. Berlin and Heidelberg, Springer-Verlag, 1966.

Leishmann, A. W. D.: Merits of reducing high blood pressure. Lancet, 1:1284, 1963.

Page, I. H., and Bumpus, F. M. (eds.): Handbook of Experimental Pharmacology. Volume XXXVII: Angiotensin. Berlin and Heidelberg, Springer-Verlag, 1973.

Page, I. H., and McCubbin, J. W. (eds.): Renal Hypertension. Chicago, Year Book Medical Publishers, 1968.

Peart, W. S.: Hypertension and the kidney. *In* Black, D. A. K. (ed.): Renal Disease. 3rd ed. Oxford, Blackwell Scientific Publications, 1972, p. 705.

Pickering, G. W.: High Blood Pressure. 2nd ed. London, J. & A. Churchill, Ltd., 1968.

Pickering, G. W.: The Nature of Essential Hypertension. London, J. & A. Churchill, Ltd., 1961.

Quinn, E. L., and Kass, E. H.: Biology of Pyelonephritis. Henry Ford Hospital International Symposium. Boston, Little, Brown & Company, 1960.

Robertson, P. W., Klidjian, A., Harding, L. K., Walters, G., Lee, M. R., and Robb-Smith, A. H. T.: Hypertension due to a renin-secreting renal tumor. Am. J. Med., 43:963, 1967.

Rose, G. A., and Blackburn, H.: Cardiovascular Survey Methods. Geneva, World Health Organization, 1968.

Stamey, T. A., and Good, P. H.: Diagnostic tools in the evaluation of renal vascular disease. *In* Brest, A. N., and Moyer, J. H. (eds.): Hypertension: Recent Advances—The Second Hahnemann Symposium on Hypertensive Disease. Philadelphia, Lea & Febiger, 1961, p. 189.

Symposium: Arterial hypertension. Arch. Intern. Med., 133:911, 1974.

Symposium: Primary hyperaldosteronism. Arch. Intern. Med., 123:113, 1969.

Veterans Administration Cooperative Study Group on Antihypertensive Agents: Effects of treatment on morbidity in hypertension. II. Results in patients with diastolic blood pressure averaging 90 through 114 mm Hg. J.A.M.A., 213:1143, 1970.

CORONARY ARTERY DISEASE

Thomas Killip

565. THE PROBLEM: ATHEROSCLEROSIS

Atherosclerosis is a disease of large and medium-sized arteries characterized by fatty deposits and thickening of the intima with disruption of the media. The aorta, its large branches such as the iliac, femoral, and carotid vessels, and the arteries supplying the heart and brain are commonly affected. Characteristically atherosclerosis progressively or abruptly interferes with blood flow; it is the leading cause of death in the United States. Deaths caused by vascular disease, specifically myocardial infarction and stroke, are more numerous than the next two leading causes, cancer and accidents, combined. Myocardial infarction and sudden death are the most common causes of vascular death. Acute myocardial infarction is responsible for 35 per cent of the deaths in the United States in males between the ages of 35 and 50. At present, a North American male has a 1 in 5 chance of having a myocardial infarct or sudden death before the age of 60. Data from many sources indicate that clinical events resulting from coronary artery disease are being recognized with increasing frequency and that the incidence has been rising for several decades.

Pathology. The advanced atherosclerotic lesion is pleomorphic and consists of accumulations of lipid, smooth muscle, fibroblasts, products of coagulation, and neovascularization in the intima of medium-sized coronary arteries. Eventually the lesion obstructs nutrient flow with consequent chronic or sudden ischemia or infarction. Although accumulation of lipid, largely cholesterol, is characteristic, proliferation of smooth muscle and fibroblasts, not normally present in the intima or media of mammalian arteries, comprises the so-called "complicated" lesion. As the focal atherosclerotic lesion increases in size, it becomes unstable. Rupture of the plaque into the lumen, intimal dissection of microscopic hematoma, or formation of thrombi and subsequent recannulation occur. Such events probably contribute to changes in the clinical state of the patient with chronic vascular disease being associated, for example, with transient cerebral ischemic attacks or unstable angina pectoris.

It is generally assumed that the atherosclerotic process begins with the *fatty streak,* a yellowish plaque visible when the affected artery is exposed. Fatty streaks have been observed in youngsters dying accidentally in the first decade. Prevalence increases rapidly with age.

The yellow streak consists of lipid deposits found mainly within intimal smooth muscle cells. How the lesion progresses from the benign fatty streak found in many mammalian species to the complex, obstructive changes of advanced atherosclerosis unique to man is unknown.

Also observed in infancy and childhood are mesenchymal lesions in the intima which show fibromuscular hyperplasia, increase in ground substance, some lipid, and disorder of elastic fibers. These lesions, found especially at bifurcations, are thought by some workers also to be precursors of atherosclerosis, but this view is not generally accepted.

Many epidemiologic surveys have demonstrated a convincing relationship between the level of dietary cholesterol, saturated fat intake, and vascular disease. How hyperlipidemia accelerates lipid deposition in the arterial system is not clear. Of the serum lipoproteins only the largest, chylomicrons, cannot pass through the endothelium into the arterial wall. In general the composition of the atheroma reflects plasma lipid content. It has been suggested that low density lipoproteins, which are characteristically found in the plaque, induce proliferation of smooth muscle cells altered to accumulate lipid. Injury to the endothelial barrier exposes the atheromatous material in the plaque to circulating platelets. This is known to induce platelet clumping and thrombus formation, leading to further damage of the vessel wall and obstruction.

Anatomy. Atherosclerosis of the coronary artery is found in the proximal segments of the medium-sized vessels, especially at branching points. Grossly the disease is segmental, although microscopic examination in advanced cases invariably reveals diffuse involvement. Lesions occur only in the vessels distributed over the surface of the heart. For reasons unknown, atheroma is not found in the penetrating or muscular branches which turn into the myocardium at right angles to the surface. Although much has been written about small vessel disease and ischemia, it is important to emphasize that the small intramuscular branches of the coronary arterial system are not involved in atherosclerosis. Small vessel involvement is said to occur in patients with diabetes mellitus, but this cannot be universally demonstrated. It is common, however, in association with various forms of muscular dystrophy.

Risk Factors. Numerous epidemiologic and clinical surveys during the past several decades have identified a series of risk factors which significantly increase the likelihood that coronary artery disease will become clinically evident. The variety of major and minor factors so far identified suggest that coronary artery disease and to the same extent cerebral vascular disease are multifactorial conditions whose probability is controlled by genetic, metabolic, anatomic, and environmental factors.

The risk of myocardial infarction increases progressively with *age* but is lower for *women* than for *men* until the sixth decade. The Framingham study and others have shown a clear association between the presence and severity of *hypertension* and occlusive vascular events. A recent Veterans Administration study revealed that persistent mild hypertension, defined as a diastolic pressure from 105 to 115 mm Hg after three days of hospitalization, was associated with increased risk of stroke and heart attack. Furthermore, treatment significantly lowered the risk of vascular disease. Curiously, although many studies have shown that reduction in occurrence of stroke is associated with effec-

tive treatment of hypertension, the same cannot be said for myocardial infarction, at least during the first three years of treatment. Although a relationship between hypertension and acceleration of atherosclerosis is well accepted, the failure to reduce the incidence of myocardial infarction after treatment emphasizes the important role of other factors in the perpetuation of the sclerotic process, once initiated.

There is overwhelming evidence that one of the most significant risk factors for atherosclerosis is elevation of *blood lipids.* This factor is most prominent in younger patients and decreases with age. An elevated blood cholesterol, of the Type IIA lipoproteinemia according to the Fredrickson et al. classification (see Ch. 817), is associated with a premature risk of extensive coronary artery disease and early myocardial infarction. Individuals, presumably homozygous for a Type II lipoproteinemia, have been reported with extraordinary high blood cholesterol and fatal myocardial infarction before age 20. A curious lesion, supervalvular aortic stenosis caused by a cholesteroloma, has also been described secondary to marked hypercholesterolemia. Elevation of triglyceride levels also carries an increased risk of myocardial infarction, whether with high cholesterol or normal cholesterol. Elevated triglyceride is frequently carbohydrate induced and associated with diabetes mellitus.

About 30 per cent of the survivors of myocardial infarction have elevated blood lipids. Among male survivors under age 40, the incidence in one study was 60 per cent. Diabetes, obesity, and hypertension are more common in those having elevated triglycerides than in those with normal blood lipids or elevation of cholesterol alone.

After an extensive survey of the relatives of patients surviving myocardial infarction, Goldstein concluded that five forms of hyperlipidemia were present: (1) a nongenetic, sporadically occurring hypertriglyceridemia, reflecting exogenous factors; (2) polygenic hypercholesterolemia, probably influenced by complex genetic and environmental interactions; and three types of monogenic hyperlipidemia: (3) familial hypercholesterolemia; (4) familial hypertriglyceridemia; and (5) an increase in both cholesterol and triglycerides, termed familial combined hyperlipidemia. Characteristically, familial hypercholesterolemia (Type II) was accompanied by early occurrence of arcus cornealis and tendinous xanthomas which could be recognized in childhood. There was no consistent relationship between the lipoprotein pattern according to the Fredrickson classification, and the apparent genetic disorder. This suggests that although the Fredrickson classification is useful clinically, it does not necessarily reflect a basic description of the genetic influences controlling lipid metabolism in patients with coronary artery disease. Goldstein estimated that in Seattle one in 150 individuals is a carrier of genes predisposing to one of the three described heritable lipid disorders.

Cigarette smoking is a prime risk factor for symptomatic coronary artery disease in the United States and Great Britain, but curiously this has not been shown to be the case in continental Europe. The tobacco, paper, and various chemicals used in the preparation and preservation of the product vary widely over the world. Such factors and their response to combustion may influence the health risk of tobacco.

Which components of the cigarette adversely affect the

cardiovascular system is subject to debate. *Nicotine* has well known vasospastic properties and releases endogenous catecholamines. This is not generally believed to be the culprit, however. Smokers have distinctly higher levels of *carbon monoxyhemoglobin* (COHb) than nonsmokers. Excessive concentration of COHb has many potential adverse effects, including reduction of available hemoglobin and a shifting of the oxyhemoglobin dissociation curve to the left. This reduces availability of oxygen in the capillary. According to Fahri, an increase in COHb concentration in blood from a normal 1 to 2 per cent to 5 to 6 per cent requires a 20 per cent increase in coronary blood flow to prevent ischemia, a requirement that could not be achieved in many patients with coronary artery disease. Increased exposure to carbon monoxide reduces exercise tolerance and decreases the threshold for pacing-induced angina in patients with coronary artery disease. Such effects have been shown under carefully controlled laboratory conditions, and also in patients with angina being driven along a Los Angeles freeway during rush hours! The possibility that carbon monoxide is an important factor in the hazard of cigarette smoking could explain the observation that, unlike the risk of cancer of the lung, the increased risk for myocardial infarction of the smoker falls rather rapidly to that of the nonsmoker after the habit is discontinued.

In addition to the so-called risk factors of dietary fat, hyperlipidemia, hypertension, and smoking discussed above, many other influences of possible importance have been identified. The association between *diabetes mellitus* and premature vascular disease, including myocardial infarction, is well known. Diabetes is commonly accompanied by hypertriglyceridemia, but how a disease expressed as glucose intolerance accelerates atherosclerosis is not understood.

Although often identified as a primary risk factor, *obesity* is not per se associated with an increased risk of coronary artery disease when coexisting hypertension or diabetes mellitus is taken into account. An increased incidence of coronary artery disease has been associated with certain *blood types,* the *hardness* of drinking water, and *hyperuricemia.* Individuals with blood types A, B, and AB have a higher incidence of myocardial infarction and angina pectoris than patients with blood type O. Communities whose residents drink *hard water* have lower death rates in general, and specifically for coronary artery disease, than do similar communities whose residents consume soft water. Water softness is a reflection of total rainfall; mortality rates in various communities have been inversely related to this factor also. That elevation of *blood uric acid* is almost as significant a marker for risk of coronary artery disease as cholesterol has long been recognized. How this factor operates is not known. Recently, excess drinking of *coffee* has been reported in patients discharged from hospital with a diagnosis of acute myocardial infarction.

Considerable debate, at times more emotional than rational, has centered on the role of *exercise* in reducing the risk of coronary disease. Vigorous exercise several times a week is postulated to enhance the growth of coronary collaterals by increasing ventricular work and myocardial oxygen demand. Many reports suggest that subjects who regularly exercise have a lower incidence of coronary events than those who are more sedentary. Although there is little doubt that such individuals may have an enhanced sense of well-being, unfortunately lit-tle of the data stands up to close scrutiny. Coronary artery disease is a slow multifactorial process developing over decades prior to clinical recognition. This, together with the difficulty of changing life styles and patterns of physical activity, makes the design of prospective studies especially difficult. It has been said that marathon running, for example, is the answer to coronary artery disease. Who ever saw an obese, hypertensive, marathon runner who was a heavy smoker? One well designed British study found that in men recording vigorous exercise during routine weekly activity, the risk of developing coronary artery disease was about one third that of a comparable group who did not. Vigorous exercise included swimming, four hours of heavy work, one hour of rapid walking in the country, or climbing 500 or more stairs a day.

Goldstein, J. L., Hazzard, W. R., Schrott, H. G., Bierman, E. L., and Motulsky, A. G.: Hyperlipidemia in coronary heart disease. J. Clin. Invest., 52:1533, 1544, 1569, 1973.
Gordon, T., and Kannel, W. B.: Premature mortality from coronary heart disease. J.A.M.A., 215:1617, 1971.
James, T. N.: Anatomy of the coronary arteries in health and disease. Circulation, 32:1020, 1965.
Kannel, W. B., Castelli, W. P., Gordon, T., and McNamara, P. M.: Serum cholesterol, lipoproteins and the risk of coronary heart disease. Ann. Intern. Med., 74:1, 1971.
Maugh, T. D., II: Coffee and heart disease: Is there a link? Science, 181:534, 1973.
Morris, J. N., Chave, S. P. W., Adam, C., Sirey, C., and Epstein, L.: Vigorous exercise in leisure-time and the incidence of coronary heart disease. Lancet, 1:333, 1973.
Ross, R., and Glomset, J. A.: Atherosclerosis and the arterial smooth muscle cell. Science, 180:1332, 1973.
Ross, R. S.: Pathophysiology of coronary circulation. The Sir Thomas Lewis lecture of the British Cardiac Society. Br. Heart J., 33:173, 1971.
Wissler, R. W.: Development of the atherosclerotic plaque. Hospital Pract., 8:61, 1973.

566. ANGINA PECTORIS

Definition. Angina pectoris is a clinical syndrome caused by inadequate oxygenation of the heart, characteristically precipitated by exertion, and relieved by rest or sublingual nitroglycerin.

Historical. Although there were several earlier reports, the condition since known as angina pectoris was masterfully described by William Heberden in 1772 in a paper entitled "Some Account of a Disorder of the Breast." The word angina refers to the sensation of strangling and anxiety which accompanies an attack. Heberden pointed out that the condition is common; that the seizure occurs while walking, especially uphill or after a meal; that the uneasiness vanishes with standing still; that prior to an attack the subjects appear perfectly well; that the pain is in the sternal area but may go to the left arm; that males past 50 are the most common victims; and that sudden death may terminate an attack.

Clinical Manifestations. *Pain.* The discomfort of angina may vary from mild to most intense. It may persist as a vague ache, and although the patient is aware of the sensation, he may continue his activities. On the other hand, once started, angina may rapidly build up to the point of intolerance, forcing the victim to stop and seek immediate relief. The pain of angina is usually not as severe as the intense precordial crushing sensation associated with acute myocardial infarction. It is usually described as pressing, boring, or gripping. The patient may feel as though a weight is on his chest. The chest feels tight, and there is often a sensation of heavy breathing. It may be difficult at times to determine whether the patient is complaining of angina, dyspnea, or both. This confusion may be partly explained by the striking alterations in ventricular function, including a sharp and reversible rise in left ventricular filling pressure, which accompany an attack of angina. Many sufferers, in describing angina, will make a fist as they grope for words to describe the discomfort. This gesture is a helpful clue.

The pain is characteristically a deep, visceral sensation—dull, aching, or heavy. Some patients do not refer to it as pain; rather they describe it as an ache or a vague awareness of discomfort. Sharp, fleeting sensations are not typical of angina. Pattients who complain of lightning pains in the anterior chest usually have some other process. Although the patient may feel that his chest is tight or squeezed so that his breath is restricted, the pain is not exaggerated by inspiratory movements. It is not searing, knifelike, or hot.

Angina may be attributed to indigestion. In some patients the sensation felt in the epigastrium is described as burning. It may be accompanied by considerable abdominal distress, including bloating and belching. The need to belch during an attack is common, and this may even give relief. Symptoms of peptic ulcer, hiatus hernia, or gallbladder disease are not uncommon in the age group suffering from angina. Clinicians have long recognized that these upper gastrointestinal conditions may precipitate attacks of angina pectoris. Intermingling of gastric and cardiac symptoms does not ease the diagnostic task.

The reaction to angina is highly variable. Those with mild discomfort may ignore the sensation and carry on normal activities, whereas others may manifest an acute fear of death. Often a strong element of denial makes obtaining an accurate history of the frequency, nature, and intensity of angina difficult. Patients with severe forms may limit activity to avoid triggering another attack. A careful history with emphasis in the frequency of attacks, the number of nitroglycerin tablets consumed, and the level of daily physical activity should enable the physician to recognize the true intensity of the condition.

The discomfort of angina is characteristically substernal. It is not felt on the surface of the chest, but may be located beneath the upper, middle, or lower portions of the sternum. Most commonly it is described in the midsternal region. The pain may also be felt beneath the precordium. It is important to emphasize that angina is seldom felt in the region of the cardiac apex. A complaint of pain localized to the apex described as "in the heart" will usually be a manifestation of a noncardiac condition. The pain may radiate widely. Typically the sensation is felt in the left arm and shoulder. It may radiate from the substernal region as intensity increases, or it may be felt predominantly in the arm, with minimal or no chest component. Usually the discomfort radiates down the medial side of the arm and may go to the fingers. Occasionally it may radiate down the right arm or both arms. A relationship between the intracardiac localization of myocardial ischemia and the pattern of pain radiation has not been established. The pain may radiate to the back, neck, or jaw, or discomfort may be localized in the intrascapular area. Occasionally, it is felt in the upper or lower abdomen. In all the areas of remote pain, the sensation retains the deep and aching character of visceral pain.

Precipitating Factors. Angina is characteristically episodic and triggered by *physical activity*. A patient may be able to predict discomfort by a specific act, for example, climbing a flight of stairs, but in other patients the effort of exertion is variable. Walking may be tolerated, but climbing a small hill may precipitate an attack. Angina is frequently induced by a heavy meal, especially if followed by exertion. Some patients are forced to change their habits and eat several small meals to avoid discomfort. Cold weather is especially prone to produce angina. Sometimes the first contact with cold air on leaving a warm room is sufficient, even though the patient is standing still. Many patients are able to walk indoors and perform labor, although they cannot do the same outdoors without discomfort.

Emotion is a well-known trigger for angina. An argument, a tense encounter, an anxiety-producing situation, or sexual excitement may induce pain. Angina may occur when the patient is resting quietly, seemingly without stimulation *(angina decubitus)*. It is thought to imply more severe disease and to have a worse prognosis than other forms. Most instances of angina decubitus are probably triggered by emotion.

Nocturnal angina may be troublesome. In this form the patient has awakened from an apparently sound sleep with angina. It is important to differentiate this condition from nocturnal dyspnea secondary to left ventricular failure, which is usually due to redistribution of interstitial water and resultant increase in plasma volume in the recumbent position. On occasion congestive failure may precipitate angina in the patient with myocardial insufficiency and inadequate coronary blood flow. It has been shown that nocturnal angina is frequently preceded by a dream in which the subject is emotionally stimulated or is exercising. The dreams are often accompanied by striking increases in respiration, heart rate, and blood pressure. In one reported example the subject dreamed he was riding a bicycle uphill, and awoke with angina.

Although most individuals will stop exertion with the onset of angina, some will carry on and "walk through" the pain. There are typically three patterns of response if exertion continues with angina. In some patients the angina eventually subsides, and physical activity can continue without discomfort. In others the pain persists, is of only moderate intensity, does not progress, and the patient is able to tolerate the level of discomfort. He continues his activity. In a third group, however, the pain becomes progressively intense and forces the subject to obtain relief by rest or medication. Most patients fall into the last category.

Duration and Relief. Anginal pain usually persists no more than three to five minutes. The duration is somewhat variable, depending on the stimulus triggering the attack. When the pain is related to exertion, such as walking, it characteristically subsides, becoming progessively less severe, if the sufferer promptly stops and rests. Most patients with angina have pain only a few times a week. Since angina characteristically occurs with exertion, especially after meals or in cold weather, many patients learn to modify their daily activity to avoid pain. To evaluate severity of symptoms the careful historian determines not only the frequency of attacks but also the pattern of daily physical and emotional effort.

Spontaneous angina decubitus or angina developing during emotional tension may be especially severe in intensity and duration. Such episodes tend to persist for 10 to 15 minutes or longer and to be of agonizing intensity. The blood pressure may rise to an extraordinary degree, with development of striking diastolic hypertension during these attacks.

Some patients with clear-cut angina complain of long periods of chest discomfort lasting an hour or more. The sensation tends to be low grade, almost at the threshold of awareness. The patient equates the sensation with angina, describing it as an ache or an annoyance, but carries on his normal activities. Exertion or emotion may precipitate a full-blown attack. It seems likely that the complaint reflects a mild, chronic myocardial ischemia. Its presence is usually a sign of advanced coronary artery disease with multiple vessel involvement. It may or may not be relieved by nitroglycerin.

Usually the characteristics of angina are reasonably constant for the individual patient. The type of stimulus, whether emotional or physical, and the intensity, frequency, radiation, and duration of the pain are fairly regular from one attack to another. Any change in pattern causing an increase in symptoms should be viewed with grave suspicion. Increase in frequency, intensity, or duration or any lowering of the threshold for triggering the pain may presage an impending coronary syndrome, also termed *unstable angina pectoris*. Both the physician and the patient should be aware of the significance of an increase in symptoms. This subject is discussed in more detail later.

Causes of Pain. Many theories have been proposed in an attempt to explain the mechanism of cardiac pain. It is most likely directly related to metabolic changes caused by ischemia. Electrocardiographic abnormalities may precede awareness of pain or may occur in absence of pain, suggesting that an accumulation of active substances to some threshold necessary to cause pain is occurring. Such substances might be H^+, K^+, and possible components of the kallikrein system. There are two networks of sensory nerve fibers in the heart: a perivascular network encircling the coronary arteries, and fibers running beside the vessels and terminating between muscle bundles. Presumably the latter are stimulated by the ischemic process.

The pain of angina pectoris and that of myocardial infarction are similar in quality. The pain of infarction tends to be more intense, and may persist for several hours. Prolonged pain implies continued ischemia, not infarction. Once death of myocardium has occurred, pain is no longer present. One explanation for the occasional sudden improvement in previously stable angina is infarction of the chronically ischemic area.

Ischemic cardiac pain and the pain of intermittent claudication presumably have a similar mechanism. Both are described as deep, visceral sensations. Both occur with increased muscular work and are relieved by rest. Both are usually secondary to obstructive vascular disease.

The nerve pathways from the myocardium travel through the superficial and deep cardiac plexus, and the thoracic cardiac nerves to the first four or five thoracic ganglia. They enter the spinal cord via the white rami of corresponding thoracic segments. Cord segments D1 to D5 also receive pain fibers from the precordium, the medial portion of the anterior surface of the arm, and the forearm. Convergence within a common anatomic pathway of nerve impulses doubtless accounts for the characteristic radiation of the pain of angina pectoris.

Physical Findings. Between attacks, patients who suffer from angina may or may not have signs of organic heart disease. During an angina episode the patient usually becomes apprehensive. He may begin to sweat. Often he will press hard on the sternum with his hands. If he has had previous experience with the medication, he is anxious to take a nitroglycerin tablet as quickly as possible.

During the attack the heart rate usually rises. The blood pressure is frequently elevated, occasionally to alarming levels. Heart sounds may become more distant. The apical impulse may be more diffuse. Careful inspection and palpation of the precordium may reveal a localized systolic bulging or a paradoxic movement, a reflection of segmental myocardial ischemia producing a localized area of noncontracting myocardium. The second sound may become paradoxically split during angina so that the components close during inspiration and widen during expiration. This reversal of the normal splitting is thought to reflect a more prolonged left ventricular ejection time during the ischemic episode, because normally the aortic valve closes before the pulmonic valve.

A *fourth heart sound* (S_4) is extremely common in patients with ischemic heart disease, especially during an attack of angina. It is so common that its absence could be interpreted as evidence against the diagnosis. Curiously this sign was usually overlooked until recently. An excellent technique for recognizing an S_4 is first to identify the A wave in superficial neck veins and then to auscultate in the appropriate areas, using a bell while watching the jugular A wave. The S_4, whether of right- or left-sided origin, will be heard synchronous with the A wave. If this technique is followed, many an apparent first heart sound will be recognized as actually an S_4.

In some patients a *systolic murmur* may appear in the region of the cardiac apex during angina. Characteristically the murmur begins in mid- or late systole after the first sound. It is rather shrill and not exceptionally loud. This murmur is ascribed to papillary muscle dysfunction secondary to localized ischemia. If the papillary muscles are involved in the ischemic process, they become incapable of holding against left ventricular pressure during systole. During the latter half of systole, the mitral valve is forced open, and regurgitation occurs. The condition is often self-limited, for the murmur may not be detected when the patient is free of pain.

Careful observation and examination of the patient during an attack of chest pain may be extremely rewarding. Detection of abnormal cardiac findings and the disappearance of the findings with the subsidence of the complaints may help considerably in establishing the diagnosis.

Electrocardiogram. It must be emphasized that the resting electrocardiogram may be entirely within normal limits in the patient who has clear-cut and indisputable angina pectoris. The electrocardiogram is more likely to be normal when the syndrome first begins. Perhaps 20 to 30 per cent of patients first experiencing angina have a normal electrocardiogram on initial examination. Neither the extent nor the distribution of coronary artery disease can be predicted from a normal electrocardiogram. In one study 16 per cent of a group of patients with greater than 50 per cent obstruction of the three major coronary arteries, as determined by selective angiography, had completely normal electrocardiograms. Of patients with total obstruction of one or more major coronary arteries, 53 per cent had abnormal Q waves, suggesting old myocardial infarction, but 5 per cent had a completely normal resting electrocardiogram.

Chronic Changes. The presence of chronic electrocardiographic abnormality does not establish a diagnosis of angina. These changes may indicate the presence of organic heart disease. The chronic abnormalities that may be present include evidence of left ventricular hypertrophy, S-T segment and T wave change, bundle branch block, or pathologic Q waves, suggesting old myocardial infarction. Abnormalities of the S-T segments or T waves in the electrocardiogram are frequently nonspecific, and one must avoid overinterpretation. It is important to know whether the patient is receiving digitalis, which will reduce T wave amplitude and produce an S-T segment depression in most leads. In the normal person the effects of digitalis may be difficult to detect in the electrocardiogram, and consist largely of some decrease in amplitude of the T wave and a very slight S-T segment depression. In the patient with organic heart disease, on the other hand, digitalization may produce more striking changes. T waves may become inverted, and S-T segments markedly depressed. A pattern of "left ventricular strain" may appear when

prior to digitalis the electrocardiogram was essentially normal.

Scarring, owing to small infarcts, may cause abnormalities of the T waves and S-T segments. Patchy fibrosis is said also to produce high frequency alterations in the QRS complex. A characteristic "ischemic" sign is said to be a flat S-T segment depression from the end of the QRS complex to the onset of the T waves. Since there are many variations of S-T segment depression and the changes are usually nonspecific, it is impossible to utilize the electrocardiogram obtained in the absence of pain to confirm the diagnosis of angina pectoris.

Significant Q waves suggesting old myocardial infarction are helpful in confirming a diagnosis of coronary artery disease. Bundle branch block patterns may be difficult to evaluate. Right bundle branch block is perhaps a more benign lesion, in terms of diagnostic implications and prognosis. Blockage of the right bundle causes a delay of terminal QRS forces, and hence does not interfere with the recognition of abnormal Q waves of myocardial infarction. It is generally held that left bundle branch block implies disease of the left ventricle, either fibrosis or coronary artery disease. The abnormality in blockade of the left bundle is a prolongation of the initial QRS vector and a change in direction. Hence the pattern

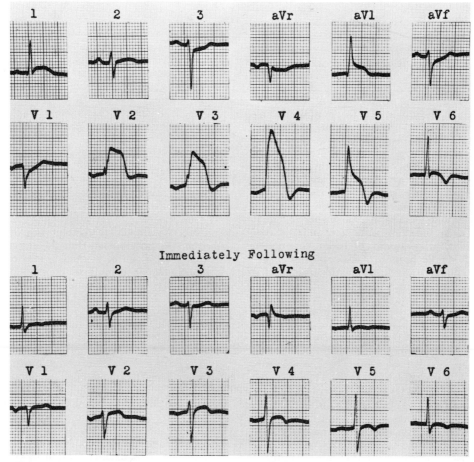

Figure 1. Electrocardiogram recorded in a 57-year-old man during an episode of angina pectoris. *Top,* During the attack. *Bottom,* After pain had spontaneously subsided. The electrocardiogram shows extensive abnormality of the S-T segments and T waves. During angina the elevation of the S-T segments in several leads and especially V₂-V₅ is characteristic of that seen in variant or Prinzmetal's angina. The electrical location of these changes suggests epicardial ischemia of the area of myocardium supplied by the left anterior descending coronary artery. The tracing obtained after angina is abnormal.

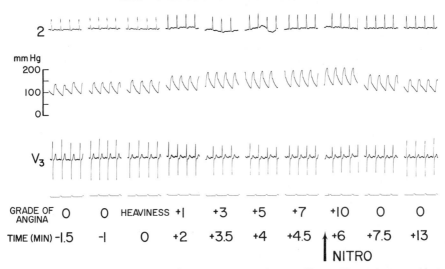

Figure 2. Physiologic changes during spontaneous angina pectoris in a 53-year-old man. The patient was able to grade the intensity of angina on a scale of 0, "no discomfort," to 10, "worst pain ever." Figure shows from top, lead 2 of electrocardiogram, brachial arterial pressure recorded directly; lead V_3 of electrocardiogram, one-second time marker, grade of angina, and time in minutes. Arterial pressure before onset of angina is 135/90 mm Hg, and heart rate is 60 beats per minute. One minute before onset of sensation of heaviness in chest, heart rate and arterial pressure have increased moderately, and slight S-T segment depression has appeared, best seen in V_3. During the next five minutes intensity of angina progressively increases, electrocardiographic changes are more marked, and blood pressure and heart rate increase. When angina is most severe, arterial pressure has risen to 210/135 mm Hg. After sublingual administration of nitroglycerin, angina is relieved within 90 seconds. Arterial pressure falls coincident with improvement of symptoms.

of old or recent infarction may be obscured in the presence of left bundle branch block by the absence of expected Q waves.

Acute Changes. An acute, self-limited, and reversible abnormality of the electrocardiogram may be recorded during an attack of angina. The electrocardiogram is abnormal in virtually all patients during angina, provided that sufficient observations with appropriate leads are obtained. The recording of an electrocardiogram continuously during an attack of chest pain may be of inestimable value in establishing the diagnosis. During angina there are dramatic changes in the so-called "ischemic" pattern, in the repolarization waves of the electrocardiogram, the S-T segment, and the T waves. Sometimes QRS changes may also appear. The R wave may increase or decrease in height, and Q waves may appear temporarily. Intraventricular conduction disturbances or bundle branch block occasionally develop. Usually the most striking electrocardiographic change during an acute attack of angina is the S-T segments and T waves. The T waves may flatten and invert. If already inverted, they may become upright. "Ischemic" S-T segments, consisting of depression of 0.1 mv or more, may appear. At times the depression is truly striking, reaching 0.4 mv or more.

In some patients the S-T segments become markedly elevated in leads with upright R waves. The changes resemble those seen in the so-called "hyperacute" stage of myocardial infarction, but promptly subside after the pain is relieved. If infarction were present, the electrocardiographic abnormality would gradually evolve rather than rapidly return to the control tracing. S-T segment elevation probably represents dominant ischemia in the subepicardial layer, whereas the more typical S-T segment depression is an expression of subendocardial circulatory and metabolic change.

Exercise Tolerance Tests. An objective assay of the cardiovascular response to exercise is an important tool in the diagnosis and evaluation of patients with suspected or known coronary artery disease or angina pectoris. The purpose of exercise is to increase body oxygen consumption and augment myocardial work. In the subject with coronary artery disease the increased cardiac oxygen demand thus induced may exceed the available supply, thereby producing myocardial ischemia as reflected in the electrocardiogram.

The *two-step exercise test of Master* is gradually being replaced by the more carefully controlled *treadmill* or *bicycle ergometer* tests. In these procedures the work of exercise is gradually increased with close electrocardiographic monitoring until fatigue, chest pain, rapid heart rate, or positive electrocardiographic changes are achieved. An important concept in exercise testing is based on the observation that the maximal heart rate during exercise can be related to maximal oxygen consumption. Under conditions of stress, the ability to transport oxygen to the tissues is a reflection of the adequacy of cardiac function and is expressed as the product of heart rate × stroke volume × arteriovenous oxygen difference. During exercise there is a general linear relationship between heart rate and oxygen uptake by the body. Thus the adequacy of an exercise test may be judged by the heart rate achieved during stress.

Maximal heart rate attained during exercise declines with age. Tables are available relating predicted maximal heart rate during exercise to sex and age. Since exercise testing to maximal heart rate is often followed by a prolonged sense of fatigue or uneasiness and might be dangerous to the patient with significant coronary artery disease, testing is usually limited in many laboratories to achieving 80 to 90 per cent of the predicted value.

The ability to attain maximal exercise in patients with angina pectoris is often limited by dyspnea, fatigue, greatly reduced endurance, or chest pain. In advanced coronary artery disease the normal increase in cardiac output, stroke volume, and even arteriovenous oxygen difference may be greatly restricted. Exercise thus may induce evidence of severe left ventricular dysfunction which is not necessarily responsive to administration of digitalis.

In the patient with coronary artery disease, an episode of myocardial ischemia induced during exercise is usually associated with the development of significant electrocardiographic abnormalities during or after the exercise. Although studies during exercise are few, the changes interpreted as "ischemic" are accompanied by evidence of anaerobic myocardial metabolism with excess lactate concentration in the coronary sinus during angina induced by pacing or isoproterenol infusion. It is not necessary to induce angina to precipitate the electrocardiographic change. The electrocardiographic patterns observed are similar to those described earlier as occurring during an episode of angina pectoris.

The hallmark of an abnormal "ischemic" electrocardiographic response to exercise is S-T segment depression or development of an S-T segment vector essentially opposite in direction to the mean QRS vector. Although many criteria have been proposed, most authorities would agree that S-T segment depression of 0.5 to 1.0 mv is of borderline significance, but that depression of greater than 1.0 mv is definitely abnormal. Significant arrhythmia or rate-related bundle branch block is also interpreted as evidence of a positive or abnormal test. These findings, however, do not necessarily reflect coronary artery disease but may be due to primary conduction abnormality.

It is important to bear in mind two essential points. First, the demonstration that a patient has an abnormal electrocardiographic response to exercise does not prove that his chest complaint is angina unless the symptom recurred during exercise and was associated with characteristic electrocardiographic change. Second, a diagnosis of ischemic heart disease owing to coronary artery abnormality as a result of a positive exercise test is inferential. Many conditions such as valvular heart disease, myocardiopathy, and diseases of the small coronary arteries may be associated with a positive test. A syndrome, discussed in greater detail below, has been described as occurring mostly in young women, and is characterized by an angina-like pain, abnormal electrocardiographic exercise tolerance test, and normal coronary arteriogram. In some patients excessive hyperventilation during exercise is associated with changes in the cardiogram, especially T wave inversion. The abnormality is apparently related to increased blood pH and decreased plasma potassium. It may be prevented by breathing 5 per cent carbon dioxide during the test and by administration of potassium salts intravenously.

The results of an exercise tolerance test must be interpreted with caution. The implications of a diagnosis of ischemic coronary artery disease are so important that there must be continued awareness of the possibility of a false positive result. The frequency of a positive maximal exercise test in normal subjects increases with age. Bruce found 12 per cent positives in the fourth decade, 18 per cent in the fifth decade, and 22 per cent in the sixth and seventh decades. What percentage of these subjects have coronary artery disease is not known. A recent study found that 65 per cent of a large group of patients with known coronary artery disease (greater than 70 per cent obstruction of one vessel determined angiographi-

cally) in whom an interpretable result was obtained had a positive treadmill test. The rate of false positivity was 8 per cent. The frequency of positive tests increased with the number of coronary arteries obstructed. Generally, greater degrees of S-T segment depression were correlated with more extensive disease. Eighty-nine per cent of patients with typical angina pectoris had significant coronary artery disease, but only 58 per cent had a positive exercise test.

Although the exercise tolerance test is a potentially dangerous manuever in a patient with severe ischemic heart disease, relatively few serious accidents have been reported. The test is contraindicated when the resting cardiogram is unstable or suggests acute ischemia or infarction. Patients with crescendo angina or frequent, severe attacks of pain, or those in whom a diagnosis of myocardial infarction is suspected should not be exercised. The test should be performed only when a defibrillator and appropriate emergency drugs are immediately available.

Pathogenesis. According to current understanding, angina pectoris develops when cardiac work, and hence myocardial oxygen need, is greater than the ability of the coronary arterial system to supply oxygen per unit time. Angina can be precipitated by an increase in cardiac work and hence oxygen need, or, conversely, angina may occur after a decrease in the oxygen supply secondary to obstruction of coronary flow or a reduction of arterial oxygen content. It most commonly results when cardiac work and hence myocardial oxygen need exceed the available oxygen supply because coronary blood flow to certain regions is restricted. Obstruction of coronary flow owing to coronary atherosclerosis is the most common anatomic finding in the presence of angina. Other conditions which greatly increase cardiac work, such as aortic stenosis, hypertrophic subaortic stenosis, and aortic regurgitation, may be associated with angina despite anatomically normal coronary arteries.

Oxygenated arterial blood is supplied by the two main coronary arteries. Coronary blood flow occurs mainly during diastole because the systolic contraction of the ventricles so increases the resistance in the coronary tree that nutrient flow is largely blocked. An adequate coronary blood flow is therefore dependent on adequate diastolic pressure. When the aortic diastolic pressure drops abruptly, as in aortic regurgitation, coronary blood flow may be severely diminished.

The oxygen content of blood obtained in the coronary sinus is the lowest in any vein draining a major organ. Usually the coronary sinus blood oxygen content, saturation, or Po_2 varies but little despite marked variations in cardiac work. Increase in myocardial oxygen consumption is met not by increased extraction from arterial blood but by increased coronary blood flow. Coronary vascular resistance is rather precisely adjusted, by mechanisms largely under metabolic control, to regulate blood flow in relation to oxygen need. Although reflex control of the coronary vasculature may be demonstrated experimentally, it is probably not an important factor in man. Many metabolites, including ADP, are vasodilators. Berne has suggested that transient excess of ADP when myocardial oxygen need increases is an important control of coronary blood flow. Thus when cardiac work and oxygen utilization increase, coronary vascular resistance falls, permitting an increase in coronary blood flow and oxygen delivery. Conversely, when oxygen demand falls, coronary vascular resistance rises, and coronary blood flow and oxygen delivery decline. Implicit in the mechanism is the maintenance of relatively constant coronary sinus oxygen levels, because changes in extraction of oxygen from arterial blood are relatively minor.

Changes in arterial P_{O_2}, as influenced by hypoxia or abnormal ventilation, may lessen myocardial oxygenation. It has been suggested that increased affinity of hemoglobin for oxygen, which would increase the oxyhemoglobin saturation or content for a given P_{O_2}, may precipitate myocardial ischemia. A number of hemoglobin variants with abnormal affinity for oxygen are now known, but their relation to ischemic heart disease has not been clarified.

Carbon monoxide may be important in myocardial ischemia. It has an affinity for hemoglobin 200 times that of oxygen, and displaces oxygen from the hemoglobin molecule; thus a given level of carbon monoxyhemoglobin reduces the blood oxygen content that can be reached even by breathing 100 per cent oxygen. The effect of carbon monoxyhemoglobin in the threshold for angina during pacing and traveling on an urban highway was discussed in Ch. 565.

Under normal conditions, myocardial metabolism is entirely aerobic, there being little capacity to maintain normal function anaerobically. A wide variety of substrates are utilized as fuels, depending on availability. These include free fatty acids, glucose, ketones, lactate, and pyruvate. Under ischemic or anaerobic conditions, glycolysis is activated through the Embden-Meyerhof cycle to derive high energy phosphate. The rate-limiting enzyme is phosphofructokinase. In mammalian hearts relatively little glycogen is available during anaerobiosis. In these circumstances pyruvate becomes the hydrogen acceptor, substituting for oxygen, and lactate is produced.

The most useful metabolic index of myocardial ischemia is demonstration of myocardial lactate production via coronary sinus sampling during angina or myocardial stress. Myocardial stress may be induced by pacing the heart at a rapid rate or by intravenous infusion of isoproterenol, which increases both heart rate and myocardial contractility, thus increasing oxygen need. Production of lactate with myocardial stress generally indicates a 90 per cent or greater occlusion of a major coronary artery.

It is difficult to obtain precise metabolic data during an episode of myocardial ischemia or angina in man. Certain animal experiments are pertinent, however. When coronary blood flow is gradually reduced but cardiac work is kept constant, a sequence of events may be identified. Myocardial extraction of oxygen is near maximal initially, so that coronary sinus P_{O_2} falls little. Coronary vascular resistance declines progressively to reach a low plateau. Further reduction in blood flow and hence oxygen delivery is followed by metabolic and physiologic evidence of ischemia. The myocardium switches from lactate extraction to lactate production. Coronary sinus blood pH falls. Potassium loss from the myocardium is detected. Electrocardiographic abnormalities appear, and the S-T segments are depressed. Ventricular performance begins to deteriorate, and left ventricular filling pressure and left atrial pressure rise.

In man, during spontaneous angina pectoris or ischemia induced by exercise, pacing, or isoproterenol, metabolic and functional changes can be detected similar to those described in animals. Lactate is produced, and potassium efflux occurs. The electrocardiogram becomes abnormal, and frequently left ventricular diastolic pressure rises. The increase in left ventricular filling pressure and hence pulmonary venous pressure probably explains the not uncommon association of dyspnea with angina in many patients.

The major determinants of myocardial oxygen consumption are heart rate, systolic tension or pressure, and contractility. In the occasional patient whose angina is made worse by digitalis, increased myocardial oxygen demand secondary to the effect of digitalis on the contractile mechanism has been postulated. Any mechanism by which heart rate, ventricular systolic pressure, or contractility is increased may induce angina. Studies during exercise or cardiac pacing have shown that patients with angina will predictably develop metabolic or electrocardiographic signs of ischemia or pain when cardiac work reaches a given value for the individual patient. Thus the level of cardiac work required to induce angina is usually reproducible under laboratory conditions.

Studies during spontaneous angina at rest have shown that the subjective awareness of pain is usually preceded by increase in heart rate and rise in blood pressure. In

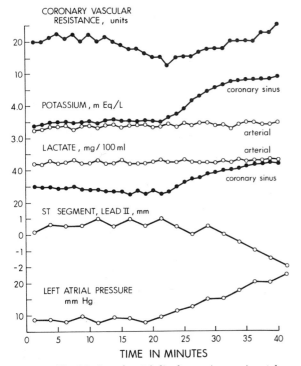

Figure 3. Physiologic and metabolic changes in experimental myocardial ischemia. A cannula is inserted into the left coronary artery, and myocardial blood flow is measured. Serial blood samples are obtained from an artery and the coronary sinus. The electrocardiogram and ventricular pressures are recorded continuously. Nutrient flow through the left coronary artery is progressively reduced in this experiment in a dog, and a series of sequential changes occurs. Coronary vascular resistance declines and reaches a minimum at 20 minutes. When coronary resistance reaches a low point, the following changes occur: onset of potassium efflux into the coronary sinus; change of myocardial metabolism from lactate utilization to lactate production; appearance of S-T segment depression in the electrocardiogram; and development of progressive rise in left ventricular filling left atrial pressure. Thus in this experiment, myocardial ischemia develops when reduction of coronary vascular resistance can no longer compensate for deficient coronary blood flow. With the onset of ischemia, there are progressive changes in myocardial cell membranes and metabolism, in the electrocardiogram, and in the function of the left ventricle. (After Case.)

some patients electrocardiographic changes appear one to three minutes before the pain, suggesting a buildup of metabolic substances prior to stimulation of pain receptors. Blood pressure usually continues to rise as the ischemic attack progresses. If the angina is not relieved by medication, the blood pressure, both systolic and diastolic, may rise to alarming levels. I have observed levels as high as 200 systolic, 150 diastolic in a patient who was normotensive between attacks.

The rise in systemic blood pressure and increase in heart rate during angina represent a potentially disastrous bio-feedback system: the higher the blood pressure and the faster the heart rate, the greater the unmet myocardial oxygen need. In patients who become severely hypertensive during angina, prompt treatment with vasodilators such as nitroglycerin or amyl nitrite is mandatory. Narcotics such as morphine will frequently relieve the pain, but usually do not lower the pressure significantly. Careful evaluation of the patient with prolonged, excruciating angina will often reveal paroxysmal hypertension, presumably in association with the pain. Adequate treatment of the pressor response will ease the angina in most instances.

The cause of the rise of blood pressure in angina is not established. It does not appear to be related to adrenocortical function. It is not initially due to pain, because the pressure usually begins to rise before pain is perceived. Although a pheochromocytoma has on occasion been suspected, there is no evidence that it is due to abnormal adrenocortical function. A chemoceptor supplied from the left descendens coronary artery has been described in dogs, and the possibility of pressor reflexes triggered by the metabolic insult of rapidly increasing local ischemia is intriguing.

The mechanism by which exposure to cold induces angina has been elucidated by recent studies. During such exposure, arterial pressure and peripheral vascular resistance reflexly rise. Cardiac work may be suddenly and sharply increased, thus inducing an ischemic attack. The exposed skin of the face is an important cold receptor triggering this reflex. This susceptibility of the face to cold may be an atavistic expression of the diving reflex found in aquatic mammals and birds. The wearing of a face mask in cold weather may reduce the frequency of angina.

Pathology. Coronary artery disease with atherosclerosis of major vessels is the most common cause of angina pectoris. Pathologic studies in patients who die almost invariably reveal extensive atherosclerosis. Blumgart showed many years ago in postmortem perfusion studies that the patient with angina has occlusion of at least one major coronary artery. Coronary arteriography has demonstrated that angina is almost invariably associated with a significant obstruction of a major coronary artery. At autopsy, the myocardium frequently also shows small scars and areas of fibrosis. This observation suggests that patients with angina may have multiple small and clinically silent myocardial infarcts.

Any condition which obstructs coronary flow or increases cardiac work may be associated with angina. *Syphilitic aortitis* is often complicated by angina, because the inflammatory process may constrict the coronary ostia. Patients with hemodynamically significant *aortic stenosis* are especially susceptible; indeed the onset of angina is an important symptom implying poor prognosis. Its presence should suggest careful evaluation of the severity of the obstructive lesion, and surgical in-

tervention should be considered. Three factors contribute to the association between angina and aortic stenosis. First, the obstructive lesion markedly increases cardiac work because of increased left ventricular systolic pressure, especially during exercise. Second, excrescences from the degenerative process of calcific aortic stenosis may obstruct the coronary ostia or cause coronary emboli. Third, patients with aortic stenosis tend to be males in the sixth or seventh decade when concomitant coronary artery disease is not uncommon.

Occasionally nonsyphilitic *aortic regurgitation* is complicated by angina. Although flow work, high cardiac output, is less costly in terms of oxygen requirement than pressure work, systolic pressure in severe aortic regurgitation is quite high. The ventricle is enlarged because of the very large stroke volume, and wall tension is increased. Diastolic pressure is correspondingly low. Coronary blood flow which occurs predominantly in diastole is reduced, and ischemic attacks may occur.

Angina is a complication of *hypertrophic subaortic stenosis*. The myocardium in this condition may be massively hypertrophied. Angina appears to be related to the markedly increased pressure – work and left ventricular wall tension – associated with this condition, because usually the coronary arteries are large and patent.

Angina is said to complicate advanced *mitral stenosis*. It is frequently difficult to separate anamnestically a sensation of chest tightness owing to acute dyspnea from that of angina. In my experience, patients with mitral stenosis and classic symptoms of angina have had concomitant coronary artery disease. It is possible that angina may reflect right ventricular ischemia in some patients with advanced pulmonary vascular change secondary to mitral stenosis.

Angina may be associated with severe *right ventricular hypertension* in congenital heart disease such as severe pulmonic stenosis, primary pulmonary hypertension, or tetralogy of Fallot. The *so-called hypercyanotic angina* or pain of pulmonary arterial hypertension is most likely right ventricular angina. There is no convincing evidence that distention of the pulmonary arteries is painful.

Anemia, hyperthyroidism, and *hypothyroidism* may be complicated by angina. In most instances there is severe pre-existing coronary atherosclerosis. The patient with myxedema may present a special problem. Restoration of a euthyroid state with thyroid medication may precipitate severe angina. There is a significant risk of acute myocardial infarction or sudden death if excessive doses of thyroid are used. Most authorities recommend a prolonged treatment period with small increments of thyroid.

Angina and Normal Coronary Arteries. Since the advent of coronary arteriography, a syndrome of angina pectoris with anatomically normal coronary arteries has been recognized. This variant amounts to 5 to 10 per cent of patients referred for arteriography. The condition occurs predominantly in young women. In some cases the history suggests classic angina. In others the story is less clear, and the physician may be uncertain about the true diagnosis, but a diagnosis of "atypical" angina is suggested. Attacks may be precipitated by exercise or emotion, but often occur spontaneously. Since current techniques for coronary arteriography can visualize vessels no smaller than 1 mm, it has been postulated that the syndrome reflects small vessel disease. Pathologic evidence is not available to support this thesis. It is also likely that a significant number of these patients do not have angina at all, and that the "atypical" pain is not cardiac in origin.

Despite the doubts raised above, there is a small group of patients who have a typical syndrome of angina pectoris and anatomically normal coronary arteries as revealed by angiography.

It is possible that occasionally obstruction of the coronary arteries is overlooked through failure to obtain high quality films or multiple views. Injection of the dye after administration of nitroglycerin may be necessary to ensure that no local obstruction exists in the coronary tree. Lactate production during stress has been observed in some of the patients with normal coronary anatomy and angina. Many patients are heavy smokers, and coronary spasm not caused by catheter trauma has been convincingly demonstrated in a small number of patients.

Raynaud's phenomenon is rarely found in association with this syndrome. Increased affinity of hemoglobin for oxygen or local metabolic abnormality has also been postulated, but confirmation is lacking.

Diagnosis. Angina pectoris is a clinical diagnosis, largely dependent on the history. In some cases the diagnosis may be established by direct observations during an attack. In the vast majority of patients, however, the diagnosis is evident to the experienced physician from the history alone, and confirmatory tests are not needed.

The electrocardiogram may be utilized to confirm the diagnosis. In doubtful cases the recording of typical electrocardiographic "ischemic" changes, as described earlier, during an attack of pain will often be diagnostic. However, use of exercise tolerance tests with electrocardiographic recording to confirm the presence or absence of angina is frequently unsatisfactory. Occurrence of pain, the patient's actual complaint, is uncommon. As discussed earlier, it is important that the test be standardized and closely monitored. A positive test, in the absence of pain, does not confirm the presence of angina. It does suggest, however, the presence of ischemic or coronary artery disease.

The response to nitroglycerin may be utilized as a critical diagnostic test. Angina pectoris is characteristically relieved in from 90 seconds to 3 minutes after sublingual administration of nitroglycerin. Failure of the symptom to be relieved promptly by nitroglycerin should cast suspicion on the diagnosis of angina. Many patients have a poor sense of timing, and cannot accurately describe the duration of an attack or the quickness of relief after medication. It is important to emphasize to the patient the necessity for accurate information before drawing the conclusion that nitroglycerin is not useful and therefore that the diagnosis is in doubt.

Coronary Arteriography. Visualization of coronary anatomy is achieved by coronary arteriography. The technique most widely used involves selective cannulation with a specially shaped catheter that is passed to the aortic root from the brachial or femoral artery. Use of the brachial artery usually requires a cut-down and incision of the vessel. After repair of the vessel, loss of the brachial pulse should occur in less than 5 per cent of patients. Utilization of larger vessels such as the femoral artery permits a percutaneous technique, as described by Seldinger, in which the vessel is punctured with a needle and a guide wire inserted. The needle is then withdrawn and a catheter advanced over the guide wire to the desired location. The wire is then withdrawn, and the catheter is flushed with heparinized saline or other fluid.

The coronary arteriogram is obtained when radiopaque dye is injected into the coronary ostia. Usually the pictures are recorded on 35 mm cine film. Several injections are filmed in various oblique views so that all vessels may be observed in multiple projections. In doubtful cases arteriograms are obtained before and after administration of nitroglycerin. The resulting vasodilation may reveal areas of obstruction not previously recognized.

Several studies have shown good correlations between the coronary arteriogram and postmortem findings. A properly performed and technically correct coronary arteriogram is believed to satisfactorily represent the anatomic configuration at the time of study. Coronary atherosclerosis is recognized by narrowing, beading, or occlusion of the arteries. Vessels as small as 1.0 mm may be demonstrated with good technique. Collateral vessels may be seen bridging obstructed areas or providing retrograde filling of a proximally obstructed artery.

At the time of the examination further information may be obtained by injecting dye into the left ventricle to obtain a left ventriculogram, and also by measurement of left ventricular end-diastolic pressure. Although the latter is influenced by many factors, including the stiffness of the ventricle, elevated levels suggesting compromised ventricular performance are frequently observed in patients with severe coronary artery disease. Myocardial contractility and size may be evaluated by scrutiny of the ventriculogram. The ejection fraction, the ratio of the volume of blood ejected during systole to the volume remaining at end-systole, may be calculated. Normally, approximately 50 to 60 per cent of the end-diastolic volume is ejected with each beat. Smaller fractions suggest myocardial disability and increased residual volume. Areas of abnormal contractility, termed *dyskinesia* or *akinesia,* owing to old scar or infarction may be observed.

The primary indication for coronary arteriography, including ventriculography, is to determine the location and extent of disease in patients being considered for coronary artery surgery and revascularization procedures. Other indications are being applied by many groups but remain controversial. They include investigation of certain electrocardiographic abnormalities such as bundle branch block or T wave inversion, especially in individuals with job security problems (e.g., airline pilots); after myocardial infarction or ischemic events in younger patients; and evaluation of a positive exercise test in the absence of symptoms.

Coronary angiograms are frequently performed to evaluate the cause of atypical chest pain. The procedure cannot establish the presence of angina; nevertheless, in some patients with incapacitating chest pain the finding of a normal coronary arteriogram can provide helpful reassurance. Attention can then be directed to symptomatic management and search for other causes of pain.

Complications of the procedure include precipitation of angina, dissection of a coronary artery, acute myocardial infarction, and asystole or ventricular fibrillation. Asystole usually responds to a blow on the chest. Atropine in several doses intravenously (0.3 to 1.0 mg) is a useful preventive in susceptible subjects. Immediate DC precordial shock usually reverts ventricular fibrillation. To be successful the shock must be applied within a few seconds of the onset of fibrillation. Mortality from coronary arteriography is approximately 0.1 to 0.5 per cent *in skilled hands.* Morbidity is largely related to complications of the arterial puncture or cut-down. Myocardial infarction may occur as a complication. The incidence depends on patient selection but should be less than 0.5 per cent.

Differential Diagnosis. Many conditions cause pain in the chest, but few if any truly mimic angina pectoris. The syndrome of angina is so characteristic in the majority of patients that errors in diagnosis are usually the result of careless history taking. In obtaining an accurate history, it is best first to allow the patient to describe his problem in his own way, and then to amplify the story by a series of questions.

Diseases of the gallbladder and gastrointestinal tract, chest wall disorders, abnormalities of the cervicodorsal spine, and pulmonary conditions may cause discomfort in the chest. Costochondral separation may be a source of confusion, but it is readily diagnosed by demonstration of exquisite point tenderness at one or more costochondral junctions on the anterior chest. Evaluation of the role of peptic ulcer disease, gallbladder abnormality, or hiatus hernia may be troublesome. Many patients with angina suffer from one or more of these conditions. It may be difficult to recognize that the patient actually has two or more complaints. Clinical experience supports the view that disease of the upper gastrointestinal tract may exacerbate angina. In some cases removal of a diseased gallbladder reduces the incidence of angina. In many patients symptoms of hiatus hernia trigger angina, especially at night; treatment with antacids and elevation of the head of the bed may give relief. Electrocardiographic changes have been reported during gallbladder attacks or symptoms from hiatus hernia. Usually these are nonspecific S-T segment or T wave changes. They probably reflect the presence of coronary artery disease and represent an abnormal response to fever or tachycardia. Reflex changes have also been postulated as causative.

Treatment. An effective plan of treatment must be based on a thorough understanding of the severity and intensity of the patient's complaint. The physician should explore carefully the circumstances in which angina occurs. Often, minor adjustments in the patient's activity will reduce the frequency of attacks. Angina often occurs repeatedly during the same activity. Avoidance of that specific activity or administration of nitroglycerin before onset will usually reduce symptoms. Should an attack occur, most patients will stop, rest, and administer a nitroglycerin tablet. Some will ignore the discomfort and continue their exertion. Progressive increase in intensity of pain usually forces the subject to stop. Occasionally the pain will improve despite continued activity. Although the development of angina usually indicates significant obstruction of one or more vessels by coronary atherosclerosis, it is important to emphasize the generally good prognosis in patients with stable angina. The patient should be encouraged to report any change in the pattern of angina promptly to his physician.

Association of angina and moderately severe depression is not uncommon. Angina may remind the patient that he is growing older, and that his activity is becoming restricted. Physician and patient should take an optimistic and realistic point of view. With appropriate therapy and some adjustment of the daily living pattern, activity may be nearly normal. Angina may persist for many years. During this time the patient may continue to work and to enjoy recreation and normal family relationships. There may be considerable anxiety, especially

on the part of the spouse, about sexual activity. The patient may reasonably be encouraged to continue those activities as long as they do not precipitate disturbing symptoms.

An essential component of management of the patient with angina is recognition by both patient and physician of the importance of identified risk factors followed by a firm outline of proposed therapy.

The evidence for an adverse effect of *smoking* on the natural history of coronary artery disease is overwhelming. Patients with coronary artery disease and angina pectoris should be urged in the strongest terms to cease smoking. Many patients who develop angina are overweight. Reduction of body mass to more normal values may be associated with clinical improvement. Significant *hypertension* should be brought under control. It is frequently useful to treat even mild diastolic hypertension, levels of 90 to 100 mm Hg, with an agent such as hydrochlorothiazide, 50 mg daily. In older patients systolic pressure may be increased because of increased vascular stiffness. Although this systolic hypertension may increase left ventricular work, treatment of systolic blood pressure elevation of itself is not usually recommended unless the condition is severe.

Occasionally angina is a manifestation of left ventricular failure; treatment of the heart failure may produce dramatic improvement. The onset of exertional dyspnea prior to the perception of pain is a clue suggesting the possibility that it is precipitated by left ventricular failure. Nocturnal angina may be a manifestation of heart failure. Rarely digitalis intensifies angina, and the drug must be discontinued. Rapid paroxysmal arrhythmia may precipitate angina even in the absence of coronary artery disease. Usually, however, angina in the presence of arrhythmia in the older patient indicates coronary atherosclerosis. Treatment aimed at prevention of the arrhythmia may forestall chest pain.

Drug Therapy. IMMEDIATE TREATMENT. *Nitroglycerin* (glyceryl trinitrate sublingual tablets) in doses of 0.15 to 0.60 mg sublingually is the single most effective agent for treatment of the acute episode in most cases. With the exception of amyl nitrite, no other agent can approach it in general usefulness. Onset of action begins in one and a half to three minutes. Relief is usually dramatic and immediate. Occasionally the patient will take a second dose a few minutes after the first for complete effect. A large number of tablets may be ingested daily with few side effects. A fullness or pounding in the head is common, but most patients tolerate this well. An occasional patient will refuse to continue the medication because of intolerable headache. Because the drug is an effective peripheral vasodilator, the individual should first test its effectiveness while sitting or lying to avoid the possibility of syncope. Nitroglycerin may lose its potency unless stored in tightly sealed glass containers. It is good therefore to advise the patient to keep small amounts only in plastic or other types of small, portable containers.

Nitroglycerin is a potent smooth muscle vasodilator. After administration, a decline in coronary vascular resistance and an increase in coronary blood flow can be demonstrated in laboratory animals and normal man. In the past it was thought that the drug relieved angina by its direct action on the coronary vascular tree. Sublingual administration of the drug probably has little primary influence on coronary vascular resistance or coronary blood flow in patients with advanced coronary artery disease. It may have an effect in small vessels, however, and the possible role of spasm of large vessels, even in the presence of extensive disease, has attracted renewed interest. Injection of nitroglycerin directly into coronary ostia in diseased vessels causes a fleeting increase in coronary flow as revealed by disappearance curves of radioactive krypton or xenon. Therapeutic effectiveness of nitroglycerin results from a complex interaction of direct cardiac and indirect systemic effects. After use of sublingual nitroglycerin there is a fall in systemic blood pressure and decrease in systemic vascular resistance. The great veins dilate, causing pooling of venous return, and cardiac output declines. The net result is a marked decrease in cardiac work. Since angina results from an imbalance between oxygen demand and oxygen delivery, any mechanism that restores a more favorable relationship by either increasing delivery (coronary blood flow) or reducing demand (cardiac work) should be helpful. Current evidence strongly suggests that an important aspect of nitroglycerin's dramatic effectiveness is its ability to rapidly reduce cardiac work, thus reversing myocardial ischemia in patients with abnormalities of the coronary arteries.

Amyl nitrite is an extremely potent vasodilator that was first used in the treatment of angina more than 100 years ago. The drug is extremely volatile; it is contained in small, 0.3 ml ampules which are crushed, and the vapor is briefly inhaled. It has a strong, clinging odor, and is best used in a room with good ventilation. Because of its potency, the drug should be applied only when the patient is lying down. The ampule is crushed and wafted under the nose two or three times. A deep breath or two is generally all that is needed to obtain an effect. If the drug is administered by a second person, caution is advised to avoid inhalation of too much drug.

Amyl nitrite causes profound peripheral arterial vasodilation. Blood pressure falls precipitously with adequate dosage. In contrast to nitroglycerin, acute administration has relatively little measurable effect on the great veins, and venous pooling is not marked. For this reason cardiac output increases considerably after inhalation of the drug. Because of these effects on peripheral resistance and flow, amyl nitrite has been utilized to evaluate certain heart murmurs, such as those associated with aortic stenosis or mitral regurgitation, and to reveal the characteristic pressure pulse in hypertrophic myocardial disease. After use of amyl nitrite, the murmur of aortic stenosis is accentuated because of the increased cardiac output, whereas the murmur of mitral regurgitation declines in intensity because of the marked drop in peripheral resistance.

The use of amyl nitrite is currently unfashionable. It is, however, extremely effective in the occasional patient with severe, persistent angina and concomitant hypertension with high levels of diastolic pressure. The hypertension may be secondary to the ischemia. In some patients with angina complicated by hypertension, amyl nitrite is the only consistently effective form of therapy.

DRUGS GIVEN TO LESSEN THE FREQUENCY OF ATTACKS. Long-acting nitrites are said to provide relief of angina throughout the day by virtue of sustained blood levels of active substances. These include *erythrityl tetranitrate* (10 to 30 mg), *pentaerythritol tetranitrate* (10 to 20 mg), and *isosorbide dinitrate* (5 to 30 mg) taken three or four times daily. Although large amounts of these drugs are dispensed and many physicians and patients are satisfied with their usefulness, objective evidence of significant prolonged clinical effect is lacking. Evaluation of the treatment of angina is difficult, because the response to therapy is often highly subjective and depends on the patient's assessment of his own symptoms. A skillful physician with positive transference from the patient may be extremely effective in managing angina, but aside from the acute effects of nitroglycerin and amyl nitrite, the role of other agents such as long-acting nitrites has been difficult to measure. A recent study of several so-called long-acting nitrites found that improvement in exercise tolerance in patients with angina persisted for only about one hour after administration of drug.

Sedation is a useful adjunct to therapy in many instances. Neither phenobarbital nor any of the many available tranquilizers have specific cardiac action in small dosage, but they may reduce anxiety and fearfulness. Alcohol in moderation may be helpful for some patients. In patients with a major component of depression, antidepressant agents such as imipramine, amitriptyline and methylphenidate may be useful.

Propranolol, a beta-adrenergic blocking agent, is effective in selected patients for reducing the frequency and severity of angina. Stimulation of the sympathetic nerves to the heart or infusion of isoproterenol intravenously increases cardiac rate and augments contractility, or the strength and velocity of the cardiac contraction. These functions are specifically blocked by propranolol, which is an important adjunct in the medical treatment of angina pectoris. Approximately two thirds of patients offered a therapeutic trial of the drug are significantly improved with a reduction in frequency and severity of angina.

Propranolol reduces heart rate and decreases myocardial contractility. Studies in man have shown that administration of the drug is associated with a fall in cardiac output and reduction in maximal dp/dt. Left ventricular and end-diastolic pressure may rise. The normal response to exercise is blunted so that the anticipated increase in heart rate and cardiac output is limited. During exertion left ventricular end-diastolic pressure in patients on propranolol may increase, suggesting impairment of myocardial function. Propranolol may induce heart block or severe bradycardia and should be used cautiously in patients with known atrioventricular conduction disturbance. The drug is contraindicated in patients with advanced forms of heart block, such as a greatly prolonged P-R interval, intermittent atrioventricular block with dropped beats, or complete heart block. As discussed subsequently, heart failure may be induced or worsened by propranolol therapy.

During treatment with propranolol, both at rest and during exercise, the product of heart rate and blood pressure (termed the *double product*) is reduced when compared to the pretreatment state at comparable levels of oxygen consumption. For a given amount of exercise, systolic pressure, heart rate, and cardiac output are lower after the drug. Tissue oxygen requirement is met by increased extraction, so atrioventricular oxygen difference across the body is higher. Thus the patient with angina treated with propranolol is able to perform more useful muscular work and to get about more before developing symptoms.

The mechanism of action of propranolol is related to its myocardial depressant effects. Myocardial oxygen need is largely controlled by systolic pressure, contractility, and heart rate. Since propranolol reduces all three, oxygen demand is lower after administration of the drug.

The drug does not increase coronary blood flow or oxygen delivery; indeed these may actually decline.

The dose of propranolol required for clinical effectiveness varies. Many patients respond well to 80 to 160 mg per day, but larger doses are sometimes needed. In treating patients with propranolol, it is best to begin with a low dose, 10 to 20 mg four times daily, and continuously increase the dosage if the drug is well tolerated in an attempt to achieve the desired therapeutic effect. Excessive dosage may induce decreased exercise tolerance owing to marked fatigue. Patients may develop heart failure on high doses of the drug, and it is common practice to administer digitalis and even mild diuretics such as hydrochlorothiazide, 25 to 50 mg daily, with appropriate potassium replacement before beginning propranolol. In some patients severe bradycardia or the development of heart block necessitates withdrawal of treatment. Propranolol is an extremely potent agent, and it must be used with caution under medical supervision. The myocardial depressant action of the drug can be demonstrated in the individual patient by noninvasive techniques. Left ventricular pre-ejection period, analyzed from the indirect carotid pulse and the phonocardiogram, is prolonged. Serial echocardiograms show an increase in width of the left ventricular minor axis after drug administration. Postural hypotension and aggravation of bronchial spasm in patients with asthma are occasional troublesome side effects.

Propranolol has many complex actions. Serum drug levels do not correlate with therapeutic effectiveness. This is not surprising for a blocking agent and probably indicates that those factors classified as "sympathetic tone" and the resting level of ventricular function are highly variable. Propranolol in vivo shifts the oxyhemoglobin dissociation curve to the right. The drug also reverses in vivo the increased aggregatability of platelets frequently observed in patients with angina. It appears to act by restoring the second stage of platelet clumping to normal. Propranolol also has a quinidine-like effect on the transmembrane action potential and is thus an antiarrhythmic. There is experimental evidence also that the drug protects myocardial glycogen stores during stress, thus increasing ability of the heart to sustain anaerobic metabolism during hypoxia or ischemia. Whether the pharmacologic effects of the drug other than its myocardial depressant action contribute to its therapeutic effectiveness in patients with angina is moot.

Surgical Treatment. Many surgical procedures have been advocated to provide additional coronary blood supply or relieve obstructed vessels. Most have been abandoned after an initial wave of enthusiasm for the lack of objective evidence of improvement and symptoms or favorable alteration of prognosis. Implantation of an internal mammary artery into a myocardial tunnel (Vineberg procedure) with various modifications was recently popular among surgeons. When the artery is implanted in an ischemic area, a network of fine anastomotic vessels gradually develops. Full development and clinical improvement usually require several months. Success varies, but angiography reveals neovascularization. Pacing studies have shown reversal of lactate production in selected cases. An acute myocardial infarction may complicate the procedure. This event could explain the immediate benefit which is sometimes observed.

During the past five years many thousands of *coronary bypass* surgical procedures have been performed in the United States in patients with coronary artery disease. There is now little doubt that this procedure is capable of providing a sizable increase in coronary blood flow around an area of coronary arterial obstruction. The procedure is technically possible because most significant obstructive lesions are segmental and proximal. Furthermore, experience has shown that a bypass graft from the aorta can be successfully anastomosed to a coronary artery as small as 1 mm in diameter. Postoperative angiograms are often impressive and have shown that the anastomoses function and provide an immediate increase in blood flow to large areas of the myocardium.

Indications for surgical revascularization of the heart focus predominantly on the relief of angina. Surgery may be considered in the patient with frequent episodes of angina which seriously hinder normal activity and are not satisfactorily responsive to medical therapy. The "ideal" candidate is one who has severe angina, risk factors that are responsive to medical treatment, proximal obstruction of major coronary arteries with good distal "run-off," normal heart size, and normal left ventricular function. The decision regarding surgery should be made by consultation between physician and surgeon. The patient's interests are best served when he is evaluated first by a physician who works closely with a cardiac surgical group and who has a continuing experience in the pre- and postoperative management of patients undergoing cardiovascular surgery.

In good risk patients, surgical mortality in the hands of experienced teams should be 3 to 5 per cent or less. Mortality is inversely related to cardiac function. Evidence of previous myocardial infarction or ventricular dysfunction sharply increases the operative risk. Congestive heart failure is not considered an indication for a bypass procedure. It is claimed by some workers that the poor ventricular contractility, elevated end-diastolic pressures, and low ejection fraction (stroke volume/end-diastolic volume) in some patients with recurrent ischemia is reversed after a successful bypass procedure. The debate on this point continues, but the author does not yet find the evidence convincing.

Recent reports suggest that after one year 65 to 80 per cent of patients undergoing surgery have complete or very good relief of angina pectoris. Approximately 85 per cent of the vein grafts remain functional after one year. Frequently an internal mammary artery will be anastomosed when technically feasible to the anterior descending coronary vessel; one-year patency rates of 95 per cent for this procedure have been reported.

After a successful bypass operation, work performed during maximal exercise is significantly increased in the patient with coronary artery disease. Appropriate dosage of propranolol has only a modest effect in comparison. Improvement in exercise tolerance has been directly related to continued patency of the bypass graft. Indeed, serial exercise testing may be utilized to assess the efficacy of the procedure. Sudden sharp reduction in exercise tolerance suggests closure of the shunt.

A troublesome problem in evaluating the bypass procedure is the apparent high *risk of myocardial infarction.* One study suggested that in the early postoperative period over 60 per cent of patients undergoing bypass had an increase in blood level of creatinine phosphokinase activity identified as myocardial in origin by electrophoresis. In contrast, less than 5 per cent of patients undergoing aortic valve replacement had such a rise. Clinical evidence of myocardial infarction postoperatively is much lower. Early reports suggested an incidence of about 20 per cent. More recently a frequency of 8 to 10 per cent has been encountered, utilizing the development of new Q waves on the postoperative electrocardiogram as criteria for diagnosis. It has been suggested that some of the electrocardiographic changes indicating new infarction are actually old infarction now revealed by the improved blood supply to an ischemic area and the generation of previously hidden QRS vector forces. A perioperative myocardial infarction could explain improvement of angina in some patients postoperatively, but would not be associated with improved maximal exercise performance.

Availability of bypass surgery is a significant therapeutic advance in the management of angina pectoris caused by coronary artery disease. Much remains to be learned before its value is fully understood. Although carefully selected patients may anticipate low surgical mortality and a good chance for relief of symptoms, the long-term effects are not yet known. How long the grafts will continue to function and whether the procedure prevents myocardial infarction or alters the prognosis in patients with angina are important questions that will require many years to answer satisfactorily.

Prognosis. Heberden wrote: "The termination of the angina pectoris is remarkable. For if no accident intervenes but the disease goes on to its height, the patients all suddenly fall down and perish almost immediately." In fact this gloomy prognosis is incorrect. An unwarranted emphasis on premature and sudden death complicating angina pectoris influences medical practice even today, particularly the impetus for newer forms of surgical treatment.

In a pioneering study, Richards, Bland, and White reported a 25 year follow-up of 500 patients with angina pectoris who entered the survey between 1920 and 1931. Annual mortality rate was slightly more than 4 per cent; 50 per cent of the patients were dead in about 12 years. Women had slightly better survival than men, an observation that has been repeatedly made. More recent workers have emphasized the adverse effect of risk factors. A Health Insurance Plan of New York study reveals an average of 1.4 per cent annual mortality in males with angina, no history of myocardial infarction, and normal electrocardiogram and blood pressure. In contrast, annual mortality in those who also had evidence of systolic hypertension was 7.4 per cent. With an abnormal electrocardiogram the risk was 8.4 per cent per year. If both factors were present, the risk was 12 per cent per year. The Framingham study has shown similar results.

Prognosis in angina pectoris is also related to the extent of coronary disease determined angiographically. Stenosis of only a single major vessel seems to have a good prognosis. An average annual mortality of 3 per cent per year has been reported in single-vessel disease unless the anterior descendens is completely occluded, in which case the mortality is approximately doubled. Annual mortality in two-vessel disease has been reported as 6 per cent, and in three-vessel disease, about 10 per cent.

Increased recognition of adverse clinical factors combined with precise anatomic and physiologic characterization in selected patients has greatly improved our understanding of prognosis in angina pectoris. Data derived from a number of clinical studies have provided a clear description of the "natural history" of angina pectoris under conservative medical management. Each ad-

dition to accepted treatment must be compared to the yardstick of prognosis as currently described. This admonition applies no less to medical than to surgical therapeutic innovations.

Variant Angina. In 1959 Prinzmetal called attention to a form of angina characterized by pain at rest and S-T segment elevation which subsides after the attack. The electrocardiogram during pain resembles that of acute myocardial infarction. Arrhythmia is not uncommon. Since most patients with angina have pain during exercise accompanied by S-T segment depression, he termed the syndrome variant angina. With the advent of routine oscillographic monitoring for patients with chest pain, variant angina has been recognized with increasing frequency.

In the laboratory animal or, as is occasionally observed, during coronary arteriography in man, occlusion of a large coronary artery produces prompt S-T segment elevation. Prinzmetal postulated that variant angina reflected organic obstruction of a major coronary artery accompanied by spasm. In exercise-induced angina and in most cases of decubitus pain, cardiac work usually increases sharply before pain and there is S-T segment depression. These EKG changes are believed to reflect subendocardial ischemia, because this layer is most vulnerable to the decreased coronary flow when left ventricular wall tension rises. Exercise performance in variant angina may be normal.

Arteriography in variant angina usually reveals high grade obstruction of a major coronary vessel. However, in some patients, with recurrent and striking changes in the electrocardiogram, the coronary angiogram has been normal. In a small number of patients with variant angina, coronary spasm not caused by catheter trauma has recently been convincingly demonstrated. It is likely that a combination of spasm and severe organic obstruction may be present in some. The prognosis in variant angina is less favorable. A high incidence of myocardial infarction and sudden death has been reported. The results of bypass surgery have been disappointing.

Aronow, W. S.: Management of stable angina. N. Engl. J. Med., 289:516, 1973.

Braunwald, E.: Determinants of myocardial oxygen consumption (Thirteenth Bowditch Lecture). Physiologist, 12:65, 1969.

Fischl, S. J., Herman, M. V., and Gorlin, R.: The intermediate coronary syndrome. Clinical, angiographic, and therapeutic aspects. N. Engl. J. Med., 288:1193, 1973.

Fulton, M., Lutz, W., Donald, K. W., Kirby, B. J., Duncan, B., Morrison, S. L., Kerr, F., Julian, D. G., and Oliver, M. F.: Natural history of unstable angina. Lancet, 1:860, 1972.

Oliva, P. B., Potts, D. E., and Pluss, R. G.: Coronary arterial spasm in Prinzmetal angina. N. Engl. J. Med., 288:745, 1973.

Parker, J. O., West, R. O., Case, R. B., and Chiong, M. A.: Temporal relationships of myocardial lactate metabolism, left ventricular function, and S-T segment depression during angina precipitated by exercise. Circulation, 40:97, 1969.

Reeves, T. J., Oberman, A., Jones, W. B., and Sheffield, L. T.: Natural history of angina pectoris. Am. J. Cardiol., 33:423, 1974.

Swan, H. J. C., Chatterjee, K., Corday, E., Ganz, W., Marcus, H., Matloff, J., and Parmley, W.: Myocardial revascularization for acute and chronic coronary heart disease. Ann. Intern. Med., 79:851, 1973.

567. ACUTE MYOCARDIAL INFARCTION

Definition. Acute myocardial infarction is a clinical syndrome resulting from deficient coronary arterial flow to an area of myocardium with eventual cellular death and necrosis. It is characterized by severe and prolonged precordial pain similar to, but more intense than, that of angina pectoris, and signs of myocardial damage, including acute electrocardiographic changes and a rise in level of certain serum enzymes.

Etiology and Pathology. Atherosclerosis of the coronary arteries is the common denominator in the overwhelming majority of patients with acute myocardial infarction. Although it is attractive to view acute myocardial infarction as the direct result of a sudden obstruction of a major coronary artery, this is not always the case. Infarction without occlusion and occlusion without infarction may be observed pathologically. An occlusion may result from an acute thrombosis, subintimal hemorrhage, or rupture of an atheromatous plaque which may initiate clot formation.

The development of coronary artery thrombi apparently depends on the time and mechanism of death. Clots in the coronary arteries have been observed in approximately 25 per cent of patients who die suddenly. Patients who survive myocardial infarction for several hours or days and then die from heart failure or cardiogenic shock manifest a high incidence of coronary thrombi; an incidence of up to 60 or 70 per cent has been reported. Often the thromboses appear younger than the associated infarction, suggesting that the myocardial damage caused the clot. In a recent report ^{125}I-labeled fibrinogen was administered to seven patients with acute myocardial infarction who subsequently died. A coronary thrombus was found in all seven at autopsy. In six the entire clot was radioactive; in the seventh there was a central portion of the thrombus without radioactivity.

Significant coronary artery disease can usually be demonstrated in the vessel directly supplying the area of infarction. Extensive collateral development may make correlation of precise myocardial and vascular relationships difficult. In the presence of collaterals, an acute arterial occlusion may not produce ischemia or infarction. If an area is dependent on collateral flow, on the other hand, a remote occlusion or a change in the balance of vascular resistance may cause infarction of an area considerably removed from the source of difficulty.

The possibility that evanescent platelet agglutination may precipitate myocardial infarction has recently attracted interest. Platelets adhere to collagen and basement membrane, and these structures may be exposed in injured vessels. Injured platelets release adenosine diphosphate and other factors which accelerate agglutination and clumping. It has been shown experimentally that injection of adenosine diphosphate causes platelet aggregation within the coronary arteries. The peripheral platelet count falls. Although platelet thrombi can be observed on microscopic sections shortly after injection of the adenosine disphosphate, the clumps are no longer apparent after ten minutes. Acute myocardial infarction can be recognized pathologically in two hours, and yet by this time the coronary arteries are not obstructed. The theory that platelets may play a role in the development of acute myocardial infarction or angina pectoris remains an intriguing but as yet unproved possibility.

A myocardial infarct is termed *transmural* when it extends from endocardium to epicardium and *nontransmural* when the necrosis does not reach the inner or outer surface. A *subendocardial* infarct involves the endocardial and subendocardial layers. In general, trans-

mural infarcts tend to be larger and are associated with more severe complications of ventricular dysfunction. Subendocardial infarcts may also be quite extensive, and are associated with occlusive disease of all three of the major coronary arteries. Since the subendocardial layer is subjected to the greatest amount of wall tension, subendocardial infarcts may result from prolonged hypotension or shock owing to noncardiac causes, and may complicate hemorrhage, anesthesia, or extensive surgical procedures.

Acute myocardial infarction is predominantly a disease of the left ventricle and the interventricular septum. Occasionally the infarct extends into the right ventricle, and the atria may also be involved. Atrial infarcts are usually not diagnosed during life; current electrocardiographic criteria are unreliable. Primary infarction of the right ventricle with severe right heart failure and tricuspid regurgitation in absence of left ventricular involvement has been described. The extent and location of the infarct depend upon the causative factors, the extent of coronary artery disease, the presence of collateral blood supply, and whether previous infarctions have occurred.

Other Causes. Coronary embolization may complicate bacterial endocarditis or left atrial thrombosis, resulting in acute infarction or sudden death. Embolization of calcified excrescences may occur in aortic stenosis. Myocardial infarction without coronary obstruction may complicate aortic stenosis if coronary perfusion pressure drops, with syncope or hypotension, when ventricular systolic work is maintained at a high level because of the fixed obstruction. Acute myocardial infarction secondary to arteritis has been described in periarteritis nodosa and acute hypersensitivity syndromes. In Marfan's syndrome, cystic necrosis of the media may involve the coronary arteries as well as the aorta. In acute aortic dissection, the separation may extend to the base of the aorta and occlude a major coronary artery. Electrocardiographic changes suggesting subendocardial ischemia or necrosis may be observed after prolonged surgical procedures, often with extensive blood loss and replacement, or secondary to hypotension or shock from a variety of causes. Coronary arteriography after recovery from myocardial infarction has revealed a small number of patients with perfectly normal coronary anatomy and no recognizable cause for the acute event.

Clinical Manifestations. The outstanding characteristic of acute myocardial infarction is severe, prolonged pain. The pain is similar to that of angina, but is more intense and persists much longer. It is usually present for at least half an hour, but may last for many hours. Nitroglycerin affords no relief or only temporarily abates the attack. The pain is usually relieved by administration of opiates, although repeated doses may be required.

The pain is described as pressing or crushing, like a deep ache inside the chest. Often patients will press on the sternum or state that it feels as though there were a great weight on the chest, such as a rock or someone sitting on it. The pain is a deep visceral discomfort, and is seldom described as sharp or stabbing. The radiation of pain is similar to that of angina; it may be felt in the right or left arm but usually the left, in the elbow and down to the fingers, in the jaw, in the back, or in the upper epigastric area. Although the symptoms have never occurred before, many patients will state that they are having a heart attack. Intense fear of impending death or doom is common. If pulmonary edema and cardiogenic shock are early complications, the pain may be obscured.

Although the typical patient with acute infarction presents with severe pain, the range of response is wide. The pain may be brief and not severe. Occasionally, an electrocardiogram will reveal evidence of acute or recent infarction without a history of pain. Patients who have associated gastrointestinal disease, such as peptic ulcer, hiatus hernia, or gallbladder disorders, may have difficulty separating the pain of infarction from that of other conditions. In patients with pre-existing angina pectoris, infarction may be heralded by a more intense episode of pain that is unrelieved by nitroglycerin or rest. Should the infarction precipitate acute pulmonary edema, the pain often becomes a minor complaint. Acute arrhythmia, especially heart block or ventricular tachycardia, may be the presenting sign. Atrioventricular dissociation is relatively common in diaphragmatic-inferior infarctions, and the first symptom may be weakness or syncope owing to marked bradycardia. Patients with severe coronary artery disease may develop myocardial infarction secondary to any prolonged circulatory disorder such as heart failure, hypertension, or arrhythmia. Sometimes it is difficult to be certain which came first, the circulatory disorder or the acute infarction.

In patients who survive to be hospitalized for acute infarction, prodromata are common. Several studies have shown that approximately two thirds of the hospitalized patients have prodromal symptoms, almost always ischemic cardiac pain, prior to the acute infarction. Prodromata are characteristically recurrent and crescendo in nature. The pain is more easily triggered, lasts longer, and is more intense than usual. Prodromata are more common in patients with angina. Any change in the pattern of previously stable angina pectoris should be viewed as possibly a forewarning of impending acute infarction. Infarcts occurring after prodromal symptoms are more likely to be anterior than posterior-inferior and nontransmural than transmural.

Physical Findings. The patient with acute infarction is usually restless, apprehensive, and in severe pain. His color may be poor, the face ashen, and the nailbeds cyanotic. Sweating is frequent, and the skin is cool. Examination of the lungs may reveal normal findings; alternatively there may be signs suggesting early heart failure or acute pulmonary edema. The heart sounds are often distant and muffled. Paradoxical splitting of the second sound has been described but is seldom detected. A fourth heart sound is almost universally present. Auscultation may reveal a soft murmur, suggesting mitral regurgitation. The pulse may be thready and the blood pressure reduced. Careful examination provides the physician with an evaluation of myocardial performance, but it can neither establish nor deny the possibility of a diagnosis of acute infarction.

Laboratory Findings. Routine laboratory examinations reveal abnormalities compatible with necrosis of tissue. The *temperature* is usually elevated for the first three to five days after acute infarction. The rise is usually modest, but occasionally the temperature becomes quite high, up to 40° C. Rarely, continued high fever, apparently caused by myocardial necrosis, threatens survival. Measures to reduce the temperature, including cooling baths and cold blankets, may be necessary.

Leukocytosis occurs regularly, but usually persists no longer than five days to a week. White counts of 12,000

to 15,000 cells per cubic millimeter with a shift to the left are usual. Counts above this level should be viewed with suspicion and possible complications assiduously sought.

Serial analysis of activity in blood of a variety of *enzymes* normally found in muscle cells is of great value in establishing the diagnosis of acute myocardial infarction. Necrosis of as little as 1 gram of myocardium will result in detectable serum enzyme rise. If the enzyme activity is not elevated in a patient suspected of having acute infarction, it is assumed that no infarction occurred or that the tissue damage was so small that it could not be recognized by current techniques. Proper interpretation of serum enzyme patterns requires measurement of enzyme activity for several days after the presumed acute infarction.

Serum creatine phosphokinase (CPK), an enzyme occurring in high concentration in heart, skeletal muscle, and brain, rises rapidly, reaching peak levels approximately 24 hours after acute myocardial infarction. Serum activity returns to normal within 72 hours. Three CPK isozymes have been identified by electrophoresis. Each is a dimer composed of two subunits of the M or B type. Brain contains BB, skeletal muscle MM, and myocardium MM and MB. Serial analysis of CPK is extremely useful in the diagnosis of acute myocardial infarction if the patient is seen within a few hours of symptoms.

Glutamic oxaloacetic transaminase (GOT) is an enzyme present in high concentration in myocardium, skeletal muscle, liver, brain, and kidney. Normal serum activity is 20 to 40 Frank-Karmen units, or 30 to 60 international units. After myocardial infarction, serum activity rises, reaching a peak in 48 to 72 hours, and gradually falling to normal by five days. Providing that liver necrosis secondary to decreased splanchnic blood flow has not also occurred, peak levels correlate with the extent of myocardial damage. Levels of over 300 Frank-Karmen units are usually associated with extensive infarction complicated by heart failure or shock. Serum GOT activity increases also in a wide variety of disorders associated with hepatic necrosis, including central necrosis of the liver, heart failure, hypotension, or shock. Narcotics such as morphine and, to a lesser extent, meperidine may cause a rise in serum activity, presumably secondary to spasm of the sphincter of Oddi. It is often useful to obtain serum glutamic pyruvic transaminase, an enzyme found predominantly in liver, to evaluate possible hepatic contribution to elevated serum GOT activity.

Lactic dehydrogenase (LDH) is found in a variety of tissues, and elevations of serum activity are usually not specific for a diagnosis of myocardial infarction.

Electrocardiogram. The electrocardiogram is extremely useful in evaluating a tentative diagnosis of acute myocardial infarction, providing that the tracing is interpreted with full knowledge of the wide variety of nonspecific factors which may induce abnormality. The hallmark of acute transmural infarction is the appearance of Q waves of sufficient amplitude and duration to be termed significant. It has been said that changes may not occur for two to five days after infarction in some patients, but this seems unlikely. Late appearance of EKG abnormality usually indicates that an impending infarction syndrome finally culminated in infarction and death of cardiac tissue. During the early state of infarction the S-T segments are markedly elevated in those leads depicting the area of infarction, with reciprocal S-T segment depression elsewhere. As the infarct evolves electrically, the S-T segments become depressed and the T waves inverted. Varying degrees of abnormality persist, although in some patients recognition of healed transmural infarction from the EKG may be difficult.

In nontransmural and subendocardial infarction, abnormalities in the EKG are primarily in the S-T segments and T waves. The S-T segments may be elevated, but are usually depressed in leads reflecting the area of infarction, and the T waves are usually inverted. Interpretation of the EKG may be difficult because of the nonspecific nature of the S-T segment and T wave change. Serial tracings over several days may be helpful, especially if the abnormalities progressively improve toward the preinfarction pattern.

Diaphragmatic or inferior infarctions are reflected in leads 2, 3, and AVF. Anterior-septal infarctions influence leads V_2 to V_4, whereas anterior-lateral infarctions involve leads V_3 to V_6. Strictly posterior infarctions are recognized by changes in V_1 and V_2. Subendocardial damage usually results in development of an S-T and T vector opposite in direction to the mean QRS vector. Left bundle branch block frequently obscures the recognition of acute infarction because of the abnormal initial QRS vector, but right bundle branch block does not. In some patients the first EKG is diagnostic. In others serial tracings and blood enzyme analysis are necessary to detect changes compatible with the diagnosis.

Diagnosis. The diagnosis of acute transmural myocardial infarction is straightforward when the patient presents with severe, crushing precordial pain lasting 30 minutes or more and the electrocardiogram reveals characteristic Q waves and S-T segment elevation of the "hyperacute" stage. Myocardial infarction, however, has a wide range of clinical manifestations, and recognition of the acute episode may be difficult.

Diagnosis is based on a clinical triad: (1) prolonged cardiac pain, more severe and longer lasting than angina; (2) abnormal electrocardiograms with a progressive evolution of pattern; and (3) rise and fall in serum enzyme activity. At least two of these should be present to support the diagnosis. In some patients pain either

does not occur or is not recognized as representing a serious illness. Denial is an important component of the initial response to the symptoms of acute infarction in many patients, making interpretation of the history difficult. As with angina, the pain may be ascribed to indigestion or other gastrointestinal complaint. When acute infarction is a complication of a surgical procedure, anesthesia, trauma, or other disease such as gastrointestinal hemorrhage, hypertension, or shock, pain may be absent. The diagnosis is then suspected from changes in the electrocardiogram, and may be corroborated by serial analysis of blood enzyme activity.

In acute transmural infarction the electrocardiogram is usually diagnostic when obtained within a few hours of symptoms. Interpretation of the electrocardiogram in nontransmural or subendocardial infarction may be difficult. Frequently the tracing was previously abnormal, and changes in the S-T segments or T waves may not be marked. The electrocardiogram may be surprisingly unrevealing in some patients with one or more previous infarctions and extensive atherosclerosis of the three major coronary vessels. Presumably the widespread yet discrete abnormalities cancel each other out on the surface electrocardiogram.

Serial assay of blood enzyme activity is most useful when the clinical story is not helpful or is imprecise. However, intramuscular injection of many drugs, including narcotics, will increase serum CPK and GOT, causing potential errors in diagnosis. Acute abnormality of the electrocardiogram followed by resolution toward normal coupled with a characteristic rise and fall of enzyme activity will usually be diagnostic. There are many situations in which it is not possible to prove or disprove the diagnosis of acute infarction, yet the wise decision may be to treat the patient as though infarction had occurred.

Differential Diagnosis. The most frequent problem is determining whether the patient has had a prolonged attack of *angina* or an infarction. Electrocardiographic abnormalities usually develop during angina, but revert to the previous pattern when the pain subsides. Fever and leukocytosis are not present. The serum enzymes do not rise after angina pectoris. Persistent electrocardio-

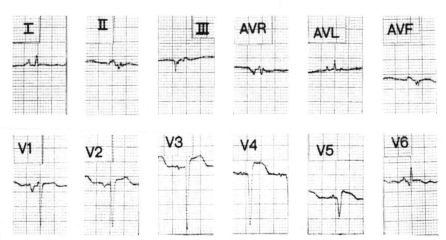

Figure 4. Large myocardial infarction with chronic heart failure. Electrocardiogram from a 66-year-old man obtained seven weeks after hospitalization for acute myocardial infarction. He had previously been in excellent health without known risk factors for cardiovascular disease. His hospital course was complicated by ventricular tachycardia, heart failure, low blood pressure, fatigue, and lassitude. Intensive treatment with antiarrhythmics, digitalis, and diuretics was required. Convalescence was prolonged. Eight weeks after the acute event, he developed an abdominal abscess from a perforated appendix and died suddenly. Electrocardiogram shows evidence of extensive transmural anterior and inferior diaphragmatic myocardial infarction.

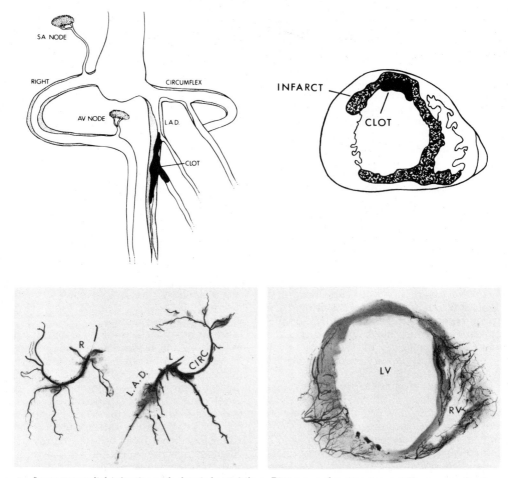

Figure 5. Large myocardial infarction with chronic heart failure. Diagrams and postmortem roentgenograms of major coronary vessels and coronal section of ventricles, obtained at autopsy from patient described in Figure 4. Coronary arteries were injected with a barium mixture and heart was fixed in formalin. Large coronary arteries were then dissected free, ventricles sectioned, and X-ray exposures obtained. Coronary artery disease in right, circumflex, and first diagonal branch of anterior descending artery is minimal. However, there is extensive involvement of left anterior descending artery with complete obstruction caused by thrombosis. Area of infarct involves anterior, septal, and posterior wall of left ventricle and septum and posterior segment of right ventricle. A mural thrombosis was present in left ventricle. Forty-four per cent of left ventricular mass was destroyed in the infarction. Extent of damage suggests continued cardiac disability had patient survived. (Courtesy of D. Alonso, M.D.)

graphic abnormality after a severe attack of angina suggests that subendocardial or nontransmural infarction has developed, especially if accompanied by changes in serum enzyme activity. Although great reliance is often placed on assay of serum enzymes, it seems likely that small, discrete infarctions may occur without detectable rise in enzyme activity.

Acute *pericarditis* may be mistaken for acute myocardial infarction. The pain of pericarditis is often made worse by deep inspiration. Relief is obtained by sitting up and leaning forward. The hallmark of pericarditis is a precordial friction rub which characteristically has three components: presystolic, early diastolic, and systolic. Faint rubs with only one or two components are often missed or mistaken for soft murmurs. The electrocardiogram in acute pericarditis shows moderate S-T segment elevation initially with upright T waves. Later the S-T segment may be slightly depressed and the T waves become inverted. Q waves do not occur in pericarditis.

Pulmonary embolus may cause chest pain and electrocardiographic changes, but the pleuritic pain is seldom suggestive of myocardial infarction. The electrocardiogram in pulmonary embolus may reveal an S₁, S₂, S₃ pattern, complete or incomplete right bundle branch block (usually evanescent), or clockwise rotation of the precordial pattern, suggesting right ventricular overload.

Other conditions which may be confused with myocardial infarction include ruptured aortic aneurysm, acute aortic dissection, acute pneumothorax, gallbladder disease, pneumonia, and acute arrhythmia. Errors in diagnosis can frequently be ascribed to inadequacies of the history and physical examination or overinterpretation of nonspecific changes in the electrocardiogram.

Unstable Angina. Onset of recurrent episodes of ischemic pain or worsening of pre-existing angina is termed unstable angina. Evaluation of symptoms is particularly troublesome when prolonged pain occurs at rest, not infrequently at night, and is accompanied by transient electrocardiographic changes. This constellation of symptoms has also been called the "intermediate syndrome," "preinfarction angina," or the "impending coronary syndrome." There is considerable controversy about prognosis and management. Recently advocates of early coronary arteriography and subsequent urgent surgical revascularization have been especially vocal.

A prospective study from Edinburgh by Oliver, Julian, and associates suggests that the prognosis is not as guarded as has been thought. Of 167 patients who developed unstable angina and were followed for several months, sudden death occurred in only 3 and acute myocardial infarction in 23. During the same period in the population under survey, about 70,000 persons at risk, there were 79 cases of sudden death and 110 of myocardial infarction. Sixty per cent of the patients with myocardial infarction had preceding unstable angina, but only a fourth of these sought medical aid. It would appear then that the major risk of unstable angina is infarction; denial or failure to recognize important symptoms is a serious problem.

Because current data are insufficient to evaluate medical or surgical therapy for unstable angina pectoris, a carefully designed random study of treatment is being carried out under the auspices of the National Institutes of Health. At this writing more than 100 patients have been randomized. No therapeutic advantage for either treatment is yet apparent, but several observations are pertinent. Angiography can be performed in unstable angina with little increase in risk. Surgical mortality is less than 10 per cent; myocardial infarction is the principal hazard occurring in both the medical and the post-surgical groups. Medical therapy generally consists of bed rest, oxygen, sedation, anticoagulants (usually), treatment of heart failure or arrhythmia, and propranolol. The results of this important study are being awaited with keen interest.

Complications. *Sudden Death.* Sudden, unexpected fatality is a common complication of acute myocardial infarction. It is currently believed that as many as 50 per cent of patients with acute infarction do not survive to reach a hospital. Early death is not related to the severity of the infarction and is most likely to occur in the

first four to six hours after onset, the frequency decreasing exponentially thereafter. Observations from monitoring units suggest that the mechanism is ventricular fibrillation in most cases, although acute heart block may be the initial arrhythmia in some.

Frequently patients do not seek medical attention until several hours after the onset of pain. The major cause of delay is failure to appreciate the significance of symptoms and denial that a problem exists. Physicians may err in evaluation of the complaint. Hospital emergency rooms, often oriented to treatment of trauma, may not move the patient into a coronary treatment system with sufficient rapidity after arrival. Cardiac arrest in the patient waiting to be evaluated for chest pain is all too common.

Arrhythmia. More than 90 per cent of patients hospitalized with acute infarction have arrhythmia, especially during the first 72 hours. Some of these are trivial, some are potentially life threatening, and some have such immediate consequences that their mere recognition should impel prompt, vigorous therapy. Abnormal rhythms may affect cardiac performance by adversely influencing ventricular rate, altering the sequence of atrial and ventricular contraction, or initiating depolarization from an abnormal focus. Of greatest importance clinically is the ventricular rate. In general if the ventricular rate is reasonable (60 to 110 beats per minute) and well tolerated, treatment of an abnormal rhythm may not be urgent. On the other hand, if the ventricular rate is either too fast or too slow, prompt correction is usually indicated. Patients with myocardial damage often have fixed stroke volumes so that minute volume, or cardiac output, is dependent upon heart rate. If the heart rate is too slow, cardiac output may fall.

A sinus rate greater than 110 beats per minute is often an ominous sign. *Sinus tachycardia* may reflect a low stroke volume or impending shock. If evidence of heart failure is present, the rate may slow after cautious ad-

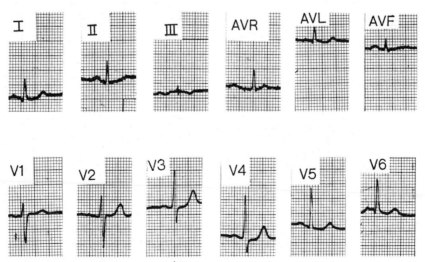

Figure 6. Crescendo angina and sudden death. Electrocardiogram obtained 24 hours before death from a 58-year-old man with stable, infrequent angina for four years. Risk factors included moderate obesity, hypertension, and history of moderate smoking. Three months previously he was hospitalized after a prolonged bout of chest pain, but a diagnosis of myocardial infarction could not be established. After this, he had progressively severe angina, including nocturnal attacks requiring several sublingual nitroglycerin tablets for relief. He was hospitalized for evaluation. Blood pressure was 125/75 mm Hg. The heart was normal on examination without evidence of failure. He continued to have intermittent episodes of chest pain at rest after hospitalization, but there was no objective evidence of myocardial infarction. On the morning of the fourth day of hospitalization he was found dead in bed. The electrocardiogram shows nonspecific S-T segment depression in most leads. The prominent R wave in leads V_1 and V_2 suggests the possibility of an old "strictly posterior" myocardial infarction.

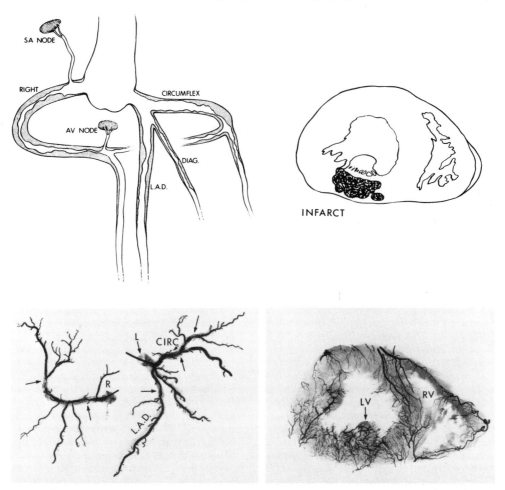

Figure 7. Crescendo angina and sudden death. Diagrams and postmortem roentgenograms of major coronary vessels and coronal section of ventricles obtained at autopsy from patient described in Figure 6. There is advanced disease of the three major coronary arteries but no complete occlusion. Neovascularization (arrow) in posterior wall of left ventricle indicates old (months) scar from myocardial infarction which was confirmed histologically. Posterior location confirms electrocardiographic interpretation. Although extent of heart disease is obvious, precise cause of death could not be determined from autopsy. (Courtesy of D. Alonso, M.D.)

ministration of digitalis. *Sinus bradycardia* occurs in 10 to 15 per cent of patients with acute infarction. Presumably it is a reflection of sinus node dysfunction secondary to alteration of blood supply, although reflex "vagotonia" has been postulated. Bradycardia is usually an early complication and lasts but a few hours. It is commonly associated with inferior wall infarction.

Arrhythmia of atrial or nodal (junctional) origin may reflect atrial infarction, the development of heart failure, hypokalemia, digitalis excess, or a combination of factors. *Atrial premature beats* are often the forerunner of sustained atrial dysrhythmia. *Atrial tachycardia* is uncommon in myocardial infarction. *Atrial fibrillation* or *flutter* occurs in about 10 per cent of patients and has a marked tendency to spontaneous reversion followed by relapse within minutes.

Prolongations of the P-R time *(first-degree block)* and Wenckebach phenomenon *(second-degree block)* are due to disorders of conduction in the region of the AV node. They are frequent complication of inferior-diaphragmatic infarctions (electrocardiographic changes in leads 2, 3 AVF) and reflect disturbance of blood supply to the AV node from the posterior surface of the heart. This form of block is almost always temporary, and improves after a few hours or a day or two. In inferior-diaphragmatic in-

farctions the normal sinus and the AV nodal pacemaker may discharge at approximately the same rate. The dominant pacemaker oscillates between the two nodes, producing AV dissociation depending on their respective rates. The QRS complex is normal in form, and the ventricular rate is usually above 55. This arrhythmia is not a form of heart block, because the normal conduction pathways will be utilized whenever a sinus node impulse arrives in the region of the AV node after ventricular repolarization. Specific treatment is not required.

Complete heart block is a dangerous and potentially lethal complication of acute myocardial infarction. It is usually associated with a large, anterior infarction. The mortality is approximately 50 per cent. In the form known as Mobitz type II, AV block develops suddenly without previous prolongation of the P-R interval or dropped beats. Direct recordings of the electrocardiogram from the bundle of His indicate that this conduction disturbance is almost always caused by bilateral bundle branch block. Prior conduction abnormality, such as right or left bundle branch block or marked by left axis deviation, is usually present. When complete heart block complicates acute infarction, the ventricular response is usually slow, and the QRS complexes are wide and bizarre. About half the patients with pre-existing bundle branch block develop acute heart block as a complication of myocardial infarction. The incidence is especially high with the QV_1-RBBB pattern. Some authorities advocate the placement of a temporary pacemaker-electrode in the right ventricle in all patients with pre-existing bundle branch block because of the danger of developing bilateral bundle branch block.

Ventricular premature beats are common in acute myocardial infarction, occurring in about 75 per cent of monitored patients. Premature beats are important because they may initiate ventricular tachycardia or ventricular fibrillation if sufficiently premature to strike the vulnerable period of the diastolic repolarization phase of the cardiac cycle. The vulnerable period occurs during the latter portion of the relative refractory period, and coincides with the ascending limb of the T wave. The more closely coupled a ventricular premature beat is to the preceding normal beat, the more likely it is to initiate tachycardia or fibrillation.

Ventricular tachycardia, defined as three or more consecutive ventricular beats, and *ventricular fibrillation* occur in about 10 per cent of patients hospitalized with acute infarction. When the rate in ventricular tachycardia is slow, the arrhythmia is usually well tolerated. With fast rates, however, the circulation rapidly deteriorates, requiring immediate emergency treatment. Ventricular tachycardia may progress to ventricular fibrillation. Fibrillation is usually heralded by preceding ventricular premature beats or tachycardia. In some instances, termed *primary* fibrillation, the arrhythmia develops suddenly without warning ectopic beats. Primary fibrillation is probably an important factor in sudden death, because its incidence is greatest in the early hours after infarction.

Physiologic Changes. Acute myocardial infarction induces regional abnormalities in cardiac contraction and adversely influences function of the heart as a whole. The left ventricle is primarily involved. Malfunction of the right ventricle is usually secondary to left ventricular failure but may occasionally reflect right ventricular infarction. In general the degree of left ventricular dysfunction reflects the extent of myocardial damage. The larger the infarct, new or old, the greater the hemodynamic abnormality. Infarction of even a small mass of myocardium is accompanied by significant increase in left ventricular filling pressure. With larger infarcts the increased filling pressure is often accompanied by signs of overt congestive failure. Damage involving more than 40 per cent of left ventricular mass is complicated by hypotension, low cardiac output, and cardiogenic shock.

It is useful to classify patients according to the presence or absence of *clinical evidence of left ventricular failure.* Mortality and the extent of hemodynamic abnormality vary directly with the severity of heart failure. Patients in Class I, no clinical evidence of heart failure, have hemodynamic performance which is essentially normal when compared with that of age-matched controls. Left ventricular diastolic pressure, however, ranges from normal (less than 12 mm Hg) to as high as 30 mm Hg without pulmonary congestion. Hospital mortality is 5 per cent owing to arrhythmia or cardiac rupture.

Class II patients have clinical evidence of mild left ventricular failure with reduced intensity of heart sounds, a third heart sound, and pulmonary rales. Left ventricular filling pressure is consistently increased; there is sinus tachycardia; stroke volume and cardiac output are reduced. Blood pressure is usually normal or slightly reduced, and peripheral vascular resistance is increased. Hospital mortality averages about 17 per cent.

Class III is defined as *pulmonary edema.* Mean left ventricular diastolic pressure is 25 mm Hg or higher, severe sinus tachycardia is the rule, and cardiac output is sharply reduced. Blood pressure may be normal or low. Mortality is 25 to 30 per cent.

Class IV, *cardiogenic shock,* develops in about 10 per cent of hospitalized patients, on the average some ten hours after the acute infarction. Shock is characterized by hypotension and signs of inadequate peripheral circulation; including cold skin, mental confusion, peripheral cyanosis, decreased urine flow, and tachycardia. Hemodynamic studies reveal marked arterial hypoxia and low stroke volume and cardiac output. A cardiac index of 1.0 liter per minute per square meter, a level barely able to support life, is not uncommon. Cardiac work is low; this factor can be related to prognosis. Progressive acidosis caused by accumulation of lactic acid is frequent. Pathologic studies have shown that fatal cardiogenic shock is characteristic of massive infarction. A combination of fresh and old scar, involving 40 per cent or more of ventricular mass, is found. Frequently also there is evidence of recent extension or reinfarction, events which have usually not been recognized clinically. Despite intensive treatment, mortality in cardiogenic shock averages about 85 per cent.

Hypoxia. Reduced arterial oxygen tension is a common complication of myocardial infarction. Po_2 in Class I patients is normal. Po_2 is reduced in classes II to IV. The degree of arterial unsaturation can be related to the clinical severity of heart failure and to the degree of elevation of left ventricular filling pressure. In one study, Po_2 in cardiogenic shock averaged 40 mm Hg, a value consistent with that observed in normal subjects at an elevation in excess of 10,000 feet. The arterial hypoxia reflects increased intrapulmonary venoarterial shunting secondary to the elevated pulmonary venous pressure and interstitial water accumulation in the lungs. Serial analysis of arterial Po_2 while the patient is breathing room air and an enriched oxygen mixture is extremely useful in management of myocardial infarction, because it provides an indirect assay of left ventricular function. Provided that primary pulmonary disease does not complicate the picture, effective treatment and recovery from the cardiac problem are accompanied by a return of arterial Po_2 to normal.

Embolism. Both systemic and pulmonary emboli may complicate myocardial infarction. Use of anticoagulants and less restrictive bed rest with attention to movement of the extremities have reduced the frequency of these hazards. Incidence of clinically recognizable episodes is currently extremely low. Pulmonary emboli from the right heart tend to be small and nonfatal, whereas those from the deep veins may be massive and cause sudden death. Systemic emboli have their source in the mural thrombi which form on the endocardium of the infarcted left ventricle.

Insufficiency of the Mitral Valve. Mitral regurgitation complicating acute infarction is usually caused by dysfunction of the papillary muscles, secondary to the ischemic process. However, it is usually not functionally significant. Heikkila reported that 30 per cent of patients with acute infarction develop murmurs of mitral insufficiency detected by repeated, daily auscultation. The murmur is usually soft and blowing, is heard at the apex, and may be holosystolic or confined to the latter half of systole. Rupture of the papillary muscle may precipitate acute and intractable pulmonary edema. The murmur is loud and holosystolic, and is usually accompanied by a systolic apical thrill. Differentiation clinically from rupture of the ventricular septum may not be easy. In the patient with refractory heart failure, emergency replacement with an artificial mitral valve may be indicated.

Cardiac Rupture. Rupture of the heart occurs in about 5 per cent of fatal cases. It is the only complication of acute infarction that is more common in women than in men. Rupture develops in transmural infarction, usually within the first ten days. Death is caused by acute hemopericardium and tamponade. The condition is characterized clinically by sudden loss of blood pressure without arrhythmia. Sinus tachycardia often persists for several minutes, although the patient is unresponsive. Occasionally the rupture is sealed by the pericardium, and survival for several months is possible.

Rupture of the interventricular septum is heralded by the appearance of a loud systolic murmur with a thrill along the left sternal border. It is seven to ten times more common than rupture of a papillary muscle. The dynamic effects depend on the size of the tear and volume of left to right shunt. Numerous reports attest to the success of surgical repair of acquired ventricular septal defect in selected cases.

Weakening of the Ventricular Wall. Aneurysm of the left ventricle results from scarring and thinning of the ventricular wall after transmural infarction. When large, the aneurysm bulges outward during systole, and this paradoxical movement may be appreciated by careful palpation of the precordium. Large aneurysms are often lined with clot, and systemic embolus is a hazard. Occasionally aneurysm of the left ventricle may be recognized on a chest film when the bulge is especially prominent. Localized disorder of ventricular contraction is common after myocardial infarction. Angiography frequently reveals unsuspected aneurysm or areas of ventricular akinesia. When the area of disordered contraction is large, the ventricle is dilated and the ejection fraction (stroke volume/end-diastolic volume) is reduced. Surgical removal of the dyskinetic muscle, often with bypass grafting to diseased coronary vessels, may improve cardiac function in selected cases.

Postinfarction Syndrome. A postinfarction syndrome, *Dressler's syndrome,* has been described, occurring a week or more after acute infarction and characterized by pericarditis with pleuritis and pleural effusions. This condition is similar to the postpericardiectomy syndrome observed after cardiac surgery. It responds dramatically to moderate doses of corticosteroids.

Treatment. The aims of treatment are (1) to make the patient comfortable, (2) to reduce the demands on the heart by maintaining the patient at rest during the healing phase, (3) to prevent complications, or (4) to treat them. Recent experiments suggest that a fifth aim, preservation of ischemic myocardium and limitation of infarct size may be feasible.

Prehospital Management. The majority of deaths from acute myocardial infarction occur before hospitalization is achieved. Two factors, a high incidence of life-threatening arrhythmia in the first few minutes or hours after the acute event, and the ubiquitous problem of misinterpretation or denial of symptoms, contribute to the early death rate. Intensive efforts to provide mobile coronary care with rapid diagnosis, treatment, and transport to hospitals have been reported from several major urban areas. Although these units have enthusiastic supporters, a careful study from Stockholm suggests that they will have little impact on survival without intense public education, because the major component of delay is failure of the victim to seek help in time.

The principles of early treatment are rapid diagnosis, alleviation of pain and apprehension, and stabilization of heart rhythm and blood pressure. Frequent ectopic ventricular beats usually respond to 50 to 100 mg of lidocaine given intravenously. Intramuscular injection of 400 mg of lidocaine will achieve a therapeutic blood level in 5 minutes and be effective for 45 minutes or more. Emergency treatment of bradycardia has become controversial. Profound slowing of heart rate and hypotension will often respond to 0.5 to 2.0 mg of atropine given intravenously in divided doses. Moderate slowing with heart rates of 60 to 65 beats per minute and an adequate blood pressure may be treated expectantly. In laboratory animals injection of atropine and the resultant increase in heart rate have been shown to enlarge the area of infarction after coronary occlusion. The administration of drugs without precise electrocardiographic control is not without hazard. In the acute situation the physician or nurse must judge what is in the best interest of the patient. Once the situation is stabilized, the patient should be transported to a hospital with adequate monitoring and resuscitative facilities.

In-Hospital Care. Serious complications of acute myocardial infarction cannot be properly managed outside the hospital. Treatment of the patient in a coronary care unit with appropriate monitoring facilities and trained personnel has reduced mortality in hospital by 30 to 50 per cent. In the well-run coronary care unit at present, hospital mortality for unselected patients with acute myocardial infarction averages 12 to 18 per cent. Despite the wide variety of electronic monitoring instruments available, the only body function which has been shown to be useful to monitor routinely and continuously is the rate and rhythm of the heart as revealed by the electrocardiogram. It is now well accepted practice to train nurses and other personnel to interpret the electrocardiogram and initiate therapy for abnormal rhythm, because the physician is only intermittently in attendance on the patient.

About a third of patients routinely admitted for coronary care will have no serious complications and recover uneventfully. Were it possible to identify these patients with low risk, hospitalization could be avoided and home care advised. Pantridge has suggested that patients hospitalized with acute myocardial infarction without significant arrhythmia and S-T segments and T wave changes only which return to normal within 48 hours can be promptly discharged to convalesce at home. A study from Bristol, England, reported that hospital mortality and home mortality in unselected patients with acute myocardial infarction were similar. It is clear, however, that both the extent of infarction and the interval from acute onset to medical intervention influence mortality and the decision to treat at home. Continued studies of the effectiveness of home treatment in selected patients will be viewed with great interest. General clinical status, suitability of home environment, and availability of medical help will affect the outcome. In the United States at present, hospitalization and monitoring in a coronary care unit for the first few days of illness are the recommended treatment for acute myocardial infarction.

Environment. The patient should be put to bed in a quiet, calm area. Rest and relaxation should be sought. Most patients prefer a single room, although this may not always be possible. Light should be subdued and noise kept to a minimum. Usually visitors are restricted during the first few days of illness. Radio, newspapers, and television are reduced to a minimum. A clock and a calendar provide the patient with considerable security and prevent a sense of isolation.

Pain and Apprehension. Morphine sulfate, 8 to 15 mg parenterally, is usually effective for pain or restlessness. In severe cases, it may be necessary to repeat the drug in smaller dosages every three to four hours. Morphine depresses respiration, reduces myocardial contractility, and is a potent vasodilator. Hypotension, which can usually be overcome by elevation of the lower extremities, or bradycardia, responsive to atropine, may develop. Meperidine, 50 to 100 mg, is also useful, although not as effective as morphine. Since intramuscular injections may elevate serum enzyme activity (CPK, GOT) and confuse diagnostic interpretation, injection into the abdominal panniculus has been recommended. The patient who is confused and restless may be suffering from cerebral dysfunction or delirium owing to heart failure or shock. It is wise therefore to be cautious in administering narcotics, especially in repeated doses.

Mood changes with apprehension are common. It is important to have a well trained, sympathetic nursing staff under the direction of an understanding physician to interpret and explain the illness and treatment. Specific treatment with barbiturates, chlordiazepoxide (Librium) or diazepam (Valium), may help.

Bowel Function. Maintenance of reasonably normal bowel function and avoidance of straining at stool are important aspects of treatment. An effective therapy is milk of magnesia, 30 ml twice daily. Dioctyl sodium sulfosuccinate (Colace), 100 mg twice daily, may be added if necessary. This program usually produces a satisfactory evacuation in midmorning. Milk of magnesia combined with cascara tends to cause bloating, cramps, and excessive flatus, as does Colace when used alone.

Smoking. Admission to a coronary unit is one of the most effective deterrents to smoking. The physician should not fail to take advantage of this opportunity.

Bed Rest. Traditional treatment has overemphasized the value of bed rest. Strict bed rest is reasonable for the first three or four days. If no serious complication develops, the patient may then be allowed modified bed rest with some activity, sitting in a chair. Use of a bedside commode is much appreciated. In an uncomplicated infarction, after a few days of chair rest, progressive ambulation may begin, to prepare the patient for discharge about three weeks after the acute attack. At home activity is gradually increased, and the patient may anticipate returning to work in six to ten weeks.

Bladder. Urinary retention resulting from bladder neck obstruction is not uncommon in older patients during prolonged bed rest. If urinary retention is suspected, the physician should not hesitate to insert an indwelling catheter with aseptic technique. After the cardiac problem has improved, definitive therapy may be undertaken if necessary.

Diet. Acutely ill patients usually have little appetite, although modest amounts of tastily prepared food may be appreciated. Usually the patient is offered a soft diet, moderately reduced in calories, 1500 to 1800, and in sodium, 2 to 3 grams (87 to 130 mEq) as soon as he wishes to eat. A number of adequate salt substitutes are available. Salt intake and the variety of food may be liberalized after the first week if no evidence of heart failure has been detected. For the overweight patient, close supervision of the convalescent period may offer an opportunity for weight reduction.

Oxygen. Hypoxia secondary to increased pulmonary venous hypertension and left ventricular dysfunction in myocardial infarction has been discussed previously. Administration of oxygen may (1) increase arterial Po_2 and (2) increase oxygen tension in the ischemic myocardium bordering the infarcted zone, thus perhaps reducing the size of infarction. Despite uncertainty about the importance of oxygen therapy, it seems reasonable to provide an atmosphere of increased oxygen to most patients during the first few days, utilizing either the Venturi mask or nasal cannula. The loose-fitting Venturi mask is comfortable and efficient. Models are available which deliver 28, 35, or 40 per cent oxygen. An oxygen tent is inefficient and expensive.

Anticoagulation. At present, with emphasis on the treatment of heart failure, early ambulation, reduced sedation, and limb movement in bed, it is apparent that the morbidity is low and the mortality essentially nil from thromboembolism complicating myocardial infarction. There is no evidence to suggest that anticoagulants influence the course of the infarction itself. The decision to use anticoagulants is largely elective. Their use should be based on the patient's past history, the quality of the supporting laboratory, and the experience of the physician with anticoagulant drugs. Recent phlebitis or embolism favors treatment. History of ulcer, bleeding tendency, signs of pericarditis, or hemorrhage would argue against anticoagulation. The most commonly used agents are Coumadin derivatives. Heparin is indicated only occasionally when thrombosis or embolism appears as a life-threatening complication.

Arrhythmia. Recognition and management of arrhythmia in acute myocardial infarction is based on a thorough understanding of electrophysiology and electrocardiography. The reader is urged to consult Ch. 569 and 570 before proceeding.

SINUS BRADYCARDIA. Reduction of the heart rate below 55 owing to failure of the normal sinus mechanism may be accompanied by evidence of low cardiac output, development of heart failure, or hypotension. Intravenous atropine, 0.5 to 1.0 mg, is usually effective. Occasionally 2.0 mg may be required. Atropine is not practical for long-term maintenance. Repeated use of the drug is limited by occasional central nervous system effects, urinary retention, and the rare precipitation of acute glaucoma. Overdosage may cause unpleasant tachycardia with consequent adverse effect in infarct size. Slowing of the sinus rate is usually temporary. Occasionally the condition persists as a manifestation of the "sick sinus syndrome," and temporary pacing with an electrode inserted into the right atrium or right ventricle is required.

ATRIAL ARRHYTHMIA. Frequent atrial premature complexes are often the harbinger of atrial fibrillation or flutter. They usually respond to digitalis. If atrial flutter and fibrillation are well tolerated, without hypotension or heart failure, they are best treated with digitalis to control the ventricular rate. If complications develop or the patient is not tolerating the arrhythmia well, DC precordial shock should be employed. Supraventricular arrhythmias are frequently recurrent, but after the acute illness subsides, spontaneous reversion is the rule.

ATRIOVENTRICULAR BLOCK. An important guide to therapy of heart block is the ventricular rate. In atrioventricular dissociation with an escape junctional rhythm, the QRS configuration is usually normal and the heart rate is well maintained. This is also true in the Wenckebach phenomenon (second degree block, Mobitz Type I). Thus treatment may be expectant. However, when there is intermittent atrial capture of the ventricle with unexpected dropped beats or complete AV block with a slow idioventricular rate characterized by wide QRS complexes (Mobitz type II), therapy is usually required. An intravenous infusion of isoproterenol may be immediately effective. Isoproterenol, 0.4 to 1.0 mg, is dissolved in 500 ml of 5 per cent glucose in water and carefully administered intravenously by slow drip. The rate of infusion and the concentration of the drug should be adjusted according to the ventricular response. Isoproterenol may induce both atrial and ventricular arrhythmia, and its use requires constant, close medical supervision.

Temporary transvenous pacemaking with an electrode catheter in the right ventricle is an effective form of therapy for a slow ventricular rate. The electrode should be activated by a battery-powered demand-type pacemaker. *Heart block* in acute myocardial infarction is almost always self-limited. Established heart block after recovery from infarction is rare. Thus if a satisfactory ventricular rate can be maintained for a few days, conduction will almost invariably resume through normal pathways, and the pacemaker catheter can then be withdrawn.

Sudden *complete heart block,* Mobitz Type II, is usually due to bilateral bundle branch block. Fifty per cent of patients with right or left bundle branch block prior to acute infarction develop bilateral bundle branch block during the acute illness. Patients with left bundle branch block have a high frequency of ventricular fibrillation. Despite widespread use of pacemakers for treatment or on standby, the mortality when complete heart block complicates myocardial infarction remains high, averaging 50 per cent.

VENTRICULAR PREMATURE BEATS; UNSUSTAINED VENTRICULAR TACHYCARDIA. The appearance of more than three ventricular premature beats per minute or bursts of ventricular contractions requires urgent treatment. In ischemia or infarction they may be forerunners of cardiac arrest, and prompt, aggressive treatment may forestall a catastrophe. The most effective and rapidly acting agent currently available is lidocaine hydrochloride intravenously in doses of 50 to 100 mg by rapid injection (bolus). The dose may be repeated in three to five minutes to achieve the desired result, obliteration of extrasystoles. When the ectopic beats have disappeared after bolus injection, a constant intravenous drip of lidocaine may be administered and the drip rate adjusted to maintain an infusion rate of 1.0 to 5.0 mg per minute. The infusion rate may be gradually reduced after several hours if there is no recurrence, and may be discontinued in 24 to 36 hours. Recurrence of extrasystoles may require extra immediate doses of lidocaine followed by an increase in the infusion rate.

Lidocaine is a local anesthetic, and it may cause sensations of body numbness or tingling or twitching of the face muscles. Large doses often cause drowsiness. Convulsions occasionally occur with excessive dosage, especially in the presence of cerebral anoxia.

If lidocaine is not effective, procainamide or quinidine sulfate may be required. Diphenylhydantoin every four to eight hours is also occasionally effective. In refractory situations, overdrive suppression with a temporary pacemaker may be tried. Overdriving shortens electrical diastole and suppresses the tendency for ectopic beats to develop.

VENTRICULAR TACHYCARDIA AND VENTRICULAR FIBRILLATION. These two arrhythmias are considered together, because ventricular tachycardia often precedes and degenerates into ventricular fibrillation. If blood pressure is maintained without circulatory collapse in the presence of ventricular tachycardia, 100 mg of lidocaine may be administered rapidly intravenously. If there is no effect within three to five minutes, DC precordial shock is applied. If blood pressure is not maintained and the patient develops clinical cardiac arrest, immediate treatment with precordial shock is mandatory.

VENTRICULAR FIBRILLATION. The proper therapy of this arrhythmia is immediate defibrillation. If the defibrillator is available, time is wasted attempting to ventilate the patient or attempting closed-chest cardiac massage. In older patients there are approximately 60 seconds in which to administer an effective shock and revert ventricular fibrillation to normal rhythm before the development of serious metabolic disturbance or brain damage. "Thump version," delivery of a sharp blow to the precordium, may be attempted for ventricular tachycardia or fibrillation. In the well run coronary care unit, defibrillation for unexpected cardiac arrest can frequently be applied by the trained nurse within 30 seconds of onset.

ASYSTOLE. Sudden, unexpected asystole is uncommon in acute infarction. Most often it is the culmination of a gradual decline in cardiac function in severe heart failure or shock. A series of thumps on the chest or closed chest cardiac massage may restore cardiac action. If an electrode catheter is in place or can be rapidly inserted, artificial pacemaking may be effective.

Pulmonary Edema. The initial manifestation of acute infarction may be sudden development of pulmonary edema. The aims of therapy are to improve cardiac function, reduce airway resistance and the work of breathing, and increase arterial oxygen tension. If the blood pressure is well maintained, the patient is propped into a sitting position. Morphine sulfate, 8 to 15 mg parenterally, is effective. Oxygen is administered, preferably by mask, in high concentration. If the patient can tolerate a tightly fitting mask, oxygen under positive pressure or with positive pressure on exhalation is useful, because the increased intrathoracic pressure impedes venous return and lowers ventricular filling pressures. Blood pressure should be carefully followed, because positive pressure inhalation is contraindicated in hypotension or shock. Rotating tourniquets impound a significant portion of the circulating blood volume in the extremities and are extremely useful. Tourniquets should be applied to three limbs tightly enough to inhibit venous return yet permit transmission of the arterial pulse, and should be rotated every 20 minutes.

Digitalis is usually not necessary in the immediate

treatment unless the condition has been precipitated by acute supraventricular arrhythmia, especially rapid atrial fibrillation or flutter. The drug is usually indicated for long-term management, and may be necessary in refractory cases. Furosemide, 40 to 80 mg, and ethacrynic acid, 50 to 100 mg, are potent diuretic agents which will initiate diuresis within 15 minutes of intravenous administration. Both are frequently used in patients with pulmonary edema. They also increase venous capacitance and have been shown to sharply reduce left ventricular filling pressure before diuresis commences. Other measures include phlebotomy of 300 to 500 ml or more, administration of aminophylline as a suppository (0.5 gram) or intravenously in a slow infusion in a dosage of 250 to 500 mg.

Heart Failure. Congestive heart failure is fairly common in acute myocardial infarction, occurring in approximately two thirds of hospitalized patients. Early signs of pulmonary congestion may be treated with diuretics or reduction of salt intake. There is strong experimental and clinical evidence to support the view that the infarcted heart has increased sensitivity to the toxic effects of digitalis. Digitalis should not be withheld when clearly indicated but should be given in smaller dosages than usual. Serum potassium level should be followed closely. Additional digitalis can always be given in cases of need. It is impossible to remove an excess.

Many different digitalis preparations are available, but it is best to avoid administration of more than one agent to a patient, as judgment about the level becomes exceedingly difficult. *Digoxin* is useful; it is rapidly absorbed and excreted with a serum half-life of about 30 hours; hence dosage depends upon frequency and route of administration. In patients who are acutely ill, the author prefers intravenous administration, as there is certainty about the time and amount given. A reasonable schedule is 0.5 mg initially intravenously, followed by 0.25 mg in six hours, followed by 0.125 mg in six hours. The total dose is conservative, but this schedule will usually avoid any problem of digitalis intoxication. For oral dosage 0.5 mg is given, followed by 0.25 mg at 6 and 12 hours, and then a maintenance schedule of 0.25 mg is given daily thereafter. *Ouabain,* available only in an intravenous preparation, has been advocated by some authorities in the treatment of heart failure complicating acute myocardial infarction. This drug has the same physiologic half-life as digoxin, and a convenient dosage schedule is as follows: 0.4 mg intravenously as an initial dose, followed by 0.1 to 0.2 mg every two hours for two or three additional doses. A detectable effect occurs within 20 minutes, with a peak action at about 2 hours.

Hypotension. If blood pressure falls, yet the patient remains alert and warm, has an adequate urine output, and is not in shock, management may be expectant. A treatable cause should be sought. The fall in blood pressure may be caused by drugs, particularly sedatives, or narcotics such as morphine. If hypotension is due to peripheral venous pooling, elevation of the lower extremities is an effective measure. Occasionally the fall in blood pressure is a reflection of reduced blood volume, and ventricular filling pressures are low. This has been observed in patients previously treated for acute pulmonary edema who then become hypotensive after brisk diuresis. The most common precipitating factor is use of potent diuretic agents such as ethacrynic acid or furosemide.

Thus when blood pressure falls, a venous pressure of less than 80 mm of saline or wedge pressure (obtained with a balloon-tipped floating catheter of the Swan-Ganz type) of less than 12 mm Hg suggests the possibility of hypovolemia. Infusion of 100 ml increments of half-normal saline or low molecular weight dextran is initiated, with careful monitoring of the ventricular filling pressure. If blood pressure increases with little or no change in venous or wedge pressure, hypovolemia is indeed present. Some patients may receive 2 or 3 liters of fluid before filling pressure increases. However, if filling pressures rise promptly as the fluid is infused, it is unlikely that hypovolemia is a contributing factor to the hypotension.

Cardiogenic Shock. The patient in shock has a systolic blood pressure less than 90 mg Hg, is usually restless, and has reduced mental awareness, cyanosis, oliguria (less than 20 ml per hour) or even anuria, and cool, moist extremities. As discussed earlier, cardiac function is severly deranged. The function of the heart as a pump is inadequate to support life. Myocardial oxygenation is insufficient, and the heart produces lactate. Progressive metabolic acidosis is a hallmark of shock, and arterial pH should be measured frequently. Mortality remains high. Autopsy almost invariably reveals massive myocardial infarction with extensive coronary artery disease.

Treatable causes such as cardiac tamponade, hypovolemia, or serious arrhythmia should be sought and vigorously managed. Tamponade may be suspected when hypotension or shock is accompanied by marked distention of the neck veins or very high venous pressure. To evaluate the possibility of hypovolemia, central venous or wedge pressure should be measured, and, if low, the response to volume replacement, as described above, carefully evaluated.

Treatment of cardiogenic shock is unsatisfactory. Isoproterenol increases myocardial oxygen demand and induces lactate production in the ischemic heart. Its overall effect in cardiogenic shock is deleterious and it is contraindicated. Norepinephrine increases peripheral vascular resistance, improves myocardial contractility, and may decrease lactate production. Despite extensive use and many eloquent testimonials, convincing evidence that infusion of norepinephrine improves mortality in cardiogenic shock is lacking. Administration of so-called alpha-blocking agents such as phenoxybenzamine or phentolamine or of large doses of adrenal corticosteroids has been advocated. Although these are apparently effective in certain types of experimental shock, there is no evidence supporting their effectiveness in cardiogenic shock secondary to acute myocardial infarction. Support of the circulation with an intra-aortic counterpulsating balloon effectively reverses myocardial lactate production, reduces left ventricular filling pressure, and increases cardiac output and coronary blood flow. Unfortunately the device does not much improve survival when applied to patients with established shock. Early use of the device when cardiac work has acutely fallen and before clinical manifestations of shock appear may be helpful. A variety of devices for applying counterpulsation externally are being developed but await critical testing.

Emotional Aspects. Anxiety, denial, and depression are almost universal in the patient with myocardial infarction. Anxiety is most prominent during the first 24 hours, when pain, fear, close medical attention, and hospitalization are intensely experienced. Denial and unrealistic evaluation of symptoms may confuse interpretation of a potentially serious illness during the first few hours or days after onset of ischemic pain.

By the third day of illness, the emotional impact of the situation, knowledge of cardiac injury, and fear of disablement engender a normal sequence of reactions characterized by *depression*. It is important for the physician and nurse to recognize that depression is almost invariable in the patient with acute myocardial infarction. Treatment with an early rehabilitation program should begin no later than the third day after hospitalization, the usual time of onset of depression. Overemphasis on bed rest and inactivity is a focus for depression and causes rapid physical "deconditioning." Beginning after the third or fourth day, the value of a thorough explanation of the illness, outline of a positive rehabilitation program, and discussion of the depression and misconceptions about illness cannot be overemphasized. It is important to include the family in these discussions. The wise physician is aware that once the acute phase of illness is passed, his most important tasks are management of depression, rehabilitation, and institution of a reasonable long-term preventive program.

Rehabilitation. Bed rest for more than a short period is deleterious. Rapid "deconditioning" results in a decrease in work capacity, an increase in heart rate during effort, and orthostatic hypotension. Depression and feelings of helplessness are intensified by bed rest. The need for prolonged bed rest or hospitalization is being vigorously re-examined. Certainly bed rest should not be prescribed without good cause. Experiments in home care in Bristol, England, suggest that some patients will do well without hospitalization. A Boston study showed that patients without complications discharged after two weeks suffer no more morbidity than those with prolonged hospitalization. Even earlier discharge has been advocated for rapidly resolving T wave infarcts.

In the patient without complications passive exercise can begin after three or four days, about the time chair rest becomes appropriate. By a week after the infarct, slow walking about, daily toilet activities, and nonstressful paperwork can commence. Current evidence suggests that the uncomplicated patient may be discharged after two to three weeks. A gradual increase in physical activity is outlined to cover the next three to six weeks at home. The majority of patients can return to former occupations from six to twelve weeks after the acute infarction. Many factors such as age, extent of myocardial injury, presence of arrhythmia or heart failure, occupation, and personal ambition will modify the rehabilitation program.

Resumption of sexual activity is of concern to patient and spouse, although the subject may not be directly broached. Folklore emphasizes a hazard of sudden death during coitus. Hellerstein points out that the risks are greatly exaggerated. The oxygen cost of sexual activity in middle-aged men with spouse of long standing is equivalent to moderate exercise such as walking briskly or climbing one or two flights of stairs. Generally, sexual activity may be resumed in parallel with other normal moderate physical exertions.

Experimental Therapy. Patients with myocardial infarction who die from heart failure or shock have less viable myocardium at autopsy than those who die from arrhythmia. Pathologic studies suggest that reinfarction

or extension may be more common than is currently recognized clinically. After recovery, cardiac performance, especially during stress, may be importantly influenced by the mass and distribution of nonischemic, normally functioning myocardium.

In a significant series of experiments, Moroko and Braunwald have demonstrated a direct relationship between reduction of the area of acute myocardial ischemia after coronary occlusion and alteration of myocardial oxygen need or delivery. Reduction of oxygen requirement is correlated with a decrease in the extent of ischemia or infarction. Thus increase in coronary perfusion or reduction of afterload with vasodilators was associated with a smaller infarction. Infusion of potassium-insulin-glucose mixtures also limited myocardial damage. Whether this resulted from metabolic, osmotic, or other effects is not known. Hyaluronidase also had a protective effect. Conversely, factors which increased cardiac work, such as tachycardia or digitalis and glucagon in the nonfailing heart, increased the apparent ischemic area.

The possibility of controlling myocardial work and hence reducing infarct size has attracted widespread interest. Clinical data supporting this concept are not yet available. Careful study in man appears to be justified, but will be dependent on development of satisfactory methods to measure infarct size. Imaging techniques, CPK curve analysis, and precordial S-T segment mapping are being applied in many centers with varying success. The importance of clinical testing is illustrated by the difficulty in evaluating the usefulness of potassium-insulin-glucose preparations which were introduced as "polarizing" solutions in the mid-1960's. Many clinical studies have been performed. Few have been able to withstand close scientific scrutiny, and no clear-cut evidence of benefit is yet available.

Prognosis. Mortality is greatest during the first few hours, before most patients reach a hospital. The risk declines rapidly from onset of the acute attack. Studies from both Belfast and Edinburgh have revealed essentially the same findings: 50 per cent of the deaths from acute myocardial infarction occur within the first 2 hours and 15 minutes after the onset of the illness. Approximately three fourths of all deaths occur within the first 24 hours. The majority of the early deaths are sudden, owing to electrical instability of the heart, and are not necessarily related to the size of the infarct or the development of heart failure.

Reliable data for total mortality outside and inside the hospital in acute myocardial infarction are difficult to obtain. Oliver observed that 42 per cent of all patients under 70 died during the first four weeks. At the end of six months the total mortality was 49 per cent. The greatest risk was incurred by women age 60 to 69, in whom the mortality was 52 per cent at four weeks and rose to 59 per cent after six months.

The patient who is admitted to hospital has already survived a considerable risk. Prognosis after recovery depends upon many factors, including age, history of previous infarctions, presence of diabetes, presence of heart failure, mental attitude, type of employment, and employment policies. Patients who have survived ventricular fibrillation and successful resuscitation have an excellent prognosis in the absence of heart failure. Persistent heart failure and frequent ventricular ectopic beats warrant a guarded prognosis. If cardiac function is well maintained six weeks after acute infarction, most patients are able to return to previous employment and a full range of normal activity. Serial evaluation of left ventricular size with a calibrated roentgenogram exposed at end-diastole at known lung volume is of considerable prognostic value. During almost one year of follow-up in one study, 8 per cent of postinfarct patients with normal heart volume died. In those with enlarged hearts, mortality was threefold higher and functional status significantly more impaired.

Alonso, D., Scheidt, S., Post, M., and Killip, T.: Pathophysiology of cardiogenic shock. Quantification of myocardial necrosis, clinical, pathologic and electrocardiographic correlations. Circulation, 48:588, 1973.

Case, R. B., Nasser, M. G., and Crampton, R. S.: Biochemical aspects of early myocardial ischemia. Am. J. Cardiol., 24:766, 1969.

Coronary Drug Project Research Group: Prognostic importance of premature beats following myocardial infarction. Experience in the Coronary Drug Project. J.A.M.A., 223:1116, 1973.

Epstein, S. E., Goldstein, R. E., Redwood, D. R., Kent, K. M., and Smith, E. R.: The early phase of acute myocardial infarction: Pharmacologic aspects of therapy. Ann. Intern. Med., 78:918, 1973.

Erhardt, L. R., Lundman, T., and Mellstedt, H.: Incorporation of ^{125}I-labelled fibrinogen into coronary arterial thrombi in acute myocardial infarction in man. Lancet, 1:387, 1973.

Fillmore, S. J., Gumaraes, A. C., Scheidt, S. S., and Killip, T.: Blood-gas changes and pulmonary hemodynamics following acute myocardial infarction. Circulation, 45:583, 1972.

Hackett, T. P., and Cassem, N. H.: The psychological adaption of myocardial infarction patients to convalescence. Heart and Lung, 2:382, 1973.

Heikkila, J.: Mitral incompetence as a complication of acute myocardial infarction. Acta Med. Scand. (Suppl.) 475:1–139, 1967.

Hellerstein, H. K., and Friedman, E. H.: Sexual activity and the post coronary patient. Arch. Intern. Med., 125:987, 1970.

Hutter, A. M., Sidel, V. W., Shine, K. I., and DeSanctis, R. W.: Early hospital discharge after myocardial infarction. N. Engl. J. Med., 288:1141, 1973.

Killip, T.: Management of arrhythmias in acute myocardial infarction. Hosp. Practice, 7:131, 1972.

Maroko, P. R., and Braunwald, E.: Modification of myocardial infarction size after coronary occlusion. Ann. Intern. Med., 79:720, 1973.

Nyquist, O.: Shock complicating acute myocardial infarction. Acta Med. Scand. (Suppl.) 536:1–72, 1972.

Scheidt, S., Ascheim, R., and Killip, T.: Shock after acute myocardial infarction: A clinical and hemodynamic profile. Am. J. Cardiol., 26:556, 1970.

Scheidt, S., Wilner, G., Fillmore, S., Shapiro, M., and Killip, T.: Objective haemodynamic assessment after acute myocardial infarction. Br. Heart J., 35:908, 1973.

Scheidt, S., Wilner, G., Mueller, H., Summers, D., Lesch, M., Wolff, G., Krakauer, J., Rubenfire, M., Fleming, P., Noon, G., Oldham, N., Killip, T., and Kantrowitz, A.: Intra-aortic balloon counter pulsation in cardiogenic shock. Report of a co-operative clinical trial. N. Engl. J. Med., 288:979, 1973.

Sobel, B. E., and Shell, W. E.: Serum enzyme determinations in the diagnosis and assessment of myocardial infarction. Circulation, 45:471, 1972.

Solomon, H. A., Edwards, A. L., and Killip, T.: Prodromata in acute myocardial infarction. Circulation, 40:463, 1969.

Weinblatt, E., Shapiro, S., Frank, C., and Sager, R.: Prognosis of men after first myocardial infarction: Mortality and first recurrence in relation to selected parameters. Am. J. Public Health, 58:1329, 1968.

Wilson, C., and Pantridge, J. F.: ST-segment displacement and early hospital discharge in acute myocardial infarction. Lancet, 3:1284, 1973.

Wolk, M. J., Scheidt, S., and Killip, T.: Heart failure complicating acute myocardial infarction. Circulation, 45:1125, 1972.

568. SUDDEN DEATH

Unexpected, rapid demise in the apparently healthy individual has recently been recognized as a major health problem. Considerable information has accumulated describing sudden death in a variety of circumstances. The perplexing problem of unexpected crib death is well known to the pediatrician. A familial syndrome of deafness, prolonged Q-T interval, and sudden death has been described. The Dalmatian coach hound suffers from a similar condition. Sudden death during or after exertion in aortic stenosis and idiopathic hypertrophic subaortic stenosis (asymmetrical septal hypertrophy, hypertrophic obstructive cardiomyopathy) is an ever-present, though statistically small, threat. Noncardiac in origin but responsive to emergency treatment is the "restaurant arrest" syndrome secondary to aspiration of a large bolus of meat with rapid asphyxia, usually associated with excess alcohol intake.

Instantaneous (a few minutes) and sudden (hours) unexpected death in the adult has been repeatedly shown to be associated with coronary artery disease in the overwhelming majority. Extensive coronary disease is the almost invariable autopsy finding in instantaneous death; evidence of acute infarction or coronary thrombosis is rare. When death occurs within a few hours of onset of symptoms, the incidence of coronary thrombosis and myocardial infarction is significantly higher.

Evidence from several epidemiologic surveys indicates that the majority of individuals who die suddenly have antemortem signs, symptoms, or significant risk factors suggesting coronary artery disease. Particular attention has focused on abnormalities of the electrocardiogram. Evidence of left bundle branch block, left axis deviation with right bundle branch block, left ventricular hypertrophy, or old infarction is associated with increased risk of sudden death. In the patient with coronary artery disease, a single ventricular premature complex recorded during routine electrocardiography or the detection of ten ventricular extrasystoles per 1000 beats is reported to increase the risk of sudden death seven- to tenfold! Despite recognition of some risk factors, there is unfortunately no information yet available on effective preventive therapy.

Many individuals who die suddenly can be resuscitated if trained personnel are available. High risk areas in hospital are the emergency room, cardiac and intensive care units, operating room, and recovery room. A long-term survival rate of 20 per cent after resuscitation has been reported from a general hospital with an intesive staff educational program. Most sudden deaths occur outside the hospital and are usually secondary to ventricular fibrillation. If life can be supported with mouth-to-mouth ventilation and closed-chest cardiac massage, defibrillation with recovery is possible.

The experience of the Seattle, Washington, community under the leadership of Alvarez and Cobb is testimony to what can be accomplished in prehospital emergency care. A system based on a rapid (two- to five-minute) response time by the fire department paramedics trained to a near-physician capability, resuscitation and defibrillation on the spot, and intense public education has proved remarkably effective. During three years, in a community of about 500,000 persons, 202 patients with cardiac or respiratory arrest outside a hospital were treated in the field, brought to a hospital, and subsequently discharged home. Seventy per cent had ventricular fibrillation. Several important observations have developed from this experience: Survival is nil if arrival of the rescue team occurs more than five minutes after the call is placed. Over 20 per cent of the successful resuscitations were initiated by lay bystanders. (Approximately 20 per cent of the Seattle population has been instructed in cardiopulmonary resuscitation.) The rate of survival has improved steadily with increasing experience and is currently about 22 per cent.

Long-term outlook in those survivors with evidence of myocardial infarction is good. When EKG criteria alone were used to diagnose acute transmural infarction, mortality after two years was 14 per cent. The survivor with no evidence of myocardial infarction has a high probability of suffering cardiac arrest again. Mortality after two years in those without infarctions was 43 per cent. These observations suggest that cardiac arrest not caused by acute myocardial infarction is likely to recur and may well be related to problems of conduction and arrhythmia in the presence of coronary artery disease without recognized ischemia.

Physicians, nurses, rescue squads, and paramedical personnel have an important obligation to maintain technical skills in cardiopulmonary resuscitation, because they may be called upon to provide or supervise emergency support of life at any time. The gratifying Seattle experience challenges medical leadership in many another community.

Cobb, L. A., and Alvarez, H.: Medic I: The Seattle system for management of out of hospital emergencies. Proceedings of National Conference in Standards for Cardio-Pulmonary Resuscitation and Emergency Cardiac Care. National Research Council, 1974.

Coronary Drug Project Research Group: Prognostic importance of premature beats following myocardial infarction. Experience in the Coronary Drug Project. J.A.M.A., 223:1116, 1973.

Eller, W. C., and Hangen, R. K.: Food asphyxiation — restaurant rescue. N. Engl. J. Med., 289:81, 1973.

Fraser, G. R., Froggat, P., and James, T. N.: Congenital deafness with electrocardiographic abnormalities, fainting attacks and sudden death: A recessive syndrome. Quart. J. Med., 33:361, 1964.

Friedman, M., Manwaring, J. H., Rosenman, R. H., Donlon, G., Ortega, P., and Grube, S.: Instantaneous and sudden deaths. Clinical and pathological differentiation in coronary artery disease. J.A.M.A., 225:1319, 1973.

Fulton, M., Lutz, W., Donald, K. W., Kirby, B. J., Duncan, B., Morrison, S. L., Kerr, F., Julian, D. G., and Oliver, M. F.: Natural history of unstable angina. Lancet, 1:860, 1972.

Kuller, L., Lilenfield, A., Fisher, R.: Sudden and unexpected deaths in young adults. J.A.M.A., 198:158, 1966.

CARDIAC ARRHYTHMIA

Anthony N. Damato

569. INTRODUCTION

Normally, the pacemaker of the heart is the sinoatrial (SA) node, which is an elongated structure (1.5 cm in length) located at the junction of the superior vena cava and the lateral border of the right atrium. In 55 per cent of cases the SA node receives its blood supply from the right coronary artery, and in 45 per cent of the cases, from the left circumflex artery. Cells of the SA node possess the property of automaticity which is responsible for the spontaneous rhythmicity of the heart beat. Automatic or pacemaker cells undergo spontaneous diastolic depolarization (phase 4 depolarization) in contrast to nonautomatic or working myocardial cells which maintain a steady diastolic or resting potential. When an automatic cell achieves threshold potential, it undergoes depolarization and serves as the excitatory or depolarizing stimulus for adjacent cells. Increasing the rate of diastolic depolarization of sinoatrial nodal pacemaker cells increases the heart rate and vice versa. The property of spontaneous diastolic depolarization can also be found in certain cells of the atrium, atrioventricular (AV) junction, bundle branches, and Purkinje network, but not in ordinary working myocardial cells. These specialized cells serve as latent or potential pacemakers of the heart, and their rate of spontaneous diastolic depolarization is normally less than that of the sinoatrial node. However, if sinus node function is depressed, latent pacemaker activity can emerge and establish an escape rhythm. At other times, certain stimuli such as digitalis excess, ischemia, or hypoxia can enhance the rate of spontaneous diastolic depolarization of latent pacemakers beyond that of normal sinus node automaticity, which results in an ectopic rhythm.

The transmission of impulses from the sinus node to the ventricles occurs along specialized conducting tissue which includes the AV node, the bundle of His (also called the common AV bundle), the right bundle branch, the left bundle branch, including its fascicular divisions, and the subendocardial Purkinje network. The bundle of His, bundle branches, and Purkinje network are commonly referred to as the His-Purkinje system or the ventricular specialized conducting system. In addition, three internodal connecting pathways (anterior, middle, and posterior internodal tracts) have been described which originate from the sinus node region and insert into different parts of the AV node. Fibers from these internodal pathways also spread in various degrees from the right to the left atrium. It has been suggested by some investigators that transmission of the sinus node impulse to the AV node and between the atria is along these specialized and preferential pathways and not by radial spread alone. Internodal pathways have also been invoked to explain some cases of short P-R interval in which it is suspected that an atrial impulse either partially or completely bypasses the AV node during its conduction to the ventricles.

The AV node lies beneath the right atrial endocardium, anterior to the os of the coronary sinus, and above the insertion of the septal leaflet of the tricuspid valve. The human adult AV node measures between 5 and 7 mm in length, and its deep surface abuts the central fibrous body of the heart. Anteriorly, the AV node is directly continuous with the bundle of His. Most of the fibers of the internodal tracts, mentioned above, enter the superior and posterior margins of the AV node, and a smaller number of fibers enter along its lateral margin. Conduction velocity within the AV node is slow (0.05 meter per second), which accounts in part for the normal physiologic AV delay that is reflected in the P-R interval. In most human hearts, the AV node receives its blood supply from the right coronary artery, which explains the association of AV nodal conduction abnormalities seen in some cases of inferior or diaphragmatic myocardial infarctions.

The anterior and deep part of the AV node becomes the common AV bundle or bundle of His in which the muscle fibers are arranged in parallel. The bundle of His penetrates the collagenous central fibrous body and lies on the upper margin of the muscular interventricular septum. At the posterior margin of the membranous interventricular septum the common bundle gives off a relatively wide left bundle branch which courses over the left side of the interventricular septum. The left bundle branch divides into anterior and posterior fascicles which enter the anterior and posterior papillary muscles, respectively. In addition, fibers from the left bundle insert directly into the interventricular septum. On the right side of the heart, the common bundle continues as a slender right bundle branch which courses over the interventricular septum and enters the anterior papillary muscle. Peripheral arborization of the right and left bundle branches constitutes the Purkinje network. In contrast to the AV node, the velocity of conduction throughout the His-Purkinje system is more rapid, being within the order of 1.0 to 3.5 meters per second.

The AV node and the proximal portion of the bundle of His are in close anatomic relationship to the tricuspid and mitral valve rings. In addition, the distal part of the bundle of His and the proximal portions of the bundle branches lie in close proximity to the noncoronary artery aortic cusp. These anatomic relationships of the AV conducting system are important to bear in mind, because inflammation, fibrosis, or calcification of the valve rings or central fibrous body may cause different types of AV block.

The P-R interval represents a combination of intra-atrial, AV nodal, and His-Purkinje conduction times. Unfortunately, the electrical activities of the sinus node, AV node, bundle of His, bundle branches, and subendocardial Purkinje network are not recorded by the surface electrocardiogram. Figure 1 presents in a schematic way the electrical events occurring during the P-R interval. The sinus node generates an impulse prior to the inscription of the P wave. As the atrial muscle is being depolarized (P wave), the sinus node impulse enters the AV node. Conduction within the bundle of His, bundle branches, and subendocardial Purkinje network occurs during the P-R segment. The QRS complex represents depolarization of the ventricular muscle.

It has become possible to record electrical activity of the bundle of His in man, using an electrode catheter which is fluoroscopically positioned in the region of the tricuspid valve. The electrode catheter records a low atrial electrogram (A), a His bundle deflection (H) which appears as a bi- or triphasic deflection within the P-R segment, and a ventricular electrogram (V) (Fig. 2). His bundle recordings permit division of the P-R interval into two subintervals, namely the A-H and H-V intervals. The A-H interval represents an approximation of AV nodal conduction time, and the H-V interval represents conduction time within the His-Purkinje system. Normal values for A-H and H-V intervals have varied slightly as reported by different investigators, but in

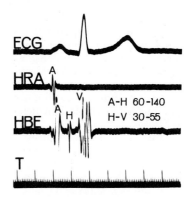

Figure 2. Tracings from top to bottom are as follows: surface EKG; a recording from the high right atrium (HRA); His bundle electrogram recording (HBE); and time lines (T) at 10 and 100 msec. A = Low atrial electrogram; H = His bundle electrogram; V = ventricular electrogram. During sinus rhythm the sequence of activation is from the high to low atrium. During retrograde conduction across the AV node, the sequence of atrial activation is reversed; the low atrial electrogram precedes the high atrial electrogram.

general are 60 to 140 msec and 30 to 55 msec, respectively. Bundle of His recordings provide a more precise method of localizing sites of AV conduction delay and block which may occur proximal to, within, or distal to the bundle of His. In addition, bundle of His recordings provide an accurate method for determining whether beats are of supraventricular or ventricular origin. Beats of supraventricular origin are preceded by His deflections with H-V intervals which are normal or greater than normal. In general, beats of ventricular origin are not preceded by His deflections.

570. ARRHYTHMIAS

SINUS ARRHYTHMIA

Sinus arrhythmia is characterized by irregular changes in the sinus rate which most often occur in relationship to the phases of respiration. The sinus rate increases at end inspiration and decreases at end expiration. The respiratory changes in sinus rate are believed to result from changes in vagal tone. Sinus arrhythmia is a normal phenomenon seen more frequently in children and young adults and tends to become less pronounced with increasing age. Electrocardiographically the P wave configuration is normal but may show slight changes in shape. The P-P intervals show cyclical increases and decreases in relation to the phase of respiration, whereas the P-R intervals remain fairly constant. Sinus arrhythmia requires no treatment.

SINUS BRADYCARDIA

Sinus bradycardia has been arbitrarily defined as a sinus rate of less than 60 per minute. It is a normal finding in a significant number of young healthy adults and is the expected finding in well trained athletes. Sinus bradycardia may result from administration of drugs such as digitalis, propranolol, morphine, reserpine, and prostigmine. Normal sinus rates return when these

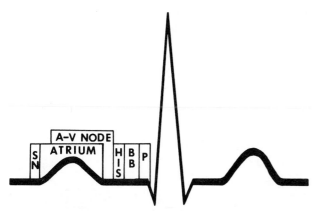

Figure 1. Schematic representation of the sequence of AV conduction in relationship to the P wave, P-R segment and QRS complex. SN = sinus node impulse; AV node = atrioventricular node; HIS = His bundle; BB = bundle branches; P = subendocardial Purkinje system. (Modified from Hoffman, B. F., and Singer, D. H.: Prog. Cardiovasc. Dis., 7:226, 1964.

drugs are withdrawn. A temporary sinus bradycardia may occur during acute diaphragmatic myocardial infarction. Usually, sinus bradycardia is associated with normal AV conduction (1:1 AV response with a normal P-R interval). In older patients AV block may signify depression of both sinus and AV nodes. Sinus bradycardia at rates of 40 per minute or less should raise the possibility of a 2:1 sinus node exit block, which is a rare phenomenon (see Fig. 4).

In general, sinus bradycardia requires no treatment. In most cases, the sinus rate shows a normal acceleration in response to exercise, atropine, or other appropriate stimuli. An inappropriate response to such stimuli raises the possibility of the sick sinus syndrome. If symptoms such as lightheadedness, syncope, congestive heart failure, or angina pectoris are the result of a low resting heart rate or inappropriate acceleration of the heart rate during stressful situations, a permanent ventricular pacemaker should be inserted.

SINUS TACHYCARDIA

For adults, sinus tachycardia is defined as a sinus rate in excess of 100 per minute. Most often, sinus tachycardia represents a normal physiologic response to stressful situations such as exercise, fright, emotional upset, fever, congestive heart failure, and hypotension. Under these conditions, the increase in sinus rate is generally associated with a normal or less than normal P-R interval, because the sympathetic stimuli causing sinus node acceleration also enhance AV nodal conduction. Vagolytic drugs, such as atropine, can also produce a sinus tachycardia. The treatment for sinus tachycardia is that of the underlying condition. Carotid sinus pressure will produce a temporary and incomplete slowing of the sinus rate which quickly returns to original levels. If sinus tachycardia is the result of congestive heart failure, digitalis will slow the sinus rate as the failure improves. However, digitalis will be ineffective in sinus tachycardias from other causes such as fever or thyrotoxicosis.

SICK SINUS SYNDROME

The sick sinus syndrome (SSS) refers to a variety of electrocardiographic abnormalities which result from dysfunction of the sinoatrial node. Included in SSS are the following:

1. Persistent, severe, or unexpected sinus bradycardia. At times, sinus bradycardia may alternate with episodes of supraventricular tachyarrhythmias, and this combination has been termed the bradycardia-tachycardia syndrome.

2. Sinoatrial block or exit block not related to drug therapy.

3. Sinus arrest (cessation of sinus rhythm) for short or long intervals, during which time either no escape rhythm arises or an atrial, junctional, or ventricular rhythm emerges.

These electrocardiographic abnormalities result because (1) the sinus node fails as an impulse generator, or (2) the sinus node impulse is delayed or blocked in its conduction out to the atrial muscle. Often, patients with SSS have an associated AV block or intraventricular conduction abnormality. The most commonly encountered symptoms in SSS are lightheadedness, dizziness, syncope, convulsions, dyspnea, fatigue, and angina pectoris.

Sinus Bradycardia

Sinus bradycardia may be the initial manifestation of SSS, and consequently not all sinus bradycardias are benign. SSS should be suspected when sinus bradycardia occurs in a symptomatic patient or is an inappropriate response to the clinical environs, such as during exercise, fever, pain, or congestive heart failure. Failure of the sinus rate to increase after atropine administration should raise the possibility of SSS, and further observations are indicated.

Bradycardia-Tachycardia Syndrome

The bradycardia-tachycardia syndrome is included in the spectrum of SSS and is characterized by sinus bradycardia alternating with episodes of atrial tachycardia, atrial fibrillation, or atrial flutter. The atrial tachycardia may be ectopic in origin or may result from AV nodal re-entry (Fig. 3). Symptoms may be related to either slow or rapid heart rates or both.

Treatment. Sinus bradycardia as a manifestation of SSS is generally, although not always, unresponsive to pharmacologic treatment. If belladonna alkaloids, atropine, or sympathomimetic amines are ineffectual in speeding up the sinus rate and the patient is symptomatic from the slow heart rate, a permanent ventricular pacemaker should be inserted. In the bradycardia-tachycardia syndrome the therapeutic problem is compounded by the fact that not only are agents such as procainamide and quinidine often ineffectual in controlling the atrial tachyarrhythmias, but these drugs may aggravate the sinus bradycardia. Likewise, digitalis,

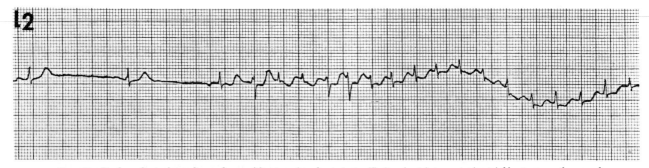

Figure 3. Bradycardia-tachycardia syndrome. After two sinus beats (rate, 45 per minute), two ectopic atrial beats occur, the second of which initiates an AV nodal re-entrant tachycardia. The initial part of the tachycardia shows aberrant ventricular conduction.

which can effectively slow the ventricular response during a period of supraventricular tachycardia, may also worsen the bradycardia. The most effective therapy to date has been the insertion of a permanent ventricular pacemaker by which the ventricular rate can be controlled and pharmacologic agents more safely administered to control the atrial arrhythmia.

SINOATRIAL BLOCK

The tissue surrounding the sinoatrial node normally imposes a conduction delay between the sinus node impulse and depolarization of the atrial myocardium. Disturbances in conduction of the sinus node impulse can take the form of first, second, or third degree SA block, all of which constitute uncommon manifestations of the clinical spectrum of SSS. Because of the inability to record the sinus node impulse in man, the diagnosis of SA block is an inferential one based primarily on the behavior of the P waves.

First Degree SA Block

In the first degree SA block the sinus node impulse is conducted more slowly out to the atrial myocardium. However, the clinical diagnosis of uncomplicated first-degree SA block cannot be made, because each sinus impulse elicits a P wave and the degree of delay is not reflected in the EKG recording.

Second Degree SA Block

Second degree SA block, like second degree AV block, has been classified into types I and II.

Type I Second Degree SA Block

In type I second degree SA block, sinoatrial conduction is of a Wenckebach type in which there is progressive conduction delay until a sinus node impulse fails to elicit a P wave. Like AV nodal Wenckebach cycles, the increment of SA conduction delay decreases throughout the cycle so that the P-P intervals progressively shorten prior to the dropped P wave. The P-P interval encompassing the dropped P wave is less than twice the P-P interval preceding the absent P wave.

Type II Second Degree SA Block

In type II second degree SA block, a sinus P wave is intermittently and unexpectedly dropped. The resultant pause is equal to twice the normal P-P interval. Atrial extrasystoles, which are hidden in the T wave and followed by a near compensatory pause, may simulate a type II SA block. In 2:1 SA block the normal sinus rate is halved. The resultant bradycardia is indistinguishable from the usual variety of sinus bradycardia unless an abrupt spontaneous doubling of the heart rate occurs (Fig. 4). Atrial bigeminy in which the ectopic P waves are masked by the T wave may simulate 2:1 SA block.

Third Degree SA Block

In third degree SA block, all the sinus impulses are blocked and there is absence of P waves. After a period of arrest, a subsidiary pacemaker located in the atrium, AV junction, or ventricles usually emerges as an escape rhythm. Third degree SA block is indistinguishable from sinus node arrest in which the pacemaker cells fail to generate impulses (Fig. 5).

ABERRATION

Ventricular aberration is defined as an alteration in the sequence of ventricular activation which results whenever an impulse of supraventricular origin is asynchronously conducted within the His-Purkinje system. Aberration results because a supraventricular impulse enters the His-Purkinje system during its refractory period. For atrial impulses the determinants of aberration include (1) the degree of prematurity of the atrial impulse; (2) the cycle length (R-R interval) preceding the premature atrial impulse; (3) the speed of AV nodal conduction; and (4) the state of recovery of excitability of the His-Purkinje system. In general, the more premature an atrial impulse, the greater the tendency for aberration to occur. Fast or relatively rapid AV nodal conduction enhances the possibility of aberration, because the premature atrial impulse can be delivered to the His-Purkinje system during its refractory period. However, at very close coupling intervals, aberrant ventricular activation may disappear if the premature atrial impulse encounters sufficient AV nodal delay that its arrival time within the His-Purkinje system is delayed and the latter is no longer refractory.

A direct relationship exists between cycle length (R-R interval) and refractoriness within the His-Purkinje system. Refractoriness of the His-Purkinje system increases with longer R-R intervals and decreases as the R-R interval shortens. A long R-R interval preceding a sufficiently premature atrial beat favors aberration, whereas de-

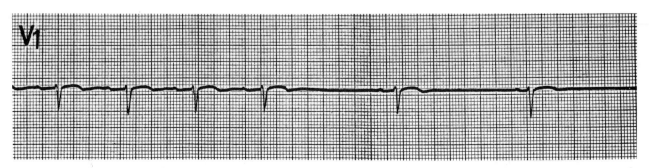

Figure 4. 2:1 SA exit block. The sinus rate is suddenly halved.

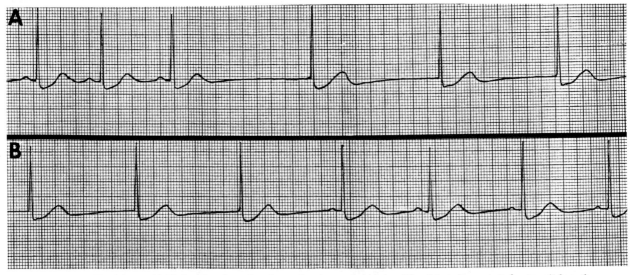

Figure 5.   Third degree SA block. After three sinus beats, the sinus node impulse either fails to be generated or to exit from the sinus node. An AV junctional pacemaker emerges, followed by resumption of sinus rhythm. During the AV junctional rhythm, the QRS complexes are similar to those of sinus origin.

creasing the preceding cycle length may abolish aberration.

Aberrant conduction involving the right bundle branch is seen more commonly than aberration involving the left bundle branch. Given the right conditions, aberrant ventricular activation can occur in normal or abnormal hearts and therefore it is not of itself a sign of heart disease. Aberrant conduction of consecutive beats during a supraventricular tachycardia can mimic a ventricular tachycardia. Examples of aberrant conduction of supraventricular impulses are shown in Figures 3, 6, 8, 9, 11, and 29.

ATRIAL EXTRASYSTOLES

Atrial extrasystoles are premature depolarizations of the atria resulting from impulses which originate in ectopic foci located anywhere within the atria. Atrial extrasystoles are also referred to as premature atrial beats, premature atrial contractions, or premature atrial systoles.

Atrial extrasystoles result in P waves (P') which are different from sinus P waves. These differences, which may be marked or subtle, are due to an altered sequence of atrial activation resulting from an ectopic origin of the depolarizing impulse.

Atrial extrasystoles may have a constant or inconstant coupling interval to the preceding sinus beat and can occur in a bigeminal or trigeminal sequence. Three or more consecutive atrial extrasystoles occurring at a rate of 100 per minute or greater constitute an ectopic atrial tachycardia.

Atrial extrasystoles occurring late in the diastolic period may be associated with little or no AV conduction delay, in which case the P-R interval will be the same as or close to that of the sinus beats. Extrasystoles of greater prematurity are almost always associated with an increased P-R interval (relative to sinus beats), which may be due to conduction delay within the AV node, His-Purkinje system, or both.

Atrial extrasystoles may result in normal or aberrant ventricular activation, the determinants of which are discussed above. Aberrant ventricular activation may mimic premature ventricular extrasystoles if the premature atrial P' wave is not recognized or is obscured within the T wave of the preceding QRS complex (Fig. 6). Atrial extrasystoles which are not conducted to the ventricles may block within the AV node or His-Purkinje system. A nonconducted atrial extrasystole may result in prolongation of the P-R interval of one or more subsequent sinus beats—a phenomenon which is called concealed conduction.

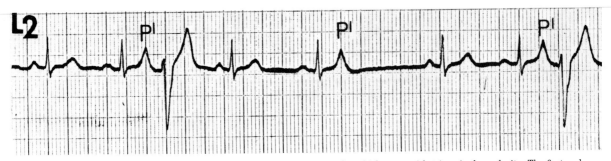

Figure 6.   The third, sixth, and ninth P waves (P') are atrial extrasystoles which occur with trigeminal regularity. The first and third atrial extrasystoles are aberrantly conducted to the ventricles. The second atrial extrasystole is blocked.

Atrial extrasystoles generally invade and prematurely depolarize the sinus node pacemaker, causing a reset of the sinus cycle which is reflected in the pause that follows the atrial extrasystole. If the delay in the appearance of the postextrasystolic sinus beat equals the prematurity of the atrial extrasystole, the pause is said to be compensatory. In a fully compensatory pause, the sum of the pre- and postextrasystolic R-R intervals equals two sinus cycle lengths. Complete compensatory pauses are uncommonly associated with atrial extrasystoles. More often, one sees postextrasystolic pauses which are incompletely compensatory; that is, the sum of the pre- and postextrasystolic pauses is less than two sinus cycles. Occasionally, one may see significant suppression of sinus node automaticity after an extrasystole.

Atrial extrasystoles are common and may occur in completely normal individuals or may be associated with various types of organic heart disease. They may presage atrial fibrillation, atrial flutter, ectopic atrial tachycardias, or AV nodal re-entrant tachycardias. Very often, patients are unaware of the presence of infrequent atrial extrasystoles, and no special treatment is required. The patient may complain of "skipped beats" and "palpitations" which are the result of the pause and forceful ventricular contraction that follow the extrasystole. Mild sedation and abstinence from alcohol, tobacco, or caffeine may be all that is required to treat occasional extrasystoles which produce mild symptoms. Quinidine sulfate is used to treat atrial extrasystoles which cause disturbing symptoms, foreshadow other atrial arrhythmias, or are unabated by conservative measures.

ATRIAL FIBRILLATION

Atrial fibrillation is a frequently encountered cardiac arrhythmia which commonly occurs in association with some form of organic heart disease. Most cases of atrial fibrillation are associated with arteriosclerotic heart disease, followed in frequency by rheumatic and hypertensive heart diseases. A high incidence of this rhythm disorder is seen in patients with thyrotoxicosis. The greater tendency for enlarged atria to fibrillate may explain the frequent occurrence of atrial fibrillation in patients with congestive heart failure and mitral valvular disease. Atrial fibrillation, usually paroxysmal in nature, can occur in apparently healthy individuals who have no detectable evidence of associated heart disease.

The exact mechanism(s) underlying the development of atrial fibrillation is uncertain. Many of its characteristics are compatible with re-entry of multiple activation fronts. However, the fact that atrial fibrillation is frequently induced by premature atrial extrasystoles suggests that alterations in automaticity also play a role in the mechanism of this arrhythmia. Factors which favor the development and perpetuation of atrial fibrillation include frequent atrial extrasystoles, increased vagal tone, and an increase in atrial muscle mass wherein significant differences in conduction and refractoriness exist in adjacent fibers. Atrial fibrillation can be precipitated by a single atrial extrasystole which occurs in the so-called vulnerable period of the atrial cycle. At sinus cycle lengths the atrial vulnerable period has been estimated to be between 180 and 300 msec after a sinus P wave.

Electrocardiographic Features. Atrial fibrillation is characterized by absence of P waves and an irregular ventricular response. Normal sinus P waves are replaced by irregular chaotic and rapid atrial impulses occurring in excess of 400 per minute. The presence or absence of P waves is best observed in leads II and V_1. Atrial fibrillation has been described as "coarse" when the baseline of the electrocardiogram presents rapid, irregular fibrillatory (f) waves of varying amplitude, and "fine" when practically no atrial activity is detected. In untreated and uncomplicated atrial fibrillation, the irregular and rapid ventricular response is generally between 110 and 160 per minute, and most or all of the QRS complexes are of normal configuration for that patient (Fig. 7).

Concealed conduction within the AV node is the major determinant of the irregular R-R cycles during atrial fibrillation. The inherent capacity of the AV node to accept and transmit impulses to the ventricles is exceeded by the rapid, irregular atrial rate in atrial fibrillation. Consequently, many atrial impulses are blocked or concealed within the AV node, thereby altering its state of refractoriness which in turn affects the conduction of subsequent impulses. Impulses which exit from the AV node and enter the His-Purkinje system almost invariably result in a ventricular response. Uncommonly is the His-Purkinje system the site of concealment. Digitalis, propranolol, or increased vagal tone increases the degree of concealment or block within the AV node and thereby slows the ventricular response. The irregular R-R intervals during atrial fibrillation predispose to the occurrence of aberrant intraventricular conduction. In atrial fibrillation the distinction between aberrant conduction and ventricular ectopy is an important one which unfortunately is made more difficult because of the absence of P waves. The diagnosis of aberrant conduction is favored (80 per cent of the time) if the beat in question (1) has a right bundle branch block pattern, (2) terminates a short cycle which is preceded by a long cycle, and (3) has initial

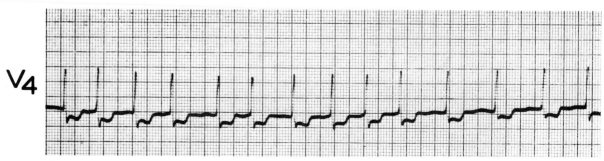

Figure 7. Untreated atrial fibrillation. There is absence of P waves with an irregular ventricular rate.

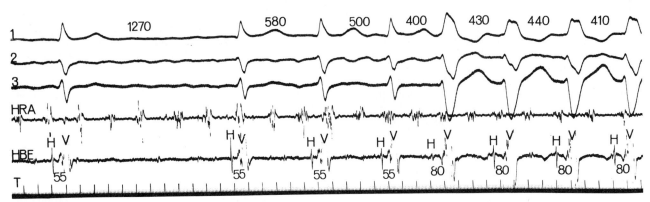

Figure 8. Atrial fibrillation with aberrant ventricular conduction. The R-R intervals are indicated above. The first four beats are the patient's normal QRS complexes with H-V intervals of 55 msec. The last four beats result from supraventricular impulses which are aberrantly conducted with a left bundle branch block pattern. The increase in H-V interval of 80 msec reflects conduction delay in the right bundle also.

vector forces which are the same as known supraventricular beats. No single criterion or combination of criteria provides absolute evidence for the origin of any beat. The distinction can be made with bundle of His recordings. In atrial fibrillation with a rapid ventricular response, aberration may persist for many consecutive cycles and may simulate ventricular tachycardia (Fig. 8). The occurrence of aberrant conduction during digitalis administration for atrial fibrillation is not a contraindication to continued use of the drug. In fact aberration usually disappears when the desired effect of ventricular slowing is achieved with digitalis. On the other hand, ventricular ectopy may signify digitalis toxicity or the presence of an additional dysrhythmic problem.

Treatment. Treatment of atrial fibrillation depends upon the urgency of the situation. If the irregular rapid ventricular response is causing severe dyspnea, hypotension, congestive heart failure, or severe anginal pain, conversion to normal sinus rhythm by DC countershock is the treatment of choice. DC countershock is contraindicated if it is suspected that digitalis intoxication is the cause of atrial fibrillation, which is uncommon. In less urgent situations, ventricular slowing is achieved with digitalis. Digoxin, 0.5 mg, is given intravenously and followed by a second dose in one half to one hour. If the ventricular rate is slowed (80 to 100 per minute), maintenance therapy of 0.25 mg digoxin per day is started. If the ventricular rate is not slowed within 2 hours of the initial dose, 0.25 mg digoxin is given every 3 to 4 hours until the desired effect is obtained. Infrequently, digitalis may convert atrial fibrillation to sinus rhythm.

Once the ventricular rate is under control, consideration is given as to whether conversion to sinus rhythm is indicated. Conversion should not be attempted in those patients who have longstanding chronic atrial fibrillation, or in whom previous conversions have been unsuccessfully maintained. In some patients with severe heart disease, the loss of atrial contribution to the cardiac output may be significant, and conversion to sinus rhythm is necessary in order to avoid intractable heart failure. Patients with atrial fibrillation of recent onset should be converted to sinus rhythm, using either DC countershock or quinidine sulfate. The maintenance dose of digitalis should be withheld for 1 to 2 days prior to DC countershock.

ATRIAL FLUTTER

Atrial flutter is characterized by a rapid, regular atrial rate between 220 and 350 beats per minute. However, there is no universal agreement about which range of atrial rates specifically defines atrial flutter and separates it from an ectopic atrial tachycardia. There can be an overlap in the lower ranges of atrial rate; some ectopic atrial tachycardias may achieve atrial rates of 220 beats per minute, whereas some cases of atrial flutter may be associated with rates of less than 220 beats per minute. Atrial flutter is almost always associated with some form of organic heart disease (coronary artery disease, cor pulmonale, rheumatic valvular disease), and rarely does it occur in normal healthy individuals. Digitalis is rarely a cause of atrial flutter. Clinical symptoms associated with atrial flutter are related primarily to the ventricular response. Atrial flutter with a 3:1 or 4:1 AV conduction ratio may result in no symptoms, and the patient may be unaware of any dysrhythmia. On the other hand, during a 2:1 or a varying AV conduction ratio, the patient may experience palpitations, shortness of breath, anginal symptoms, or congestive heart failure.

Electrocardiographic Features. The following are the commonly found electrocardiographic features associated with atrial flutter: (1) the atrial rate is between 220 and 350 beats per minute; (2) the P waves are broad, bizarre atrial deflections which have been termed F waves; (3) leads II, III, and AVF show a "sawtooth effect with absence of an isoelectric period between flutter waves." One flutter wave appears to be merging directly with the next. The "sawtooth" effect may be absent in lead I and left-sided chest leads (V_5,V_6); (4) in most cases of atrial flutter, atrial activation is in a caudocranial direction; and (5) some degree of AV block exists which may be fixed, alternating, or variable. Many of the characteristic features associated with atrial flutter are presented in Figure 9.

A 1:1 AV response in atrial flutter is very uncommon, because atrial rates of 220 or greater generally exceed the inherent transmission capacity of the AV node. The presence of atrial flutter with a suspected 1:1 AV response should raise the possibility of an accessory or anomalous AV pathway such as exists in the Wolff-Parkinson-White syndrome. Conduction ratios of 2:1 or 4:1 are more commonly observed. Effective vagotonic maneuvers such as carotid sinus pressure temporarily

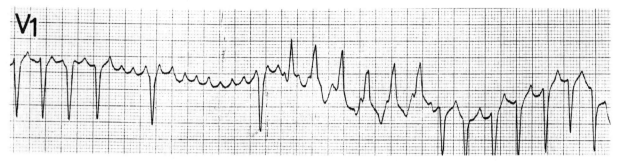

Figure 9. Atrial flutter with varying degrees of AV block. In the middle of the tracing, a period of high degree AV block occurs, during which time the atrial flutter waves are more easily identified. The second to the sixth beats after the long pause are aberrantly conducted with a right bundle branch block pattern.

increase the degree of AV block, permit a more positive identification of the atrial flutter waves, and do not significantly affect the atrial flutter rate. At times an increase in vagal tone which causes a shortening of atrial refractory period may convert atrial flutter to atrial fibrillation. By a similar mechanism, digitalis may convert atrial flutter to fibrillation.

Treatment. Direct current countershock is very effective in converting atrial flutter to sinus rhythm and is often the treatment of choice. Conversion can be achieved with low energy discharges. Direct current countershock is certainly the treatment of choice when the ventricular response is rapid and the patient is symptomatic.

Digitalis and quinidine sulfate are the primary drugs used in the treatment of atrial flutter. Depending upon the urgency of the situation, digitalis may be given intravenously or orally. Its main function is to increase the degree of AV nodal block and to slow the ventricular rate. Rarely does digitalis convert atrial flutter directly to sinus rhythm; it may, however, convert flutter to atrial fibrillation, whereupon withdrawal of digitalis may re-establish sinus rhythm or atrial flutter may resume. Once the ventricular rate is controlled with digitalis, quinidine sulfate is given orally to convert the atrial flutter to sinus rhythm. It is preferred not to give quinidine initially without first digitalizing the patient, because quinidine may slow the atrial flutter, enhance AV nodal conduction, and precipitate dangerously rapid ventricular rates. If digitalis and quinidine are the primary therapies and prove to be unsuccessful, cardioversion by direct current countershock can be used but only after digitalis has been withheld for several days, because countershock and excessive amounts of digitalis may precipitate more serious ventricular dysrhythmias.

PAROXYSMAL ATRIAL TACHYCARDIA

Paroxysmal atrial tachycardia (PAT) is a relatively common arrhythmia. Two forms are recognized which differ in etiology, underlying mechanism, and therapeutic approach. One form of PAT results from sustained reciprocation or re-entry within the AV node, and the other results from ectopic atrial foci.

PAT Due to Sustained Reciprocation or Re-entry Within the AV Node

This form of atrial tachycardia is the more common of the two. It is seen in all age groups and frequently occurs

in the absence of any clinically detectable heart disease. Characteristically, these tachycardias begin and terminate abruptly. During the tachycardia the patient may be keenly aware of a rapid heart rate and may complain of a fluttering within the chest or palpitations. Other associated symptoms include dyspnea, lightheadedness, or diaphoresis. Syncope may occur upon termination of the tachycardia if a sufficiently long pause follows prior to re-establishment of sinus rhythm or the occurrence of an escape beat. In patients with coronary artery disease, episodes of PAT may produce angina pectoris and significant S-T segment depression.

Electrocardiographic Features. Sustained re-entry within the AV node is almost always initiated by an atrial extrasystole. It is uncommon for this type of tachycardia to be precipitated by a ventricular extrasystole. If an atrial extrasystole encounters sufficient antegrade delay within the AV node (as indicated by a prolonged P-R or A-H interval), the impulse may at some point enter a nonrefractory pathway within the AV node and may be retrogradely transmitted back to the atria. If the retrogradely conducted impulse finds the antegrade pathway recovered, it may re-enter it, and the sequence is repeated, resulting in sustained reciprocation and a paroxysmal atrial tachycardia (Fig. 10).

During the reciprocating tachycardia, the atria are retrogradely activated. The P waves are inverted in leads II, III, and AVF and most often occur during the inscription of the QRS complex or the S-T segment. In some cases the retrograde P waves are located on the descending limb of the T wave or within the T-P segment and thereby mimic an ectopic atrial tachycardia with first degree heart block. The rate of these tachycardias is generally between 150 and 250 per minute. Aberrant conduction may occur for the first few beats or may persist for the entire episode of the tachycardia (Fig. 11). If aberration persists throughout the duration of the tachycardia, differentiation from ventricular tachycardia may be difficult.

Perpetuation of a reciprocating tachycardia depends primarily upon a balance of refractoriness and conduction between the reciprocating limbs within the AV node. Consequently, any intervention which alters AV nodal conduction or refractoriness can terminate these tachycardias. Abrupt termination of these tachycardias can be achieved by increasing vagal tone with carotid sinus massage, gagging, Valsalva maneuvers, or raising the blood pressure. Propranolol and digitalis, both of which increase AV nodal conduction and refractoriness, have been used successfully to treat AV nodal reciprocating tachycardias.

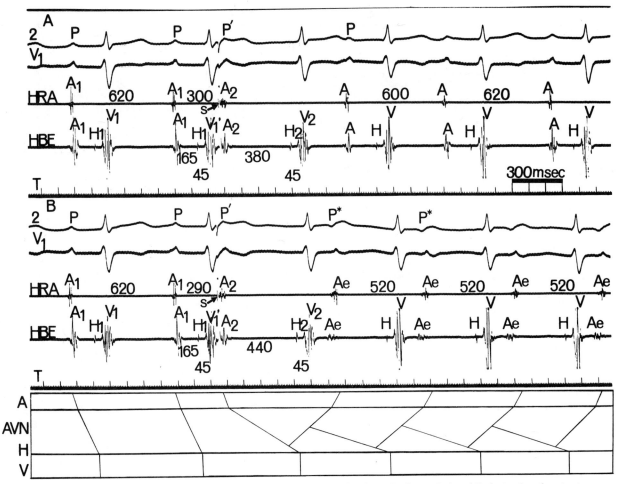

Figure 10. Re-entry within the AV node resulting in a paroxysmal atrial tachycardia. In panels A and B, the tracings from top to bottom are as follows: electrocardiographic leads 2 and V_1, a high right atrial electrogram (HRA), His bundle electrogram (HBE), and time lines at 10 and 100 msec. In each panel the first two beats are of sinus node origin with upright P waves in lead 2, a high to low sequence of atrial activation, AV nodal conduction time of 165 msec, and His-Purkinje conduction time of 45 msec. In panel A, a premature atrial depolarization (P' or A_2), introduced 300 msec after the last sinus beat (A_1), is conducted within the AV node with a delay of 380 msec; after activation of the ventricles, sinus rhythm resumes. In panel B, a slightly earlier atrial extrasystole (P' or A_2) encounters greater AV nodal delay as indicated by an A-H interval of 440 msec, which for this patient was sufficient to initiate an AV nodal re-entrant or reciprocating tachycardia at a cycle length of 520 msec. Note that the sequence of atrial activation is from the low to the high right atrium and the P waves are inverted in lead 2. Atrial activation during the reciprocating tachycardia is indicated by P* on the surface EKG's and by Ae on the intracardiac recordings. The lower part of panel B depicts the events in the form of a ladder diagram.

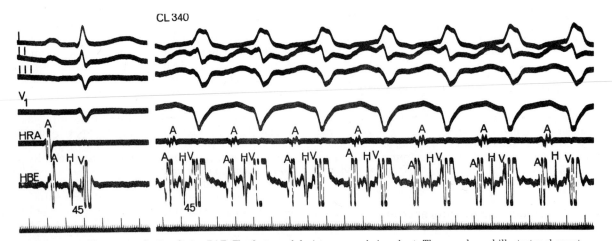

Figure 11. Aberrant conduction during PAT. The first panel depicts a normal sinus beat. The second panel illustrates aberrant conduction of a left bundle branch type during AV nodal re-entry which was initiated by a single atrial extrasystole. Note the low to high sequence of atrial activation during the PAT and the normal H-V interval (45 msec) associated with the aberrant beats.

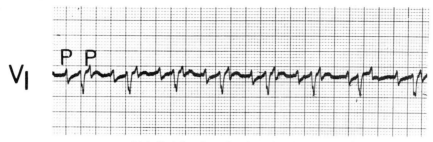

Figure 12. Digitalis-induced atrial tachycardia with 2:1 AV block.

Prophylactic therapy should be directed toward eliminating atrial extrasystoles, which are the most frequent initiating cause. For this purpose quinidine sulfate is given orally every four to six hours. Digitalis may be added to the therapeutic regimen if required.

Ectopic Atrial Tachycardia

Areas within the atria but outside the sinus node can serve as the pacemaker of the heart. Depolarization of the atria by an ectopic atrial pacemaker in excess of 100 beats per minute constitutes an ectopic atrial tachycardia. The atrial rates of most ectopic tachycardias are between 150 and 220 per minute. The tachycardias may be sustained for long periods of time or occur in paroxysms lasting seconds to hours. Ectopic atrial tachycardias can occur in all forms of heart disease. They may occur in association with digitalis toxicity, chronic obstructive lung disease, or enlarged diseased atria, or may be associated with no apparent heart disease.

Electrocardiographic Features. In ectopic atrial tachycardias the configuration of the P waves is different from that of sinus beats. If all the ectopic P waves are of the same size and shape, it is called unifocal ectopic atrial tachycardia. A multifocal ectopic tachycardia is one in which the ectopic atrial impulses arise from different parts of the atria, and consequently the configuration of P waves varies.

Depending upon the atrial rate and the capacity of the AV node to transmit impulses to the ventricle, ectopic atrial tachycardias may be associated with 1:1 AV conduction with normal or prolonged AV conduction times, AV nodal Wenckebach cycles, or 2:1 AV block. Digitalis toxicity is a frequent cause of rapid unifocal ectopic atrial tachycardias with 2:1 AV block (Fig. 12). Multifocal ectopic atrial tachycardias are frequently associated with chronic obstructive lung disease or marked atrial disease and may precipitate atrial fibrillation (Fig. 13).

The differentiation between paroxysmal atrial tachycardias caused by AV nodal re-entry from a unifocal ectopic tachycardia may at times be difficult. Tachycardias associated with inverted P waves in leads II, III, and AVF favor re-entry within the AV node as the mechanism but do not exclude a rhythm of ectopic origin. Upright P waves in these same leads strongly suggest an ectopic tachycardia. If the configuration of the P waves during the tachycardia is the same as the initiating atrial extrasystole, ectopy is favored, especially if the P waves are upright in leads II, III, and AVF. If the initiating atrial extrasystole is upright in II, III, and AVF and inverted in these same leads during the tachycardia, re-entry is likely. Abrupt termination of the atrial tachycardia by carotid sinus massage or an electrically induced atrial extrasystole favors a mechanism of AV nodal re-entry. These maneuvers generally produce a temporary slowing or pause in the ectopic atrial tachycardia, followed by resumption of its inherent firing rate.

Treatment. The treatment of digitalis-induced ectopic atrial tachycardias is withdrawal of the cardiac glycoside and administration of potassium supplements. Treatment of ectopic tachycardias in patients with chronic obstructive lung disease should first be directed toward correcting hypoxemia, hypercapnia, or acid-base or other metabolic imbalances, which frequently are present and are the initiating cause of these rhythm disturbances. Ectopic atrial tachycardias of other causes should be treated with either quinidine or procainamide.

VENTRICULAR EXTRASYSTOLES

Ventricular extrasystoles (ventricular premature beats, contractions, or systoles) are a common occurrence in patients with and without heart disease. In young healthy individuals, the incidence varies between 0.5 and 2.0 per cent. They may be caused by emotional stress, tobacco, alcohol, caffeine, anoxia, sympathomime-

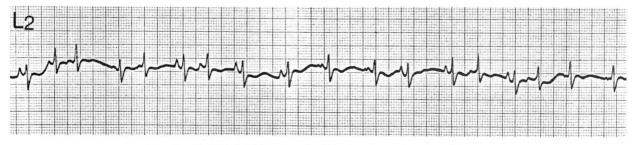

Figure 13. Multifocal atrial tachycardia. Note changing configuration of P waves.

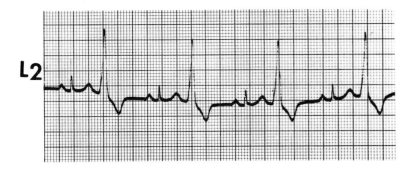

Figure 14. Ventricular bigeminy. A single premature ventricular extrasystole is coupled at a constant interval to each sinus beat.

tic drugs, or exercise. They are associated with all forms of heart disease and occur frequently (up to 80 per cent) in patients with acute myocardial infarction. Digitalis excess is a common cause of ventricular extrasystoles, especially if hypokalemia is present. Patients with occasional or even frequent ventricular extrasystole may be completely unaware of their presence. On the other hand, some patients complain of "pauses," "palpitations," or "thumping" in the chest.

Electrocardiographic Features. Ventricular extrasystoles are characterized by wide QRS complexes (0.12 sec) with S-T and T wave changes. They may occur early or late in the cardiac cycle and very often have a constant coupling interval to the preceding sinus beat. The coupling interval is considered constant if the variation is within 0.08 sec (80 msec). A single ventricular extrasystole occurring after each sinus beat is referred to as ventricular bigeminy (Fig. 14). The term trigeminy refers to repeat cycles of either two sinus beats followed by a single extrasystole or one sinus beat followed by two consecutive ventricular extrasystoles.

Recurrent ventricular extrasystoles which always exhibit the same QRS morphology are referred to as unifocal in origin (arising from the same ectopic focus), whereas recurrent extrasystoles of different morphologies are termed multifocal in origin. Ventricular extrasystoles can arise anywhere within the bundle branch–Purkinje network. Extrasystoles arising from the left side of the conduction system result in QRS complexes which resemble right bundle branch block

patterns, and those arising from the right side result in QRS complexes resembling a left bundle branch block pattern. Infrequently, extrasystolic impulses may arise high in one of the bundle branches, close to the bundle of His, and conduct with slight asynchrony down both bundle branches, resulting in narrow QRS complexes.

Most ventricular extrasystoles occur late in the cardiac cycle, i.e., after completion of the T wave of the preceding sinus beat, and are frequently coupled to the preceding sinus beat by a fairly constant interval. Less commonly, ventricular extrasystoles occur in early diastole, near the peak of the T wave or on its descending limb. This has been called the R on T phenomenon; it may reflect a very serious situation, because extrasystoles occurring near the so-called vulnerable period of the ventricle may lead to ventricular tachycardia or ventricular fibrillation.

Ventricular extrasystoles may be associated with various types of retrograde conduction patterns. The more common of these patterns include the following:

1. Complete retrograde conduction may occur across the AV conducting system, resulting in premature retrograde depolarization of the atria with inverted P waves in leads II, III, and AVF.

2. The extrasystolic impulse may retrogradely block within the AV node. This may result in the phenomenon of retrograde concealed conduction in which the next sinus impulse either is blocked or conducts with a P-R interval longer than sinus beats (Fig. 15).

3. During prolonged retrograde AV nodal conduction

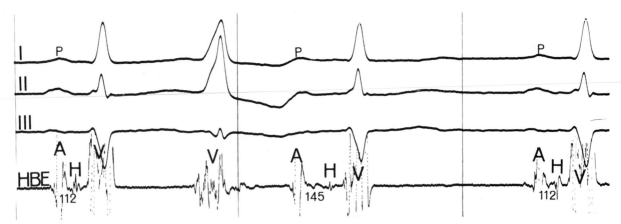

Figure 15. Retrograde AV nodal concealed conduction caused by a ventricular extrasystole. Note absence of His deflection preceding the second QRS complex. The ventricular extrasystolic impulse retrogradely penetrates the AV node and leaves it partially refractory to the second sinus P wave, which is conducted with a longer P-R interval. The delay in conduction is localized to the AV node, as indicated by an A-H interval of 145 msec compared to normal values of 112 msec.

delay, the extrasystolic impulse may reciprocate within the AV node and return to the ventricles, producing a ventricular echo beat (see Fig. 19).

4. Very premature extrasystolic impulses may retrogradely block within the His-Purkinje system. This type of retrograde conduction pattern cannot be determined from the electrocardiogram.

Treatment. The treatment of ventricular extrasystoles depends upon their cause, the underlying cardiac condition, severity of symptoms, their frequency, the coupling interval, and whether they are unifocal or multifocal in origin.

Ventricular extrasystoles which are related to emotional upsets, tobacco, alcohol, or sympathomimetic drugs may require only reassurance, mild sedation, or abstinence. Withholding of digitalis therapy for one or more days, in conjunction with oral potassium supplements, may be all that is necessary to treat extrasystoles caused by excess digitalis.

Ventricular extrasystoles occurring during an acute myocardial infarction require antiarrhythmic therapy. Therapy is urgently indicated if the extrasystoles have a close coupling interval, occur at a rate of five or more per minute, or are multifocal in origin. Irrespective of the underlying cardiac condition, antiarrhythmic therapy is indicated for ventricular extrasystoles which demonstrate the R on T phenomenon, are multifocal in origin, or occur consecutively in pairs.

VENTRICULAR TACHYCARDIA

Three or more consecutive beats occurring at rates greater than 100 per minute and arising from a focus located below the bundle of His constitute an episode of ventricular tachycardia. Most ventricular tachycardias occur at rates between 120 and 180 beats per minute; they may occur in paroxysms lasting a few seconds to several minutes or may persist for hours or days. Ventricular tachycardia is almost always associated with some form of organic heart disease, the most common being arteriosclerotic, rheumatic, and hypertensive heart diseases. As many as 50 per cent of patients with acute myocardial infarction may have one or more episodes of ventricular tachycardia of varying duration. Toxic doses of digitalis are a common cause of ventricular tachycardia. Other precipitating causes of paroxysmal ventricular tachycardia include hypoxia, hypokalemia, exercise, drugs (such as epinephrine, quinidine, and procainamide), cardiac catheterization of either the right or left heart, and anesthetic agents (cycloproprane, chloroform). Ventricular aneurysms may be the cause of recurrent or drug-resistant ventricular tachycardias.

Paroxysmal ventricular tachycardia has been reported to occur in young patients (less than 30 years old) in whom no evidence of heart disease could be detected. In this group, some attacks have been demonstrated to occur during exercise or emotional stress, implying a relationship between increased sympathetic tone and the ventricular dysrhythmia. In other patients, no precipitating factor could be demonstrated.

Electrocardiographic Features. In ventricular tachycardia, the QRS complexes are wide (0.12 sec or greater) and bizarre, recurring regularly at rates over 100 per minute (usually 120 to 180). Since the pacemaker is located below the bundle of His (i.e., within the bundle branches or Purkinje network), ventricular tachycardia is characterized electrophysiologically by the absence of a His bundle electrogram preceding the onset of ventricular activation. The bundle of His is retrogradely activated, and although in most cases it is not discernible, it is located within the ventricular electrogram. Initiation of the tachycardia may begin with a premature ventricular beat occurring close in time to the peak of the T wave of a preceding sinus beat; at other times, the initiating beat is located at the end of or after inscription of the T wave. Once initiated, ventricular tachycardia may be continuous for long periods of time or intermittent with one or more sinus beats interspersed (Fig. 16).

Often, it is extremely difficult to define the pattern of atrial activity during episodes of ventricular tachycardia from standard electrocardiographic tracings. Esophageal or intra-atrial recordings can be quite helpful in defining the frequency of atrial activity and its relationship to the QRS complexes.

During ventricular tachycardia, the atria may be dissociated from the ventricles, in which case independent P waves will be observed. At other times, various degrees of retrograde capture of the atria will occur (1:1, 2:1 retrograde Wenckebach cycles) (Fig. 17). If discernible, the P waves would be inverted in leads II, III, and AVF during retrograde activation of the atria.

An important and sometimes difficult clinical problem is the differentiation of supraventricular tachycardia with aberration from ventricular tachycardia. A comparison of Figures 11 and 17 demonstrates the value of His bundle recordings in making this distinction. In the former, a His deflection with a normal or greater than normal H-V interval precedes ventricular activation, whereas in the latter there is absence of a His electrogram preceding ventricular activation.

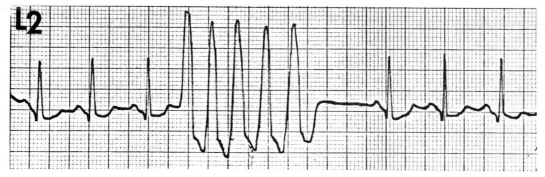

Figure 16. A short episode of a unifocal ventricular tachycardia interspersed between periods of sinus rhythm.

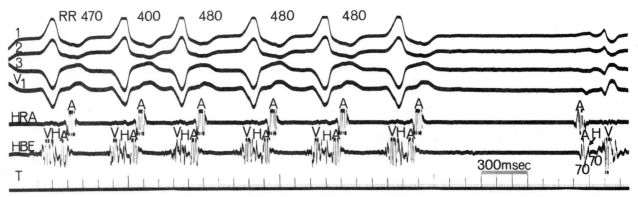

Figure 17. Ventricular tachycardia showing a left bundle branch block pattern and 1:1 retrograde conduction. Note the absence of a His deflection preceding ventricular activation. A retrograde His deflection can be seen within the ventricular electrogram. A low to high sequence of atrial activation occurs during retrograde atrial depolarization. The last beat is a sinus beat which occurs after spontaneous termination of the tachycardia. These results should be compared with those of Figure 11.

From the electrocardiographic point of view the presence of fusion beats during a sustained tachycardia provides strong supportive evidence that the rhythm in question is of ventricular origin. Fusion beats refer to partial activation of the ventricles by both supraventricular and ventricular impulses. During ventricular tachycardia, fusion beats may result because the atria are dissociated from the ventricles, and a sinus impulse occurring at an appropriate time in the cardiac cycle penetrates the AV conducting system and partially activates the ventricles; or during retrograde Wenckebach cycles, the impulse may reciprocate within the AV node and return to the ventricles, resulting in partial activation of that chamber. Complete activation or capture of the ventricles by either of the aforementioned mechanisms may terminate the tachycardia for one or more cycles, during which time sinus beats may appear, after which the tachycardia usually resumes.

A diagnosis of ventricular tachycardia is favored if one can discern independent atrial activity at a rate slower than the ventricular rate. On the other hand, supraventricular tachycardia with aberration is favored if carotid sinus pressure or other vagal maneuvers abruptly terminate the tachycardia.

Treatment.   The choice and urgency of treatment for ventricular tachycardia depends on a number of factors, including its cause, the age and general condition of the patient, the severity and type of the underlying heart disease, blood pressure, and the state of consciousness. Causative factors such as hypoxia, hypokalemia, or other metabolic imbalances must be recognized and corrected.

DC countershock and drug therapy are the two commonly used methods for treating ventricular tachycardia. DC countershock is generally reserved for emergent situations in which the ventricular dysrhythmia is continuous or causes profound hemodynamic disturbances, or when drug therapy is ineffective. DC countershock is not the preferred treatment for ventricular tachycardias caused by digitalis toxicity.

Lidocaine is the most commonly used drug for the conversion of ventricular tachycardia to sinus rhythm. It is administered intravenously as a 100 mg bolus which can be repeated in two to three minutes if the initial injection is totally or partially ineffective. After suppression of the arrhythmia, lidocaine may be given as a continuous intravenous drip of 1 to 3 mg per minute. Occasionally, higher concentrations (4 mg per minute) are required. Approximately, 90 per cent of ventricular tachycardias can be suppressed at lidocaine blood levels of 2 to 4 μg per milliliter. The more common side effects of lidocaine include drowsiness, paresthesias, decrease in auditory acuity, agitation, and convulsions. Since lidocaine is metabolized by the liver, lower doses of the drug may cause side effects in patients with hepatic dysfunction.

Intravenous procainamide is also highly effective in the treatment of ventricular tachycardia. The drug can be administered at a rate of 25 to 50 mg per minute until either the tachycardia is terminated or 1000 mg has been administered. Most ventricular tachycardias are suppressed at blood concentrations of 4 to 8 μg per milliliter. Occasionally, higher concentrations are required. Continued suppression of the tachycardia can be achieved by a continuous intravenous drip at a rate of 2.5 mg per minute. Procainamide, like most antiarrhythmic drugs, may cause significant hypotension after intravenous administration, especially if the underlying myocardial dysfunction is severe. At other times, the arrhythmia is the cause of a lowered blood pressure which improves when normal sinus rhythm is restored.

If lidocaine and procainamide are ineffective in controlling the arrhythmia, one can use diphenylhydantoin, propranolol, or quinidine sulfate. On occasion, a combination of drugs is required.

If ventricular tachycardia is associated with an underlying complete or high degree of AV block, an electrode catheter should be positioned within the right ventricular cavity and endocardial pacing initiated immediately upon terminating the ventricular tachycardia with drug therapy. This is required because effective drug therapy may suppress all idioventricular pacemaker activity and ventricular asystole may ensue.

ACCELERATED IDIOVENTRICULAR RHYTHMS

Accelerated idioventricular rhythms (AIVR) is a term applied to ectopic ventricular rhythms with rates intermediate between idioventricular escape rhythms (30 to 40 per minute) and ventricular tachycardia (120 to 180 per minute). Most frequently the rates are between 75 and 100 per minute. Accelerated idioventricular

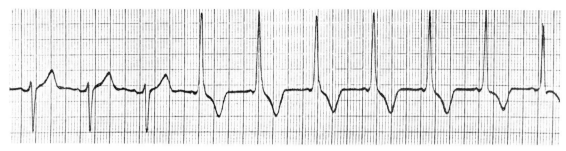

Figure 18. Accelerated idioventricular rhythm which begins just prior to the fourth sinus P wave. The rates of the sinus node and idioventricular pacemakers are nearly identical, thereby resulting in a period of isorhythmic AV dissociation.

rhythms are commonly associated with myocardial infarction or digitalis toxicity. Current thinking holds that AIVR represents an enhancement of the normal escape rhythm of latent ventricular pacemakers. Like other ventricular rhythms, the QRS complexes are bizarre and wide (0.12 sec). The rate of the AIVR is usually close to that of the sinus rate, and consequently it becomes manifest when sinus rhythm is slowed by increasing vagal tone (carotid sinus massage) or premature atrial extrasystoles, or when some degree of AV block develops. AIVR usually begins late in the cardiac cycle, and it may start with a fusion beat (Fig. 18). If dissociation between the atria and ventricles is present, fusion beats may occur frequently. If 1:1 retrograde conduction occurs, the AIVR may persist for long periods of time (Fig. 19). In some patients, episodes of AIVR (75 to 100 per minute) and ventricular tachycardia (120 to 180 per minute) coexist. Treatment of AIVR is the same as that of ventricular tachycardia. Also, acceleration of the sinus rate by atropine or atrial pacing can and usually does suppress AIVR.

BIDIRECTIONAL TACHYCARDIA

Bidirectional tachycardia is an infrequently encountered arrhythmia which is characterized by (1) rapid regular rate of 140 to 180 beats per minute, (2) alternating rightward and leftward axis shifts in the frontal plane, and (3) a constant right bundle branch block pattern in lead V_1. Most bidirectional tachycardias occur in the presence of severe myocardial disease and digitalis toxicity and are associated with a poor prognosis. Two different mechanisms have been proposed to explain the electrocardiographic pattern of bidirectional tachycar-

dia. One suggested mechanism is that bidirectional tachycardia originates from a supraventricular tachycardia in which there is permanent aberrant conduction within the right bundle branch along with alternating aberrant conduction in the two divisions (anterior and posterior fascicles) of the left bundle branch. The other mechanism, confirmed by His bundle recordings, indicates that bidirectional tachycardia results from an ectopic focus located in the left ventricle, which would account for the permanent right bundle branch block pattern observed (Fig. 20). It is as yet unclear whether the alternating rightward and leftward axis shift is the result of alternating routes of ventricular activation by a single ectopic left ventricular focus or alternating discharge of two separate left ventricular foci. The treatment of bidirectional tachycardia is withdrawal of digitalis and administration of potassium and an antiarrhythmic agent such as lidocaine or diphenylhydantoin.

VENTRICULAR FIBRILLATION

Ventricular fibrillation consists of rapid, disorganized, multifocal depolarizations of the ventricular myocardium. The absence of rhythmic coordinated muscular contractions produces a loss of the pumping action of the heart and causes a precipitous fall of the blood pressure to zero levels and unconsciousness. Ventricular fibrillation is most often seen in patients with significant underlying cardiac disease, especially ischemic heart disease. It may also occur in patients without clinical or pathologic evidence of heart disease. It may accompany digitalis toxicity, especially if hypokalemia or other metabolic imbalances are present. Quinidine sensitivity or

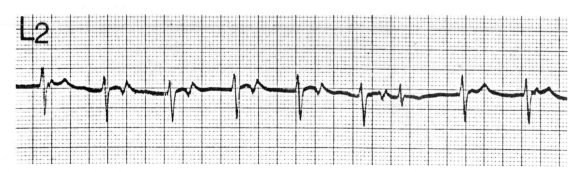

Figure 19. Accelerated idioventricular rhythm associated with retrograde Wenckebach type conduction to the atria. The sixth ventricular impulse re-enters within the AV node and is antegradely conducted back to the ventricles, resulting in a ventricular echo beat (seventh QRS complex).

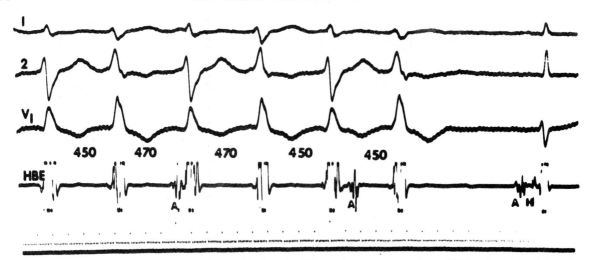

Figure 20. Bidirectional ventricular tachycardia. The first six QRS complexes show a persistent RBBB pattern in lead V_1 and alternating left and right axis deviation in lead 2. The ventricular origin of these beats is indicated by absence of a His deflection preceding the QRS complex. Ventricular activity is dissociated from atrial activity. The last beat shows a normally conducted atrial impulse with normal A-H and H-V intervals. (From Kastor, J. A., and Goldreyer, B. N.: Circulation, *48*:897, 1973. Copyright 1973, American Medical Association.)

toxicity may also be the cause of ventricular fibrillation. Ventricular extrasystoles occurring within the so-called vulnerable period of the ventricles (R on T phenomenon) may initiate ventricular fibrillation (Fig. 21).

The treatment of ventricular fibrillation must be prompt and decisive. The patient must be ventilated and defibrillated, using DC countershock at 400 watt-seconds.

AV DISSOCIATION

AV dissociation is a general term which describes any rhythm in which the atria and ventricles are independently activated by different pacemakers discharging at similar or dissimilar rates. The atria may be activated by either the sinus node or an ectopic atrial pacemaker, whereas the ventricles may be under the control of either a junctional or an idioventricular pacemaker. AV dissociation may occur with an essentially intact AV conduction system and may be of short duration, lasting for one or a few cardiac cycles, or it may persist for much longer periods. AV dissociation may be caused by (1) acceleration of a junctional or idioventricular pacemaker (Fig. 18), (2) slowing of an atrial pacemaker accompanied by an escape rhythm located in either the AV junction or ventricles, or (3) SA or AV block accompanied by an escape rhythm (Fig. 5).

Isorhythmic AV dissociation is one type of dissociated rhythm in which (1) the atria and ventricles are controlled by independent pacemakers discharging at equal or nearly equal rates, and (2) the P waves remain in close proximity to the QRS complexes; they may precede, occur simultaneously with, or follow the QRS complex. An example of isorhythmic AV dissociation in which the ventricles come under control of a junctional pacemaker is shown in Figure 22. As the atrial cycle length increases, the ventricles come under control of a junctional pacemaker, and the P waves which remain under control of the sinus node appear to be "marching" into the QRS complex. The P wave may appear to the right of the QRS complex and maintain a fixed R-P relationship, during which time the atria may remain under control of the sinus node or be retrogradely activated by the junctional pacemaker. After a variable period of time, acceleration of the sinus rate occurs, the P waves reappear in front of the QRS complex, and sinus rhythm is re-established. Sinus acceleration results from changes in baroreceptor activity, consequent to changes in arterial pressure or the effect of right atrial stretch, or both. Acceleration of the sinus rate is dependent upon the magnitude of these accelerating influences and the responsiveness of the sinus node.

JUNCTIONAL RHYTHMS

Traditionally, AV nodal rhythms have been described as arising from the upper, middle, or lower portions of the AV node. This classification has been based primarily on the relationship of inverted P waves (leads II, III, AVF) to the QRS complex. In upper AV nodal

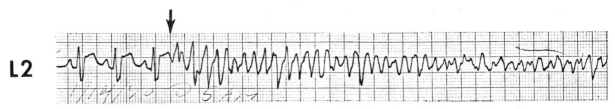

Figure 21. Ventricular fibrillation initiated by a rapid burst of ventricular activity (arrow).

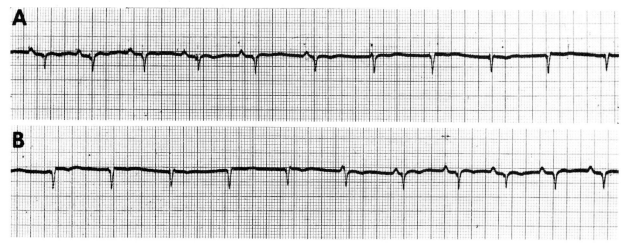

Figure 22. Isorhythmic AV dissociation. After the first five sinus beats, the sinus rate slows and an AV junctional pacemaker emerges, starting with the sixth QRS complex. The atria continue to be activated by the sinus node, and the P waves are obscured within the QRS complex. In the bottom strip, accelerating forces cause an increase in the sinus node rate and sinus rhythm is re-established.

rhythms the inverted P wave precedes the QRS complex, whereas in middle or lower AV nodal rhythms the P wave occurs simultaneously with or follows the QRS complex, respectively. It has been recommended that the terms "junctional" or "AV junctional rhythms" replace that of "AV nodal rhythms," because (1) experimentally it has been difficult to consistently and convincingly demonstrate pacemaker activity (phase 4 depolarization) in all three regions of the AV node and (2) pacemaker activity in other areas of the heart (coronary sinus, left atrium, and bundle of His) can result in electrocardiographic patterns similar to those ascribed to AV nodal rhythms.

AV junctional rhythms are primarily escape rhythms with rates usually in the range 40 to 70 per minute. They become manifest if there is (1) significant sinus slowing, (2) AV block, or (3) SA block. If the discharge rate of the sinus node falls below that of a subsidiary junctional pacemaker, as may occur during sinus bradycardia or after premature discharge of the sinus node by an extrasystolic impulse, an area within the AV junction can take over as the pacemaker of the heart. In similar fashion, an escape junctional rhythm can emerge when sinus node impulses fail to conduct to surrounding atrial myocardium such as occurs in SA block (Fig. 5). Escape junctional rhythms also occur during AV block in which supraventricular impulses block in the AV node and proximal to the site of a junctional pacemaker (see Fig. 35). In complete AV block in which the nonconducted atrial impulses block below the bundle of His, the escape rhythms are located below the AV junction (idioventricular pacemaker). AV junctional rhythms result in QRS complexes which are similar to those of sinus rhythm.

SYNDROME OF SHORT P-R INTERVAL, NORMAL QRS COMPLEXES, AND SUPRAVENTRICULAR TACHYCARDIAS
(Lown-Ganong-Levine Syndrome)

The syndrome of short P-R interval (0.12 sec or less), normal QRS complexes (0.10 sec), and paroxysmal supra-

ventricular tachycardias is known as the Lown-Ganong-Levine syndrome. The mechanisms responsible for both the short P-R interval and the tachycardias have remained obscure. Several theories, based primarily on anatomic considerations, have been proposed to explain the short P-R interval. The most popular theory centers about the presence of specialized internodal pathways by which atrial impulses can partially or completely bypass the AV node. Recent electrophysiologic studies, using His bundle recordings and atrial pacing techniques, have shown that most cases of short P-R interval are associated with AV nodal conduction times which are at the lower range of normal values. The A-H intervals were 60 to 80 msec, whereas H-V intervals were between 30 and 55 msec. In addition, in most patients when the right atrium was stimulated at progressively increasing rates, the expected A-H interval increases were qualitatively similar to, but quantitatively less than, that observed for subjects with normal P-R intervals. In only an occasional patient with a short P-R interval was the A-H interval found to be less than 60 msec or did the A-H interval not increase as the paced atrial rate was increased. These limited data suggest that most cases of short P-R interval are due to an abbreviated AV nodal conduction time which could be due to (1) atrial impulses partially bypassing the AV node (? specialized internodal tracts), (2) an anatomically small AV node, (3) preferential intranodal pathways, or (4) a combination of these. In only occasional patients are the electrophysiologic data compatible with a complete bypass of the AV node, accounting for the short P-R interval. It should be pointed out that prolonged periods of isorhythmic AV dissociation can mimic a short P-R interval with normal QRS complexes. Studies to date have shown that AV nodal re-entry is a common mechanism for the paroxysmal supraventricular tachycardias in this syndrome.

WOLFF-PARKINSON-WHITE SYNDROME

The electrocardiographic pattern of the Wolff-Parkinson-White syndrome is characterized by a short P-R interval (less than 0.12 sec) and a widened QRS

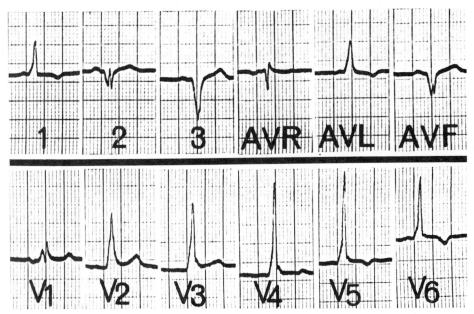

Figure 23. Wolff-Parkinson-White syndrome, showing Type A QRS complexes. The delta wave can be seen in almost all leads. The precordial leads resemble a right bundle branch block pattern. In leads 2, 3, and AVF the delta wave produces a Q wave which mimics a diaphragmatic myocardial infarction.

complex, starting with an initial delta wave. This abnormal electrocardiographic pattern occurs in approximately 0.1 to 0.4 per cent of routine tracings. A significant number of patients exhibiting this pattern have episodes of supraventricular tachycardia. Other terms used to describe this phenomenon include anomalous AV excitation, ventricular pre-excitation, and accessory AV conduction.

Over the years, many hypotheses have been put forth to explain the electrocardiographic findings in this syndrome. Currently, there is anatomic as well as electrophysiologic evidence indicating that atrial impulses pre-excite the ventricles via accessory bypass tracts composed of myocardial fibers which connect the atria and ventricles. These bypass tracts are referred to as bundles of Kent. Atrial impulses are simultaneously conducted to the ventricles via the normal AV nodal His-Purkinje conducting system and the accessory pathway. AV con-

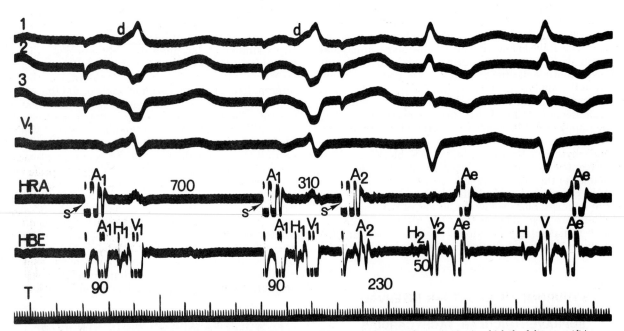

Figure 24. The first two QRS complexes show a Wolff-Parkinson-White type of ventricular excitation in which the delta wave (d) in leads II and III mimics a diaphragmatic myocardial infarction. Atrial impulses are also conducted along the AV nodal His-Purkinje system; bundle of His activation occurs at about the time of the onset of the delta wave. The third P wave (A₂) is premature and finds the accessory pathway refractory. Exclusive conduction along the AV nodal His-Purkinje system results in normal ventricular activation, followed by a re-entrant supraventricular tachycardia. Note the absence of electrocardiographic evidence of myocardial infarction.

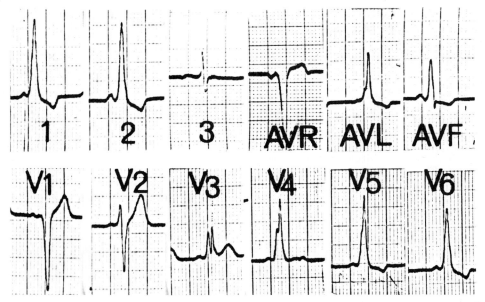

Figure 25. Type B QRS complexes of the Wolff-Parkinson-White syndrome in which the precordial leads resemble a left bundle branch block pattern.

duction via the latter results in shortening of the P-R interval, and pre-excitation of the ventricle produces the delta wave. In most cases, the QRS complex in the Wolff-Parkinson-White syndrome represents fusion activation, the delta wave being an expression of ventricular excitation via the accessory pathway, and some part of the remaining portion of the QRS the result of excitation via the normal AV nodal His-Purkinje conducting system. If significant delay or block exists within the AV nodal His-Purkinje pathway, the QRS complex may represent one of total pre-excitation. Alternatively, if AV nodal conduction time is shortened, as may occur with increased sympathetic tone or during an isoproterenol infusion, activation of the ventricles by the AV nodal His-Purkinje system is increased and the QRS tends toward normalization. Anomalous AV excitation may be always present during sinus rhythm, or it may intermittently alternate with periods of normal activation. At times, anomalous AV excitation may mimic the electrocardiographic pattern of a myocardial infarction (Fig. 23). Bundle of His recordings in conjunction with atrial pacing techniques can establish the correct diagnosis (Fig. 24).

The syndrome has been divided into two major groups, types A and B. In type A the accessory bundle crosses the AV sulcus on the left side, causing pre-excitation of the base of the left ventricle. The vector of the delta wave is directed anteriorly in all precordial leads (upright in V_1 V_6), and the QRS pattern resembles right bundle branch block pattern (Fig. 23). In type B, the accessory bundle pre-excites the lateral margin of the right ventricle and the initial delta forces are directed leftward and posteriorly, producing a biphasic or negative delta wave in V_1 and QRS complexes resembling the left bundle branch block pattern (Fig. 25). Intermediate forms of these two major categories exist. Early activation of the base of the left ventricle in type A Wolff-Parkinson-White syndrome and of the lateral margin of the right ventricle in type B Wolff-Parkinson-White syndrome has been confirmed by epicardial mapping studies performed at the time of cardiac surgery.

Supraventricular Tachycardias in Wolff-Parkinson-White Syndrome

Between 25 and 70 per cent of patients with Wolff-Parkinson-White type QRS complexes have episodes of supraventricular tachycardia, and most of these appear to be re-entrant in nature. However, it should be noted that atrial tachycardias which are ectopic in origin may also occur in these patients. Most re-entrant tachycardias occurring in the patients with the Wolff-Parkinson-White syndrome have normal QRS complexes with long P-R intervals and are initiated by premature atrial beats. Less commonly are re-entrant tachycardias associated with pre-excitation type QRS complexes.

There are two possible mechanisms to explain re-entrant supraventricular tachycardias with normal QRS complexes in patients with the Wolff-Parkinson-White syndrome. If a closely coupled premature atrial beat finds the accessory pathway refractory to antegrade conduction, it may traverse the AV nodal His-Purkinje conducting system (usually with some delay) and activate the ventricles, producing a normal QRS complex. If sufficient time has elapsed to permit recovery of excitability of the accessory pathway, retrograde conduction back to the atria will occur via the accessory pathway. If, after atrial activation, the AV nodal His-Purkinje conducting system has recovered, activation of the ventricles will follow and a self-sustaining re-entrant tachycardia will result. Alternatively, a re-entrant supraventricular tachycardia with normal QRS complexes could be initiated by a premature ventricular beat which was retrogradely blocked within the His-Purkinje AV nodal conducting system but which retrogradely activated the atria via the accessory pathway. Recovery of excitability of the AV nodal His-Purkinje conducting system would allow antegrade conduction to ventricles to follow retrograde activation of the atria; if the process is repetitive, a sustained tachycardia with normal QRS complexes will result.

The second mechanism involved in producing re-entrant supraventricular tachycardias with normal QRS complexes is one in which reciprocation or re-entry occurs only within the AV node; the accessory pathway, although present, is not utilized in the re-entrant process. This type of re-entry is the same as that occurring in patients who have paroxysmal atrial tachycardia without Wolff-Parkinson-White complexes.

Re-entrant supraventricular tachycardias with pre-excitation type QRS complexes result when antegrade conduction occurs via the accessory pathway and the impulse is retrogradely returned to the atria via the AV nodal His-Purkinje pathway.

A potentially life-threatening situation may occur in patients with the Wolff-Parkinson-White syndrome who develop atrial fibrillation. Rapid irregular activation of the ventricles via the accessory pathway exclusively or both pathways simultaneously may lead to ventricular fibrillation.

Treatment. Most re-entrant tachycardias associated with the Wolff-Parkinson-White syndrome respond to vagotonic maneuvers such as carotid sinus stimulation, the Valsalva maneuver, eyeball pressure, or elevation of blood pressure. Increased parasympathetic tone alters the re-entrant pathway by increasing refractoriness and delaying conduction within the AV node. Similarly, digitalis and propranolol can terminate re-entrant tachycardias by the same mechanism. DC countershock is reserved for those tachycardias which (1) are resistant to vagotonic maneuvers and require excessive amounts of drug therapy, or (2) are associated with very rapid ventricular responses. If, during atrial fibrillation, excitation of the ventricles occurs in part or totally through the accessory AV pathway, DC countershock should be applied immediately in order to avoid the possibility of ventricular fibrillation.

Prophylactic therapy should be directed at suppressing atrial extrasystoles which are a very common initiating cause of re-entrant tachycardias in the Wolff-Parkinson-White syndrome. Quinidine sulfate should be given for this purpose. In some cases quinidine given in combination with digitalis or propranolol is more effective. Less commonly, when ventricular extrasystoles are the initiating cause of the re-entrant tachycardias, procainamide is the drug of choice.

A small percentage of patients with the Wolff-Parkinson-White syndrome have frequent severe episodes of supraventricular tachycardia which, in addition to causing disabling symptoms, are resistant to control by drug therapy alone. An operative procedure has been devised for surgically interrupting the anomalous atrioventricular bypass tract which in some reported cases has effectively terminated the recurrence of tachycardias. Surgical therapy in these very selective patients requires that the region of the anomalous bypass tract be localized by epicardial mapping studies.

DISORDERS OF AV CONDUCTION
First Degree Heart Block

In adults a P-R interval of more than 0.20 sec constitutes electrocardiographic evidence of first degree heart block which most commonly (90 per cent or more) is due to conduction delay occurring within the AV node. First-degree heart block in the presence of normal QRS complexes is almost always due to AV nodal conduction delay, an example of which is presented in Figure 26. Bundle of His recordings reveal that the A-H interval was prolonged at 310 msec and His-Purkinje conduction time was within normal limits at 39 msec.

Drugs such as digitalis and propranolol cause P-R prolongation by delaying conduction within the AV node. Neither drug affects conduction within the His-Purkinje system to any significant degree. The A-H interval returns to normal when these drugs are discontinued. At times, first degree AV nodal block may alternate with periods of type I second degree AV block or 2:1 AV block. In general, no specific treatment for first degree AV block is required. In most patients an increase in sympathetic tone, such as occurs during exercise or vagal blockade by atropine (0.5 to 1.0 mg intravenously), causes a decrease in the A-H interval concomitant with an increase in sinus rate so that 1:1 AV conduction is maintained.

His-Purkinje Delay

Less commonly, first degree heart block is due solely to conduction delay within the His-Purkinje system. Figure 27 is an example of P-R prolongation and right bundle branch block in which AV nodal conduction (A-H interval) is within normal limits and His-Purkinje conduction time (H-V interval) is markedly prolonged at 90 msec. The presence of a prolonged H-V interval is almost always associated with a bundle branch block pattern or widened QRS complex. However, not all patients with a bundle branch block pattern have prolonged H-V intervals. A prolonged H-V interval (greater than 60 msec) in the presence of a bundle branch block pattern usually indicates that there is conduction delay within the contralateral bundle. In asymptomatic patients, no specific treatment is required.

AV Nodal Plus His-Purkinje Conduction Delay

First degree AV block may be due to conduction delays in both the AV node and His-Purkinje system.

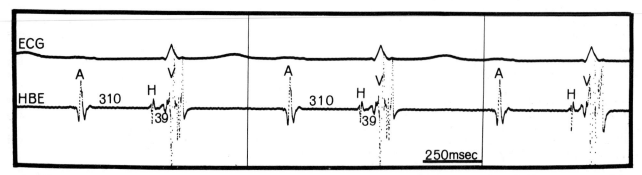

Figure 26. First degree heart block due to AV nodal delay.

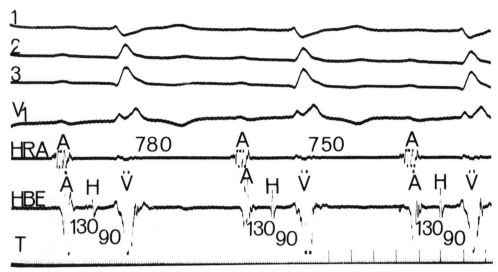

Figure 27.   First degree heart block due to a prolonged H-V interval (90 msec) in a patient with right bundle branch block.

Intra-His Bundle Delay

Conduction delay occurring within the bundle of His itself can cause a prolongation of the P-R interval. However, this is an uncommon cause of first degree heart block.

Second Degree AV Block

Second degree heart block has been classified into two types. Type I second degree heart block (Wenckebach phenomenon, Mobitz type I AV block) is electrocardiographically characterized by a progressive prolongation in the P-R interval preceding a nonconducted atrial beat. After the nonconducted P wave, the P-R interval is shorter. Type II second degree AV block (Mobitz II) is electrocardiographically characterized by a constant P-R interval preceding an unexpected nonconducted atrial impulse.

Type I Second Degree AV Block

The electrocardiographic pattern of type I second degree AV block can result from Wenckebach type conduction occurring within (1) the AV node, (2) the bundle of His itself, or (3) the bundle branch–Purkinje system. Delay in the AV node is by far the most common cause (more than 90 per cent) of type I AV block. The next most common site is the bundle branch–Purkinje system, and the least common is the bundle of His itself.

Classically the AV nodal Wenckebach phenomenon is depicted as one in which the greatest increment in P-R interval occurs with the second beat of the Wenckebach cycle and thereafter progressively diminishes. This re-

sults in a decreasing R-R interval in the presence of increasing P-R intervals. Some AV nodal Wenckebach cycles do not follow this classic pattern, and the greatest increment in P-R interval may occur with the last conducted beat. Also, one may observe little or no change in the P-R interval for several beats throughout the cycle.

Figure 28 is an example of type I second degree AV block resulting from progressive conduction delay and block within the AV node. Type I AV block in the presence of normal QRS complexes is almost always AV nodal in origin. At times, the second beat of the Wenckebach cycle may be aberrantly conducted to the ventricles. Aberrant conduction is favored by the fact that the nonconducted atrial impulse of the preceding Wenckebach cycle results in a long R-R interval. In a 3:2 AV nodal Wenckebach cycle, aberrant conduction of every second beat may simulate a ventricular bigeminy, especially if the P wave of the aberrant beat is obscured by the T wave of the preceding QRS complex (Fig. 29).

Type I AV block occurring within the AV node may be associated with inferior wall myocardial infarctions or excessive digitalis administration, and in both of these situations the block is generally reversible. Small doses of atropine, which enhances AV nodal conduction, usually re-establish 1:1 AV conduction. However, in some cases atropine may increase the sinus rate without appreciably affecting AV nodal conduction, and higher degrees of AV block (2:1, 3:1) may result. In type I AV block of AV nodal origin, the ventricular rate is seldom slow enough to warrant aggressive drug therapy or temporary right ventricular endocardial pacing.

The electrocardiographic pattern of type I second degree AV block can also result from Wenckebach type conduction occurring within the His-Purkinje system, as

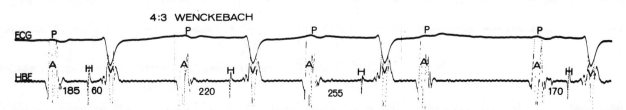

Figure 28.   Type I second degree AV block due to progressive conduction delay and block within the AV node.

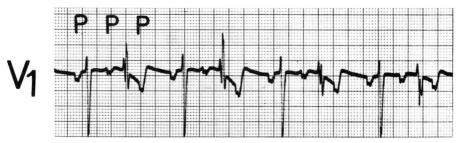

Figure 29. A 3:2 AV conduction during type I second degree AV block within the node, in which every second beat of the Wenckebach cycle is aberrantly conducted with a right bundle branch block pattern.

illustrated in Figure 30. During 3:2 AV conduction in the presence of a fixed right bundle branch block pattern, a small increase in the P-R interval precedes a nonconducted P wave. The H-V interval increases from an initially abnormal value of 60 msec to 100 msec, indicating progressive conduction delay within the left bundle branch and the third P wave blocks within the His-Purkinje system. Patients exhibiting the findings illustrated in Figure 30 will also have intermittent periods of high degree (e.g., 2:1, 3:1) AV block within the His-Purkinje system, which accounts in part for their symptoms of fatigue, dizziness, and even syncope. Also, these patients almost invariably go on to develop complete AV block within the His-Purkinje system.

In the presence of a fixed bundle branch block pattern, the distinction, based solely on the EKG tracings, between type I second degree AV block occurring within the AV node and that of His-Purkinje origin may be quite difficult. In general, although not always, the increase in P-R interval from the first to the last of the conducted beats is significantly less in a His-Purkinje Wenckebach cycle than in an AV nodal Wenckebach cycle. However, when AV nodal Wenckebach type conduction is superimposed on a pre-existing first degree AV nodal block, the difference in P-R interval changes from the first to the last of the conducted beats may be of the magnitude seen with His-Purkinje Wenckebach cycles.

The least common site for the occurrence of Wenckebach type conduction is within the bundle of His itself (Fig. 31). This phenomenon is characterized by the re-

cording of two His deflections (H and H′), which signifies intra-His bundle conduction delay. As the P-R interval increases, the H-H′ interval increases, and the nonconducted atrial impulse of the Wenckebach cycle is followed by only a single His deflection (H).

Type II Second Degree AV Block (Mobitz II)

Type II second degree AV block occurs less commonly than type I; it is almost always associated with a bundle branch block pattern and is a forerunner to complete AV block. The AV conduction ratio may be 3:2, 4:3, 5:4, and so forth, and the P-R intervals preceding the nonconducted atrial beat are constant. His bundle recordings have consistently demonstrated that the site of block is within the His-Purkinje system. Figure 32 is a typical example of type II second degree AV block; a left bundle branch block pattern is present, and 3:2 AV conduction progresses to 2:1 AV block. The third P wave, which is unexpectedly blocked within the His-Purkinje system, is preceded by constant P-R intervals. A prolonged H-V interval of 76 msec in the presence of left bundle branch block indicates that a significant conduction delay also existed in the right bundle branch system.

In patients with type II second degree AV block, acceleration of the atrial rate by atropine, exercise, or atrial pacing generally leads to an increase in the degree of AV block within the His-Purkinje system. Lightheadedness, dizziness, fatigue, syncope, convulsions, and congestive heart failure are common symptoms and signs associated

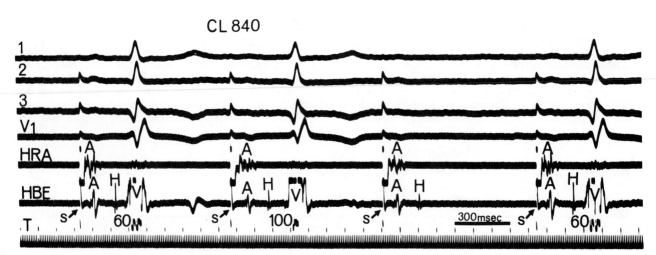

Figure 30. Type I second degree AV block within the His-Purkinje system.

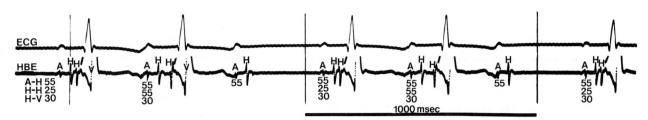

Figure 31. A 3:2 AV conduction and Type I second degree AV block occurring within the bundle of His itself. The H-H′ interval increases from 25 to 55 msec, and the third P wave, which is followed by only an H deflection, blocks within the bundle of His.

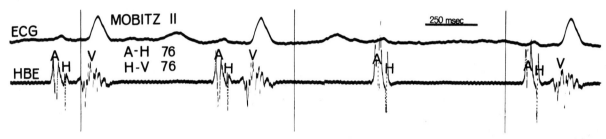

Figure 32. Type II second degree AV block in a patient with left bundle branch block and 3:2 AV conduction which progressed to 2:1 AV block. The third P wave is blocked within the His-Purkinje system.

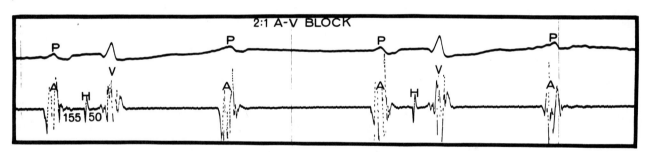

Figure 33. 2:1 AV nodal block in a patient with normal QRS complexes.

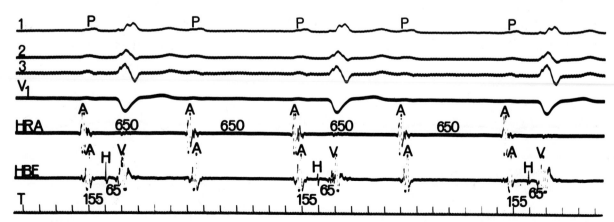

Figure 34. Patient with left bundle branch block and 2:1 AV nodal block. Both the A-H and H-V intervals (155 and 65 msec, respectively) of the conducted beats are prolonged.

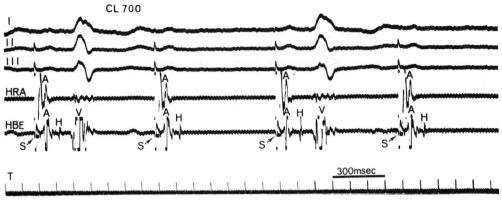

Figure 35. Patient with left bundle branch block and 2:1 AV block within the His-Purkinje system. Each of the nonconducted atrial impulses is followed by a His deflection. The H-V intervals of the conducted beats are prolonged.

with type II AV block. The demonstration of type II AV block requires that a permanent ventricular pacemaker be inserted, because this form of block almost always progresses to complete AV block within a relatively short period of time.

During complete AV block, atrial impulses continue to block within the His-Purkinje system, and the ventricles come under the control of an idioventricular pacemaker discharging at a rate of 35 to 50 per minute (see Fig. 37). It is not unusual for patients with type II AV block which progresses to complete AV block to demonstrate 1:1 retrograde conduction during ventricular pacing at a rate faster than the sinus rate. This is called unidirectional block.

2:1 AV Block

Like all other forms of AV block, 2:1 AV block may result from lesions in the AV node, bundle of His, or bundle branch–Purkinje system.

A fixed 2:1 AV block in the presence of normal QRS complexes is almost always due to AV nodal block, and the nonconducted P waves are not followed by bundle of His deflections (Fig. 33). The P-R interval of the conducted atrial impulses may be normal or prolonged. Uncommonly, 2:1 AV block with normal QRS complexes is due to block within the bundle of His itself. Each of the nonconducted atrial impulses is associated with a bundle of His deflection, and the P-R intervals of the conducted beats are normal.

In 2:1 AV block with a bundle branch block pattern, the localization of block by electrocardiographic record-

ings alone is difficult. In our experience, block within the His-Purkinje system is slightly more common than AV nodal block. The two forms of block are illustrated in Figures 34 and 35.

Third Degree AV Block

Third degree AV block (also referred to as complete AV block) may result from lesions located in the AV node, bundle of His, or bundle branch–Purkinje system.

In third degree AV nodal block (Fig. 36), atrial impulses are blocked within the AV node. The bundle of His usually emerges as the subsidiary or escape pacemaker, activating the ventricles at a rate of 40 to 60 per minute. Each QRS complex is preceded by a single His bundle deflection, and in general both the QRS complex and H-V intervals are the same as prior to the occurrence of AV block. Patients with complete AV nodal block and a junctional pacemaker (bundle of His) may remain asymptomatic for relatively long periods of time, and therefore the mere presence of complete AV block is not an indication for pacemaker therapy. Junctional pacemakers generally increase their discharge rate in response to exercise or after administration of atropine.

Complete AV block within the bundle of His itself is characterized by nonconducted atrial impulses which are followed by a His bundle deflection (H) and QRS complexes which are preceded by His bundle deflections (H'). The QRS complexes may be normal or abnormal and the H'-V intervals normal (30 to 55 msec) or greater than normal. It is believed that the junctional pacemaker is located within the bundle of His but distal to the site of

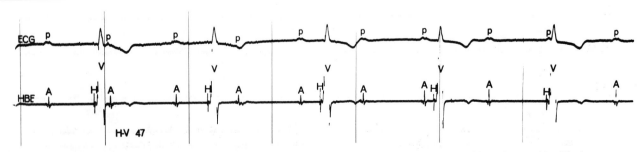

Figure 36. Third degree AV block. Atrial impulses are blocked within the AV node and dissociated from the ventricles. The latter come under control of a bundle of His pacemaker. H-V interval of 47 msec is within the normal range.

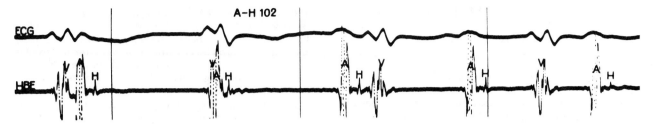

Figure 37. Third degree AV block within the His-Purkinje system. Nonconducted atrial impulses are followed by His bundle deflections. The wide QRS complexes come under control of a subjunctional pacemaker and are not preceded by bundle of His deflections.

block. These patients may not demonstrate acceleration of their ventricular rates in response to exercise or atropine. This would not be surprising if the process which caused the intra-His bundle block also affected the autonomic innervation of the common bundle. In these cases of determination for pacemaker, therapy depends upon the patients' symptoms.

Complete AV block distal to the bundle of His is characterized by nonconducted atrial impulses which are followed by His bundle deflections and abnormal QRS complexes which are not preceded by His bundle deflections (Fig. 37). The subsidiary pacemaker is located somewhere within the bundle branch–Purkinje system, and its discharge rate is generally between 35 and 50 per minute. These patients are almost always symptomatic (fatigue, dyspnea, dizziness, syncope, congestive heart failure) and require permanent ventricular pacemaker therapy.

Simulated Type II Second Degree AV Block

The electrocardiographic pattern of type II second degree AV block can be simulated when subtle increases in AV nodal delay are superimposed on a pre-existing first degree AV nodal block, as shown in Figure 38. During sinus rhythm and first degree heart block caused by AV nodal delay, the fourth P wave appears unexpectedly blocked and preceded by constant P-R intervals. However, His bundle recordings at rapid paper speeds (150 mm per second) reveal that a slight increase in the A-H interval preceded the fourth P wave which is blocked in the AV node. The electrophysiologic findings are consistent with a type I second degree AV block of the AV node and not a type II block within the His-Purkinje system. Small increases in AV nodal conduction can result from either spontaneous fluctuations in vagal tone or changes in the P-P cycle length. It is apparent that the small

changes in AV nodal conduction, depicted in Figure 38, would not be appreciated on standard EKG recordings at paper speeds of 25 mm per second. Thus caution should be exercised in making the diagnosis of type II AV block in the presence of an underlying first degree AV block. However, the fact that the patient had normal QRS complexes would argue against the diagnosis of type II AV block, because the latter is generally associated with bundle branch block patterns. In addition, atropine may help in distinguishing the site of block. In type I AV block, atropine shortens the P-R interval and 1:1 AV conduction is established at a faster sinus rate. In type II block, atropine would have a tendency to increase the degree of AV block at a faster sinus rate, because atropine does not directly effect conduction within the His-Purkinje system.

Functional or Physiologic AV Block

At sinus rates of 60 to 100 per minute, the spontaneous occurrence of various types of AV block usually represents an abnormal response of the AV conducting system. On the other hand, acceleration of the atrial rate in resting subjects, such as may occur with atrial flutter, with an ectopic atrial rhythm, or during electrical stimulation of the atrium, can result in various degrees of AV block which may be considered physiologic or functional in nature. Normally, the autonomic nervous system mediates a fine balance between atrial rate and AV nodal conduction. During exercise or other stressful situations, sympathetic stimulation simultaneously increases sinus rates and enhances AV nodal conduction so that there occurs little or no change in the P-R interval. During nonsympathetically mediated increases in atrial rate, the capacity of the AV node to transmit impulses to the ventricles is exceeded and a functional AV nodal block ensues.

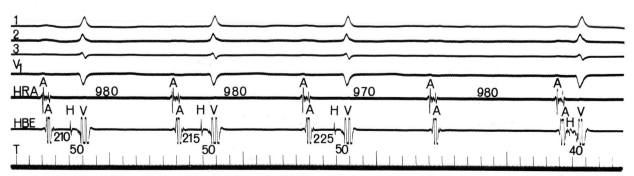

Figure 38. Subtle AV nodal Wenckebach type of conduction simulating type II second degree AV block. The P-P intervals are constant. During 4:3 AV conduction, the A-H interval increases only 15 msec prior to the fourth P wave being blocked in the AV node.

PERICARDITIS*

Patrick J. Hogan

571. INTRODUCTION

Inflammation of the pericardium results in deposition of inflammatory cells over the serosal surface and, depending on the cause, a variable amount of serous, fibrinous, purulent, or hemorrhagic exudate. The character, amount, and rate of formation of this exudate determine whether acute fibrinous pericarditis, pericardial effusion, cardiac tamponade, or constrictive pericarditis will develop. The pericardium is involved by a variety of etiologic agents, but rarely is it the sole structure reflecting underlying disease (see accompanying table). The diagnosis of pericarditis is consequently incomplete until the clinician has determined the precise cause with its relatively predictable subsequent clinical course and specific therapeutic demands.

572. ACUTE FIBRINOUS PERICARDITIS

Clinical Manifestations. The most reliable signs of acute pericarditis are chest pain, friction rub, and elec-

*The assistance of Dr. Henry D. McIntosh in the preparation of this chapter is gratefully acknowledged.

Classification of Pericardial Disease

I. Inflammatory
  A. Acute pericarditis
    1. Nonspecific (idiopathic)
    2. Infectious
      a. Viral (coxsackievirus, echovirus, cytomegalovirus, influenza, Epstein-Barr)
      b. Bacterial
      c. Tuberculous
      d. Mycotic (histoplasmosis, actinomycosis, nocardia)
      e. Other (protozoal, mycoplasmal, spirochetal)
    3. Associated myocardial infarction
    4. Traumatic
      a. Penetrating or nonpenetrating injury to thorax
      b. Postmyocardial infarction syndrome
      c. Postpericardiotomy, postcardiotomy
    5. Connective tissue disorders (systemic lupus erythematosus, progressive systemic sclerosis, rheumatoid arthritis, rheumatic fever)
    6. Allergic and hypersensitivity diseases (serum sickness, penicillin, drugs)
    7. Metabolic disorders (uremia, myxedema, gout)
    8. Physical and chemical agents
      a. Postirradiation
      b. Postanticoagulation
  B. Chronic pericarditis
    1. Chronic pericardial effusion
    2. Chronic adhesive pericarditis
    3. Chronic constrictive pericarditis
II. Neoplastic
  A. Benign (teratoma, fibroma, angioma, lipoma)
  B. Malignant
    1. Primary (mesothelioma, sarcoma)
    2. Secondary (lung, breast, other)
    3. Leukemia and lymphoma
III. Congenital
  A. Pericardial cysts and diverticula
  B. Complete or partial absence of pericardium

trocardiographic (EKG) changes. Pericardial *pain* is usually abrupt, sharp, and severe, with a wide area of radiation to the neck, back, and left shoulder and, rarely, to the arm. Characteristically, it is parasternal, exacerbated by deep inspiration and recumbency, and relieved by sitting or leaning forward. The severity, location, and radiation of the pain may be strikingly similar to that of myocardial infarction, although, in the young, its epigastric location can suggest an acute abdominal disorder. Chest pain may be constant, trivial, or even totally absent, as is often the case in later stages of tuberculous or uremic pericarditis. Most patients are dyspneic and febrile, and complain of malaise, weakness, chills, or other symptoms reflecting the primary disorder.

On physical examination these patients appear anxious and restless, and are either sitting or leaning forward. They are generally febrile and tachycardic, particularly so with idiopathic and suppurative pericarditis. Heart sounds are of normal intensity unless muffled by large effusions. *Friction rubs,* the hallmark of pericarditis, result from inflammation of the pericardial surface, and are often well localized to the lower left parasternal area where they may be palpable (*pericardial fremitus*). These "grating" or "leathery" high frequency sounds exhibit marked changes in intensity, timing, and duration, and vary with phases of respiration and body position. Roughly half are augmented or are equally loud in inspiration and hence often confused with pleural or pleuropericardial rubs. Typically, rubs consist of three or two components, less often of one. The ventricular systolic component is generally the loudest; it may extend throughout systole, and is easily confused with adventitious sounds or systolic murmurs. The persistence of a rub longer than two to three weeks suggests a uremic, tuberculous, or neoplastic origin.

Laboratory studies reflect systemic reaction to pericardial inflammation and often suggest or confirm the presence of the primary underlying disease. Myocardial enzymes are normal or only slightly elevated. X-ray may demonstrate evidence of the primary disease; a pericardial effusion can be appreciated once 200 ml or more of fluid has collected. Electrocardiographic abnormalities are seen in 90 per cent of patients with acute pericarditis, but pathognomonic serial changes are observed in less than 50 per cent of such patients. Characteristically, in standard and lateral precordial leads, there is an initial S-T segment elevation, often with an upward concavity, that persists for a few days to several weeks. As the subepicardial muscle injury subsides, the S-T segment elevation disappears, the P-R segments may become displaced, and the T waves diminish and progressively invert owing to repolarization delay. The notched or inverted T waves generally return to normal by three months, but may be persistent in conditions that cause adhesive or constrictive pericarditis. Absence of Q waves and reciprocal S-T segment depression, plus the notable concavity of the upward S-T segment elevation, helps make the important electrocardiographic differentiation between acute pericarditis and myocardial infarction. Rhythm disturbances, predominantly atrial fibrillation or flutter, are seen in 10 per cent of patients with pericarditis, most likely a consequence of the proximity of the sinus node to the inflamed pericardium.

Differential Diagnosis. The diagnosis can be made with considerable certainty when a young man suddenly develops chest pain, later exacerbated by inspiration and relieved by sitting forward, and demonstrates a loud friction rub and characteristic serial EKG changes without Q waves, with normal serum myocardial enzymes, and with a normal or rapidly enlarging cardiac silhouette on chest x-ray. More commonly, the differentiation of pericarditis from myocardial infarction, dissecting aneurysm, pneumonia, pulmonary emboli, pleurisy, pneumothorax, mediastinitis, intercostal neuralgia, and acute pericardial fat necrosis may not be immediately apparent. Once the diagnosis of pericarditis has been established, the clinician must then attempt to determine the cause with its specific prognostic and therapeutic implications.

573. INDIVIDUAL VARIETIES OF PERICARDITIS

IDIOPATHIC (NONSPECIFIC) PERICARDITIS

Despite the prevailing suspicion of a viral, autoimmune, or hypersensitive cause, this clinical syndrome by definition remains of questionable and presumably diverse origin. The diagnosis is made only after carefully excluding known causes of acute pericarditis. Acute idiopathic pericarditis is largely a disease of males in the third or fourth decade, although it is certainly seen over a wide spectrum of ages and in females. A history of preceding upper respiratory infection can be elicited in one third to two thirds of these patients. They generally note a sharp, "sticking," retrosternal pain, often of maximal intensity within 24 hours, that is markedly influenced by respiratory changes. The majority of these previously healthy individuals are usually mildly toxic, but a few have high fevers. A transient rub is present, more often than not with a small serous pericardial effusion. Moderate leukocytosis is common; leukopenia and anemia are rare. Pneumonitis and pleural effusions are noted on x-ray one third of the time, occasionally accompanied by evidence of congestive heart failure. The EKG is nearly always abnormal, consistently demonstrating the typical evolutionary changes of pericarditis. The major symptoms of this syndrome generally respond to bed rest and analgesics, and usually resolve by one to three weeks. A quarter of these patients suffer recurrences of their symptoms months to years later with a generally shorter and less severe course. Rare fatalities have been reported to be due to cardiac tamponade, occasionally precipitated by anticoagulation. Although an occasional patient will have a protracted course, development of constrictive pericarditis is decidedly rare and should raise the possibility of an underlying tuberculous or collagen-vascular process.

VIRAL PERICARDITIS

The consistent recovery of certain enteroviruses from cardiac tissue in perimyocarditis strongly suggests a pathogenic correlation. Although other viruses have been isolated, for practical purposes viral carditis is mainly associated with coxsackievirus infection, primarily type B and rarely type A. Systemic manifestations of viral disease such as myalgias and arthralgias are common and accompany the typical pain, fever, and friction rub. Rubelliform rash or lymphadenopathy may be present. Pleural effusions are very frequent, and pleurodynia is present 25 per cent of the time. An en-

larged cardiac silhouette is the rule, and congestive heart failure has been noted in perhaps a quarter of these patients. The increased incidence of conduction disturbances, occasional transient Q waves, and higher myocardial enzyme elevations reflect the more significant myocardial involvement seen with viral pericarditis. A fourfold rise in neutralizing antibody titer or isolation of the virus in tissue culture confirms the diagnosis. Treatment of viral pericarditis is essentially the same as for idiopathic pericarditis, namely rest and analgesics; steroid therapy should be reserved for clearly refractory patients, particularly in life-threatening situations. The immediate prognosis depends on the degree of accompanying myocarditis.

PERICARDITIS OF ACUTE MYOCARDIAL INFARCTION

Pericarditis complicates acute myocardial infarction in one of five cases. Large effusions are exceptional and suggest an underlying diffuse pericarditis, whereas hemorrhagic effusions suggest the ominous complications of myocardial rupture or excessive anticoagulant therapy. Pericardial pain or friction rubs generally occur during the second to fourth day, rarely as early as the first or as late as the tenth day. These transient rubs are limited in extent, and are best appreciated at the apex or medial to the sternum. Fever and tachycardia may coincide with the rub, or may continue on from the time of the initial infarction. This self-limited process usually requires little therapy other than analgesics and occasionally anti-inflammatory agents such as aspirin or indomethacin; steroids are rarely needed. To avoid the development of cardiac tamponade or hemopericardium, anticoagulants should be withheld in the presence of a diffuse rub or with evidence of a large or enlarging effusion or ventricular aneurysm.

POSTCARDIAC INJURY SYNDROME

The common association of fever, pericarditis, and pleuritis that follows a latent period after injury to the heart or thorax has prompted many investigators to consider that the postmyocardial infarction syndrome, postpericardiotomy syndrome, post-traumatic pericarditis, and even idiopathic pericarditis may be subsets of a syndrome with a common pathogenic basis. Trauma or injury of some kind to the pericardium, myocardium, or both appears to be essential; the possibility of reactivation of latent virus infections is proposed by some. The common association of elevated titers of heart antibodies with serositis and arthritis is supportive, if indirect, evidence for an immunologic cause. However, these antibodies may represent a nonspecific response to traumatized or infarcted tissue.

Postmyocardial Infarction Syndrome
(Dressler's Syndrome)

In 1 per cent of cases of myocardial infarction, pericarditis develops late, has a prolonged course, or recurs. This syndrome normally develops 2 to 12 weeks after the infarction. Pericardial pain precedes or occurs simultaneously with the prolonged, recurrent fever that characterizes this disorder. Pericardial and pleural effusions are common, as is patchy pneumonitis. Tamponade is rare. The EKG may be helpful if typical features of pericarditis are present, but this is unusual. The characteristic pain, friction rub, and fever occurring several weeks to months after a myocardial infarction in the presence of pleural effusion and pneumonitis help make the necessary differentiation from pulmonary emboli or recurrent or extending myocardial infarction. The symptoms generally respond to analgesics, anti-inflammatory drugs, and reassurance; however, steroids may be required. Once instituted, it is often difficult to avoid rebound of symptoms when steroids are tapered. Anticoagulants are contraindicated once this diagnosis is made, because of the more diffuse pericarditis and extensive effusion seen with this disorder.

Post-thoracotomy-Pericardiotomy Syndrome

Approximately 10 per cent of post-thoracotomy patients will develop a delayed febrile response one week to several months after surgery, with signs and symptoms of pericarditis and often with pleural or pericardial effusion. Typically, the pain, fever, rub, and effusion follow a benign and self-limited course. The timing of this syndrome demands close scrutiny to rule out more significant postoperative complications such as pulmonary infarction, atelectasis, or hemopericardium. Bed rest, sedation, and analgesics are important adjuncts to therapy. Steroids effect prompt cessation of symptoms but must be used with particular caution in this setting in which infections are commonplace. This syndrome recurs often and on occasion has persisted intermittently for periods of several years.

COLLAGEN VASCULAR DISEASES AND PERICARDITIS

Systemic Lupus Erythematosus

Lupus pericarditis accounts for less than 5 per cent of all types of pericarditis, yet it may be clinically evident in up to 40 per cent of documented cases of systemic lupus erythematosus (SLE). Pericarditis may precede the more common signs and symptoms of lupus by a considerable time period, often resulting in a misdiagnosis of rheumatic or idiopathic pericarditis. This diagnosis is facilitated by the demonstration of a positive lupus preparation or antinuclear antibody test in serum or more rarely in the pericardial fluid itself. These patients generally respond to steroids, often needed in large doses for prolonged periods. Aside from an increased incidence of congestive heart failure, there is no apparent prognostic significance to the development of pericarditis in SLE over and above that of the primary disease process.

Rheumatoid Arthritis

Clinical evidence of acute pericarditis is uncommon in patients with rheumatoid arthritis (RA), but surgical and postmortem specimens indicate that a nonspecific fibrinous inflammation resulting in adhesive pericarditis has occurred in one of two RA patients. Pericarditis is typical of the extra-articular features of rheumatoid arthritis, in that it occurs in patients with significant, well documented peripheral arthritis, usually having subcutaneous nodules and high titers of rheumatoid factor. Fever, leukocytosis, anemia, and an elevated sedimentation rate give evidence of the active inflammatory process commonly associated with the development of pericarditis. Friction rub is normally present, and signs of pleural effusion and congestive failure are not uncommonly detected. The fluid in rheumatoid pericardial effusion, like that of rheumatoid pleural effusion, is characterized by a markedly low concentration of glucose, elevated LDH enzymes, elevated gamma globulin, and decreased hemolytic complement and complement components. Cytologic examination may demonstrate giant round or oval multinucleated cells, thought by some to be pathognomonic of this disorder. Rheumatoid pericarditis is a low-grade inflammatory process that usually pursues a short course and requires minimal therapy. Steroids predictably reverse the pericardial symptoms of these patients, but may have little or no effect on the articular symptoms. Rare cases of rheumatoid pericarditis have developed into constrictive pericarditis despite steroid intervention.

UREMIC PERICARDITIS

Formerly regarded as a sign of imminent death, pericarditis is now an expected manifestation of uremia. The introduction of hemodialysis has significantly altered the natural history, clinical features, and therapy of uremic pericarditis. Previously, other symptoms and signs of uremia overshadowed the infrequent chest pain, insignificant friction rubs, rare nonspecific EKG findings, and small fibrinous effusions that characterized uremic pericarditis. Now, the 10 to 15 per cent of patients who develop uremic pericarditis while on hemodialysis complain of significant pain and fever, have loud friction rubs, and manifest large, often hemorrhagic, pericardial effusions with pronounced EKG changes and rhythm disturbances. These patients are often hypotensive during dialysis, have frequent arrhythmias, and have cardiomegaly on x-ray, with elevated venous pressure with or without evident pericardial effusion. Heart failure and pulmonary congestion are not uncommon and give evidence of the severity of underlying myocardial damage that occurs with uremic pericarditis. The precise cause of both fibrinous and hemorrhagic pericarditis in uremia remains obscure. The level of renal function does not differentiate between those patients who will or will not develop pericarditis or hemorrhagic effusion. The apparent protection afforded by more intense hemodialysis suggests that dialyzable compounds play an etiologic role in the development of this syndrome. Cardiac tamponade and subsequent constriction are seen with increased frequency after the institution of hemodialysis, presumably reflecting the increased bleeding tendency and qualitative platelet abnormalities of chronic uremia and technical anticoagulation problems of the hemodialysis procedure. It is vital to recognize the development of these syndromes and not attribute a falling glomerular filtration rate (GFR) to terminal renal failure, rather than to an altered cardiac output resulting from pericardial disease which may be correctable. The development of uremic pericarditis is an indication for initiating or increasing hemodialysis. This therapeutic technique will prevent the occurrence or reoccurrence of pericarditis in two thirds of uremic patients. Recurrent pericarditis and effusion, particularly with hypotension or evidence of tamponade, requires at least pericardiocentesis, but more often will require pericardiectomy.

PURULENT PERICARDITIS

Pyogenic pericarditis demands early recognition and specific, aggressive therapy to avoid its lethal consequences. The clinical signs of pericarditis may significantly postdate the initial infection, may be overshadowed by the primary focus, or may be altered by intervening antimicrobial therapy. Purulent pericarditis generally occurs as a consequence or complication of other diseases, particularly mediastinal or pulmonary infection. Pneumonia, empyema, or other thoracic infections most commonly invade the pericardium by direct extension, often after penetration of the thorax and pericardium during surgery or by trauma. Septicemia from distant skin, soft tissue, or bone infections is less often responsible for this syndrome, and subdiaphragmatic abscesses rarely so. Pericarditis occurs more than 10 per cent of the time in fatal bacterial endocarditis, and may accompany myocardial abscesses. Dyspnea, fever, tachycardia, and chest pain are prominently present in adults. Cardiomegaly is frequent, often with muffled heart sounds and pulsus paradoxus, attesting to the usual presence of an accompanying significant effusion. A friction rub or classic EKG pattern is absent in more than half of these patients and should not impede a diagnostic and often therapeutic pericardiocentesis. Appropriate antimicrobial drugs and surgical drainage have led to gratifying results. *Pneumococcal* pericarditis, formerly the prototype of purulent pericarditis, is now rarely seen, and is nearly always due to untreated pneumonia or associated empyema. *Staphylococcal* pericarditis, often hospital acquired, usually arises from a remote focus of infection, and pursues a devastating clinical course. It is renowned for complicating a variety of surgical procedures, particularly open heart surgery. Gram-negative organisms, including Pseudomonas, Proteus, *E. coli*, and Klebsiella, involve the pericardium, especially in the immunosuppressed patient. Meningococcus, with or without meningitis, and gonococcus can infect the pericardium in the untreated patient, often with massive effusion. The systemic mycoses *histoplasmosis, actinomycosis, and aspergillosis* have caused purulent pericarditis, but more often result in a granulomatous reaction, occasionally with resultant constrictive pericarditis. *Amebiasis* of the left lobe of the liver has involved the pericardium by simple contiguity or by direct rupture into the pericardial space. Creation of a pericardial window with pleural drainage or pericardiectomy is mandatory with purulent pericarditis and usually eliminates the possibility of constrictive pericarditis developing subsequently.

TUBERCULOUS PERICARDITIS

Tuberculous pericarditis occurs in 5 to 10 per cent of tuberculous patients. It accounts for up to one tenth of all cases of acute pericarditis and a significantly larger percentage of cases of constrictive pericarditis. It shares with the other forms of pericarditis a characteristic male predominance, usually appearing between the second and sixth decade, but is peculiar in its racial predisposition, occurring perhaps 10 to 12 times more commonly in blacks than in whites. The pericardium may appear as the sole or primary site of tuberculous involvement, but it is probably always secondary to tuberculous infection elsewhere. Obvious pulmonary or pleural tuberculous manifestations are detected in half these patients. In nearly all clinically recognized cases, there is retrograde tuberculous extension from pleural, pulmonary, or mediastinal lymph nodes. The onset of symptoms may be sudden, but generally these symptoms occur insidiously. Unexplained cardiomegaly may be the initial indication of disease, and dyspnea, cough, and chest pain are common, particularly with large effusions. High spiking temperatures are noted in the acute phase, but more commonly low-grade fever, weakness, fatigue, night sweats, and transient arthralgia are noted. It is not rare for patients with this disease to present initially with symptoms of constrictive pericarditis or cardiac tamponade.

The diagnosis is established by determining that pericarditis exists in the presence of pulmonary or extrapulmonary tuberculous lesions. The absence of x-ray evidence of tuberculosis by no means excludes this diagnosis. Under optimal circumstances it is possible to culture the mycobacterium, or to verify the diagnosis by pericardial biopsy in about half the patients in which the condition is suspected. Nevertheless, tuberculous pericarditis should be high on the list of diagnostic possibilities if a positive tuberculin reaction is present with evidence of pericarditis, particularly with weight loss, fever, night sweats, and massive or rapidly occurring sanguineous or hemorrhagic effusion. Triple therapy with isoniazid, streptomycin, and rifampin or ethambutol is required for 18 to 24 months. Most authorities recommend a brief trial of steroids to decrease the toxic manifestations of this disease and to diminish inflammatory exudation. If symptoms of constriction persist for six weeks, or if there is no evidence of chemotherapeutic response by six months, these patients should undergo pericardiectomy.

574. PERICARDIAL EFFUSION

Pericardial effusion can occur with any variety of acute pericarditis, or can accompany hepatic, renal, or cardiac failure or other conditions complicated by anasarca. Rarely the effusion may persist for many years, and such patients have been misdiagnosed as having chronic congestive heart failure. Chronic effusion has been associated with a variety of systemic disorders such as myxedema, collagen diseases, and chronic anemia. Some cases are idiopathic, with the pericardial fluid having markedly elevated protein and excessive "cholesterol" crystals.

Pathophysiology. The sudden accumulation of even a few hundred milliliters of blood in the pericardium may impair cardiac filling to the point of arterial hypotension, syncope, or sudden death. In contradistinction, several liters of fluid may gradually accumulate in myxedema or tuberculous or idiopathic pericarditis and may fail to elicit recognizable signs or symptoms. Other determinants of the physiologic response to pericardial effusion include the type of fluid, the size and compliance of the pericardial sac, the functional competence of the underlying myocardium, and the status of the visceral pericardial lymphatics and right heart venous drainage.

Physical Findings. The clinical detection of less than 200 to 300 ml of pericardial fluid in the absence of cardiac compression may be impossible. Larger amounts of fluid, especially if rapidly acquired, can be determined reliably by physical examination. Such patients are anxious, dyspneic, tachycardic, and diaphoretic and often assume the upright position. Depending on the compression caused by the pericardial accumulation, the pulses may be normal, depressed, or paradoxical; the neck veins may be normal or elevated. The heart sounds are of normal intensity, and friction rubs are commonly heard despite the presence of large effusion. Repeated examination, particularly in the prone position, may disclose muffling of the heart sounds. The cardiac apical impulse may be weak or absent; its detection medial to the left border of cardiac dullness is diagnostically helpful. A distinctive flatness to percussion that extends laterally beyond the apex or to the right of the sternum, that extends to the lower half of the sternum, or that expands to the second or third left intercostal space on recumbency is similarly a useful sign. Another helpful, if uncommon, indicator of pericardial effusion is the development of an area of dullness under the angle of the scapula generally associated with bronchial breath sounds, referred to as *Ewart's sign*. This sign is due to compression of the lung and can occasionally result from marked cardiomegaly.

Laboratory Studies. The *EKG* may be normal or, more commonly, may demonstrate nondiagnostic changes. The association of low QRS voltage and pericardial effusion has long been appreciated. It is not an invariable finding, but any diminution of voltage in patients with acute pericarditis suggests the development of an effusion. With large effusions and tachycardia, a regular alternating QRS voltage may be recorded (*electrical alternans*). This is thought to result from the oscillatory movements of the heart cushioned from mediastinal and pulmonary restraints by the pericardial effusion. Total electrical alternans of both P and QRS waves is seen only with very large effusions, usually with cardiac tamponade. The most reliable and earliest *radiologic sign* of pericardial effusion is the demonstration of an abrupt, symmetrical increase in the cardiac silhouette on serial roentgenograms, especially in the absence of congested lung fields. The normal contour of the left heart border may straighten, or the right cardiophrenic junction may bulge convexly. With widening and obliteration of the outline of the great vessels and general loss of angular curves, the heart assumes a characteristic "pear" or "flask" configuration. The *fluoroscopic* demonstration of decreased ventricular pulsations is helpful, and is quite specific if these pulsations are totally absent. The demonstration of the epicardial fat line well inside the cardiac contour with image intensification is another indication of the presence of pericardial fluid. All these roentgenographic signs are helpful but are rarely totally definitive in distinguishing pericardial effusion from cardiac hypertrophy, dilatation, or variations of the normal cardiac silhouette. Conclusive differentiation between them often requires the use of some form of contrast: positive contrast with angiographic techniques, negative contrast with carbon dioxide, or gamma-emitting radioisotopes. *Echocardiography* has proved to be a safe, simple technique that permits accurate diagnosis and monitoring of pericardial effusions. When fluid separates the ventricular epicardium from the posterior or anterior pericardium, a distinctive motionless echo interface can be detected. The echo-free space between the epicardium and pericardium roughly estimates the amount of peri-

cardial effusion. The echocardiogram can supply additional information relating to cardiac size and contractility. Most centers now initially use this diagnostic mode and resort to further angiographic verification when echoes are technically difficult or the results confusing.

575. CARDIAC TAMPONADE

Etiology. When intrapericardial pressure rises sufficiently to impede ventricular filling and myocardial contractility, cardiac compression or *tamponade* exists. Essentially anything that causes pericardial inflammation or injury can result in tamponade, depending on the tempo and duration of the inciting process. Overwhelming exudation from pyogenic, tuberculous, or neoplastic pericarditis, or the exuberant transudation of lupus, rheumatic, or even idiopathic pericarditis has caused tamponade. More commonly, tamponade occurs with the sudden development of intrapericardial hemorrhage or the transformation of a pre-existing effusion into hemopericardium. Contusion, laceration, or rupture of the heart or great vessels, hemorrhagic complications of uremic or neoplastic pericarditis, and the excessive administration of anticoagulants have all led to cardiogenic shock from tamponade.

Pathophysiology. The presence of large pericardial effusions in the absence of cardiac compression may cause no hemodynamic impairment; but once the pericardium becomes indistensible, further increments of fluid cause severe restriction of diastolic expansion by the myocardium. Pericardial compression of the right atrium interferes with venous inflow, resulting in a back-up or pooling of venous blood causing elevated central venous pressures. Both ventricles are similarly compromised by decreasing compliance, with elevated end-diastolic pressures and reciprocally depressed end-diastolic volumes resulting in decreased stroke volumes and cardiac output. Compensatory tachycardia and vasoconstriction may initially support the circulation; but once the fluid accumulation proves inexorable, the stroke volume decreases further and the elevated heart rate alone becomes insufficient to maintain cardiac output. In the face of escalating tachycardia with decreased diastolic filling periods, lowered aortic pressures, and increasing compression on the myocardium and coronary vessels, coronary insufficiency and eventual myocardial necrosis become inevitable, resulting in decreased myocardial performance and an even further decreased stroke volume. The unsupported venous pressure then falls and diastolic filling substantially decreases, causing this vicious cycle to perpetuate itself, leading eventually to total circulatory collapse.

Physical Findings. The dramatic appearance of patients with tamponade should impress the clinician with the necessity for rapid diagnosis and decisive therapy. When first seen, these patients may be comatose and in profound shock, particularly in cases of acute hemopericardium; but more often they appear anxious, pale or cyanotic, and dyspneic, sitting or leaning forward and often giving a history of antecedent pericarditis. Such patients are characteristically hypotensive, with marked venous distention and no evidence of cardiac enlargement (Beck's triad), and usually demonstrate paradoxical pulse and narrowed pulse pressure.

Pulsus paradoxus is defined as a drop in systolic blood

pressure of more than 10 mm Hg on quiet inspiration. Demonstration of this pulse deficit at the bedside can be a valuable clue to the presence of cardiac compression, particularly if accompanied by elevated venous pressures that distend or fail to collapse on inspiration. Virtually always present with cardiac tamponade, this sign is similarly seen in some cases of constrictive pericarditis. With normal inspiration there is a decrease in intrathoracic pressure, and the right heart pressures decline accordingly with the lowered intrapleural pressure. This results in augmented right ventricular filling by virtue of the increased gradient between the extrathoracic veins and the right chambers of the heart. Coincident with the more negative intrathoracic pressure, there is a redistribution of blood to the more compliant pulmonary veins and left atrium at the expense of decreased filling of the less compliant left ventricle. These mechanisms account for the physiologic lowering of both systolic and pulse pressure during inspiration when intrapleural pressure is minimal. With the development of cardiac tamponade, these normal respiratory variations become amplified and acquire pathologic significance. As the right ventricle distends during inspiration with tamponade, there is competition for the limited available space in the pericardium, resulting in an intrapericardial pressure rise with subsequent compromise of the left ventricular output and systemic arterial pressure. Other factors of varying significance include inspiratory descent of the diaphragm, causing traction in the already taut pericardium; heightened inspiratory pooling of blood in the lungs and right heart, accounting for decreased left ventricular ejection; and interference by the tense pericardial sac with the transmission of intrathoracic pressures to the left ventricle, resulting in a decreased effective filling pressure with pooling of the blood in the pulmonary veins. This sign is not pathognomonic of pericardial tamponade and is more commonly associated with obstructive airway disease. Prominent engorgement of neck veins should suggest cardiac tamponade and help distinguish it from other conditions of shock. Inspiratory augmentation of cervical venous waves and the precipitous pulse collapse of these veins are further evidence of tamponade. The lung fields are surprisingly clear, with Ewart's sign occasionally observed. Percussion and palpation of the heart are typically unremarkable, whereas with auscultation the heart sounds are often distant or frankly muffled, with a notable absence of gallops or murmurs. Diastolic sounds and friction rubs are generally not heard. Liver tenderness and enlargement may be the initial signs of tamponade. Manual compression of the liver with cervical venous distention (positive *hepatojugular reflux*) is further indirect evidence of tamponade. Ascites may be prominent with chronic tamponade, but edema is rarely noted in either acute or chronic tamponade.

Laboratory Studies. Cardiac tamponade is primarily a clinical diagnosis, and laboratory studies, although they may be supportive, are of secondary value and are rarely diagnostic in themselves. EKG findings are usually nonspecific, but occasionally demonstrate typical changes of acute pericarditis. S-T segment changes that revert after pericardiocentesis suggest that tamponade was present, causing subendocardial ischemia. Electrical alternans and low QRS voltage are suggestive, but do not help differentiate effusion from tamponade. Total electrical alternans of the P, QRS, and T waves is said to be virtually diagnostic of acute tamponade. In view of the fact that acute tamponade can be produced by small effusions that are radiologically indistinct, a normal-sized cardiac silhouette in no way excludes this diagnosis. Fluoroscopy or angiography may document an effusion in a majority of patients, but does not distinguish effusion from tamponade.

Pericardiocentesis. Pericardiocentesis becomes mandatory when tamponade causes hypotension, pulse pressure less than 20 mm Hg, central venous pressure greater than 20 cm H_2O, pulsus paradoxus greater than 50 per cent of the pulse pressure, or shock. The subxiphoid-subcostal approach is preferred as a safe, anatomically well defined position which avoids the pleural space and is more likely to yield small amounts of dependent pericardial fluid. A large-bore, short-beveled needle attached to the precordial or exploring lead is advanced, with continuous EKG monitoring, upward under the rib cage and medially toward the right shoulder until fluid is returned. Should inadvertent contact with the atria or ventricle be made, cardiac pulsations can be felt and indicated electrocardiographically by S-T segment elevation or runs of premature atrial or ventricular contractions. It is vital to recognize myocardial puncture in order to avoid myocardial or coronary laceration, air embolism, catastrophic arrhythmias, or excessive aspiration of intravascular fluid in an already hemodynamically compromised patient. Once the aspiration needle has been correctly positioned, enough fluid should be removed to demonstrate at least overt hemodynamic improvement, often a quantity as small as 50 to 100 ml. This fluid should always be submitted for culture and cytologic examination.

Treatment. All patients with acute pericarditis or effusion require repeated physical examinations with serial x-rays and careful monitoring of vital signs for manifestations of cardiac tamponade. If aspiration attempts prove unsuccessful or fail to relieve the tamponade, surgical exploration with pericardiectomy or creation of a pericardial window should be undertaken without delay, especially in situations of trauma or after cardiac surgery. If the pericardial fluid cannot be evacuated immediately, the circulation must be stabilized by the maintenance and expansion of venous blood volume. Vasopressors and digitalis are often ineffective in this setting, but isoproterenol has been consistently helpful, provided the heart rate is sufficiently slow and the central venous pressure well maintained.

576. CONSTRICTIVE PERICARDITIS

Recovery from pericarditis can be complicated by the development of chronic pericardial effusion, adhesion, or constriction.

Adhesive pericarditis may develop between the visceral and parietal pericardium, the pericardium and myocardium, or the pericardium and neighboring mediastinal structures. Adhesive pericarditis, by and large, causes negligible circulatory disturbances. *Constrictive pericarditis* ensues once the adherent layer of the pericardium becomes thickened and fibrosed to the extent of myocardial encasement and impairment of diastolic filling. Although constrictive pericarditis was formerly considered to be a common sequela of tuberculosis, more recent surveys have been unable to identify any consistent etiologic agent. Pyogenic pericarditis, particularly staphylococcal or pneumococcal, often results in subacute and chronic constrictive pericarditis, as does idiopathic and viral pericarditis. Trauma to the heart, neoplastic invasion or irradiation of the pericardium, and uremia, all conditions associated with hemorrhagic pericarditis, have been associated with the development of this syndrome.

Pathophysiology. Many factors contribute to the altered physiology of constrictive pericarditis, not the least of which being the degree and location of fibrosis interfering with ventricular diastolic filling. Usually the restrictive scar tissue involves both ventricles equally, resulting in a typical "small, quiet" heart. On occasion it may selectively surround a single ventricle, atria, great vessels, or vena cava. Such patients may have compensatory enlargement of the heart, particularly if there is some associated myocardial or valvular disease. Persistence of this syndrome after surgical failure to adequately liberate each ventricle emphasizes how hemodynamically significant localized pericardial constriction can be. Variable myocardial fibrosis and disuse atrophy accompanying pericardial fibrosis add to the hemodynamic burden imposed by impaired diastolic filling.

Clinical Manifestations. Signs and symptoms suggestive of right heart failure develop in this syndrome, predictably in young or middle-aged adults of either sex, who often have a recent or remote history of pericarditis. Some patients complain of relatively acute exertional dyspnea, abdominal swelling, or peripheral edema occurring over a matter of weeks to months. Other patients notice the insidious progression of weakness and fatigability, slight breathlessness, epigastric discomfort, or a tendency for fluid retention occurring over many years. Abdominal swelling and discomfort caused by tender hepatomegaly and accumulated ascitic fluid are prominent features of this syndrome that usually antedate and overshadow any peripheral edema. Subtle signs of left heart failure, such as dyspnea occurring only with exertion, or gradually increasing orthopnea, are often elicited and generally tend to be progressive. Paroxysmal nocturnal dyspnea and pulmonary edema are not usual features of this syndrome.

The cervical veins are obviously engorged and highlight the cardiogenic origin of the ascites, hepatomegaly, and edema that generally bring this disorder to medical attention. Careful examination of the swollen jugular venous pulse reveals a marked diastolic collapse or prominent "Y" descent. The magnitude and volume of the arterial pulse are normally decreased; pulsus paradoxus is not common. Examination of the lungs may reveal modest pulmonary congestion and, generally at some stage of the disease, signs of pleural effusion. Sometimes there is an early diastolic tap or shock caused by the rapid inflow of blood against an indistensible ventricle. On auscultation the heart sounds may be distant, with mid- to late systolic clicks frequently heard. A loud snapping, apical, high-pitched diastolic sound (pericardial knock), occurring 0.09 to 0.12 second after aortic valve closure, helps confirm this diagnosis. This sound coincides with the "Y trough" and palpable diastolic shock, reflecting termination of rapid inflow of blood by the sudden pericardial impediment to the dilating ventricle. Prominent, tender hepatomegaly, ascites, and splenomegaly have more than once caused the erroneous diagnosis of hepatic cirrhosis.

Laboratory Studies. Characteristic but nondiagnostic electrocardiograms are present in nearly all cases of chronic constrictive pericarditis. The EKG most commonly demonstrates decreased QRS voltage, flattened or inverted T waves, broad or notched P waves, and, often, right axis deviation. These changes usually persist after pericardiectomy and are undoubtedly attributable to subepicardial fibrosis and myocardial atrophy. Electrical alternans does not occur in the absence of a significant effusion. Arrhythmias are seen 40 per cent of the time, with atrial fibrillation most consistently recorded. The heart on chest x-ray may appear small, normal, or slightly enlarged. Fluoroscopy typically reveals diminished cardiac pulsations, dilated superior vena cava, abrupt, early diastolic dilatation, and straight left and right heart borders, with a small to absent aortic knuckle. *Pericardial calcification* signifies the presence of pericardial adhesion but not necessarily constriction. Although not pathognomonic, this valuable sign can be detected in over 75 per cent of the cases of chronic constriction if carefully sought. Angiography may delineate the presence of a thickened, rigid atrial wall, slowed circulation, and possible right or left atrial enlargement. The *echocardiographic* confirmation of diminished ventricular volumes, enlarged atrium, and thickened, immobile posterior wall with impaired contraction affords corroborative evidence of pericardial constriction. Hepatic function tests, particularly the Bromsulphalein test, become abnormal with progressive, passive liver congestion. Hypoalbuminemia, normal or elevated globulins, and albuminuria, as well as other results associated with protein-losing enteropathy, can accompany this syndrome. At cardiac catheterization the right atrial pressure is invariably elevated and is usually equaled by that of the left atrium, as well as the right and left ventricular end-diastolic, pulmonary artery diastolic, and wedge pressures. Prominent atrial "X" and "Y" descents result in a distinctive "M" or "W" pressure tracing. Right ventricular pressures reflect an abrupt termination of this "Y" descent by an early diastolic dip with a rapid rise to an elevated diastolic pressure plateau, notably more than a third that of the pressure recorded at end-systole. This "square root" pattern with its high end-diastolic pressure and compromised stroke volume is duplicated, as expected, in left ventricular pressure tracings. The cardiac output is usually normal at rest, and there is diminished response to exercise. Similar hemodynamic changes have been recorded with severe myocardial failure, usually biventricular, from a variety of causes. Differential diagnosis can be difficult at times.

Treatment. The definitive treatment of constrictive pericarditis consists of adequate surgical decortication. Symptoms or signs of excessive fatigue, dyspnea, edema, or ascites and evidence of depressed cardiac output, impaired diastolic filling, or hepatic congestion are indications for surgical intervention. Ideally this should be performed before obliteration of the pericardial space has occurred; before hepatic dysfunction, protein-losing enteropathy, or nephrotic syndrome has developed; and before the myocardium and great vessels become inextricably fibrotic and calcified. Surgical results, previously dismal, have improved substantially to an expected 10 to 12 per cent perioperative mortality and 5 per cent late mortality. Factors that determine the surgical outcome include the duration of the disease, age of the patient, character of the constrictive tissue, atrial fibrillation, ability to establish a cleavage plane at the time of surgery, and, most important, the presence and degree of cardiomyopathy or dilatation. Patients who have had pericarditis for a long time, with marked myocardial atrophy from longstanding constriction, may experience only minimal improvement, or may require very long recuperative periods.

Bishop, L. H., Jr., Estes, E. H., Jr., and McIntosh, H. D.: The electrocardiogram as a safeguard in pericardiocentesis. J.A.M.A., 162:264, 1956.

Comty, C. M., Cohen, S. L., and Shapiro, F. L.: Pericarditis in chronic uremia and its sequels. Ann. Intern. Med., 75:173, 1971.

Cortes, F. M. (ed.): The Pericardium and Its Disorders. Springfield, Ill., Charles C Thomas, 1970.

Dressler, W.: The postmyocardial infarction syndrome. A report on forty-four cases. Arch. Intern. Med., 103:28, 1959.

Ellis, K., and King, D. L.: Pericarditis and pericardial effusion. Radiol. Clin. North Am., 9:393, 1973.

Feigenbaum, H.: Echocardiographic diagnosis of pericardial effusion. Am. J. Cardiol., 26:475, 1970.

Fowler, N.: Cardiac Diagnosis. New York, Harper & Row, Publishers, 1968, p. 593.

Franco, A. E., Levine, H. D., and Hall, A. P.: Rheumatoid pericarditis. Ann. Intern. Med., 77:837, 1972.

Holt, J. P.: The normal pericardium. Am. J. Cardiol., 26:455, 1970.

Koontz, C. H., and Ray, C. G.: The role of Coxsackie Group B virus infections in sporadic myopericarditis. Am. Heart J., 82:750, 1971.

Schepers, G. W.: Tuberculous pericarditis. Am. J. Cardiol., 9:248, 1962.

Shabetai, R., Fowler, N. O., and Guntheroth, W. G.: The hemodynamics of cardiac tamponade and constrictive pericarditis. Am. J. Cardiol., 26:480, 1970.

Spodick, D. H.: Acute cardiac tamponade. Pathologic physiology, diagnosis, and management. Progr. Cardiovasc. Dis., 10:661, 1967.

Spodick, D. H.: Chronic and Constrictive Pericarditis. New York, Grune & Stratton, 1964.

Spodick, D. H.: Diagnostic electrocardiographic sequences in acute pericarditis. Circulation, 48:575, 1973.

Thadani, U., Chopra, M. P., Aber, C. P., and Portal, R. W.: Pericarditis after acute myocardial infarction. Br. Med. J., 2:135, 1971.

Wood, P.: Disease of the Heart and Circulation. 3rd ed., Philadelphia, J. B. Lippincott Company, 1968, p. 762.

DISEASE OF THE MYOCARDIUM

Wallace Brigden

577. INTRODUCTION

General Considerations. Many diseases of the heart are initiated by mechanical faults concerned with valve defects, deprivation of fuel supplies, or increased cardiac work. The myocardium, although showing remarkable reserves, is eventually secondarily affected in these conditions, and its failure often finally determines the course of events. These chapters are concerned with those rather less common conditions which are primarily localized in the myocardium leading to defective muscle function and its final failure.

These primary myocardial diseases are probably much more common than is generally recognized. Their true incidence is unknown, because serious investigation into these disorders has developed only in the last two or three decades. Furthermore, diagnostic errors are common not only because physical signs are often inconspicuous, but also because symptoms and signs may suggest one of the more well known disorders which affect the heart of man. The incidence of primary myocardial diseases is greatly affected by socioeconomic and geographical factors, and it happens that primary myocardial diseases are most common in developing parts of the world such as central Africa where sophisticated medical care with modern diagnostic methods is thinly spread.

Innumerable terms have been used for these disorders, but most are unsatisfactory and must remain so until the etiologic processes are fully understood. Primary myocardial disease indicates a process often of obscure etiology which is localized in the myocardium; cardiomyopathy indicates a somewhat wider range and includes processes which, although dominantly affecting the myocardium, may be of a generalized nature. Myocarditis, in keeping with usage of the suffix, should be restricted to disorders of an infectious or inflammatory nature. Myocardosis is an unsatisfactory term sometimes used to embrace all the noninflammatory processes. Classification is as unsatisfactory as terminology and for similar reasons. However, it is apparent that the myocardium may be damaged by any of the known disease processes which affect man; thus genetic, infective, metabolic, nutritional, and immunologic disorders may be found among the causes of cardiomyopathy. It would be rational, in such a classification, to include muscle disease resulting from vascular disorders, but habit and the magnitude of the problem have naturally led to isolation and separate consideration of coronary disease. However, there are rare cases of diffuse small vessel coronary occlusion which result in diffuse myocardial fibrosis causing clinical features which resemble other forms of cardiomyopathy. The following features concern primary myocardial disease in general.

Clinical Manifestations. The primary myocardial diseases present in diverse ways and their clinical features depend on the site, extent, and nature of the myocardial disorder and consequent disturbance of hemodynamics. Almost any of the symptoms and signs of heart disease (and any combination thereof) which arise in the whole field of heart disease may occur in the cardiomyopathies.

Dyspnea is the most common symptom. All forms are met, but since most myopathies dominantly affect the left ventricle, orthopnea and nocturnal asthma are common. *Syncope* is especially likely to occur in those forms of myocardial disease which cause heart block and paroxysmal arrhythmia; it may also result from effort when there is outflow tract obstruction (see Ch. 578), as in other obstructive disorders of the cardiovascular system. *Cardiac pain* is not common, but when it occurs an erroneous diagnosis of coronary disease is often made. True angina is a feature of idiopathic hypertrophic subaortic stenosis (see Ch. 578). Myocarditis, possibly when associated with pericarditis, may cause prolonged cardiac pain. Hepatic pain arising and increasing during effort may superficially resemble angina pectoris. *Palpitation* from frequent extrasystoles or other arrhythmia is common, especially in the familial forms, in alcoholic cardiomyopathy, and in myocarditis. Occasionally a primary muscle disorder may masquerade as an innocent paroxysmal tachycardia in the early stages of the disease process.

Physical examination and cardiovascular investigation may show any one of a number of dynamic disturbances which depend on the site and nature of the pathology. These may be classified in various ways. A division into congestive, constrictive, and hypertrophic (including obstructive) types, depending on the dominant hemodynamic derangement, has been suggested. From increasing experience with these conditions, it is clear that although there are such clear-cut hemodynamic disorders, there is also much overlap. However, the hypertrophic obstructive type is sufficiently discrete to be considered a separate and possibly single disease entity (see Ch. 578).

Chronic hypokinetic heart failure (congestive type) occurs in many forms of primary myocardial disease, but is probably most common in postinflammatory cardiomyopathy, active myocarditis, and familial cardiomegaly. The heart is very large and relatively "quiet" on fluoroscopy, and lung fields are often clear owing to right ventricular failure. All signs point to a chronic low cardiac output. At *necropsy* the heart weight is usually well above average, but the ventricular wall may appear thinner than normal because of the great dilatation. Macroscopic appearances of the muscle vary from normality to patchy fibrosis, and even large areas of damage may be found. Mural thrombi in varying stages of organization are common.

"Constrictive" forms of cardiomyopathy are not uncommon and cause confusion with constrictive pericarditis. This disorder is produced by restriction of ventricular filling because of diminished compliance of thick abnormal muscle or because of obstruction at the atrioventricular valves by masses of ventricular myocardium, or by massive endocardial thrombi and fibrosis (see Endomyocardial Fibrosis in Ch. 583). However, in many cases of cardiomyopathy the resemblance to constrictive pericarditis is relatively superficial. The venous pressure is high, an early diastolic sound is usual, and the right ventricular pressure curve shows a sharp early diastolic dip coincident with the *y* descent and a late diastolic plateau of the JVP. The *x* descent of the venous pulse (or RA pressure pulse) is usually shallow in primary myocardial disease in contrast to constrictive pericarditis. Furthermore, the electrocardiogram in constrictive cardiomyopathy usually shows a very abnormal QRS-T, whereas in constrictive pericarditis the QRS tends to remain near normal. However, the greatest diagnostic difficulty arises in some forms of endomyocardial fibrosis when the bulk of the muscle mass may be relatively normal, resulting in a nearly normal QRS complex. Calcification of the pericardium is absent, but difficulty may arise when there is myocardial or endomyocardial calcification. Cardiac amyloidosis and the African form of endomyocardial fibrosis often cause features of the constrictive syndrome.

Burch, G. E. (ed.): Cardiomyopathy. *In* Cardiovascular Clinics, Vol. 4. Philadelphia, F. A. Davis Company, 1972.

Goodwin, J. F.: Clarification of the cardiomyopathies. Mod. Concepts Cardiovasc. Dis., 41:41, 1972.

Mattingly, T. W.: Clinical features and diagnosis of primary myocardial disease. Mod. Concepts Cardiovasc. Dis., 30:677, 683, 1961.

578. HYPERTROPHIC CARDIOMYOPATHY

A group of patients have primary myocardial disease which is essentially of a hypertrophic nature. This hypertrophy may be of such magnitude that it causes dynamic derangement of an *obstructive nature* which may embarrass inflow to, or outflow from, either ventricle. The clinical features, laboratory findings, and pathologic changes are sufficiently uniform to justify consideration of this condition as a single disease entity variously known as *asymmetrical hypertrophy, idiopathic hypertrophic subaortic stenosis,* and *hypertrophic obstructive cardiomyopathy.* The cause is unknown, but in at least 30 per cent of patients there is a strongly positive family history of the same disease.

Pathology. Necropsy shows great ventricular hypertrophy which is often asymmetrical, and the ventricular cavity tends to be obliterated. The heart weight is always above normal and often greatly so. Diffuse fibrosis may be apparent, but large areas of fibrosis are not usually seen. The microscopic picture is of a bizarre arrangement of large muscle fibers separated by connective tissue. Fibrosis is common in the center of the muscle bundles. Using histochemical methods and electron microscopy, Pearse found widespread dystrophy of grossly hypertrophic muscle fibers accompanied by glycogen storage and mitochondriosis. There are also abnormal shortness of myofibers, proliferation of connective tissue with functional hyperplasia of arterioles and capillaries, and a proliferation of sympathetic nerve fibers (sympathosis) with consequent noradrenosis. At the electron microscopic level there is a close resemblance of cardiomyopathic fibers to normal atrial fibers; thus there is a possibility that developmental abnormality lies behind the syndrome. However, the proliferation of the sympathetic nerves may indicate a primary role of the autonomic nervous system.

Etiology. It is clear that many patients with hypertrophic obstructive cardiomyopathy have familial cardiomyopathy (see Ch. 579); however, in many cases there is no evidence of a familial disorder. A real division into familial and nonfamilial groups is supported by a different sex incidence which appears to be equal in the familial form, whereas males predominate in the nonfamilial forms. Furthermore, sudden death is much more common in the familial disease. It is possible that obstructive features may develop in any condition causing extreme ventricular hypertrophy associated with long survival. Thus it appears to be most common in congenital cardiomyopathy. Its rare appearance in such conditions as hypertensive heart disease and aortic valve disease is possibly due to the limited "natural history" imposed by other factors such as coronary disease.

Clinical Manifestations. The clinical features and diagnosis of this condition are discussed in Ch. 560.

Natural History. Many patients are apparently asymptomatic for many years. Even those with severe symptoms may undergo a period of remission, and symptoms may remain unchanged over a long period. Prognosis is difficult, but it appears to be less serious than might be anticipated from the severity of symptoms and signs. Sudden death is most likely to occur in the familial form and may occur in asymptomatic patients as well as in incapacitated ones.

Treatment. There is no effective treatment, but long-term medication with propranolol is under investigation. Restriction of physical activity should be advised as this may provoke arrhythmia, and it is known that the pressure gradient is increased by effort. A prolonged rest with sodium restriction or thiazide diuretics may help those with dyspnea or other evidence of heart failure. Digitalis is not advisable. Beta-adrenergic blocking drugs should be beneficial, but long-term results of treatment with these drugs are not available. *Surgical treatment* is indicated for patients with serious progressive symptoms from obstruction. Operative relief by resection of obstructing muscle or myotomy can be consistently accomplished even in severely ill patients, and survivors show striking symptomatic and hemodynamic improvement. Complete heart block is sometimes a complication of the operation, and postoperative left bundle branch block is usual though not invariable, but is not essential for a good result.

Braunwald, E., Lambrew, C., Morrow, A., Pierce, G., Rockoff, S. D., and Ross, J.: Idiopathic hypertrophic subaortic stenosis. Circulation (Suppl.), 1964.

Spodick, D. H.: Hypertrophic obstructive cardiomyopathy. Cardiovasc. Clin., 4:133, 1972.

579. FAMILIAL CARDIOMYOPATHY

Some forms of primary myocardial disease are perhaps best regarded as congenital cardiomyopathy. These include so-called *idiopathic familial cardiomegaly, obstructive cardiomyopathy* (idiopathic hypertrophic subaortic stenosis), some forms of *endocardial fibroelastosis,* and certain hereditary neuromuscular disorders which also involve the myocardium.

Familial cardiomyopathy may be a single disease entity which presents in a variety of ways, including hypertrophic obstructive disorder (see Ch. 578), congestive cardiac failure, and dysrhythmia. In some cases there is evidence of inheritance as a mendelian dominant, and transmission appears most commonly through the female parent, possibly because males die at a younger age; but there is no evidence of sex linkage. Birth order is not important, as most pedigrees suggest an erratic distribution in the family. It has been suggested that this may be the same disease as the cardiomyopathy associated with familial muscular dystrophies and ataxias, but the history of families with primary cardiomyopathies does not generally reveal other members with neuropathy. However, cardiomyopathy may be apparent before the development of neurologic features in Friedreich's ataxia and in myotonia, and a few families affected by neuropathy have been reported with some members having cardiomyopathy alone. It has also been suggested that familial heart disease is a result of intrauterine myocarditis from an infection such as toxoplasmosis, but the evidence for this is poor. Organisms have not been found in the myocardium in familial cardiomegaly, although inflammatory reactions have been reported, and, on a priori grounds, it is unlikely that latent infection could persist through many generations, or be transmitted through the male as it is in some affected families.

At necropsy the heart is often very large, and heart weights tend to be greater in this condition than those found in other cardiomyopathies. Histologic examination shows giant fibers with vacuolation and varying amounts of fibrous tissue. Electron microscopy and histochemistry show interesting and possibly specific features at least in the variety presenting as subaortic obstructive myopathy.

The symptoms of familial cardiomyopathy include palpitation from arrhythmia, giddy attacks and syncope, either from arrhythmia or after effort in obstructive cardiomyopathy, and dyspnea from varying degrees of heart failure. The age at onset of symptoms is variable, but it is usually between 5 and 30 years. Pregnancy may precipitate heart failure in the last trimester or early in the puerperium, thus leading to an erroneous diagnosis of "puerperal cardiomyopathy." Sudden death in pre-

viously asymptomatic individuals is not uncommon and has been recorded in most writings on the subject. Various arrhythmias have been described in this condition, including atrial fibrillation, atrial flutter, multiple ventricular extrasystoles, and heart block.

As in other cardiomyopathies the electrocardiogram is not specific, but gross conduction defects, left ventricular preponderance, and widespread Q waves are common. Radiology provides no special evidence in diagnosis, but some degree of cardiomegaly is usual, the left ventricle being most commonly affected. The left atrium is selectively enlarged when mitral valve regurgitation is a feature as in some cases. Angiography may show the characteristic appearance of left ventricular outflow tract obstruction in a minority; in others there is ventricular dilatation.

There is no specific treatment for familial cardiomyopathy. Arrhythmias are usually difficult to control. However, the poor prognosis of patients in heart failure may be considerably improved by prolonged rest, a low salt regimen, thiazide diuretics, and indefinite restriction of physical activity. Considerable reduction in heart size may be achieved by these means. Surgical treatment may be indicated when there is dominant left ventricular outflow obstruction (see Ch. 578).

Emanuel, R.: Familial cardiomyopathies. Postgrad. Med. J., 48:742, 1972.

Whitefield, A. G. W.: Familial cardiomyopathy. Quart. J. Med., 30:119, 1961.

580. INFLAMMATORY OR INFECTIVE CARDIOMYOPATHY (Myocarditis)

The term "myocarditis" should be restricted to inflammatory disease of the myocardium. Clinicians have been reluctant to diagnose myocarditis, but there is no doubt that the myocardium may be damaged in many different infections of viral, rickettsial, bacterial, protozoal, and even metazoal origin. Myocarditis is mainly incidental in the course of a generalized infection and remains relatively unimportant. However, it may dominate the clinical picture and determine the outcome of the disease, and sometimes it appears to be "isolated" with no evidence of generalized infection. Fatal heart failure and sudden death may result from severe myocarditis, but most attacks are probably subclinical or mild and are easily overlooked by the unwary. The long-term effects of such infection may lead to myocardial damage and fibrosis, but such sequelae are difficult to investigate and prove. It is probable that idiopathic myocardial hypertrophy, diffuse myocardial fibrosis, subendocardial fibrosis, and idiopathic cardiomyopathy are in some instances the residue of previously unrecognized acute or subacute myocarditis. Such sequelae may follow any type of myocardial inflammation.

Fiedler's myocarditis is not a specific disease, and the eponym should be dropped. The lesions found in the heart muscle in hypersensitivity diseases, serum sickness, diseases of connective tissue, hypokalemia, and many other states without evidence of an infectious inflammatory nature are not classified here as myocarditis.

Clinical Manifestations. Clinical manifestations include almost the whole range of symptoms and signs found in heart disease. They clearly depend on the nature of the infection, the severity and site of the myocardial damage, the resistance of the host, the capacity of the damaged myocardium to recover, and other associated factors such as anemia, nutritional status, and the presence or absence of pre-existing cardiovascular disease.

In acute cases substernal discomfort and even pain (possibly caused by accompanying pericarditis) are common. Dyspnea will depend on the degree of damage to left ventricular function. The most frequent physical signs of myocarditis are tachycardia, dysrhythmia, gallop rhythm, and evidence of developing congestive cardiac failure. The electrocardiogram provides good evidence of myocardial damage; it may show evidence of myocarditis before enlargement of the heart is seen on x-ray or before physical signs of abnormality appear.

Viral Myocarditis. Poliomyelitis, measles, mumps, viral pneumonias, encephalitis, infectious hepatitis, psittacosis, choriomeningitis, influenza A, rabies, varicella, and infectious mononucleosis may be complicated by myocarditis, but proof of direct viral invasion is almost invariably lacking. However, during the past decade there have been many reports of *Coxsackie Group B* myocarditis in infants and children, and, as in suckling mice, it was thought that the virus was especially cardiotropic at this age. Coxsackie myocarditis does not produce a specific histologic picture, but interstitial edema, infiltration with mononuclear cells, and areas of myocardial necrosis are usual. The criteria for the diagnosis of a Coxsackie myocarditis, apart from the evidence of myocardial disease, are the isolation of the virus from blood, feces, or throat swabbings, and the demonstration of a rising titer of neutralizing antibodies against the virus recovered from a patient. Pericarditis is the most common manifestation of Coxsackie carditis in adults.

Myocarditis is a common feature in *poliomyelitis* and its prevalence probably varies in different epidemics. Histologic examination may show capillary dilatation and perivascular infiltration with lymphocytes and polymorphonuclear leukocytes, and in some cases the myocardial fibers are necrotic. The lesions are similar to those found in influenza A infection and are probably produced by the direct invasion of the poliomyelitis virus which has been recovered from human heart muscle by transfer to monkeys. Some myocardial damage may be due to the anoxia which occurs in most cases prior to death.

Although many filterable viruses—possibly all of those which cause disease in man—may cause myocarditis, it is probable that other factors which impair myocardial metabolism make the myocardium susceptible to infection. Pre-existing disease, anoxia, digitalis, steroids, alcohol, and electrolyte disturbances are possible determinants. Indeed, it has been shown in laboratory animals that those procedures which reduce the supply of oxygen to the heart result in a high incidence of myocardial lesions in laboratory animals infected with Virus III. Furthermore it is possible that in some viral diseases the mechanism of heart damage may concern biochemical disturbances, lesions of the central nervous system, or autoimmune reactions rather than direct viral invasion.

Bacterial Myocarditis. Bacterial myocarditis rarely if ever occurs in isolation. The incidence of pyogenic myocarditis has fallen with the use of antimicrobials for all bacterial infections. Myocarditis associated with bacterial endocarditis remains an important component of the disease—indeed, late-developing heart failure after cure of the infection is in some cases due to myocardial damage rather than to increased valve disease.

The most important effect of specific bacterial infection is by an indirect action of which rheumatic carditis and diphtheritic myocarditis are the well known common examples. Streptococcal fever may cause a myocarditis (other than rheumatic); diffuse parenchymatous and focal interstitial reactions have been observed. Although clinical evidence may suggest that recovery is complete, it is possible that healing may result in fibrosis which, with hypertrophy, appears as a chronic cardiomyopathy many years later.

Diphtheritic Myocarditis. Diphtheritic myocarditis, although now uncommon, remains the most serious sequel of diphtheritic infection, and is responsible for more than half the deaths from diphtheria. Myocardial cells are primarily damaged, but an interstitial reaction occurs which may be a nonspecific response to muscle death. The clinical picture varies in intensity, and in severe cases the development of hypokinetic failure or severe hypotension carries a bad prognosis. The electrocardiogram shows various abnormalities. Conduction defects are especially common, and complete heart block may lead to Adams-Stokes syndrome.

Toxoplasma Myocarditis. Toxoplasmosis may involve the heart in both its congenital and acquired forms. The organism has been observed in heart muscle in the acquired generalized form and, although myocarditis is usually part of the generalized illness, it may be the presenting and dominant feature of the disease. There are several well documented fatal cases of toxoplasmic myocarditis, the diagnosis being proved by finding the organism on histologic examination or by inoculation of heart muscle into a mouse. It has been suggested that some cases of familial cardiomyopathy are due to toxoplasmosis; pregnancy may reactivate toxoplasmosis in the mother, resulting in fetal infection. It is thus clear that in cases of subacute myocarditis, familial cardiomegaly, or isolated chronic cardiomyopathy, the possibility of toxoplasmosis should be considered although proof is generally unobtainable.

Trichinosis. It is known that the heart muscle may be infected in trichinosis. The parasite may be seen in heart muscle, but this is unusual even in cases in which there has been evidence of myocarditis in life. Trichinosis may be mistaken for rheumatic fever because of arthralgia, fever, epistaxis, and electrocardiographic abnormalities; ventricular ectopic beats are common. These signs of myocarditis may disappear with the administration of corticotrophin or cortisone, which probably suppresses the inflammation after invasion by the larvae which later became encysted.

Trypanosomiasis. The myocardium may be damaged in both the acute generalized and chronic forms of infection with *Trypanosoma cruzi* (Chagas' disease). Interstitial myocarditis and even extensive necrosis of muscle may be found in the acute form. Chagas' disease should be regarded as an essentially cardiotropic infection by the trypanosome. The acute form occurs mainly in infants and children, and the heart is affected in most cases. In chronic cases, arrhythmias and conduction defects are especially common. Sometimes chronic lesions of the heart are associated with megaesophagus, and men between 20 and 50 are more often affected than women. As in other forms of myocarditis, it is probable that the healing process is associated with fibrosis and hypertrophy of undamaged muscle, although even in chronic cases some degree of inflammatory reaction persists.

Giant Cell Myocarditis. Giant cells occur in the granulomas caused by tuberculosis, syphilis, and some fungal infections, but there seems to be a distinct form of giant cell myocarditis unassociated with these conditions. This rare disease affects young adults and affects the sexes equally. An acute onset of heart failure is followed by a rapidly deteriorating fatal course. At necropsy only the heart is affected. The myocardium shows a lymphocytic reaction with occasional eosinophils and a variable number of multinucleate giant cells. The etiology is quite obscure, and there is no known specific treatment.

Treatment. The management of acute myocarditis concerns the causal disease process (if known) and the heart disease per se. The former is dealt with in the appropriate chapters of this book. From the cardiac point of view, absolute rest is indicated for any form of active myocarditis, and rest should be continued until clinical and laboratory evidence indicates that active myocarditis has subsided. Heart failure demands treatment by routine methods as soon as the most minimal evidence appears. A slight elevation of venous pressure, the presence of a gallop sound, or venous congestion on x-ray is an indication for the use of a thiazide diuretic, and a maintenance dose of digitalis should be given providing that there is no electrocardiographic sign of developing heart block. A light diet with sodium restriction is an obvious requirement. Adrenal corticosteroids have a favorable effect in myocarditis associated with rheumatic fever and other hypersensitivity forms of myocarditis, but indications for their use in isolated myocarditis and the infectious forms mentioned above are not clear. However, because occasional favorable effects have been observed, a trial is indicated when activity of the myocarditis is not subsiding with rest or when a life-threatening deterioration develops.

Burch, G. E., and DePasquale, N.: Viral Myocarditis. Cardiomyopathies. Ciba Foundation Symposium, 1964, p. 376.
Case Records of the Massachusetts General Hospital: Giant cell myocarditis. N. Engl. J. Med., 287:296, 1972.
Dilling, N. V.: Giant cell myocarditis. J. Pathol., 71:295, 1956.
Gore, I., and Saphir, O.: Myocarditis. Am. Heart J., 34:827, 1947.
Webster, R. H.: Cardiac complications of infectious mononucleosis. Am. J. Med. Sci., 234:62, 1957.
Wenger, N. K.: Infectious myocarditis. Cardiovas. Clin., 4:167, 1972.
Whitehead R.: Isolated myocarditis. Br. Heart J., 27:220, 1965.

581. NUTRITIONAL CARDIOMYOPATHY

The association of myocardial disease and malnutrition has been recognized for a long time. Several distinct but overlapping syndromes have been described, and it is probable that multiple factors are involved in most cases. Mixed vitamin deficiencies, repeated infection and infestation, disturbed immunologic mechanisms, anemias, hypoproteinemia, hypomagnesemia, and hypokalemia are some known factors, and no doubt there are many unknowns which may cause disturbed myocardial function. Thus exact pathogenesis remains obscure in most cases.

In Africa two distinct syndromes of nutritional heart disease have been recognized. A *form of hypokinetic heart failure occurs in the Bantu,* which is reversible when an adequate mixed diet is given, although in the most seriously affected patients deterioration continues in spite of treatment. At necropsy there are hepatic cirrhosis and patchy fibrosis in the heart without hydropic change. A second form occurs in *kwashiorkor* which is due to protein deficiency in the growing child after weaning, and, as in other severe nutritional disorders, recovery occurs when the condition is treated early enough.

Beriberi causes the most well known form of nutritional cardiomyopathy, but this disease is relatively rare among the more affluent peoples of the world. Beriberi heart disease, although occurring in alcoholics, is perhaps the least common form of myocardial disease associated with alcohol. It has been known for a long time that not all patients with beriberi have a hyperkinetic circulatory state; indeed some investigations have shown that chronic myocardial disease with hypokinetic heart failure is more common. Some confusion arises here from the use of the term "beriberi," which should be restricted to patients with a hyperkinetic circulatory state and with a clear response to thiamin.

Potassium deficiency may cause cardiomyopathy. Myocardial damage and patchy necrosis result in some animals from being fed potassium-deficient diets. Similar abnormalities have been found in man; after chronic potassium deficiency extensive myocardial fibrosis has been found in the absence of coronary disease. A low potassium level should be corrected completely if permanent myocardial injury is to be avoided.

Alcoholic Cardiomyopathy. Perusal of case histories presented in the many papers on noncoronary myocardial disease reveals a frequent mention of alcohol, sometimes ignored by the authors. A causal relation has, however, long been recognized, with varying degrees of conviction, by many writers. It is now clear that there is an association in some patients between a longstanding high consumption of alcohol and the development of cardiomyopathy.

Adult males are most commonly affected, and three clinical syndromes which depend on the dominant derangement of circulatory function at any one time have been recognized. *Cardiac beriberi* (thiamin-responsive disease) is the least frequent and least serious disorder, occurring especially in very heavy beer drinkers (not averse to spirits as well) who have an additional adverse nutritional status for economic, psychiatric, or gastrointestinal reasons. Therapeutic response to vitamin B_1 and withdrawal of alcohol is effective, but relapse occurs on resumption of previous habits. A chronic myocardial fault may be indicated by persistent abnormality in the electrocardiogram. *Arrhythmia*—especially atrial fibrillation—with or without varying degrees of heart failure is probably the most common mode of presentation in alcoholic cardiomyopathy. The ventricular rate tends to be fast, and multifocal ventricular ectopies are common. Fast heart rates, frequent ventricular extrasystoles, cardiomegaly, and abnormal QRS-T complexes in the electrocardiogram distinguish the condition from so-called idiopathic atrial fibrillation. Treatment with digitalis, diuretics, and conversion of the rhythm meets with varying degrees of success. Reasonable health may be maintained if total abstinence is observed, especially when the development of an arrhythmia with accompanying palpitation draws attention to alcoholic heart disease before irreversible damage has been done.

A few patients present with *hypokinetic heart failure,* cardiomegaly, and electrocardiographic evidence of severe myocardial disease. Response to treatment is poor, and an episodic downhill course is usual.

The electrocardiogram in alcoholic cardiomyopathy shows a wide range of abnormality as in other forms of myocardial disease. A normal or nearly normal electrocardiogram strongly supports a diagnosis of beriberi heart disease. There is a fairly close correlation between the degree of cardiographic abnormality and the severity of the myocardial disease as judged by heart size and response to treatment. Mild polycythemia, which is probably a response to low-grade chronic cardiac insufficiency, and low serum cholesterol levels, probably the result of dietary replacement by ethanol, are common findings. Differential diagnosis may be difficult. "Silent" coronary occlusion, "fallen" hypertension, and thyrotoxicosis (because of tremor, atrial fibrillation, tachycardia, and low cholesterol) are common errors.

Necropsy shows moderate left ventricular hypertrophy and small areas of macroscopic fibrosis. Microscopically there are scattered small areas of muscle degeneration, showing fibrosis or recent necrosis with a slight cellular reaction. The histochemical findings show an accumulation of neutral lipid in the myocardial fibers and varying degrees of mitochondrial damage. These findings are nonspecific and indicate a process of chronic myocardial degeneration, the end result of which is cell death and healing by fibrosis. There is some evidence that electron microscopy may show more specific features.

It is clear that there is some causal relationship between a high consumption of alcohol and myocardial disease, but the pathogenesis of the lesion and the nature of individual susceptibility remain obscure. The following theories merit consideration: (1) That alcohol acts as a direct myocardial toxin; however, there is little evidence for this and it would not explain great variation in individual and organ susceptibility. (2) That alcohol exhausts thiamin and resources, but few patients are helped by thiamin therapy, and the clinical features are unlike those of thiamin depletion. (3) That alcohol causes hypomagnesemia and thence hypokalemia; certainly histologic appearances are similar to those produced by hypokalemia, which may be associated with magnesium depletion known to occur in some alcoholics. (4) That alcoholic injury to the myocardium provides conditions for viral invasion. (5) That myocardial necrosis caused by alcohol in one way or another initiates an autoimmune process which is self-perpetuating; however, none of the usual clinical features of hypersensitivity are found.

Cobalt-Beer Cardiomyopathy. A fulminating form of heart failure in heavy beer drinkers was first described in Quebec and subsequently in other cities, notably Omaha and Minneapolis. This curious syndrome, which appeared between 1964 and 1967, has been shown to be due to the addition of trace amounts of cobalt (0.5 to 1.5 ppm) to certain beers as a foaming agent. This condition differs from chronic alcoholic cardiomyopathy in the abrupt onset and severity of heart failure; indeed, cardiogenic shock soon caused fatality in some patients. Polycythemia and pericardial effusion are common features. The mortality for the acute illness seems to be between 15 and 20 per cent. Most survivors have evidence of continuing myocardial disease, although a few appear to make a complete recovery.

Examination of the myocardium from necropsy or biopsy material shows abnormalities of myofibrils, mitochondria, and sarcoplasmic reticulum. Significantly the swollen mitochondria contain particles of a cobalt protein complex. It seems probable that the cardiotoxicity of cobalt is conditioned by previous myocardial injury from alcohol or protein malnutrition, or both.

Treatment. Total abstinence is indicated. A first attack of heart failure should respond well to routine measures, but relapse is inevitable unless rest is prolonged and alcohol avoided altogether. When there is atrial fibrillation, an attempt at conversion by DC countershock after treatment of heart failure, and under anticoagulant therapy, should be made. Excellent recovery, even in patients with longstanding heart failure and cardiomegaly, has been achieved by prolonged bed rest under sanatorium conditions.

Alexander, C. S.: Cobalt beer cardiomyopathy. Am. J. Med., 53:395, 1972.
Brigden, W.: Alcoholic cardiomyopathy. Cardiovasc. Clin., 4:187, 1972.
Burch, G., Walsh, J., Ferrans, V., and Hibbs, R.: Prolonged bed rest in the treatment of the dilated heart. Circulation, 32:852, 1965.
Morin, Y. C., Foley, A. R., Martineau, G., and Roussel, J.: Quebec beer drinkers' cardiomyopathy, 48 cases. Can. Med. Assoc. J., 97:881, 1967.

582. CARDIAC AMYLOIDOSIS

Cardiac amyloidosis usually appears in primary amyloid; it also occurs in some 15 per cent of patients with myelomatosis, and accounts for between 5 and 7 per cent of all forms of isolated noncoronary myocardial disease in adults. The sexes are equally affected. Small amounts of amyloid may be found in perhaps 2 per cent of elderly hearts (in patients over age 60), but cardiac amyloidosis of sufficient severity to cause death from heart failure is a relatively rare disease; however, some 50 per cent of patients with primary amyloidosis die of heart failure.

Pathology. At necropsy the heart weight is usually moderately increased. Any structure in the heart may be the site of amyloid deposition, and the amount may vary from an occasional small nodule or vascular cuff to almost total replacement of the myocardial mass. The pericardium is frequently affected, and small nodules may be seen on its surface. Occasionally both layers are diffusely thickened and gray. Histologic examination may show perivascular amyloid in the small vessels of the epicardial fat. In patients who have died from heart failure, the greatest amount of amyloid is found in the myocardium, both atria and ventricles being frequently affected. The muscle is curiously stiff, and presumably this diminished compliance of the ventricular mass is the main factor in creating the hemodynamic features of restricted ventricular filling which closely resemble those of constrictive pericarditis. Histologically the muscle cells appear surrounded by rings of amyloid apparently deposited on the cell surface or in the perivascular reticulum of the interstitium. In most severely affected hearts the muscle fibers appear atrophic, necrotic, completely replaced by amyloid, or actually transformed into amyloid substance. Hypertrophic fibers, presumably responsible for the increased heart weight, may be seen in less damaged areas. The valves are occasionally affected.

Clinical Manifestations. Most patients with cardiac amyloidosis are over 50 years old, and the sex distribution is about equal. The majority present with insidious heart failure, although occasionally palpitation or syncope resulting from arrhythmia may be the first symptom. Cardiac pain may occur, and when it is associated with the finding of abnormal Q waves in the cardiogram, an erroneous diagnosis of coronary disease may be made. Effort dyspnea is the most common symptom, but it may be conspicuously absent in patients with the "constrictive" syndrome, which occurs when both sides of the heart are equally affected. Paroxysmal nocturnal dyspnea develops when disease mainly affects the left side of the heart. Uneven deposition of amyloid within the heart may affect the clinical features. Thus deposition in papillary muscle and the mitral valve may cause left atrial enlargement and even a mitral diastolic murmur, although murmurs are absent in most cases. Arrhythmia, including atrial fibrillation and nodal and ventricular extrasystoles, and various degrees of heart block are not uncommon. Deposition of amyloid in the lung parenchyma and small vessels may increase dyspnea from heart failure, and possibly cause obstructive pulmonary hypertension.

Diagnosis is helped by finding evidence of amyloid in other organs. Macroglossia and infiltration of the base of the tongue may cause difficulty in speaking and swallowing. Cutaneous manifestations are important from the diagnostic point of view and include purpura, papules, and localized nodular deposits. The central nervous system is usually unaffected, but a few patients have presented with minor degrees of peripheral neuropathy. Hoarseness may be due to amyloid infiltration of the larynx, and biopsy of a vocal cord nodule has led to correct antemortem diagnosis. Although clinical evidence of renal disease is uncommon in patients with dominant cardiac amyloidosis, the kidneys are affected in about one third of cases at necropsy. Diarrhea, meteorism, and gastrointestinal bleeding may result from gastrointestinal amyloid, but this is rare in primary cardiac amyloid.

The electrocardiogram is always abnormal in clinically significant cardiac amyloid. The findings, although not specific, are perhaps more suggestive of the nature of the underlying disease than in most other forms of cardiomyopathy. P waves are often small, and the P-R interval may be prolonged. The most characteristic abnormalities are low voltage of the QRS-T complex, especially in the frontal plane leads, and abnormal Q waves indicating extensive myocardial disease. Both forms of bundle branch block have been reported, and T waves are almost invariably flat or inverted. Cardiac catheterization may show great elevation of both right and left atrial pressures as in other forms of severe myocardial failure. Restricted ventricular filling (probably owing to diminished compliance of ventricular myocardium) and diminished contractility result in low arterial pulse pressures and a low cardiac output. As a reasonably accurate assessment of hemodynamic status can be made at the bedside, there seems little indication for cardiac catheterization, for the findings are not specific. Confirmation of diagnosis is best obtained by biopsy of some accessible part that appears to be affected, but even a "positive" specimen may be misinterpreted or missed because of the variable tinctorial character of amyloid. The Congo red test is positive in less than 50 per cent of the patients in whom it has been performed. Hypoproteinemia and hyperglobulinemia (moderate increase in alpha-2 and gamma-fractions) support a diagnosis of amyloid, but as serum protein studies are abnormal in only 15 per cent of cases they do not provide much help in diagnosis.

The outlook for patients with clinical cardiac amyloidosis is uniformly bad. Progressive heart failure usually leads to death in less than two years. Rest, digitalis, and diuretics may improve heart failure temporarily, but the response is mostly unsatisfactory. Various treatments have been suggested, including large doses of liver, ascorbic acid, corticotrophin, and coritisone, but none has been clearly effective.

Brigden, W.: Cardiac amyloidosis. Prog. Cardiovasc. Dis., 7:142, 1964.
Buerger, L., and Braunstein, H.: Senile cardiac amyloid. Am. J. Med., 28:357, 1960.

583. OTHER CARDIOMYOPATHIES

Endomyocardial Fibrosis. Minor degrees of endocardial fibrosis are common in myocardial disease but this should not be confused with an obscure cardiopathy which occurs commonly in tropical Africa and sporadically elsewhere. It is characterized by extensive endocardial and subendocardial fibrosis. The disease appears to be a specific entity, but its etiology remains unknown. Indirect evidence suggests that it is of an infectious nature, the organism or its vector being responsible for the geographical distribution of the disease (Parry). Malnutrition is not likely to be a factor, for this disease occurs in well-fed Africans, and it has been seen in well nourished expatriates from Africa residing in the United Kingdom.

At necropsy the cavities of either or both ventricles are partially obliterated by dense fibrous tissue which may be organized into a dense white thick lining. Fibrous tissue may bind papillary muscles and chordae to the posterior wall of the ventricle, producing gross mitral reflux.

The clinical manifestations are varied and depend on which ventricle is most severely affected. Insidious heart failure of a "constrictive" type results from uniform biventricular disease. Dominant left ventricular disease may present with symptoms of left ventricular failure with or without severe mitral reflux. A few patients develop severe reactive pulmonary hypertension which dominates the clinical picture. Pure right ventricular disease is not uncommon, and its features have been described by Abrahams (1962). Ascites and hepatomegaly without peripheral edema are usual, the jugular venous pressure is very high, and roentgenography shows an aneurysmal right atrium.

There is no specific treatment. Routine treatment of heart failure may delay the inevitable deterioration which occurs in this extraordinary disease.

Löffler's Fibroplastic Endocarditis. See Ch. 108.

Sarcoidosis. See Ch. 102.

Peripartum Cardiomyopathy (Puerperal Myocarditis). Peripartum cardiomyopathy is probably not a single disease entity. It describes a condition of heart failure arising in the last trimester of pregnancy or the puerperium and is due to idiopathic myocardial disease. It is unrelated to toxemia of pregnancy but may be difficult to differentiate from "silent" pulmonary thromboembolism; however, the heart failure tends to be mainly of left ventricular origin. It is probable that the late stages of pregnancy and/or the metabolic effects of involution in the puerperium in some unknown way have an adverse effect on hitherto asymptomatic myocardial disease. Clinical recovery is usual, but the electrocardiogram usually reveals the continuation of myocardial disease. Furthermore, subsequent pregnancies are likely to be followed by heart failure. No specific treatment is known.

Myocardial Disease and Neurologic Disorders. Friedreich first recorded that the heart was affected in the congenital neurologic disorder named after him. This finding has since been amply confirmed; indeed, some have considered that the disease is as much an affection of the heart as of the nervous system. The left ventricular myocardium is the site of degenerating fibers, interstitial fibrosis, and hypertrophy. The electrocardiogram may be abnormal in infancy before neurologic features appear. Furthermore, the author of these chapters has seen cardiomyopathy without neurologic manifestations in a man whose several adult siblings suffered from ataxia. Arrhythmias and congestive cardiac failure are the usual outcome.

Myocardial disease also occurs in association with the *myotonic dystrophies.* Cardiac manifestations may arise at any time in the natural history of the disease, and arrhythmia is the most common presenting feature.

Boyer, S. H., Chisholm, A. W., and McKusick, V. A.: Cardiac aspects of Friedreich's ataxia. Circulation, 25:493, 1962.

Burch, G. E., and Walsh, J. J.: Postpartal heart disease. Arch. Intern. Med., 108:817, 1961.

Emanuel, R.: Cardiomyopathy and neuromyopathic disorders. Proc. R. Soc. Med., 65:939, 1972.

Parry, E., and Abrahams, D.: The natural history of endomyocardial fibrosis. Quart. J. Med., 34:383, 1965.

Perloff, J.: Cardiomyopathy associated with heredofamilial neuromyopathic diseases. Mod. Concepts Cardiovasc. Dis., 40:23, 1971.

584. TUMORS OF THE HEART

Primary tumors of the heart are rare but important, because the majority may be cured by surgery. *Myxomas* are the most common; they are benign in the oncologic sense, but malignant insofar as they cause death by obstruction or embolism. *Rhabdomyoma, fibroma,* and *lipoma* are other very rare benign tumors. Malignant *sarcomas* are also rare and may arise from any part of the heart or pericardium.

Myxomas are of special interest not only because they are the most common and can be cured, but also because of their clinical features, which mimic other diseases and pose difficult problems in diagnosis. They may occur at any age. Myxomas arise from atrial endocardium, most commonly in the left heart, and produce features resulting from obstruction, a generalized systemic disturbance, or peripheral embolism. Obstruction at the atrioventricular valves may cause signs resembling mitral or tricuspid stenosis, but because these tumors may move, the symptoms and signs characteristically vary from time to time. Acute transient obstruction may be caused by a change in posture, leading to syncope, and there may be a periodic change in venous congestion of the lung. Occasionally the mitral valve cusps may be kept open in systole, leading to an erroneous diagnosis of valvar mitral reflux. In one patient we have seen the development of severe pulmonary hypertension presumably caused by chronic obstruction of pulmonary veins. Systemic symptoms probably resulting from an abnormal immunologic response to the tumor may sometimes dominate the clinical picture. They comprise vague aches and pains, low-grade fever, anemia, raised sedimentation rate, and abnormal serum proteins. When present, these features may lead to an erroneous diagnosis of bacterial endocarditis or collagen disease. Sudden embolism of a major artery may be the presenting feature, and diagnosis has been made on histologic examination of emboli removed at emergency surgery. Right atrial myxomas may produce signs of tricuspid valve obstruction or recurrent pulmonary emboli and polycythemia. We have seen one with features resembling rheumatoid arthritis and anemia which disappeared after successful removal of the tumor.

The diagnosis of myxoma depends first on the physician's being sensitive to the possibility in a patient with unexplained dyspnea, hints of mitral valve disease without hard evidence, and/or the systemic features mentioned above. Thereafter a firm diagnosis may be readily established by echocardiography and selective angiocardiography; the former shows characteristic echos behind the valve leaflet, whereas the latter is confirmatory in showing an atrial filling defect. Occasionally these tumors develop calcification which may be seen on x-ray.

Treatment is by removal under cardiopulmonary bypass. Successful surgery is followed by rapid resolution of the mechanical and immunologic features.

Metastatic tumors in the heart are much more common than primary ones. Various necropsy series in malignant disease place the incidence between 10 and 20 per cent. Bronchial cancer accounts for one third; breast and esophageal neoplasms are other common sources. Pericarditis with effusion is the usual mode of presentation; indeed, this occasionally provides the first evidence of malignant disease.

Goodwin, J. F.: Diagnosis of left atrial myxoma. Lancet, 1:464, 1963.

Hambling, S. M.: Metastatic cancer to the heart. Circulation, 22:474, 1960.

Hudson, R. E. B.: Tumours of the heart. *In* Cardiovascular Pathology. Vol. 2. London, Edward Arnold, Ltd., 1965, p. 1563.

Selzer, A., Sakai, F. J., and Popper, R. W.: Protean manifestations of tumors of the heart. Am. J. Med., 52:9, 1972.

DISEASES OF THE AORTA

J. Willis Hurst

585. ELONGATION AND KINKING OF THE AORTA

Medial sclerosis (*Mönckeberg's sclerosis*) is one of the most common disease processes affecting the larger arteries. In this condition the media shows varying degrees of loss of muscular and elastic tissue along with calcification.

The cause of medial sclerosis is not known, but it begins in middle life and increases with advancing age. The abnormality of the media causes the vessels to elongate and is responsible for the firm and tortuous nature of the temporal, brachial, and radial arteries observed in some middle-aged and most elderly people. This process in itself does not lead to occlusion or rupture of a vessel. The disease may be associated with atheromatous changes in the media, which, of course, may lead to more serious complications.

The decrease in elastic and muscular elements of the media, with or without calcification, causes systolic hypertension. The aorta, as well as the visible peripheral

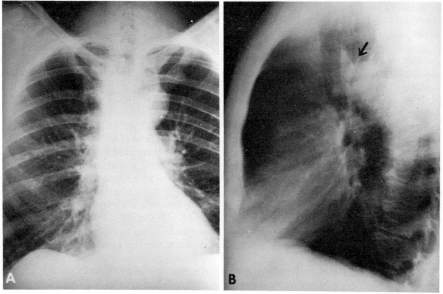

Figure 1. Posteroanterior *(A)* and lateral *(B)* roentgenograms of the chest showing an "elongated" aorta with pseudocoarctation.

arteries, becomes long and tortuous. The abnormality and the medical calcification may be detected on a roentgenogram of the chest. The elongated aorta may simulate an aneurysm. The esophagus tends to follow the course of the aorta because it is bound intimately to it. Accordingly, when the aorta takes an unusual course because of the effects of medial sclerosis, the barium-filled esophagus will be seen to do the same when viewed under the fluoroscope or on the roentgenogram of the chest. The unusual path taken by the esophagus in such cases may simulate posterior displacement of that structure by the heart.

The aortic arch may elongate until it becomes kinked or folded downward in the region of the ligamentum arteriosum. The condition is called *pseudocoarctation.* There may be mild obstruction in rare cases (Fig. 1). This abnormality can resemble mediastinal tumor. An aortogram may occasionally be needed for its identification.

Elongation of the aortic arch combined with similar changes in the brachiocephalic arteries may cause pulsating masses in the base of the neck which simulate aneurysms. This is most commonly found on the right side. Arteriography usually reveals twisting, coiling, or looping of the innominate, subclavian, or common carotid artery. This is sometimes called the *innominate loop.* Once diagnosis is established, the lesion has little significance, but it may rarely result in some deviation of the esophagus or trachea which produces annoying, though not disabling, symptoms.

Robbins, S. L.: Pathology. Philadelphia, W. B. Saunders Company, 1967, pp. 578 ff.

586. ANEURYSM OF THE AORTA

Definition. An aneurysm is a localized or diffuse enlargement of an artery. When one or all of the layers of the aorta make up the sac of the aneurysm, it is called a *true aneurysm.* When the aorta is injured by trauma or infection, a pulsating hematoma may develop owing to destruction of the wall of the vessel. Perivascular clot and connective tissue make up the wall of the enlargement, and the condition is called a *false aneurysm.* A *saccular aneurysm* has a pouchlike appearance and appears to be a sac attached to the side of the aorta. A *fusiform aneurysm* is spindle-shaped and involves the entire circumference of the aorta. The terms *saccular* and *fusiform* are used for clinical designation, whereas the terms *true* and *false* are pathologic designations.

Etiology. Aneurysms of the aorta may be due to atherosclerosis, syphilis, medial cystic necrosis, trauma, infection (mycotic aneurysm), and congenital vascular disease. The discussion dealing with atherosclerotic and syphilitic aneurysms of the aorta will make up the major portion of this chapter. Inasmuch as dissecting aneurysm, traumatic aneurysm, mycotic aneurysm, and aneurysms of the sinuses of Valsalva have many unique features, they will be discussed separately.

Pathogenesis. Although the pathologic processes associated with production of aortic aneurysm are varied, certain factors are common to all. The media of the normal aorta must remain intact in order for the aorta to withstand the systolic blood pressure. When the media is damaged, there is progressive dilatation at the weakened area and an aneurysm gradually develops. Once an aneurysm develops it tends to increase gradually in size, being restrained only by blood clots and scar tissue; hence, there is the likelihood that the aneurysm may finally rupture.

Incidence. The incidence of aneurysms at autopsy is approximately 2 per cent. The majority of aortic aneurysms are found in patients between 40 and 70 years of age, and the incidence is higher in men than in women. Syphilitic aneurysms of the arch of the aorta are still found, but are fortunately decreasing in frequency. Today most aneurysms of the aorta seen in the United States are due to atherosclerosis, regardless of location, even those of the ascending aorta.

Clinical Manifestations. The signs and symptoms depend upon the size and location of the aneurysm. Venous distention and edema of the face, neck, and shoulders may develop when an aneurysm compresses the superior vena cava. Impingement on the trachea and bronchi may produce cough and dyspnea, and compression of the esophagus can produce dysphagia. An aneurysm may impair the function of the recurrent laryngeal nerve and cause hoarseness. A syphilitic aneurysm of the first portion of the aorta may erode the sternum (Fig. 2). Severe pain may occur when a syphilitic aneurysm of the arch and early descending aorta erodes the vertebra and ribs. Death may be the result of hemorrhage into the trachea, bronchi, pleural space, or pericardium. An atherosclerotic aneurysm of the abdominal aorta may cause no symptoms until rupture occurs. The patient or his physician may discover the aneurysm because of a pulsating mass in the abdomen. The aneurysm may cause pain in the upper portion of the abdomen, the lower portion of the back, the groin, and occasionally in the testicles. The mechanism of such pain may be associated with rupture, sudden enlargement, or a small leak into the retroperitoneal space. The pulsating mass, usually felt without difficulty, may extend from above the umbilicus into the pelvis. The mass may be nontender and movable, but tends to become tender and fixed when there has been recent symptomatic enlargement.

A thoracic aortic aneurysm can usually be identified on posteroanterior and lateral roentgenograms of the chest. The pulsation of the mass can be studied during fluoroscopic examination. Pulsations may be absent, however, because thrombosis in the aneurysm may prevent movement. Since some solid tumors located adjacent to the heart appear to pulsate, it is occasionally necessary to resort to aortography in order to differentiate an aortic aneurysm from a tumor. An abdominal aneurysm can often be identified in the ordinary roentgenogram of the abdomen (particularly in the lateral view) because calcification of the aortic wall is frequently present. Aortography may be needed to establish the diagnosis.

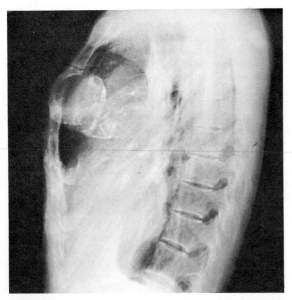

Figure 2. Lateral roentgenogram of the chest showing the erosion of the sternum by a syphilitic aortic aneurysm.

Prognosis and Complications. Aortic aneurysm is a serious disease with poor prognosis. According to Estes, one third of patients with atherosclerotic aneurysm of the abdominal aorta die within a year after the diagnosis is made. Three fourths of the patients die within five years after diagnosis, usually from rupture. Kampmeier's study of aneurysms of the thoracic aorta indicated that the average duration of life, after the onset of symptoms, was six to eight months, and De Bakey found that over 90 per cent of patients with aneurysms of the thoracic aorta died within five years.

Aneurysm results in increased lateral pressure, so that the natural history of an aneurysm in the body cavity is one of progressive though highly variable expansion. Rupture is almost inevitable if the patient survives long enough. Patients with aneurysm, however, usually have significant coexisting diseases which modify this outlook. Thus many patients do die of causes other than rupture of the aneurysm with exsanguination. Nevertheless, because the aneurysm is potentially lethal, it is correct to recommend aneurysmectomy in most instances. Naturally, the threat of rupture is greater when the aneurysm is larger. An appropriate dividing line appears to be a transverse diameter of 6 cm. Complications with smaller aneurysm are infrequent except for the fact that smaller ones usually become larger. Turbulence in an aneurysm results in platelet and fibrin thrombi which are a source of peripheral arterial emboli.

Treatment. There is no medical treatment for aortic aneurysms. The discovery of an aortic aneurysm forces one to consider resection of the lesion and replacement by a plastic prosthesis. When an aneurysm of the abdominal aorta is found and the patient has no other recognizable disease, surgical resection is usually possible; the operative mortality is less than 5 per cent in many medical centers. When the patient is older than average, say in the eighth decade of life, or when there is clear evidence of heart, cerebrovascular, renal, or other serious disease, the operative mortality may be 25 per cent or more. It is obvious also that, if such a patient survives the operation, his life expectancy will be less than that of a normal person because of the underlying disease. Generally speaking, then, aneurysms of the abdominal aorta that have a transverse diameter of 6 cm or greater should be surgically resected regardless of symptoms. Aneurysms of the abdominal aorta that are smaller than this must be carefully observed for change in size. Resection should not be attempted for asymptomatic lesions if the patient has associated disease that will shorten his life anyway or will greatly increase the operative risk. The mortality of untreated ruptured aneurysm is 100 per cent. Accordingly, if the aneurysm has actually ruptured or if symptoms suggest that rupture may be imminent, operation should be attempted even though the operative risk is high.

Surgical treatment of aneurysms of the thoracic aorta carries a higher operative mortality rate than that for aneurysm of the abdominal aorta. Even in expert hands the operative mortality is about 30 per cent. A saccular aneurysm can at times be resected at its neck and the wall of the aorta repaired. Fusiform aneurysms are more difficult to resect. The mortality varies with the location of the aneurysm. Although it is possible to resect an aneurysm of the entire aortic arch, the death rate from the procedure is very high. Techniques have been developed that prevent cardiac strain and provide blood to the heart, brain, spinal cord, and kidneys, while the aorta is occluded, using extracorporeal circulation, temporary bypass shunts, and hypothermia. The prognosis of thoracic aneurysm is so grave that one is forced to consider resection of the lesion despite the high operative mortality. Accordingly, if resection seems technically possible and no serious associated disease precludes the procedure, an attempt should be made.

De Bakey, M. E.: Surgical treatment of the diseases of the aorta and arteries. *In* Hurst, J. W. (ed.): The Heart. 3rd ed. New York, McGraw-Hill Book Company, 1974, p. 1666.

De Bakey, M. E., et al.: Aneurysm of abdominal aorta: Analysis of results of graft replacement therapy one to eleven years after operation. Ann. Surg., 160:622, 1964.

Estes, J. E., Jr.: Abdominal aortic aneurysm: A study of 102 cases. Circulation, 2:258, 1950.

Lord, J. W., Jr., and Imparato, A. M.: The abdominal aortic aneurysm. Its importance to the internist. J.A.M.A., 176:93, 1961.

Szilagyi, D. E., et al.: Contribution of abdominal aortic aneurysmectomy to prolongation of life. Ann. Surg., 164:678, 1966.

DISSECTING ANEURYSM

Definition. Dissecting aneurysm of the aorta is really a dissecting hematoma. Blood enters the wall of the aorta and splits the media of the vessel.

Etiology and Pathology. Medial cystic necrosis is usually considered to be the abnormality responsible for dissecting aneurysm. Actually the problem is complex, because dissecting aneurysm may occur when medial cystic necrosis is absent or slight, or, on the other hand, medial cystic necrosis may be found without dissection. The cause of medial cystic necrosis is not known. It is considered by some to be a nonspecific change in the aorta in response to hemodynamic stresses. The disease process is usually most severe in the ascending aorta and decreases progressively toward the distal aorta, but may be extensive throughout the aorta and major vessels.

Dissecting aneurysm and rupture of the aorta can be produced experimentally by feeding growing rats. *Lathyrus odoratus* (sweet pea) meal, which contains B-aminopropionitrile. The rats develop skeletal abnormalities and medial degeneration of the aorta.

Dissecting aneurysm is common in *Marfan's syndrome*. This condition is characterized by severe medial cystic necrosis, which, like the remainder of the syndrome, is genetically determined. In fact, some persons with dissecting aneurysm may appear normal, yet are found in a family group whose other members have typical Marfan's syndrome. In addition, the incidence of dissecting aneurysm seems to be increased in patients with skeletal deformities, e.g., scoliosis, pigeon breast, and funnel depression of the thorax.

The relation of *hypertension* to dissecting aneurysm is not clear. Although hypertension is frequently associated with dissecting aneurysm, it is notable that the younger the patients in a series, the larger is the proportion without hypertension. Some believe that hypertension, by increasing hemodynamic stresses on the aorta, accelerates the development of medial cystic necrosis.

Dissecting aneurysm may occur during *pregnancy;* many case reports are available emphasizing this point. Patients with *coarctation of the aorta* may die of dissecting aneurysm. Dissecting aneurysm has also been reported to be associated with *aortic stenosis* and with *myxedema.*

Atheromatous disease of the aorta is not the direct cause of medial cystic necrosis, although the two diseases may occur together. Occasionally bleeding into the media of the aorta may originate at the edge of an atheromatous ulcer. Syphilis is not the cause of medial cystic necrosis, and the syphilitic process does not prevent dissection in situations in which both diseases occur together. Other lesions, such as an aortic abscess, may initiate dissection of the aorta.

De Bakey classified dissecting aneurysm into three types. Type I begins as a transverse tear in the intima of the ascending aorta and extends distally for a variable distance. Type II is said to be present when the dissection is confined to the ascending aorta. Type III is used to signify the condition when the process begins distal to the arch vessels. When the dissection proceeds distal to the intimal tear it may also involve the branches of the aorta and may re-enter the lumen of the aorta some distance from the .origin. (This can produce a double-barreled aorta). Occasionally an intimal tear is absent; this has led to speculation that an intramural hematoma developed because the vasa vasorum ruptured as a result of medial cystic necrosis. Some have extended the reasoning to state that the intimal tear itself occurred because the media supported it so poorly. Braunstein's study refutes this idea and supports the concept that dilatation and hypertension promote the intimal tear by increasing the tension on the intima of the aorta.

Incidence. Dissecting aneurysm of the aorta is far less common but far more serious than myocardial infarction. Men are affected twice as often as women except in the advanced age groups. The peak incidence is in the fourth to seventh decades. Type I dissection is more common than Type III dissection, and Type II is comparatively rare.

Clinical Manifestations. The clinical features and prognosis associated with dissecting aneurysm are determined by the anatomic derangement which characterizes the three types of the condition. Dissecting aneurysm is frequently mistaken for and treated as myocardial infarction. It can be misdiagnosed as pulmonary embolism. In view of the fact that the arteries supplying blood to the brain and cord, the abdominal viscera, and the extremities branch off the aorta, it must be borne in mind that dissecting aneurysm can mimic cerebrovascular accident, acute abdominal crises, or peripheral vascular occlusions. The following points are useful in differential diagnosis:

Pain. Although the majority of patients with dissecting aneurysm of the aorta have chest pain, it is now clear that some do not. Painless dissection occurs especially with Marfan's syndrome. It must be remembered that a severe neurologic deficit, caused by the dissection, may prevent the patient from giving a history of pain. The patient usually experiences severe anterior chest pain, however, and it is for this reason that the condition is frequently misdiagnosed as myocardial infarction. Dissecting aneurysm should be considered under the following circumstances: when the chest pain is excruciating and when considerable morphine is needed for relief; when the pain is maximal at the onset rather than gradually increasing, as it frequently does with myocardial infarction; when the pain radiates to the back or predominates in the back; when the pain is widespread and radiates to the abdomen, legs, head, and neck; and when the pain shifts to a lower level in the body as the dissection extends.

Pain may be the only manifestation of the condition in patients with Type II dissection, whereas patients with Types I and II are likely to have pain plus other physical abnormalities.

Level of Blood Pressure. Although the patient may have the appearance of being in shock, with anxiety, pallor, sweating, tachypnea, and tachycardia, the blood pressure is elevated in most patients with dissecting aneurysms. This occurs because many patients have hypertension prior to the catastrophic event and there may be an increase in blood pressure during dissection as a result of severe pain. In addition, the heart may function well in such circumstances, unlike myocardial infarction, in which a portion of the myocardium is destroyed. Marked elevation of systemic blood pressure is more common in patients with Type III dissection as compared with those with Type I dissection. Shock levels of blood pressure are seldom observed in patients with Type III dissection but may be seen in 20 per cent of patients with Type I dissection.

Arterial Pulsations. The carotid, brachial, radial, and femoral arteries must be palpated repeatedly for change in pulsation. Absence or inequality of pulsations is an important clue and indicates arterial occlusion. The degree of pulsation may vary from hour to hour because of arterial spasm. When signs and symptoms of peripheral arterial occlusion occur within a few hours after chest pain, dissecting aneurysm should be considered rather than myocardial infarction, because an embolic episode resulting from infarction is delayed until several days after the onset of chest pain. Alteration of the pulsation of the various arteries is more common in patients with Type I dissection than in those with Type III dissection.

Aortic Regurgitation. The murmur of aortic regurgitation may be heard in about one third of patients with dissection of the aorta. It is more common in patients with Type I dissection. Aortic regurgitation occurs because the integrity of the aortic ring is altered and because the support of the aortic valve cusps may be destroyed. On rare occasions a peculiar fluttering sound can be heard in diastole, probably caused by a piece of the intima vibrating in the bloodstream during diastole. Chest pain followed by the development of aortic regurgitation should suggest dissecting aneurysm.

Pulsation of the Sternoclavicular Joint. Pulsation of the right or left sternoclavicular joint may be noted in dissecting aneurysm. This unusual pulsation can also be produced by other types of aortic aneurysms. A rare cause of right sternoclavicular pulsation is an anomalous right aortic arch.

Neurologic Abnormalities. Neurologic abnormalities are common and result from decreased blood flow to the brain and cord associated with shock or obstruction of the arteries by the dissecting hematoma. Neurologic complications are more often associated with Type I dissection. Coma, hemiplegia, confusion, and visual disturbances may occur. Weakness and even paralysis of the lower extremities may be caused by ischemia of the spinal cord or ischemia of the legs. The weakness may be associated with pain, paresthesia, and sensory and reflex changes in the extremities. Severe chest pain accompanied by severe weakness of the lower extremities should always suggest the possibility of a dissecting aneurysm.

Abdominal Findings. When abdominal symptoms predominate in a patient with dissecting aneurysm, laparotomy may be performed because of the diagnosis of "acute abdomen." At operation, the bowel, gallbladder, or other organs are found to be ischemic or blood is found leaking into the abdominal cavity.

When the renal arteries are involved, hematuria, suppression of urine flow, and the aggravation of hypertension by renal ischemia may result.

Cardiovascular Findings. A pericardial friction rub may be noted. Such a finding does not invariably mean that the aorta has dissected into the pericardial space, because a rub may occur when the beads of blood surrounding the injured vasa vasorum of the ascending aorta leak into the pericardial space. (The pericardium encloses a small part of the aorta). Neck veins may be distended because of superior vena caval obstruction or because of bleeding into the pericardial space with subsequent cardiac tamponade. The latter is almost always followed by death. The precordial thrust may be large and sustained because of left ventricular hypertrophy owing to previously existing hypertension. Aortic regurgitation has already been mentioned. The electrocardiogram may show left ventricular hypertrophy, nonspecific S-T and T changes, rhythm disturbances, and pericarditis. Dissection of the coronary arteries may cause myocardial infarction and death.

Roentgenographic Findings. Enlargement of the aortic shadow is the most common roentgenographic sign of dissecting aneurysm (Fig. 3). Unfortunately the roentgenogram must be made with the patient recumbent because of his critical state. Bedside techniques for roentgenography of the chest produce considerable distortion of the heart and great vessels, thereby making accurate interpretation of a wide upper mediastinum difficult. Progressive enlargement of the aorta over a period of days or weeks may be noted. Occasionally the width of the aortic wall may be identified if intimal calcification is present, thereby marking the internal limit of the aortic wall. When a hematoma is present, the wall thickness is greater than the normal 2 to 3 mm. In many instances aortography may be needed to determine the presence and extent of dissection (Fig. 4). Modern aortographic techniques have assisted in clarifying the clinical spectrum of this condition. The identification of Type III dissection has improved considerably since the development of aortography.

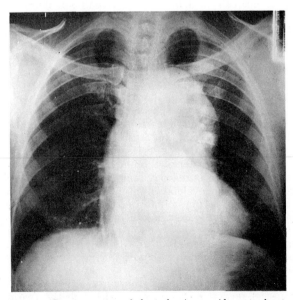

Figure 3. Roentgenogram of chest showing a wide aorta due to a dissecting aneurysm.

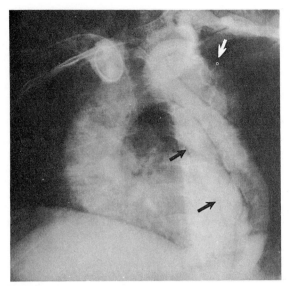

Figure 4. Aortogram showing a "double lumen" aorta secondary to dissecting aneurysm.

Laboratory Findings. Leukocytosis may develop in a few hours and may reach 25,000 cells per cubic millimeter. Anemia may develop, and hyperbilirubinemia may occur occasionally. Urinalysis may show erythrocytes, albumin, casts, and gross hematuria because of renal artery occlusion.

Prognosis. Dissection of the aorta is a serious disease and is usually fatal within hours or days. The natural history of dissecting is poorly understood, and this fact makes it difficult to assess therapeutic intervention. In one report (Lindsay and Hurst) of 62 patients, the initial and long-term survival was far better in patients in whom the ascending aorta was spared by the disease process. No patients in this series in whom the ascending aorta (Type I) was involved survived more than 3 weeks, whereas 8 of 19 patients whose disease began distal to the arch of the aorta (Type III) were known to survive 6 to 69 months.

Death is usually due to hemopericardium and cardiac tamponade, hemothorax, hemomediastinum, retroperitoneal hemorrhage, myocardial infarction, shock, neurologic abnormalities, congestive heart failure, renal failure, and, rarely, gangrene of the bowel.

Treatment. The treatment of patients with dissecting aneurysm is unsatisfactory. Pain must be relieved with opiates, blood should be replaced when needed, and oxygen may be administered. Anticoagulants are absolutely contraindicated. Wheat, Palmer, et al. have pioneered in the use of drugs to reduce the arterial blood pressure and pulsatile forces in patients with dissecting aneurysm. Trimethapan, guanethidine, α-methyldopa, and parenteral reserpine may be used to lower the systolic blood pressure to 100 to 120 mm of mercury as quickly as possible. It may not be possible to use such therapy when the blood pressure is already low, when ventricular arrhythmias are present, or when oliguria is present. Propranolol hydrochloride can be used to diminish the force of ventricular contraction and pulsatile force of aortic flow. It may be used alone or with other agents in doses of 1.0 mg intramuscularly every four to six hours. After the acute phase is over, oral medication may be used. This drug produces little change in arterial

pressure and may be quite useful in normotensive patients with aortic dissection and in the long-term management. It is now clear that this form of treatment decreases the degree of pain, may decrease the extent of dissection, and favorably alters the mortality rate.

Operation is not indicated during the acute stages of disease because the risk is prohibitive, although it is occasionally attempted if a limb appears to be dying from lack of blood supply or if there appears to be a slow leak from the aorta. After several days, when the dissection is presumed to be no longer progressing, operation may be considered. On rare occasions the dissection may be well localized, and excision with aneurysmorrhaphy may be possible. A re-entry passage may be created into the true lumen of the descending aorta, and the false lumen can be obliterated by suture. When possible, it seems wise to use some form of excisional therapy and aortic replacement with the use of left atriofemoral bypass perfusion, external bypass graft, or hypothermia. Aortic regurgitation has occasionally been corrected by means of a Starr-Edwards ball-valve prosthesis. The operative mortality experienced by the De Bakey team is about 25 per cent. Follow-up observations for more than five years reveal that many vascular problems have occurred in the group of survivors.

The treatment of dissecting aneurysm is now being studied in many medical centers. The trend in therapy seems toward a combination of drug therapy and surgical therapy. Unfortunately the treatment remains unsatisfactory.

Braunstein, H.: Pathogenesis of dissecting aneurysm. Circulation, 28:1071, 1963.
De Bakey, M. E., Henley, W. S., Cooley, D. A., Morris, G. C., Crawford, E. S., and Beall, A. C.: Surgical management of dissecting aneurysms of the aorta. J. Thorac. Cardiovasc. Surg., 49:130, 1965.
Hirst, A. E., Johns, V. J., Jr., and Kime, S. W., Jr.: Dissecting aneurysm of the aorta. A review of 505 cases. Medicine, 37:217, 1958.
Lindsay, J., Jr.: Diseases of the aorta. *In* Hurst, J. W. (ed.): The Heart. 3rd ed. New York, Mc-Graw-Hill Book Company, 1974, p. 1586.
Lindsay, J., Jr., and Hurst, J. W.: Clinical features and prognosis in dissecting aneurysm of the aorta: A reappraisal. Circulation, 35:880, 1967.
Lindsay, J., Jr., and Hurst, J. W.: Drug therapy of dissecting aortic aneurysms: Some reservations. Circulation, 37:216, 1968.
Lindsay, J., Jr., and Hurst, J. W.: Dissecting aneurysm of the aorta. J.A.M.A., 217:1533, 1971.
Shuford, W. H., Sybers, R. G., Weens, H. S., Lindsay, Jr., and Hurst, J. W.: Aortographic findings in dissecting aneurysm of the aorta. Am. J. Cardiol., 24:111, 1969.
Wheat, M. W., Jr., Palmer, R. F., Bartley, T. D., and Seelman, R. C.: Treatment of dissecting aneurysms of the aorta without surgery. J. Thorac. Cardiovasc. Surg., 50:364, 1965.

TRAUMATIC ANEURYSM

Injury of the aorta may be caused by penetrating wounds or by blunt trauma. Damage to the thoracic aorta may be produced by injuries that do not produce rib fractures. The most common cause of such injuries is automobile, motorcycle, and helicopter accidents.

Ruptures and tears with subsequent aneurysm formation are usually found at points where the aorta is relatively fixed in position—just distal to the origin of the left subclavian artery at the site of the ligamentum arteriosum, and in the ascending aorta just beyond the aortic valve. When a severe accelerative or decelerative force is sustained, the remainder of the aorta moves more freely than the fixed points, producing an injury to the vessel. An injury to the aorta that tears all layers of the aorta causes death, but when the tear involves only the intima it may cause only a hematoma in the media or, on rare occasion, a dissecting aneurysm.

A small leak from the aorta may cause mediastinal hemorrhage, which may be diagnosed by the mediastinal widening in chest roentgenograms. An aortogram should be done promptly if aortic rupture is suspected. When immediate surgery is not carried out, repeat roentgenograms of the chest should be made in such cases in order to detect the appearance of aortic aneurysm, which may become visible in a few days to several weeks. The aneurysm may be noted first on a routine chest film made years after the injury.

Resection is usually indicated for traumatic aneurysms of the aorta. Since this type of aneurysm is not necessarily related to other diseases, the general vascular status in patients is frequently good. Accordingly, the operative risk for the resection of traumatic aneurysms is less than it is for other kinds of aneurysms.

An unexplained aneurysm, discovered on x-ray of the chest, in the region of the left subclavian artery may be the result of old trauma.

De Bakey, M. E., and Crawford, S. E.: Surgical considerations of acquired diseases of the aorta and major peripheral arteries. I. Aortic aneurysms. Mod. Concepts Cardiovasc. Dis., 28:557, 1959.

Goyette, E. M., Blake, H. A., Forsee, J. H., and Swan, H.: Traumatic aortic aneurysms. Circulation, 10:824, 1954.

Symbas, P. N.: Traumatic rupture of the aorta. Ann. Surg., 178:6, 1973.

Symbas, P. N.: Traumatic injuries of the heart and great vessels. Springfield, Ill., Charles C Thomas, 1972.

MYCOTIC ANEURYSM

Mycotic aneurysm of the aorta may be associated with bacterial endocarditis, septicemia, or the extension of a neighboring abscess into the aortic wall. Perdue and Smith have emphasized that patients in the older age group may have mycotic aneurysms at the site of atherosclerotic ulceration or aneurysm of the aorta. Microscopic examination of the vessel wall shows inflammatory cells and destruction of tissue. The offending organisms include streptococci, staphylococci, and salmonellae.

Mycotic aneurysm or suppurative arteritis caused by salmonellae is being recognized more frequently than before. Sower and Whelan have reported that three types of vascular lesions may be produced by salmonellae: (1) a diffuse suppurative arteritis with rupture and the development of a saccular or false aneurysm; (2) a focal arteritis with the formation of a mycotic aneurysm and rupture; or (3) a secondary infection superimposed upon a pre-existing arteriosclerotic aneurysm. A normal vessel can be involved when an infected embolus becomes lodged on its wall, or organisms gain access to the vessel wall through the vasa vasorum. The vessels involved in many of the reported cases have had pre-existing lesions, including dissecting aneurysm, atherosclerosis, and syphilis.

Once a mycotic aneurysm of the aorta has developed, surgical resection offers the only possibility of cure, and prolonged antimicrobial therapy must be provided.

Allen, E. V., Barker, N. W., and Hines, E. A.: Peripheral Vascular Diseases. 3rd ed. Philadelphia, W. B. Saunders Company, 1962.

Perdue, G. D., Jr., and Smith, R. B., III: Surgical treatment of mycotic aneurysms. South. Med. J., 60:848, 1967.

Sower, N. D., and Whelan, T. J.: Suppurative arteritis due to salmonella. Surgery, 52:851, 1962.

ANEURYSMS OF THE SINUSES OF VALSALVA

An aneurysm of one of the sinuses of Valsalva may be due to syphilitic aortitis, bacterial endocarditis, medial cystic necrosis, or a congenital defect. The lesion is described in Ch. 553.

587. SYPHILIS OF THE AORTA

Syphilis is described in Ch. 246. The discussion here is confined to its effect on the aorta (and the heart). Aneurysm of the aorta caused by syphilis has been described in Ch. 586.

Pathology. Although syphilitic myocarditis, gummas of the myocardium, and syphilitic involvement of the coronary arteries are known to occur rarely, it is safe to assume that the aorta is always involved in cardiovascular syphilis. Syphilitic aortitis begins with perivascular inflammation of the vasa vasorum in the adventitia. Treponemas subsequently invade the media via the lymphatics, producing medial inflammation and destruction. The ensuing fibrous proliferation results in intimal wrinkling and the characteristic "tree bark" appearance. It seems likely that many of the lesions of the aorta just described are secondary to changes that have occurred in the vasa vasorum that result in a diminished blood supply to the aorta itself. As a rule, the pathologic process is limited to the thoracic portion of the aorta. Gummatous lesions of the aorta may occur, but they are not common.

Clinical Manifestations. Uncomplicated syphilitic aortitis is difficult to diagnose during life. There are no reliable clinical signs that allow one to make a diagnosis. The majority of patients who have had inadequate treatment of syphilis during its early stages show syphilitic aortitis at autopsy. Diagnosis of uncomplicated aortitis is not based on signs and symptoms.

Syphilitic aortitis may lead to *dilatation of the aorta*. This almost always occurs in the ascending portion, and no symptoms are produced by it. There are no clearly diagnostic physical findings. It has long been said that the second heart sound is accentuated and has a tambour-like quality when there is syphilitic aortitis. Dilatation of the aorta secondary to systemic hypertension or atherosclerosis can also be associated with a loud second heart sound. Since these diseases are far more common than dilatation of the aorta caused by syphilis, the sign is not of diagnostic value. Dilatation of the ascending aorta may produce a nonspecific systolic murmur in the aortic area. Visible and palpable pulsations in the upper parasternal region may be noted. When there is moderate dilatation or aneurysmal formation of the ascending aorta, pulsation of the right or left sternoclavicular joints may be detected (see Fig. 2). When the ascending aorta is dilated, the upper parasternal dullness may be wider than normal.

Dilatation of the ascending aorta may be detected at fluoroscopic examination of the heart and aorta and on roentgenograms of the chest utilizing the oblique positions. Unfortunately, it is not easy to state when the aorta has attained definitely abnormal size. The width of the root of the aorta can be studied far more adequately by angiocardiography. This is not always needed, but it may occasionally be justified. The surest sign of syphilitic aortitis is calcification of the early portion of the ascending aorta (Fig. 5). About one fifth of the cases of

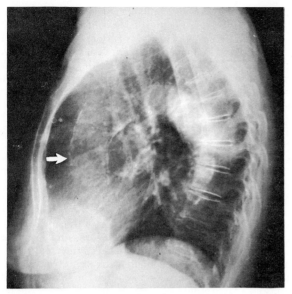

Figure 5. Lateral roentgenogram of chest showing calcification of the early portion of the aorta. This type of calcification is characteristic of atherosclerosis superimposed on syphilitic aortitis.

The surgical correction of aortic regurgitation with the use of a prosthetic aortic valve is discussed in Ch. 561.

Syphilitic aortitis may cause *narrowing of the ostia of the major arterial branches* of the thoracic aorta. There may be diminished pulsation of the carotid arteries, and the blood pressure and pulsations of the upper extremities may be altered (see Ch. 591). Narrowing of the coronary ostia, when mild, causes no symptoms. Angina pectoris in patients with syphilitic aortitis is usually due to a combination of factors, including narrowed coronary ostia, the hemodynamic effects of aortic regurgitation, the increased demand of associated left ventricular hypertrophy, congestive heart failure, and associated coronary atherosclerosis. Angina pectoris in this clinical setting may be more severe and less responsive to nitroglycerin than usual. Myocardial infarction is an uncommon autopsy finding in patients with cardiovascular syphilis, but prolonged chest pain and sudden death are not rare. It is not wise to make a diagnosis of isolated coronary ostial disease caused by syphilis with no other evidence of syphilitic aortitis. Coronary atherosclerosis is so common that it is likely to be the cause of angina pectoris in such cases.

Rimsa, A., and Griffith, G. C.: Trends in cardiovascular syphilis. Ann. Intern. Med., 46:915, 1957.

syphilitic aortitis have the sign. The calcification is actually due to the atherosclerosis of the aorta. Ordinarily calcification of the intima of the aorta caused by atherosclerosis is seen roentgenographically in the aortic knob. The atherosclerotic process seems to increase in the root and ascending portion of the aorta where the syphilitic process is most severe. Calcification of the early portion of the aortic arch may also occur in patients with giant cell arteritis of unknown cause.

Aortic regurgitation, the most frequent complication of syphilitic aortitis, is mainly due to the dilatation of the aortic ring. The syphilitic process also extends into the base of the valve leaflet. The result is separation of the valve commissures and deformity of the cusps. This deformity, plus the dilated aortic ring, produces aortic regurgitation. Aortic stenosis never develops as a result of syphilis, and a systolic murmur in such patients is due to "turbulent" blood flow.

Aortic regurgitation caused by syphilis usually appears between the ages of 35 and 50. Men have the condition far more often than women. It occurs in about half of all cases of cardiovascular syphilis. The murmur of aortic regurgitation may be louder to the right of the mid-sternal area than to the left. An Austin Flint murmur is commonly heard at the apex. The cooing diastolic murmur caused by a retroverted aortic cusp may occur.

The signs and symptoms of aortic regurgitation caused by syphilis depend upon the degree and duration of the abnormality. Symptoms and signs of heart failure are likely to ensue within three to four years after aortic regurgitation is discovered. Heart failure may develop gradually or may be heralded by acute pulmonary edema. Therapy may be beneficial for a time and a few patients survive more than a decade after heart failure has developed, but the majority do not live more than a few years. Sudden and unexpected death may occur in patients with severe aortic regurgitation.

Treatment. The treatment of heart failure is discussed in Ch. 541.

588. THROMBOSIS OF THE TERMINAL AORTA

Thrombosis of the terminal aorta may occur suddenly or may develop gradually, usually on atheromatous lesions. Most often it occurs in males between the ages of 40 and 65, although it has occurred at a younger age.

Sudden thrombosis of the terminal aorta may simulate embolic obstruction when the aortic lumen has been almost normal in size prior to the formation of the clot (see Ch. 589). If sudden thrombosis is superimposed on a partially obstructed aorta, the signs and symptoms may be less severe because collateral circulation has had time to develop prior to the acute thrombosis. Pain and weakness of the lower extremities may occur after sudden thrombosis of the aorta. The pain may radiate to the lower back and inguinal regions. The arterial pulses below the obstructed area are absent. The legs may be pale, mottled, cyanotic, or white, and signs of shock may be present. It may be impossible to differentiate a saddle embolus to the aortic bifurcation from sudden thrombosis of the terminal aorta. When a heart lesion is present that could be the source of an embolus, the diagnostic scale tips in that direction.

When thrombosis of the aorta occurs with normal aortic lumen, the outlook is poor. The treatment is similar to that of saddle embolus. When thrombosis of the aorta occurs in a partially occluded aorta with a better collateral circulation, the outlook may be somewhat less grave. Surgical resection and grafting of the occluded portion of the aorta is usually indicated as an emergency procedure.

Gradual thrombosis of the terminal portion of the aorta has been called *Leriche's syndrome.* This condition differs from sudden occlusion of the aorta and is far more common. The patient feels distress produced by walking and relieved by rest. The discomfort develops in the thighs, hip region, or buttocks and represents intermittent claudication at a high level. Sexual impotence is a frequent associated symptom in male patients. The arterial pulses are absent or decreased in the lower extremities. Feeble pulsations are sometimes found when collateral circulation has developed to a moderate degree. Bruits may be heard over the abdominal aorta and over the iliac and femoral arteries. Atrophy of leg muscles may develop in time. Many patients with Leriche's syndrome have good nutrition of the skin of the extremities because of the adequate collateral circulation that develops when the vascular obstruction is high. In fact, the good prognosis with regard to limb survival should be emphasized. Some patients do have coldness, pallor, cyanosis, trophic changes of the legs, and rarely, gangrene of the feet, but it is likely that the smaller peripheral vessels are also diseased when these signs of arterial insufficiency are present. Many cases of Leriche's syndrome are misdiagnosed as osteoarthritis of the lumbosacral spine or hip, ruptured intervertebral disc, or bursitis of the hip. The majority of these patients die as a result of cerebral or coronary atherosclerosis. Rarely, the renal arteries may become occluded by cephalad extension of the aortic thrombus.

Aortography is not usually needed to make the diagnosis of thrombosis of the aorta. It is useful, however, in determining the site and extent of the obstruction, estimating the collateral circulation, and determining the amount of disease in the distal vessels. The modern contrast media and newer techniques have made aortography much safer than formerly.

The usual conservative therapy for chronic occlusive peripheral vascular disease is indicated. Surgical treatment is indicated when the intermittent claudication is severe enough and disabling enough to justify the mortality and morbidity risk of such treatment. Recognizable cerebral, coronary, and other serious diseases are usually contraindications to operation. Three operative procedures are utilized; thromboendarterectomy, excision with graft replacement, and bypass graft. The operative risk reported by De Bakey is only about 2.5 per cent, and relief of symptoms and restoration of pulses were obtained in 96 per cent of cases. Operation on the aorta of course does nothing to prevent the complications of cerebral and coronary atherosclerosis in these patients.

De Bakey, M. D., and Crawford, S. E.: Surgical considerations of acquired diseases of the aorta and major peripheral arteries. III: Atherosclerotic occlusive vascular disease. Mod. Concepts Cardiovasc. Dis., 29:571, 1960.

Juergens, J. L., Barker, N. W., and Hines, E. A.: Arteriosclerosis obliterans: Review of 520 cases with special reference to pathogenic and prognostic factors. Circulation, 21:188, 1960.

Leriche, R., and Morel, A.: The syndrome of thrombotic obliteration of the aortic bifurcation. Ann. Surg., 127:193, 1948.

Massarelli, J. J., Jr., and Estes, J. E.: Atherosclerotic occlusion of the abdominal aorta and iliac arteries: A study of 105 patients. Ann. Intern. Med., 47:1125, 1957.

Perdue, G. D., Long, W. D., and Smith, R. B., III: Perspective concerning aorto-femoral arterial reconstruction. Ann. Surg., 173:940, 1971.

589. EMBOLISM AT THE BIFURCATION OF THE AORTA

An embolus lodging at the bifurcation of the aorta is called a *saddle embolus*. Perhaps no more than 5 per cent

of all systemic arterial emboli lodge at this point; but when one does, a true emergency is created.

Large emboli almost always originate in the heart. In patients with rheumatic heart disease who have mitral valve disease and a dilated left atrium, left atrial clots may be the source of emboli. Emboli are more often associated with mitral stenosis than with mitral regurgitation. They occur with higher frequency when there is atrial fibrillation rather than normal sinus rhythm. The presence of heart failure does not seem to increase the frequency of emboli from this source. Occasionally an embolus seems to be related to a change in cardiac rhythm from atrial fibrillation to normal sinus rhythm. An embolus may follow mitral valve surgery. A large, friable, left ventricular thrombus may develop secondary to myocardial infarction, and it may break off and be swept by the blood to the bifurcation of the aorta, where it lodges. This has occurred with decreasing frequency since anticoagulants have been used in the treatment of myocardial infarction. Emboli can occur from such a source a week or several weeks after the myocardial infarction. The presence of heart failure increases the possibility of left ventricular thrombosis and peripheral emboli in such cases. The emboli related to bacterial endocarditis are usually too small to cause a saddle embolus. Rarely an embolus may arise from the systemic veins and pass through an atrial septal defect into the systemic arteries. Thrombi in aortic aneurysms or on ulcerated atherosclerotic lesions of the aorta may be the source of emboli.

Although a rather large clot is required to produce a saddle embolus, the clot need not be as large as the aorta itself. Edema of the aortic wall and intense arterial spasm of the involved collateral vessels occur very quickly after an embolus. These factors, along with secondary thrombosis, can convert a partial block into a complete one.

Clinical Manifestations. Pain in the legs usually develops suddenly, but may come on gradually. Abdominal or sacral pain may occasionally predominate. Paresthesia, anesthesia, and muscular weakness of the lower extremities may follow the pain or may develop without pain. The clinician must be alert when a patient with reason for peripheral arterial embolus complains that his leg has "gone to sleep." The skin of the lower extremities may be cold, pale, mottled, or cyanotic. Pulsations of the femoral, popliteal, posterior tibial, and dorsalis pedis vessels are usually not felt. Saddle embolus of the aorta must be differentiated from thrombosis of the terminal aorta and thrombophlebitis with associated severe arterial spasm.

It should be emphasized that more distal peripheral emboli may proceed or follow the embolus to the bifurcation of the aorta.

Patients with saddle block embolus frequently die or lose a limb unless embolectomy can be performed promptly. Even with surgical intervention the mortality is high, especially when the embolus occurs subsequent to myocardial infarction. The technique described by Cranley et al., using an "embolectomy catheter" with a balloon, has been employed with moderate success. Heparin should be administered as soon as the diagnosis of arterial embolism is made. Heparin and drugs useful for long-term anticoagulation should be used postoperatively. At times, cardiac valve abnormalities should be corrected surgically when they are thought to be responsible for the intracardiac thrombi.

Cranley, J. J., Krause, R. J., Strasser, E. S., Hafner, C. D., and Fogarty, T. S.: Peripheral arterial embolism: Changing concepts. Surgery, 55:57, 1964.

Crave, C.: Embolism to the bifurcation of the aorta. N. Engl. J. Med., 258:359, 1958.

Deterling, R. A.: Acute arterial occlusion. Surg. Clin. North Am., 46:587, 1966.

Fogarty, T. J., and Cranley, J. J.: Catheter technic for arterial embolectomy. Ann. Surg., 161:325, 1965.

Whitman, E. J., and McGoon, D. C.: Surgical management of aorto-iliac occlusive vascular disease. J.A.M.A., 179:923, 1962.

590. THE AORTA AS A SOURCE OF MICROEMBOLI

Perdue and Smith have emphasized that disease of aorta may be a source of atheromatous microemboli. They report that fragmentation of atheromatous plaques or dislodgment of debris from aneurysm or ulcerated areas in the aorta and larger arteries may cause distal emboli of various sizes. The small arterioles may be obstructed by the particles themselves or by an inflammatory response to cholesterol crystals and subsequent thrombosis and fibrosis.

Autopsy reports have indicated that renal lesions (with or without the acute development of hypertension), acute pancreatitis, and gastrointestinal ulceration and bleeding can be the result of microemboli. When multiple organs are involved, the clinical picture may resemble that of collagen disease.

Cerebral and retinal emboli may be associated with multiple system emboli. Atheromatous emboli to the extremities may simulate primary occlusive disease of the peripheral arteries. An embolic cause is suggested when myalgia and muscle tenderness occur in association with skin changes of lividity, necrosis, and ulceration with or without evidence of associated occlusive arterial disease. Some clinical investigators have concluded that a search for cholesterol crystals in random muscle biopsy may assist one in identifying the exact cause of the occlusive disease.

The microemboli may occur spontaneously, but may also occur when a diseased aorta is manipulated at the time of surgery or after catheter aortography.

Heparin and corticosteroids have been used in some patients with microemboli to the extremities. At times an aortogram is indicated in an effort to find the origin of the emboli. The recognition and treatment of surgically curable lesions eliminates the primary sources and prevents recurrences.

Crane, C.: Atherothrombotic embolism to lower extremities in arteriosclerosis. Arch. Surg., 94:96, 1967.

Haygood, T. A., Fesset, W. J., and Strange, D. A.: Atheromatous microembolism simulating polymyositis. J.A.M.A., 203:135, 1968.

Perdue, G. D., Jr., and Smith, R. B., III: Atheromatous microemboli. Ann. Surg., 169:954, 1969.

591. THE AORTIC ARCH SYNDROME

The term "aortic arch syndrome" is given to a group of disorders leading to occlusion of the vessels arising from the arch of the aorta. (The term "pulseless disease" is often used synonymously with the term "aortic arch syndrome.") The disease may be due to nonspecific arteritis (*Takayasu's disease*). It may be due to the obstructive lesions found in arteries associated with *supravalvular aortic stenosis.* Years ago *syphilitic arteritis* was a common cause of the obstructive lesions of the vessels arising from the aortic arch. Today the majority of patients seen in the United States with pulseless disease are in the middle and older age groups, and the pathologic lesion causing the occlusive disease of the arteries is almost invariably *atherosclerosis.* The signs and symptoms associated with obliterative disease of the vessels arising from the arch of the aorta are predictable when one considers the blood supply of the brain, eyes, face, and arms.

The rare disease known as *Takayasu's disease* has been observed as early as age 11 and as late as age 64. The diagnosis is usually made during the third decade of life. For unexplained reasons, most patients with the syndrome are females. Reports from many countries prove that the condition is not confined to Japan, as it was once thought to be. The clinical features include vertigo; syncope; convulsions; aphasia; headache; transient cerebral ischemia resulting in hemiplegia or hemiparesis; absence of palpable carotid arteries on one or both sides; transient episodes of blindness; amblyopia; rapidly developing cataracts; retinal atrophy or pigmentation; photophobia; optic atrophy; atrophy of the iris; sluggish blood flow in the retinal vessels; decreased intraocular arterial pressure; muscular atrophy of the face; thin pigmented skin of the face; ulcerated nose and palate; claudication of muscles of mastication; decreased or absent audible blood pressure in the arms and increased blood pressure in the lower extremities (hence the term "reversed coarctation"); diminished or absent subclavian, brachial, and radial pulses; decreased to absent blood pressure in arms and legs; claudication of upper extremities; palpable collateral arteries in the neck and intercostal spaces; rib notching; and continuous murmurs in the neck and upper chest. Calcification of the intima of the ascending aorta, aortic regurgitation, angina pectoris, and myocardial infarction may occur. The blood pressure in the aorta may be quite high for several reasons, and yet the blood pressure as measured in the extremities may be low. This multitude of symptoms and signs can be kept in mind if one remembers that they are associated with ischemia of the brain, eyes, face, and upper extremities. Leukocytosis and elevated sedimentation rate are common.

Histologically the lesions are characterized by an arteritis of all layers of the involved vessels with giant cell infiltration and obliteration of the lumen. The pathologic process is usually limited to the innominate, subclavian, and carotid arteries as well as the coronary ostia. It has also been observed to involve the thoracic and abdominal aorta and the mesenteric arteries.

Patients with this syndrome usually die of cerebral ischemia or heart disease. No figures are available to indicate the average length of life after onset of the disease. After the onset of symptoms, patients have lived from 1½ to 14 years. Long-term anticoagulant treatment has been recommended in an effort to prevent arterial thrombosis. Surgical treatment, including endarterectomy, local resection, and vessel grafts, may be applicable in suitable cases.

Cheitlin, M. D., and Carter, P. G.: Takayashu's disease. Unusual manifestations. Arch. Intern. Med., 116:283, 1965.

Judge, R. D., Currier, R. D., Gracie, W. A., and Figley, M. M.: Takayasu's arteritis and the aortic arch syndrome. Am. J. Med., 32:379, 1962.

Kalmansohn, R. B., and Kalmansohn, R. W.: Thrombotic obliteration of the branches of the aortic arch. Circulation, 15:237, 1957.

Shimizu, K., and Sano, K.: Pulseless disease. J. Neuropathol. Clin. Neurol., 1:37, 1951.

Vinijchaikul, K.: Primary arteritis of the aorta and its main branches (Takayasu's arteriopathy): A clinicopathologic study of eight cases. Medicine, 43:15, 1967.

592. RHEUMATOID AORTITIS

Aortitis may be recognized in a small percentage of patients with rheumatoid arthritis. A rheumatoid etiology for aortic regurgitation is especially likely when there is rheumatoid spondylitis, uveitis, or psoriasis. Complete heart block may occur when the atrioventricular conduction tissue in the heart is involved by the disease process. Heart failure may result from the aortic regurgitation. When the murmur of aortic regurgitation develops during an exacerbation of rheumatoid arthritis, particularly in the presence of uveitis, it is considered to be diagnostic of rheumatoid aortitis and aortic valve disease. Aortic regurgitation caused by rheumatoid aortitis and aortic valve disease is differentiated from syphilitic heart disease when the serologic tests for syphilis are negative and when the murmur occurs at an early age in a patient with rheumatoid arthritis.

Although the clinical features of rheumatoid aortitis and aortic valve disease are similar to the findings in rheumatic heart disease, the pathologic findings are more distinctive. The cusps of the aortic valve do not fuse at the commissures as they do in rheumatic aortic valve disease. Plaquelike lesions of the aortic intima near the valve commissures found in rheumatoid aortitis have not been observed in rheumatic fever. The lesions in the aorta usually do not extend beyond the ascending portion of the vessel. The entire clinical and pathologic picture forces one to support the idea that rheumatoid aortitis is a specific complication of rheumatoid arthritis.

When surgical treatment for aortic regurgitation is deemed necessary in patients with rheumatoid spondylitis, the newest surgical techniques, including the placement of a Starr-Edwards prosthetic valve, can be utilized. A cardiac pacemaker may be needed for heart block.

Clarke, W. S., Kulka, J. P., and Bauer, W.: Rheumatoid aortitis with aortic regurgitation; An unusual manifestation of rheumatoid arthritis (including spondylitis). Am. J. Med., 22:580, 1957.

Cobbs, B. W., Jr.: Clinical recognition and medical management of rheumatic heart disease and other acquired valvular disease. In Hurst, J. W. (ed.): The Heart. 3rd ed. New York, McGraw-Hill Book Company, 1974, p. 826.

Graham, D. C., and Smythe, H. S.: The carditis and aortitis of ankylosing spondylitis. Bull. Rheum. Dis., 9:171, 1958.

593. OTHER CAUSES OF AORTITIS

Aortitis may develop in association with a variety of conditions. These include scleroderma and Hodgkin's disease.

Giant cell arteritis may involve the aorta and produce the aortic arch syndrome, aneurysm of the ascending aorta, aortic regurgitation, and dissecting aneurysm. This condition is being recognized with increasing frequency.

Behçet's syndrome, consisting of mouth and genital ulcerations, blindness, central nervous system involvement, thrombophlebitis, and arterial involvement, may be associated with aortic aneurysms.

Austin, W. G., and Blennerhassett, J. B.: Giant cell aortitis causing an aneurysm of the ascending aorta and aortic regurgitation. N. Engl. J. Med., 272:80, 1965.

Fraumeni, J. F., Jr., Herweg, J. C., and Kissane, J. M.: Panaortitis complicating Hodgkin's disease. Ann. Intern. Med., 67:1242, 1967.

Hills, E. A.: Behçet's syndrome with aortic aneurysms. Br. Med. J., 4:152, 1967.

Hunder, G. G., Ward, L. E., and Burbank, M. K.: Giant-cell arteritis producing an aortic arch syndrome. Ann. Intern. Med., 66:578, 1967.

Roth, L. M., and Kissane, J. M.: Panaortitis and aortic valvulitis in progressive systemic sclerosis (scleroderma). Am. J. Clin. Pathol., 41:287, 1964.

594. CONGENITAL ANOMALIES OF THE AORTA

A right aortic arch may occur as an isolated and asymptomatic abnormality. It may produce pulsation of the right sternoclavicular joint and is usually identified on the chest roentgenogram. The anomaly may be associated with other cardiovascular defects. For example, 25 per cent of patients with tetralogy of Fallot and truncus arteriosus and 5 per cent of patients with tricuspid atresia have the aortic arch on the right side.

The right subclavian artery may arise from the descending aorta (aberrant right subclavian artery). The anomaly may be unassociated with other abnormalities, but an association with tetralogy of Fallot has been reported. The vessel passes posterior to the esophagus and for this reason is usually identified by observing an indention of the barium-filled esophagus during fluoroscopy. This anomaly is occasionally associated with a large aneurysmal diverticulum of the aorta (Kommerell's diverticulum). An aberrant right subclavian artery is found in approximately 1 per cent of routine barium studies of the esophagus. It is almost always asymptomatic but has been claimed to cause dysphagia on rare occasions. Aneurysmal dilatation and rupture of an aberrant subclavian artery have been reported.

A number of vascular anomalies of the aortic arch may contrive to encircle the esophagus and trachea and produce a vascular ring. Although many varieties of rings are possible, the two common types are double aortic arch and right aortic arch with retroesophageal segment with a left-sided ligamentum arteriosum. Vascular rings may produce noisy respiration, brassy cough, recurrent pulmonary infections, and dysphagia during early life. Infants may be more comfortable with the neck hyperextended. The vascular abnormality may be suspected in a routine roentgenogram of the chest if the air column of the trachea is constricted at the proper location. More often the condition is identified by fluoroscopic examination of the barium-filled esophagus. More exact delineation of the vessels can be accomplished by aortography (Fig. 6). When obstructive lesions are severe, surgical correction is indicated.

Atresia of the aortic arch may be the cause of heart failure during the first few days of life. In fact, heart failure at this age is a clue to the diagnosis. Death usually occurs in a few days to weeks. On rare occasions pulmonary arteriolar disease protects the lungs and prolongs survival time. The atretic area is usually located be-

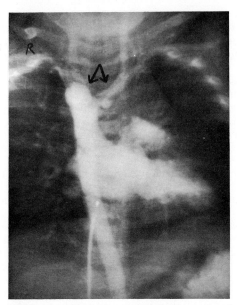

Figure 6. Angiocardiogram showing double aortic arch.

tween the left common carotid artery and the ductus arteriosus. Arterial unsaturation is found in the lower extremities.

Supravalvular aortic stenosis may be misdiagnosed as ordinary valvular aortic stenosis. This less common condition occasionally occurs as a familial trait and is characterized by unusual facies, occasional mental retardation, a pressure difference in the two arms (lower in left arm), obstructive lesions of the vessels arising from the aortic arch (including obstruction of the coronary arteries), associated pulmonary stenosis, multiple pulmonary artery stenoses, and hypercalcemia, in addition to the murmur of aortic obstruction. Surgical correction of this condition is not entirely satisfactory since multiple abnormalities may be present.

COARCTATION OF THE AORTA

This is described in Ch. 552.

Blake, H. A., and Manion, W. C.: Thoracic arterial arch anomalies. Circulation, 26:251, 1962.

Brinsfield, D. E., and Wedwards, F. K.: Clinical recognition and medical management of congenital heart disease. *In* Hurst, J. W. (ed.): The Heart. 3rd ed. New York, McGraw-Hill Book Company, 1974, p. 683.

Stewart, J. R., Kincaid, O. W., and Edwards, J. E.: An Atlas of Vascular Rings and Related Malformation of the Aortic Arch System. Springfield, Ill., Charles C Thomas, 1964.

594a. TUMORS OF THE AORTA

Primary malignant tumors of the aorta may present a clinical picture suggesting herniated nucleus pulposus, renal colic, peripheral vascular disease, coarctation of the aorta, or Leriche's syndrome. The tumor may originate in the arch of the aorta or thoracic aorta but may originate in the thoracoabdominal aorta or abdominal aorta. The tumors, which may be spindle cell sarcoma, giant cell sarcoma, malignant endothelioma, fibromyxosarcoma, or leiomyosarcoma, metastasize widely to the kidney, spleen, vertebra, mesentery, skin, and pleura.

Hypertension, which may begin abruptly, has occurred in about a quarter of the patients.

The medical and surgical management of patients with malignant tumors of the aorta is quite limited, and death usually occurs a short while after the first symptoms appear.

Stevenson, J. E.: Primary malignant tumor of the aorta. Am. J. Med., 51:555, 1971.

DISEASES OF THE PERIPHERAL VESSELS

Jay D. Coffman

595. PERIPHERAL VASCULAR DISEASES DUE TO ORGANIC ARTERIAL OBSTRUCTION

ARTERIOSCLEROSIS OBLITERANS

Definition. Arteriosclerosis obliterans is caused by arteriosclerotic narrowing or obstruction of large and medium-sized arteries supplying the extremities; symptoms and signs are produced by ischemia.

Etiology. The etiology of arteriosclerosis is discussed in Ch. 723.

Incidence. Arteriosclerosis obliterans is the leading cause of obstructive arterial disease of the extremities after age 30. The lower extremities are involved most commonly; the superficial femoral artery is affected by stenosis or obstruction in approximately 90 per cent of patients. The aortoiliac and popliteal areas are the next most common sites. The greatest incidence of superficial femoral and more distal arterial disease occurs in the seventh decade, but aortoiliac disease has its peak a decade earlier. The disease is more common in males than in females, especially before the menopause (about 9:1). Patients with diabetes mellitus develop arteriosclerosis obliterans more frequently and at an earlier age than nondiabetics. Diabetics have the same incidence of femoropopliteal disease but a greater frequency of vessel involvement between the knee and ankle than nondiabetics. In patients with isolated aortoiliac disease, high plasma cholesterol and total lipids are frequent findings, but diabetes mellitus is not.

Pathology. It should be emphasized that the stenotic or occlusive process is usually segmental, for surgical therapy depends on this characteristic; however, the intima also displays widespread arteriosclerotic changes proximal and distal to the segmental lesion. Although the occlusive or stenotic lesions causing symptoms are usually proximal to the knee, the incidence of lower leg arterial occlusions is high (45 per cent in some surveys) and rises steeply with increasing age. Of the vessels in the calf, the posterior tibial artery is most often affected. A specific lesion of arteriolar and capillary endothelial proliferation has been described in diabetes by some investigators but has not been found by others. In patients with diabetes the development of indolent ulcers in the presence of adequate pulses may be due to diabetic neuropathy and not to small vessel disease.

Pathophysiology. Symptoms and signs are produced by inadequate oxygenation of the tissues distal to the arterial lesion, secondary to the decrease in blood flow or pressure at rest or during exercise. Large and medium-sized arteries must have a decrease in cross-sectional area of 70 to 90 per cent before a decrease in blood flow or pressure occurs at rest; during exercise a 60 per cent decrease may suffice. The critical stenosis diameter which decreases flow or pressure is dependent on the velocity of flow and therefore the peripheral resistance; the length of the stenotic segment has a lesser effect. Factors affecting peripheral resistance are discussed below. In patients who develop ischemic symptoms only during exercise, the calf blood flow may be normal at rest; however, during exercise the blood flow may stop or be abnormally slow. The decreased blood pressure in the artery distal to the obstructing lesion allows the force of the contracting muscle during exercise to partially or completely obstruct arterial flow. Also, if full vasodilatation (reactive hyperemia) is produced in an involved limb, the total blood flow is usually much less than in the normal limb.

Although all the vessels of a system contribute to its total resistance, the arterioles and precapillary sphincters are of greatest importance. Peripheral resistance is regulated reflexly by the sympathetic nervous system and locally by the formation of vasodilator metabolites. Activity of the sympathetic nervous system usually causes cutaneous vasoconstriction, thereby increasing peripheral resistance. This normal activity, i.e., reflex vasoconstriction when exposed to cold, can be harmful to an ischemic extremity. Removal of vasoconstrictor activity in an extremity results in vasodilatation. Blood vessels in skeletal muscle also are affected by sympathetic activity but only to a very limited extent during exercise when vasodilator metabolites are active.

Blood supply to the limb distal to an obstructing or stenotic arterial lesion is via collateral blood vessels. Most of these collaterals are present in the normal limb but unused until an obstruction occurs; many appear almost immediately after an acute arterial occlusion, but others form more gradually over a period of months. Little is known concerning the reactivity of the collateral vessels in man; in animals, exercise and systemic blood pressure elevation decrease collateral vessel resistance, whereas a decrease in systemic blood pressure increases collateral vascular resistance. Blood flow can be increased through collateral vessels in man by raising the systemic blood pressure.

Clinical Manifestations. The most common symptom of arteriosclerosis obliterans is *intermittent claudication* (intermittent limping). The patient experiences cramping pain, tightness, numbness, or severe fatigue in the muscle group being exercised. The amount of exercise producing the pain is relatively constant in each patient, and the pain is relieved promptly by rest. In a few patients, pain may disappear on further walking, perhaps because of an unconscious slowing of gait. Intermittent claudication is most frequent in the calf muscles because femoral artery disease is so common. However, even in more proximal lesions (aortoiliac disease) the calf is the most common site of claudication because these muscles do the most work in walking. Low back, buttock, thigh, and foot claudication may also occur; the site of the symptoms localizes the obstructing lesion proximally.

Rest pain is the other important symptom of obstructive arterial disease. Rest pain is a grave sign indicating that the blood supply is not sufficient even for the small nutritional requirements of the skin. It may be localized to one or more toes but often has a stocking distribution. The latter distribution means that ischemic neuritis is not usually the cause of rest pain. Rest pain is worse at night and is relieved somewhat by dependency and by cooling.

Other symptoms of arteriosclerosis obliterans include coldness, numbness, paresthesias, and color changes in the involved extremity.

Examination of the patient with intermittent claudication reveals diminished or absent pulses below the site of obstruction. Although the dorsalis pedis pulse may be absent congenitally in more than 10 per cent of people, the posterior tibial pulse is absent in only 2 per cent, and both pulses in approximately 0.5 per cent. If pulses are palpable in the presence of an obstructive lesion, exercise will make the pulses disappear; this is often a valuable diagnostic test. If pulses cannot be detected with the fingertips, an oscillometer is often useful. The oscillometer gives a qualitative measure of the pulse beneath a blood pressure cuff. It will reveal pulsations in the presence of edema and obesity when vessels are too deep to be palpated, and sometimes when vasospasm rather than complete obstruction is present. Marked differences in oscillometric readings between two limbs at symmetrical positions or between different levels on the same limb are important. The second important part of the examination is to listen with the stethoscope over the aorta and peripheral arteries. The presence of a systolic or continuous bruit indicates a proximal obstructive or stenotic lesion; a continuous bruit denotes a very low diastolic pressure distal to the obstruction and therefore an inadequate collateral blood flow.

Examination may also reveal signs of ischemia. Distal to an arterial obstruction, the limb is often cool when compared with the proximal part of the same extremity or the symmetrical part of the opposite extremity. Skin temperature may vary widely in health, and even profound coldness, if present in all extremities, particularly in a cool environment, may be physiologic. Severe coldness that persists in a warm environment is usually abnormal, and, if unilateral, definitely abnormal. A warm extremity with normal color but absent pulses means collateral blood flow is adequate. The involved extremity may also show color changes: pallor, owing to a markedly decreased blood flow; cyanosis, caused by a diminution in blood flow not sufficient to cause blanching of the skin; rubor, a persistent red or reddish-blue discoloration of a cold extremity secondary to persistent dilatation of the cutaneous capillaries and venules owing to injury from anoxemia. Trophic changes may develop: the subcutaneous tissue becomes puffy and thickened; the skin becomes dry, atrophic, shiny, and tightly drawn with an absence of hair; and the toenails become hard, brittle, thickened, ridged, and deformed. Indolent ulceration and gangrene indicate severe local ischemia. Ischemic ulcers on the toes, and sometimes over the anterior and lateral lower calf, are usually quite painful and sensitive.

Isolated aortoiliac disease (Leriche's syndrome) produces a characteristic picture. Intermittent claudication of the low back, buttock, thighs, or calves may be present. Global atrophy of the limbs and pallor of the legs and feet are frequent findings. Other trophic changes are usually absent; if present, concomitant femoropopliteal disease is often found. Hypertension may be present in the upper extremities; impotence has been emphasized as a symptom but is not frequent. All pulses are usually absent in the legs, but weak femorals may be felt if the collateral circulation is well developed or if the occlusive process is only partial. A systolic murmur is often heard over both femoral arteries and lower abdomen.

Diagnosis. By careful palpation of pulses and auscultation for bruits, the diagnosis and site of obstruction or stenosis are easily determined in most patients. The presence of coldness, discoloration, and trophic changes indicates the degree of ischemia. A triad of tests can be used to evaluate the degree of ischemia and collateral circulation. With the patient supine, the involved limb is raised to a 45 degree angle. Normally the plantar surface remains pink; pallor indicates a deficient blood supply. If pallor occurs only after ankle exercise, the circulation is not as compromised. Then the patient sits up quickly, allowing the extremities to assume a dependent position, and flushing and filling of the veins of the feet are timed. Flushing should occur immediately; veins should fill in about 10 seconds. Flushing and venous filling times of greater than 20 and 30 seconds, respectively, denote a severely ischemic limb with inadequate collateral circulation. These tests should be performed in a warm room to rule out vasospasm; varicosities invalidate the venous filling time. The use of a Doppler to measure systolic blood pressure in the dorsalis pedis and posterior tibial arteries with the pneumatic cuff on the thigh and then at the ankle is especially helpful in diagnosing obstructive disease (the pedal pressures should be equal to or higher than the brachial artery pressure) and its site. A pressure less than 30 mm Hg indicates very severe ischemia and often presages gangrene.

The presence or absence of calcification by x-ray of the extremities is usually meaningless. *Arteriography* may be necessary if the diagnosis is in doubt. It is always performed if surgery is being considered to reveal the exact location and extent of the obstructive lesion and the collateral circulation. In doubtful cases, an exercise test may be performed while blood flow is measured by the disappearance of a radioisotope (^{131}I, ^{133}Xe) from the involved muscle. During exercise the disappearance rate either stops or is abnormally slow in claudicators compared with that in normal subjects. The postexercise disappearance rates are also usually abnormal in obstructive arterial disease. Postexercise or postischemic flow can also be measured with a plethysmograph, but there is some overlap of values between claudicators and normal persons. A variety of equipment has been used to demonstrate the small, rounded pulse with a slow upstroke and downstroke and absent dicrotic notch, or to show the decrease in systolic pressure below an obstructing or stenotic lesion. These tests can be valuable, but it is important that the "normal ranges" are first established for the particular combination of methods or procedures used.

Intermittent claudication may occur in *severe anemia* and in *McArdle's syndrome;* both are easily distinguished from arteriosclerosis obliterans by the presence of normal pulses. The pain of *arthritis* may radiate to the thighs or calves, but is present at rest and not usually worse with exercise. *Arterial embolism* pain does not develop as insidiously as arteriosclerotic ischemic symp-

toms. In occasional patients with *lumbar disc, spinal canal, or cauda equina disease,* pain may occur only with exercise; also vasospasm may be intense so that distal pulses cannot be felt. Usually neurologic signs are present or appear with exercise. Even large vessel pulsations may disappear in patients taking *vasoconstrictive drugs* (see Ergotism and Methysergide Toxicity in Ch. 596); patients should be carefully questioned concerning the use of these drugs.

Ischemic ulcers resulting from arteriosclerosis obliterans must be differentiated from ulcers that occur in patients with hypertension *(Hines' ulcers).* In hypertensive ischemic ulcers, pulses in the leg and foot are normal, and signs of ischemia are absent elsewhere in the extremity. The hypertensive ulcer is most commonly located on the lateral aspect of the leg or ankle, but arteriosclerotic ulcers are usually on the toes. Hypertensive ulcers are more common in females and are extremely painful. They begin as a purplish plaque which develops into a hemorrhagic bleb; the bleb then ulcerates, leaving a lesion with purplish red margins.

Prognosis. Often intermittent claudication is the first symptom of generalized arteriosclerotic vascular disease, and most patients die eventually from myocardial infarctions or cerebrovascular accidents. Seventy to 90 per cent of patients with femoral artery disease remain stable in their symptoms or improve over a nine-year follow-up period. If diabetes mellitus is present, the prognosis is grave, for progression of the disease almost always occurs. The prognosis after surgical revascularization appears good in large vessel (aortic or femoral artery) disease.

Treatment. If the patient has only intermittent claudication with a normal-appearing limb, he should be treated conservatively. He will be able to walk farther without pain if he slows his gait and loses excess weight. Tobacco should never be used in any form, for it causes cutaneous vasoconstriction via the sympathetic nervous system. The patient is advised to exercise frequently to the development of pain but to rest until the pain totally disappears. It is hoped that exercise will stimulate further growth of collateral blood vessels, but proof is lacking for this point. Although studies are not yet available to demonstrate that treatment of the common forms of hyperlipoproteinemias (Types 2 and 4) will prevent or improve arteriosclerotic lesions, they may be a contributing factor and should be sought and treated if present (see Ch. 819). Patients should protect their limbs from cold or trauma; careful attention to keep the skin scrupulously clean, dry, and soft is important. Even minor infections such as the dermatophytoses may produce problems. Toenail trimming should be done regularly and with care.

If the claudication is found to be progressively worse over a six-month to two-year observation period, if it interferes seriously with the patient's daily activity, or if even minor ischemic symptoms such as numbness or paresthesias are present, *surgery* should be considered. Since the lesion is often localized and segmental, restoration of circulation beyond segmental stenotic or obstructive areas by graft bypass or thromboendarterectomy is the treatment of choice. Currently autogenous saphenous vein grafts are used most frequently because the incidence of thrombosis is less than with grafts made of synthetic materials. Often patch grafts are used on one portion of the vessel. Thromboendarterectomy is performed when there is minimal medial and adventitial involvement of the artery by the sclerotic process. Bypass grafts are favored over excision and graft replacement, because collateral circulation is not destroyed with the bypass method. Before a grafting procedure can be performed, arteriography must be done to determine that there are patent vessels below the obstruction ("good runoff"). However, connection of a graft to an "isolated" popliteal segment (no calf vessels patent) may produce good results with healing of trophic lesions. Vein grafts have been connected to distal arteries in the lower calf and foot in attempts to save ischemic, even gangrenous, feet. In patients with aortoiliac disease who cannot undergo major surgery, subcutaneous axillofemoral or, if one femoral is patent, femorofemoral grafts have been a very successful innovation. In patients with more than one obstructing lesion in the vessels supplying an extremity, correction of the most proximal obstruction often produces relief of symptoms. The success of a surgical attack on involved vessels is proportional to the size of the vessel involved; aortoiliac operations have a 90 per cent or better success rate; femoropopliteal, 70 to 80 per cent; and posterior tibial artery, 50 per cent.

If surgery cannot be performed because of poor runoff or other serious disease, and rest pain or gangrene is present, rest in bed is essential. The affected extremity should be kept 20 to 30 degrees below the horizontal, for the dependent position increases blood flow and pressure and occasionally is the only position the patient can tolerate. If edema is present, the extremity should be kept horizontal but never elevated. External local warmth, if used at all, is best applied by means of a thermoregulated cradle kept at a temperature below 38° C (100.4° F). Direct application of external heat should never be used, because ischemic tissue blisters and burns at much lower temperatures than normal tissue. Rest pain may require the use of aspirin, phenobarbital, propoxyphene (Darvon), pentazocine (Talwin), or even narcotics. Ulcers caused by ischemia are treated the same as rest pain; warm saline soaks should be used to keep the ulcer open, moist, and clean. Enzymatic debridement is not advised because of possible local allergic reactions. If infection is present, the appropriate systemic and local antimicrobial drug should be used as determined by culture and sensitivity tests.

Preganglionic lumbar sympathectomy may be performed to increase skin blood flow when ulcers, rest pain, or small areas of gangrene are present. Before surgery, it must be demonstrated that the sympathetic nervous system is intact in the extremity, especially in diabetics in whom peripheral neuropathy sometimes produces an autosympathectomy. To assess sympathetic activity in an extremity, plethysmographic foot blood flow, toe pulse, or skin temperature may be measured before and after a procedure to remove sympathetic activity. Methods used to remove sympathetic activity are (1) a warm environment, (2) local anesthesia of sympathetic ganglia, (3) local anesthesia of appropriate mixed nerves, (4) spinal anesthesia, or (5) autonomic blocking agents. An increase in the parameter being measured after one of these procedures indicates that a sympathectomy may be beneficial. Sweating of the involved extremity is also an indication of sympathetic activity. Although superficial ulcers often heal after the operation, sympathectomy alone rarely improves intermittent claudication.

Arteriosclerotic *gangrene* often necessitates *amputation* of the limb. In the presence of gangrene with ascending infection (advancing lymphangitis, fever, and leukocytosis), antimicrobial chemotherapy is indicated. Prompt amputation must be considered, because the efficacy of the antimicrobial agents may be limited by the ischemia of the affected tissues and by local necrosis. The level of amputation is determined by palpable pulses and the presence of warm viable tissue of good color. The percentage of patients who become ambulatory after amputation is much higher with below-the-knee than above-the-knee operations.

Vasodilator drugs and agents are widely advertised but have little, if any, place in the treatment of arteriosclerosis obliterans. They are consistently ineffective in relieving intermittent claudication but may increase muscle or skin blood flow at rest in some patients. The efficacy of drugs with prolonged vasodilator action depends upon the degree to which structural disease has rendered the peripheral arteries rigid and incapable of dilatation; it has yet to be shown that they are active on the collateral vessels. Vasodilator drugs often lower systemic blood pressure so that flow to the ischemic limb may be decreased; even intra-arterial administration has been shown to decrease foot flow in some patients.

Long-term anticoagulation has also been recommended for treatment of arteriosclerosis obliterans, but conflicting results have been reported. Fibrinolytic therapy with intravenous streptokinase has been evaluated for chronic arterial occlusive disease, and a few patients, especially those with a recent onset of symptoms, have benefited.

Coffman, J. D.: Peripheral collateral blood flow and vascular reactivity in the dog. J. Clin. Invest., 45:923, 1966.

Coffman, J. D., and Mannick, J. A.: An objective test to demonstrate the circulatory abnormality in intermittent claudication. Circulation, 33:177, 1966.

Coffman, J. D., and Mannick, J. A.: Failure of vasodilator drugs in arteriosclerosis obliterans. Ann. Intern. Med., 76:35, 1972.

Cooke, T. D. V., and Lehmann, P. O.: Intermittent claudication of neurogenic origin. Can. J. Surg., 11:151, 1968.

Davis, R. C., O'Hara, E. T., Mannick, J. A., Vollman, R. W., and Nasbeth, D. C.: Broadened indications for femorofemoral grafts. Surgery, 72:990, 1972.

Gaskell, P., and Becker, W. J.: The erect posture as an aid to the circulation in the feet in the presence of arterial obstruction. Can. M. Assoc. J., 105:930, 1971.

Levy, R. I., Fredrickson, D. S., Shulman, R., Bilheimer, D. W., Breslow, J. L., Stone, N. J., Lux, S. E., Sloan, H. R., Krauss, R. M., and Herbert, P. N.: Dietary and drug treatment of primary hyperlipoproteinemia. Ann. Intern. Med., 77:267, 1972.

Mannick, J. A., and Coffman, J. D.: Ischemic Limbs. New York, Grune & Stratton, 1973.

Schadt, D. C., Hines, E. A., Jr., Juergens, J. L., and Barker, N. W.: Chronic atherosclerotic occlusion of the femoral artery. J.A.M.A., 175:937, 1961.

Verstraete, M., Vermylen, J., and Donati, M. D.: The effect of streptokinase infusion on chronic arterial occlusions and stenoses. Ann. Intern. Med., 74:377, 1971.

THROMBOANGIITIS OBLITERANS
(Buerger's Disease)

Definition. Thromboangiitis obliterans is an obliterative vascular disease or syndrome, probably inflammatory in type, affecting chiefly the peripheral arteries and veins. Identified first as endarteritis obliterans (von Winiwarter, 1879), it was described more fully and given its present name by Buerger (1908).

Incidence. All races are subject to thromboangiitis obliterans, but the greatest incidence is in the Ashkenazic Jews, of whom 20 in 100,000 develop the disease compared with 7 or 8 per 100,000 in the general population. The disease is also common in the Orient. The incidence of the disease in the United States has decreased markedly in the last two decades. Men are affected far more frequently than women, in a ratio of about 75 to 1. Thromboangiitis obliterans has been observed at all ages but occurs most frequently between 20 and 45.

Etiology. Although many agents, toxic and infectious, have been suggested, no etiology has received general acceptance. Cigarettes are used moderately or excessively by many, but not all, patients with thromboangiitis obliterans and have been thoroughly investigated as a causative agent, for smoking aggravates the disease. An increased skin sensitivity to tobacco has been reported by some investigators but not found by others. The higher carboxyhemoglobin levels observed in smokers have been proposed as an etiologic factor by increasing the affinity of hemoglobin for oxygen. Recent research has been directed at a thrombotic etiology; the thromboplastin generation test has been reported abnormal, and higher levels of heparin precipitable fraction of fibrinogen in plasma have been found in patients with thromboangiitis obliterans than in normal persons or patients with arteriosclerosis obliterans. A rise in adhesive platelet counts has also been described in the disease and apparently correlates with tobacco smoking.

Considerable skepticism has been expressed that this disease is an entity different from arteriosclerosis occurring in young people. Evidence has been presented that its clinical and pathologic pictures are specific; however, it may be a syndrome with more than one cause.

Pathology. The lesions are segmental in that diseased sections of arteries or veins are separated by normal areas. In the acute stage cellular proliferation of the intima is accompanied by the formation of red thrombi in small and medium-sized vessels, but the internal elastic lamina usually remains intact. Polymorphonuclear leukocytes, lymphocytes, and giant cells infiltrate all coats of the artery and extend into the thrombus. The formation of sterile microabscesses within the thrombi is a specific finding in this disease. Additional segments of artery or vein are involved acutely at intervals from days to years; hence, a single long artery may exhibit many stages, ranging from the acute picture to dense scar formation. Late stages cannot be distinguished pathologically from arteriosclerosis obliterans.

Pathophysiology. The disease is characterized by alternating periods of activity and quiescence. Depending upon the time relation between the developing occlusion and compensation by collateral circulation, the onset and course vary from insidious to fulminant. Usually occlusion gradually outstrips the developing collateral circulation, and definite peripheral ischemia brings the patient under medical care within one to four years after the first mild symptoms appear. The disease often has an initially more active course of six to twelve years, and then advances much less rapidly; at this stage it is very difficult to differentiate from arteriosclerosis obliterans.

Clinical Manifestations. The typical patient with thromboangiitis obliterans is a young male who smokes cigarettes, presents symptoms of peripheral vascular ischemia, and may have a history of thrombophlebitis. The lower extremities are affected most commonly, and the most frequent presenting complaint is persistent coldness of the limbs. The upper extremities are involved in more than 70 per cent of patients (sometimes without symptoms), the digital arteries being affected more frequently than the ulnar or radial. Raynaud's phenomenon, hyperhidrosis, and ulcers of the digits are common.

In comparison with other vascular diseases, the pain is often excruciating. Migratory thrombophlebitis may precede or accompany arterial involvement and occurs in approximately 40 per cent of patients. Tender, red, elevated areas about 1 cm in diameter appear suddenly in the skin near the valves of small, superficial veins and gradually disappear during two to three weeks, to be followed after irregular intervals by new lesions. Other symptoms and signs (intermittent claudication, rest pain, ulcers, gangrene) are the same as in arteriosclerosis obliterans except that femoral artery disease is less frequent and aortoiliac, rare. Thromboses of the mesenteric, coronary, cerebral, and renal arteries have been described but are uncommon.

Diagnosis. The diagnosis may be suspected when a young male presents with peripheral vascular insufficiency and thrombophlebitis, but it can be definitely proved only by biopsy of an active lesion. The age group, sex, thrombophlebitis, frequent involvement of upper extremities, Raynaud's phenomenon, and normal blood cholesterol and glucose tolerance test help differentiate the disease from arteriosclerosis obliterans. Arteriography can be helpful in demonstrating normality of vessels between lesions, absence of atheroma, a characteristic tree root configuration of the collateral vessels around the point of abrupt occlusion, and asymptomatic involvement of the upper extremities. Since Raynaud's disease is rare in men, affects the upper extremities more severely, and does not obliterate arterial pulsation at the wrist or ankle, it should not be confused with Raynaud's phenomenon in thromboangiitis obliterans. Migratory thrombophlebitis without symptoms or signs of arterial involvement cannot be diagnosed as thromboangiitis obliterans unless histologic proof is obtained.

Prognosis. The prognosis for life is good, but amputation of extremities is common, especially in the fulminant form. In the late stages, the prognosis and course are similar to arteriosclerosis obliterans.

Treatment. The treatment is the same as that outlined for arteriosclerosis obliterans, but it is imperative that tobacco never be used in any form. Nicotine produces transient vasoconstriction and probably favors extension of the disease. Bilateral preganglionic sympathectomy has been advocated for established, gradually advancing thromboangiitis obliterans, especially if vasospasm is prominent. This major operation is not indicated in mild cases responding well to medical treatment or in advanced cases with massive gangrene. Opinion is still divided concerning the usefulness of sympathectomy in this disease. In thromboangiitis obliterans resistance to infection is fairly high and collateral circulation usually good, so that minor amputations may be performed more safely than in arteriosclerotic gangrene.

Astrup, P., Hellung-Larsen, P., Kjeldsen, K., and Mellemgaard, K.: The effect of tobacco smoking on the dissociation curve of oxygen hemoglobin. Scand. J. Clin. Lab. Invest., 18:450, 1966.

Barker, N. W.: Diagnosis and treatment of thromboangiitis obliterans (Buerger's disease). Minnesota Med., 39:303, 1956.

Craven, J. L., and Cotton, R. C.: Haematological differences between thromboangiitis obliterans and atherosclerosis. Br. J. Surg., 54:862, 1967.

Goodman, R. M., Elian, B., Mozes, M., and Deutsch, V.: Buerger's Disease in Israel. Am. J. Med., 39:601, 1965.

McKusick, V. A., Harris, W. S., Ottesen, O. E., Goodman, R. M., Shelley, W. M., and Bloodwell, R. D.: Buerger's disease: A distinct clinical and pathologic entity. J.A.M.A., 181:5, 1962.

Wessler, S., Ming, S. C., Gurewich, V., and Freiman, D. G.: A critical evaluation of thromboangiitis obliterans. N. Engl. J. Med., 262:1149, 1960.

Williams, G.: Recent views on Buerger's disease. J. Clin. Pathol., 22:573, 1969.

ARTERIAL EMBOLISM

Definition. Fragments of centrally located thrombi or atheromatous material may embolize and occlude large or small peripheral blood vessels.

Etiology. Emboli usually originate from mural or valvular thrombi in the left side of the heart (atrium or ventricle), less commonly from an atheromatous ulcer in the aorta or a more peripheral artery, and from thrombi in aneurysms. Paradoxical emboli originate from the right side of the heart and pass through a patent foramen ovale. Most emboli occur in association with myocardial infarction, atrial fibrillation, mitral valve disease, chronic congestive heart failure, or endocarditis. With the advent of surgical replacement of heart valves, prostheses have become a common source of emboli.

Pathophysiology. Emboli lodge at bifurcations of arteries and at narrowed arteriosclerotic areas. The most common site is at the junction of the femoral artery with the profunda femoris; emboli at the origin of the iliac arteries from the aorta (*saddle emboli*) are also frequent. The embolus stops blood flow through the artery and is followed within a few hours by secondary progressive arterial thrombosis below and sometimes above the point of obstruction. Secondary vasospasm has been assumed to be an important factor causing ischemia of the affected extremity, but convincing experimental evidence has not been presented to support this theory. The amount of muscle and skin ischemia that occurs depends on the degree of collateral circulation development.

Pathology. Emboli from the heart or aneurysms show the same pathology as the parent thrombi. Emboli lodged in arteries usually organize by the ingrowth of connective tissue, and later recanalization may occur. However, fragmentation of the embolus before organization is not uncommon with fragments lodging in more distal vessels. Emboli that originate from friable, ulcerated atheromatous lesions produce either large vessel obstruction by amorphous debris or arteriolar and capillary blockage by a variable combination of cholesterol crystals and lipoid material. The cholesterol crystals incite an inflammatory response which leads to fibrosis and complete vessel obstruction.

Clinical Manifestations. In approximately half of patients, there is the sudden onset of severe pain in the extremity distal to the site of embolization. The other cases have an insidious beginning over one to several hours; numbness and paresthesias may precede the pain. Pain is present in 80 per cent of patients and may become excruciating within one or two hours, particularly if the patient exercises the limb. Paresthesias occur in about 60 per cent of cases, and 20 per cent develop muscular weakness or actual paralysis. With an aortoiliac embolus, fainting, nausea, vomiting, and abdominal pain may precede a shocklike state.

Examination of the involved extremity reveals pallor and coldness, sharply demarcated distal to the site of embolization, viz., at the inguinal ligaments or sometimes as high as the umbilicus in saddle embolus, at the lower third of the thigh in femoral artery embolus, and at midcalf in popliteal artery embolus. Arterial pulses are absent below the embolus by palpation or oscillometry. In the arms, because of the easy palpability of the brachial artery, the site of embolus lodgment can be determined by the disappearance of the pulse. Occasionally there is tenderness directly over the embolus in an artery. The extremity may also show collapsed veins, decreased to absent reflexes and sensation, and weakness and paralysis. Later the initial pallor changes to a blotchy cyanosis. If collateral circulation is good, the extremity soon shows signs of improvement in color and temperature, but muscle tenderness and pitting edema may develop. If the collateral circulation is inadequate, massive gangrene follows with bleb formation, spotty vermilion discoloration of the skin, and mummification.

Large emboli from thrombi or amorphous atherosclerotic debris show the aforementioned picture. Smaller emboli may produce only local digital cyanosis with or without pain. Atheromatous microemboli (cholesterol crystals and lipoid material) may produce sudden leg pain, tender muscles, cool legs with pulses, petechiae, livedo reticularis, and plaquelike reddened elevations of the skin. Pedal pulses may disappear later in this syndrome. The spontaneous appearance of painful dusky discoloration of a toe or toes in the presence of pulses should suggest atheromatous microembolism.

Diagnosis. The diagnosis of embolization is not difficult in the patient with the acute onset of a painful, ischemic extremity who demonstrates a source for embolus formation. Acute arterial thrombosis can be distinguished from an embolus only by the presence or absence of underlying etiologies; absent or decreased arterial pulsations in the opposite limb support a diagnosis of acute thrombosis. Patients with acute iliofemoral thrombophlebitis sometimes have no palpable pulses in the affected extremity and may show signs resembling those of arterial embolus. Detection of a feeble pulse by oscillometry, distended veins, and massive edema of the extremity helps rule out embolus. In patients with symptoms and signs of embolization or microembolization and normal pulses, angiography must be performed to look for ulcerative atherosclerotic lesions or aneurysms in the proximal large vessels. Microembolization is often confused with polymyositis or polyarteritis nodosa; muscle biopsy may be necessary to demonstrate the cholesterol crystals.

Prognosis. The prognosis in acute arterial embolization depends on several factors, including size of vessel affected, age of patient, collateral blood supply, and speed of treatment. The larger the artery involved, the worse the prognosis without treatment. Gangrene is much more common after the age of 60 years, probably because of concomitant arteriosclerotic involvement of the blood vessels and collaterals. The development of collateral circulation is very important, for sufficient collaterals may save a limb without treatment. The presence of patent companion vessels, e.g., around the elbow, gives a favorable outlook. The earlier an embolus can be removed surgically, the better the prognosis for survival of the severely ischemic limb.

With any method of treatment, the mortality in most studies is usually greater than 20 per cent, owing to the underlying disease and recurrent embolization to vital areas. The incidence of embolus recurrence is very high. After either medical or surgical treatment, limb incapacity from muscle fibrosis with tendon shortening or intermittent claudication is common.

Treatment. Although embolectomy should restore the normal physiology and is strongly recommended in the surgical literature, conservative medical management often gives as good end results. The exception is emboli at the aortic bifurcation, when surgery is the optimal treatment. When the patient is first seen, treatment should be instituted to improve blood flow to the extremity, and a vascular surgeon should be immediately called in consultation. Anticoagulation with heparin should be started at once to prevent thrombus formation below and above the embolus, and further embolization (long-term anticoagulation is usually indicated to prevent recurrent emboli). Early studies indicate that thrombolytic therapy with streptokinase may be valuable in acute embolization in about one third of patients; such therapy is given intravenously and must be followed by adequate anticoagulation (see Ch. 545). The limb should be positioned in 15 degree dependency and adequate analgesics given to relieve the pain. The affected limb should be kept comfortably warm, as in a thermoregulated (30 to 34° C, 86 to 93.2° F) cradle, and the body and uninvolved extremities warmed in an effort to produce reflex vasodilatation in the involved limb. Every precaution should be taken to prevent burning during heat application; ischemic limbs burn at much lower temperatures than normal limbs. Lumbar sympathetic block by paravertebral injection of procaine or xylocaine has been recommended to relieve vasoconstrictor tone and vasospasm if present; if used it should be performed before anticoagulation.

If conservative medical therapy is not effective in greatly improving the extremity in two to four hours and the underlying condition of the patient will allow surgery, embolectomy is indicated. Early diagnosis is essential as the greatest success with embolectomy is within eight to ten hours of the incident. In recent years, embolectomy has been performed longer than 48 hours after the acute insult with some success, although less than with earlier operations. Muscle tenderness and edema often occur after embolectomy and may be mistakenly diagnosed as thrombophlebitis. In cases presenting with gangrene, amputation is usually necessary. In atheromatous embolization or emboli from aneurysmal thrombi, surgical attack on the proximal lesion may be successful in preventing further emboli.

Amery, A., Deloof, W., Vermylen, J., and Verstraete, M.: Outcome of recent thromboembolic occlusions of limb arteries treated with streptokinase. Br. Med. J., 4:639, 1970.
Baird, R. J., and Lajos, T. Z.: Emboli to the arm. Ann. Surg., 160:905, 1964.
Eliot, R. S., Kanjuh, V. I., and Edwards, J. E.: Atheromatous embolism. Circulation, 30:611, 1964.
Haygood, T. A., Fessel, W. J., and Strange, D. A.: Atheromatous microembolism simulating polymyositis. J.A.M.A., 203:423, 1968.
Jacobs, A. L.: Arterial embolism in the limbs. Edinburgh, E. & S. Livingstone, Ltd., 1959.
Silverblatt, C. W., Wasserman, F., and Wolcott, M. W.: Pulmonary artery embolism and paradoxical embolization. Arch. Intern. Med., 107:105, 1961.
Szekely, P.: Systemic embolism and anticoagulant prophylaxis in rheumatic heart disease. Br. Med. J., 1:1209, 1964.
Wessler, S., Sheps, S. G., Gilbert, M., and Sheps, M. C.: Studies in peripheral arterial occlusive disease. III. Acute arterial occlusion. Circulation, 17:512, 1958.

PERIPHERAL ARTERITIS AND GANGRENE IN SYSTEMIC INFECTIONS

Symptoms and signs of peripheral vascular disease, mild or severe, appear occasionally as complications in bacterial, viral, rickettsial, and fungal infections. Bacterial arteritis and abscess of the wall of an artery are uncommon complications of bacterial endocarditis and septicemias and may lead to hemorrhagic lesions or aneurysm formation. The rickettsial diseases, especially typhus and Rocky Mountain spotted fever, may cause endothelial proliferation of the arterioles, capillaries, and

venules followed by degeneration and necrosis of the media; thrombosis of larger arteries may occur rarely. In infectious arteritis with direct vascular involvement, signs of subacute or acute arrest of peripheral blood flow occur with necrosis of skin and sometimes massive gangrene. However, peripheral ischemia may be transitory and, in large part, vasospastic. Gangrene of the extremities may follow acute infectious conditions, such as pneumonia and gastroenteritis, especially in children; the cause is unknown.

Tuberculosis of the peripheral arteries is rare, but occasionally metastatic infection or embolism produces panarteritis or endarteritis with fully developed tubercles in thrombosed vessels. Direct involvement by extension from adjacent tuberculous lesions, although common in centrally located vessels, is rare in the extremities.

Syphilis may diminish peripheral circulation by producing periarteritis, obliterative intimal hyperplasia, or panarteritis, but the media is much less affected than in the large arteries. True gummas have been found in the vessels of gangrenous limbs. Peripheral vascular complications of syphilis are more common in men than in women. Peripheral ischemia, vasospastic or organic, appears insidiously or suddenly, but gangrene is rare. Active antisyphilitic therapy usually arrests the acute progress of the disease and relieves vasospasm, but organic occlusion remains.

Collins, R. N., and Nadel, M. S.: Gangrene due to the hemolytic Streptococcus—a rare but treatable disease. N. Engl. J. Med., 272:578, 1965.
Derick, C. L., and Hass, G. M.: Diffuse arteritis of syphilitic origin. Am. J. Path., 11:291, 1935.
Koten, J. W.: Peripheral gangrene in infancy and childhood. Br. Med. J., 3:798, 1967.
Learmouth, G. E.: Gangrene of the lower extremities complicating scarlet fever. Can. Med. Assoc. J., 15:69, 1925.
Slaughter, W. H.: Symmetrical gangrene of malarial origin. J.A.M.A., 86:1607, 1926.

SHIN SPLINTS AND ANTERIOR TIBIAL COMPARTMENT SYNDROMES

The anterior tibial compartment is a closed space in which the muscles and blood vessels are surrounded by nonexpanding fascia and bone. Swelling of the tissues in this compartment can cause mild to severe complications.

Shin splints is a frequently encountered syndrome of pain and discomfort in the lower anterior part of the leg after repetitive, unusual exertion. The syndrome is presumably a result of ischemia from an abnormally high tissue pressure compressing the blood vessels. It often occurs in athletes or dancers early in the season. The pain in the front of the legs occurs during or after exercise and is only slowly relieved by rest. Tenderness is most frequent at periosteal attachments of the muscles to the tibia or interosseous membrane. Mild swelling and a slight rise in local skin temperature may be present. When the pain is reproduced by repeated dorsiflexion of the foot against resistance, the anterior tibial muscles become very hard and bulge prominently; a pulsation may become visible over the front of the legs. Arterial pulses are normal. Treatment consists of rest of the muscles, supportive strapping, and a program of graduated exercise.

The *acute anterior tibial compartment syndrome* is a

rare condition caused by the rapid onset of ischemic necrosis of muscles in the anterior tibial space. Swelling of the muscles compresses muscles, nerves, and blood vessels. The cause is unknown, but there is usually a history of excessive exertion. A dull, aching pain which becomes progressively severe is the major symptom; it is unrelieved by rest and sometimes by analgesics. Extreme tenderness is present over the entire anterior tibial compartment, and the fascia rapidly becomes tense and boardlike. The skin becomes glossy, erythematous, and edematous as muscle necrosis occurs; a slight fever and leukocytosis may be present. Loss of dorsiflexion of the great toe and foot then occurs, and sensation may be lost between the first and second toes (deep peroneal nerve compression). The dorsalis pedis pulse may be present or absent. Treatment must be immediate and involves surgical decompression of the anterior tibial compartment by fasciotomy. If treatment is delayed, complete necrosis of the muscles occurs with a resultant permanent footdrop.

A *chronic anterior tibial compartment syndrome* also has been described with pain similar to intermittent claudication in the front of the lower leg on severe exertion but not with ordinary walking. The discomfort disappears with rest. Tenderness is present over the entire compartment when the pain occurs; arterial pulses are normal. The syndrome is thought to be due to an abnormally small compartment. Treatment is usually unnecessary, but a fasciotomy will relieve the symptoms.

French, E. B., and Price, W. H.: Anterior tibial pain. Br. Med. J., 2:1290, 1962.
Leach, R. E., Zohn, D. A., and Stryker, W. S.: Anterior tibial compartment syndrome. Arch. Surg., 88:187, 1964.
Slocum, D. B.: The shin syndrome. Am. J. Surg., 114:875, 1967.

596. PERIPHERAL VASCULAR DISEASE DUE TO ABNORMAL VASOCONSTRICTION OR VASODILATATION

RAYNAUD'S PHENOMENON AND DISEASE

Definition. Raynaud's phenomenon is a syndrome characterized by paroxysmal, bilateral ischemia of the digits induced by cold or emotional stimuli and relieved by heat.

Etiology. Raynaud's phenomenon may be secondary to an underlying disease or anatomic abnormality, but the most common cause is *Raynaud's disease,* which is of unknown etiology. It is less common before puberty and after age 40 but may occur at any age. Women are affected more frequently than men (5:1). Raynaud concluded from his early studies (1862, 1874) that excessive sympathetic activity was responsible for the attacks, but Lewis found that the digital vessels were abnormally reactive to local cold. Since ischemic attacks can still be induced after sympathectomy, it may be concluded that there is a local fault in the blood vessels in Raynaud's disease which is aggravated by the normal degree of reflex sympathetic nervous activity. However, about a dozen cases of Raynaud's phenomenon associated with pulmonary hypertension have been reported, suggesting that a neurohumoral mechanism may be operative in causing both syndromes.

Raynaud's phenomenon may occur in occlusive arterial disease (thromboangiitis obliterans, arteriosclerosis obliterans, arterial emboli), collagen disease (especially scleroderma), after trauma (pneumatic hammer disease, injuries to pianists or typists, after gangrene from any cause), drug intoxication (ergot, methysergide), blood dyscrasias (cryopathies, cold hemagglutinins), and neurogenic lesions (thoracic outlet compression syndromes, poliomyelitis, syringomyelia, causalgia). In Raynaud's phenomenon from secondary causes, the syndrome is caused usually by irritation of the sympathetic nerves, pathologic alterations in the small blood vessels, or sludging and agglutination of red blood cells.

Pathologic Physiology. The paroxysmal ischemia of the digits is due to constriction of the digital and palmar or plantar arteries; initial pallor indicates that vasoconstriction involves the small cutaneous vessels. Later the digital capillaries and venules become dilated, and the slowed blood flow allows the hemoglobin to release more of its oxygen, producing cyanotic, cold digits. When the vasconstriction is relieved, blood flow increases greatly (reactive hyperemia), imparting a red color to the previously ischemic digits. Total and capillary fingertip blood flow are smaller in patients with Raynaud's phenomenon and disease than in normal subjects. With a cooling stimulus, patients show a significant decrease in fingertip capillary flow not seen in normal subjects.

Pathology. In the early stages of the disease, the blood vessels are histologically normal. Later, in progressive cases, the intima is thickened and the muscular coats of the arteries are hypertrophied. Eventually thrombosis of small arteries may occur and focal gangrene of the digital tips may form, although elsewhere the arteries are still histologically normal or show only slight hypertrophy.

Clinical Manifestations. In typical Raynaud's phenomenon, the fingers of both hands blanch on exposure to cold and then may turn cyanotic; sometimes only cyanosis occurs. During recovery, a bright red color (reactive hyperemia) replaces the cyanosis. During the ischemic phase, the digits are cold, numb, and covered with perspiration. In the reactive hyperemia phase, throbbing pain, tingling, swelling, and a rise in skin temperature are found. The digits are affected to different levels in each patient (sometimes extending to the wrist), but the terminal phalanges are always most severely involved. Initially, attacks may be unilateral and involve only one or two digits, but they soon become bilateral and may be induced by emotional upsets as well as by cold exposure.

In Raynaud's disease, the onset is usually gradual with attacks only in the winter. Attacks may be rare, or they may occur several times a day; they may last a few minutes in mild cases to two hours or more in severe cases. They end spontaneously or can be terminated by immersing the hands in warm water. Between episodes, the digits are normal or, in severe cases, mildly cyanotic.

The hands alone are affected in half the cases, hands and feet in the remainder; nose, cheeks, ears, and chin are affected much more rarely. The course of the disease varies; after onset it may persist indefinitely in mild form, improve spontaneously, or become more severe. In the small number of cases that are progressive, the attacks become more frequent, persist during the summer, and last longer; finally, mild cyanosis may be present constantly.

Trophic changes appear in progressive cases, usually one to four years after onset. The fingers become thin and tapering and their skin smooth, shiny, less mobile, and eventually tightly stretched (sclerodactyly). The nails grow slowly and are ridged or curved. Recurrent infections, blisters, and small areas of local cutaneous gangrene appear on the fingertips, but gangrene of a whole digit is rare. The gangrenous areas are extremely painful and, on healing, leave tiny depressed scars.

Diagnosis. Criteria which should be present in patients with Raynaud's phenomenon in order to diagnose Raynaud's disease include (1) absence of any disease or anatomic abnormality to which paroxysmal digital ischemia might be secondary; (2) digital pallor or cyanosis occurring in intermittent attacks, induced by cold or emotion and followed by recovery with reactive hyperemia; (3) symmetrical or bilateral involvement of digits; and (4) gangrene, if present, usually limited to small areas of skin. Previously, presence of symptoms for two years with no evidence of an underlying cause had been considered a fifth diagnostic point; however, Raynaud's phenomenon may precede the diagnosis of scleroderma by 12 years. It is probably unsafe to diagnose the idiopathic disease in the presence of an elevated sedimentation rate or minor symptoms or signs suggestive of an underlying disease (arthralgias, telangiectasis). Raynaud's phenomenon is diagnosed by discovering an underlying disease or condition known to cause attacks.

Raynaud's disease and phenomenon are distinguished from acrocyanosis by the intermittency of attacks. The cyanotic, cold, and edematous limb affected by poliomyelitis or other diseases causing paralysis is also persistent in nature. The cause of sudden "bilateral gangrene of the digits" (Lewis), which appears rarely in children or young adults without previous attacks of discoloration and without cold exposure, is unknown. The fingers, toes, nose, and ears become permanently cyanotic, and within a few days gangrene develops in the distal phalanges of one or more fingers, often symmetrically and bilaterally. The gangrene is extensive and is due to sudden thrombotic occlusion of the final end branches of the digital arteries. The relationship of this syndrome to Raynaud's disease is uncertain, although typical cyclic color changes may appear during the healing stage.

Prognosis. Mild cases of Raynaud's disease improve slowly or remain stationary for years, and the attacks, being few and avoidable, are merely an inconvenience. In a large series of cases, the disease caused no deaths and very little disability; amputations of terminal phalanges were necessary in only 0.4 per cent, and the phenomenon improved or disappeared in 46 per cent. The progressive form, with recurring infection and local gangrene, becomes increasingly painful and disabling, usually despite treatment, but only rarely results in the loss of more than the distal phalanges. The prognosis for secondary Raynaud's phenomenon depends on the underlying cause. Generalized scleroderma and rheumatoid arthritis, which are frequently associated with Raynaud's phenomenon, may produce extreme deformity and disability.

Treatment. Mild cases of Raynaud's disease with infrequent attacks limited to cold exposure, and without trophic changes or gangrene, may be relieved by reassurance, sedatives or tranquilizers, and protection from cold exposure. Smoking has been shown to produce cutaneous vasoconstriction, and the use of tobacco should therefore be avoided. Rauwolfia products in continued small oral doses (reserpine, 0.25 to 0.5 mg daily) will often decrease the severity and frequency of attacks. If necessary, a vasodilator drug (tolazoline long-acting tablets, 80 mg every 12 hours) can be added to the therapeutic regimen. The addition of thyroid substances and androgens has been recommended but helps little, if any.

Vasoconstrictor tone caused by sympathetic nervous system activity is an important factor in bringing on and maintaining attacks of digital ischemia, whether or not the local arteries are abnormally reactive to cold. Removal of vasoconstrictor impulses by regional sympathectomy may be of benefit for the progressive type of Raynaud's disease with indolent ulcers or local gangrene. The success of the sympathectomy depends upon the extent to which the normal capacity for vasodilatation is preserved, as shown by the vasodilator response to body warming or sympathetic ganglion nerve block with lidocaine. In early Raynaud's disease of the lower extremities, lumbar sympathetic ganglionectomy gives complete relief of symptoms. For the upper extremity, preganglionic cervicodorsal sympathectomy is the operation of choice but usually is of temporary (six months to two years) benefit.

The treatment of Raynaud's phenomenon secondary to an underlying disease or anatomic abnormality is directed at the secondary causes. Sympathectomy is of little or no benefit in scleroderma or arthritis but may be helpful in Raynaud's phenomenon secondary to pneumatic hammer disease or causalgia (reflex sympathetic dystrophy).

Baddeley, R. M.: The place of upper dorsal sympathectomy in the treatment of primary Raynaud's disease. Br. J. Surg., 52:426, 1965.

Coffman, J. D., and Cohen, A. S.: Total and capillary fingertip blood flow in Raynaud's phenomenon. N. Engl. J. Med., 285:259, 1971.

Farmer, R. G., Gifford, R. W., Jr., and Hines, E. A., Jr.: Raynaud's disease with sclerodactylia: a follow-up of seventy-one patients. Circulation, 22:13, 1961.

Gifford, R. W., Jr., and Hines, E. A., Jr.: Raynaud's disease among women and girls. Circulation, 16:1012, 1957.

Guntheroth, W. G., Morgan, B. C., Harbinson, J. A., and Mullins, G. L.: Raynaud's disease in children. Circulation, 36:724, 1967.

Lewis, T., and Pickering, G. W.: Observations upon maladies in which the blood supply to digits ceases intermittently or permanently, and upon bilateral gangrene of digits; observations relevant to so-called "Raynaud's disease. Clin. Sci., 1:327, 1934.

Mannick, J. A., and Coffman, J. D.: Ischemic Limbs. New York, Grune & Stratton, 1973.

Winters, W. L., Jr., Joseph, R. R., and Learner, N.: "Primary" pulmonary hypertension and Raynaud's phenomenon. Arch. Intern. Med., 114:821, 1964.

ACROCYANOSIS

Acrocyanosis (Croq, 1896; chronic acro-asphyxia, Cassirer, 1900) is a symmetrical cyanosis of the hands and, less commonly, the feet with few or no symptoms and no complications.

Etiology and Pathology. It is primarily a vasospastic disturbance of the smaller arterioles of the skin of unknown cause, but is probably due to local cold sensitivity. When compared with normal digits, acrocyanotic digits have a heightened arteriolar tone at average room temperature. Secondary dilatation of the capillaries and the subpapillary venous plexus occurs, and the slower blood flow allows the hemoglobin to release a greater part of its oxygen content, accounting for the blue color. Acrocyanosis occurs without special age or sex incidence, and may be associated with various endocrine disorders or asthenias as well as with certain anxiety states. No specific pathology has been described.

Clinical Manifestations. Patients usually present with an unevenly blue and red discoloration of the skin which may extend from the digits to the wrists and ankles but is most intense distally. The digits are also persistently cold and sweat profusely. Puffiness of the digits and mild hypesthesia may be present, but other trophic changes are rare. The cyanosis is intensified by cold or emotional upsets and is relieved by warmth.

Diagnosis. Acrocyanosis can be distinguished from Raynaud's disease by the persistent nature of the discoloration. The presence of normal arterial pulses rules out obstructive arterial disease. Since the discoloration is limited to the hands and feet and disappears when the extremities are warmed, it should not be confused with various types of generalized cyanosis.

Treatment. Except for reassurance, treatment is usually unnecessary. Possible endocrine abnormalities should be investigated. To prevent reflex sympathetic vasoconstriction, general body protection from cold, as well as local measures, helps to decrease the intensity of the discoloration. For cosmetic reasons, vasodilator drugs (tolazoline long-acting tablets, 80 mg every 12 hours, or nicotinyl alcohol, 50 mg every 6 hours) may be used. Sympathectomy is helpful but seldom warranted.

Elliot, A. H., Evans, R. D., and Stone, C. S.: Acrocyanosis: A study of the circulatory fault. Am. Heart J., 11:431, 1936.

Larsson, Y.: The vasoconstrictor tone of the cutaneous arterioles in acro-asphyxia, hypertension, and in the cold pressor test. Acta Med. Scand. (Supp. 206), 130:146, 1948.

Lewis, T., and Landis, E. M.: Observations upon the vascular mechanism in acrocyanosis. Heart, 15:229, 1930.

Lottenbach, K.: Vascular response to cold in acrocyanosis. Helv. Med. Acta, 33:437, 1966.

ERGOTISM AND METHYSERGIDE TOXICITY

Definition. Intense vasoconstriction of small and large blood vessels, producing symptoms and signs of peripheral vascular ischemia, may result from the ingestion of ergot or methysergide.

Etiology. Ergotism results from the use of ergot-containing drugs or the ingestion of bread made from rye or wheat infected with the ergot fungus (*Claviceps purpurea*). It formerly occurred in epidemic form, but is now seen only sporadically (due to the fungus), or after the repeated administration of ergotamine (Gynergen, Cafergot) for migraine or pruritus or of ergot in abortion. Methysergide is a synthetic serotonin antagonist useful in the treatment of migraine headaches. Approximately 7 per cent of patients develop peripheral vascular symptoms or signs with methysergide ingestion, usually after large doses, although as little as 1 mg has caused symptoms in some patients.

Pathophysiology and Pathology. Both drugs induce large and small blood vessel vasoconstriction. Ergot induces vasoconstriction by a direct action on vascular smooth muscle and can lead to secondary intimal hyperplasia and thrombosis. Gangrene may result if thrombosis occurs. The pathology of methysergide toxicity is unknown as is the mode of action, but it does potentiate the effect of catecholamines on blood vessels.

Clinical Manifestations. *Acute ergotism* produces diarrhea, colic, and vomiting, followed by headache, vertigo, paresthesias, convulsive seizures, and occasionally gangrene of the digits, nose, and ears. It is rarely seen with the drug ingestion. In *chronic intoxications,* intermittent claudication, muscle pains, numbness, coldness and pallor of the digits, and even Raynaud's phenomenon may

occur. Examination reveals only cool, pale digits or mottling of the skin with normal or decreased arterial pulsations; however, complete absence of medium- and large-vessel pulsations in the extremities may occur. Gangrene may develop in the severe cases. A similar picture of peripheral vascular ischemia may follow methysergide ingestion. Abdominal angina, angina pectoris, and cerebral ischemic symptoms have also been caused by these drugs. Methysergide has been implicated as an etiologic agent in periureteral or retroperitoneal fibrosis which can extrinsically obstruct arteries and veins.

Diagnosis. The diagnosis is made from the history of drug ingestion associated with symptoms and signs of peripheral ischemia. Arteriography characteristically shows diffuse or segmental narrowing of large arteries and often very constricted distal vessels with collateral vessels present. Arteriosclerosis obliterans, Raynaud's disease, and acrocyanosis are differentiated from ergotism and methysergide toxicity by the history of drug ingestion and by arteriography.

Prognosis. The prognosis is excellent if gangrene has not appeared before treatment and if drug administration is stopped.

Treatment. Treatment involves anticoagulation to prevent thromboses and the use of vasodilators, e.g., tolazoline, 25 mg, intra-arterial or intravenous, to counteract the vasoconstriction. Body warming is recommended to produce reflex vasodilatation in the involved extremities, but is often unsuccessful as is vasodilator drug therapy. With avoidance of the offending drug, the vasoconstriction usually subsides in one to three days. Sympathetic nerve block or sympathectomy may be necessary in pregangrenous or gangrenous cases.

Cranley, J. J., Krause, R. J., Strasser, E. S., and Hafner, C. D.: Impending gangrene of four extremities secondary to ergotism. N. Engl. J. Med., 269:727, 1963.

Graham, J. R.: Methysergide for prevention of headache. N. Engl. J. Med., 270:67, 1964.

Rackley, C. E., Mengel, C. E., Pomerantz, M., and McIntosh, H. D.: Vascular complications with use of methysergide. Arch. Intern. Med., 117:265, 1966.

Richter, A. M., and Banker, V. P.: Carotid ergotism. Radiology, 106:339, 1973.

ERYTHROMELALGIA
(Erythermalgia)

Definition. Erythromelalgia (Mitchell, 1872) is a rare syndrome of paroxysmal, bilateral vasodilatation of the feet and, less often, the hands, associated with burning pain, increased skin temperature, and redness of the skin.

Etiology and Pathology. The cause is unknown. It has occurred as an hereditary affliction. Increased blood flow is usually present, but symptoms may occur in a limb in which the arteries are occluded by a blood pressure cuff. Therefore it is thought that there is a hypersensitivity of the skin to heat or tension. No uniform pathologic condition has been found, but data are scarce. The syndrome occurs without special age or sex incidence.

Clinical Manifestations. The patient with erythromelalgia complains of attacks of bilateral burning pain, superficial or deep, involving circumscribed areas on the soles or palms, the entire foot or hand, or even the whole extremity. The attacks follow stimuli that normally induce only physiologic peripheral vasodilatation or engorgement such as local heat, a warm environment, exercise, standing, or simple dependency of the extremity. The onset is gradual, and symptoms may remain mild for years or may become so severe and continuous that total disability results. Examination during an attack (which may be produced by exposure to a 32 to 36° C environment) usually reveals that the affected skin is hot and red and often sweats profusely; arterial pulsations are normal. Trophic changes, gangrene, and ulceration do not occur, but swelling may be present.

The syndrome may be either idiopathic or secondary to *polycythemia vera* or *hypertension*. The condition may precede the polycythemia by as long as 12 years. Secondary erythromelalgia occurs more commonly in an older age group, is more often unilateral, and produces pain of lesser intensity than idiopathic erythromelalgia.

Diagnosis. Arteriosclerosis obliterans may produce localized and often unilateral burning pain and redness but, unlike erythromelalgia, is not associated with normal pulses or a rise in skin temperature. Neuritis, infectious ganglionitis, and poisoning by thallium, lead, or arsenic may produce painful peripheral hyperemia. Chronic inflammatory states produce in the skin a "susceptible state" with diminished capillary and arteriolar tone. Burning pain (erythralgia, Lewis) is then induced by mild grades of heat, cold, friction, and congestion that leave normal skin unaffected. A temporary reactive vasodilatation of the cutaneous vessels also normally occurs after prolonged exposure to cold in response to a histamine-like substance liberated by local tissue damage (Lewis). This is easily distinguished from erythromelalgia by the history.

Treatment. Attacks can be avoided or aborted by rest, elevation of the extremity, and cold applications. Aspirin (0.6 gram orally) quickly relieves pain in some cases, and the remarkable response is of diagnostic value. Vasoconstrictor agents such as ephedrine (25 mg orally) may be useful; methysergide (1 to 4 mg orally) has also produced relief. Even vasodilator agents (isoproterenol, nitroglycerin) have been reported to be helpful. Contrast baths, using heat below the threshold for pain, often afford considerable but temporary relief. Severe attacks require liberal doses of sedatives, and the therapy is generally unsatisfactory. Occasionally section or alcohol injection of peripheral nerve is required; sympathectomy has been successful in the treatment of three cases.

Prognosis. The prognosis in idiopathic erythromelalgia is guarded, because the severe pain may become disabling. Prognosis of secondary cases depends on the underlying disease; treatment of polycythemia often relieves the symptoms.

Babb, R. R., Alarcon-Segovia, D., and Fairbairn, J. F., II: Erythermalgia. Review of 51 cases. Circulation, 29:136, 1964.
Catchpole, B. N.: Erythromelalgia. Lancet, 1:909, 1964.
Cross, E. G.: The familial occurrence of erythromelalgia and nephritis. Can. Med. Assoc. J., 87:1, 1962.
Lewis, T.: Clinical observations and experiments relating to burning pain in extremities and to so-called "erythromelalgia" in particular. Clin. Sci., 1:175, 1933.
Telford, E. D., and Simmons, H. T.: Erythromelalgia. Br. Med. J., 2:782, 1940.

597. PERIPHERAL VASCULAR DISEASES DUE TO EXPOSURE TO COLD

Exposure to cold induces vasoconstriction by a direct action on blood vessels and also by reflex sympathetic nervous system activity. Cold application to the forehead or to one extremity stimulates vasoconstriction in all extremities. The decreased blood flow and local anoxia may lead to tissue damage, depending on the degree and duration of exposure and the susceptibility of the patient.

Even brief exposure to nonfreezing cold is followed in sensitive persons by an exaggerated and prolonged type of reactive vasodilatation, low-grade edema, and tingling pain. Similar exposure in more susceptible patients produces pronounced edema of the angioneurotic or urticarial type on exposed areas; even mucous membranes may be involved on ingesting cold substances. A systemic reaction with increased pulse rate, decreased blood pressure, flushing of the face, and even syncope may accompany the edema. After swimming in cool water, this reaction has proved fatal in some instances. Familial cases of cold urticaria have been described; this is a milder condition not affecting mucous membranes. A histamine-like substance has been shown to be released and is measurable in the urine in about 50 per cent of patients. The passive transfer of cold urticaria has been demonstrated with both IgE and IgM fractions of patients' serum. Diagnosis is made by exposure of a hand or arm to 12 to 14° C (53 to 57° F) water; edema will develop during or after exposure. Antihistamines or cyproheptadine (Periactin, 4 mg three times a day) may be of use in the treatment of cold sensitivity, but protection of the patient from cold exposure is most important.

Tindall, J. P.: Cold urticaria. Postgrad. Med., 50:133, 1971.
Wanderer, A. A., and Ellis, E. F.: Treatment of cold urticaria with cyproheptadine. J. Allergy Clin. Immunol., 48:366, 1971.
Wanderer, A. A., Maselli, R., Ellis, E. F., and Ishizaka, K.: Immunologic characterization of serum factors responsible for cold urticaria. J. Allergy Clin. Immunol., 48:13, 1971.

IMMERSION FOOT
(Trench Foot)

Definition. Immersion foot is due to prolonged exposure of the extremities to water; syndromes characterized only by painful, swollen feet or hands to the more serious manifestations of muscle necrosis, ulceration, and gangrene may result.

Etiology. Although prolonged exposure (greater than 48 hours) to dampness or water is the important factor in the production of immersion foot, immobility and dependency of the lower extremities, constricting garments, chilling of the body, trauma, exhaustion, or dehydration, and, in some instances, semistarvation with deficient intake of protein and vitamins are often contributing causes. Two types, cold water and warm water (tropical) immersion foot, exist and present different clinical pictures. The combination of wetness plus cold (not necessarily freezing) temperatures produces the most serious condition.

Pathophysiology. The factors causing cold water immersion foot tend to decrease blood flow to the extremities. Vasoconstriction is caused by direct and reflex cold stimulation; actual cellular damage and the ensuing hyperemia are important in producing the clinical and pathologic picture. Persistent local anoxia leads to tissue necrosis and injures the capillary walls. Capillary filtration increases remarkably, and plasma and protein pass freely into the interstitial tissue, producing a tense edema. The resultant increased viscosity of the blood leads to stasis and occlusion of small vessels. The local anoxia may also produce wallerian degeneration of the nerves in the affected area.

Warm water immersion foot is thought to be caused by waterlogging and swelling of the stratum corneum together with abrasion from footwear. *Pseudomonas aeruginosa* can usually be cultured from the affected areas and may contribute by digesting human callus with its proteolytic enzymes.

Pathology. The early pathologic picture of the cold type has not been studied. In late stages, a nonspecific picture of vascular occlusion, desquamation of skin, deep fibrosis, and superficial gangrene is seen. The nerves may be embedded in contracting fibrous tissue, and fibrosis of the media of arterioles and venules is present. The pathologic features of the severe, warm-water type are a lymphocytic infiltration, diapedesis of red blood cells, and swelling and proliferation of the endothelial lining of capillaries in the upper dermis.

Incidence. Cold water immersion foot is common in most wars and is seen in training camps where appropriate conditions exist. Non-Caucasians are thought to be more susceptible to the disease, perhaps on the basis of acclimatization.

Clinical Manifestations. At the time of rescue from sea, or when first seen in trench warfare, cold water immersion foot often presents as pulseless, cold, red feet with a sock distribution of hypesthesia or anesthesia. The condition may develop insidiously with only numbness, paresthesias, and slight swelling as long as the tissues are supported by boots or shoes. As soon as the support is removed, edema, tingling, itching, and severe pain occur. The skin later becomes mottled yellow, blue, or black. This is called the prehyperemic stage and lasts a few hours to a few days. A hyperemic stage follows, characterized by red, hot, dry feet, burning paresthesias, and intense pains, shooting or stabbing in nature. Pulses are now bounding. Edema increases with formation of blisters, which may weep serous fluid and then slowly heal. In severe cases, muscle weakness and wasting, ulcerations, and gangrenous patches develop. Gangrene is often superficial, and the necrotic skin sometimes sheds in large pieces, leaving healthy skin beneath. Even in the absence of gangrene, extensive exfoliation is common. This stage lasts one to ten weeks, depending on the grade of initial injury.

The recovery stage (posthyperemic) blends indistinguishably with the hyperemic stage; there is a return of vascular tone with restoration of normal skin color and temperature. Recovery may be complete in mild cases within two to five weeks, but severe cases often require three to twelve months. A few patients show late sequelae such as sensitivity to cold with Raynaud's phenomenon; general or marginal hyperhidrosis; paresthesias that are increased by warmth, dependency, or exertion; rigid toes caused by fibrosis of muscles; contracted joints in the feet and toes; or painful, indolent ulcers of the digits or their stumps.

Warm water immersion foot presents with painful and extremely tender feet, especially over pressure areas. Wrinkled, white, convoluted plantar surfaces and even maceration are seen on examination in the mild syndrome. In the more severe cases, one also finds pronounced erythema and edema of the ankles and dorsal aspects of the feet; fever and femoral lymphadenopathy may occur. During healing, these patients develop diffuse ecchymoses, vesicles, and a maculopapular rash.

Symptoms and signs subside within a week, usually leaving no residua.

Prophylaxis. Drying of the feet overnight is the best method to prevent immersion foot. Avoidance of constricting clothing, prolonged dependency, or immobility; frequent rest periods; and several changes of clothes and boots will also help. If these conditions are impractical, application of silicone grease once a day will reduce the incidence of the affliction.

Treatment. In the prehyperemic stage bed rest and body warming are important. It is probably best to keep the extremities at heart level until pulses are present. Treatment of the hyperemic stage consists of complete bed rest, cooling of the hyperemic tissues to control pain and edema, keeping the body warm, elevation of the extremities above heart level, and correction of dietary deficiencies. If cleansing is necessary, light washing with dilute hexachlorophene solution may be used. Infected tissue and epidermophytosis should be treated with appropriate agents. For cooling, it may be sufficient to expose the extremities to room air, but sometimes electric fans with water sprays or ice bags are needed. With cooling, pain is usually relieved in a few hours, but in some instances it is necessary to discover an optimal temperature, because too low a temperature may again produce pain. Analgesics must be used. Tobacco smoking is prohibited. The patient is ready to walk when edema does not occur on dependency.

Sympathectomy has not been helpful in the hyperemic stage but appears to improve late sequelae such as chronic painful ulcers, persistent vasospasm, and hyperhidrosis.

The treatment of warm water immersion foot involves bed rest with extremity elevation until edema and pain entirely disappear. Other measures are usually unnecessary; the symptoms and signs disappear in one to seven days.

Allen, A. M., and Taplin, D.: Tropical immersion foot. Lancet, 2:1185, 1973.

Clayton, A. J. W.: Twenty-one cases of immersion foot. Med. Ser. J. Canada, 23:857, 1967.

Lange, K., Weiner, D., and Boyd, L. J.: The functional pathology of experimental immersion foot. Am. Heart J., 35:238, 1948.

Montgomery, H.: Experimental immersion foot; review of physiopathology. Physiol. Rev., 34:127, 1954.

White, J. C.: Vascular and neurologic lesions in survivors of shipwreck. I. Immersion foot syndrome following exposure to cold. II. Painful swollen feet secondary to prolonged dehydration and malnutrition. N. Engl. J. Med., 228:211, 1943.

CHILBLAIN AND PERNIO

Chilblain and pernio (*erythrocyanosis*) occur commonly in patients, especially females, with a history of cool limbs in summer as well as winter. The etiologic and pathogenic factors are unknown, but the disease is seen only in cold, damp climates. However, it is much more frequent in England than in areas of the United States with comparable climates.

Acute chilblain occurs on the dorsum of the digits, hands, or feet as localized, warm, red, intensely pruritic swelling that may disappear spontaneously in a few days. Pernio is probably the same disease but involves the lower parts of the legs, especially in women who, because of their mode of dress, do not adequately protect their legs from cold weather. Rarely, indolent lesions, dull red or violaceous, proceed to painful bleb formation.

The blebs contain blood-stained serous fluid and often lead to ulcer formation.

In some patients exposed repeatedly to cold, recurrent and chronic lesions, often appearing in crops, may develop. The lesions are erythematous and ulcerative and may leave residual scarring, fibrosis, and atrophy of the skin and subcutaneous tissues. The disease is more active during the cooler months and subsides in warm weather. Bilateral and symmetrical parts of the extremities are involved. This state is called chronic chilblain or pernio (erythrocyanosis frigida crurum).

Treatment is nonspecific. Corticosteroid creams may be used for itching and inflammation, antimicrobials for sepsis. Reserpine (0.25 mg orally daily) has been reported to ameliorate the disease.

Eskell, J.: Reserpine in the treatment of chilblains. Practitioner, 189:792, 1962.

Lewis, T.: Observations on some normal and injurious effects of cold upon the skin and underlying tissues. II. Chilblains and allied conditions. Br. Med. J., 2:837, 1941.

McGovern, T., Wright, I. S., and Kruger, E.: Pernio: A vascular disease. Am. Heart J., 22:583, 1941.

Thomas, E. W. P.: Chapping and chilblains. Practitioner, 193:755, 1964.

FROSTBITE

Definition. Frostbite is due to freezing of tissues which may result in damage to skin, muscle, blood vessels, and nerves.

Etiology. Superficial freezing of tissues evidently begins when the temperature of deeper tissues reaches about 10° C (50° F). During the Korean War, most cases of frostbite occurred at −6.5° C (20° F) or below, after 7 to 18 hours' exposure. High winds, dampness, and general chilling of the body make frostbite more likely at above-freezing temperatures. Predisposing factors include any type of peripheral vascular insufficiency, improper clothing, exhaustion, and previous cold injury. Lack of acclimatization and geographic origin have also been implicated; the black race is more susceptible to frostbite. Most frostbite is of the slow freezing type, but a rapid frostbite (occurring in a few minutes) takes place at high altitudes with extremely low temperatures and has a predilection for the extremities rather than the face and ears.

Pathophysiology. Whether actual tissue freezing or decreased blood flow from vasoconstriction is most important in producing cell injury is unknown. Damage is probably due to a combination of direct freezing with the formation of extracellular ice crystals, inducing dehydration of cells, and to intense vasoconstriction. The vasoconstriction is due to direct cold exposure of the tissues but may also involve reflex vasoconstriction from chilling of other body areas. The reduced blood flow leads to capillary stasis and arteriolar and capillary thromboses. Capillary permeability is increased and results in edema formation.

Pathology. The pathologic findings vary with the stage of the disease and the depth of tissue affected. In early stages, low-grade vasculitis and inflammation in all tissues are seen. Later the skin is atrophied and may be keratinized, muscle is necrosed and shows waxy degeneration, arterioles and capillaries are thrombosed, and nerves demonstrate fibroblastic proliferation and neurolysis.

Clinical Manifestations. The first indication of frostbite is often a sharp, pricking sensation that draws attention to a yellowish-white, numb area of hardened skin. However, cold itself produces numbness and anesthesia that may allow freezing of tissue without warning. When the freezing is superficial, thawing leads to local reddening and wheal and flare formation. When freezing involves deep tissues, subcutaneous edema occurs with thawing, followed by formation of vesicles and bullae. A hyperemic, reddish zone may be apparent between frozen and normal tissue. As the edema subsides in a day or two, necrosis and gangrene may become evident. However, it may take two to three months before final demarcation between viable and dead tissue can be ascertained. In the healing phase, a black eschar usually covers the area.

The traditional classification of frostbite has been from first to fourth degree, depending on the depth of tissue injury. Since the true extent of tissue damage cannot be judged on initial examination, a simpler classification of superficial and deep frostbite is more practical. The prognosis depends on the depth of freezing, as superficial cases usually have no sequelae, although deep freezing may finally end in amputation.

Prophylaxis. Frostbite is preventable and occurs rarely among those who have been instructed how to protect themselves. Prophylactic measures include observance of each other for signs of frostbite; wearing adequate, loose fitting, dry clothing and mittens; exposure for only brief periods when exercise is not possible; and avoidance of smoking before and during exposure. Feet and socks should be kept dry.

Treatment. Superficial frostbite can be treated immediately by rewarming; affected areas on the face and ears can be warmed with the hands, hands can be placed in the axillae, or frostbitten parts can be warmed on the exposed torso of a partner. Frostbitten areas should not be rubbed with snow or exercised.

Treatment of deep frostbite should be delayed until adequate facilities for rewarming are available. Therapy should always be very conservative, because the depth of tissue damage is difficult to ascertain, sometimes for months. It is best to rewarm the tissues as rapidly as possible in 40 to 44° C water (104 to 111° F). Massage, exposure to too high temperatures, and reactive hyperemia should be avoided because they tend to increase pain and edema. Analgesics usually are needed during rewarming. After rewarming, which usually requires about 20 minutes, the frostbitten area is exposed to room air (21 to 26° C, 70 to 78° F). Although pressure dressings may be used, the open method with sterile surroundings is usually preferred. Vesicles, bullae, and eschars are left untouched. Antimicrobial drugs are indicated if infection is present. Tobacco smoking should be prohibited. Regional sympathectomy has been reported as beneficial, both clinically and experimentally, if performed at an optimal time of 24 to 48 hours after frostbite occurs. Sympathectomy may conserve tissue and lead to earlier demarcation, cessation of pain, and healing of tissue.

Eventual recovery is usually surprisingly good, the black eschar peeling off to leave normal tissue beneath. Sensitivity to cold, paresthesias, and a predilection to repeated frostbite often persist. In severe frostbite, fibrosis of tissue may lead to disability, and gangrenous extremities may require amputation.

Golding, M. R., Martinez, A., DeJong, P., Mendosa, M., Fries, C. C., Sawyer, P. N., Hennigar, G. R., and Wesolowski, S. A.: The role of sympathectomy in frostbite, with review of 68 cases. Surgery, 57:774, 1965.

Lapp, N. L., and Juergens, J. L.: Frostbite. Mayo Clin. Proc., 40:932, 1965.

Meryman, H. T.: Tissue freezing and local cold injury. Physiol. Rev., 37:233, 1957.

Washburn, B.: Frostbite. What it is, how to prevent it, emergency treatment. N. Engl. J. Med., 266:974, 1962.

598. PERIPHERAL VASCULAR DISEASES DUE TO ABNORMAL COMMUNICATIONS BETWEEN ARTERIES AND VEINS

ARTERIOVENOUS FISTULA

Definition. Arteriovenous fistulas are abnormal communications, single or multiple, between arteries and veins by which arterial blood enters the veins directly without transversing a capillary network.

Etiology. Arteriovenous fistulas created to facilitate renal dialysis are the most common fistulas. Acquired arteriovenous fistulas, usually single and saccular, may develop after a bullet or stab wound involving an artery and a contiguous vein. Fistulas of the iliac vessels may occur after surgery for intervertebral disc disease. Congenital fistulas are present from birth and are usually multiple; they result from defects in differentiation of the common embryologic anlage into artery and vein. There is no special sex incidence, and any part of the body may be involved.

Pathophysiology. Arterial blood, following the path of least resistance, flows directly into the vein, bypassing the corresponding capillary bed. The arterial pressure is transmitted to the venous side of the fistula; the distal vein pressure is increased, but the proximal vein pressure may actually be negative during systole owing to the high velocity of blood flow. The elevated venous pressure leads to the development of varicose veins and venous stasis changes in the limb. Increased blood flow makes the tissues near the fistula abnormally warm, and diminished flow distal to the fistula may produce peripheral coldness and trophic changes. Large fistulas impose a burden on the heart; the cardiac output must be increased above normal by an amount proportional to the size of the fistula in order to maintain the general circulation. Total blood volume may be increased. The low peripheral resistance of the involved area tends to decrease diastolic and increase systolic and pulse pressures systemically. Large fistulas may lead to cardiac decompensation. Even the small fistulas created for renal dialysis have been shown to induce a small increase in cardiac output and heart rate with a decrease in peripheral resistance.

Pathology. In the region of the fistula, the intima and media of the involved veins become thickened, and newly developed elastic fibers appear. The arteries show a thinning of their walls with loss of elastic tissue and muscular fibers in the media.

Clinical Manifestations. Patients complain of aching pain, edema, varicosities, or hypertrophied extremities. Occasionally, cardiac symptoms such as palpitation, substernal pain, and dyspnea on exertion are present. Examination reveals tortuous, dilated superficial veins in the extremity, and venous pulsation can be felt unless the fistula is small and deeply placed. In congenital fistulas, the skin temperature is usually elevated locally but decreased distal to the fistulas, although in acquired lesions, the temperature of the digits may be greater than in the opposite normal limb. A bruit and thrill are common over acquired fistulas; the bruit lasts throughout systole and diastole and has a coarse, machinery-like quality. The tissues near the fistula may be tender, edematous, and either red or slightly cyanotic. The circumference of the extremity is increased by edema or true hypertrophy, but bony structures are hypertrophied only if the fistula was present before epiphyseal closure. Stasis pigmentation and chronic indurative cellulitis with or without indolent ulceration may be present distal to the fistula. In contrast to the postphlebitic limb in which ulcers form around the medial malleolus, the ulceration of fistulas may affect the distal parts of the foot. Rarefaction of bone in the extremity may also occur. Temporary compression of the artery supplying a large fistula diminishes the heart rate (*Branham's sign*) and may be a helpful diagnostic sign.

Diagnosis. If the diagnosis cannot be made from the clinical manifestations, other examinations may be helpful. The oxygen saturation of blood removed from fistula veins will be found to be greater than that of blood removed from corresponding veins in the opposite extremity. Arteriography will reveal the lesion, its location, and the number and size of communications. Edema of one or both extremities after surgery for intervertebral disc disease should suggest the possibility of a fistula. Thrombophlebitis and the postphlebitic extremity can be distinguished from fistulas by the oxygen studies and arteriography.

Prognosis. The prognosis of acquired and single congenital fistulas is good after surgical repair. In acquired iliac vessel fistulas, congestive heart failure develops in two thirds of patients, and immediate repair is important. Without surgical repair, which is often not possible in multiple fistulas, the outlook is for a chronically swollen limb with varicosities, stasis pigmentation, and ulceration. Bacterial infection of acquired fistulas occurs but is rare.

Treatment. Single fistulas can be repaired surgically by re-establishing the continuity of the involved artery and vein walls by a variety of procedures (arteriorrhaphy, end-to-end suture, grafting). Ligation of the involved artery and vein leads to a high incidence of arterial and venous insufficiency of the extremity and should be avoided if possible. If the arterial supply depends upon a large anomalous artery, ligation of this vessel, followed by sclerosing injections of the dilated veins, may be effective. Multiple fistulas are much less amenable to surgery. Ulcers, edema, and pain may be relieved by wearing elastic bandages or stockings; pressure on the veins encourages blood flow to follow the arterial pathway. Amputation is required for large inoperable fistulas producing cardiac decompensation or gross deformity.

Binak, K., Regan, T. J., Christensen, R. C., and Hellems, H. K.: Arteriovenous fistula: Hemodynamic effects of occlusion and exercise. Am. Heart J., 60:495, 1960.

Johnson, G., Jr., and Blythe, W. B.: Hemodynamic effects of arteriovenous shunts used for hemodialysis. Ann. Surg., 171:715, 1970.

Lawton, R. L., Tidrick, R. T., and Brintnall, E. S.: A clinicopathologic study of multiple congenital arteriovenous fistulae of the lower extremities. Angiology, 8:161, 1957.

Nickerson, J. L., Elkin, D. C., and Warren, J. V.: The effect of temporary occlusion of arteriovenous fistulas on heart rate, stroke volume, and cardiac output. J. Clin. Invest., 30:215, 1951.

Spittell, J. A., Jr., Palumbo, P. J., Love, J. G., and Ellis, F. H., Jr.: Arteriovenous fistula complicating lumbar disk surgery. N. Engl. J. Med., 268:1162, 1963.

Wakim, K. G., and Janes, J. M.: Influence of arteriovenous fistula on the distal circulation in the involved extremity. Arch. Phys. Med. Rehabil., 39:431, 1958.

GLOMANGIOMA OR GLOMUS TUMOR

Definition. Glomangioma or glomus tumor designates painful enlargement of a glomus body.

Pathology. The pathology consists of hypertrophy of the glomus body which contains an arteriovenous anastomosis with its associated smooth muscle coat, nonmyelinated nerve fibers, and connective tissue. Histologically, the lesion is encapsulated, occasionally diffuse but never invasive, and contains numerous epithelioid cells with no inflammatory cells.

Clinical Manifestations. Glomus tumors are extremely tender but inconspicuous subcutaneous nodules which develop slowly during adult life. Pain may be present before the nodule becomes visible. They are found in various parts of the upper and lower extremities, but most frequently (30 per cent) beneath the fingernail. The diameter of the tumor is usually only a few millimeters. The nodule has a flat or slightly raised surface with reddish-blue to purplish discoloration. Excruciating burning or shooting pain, both local and referred up the extremity, occurs spontaneously or is produced by the slightest pressure. Hyperhidrosis, abnormal vasomotor activity, increased skin temperature, and tissue atrophy in the involved limb may be present. Heat, cold, and even contact with clothing may become intolerable so that protection is required continuously day and night. In glomus tumors beneath nails, a small excavation of the phalanx from erosion by the tumor can often be seen by roentgenography.

Treatment. Surgical excision leads to complete and immediate relief without recurrence.

Bailey, O. T.: The cutaneous glomus and its tumors—glomangiomas. Am. J. Path., 11:915, 1935.

Cooke, S. A. R.: Misleading features in the clinical diagnosis of the peripheral glomus tumor. Br. J. Surg., 58:602, 1971.

Horton, C., Maguire, C., Georgiade, N., and Pickrell, K.: Glomus tumors: An analysis of 25 cases. Arch. Surg., 71:712, 1955.

599. DISEASES OF THE PERIPHERAL VEINS

THROMBOPHLEBITIS

This subject is discussed in Ch. 544.

VARICOSE VEINS AND THE POSTPHLEBITIC SYNDROME

Definition. Varicose veins are distended, tortuous veins with incompetent valves. The postphlebitic syndrome denotes the chronically swollen extremity with trophic changes secondary to chronic venous stasis; despite the name, a previous history of thrombophlebitis is often not obtainable.

Etiology. Varicose veins are considered to be caused either by congenitally defective valves or by a condition that deforms valves or obstructs venous outflow over long periods of time. Varicosities resulting from congenital defects may develop early in life. Thrombophlebitis may lead to the formation of varicosities by deformation or destruction of venous valves and venous obstruction. Pregnancy, ascites, abdominal tumor, excessive weight or height, and prolonged weight bearing are all considered accelerating factors which cause increased venous pressure in the legs, distention of veins, and finally incompetency of valves. A generalized abnormality of the veins has been suggested as a predisposing factor. An increased forearm vein distensibility and a decreased amount of collagen and hexosamine in uninvolved veins have been demonstrated in patients with lower extremity varicosities; however, genetic evidence is not substantial. Since the majority of patients do not have obvious causes and varicose veins are an affliction of Western civilization, other factors in our society have been sought. The constipation associated with the Western countries' low-residue diet has been proposed as a frequent etiologic factor in varicosities. Emphasis is placed on the association of varicosities with hemorrhoids and diverticulosis, as a result of either increased intra-abdominal pressure during bowel movements or local pressure exerted by the bowel on intra-abdominal structures.

Incidence. Varicose veins are very common, appearing in approximately 40 per cent of women; the incidence is less in men. The saphenous veins in the lower extremities are most frequently affected.

Clinical Manifestations. The dilated, tortuous, sacculated varices are easily visible. Some patients with extensive superficial varicosities have no other symptoms or signs, but others have aching pain or easy fatigability of the calf muscles and edema after weight bearing. The edema usually disappears with bed rest overnight. Rarely the varicosities are so large that postural hypotension may result from pooling of blood in the lower extremities. When the communicating or deep veins are incompetent, symptoms and signs are more common. Chronic venous insufficiency is manifested by edema, which may later become fibrosed to produce a brawny induration. Extravasation of blood locally may cause a brownish pigmentation; an itchy, eczematoid rash may appear in the area. Finally the skin may ulcerate, producing an indolent, nonpainful lesion, usually above the medial malleolus near a palpable, incompetent communicating vein. This picture of chronic swelling and stasis dermatitis is called the postphlebitic syndrome. Arterial pulses are normal. When the deep venous system is blocked, pain similar to intermittent claudication may rarely occur.

Diagnosis. The diagnosis can be made from the clinical picture. Retrograde flow of blood past incompetent valves can be demonstrated by the Trendelenburg test and its variations. The leg of the recumbent patient is elevated to empty the veins, and then a tourniquet is applied to occlude the superficial veins. The patient quickly assumes a standing position, the tourniquet is released, and the veins will become distended immediately if back flow is present. If two tourniquets are applied and left in place when the patient stands, filling of the saphenous veins between the tourniquets indicates an incompetent communicating vein. Application of the tourniquets to different levels on the limb can delineate exactly the sites of vein pathology. Venography may be used in doubtful cases or to be certain the deep venous system is patent. In a patient with varicosities and edema, other causes of edema, e.g., cardiovascular and renal disease, should be investigated.

Prognosis. The prognosis for simple superficial varicose veins is good with treatment. Once the postphlebitic syndrome has developed, progressive disability usually can be expected despite treatment.

Treatment. Uncomplicated varicose veins respond well to support with elastic stockings or bandages to prevent progression. Panty girdles should never be worn. Frequent periods of elevation of the extremity above heart level, high ligation with stripping of the saphenous veins, and injection of sclerosing solutions may become necessary to prevent or treat the postphlebitic syndrome. However, since saphenous veins may be needed for arterial (coronary or peripheral) surgery, stripping should be performed only when absolutely unavoidable. Venous stasis ulcers are treated with sponge rubber pressure dressings or gelatin boots; local or systemic antimicrobials are indicated if infection is present. Sometimes the entire fibrosed area must be removed and a skin graft applied to heal an indolent ulcer.

Alexander, C. J.: The theoretical basis of varicose vein formation. Med. J. Aust., 1:258, 1972.

Bauer, G.: Pathophysiology and treatment of the lower leg stasis syndrome. Angiology, 1:1, 1950.

Burkitt, D. P.: Varicose veins, deep vein thrombosis, and haemorrhoids: Epidemiology and suggested etiology. Br. Med. J., 2:556, 1972.

Fegan, W. G.: Conservative treatment of varicose veins. Prog. Surg., 11:37, 1973.

Mullarky, R. E.: The Anatomy of Varicose Veins. Springfield, Ill., Charles C Thomas, 1965.

Thurston, O. G., and Williams, H. T. G.: Chronic venous insufficiency of the lower extremity. Arch. Surg., 106:537, 1973.

Wood, J. E.: The Veins. Boston, Little, Brown & Company, 1965.

600. DISEASES OF THE PERIPHERAL LYMPHATIC VESSELS

Lymph is formed by the transudation of plasma through capillary walls into tissue spaces. The plasma that is not reabsorbed into the venular end of the capillaries is collected by a rich intercellular network of tiny lymphatic vessels. These vessels possess semilunar valves and become larger as they convey lymph to the regional lymph nodes; then the lymph travels through trunk lymphatics to the thoracic duct and finally to the left internal jugular vein. In the extremities, there are superficial and deep lymphatic systems which probably are joined by communicating vessels. The flow of lymph depends on intrinsic, rhythmic contractions of the lymph vessels, muscular contraction, respiratory movements, and, to a certain extent, gravity. The lymphatic vessels are responsive to sympathetic nerve stimulation, but the functional significance of this is not known.

LYMPHEDEMA

Definition. Lymphedema is a form of chronic unilateral or bilateral edema of the extremities caused by the accumulation of lymph secondary to abnormalities or blockage of the lymph vessels or pathologic conditions of the lymph nodes.

Etiology. Primary lymphedema may be a hereditary disease or may occur sporadically. Various classifications exist according to whether the lymphedema is present at birth (*congenital*), appears at or near puberty (*praecox*), occurs after age 35 (*tarda*), or is familial and congenital (*Milroy's disease*). The mode of inheritance is probably dominant but has not been thoroughly investigated. An increased incidence occurs in ovarian dysgenesis syndromes. Primary lymphedema affects females predominantly (about 8:1); the onset of the disease occurs before age 40 in more than 90 per cent of cases.

Secondary lymphedema is most commonly caused by inflammation and follows recurrent lymphangitis (see below). In tropical and subtropical regions, filariasis often leads to lymphedema. Neoplasms are the second most common cause either by invasion or compression of lymph vessels or nodes. Surgical removal of lymph nodes and the fibrosis that follows irradiation may also cause lymphedema. Secondary cases have no special sex incidence and are uncommon before age 40.

Pathology. Examination of primary lymphedematous limbs by lymphangiography has revealed aplasia, hypoplasia, or hyperplasia (varicosities) of the lymphatic vessels. The lymph nodes may also be aplastic or hypoplastic, producing an obstructive type of lymphedema. No specific pathologic picture has been correlated with the current classification system, but the few cases of Milroy's disease examined have revealed aplasia (or absence) of the lymphatic vessels. There is some indication that lymphedema may be part of a generalized defect in lymphatic vessels. Patients with lymphedema have been reported to have chylous pleural effusions, chylous ascites, and even intestinal lymphangiectasis. A syndrome of yellow nails, recurrent pleural effusion, and lymphedema occurs and is believed to be secondary to lymphatic abnormalities in each area. Another familial syndrome of recurrent intrahepatic cholestasis and lymphedema exists, the cholestasis probably being caused by defective hepatic lymphatic vessels. In secondary lymphedema, innumerable small, irregular lymphatics are usually seen beside normal or tortuous, sometimes varicose, vessels.

Clinical Manifestations. Primary lymphedema is usually gradual in onset and asymptomatic; the distal portion of the extremity or whole extremity, or even a portion of the trunk, may increase in size. The edema is soft and pitting at first and disappears with treatment but later becomes firm and nonpitting, and cannot be relieved completely by treatment. At this stage, the skin becomes thickened and resists wrinkling; hair follicles are prominent. The lower extremities are involved most often; about half the patients develop bilateral swelling. The edematous tissue is especially susceptible to episodes of lymphangitis and cellulitis, which add to the deformity.

Secondary lymphedema is seldom bilateral. Lymphedema of the inflammatory type follows recurrent episodes of lymphangitis. Each attack leaves more residual edema after the inflammation subsides. The skin finally becomes thick, coarse, folded, and hard so that the eventual deformity may be extreme (elephantiasis). Secondary lymphedema resulting from neoplasm and other noninflammatory causes produces painless swelling of an extremity. Painless swelling of an extremity in an elderly male must be considered secondary to carcinoma of the prostate until proved otherwise.

Diagnosis. Painless chronic swelling of an extremity suggests the diagnosis of lymphedema. Differentiation from venous insufficiency may be made by the lack of prominent veins, stasis dermatitis, and ulceration; lymphangiography and venography may be necessary. Mixed lymphangiomatous and hemangiomatous malformations that cause enlarged limbs can be diagnosed by the obvious tumor mass. In lipodystrophy, lymphangiography is necessary to delineate the normal lymphatics displaced by the lipomatous masses.

Prognosis. Primary lymphedema usually progresses inexorably to a chronically swollen limb or limbs despite treatment. However, the lymphedema associated with gonadal dysgenesis may disappear spontaneously in months to years. Secondary lymphedema caused by infection may be controlled with adequate treatment. The prognosis is that of the underlying disease in other causes.

Treatment. In primary lymphedema, the most important aim of therapy is to keep the involved extremities free of edema in order to prevent fibrosis and recurrent infection. Frequent elevation of the extremity (including sleeping with the extremity above the heart level), elastic support applying graded pressure from the foot proximally when ambulatory, low sodium diet, and diuretics are usually necessary. Local infection and obvious lesions, such as epidermophytosis, should be eradicated. Surgical attack in advanced cases with fibrosis and resistant edema (Kondoleon operation and its modifications) has produced some relief but is usually disappointing.

Dilley, J. J., Kierland, R. R., Randall, R. V., and Shick, R. M.: Primary lymphedema associated with yellow nails and pleural effusions. J.A.M.A., 204:670, 1968.
Gough, M. H.: Primary lymphedema: Clinical and lymphangiographic studies. Br. J. Surg., 53:918, 1966.
Hall, J. G.: The flow of lymph. N. Engl. J. Med., 281:720, 1969.
Kinmonth, J. B.: The Lymphatics: Diseases, Lymphography and Surgery. Baltimore, Williams and Wilkins Company, 1972.
Sigstad, H., Aagenaes, Ø., Bjorn-Hansen, R. W., and Rootwelt, K.: Primary lymphoedema combined with hereditary recurrent intrahepatic cholestasis. Acta Med. Scand., 188:213, 1970.
Smith, R. D., Spittell, J. A., Jr., and Schirger, A.: Secondary lymphedema of the leg: Its characteristics and diagnostic implications. J.A.M.A., 185:80, 1963.
Stone, E. J., and Hugo, N. E.: Lymphedema. Surg. Gynecol. Obstet., 135:625, 1972.

LYMPHANGITIS

Definition. Lymphangitis is an acute or chronic inflammation, usually pyogenic, of the lymphatic vessels.

Etiology. In the majority of cases of lymphangitis the hemolytic Streptococcus is the infecting agent; second most common is the coagulase-positive Staphylococcus. The bacteria enter the skin via areas of local trauma, trichophytosis, or arterial ischemic or venous stasis ulcers, although a portal of entry cannot always be discovered. Infection then spreads by the lymphatic vessels to the local lymph nodes; an accompanying diffuse cellu-

litis of the extremity is often present. An immune response to previously present bacteria or their products has been postulated as a cause of lymphangitis when an organism cannot be isolated, but proof of this is lacking.

Pathology. Acute, subacute, or chronic inflammation is found in the subcutaneous tissues and regional lymph nodes.

Clinical Manifestations. Attacks of lymphangitis may be ushered in by malaise, headache, nausea, vomiting, and shaking chills followed by fever. Systemic symptoms, however, may not be present. Red streaks appear in the affected extremity, originating at the portal of entry and following the pathway of lymphatic vessels. Regional lymph nodes are usually enlarged and tender. There may be a surrounding area of cellulitis with tenderness and red discoloration in the lower part of the extremity, which is usually swollen with a soft, pitting edema.

Diagnosis. The clinical picture is usually typical and allows the diagnosis to be made easily. A leukocytosis is often present. The inciting organism should be sought by culturing the portal of entry if obvious or by needle puncture of the subcutaneous tissues. A difficult diagnosis to rule out is acute thrombophlebitis, especially when a diffuse cellulitis is present, for symptoms and signs are similar; it is often wise to administer therapy for both diseases simultaneously.

Prognosis. For an initial attack in a limb without underlying disease, the prognosis with treatment is excellent. However, some patients have recurrent attacks, often mild, which can lead to the development of lymphedema. In recurrent cases, the limb may remain somewhat larger after each attack.

Treatment. Systemic antimicrobial drugs should be administered as indicated by culture (and sensitivity studies if necessary). If no organism is cultured, penicillin should be given because the Streptococcus is so commonly the etiologic agent. Drainage of any focus of origin is also extremely important. Adjunctive measures include rest, elevation of the extremity above heart level, and warm wet dressings. Possible fungal infections in the feet and causes of secondary lymphedema should be sought. When attacks subside, elastic support should be worn on the extremity for three months to prevent residual swelling. In recurrent cases, either with or without underlying lymphedema, prophylactic long-term antimicrobial therapy should be instituted. Lymphangitis is especially dangerous in the ischemic tissues of patients with obstructive arterial disease; only under these unfavorable conditions is prompt amputation sometimes required.

Babb, R. R., Spittell, J. A., Jr., Martin, W. J., and Schirger, A.: Prophylaxis of recurrent lymphangitis complicating lymphedema. J.A.M.A., 195:871, 1966.
Edwards, E. A.: Recurrent febrile episodes and lymphedema. J.A.M.A., 184:858, 1963.

Part XIII
RENAL DISEASES

601. INTRODUCTION: ROLE OF THE KIDNEY IN HEALTH AND DISEASE

D. N. S. Kerr

EXCRETION

The prime function of the kidney is to excrete the surplus water and nonmetabolized solute in the diet, as well as the nonvolatile end products of metabolism, in such a manner as to preserve a constant internal environment. The major constituents of the urine are water, urea, sodium, chloride, potassium, phosphate, and creatinine; but several hundred substances can be identified in urine, and the excretion of many minor constituents is essential to health. The minimal urine volume is determined by the osmotic load, of which urea, sodium, and chloride are the main determinants. A subject taking a low protein, low salt diet can survive on a daily urine output of only 200 ml, whereas the steak and salt addict must excrete well over the conventional 500 ml per 24 hours. In a temperate climate a subject with normal renal function can preserve a nearly constant extracellular fluid volume and chemical composition on a sodium intake which can vary one hundred fold, or on a water intake of from less than 1 liter to more than 10 liters per 24 hours.

These extremes of renal function are rarely required in modern living. The average citizen keeps his water intake within narrow limits of 1 to 2 liters per day, and his sodium and protein intake do not vary any more widely from day to day. His kidneys are stressed only occasionally at a celebration night in the bar or during illness involving fever, water deprivation, vomiting, and diarrhea. If his kidneys are slowly destroyed by disease, he may continue to live a comfortable life and hold down a demanding job until about 90 per cent of his excretory function is lost, provided he continues his normal routines and does not challenge his kidneys by dietary aberration, intercurrent illness, or the consumption of medications which contain drugs or electrolytes he cannot readily excrete. Apparently those mechanisms which control excretion in health can be adapted very successfully to achieve the same end while the nephron population is declining. The nature of these control mechanisms and their modification in disease are subjects of intensive research and lively controversy.

Water excretion is controlled mainly by the secretion from the neurohypophysis of antidiuretic hormone, which affects the permeability of the distal tubule. The osmotic load per nephron is a second mechanism controlling water excretion, of particular importance when intake is low. Alteration in glomerular filtration rate (GFR) was once regarded as the first mechanism controlling sodium excretion, but it now seems unlikely that it plays a major part in health. There is some evidence, discussed in Ch. 603, that the patient in chronic renal failure does utilize alterations in GFR to achieve sodium

balance. Aldosterone is a second important control mechanism, but it cannot be responsible for more than the fine control of sodium excretion. The remaining mechanisms controlling the tubular reabsorption of sodium and chloride are still uncertain; they may include the colloid osmotic pressure and hydrostatic pressure of peritubular capillaries and an unidentified natriuretic hormone. These and other possibilities are lumped together in imprecise nephrologic jargon as *"third factor."*

One of the most remarkable adaptations to chronic renal disease is an increase in the proportion of filtered sodium which is excreted in the urine, from the normal 0.5 to 1 per cent up to 20 per cent or more in late renal failure. An increased osmotic load per nephron and suppression of aldosterone secretion may play a part in this adaptation, but much of the change has yet to be accounted for. Presumably "third factor" is altered in the appropriate direction. The feat may not be achieved without some cost. Bricker has suggested that many of the symptoms of renal failure may be the result of overproduction of hormones to achieve such compensation, rather than the effect of more direct mechanisms such as the retention of waste products. He illustrates this "trade-off hypothesis" with an example that is better understood than sodium excretion. Phosphate is retained as glomerular filtration falls, depressing plasma-ionized calcium concentration and stimulating parathyroid hormone secretion. This corrects plasma phosphate until late in the course of renal failure but at the cost of causing osteitis fibrosa. Another effect of increased parathyroid hormone secretion is to produce a renal bicarbonate leak which contributes to "renal acidosis."

There is a limit to the loss of renal function which can be compensated in this manner. In chronic renal disease it is reached when GFR falls to about 10 per cent of normal, at which point symptoms often become prominent even on normal diet and undisturbed routine. When excretory function is lost suddenly, as in bilateral ureteral obstruction, cortical necrosis, or fulminant glomerulonephritis, no compensation is possible, and death may occur within a few days from intoxication with water (convulsions), salt and water (pulmonary edema), or potassium (cardiac arrest). Only if the intake is regulated to prevent these disasters does the patient survive long enough to suffer from the retention of metabolic end products. Which of these waste products harm him and in what way are still topics of which we are surprisingly ignorant. Ultimately any of them would prove toxic; if there were no alternative pathway of excretion it would accumulate until it caused cell death or the patient turned, like Lot's wife, into a pillar of crystallized solute. However, it remains uncertain which of these compounds in practice achieve toxic concentrations in human disease. Even the contribution of urea to the symptoms of uremia is undecided, although it is probably small. Creatinine is declared innocent by almost every commentator even though it accelerates autohemolysis in vitro. Guanidines, phenols, amines, and sulfate have been blamed for some symptoms by some authors. When an alternative, unphysiologic pathway of excretion is provided through the peritoneum or the artificial kidney, small molecules are removed preferentially, and "middle molecules" of molecular weight 300 to 1500 are retained. There is a burgeoning literature attributing uremic symptoms, particularly those in the nervous system, to these unidentified compounds, but the case is far from proved and their role, if any, in unmodified renal failure is largely unexplored.

The glomerulus has only one function – production of glomerular filtrate. *Glomerular disease* is therefore manifest as acute or chronic renal failure or through a leak of protein and cells in the filtrate. *Tubular function* is much more complex, involving many different enzyme systems in active transport. One would therefore expect to find a number of syndromes associated with enzyme deficiencies in the tubules, the result of inherited defects and intoxications. This proves to be the case; many defects of amino acid, dextrose, phosphate and uric acid reabsorption, hydrogen ion excretion, and end-organ responsiveness to individual hormones are recognized. They have provided invaluable insight into renal physiology and are often rewarding conditions to treat, but numerically they make up a very small part of clinical nephrology, compared with glomerular disease and whole nephron failure.

BLOOD FLOW

The kidneys receive a quarter of the cardiac output. Renal blood flow varies little during sedentary activity, but it falls during strenuous exercise, in hypovolemia, and in many pathologic states such as cardiac or hepatic failure. Infusion of vasodilator drugs such as acetylcholine, papaverine, and dopamine increase renal blood flow by up to 100 per cent. Over a wide range of blood flow in these conditions glomerular filtration rate is kept almost constant. This autoregulation has been attributed to balanced control of tone in the afferent and efferent arterioles, maintaining constant glomerular capillary pressure, but it is now apparent that intraglomerular pressure varies appreciably and is balanced by other mechanisms such as compensatory rise in proximal tubular pressure.

Radiokrypton studies show four components in the blood flow pattern through the kidney. There is a fast flow through the outer cortex and progressively slower streams through inner cortex, outer medulla, and papilla. Outer cortical nephrons have short Henle loops and are concerned primarily with excretion; inner cortical nephrons have long loops which maintain the high osmolality of the papilla and permit urinary concentration. Outer cortical ischemia is accompanied by sodium retention, e.g., in prerenal uremia or hepatic failure; renal vasodilatation causes sodium and water loss, e.g., in one phase of endotoxic shock. Alterations in the pattern of renal blood flow do not appear to be important in physiologic control of water and electrolyte excretion, but they probably play an important part in many diseases.

ENDOCRINE FUNCTION

The kidney has at least three endocrine functions: secretion of renin, erythropoietin, and the active metabolites of vitamin D; medullary prostaglandins and unidentified intrarenal hormones may also be important endocrine secretions, but the evidence is inconclusive.

Renin, an enzyme which has been obtained almost pure from the pig, has a molecular weight of about 40,000. It acts on a substrate in plasma to produce the decapeptide angiotensin I which is split by a converting enzyme, mainly in lung capillaries, to form the active octapeptide angiotensin II. Angiotensin II stimulates the adrenal to produce aldosterone, and this appears to be its main physiologic function. It is not the only control mechanism. After bilateral nephrectomy, the output of aldosterone responds to changes in plasma potassium, probably from a direct action on the adrenal, and it rises with a fall in plasma sodium. The latter phenomenon is unexplained. However, in health, aldosterone secretion rate is probably controlled mainly by angiotensin II, and this in turn is determined by the secretion rate of renin, because the supply of substrate, converting enzyme, and angiotensinases is seldom rate limiting. Renin is produced in the juxtaglomerular apparatus, which comprises the macula densa of the distal convoluted tubule, the lacis cells continuous with the mesangium, and specialized cells of the afferent arteriole. Consequently, alterations in tubular fluid composition and/or vascular stretch have been suggested as stimuli for renin secretion. The output of renin is increased by sodium depletion, hypovolemia, stimulation of sympathetic nerves or secretion of catecholamines, adoption of the upright posture, and several drugs, including diuretics and antihypertensives. It is decreased by the administration of mineralocorticoids or beta-blockers. Consequently, withdrawal of drug therapy and controlled conditions of posture and freedom from stress are required for studies of renin in disease.

In concentrations higher than those usually found in the plasma in health, angiotensin II is a powerful vasoconstrictor which has direct actions on the tubule. Hypersecretion of renin is important in at least two disease states: hypertension caused by renal artery stenosis; and the severe hypertension, resistant to sodium and water removal, found in a small minority of patients with bilateral renal disease maintained on regular hemodialysis. After bilateral nephrectomy, loss of renin secretion produces surprisingly few ill effects, but some patients suffer troublesome postural hypotension.

Erythropoietin is a glycoprotein, or proteins, produced in the kidney which stimulates committed stem cells in the bone marrow to produce normoblasts. It has proved very difficult to isolate, assay, label, and study physiologically. Its molecular weight is uncertain, but is probably between 10,000 and 60,000. Its site of origin is equally doubtful, but it can be extracted from both medulla and cortex. Its action is enhanced by normal plasma, and it may, like renin, require a plasma substrate. Erythropoietin output is increased by renal hypoxia, e.g., at high altitudes, in cyanotic heart disease, and in chronic lung disease. Plasma erythropoietin is high in all forms of anemia except that of renal disease. Androgens increase the hemoglobin concentration, partly by stimulating erythropoietin output, and estrogens block the action of erythropoietin. A rare form of polycythemia is associated with overproduction of erythropoietin from renal tumors or cysts, and erythropoietin lack is one of several factors producing the anemia of renal failure. This anemia is aggravated by bilateral nephrectomy, suggesting that even shriveled remnants of kidney produce useful amounts of the hormone.

The kidney is the only organ which converts *25-*

hydroxycholecalciferol to its very active *1,25-dihydroxy metabolite.* The output of this hormone is increased by hypocalcemia, which acts via parathyroid hormone secretion, and by hypophosphatemia; 1,25-HCC stimulates calcium and phosphate absorption from the gut and mobilization from the bones, correcting the plasma calcium and phosphate. Trihydroxy metabolites of vitamin D are also produced in the kidney and may have a similar effect. Osteomalacia is a characteristic feature of severe, longstanding renal osteodystrophy, and it is tempting to attribute this to lack of 1,25-HCC. However, it is not yet certain that 1,25-HCC mediates the healing effect of vitamin D on osteomalacia, and some patients with bilateral nephrectomy have bones which are normal clinically, radiologically, and histologically.

THE CLASSIFICATION OF RENAL DISEASE

This topic has obsessed nephrologists and puzzled students for more than a century. The traditional medical textbook presents a series of diseases, each with a specific etiology, and with pathogenesis, pathology, clinical features, and treatment that proceed from it in logical order. The cause of many renal diseases is unknown, and it is probable that many different etiologic agents can initiate some pathogenic mechanisms, e.g., the formation of immune complexes of the right size to lodge in the glomerular filter. It is therefore necessary to attach to each patient a series of diagnoses at different levels: etiologies, pathogenic mechanisms, pathology (morphologic and functional), and clinical features. The first of these is plural, because two or more factors are often necessary for the development of a renal disease. It is likely that only some individuals have the necessary immunologic constitution to develop glomerulonephritis when exposed to the appropriate organism; and whereas many women (perhaps all) admit bacteria into their bladders, only a minority with impaired defense mechanisms, e.g., refluxing ureters, develop pyelonephritis.

Ideally the nomenclature should indicate at what level a diagnosis has been made. A child with hematuria, oliguria, edema, and hypertension should be labeled as having "acute nephritic syndrome." When the pathology has been confirmed and the streptococcal origin has been demonstrated from a rising antistreptolysin-O titer, he merits the full diagnosis of "poststreptococcal acute glomerulonephritis." Since the pathogenesis of this disease is believed always to involve the formation of immune complex, a pathogenetic diagnosis is unnecessary. However, when a similar syndrome is seen in the absence of streptococcal infection and the role of immune complexes can be inferred from the presence of cryoglobulins in plasma, a fall in serum complement, deposition of complement fractions and immunoglobulins in the glomerulus, and "humps" on the basement membrane, "immune complex nephritis of unknown etiology" is a legitimate title and a pointer to possible therapy.

Logical terminology is cumbersome, and the habits of a lifetime are not easily broken. Consequently the chapters which follow preserve some traditional usages which are not strictly logical. However, in these chapters more space is devoted to the description of clinical syndromes, states of disordered function, and pathogenic mechanisms than to individual diseases.

602. INVESTIGATION OF RENAL FUNCTION

D. N. S. Kerr

The common effects of disease on the function of the renal parenchyma are increased excretion of protein, alteration in the formed elements in the urine, reduction in renal blood flow and glomerular filtration rate, impairment of tubular reabsorption and secretion, alteration in the secretion rates of erythropoietin and renin, and disordered metabolism of vitamin D. Accurate study of these functions is an essential part of renal research, but most of the precise methods are too demanding or too tedious for routine clinical use. Plasma renin and angiotensin assays are employed almost exclusively in the investigation of hypertension. Assay of erythropoietin is still too imprecise and difficult to be of use outside research laboratories, and measurement of plasma 1,25-hydroxycholecalciferol is available in only a few centers in the world. Individual tubular functions, other than concentrating power, are tested in the investigation of renal tubular acidosis, other inherited and acquired tubular disorders, and renal calculous disease, and the appropriate tests are described in the chapters dealing with those subjects.

The study of proteinuria and urine microscopy are important in differential diagnosis. Measurement of glomerular filtration rate has little value in diagnosis, except in distinguishing early renal disease from physiologic states such as postural proteinuria, but is important in following the progress of disease and the response to treatment. Renal blood flow would be of some value diagnostically were it not so difficult to measure. Concentrating ability has been used more as a test for early renal damage than as one of specific tubular function, but in the latter role it has a limited value in differential diagnosis.

Proteinuria. The urine of normal adults contains about 40 to 100 mg of protein per 24 hours during sedentary activity. The very low concentrations in normal urine are difficult to measure accurately, and the mean figure quoted varies widely. Conventionally the upper limit of normal is taken as 150 mg per 24 hours in the ambulant subject and 0.03 mg per minute during short collection periods in recumbency. The most sensitive screening test for urinary protein is the formation of a white cloud on heating filtered urine saturated with sodium sulfate and acidified with a few drops of 3 per cent acetic acid; this detects about 5 to 10 mg per 100 ml as a faint trace. A definite positive with any clinical test therefore indicates a protein concentration higher than the normal should achieve under resting conditions, and "proteinuria" has been accepted as the term to describe excessive proteinuria.

All such screening tests have a considerable observer error. The formation of a cloud with 25 per cent salicylsulfonic acid and the appearance of a green color on paper impregnated with bromophenol blue and a buffer (Albustix, Labstix) are much simpler than the heat test, and this compensates for their slightly lower sensitivity. All three tests give a very crude guide to the concentration of protein, the +, ++, +++, and ++++ corresponding roughly to 30, 100, 300, and 1000 mg per 100 ml in the case of bromophenol blue. However, the middle part of the range has poor reproducibility, and a more accurate test is necessary even for general medical use. A turbidimetric method, using salicylsulfonic acid, can be performed in the ward laboratory, the sample being compared with an albumin standard. It underestimates globulins but is sufficiently accurate for clinical purposes. An automated biuret method is more satisfactory, but interfering substances must be removed for really accurate results.

Normal urinary protein contains at least 30 components, the largest of which is a high molecular weight mucoprotein called *Tamm-Horsfall protein,* which originates in the cells lining the ascending limb of Henle's loop and the macula densa segment of the distal convoluted tubule. Precipitation of this protein in the distal tubule forms the basis of renal casts. Other components include most of the plasma proteins of small molecular weight, with albumin the most prominent, and several proteins derived from the prostate and seminal vesicles. The normal glomerulus has been shown to have a high selectivity, i.e., to filter predominantly small colloid molecules, by studies with graded dextrans.

Increased protein excretion occurs with heavy exertion, fever, heart failure, and operative trauma without any known changes in renal structure or permanent change in renal function. Proteinuria from these sources is usually under 500 mg per 24 hours and rarely over 1 gram per 24 hours; its major component is albumin and its presumed origin, the glomerular filtrate. Proteinuria is detected in about 5 per cent of children and adolescents at school medical examinations; the majority of the "positives" prove to have benign exercise or postural proteinuria. Nearly all adolescents and about 50 per cent of young adults can produce proteinuria by adopting a lordotic position, e.g., bent backward over a chair. The proteinuria may be heavy but has no pathologic significance. A smaller proportion (about 5 per cent) of adolescents and a few young children and young adults develop proteinuria simply from standing erect. During prolonged standing the proteinuria may become quite heavy—up to 14 mg per minute has been recorded—but over 24 hours the loss is usually below 1 gram, rarely exceeds 2 grams, and virtually never causes nephrotic syndrome. This *orthostatic proteinuria* in an adolescent or young adult is nearly always benign and often disappears around the age of 20. However, before making the diagnosis and reassuring the patient, it is important to confirm that the proteinuria consistently disappears on recumbency and that there is no other evidence of renal disease. The patient should be asked to empty his bladder immediately before retiring and to collect a urine sample as soon as he rises on three convenient days. He should collect three afternoon samples for comparison. If there is no proteinuria in the morning samples, proteinuria in some of the afternoon samples, a 24-hour excretion of less than 1 gram, a normal plasma urea and creatinine, and no abnormality in the urine deposit on three careful examinations, a confident diagnosis of benign orthostatic proteinuria can be made.

Lordotic and postural proteinuria are generally attributed to temporary obstruction of the renal venous outflow, but their origin within the kidney is uncertain. The proteinuria is unselective (see below), but glomerular permeability is normally selective as judged by the dextran test, suggesting that some of the larger proteins originate below the glomerulus. However, studies with labeled proteins suggest that most of the protein passes

through the glomerulus, and transient changes in the podocytes, similar to those found in childhood nephrosis, have been shown in a few patients with orthostatic proteinuria.

Persistent proteinuria is always pathologic. Even if there is no other evidence of renal disease, biopsy usually reveals glomerular or vascular disease. Pathologic proteinurias can be subdivided by concentrating urine (when necessary) and examining it electrophoretically and by immunologic methods. A characteristic pattern, with only a small proportion of albumin, large components of alpha$_1$, alpha$_2$, and beta$_1$ globulins, and an abnormally high proportion of beta$_2$ microglobulin, is found in patients with active pyelonephritis, medullary cystic disease, congenital tubular disorders, Wilson's disease, hypokalemic nephropathy, sarcoidosis, some toxic nephropathies, including the Balkan nephropathy, and some forms of transplant rejection. It is referred to as "tubular proteinuria" and rarely exceeds 1 gram per 24 hours. In some forms of myelomatosis, the light chains of the abnormal immunoglobulins, being small enough to pass through the glomerular filter easily, appear in the urine as *"Bence Jones proteinuria."* All other patterns of proteinuria are attributed to increased permeability of the glomerular filter. The normal glomerulus allows macromolecules to enter the filtrate at a rate proportional to the logarithm of their molecular size (Fig. 1). This relationship still holds approximately when the glomerulus becomes excessively leaky, but the slope of the graph varies according to the disease. In nephrotic syndrome with minimal change (childhood nephrosis) it remains steep, so that only the smaller plasma proteins such as albumin appear in the urine in detectable quantities (Fig. 2). In several diffuse diseases of the glomeruli, including membranous glomerulonephropathy and amyloidosis, the graph is less steep, and very large molecules such as alpha$_2$ macroglobulin can be detected in the urine. Proliferative glomerulonephritis occupies an intermediate position, but yields rather variable results. This is probably due to the

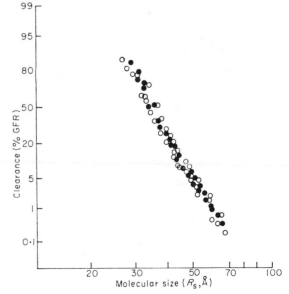

Figure 1. Relationship between the molecular size and the glomerular clearance of large polymers (○ = allyl-dextran; ● = polyvinylpyrrolidone) in normal rabbits. (From Hardwicke, J., et al.: Clin. Sci., 34:509, 1968.)

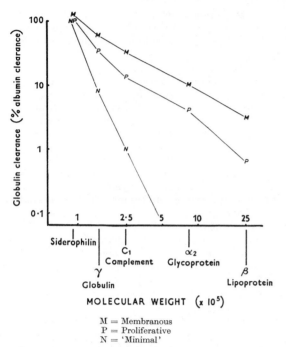

M = Membranous
P = Proliferative
N = 'Minimal'

Figure 2. Relationship between molecular weight and relative clearance of plasma proteins in the three main types of nephrotic syndrome. (From Blainey, J. D., et al.: Quart J. Med., 34:235, 1959.)

patchy nature of the lesion; tests of selectivity based on proteins in plasma and urine exaggerate the loss of selectivity in this condition, probably because protein is reabsorbed in the tubules of the least affected nephrons. A simplified test for selectivity of proteinuria in which transferrin and IgG or alpha$_2$ macroglobulin are measured in serum and urine with the aid of immunoplates is now a standard laboratory test much simpler than electrophoresis of concentrated urine. Its main value is in the nephrotic syndrome of childhood in which selective proteinuria makes a response to corticosteroids so likely that renal biopsy may often be avoided.

Urine Microscopy. Midstream urine should be collected at a time when it is likely to be concentrated, using the same precautions as for culture. It should be handled by a constant technique, e.g., by centrifuging 10 ml at 3000 rpm for five minutes and resuspending the sediment in the last 0.5 ml of urine. When many urines are examined, an acceptable alternative is to allow the urine to settle in a test tube for an hour and withdraw the sediment with a Pasteur pipette. A well spread thick drop should be examined under low power for casts and crystals, and a thin film under high power for red cells, white cells, and bacteria and for the exact identification of casts. Red and white cells are often confused under low power even by experienced observers, but the most common error in microscopy is omission of the initial thick drop examination and consequent failure to recognize casts. The microscope must be well maintained and equipped with a variable illuminator and preferably a polarizer. A medium power high enough to permit identification of casts in the thick drop is an added advantage.

Red cells are normally excreted at a rate of about 150 to 300,000 per 24 hours, with an approximate upper limit of 1 million per 24 hours or 1000 per minute in

short collections. Only an occasional red cell should be seen on qualitative microscopy as described above. White cells are excreted at an average of about 70,000 per hour in both sexes, but this applies only to urine entirely free from contamination in the female. If there has been much contamination with vaginal secretion, as indicated by large numbers of squamous epithelial cells, leukocyturia cannot be interpreted unless it is extremely heavy. The upper limit of normal leukocyte excretion is 200,000 per hour, which yields one or two leukocytes per high-power field in qualitative microscopy of a concentrated urine. Leukocytes are difficult to distinguish from nonsquamous epithelial cells from the renal tubules, and the two are usually counted together. The increase in leukocyte excretion after pyrogen injection or prednisolone has been proposed as a test for chronic pyelonephritis, but it is so difficult to obtain noncatheter, timed urine samples from females free from vaginal contamination that it is seldom employed in practice. Qualitative examination for leukocytes is nonetheless of great importance in the detection of urinary infection, renal tuberculosis, and analgesic nephropathy.

Hyaline casts consist of precipitated Tamm-Horsfall protein only; they have a refractive index close to that of urine and are easily missed if the illumination is too high. Up to 10,000 per 24 hours are excreted by normal subjects, but at this rate only a very occasional one is seen even on the thick drop under low power. Numerous hyaline casts are seen in nearly all renal diseases associated with glomerular proteinuria; hyaline casts with few or none of the other varieties described below are seen in benign essential hypertension and nephrotic syndrome with minimal change. Hyaline casts are mainly of roughly constant diameter corresponding to the lumen of the distal convoluted tubule, but short thick casts, formed in the collecting duct, are seen in chronic renal failure and recovering tubular necrosis or glomerulonephritis. Misshapen, long, and branching casts are formed in the late stages of chronic renal diseases, particularly chronic nephritis, reflecting the distorted shape of some nephrons.

Granular casts are speckled or barred owing to the presence of immunoglobulin aggregates in a matrix of Tamm-Horsfall protein. Lightly speckled casts may appear in normal urine after strenuous exercise or during fever; when present in the resting afebrile subject, they nearly always indicate renal pathology but do not point to any particular disease. Densely granular casts, which may appear almost black on microscopy and which are readily confused with red cell casts, are always a sign of disease and are commonly found in active glomerulonephritis, lupus nephritis, malignant hypertension, and renal amyloidosis. Deeply pigmented granular casts are found in association with hemoglobinuria and in the brown urine that is often excreted in the early stages of acute renal failure. Bile-stained granular casts are excreted in large numbers by patients with obstructive jaundice, often without any other evidence of renal dysfunction.

Red blood cell casts have greater diagnostic significance than any other variety. They indicate glomerular bleeding and are excreted in very large numbers in the acute phase of poststreptococcal glomerulonephritis. Smaller numbers are excreted in other forms of glomerulonephritis, notably membranoproliferative nephritis and the focal nephritis of Henoch-Schönlein syndrome and polyarteritis, and in malignant hypertension. They are said to have a reddish tinge, but this is rarely found and is confined to casts with very numerous red cells. Usually they have a greenish tinge under tungsten light. They are readily distinguished from other cellular casts because the red cells are incorporated in the matrix; this can be confirmed by focusing up and down through the cast under medium or high power. *Leukocyte casts* are typical of active pyelonephritis; they are rarely found in chronic pyelonephritis with sterile urine, in which the deposit contains only a few leukocytes if the patient is normotensive. *Epithelial cell casts* are typical of acute tubular necrosis but may be found in active glomerulonephritis, which is often an important differential diagnosis. *Fatty casts,* staining red with Sudan III and showing "Maltese crosses" in polarized light, accompany heavy proteinuria and are probably due to the leakage of lipoproteins through the glomerular filter. Free fat globules and oval fat bodies—degenerate tubular cells in which the "Maltese crosses" of cholesterol esters are best demonstrated—are also typical of nephrotic syndrome.

The recognition of casts is a very important step in establishing the existence of renal disease; they are particularly helpful in the investigation of proteinuria and hematuria, indicating a probable renal cause for the latter. They have a limited usefulness in distinguishing between different renal diseases and have some value in following the activity of disease. The disappearance of red cell casts and dense granular casts from the deposit as malignant hypertension is controlled points to essential hypertension as the primary disease. Once the diagnosis is established, however, cast excretion has little additional prognostic value. Excessive excretion of hyaline and lightly granular casts can continue for decades in inactive disease such as treated essential hypertension, gouty nephropathy, or nonprogressive chronic glomerulonephritis.

Glomerular Filtration Rate. If a substance is filtered at the glomerulus in proportion to plasma water and is not reabsorbed or secreted by the tubule, it can be used to estimate glomerular filtration rate (GFR) because the excretion rate is then determined only by the plasma level and the GFR.

GFR (clearance rate of marker substance) =
$$\frac{\text{excretion rate}}{\text{plasma level}}$$

The one universally accepted marker substance is *inulin,* a mixture of fructose polymers with an average molecular weight of about 5200, but it has the disadvantages of being a variable mixture, of having a low solubility, and of hydrolyzing to fructose during the boiling necessary to dissolve it. The analytic methods for inulin are also difficult. Polyfructosan, with a narrow range of molecular weight and better solubility, is probably superior but less familiar. Any exogenous substance used for measurement of GFR must be infused at a constant rate for long enough to allow complete stabilization of the blood level, and then continued until several urine samples can be obtained of sufficient volume to minimize bladder-emptying errors. Consequently accurate measurement of GFR with inulin, without bladder catheterization, takes four to six hours, and is unsuitable for routine clinical use. The need for urine collection can be eliminated if the constant infusion is continued long enough to ensure that plasma levels are completely stable; the infusion rate is then assumed to equal the urinary excretion rate,

the very small extrarenal loss of inulin being ignored. The technique has some popularity in pediatrics.

Several substances more easily measured than inulin are available; they are not protein bound, are freely filtered, and are little affected by tubular secretion or reabsorption. EDTA labeled with ^{51}Cr is the most popular, but ^{131}iodine labeled inulin and diacetrizoate are also in use. As all these substances have a very low rate of extrarenal excretion, they can be used to measure GFR approximately by a single injection technique. After an initial delay for equilibration in its volume of distribution, the plasma level of the marker substance falls exponentially, and the slope of the line is a measure of GFR. This technique gives a reproducibility of about ±5 per cent using multiple plasma samples, and a little poorer result using an external counter to avoid blood sampling. The method is now provided by many hospital physics departments on a routine basis, and is sufficient for clinical purposes, as the GFR is in any case subject to a diurnal variation of about ±10 per cent, reaching its peak in the afternoon and its trough during the night; it is also readily disturbed by exercise or emotional disturbance.

The most popular rough estimate of GFR is the endogenous *creatinine clearance,* using a 24-hour urine collection and a single plasma sample. If renal function is stable, the plasma sample can be drawn at any time in the collection period, because plasma creatinine varies little during the 24 hours in these circumstances. In outpatient investigation it is even permissible to draw the blood sample a few hours after the end of the collection period. The automated technique used in most hospitals, based on the Jaffé reaction, measures creatinine plus some of the creatinine-like chromogen, but its reproducibility is better than that of the manual methods measuring true creatinine. Even with the automated method there is a high interlaboratory variation in quality control surveys, particularly when the result is close to normal. This reflects the difficulty in measuring plasma creatinine accurately in the normal range. The analytical error alone is of the order of ± 10 per cent, so small changes in creatinine clearance should not be overinterpreted when they are close to normal. Important additional sources of error are loss of urine during defecation, mistiming of collection, incomplete bladder emptying, and washout effects caused by the consumption of diuretics or fluctuations in fluid intake. Careful instruction and good patient cooperation are needed for meaningful results. Two or three consecutive collections are preferable, to compensate for bladder-emptying errors. Creatinine clearance considerably and unpredictably overestimates GFR in nephrotic syndrome, after renal transplantation, and in terminal renal failure, probably because of tubular secretion of creatinine.

The plasma creatinine concentration is determined by the production rate, which is largely a reflection of muscle mass, and the excretion rate, which is roughly proportional to GFR. In a patient whose muscle mass is not changing rapidly, alterations in plasma creatinine are determined almost exclusively by changes in GFR; diet and fluid intake have very little effect. When plasma creatinine is greater than 1.0 mg per 100 ml its estimation presents few difficulties, and it is a much more convenient and reproducible test than creatinine clearance. It is therefore used by most nephrologists as their day-to-day guide to the progress of renal function. The relationship to GFR is hyperbolic; a large change in GFR produces a small change in plasma creatinine close to the normal range, whereas a small change in GFR causes a large change in plasma creatinine in late renal failure.

Although plasma creatinine is of pre-eminent importance in following renal function, it cannot be readily converted into an estimate of GFR, owing to the wide differences in muscle mass between individual patients. This limits its usefulness in confirming normal renal function. A raised plasma creatinine always indicates a depression in GFR, temporary or permanent, but a normal plasma creatinine does not exclude renal disease unless the patient's muscle mass is obviously normal, e.g., the young athlete with exertional proteinuria. The prediction of GFR from plasma creatinine can be improved if allowance is made for age and sex, which are two major determinants of muscle mass. The calculation is particularly useful when drug therapy is required by the patient with renal impairment; an accurate, recent estimate of GFR is usually unavailable, but a plasma creatinine can be obtained within the hour and used to calculate the required dose. A formula for calculating GFR from plasma creatinine, with correction factors, is shown in Table 1. It is only valid if plasma creatinine is stable, and this should be confirmed during the first 12 to 24 hours of drug therapy.

Plasma urea has been used as the main guide to renal function by the majority of general physicians and surgeons at least until the last few years, but it is a poor guide. Under stable conditions of diet, lean body mass, and fluid intake, it has a roughly hyperbolic relationship to GFR in the same manner as plasma creatinine, but the curve is distorted in severe renal failure by a rise in urea clearance relative to GFR (reaching almost 100 per cent when GFR is below 5 ml per minute) and by extrarenal removal of urea. However, these stable conditions are not common in clinical practice, and plasma urea is readily affected by variations in protein intake and in net body catabolism or anabolism caused by trauma, infection, inactivity, refeeding, the anabolic phase after illness, and drug therapy, particularly corticosteroids. It takes about two weeks for the plasma urea to stabilize under constant conditions in the metabolic ward. Plasma urea is affected by fluid intake; it falls during a water diuresis and fluctuates appreciably during the 24 hours under the influence of food and drink. Many laboratories now provide a plasma creatinine result

gratis when a plasma urea is requested, in the hope of educating doctors to use the better estimate of renal function. However, plasma urea retains some usefulness as an index of retention of the compounds produced in response to protein ingestion. The ratio of plasma urea and plasma creatinine has some diagnostic significance. Plasma urea rises preferentially during water or sodium and water depletion, whereas plasma urea and creatinine rise together in established acute renal failure.

Renal Blood Flow. Renal blood flow can be estimated by dye dilution methods or by the elution curve of radiokrypton if the renal artery and vein are catheterized. These techniques are sometimes employed clinically after renal transplant when fine catheters can be left in the donor organ at operation and kept in situ during the first few weeks. A fall in renal blood flow is probably the first detectable sign of rejection of a homograft. In other situations renal plasma flow is usually measured as the clearance rate of para-aminohippurate (PAH) on the assumption that PAH is both filtered at the glomerulus and secreted by the tubules so that it is cleared almost completely from the plasma in a single passage through the kidney. PAH is easy to measure accurately, and it equilibrates in the body more rapidly than inulin so the performance of PAH clearance is relatively simple. In the normal subject the removal of PAH from blood traversing the kidney is about 92 per cent, which is near enough to the theoretic 100 per cent to make the test useful; it has been employed to show that renal blood flow varies more widely than GFR with exercise and emotion but has about the same and parallel diurnal variation. In renal disease the extraction ratio of PAH may be well below 92 per cent, so PAH clearance cannot be equated with renal plasma flow unless the extraction ratio can be measured simultaneously with the aid of a renal vein catheter—seldom a justifiable clinical procedure.

Glomerular filtration rate and renal blood flow are both related to body size, and surface area has been found to correlate with them most closely in the adult. They are therefore corrected to a standard surface area of 1.73 square meters before comparison with the normal range. This correction is of course unnecessary when they are used serially to follow the progress of disease. In infants under one year the GFR and renal blood flow are low in relationship to surface area, but this is probably a reflection of the high surface area of the infant rather than of a reduced renal reserve. On other criteria, e.g., using body volume as a standard, the GFR reaches adult proportions at about one month. Both GFR and renal blood flow rise in pregnancy, reaching a peak at about 36 weeks, so it is essential to compare results in pregnancy with the normal range for the same stage of gestation. Glomerular filtration rate and renal plasma flow both decline with age. In men, mean GFR falls from about 125 ml per minute at age 40 to about 60 ml per minute at age 90 in a roughly linear manner but with a wide scatter. The fall with age in women is not so well documented and is probably slower. Normal ranges at different ages are illustrated by Wesson.

Urinary Concentrating Power. The ability to concentrate urine is impaired as the population of nephrons declines with disease, and it is seldom worthwhile testing concentrating power at a GFR less than 20 ml per minute. It is impaired disproportionately by any disease affecting the loop of Henle or the collecting duct. The concentration test has often been described as a sensitive

TABLE 1.   Calculation of Creatinine Clearance
from Corrected Serum Creatinine*

$$\text{Creatinine clearance per 1.73 sq m} = \frac{64.56}{\text{Corrected serum creatinine}} - 0.55$$

Corrected serum creatinine is calculated by multiplying observed serum creatinine by a correction factor from the table below:

Age (Years)	Males	Females
30	0.68	0.76
40	0.74	0.86
50	0.80	0.97
60	0.87	1.09
70	0.94	1.24
80	1.03	1.40

*Relationship calculated from the data of Nielsen et al., 1973.

index of early renal damage, but the reproducibility is so low and the normal range so wide that it cannot be more than a crude index. To obtain maximal concentration reliably, it is necessary to deprive the patient of fluid for more than 24 hours, which makes the test inapplicable to outpatients and dangerous to those in renal failure. Four simpler tests are therefore used to give a rough idea of concentrating ability. (1) *Early morning urine;* if one or more of several early morning samples, taken without special precautions, have an osmolality over 700 mOsm per liter, it is unlikely that there is an important defect in urinary concentration. (2) The *16-hour test;* fluid is withheld from 4 P.M. and a dry supper administered. The bladder is emptied at 10 P.M. and all samples collected until 8 A.M. Breakfast and morning drinks are not given until 8 A.M. One of the samples should have an osmolality of 700 mOsm per liter or greater. (3) *Pitressin tannate test;* fluid is withheld from 6 P.M.; 5 units of pitressin tannate in oil, well warmed and shaken, is given intramuscularly at 8 P.M.; the bladder is emptied at 10 P.M. and all samples collected until 10 A.M., when a late breakfast is provided. This gives results close to those of a 24-hour fast, the difference being negligible in patients with impaired concentrating ability. (4) The *16-hour test* can be *improved by the administration of a short-acting diuretic* such as furosemide, 40 mg, at the start of fluid deprivation.

Traditionally urine specific gravity has been used as the criterion of urinary concentration, but as it bears an inconstant relationship to osmolality (which is the best measure of the work of concentration), particularly in the presence of proteinuria, glycosuria, and some exogenous substances such as contrast media, it should now be abandoned in favor of osmolality, which can be measured more accurately on a much smaller sample and, with modern instruments, almost as quickly. An osmolality of 700 corresponds roughly to a specific gravity of 1.020.

Heinemann, H. O., Maack, T. M., and Sherman, R. L.: Combined clinical and basic science seminar: Proteinuria. Am. J. Med., 56:71, 1974.

Morrison, R. B. I.: Urinalysis and assessment of renal function. *In* Black, D. A. K. (ed.): Renal Disease. 3rd ed. Oxford, Blackwell, 1973, Chapter 9.

Nielsen, B., Sørensen, A. W. S., Szabo, L., Pedersen, E. A., and Scharff, A.: Kanamycin serum half-life and renal function: Age and sex. Dan. Med. Bull., 20:144, 1973.

Relman, A. S., and Levinsky, N. G.: Clinical examination of renal function. *In* Strauss, M. B., and Welt, L. G. (eds.): Diseases of the Kidney. 2nd ed. Boston, Little, Brown & Company, 1971, Chapter 3.

Spencer, E. S., and Pedersen, I.: Hand Atlas of the Urinary Sediment. Copenhagen, Munksgaard, 1971.

Wesson, L. G., Jr.: Physiology of the Human Kidney. New York, Grune & Stratton, 1969.

603. CHRONIC RENAL FAILURE

D. N. S. Kerr

ETIOLOGY

The major causes of renal failure, and some of the minor ones, are set out in Table 2 in a manner intended to aid differential diagnosis. Diseases in the first group usually present with features of renal disease, although extrarenal manifestations such as tuberculous epididymitis or back pain with retroperitoneal fibrosis may

TABLE 2. A Clinical Classification of the Causes of Chronic Renal Failure

1. *Local causes:*
   Diseases in which the kidneys are predominantly involved and in which the presenting features are usually those of renal disease
   - Proliferative glomerulonephritis
   - Membranous glomerulonephropathy
   - Chronic pyelonephritis
   - Tuberculous pyelonephritis
   - Renal calculi
   - Congenital nephritis
   - Polycystic disease
   - Medullary cystic disease
   - Renal hypoplasia
   - Renal tubular acidosis
   - Balkan nephropathy
   - Upper urinary tract obstruction
     - Hydronephrosis
     - Retroperitoneal fibrosis
     - Neoplasm

2. *Lower urinary tract obstruction:*
   Presenting features often those of bladder dysfunction, but may present in renal failure
   - Prostatic enlargement
     - Adenoma
     - Neoplasm
   - Urethral stricture
   - Urethral valves
   - Bladder neck obstruction
   - Neurogenic bladder

3. *Systemic diseases and intoxications:*
   a. In which renal failure is not infrequently a presenting feature
   - Malignant essential hypertension
   - Polyarteritis nodosa
   - Disseminated lupus erythematosus
   - Primary and secondary amyloidosis
   - Analgesic overconsumption
   - Potassium deficiency
   - Hypercalcemia
   - Cystinosis
   - Oxalosis
   - Consumption coagulopathies
     - Hemolytic-uremic syndrome
     - Thrombotic thrombocytopenic purpura
     - Postpartum renal failure
   - Lead or cadmium poisoning

   b. In which renal failure is usually a late feature or overshadowed by other manifestations
   - Benign essential hypertension
   - Atheroma
   - Systemic emboli
     - Subacute bacterial endocarditis
     - Rheumatic heart disease
   - Gout
   - Diabetes
   - Heart failure
   - Cirrhosis

provide a clue. Many diseases in Groups 2 and 3a will be identified by involvement of the bladder or of some other system, and most of those in Group 3b should be recognized readily from other features of the disease, although renal failure may occasionally be a presenting feature. If a full history and examination fail to reveal a systemic cause for chronic renal failure, the most likely possibilities are in Groups 1 and 3a.

Selection of the most appropriate diagnostic aids is helped by a knowledge of the relative frequency of the diseases listed in Table 2, some of which are rare. Unfortunately death certification statistics are not a reliable source of this information. They have been repeatedly contradicted by more accurate surveys of living patients, and they provide some information that stretches credulity. An example is shown in Figure 3. The data are from England and Wales, but the trends were observed in many developed countries. Between 1950 and 1966, the reported mortality from urinary infection trebled, and pyelonephritis appeared to displace glomerulonephritis as the leading renal cause of death. This seems improbable at a time when increasingly effective urinary antiseptics were introduced and there was no effective treatment for glomerulonephritis. The anomaly is partly explained by the changing age structure of the population; three quarters of all deaths from urinary infection, but only half those from nephritis and nephrosis, occur after the age of 65. However, the aging population alone cannot account for the dramatic changes reported. The main explanation is probably a change in habits of certification as doctors became more aware of chronic pyelonephritis after the introduction of midstream culture and the campaign against the catheter. The pendulum swung too far and pyelonephritis was overdiagnosed. It is now swinging back and has done so abruptly in Scotland, where a national survey of renal disease led to more accurate diagnosis from about 1969.

An alternative source of information is provided by the annual reports of the transplant and dialysis registries. They give little information on the extremes of life and they are subject to some selection, but they are our best guide to the incidence of disease in children and young and middle-aged adults. European statistics are quoted in Table 3, which shows the relative importance of the main disease in each group; American and Australasian experience is similar. Essential hypertension is certainly underrepresented in these statistics as a cause of renal failure. Malignant hypertension of rapid onset in young adults causes afferent arteriolar necrosis and renal failure, with kidneys of normal size which are not easily confused with those of glomerulonephritis. More slowly progressive severe hypertension causes medial and intimal thickening of interlobular arteries and hyaline degeneration of afferent arterioles which leads to diffuse scarring of the kidney. In its late stages this hypertensive nephrosclerosis may be difficult to distinguish from chronic glomerulonephritis with secondary hypertension. The effects of hypertension merge into those of atheroma, which frequently complicates hypertension but which also occurs in normotensive subjects. Atheroma of the renal arteries may cause renal hypertension, atheroembolism, or thrombosis with infarction,

TABLE 3. Main Causes of Renal Failure in Children and Young and Middle-Aged Adults*

	Adults (%)	Children (%)
Glomerulonephritis	55.7	52.1
Pyelonephritis	21.2	19.9
Polycystic disease	7.5	2.6
Renal vascular disease	4.4	2.0
Drug nephropathy	2.9	0.2
Congenital nephritis	1.5	6.2
Congenital hypoplasia	1.5	9.3
Other	5.3	7.7

*Data of the European Dialysis and Transplant Registry.

any of which will hasten the decline in renal function. Methods of data collection used by the renal registries discourage these diagnoses, and patients with hypertension or atheroma tend to be misclassified as having glomerulonephritis.

Gout does not figure individually in Table 3, although it is a fairly common disease which is usually accompanied by histologic damage in the kidney and which has been said to terminate in renal failure in 18 to 30 per cent of cases. This is an overstatement based on selected hospital patients. The very few patients with gout who reach dialysis and transplant units do so in middle age, usually beyond the age of 40.

INVESTIGATION OF CHRONIC RENAL DISEASE

Investigation has four objectives: recognition of the primary disease, assessment of the degree of renal failure, detection of any aggravating factors, and exploration of other medical and social problems which may have a bearing on the treatment of renal disease.

Recognition of the Primary Disease. It is the plea of every nephrologist that patients with chronic renal disease be referred early, when pyelography is particularly informative and renal biopsy can be performed without the hazards of uremia, hypertension, and small fibrotic kidneys. At this stage diagnosis of the primary renal disease is usually straightforward and worthwhile. When patients first present in established renal failure, exact diagnosis is more difficult. High-dose pyelography may still provide a good deal of information, but fine details of the calyceal pattern cannot be expected; if renal biopsy is performed, it may be difficult to interpret in an "end-stage kidney." Nonetheless, considerable information can still be obtained, and it is important, even in late renal failure, to recognize several reversible causes and some conditions which will influence later decisions about dialysis and transplantation. Correction of urinary obstruction, removal of calculi, and withdrawal of analgesics from patients with analgesic nephropathy may all arrest a decline in renal function and occasionally reverse it. Retroperitoneal fibrosis often improves, spontaneously or with steroid therapy, after withdrawal of methysergide and is also amenable to surgery. Lupus nephritis reponds to corticosteroid and other immunosuppressive agents, and gouty nephropathy may improve with allopurinol therapy. The demonstration of a normal bladder and competent ureterovesical valves is an important preliminary to transplant in patients with chronic pyelonephritis who may therefore require micturating cystography at a stage when surgery for reflux

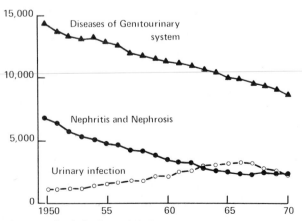

Figure 3. Crude death rate from diseases of the genitourinary tract in England and Wales (population approximately 50 million).

would not otherwise be contemplated. The recognition of oxalosis, cystinosis, and mesangiocapillary nephritis has important implications, because all may recur in a grafted kidney, whereas Fabry's disease may be a specific indication for transplantation, because it replaces the missing enzyme.

The *history* should include a lifelong survey of previous renal complaints, occupations, and drug consumption. Specific inquiry should be made about symptoms suggestive of urinary obstruction and the intake of analgesics, other phenacetin-containing drugs, and methysergide, because these are often overlooked by the patient. The family history should include specific inquiry about renal disease, hypertension and its sequelae, gout, collagenoses, preeclampsia, and deafness. Comprehensive history-taking is aided by a self-administered questionnaire; even experienced clinicians often omit vital questions when relying on memory alone. The facets of physical examination and general medical investigation that may be important compose most of the physician's repertoire. Among the physical signs that should be sought are those indicating longstanding uremia (skin pigmentation and excoriation, a brown arc under the nail margins, tissue-wasting, neuropathy), hypertension (retinopathy, cardiac enlargement), atheroma (peripheral pulses, murmurs in main vessels), disturbed calcium metabolism (band keratopathy, pseudoclubbing, proximal muscle weakness), and collagenoses (joint deformity, arteritic skin lesions).

Investigations should include qualitative tests for glycosuria and hematuria and a quantitative test for proteinuria; pH of early morning urine; urinary microscopy and midstream culture; plasma or serum urea, creatinine, sodium, potassium, chloride, bicarbonate, urate, calcium, phosphate, alkaline phosphatase, total protein, and electrophoresis; and straight roentgenography of the renal tract. Chest roentgenogram, electrocardiogram, serum magnesium, and creatinine clearance should also be included in the initial screening, but not for the sake of differential diagnosis. If the renal size is not obvious from the straight roentgenogram, it is often revealed by tomography. *High dose or infusion pyelography,* with *renal tomograms* and late films up to 24 hours, usually provides some information about the calyceal pattern down to a GFR of about 5 ml per minute and gives an idea of renal size, shape, and quantity of peripelvic fat down to a GFR of about 2 ml per minute. It is particularly helpful in the diagnosis of urinary obstruction and polycystic disease, even at a very late stage in renal failure.

Proteinuria exceeding 3 grams per 24 hours is unusual in chronic pyelonephritis, analgesic nephropathy, benign hypertension, urinary obstruction, calculous disease, renal tubular acidosis, and polycystic disease; it is usual or common in chronic proliferative glomerulonephritis, membranous glomerulonephropathy, amyloidosis, diabetic nephropathy, polyarteritis, disseminated lupus erythematosus, and malignant hypertension. Glomerular proteinuria diminishes as GFR falls, but heavy proteinuria may still be encountered in terminal renal failure, and the consequent derangements of plasma protein may persist for several weeks after the start of regular hemodialysis. Mild hypoproteinemia accompanies fluid overload in many forms of chronic renal disease, but severe hypoproteinemia (below 5 grams per 100 ml), particularly if accompanied by a nephrotic electrophoretic pattern and hypercholesterolemia, strongly suggests that heavy proteinuria was present in the recent past, even if it is no longer demonstrable.

Red cell *casts in the urinary deposit* in chronic renal failure suggest one of the progressive forms of glomerulonephritis (e.g., crescent nephritis, mesangiocapillary nephritis, the renal lesion of subacute bacterial endocarditis), including the collagenoses or malignant hypertension. Numerous dense granular casts are encountered in these conditions and in amyloidosis and diabetic nephropathy. They are seldom found in chronic pyelonephritis or analgesic nephropathy, in both of which an increased output of white cells is often the only abnormality of microscopy. Hyaline casts predominate in membranous glomerulonephropathy and benign essential hypertension.

Hyperchloremic acidosis accompanies urinary diversion into the bowel. If the lower urinary tract is intact, it should suggest chronic pyelonephritis, analgesic nephropathy, renal tubular acidosis, or polycystic disease, although it may be encountered in other renal diseases. *Hypercalcemia* is occasionally found in secondary hyperparathyroidism, but it should always raise the suspicion that the hypercalcemia is the cause of the renal failure and not vice versa. *Serum electrophoresis* and search for Bence Jones protein in urine will detect most examples of renal failure caused by myelomatosis, but specific immunologic tests for light chains are sometimes required. Immunoelectrophoresis may be required to demonstrate the monoclonal gammopathies that underlie most cases of "primary" renal amyloid—one of the diseases that most frequently elude detection until renal biopsy is performed.

Very large kidneys are typical of obstruction or polycystic disease. Renal failure with *kidneys of normal size* should always alert the clinician to the possibility of acute rather than chronic renal failure, although amyloidosis, crescent nephritis, and membranous glomerulonephropathy may all reach the end stage without much contraction of the kidney. *Small symmetrical kidneys* with preservation of the calyceal pattern are found in many chronic renal diseases, notably most forms of glomerulonephritis. Chronic pyelonephritis is confirmed by *asymmetrical and irregular scarring,* with clubbing and outdrawing of the calyces; in late renal failure, when calyceal detail is poor, a gross increase in peripelvic fat on the tomograms is a helpful sign. Typical findings in analgesic nephropathy are small kidneys with scalloped outlines—sometimes misinterpreted as fetal lobulation—and clubbed calyces corresponding to the sloughed papillae. Rare but diagnostic signs are calcification of papillae and encirclement of separated papillae by contrast medium ("ring sign"). The pyelogram may, however, remain normal until late in the disease. Passage of separated papillae causes attacks of renal colic and may permit firm diagnosis by histologic examination of a soft black "calculus."

Urinary *infection* is still present in about half the patients with chronic pyelonephritis currently seen in renal failure; it is also a common accompaniment of calculous disease, analgesic nephropathy, and lower urinary tract obstruction, but is probably no more common in other renal diseases than in the general population. Nonetheless, all patients with chronic renal disease should be screened for urinary infection by the culture of at least three midstream urines at a time when no antimicrobial drugs are being, or have recently been, administered.

Assessment of the Degree of Renal Failure. An initial measurement of GFR should be made by one of the techniques discussed in Ch. 602. Thereafter serial measurement of serum creatinine is the most useful and practical guide to changes in renal function.

Detection of Aggravating Factors. Glomerular filtration rate may be depressed by hypovolemia from renal sodium loss, vomiting and diarrhea, systemic infections, surgery, trauma, hemorrhage, urinary infection, sudden reduction of longstanding hypertension, rapid rise in blood pressure, and administration of nephrotoxic drugs. The production rate of urea and other metabolic end products may be increased by excessive protein intake, tissue wasting from starvation, infection, trauma and surgery, resorption of hematoma, bleeding into the gut, and administration of corticosteroids or tetracyclines.

These aggravating factors should be sought and corrected in every patient seen for the first time in chronic renal failure, and no subsequent deterioration should be blamed on the primary disease until they have been excluded as contributory factors. When doubt exists, the patient should be kept alive for several weeks, if necessary by peritoneal dialysis or hemodialysis, to provide time for investigation and for his recovery from complications.

Investigation of Other Medical and Social Problems. This is an essential part of the management of any chronic disease, but it is particularly important in chronic renal failure because regular dialysis and transplantation place heavy demands on the patient's physical and social resources. A full social report should be carried out at the time of diagnosis and updated as the need for dialysis becomes imminent, so that such factors as rehousing and home adaptations can be planned well in advance. Family planning should be discussed and sterilization procedures carried out before advanced renal failure adds to their hazards; they are best performed on the affected partner in young couples, because five-year survival on dialysis and transplantation is still of the order of 70 to 80 per cent, so remarriage of the unaffected partner is a considerable possibility. A dental survey should be arranged so that extractions can be performed before intermittent anticoagulation and immunosuppressive therapy become necessary, and regular conservative dental care should be maintained thereafter. Indigestion should be thoroughly investigated and surgery for peptic ulcer considered before transplantation makes corticosteroid therapy essential.

As renal failure advances, regular search should be carried out for the complications discussed below, notably hypertension and its sequelae, neuropathy, myopathy and encephalopathy, pericarditis, bone disease, anemia, sexual dysfunction, and electrolyte disturbances. This tedious and repetitive work can be aided by regular completion of a self-administered questionnaire and a structured physical examination and biochemical screen, guided by a checklist. A problem-oriented summary of all the medical and social problems in the front of the case record is an invaluable adjunct to management.

THE PATHOPHYSIOLOGY OF CHRONIC RENAL FAILURE

Chronically diseased kidneys often support life in comfort until about 90 per cent of their glomerular filtration has been lost, and they maintain some sort of life until 97 to 99 per cent has gone. This statement applies to most of the conditions listed in Table 2 and is the justification for considering them together. It implies that even in the late stages of disease the kidneys retain some ability to respond to the demands of the body by varying the output of water and important solutes. The most popular explanation for this response of the diseased kidney to physiologic stimuli is the "intact nephron hypothesis."

According to this theory the deformed nephrons seen in histologic preparations and nephron dissections are largely nonfunctional; excretory function is maintained by a remnant of surviving nephrons in which both glomerulus and tubule have escaped irreparable damage. In these nephrons the glomerulus produces an increased volume of glomerular filtrate. Hypertrophy of the tubule enables it to handle this extra filtrate within limits, but the additional solute load causes an osmotic diuresis which has the same effects as a saline or urea diuresis in the normal subject. Urine is produced at a nearly constant rate throughout the 24 hours, at an osmolality which is eventually fixed around 300 mOsm per kilogram (specific gravity, SG, about 1.010) — a state referred to as isosthenuria. This condition becomes established only when the GFR is reduced to about a quarter of normal. It results in nocturia, one of the most common symptoms of early renal failure (but one which often fails to alert the patient to his condition; the accompanying polyuria leads to thirst, and the nocturia is blamed on an increased consumption of fluid in the evenings).

There is substantial evidence in support of the intact nephron hypothesis, and the events outlined in the preceding paragraph probably underlie most of the adaptations to chronic renal failure. However, there are important exceptions. The grotesquely deformed nephrons of polycystic disease retain some excretory function, and the same may apply to other renal diseases. Those conditions in which medullary damage is a prominent feature — particularly chronic pyelonephritis, analgesic nephropathy, and medullary cystic disease — are often characterized by severe polyuria with hypotonic urine, suggesting that many functioning nephrons have lost their concentrating mechanism, and there is other evidence of impaired distal tubular function in these patients. At the other end of the scale are diseases such as rapidly progressive nephritis, in which glomerular damage is widespread and roughly uniform in time, which do not pass through an isosthenuric phase, so that patients may enter the terminal stage of renal failure without ever having experienced nocturia.

Water. Polyuria commonly accompanies isosthenuria. It reaches a peak while the GFR is declining through the range 25 to 5 ml per minute, then gives way to oliguria in the preterminal phase of chronic renal failure, except in a minority of patients with predominant medullary damage who remain polyuric to the end. Thirst is a constant accompaniment of polyuria, and if the patient has free access to water he will usually maintain his water balance with reasonable accuracy. The once popular practice of "pushing fluids" to reduce the plasma urea is unnecessary and potentially dangerous. Thirst is sometimes excessive, because dryness of the mouth is common in late renal failure. This symptom is occasionally due to overbreathing from acidosis, but is usually the result of an unexplained reduction in salivary flow.

Large water loads are excreted more slowly than in

the normal subject; hyponatremia follows their ingestion for several hours; convulsions are occasionally precipitated. Conversely, obligatory water loss through the kidneys is increased, and patients are therefore sensitive to water deprivation, caused by drowsiness or vomiting.

Sodium. The excretion of most solutes can only be varied over a restricted range in renal failure. The patient remains in reasonable health if his intake is adjusted to the ability of his kidneys to excrete, but he faces trouble if it is close to one of the extremes tolerated by normal persons. The hormonal mechanisms which maintain sodium homeostasis in health with remarkably little change in extracellular fluid (ECF) volume become inadequate as renal function declines. Changes in sodium intake produce alterations in ECF, and plasma volume and fluctuations in GFR acquire an important role in sodium homeostasis. A patient with chronic renal failure placed on a very low sodium diet, e.g., the traditional 22 mEq per day, is often unable to reduce his sodium output by hormonal control alone because of the osmotic diuresis in his surviving nephrons. He goes into negative sodium balance and excretes a corresponding volume of water; his extracellular fluid volume, plasma volume, and GFR all fall. This reduces the osmotic load per nephron and permits more avid sodium retention. Sodium balance is re-established at the price of some decline in glomerular filtration rate.

If the patient is now placed on a high-sodium intake, he passes into positive sodium balance, retaining water in proportion, expanding his extracellular fluid volume, and raising his GFR. This increases the osmotic load per nephron until sodium output again equals intake. This new equilibrium is achieved at the price of an expanded extracellular fluid volume, which may be detectable as peripheral or pulmonary edema and which is often interpreted by the clinician as heart failure. Quite often, however, several liters of tissue fluid are accommodated without overt edema; the overloaded subcutaneous tissue conceals the wasting of muscle and fat characteristic of chronic renal failure, giving the patient a false appearance of adequate nutrition, which is rapidly corrected when his surplus fluid is removed at the start of regular dialysis.

A fortunate minority of patients remain normotensive even when grossly edematous, but the majority develop hypertension when their ECF is overexpanded. In the animal with experimental chronic renal failure, the initial event is a rise in cardiac output followed by a compensatory increase in peripheral resistance and a fall in cardiac output; there is accumulating evidence that this sequence of events is followed in man. Soon after the hypertension develops, the events can be reversed by removing the surplus ECF and preventing its reaccumulation by dietary restriction. This is the treatment employed when the patient becomes dependent on regular hemodialysis. Control of hypertension may be followed by the disappearance of any remaining excretory function, which is unimportant at this juncture. At an earlier stage in renal failure the same control of blood pressure can often be achieved with diuretics and low sodium diet, but at the cost of some reduction of GFR. There is therefore no ideal sodium intake for an individual in chronic renal failure; he must often choose between being normovolemic and normotensive with a low GFR or edematous and hypertensive with a higher GFR. In those countries where the majority of young and middle-aged patients will be offered dialysis and transplanta-

tion, it is better to err on the side of sacrificing GFR to blood pressure control; a well-preserved vascular tree is a much better asset than a few extra months of conservative treatment of renal failure.

As GFR declines to a few milliliters per minute, the proportion of filtered sodium excreted in the urine must rise if sodium balance is to be maintained. The normal subject excretes only about 1 per cent of his filtered sodium, but in terminal renal failure some patients lose about 30 per cent of the filtered sodium in their urine—about the same as a normal subject under maximal osmotic diuresis. However, a substantial proportion are unable to approach this theoretic maximum, and they can be maintained in sodium balance only by severe dietary restriction or high-dose diuretic therapy. Their hypertension is accordingly difficult to control, and regular hemodialysis may be required for control of blood pressure before being required on other grounds. Low sodium dieting in this group can be inadvertently vitiated by the use of medicines; indigestion mixtures and antidiarrheal preparations, e.g., magnesium trisilicate mixture NF and kaolin and morphine mixture NF, are the main offenders, providing 20 to 40 mEq of sodium per day at standard dosage.

At the other extreme a minority of patients excrete a high proportion of their filtered sodium even in early renal failure, and are liable to become sodium depleted if they fail to keep up a high dietary intake. The condition is sometimes referred to as "salt-losing nephritis," but it is not a separate pathologic entity. The syndrome may be encountered in analgesic nephropathy, polycystic disease, or occasionally chronic pyelonephritis. The most common cause in childhood and early adult life is probably medullary cystic disease. The patients are often pigmented and may be thought to have Addison's disease. A helpful point in differentiation is the almost invariable presence of hyperchloremic acidosis in those with renal disease. Most of these patients are normotensive and tolerate dietary sodium supplements (usually as sodium bicarbonate or citrate, liberal condiment, and slow-release sodium tablets) without trouble. Postural hypotension is an early sign of inadequate sodium intake, and hypertension or edema indicates an excess. A few unfortunate patients live on a knife edge between sodium depletion and overload, and require careful control. Sodium depletion makes the patient unduly susceptible to potassium intoxication.

Potassium. Hypokalemia is found in a minority of patients with early renal failure. It is usually caused by diuretic therapy, diarrhea, vomiting, or purgation, but is sometimes due to spontaneous potassium loss in the urine. In a very few patients potassium loss is sufficient to cause severe hypokalemia and muscular paralysis. The condition has been called "potassium-losing nephritis," but is not a separate disease; it is an unusual manifestation of chronic pyelonephritis, renal tubular acidosis, ureterosigmoid anastomosis, and very occasionally other renal diseases. Excessive sodium and calcium loss in the urine sometimes coexist. When the potassium leak is an isolated defect, differentiation from Conn's syndrome can be difficult; a hyperchloremic acidosis strongly suggests a renal cause and a complete response to spironolactone an aldosteronoma, but diagnosis has sometimes awaited adrenal exploration.

During most of the course of renal failure most patients maintain normal plasma potassium, and their potassium excretion varies with their intake. As renal failure advances, potassium excretion may exceed the filtered potassium, presumably as a result of increased exchange for sodium in the distal tubule aided by the osmotic diuresis. However, the maximal capacity to excrete potassium is impaired even in early renal failure. An oral or intravenous dose causes an excessive rise in plasma potassium, which is corrected only over an extended period. Dangerous hyperkalemia may therefore follow endogenous release of potassium after hemolysis, trauma, or infection, or its administration medicinally or in stored blood. Deaths have resulted from the use of potassium citrate in chronic urinary infection (in which it is of doubtful value), and care must be exercised in prescribing potassium supplements, amiloride, and spironolactone during diuretic therapy.

Hyperkalemia is common in terminal renal failure; at this stage even dietary ingestion of excess potassium as instant coffee, fruit, fried potatoes, meat, and meat products can be hazardous. Occasional patients complain of muscle weakness or paresthesias when the plasma potassium reaches dangerous levels (over 7 mEq per liter), but the majority are unaware of the condition until cardiac arrest occurs. The only warning signs are those detected by electrocardiography—flattened P wave, widened QRS complex, and peaked T wave.

In patients with a potassium leak, hypokalemia usually reflects severe depletion of total body potassium, but in other situations in renal failure the plasma level is not a reliable guide to body stores. Plasma potassium rises in acidosis and falls rapidly when this is corrected with sodium bicarbonate, without appreciable change in body potassium. Some hyperkalemic patients in terminal renal failure or on regular dialysis have diminished total body potassium, but this may be a reflection of reduced muscle mass rather than cellular potassium deficiency and is not to be regarded as an indication for potassium therapy.

Magnesium. Mild asymptomatic hypomagnesemia is not uncommon in early renal failure. It is due to an increased fecal loss which is accentuated by high calcium diet, because calcium and magnesium compete for the same absorptive mechanism. Hypomagnesemia of more than slight degree is usually due to diuretic therapy.

For most of the course of renal failure serum magnesium is usually normal, but hypermagnesemia appears with increasing frequency when the GFR falls below 30 ml per minute, and is the rule in terminal renal failure. Serum magnesium rises in the presence of acidosis or tissue trauma and is increased by the administration of vitamin D or its analogues; very high levels (over 3.5 mEq per liter) are nearly always due to administration of magnesium salts as antacids, purgatives, or enemas (magnesium is well absorbed from the colon). Little is known about total body magnesium in chronic renal failure, but severe magnesium depletion has been reported in the presence of hypermagnesemia.

Spontaneous hypermagnesemia impairs nerve conduction time but probably plays no part in the development of neuropathy and may even protect against it; it is probably not responsible for any of the symptoms of renal failure. The very high levels (3.5 to over 8 mEq per liter) that have followed magnesium medication or the use of hard water for hemodialysis have produced drowsiness, light coma, muscle weakness, and skin irritation.

Hydrogen Ion. Nonrespiratory acidosis virtually always develops during the progression of chronic renal failure, though it can be reversed temporarily by vomiting. In patients without predominant medullary damage it becomes pronounced only after the GFR falls below about 20 ml per minute. A renal bicarbonate leak can be demonstrated in many patients with chronic renal failure when their plasma bicarbonate level is restored to normal with sodium bicarbonate. When the bicarbonate infusion is stopped, renal excretion of bicarbonate continues until the plasma bicarbonate falls again to its previous level. This resetting of the plasma level at which a bicarbonate leak occurs is also encountered in primary hyperparathyroidism, and it has been attributed to hypersecretion of parathyroid hormone in renal failure.

As renal acidosis progresses, urine becomes more acid, eventually reaching a pH of about 5—close to the minimum achieved by normal subjects after acid loading. This does not imply normal urinary acidification, as the patient achieves this urine pH at a much lower plasma bicarbonate level than normal. Moreover he excretes a considerably smaller quantity of hydrogen ion at any given urinary pH than normal. This is mainly due to a defect in ammonia production shown by a lower excretion of ammonium. Titratable acidity is normal or slightly reduced for the urine pH, because the main buffers (monohydrogen phosphate and creatinine) are excreted in nearly normal amount until late in renal failure.

It is now possible to calculate with fair accuracy the hydrogen ion produced by a stated diet. It is derived mainly from the oxidation of sulfur-containing amino acids to sulfuric acid, the hydrolysis of phosphate esters to phosphoric acid, the metabolism of purines to uric acid, and the production of intermediary acids during carbohydrate metabolism. Balance studies show that patients in renal failure excrete only about three quarters of their acid production, retaining 10 to 20 mEq of hydrogen ion per day. In spite of this, their plasma bicarbonate level changes very slowly; the extra acid is believed to be neutralized by calcium carbonate in bone. This probably accounts in part for the negative calcium balance in renal failure, and may be a factor in the genesis of renal bone disease.

Respiratory compensation for the acidosis occurs in a predictable manner if there is no lung disease, the uremic subject behaving in the same manner as a normal subject ingesting ammonium chloride. Pa_{CO_2} falls by about 1.2 mm Hg for every 1 mEq per liter fall in plasma bicarbonate. This does not completely correct the blood pH, which falls in a roughly linear relationship to the plasma bicarbonate, reaching the lower limit of normal (7.35) when the plasma bicarbonate is about 15 mEq per liter. In terminal renal failure the plasma bicarbonate falls below 10 mEq per liter and there is deep sighing (Kussmaul) respiration which produces a low Pa_{CO_2}, but blood pH is well below the normal range. Any interference with respiratory compensation by chest infection, pulmonary edema, heavy sedation, or coma leads to a rapid increase in the acidosis, and the plasma bicarbonate then ceases to be a reliable guide to the severity of the condition.

Rapid correction of extracellular acidosis by fast hemodialysis or infusion of sodium bicarbonate is followed by a respiratory alkalosis which persists for up to 24 hours. Bicarbonate diffuses slowly into the CSF, which therefore remains acid and continues to stimulate the respiratory centers on the anterior surface of the medulla, inappropriately lowering the Pa_{CO_2}.

The *genetic forms of renal tubular acidosis* have been divided into a *proximal type,* usually found in infants and caused by incomplete reabsorption of bicarbonate in the proximal tubule, and a *distal type,* caused by inability of the distal tubule to maintain a low pH. In both types, urinary pH remains high (typically over 6.0) in the presence of an acidosis. A distal type of renal tubular acidosis is found in analgesic nephropathy, some cases of chronic pyelonephritis, calculous disease, and polycystic disease, and as a manifestation of tubular damage in Sjögren's syndrome, disseminated lupus, and amyloidosis. Both proximal and distal tubular types are encountered after renal transplantation. In these diseases urinary pH remains higher than in other renal disease at the same level of GFR. The fall in plasma bicarbonate is then accompanied by a rise in plasma chloride which may exceed 110 mEq per liter. Presumably when there is a reduced bicarbonate concentration in glomerular filtrate, some other anion must be reabsorbed with sodium; in early renal failure the readily available anion is chloride. Hyperchloremic acidosis therefore indicates impairment of hydrogen ion excretion greater than would be expected from loss of nephrons alone. A striking hyperchloremic acidosis is found after urinary diversion into the bowel, particularly the sigmoid colon, and is attributed to the action of bowel mucosa on retained urine, compounding the effect of the commonly associated pyelonephritis. When acidosis develops late in renal failure, plasma chloride is usually normal or depressed, the anion concentration being made up by retained sulfate and phosphate.

Calcium and Plasma Phosphate. Renal *calcium excretion* falls early in renal failure, before there is any drop in serum calcium, probably as a reflection of the fall in GFR. However, tubular reabsorption also decreases so that calcium excretion declines more slowly than GFR. In very early renal failure, intestinal absorption of calcium is normal; but as the GFR falls below about half normal, intestinal absorption is progressively impaired, and in late renal failure there may be net intestinal excretion of calcium. At this stage urinary calcium excretion has usually fallen to less than 100 mg per day, but over-all negative calcium balance is usual and is not corrected by regular hemodialysis, in spite of the absence of urinary excretion, unless calcium is effectively infused into the patient by the use of a high calcium dialysate. Positive calcium balance can be restored by the administration of *vitamin D* (1 to 2.5 mg per 24 hours) or its metabolites and analogues *25-hydroxycholecalciferol, 1-alpha-hydroxycholecalciferol* (up to 5 μg per 24 hours), or *dihydrotachysterol* (0.25 mg per 24 hours) by mouth. The natural hormone 1,25-dihydroxycholecalciferol is poorly absorbed by mouth but readily restores positive calcium balance in a dose of 1 to 3 μg per 24 hours by injection. These more potent derivatives of vitamin D are increasingly used in place of the parent compound because they are less subject to storage in body fat and to the "therapeutic overshoot" that results with vitamin D. Normal calcium balance is restored by renal transplantation if renal function is close to normal and steroid therapy is not excessive.

Serum calcium declines in late renal failure, often reaching 6 mg and occasionally 4 mg per 100 ml, when cataract formation is a hazard. The proportion of total serum calcium which is ionized and complexed is increased so that ultrafilterable calcium remains close to normal until serum calcium is depressed below about 8 mg per 100 ml. Even in the presence of very low serum calcium, which must be accompanied by a fall in ionized calcium, tetany is unusual in renal failure. It may be precipitated by the infusion or ingestion of sodium bicarbonate or lactate to correct acidosis, and may then be accompanied by grand mal seizures. However, the common forms of muscle cramp, muscle twitching, and convulsion seen in terminal uremia are probably not related to the serum calcium, and are seldom alleviated by calcium infusion.

Hypercalciuria accompanying the hypercalcemia of parathyroid adenoma, sarcoidosis, and hypervitaminosis D disappears when renal failure develops, but the hypercalciuria of renal tubular acidosis, medullary cystic disease, and other tubular disorders may persist in the presence of renal failure. A high urinary calcium is also found in a minority of patients with medullary damage, usually in association with a sodium leak.

Plasma phosphate remains in the normal range until the GFR has fallen to about 30 ml per minute. This is the result of a normal urinary phosphate excretion in the face of a falling GFR, probably owing to the elevated plasma parathormone level, which in late renal failure reaches about ten times the normal level. The rise in plasma phosphate which occurs in late renal failure bears no constant relationship to the simultaneous changes in serum calcium. Patients on regular hemodialysis maintain nearly stable serum calcium in the face of wide fluctuations in plasma phosphate, and those receiving vitamin D may experience a simultaneous rise in plasma phosphate and serum calcium.

Bone Disease. Bone disease is a clinical problem to about 5 per cent of patients reaching the end stage of chronic renal failure, but radiologic abnormalities can be detected in 30 per cent, and bone histology is abnormal in 90 per cent. Growing children are more susceptible than adults to the development of symptomatic bone disease, and it was in adolescents that "renal rickets" was originally described in the last century. The term is a misnomer, because the resemblance to nutritional rickets is only superficial; bone histology reveals a mixed picture of osteitis fibrosa and impaired ossification of cartilage, with the former often predominating even though radiograms resemble those of rickets. Until recently it was believed that osteomalacia developed early in renal failure to be replaced at a later stage by osteitis fibrosa. It is now apparent that osteitis fibrosa is an almost invariable accompaniment of chronic renal failure unless special measures have been taken to prevent it, whereas osteomalacia develops only in a minority of patients, particularly those with slowly progressive renal failure caused by obstructive uropathy, chronic pyelonephritis, renal hypoplasia, and analgesic nephropathy. It is uncertain whether the underlying disease is important in any other respect, but it has been pointed out that these are diseases with a particular proneness to acidosis.

Secondary hyperparathyroidism, shown by proliferation of both osteoclasts and osteoblasts, scalloping, and bone marrow fibrosis, correlates well with the size and cellularity of the parathyroid glands and with the circulating level of parathyroid hormone. Only when histologic changes are severe do the radiologic signs appear—subperiosteal erosions, best seen in the phalanges; "rugger jersey" spine (density of the upper and lower margins of the vertebrae); "pepper pot" skull, and erosion of the outer ends of the clavicles. Bone pain and pathologic fractures are unusual until radiologic change is far advanced. Metastatic calcification occurs, first in the larger vessels, and then in small peripheral vessels, periarticular tissues, and skin. Rarely an ischemic myopathy results from vascular calcification. Metastatic calcification in the cornea produces band keratopathy, best seen with a slit lamp but often visible with the +30 lens of the ophthalmoscope when viewing from the side. "Red eye"—irritation and conjunctivitis—may accompany conjunctival calcification but is an inconstant symptom.

The main stimulus to the parathyroid glands is phosphate retention which probably acts by temporarily depressing plasma ionized calcium. Plasma parathyroid hormone concentration can be restored to normal and osteitis fibrosa healed by dietary phosphate restriction or administration of aluminum hydroxide gel by mouth. Excessive use of the latter can cause phosphate depletion and produce osteomalacia. Suppression of hyperparathyroidism is aided by administration of oral calcium carbonate (1 to 2 grams, three times a day), but in combination with aluminum hydroxide it readily produces hypercalcemia. Metastatic calcification occurs particularly when the $Ca \times P$ concentration product exceeds 70, so regular estimation of serum calcium and phosphate is essential during such manipulations. Serum alkaline phosphatase and hydroxyproline are consistently raised in secondary hyperparathyroidism.

Regular hemodialysis has a variable effect on hyperparathyroidism. In some medical centers the disease slowly heals; in others it progresses, the difference probably reflecting the enthusiasm with which plasma phosphate levels are controlled. After renal transplantation, hyperparathyroidism resolves over a period of 6 to 12 months on biochemical and radiologic criteria, provided that renal function is satisfactory. In a few patients there is persistent hypercalcemia which has been attributed to autonomous "tertiary" hyperparathyroidism. A more likely explanation is that very large parathyroid glands involute slowly, and while they remain large they are not as readily suppressed as normal glands.

Pruritus is common in patients with hyperparathyroidism and is attributed to calcium phosphate deposition in skin. It sometimes resolves with control of plasma phosphate and is regularly relieved by parathyroidectomy.

Osteomalacia is uncommon in the United States but a major problem in some centers in Britain, particularly after the start of regular dialysis. The difference is probably due to variations in sunshine exposure and vitamin D intake which produce borderline vitamin D deficiency in northern Britain in winter. Even though the damaged kidneys cannot make 1,25-dihydroxycholecalciferol, the accumulation of the precursor 25-hydroxycholecalciferol has some antirachitic action and probably protects patients with a high intake or production of vitamin D. Looser zones and pathologic fractures are much more common in osteomalacia than in osteitis fibrosa, and bone pain is a more prominent symptom. Proximal muscle weakness (myopathy) is commonly present.

Osteosclerosis is often shown by bone biopsy on a membrane bone such as the iliac crest and is occasionally seen on radiograms. Since the patients are in negative calcium balance, the sclerosis is presumably caused by redistribution of bone. During regular dialysis there is often a very rapid loss of skeletal calcium, and osteosclerosis rapidly gives way to osteoporosis.

All the lesions of renal osteodystrophy—osteitis fibrosa, osteomalacia, osteosclerosis, and osteoporosis—can occur simultaneously or successively in the same patient.

Trace Elements. Regular hemodialysis has permitted study of the role of trace elements in the manifestations of renal failure. Many trace elements are present in tap water, and they may accumulate in anuric patients exposed to large volumes of dialysis fluid made from raw water. Fatal copper poisoning has resulted from solution of copper pipes by acid dialysis fluid, and zinc uptake has resulted from the use of zinc oxide plaster on coils. During renal failure plasma fluoride may rise to two or three times the range for normal subjects in areas where tap water is fluoridated, and it rises to about 100 times the control value after some years of regular dialysis in these areas. An association with renal bone disease in dialyzed patients has been suggested, but the evidence is not conclusive.

Sulfate. Sulfate is produced from the metabolism of sulfur-containing amino acids and is therefore in approximate proportion to protein ingestion. The plasma sulfate level rises as GFR declines, roughly parallel with plasma urea. Sulfate retention is not the direct cause of any known symptom of renal failure.

Urea and Ammonia. *Urea* diffuses into all body secretions. If the plasma level is very high, it occasionally crystallizes out of sweat, leaving "urea frost" on the skin. The breakdown of urea to ammonia in a dry and crusted mouth is probably the cause of the unpleasant taste and "uremic odor" of terminal renal failure.

In normal subjects about 20 per cent of the daily production of urea is secreted into the gut and broken down by bacteria to ammonia and carbon dioxide. The *ammonia* is reabsorbed and resynthesized into urea in the liver. In chronic renal failure the proportion of urea production removed extrarenally may rise as high as 80 per cent; most of this is probably broken down and resynthesized to urea, as in the normal person. However, ammonia can be used as a substrate for the synthesis of amino acids, and a patient in renal failure who has an adequate supply of essential amino acids, but an over-all protein deficiency, will utilize a considerable proportion of the ammonia released in his gut for protein synthesis; this observation is the basis of the Giordano-Giovannetti dietary regimen. Even in terminal renal failure the large supply of ammonia from the gut does not elevate the blood ammonia level of peripheral blood, which is usually subnormal. However, simultaneous hepatic and renal failure cause a rapid rise in blood ammonia and the early onset of coma.

Urea was long regarded as nontoxic, but the Giovannetti diet, which reduces plasma urea without much change in other plasma constituents, relieves nausea, vomiting, and diarrhea and raises the hemoglobin level. Ammonia released by bacteria from urea in the gastrointestinal tract has been blamed for vomiting, hematemesis, and uremic ulceration of the gut, but there are alternative explanations for these symptoms and signs.

Uric Acid. A rise in plasma urate level begins very early in chronic renal disease, but it is so slight that the level becomes consistently abnormal only when the GFR falls to about 15 ml per minute. This stability of the plasma urate in the face of a normal production rate and a declining GFR is the result of increased distal tubular secretion of urate and increased uricolysis in the gut. In late renal failure there is a further increase in fractional urate clearance so that plasma urate rises less steeply than plasma urea or creatinine. Levels at least as high as those in gout are often encountered in terminal renal failure, but secondary gout is rare except in lead nephropathy, obstructive uropathy, and analgesic nephropathy, or during regular dialysis. Urate crystals are often found in the kidneys of patients with secondary hyperuricemia, and may accelerate the decline in renal function.

Plasma urate correlates much better than plasma urea with the onset of uremic pericarditis, but urate crystals are not found in the inflamed pericardium, and pericarditis is a rare complication of primary gout.

Carbohydrate. More than 50 per cent of patients in late renal failure have *glucose intolerance* as severe as in mild diabetes but with a normal fasting blood dextrose and often without glycosuria. It is not a cause of symptoms unless a large dose of glucose is administered during intravenous therapy, peritoneal dialysis, or hemodialysis, when severe hyperglycemia can be provoked. Fructose, galactose, and sorbitol tolerance are normal, showing that there is no defect in hepatic glycogenesis. Plasma insulin levels are appropriate to blood sugars, or nearly so, and there is a reduced response to injected insulin, implying peripheral antagonism to insulin action. Plasma growth hormone levels are usually normal, and potassium deficiency is only occasionally implicated. Glucose tolerance returns to normal after one or two weeks of adequate dialysis, suggesting the presence of a dialyzable insulin antagonist.

Lipids. Total plasma lipids are raised in late renal failure, mainly owing to a rise in triglycerides; phospholipids and cholesterol are normal or slightly elevated. There is a consistent rise in pre-β lipoproteins. More striking elevation in plasma lipids is found in those who remain nephrotic in renal failure. Hyperlipidemia may act synergistically with hypertension to produce a high incidence of atheroma in older patients with renal failure.

Other Compounds Implicated in Uremia. "Uremia" comprises those symptoms and signs of renal failure which are not explained by water and electrolyte imbalance or hypertension. Most of these features correlate only approximately with the plasma levels of urea, creatinine, uric acid, and other substances that have been thoroughly investigated. Current contenders for the role of "uremic toxins" include *guanidines, amines,* and *phenolic acids.* They are difficult to measure accurately, and it is uncertain whether they correlate with symptoms any more closely than urea, but some of them, e.g., methylamine and methylguanidine, produce convulsions, coma, vomiting, and other uremic symptoms in laboratory animals at concentrations found in uremic plasma. "Middle molecules"—substances of molecular weight 300 to 1800, probably predominantly polypeptides—accumulate in patients on regular hemodialysis, as they are poorly dialyzable through conventional membranes, but they are also present in excess in untreated uremia. They have been blamed for some of the features of renal failure, notably neuropathy and encephalopathy, but without conclusive proof.

Many of the symptoms of renal failure are mimicked by the side effects of drugs that accumulate when GFR is depressed. The claims that "the best thing you can do for a uremic is to stop all his drugs" has a germ of truth.

CLINICAL FEATURES OF RENAL FAILURE AND THEIR TREATMENT

Plan of Management in Irreversible Renal Failure

Patients without extensive vascular disease and with no systemic disease which threatens life should receive conservative management on a moderately restricted (40-gram protein) diet until the first incapacitating symptoms of uremia begin to appear or until working time is lost—usually when the GFR is around 5 ml per minute. Regular hemodialysis should then be instituted until a well-matched cadaver transplant is available. If this plan is followed, these patients sacrifice a few months of independence in increasing discomfort, but escape most of the clinical features listed below and should require therapy only for hypertension and, in some cases, bone disease. Their treatment must be planned well in advance of the crises. An arteriovenous fistula should be inserted many months before it is required so that it is available for dialysis during intercurrent illness and is well developed when required. The blood group, tissue type, and calculated chance of a well matched cadaver donor should be recorded on the case record, because they influence decisions such as the choice of home or hospital dialysis. Home adaptations should be completed before training begins so that a minimum of time is lost from work; the uremic patient has a precarious hold on his employment. The following description applies mainly to those patients for whom definitive treatment is not available.

Skin. Pruritus is common and often distressing. It is particularly associated with secondary hyperparathyroidism, but occurs in the absence of radiologic bone disease; it is sometimes caused by sensitivity to *Candida albicans.* The skin is often dry, flaky, and affected by erythematous and maculopapular rashes which become excoriated with scratching. Pigmentation, which is common in slowly progressive renal failure, is due to melanin and urochromes.

Itching occasionally responds to oral aluminum hydroxide gel. Phenothiazine antipruritics are not very effective, and their cumulation in renal failure causes mental blunting and parkinsonism; oculogyric crises are sometimes misinterpreted as uremic fits. Hydrocortisone cream is useful in areas of skin rash.

Gastrointestinal Tract. Dry mouth, metallic taste, and uremic odor can be helped a little by chewing gum. Anorexia is a common early symptom, progressing to nausea and vomiting. Vomiting is sometimes effortless and unexpected, but in the terminal stage continuous dry retching becomes a distressing feature. The disorder responds to the Giovannetti diet, provided that an anorexic patient can be persuaded to eat it. Preliminary treatment with peritoneal dialysis and intravenous feeding may be required until appetite returns. Antiemetics are of little value in restoring appetite, but they do have a role in controlling the retching of terminal uremics for whom no better treatment is available. Metoclopramide, 10 mg, or prochlorperazine, 10 mg, three times a day may be tried orally, but can be given intramuscularly in the same dosage if necessary. Thiethylperazine, 10 mg, can be given as a suppository. In the last resort, stupor caused by large doses of chlorpromazine is preferable to continuous retching.

Diarrhea is often described as a feature of chronic

renal failure, but it is seldom encountered before the very last stages of the illness unless produced by antihypertensives, antimicrobial drugs, or the high vegetable content of some Giovannetti diets. Constipation is a much more common complaint.

There is probably an increased incidence of hematemesis and melena in uremic patients even before they are subjected to intermittent anticoagulation for hemodialysis. Autopsy used to reveal ulceration of nasopharynx, mouth, stomach, or bowel in about a quarter of all uremics, but these features are now uncommon.

Nutrition and Growth. Anorexia and vomiting cause inadequate caloric intake, leading to wasting of fat and muscle. Dry, straggly, and depigmented hair is common in malnourished uremics. Gain of weight and improvement in hair texture occur during adequate hemodialysis and, to a lesser extent, during successful Giovannetti dieting.

Children with a GFR below about 20 per cent of normal have impairment of growth and are often below the third percentile for height. Bone age is retarded, and a late growth spurt may occur during adequate dialysis or after transplantation. Loss of height is often accentuated by bone bending owing to renal rickets. Bone growth and gain in height are promoted by high caloric feeding.

Endocrine Function. The onset of puberty is delayed by several years in children with renal insufficiency. In adults, libido and potency decline in the last few months of the illness in males. Libido is depressed, ovulation suppressed, and amenorrhea common in females. However, contraception is advisable, because pregnancy can occur late in renal failure, and is associated with decline in renal function, increased hypertension, slow fetal growth, and high fetal mortality. As a general guide, pregnancy is hazardous and unlikely to produce a live child if the plasma urea is consistently raised on a normal diet and hypertension is present in the first trimester. It is usually uneventful for mother and child if the renal disease is static or slowly progressive and the plasma urea and the blood pressure are normal at the start of pregnancy. Immunologic tests for pregnancy often give false positives in the presence of proteinuria.

Hypertension. Hypertension develops at some stage in more than 80 per cent of patients with chronic renal failure. It is associated with sodium and water retention; plasma renin is usually normal except in malignant hypertension. The complications are similar to those of any type of hypertension, but a malignant phase and resistance to drug therapy are more common in renal failure. After the primary disease, hypertension is the most important determinant of survival; it leads to a vicious spiral of declining renal function, further sodium retention, and rising blood pressure. The aim of treatment should be the restoration of normal blood pressure in all postures. This demands persistence and close supervision — weekly outpatient visits for many months in resistant cases.

Methyldopa is a common first choice, in a starting dose of 250 mg twice daily increased every few days. Side effects appear at a lower dose in renal failure than in essential hypertension as it is partly dependent on renal excretion, and depression and drowsiness are common if the dose exceeds 2 grams per day. Many patients are uncontrolled by this dose and require one of the sympathetic blockers — bethanidine, debrisoquine, or guanethidine — all in an initial dose of 10 mg daily and with increments every few days. These drugs all produce incapacitating postural and exercise hypotension if supine blood pressure is restored to normal. It is a salutary experience to check blood pressure of the patient supine, standing, and after exercise at each examination.

Propranolol reduces blood pressure without postural change and suppresses renin secretion. The initial dose is 10 mg three times a day, and it can be increased to 320 mg per day or more. Heart failure or bronchial asthma is occasionally precipitated; bradycardia below 50 per minute calls for a reduction in dose. Oxprenolol is an alternative which may be less likely to cause cardiac failure.

Thiazide diuretics lose their diuretic — and probably their antihypertensive — action below a GFR of about 15 ml per minute. Furosemide, bumetanide, and ethacrynic acid in high doses still produce a diuresis down to a GFR of about 3 ml per minute; ethacrynic acid occasionally causes deafness in renal failure. Furosemide is given in an initial dose of 40 to 80 mg daily and is increased until adequate diuresis is obtained. In terminal renal failure a daily dose of 1 to 2 grams may be required. No antihypertensive effect is exerted without a diuresis. Hypokalemia can occur even in renal failure, and potassium supplements may be required; regular estimation of plasma potassium is essential.

Diazoxide is a thiazide derivative without diuretic action which probably lowers blood pressure by direct vasodilatation. It can be given intravenously (200 mg) or orally (200 mg three times a day, increasing as necessary) and has proved very effective in controlling hypertension resistant to all conventional drugs. It causes hyperglycemia and may precipitate frank diabetes mellitus, but this can be controlled with sulfonylureas while diazoxide is continued.

Minoxidil is a new drug with actions similar to those of diazoxide but without the same risk of hyperglycemia; it is not yet available in Britain.

Clonidine (0.1 to 0.5 mg three times a day) has an unexplained action similar to that of methyldopa, with the side effects of drowsiness and dry mouth.

Edema. Edema may be due to hypertensive heart failure, impaired sodium and water excretion, or nephrotic syndrome. The last should be recognized by the heavy proteinuria, the electrophoretic pattern, and the hyperlipidemia, as it may call for high protein feeding except in late renal failure. Heart failure and salt and water retention are difficult to distinguish, but the treatment is the same — sodium and water restriction plus diuretics if necessary. Cardiac glycosides confer little benefit if rhythm is normal, and are dangerous when plasma potassium is varying, particularly during dialysis which removes potassium faster than the glycosides. If they are employed, the dose should be reduced by about a third to compensate for the loss of renal excretion, but they are best avoided except in atrial fibrillation.

Pulmonary edema is a common complication of renal failure with hypertension; it is characterized by attacks of nocturnal dyspnea, basal crepitations, and "bat's wing" perihilar shadows on chest roentgenograms. After repeated attacks the lung becomes infiltrated with macrophages and the fibrous septa thickened, a condition sometimes called "uremic lung" in this situation, but it is essentially the same as the "hexamethonium lung" of inadequately treated essential hypertension. Vital capacity, forced expiratory volume, and diffusing capacity are all reduced, particularly the last. Acute pulmonary edema responds rapidly to fluid removal by diuretics, peritoneal dialysis, or hemodialysis.

Pericarditis. Pericarditis was once the harbinger of death. It occurred in about half the patients dying of chronic renal failure, and they seldom survived its onset by more than two months. It is now a sign that dialysis has been delayed or ineffective and calls for urgent treatment.

The onset is usually signaled by pain, which is often felt on the left side of the chest on inspiration for the first few hours, but may be central from the start. Pain is frequently severe, mimicking myocardial infarction, but it may appear after the friction rub and disappear long before it. The friction rub is usually loud, generalized, and palpable, and it may persist when the pericardial cavity contains half a liter of fluid and fatal tamponade is imminent. Tamponade was rare until the 1960's, but became a major cause of death in the early weeks of regular hemodialysis when this was instituted late. The important signs are falling blood pressure and pulse pressure, paradoxic fall in blood pressure with inspiration, cold, poorly perfused extremities, and raised jugular venous pressure. Paradoxic movement of the neck veins is a late and inconstant sign. On chest roentgenogram the typical globular shape of the heart may be seen in first attacks, but recurrent pericarditis produces a dense fibrous parietal pericardium which alters little in shape when fluid accumulates. The effusion can be confirmed by an ultrasonic scan, by superimposing a radioalbumin scan on the chest film or passing a cardiac catheter into the right atrium to demonstrate that the edge of the cardiac shadow is beyond the atrial wall. The fluid should be removed by paracentesis, repeatedly if necessary, and intensive dialysis should be instituted; many authors favor early pericardectomy. Hemorrhagic effusion is the rule in uremia. The hematocrit of the aspirated effusion is usually about half that of circulating blood.

In the acute stage there is a fibrinous exudate over the visceral pericardium. After several attacks, sometimes after a single attack, an adherent pericardium thickens and within a few months to a few years produces constrictive pericarditis, usually without calcification, which must be treated surgically. The whole affected pericardium should be stripped off the heart.

Other Cardiovascular Effects. Deposits of calcium phosphate are found in the heart in severe hyperparathyroidism, and calcium oxalate and urates are deposited after some months of inadequate regular hemodialysis. Sudden cardiac arrest or arrhythmias result from deposition in the conducting tissue.

Anemia. Anemia is so nearly universal in chronic renal failure that a uremic patient with a normal hemoglobin must be presumed to have acute renal failure until proved otherwise. Red cells are normochromic or have a slightly reduced MCHC, about 30 to 31. The major cause is a reduction in plasma erythropoietin level which results in relative hypoplasia of the marrow. The red cell precursors in the marrow are normal or slightly increased, the reticulocyte count, when corrected for red cell count, is one to four times normal, and radioiron transit time through the marrow is normal or reduced; but in each case the level of activity is well below that which occurs in anemia of the same degree from other causes.

Uncommon exceptions to this rule are a few patients with urinary obstruction, renal artery stenosis, and polycystic disease who overproduce erythropoietin and maintain a normal or even increased hemoglobin in early renal failure. Polycystics as a group have significantly higher hemoglobins than other patients with renal failure throughout the course of the illness and into their experience of regular hemodialysis.

Mild degrees of folate deficiency can be demonstrated by leukocyte lobe counts and marrow morphology in a minority of patients in late renal failure, but response to folic acid is slight. Deficiency of folic acid and pyridoxine, which are dialyzable, and deficiency of iron become important after the start of regular hemodialysis.

Uremia may be responsible for some of the marrow hypoplasia. Improvement in erythropoiesis occurs during regular hemodialysis. Bilateral nephrectomy causes fall in hemoglobin, but a stable hematocrit can eventually be maintained.

An important effect of uremia is the occurrence of mild hemolysis. Red cell life is shortened to about half normal when the blood urea exceeds 200 mg per 100 ml. Burr cells, helmet cells, and other misshapen red cells appear in the blood film as uremia increases. An improvement in red cell survival and hemoglobin level occurs when plasma urea is lowered by the Giovannetti diet. Much more striking hemolysis and deformation of red cells occur in malignant hypertension and in association with several diseases that cause renal failure, such as thrombotic thrombocytopenic purpura.

Anemia becomes a major cause of symptoms in uremia only when the hemoglobin falls below about 7 grams per 100 ml. It is then responsible for dyspnea, may precipitate angina and claudication, and produces ejection systolic murmurs, raised cardiac output, and elevated venous pressure.

Two groups of drugs will raise the hemoglobin level in chronic renal failure by a modest 1 to 3 grams per 100 ml. Salts of cobalt probably act by inducing tissue anoxia, and have therefore been condemned as illogical and dangerous; cardiac failure and impaired thyroid function may develop. Androgens and related anabolic steroids increase the hemoglobin level of normal women in small doses and normal men in larger doses. They act on the marrow directly, as well as through an increased output of renal erythropoietic factor. Success has been claimed in the anemia of renal failure in patients of both sexes, with and without kidneys and before and after regular hemodialysis. Testosterone propionate, 150 mg intramuscularly per week, may be given in men, and it may incidentally help to restore flagging libido. Priapism is a risk, particularly in those on overnight hemodialysis. In females nonicterogenic steroids of low androgenicity, such as nandrolone decanoate, 25 mg intramuscularly per three weeks, seldom cause troublesome side effects, and their anabolic effect at least is well established. Patients should be warned to report hair growth and skin thickening, which are reversible, because the voice change which follows them may be permanent.

Transfusion was once the mainstay of treatment. Packed red cells are given in small volume (200 to 500 ml) with particular caution if the patient is hypertensive. The fear that a rise in hematocrit might imperil renal function by reducing renal plasma flow has been dispelled in clinical trial; renal function declines only if heart failure is precipitated by overtransfusion. However, the benefit is short lived; donor cells have the same shortened life span as the patient's own red cells, and erythropoiesis is depressed by even a small transfusion. Transfusion should be avoided if possible, and only blood negative for hepatitis B associated antigen should be used. A hemoglobin level compatible with reasonable activity can be maintained without transfusion during regular hemodialysis if blood losses are kept to a minimum; after successful transplantation the hemoglobin rises to, or even above, normal. Symptomatic anemia in a patient destined for regular dialysis or transplantation is therefore an indication for expediting definitive treatment. Hypersplenism has been described, particularly in patients on regular dialysis. Splenectomy raises hemoglobin and white cell counts.

Bleeding Tendency. A hemorrhagic tendency is common in late renal failure. Epistaxis, menorrhagia, gastrointestinal hemorrhage, and excessive bleeding or bruising after trauma are common manifestations; purpura is unusual. Whole blood clotting time and prothrombin time are usually normal, although deficiencies of factors V and VII are occasionally described. The total platelet count is normal or slightly reduced, and the life span of platelets is normal; but defects of platelet function can usually be detected and are thought to be the major cause of uremic bleeding. The proportion of sticky platelets is reduced, platelet aggregation with ADP impaired, the prothrombin consumption test abnormal, and platelet factor III availability decreased. The bleeding time is often prolonged, but a modification of the Ivy test, using multiple punctures and measurement of blood loss, may be required to demonstrate it. The platelet defect is roughly proportional to plasma urea, is corrected when plasma urea is reduced by dialysis or low protein diet, and can be reproduced in normal persons by feeding urea, but it is not produced by addition of urea to blood in vitro.

Plasma fibrinogen level is usually raised in renal failure, the mean elevation being about 30 per cent, and this is probably responsible for the characteristic rise in erythrocyte sedimentation rate. Plasma fibrinolytic activity is depressed, as indicated by a prolonged euglobulin lysis time, but fibrin degradation products can often be demonstrated in plasma, suggesting excessive intravascular deposition and removal of fibrin. As the kidney is a major source of plasminogen activator, it is tempting to attribute the reduced blood fibrinolytic activity in renal failure to the loss of renal mass, but this is probably not the true explanation, because regular hemodialysis restores the fibrinolytic activity to normal, even after bilateral nephrectomy. Plasma fibrinogen also returns to normal during regular dialysis.

Troublesome bleeding in uremia is best controlled by peritoneal dialysis or hemodialysis with reduced, or regional, heparinization. Infusion of inhibitors of fibrinolysis, such as aminocaproic acid (EACA) in an initial dose of 100 mg per kilogram of body weight over four hours, is helpful if local measures and dialysis fail to control bleeding externally or into the gut. It should be used only in dire emergency for bleeding into the urinary tract or internal cavities because of the risk of producing indissoluble clot.

Infection. Susceptibility to bacterial infection is characteristic of uremia; it is the main cause of death in acute renal failure and a major source of morbidity in chronic renal failure. The neutrophil count is normal and rises normally in response to infection, but the ability of the cells to ingest and kill bacteria is impaired. Total serum immunoglobulins are normal, unless reduced by the primary disease or by heavy proteinuria, and the anamnestic response to antigens such as tetanus toxoid is normal, but the appearance of antibodies to new antigens is delayed and their titer low, at least in laboratory animals. The Mantoux and similar tests show impairment of delayed hypersensitivity which is not corrected by regular hemodialysis. The circulating lymphocyte count is reduced. The prolonged tolerance of homografts in uremia is further evidence of altered cellular immunity.

Two common and important problems in renal failure are colonization of the nose and other carrier sites by staphylococci, leading to recurrent infection of the operation wounds and arteriovenous shunts, and infection with *Candida albicans.* Both are encouraged by repeated exposure to antimicrobials and the hospital environment, and may reflect this rather than a specific vulnerability of the uremic patient. On the tongue and buccal mucosa, Candida forms painful white plaques which may make eating almost impossible and which are the usual cause of "uremic ulceration of the mouth." It spreads to the esophagus, causing dysphagia and a moth-eaten appearance on barium swallow. In the gut it causes diarrhea, and may produce generalized allergic rashes as well as pruritus ani. In the vagina it causes discharge and pruritus vulvae.

Strenuous efforts should be made to identify the causative organisms before starting antimicrobial therapy and to follow the change in the bacterial flora during treatment. In seriously ill patients it is worthwhile swabbing the usual carrier sites and wounds and culturing sputum, blood, urine, and stool every few days in an effort to keep one jump ahead of the bacteria. Pathogens found in the nose on Monday are likely culprits in a pneumonia or wound infection developing on Friday; their antimicrobial sensitivities can guide therapy during the first 48 hours while the new invaders are being identified.

If the causative organism can be identified, narrow-spectrum antimicrobials should be employed when there is a choice. If broad-spectrum therapy is needed, and in all seriously ill uremics receiving antimicrobials, antifungal agents, e.g., nystatin suspension, 500 mg four times a day, should be given orally to prevent Candida superinfection, and particular care should be taken with mouth toilet. Established Candida infection of mouth and esophagus should be treated with amphotericin lozenges (10 mg) sucked continuously, at a rate of 10 to 20 per day. If response is slow, the lesions should be painted with gentian violet solution, 1 per cent, three times a day.

The loading dose of antimicrobials is unchanged in renal failure, but the size or spacing of maintenance doses must be adjusted to renal function (Table 4). When the drug is wholly dependent on excretion by glomerular filtration, the blood level produced by a standard regimen will vary up and down with the alterations in GFR that commonly occur in the course of infections in renal failure. If the drug has a low margin of safety, e.g., all ototoxic antimicrobials, the dose should be adjusted daily on the basis of blood antimicrobial measurements; these can now be performed in most hospital laboratories, and the results are available within 24 hours, provided that only one or two drugs are used at a time.

Peripheral Neuropathy. Nerve conduction slows with uremia, falling to about half normal in the legs in terminal renal failure; the arms are less affected. The abnormality is gradually reduced during regular hemodialysis and corrected by successful transplant. Hypesthesia of the feet and diminished ankle jerks can often be detected in the most severely affected patients, but they seldom

TABLE 4.   Maintenance Dose of Antimicrobials in Renal Failure

Group 1. Mainly excreted or metabolized by nonrenal routes. Must be given in normal dosage for therapeutic effect.
   Fusidic acid
   Chloramphenicol

Group 2. Major pathway of nonrenal excretion or metabolism. Normal dosage schedule may be used for a day or two, but some reduction in dosage is desirable.

Methicillin	Erythromycin
Cloxacillin	Sulfadimidine
Flucloxacillin	Carbenicillin
Ampicillin	Doxycycline
Amoxycillin	Cephalexin

Group 3. Predominantly renal excretion. Some dosage reduction is desirable from the start. Space doses (of normal size) more widely than usual, but not more than 24 hours apart.

Penicillin G	Co-trimoxazole
Cephaloridine	Nalidixic acid
Cephalothin	Isoniazid
Lincomycin	Ethambutol
Clindamycin	Rifampicin

Group 4. Mainly renal excretion and toxic effects during cumulation. Major adjustment of dosage required; daily monitoring of blood antibiotic concentration required.

Kanamycin	Vancomycin
Gentamicin	Para-aminosalicylate
Polymyxin B	Amphotericin
Colomycin	
Streptomycin	

Group 5. Contraindicated in renal failure.
   Nitrofurantoin
   All tetracyclines except doxycycline
   Long-acting sulfonamides

cause spontaneous complaint, and severe neuropathy was rare until the advent of regular hemodialysis. The first symptom is usually numbness of the toes and feet, sometimes accompanied by unpleasant tingling and burning. Ascending anesthesia, areflexia, and muscle weakness may progress rapidly over a few days or weeks to quadriplegia. The condition may deteriorate during the first few weeks of regular hemodialysis, particularly if rapid fluid removal is necessary; the most disabling permanent neuropathies have occurred during inadequate hemodialysis. Sural nerve biopsy shows axonal degeneration and segmental demyelination.

The incidence of fulminant uremic neuropathy varies between geographic centers. This is partly explained by local fashions in drug therapy; nitrofurantoin is an important cause of neuropathy in the uremic, and the onset of symptoms demands a careful review of drug therapy.

The only effective treatment is intensive hemodialysis—30 to 40 hours per week on the Kiil dialyzer or its equivalent. Multivitamin supplements, including thiamin, pyridoxine, and hydroxycobalamin, are usually given to protect against any deficiency caused by anorexia, diet, or dialysis, but they have no therapeutic effect. All but the most advanced cases of neuropathy remit completely within a few months of successful transplant.

The tingling and numbness of neuropathy must be distinguished from the similar symptoms produced by hypocalcemia, which are usually precipitated by feeding sodium bicarbonate, and from Raynaud's phenomenon. The latter is common in renal failure, particularly in patients whose hypertension has been controlled by sodium and water removal.

Myopathy.   A proximal myopathy accompanies renal osteomalacia and may occur with severe osteitis fibrosa. It may be severe enough to produce a waddling gait and prevent stair-climbing. Wasting is slight and tendon reflexes paradoxically brisk. This rare syndrome becomes more common after the start of regular hemodialysis in those centers where bone disease is a major problem.

Cramps.   Muscle cramps in the calves, thighs, and flexors of the toes are common in early renal failure, particularly at night. They may also occur in the upper limbs and during the day when they are precipitated by stretching, awkward posture, or repetitive exercise such as knitting. They accompany sodium depletion or dehydration through the artificial kidney, and are then relieved by infusion of saline, but they also occur commonly in the absence of any specific electrolyte abnormality. Nocturnal cramps are alleviated by a nightly dose of quinine sulfate, 300 mg orally.

Other Nervous and Muscular Symptoms.   *Muscle twitching* affects single muscles or groups in late renal failure. It wakes the patient as he dozes off, and, when severe, interferes with activities such as writing or holding a cup. Flapping tremor, which is demonstrated by dorsiflexing the wrist of an outstretched arm, is due to a similar sudden involuntary relaxation of muscle groups. A common complaint, probably of central origin, is *restlessness of the limbs,* particularly the legs. The limbs or the whole body must be moved to relieve an uncomfortable feeling which the patient finds it hard to describe. The symptom is at its worst during the first hour after lying down to sleep. It may be accompanied by a feeling as of insects crawling under the skin—a sensation so unpleasant that it may be described as a pain. This dysesthesia and restless limbs may be precursors of a state of extreme hyperexcitability and muscular overactivity, seen at its worst in patients undertreated by peritoneal or hemodialysis, which is rapidly fatal unless treated by intensive dialysis. As a symptomatic measure, diazepam, 5 to 10 mg intravenously, is effective and may be repeated every four hours.

Persistent *hiccup* is common in terminal renal failure, and it occasionally affects a patient at an earlier stage, exhausting him over the course of a few days. There is no really effective treatment short of very heavy sedation, but chlorpromazine, 25 mg orally three times a day, will sometimes abort an attack.

Insomnia is common and, although sometimes caused by restless limbs or pruritus, it often persists beyond the first hour in bed when these are at their worst. It is accompanied by lethargy during the day and may represent reversal of normal sleep rhythm. Recourse to nocturnal sedatives is often necessary; barbiturates, nitrazepam, and methaqualone are currently most popular and about equally effective. They are given in full dosage, and all but the longest-acting barbiturates are well tolerated without troublesome hangover in spite of the fact that they all depend partly on renal excretion.

Tiredness is almost universal in uremia, although the level at which it occurs is variable; some patients are active in business with a blood urea over 200 or even 300 mg per 100 ml. Its causes include sleep disturbance, anemia, hypertensive heart failure, muscle weakness, and drug side effects, but there is probably a specific effect of uremia that is noticeably relieved by the first one or two hemodialyses.

Increased *mental fatigability* may begin early in renal

failure and is succeeded by loss of concentration, reduced performance at mental arithmetic and other demanding skills, impaired memory, and in terminal renal failure by drowsiness, disorientation, stupor, and coma. Episodes of toxic psychosis with confusion, hallucinations, delusions, and intervals of insight are particularly associated with infections and pericarditis in late renal failure. Major electroencephalographic changes accompany these severe mental symptoms; spike potentials occur sporadically in bursts, and slow waves come to dominate the recording, the mean frequency falling as low as 2 or 3 per second. Toxic *psychosis* and *confusion* respond to intensive peritoneal or hemodialysis, but some caution must be exercised during initial treatment. A "disequilibrium syndrome" of headache, vomiting, confusion, coma, and convulsions with further deterioration of the EEG occurs when patients with severe uremia are treated by rapid dialysis. It was a common and sometimes fatal problem in the days when hemodialysis was instituted at a blood urea of 400 mg per 100 ml with large membrane area machines. It has almost disappeared from those centers at which dialysis is performed early and at a reasonable pace, and is there encountered almost exclusively in the treatment of already confused patients with chronic renal failure. It is attributed to cerebral edema caused by the removal of osmotically active substances—urea and in some cases sodium and chloride—from the extracellular compartment. A shift in the oxygen dissociation curve resulting from correction of acidosis, causing hypoxia, may be an additional explanation. It can be prevented by using a slow method of dialysis, e.g., peritoneal dialysis, for the first 24 to 48 hours and by inducing a compensatory hyperglycemia. This is achieved by using dialysis fluid with an increased dextrose content and monitoring blood sugar every few hours. The main dangers of the syndrome are convulsions and inhalation of vomitus; anticonvulsants should be given prophylactically and the stomach kept empty with the aid of a gastric tube.

Convulsions. Convulsions can be precipitated in terminal renal failure by a variety of alterations in plasma composition, of which water intoxication is the most common. Intravenous therapy should be planned to correct abnormalities slowly. However, the most important precipitant is severe hypertension, which is responsible for about two thirds of all uremic fits and for nearly all such episodes in early renal failure. Acute hypotension initiates some fits, particularly in the course of hemodialysis. In terminal renal failure convulsions may occur without any obvious precipitant. They are usually of grand mal type, occasionally jacksonian. They often recur in rapid succession, and carry a formidable mortality from asystole or ventricular fibrillation. They are a dire medical emergency and must be controlled rapidly, by anesthetizing the patient and maintaining him on a respirator if necessary. Usually they can be managed less drastically with intravenous diazepam, 10 mg, or sodium amylobarbitone, 125 to 250 mg, repeated every hour or two initially. If fits recur, sedation should be heavy enough to allow the insertion of an intratracheal tube, as it is vital to prevent anoxia; the stomach should be aspirated hourly. Intravenous sodium phenytoin, 200 mg, should be given at the start and may be repeated two or three times in the first 24 hours. Maintenance therapy with phenobarbitone, 60 to 120 mg daily, and sodium phenytoin, 50 to 100 mg three times a day, should be continued until definitive treatment for uremia has begun.

Phenobarbitone and phenytoin accumulate in renal failure, and their blood levels should be checked if the patient develops depression, drowsiness, or mental blunting. Severe hypertension should also be corrected as an emergency. A useful regimen is hydralazine, 20 to 40 mg intramuscularly hourly until the blood pressure is controlled, if an initial test dose of 10 mg is well tolerated. Methyldopate hydrochloride, 250 to 1000 mg every 6 hours by infusion, acts more slowly, reducing blood pressure over 6 to 12 hours. Diazoxide, 200 mg intravenously, is effective within an hour or two.

The brain of a patient dying in uremia shows areas of nerve cell depopulation in addition to the acute neuronal damage, scattered petechiae, and edema attributable to uremia or convulsions. Some permanent decline in cerebral function probably occurs if the patient survives, and one survey suggested an average drop of 10 to 15 per cent in IQ in a group treated by regular hemodialysis. However, the most striking examples of failing intelligence and impoverished personality are seen in hypertensive patients; these probably reflect vascular damage in the brain rather than the effects of uremia.

Ocular Manifestations. The most important changes in the eye are those of *hypertensive retinopathy*. In spite of many references to "albuminuric retinopathy" there are no features that distinguish these changes from those of hypertension in the patient with normal renal function. Visual acuity is usually impaired in the presence of papilledema, and scotomas corresponding to large hemorrhages may be noticed by the patient. Control of hypertension is followed in sequence by the clearing of hemorrhages, resolution of papilledema, and disappearance of exudates, the macular star often persisting for some months after blood pressure is normal. Vision usually returns to nearly normal, but some patients are left with optic atrophy and permanent loss of acuity.

Retinal detachment, usually of globular shape in the lower half of the eye, occurs in patients with severe hypertensive retinopathy, renal failure, and fluid overload; hypertension is probably the most important precipitant, but the condition often resolves spontaneously even if the blood pressure is poorly controlled. It is due to serous effusion below the retina. Resolution is usually complete if hypertension and fluid overload are treated rapidly by dialysis.

"Red eyes" in renal failure are caused by conjunctival vasodilatation and are described above.

Pancreatitis. Pancreatitis is common in renal failure. A modest rise in serum amylase can occur from renal failure alone.

Wound Healing. Wound healing is impaired, and incisional hernia is common. Stitches should be retained for an extra week.

Low Protein Diet. Diet is used solely as a symptomatic measure. It is important that the treatment should be more tolerable than the disease and that it should improve the patient as well as his biochemical data. A common fault is the prescription of diet before it is really needed. The only symptoms consistently relieved are anorexia, nausea, and vomiting, although improvement in mental symptoms, muscle twitching, and pruritus are described often enough to suggest that they are genuine.

With 40 grams of predominantly first-class protein per day a diet can be constructed with a calorie content sufficient for light work which is reasonably attractive to patients with some culinary skill and an adventurous palate. Extra calories for heavy workers can be provided in electrolyte-free carbohydrate supplements such as Hycal or Caloreen which are less sweet than natural carbohydrates and can be disguised in other food.

The diet is much less attractive when simultaneous restriction of sodium, potassium, or water becomes necessary. It is expensive, involves a change from traditional food, and is unacceptable to other members of the family. It is rarely consumed conscientiously unless supported by detailed initial training and prolonged follow-up with dietary counseling by medical staff as well as dietitians. Poorly instructed patients, fobbed off with a diet sheet, merely consume a calorie-deficient, truncated version of their normal diet.

A 40-gram protein diet should be started when symptoms first develop on free diet—a variable point in the course of renal failure, but on average at a GFR of about 10 ml per minute. When these symptoms recur on the 40-gram diet, a diet containing only 18 grams of protein will maintain nitrogen balance after an initial period of nitrogen loss, reduce plasma urea, and relieve many uremic symptoms, if at least two thirds of the protein is first class, providing a high proportion of essential amino acids and sufficient caloric content. This is achieved in the *Giordano* or *Giovannetti diet* by using cereals, from which most of the protein has been removed, as calorie sources and egg with a little milk or meat to provide the protein. This high egg content makes the diet nauseating to some, and acidosis is increased by the metabolism of phospholipids in yolk. Bread and spaghetti made from protein-free flour are stodgy and flavorless. Many modifications have been devised to suit local tastes. Egg white can be baked into the bread to improve its texture. Potatoes have a better amino acid mixture than cereals and can be used without protein extraction, but their potassium content must be reduced by preboiling. With ingenuity the diet can be made just tolerable to most patients with GFR down to 3 ml per minute, but even its conscientious use adds only a few months to the average life span of the patient in renal failure. If facilities for dialysis and transplantation are available, this short respite does not justify the effort involved.

Bennett, W. M., Singer, I., and Coggins, C. H.: Guide to drug usage in adults with impaired renal function. J.A.M.A., 223:991, 1973.
Bergström, J., Furst, P., Josephson, B., and Norée, L. O.: Factors affecting the nitrogen balance in chronic uremic patients receiving essential amino acids intravenously or by mouth. Nutr. Metab., 14:(Suppl., p. 162), 1972.
Blagg, C. R., and Scribner, B. H.: Diet, drugs and dialysis in the management of renal failure. In Edwards, K. D. G. (ed.): Drugs Affecting Kidney Function and Metabolism. Basel, Karger, 1972.
Boulton-Jones, J. M., Vick, R., Cameron, J. S., and Black, P. J.: Immune responses in uremia. Clin. Nephrol., 1:351, 1973.
Chantler, C., and Holliday, M. A.: Growth in children with renal disease with particular reference to the effects of calorie malnutrition: A review. Clin. Nephrol., 1:230, 1973.
Coburn, J. W., and Norman, A. W.: Role of the kidney in the metabolism of calciferol (vitamin D). Clin. Nephrol., 1:273, 1973.
Dathan, J. R. E., Johnson, D. B., and Goodwin, F. J.: The relationship between body fluid compartment volumes, renin activity and blood pressure in chronic renal failure. Clin. Sci., 45:77, 1973.
David, D. S.: Dietary treatment of renal failure. Am. Heart J., 86:1, 1973.
Davies, D. L., Schalekamp, M. A., Beevers, D. G., Brown, J. J., Briggs, J. D., Lever, A. F., Medina, A. M., Morton, J. J., Robertson, J. I. S., and Tree, M.: Abnormal relation between exchangeable sodium and the renin-angiotensin system in malignant hypertension and in hypertension with chronic renal failure. Lancet, 1:683, 1973.
DeFronzo, R. A., Andres, R., Edgar, P., and Walker, W. G.: Carbohydrate metabolism in uremia: A review. Medicine (Baltimore), 52:469, 1973.
Goldsmith, R. S., Furszyfer, J., Johnson, W. J., Fournier, A. E., Sizemore, G. W. and Arnaud, C. D.: Etiology of hyperparathyroidism and bone disease during chronic hemodialysis. III. Evaluation of parathyroid suppressibility. J. Clin. Invest., 52:173, 1973.
Hosking, D. J., and Chamberlain, M. J.: Calcium balance in chronic renal failure. Quart. J. Med., 42:467, 1973.
Kodicek, E.: The story of vitamin D. From vitamin to hormone. Lancet, 1:325, 1974.
Massry, S. G., Friedler, R. M., and Coburn, J. W.: Excretion of phosphate and calcium. Arch. Intern. Med., 131:828, 1973.
Milne, M. D. (ed.): Management of renal failure. Br. Med. Bull., 27:No. 2, 1971.
Peacock, M., Gallagher, J. C., and Nordin, B. E.: Action of 1-alpha-hydroxy vitamin D₃ on calcium absorption and bone resorption in man. Lancet, 1:385, 1974.
Popovtzer, M. M., Katz, F. H., Pinggera, W. F., Robinette, J., Halgrimson, C. G., and Butkus, D. E.: Hyperkalemia in salt-wasting nephropathy. Arch. Intern. Med., 132:203, 1973.
Reidenberg, M. M.: Renal Function and Drug Action. Philadelphia, W. B. Saunders Company, 1971.

604. ACUTE RENAL FAILURE

Neal S. Bricker

Definition. Acute renal failure is a clinical syndrome characterized by a sudden decrease in glomerular filtration rate, often to values of less than 1 to 2 ml per minute. Acute renal failure is usually associated with oliguria (urine volumes of less than 400 ml per day), and is always associated with biochemical consequences of the reduction in glomerular filtration rate such as a rise in blood urea nitrogen (BUN), and serum creatinine concentrations. The occurrence of other abnormalities in body fluids such as metabolic acidosis, hyperkalemia, hyperphosphatemia, and hypocalcemia will depend upon the duration and severity of the renal failure, the nature and severity of any underlying injury or disease process, and the nature and intensity of treatment.

Acute renal failure so defined encompasses many different forms of disease with widely varying pathogeneses, natural histories, and prognostic implications. For example, a sudden decrease in glomerular filtration rate may occur in association with profound reduction in effective extracellular fluid volume or fall in blood pressure, and may be readily reversible by volume expansion or blood pressure elevation. More commonly acute renal failure is due to intrinsic disease of the renal parenchyma; but some forms are ultimately (albeit not immediately) reversible, and others are not. Finally, this syndrome may occur in consequence of urinary tract obstruction or occlusion of the renal arteries or veins.

Because of the diversity of etiologic and pathogenetic events which can culminate in acute renal failure; because recognition of the immediately reversible forms of the syndrome can lead to prompt restitution of normal renal function, whereas failure of recognition may lead to persistence of renal failure, increasingly severe manifestations of uremia, and, in some instances, permanent nephron destruction; because the syndrome is so frequently superimposed upon major injuries or serious systemic disease; and because a substantial percentage of patients will survive their disease if therapy is dedicated and skillful, this group of abnormalities stands among the most challenging problems in clinical medicine.

The discussion in this chapter will deal principally with one form of acute renal failure, *acute tubular necrosis*. Other types of the syndrome will be considered, but primarily as they relate to the differential diagnosis of acute tubular necrosis.

Acute tubular necrosis is defined as a special form of

acute renal failure caused by an intrinsic abnormality of the renal parenchyma that is potentially reversible after an interval ranging from several days to several weeks. Although the term acute tubular necrosis may not reflect accurately the basis of the lesion or even its pathologic concomitants, and although other names have been used or proposed (e.g., lower nephron nephrosis, tubulo-interstitial nephritis, and vasomotor nephropathy), the designation acute tubular necrosis (or ATN) will be retained in this chapter because it remains the most commonly used expression and because none of the other terms have gained more widespread acceptance. Acute tubular necrosis may follow exposure to a nephrotoxic drug or to a primary extrarenal injury or disease, especially when attended by hypotension; occasionally it may appear without an obvious predisposing abnormality. Most characteristically there is a period of oliguria, followed by gradually increasing rates of urine flow, culminating in a period of polyuria. Recovery of renal function toward the pre-illness level then occurs in patients who survive.

Causes of Acute Renal Failure. *Acute Tubular Necrosis.* NEPHROTOXIC DRUGS OR CHEMICALS. Acute tubular necrosis may follow exposure to a host of different chemical agents, some when administered in therapeutic doses. Sulfonamides and many of the commonly used antimicrobial drugs, including gentamicin, kanamycin, streptomycin, colistin, cephaloridine, amphotericin, bacitracin, neomycin, vancomycin, and polymixin, have been incriminated as the causal agents in the induction of acute tubular necrosis. ATN has occurred after exposure to organic iodonated x-ray contrast media and after the use of the anesthetic methoxyflurane. It may also follow either accidental or intentional exposure to a variety of nephrotoxic agents. Included among these are organic solvents (especially carbon tetrachloride and tetra-chloroethylene); ethylene and diethylene glycol; inorganic mercurials and other heavy metals, including bismuth, uranium, lead, and, rarely, organic mercurials; methyl alcohol; and massive doses of salicylates and paraldehyde. This subject is dealt with in greater detail in Ch. 626.

SYSTEMIC INJURY OR ILLNESS. Acute tubular necrosis may follow severe trauma such as crushing injuries or major operative procedures, especially when blood loss and/or hypotension occur. It may occur in association with rhabdomyolysis and myoglobinuria of any cause, including heat stroke and overdosage with heroin and probably intravenous methadone. It may also follow severe febrile illnesses, gram-negative or, less frequently, gram-positive sepsis, profound and sustained lactic acidosis, major losses of extracellular fluid volume, or major translocations of this volume, into gut, soft tissues, and skin (in burns). Acute tubular necrosis may develop in the course of complicated pregnancies, particularly when hemorrhage or hypotension occurs. It may follow an incompatible blood transfusion and, occasionally, intravascular hemolysis resulting from other mechanisms. In most of the foregoing entities, one or more of the following events frequently occurs: (1) profound depletion of actual or effective extracellular fluid volume, (2) hypotension, or (3) hemoglobinuria or myoglobinuria.

ACUTE TUBULAR NECROSIS OCCURRING DE NOVO. Rarely, the disease occurs without known exposure to any nephrotoxic agent and in the absence of a detectable fall in blood pressure, obvious change in circulatory dynamics, loss or translocation or extracellular fluid vol-

ume, intravascular hemolysis, or myoglobinuria. Indeed, it may in some instances occur without any apparent predisposing illness or injury and in an apparently healthy individual.

Other Parenchymal Diseases. BILATERAL RENAL CORTICAL NECROSIS. Cortical necrosis may be diffuse or patchy. In the former instance, acute renal failure is severe, and may be characterized by total anuria. In patchy cortical necrosis, the occurrence and severity of the renal failure will depend upon the extent of cortical destruction. Return of enough renal function to support life is unusual (but may occur) in patients with diffuse bilateral cortical necrosis; it is not infrequent in patients with patchy cortical necrosis.

GLOMERULITIS. Severe acute renal failure may be seen occasionally in poststreptococcal acute glomerulonephritis, particularly in the adult. Acute renal failure may also be seen in the acute glomerulitides associated with systemic lupus erythematosus, hypersensitivity angiitis, polyarteritis nodosa, rapidly progressive glomerulonephritis, Henoch-Schönlein purpura, Goodpasture's syndrome, thrombotic thrombocytopenic purpura, the hemolytic-uremic syndrome, and malignant nephrosclerosis. It may also be seen in accelerated scleroderma in which the predominant site of involvement is in the small arterioles of the kidney.

PAPILLARY NECROSIS. Renal papillary necrosis appears classically in patients with diabetes mellitus, urinary tract obstruction (especially when accompanied by severe pyelonephritis), and sickle cell anemia, as well as in patients who have ingested excessive quantities of phenacetin and possibly other analgesic drugs. The severity of the renal failure, as well as the potential for ultimate recovery, will depend upon the number of renal papillae that escape destruction.

END-STAGE CHRONIC RENAL DISEASE. Acute renal failure may occur under two circumstances in patients with chronic progressive renal disease: (1) when the nephron population diminishes below a critical level and oliguria supervenes; and (2) when an acute complicating process (such as extracellular fluid volume depletion, acute glomerulitis, or urinary tract obstruction) results in a sudden but potentially reversible decrement in renal function from the previous steady-state level.

MISCELLANEOUS FORMS OF PARENCHYMAL INVOLVEMENT. Severe *hypercalcemia* may be associated with the rapid onset of acute renal failure. In most instances the rising BUN is accompanied by polyuria rather than oliguria; but occasionally, particularly with extremely high levels of serum calcium, urine volumes may fall to the oliguric range. *Hyperuricemia* can lead to acute renal failure when the plasma levels increase very rapidly and to concentrations in excess of 15 to 20 mg per 100 ml. The renal failure presumably is due to intrarenal obstruction caused by deposition of uric acid precipitates in collecting ducts and the renal papillae. Renal failure may occur during the course of *multiple myeloma*. In some instances this is the result of severe (but reversible) hypercalcemia; the disease may also follow a period of fluid deprivation, usually for purposes of performing intravenous pyelography, in patients with Bence Jones proteinuria. The renal failure is presumed to be due to the inspissation of proteinaceous materials in the tubular lumina. Wheter the x-ray contrast media per se play a role in this form of the disease is not clear. Another cause which is being seen with increasing frequency is *homograft rejection* in transplanted kidneys. Treatment of the rejection often results in reversal of the acute renal failure. However, patients receiving transplanted kidneys, particularly from cadaveric sources, are also prone to the development of acute tubular necrosis.

Occlusion of the Renal Arteries or Veins. Acute interruption of the blood supply to the kidneys may occur after embolization, in situ thrombosis, or dissection of the aorta. For renal failure to occur, virtually the entire nephron population of both kidneys must be deprived of blood supply, and, with the exception of aortic surgery, when "sludge" may flow into both renal arteries during or after release of aortic clamping or extensive athereoembolization, arterial occlusion is an unusual cause of the renal failure. Bilateral renal vein thrombosis is also an unusual cause of the disease, for the involvement must be bilateral (if there are two kidneys), and the luminal occlusion must be complete or virtually complete.

Hemodynamic Alterations (Prerenal Azotemia). Prerenal azotemia is a reversible abnormality characterized by a functional reduction in glomerular filtration rate per nephron. The latter may be secondary to a decrease in mean arterial blood pressure and/or to intrarenal vascular adjustments initiated by marked depletion of effective extracellular fluid volume. This loss may be extracorporeal, or it may represent a sequestration of fluid in areas of the body such as the intestine (after major surgical procedures), or skin bullae (in burns). If prerenal azotemia is not recognized promptly and treated, it may lead to the development of acute tubular necrosis.

Hepatorenal Syndrome. Acute renal failure may occur in the course of severe hepatic failure, usually in association with incipient or overt hepatic encephalopathy. In some instances it is due to acute tubular necrosis; but it may also be due to the hepatorenal syndrome, an abnormality that typically is irreversible. The etiology and pathogenesis of the syndrome are unknown, and there are no characteristic pathologic changes in the kidneys. From a pathophysiologic point of view, the hepatorenal syndrome has functional characteristics (to be described under Pathologic Physiology) which simulate those of prerenal azotemia and clearly differentiate the abnormality from acute tubular necrosis.

Urinary Tract Obstruction. For obstruction of the urinary tract to produce acute renal failure, the obstructing process must interfere with the flow of urine from the vast majority of nephrons. Thus if the obstructing lesion is at or above the ureterovesical junction, it must be bilateral if both kidneys are functioning.

Pathogenesis of Acute Tubular Necrosis. Several theories have been proposed for the pathogenesis of acute tubular necrosis. Each has its proponents, and there are at least some supporting experimental data in animals. But for each, contradictory evidence has also accrued; and for none is there universal acceptance.

The most prominently considered theories are the following: (1) *Obstruction of tubular lumina* secondary to inspissated debris; the debris may be composed of hemoglobin or myoglobin, or of sloughed epithelial cells and protein. (2) *A profound reduction in glomerular filtration rate per nephron,* with or without tubular obstruction. The decrease in glomerular filtration rate would be sufficiently severe to eliminate the great majority of nephrons from the urine-forming group, and would presumably affect the cortical nephrons preferentially. Both

the renin-angiotensin system and an intrinsic change in glomerular permeability have been incriminated in the production of the drastic fall in single nephron glomerular filtration rate; but for the former the data are conflicting, and for the latter the evidence is preliminary and incomplete. (3) *"Back-leak" of tubular fluid into the renal interstitium through areas of discontinuity in the tubular walls.* The accumulation of tubular fluid in the interstitium would result in obstruction of contiguous nephrons. Back-leak could occur with or without nephron obstruction and with or without a decrease in glomerular filtration rate per nephron.

Essential to each of the hypotheses is damage to the tubular epithelial cells. The proponents of tubular obstruction believe that the damaged cells contribute to the luminal occlusion. Proponents of the reduced glomerular filtration rate thesis secondary to activation of the renin-angiotensin system view the damage as impairing sodium reabsorption in proximal tubules. An increase in volume or sodium concentration of tubular fluid reaching the macula densa would follow. The sensors in the macula densa, in turn, would initiate the release of renin from the juxtaglomerular granules, and the renin would lead to high local concentrations of angiotensin. Finally the angiotensin would produce vasoconstriction of the afferent arteriole and a decrease in glomerular filtration rate. A reduction in single nephron GFR secondary to impaired glomerular permeability would also require tubular damage, for, as will be discussed under Pathologic Physiology, a decrease in GFR without any change in the integrity of tubular function should produce the physiologic changes of prerenal azotemia rather than those of acute tubular necrosis. In the "back-leak" hypothesis, damage to the epithelial cells and basement membranes would account for the discontinuity of the tubular walls, and thus the cycling of tubular fluid from nephron lumina into interstitial spaces.

In at least some forms of experimental acute tubular necrosis, there is little evidence of widespread cast formation, of diffuse tubular dilatation, or of increase in intratubular pressure in individual surface nephrons. Thus distal tubular obstruction is not a universal phenomenon. Moreover, direct measurement of glomerular filtration rate in single nephrons indicates that a primary or at least causal reduction in the filtration rate is not universal. Finally in some models, inulin injected directly into proximal tubules has been recovered essentially completely in the urine, thus indicating that back-leak is not universal. The ambiguity, in all probability, relates to the fact that many different techniques have been used to produce acute tubular necrosis in the animal; and there may be differences in pathogenesis among these entities. Hence, it is conceivable that tubular obstruction, reduction in single nephron glomerular filtration rate, and back-leak may contribute either alone or in combination to the pathogenesis of the acute renal failure in the laboratory animal. But acute tubular necrosis in man also arises in a wide spectrum of circumstances and after a multiplicity of different insults; and it is equally conceivable that there is more than one pathogenetic pathway leading to the development of the human disease.

Pathology. On gross examination, kidneys with acute tubular necrosis appear enlarged and swollen. On cut section they exhibit a pale cortex and a dark congested medulla. Microscopically the changes are largely confined to the tubules, and neither the glomeruli nor the vessels show consistent abnormalities. The changes in the tubular epithelia tend to be scattered and nonuniform, and in some cases no abnormalities can be seen on light microscopy. Usually, however, the proximal tubular epithelia tend to appear flattened, and mitotic figures may be seen. Frank necrosis may be observed in the proximal tubule, particularly after exposure to a nephrotoxic agent. The distal tubules appear dilated, and the epithelia are low and basophilic with dense staining nuclei and occasional mitotic figures. Casts of varying types may appear within the distal segments of the nephrons. Tubular basement membranes may be disrupted in scattered areas in non-nephrotoxic acute tubular necrosis, but this change is unusual when the disease is secondary to a nephrotoxic drug. Within several days of the onset of acute tubular necrosis, round cell infiltration and edema of the interstitial spaces occur in most cases. The edema may become quite pronounced in overhydrated patients.

Electron microscopic examination has revealed structural alterations in the mitochondria of tubular epithelial cells, loss of the microvilli in the proximal tubular epithelia, and loss of endoplasmic reticulum; there may also be disruption of continuity of the tubular basement membrane. However, the glomeruli have shown no consistent lesion that could provide a morphologic basis for a decrease in glomerular permeability.

Pathologic Physiology of Acute Tubular Necrosis. With normal renal function, less than 1 per cent of the water filtered at the glomeruli is ordinarily excreted in the urine, and only about 0.5 per cent of the filtered sodium is excreted on an average salt intake. In a typical patient with oliguric acute tubular necrosis, from 10 to 20 per cent of the filtered water and from 5 to 10 per cent of the filtered sodium are excreted. Considering the marked decrease in total kidney glomerular filtration rate, these increased *fractional* excretion rates are appropriate in direction; however, the changes are much less marked than in patients with chronic renal failure. For example, a patient with chronic uremia and a filtration rate of 1 ml per minute may excrete 50 per cent or more of the filtered water and sodium. The consequences of these excretory patterns are as follows: At a glomerular filtration rate of 1 ml per minute, the patient with acute tubular necrosis will typically excrete less than 300 ml of urine and less than 20 mEq of sodium per day, whereas the patient with chronic renal disease may excrete 1 liter or more of urine and as much as 100 mEq of sodium per day.

Two questions about the patterns of salt and water excretion in acute tubular necrosis thus emerge: (1) Are the increments in fractional salt and water excretion regulatory in nature or are they fortuitous consequences of intrinsic damage to the tubular epithelial cells? (2) Why are the responses not greater? Does it take time to build up natriuretic forces in a patient with uremia; or do the functioning nephrons in acute tubular necrosis fail to respond to these forces, either because the tubular epithelial cells are damaged or because single nephron glomerular filtration rate is too low? To date, the answer to these questions is not available. However, the fact that patients with acute tubular necrosis do spontaneously excrete a moderately high percentage of filtered water and filtered sodium (regardless of the mechanism) provides a clear explanation for "nonoliguric" tubular necrosis and for certain

of the characteristics of the diuretic phase of the disease.

In most patients with the disease, the glomerular filtration rate (as estimated by endogenous creatinine clearance) drops to values of 1 ml per minute or less. Such patients are oliguric. However, in some patients the drop in the filtration rate is not as severe, and values may not fall below 3 to 5 ml per minute. Urea synthesis will still far exceed urea excretion, and the BUN will rise progressively. Creatinine and phosphate concentrations also will rise, and acidosis and hyperkalemia may develop. The patient thus may develop all the symptoms and signs of acute uremia. However, if 20 per cent of the filtered water is excreted at a glomerular filtration rate of 4 ml per minute, urine flow will be almost 1200 ml per day and sodium excretion may exceed 60 mEq per day. Hence there will exist a seeming paradox wherein the patient will present with stigmata of mounting uremia but with urine volumes that are not reduced, i.e., nonoliguric acute tubular necrosis.

A similar physiologic basis exists for the continued rise of the BUN during the first few days of the diuretic phase of oliguric acute tubular necrosis. If 20 per cent of the filtered water is excreted, urine volumes may exceed 1.5 to 2 liters per day before the glomerular filtration rate becomes high enough to allow for the filtration (and thus the excretion) of an amount of urea equal to that produced. The more catabolic the patient is, the higher must be the filtration rate (and the rate of urine flow) before the BUN will start to decline.

As the GFR increases progressively during the recovery phase of acute tubular necrosis, urine volumes may rise to very high levels. Three factors appear to have a profound influence on the magnitude of the diuresis. The first is the degree to which urea and other endogenous solutes accumulate in the blood during the oliguric phase. If urea is allowed to accumulate in body fluids rather than being removed by repeated dialysis, the retained solute will be excreted as the filtration rate rises toward normal. And because the urine remains isosmotic in acute tubular necrosis, every 300 mOsm of extra solute excreted will obligate the excretion of approximately a liter of water. If the BUN concentration is lowered by 20 mg per 100 ml in a 24-hour period via excretion in the urine, approximately 18 grams of urea (equal to 300 mOsm) will be excreted in a 70-kg man, and this will increase the 24-hour urine volume by about 1 liter.

The second factor that may influence the magnitude of the diuresis is the degree of expansion of extracellular fluid volume. If effective extracellular fluid volume is supernormal, natriuretic forces will be mobilized, and as the diuretic phase proceeds, the nephrons will respond to these forces and excrete an increasing fraction of filtered sodium and water. This phenomenon can lead to a vicious cycle wherein urine volume and solute excretion increase in consequence of fluid volume expansion, and the rate of fluid administration in turn is increased to keep up with the rising urine volumes.

The third factor which will influence importantly the magnitude of the diuresis is the rate of recovery of tubular reabsorptive capacity.

Clinical Manifestations. When there is an inciting event, the onset of acute renal failure follows the insult by an interval varying from hours to as long as two days. The oliguric phase may last from a few hours to three or more weeks, and in some instances it appears not to occur at all. The diuretic phase lasts from a few days to a week or longer. The recovery phase is characterized by a progressive rise in glomerular filtration rate and restoration of renal responsiveness to the volume needs of the organism. With recovery, renal function is restored toward the pretubular necrosis level, but in most patients some permanent nephron loss probably occurs.

The presenting picture is usually that of an oliguric patient with a rising concentration of blood urea and creatinine. If the oliguria has been present for some period of time and if salt and water intake have continued unabated, or if an effort was made to restore normal renal function by overzealous fluid administration, salt and water retention, occasionally of massive proportions, may be present. Hyperkalemia may also be present when the patient is first seen. In untreated patients, the symptoms and signs of uremia may develop rapidly, and if there is an underlying injury or illness, the total constellation of clinical abnormalities will reflect the primary disease plus the superimposed manifestations of advancing uremia.

Uremia in acute tubular necrosis may affect many organ systems. *Gastrointestinal manifestations* include anorexia, nausea, and vomiting; if water must be restricted, thirst may become a disturbing symptom. *Central nervous system manifestations* include asterixis, subtle to overt changes in mentation (including organic psychosis), convulsions, and coma. *Cardiovascular changes* include an increase in cardiac output, presumably resulting from anemia and acidosis and, when present, hypervolemia, an increase in blood pressure in some patients, acute left ventricular failure in patients who are markedly hypervolemic, and pericarditis. Electrocardiographic changes are principally those of hyperkalemia, and may include the successive development of tall peaked tent-shaped T waves, prolongation of the P-R interval, prolongation of the QRS interval, disappearance of P waves, and ultimately disintegration of the electrocardiographic pattern with a so-called sine wave appearance. For any given level of elevation of plasma potassium concentration, the cardiotoxic effects tend to be greater when either severe acidosis or hyponatremia is also present.

Therapy will exercise a profound influence on the clinical course of acute tubular necrosis. If dialysis is performed early and at frequent intervals, the patient may progress through the entire course of his illness with few symptoms or signs attributable to the renal failure and without the burden of severe dietary restrictions. If the patient is treated with optimal conservative therapy, but without dialysis, he will develop progressive manifestations of uremia, and moreover will be required to restrict markedly his fluid intake and protein intake. He also may require special treatment for preventing a dangerous rise in plasma potassium concentration. The diuretic phase will be more exaggerated. *In all instances the clinical course is influenced greatly by the nature and severity of any underlying illness or injury.* Patients with acute tubular necrosis need no longer die of uremia, but many, unfortunately, continue to die of the underlying abnormality that precipitated the renal failure.

During the recovery phase patients not infrequently exhibit reactive mental depression. They also may require a long period of recuperation, particularly if catabolism has been severe. Finally, at the end of the diuretic phase, body weight may be substantially less than the clinical estimate of dry weight. This reflects the fact that lean body mass often decreases far more than is suspected during the course of the illness, and the decrease is masked by unrecognized extracellular fluid volume expansion.

Treatment. The treatment of the renal failure in acute tubular necrosis is best accomplished by early and frequent dialysis. Either peritoneal or hemodialysis may be employed. If hemodialysis is preferred or is required because peritoneal dialysis is contraindicated, an arteriovenous shunt may be placed in an extremity at the beginning of the illness to facilitate dialysis on a daily or every-other-day basis. When frequent dialysis is employed, only modest salt and water restriction is needed, and a moderate amount of protein, e.g., 40 to 60 grams per day, may be allowed in the diet. However, when dialysis is not used on a frequent basis, the amount of water, sodium, and potassium must be regulated carefully so as to minimize chemical and volumetric abnormalities of body fluids.

The standard principles of management in a patient who is not dialyzed repeatedly include fluid restriction sufficient to effect the loss of approximately half a pound of body weight per day. In general this amounts to the administration of 400 to 500 ml of fluid plus the amount lost in the urine and gastrointestinal tract. Excessive fluid administration carries the risk of inducing congestive heart failure and pulmonary edema. If the patient is able to take food by mouth, a diet providing approximately 2000 calories which is potassium and protein free and essentially sodium free is recommended; there are some observers, however, who favor the inclusion in the diet of a small amount of protein (ca. 20 grams per day), containing the minimal daily requirements of essential amino acids. If parenteral alimentation is necessary, it is the general practice to infuse dextrose (at least 100 grams per day) and vitamins; but the caloric requirements may also be partially fulfilled by intravenous fat emulsions. When glucose is administered, it must usually be given as a hyperosmotic solution because of the requirement for fluid restriction. Precautions are required to prevent venous thrombosis and infection of the venous catheter.

Particular attention may be necessary to prevent the development of progressive hyperkalemia. The administration of a potassium-binding resin either by mouth or by enema two to four times daily will generally serve to prevent serious elevations of plasma potassium concentrations.* If marked hyperkalemia is present when the patient is first seen, intravenous glucose and insulin, sodium bicarbonate, or calcium chloride all will protect temporarily against the cardiotoxic effects of potassium. But potassium exchange resins and/or dialysis, both of which remove potassium from the body, should be initiated promptly to prevent the recurrence of hyperkalemia. Metabolic acidosis can generally be corrected and controlled by dialysis. If dialysis is not available, or the acidosis progresses despite dialysis, the administration of $NaHCO_3$ in carefully regulated amounts is indicated to keep the plasma bicarbonate concentration above 15 mEq per liter. Hyponatremia can best be controlled by preventing progressive water retention and can best be corrected by dialysis. *Hyponatremia should not be treated by the administration of hypertonic saline.* Anemia will develop routinely in the course of acute tubular necrosis,

---

*The resin generally used in the United States is a sodium cycle resin (Kayexalate), and in a standard dose of 15 to 60 grams per day over 30 mEq of Na may be released into the gastrointestinal tract. To obviate sodium retention, part or all of the resin may be given as a calcium cycle resin if the latter is available.

and ordinarily no effort should be made to maintain the hematocrit in excess of 20 volumes per 100 ml. If blood transfusion does become necessary because of a progressive fall in hematocrit or cardiovascular complications, packed red blood cells using fresh blood should be employed. In treating hemorrhage, fresh whole blood may be preferable. Hyperphosphatemia may occasionally become very pronounced, and may be attended by the development of hypocalcemia. The latter ordinarily does not produce manifestations of tetany; but if ionized calcium concentrations become reduced inordinately, as may occur if the patient becomes alkalotic from the infusion of bicarbonate in excessive amount or from vomiting, tetany and even seizures may develop. Hyperphosphatemia is best controlled by protein restriction and/or frequent dialysis, but the administration of phosphate-binding gels, e.g., aluminum hydroxide gel, 30 to 60 ml every six hours by mouth may be of great value.

All drugs from antimicrobials to digitalis glycosides must be administered with full knowledge of their route of degradation and excretion. Drugs which are not detoxified, metabolized, or excreted by the kidney may be given in full dosage. But these are the exception rather than the rule. Most drugs, including many antimicrobials, will have to be given in reduced amounts and at prolonged intervals. It is tragic indeed to have a patient recover from acute tubular necrosis only to have a permanent vestibular or auditory defect owing to streptomycin or kanamycin toxicity. Digoxin is the most widely recommended digitalis glycoside, although some authorities prefer digitoxin. If digoxin is employed, a digitalizing dose of 1.5 to 2.0 mg and a maintenance dose of 0.125 mg daily will provide a therapeutic effect without toxicity in most adult patients with acute tubular necrosis.

If the renal failure is treated satisfactorily, the outcome will depend almost entirely upon the natural history of any underlying illness or injury. Thus the intensity of treatment of a surgical wound, an area of necrotic tissue, or a burn should not be diminished because of the existence of acute tubular necrosis; quite the contrary: any delay in appropriate treatment may compromise the patient's chances of survival. Removal of necrotic tissue is, if anything, more urgent in the patient with acute renal failure than in the patient with normal renal function; and surgical procedures, even major ones, are not contraindicated if they are considered to have lifesaving importance. Finally, although prophylactic antimicrobial drugs are contraindicated, infection must be treated promptly with the correct drugs but with prorated dosages. In the same context, careful attention must be given to avoiding the introduction of secondary infection. Thus after the first day of the disease, the use of a bladder catheter solely to monitor urine volumes is not justified, and intravenous catheters should be treated aseptically and never left in place for more than three days. Skin care, with special attention to the prevention of pressure sores, is an essential component of rational and effective therapy.

Differential Diagnosis. The fact that the patient with acute tubular necrosis characteristically excretes a relatively large percentage of filtered salt and water may be very helpful in differentiating the disease from the oliguric states associated with volume depletion, hypotension with a readily reversible decrease in effective filtration pressure, acute glomerulitis, and the hepatorenal syndrome.

As indicated previously, a normal person with normal salt and water intake will excrete less than 1 per cent of his filtered sodium and water. If extracellular fluid volume depletion occurs, the appropriate response is to *decrease* fractional salt and water excretion. If volume losses are profound, the glomerular filtration rate may fall markedly, in which case the patient will present not only with oliguria but with a rising level of BUN and creatinine. Thus he will fulfill the criteria for acute renal failure. But in contrast to the patient with acute tubular necrosis, the patient with volume depletion will typically excrete less than 5 per cent of his filtered water, and may excrete urine which is virtually free of sodium. A similar picture evolves early in the course of a severe glomerulitis and in the hepatorenal syndrome.

The urine/plasma (U/P) creatinine ratio is a readily available test for estimating the fraction of filtered water excreted. The accompanying table compares the U/P ratios with the fractional rate of water excretion. A U/P ratio of 10 indicates that approximately 10 per cent of the filtered water is excreted. A U/P ratio of 5 is equivalent to the excretion of 20 per cent of the filtered water, and a ratio of 2 signifies the excretion of 50 per cent of the filtered water. In acute tubular necrosis, creatinine U/P ratios typically range between 5 and 10, and rarely exceed 20. In extracellular fluid volume depletion, acute glomerulitides, and the hepatorenal syndrome, creatinine U/P ratios typically exceed 10, and often are well above 20. The urinary sodium concentration (U_{Na}) in acute tubular necrosis typically exceeds 20 mEq per liter, and in most patients ranges from 40 to 90 mEq per liter. In volume depletion, acute glomerulitis, and the hepatorenal syndrome, U_{Na} is usually less than 20 mEq per liter, and often is less than 10 mEq per liter. Calculation of the fraction of filtered sodium excreted may also be very helpful. This value is equal to the U/P ratio for sodium divided by the U/P ratio for creatinine and expressed as a percentage. In acute tubular necrosis, 5 per cent or more of the filtered sodium typically is excreted; in volume depletion, acute glomerulitis, and the hepatorenal syndrome, less than 5 per cent and often less than 2 per cent of the filtered sodium is excreted. In chronic end-stage renal disease, the values will depend upon the glomerular filtration rate and the salt intake; but at a GFR of 2 ml per minute and with an average salt and water intake (approximately 7 grams of salt and 1 liter of water per day), about 30 per cent of the filtered salt and water is excreted.

The creatinine U/P ratio, U_{Na}, and the U/P Na U/P creatinine ratio are thus of help in the differential diagnosis of acute renal failure. But there are substantial gray zones where the patterns overlap, and these biochemical values must in all instances be viewed in light of the historical and clinical findings. There are also

The Relationship Between Creatinine Urine/Plasma (U/P) Ratios and the Percentage of Filtered Water Excreted

Creatinine U/P ratio	Per Cent Filtered H$_2$O Excreted
100	1
50	2
20	5
10	10
5	20
2	50

sources of error in utilizing the biochemical values. One of these is that acute renal failure secondary to volume depletion may progress to acute tubular necrosis; and if the urine examined was produced prior to the advent of acute tubular necrosis, it will be low in sodium and have a high creatinine U/P ratio. Another source of error exists in a patient with true acute tubular necrosis in whom there is a profound stimulus to sodium retention. For example, in acute tubular necrosis associated with burns, the translocation of extracellular fluid into the affected areas results in a striking decrease in effective ECF volume. The patient thus may present with oliguria, a glomerular filtration rate below 1 ml per minute, a creatinine U/P ratio of less than 10, but virtually no sodium in the urine. A low U_{Na} has also been observed in acute tubular necrosis after cardiac surgery and mercury poisoning.

Error in using the creatinine U/P ratio and U_{Na} may also occur in patients with glomerulitis, after the occurrence of compensation but before the filtration rate rises appreciably. After enough salt and water have been retained to expand extracellular fluid volume appreciably, natriuretic forces may be mobilized and fractional reabsorption of sodium (and water) in the urine-forming nephrons may be markedly depressed. Thus creatinine U/P ratios may fall below the 10 to 20 range and U_{Na} may be high. When acute renal failure is superimposed on underlying chronic renal disease, e.g., from volume depletion or acute glomerulitis, the creatinine U/P ratio may remain low, and the U_{Na} high.

Other Aids in Differential Diagnosis. URINE VOLUME. Total anuria is very rare in acute tubular necrosis unless it is due to the ingestion of bichloride of mercury. Total anuria is seen in severe acute glomerulitis, bilateral cortical necrosis, and urinary tract obstruction. If there is a history of an abrupt change in urine volume from very low to high levels in a short period of time, or if there are alternating periods of oliguria and polyuria, obstruction is strongly suggested.

URINARY SEDIMENT. Red blood cell casts are unusual in acute tubular necrosis (but they occur) and are the rule in glomerulitides (but they may be absent). Qualitative measurements of protein in urine in the disease rarely exceed 1 to 2+ in acute tubular necrosis, whereas they often are 3 to 4+ in glomerulitides.

URINE OSMOLALITY. The osmolality of the urine is the same as that of the plasma in patients with tubular necrosis. In patients with severe volume depletion, glomerulitides, and the hepatorenal syndrome, the urine may occasionally be hyperosmotic to the plasma. *Consequently isosmotic urine is not of value in differential diagnosis, although hyperosmotic urine favors volume depletion, acute glomerulitis, and the hepatorenal syndrome, and virtually excludes acute tubular necrosis.*

RESPONSE TO MANNITOL, FUROSEMIDE, OR VOLUME EXPANSION. A limited increase in urine volume may occur in the disease after mannitol infusion, furosemide administration, or volume expansion. However, unless the increase is progressive and is attended by a substantial rise in glomerular filtration rate, repeated administration of either mannitol or furosemide or continuous infusion of a synthetic extracellular fluid solution is contraindicated in patients with acute renal failure of unknown variety. The differential diagnostic implications of a small increase in urine volume and sodium excretion after the administration of potent diuretics such as furosemide are not yet clear; but large increments in urine volume point away from the diagnosis of acute tubular necrosis.

Prognosis. In uncomplicated cases of acute tubular necrosis, in which there is no serious underlying disease and treatment is optimal, survival rates in excess of 70 to 80 per cent are common. On the other hand, when there is a serious underlying disease or injury, the death rate exceeds 50 per cent, and in severely traumatized patients may exceed 70 per cent. Judging from the experience in the Vietnam war, as contrasted with the Korean war, the speedy evacuation of wounded and rapid treatment of blood loss and shock will substantially reduce the incidence of acute tubular necrosis; but unfortunately once it does develop, the mortality rate among wounded patients requiring hemodialysis remains at about 70 per cent.

Prevention. The likelihood of occurrence of acute tubular necrosis after a given insult is influenced by the composite physiologic adversities. Thus the better the supportive therapy, the lower should be the incidence of the disease. The war experience just cited supports this view.

The role of mannitol in preventing acute tubular necrosis is uncertain. Some observers have favored the view that administration of mannitol to an oliguric patient will confer a substantial degree of protection by eliminating the contribution of luminal obstruction to the disease. However, at the very least, obstruction is not a universal factor in its pathogenesis; moreover, it can be induced in the laboratory animal with myoglobinuria despite the presence of high rates of urine flow per nephron. Mannitol may also increase renal blood flow, and conceivably some protective effect could derive from this. But it seems most reasonable to confine the use of mannitol chiefly to patients in whom there is an increase in the creatinine U/P ratio and a decrease in urinary sodium concentration, but no evidence of hypervolemia. The mannitol should be administered only for a limited period of time and in an amount not to exceed 25 to 50 grams; if no substantial rise in glomerular filtration rate and/or urine flow occurs, its use should not be continued. The role of furosemide in preventing the development of acute tubular necrosis also has not been established, and repeated administration of high doses of this drug is contraindicated.

In patients with extracellular fluid volume depletion and oliguria, volume repletion should be effected as expeditiously as possible. When hypotension exists, this also should be corrected as rapidly as possible. The use of sodium bicarbonate intravenously in patients with intravascular hemolysis is of dubious value.

The early recognition of urinary tract obstruction is of importance not only for the prompt reversal of acute renal failure, but also for the prevention of progressive nephron destruction. When obstruction is suspected in a patient with acute renal failure, either bladder catheterization or unilateral ureteral catheterization should be performed without delay.

Flamenbaum, W.: Pathophysiology of acute renal failure. Arch. Intern. Med., 131:911, 1973.

Franklyn, S. S., and Maxwell, M. H.: Acute renal failure. *In* Maxwell, M. H., and Kleeman, C. R. (eds.): Clinical Disorders of Fluid and Electrolyte Metabolism. New York, McGraw-Hill Book Company, 1972.

Merrill, J. P.: Acute renal failure. *In* Strauss, M. B., and Welt, L. G. (eds.): Diseases of the Kidney. Boston, Little, Brown and Company, 1971.

Muehrcke, R. C.: Acute Renal Failure: Diagnosis and Management. St. Louis, C. V. Mosby Company, 1969.

TREATMENT OF IRREVERSIBLE RENAL FAILURE BY TRANSPLANTATION AND DIALYSIS*

605. INTRODUCTION

Priscilla Kincaid-Smith

Renal transplantation and intermittent dialysis have become established as successful methods of treatment for irreversible renal failure over the last 10 to 15 years. There are few medical reasons for a definitive choice between dialysis and transplantation, and both offer reasonable success rates and good rehabilitation. From the patient's point of view a successful transplant offers a more independent life and avoids anemia, which is the major disadvantage of maintenance dialysis. Furthermore cadaveric transplantation is the only practical approach for a country wishing to accept and treat all medically suitable patients with irreversible renal failure and to avoid the allocation of very considerable financial and medical resources to treatment by dialysis.

An integrated program for patients with irreversible renal failure, utilizing both dialysis and transplantation, has evolved in the last few years. Such an approach is based on an initial choice made by patient and physician together. The medical commitment is to maintain the highest quality of life possible for each patient. Successful transplantation will usually remain the ultimate goal, but dialysis is carried out preferably in such a way that it can continue indefinitely if the need arises. Transplantation is carried out on optimally fit patients and is not regarded as a treatment for "failed" dialysis. Grafts are removed early if function is poor or deteriorating, and immunosuppression is not used to excess. Failed transplants are returned to dialysis to await another transplant should it be indicated. This integrated approach allows maximal use of available cadaver kidneys and in addition achieves an improved patient survival rate. This approach in the last three years at the Royal Melbourne Hospital has resulted in a two-year patient survival of 80 per cent, four fifths of whom have a functioning cadaveric renal transplant.

Progress in clinical transplantation has proved disappointingly slow. Tissue typing assists the selection of living related donors but does not help in the majority of cadaveric donors. Organ preservation is now widely used and allows elective surgery and better preparation and selection of recipients. There has been a worldwide increase in patient survival, particularly in cadaveric transplantation (Table 1). Isolated units and some national programs, for example, that in Australia, report significantly better results than the worldwide experience.

THE PROBLEM OF IRREVERSIBLE RENAL FAILURE IN THE COMMUNITY

The provision of services to the community has recently been reviewed by Kerr. No country has yet reached an equilibrium in providing services for patients with irreversible renal failure in which the number of patients presenting for treatment equals those dying after treatment with dialysis or transplantation. It is notable that in Denmark and Australia, where cadaveric transplantation has been the major goal, twice the number of patients have been accepted for treatment and are alive as in countries where the major effort has gone toward dialysis (Table 2).

The most significant factor in determining the need for facilities is the number of patients presenting for treatment. This number is age dependent, because renal failure is common above the age of 55. The other significant variable is "medical suitability." The criteria for medical acceptance have widened with experience, and there are now few absolute contraindications for either dialysis or transplantation. Estimates of the number of patients requiring treatment have varied from 25 to 75 per million per year, depending on the upper age limit. The figures of 35 per million of the population per year with an upper age limit of 55 and 50 per million per year for patients up to 65 years of age are probably accurate for most communities.

Utilizing published survival data for dialysis and transplantation and making reasonable assumptions in keeping with an integrated program, Kerr has calculated that approximate equilibrium could be achieved after 12 years (Table 3). These figures provide a valuable guide to physicians and administrators in planning the community requirements.

Transplantation costs approximately equal those of home dialysis in the first year but thereafter have been estimated to be a quarter of those of maintenance dialysis at home. Countries with transplantation as the major goal may therefore expect to save about US$500,000 per year per million of population (based on Australian cost estimates applied to Table 3), compared with countries where the major goal is home dialysis.

A program based on cadaveric transplantation is dependent on an adequate supply of donor kidneys and a

*The assistance of Dr. T. H. Mathew in preparation of this article is gratefully acknowledged.

TABLE 1. Patient and Graft Survival, 1968 and 1971 — Primary Cadaveric Transplants (10th Report of Human Renal Transplant Registry)

	One Year			
	% Living		% Functioning	
1968	58	(58)	46	(39)
1971	68	(88)	46	(69)

Royal Melbourne Hospital data are shown in parentheses.

TABLE 2. Dialysis and Transplant Survivors per Million Population on December 31, 1971*

		Rate Per Million		
Country	Population (Millions)	On Dialysis	With Graft	Total
Denmark	4.9	29	41	70
Australia	12.9	20	38	58
France	50.8	31	6	37
Britain	55.7	21	9	30

*Data from EDTA, 1971 and Australian National Hemodialysis and Transplant Survey.

TABLE 3.　Approximate Equilibrium Population of Dialysis and Transplant Patients Expected from Current Survival Rates at Two Different Rates of Admission*

Treatment	Admission Rate 25 Million/Year		Admission Rate 50 Million/Year	
	Annual Cohort	Equilibrium Population	Annual Cohort	Equilibrium Population
Live donor graft	2.5	18	5	35
Home dialysis	18	32	22.5	40
Hospital dialysis	4.5	8	22.5	37
Cadaver graft	20	97	39	189
		155 million†		301 million†

*From Kerr, D. N. S.: Kidney Int., 3:197, 1973; with permission.
†The calculations are based on many simplifying assumptions and should be used only as a rough guide.

reasonable success rate. The Australian experience has proved encouraging in both these areas, with a donor procurement rate of 9 (18 kidneys) per million per year and a two-year graft survival of 62 per cent with primary cadaveric transplants (compared to the Human Renal Transplant Registry report of 46 per cent). Factors contributing to the high donor procurement and graft success rate are discussed below.

PREVENTION OF IRREVERSIBLE RENAL FAILURE

A program which aims to treat irreversible renal failure in the community must include adequate provision for prevention. Irreversible renal failure can be prevented by the application of available methods of treatment to renal disease and improvement of present methods of treatment through research. All major renal units should include facilities for research and for adequate diagnosis and treatment of renal disease and renal failure at all stages. Even by applying present methods of prevention and treatment, the numbers requiring dialysis and transplantation may decrease substantially. Detection and treatment of asymptomatic bacteriuria and hypertension are very likely to reduce the numbers presenting with chronic renal failure. Glomerulonephritis is the most common cause of irreversible renal failure; although treatment of this condition has usually proved ineffective, promising results with newer forms of treatment, including immunosuppression and anticoagulants, have been reported. Analgesic nephropathy, a totally preventable disease, is at present contributing 18 per cent of all patients presenting for dialysis and transplantation in Australia. This disease, which results from prolonged high doses of proprietary "over-the-counter" analgesic drugs, would disappear completely if abuse could be stopped by public education or if such preparations were available only on prescription.

606. RENAL TRANSPLANTATION
Priscilla Kincaid-Smith

The value of renal transplantation in identical twins was established 20 years ago; however, despite the sur-

prising success of some of Hume's cadaver transplants in 1955, many years passed before transplantation became accepted as an effective means of treatment in chronic renal failure. Early deaths were mainly due to immunosuppressive methods, including total body irradiation; clinical success dates from the introduction of azathioprine in 1962. This drug remains the major immunosuppressive agent used in renal transplantation.

SELECTION AND PREPARATION OF PATIENTS

The selection of patients with irreversible renal failure who are suitable for renal transplantation poses few problems if adequate dialysis facilities exist and the invidious situation of competition for places is thus avoided.

Relative contraindications include old age, metastatic carcinoma, psychosis, active infection (e.g., tuberculosis), and severe cerebral, myocardial, or peripheral vascular disease. Patients with diabetes, inactive tuberculosis, coronary artery disease, multisystemic disease such as systemic lupus erythematosus, chronic obstructive lung disease, and peptic ulceration have all had successful transplants.

Age alone is not a contraindication to transplantation, because transplants have been performed in neonates and in those over the age of 80. Patient survival decreases in both low and high age groups. More important than chronologic age is the quality of life which can be achieved by the patient under consideration after a successful graft.

Transplantation in the very young poses problems relating to size of vessels, lack of growth, and difficulties in social adjustment. Dialysis in this age group introduces further problems such as fluid and diet restriction and long hours of dialysis, and does not avoid the problems of growth and social adjustment. Children over age eight who weigh 20 kg or more pose fewer problems; with reduction in dose and the use of alternate-day steroid regimens, growth, sometimes with impressive spurts, has been reported.

In Fabry's disease and cystinosis, transplantation may allow correction or alleviation of specific enzyme defects; however, the success of transplantation in these conditions may be due to improved renal function alone. In the congenital nephrotic syndrome transplantation appears to be "curative," whereas in hyperoxaluria the defect persists and has led to early graft loss.

There is no medical state (except for steroid-related psychosis) for which dialysis is definitely indicated and transplantation not. Advanced vascular disease has been suggested as a contraindication to transplantation, but it is the most common cause of death on dialysis and makes blood vessel access difficult. Reported experience with hyperoxaluria patients on dialysis is poor, and survival in diabetes is worse than with transplantation.

Immunologic sensitization to transplantation antigens may make the selection of a suitable kidney more difficult; but if an appropriate donor can be found, transplantation is not contraindicated.

The patient must be optimally fit at the time of transplantation in order to have every chance of surviving the stresses and complications of surgery, high steroids, and immunosuppression. Hypertension must be effectively controlled, the heart size returned toward normal, calcium and phosphate abnormalities rectified, anemia improved as far as possible, and infection eradicated. Preparatory surgery such as bilateral nephrectomy, ileal bladder construction, and peptic ulcer surgery may be necessary. Careful attention to patient preparation may be a major factor in the increased graft and patient survival rate achieved in Australia.

Bilateral nephrectomy carries a predictable morbidity and mortality and is only indicated when the patient's own kidneys may contribute to subsequent graft failure or death. Atrophic pyelonephritis and persistent active infection, as in some polycystic kidneys and in association with calculi, require bilateral nephrectomy. Patients with anti-GBM antibody mediated glomerulonephritis have been transplanted successfully with kidneys in situ. The case for leaving kidneys intact is compelling in an integrated program which may involve long periods on dialysis. This will significantly minimize anemia and fluid restriction and may permit clearance of "middle molecules" which may be of value.

DONOR PROCUREMENT

An adequate supply of cadaveric donors can be achieved only with cooperation and understanding between the public and physicians. To achieve HL-A phenotype identical and ABO compatible cadaver donors for a pool size of 500 recipients and an average waiting time of six months, Kountz has estimated the necessity for 50 donors per month. This recruitment rate is not an unrealistic target even for large geographic areas, because Australia has consistently recruited one donor per month per 1.5 million of population over the last four years.

Any patients under the age of 65 to 70 years who have basically normal renal function and have no evidence of malignancy (excluding cerebral tumor) are potential donors. Systemic or urinary infection, severe hypertension, and renal disease are not acceptable in the donor. Urine flow must exceed 30 ml per hour up to one hour before death. Despite these liberal criteria, the vast majority of donors have in practice come from patients with head injuries or spontaneous intracerebral vascular catastrophes.

ORGAN PRESERVATION

Although kidneys can be successfully stored by simple flushing with a hyperosmolar solution followed by immersion in saline slush for up to 10 to 12 hours, pulsatile perfusion with oxygenated plasma at 10° C for 24 hours is associated with little deterioration in graft function. The advantages of perfusion are the performance of elective surgery at a time convenient to the patient and to the medical and surgical staff, as well as more detailed cross-matching and tissue typing and better preparation of the patient.

CADAVER VERSUS LIVE DONOR

There is a clear improvement in graft survival rate using living related donors with only one haplotype difference or no difference between donor and recipient. Experience with "HL-A identical" siblings has been very good. If both haplotypes are nonidentical, results are no better than those of cadaveric transplantation, and most units no longer transplant in this situation.

The data in "HL-A identical" siblings are so impressive that the results should be actively pointed out to families for their consideration.

The over-all trend is toward cadaveric transplantation.

HISTOCOMPATIBILITY TESTING

There is now general agreement that a single autosomal gene complex constitutes the major histocompatibility system (HL-A) in man. This system includes at least two closely linked loci (first locus or LA and second locus or Four) whose alleles determine serologically defined antigens. The system also includes other loci which have been detected so far only by in vitro lymphocyte response studies in mixed lymphocyte culture tests. Each individual has four serologically defined antigens, two of which (one LA and one Four locus antigen) are inherited en bloc from each parent. The chromosomal segment carrying these closely linked loci is called a haplotype. Each child receives one haplotype from each parent, and both antigens associated with each parental haplotype are detectable in the child.

Skin and renal grafts in man have verified the importance of the HL-A system in determining histocompatibility, and, as discussed above, HL-A matching allows definite prognostic implications for the living related donor-recipient pair. For the cadaveric situation, however, the multiplicity of antigens (15 of which have now been identified on the first locus and 25 on the second) has meant that in practice it is rare to achieve four antigen (or full house) identity between donor and recipient. With the most frequent phenotypes the chance of finding an HL-A identical donor is approximately 1 in 100, and with the less frequent phenotypes it may be as little as 1 in 100,000. Initial hopes that partial identity, or sharing of one, two, or three antigens by donor and recipient, might also lead to a more favorable graft outcome have not been realized. Most reports suggest that there is a significant difference between four antigen identity and the remainder, but do not show a grade of success relating to antigen identity. In practical terms this has led to the recommendation that tissue typing should not be used as the basis for cadaver kidney distribution except in the case of four antigen identity. This has led to the establishment of large kidney donor sharing programs in order to increase the likelihood of perfect matching; however, the rarity of these matches means that they can make little impact on the over-all results of cadaver transplantation.

The further contribution of HL-A typing to cadaveric transplantation has been its use as a means to detect sensitization to HL-A antigen. Such sensitization may arise through previous blood transfusion, pregnancy, or prior transplantation. The demonstration of donor-specific cytotoxic antibodies in the recipient, referred to as a positive direct cross-match, is generally regarded as a contraindication to transplantation and is associated with a 95 per cent failure rate caused by hyperacute rejection. Poorer results in patients demonstrating non-donor-specific HL-A antibodies (with a negative direct lymphocytotoxicity cross-match) have led to the suggestion that this group of antibody formers may be an immunologically active or "responder" group. The ability of such patients to produce antibodies to blood transfusion may reflect a broader ability to mount a strong immune attack on a future transplant. In this sensitized group, HL-A matching has been shown by some workers to correlate better with graft outcome. Future work may lead to the identification of a responder group in whom only full antigen identity with cadaveric transplantation or identical sibling transplantation should be performed, and of a nonresponder group in whom HL-A typing of donors is unimportant.

PATHOLOGIC FEATURES OF REJECTION

Although intense cellular infiltration is a prominent feature in the unmodified rejection reaction seen in animals, this is not a prominent feature in patients in whom rejection is modified by treatment with steroids and azathioprine. The major lesions seen in renal allografts in man are in the vessels and they involve all blood vessels from the main artery and vein to the glomerular capillaries and intertubular sinusoids.

Polymorphonuclear leukocytes may accumulate within the blood vessels of the allograft within minutes, and so-called "hyperacute" rejection, with very florid thrombotic vascular lesions, may develop within hours or days of grafting. Such patients probably have preformed humoral antibody in their serum which conventional screening methods failed to detect. The vascular lesions of hyperacute rejection are similar to those occurring in acute and chronic rejection. The differences between the three are differences of degree and rate of progress, but the essential pathogenesis of lesions seen in vessels in serial percutaneous biopsies is similar. Platelet and fibrin thrombi may be demonstrated within vessels of all sizes in the acute stages, and the glomerular and vascular lesions seen months or years after transplantation represent the residual lesions that follow these thrombotic lesions. This process of "organization" may result in lesions which resemble atheroma and cause stenosis of the main renal artery. Intimal proliferation causes narrowing of interlobar, arcuate, and interlobular arteries and of arterioles. Glomerular capillaries show changes which closely mimic those of mesangiocapillary glomerulonephritis and make the distinction between late rejection and glomerulonephritis difficult.

Rejection poses the most danger during the first three months; subsequently severe acute rejection is rare, but episodes of rejection may occur as long as several years after transplantation. In a controlled trial, anticoagulation and antithrombotic drugs appear to affect the histologic lesions but have not shown any effect on graft function during the first three years.

NATURAL HISTORY OF PATIENTS WITH RENAL ALLOGRAFTS

Early Course

Although urine flow usually commences promptly with well-prepared live donor kidneys, a period of oliguria is common in cadaveric transplantation. Prompt urine flow will occur if warm ischemic times are kept to less than one hour and cold ischemic time to a minimum. Early good renal function avoids dialysis and facilitates

the early diagnosis of rejection, but initial oliguria does not alter the long-term outcome.

In the absence of complications, the patient may be ambulant on the second day and discharged from hospital between the fifth and tenth postoperative days. Daily outpatient attendance for review of renal function and detection of rejection and complications is essential during the first three to four weeks. Visits are gradually reduced in frequency to once a week at three months and once a month at a year and thereafter. Close and intense supervision in the first weeks and months is probably the major factor responsible for higher success rates in some programs.

Return to full activities is achieved in over 90 per cent of patients at about two months, and this coincides with the spontaneous restoration of a normal hemoglobin.

Rejection crises occur in the majority of cadaver transplants and may even occur with identical sibling live donor kidneys. Although a number of techniques such as urinary FDP's, I^{131} fibrinogen uptake, urinary enzyme levels, urine cell counts, hyperchloremia, induced lymphocyte transformation, urinary electrolyte patterns, and scanning techniques have all been suggested to give advance warning of rejection, alteration of renal function as judged by an elevation of the serum creatinine remains the mainstay of diagnosis. The urinary sodium is the only additional test that is reliable, easy to perform, and may precede the rise in creatinine by one to two days. Fever, leukocytosis, local pain, and systemic symptoms are late features and correlate much better with a local complication such as a perirenal hematoma or a urinary leak.

The majority of rejection crises can be reversed by increased steroid dosage, and heparin may be of benefit.

It is important that immunosuppression and steroids should not be pushed to excess with consequent severe morbidity and mortality from infection and marrow depression. Azathioprine should be reduced in dosage when renal function is abnormal rather than increased. Consistent elevation of the serum creatinine above a level of 6 mg per 100 ml after the first four weeks results in high morbidity and mortality and is an indication for graft removal.

The best guide to graft prognosis is percutaneous renal biopsy, which is simple and safe owing to the fixed and superficial position of the kidney. The histologic appearance assists in the diagnosis of the cause of acute functional deterioration and may lead to the diagnosis of renal artery stenosis or obstruction if the histologic features of rejection are not sufficient to account for the deterioration in function.

Early Complications

Persistent Nonfunction of Renal Allograft

If the serum creatinine is not falling a month after transplantation, severe rejection, major vessel thrombosis, or nonviability is likely and the graft should be removed, but obstruction to urine flow must always be excluded, and a biopsy is helpful before the graft is removed.

Urinary Leakage

The incidence of urinary leaks leading to fistula formation or obstruction from a urine collection is only about 5 per cent if careful attention is paid to preserving ureteral blood supply and to surgical technique. Early surgical intervention in established urinary fistula reduces the morbidity from infection, although a fistula will usually close spontaneously in four to six weeks.

Lymphocele

Interruption of lymph channels during graft insertion may lead to lymph collections around the kidney or to fistula formation. Meticulous attention must be paid to ligation of all visible lymph channels at the time of initial operation. Marsupialization of the lymphocele into the peritoneal cavity may be necessary if leakage persists and collections recur.

Urinary Infection

Seventy-five per cent of all patients will have a urinary infection in the first three postoperative months, and in a few it will be recurrent. The patient who refluxes up the transplanted ureter often shows deterioration of function accompanying reflux and is at high risk from septicemia; but in the absence of reflux, infections are easily eradicated by conventional antimicrobial treatment. Preliminary data suggest that reflux in the absence of infection may cause scarring in the transplanted kidney.

Hypertension

Hypertension may be difficult to control during severe acute rejection, and intravenous diazoxide administration may be necessary. The majority of successful cadaveric transplants are hypertensive, but control of the blood pressure is easily achieved. An increase in dose requirements or the development of severe hypertension is an indication for renal arteriography to exclude renal artery stenosis. Tight renal artery stenosis occurring just distal to the anastomosis is common, and correction may cure hypertension and improve renal function.

Other Infections

The patient receiving immunosuppressive agents is particularly liable to develop infections, most especially those fungal and viral infections for which man requires an intact "T" cell lymphocyte population to ensure an adequate resistance. Cytomegalic virus, herpes simplex and zoster, Pneumocystis carinii, Listeria, Nocardia, actinomycoses, and other unusual infections may be fatal. Most infections can be treated; early diagnosis, a high index of clinical suspicion, and sophisticated microbiologic facilities are essential for optimal results.

Bacteria are more likely to cause serious infection, and death from an overwhelming septicemia can occur within hours.

Respiratory Distress Syndrome

A syndrome of progressive dyspnea, cyanosis, with or without fine crepitations at the lung bases, an alveolar capillary block, and diffuse mottling and opacity on chest x-ray has been described. Progressive hypoxia with death in one to three weeks from presentation is the rule. The suggestion that this "transplant lung" syndrome is immunologic in origin seems unlikely because path-

ogenic organisms such as Pneumocystis carinii and cytomegalic virus are almost always found, and an identical syndrome is seen in immunosuppressed patients without a renal transplant.

Aseptic Necrosis of Bone

This disabling complication usually affects the hip joint and may be bilateral. Its incidence correlates with prolonged or high doses of steroids, rapid reduction of steroid dose, and secondary hyperparathyroidism.

Other Steroid Complications

Any of the well-recognized complications of steroid therapy such as peptic ulceration, diabetes, and cataract formation may develop after transplantation.

Late Course

The long-term prognosis for patients completing one year with normal or near normal renal function is excellent; however, there is a continuing slow rate of loss of grafted kidneys and mortality (see accompanying figure). Slow deterioration of renal function may be due to the chronic rejection, recurrence of glomerulonephritis, or other disease. Vesicoureteral reflux may contribute progressive "atrophic pyelonephritic" lesions in the absence of infection. In some patients the kidney is both histologically and functionally normal five or more years after a cadaver graft.

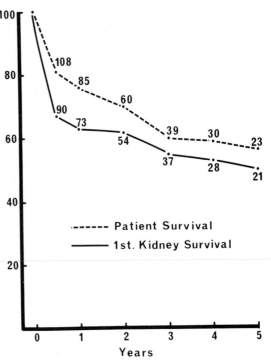

Cumulative survival of patients who received cadaveric renal allografts at the Royal Melbourne Hospital between April 1965 and April 1970. There are no exclusions. Beyond five years, numbers in the groups are small. Few grafts failed between one year and five years after transplantation, even though this figure includes early experience when results were not as good as they are at present.

Chronic Rejection

Progressive ischemia of the kidney caused by the vascular lesions affecting small and large vessels, along with glomerular capillary change identical to that seen in mesangiocapillary glomerulonephritis, characterizes chronic rejection. Deterioration of renal function is slow and occurs over several years. European experience suggests that there is a correlation between chronic rejection and the number of pretransplant blood transfusions.

Recurrent Glomerulonephritis

A true recurrence of an identifiable type of glomerulonephritis is unusual but has been described in focal and segmental hyalinosis, antiglomerular basement membrane antibody-mediated glomerulonephritis, IgA-IgG glomerulonephritis, "dense deposit" disease, and hypocomplementemic mesangiocapillary glomerulonephritis, including lobular glomerulonephritis. Unless a histologic marker is present, it may be very difficult to separate changes caused by rejection from those of glomerulonephritis, particularly as the change is usually of the mesangiocapillary type. Minor degrees of mesangiocapillary change always accompany rejection lesions identical with those of mesangiocapillary "recurrent" glomerulonephritis and may occur in a patient who had chronic pyelonephritis or some other "nonglomerular" cause of end-stage renal failure. Transplantation is not contraindicated in any form of glomerulonephritis, because the incidence of significant "recurrence" is low in the first five years and deterioration in the function of the affected transplant is often slow. Sometimes the same morphologic lesion which recurs progresses much more slowly in the transplanted kidney than it did when it caused renal failure prior to transplantation.

Malignancy in the Transplant Recipient

There is little doubt the the incidence of malignancy is increased significantly in transplanted patients, presumably as a result of immunosuppression. There is a 5 to 6 per cent chance of a cancer's developing within a few years of transplantation. Of reported cases 61 per cent have been epithelial in origin and 39 per cent mesenchymal. Skin, lip, and cervix have been the sites of the most common epithelial tumors, and reticulum cell sarcoma, often of the central nervous system, is the most common mesenchymal tumor. It appears that the risk of cancer is increased by 20 to 40 times. This complication may prove to be a major limiting factor in transplantation.

Treatment

Treatment regimens vary considerably from center to center. Azathioprine and steroids remain the major agents used for immunosuppression, although steroids may be avoided in "identical" sibling grafts, and cyclophosphamide is a reasonable alternative to azathioprine.

Antilymphocyte Sera

Despite the experimental evidence of the effectiveness of antilymphocyte serum, doubt still remains regarding its benefit to graft survival in man. Controlled trials are few; none have shown a statistically significant improvement in survival, and most have failed to demonstrate any difference. The problems of hypersensitivity and thrombocytopenia have been overcome by the use of goat antisera, but concern has been expressed about an increased incidence of exotic infections as a delayed complication. The role of antilymphocyte serum in clinical transplantation awaits clarification by further controlled trials, but it seems unlikely to prove a major advance in transplantation.

Fate of Secondary Transplants

The results of multiple transplantation, particularly with repeated cadaveric donors, have been disappointing. The American College of Surgeons' Renal Transplant Registry (1972) shows a 26 per cent two-year survival. However, isolated units are achieving much better success rates, to as high as 75 per cent graft survival at one year. The major factor is presumably sensitization from the first graft; with careful selection of the second kidney, retransplantation remains justifiable. The avoidance of disparate antigens which were present on the first kidney, particularly HL-A2, careful cross-matching using donor spleen or lymph node cells which increase the sensitivity of the test, and an insistence on three or more shared antigens may increase second graft survival. In an integrated program in which home dialysis is available, the time needed to achieve these requirements in a second donor is not a problem. Splenectomy has now been shown in a large series to be ineffective in prolonging the function of a second transplant.

A. L. G. Therapy and Standardization Workshop. Behring Institute Mitteilungen No. 51, September 1972.

Australian National Renal Transplantation Survey: Second report by a Subcommittee. Med. J. Aust., 2:605, 1971.

Brunner, F. P., Gurland, H. G., Harlem, H., et al.: Combined report on regular dialysis and transplantation in Europe II, 1971. Proc. E.D.T.A., 9:3, 1972.

Kerr, D. N. S.: Provision of services to patients with chronic uremia. Kidney Int., 3:197, 1973.

Kincaid-Smith, P.: The pathogenesis of the vascular and glomerular lesions of renal allografts and their modification by antithrombotic and anticoagulant drugs. Alsian Ann. Med., 19:201, 1970.

Kountz, S. L.: Clinical transplantation—an overview. Transplant. Proc., 5:59, 1973.

Penn, I., and Starzl, T. E.: Immunosuppression and cancer. Transplant. Proc., 5:943, 1973.

Stewart, J. H., Topp, N. D., Martin, S., et al.: The costs of domiciliary maintenance dialysis. Med. J. Aust., 1:156, 1973.

Tenth report of the Human Renal Transplant Registry. J.A.M.A., 221:1495, 1972.

607. DIALYSIS

Constantine L. Hampers

The process of dialysis is based on simple physical concepts. Essentially, it involves the separation of two fluid compartments by a semipermeable membrane which can be viewed as having finite holes. Materials of low molecular weight can cross from one side of the membrane to the other toward decreasing concentration gradients. Larger particles, such as protein molecules and red blood cells, cannot traverse the membrane. In the case of peritoneal dialysis, the "membrane" is the peritoneum which is separating the dialysate fluid (in the peritoneal cavity) from the interstitial fluid surrounding the peritoneal membrane. With hemodialysis, the "membrane" is a synthetic material such as cellophane or cuprophan which separates blood from the dialysis bath.

PERITONEAL DIALYSIS

Peritoneal dialysis is a well-established technique in most general hospitals. Its use, however, is primarily reserved for the treatment of reversible renal failure, and it has not been widely instituted on a repetitive basis for management of the patient with chronic renal failure. However, the development of permanent peritoneal catheters which do not require repeated punctures of the abdomen with each treatment and the ability to produce dialyzing fluid economically have rekindled some interest in long-term maintenance of patients by this means.

The procedure requires insertion of a catheter into the peritoneal cavity, usually in the midline. Where permanent catheters are used, an attempt is made to separate the entrance into the peritoneal cavity by some distance (subcutaneously) from the exit site from the skin. The location of the insertion of the catheter need not necessarily be midline, and under special circumstances it can be placed in almost any area of the abdominal wall. Strict asepsis when inserting the catheter and throughout the entire procedure is of the greatest importance, because peritonitis is the most common complication of peritoneal dialysis. There appears to be an indirect relationship between infection and the fastidiousness of technique utilized in manipulating the catheter.

A "routine" peritoneal dialysis will last between 12 and 48 hours, depending upon the individual needs. One or 2 liters of peritoneal dialyzing fluid (commercially available and containing electrolytes in their proper concentrations) is allowed to run into the peritoneal cavity as rapidly as possible, usually five to ten minutes. The dialysate remains in the abdomen for 15 to 60 minutes ("dwell time") in order for the transfer of solutes to take place. The fluid is then drained out by gravity flow, and the cycle is repeated. This procedure is continued until the desired effect is accomplished. The reason for the variation in dwell time depends upon what one needs to accomplish. The most efficient length of time for the removal of solutes, such as urea or creatinine, is 30 to 60 minutes, and this is the period generally utilized. Automatic cycling machines are available which can be set to adjust the dwell time and reinstill fresh dialysate as required. When peritoneal dialysis is performed for the alleviation of gross overhydration, the dwell time may be considerably shortened, because the transfer of water across the peritoneum is rapid and is accomplished within a few minutes of the instillation of a hyperosmolar (4.5 per cent) glucose solution into the peritoneal cavity.

Some patients have been taught to perform peritoneal dialysis at home. They usually undergo dialysis for 12 to 18 hours twice a week. When maximally automated, this can be done overnight while the patient is asleep. Although some centers have utilized this method repeatedly in the same patient for a period of years, in most hands it has been unsatisfactory. The various prosthetic devices for access to the peritoneum are limited by propensity to infection.

HEMODIALYSIS

Hemodialysis was applied to animals by Abel, Rountree, and Turner, in 1913, with the use of a collodion dialyzing membrane. Its application in clinical medicine, however, was not attempted until the mid-1940's when Willem Kolff, working in Europe, applied the procedure to man. Despite the fact that hemodialysis was successfully utilized for the treatment of acute renal failure for a number of years, it was not applied repetitively for patients with chronic renal failure until the late 1950's. The major breakthrough in its use for the patient with end-stage kidney disease was the development of a prosthetic arteriovenous bypass which could be used for repeated access to the circulation. Prior to this, each dialysis required a fresh arterial and venous cutdown.

The type of access to the circulation has been modified somewhat, and presently there are two methods. Arteriovenous shunts are generally constructed of Teflon connected subcutaneously to a Silastic tube. The Silastic tube exits from the skin and remains extracorporeal. It can be disengaged for attachment to the machine. A second type of access (which is the most popular today) is the arteriovenous fistula. The fistula is made by surgically creating a window between a peripheral artery and vein, usually in the forearm; this results in the arterialization of the peripheral veins. After a few days to a few weeks, the veins become prominent and can be easily identified for venipuncture. Two large needles (15 gauge) are inserted into the arterialized veins with each dialysis. The arteriovenous fistula has the advantage of requiring little foreign material and thereby reduces the risk of infection. In addition, because no prosthetic material of any kind is present between dialyses, it allows the patient more freedom with the use of the extremity and eliminates the possibility of accidental dislodging of the access, as may occur with the shunt.

Arterial venous shunts or fistulas are usually placed in the upper extemity but can, under special circumstances, also be placed in the leg. The life of the access tube is variable, depending on individual patient factors, but some patients have kept the original access for a number of years.

TYPES OF ARTIFICIAL KIDNEYS

A hemodialysis system is composed of two basic units. The first is the exchanger and is that portion of the system in which mass transfer occurs. The basic components are a blood compartment, a dialysate compartment, and an intervening semipermeable membrane. The second portion of the system is a device which functions to deliver fresh dialysate of suitable composition to the exchanger. Exchangers in common clinical use today fall into three basic types: coil, parallel plate, and hollow fiber.

A *coil dialyzer* is constructed from one or more membrane tubes which are concentrically wound with an intervening membrane support. Blood passes through the tubes and the dialysate is pumped through the supporting structure over the outside of the blood conduits. The high velocity of dialysate flow and the turbulence created by the supporting structure are sufficient to reduce the dialysate side fluid film mass transfer resistance to very low levels. By and large, coils are highly efficient devices which may yield a urea dialysance (clearance) of up to 160 ml per minute at a blood flow rate of 200 ml per minute. Coils operate at relatively high pressure, and a blood pump is required for their use.

Parallel plate exchangers were among the earliest dialyzers to achieve clinical use, and a variety of permutations on the basic design have been described. A dialyzing membrane is stretched over a supporting structure. Another membrane is placed on top of the first, and blood ports are placed at either end of the dialyzer between the membranes. Another support is placed on top of the second membrane. Blood flows between the membranes while dialysate flows between the support structures and the membrane. The mass transfer performance of these devices has not been as impressive as that observed with coils. Generally, the number of hours per week required to achieve the same clinical results is longer than with coil devices. Dialysance of urea at blood flow rates of 200 ml per minute is only 120 to 130 ml per minute. Blood flow resistance in parallel plate dialyzers is usually small so that they can be operated without a pump when used in a patient with an arteriovenous shunt.

The *hollow fiber kidney* employs 10,000 to 15,000 fibers with an internal diameter of 200 to 250 μ as a dialyzing surface. From an engineering point of view, this configuration represents an optimal design. The narrow channels allow a minimal blood fluid film resistance and a maximal surface area to blood volume ratio. The device has extremely stable dimensions and is, for all practical purposes, noncompliant. Mass transfer capability approaches that achievable with coil-type devices. The most significant problem with this device is clotting in the hollow fibers.

It should be pointed out that all types of artificial kidneys are adequate and the choice depends on the experience and prejudices of the physician in charge.

SELECTION AND CARE OF THE PATIENT

Many factors enter into the type of treatment to be provided. These include the patient's age, availability of a suitable living kidney donor, patient motivation and ability to cooperate, support for the patient at home, the presence or absence of a spouse and the spouse's occupation, patient intelligence, in some instances financial resources, and, finally but equally important, the patient's own preference. It has been our feeling, as well as that of most others, that the availability of a suitable and willing living donor should make transplantation the treatment of choice for the young and middle-aged. Recognizing the hazards of arbitrary age limits, we nevertheless tend not to recommend transplantation in patients over age 55. There are some, however, who feel that the use of living donors is inappropriate and that transplantation should take place only when cadaveric material is available. In our hands, when a suitable living donor is not available and the patient is seemingly an appropriate candidate for home dialysis, this then becomes the next most preferred method of treatment. In general, dialysis and transplantation should be considered as complementing procedures used together to offer the best type of therapy for each patient. An attempt to separate these procedures into an either/or category is a disservice to the patient.

It is most desirable to select patients for maintenance hemodialysis and transplantation prior to their actual need for therapy. As chronic renal failure develops and the serum creatinine rises to 10 mg per 100 ml or above, it is usually appropriate to plan for dialysis. When patients begin to show signs of being unable to perform adequate business, social, or personal functions because of

mounting azotemia, dialysis should be considered. It is clear that the complications of uremia are considerably more difficult to correct than they are to prevent.

Once a patient is selected for a dialysis/transplantation program, access to the circulation needs to be established. In cases in which arteriovenous fistulas are to be utilized, some lead time should be allowed for development of the access. Often a fistula can be created months prior to actual need. In the case of shunts, a few days to a week should be allowed prior to use.

When patients are severely uremic at the time of initial dialysis, complications are more likely to ensue, and considerably more caution should be exercised in treatment. In this setting, peritoneal dialysis may be employed to more gradually correct the uremic syndrome. The most common complication seen with initiation of dialysis is the *"disequilibrium" syndrome*. These manifestations are more likely to appear when the patient has undergone very efficient dialysis; they are most common in the elderly; however, they may occur at any time, even after the most gentle dialyses. The cause of this syndrome is not wholly clear. Available data suggest that a rapid lowering of serum osmolality plays a major role in the neurologic manifestations seen. With an acute reduction in osmolality which may occur with the removal of urea and/or other ions, there may be insufficient time for equal reduction in the cerebrospinal fluid. Because of the slow transport of urea and/or some other as yet unidentified substances across the "blood-brain barrier," an osmotic gradient is produced in which water moves from the blood and extracellular fluid into the central nervous system. A "reverse osmotic effect" is produced, and water moves down the gradient into the central nervous system. The symptoms seen in the patient are headache, nausea, vomiting, restlessness, agitation, rising blood pressure, confusion, and, in severe cases, grand mal seizures. Anticonvulsants may be given prophylactically to patients who are at high risk. Fortunately, the syndrome tends to subside after 12 to 24 hours.

Once a patient has begun dialysis therapy and has been stabilized, the procedure is usually performed on a regular basis three times per week. The number of hours required for each treatment depends on the size of the patient and the type of dialyzer utilized. Some centers dialyze two times per week, but the majority of experience would indicate that this is inadequate.

Where a patient receives his dialysis depends somewhat on long-term plans for transplantation as well as the medical or social factors surrounding him. Most centers agree that a hospital setting is not proper for long-term dialysis. The high cost and acute problems associated with the hospital dialysis unit make it unattractive for long-term care. When the home environment is stable and a suitable family member can cooperate, *dialysis at home* is the treatment of choice. In this situation, a family member is trained to operate the artificial kidney along with the patient, and the pair then perform the treatments in the home setting. The use of home dialysis requires a suitable home atmosphere and an emotionally stable patient and spouse. The advantage, in addition to whatever savings may be effected, is the maximal rehabilitative potential of such an environment.

An alternative to home dialysis is dialysis performed in a *limited care center* or a self-dialysis type of facility. Here, costs can be kept to a minimum while providing the patient his treatment in a noninstitutionalized setting. Limited care facilities are especially useful when the patient need be dialyzed for only a short period of time prior to transplantation. In these instances, even when home dialysis can be performed, it may not be feasible to train the family for only one or two months of dialysis in preparation for transplantation. Home dialysis has also been found unsuitable for programs which deal with disadvantaged communities in which motivation and proper home environment are lacking. The number of patients entering a chronic program who can be successfully treated at home varies, depending, among other things, on location. Estimates run as high as 85 per cent in some middle-class rural areas and as low as 10 per cent in urban ghetto populations.

MEDICAL PROBLEMS OF CHRONIC DIALYSIS

Hematologic. Patients maintained with the artificial kidney invariably show some degree of *anemia*. The degree of anemia varies and may be in some way related to the type of renal disease present. Patients with polycystic kidney disease tend to run higher hematocrits than those with other diseases.

The problems of anemia are compounded in the dialysis patient by some blood loss during the procedure. Loss of red cells left in the dialyzer at the close of the treatment may aggravate the anemia. Similarly, care should be taken to keep the laboratory evaluation of the patient to a minimum, because repeated blood testing can only contribute to the anemia. Since there is some evidence to indicate that, in addition to a lack of production of erythrocyte stimulating factor (ESF), the uremic marrow is unresponsive to the effects of ESF, one might expect that severely uremic patients may be benefited by chronic dialysis. This is the case, and most individuals can be maintained without the need for transfusions even though they do not have normal hematocrits. This must be individualized, however, depending on the accompanying symptoms produced by the anemia. In young patients, hematocrits as low as 12 to 14 vol per 100 ml can be tolerated without difficulty. In the older patient with cardiovascular difficulties, it may be necessary to tranfuse weekly. Since hepatitis can be a significant complicating factor in a hemodialysis unit, decision to use transfusion should be considered carefully.

Peripheral Neuropathy. There has been increasing awareness of peripheral nerve dysfunction in uremia. The neurologic involvement when it occurs is typically symmetrical, beginning distally at the toes and spreading up the leg. Upper extremity involvement, seen only when there is severe lower extremity involvement, develops insidiously and in the majority of patients is manifested solely by reduction in nerve conduction velocity. Only in its severe stages are there clinical symptoms. The neuropathy may cause pain and paresthesias of the lower extremities, marked sensitivity to touch, and a "burning" feeling. Although sensory manifestations of the disease may initially predominate, there may be a significant motor component as well. The presence of peripheral neuropathy is a clear indication for beginning treatment. In addition, peripheral neuropathy has been adjudged by some to be a manifestation and a consequence of inadequate dialysis. A significant percentage of patients referred to maintenance dialysis centers already have demonstrable neuropathy, at least

as measured by nerve conduction velocity. The incidence and severity of neuropathy usually depend upon the timeliness of the referral for dialysis, and neuropathy is much less common when dialysis is instituted three times per week than when the patient is treated only twice a week.

Cardiovascular. *Hypertension* is a common accompaniment of chronic renal failure, and the majority of patients presenting to a dialysis program have elevated blood pressure. Approximately 80 to 85 per cent of these can be managed without antihypertensive medication simply by careful attention to salt and water balance. Ultrafiltration with the artificial kidney and dietary restriction of salt and water are mandatory. Despite fluid control, however, a small number of patients continue with hypertension and require antihypertensive medications. An even smaller group with malignant hypertension cannot be controlled with dialysis and antihypertensive drugs at all. In the latter case, which is generally accompanied by a markedly elevated peripheral renin concentration, bilateral nephrectomy can be curative. Since the renin-angiotensin-aldosterone system has been incriminated in the hypertension associated with renal disease, this beneficial effect of nephrectomy is not surprising. It should be pointed out, however, that bilateral nephrectomy as a treatment for uncontrollable hypertension should be a last resort. Aside from the hazards of the surgical procedure, the anephric state usually complicates the dialysis treatment by imposing stricter dietary fluid controls upon the patient and results in a more severe anemia. Totally anephric patients tend to run lower hematocrits and require more transfusions than do others with their kidneys in situ.

Pericarditis, which is a common manifestation of untreated uremia, may occasionally occur in patients undergoing chronic dialysis. In our experience, pericarditis is usually associated with a stressful situation such as surgery or infection, and we have regarded it as an indication for increasing dialysis time. However, there are a few patients who develop pericarditis despite what is apparently adequate dialysis and without evidence of stress. The importance of pericarditis in dialysis patients, aside from the symptoms they may produce, lies with the potential development of *pericardial tamponade.* Inasmuch as patients are anticoagulated with each dialysis, an inflamed pericardium may bleed heavily, producing tamponade. This can be an emergency which requires pericardiocentesis and, if recurrent, pericardiectomy. If the patients are seen frequently prior to dialysis and a pericardial friction rub is detected, one can adjust the dialysis procedure with regional heparinization and lessen the risk of bleeding.

Congestive heart failure is commonly seen in patients on dialysis and is most often related to volume overload. The problem is most severe in patients with underlying coronary artery disease or hypertension but may occur in anyone who is markedly overhydrated. The physician must work with the dietician to impress upon the patient the importance of dietary control of salt and water.

Skeletal System. There seems little doubt that defective absorption of calcium from the gut is one of the prime factors resulting in the abnormal calcium metabolism of chronic renal failure, and this is not totally corrected with long-term hemodialysis. In addition, deranged metabolism of vitamin D seems to play a major role.

The main circulating form of vitamin D_3 is 25-hydroxycholecalciferol (25-HCC), and this is produced by hydroxylation in the liver from the parent substance. When the plasma calcium is low, 25-HCC is further metabolized in the kidneys to 1,25-dihydroxycholecalciferol (1,25-DHCC); when the plasma calcium is high, it is metabolized to 21,25-dihydroxycholecalciferol. The 1,25 derivative is the most active form of the vitamin so far discovered. After production by the kidneys, it is taken up by the intestines and bones. Therefore the kidneys may be regarded as endocrine organs producing a calcium-regulating hormone at a rate dependent on the serum calcium. Alterations in metabolism of vitamin D or its hydroxylated metabolites in uremia may result in accumulation of structurally related abnormal metabolites which compete with 1,25-DHCC for receptor sites in specific target organs. The end result in bone is decreased or defective mineralization of collagen, probably secondary to maturation arrest of collagen tissue. The combination of defective calcium absorption, abnormal vitamin D metabolism, and hyperphosphatemia accompanying decreased excretory function may all serve to depress serum calcium which in turn stimulates parathyroid hormone secretion. In clinical practice, patients being maintained by dialysis may histologically show osteomalacia, osteitis fibrosa cystica, and/or osteosclerosis.

It seems important to control serum phosphate levels in patients on chronic dialysis in order not to further suppress serum calcium levels, and this is usually done by giving phosphate binders orally. If serum phosphate is excessive, one may see precipitation of calcium salts in ectopic sites such as blood vessel walls or soft tissues.

The vast majority of patients with severe renal failure and almost all individuals who have been maintained with the artificial kidney for a long period show some evidence of parathyroid hyperplasia and histologic evidence of early bone resorption. Fortunately, only a small percentage of these develop clinical abnormalities of bone metabolism which require specific treatment.

It is helpful to divide renal osteodystrophy into two categories: osteomalacia and osteitis fibrosa cystica. Pathologic examination of bone in uremia, however, may show a mixture.

Treatment of the patient with marked parathyroid hyperfunction as manifested by progressive disability seems to be subtotal parathyroidectomy. By removing all but half of the smallest parathyroid gland, one may reverse or at least arrest the progression of hyperparathyroidism. Therapy with vitamin D and calcium in the postoperative period is optional but usually helpful.

In patients with less severe signs of hyperparathyroidism one may attempt to overcome vitamin D resistance by supplementing higher doses of the vitamin along with oral calcium. Dihydrotachysterol along with control of serum phosphate by use of antacids may be effective in preventing further progression of the disease. Further discussion of renal osteodystrophy may be found in Ch. 890.

Infection. Peritonitis is the most common complication in patients being maintained with peritoneal dialysis. Usually physical signs of peritonitis are evident, although they may be modified considerably, depending on the extent of the infection and the severity of the uremia. Gram-negative infections are, in our experience, the most common, although many organisms may be responsible. It is not always necessary to discontinue peritoneal dialysis because of peritonitis. Despite the fact that the catheter is a "foreign body," it is frequently possible to treat the peritonitis with the appropriate antimicrobials instilled into the peritoneal dialyzing fluid (and systemically administered if required) while continuing the dialysis. Salvaging the catheter is particularly important when permanent prosthetic devices are being used.

Infections commonly occur in patients being treated with the artificial kidney, and a whole spectrum of infectious diseases is seen. By all odds the most common site of infection is at the access to the circulation and is usually localized. Patients with arteriovenous shunts (i.e., permanent foreign bodies) have the highest incidence. Infection may also be seen, however, with an arteriovenous fistula. The most common reason for the infection is faulty technique in handling the shunt or fistula. The Staphylococcus is the predominant organism cultured, but, as in peritonitis, a wide range of organisms can be seen. Depending, of course, on the severity of the infection, one need not necessarily remove the access, and the majority of these incidents can be treated with local measures and systemic antimicrobials. We have had the impression that once an access (especially an arteriovenous shunt) is infected, its longevity is limited, but this is difficult to quantitate. Occasionally septicemia may occur from shunts and fistulas and must be treated vigorously. Usually the site of infection is obvious, but occasionally an endarteritis may be present as a site of a "seeding" and is not clinically apparent. In some cases acute or subacute bacterial endocarditis may occur, although this is unusual. In more than 500 patients treated with the artificial kidney over the last five years, we have seen endocarditis only three times. The treatment of this complication is discussed in Ch. 192.

It goes without saying that the responsible organism must be identified in cases of infection and treated appropriately. One must be aware, however, of the limited excretory ability of these patients and how this relates to the use of antimicrobial drugs. Administration should be modified to take into account the lack of kidney function and the dialyzability of the individual drug (see Ch. 268).

One of the most feared problems which may occur in a dialysis unit is *hepatitis*. Every precaution should be exercised to reduce its incidence in both patients and staff. In the United States a survey of a number of dialysis units disclosed the incidence of hepatitis infection for center-based patients and staff to be 4.4 cases and 3.4 cases, respectively, per 100 persons at risk. It is of interest that almost 70 per cent of the hemodialysis patients were anicteric; many would not have been detected if periodic screening for hepatitis B antigen or liver function tests had not been performed routinely. The hemodialysis patient seems to tolerate hepatitis quite well and usually recovers. However, the disease in staff members may be fulminant, and a number of deaths have been reported. It is essential that a hemodialysis unit take every precaution to protect the staff and patients from this infection.

General Comment. No matter how well adjusted or how well dialyzed a patient may be, it must be acknowledged that he is not totally well. In addition to low level uremia and chronic anemia, he is confronted regularly with the time-consuming dialysis, limitations in diet, and whatever hemodynamic instability may be caused by the procedure itself. Despite, this, however, many patients can lead productive and comfortable lives. Some need to change their type of vocation since they are not capable of doing heavy manual labor. Sedentary occupations can be performed quite effectively, however. The patient on dialysis also has to come to grips with the real and psychologic dependence on the machine. Travel is much less available to him, and he must constantly arrange travel schedules with a back-up dialysis facility in mind. There are organizations which do provide dialysis patients with a list of units in various locations, and this has been a great help. In short, life on dialysis, although adequate and productive, is not optimal and is at the very best a compromise. Its use in combination with an active transplantation program offers the patient a number of treatment choices, and seems the best approach. Although, as pointed out, the quality of life achieved with the artificial kidney does not approach that possible with a well-functioning transplanted kidney, differences in mortality and morbidity with both procedures must be considered. In a well-run, carefully monitored dialysis program, the yearly mortality rate may be as low as 5 per cent, and this needs to be measured against the higher mortality rate which may occur with some forms of transplantation. The decision as to which modality or combination of modalities of therapy is employed must be made considering all these factors.

Abel, J. J., Rountree, L. G., and Turner, B. B.: On the removal of diffusible substances from circulating blood by means of dialysis. Trans. Assoc. Am. Physicians, 23:51, 1913.

Bailey, G. L. (ed.): Hemodialysis—Principles and Practice. New York, Academic Press, 1972, p. 496.

Garibaldi, R. A., Forrest, J. N., Bryan, J. A., Hanson, B. F., and Dismukes, W. E.: Hemodialysis-associated hepatitis. J.A.M.A., 225:384, 1973.

Hampers, C. L., Schupak, E., Lowrie, E. G., and Lazarus, J. M.: Long-term Hemodialysis. 2nd ed. New York, Grune and Stratton, 1973.

GLOMERULAR DISEASE

O. M. Wrong

608. INTRODUCTION

Diseases which affect glomeruli display such important features in common that they can usefully be considered together and contrasted with diseases commencing in other parts of the kidney. Numerically, glomerular disease accounts for approximately half of the patients with severe renal disease seen in most communities and over two thirds of the patients accepted for renal replacement by units undertaking intermittent hemodialysis or renal transplantation.

Each glomerulus consists of a complex branching system of capillaries; thus, even though these capillaries are highly specialized, glomerular disease can be regarded as a form of capillary disease. In many forms of glomerular disease small blood vessels in other parts of the body are also diseased, but because the glomerular circulation is particularly vulnerable to pathologic insult the effects of renal damage may dominate the clinical picture. Many glomerular diseases, particularly the inflammations, are the result of antigen-antibody reactions; in others the glomeruli are infiltrated with abnormal deposits, e.g., diabetic renal disease, amyloid, Fabry's disease.

Most forms of glomerular disease are macroscopically diffuse, affecting equally the cortex of both kidneys, and one part of the cortex as severely as another. Consequently the small amount of material which can be removed by percutaneous renal biopsy usually yields a histologic picture which is representative of the kidneys as a whole, and this investigation has been valuable in both diagnosis and study of the natural history of glomerular disease. Histologically glomerular lesions may be *generalized* (i.e., involving all glomeruli), or *focal* (involving only some); within a glomerulus a lesion may be either *diffuse* (affecting the whole glomerulus) or *segmental* (affecting only a portion of the glomerulus). These topographic distinctions are of help in categorizing glomerular disease further.

Proteinuria. Increased loss of protein in the urine, in excess of the 30 to 130 mg per day excreted normally, is almost invariable in glomerular disease; it is a direct result of increased glomerular permeability to plasma proteins caused by the disease process. The amount of protein lost in the urine may be much greater than in other forms of renal disease; losses of more than 3 grams per day are not seen except in glomerular disease, and this finding therefore has great diagnostic value. The main urinary protein is always albumin, but variable amounts of the other plasma proteins are also lost, depending on the type of disease. When urinary protein losses of more than 5 grams a day persist, hepatic synthesis may not be able to increase sufficiently to maintain the serum albumin, and hypoalbuminemic edema may result. The triad of proteinuria, hypoalbuminemia, and edema is known as *nephrotic syndrome,* and is discussed in detail in Ch. 609.

Hypertension. Hypertension may complicate any form of renal disease, but is particularly common and severe in glomerular disease, although even here it is not invariable. It is now known that renal hypertension has at least two causes: (1) increased secretion of renin by the juxtaglomerular apparatus (JGA), and (2) increased extracellular fluid and blood volume caused by diminished renal ability to excrete salt and water, e.g., the "renoprival" hypertension that follows bilateral nephrectomy. Both factors play a part in the hypertension of glomerular disease, but their relative contributions differ from case to case. The JGA may be directly involved or rendered ischemic by the primary disease, and hypertension may be caused by the resultant hypersecretion of renin. When glomerular disease has resulted in renal failure, hypertension analogous to renoprival hypertension may develop simply from failure to excrete salt and water. The development of severe hypertension in glomerular disease is an ominous sign, as it leads to further damage from the effects of high blood pressure on the renal circulation. Prompt control of hypertension is therefore of vital importance in the care of such patients.

Tubular Defects. Evidence of tubular dysfunction occurs early in the clinical course of many types of renal disease, e.g., analgesic nephropathy, polycystic disease, and obstructive uropathy. In such conditions renal acidosis, or renal wasting of sodium or water, may develop when there is still little reduction in glomerular filtration rate. In primary glomerular disease these defects are rarely seen until renal failure develops, with serum creatinine raised above 3 to 5 mg per 100 ml, and even then marked tubular abnormalities are rare. The acidosis is less severe than occurs in tubular syndromes with similar degrees of renal failure, and is not usually hyperchloremic in type. Urinary concentrating ability is impaired, but the defect is usually an obligatory isosthenuria rather than the hyposthenuria seen in some tubular syndromes. Experiments involving dietary sodium depletion have shown that patients with glomerular disease are often unable to reduce urinary losses of sodium as efficiently as normal subjects, but their obligatory losses are usually well below the amounts supplied by their diet, and it is exceptional for a sodium supplement to be required.

In clinical practice use of the aforementioned principles will usually distinguish glomerular disease from other forms of renal disease. However, it is frequently difficult to distinguish between different forms of glomerular disease, even with the assistance of all modern diagnostic laboratory aids. To some extent this is the result of artificial distinctions between so-called disease entities, which may represent merely groups of commonly associated clinical features, rather than the results of distinct etiologic processes. But the problem is also due to the very limited way in which glomeruli can respond to different pathologic insults, which means that the same histologic and clinical picture may result from several different pathologic processes.

609. NEPHROTIC SYNDROME

Definition. In the first half of this century the term *nephrosis,* introduced by Müller in 1905, was widely used in at least two quite different senses: (1) as a descriptive histopathologic term for renal disease without an inflammatory component, and (2) to describe the clinical picture caused by heavy urinary protein losses. Much confusion was caused by this double use, and as a result the word has been largely abandoned. By general agreement the term *nephrotic syndrome* has been adopted for the second of these meanings, and refers to the *clinical association of heavy proteinuria, hypoalbuminemia, and generalized edema.* It is further understood that the

TABLE 1. Causes of Nephrotic Syndrome

Autoimmune forms of primary glomerular disease (see Table 2, Ch. 610)
Glomerular involvement in connective tissue diseases
  Systemic lupus erythematosus
  Polyarteritis
  Anaphylactoid purpura
  Goodpasture's syndrome
  Hemolytic-uremic syndrome
Familial nephritis
Congenital nephrotic syndrome
Glomerular involvement in other systemic diseases
  Quartan malaria
  Schistosomiasis
  Secondary syphilis
  Accelerated hypertension
  Diabetic glomerulosclerosis
  Amyloidosis
Mechanical causes
  Renal vein thrombosis
  Constrictive pericarditis
  Obstruction of inferior vena cava
  Sickle cell anemia
Toxins
  Mercury, organic or inorganic
  Gold
  Allergy to pollen, insect bites, snake venom, plant toxins, vaccines
  Serum sickness
Drug hypersensitivity
  Trimethadione and paramethadione, perchlorate, probenecid, penicillamine, sulfonamides, etc.
Miscellaneous
  Toxemia of pregnancy
  Renal transplant

plasma albumin is low as a result of urinary albumin loss, and the edema is the result of the altered Starling capillary forces caused by the consequent low plasma oncotic pressure. In general these criteria are not fulfilled unless at least 5 grams of protein a day are lost in the urine at some time in the course of the disease and the plasma albumin is less than 3 grams per 100 ml.

The aforementioned definition does not include reference to renal excretory failure, to hypertension, or to hypercholesterolemia. At various times attempts have been made to include one or another of these features as obligatory items in the definition, particularly hypercholesterolemia. However, the advantages of simplicity are lost if the definition includes features not closely linked causally, such as hypertension and renal failure, or of which the mechanism is uncertain, such as hypercholesterolemia.

Etiology. The nephrotic syndrome has many causes. Table 1 shows those that have been fully substantiated. The list includes almost all recognized forms of glomerular disease, and *only* forms of glomerular disease, for urinary protein losses in other forms of renal disease are not gross enough to give rise to hypoalbuminemia. (It has sometimes been claimed that pyelonephritis can give rise to the nephrotic syndrome, but the patients referred to have probably had glomerular disease complicated by pyelonephritis.) The most important items in Table 1 are separately described in the text; in some of the others the glomerular morphology has not been fully established. There is some overlap between parts of the table; thus the nephrotic syndrome caused by various foreign proteins can be due to a proliferative glomerulonephritis or minimal change disease, and that seen in renal transplants may have either a proliferative or a membranous picture. Drug hypersensitivity may cause nephrotic syndrome as part of an allergic vasculitis (sulfonamides), an immune-complex glomerulonephritis (penicillamine), or minimal change disease (probenecid).

Many of the causes listed give rise to transient nephrotic syndrome which in itself is neither a diagnostic nor a therapeutic problem. Persistent nephrotic syndrome, on the other hand, is a major diagnostic and therapeutic problem to all who deal with renal disease. In Europe and North America about 75 per cent of cases are caused by three idiopathic types of glomerular disease – minimal change disease, membranous disease, and the various types of chronic proliferative glomerulonephritis. The frequency of these three types varies between centers, partly because of variations in classification of cases with mixed membranous and proliferative change, but in most centers minimal change disease causes the majority of cases in children and one fifth to one third of adult cases. The proliferative varieties of glomerulonephritis are slightly more common than membranous disease except in elderly men. The main causes of the disease in the remaining 25 per cent of nephrotics who do not have idiopathic glomerular disease are diabetic glomerulosclerosis, amyloidosis, various forms of focal glomerulonephritis (including lupus erythematosus and anaphylactoid purpura), and renal vein thrombosis.

Clinical Manifestations. Generalized edema, often accompanied by ascites and pleural effusions, is the sine qua non of the nephrotic syndrome. The edema is primarily due to the reduced plasma oncotic pressure caused by hypoalbuminemia, but numerous other factors, such as salt intake and mineralocorticoid activity, contribute to its development, and because of these there is no predictable relationship between the amount of edema and the level of the plasma albumin. The sequence giving rise to edema is shown in Figure 1. In children gross edema of the face may develop early in the course of the disease, but in adults the legs are usually most affected. In severe cases the weight of the body may be increased by 50 per cent simply from accumulation of edema fluid.

Hypertension is present in some patients, but its presence depends on the type of glomerular disease. The low plasma volume which results from a very low plasma albumin may occasionally cause severe vascular collapse with hypotension. Protein malnutrition caused by the high urinary losses may lead to muscle wasting (often obscured by the generalized edema) or growth retardation in children. Increased opacity of the nails (leukonychia) is often present, and occasionally it is possible to estimate how long the nephrotic syndrome has existed by the position of the discolored area.

Urine may be scanty while edema is accumulating, and contains more than 5 grams of protein a day. The feature of the urinary deposit and degree of renal impairment depend on the underlying glomerular pathology, but transient renal failure may occur from hypovolemia or tubular damage without implying a destructive glomerular disease. Children with nephrotic syndrome

sometimes develop evidence of multiple renal tubular defects, with renal glycosuria, aminoaciduria, and a potassium-losing tendency.

Plasma albumin is invariably reduced below 3.0 grams per 100 ml. The usual value is between 1.0 and 3.0 grams per 100 ml, but occasionally concentrations as low as 0.5 gram per 100 ml are seen; in such cases signs of hypovolemia (particularly postural hypotension) are common, and the edema is often resistant to treatment. The plasma proteins other than albumin may be normal, but electrophoresis often shows a decrease in alpha$_1$ and gamma globulins, and an increase in alpha$_2$ and beta globulins which is mainly due to increases in alpha-glycoprotein and beta lipoprotein. The concentrations of the relatively small molecular weight transferrin and ceruloplasmin are reduced, whereas fibrinogen concentrations are increased.

The other characteristic chemical change in the blood is hyperlipidemia. This involves not only cholesterol, the most easily measured plasma lipid, but all the major lipid components of plasma, including triglycerides and phospholipids. Plasma cholesterol may rise to 1500 mg per 100 ml, but the level of this and of the other lipids varies considerably, even in patients with the same type of nephrotic syndrome. Little prognostic or diagnostic value can be attached to the determination except that marked elevations appear to be less common in lupus erythematosus than in other forms of the nephrotic syndrome. The mechanism of the hyperlipidemia is obscure, but seems intimately linked to the low albumin concentration. Nephrotic hyperlipidemia appears to carry an increased risk of premature generalized atheroma.

Differential Diagnosis. Two complex investigations, *renal biopsy* and *differential protein clearances,* have proved of great value in establishing the morphologic diagnosis in individual cases. Nephrotic syndrome is now one of the main indications for renal biopsy. The diseases that cause the syndrome are nearly always diffuse, so that needle biopsy yields a representative picture. The procedure is not usually technically difficult unless the kidneys are small, which is unusual. Frequently it is possible to base treatment and prognosis on the histologic findings. This matter is discussed under the various disease headings, and will not be further elaborated here.

The diagnostic value of differential protein clearances was largely established by Squire and his colleagues (for references, see under minimal change glomerular disease). The principle is that the abnormal glomerulus in nephrotic syndrome permits the passage of increased amounts of protein, and that the selective pattern of this permeability varies in different diseases. Some glomerular diseases permit only the smaller proteins, e.g., albumin and transferrin, to escape in the urine (selective), whereas in others all the plasma proteins are found (nonselective). A crude idea of glomerular permeability can be obtained by electrophoresis of the urine; a highly selective proteinuria consists almost entirely of albumin with small peaks of alpha$_1$ and gamma globulin, whereas a nonselective proteinuria shows an electrophoretic pattern similar to that of normal plasma. However, electrophoresis is an unsatisfactory method for the study of glomerular selectivity, for the electrical charge and molecular weight of proteins are not closely related, and more satisfactory results can be obtained by measurement of individual proteins. A useful indication of selec-

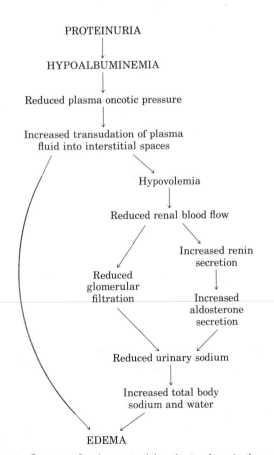

Increased glomerular permeability to
large molecules

PROTEINURIA

HYPOALBUMINEMIA

Reduced plasma oncotic pressure

Increased transudation of plasma
fluid into interstitial spaces

Hypovolemia

Reduced renal blood flow

Increased renin
secretion

Reduced
glomerular
filtration

Increased
aldosterone
secretion

Reduced urinary sodium

Increased total body
sodium and water

EDEMA

Figure 1. Sequence of main events giving rise to edema in the nephrotic syndrome.

tivity, suggested by Cameron and Blandford, is the ratio of the clearance of IgG to that of transferrin; in highly selective proteinuria, values below 0.15 are obtained. The major cause of a highly selective proteinuria is minimal change glomerular disease, which carries a good prognosis and usually responds well to steroids. The forms of nephrotic syndrome likely to be confused with this disease, which have a much worse prognosis and do not satisfactorily respond to steroids, i.e., membranous and proliferative glomerular disease, show poor selectivity in their pattern of protein excretion. There appear to be only two exceptions to the general rule that a highly selective proteinuria indicates a good prognosis, and both are uncommon—congenital nephrotic syndrome, a rare and invariably fatal disease, and occasional cases of renal amyloidosis.

Treatment. *Glomerular Lesion.* Treatment of the underlying glomerular disease of the common causes of nephrotic syndrome will be discussed under specific glomerular diseases. In general it is unsatisfactory, but exceptions will be mentioned as they arise.

Treatment of the Nephrotic Syndrome. Gross edema carries an appreciable morbidity and mortality, mainly from infection and the effects of immobility, and patients appear to be improved both physically and psychologically when treatment leads to its disappearance. But although the cause of the edema is the low serum albumin, there is no practicable way of increasing plasma albumin while urinary protein losses persist. *High protein diets* have been advocated for years; occasionally they cause a marginal increase in plasma albumin, but usually their only obvious effect is to increase urinary protein losses. Moreover, protein is the most costly item of the diet, and many patients are unable to take a high protein diet because of its expense. *Intravenous protein,* given as salt-poor human albumin, is occasionally of value in the treatment of hospital patients with circulatory collapse caused by hypovolemia, or to initiate diuresis in a patient with refractory edema, but it produces a transitory effect and is impractical for long-term treatment.

The most important factor in treatment is the proper use of *diuretics.* Except in cases of profound hypoalbuminemia, or when the syndrome is complicated by severe renal failure, edema can nearly always be controlled by diuretics alone. The diuretic regimen required varies from patient to patient; in general oral agents are best, and it is wise to start treatment with a relatively gentle drug, such as a thiazide, and only use the more powerful diuretics, e.g., furosemide and ethacrynic acid, if initial treatment fails to produce diuresis. Potassium deficiency usually arises in patients given diuretics more than three times a week, and should be prevented by the simultaneous administration of potassium supplements or of potassium-sparing diuretics, such as spironolactone or amiloride; however, in renal failure potassium depletion is seldom a problem, and these measures should be avoided as they can precipitate hyperkalemia. Disappearance of edema can be hastened by combining diuretics with a low sodium intake (as low as 20 mEq per day), but this step is not usually necessary except in advanced renal failure.

Modern diuretics are now so efficient that there is no longer a place for local fluid removal by abdominal paracentesis or Southey's tubes, although occasionally benefit may be obtained by aspiration of pleural effusions if these do not disappear rapidly.

When assessing the progress of a patient with nephrotic syndrome, the most useful guides are the presence or absence of edema, body weight, 24-hour urinary proteins, and serum albumin, and decisions regarding changes in treatment can be taken only with this information. Even when there is no effective treatment for the glomerular lesion per se, it is often found that proteinuria varies spontaneously over a wide range, and it may be possible to reduce or stop the use of diuretics as plasma albumin rises to a level at which edema no longer occurs. When diuretics are required, the mistake must not be made of pushing treatment to the point at which the patient suffers severe postural hypotension, and it may be good judgment to allow mild edema to persist, particularly when the serum albumin is below 1.0 gram per 100 ml.

Nephrotic syndrome is usually a chronic state, and it is wise therefore to encourage patients to follow their normal activities as far as possible. Frequently the physician will be asked about possible risks of pregnancy. The dangers depend largely on the nature of the underlying renal disease and the risk that because of this the pregnancy will be complicated by hypertension and placental insufficiency. Hypoalbuminemic edema does not per se contraindicate pregnancy (although edema frequently gets temporarily worse during pregnancy), and many women with nephrotic syndrome, particularly that resulting from minimal change glomerular disease, have completely normal pregnancies.

Cameron, J. S., and Blandford, G.: The simple assessment of selectivity in heavy proteinuria. Lancet, 2:242, 1966.
Edwards, K. D. G.: Antilipaemic drugs and nephrotic hyperlipidaemia. *In* Edwards, K. D. G. (ed.): Drugs Affecting Kidney Function and Metabolism. Basel, S. Karger, 1972, p. 370.
Robson, J. S.: The nephrotic syndrome. *In* Black, D. A. K. (ed.): Renal Disease. 3rd ed. Oxford, Blackwell Scientific Publications Ltd., 1972, p. 331.

610. GLOMERULONEPHRITIS

Definition. The term "glomerulonephritis" has usually been applied to forms of glomerular disease characterized by an inflammatory reaction, with leukocyte infiltration and cellular proliferation of the glomeruli. However, in recent years it has become clear that most forms of glomerular inflammation are caused by immune injury; this chapter has therefore been expanded to include some types of glomerular disease, e.g., minimal and membranous glomerulopathies, which strictly are not glomerular inflammations at all but also appear to be the results of immune glomerular injury.

Etiology. Repeated attempts to isolate microorganisms from the lesions of glomerulonephritis have failed, and these diseases are not considered to be the direct result of bacterial invasion of the kidneys. It is more difficult to exclude the role of viruses, but at present there is no good evidence that any form of human glomerulonephritis is caused by the presence of viruses in the glomeruli.

The detailed pathogenesis of glomerulonephritis is still obscure, but there is considerable evidence that an antigen-antibody reaction plays a major part in initiating the glomerular lesions in most forms of glomerulonephritis. The evidence can be summarized as (1) demonstration by immunofluorescence and electron microscopy of complexes of antigen-antibody and complement either on or within the glomerular basement membrane in many forms of glomerulonephritis; (2) marked lowering of various fractions of serum complement in many cases; (3) experimental production of glomerular lesions resembling human glomerulonephritis by injections either of antikidney antibodies prepared from other species or of nonspecific antigen or antigen-antibody complexes.

Two main types of immune injury appear to be etiologically important in glomerulonephritis. In the first of these, antibodies are directed against the glomerular basement membrane (anti-GBM nephritis) which becomes the seat of a reaction involving antigen (GBM), antibody, and complement, leading to polymorphonuclear infiltration, cellular proliferation, and fibrin deposition, with eventual crescent formation and obliteration of the glomerular space. Antibody (IgG) and complement can be shown by immunofluorescence to be deposited in a fine continuous line along the basement membrane of every capillary loop (Fig. 2). This type of immune injury appears to account for most cases of Goodpasture's syndrome and some cases of rapidly progressive proliferative glomerulonephritis and renal transplant nephritis.

The second and more common type of immune glomerular injury, immune complex disease (ICD), does not involve antibodies directed against renal tissues. The glomeruli are damaged by immune complexes which arise in the circulation from interaction of antibody with antigens of extrarenal origin. These complexes are deposited in the glomeruli in close relation to the basement membrane. Antigen-antibody complexes arising from relative antigen excess are particularly liable to cause glomerular injury, as they are relatively small and are not removed by the reticuloendothelial system as rapidly as larger complexes. Once deposited in the glomeruli, antigen-antibody complexes activate complement, leading to an acute inflammatory reaction, with polymorphonuclear infiltration and fibrin deposition. Immunofluorescent studies show irregular granular staining for gamma globulin and complement along the basement membrane (Fig. 3), a pattern distinct from the smoothly linear deposition seen in anti-GBM disease (Fig. 2). Under the electron microscope complexes appear as electron-dense masses arising from the basement membrane, usually on

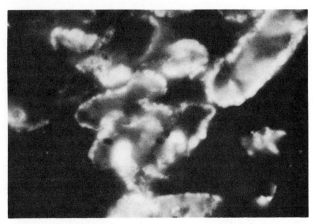

Figure 3. Granular glomerular deposition of IgG in a patient with idiopathic membranous disease. (× 1050.) (Courtesy of Dr. D. J. Evans.)

its epithelial surface. Examples of this type of glomerular disease are lupus nephritis (in which the antigen is DNA), poststreptococcal nephritis (streptococcal antigen), glomerulonephritis with glomerular deposition of Australia antigen, and the nephritis of both quartan malaria and infective endocarditis. However, in most cases of immune complex disease, it has not yet been possible to identify the responsible antigen.

It may eventually prove possible to devise a classification of glomerulonephritis entirely in immunologic terms, but this is not yet practicable. Renal immunology is still in its infancy, and there are many unanswered questions—for example, the role of deficiencies in the immune response of the host, the parts played by complement fixation and cell-mediated immunity, and the importance of damaged renal tissues as antigens promoting a further immunologic reaction. The classification used here (Table 2) is therefore based primarily on clinical and morphologic criteria.

Platelet aggregation in glomerular capillaries and fibrin deposition in the glomerulus and glomerular space occur in inflammatory forms of glomerular disease and potentiate immunologic damage. The presence of fibrin deposition can be suspected from the finding of fibrin degradation products in the urine; when intravascular coagulation is marked, and particularly when the renal disease is part of a generalized small vessel disease, fragmented and distorted red cells may appear in the peripheral blood and occasionally the full picture of a microangiopathic hemolytic anemia, with a lowered platelet count, increased platelet turnover, and reduced plasma fibrinogen.

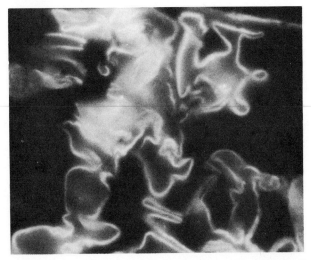

Figure 2. Linear glomerular deposition of IgG in a patient with Goodpasture's syndrome. (× 1050.) (Courtesy of Dr. D. J. Evans.)

TABLE 2. Classification of Glomerulonephritis

1. Minimal change glomerular disease
2. Focal glomerulosclerosis
3. Idiopathic membranous glomerular disease
4. Proliferative glomerulonephritis
   a. Acute poststreptococcal glomerulonephritis
   b. Acute glomerulonephritis caused by other infections
   c. Glomerulonephritis in infective endocarditis
   d. Mesangiocapillary glomerulonephritis
   e. Focal glomerulonephritis with recurrent hematuria
   f. Other varieties of proliferative glomerulonephritis
5. Renal involvement in connective tissue diseases

Logical therapeutic attempts to interrupt the immunologic processes responsible for glomerulonephritis, as well as their immediate consequences, have included cytotoxic drugs, such as the nitrogen mustards, cyclophosphamide, and azathioprine, to reduce antibody formation; steroids or other anti-inflammatory agents to reduce the effects of immune injury on the kidney; and anticoagulants to lessen platelet and fibrin deposition. Such rational forms of therapy have in general proved disappointing; the occasional successes are mentioned when appropriate.

Brain, M. C., Dacie, J. V., and Hourihane, D. O.: Microangiopathic haemolytic anaemia: The possible role of vascular lesions in pathogenesis. Br. J. Haematol., 8:358, 1962.

Dixon, F. J.: The pathogenesis of nephritis. Am. J. Med., 44:493, 1968.

Fish, A. J., Michael, A. F., and Good, R. A.: Pathogenesis of glomerulonephritis. In Strauss, M. B., and Welt, L. G. (eds.): Diseases of the Kidney. 2nd ed. Boston, Little, Brown & Company, 1971, p. 373.

Germuth, F. G., and Rodriguez, E.: Immune Complex Deposit and Antibasement Membrane Disease. Boston, Little, Brown & Company, 1973.

Peters, D. K.: The kidney in allergic disease. In Gell, P. G. H., Coombs, R. R. A., and Lachmann, P. J. (eds.): Clinical Aspects of Immunology. 3rd ed. New York, Oxford University Press, 1974.

MINIMAL CHANGE GLOMERULAR DISEASE
(Lipoid Nephrosis)

Definition. This is a glomerular disease causing heavy proteinuria, characterized by absence of obvious histologic glomerular changes on light microscopy.

The term "lipoid nephrosis" was introduced by Munk in 1913, and refers to the presence of fat bodies in the urine and fatty change in the tubular cells. These changes are now known to be the result of a glomerular protein leak, but with the light microscope it is not usually possible to see glomerular abnormalities, and it was not until the advent of the electron microscope that glomerular changes were shown to be invariably present. Hamburger's suggestion that the term "minimal change" should be used to describe the glomerular lesions has been widely followed.

Etiology, Incidence, and Pathology. The frequent association with allergic conditions such as asthma and sensitivity to foreign proteins, and the dramatic response induced by steroids, have suggested to some that the condition is a form of IgE-mediated immune glomerular injury, but this has not been convincingly demonstrated.

The disease is most common in infancy and childhood, a fact largely responsible for the good prognosis of the nephrotic syndrome in childhood. The peak incidence is between three and four years, but no age is exempt. Males are affected more often than females, in a ratio of 3:2. In adults lymphoma elsewhere in the body, particularly Hodgkin's disease, has sometimes been reported in association with this type of renal disease, but the causal connection between the two conditions has not been explained.

Light microscopy usually shows no glomerular abnormalities, but there may be occasional small areas of glomerular proliferation or adhesions to Bowman's capsule. The tubules usually show protein casts and doubly refractile lipid vacuoles in the cells of the proximal tubule; edema of the interstitium is often present and may cause considerable renal enlargement. The electron microscope invariably shows changes in the glomeruli, consisting of swelling and fusion ("smudging") of the foot processes of the epithelial cells on the outer side of the basement membrane. The basement membrane itself usually has a normal appearance, but sometimes contains small vacuoles or shows irregular thickening.

Until recently the view was widely held that this form of renal disease represented an early form of glomerulonephritis which would eventually show destructive glomerular changes. This view is no longer tenable; serial renal biopsies have shown that the glomerular lesions do not usually progress; indeed, they disappear after a spontaneous or steroid-induced clinical remission. The few patients who do not remit appear to have a different condition to start with—either an early form of membranous glomerulopathy, which should be detected by electron microscopy, or focal glomerular sclerosis (described subsequently) which usually produces a nonselective proteinuria.

Despite the absence of gross changes in the basement membrane on light microscopy, it is likely that the protein leak is the result of change in the basement membrane itself. The change in the foot process is probably caused by the presence of protein within Bowman's space, for identical appearance can be produced in animals by intravenous injection of proteins which cross the glomerular filter. This histologic appearance is also a feature of other forms of glomerular disease with heavy proteinuria, and is in no way specific for minimal change glomerular disease, although here it is the only constant glomerular finding.

The permeability characteristics of the glomerulus in this disease have been well worked out (Squire, Blainey, Hardwicke, and Soothill). The urinary proteins consist almost entirely of the plasma proteins of lower molecular weight, particularly albumin (molecular weight 68,000) and transferrin (90,000), whereas plasma proteins of larger size, such as beta-lipoprotein (molecular weight up to 2,500,000) are almost completely absent. The same pattern of glomerular permeability can be demonstrated after intravenous injection of dextrans of different molecular sizes, when only the smaller molecules are found in the urine. The glomerular protein leak is thus highly selective, whereas in almost all other forms of glomerular disease the leak is nonselective, or poorly selective, in that plasma proteins of every molecular size are found in the urine.

Clinical Manifestations. The most common first symptom is edema, which develops insidiously and often reaches mammoth proportions. Examination at this stage reveals all the characteristics of the nephrotic syndrome: heavy proteinuria (more than 5 grams per day), hypoalbuminemia, and usually hypercholesterolemia. The urine sediment contains hyaline, granular and fatty casts, and occasional red cells; red cell casts are not found. The plasma urea and creatinine are usually normal; however, azotemia is not uncommon in the early stages of the disease, and rarely transitory oliguric renal failure develops—perhaps the result of hypovolemia or obstruction of tubules by protein casts.

The disease has a remarkable tendency to remit. This may take place spontaneously, may follow systemic infections such as measles, or may result from treatment with steroids or cytotoxic drugs. Remissions are usually complete, with disappearance of all signs, but partial remissions with continuing mild proteinuria are also common. Relapses are unfortunately frequent, and may exactly replicate the initial attack. Repeated relapses may occur over a period of many years (over 20 years in one case personally known to the author) without deterioration in renal excretory function or the appearance of destructive changes in the glomeruli.

Treatment. The chief hazard lies in the complications of edema, particularly infection, which have been greatly reduced by modern diuretics and antimicrobial drugs. Before the advent of penicillin, pneumococcal peritonitis was a common cause of death, but this is now very rare. Treatment of edema is discussed in connection with the nephrotic syndrome. Two other hazards of the disease require mention. Hypogammaglobulinemia, owing partly to reduced synthesis and partly to urinary losses of gamma globulin, itself carries a risk of infection; hypercholesterolemia, as in other forms of nephrotic syndrome, may eventually lead to early atheroma and a predisposition to arterial thrombosis.

This is one of the very few forms of glomerular disease in which the underlying glomerular fault can be remedied by treatment. When given steroids or corticotrophin (ACTH), most patients rapidly lose their proteinuria and all other signs, usually within two to six weeks of the start of treatment. Serial renal biopsies have shown that the glomerular foot processes simultaneously return to normal. It is not known how adrenal steroids exert this remarkable effect, and the dose required varies from case to case, usually being in the range of 20 to 60 mg of prednisolone, or equivalent, daily. Relapses often follow withdrawal of steroids, even when the dose has been reduced very gradually.

Treatment with steroids should not be lightly undertaken. It must be realized that this is the only form of nephrotic syndrome which shows a satisfactory response at all frequently, and that this treatment has definite dangers. The diagnosis should not rest on clinical manifestations alone, but should be based on the appearances of renal biopsy and on the finding of a highly selective proteinuria. In children, in whom high doses of steroids are less dangerous, and in whom most cases of nephrotic syndrome are caused by this process, it is justifiable to commence steroids without the evidence of renal biopsy or protein clearances, provided that treatment is gradually withdrawn if no effect is seen within six weeks. Conversely, in a few elderly patients, even those who have been shown by renal biopsy to have the disease, the risks of long-continued steroids, particularly peptic ulcer, may be greater than the risks of nephrotic syndrome, provided that edema can be satisfactorily controlled.

Once a decision is made to employ steroid treatment, it is wise to begin with a high dose, e.g., 60 to 80 mg of prednisolone per day in an adult, or 40 to 60 mg in a child. This should be maintained for three to six weeks and then reduced to a maintenance dose of one half to two thirds the original dose if a satisfactory response (disappearance or marked lessening of proteinuria) occurs; if not, the treatment should be gradually withdrawn. Maintenance treatment should be continued for three to six months; then periodic attempts can be made to reduce dosage further or stop altogether; if clinical relapse occurs, it will be necessary to increase the dose temporarily.

Troublesome side effects of steroids are common, but there is some evidence that they can be prevented or lessened by giving steroids on alternate days, without loss of therapeutic effect. It is unwise to regard complete abolition of proteinuria as the sole aim of treatment, for in some cases this requires an unacceptably high dose of steroids, whereas a much smaller dose will sufficiently

lessen proteinuria to return the plasma albumin to normal and so remove the risk of edema.

The most difficult patients to treat are those who become steroid dependent, relapsing as soon as the dosage is reduced or after intercurrent infections, yet developing severe side effects of steroid overdose. These patients are usually children, in whom retardation of growth is the most troublesome complication. In such cases ACTH may be preferable to steroids, because there is evidence that it has less effect in retarding growth. Alternatively, prolonged remission may be obtained by the use of cytotoxic drugs, of which cyclophosphamide and chlorambucil have been the most successful.

Barratt, T. M., and Soothill, J. F.: Controlled trial of cyclophosphamide in steroid-sensitive relapsing nephrotic syndrome of childhood. Lancet, 2:479, 1970.

Black, D. A. K., Rose, G., and Brewer, D. B.: Controlled trial of prednisone in adult patients with the nephrotic syndrome. Br. Med. J., 3:421, 1970.

Connolly, M. E., Wrong, O. M., and Jones, N. F.: Reversible renal failure in idiopathic nephrotic syndrome with minimal glomerular changes. Lancet, 1:665, 1968.

Farquhar, M.: Ultrastructure of the nephron disclosed by electron microscopy. A review of normal and pathologic glomerular ultrastructure. In Metcoff, J. (ed.): Proceedings, 10th Annual Conference on the Nephrotic Syndrome. New York, National Kidney Disease Foundation, 1959, p. 2.

Hardwicke, J., and Soothill, J. F.: Proteinuria. In Black, D. A. K. (ed.): Renal Disease. 2nd ed. Oxford, Blackwell Scientific Publications, Ltd., 1967, p. 252.

Squire, J. R., Blainey, J. D., and Hardwicke, J.: The nephrotic syndrome. Br. Med. Bull., 13:43, 1957.

FOCAL GLOMERULOSCLEROSIS
(Segmental Hyalinosis)

Definition, Pathology, and Incidence. This form of glomerular disease is characterized by focal and segmental areas of glomerular sclerosis, usually commencing in the juxtamedullary glomeruli and gradually spreading to involve other parts of the kidney, with eventual renal failure. The condition has only recently been demarcated from other varieties of glomerulonephritis. The cause is obscure, but affected glomeruli have been shown to contain deposits of complement and gamma globulin. There is evidence that patients treated by renal transplantation may develop the disease in the transplanted kidney.

Incidence and Clinical Course. The incidence of the disease is unknown, for it is still frequently confused with minimal change glomerular disease, benign recurrent hematuria, and various other types of proliferative glomerulonephritis. It most commonly presents in children or adolescents, with nonselective proteinuria, often gross enough to cause nephrotic syndrome, or recurrent macroscopic hematuria. Renal biopsy may not sample the affected glomeruli, thus giving rise to a false diagnosis of minimal change glomerular disease. No treatment is known to definitely alter the course of the disease, but the progression to renal failure usually takes many years.

Churg, J., Habib, R., and White, R. H. R.: Pathology of the nephrotic syndrome in children. Lancet, 1:1299, 1970.

IDIOPATHIC MEMBRANOUS GLOMERULAR DISEASE
(Epimembranous Nephritis)

Definition. This is a glomerular disease of obscure cause, characterized by thickening of the capillary basement membrane, without cellular infiltration. The condition is often called "membranous glomerulonephritis," but this term is inappropriate inasmuch as there is no histologic evidence of glomerular inflammation.

Etiology, Incidence, and Pathology. The finding of granular deposits of IgG and complement on the thickened basement membrane has led to the suggestion that it is a form of immune-complex disease.

The disease affects all ages, but is most common in adults; males are affected more often than females, particularly in middle age and later life.

Histologically it can be recognized with the light microscope by a more or less uniform thickening of the capillary basement membrane of every glomerulus. This is often obvious in sections stained with hematoxylin and eosin, but is particularly apparent in thin sections (less than 2μ) stained with periodic acid–methenamine–silver. The thickening may be so marked that the capillary lumen is reduced in caliber or obliterated, but there is no increase in glomerular cellularity. Under the electron microscope the basement membrane is thickened, vacuolated, and irregular; arising from its epithelial side, under the fused foot processes of the epithelial cells, are electron-dense granules which can be shown by immunofluorescence (Fig. 3) to contain IgG and complement. These findings are very similar to those in some forms of proliferative glomerulonephritis, except for the absence of a cellular reaction, and the suggestion has been made that this is a similar type of immune-complex disease, but without involvement of cell-mediated immunity.

An association of membranous glomerular disease with malignancy arising outside the kidneys (especially bronchus and gut) has been reported, suggesting that in these cases the renal disease is caused by immune complexes of host antibody and tumor antigen.

The membranous form of glomerular disease is generally believed to be distinct from other forms, not merely a stage in the evolution of another process. This view is supported by serial renal biopsies, which have shown a worsening in the glomerular alterations with time but no real change in nature.

Clinical Manifestations. Membranous glomerular disease usually presents with nephrotic syndrome, less often with asymptomatic proteinuria, renal hypertension, or chronic renal failure. All features of the nephrotic syndrome may be found, but the condition may be distinguished from minimal change glomerular disease by higher average age of patients, frequent presence of hypertension and renal failure, nonselective nature of the proteinuria, and rarity of clinical remission. Microscopic hematuria is slightly more common than in minimal change glomerular disease, but hypercholesterolemia is less frequent.

The disease runs a slowly progressive course; usually many years elapse before renal failure is a serious problem. Very occasionally a fulminant course is followed, oliguric renal failure developing within a few months of onset. No treatment is known to alter the course of the disease, although there have been occasional reports of remission after use of steroid or cytotoxic drugs. It is difficult to evaluate the role of these treatments, and the few properly controlled trials that have been reported have shown no evidence of benefit. Spontaneous clinical remissions occur but are rare, in most cases only temporary and not accompanied by change in the histologic features. When the disease is associated with carcinoma, remission may follow successful removal of the tumor.

Franklin, W. A., Jennings, R. B., and Earle, D. P.: Membranous glomerulonephritis. Long-term serial observations on clinical course and morphology. Kidney Int., 4:36, 1973.
Gluck, M. C., Gallo, G., and Lowenstein, J.: Membranous glomerulonephritis. Evolution of clinical and pathologic features. Ann. Intern. Med., 78:1, 1973.

PROLIFERATIVE GLOMERULONEPHRITIS

Definition. This term strictly covers all diseases in which cellular proliferation affects the glomeruli, but is most conveniently restricted to those in which renal involvement is not part of the vasculitis of systemic disease (e.g., lupus erythematosus).

Etiology. Until quite recently it was widely believed that most cases were poststreptococcal in origin. This view is now clearly recognized as incorrect; it is difficult to know the true proportion, but in adults less than 25 per cent appear to have disease of this cause.

The group is heterogeneous, but immune renal injury probably plays a part in all forms. Some cases of rapidly progressive disease show linear deposition of IgG and complement in the glomeruli, and are probably examples of anti-GBM nephritis. Immune-complex injury appears to be responsible for poststreptococcal nephritis, the nephritis caused by other acute infections and infective endocarditis, and that caused by chronic quartan malaria. In many other cases the immunofluorescent findings are those of immune-complex disease, but the nature of the antigen is unknown. Often patients come to medical attention late in the course of their disease, when evidence of the original immune glomerular injury can no longer be found.

Acute Poststreptococcal Glomerulonephritis

This is the best documented and most understood form of proliferative glomerulonephritis. Although its course is complex and variable, it does demonstrate almost all the possible features of glomerular disease, and therefore has served in the past as the usual starting point and reference in discussing glomerulonephritis. To some extent this emphasis has been unfortunate in that it has tended to delay recognition of the many forms of glomerulonephritis which are unrelated to the Streptococcus and are now becoming relatively more important because of the falling incidence of streptococcal infection. However, the disease is still common enough to deserve emphasis in its own right.

Etiology. In 1836 Richard Bright recognized that acute glomerulonephritis usually followed an infection, particularly scarlet fever. Since then scarlet fever has become much less common, and the incidence of post-scarlatina nephritis has likewise fallen. It is now recognized that acute nephritis can follow streptococcal infection in any part of the body, although the pharynx is the usual site, and is unrelated to the production of erythrotoxin by the organism. Only certain strains of Streptococcus are "nephritogenic" (capable of initiating nephritis); all the offending organisms are Group A hemolytic streptococci, and the majority are of Type 12. Other less common nephritogenic strains are Types 1, 4, 25, 41, 49 (Red Lake strain), and 57; the last two have

been incriminated in outbreaks of streptococcal pyoderma causing nephritis.

Symptoms of acute glomerulonephritis do not usually
develop until 7 to 20 days after the streptococcal infection, by which time the patient appears to have recovered from the local infection. Transitory mild proteinuria and microscopic hematuria are common during the
initial streptococcal infection, particularly in persons
who subsequently develop clinical nephritis, but it is not
clear whether these are the first manifestations of
nephritis or merely represent the urinary changes common in any severe infection.

Coincident with the development of nephritis there is
a marked reduction in serum complement, apparently
caused by its deposition in the kidney. Immunofluorescent studies during the acute stage of the disease show
irregular staining for complement and gamma globulin,
particularly IgG, within the glomeruli, and electron
microscopy reveals electron-dense deposits, corresponding to this immunofluorescence, on the epithelial
side of the glomerular basement membrane. These findings indicate that the disease is an immune-complex
form of renal injury, but it is not known why only certain
strains of streptococci can provide the necessary antigenic stimulus. Antigenic similarities between the
glomerular basement membrane and Streptococcus have
been demonstrated, but the weight of evidence is against
this being a form of anti-GBM nephritis.

Incidence.   Acute poststreptococcal nephritis occurs in
all parts of the world. Males are affected about twice as
frequently as females. No age is exempt, but the disease
is particularly common in children and adolescents,
perhaps because of the increased risk of acquiring a
streptococcal infection from exposure at school. In temperate climates it is most common in winter, when streptococcal infections are at their peak. The relationship of
acute nephritis to certain streptococcal strains explains
some epidemiologic features of the disease, such as its
tendency to cause small epidemics in homes or schools,
as well as the variations in incidence in persons known
to have had streptococcal infections—from nil with a
non-nephritogenic strain to as high as 40 per cent with a
strain known to be nephritogenic. By contrast the incidence of rheumatic fever in those with streptococcal infections who have not previously had the disease is fairly
constant at 2 to 3 per cent.

Pathology.   The disease is rarely fatal, and most
knowledge of its pathology comes from material obtained
by biopsy. The occasional necropsy has shown symmetrical renal enlargement and pallor of the cortex. Histologically the glomeruli are nearly all similarly affected, with
enlargement of the whole glomerulus and marked increase in the number of nucleated cells, consisting
mainly of endothelial and mesangial cells and mononuclear leukocytes, although polymorphonuclears may also
be found. Epithelial cell proliferation is usually not
prominent. The glomerular lobules are swollen and relatively bloodless, with reduced capillary lumina and occasional necrotic and thrombosed capillary loops. The
transitory renal failure of the acute phase of the disease
is the result of these changes, rather than obliteration of
Bowman's space by epithelial crescents.

During resolution the last feature to remain is hypercellularity, most marked in the vicinity of the glomerular stalk or mesangium, which may be detectable several
months after apparently complete clinical recovery. This
change, though typical of resolving poststreptococcal

glomerulonephritis, does occur in some other forms of
proliferative glomerulonephritis, and its presence cannot be regarded as conclusive evidence of an earlier poststreptococcal disease.

Clinical Manifestations.   Most patients have a fairly
clear history of preceding streptococcal infection.
Usually it is a pharyngitis which has been sufficiently
severe to keep the patient away from school or work, but
occasionally the infection lies elsewhere—for example,
an otitis media, a leg ulcer, or a surgical wound. Sometimes the infection can only be demonstrated by a positive bacteriologic culture, or presumed from the finding
of a raised antistreptolysin O titer.

The patient has usually recovered from the initial infection when manifestations of nephritis appear, some 7
to 20 days after onset of the original infection. The most
common presenting symptom is edema, noted particularly in the face on first arising. Hematuria is also a common first symptom; usually the urine has a smoky
brown color, but occasionally it is frankly blood stained.
Less commonly the patient complains of reduced urine
output, or of bilateral dull loin pain, which is probably
caused by stretching of the renal capsules.

It is important to note that the edema present at the
onset of the disease is invariably caused by fluid retention, which itself is the result of reduced renal excretion
of salt and water. In an adult of average size the presence
of generalized edema implies a weight gain of at least 5
kg. At this stage patients have not lost enough protein in
the urine to develop hypoalbuminemic edema (nephrotic
syndrome), although this complication may develop
later; nor is there good evidence for the earlier views
that the edema of acute nephritis is caused either by
increased capillary permeability or by heart failure.

Vague malaise, nausea, and headache are common in
acute nephritis, but fever is unusual, and patients do not
usually feel really ill, although often distressed by the
appearance of edema. In mild cases they may be quite
asymptomatic; the disease may be picked up only by examining the urine of a person known to have had a
recent streptococcal infection.

Physical examination usually shows generalized
edema and mild hypertension of the order of 140 to 160
systolic, 90 to 110 diastolic. Very occasionally hypertension is severe, with retinal hemorrhages and exudates,
papilledema, or hypertensive encephalopathy. In general, the degree of hypertension is in proportion to the
amount of edema. Fluid retention, if marked, may lead
to the signs of congestive cardiac failure, with cardiac
enlargement and triple rhythm, venous engorgement,
hepatic distention, and gross pulmonary and systemic
edema.

Urinary output is usually reduced, although the reduction is often not noticed by the patient. Complete
suppression of urine is rare, and indicates a very severe
attack of nephritis; this complication may develop
within a few days of the onset, or urinary output may
gradually fall to nothing over several weeks. As might
be expected, fluid retention is particularly severe in such
cases, and unless rigid restriction of sodium and water
has been instituted, edema and hypertension are particularly marked. Unless renal function returns rapidly,
symptoms of renal failure eventually appear, with nausea and vomiting, twitching and pruritus, acidotic respirations, and progressive anemia.

Urine.   Urinary concentration is usually in the range
of 350 to 600 mOsm per kilogram (corresponding to a

specific gravity of 1.010 to 1.017) when correction is made for a protein content, but appears more concentrated because of the presence of red cells. Moderate quantities of protein are present, and occasionally mild renal glycosuria occurs. The urinary sediment contains large numbers of red cells and leukocytes, particularly the former, and a smaller number of renal tubular cells. Casts, particularly the granular variety, are also present; erythrocyte and hemoglobin casts indicate bleeding from the glomerulus and are particularly helpful in diagnosis.

Laboratory Tests. Mild renal failure, with plasma creatinine values of 1.5 to 4.0 mg per 100 ml, is very common in the initial stage of the disease. In the rare case of severe renal failure, the biochemical sequelae are similar to those of renal failure from other causes except that hyperkalemia seems particularly common, probably because these patients are usually previously fit and active young people who rapidly lose muscle mass during their illness.

A nephritogenic strain of Streptococcus can be cultured from the pharynx of many patients, except those treated with effective antimicrobial drugs, even when all clinical evidence of local infection has disappeared. Occasionally cultures taken from the throats of other members of the family will reveal the presence of a nephritogenic organism when this can no longer be cultured from the patient's own throat.

The serum antistreptolysin O titer is usually raised, indicating recent streptococcal infection, but the titer may fall rapidly to normal and so pass unnoticed, or it may not rise at all if the streptococcal infection is rapidly aborted by the use of antimicrobials. Unfortunately, as has been pointed out by Rammelkamp, not all nephritogenic strains of streptococci produce streptolysin O (nor do they invariably cause beta-hemolysis in culture), and so detection of the preceding streptococcal infection by this means may be difficult. The serum titer of type-specific antibody to streptococcal M antigen is more difficult to measure, but remains raised for considerably longer after a streptococcal infection (often for years), and has the added advantage of indicating whether an infection was caused by a strain known to be nephritogenic. A marked drop in serum complement is characteristic of acute poststreptococcal nephritis, but this finding is not diagnostic because it may occur in other forms of nephritis, e.g., systemic lupus erythematosus and the nephritis of bacterial endocarditis, and few laboratories can provide the measurement as a routine.

The erythrocyte sedimentation rate is moderately raised. The hemoglobin concentration is usually slightly reduced (to 11 to 12 grams per 100 ml) as a result of dilution.

Course and Prognosis. Diuresis usually starts 7 to 14 days after the onset of symptoms, and over the space of two days the patient loses edema and hypertension. Renal clearances and the plasma creatinine concentration return to normal, but microscopic hematuria and proteinuria persist longer, and may not disappear for weeks or months. During this period clinical relapses may occur, particularly at the time of other respiratory infections.

Occasionally urinary losses of protein during the first few weeks are sufficiently large to cause hypoalbuminemic edema, which at first reveals itself when renal excretory function improves and the expected diuresis does not materialize. Although the development of nephrotic syndrome is of grave import if it first appears after several months, its rapid appearance at this early stage of the disease does not necessarily carry a bad prognosis, and patients with this syndrome may recover completely within the next few weeks.

It is difficult to ascertain what proportion of patients recover completely, for hospital series are weighted by the more severe cases. Most estimates state that over 90 per cent of children and about 60 per cent of adults eventually make a full clinical recovery. These figures may be unduly pessimistic, because many of the published series have included patients, who, with the benefit of more recent advances of glomerular immunofluorescence and electron microscopy, might not now be classified as having poststreptococcal nephritis.

In the early years of this century, poststreptococcal nephritis in the acute stage caused death in about 5 per cent of patients. Death was usually due to pulmonary edema, the complications of hypertension, or intercurrent infections. Nowadays these complications can usually be prevented, and most fatalities are the result of acute renal failure with anuria or severe oliguria. Patients can be kept alive by peritoneal dialysis or hemodialysis, and many so treated, particularly children, experience return of renal function after days or weeks. If renal recovery does not ensue or is inadequate to maintain life, and renal biopsy shows irrecoverable glomerular damage, they may be treated by intermittent hemodialysis or renal transplantation.

Unfavorable features which suggest that satisfactory recovery will not take place are (1) delayed or absent diuresis; (2) persistent renal failure; (3) persistent hypertension; (4) prolonged or increasing proteinuria, often leading to nephrotic syndrome; (5) a persistently lowered plasma complement; and (6) severe changes in the renal biopsy, particularly obliteration of Bowman's space by epithelial crescents and disappearance of glomerular capillaries.

Patients who recover from acute glomerulonephritis are not immune to second attacks, but these are uncommon because of the development of type-specific antibodies which protect against infection by the original strain of Streptococcus and exert an effect for many years. Some apparent second attacks of acute poststreptococcal glomerulonephritis are in reality exacerbations of a longstanding chronic glomerulonephritis.

Differential Diagnosis. The condition most easily confused with acute poststreptococcal nephritis is exacerbation of a subacute or chronic glomerulonephritis, with transitory hematuria and further reduction in renal function. Such exacerbations may be precipitated by many different infections, even those caused by viruses, but are particularly common after streptococcal infections; in the absence of previous evidence of renal disease, this situation closely resembles an initial attack of poststreptococcal nephritis. This diagnostic problem is now rather infrequent, probably because of the declining incidence of streptococcal infections.

The transient proteinuria and microscopic hematuria that accompany many severe systemic infections may also be mistaken for poststreptococcal nephritis, but these signs occur at the height of the infection and are not usually associated with other features of renal disease.

It may be difficult to distinguish acute poststreptococcal nephritis from other forms of acute glomerulonephritis, such as Henoch-Schönlein nephritis (which may also be precipitated by a streptococcal infection), systemic lupus erythematosus, the microscopic form of polyarteritis nodosa, recurrent focal nephritis with hematuria, and the nephritis of bacterial endocarditis. Here the physician will be guided by features suggesting systemic involvement and by evidence of recent streptococcal infection. Renal biopsy may also help by showing a glomerular lesion more focal than that of poststreptococcal nephritis.

Less often, acute poststreptococcal nephritis may be confused with primary malignant hypertension, with various forms of hemolytic anemia with hemoglobinuria, or with acute tubular necrosis, particularly when the latter is precipitated by a systemic infection.

Treatment. It has not been convincingly shown that any form of treatment alters the course of the glomerular lesion, but individual manifestations and complications frequently require treatment.

Infection. In the acute stage of nephritis, penicillin is usually given either by mouth or by injection to eradicate any remaining streptococcal infection. This treatment has much to commend it, but there is no evidence that it alters the subsequent evolution of the glomerular disease. Penicillin should also be used prophylactically to treat close contacts, particularly members of the family who may have contracted streptococcal infection from the patient, unless this possibility is excluded by bacteriologic tests. Oral penicillin V (phenoxymethyl penicillin, 250 mg twice a day) is often recommended after attacks of acute nephritis to reduce subsequent respiratory infections which might cause exacerbations of nephritis; if used, it is best continued through the next winter season when streptococcal infections are more widespread. (The question of prophylaxis against streptococcal infections is further discussed in Ch. 190.)

Edema. Fluid retention during the oliguric phase of the disease should be prevented by careful attention to body weight. Salt and fluids should be restricted if edema is present or a weight gain of more than 2 to 3 kg occurs. In these circumstances oral fluids should be limited to no more than 500 ml per day, plus a volume equal to the urine output of the previous day, and dietary sodium should be reduced as far as possible, preferably to 20 mEq per day. If severe edema is already present, or develops despite these measures, a diuresis may occasionally be obtained by oral diuretics, particularly furosemide in doses of 40 to 1000 mg twice a day. Digitalis is ineffective, despite the presence of many classic features of congestive cardiac failure, because the circulatory troubles are due to excess of extracellular fluid, and not to a primary cardiac cause. In the rare case in which fluid overload threatens life and diuresis cannot be obtained by drugs, the excess fluid should be removed by dialysis.

Uremia. There is no convincing evidence that dietary protein influences the course of the glomerular lesion, but early in the disease it is wise to restrict protein intake moderately (40 to 70 grams per day) until it is clear that the patient is not likely to develop renal failure. Patients who do develop severe renal failure should be treated by more drastic protein restriction, with or without some form of dialysis, as described in Ch. 605 to 607.

Hypertension. If fluid retention is carefully controlled, there is usually no need to treat hypertension specifically. But the patient with severe fluid overload may require treatment for hypertensive encephalopathy with convulsions, or retinopathy with failing vision; in these emergencies parenteral hydralazine, reserpine, or diazoxide is the drug of choice.

Other Drugs. Steroids, anticoagulants, and cytotoxic drugs, either alone or in various combinations, have been used in the acute stage of the disease, particularly in patients with severe renal failure, but there is no good evidence that they alter the outcome.

Rest. In the acute stage of the disease bed rest is advisable. The patient does not usually wish to be active, and the recumbent position facilitates diuresis. Once macroscopic hematuria, edema, and hypertension have disappeared and the plasma creatinine has returned to normal, the value of rest is uncertain. Many authorities recommend that bed rest continue as long as proteinuria is diminishing, but there is no evidence that this alters the course of the disease, and it may be impractical or economically disastrous for the patient whose proteinuria persists for months.

Continued Observation. Because of the difficulty in deciding when a patient has recovered from the disease, it is valuable to follow all patients until at least a year after the last clinical evidence of nephritis. Frequent determinations of blood pressure, urinary proteins and sediment, and plasma creatinine and creatinine clearances are the most useful indications of disease activity. The purpose of this follow-up is to observe any exacerbation of the disease, so that renal failure, nephrotic syndrome, or hypertension can be immediately recognized and treated. Acute urinary infections, which are not uncommon in such patients, can also be recognized and treated.

Bright, R.: *In* Osman, A. A. (ed.): Original Papers of Richard Bright on Renal Disease. London, Oxford University Press, 1937.

Dodge, W. F., Spargo, B. H., Travis, L. B., Srivastava, R. N., Carvajal, H. F., Debeukelaer, M. M., Longley, M. P., and Menchaca, J. A.: Poststreptococcal nephritis. A prospective study in children. N. Engl. J. Med., 286:273, 1972.

Heptinstall, R. H.: Pathology of acute glomerulonephritis. *In* Strauss, M. B., and Welt, L. G. (eds.): Diseases of the Kidney. 3rd ed. Boston, Little, Brown & Company, 1971, p. 405.

Levy, J. E., Salinas-Madrigal, L., Herdson, P. B., Pirani, C. L., and Metcoff, J.: Clinico-pathologic correlations in acute poststreptococcal glomerulonephritis. Medicine, 50:453, 1972.

Rammelkamp, C. H., and Earle, D. P.: Pathogenesis of chronic glomerulonephritis. *In* Ingelfinger, F. J., Relman, A. S., and Finland, M.: Controversy in Internal Medicine. Philadelphia, W. B. Saunders Company, 1966, p. 331.

Schwartz, W. B., and Kassirer, J. P.: Clinical aspects of acute poststreptococcal glomerulonephritis. *In* Strauss, M. B., and Welt, L. G. (eds.): Diseases of the Kidney. 3rd ed. Boston, Little, Brown & Company, 1971, p. 419.

Zabriskie, V., Utermohlen, V., Read, S. E., and Fischetti, V. A.: Streptococcus-related glomerulonephritis. Kidney Int., 3:100, 1973.

Acute Glomerulonephritis Caused by Other Infections

Frequently patients with acute glomerulonephritis show no evidence of a preceding streptococcal infection, even though in almost every other way their disease is typical of poststreptococcal nephritis. It is impossible to be sure that any patient has not had a streptococcal infection, and probably many of these patients have had an infection which cannot be detected in retrospect. However, it is now recognized that an acute glomerulonephritis may follow infections caused by microorganisms other than streptococci. It seems likely, from a consideration of the pathogenesis, that an acute immune complex type of nephritis in humans may, like the experimental model, be precipitated by exposure to a variety of foreign proteins, which need not be exclusively of infective origin.

When pneumococcal pneumonia was a common disease, before the advent of antimicrobial drugs, it was frequently reported to be a cause of acute glomerulonephritis. The disease was similar to the poststreptococcal variety, except that the latent interval was shorter and fluid retention and hypertension were less apparent. In most instances the possibility of a complicating streptococcal infection was not adequately excluded, and there must be doubt as to the existence of such an entity.

Acute glomerulonephritis has also been reported after typhoid fever and diphtheria and after many virus infections such as mumps, measles, chickenpox, infective hepatitis, mononucleosis, and infections with echovirus and adenovirus. Although in many instances a complicating streptococcal infection has not been excluded, the number of these reports is so great that it is difficult to accept that they all represent cases of poststreptococcal nephritis. In several recent cases a renal biopsy has been obtained or the patient has come to necropsy, and glomerular changes very similar to those of poststreptococcal nephritis have been found.

The concept of an acute diffuse glomerulonephritis which results from nonstreptococcal infections has thus been established, but it should be emphasized that nephritis is much rarer after these infections than it is after infections with nephritogenic strains of group A streptococci.

The natural history of glomerulonephritis caused by other than streptococcal infections is not fully known. The disease appears to behave like poststreptococcal nephritis in that the majority of patients recover completely, but a few are left with a continuing process with progressive impairment of renal function, which may be complicated by nephrotic syndrome of severe hypertension.

Glomerulonephritis in Infective Endocarditis

The subacute glomerulonephritis that complicates endocarditis has often been regarded simply as a form of acute glomerulonephritis caused by streptococcal infection. This view is misleading for several reasons: (1) The viridans streptococci do not cause nephritis when they invade other parts of the body; (2) it has been increasingly realized, perhaps because of longer survival, that patients with other forms of infective endocarditis (e.g., pneumococcal, *H. influenzae,* and fungal) also develop glomerulonephritis. The usual alternative hypothesis, that the disease is caused by bacterial embolization to the glomeruli, would explain the focal type of glomerulonephritis which is sometimes seen, but not the more usual diffuse glomerulonephritis nor the fact that bacteria cannot be demonstrated in the glomeruli. Recent immunofluorescent and electron microscope studies have shown granular deposits of IgG and complement, and more rarely fibrin, in the glomeruli of patients with diffuse glomerulonephritis associated with endocarditis caused by a variety of organisms, findings strongly suggesting immune-complex disease.

Patients with infective endocarditis do not usually show evidence of glomerulonephritis until they have had infection for several weeks. The condition presents with hematuria and proteinuria, and less frequently with impairment of renal function, which is often first mistakenly attributed to severe cardiac failure and resulting reduced renal perfusion. Hypoalbuminemic edema and hypertension have not been features of most reports. Severe renal failure is seldom seen except in patients in the terminal stages of a prolonged endocarditis.

In most cases the diagnosis presents no difficulty because the symptoms and signs of the underlying endocarditis are prominent. Rarely this is not so, and the disease may be confused with diffuse forms of vasculitis, such as periarteritis or systemic lupus, because of fever and evidence of a systemic disease, necrotic and hemorrhagic skin lesions, or renal biopsy findings of a mixed focal and generalized glomerulonephritis. In such patients the true diagnosis may only be revealed by repeated blood culture, by the finding of splenomegaly, or by evidence of a cardiac lesion.

At present there is insufficient information on the natural history of the glomerulonephritis after successful treatment of the causative endocarditis, but it is unlikely that complete healing occurs in those with extensive glomerular disease.

Gutman, R. A., Striker, G. E., Gilliland, B. C., and Cutler, R. E.: The immune complex glomerulonephritis of bacterial endocarditis. Medicine, 51:1, 1972.

Mesangiocapillary Glomerulonephritis
(Membranoproliferative Glomerulonephritis)

Definition. This disorder is a form of chronic glomerulonephritis, only recently demarcated, in which glomerular mesangial cells are increased and capillary walls are irregularly thickened. There is marked and persistent reduction in serum C3 complement.

Etiology and Pathology. The reduction in complement is more persistent than in other forms of glomerulonephritis, and is not the result of deposition in the glomeruli, as it is unrelated to disease activity and persists after nephrectomy. There is evidence of an alternate pathway of C3 metabolism, caused by an abnormal factor of nonrenal origin (C3 "nephritic" factor, or C3 NeF) which in vitro breaks down C3 by a mechanism which does not involve the normal early components of complement activation. The fact that renal transplants can become affected by the disease suggests that a continuing systemic abnormality, perhaps involving the complement system, is responsible for the nephritis.

Immunofluorescence shows granular deposits of complement and properdin in glomerular capillaries; less often IgG and fibrin can be demonstrated. Histologic examination shows increased thickness of the basement membrane of peripheral glomerular capillaries, with some deposits on the endothelial sides of the basement membrane and narrowing of capillary lumina. Mesangial cells are increased in number, and their proliferation throughout the kidney may give the appearance of a lobular nephritis; there are occasional granulocytes.

Clinical Manifestations. Older children and young adults are most often affected. The disease may present with symptomless hematuria, proteinuria, or nephrotic syndrome, or rarely as an acute nephritis, although there is seldom a prior streptococcal infection. The course is slowly downhill, with episodes of hematuria and nephrotic syndrome, persistent hypocomplementemia, and gradual renal failure, apparently uninfluenced by any treatment. The average duration, from diagnosis to death or maintenance dialysis, is about ten years. In view of reports of involvement of renal homografts by the disease, maintenance dialysis is preferable to transplantation as a form of renal replacement.

Lancet Annotation: Pathways in complement activation. Lancet, 1:473, 1973.
Mandalenakis, N., Mendoza, N., Pirani, C. L., and Pollak, V. E.: Lobular

glomerulonephritis and membranoproliferative glomerulonephritis. Medicine, 50:319, 1972.

West, C. D., Ruley, E. J., Forristal, J., and Davis, N. C.: Mechanisms of hypocomplementemia in glomerulonephritis. Kidney Int., 3:116, 1973.

Focal Glomerulonephritis with Recurrent Hematuria
(Essential or Benign Hematuria)

The term *focal nephritis* has often been used in the European literature to designate a form of renal disease characterized by repeated attacks of profuse hematuria after systemic infection, leaving little residual renal damage. The renal lesion is a focal glomerular inflammation, but the disease clinically has little in common with other forms of focal glomerulonephritis, such as the renal lesions of polyarteritis or lupus erythematosus.

Clinical Manifestations. The disease is most common in the second and third decades of life, and affects males much more frequently than females. Rarely other members of the family may be affected. The characteristic features are recurrent attacks of hematuria, which usually start about the age of puberty and continue at the rate of several a year for as many as 20 or 30 years. Attacks may occur without obvious precipitating cause, but most often follow a febrile illness or, less frequently, surgical operation or some strenuous unaccustomed exertion. Unlike poststreptococcal nephritis, hematuria may develop within a few hours of the evidence of systemic infection, and is seldom delayed more than two days; it is often heavier than that which occurs in poststreptococcal nephritis, and may be accompanied by renal pain. There is no constant relationship to group A streptococci or to any particular form of infection. Often the manifestations of the precipitating illness (usually an evanescent pyrexia and myalgia) are so slight that this cannot be diagnosed with certainty.

Even during the attack of hematuria it is unusual for hypertension, renal failure, or edema to develop, although the urinary deposit is characteristic of an acute glomerulonephritis. Renal biopsy discloses focal areas of glomerular proliferation, usually affecting only a segment of a glomerulus here and there. The glomerular lesions are similar to those of Henoch-Schönlein purpura, but are usually less diffuse, and, like them, they show immunofluorescence to IgA. Complement and IgG can also be shown, and the deposits tend to have a mesangial distribution.

Prognosis. At first the urine clears completely after each attack, but in older patients mild proteinuria and microscopic hematuria may persist between attacks. The disorder is usually regarded as benign, because renal failure and hypertension do not commonly develop. However, occasionally these complications develop; more rarely still, the nephrotic syndrome is seen, and in such patients renal biopsy shows that the glomerular lesions, although still focal, have resulted in very severe glomerular destruction.

Management. The history is so distinctive that a diagnosis can usually be made with confidence from this alone. However, it is often valuable to demonstrate the characteristic histology by renal biopsy, either in order to reassure the patient that he has a form of renal disease that does not usually shorten life, or to put an end to repeated urologic investigations performed in an attempt to explain the hematuria.

Patients with the syndrome should be advised to avoid infections or any activities which they know are liable to precipitate an attack. Penicillin prophylaxis, to reduce bacterial respiratory infections, is often tried, but the results have been disappointing. The usual benign course of the condition does not justify routine use of steroids, nor is there any evidence that they influence the disease. Prolonged follow-up is advisable, because the course is not invariably benign and some of the long-term complications (e.g., hypertension and renal failure) require treatment.

Rapoport, A., Davidson, D. A., Deveber, G. A., Ranking, G. N., and McLean, C. R.: Idiopathic focal proliferative nephritis associated with persistent hematuria and normal renal function. Ann. Intern. Med., 73:921, 1970.

Roy, L. P., Fish, R. A., Vernier, R. L., and Michael, A. F.: Recurrent macroscopic hematuria, focal nephritis, and mesangial deposition of immunoglobulin and complement. J. Pediatr., 82:767, 1973.

Other Varieties of Proliferative Glomerulonephritis

Many cases of proliferative glomerulonephritis do not fit clearly into one or other of the categories so far described. Although some are probably poststreptococcal in origin, this is no longer believed to be the cause in most cases.

Extracapillary Glomerulonephritis with Epithelial Crescents (Fig. 4). This type of glomerulonephritis is only rarely of poststreptococcal origin, and is often of anti-GBM type, showing linear glomerular immunofluorescence for IgG and complement. Epithelial proliferation leads to the formation of crescents which fluoresce for fibrin and obliterate Bowman's space. The course is often fulminating, justifying the title "rapidly progressive glomerulonephritis," but occasionally the disease appears to become stationary or only slowly progressive. Children are rarely affected, but the condition is a frequent type of glomerular disease at all other ages.

Clinical presentation is with hematuria, nephrotic syndrome, renal hypertension, or oliguric renal failure. No treatment is known to definitely alter the course of the disease; there is good rationale for the use of anticoagulants to reduce crescent formation, but there is no convincing evidence that they improve survival.

Endothelial Glomerulonephritis. When cells from within the glomerulus (endothelial and mesangial cells) proliferate, the histologic changes are those of a lobular nephritis, with fusion of glomerular capillary loops, but without marked adhesion formation between the visceral and parietal layers of Bowman's capsule (Fig. 5). This pathologic picture is much more common than the extracapillary type of glomerulonephritis, but mixed types are also frequent. Some appear to be the result of a streptococcal infection, but in others this cause can be excluded with confidence.

The usual clinical presentations are with recurrent hematuria, nephrotic syndrome, or renal hypertension. Renal failure is not a prominent early feature, but it eventually develops after months or years as a result of progressive glomerulosclerosis. The disease frequently appears to remain unchanged for long periods, and renal function may even improve spontaneously, particularly in poststreptococcal cases. This is the histologic variety of glomerulonephritis to which the descriptive name *chronic glomerulonephritis* can most suitably be applied.

Although mixtures of types of glomerular disorders occur, in any one patient the renal condition usually runs true to type, the histology as shown by serial biop-

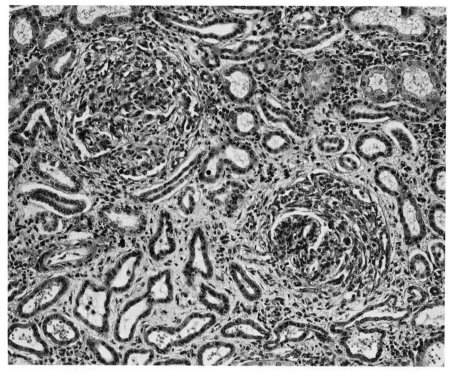

Figure 4. Abundant crescent formation in a 13-year-old girl with rapidly progressive glomerular nephritis. No good history of streptococcal infection was obtained. (H & E; × 150.) (From Heptinstall, R. H.: Pathology of the Kidney. Boston, Little, Brown & Company, 1966.)

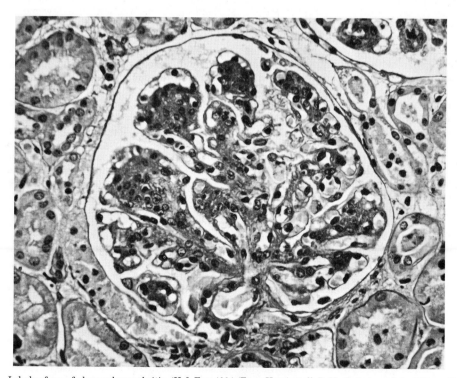

Figure 5. Lobular form of glomerular nephritis. (H & E; × 400.) (From Heptinstall, R. H.: Pathology of the Kidney. Boston, Little, Brown & Company, 1966.)

sies retaining its characteristics despite evolution of the disease.

In longstanding proliferative glomerulonephritis there may be little or no remaining cellular proliferation in the glomeruli, many of which are destroyed by fibrosis while the remainder show adhesions and segmental scarring. The atrophy of tubules rendered ischemic by glomerular destruction leads to gross renal shrinkage and distortion of renal architecture. Hypertensive damage, involving arterioles and arteries, is usually present and may lead to further ischemic atrophy. The final picture is difficult to distinguish from end-stage renal disease caused by other types of glomerular disease (e.g., membranous glomerular disease) and can even be confused with diseases which are not primarily glomerular, such as hypertensive nephropathy or chronic pyelonephritis.

Cameron, J. S.: The natural history of glomerulonephritis. *In* Black, D. A. K. (ed.): Renal Disease. 3rd ed. Oxford, Blackwell Scientific Publications, 1972, p. 295.

611. RENAL INVOLVEMENT IN CONNECTIVE TISSUE DISEASES

Many generalized diseases of connective tissue may cause glomerular disease which may be difficult to distinguish, on either clinical or histologic grounds, from other forms of glomerulonephritis.

Systemic Lupus Erythematosus. Some 50 to 75 per cent of patients with this condition develop renal disease at some time. It is an example of immune-complex glomerular injury, the complexes consisting of DNA (antigen), IgG, and complement. Glomerular involvement takes several forms: (1) segmental areas of glomerulitis, with hypercellularity and thickening of the basement membrane; (2) a membranous type of glomerulopathy without cellular proliferation; and (3) a diffuse proliferative glomerulonephritis with cellular proliferation, areas of glomerular necrosis, and crescent formation. These changes are not specific for lupus erythematosus, but their appearance in a patient with serologic and systemic evidence of that disease is sufficient to establish the cause of the glomerular lesion.

Renal involvement may be manifested clinically as a symptomless proteinuria which remains unchanged for months or years, with nephrotic syndrome, or with a severe progressive acute glomerulonephritis. Once renal failure has developed, the course is usually one of steady deterioration, leading to death in renal failure within a few months unless the patient is put on a renal replacement program. Steroids in high dosage (45 mg or more of prednisolone daily) have long been used in the treatment of active forms of lupus, and there is a strong impression that they produce benefit in the nephritis, although this has never been the subject of a properly randomized clinical trial. Patients with localized areas of glomerulitis appear to do best, whereas there is little evidence of benefit in those with diffuse proliferative glomerulonephritis. Various cytotoxic drugs (especially the nitrogen mustards and azathioprine) have also been used, but the number of patients reported has not been sufficient to decide on the benefit of such treatment.

Periarteritis Nodosa. Small arteries of the kidney may be affected, leading to macroscopic infarcts of the renal

substance, or there may be the microscopic form first described by Davson, Ball, and Platt, in which glomerular arterioles and capillaries are involved, leading to a proliferative glomerulonephritis which closely resembles other types of this disease but usually shows a more segmental pattern.

Although the systemic manifestations of the disease may affect any organ of the body, skin involvement seems particularly common in those with renal disease, and is often manifested as small tender areas, 2 to 4 mm across, representing infarcts in the pulp of the fingers and toes. Subungual splinter hemorrhages, if numerous, may have the same significance. However, it is not uncommon for renal disease to be the sole clinical manifestation of a polyarteritis.

The renal presentation may be that of a repeated renal infarction with local pain and hematuria, of an acute oliguric nephritis, or of chronic glomerulonephritis with proteinuria and steady reduction in renal function. Renal hypertension is common.

Usually the course is progressive deterioration, particularly in those with the microscopic form of the disease. Large doses of steroids appear to halt the progress of the disease in a small proportion of cases, and steroid-induced remissions of several years have been recorded. Rarely the disease appears to become stationary spontaneously, or there may even be temporary periods of improved renal function.

Wegener's Granulomatosis. This entity is discussed in Ch. 105. The renal lesions may contain small granulomas in relation to blood vessels in glomeruli; otherwise the kidney disease cannot be distinguished from classic polyarteritis.

Although it may be months or years before the syndrome is complicated by renal involvement, the progression of the renal disease is usually rapid once it appears, leading to uremia within a few months. Steroids have been used in treatment, with little effect, but more recently encouraging results have been obtained with cytotoxic drugs, particularly cyclophosphamide, the renal disease either becoming stationary or showing actual improvement. No controlled trial of this treatment has been reported, but the course of the untreated renal disease is so uniformly bad that this treatment is worthy of trial.

Anaphylactoid Purpura (Henoch-Schönlein Syndrome). In anaphylactoid purpura hematuria may be caused by bleeding from the mucosal surface of the ureters, bladder, or urethra. Occasionally, however, anaphylactoid purpura causes a true glomerulonephritis, which clinically resembles a poststreptococcal acute glomerulonephritis. This resemblance is enhanced if the disease follows a streptococcal infection, as is often the case. However, serum complement is not diminished, and renal biopsy shows focal rather than diffuse glomerulonephritis. The glomerular lesions are unusual in that they may show deposits of IgA on immunofluorescence, often accompanied by fibrin. It is generally believed, although the evidence is not convincing, that complete renal recovery is less common than after a poststreptococcal nephritis; but it must be remembered that recurrent attacks of anaphylactoid purpura are common, and the possibility of permanent renal damage may be greater for that reason. The course of the disease in patients whose glomerulonephritis does not resolve completely is very like that of other forms of glomerulonephritis, except that the nephrotic syndrome appears to be less common.

Goodpasture's Syndrome (Lung Purpura and Nephritis). Goodpasture's syndrome is a form of acute progressive glomerulonephritis accompanied by massive capillary hemorrhage into the lungs. The primary cause is unknown, but the glomerulonephritis appears to be caused by circulating anti-GBM antibodies (see Fig. 2) which also react with the basement membrane of the pulmonary alveoli. Histologically the renal lesion is difficult to distinguish from other forms of acute proliferative glomerulonephritis, except that it may initially show focal features. Within a few weeks the glomerular disease usually becomes generalized, with glomerular obliteration by epithelial crescents. The lungs show massive confluent alveolar hemorrhage, identical with that seen in the rare condition *idiopathic pulmonary hemosiderosis;* the pulmonary capillaries show patchy basement membrane changes, but it is usually difficult to see changes gross enough to account for the amount of blood in the alveoli.

No age is exempt, but the disease is most common in the second and third decades, and males are affected three or four times as often as females. The first symptom is usually recurrent hemoptysis, and only after days or weeks do manifestations of nephritis occur, most often hematuria. The pulmonary hemorrhage is often very severe, with symptoms and signs of acute blood loss; after repeated episodes an iron deficiency anemia may appear, owing to a sequestration of large amounts of iron in the lungs as hemosiderin. Occasionally the first manifestations are those of subacute glomerulonephritis, and only after several weeks does pulmonary hemorrhage indicate the presence of a generalized disease.

In most cases the renal lesion progresses rapidly to total glomerular destruction, often passing through a nephrotic phase, and leading to uremia within a few weeks or months of the onset of symptoms. Death may also result from pulmonary hemorrhage, either from asphyxia or acute blood loss. Treatment is usually without influence on the course of the disease, although there have been reports of long remissions after treatment with steroids. Hemorrhage into the lungs sometimes ceases after bilateral nephrectomy, and in cases in which lung hemorrhage is life-threatening this drastic form of treatment, combined with maintenance hemodialysis or renal transplantation, may have to be considered.

Hemolytic-Uremic Syndrome. This affects infants and young children and, less frequently, young adults. It is characterized by thrombocytopenia, microangiopathic hemolytic anemia, and acute progressive renal failure. Histologically the renal lesion is a proliferative glomerulonephritis, less frequently a patchy cortical necrosis.

The hematologic manifestations appear to be secondary to vasculitis, which may be generalized or confined to the glomeruli. Minor degrees of the same blood changes are common in all forms of acute glomerulonephritis, or diffuse small vessel vasculitis, and for this reason many authorities do not accept the hemolytic-uremic syndrome as a separate disease entity, but regard it as a syndrome with many causes, including poststreptococcal nephritis and polyarteritis. However, because the condition has sometimes occurred in small local outbreaks and is much more common in some communities, e.g., Argentina and Chile, than in others, it has been suggested by some that there might be an infective basis.

The condition often starts with evidence of acute gastroenteritis with bloody diarrhea, but whether this is infective or due to vascular lesions in the bowel is uncertain. Fever, pulmonary symptoms, cutaneous purpura, and neurologic features (especially convulsions and coma) are common. It is difficult to ascertain in an individual case whether the diffuse organ involvement is caused by underlying vasculitis or by local hemorrhage resulting from the thrombocytopenia, which is often profound.

Renal involvement is shown by hematuria and the rapid development of oliguric renal failure, without clinical remissions. Milder cases occur, but when renal failure develops it seldom improves; the few recoveries that have been reported have often followed treatment with steroids or heparin.

The Kidney in Systemic Sclerosis (Scleroderma). Although systemic sclerosis may affect the kidney, it is unusual among connective diseases in that it does not cause glomerulonephritis. Instead there is a slowly progressive obliteration of renal arteries of interlobular size or smaller, and of the renal arterioles, morphologically identical to the vascular involvement of other organs. Histologically the vascular changes closely resemble those of malignant hypertension and radiation nephritis. The usual clinical manifestations, if indeed there are any, include mild proteinuria, slowly progressive renal failure, and renal hypertension, which may be severe. Treatment of hypertension may be required, but otherwise there is no treatment for the renal lesion.

Benoit, F. L., Rulon, D. B., Theil, G. B., Doolan, P. D., and Watten, R. H.: Goodpasture's syndrome. A clinicopathologic entity. Am. J. Med., 37:424, 1964.

Clarkson, A., Lawrence, J., Meadows, R., and Seymour, A.: The haemolytic uraemic syndrome in adults. Quart. J. Med., 39:227, 1970.

Lieberman, E.: Hemolytic-uremic syndrome. J. Pediatr., 80:1, 1972.

Meadow, S. R., Glasgow, E. F., White, R. H. R., Moncrieff, M. W., Cameron, J. S., and Ogg, C. S.: Schönlein-Henoch nephritis. Quart. J. Med., 41:241, 1972.

Pollak, V. E., Pirani, C. L., and Schwartz, F. D.: The natural history of the renal manifestations of systemic lupus erythematosus. J. Lab. Clin. Med., 63:537, 1963.

Walker, W. G., Harvey, A. M., and Yardley, J. H.: Renal involvement in myeloma, amyloidosis, systemic lupus erythematosus, and other disorders of connective tissue. *In* Strauss, M. B., and Welt, L. G. (eds.): Diseases of the Kidney. 3rd ed. Boston, Little, Brown & Company, 1972, p. 825.

612. HEREDITARY NEPHRITIS
(Alport's Syndrome)

Definition. Hereditary nephritis is a form of hereditary renal disease, characterized histologically by glomerulonephritis and interstitial nephritis, frequently associated with nerve deafness.

Genetic Aspects and Incidence. The disease is inherited as an autosomal dominant. Males and females are approximately equally affected, but the disease usually takes a more serious form and is manifest at an earlier age in men. Patients with renal disease frequently have nerve deafness, and some members of the family may have deafness with normal renal function. Ophthalmologic defects, such as cataracts and lenticonus, occur less frequently.

Several hundred cases have been reported, but it is very difficult to make the diagnosis in sporadic cases or in families without deafness, and the true incidence is probably many times greater.

Etiology and Pathology. The nature of the underlying defect is unknown. Histologically the renal lesion may be a chronic proliferative glomerulonephritis, often with segmental glomerular lesions; in other patients the glomeruli appear normal, but there is an extensive interstitial nephritis which resembles pyelonephritis or analgesic nephropathy. Most writers have remarked on the fat-laden foam cells in the interstitium, but these are common in other forms of renal disease, and their presence cannot be regarded as diagnostic.

Clinical Manifestations. The first symptom is usually hematuria, often noticed in childhood, and frequently preceded by a systemic infection. Proteinuria is usually present, but is seldom severe enough to cause the nephrotic syndrome. Occasionally frank attacks of pyelonephritis occur, with positive urine cultures. The usual course is slow deterioration in renal function, often with hypertension, leading to renal failure in the third to fifth decade. Nerve deafness can develop at any age; initially it affects high tones predominantly, and may be unsuspected until revealed by audiometry.

Diagnosis. The diagnosis is often difficult because no single known feature of the disease is absolutely diagnostic. The most helpful features are nerve deafness in the patient or immediate relatives and familial renal disease. However, to be convincing, the family history should include more than one generation, for the presence of glomerulonephritis in several sibs might be the result of simultaneous infection with a nephritogenic Streptococcus during earlier childhood. Sporadic cases may be confused with other forms of chronic glomerulonephritis, with the syndrome of focal nephritis and recurrent hematuria described above, or with familial renal tubular defects which are occasionally associated with nerve deafness.

Treatment. No treatment is known to alter the progress of the renal disease, but patients may require treatment for urinary infections, for renal hypertension, or for symptomatic renal failure.

Perkoff, G. T.: Hereditary chronic nephritis. *In* Strauss, W. B., and Welt, L. G. (eds.): Diseases of the Kidney. 3rd ed. Boston, Little, Brown & Company, 1971, p. 1275.

613. RENAL VEIN THROMBOSIS

Increased renal pressure can give rise to heavy proteinuria alone or to all the manifestations of the nephrotic syndrome. This association has occasionally been reported in constrictive pericarditis, congestive cardiac failure, or thrombosis of the inferior vena cava, but it is more often the result of thrombosis of the renal veins.

There are five main varieties of renal vein thrombosis:

1. Thrombosis of the inferior vena cava with secondary involvement of the renal veins. Usually patients have a history of deep venous thrombosis of the legs or repeated pulmonary emboli. The full clinical picture of inferior vena caval obstruction, with conspicuous superficial and anastomotic veins, takes time to develop and is not always apparent.

2. Renal vein thrombosis associated with pregnancy. The cause of the association is unknown; it may be the result of stasis of the blood in the renal veins, caused by pressure of the gravid uterus, or a manifestation of the thrombotic tendency of pregnancy.

3. Obstruction of the renal veins or inferior vena cava by external pressure or neoplasm. Renal carcinoma, which often grows along the lumen of the renal veins, is one of the common causes in this category.

4. Renal vein thrombosis secondary to primary renal disease. This is the most common type of renal vein thrombosis. The main predisposing factor to thrombosis is probably a reduced renal blood flow. Thrombosis, usually bilateral, starts in the renal vein radicles, and only later extends to the main renal veins, whence parts of the thrombi may break away and cause pulmonary emboli. Although patients with many different types of renal disease are at risk, the condition appears to be particularly common as a complication of renal amyloidosis.

5. Primary renal vein thrombosis. This may complicate acute gastroenteritis, particularly in infants, perhaps as a result of increased blood viscosity caused by saline depletion, or there may be no obvious predisposing cause.

Pathology. When renal vein thrombosis is sudden and complete, as in the primary variety in children, the result is hemorrhagic infarction of the kidney. More often thrombosis is slowly progressive, allowing time for an anastomotic circulation to develop. The kidney is enlarged as a result of interstitial edema. The glomeruli show surprisingly little histologic change, and in some cases are virtually normal or merely enlarged. However, there is usually a mild diffuse thickening of the capillary basement membrane which resembles idiopathic membranous disease, even under the electron microscope, except that the thickening tends to be less marked. The glomerular capillaries are widely patent, and often show margination of leukocytes. There may be considerable tubular atrophy and interstitial cellular infiltration. None of these histologic changes are absolutely specific, and the findings on renal biopsy are not usually diagnostic except on the rare occasion when the biopsy includes a thrombosed vein.

Clinical Manifestations. Local pain and swelling may result from edema of the kidney with stretching of the renal capsule. Other clinical features depend very much on the cause of the thrombosis, but two developments are usual — nephrotic syndrome and renal failure. In patients who already have these features because of primary renal disease, there is sudden deterioration which often enables the diagnosis to be suspected. In patients without primary renal disease the picture is very similar to the insidious onset of the nephrotic syndrome of idiopathic membranous disease, and no doubt many patients are incorrectly so diagnosed; features which should arouse suspicion are severity of the nephrotic syndrome (protein losses of 40 to 80 grams a day may occur), the presence of local pain, coincident development of renal failure early in the course, pulmonary emboli, caval thrombosis, and the finding of marked interstitial edema and cellular infiltration in the renal biopsy.

Radiology may make a significant contribution to diagnosis. Venography of the inferior vena cava may show obstruction to this vein, thrombi protruding into the cava from the orifices of the renal veins, or reduced streaming of blood from the renal veins; when combined with the Valsalva maneuver, in which caval blood usually refluxes into the renal veins, phlebography may reveal obstruction to the main renal veins or filling of an anastomotic venous circulation.

Prognosis. In those with underlying renal disease the outlook for renal recovery is grave, and even with all modern resources these patients usually die unless treated with a renal replacement program.

In those without prior renal disease the prognosis is

less serious, although renal failure, gross nephrotic syndrome, and the risk of pulmonary embolization are all hazards. Fortunately renal function usually improves eventually, because of either recanalization or the development of anastomoses, but further attacks of renal vein thrombosis may occur. Renal hypertension is not usually a problem, but there is a risk of secondary pyelonephritis. In patients who survive, the features of nephrotic syndrome gradually relent, although they may take years to disappear.

Treatment. Nephrectomy is often recommended in acute renal vein thrombosis of childhood when the disease is unilateral; the value of the operation is controversial, but its proponents claim that the removal of the infarcted organ may prevent local infection or hypertension, and may reduce the spread of thrombosis. In adults nephrectomy has not been popular, although it is reasonable to believe that it would cure the nephrotic syndrome in the rare cases of unilateral renal vein thrombosis. The main aspects of treatment are anticoagulation, which needs to be continued for very long periods, treatment of the complicating nephrotic syndrome and renal failure, and, when necessary, the use of some form of dialysis.

Harrison, C. V., Milne, M. D., and Steiner, R. E.: Clinical aspects of renal vein thrombosis. Quart. J. Med., 25:285, 1956.

Rosenmann, E., Pollak, V. E., and Pirani, C. L.: Renal vein thrombosis in the adult. A clinical and pathological study based on renal biopsies. Medicine, 42:269, 1968.

614. RENAL CHANGES IN OTHER SYSTEMIC DISEASES

DIABETES MELLITUS

Although the renal complications of diabetes mellitus include capillary necrosis and pyelonephritis, the most serious and relentlessly progressive lesion is *intercapillary glomerulosclerosis (Kimmelstiel-Wilson lesion)* in which nodular deposits of eosinophilic material arise within the lobules of the glomerular tuft, and are associated with diffuse mesangial thickening, obliteration of the basement membrane, and gradual obliteration of the glomerular capillaries.

Glomerular lesions may be present in the prediabetic state, but it is unusual for them to give rise to clinical features until after the development of overt diabetes, and they are first seen most commonly in patients who have been known to have had diabetes for at least 10 to 15 years. Although the pathogenesis of the lesions is not clear, it seems likely that they are part of a generalized small vessel change which is also responsible for diabetic retinopathy and neuropathy. These three complications of diabetes are often found together; in particular, patients with renal disease almost invariably have retinal complications. There is no good evidence that careful control of diabetes influences the development of the glomerular lesion.

Patients with known diabetes usually have their urine tested frequently, and the first sign of glomerulosclerosis is therefore apt to be proteinuria, which may persist unchanged for years. Sooner or later the proteinuria increases and gives rise to the nephrotic syndrome. From then on the course is more rapidly progressive, with steady deterioration in renal function, leading within

months to renal failure, often accompanied by severe hypertension. No treatment is known to alter the course of the renal disease. Patients with end-stage uremia may be kept alive by intermittent hemodialysis, but are often not considered suitable for renal transplantation because of the difficulty experienced in controlling diabetes in patients given large doses of steroids. The nonrenal complications of diabetes, particularly the blindness from proliferative retinitis, are apt to cause difficulties even with maintenance hemodialysis.

Churg, J., and Dolgen, H.: Diabetic renal disease. *In* Strauss, W. B., and Welt, L. G. (eds.): Diseases of the Kidney. 3rd ed. Boston, Little, Brown & Company, 1971, p. 873.

AMYLOIDOSIS

Although systemic amyloidosis exists in several different forms that tend to affect different groups of organs, all forms are liable to attack the kidney, and renal failure is the most common cause of death from amyloidosis.

In the early stages renal amyloid causes considerable renal enlargement, but later the kidneys shrink to normal or subnormal size. The glomeruli and small arteries are the usual sites of deposition; tubules are affected less often. Glomerular involvement histologically resembles that of idiopathic membranous disease, except that the lesions are more nodular and often appear to be on the capillary side of the basement membrane. Renal amyloid usually stains well with Congo red, methyl violet, or thioflavine T; occasionally it does not take up these dyes and then can only be recognized with certainty by the electron microscope, which shows a characteristic fibrillary structure with a periodicity of 80 to 100 Å.

The first sign of amyloid is usually proteinuria, which may persist unchanged for years, but it occasionally disappears temporarily. More severe renal involvement causes nephrotic syndrome or renal failure. It was formerly believed that renal amyloidosis does not cause hypertension; this view is incorrect, although hypertension may be less common than in other forms of glomerular disease. Renal vein thrombosis is a very serious complication of amyloidosis, and should be suspected whenever a patient suddenly develops oliguric renal failure or marked worsening of nephrotic syndrome.

Although it is widely believed that cure or surgical removal of sepsis leads to regression of secondary amyloid, this is not a common event as far as the kidney is concerned, and amyloid may persist or accumulate further despite removal of the cause. Certainly it is not justifiable to submit patients to heroic surgery, which would not otherwise be warranted, simply because of the existence of amyloid. Treatment of nephrotic syndrome and renal failure caused by amyloid follows conventional lines. The value of prophylactic anticoagulants in preventing renal vein thrombosis is uncertain.

Very occasionally patients show a sodium-losing tendency and require a small salt supplement. This feature, so unusual in glomerular disease generally, may here be the result of deposition of amyloid in the adrenal cortex or distal renal tubules. Rarely other tubular syndromes, including nephrogenic diabetes insipidus and renal tubular acidosis, have been encountered in renal amyloidosis with unusually severe tubular involvement.

Patients with severe uremia from amyloidosis are eligible for intermittent hemodialysis, but they may be unsuitable for renal transplantation because of the danger that the steroids and cytotoxic drugs given to suppress transplant rejection lead to a flare-up of the original sepsis.

Triger, D. R., and Joekes, A. M.: Renal amyloidosis—a fourteen year follow-up. Quart. J. Med., 42:15, 1973.

615. BENIGN POSTURAL PROTEINURIA
(Orthostatic Proteinuria)

Benign postural proteinuria is a condition in which proteinuria occurs in the erect or lordotic position but disappears in recumbency, and in which there is no other clinical evidence of renal disease.

The condition—hardly a disease—appears to be most common in children and young adults, particularly men, although to some extent this distribution may be the result of their more frequent urine examinations. The condition is usually discovered at a routine medical examination for employment or medical insurance, and its incidence has been stated to be as high as 2 to 3 per cent in military recruits.

Characteristically the proteinuria cannot be demonstrated by conventional tests (Albustix or salicylsulfonic acid) in urine passed during recumbency, and is therefore absent from the urine passed immediately on waking in the morning, but it reappears after standing or placing the patient in a lordotic position while still recumbent. It is widely believed, though not proved, that subjects with this condition have a more marked lumbar lordosis on standing than the average for the population.

Postural proteinuria has long been regarded as a functional condition in which there is no morphologic abnormality in the kidney. Recent studies by Robinson and his colleagues, and others, have shown that this is untrue, for renal biopsy in a series of cases fulfilling the aforementioned criteria showed histologic glomerular lesions in the majority. A few cases showed glomerular lesions typical of some well-recognized type of glomerular disease, particularly membranous disease, but in most patients the lesions were mild and segmental, and were not sufficiently marked to merit classification as any form of glomerulonephritis. A follow-up examination ten years later showed that no subject had developed overt clinical renal disease, and that 50 per cent had lost their proteinuria, thus confirming the general belief that the condition is benign.

Benign postural proteinuria is clinically important for two main reasons: (1) It may interfere with employment of young subjects on the threshold of their adult life, because of the mistaken belief that their proteinuria is due to serious renal disease; and (2) this diagnosis may be incorrectly made in patients with more sinister types of glomerulonephritis in whom the proteinuria is increased by standing. For these reasons it is wise to submit subjects suspected of the condition to a full clinical examination, with urine microscopy (the deposit is normal in postural proteinuria), determination of creatinine clearance, and intravenous pyelography. Renal biopsy is not indicated unless abnormalities are revealed by the initial investigations. Selective protein clearances are of no value, as they show poor selectivity in this condition.

Robinson, R. R.: Idiopathic proteinuria. Ann. Intern. Med., 71:1019, 1969.

Thompson, A. L., Durrett, R. R., and Robinson, R. R.: Fixed and reproducible orthostatic proteinuria. VI. Results of a 10-year follow-up examination. Ann. Intern. Med., 73:235, 1970.

616. RENAL DISEASE IN PREGNANCY
Thomas F. Ferris

Because pregnancy is occasionally associated with edema, hypertension, and proteinuria, pre-existent renal disease in a pregnant woman has traditionally been viewed with alarm. However, the majority of women with renal disease can, with proper medical care, have an uncomplicated pregnancy. In most women, pregnancy does not worsen renal disease or adversely affect the ultimate prognosis.

GLOMERULONEPHRITIS

The development of *acute glomerulonephritis* during pregnancy usually results in fetal death. Differentiation between acute glomerulonephritis and preeclampsia may be difficult if the disease occurs late in pregnancy, but the presence of microscopic hematuria with cellular and hyaline casts is most consistent with glomerulonephritis. The treatment of the disease is similar to that in the nonpregnant patient, with careful control of blood pressure and fluid balance. The danger of pregnancy in women with *chronic glomerulonephritis* is increased incidence of preeclampsia. When proteinuria is the only manifestation of chronic glomerulonephritis, the incidence of preeclampsia is 35 per cent, with fetal survival around 80 per cent. If azotemia and hypertension precede the pregnancy, the incidence of preeclampsia rises to over 75 per cent, with fetal survival less than 40 per cent. The level of azotemia and hypertension best correlates with the risk of preeclampsia and fetal loss. Control of hypertension throughout pregnancy and careful observation of BUN, creatinine, and uric acid, particularly in the last trimester, are essential for a successful pregnancy. When preeclampsia develops early, termination of the pregnancy is indicated, because there is little chance for fetal survival in this group, and the renal disease may worsen.

PYELONEPHRITIS

Acute pyelonephritis occurs in approximately 1 per cent of pregnant women, but in 30 per cent of women who have bacteriuria greater than 100,000 organisms per milliliter on their first prenatal visit. The incidence of bacteriuria is no greater in pregnancy, but the higher incidence of pyelonephritis is attributable to the dilatation of the urinary tract which occurs with pregnancy and which results in stasis and incomplete emptying. Two thirds of all cases of pyelonephritis during pregnancy can be prevented by treatment of asymptomatic bacteriuria. The relationship between asymptomatic bacteriuria, prematurity, fetal loss, and preeclampsia is unclear, because patients with chronic renal disease are more apt to have bacteriuria.

SYSTEMIC LUPUS ERYTHEMATOSUS

The course of systemic lupus erythematosus is varied during pregnancy. Most patients either have no change or an improvement in the symptoms of the disease. Aggravation of lupus seems to occur more frequently post partum. Whether this is a specific effect of the pregnancy or of demands made on the new mother is unclear. The course of lupus nephropathy during pregnancy is similar to that of chronic glomerulonephritis; patients with hypertension and azotemia preceding pregnancy have an increased incidence of preeclampsia, whereas patients with normal renal function usually have uncomplicated pregnancies.

POSTPARTUM RENAL FAILURE

The rapid development of renal failure has been reported to occur from one to ten weeks post partum with findings at autopsy of malignant nephrosclerosis. Evidence of intravascular coagulation is found in some patients with thrombocytopenia, fibrin degradation products in the serum, and findings on renal biopsy of interarteriolar and interglomerular thromboses. The disease has been termed "postpartum hemolytic-uremic syndrome" by some; its cause may have a relationship to preeclampsia in which fibrin deposits are present in glomeruli and evidence of a consumptive coagulopathy is occasionally seen. There is some evidence that anticoagulant therapy may be of benefit in postpartum renal failure.

TOXEMIA OF PREGNANCY

Toxemia of pregnancy is a disease occurring in late pregnancy, characterized by hypertension, edema, and proteinuria. Historically, convulsions have been the hallmark of toxemia, and the disease has been divided into eclampsia (Greek, eclampsis: a sudden flash) and preeclampsia, based upon whether a convulsion has occurred. Although the presence of convulsions is usually indicative of severe disease, separating toxemia on this basis does not imply different causes, and may have no more validity than separating other hypertensive processes associated with convulsions, e.g., acute glomerulonephritis and malignant hypertension.

Incidence. The disease occurs in 5 to 10 per cent of pregnancies, but the reported incidence depends upon criteria used to make the diagnosis and on the population studied. Hypertension alone has been reported to occur during the first pregnancy in 25 per cent of women in Great Britain. There is a bimodal frequency of the disease, with peak incidences in young primiparous women and in multiparous women over 35. Toxemia is more common with pre-existing renal disease, hypertension, and diabetes, with twin pregnancies, and in black women.

Clinical Manifestations. The usual sequence of manifestations is edema and hypertension followed by proteinuria; occasionally proteinuria precedes hypertension. Because normal pregnancy is characterized by reduction in blood pressure, particularly in the second trimester, blood pressures higher than 130 systolic and 80 diastolic should be considered abnormal during pregnancy. Diastolic hypertension is more striking than systolic with toxemia, and systolic blood pressures greater than 180 to 200 mm Hg usually indicate that preceding hypertensive disease existed. Toxemia typically begins after the thirty-second week of pregnancy, but may occur as early as the twenty-fourth week, particularly in women with pre-existing renal disease or hypertension. It can occur during the first trimester with a hydatidiform mole. Excessive weight gain during pregnancy predisposes to its development, probably through mechanisms similar to those associating obesity with hypertension; but sudden weight gain is caused by edema. The edema is similar to that seen in acute glomerulonephritis, with prominent distribution in the periorbital region, hands, and ankles. Headache, visual disturbances, or midepigastric pain are frequent symptoms. On funduscopic examination, segmental arteriolar narrowing and a wet glistening retina ("retinal sheen") are often seen. The presence of increased light reflex and tortuosity of the arterioles points to hypertensive disease having preceded the toxemia. Retinal hemorrhages and exudates are rare. The spinal reflexes may be hyperactive, and are important parameters to follow in assessing the degree of central nervous system excitability. Proteinuria ranges from trace amounts to levels seen in the nephrotic syndrome, 5 to 10 grams per 24 hours. Microscopic examination of the urine may reveal a few red blood cells, but significant hematuria or pyuria is more consistent with the presence of a primary renal disease. Although reduction in glomerular filtration occurs with toxemia, azotemia is seldom prominent because of the increase in glomerular filtration accompanying pregnancy. The low blood urea nitrogen (9±2 mg per 100 ml) and creatinine (0.75±0.2 mg per 100 ml) in late pregnancy are indicative of this increase, and even with a 50 to 75 per cent fall in glomerular filtration, the blood urea nitrogen and creatinine can remain within the normal range. A disproportionate reduction in urate clearance occurs in toxemia so that hyperuricemia usually precedes the development of azotemia.

Pathogenesis. The cause of toxemia is unknown. Nonspecific changes have been described in the liver, brain, heart, and adrenals, but renal biopsies have demonstrated consistent findings. The glomeruli are swollen, and the glomerular lumen is occluded by cytoplasmic swelling of the endothelial cells. Electron microscopy may reveal focal basement membrane thickening, and immunofluorescent studies have demonstrated fibrin deposits in glomeruli. These glomerular changes are distinctive for toxemia and are not seen in other hypertensive diseases.

The mechanism of the hypertension is unclear. Salt retention, caused by the reduction in glomerular filtration rate, might exacerbate the hypertension but alone would not cause it. The similarity of uterus and kidney in containing both renin and prostaglandins is of interest, because there is clinical evidence to suggest uterine ischemia as a factor in the pathogenesis of toxemia. If renin is involved, the sequence of events resulting in hypertension has not been elucidated. Plasma renin is not elevated in toxemia, but since extracellular fluid expansion and increased sensitivity to angiotensin simultaneously occur, the effect of a specific level of plasma renin on blood pressure is difficult to evaluate. Any explanation of the pathogenesis of toxemia must account not only for hypertension but also for the renal pathology and central nervous system excitability which are disproportionate to the magnitude of the hypertension.

Treatment. Control of weight gain during pregnancy and the use of diuretics when edema appears reduce the incidence of complete expressions of the disease. With the onset of toxemia, bed rest, salt restriction, diuretics, and sedation constitute the initial therapy. If hypertension does not abate, antihypertensive drugs should be instituted. For immediate control of the blood pressure intravenous hydralazine (Apresoline), 25 to 40 mg in 500 ml dextrose and water, diazoxide, 300 mg, or methyldopa (Aldomet), 500 mg, have been efficacious. Magnesium sulfate has been widely used in toxemia, because it has both a depressant effect upon the central nervous system and a mild antihypertensive action. Barbiturates are useful in controlling central nervous system hyperexcitability, and should be used if convulsions appear imminent. The definitive therapy is termination of the pregnancy, and, provided that the fetus is viable, this should be accomplished as soon as the patient's condition is stable. When fetal size makes viability of concern, control of the disease with antihypertensive drugs and diuretics may allow time for further fetal development. If proteinuria or azotemia persists despite therapy, delivery should be accomplished; there is little evidence that fetal growth occurs in the face of persistent toxemia. Eclampsia is sufficient reason for inducing delivery, because convulsions significantly increase maternal and fetal mortality.

Prognosis. Maternal death with toxemia is now rare. Blood pressure usually returns to normal within two weeks after delivery, although the proteinuria may persist longer. However, women who develop toxemia have a higher incidence of hypertension in later life, and the role toxemia plays in its development has been a subject of concern and controversy. The unresolved question is whether toxemia causes subsequent hypertension or simply occurs more frequently in women with latent hypertension. In women having toxemia with a multiparous pregnancy, two findings favor an underlying hypertensive diathesis as a factor in the toxemia. First, the incidence of late hypertension is greater after multiparous than primiparous toxemia; indeed, in white women with eclampsia, a higher incidence of late hypertension can be demonstrated only after a multiparous toxemia. Second, the recurrence of toxemia with subsequent pregnancies is over 50 per cent after multiparous toxemia, but only 25 per cent in women developing toxemia with the first pregnancy.

Eastman, N. J. (ed.): Williams Textbook of Obstetrics. 13th ed. New York, Appleton-Century-Crofts, 1966.

Sheehan, H. L., and Lynch, J. B.: Pathology of Toxaemia of Pregnancy. Baltimore, Williams & Wilkins Company, 1973.

617. URINARY TRACT INFECTIONS AND PYELONEPHRITIS

Calvin M. Kunin

Definition. The phrase urinary tract infection is a broad term used to describe both bacterial colonization of the urine and invasion of structures in any part of the urinary tract. Urine is ordinarily sterile. Colonization of the urine, that is, multiplication of large numbers of bacteria in the urine, is often difficult to distinguish from actual tissue invasion eliciting a host response, because of the frequent tendency of urinary tract infections to exhibit either few or no symptoms. This phenomenon is known as *asymptomatic bacteriuria.* At any given point in time, an individual may have bacteriuria alone, or bacteriuria with silent tissue invasion, or bacteriuria accompanied by signs of inflammation of the bladder *(cystitis)* or kidneys *(pyelonephritis).* Infections of the structures of the urinary tract are usually accompanied by colonization of the urine which bathes the kidney, ureter, bladder, and urethra. Thus bacteriuria is the most common denominator of urinary tract infections. Bacteriuria may be absent, however, when the infected focus is not contiguous with the urine as in early lesions of hematogenous pyelonephritis, when there is marked obstruction of the affected portion of the tract or when it is masked by antimicrobial therapy. Bacteriuria does not necessarily indicate that the patient has pyelonephritis or cystitis. Rather, it is an important and generally reliable laboratory finding that indicates an abnormal situation, reflecting either the presence of, or potential for, infection of the urinary tract. It is an excellent guide to early diagnosis and evaluation of therapy, because signs and symptoms of infection may be absent or disappear without bacteriologic cure.

The term *pyelonephritis* refers to immediate and residual effects of bacterial infection in the kidney. The clinical manifestations are generally conceived of as existing in two forms: *acute pyelonephritis,* an active pyogenic infection, usually accompanied by local and systemic symptoms of infection; and *chronic pyelonephritis,* wherein the principal manifestations are caused by the injury sustained in preceding active infections. Actually, considerable uncertainty exists regarding the relationship between acute and chronic pyelonephritis in patients in whom no structural or neurologic abnormality affecting the urinary tract can be detected. For example, many patients known to have had multiple attacks of acute pyelonephritis show no indication of progression to chronic pyelonephritis even after intervals of many years. Furthermore, comparatively few patients thought to have chronic pyelonephritis give a history of acute infection of the urinary tract. The possibility exists therefore that some cases of the disease we are now calling "chronic pyelonephritis" result from something other than bacterial infection of the kidney. Reasons for this uncertainty include inadequacy of diagnostic procedures for diagnosis of chronic pyelonephritis and erroneous interpretation of bacteriologic findings. A large part of the problem is due to the fact that a variety of other disease states can produce renal lesions that mimic pyelonephritis (see Ch. 618).

The normal urinary tract is free of bacteria except near the external urethral meatus. In both sexes, some organisms are normally present in the distal urethra. These are usually similar to the flora of the skin, and frequently consist of staphylococci and diphtheroids. Urine is a variable culture medium, depending upon pH, tonicity, and its constituents. High concentrations of urea, low pH, hyperosmolality, and products of dietary organic acids are generally unfavorable to bacteria. In addition, the dynamics of urine flow, or washout, and antibacterial properties of the lining membrane of the urinary tract appear to be important defense mechanisms.

The large bowel is considered to be the reservoir of most of the bacteria that invade the urinary tract because of the high frequency of aerobic coliforms found in urinary tract infection. Several possible pathways from the lumen of the intestine to the urinary passages and kidney can be postulated. There has been some dispute regarding their relative importance. The principal possibilities are the hematogenous, the lymphatic, and the "ascending" routes. The "ascending" pathway, involving migration of bacteria from the anus to the periurethral zone and through the urethra to the bladder, is the most favored at present. This route can be demonstrated experimentally, particularly in the presence of obstruction or of a foreign body. It also fits in well with the very much higher rate of urinary infections in the female, whose urethra is shorter than that of the male, and with the marked frequency of urinary infections associated with instrumentation of the urethra and bladder. Clear instances of the hematogenous origin of urinary infection have been demonstrated, particularly in the presence of staphylococcal or gram-negative bacteremia, but these are relatively less common.

Pathology. Knowledge of the pathologic process is meager because uncomplicated acute pyelonephritis does not lead to death. Nevertheless, on the basis of occasional chance opportunities and experiments in animals, it is possible to describe the probable form of the lesion with reasonable assurance. One or both kidneys may be affected. The lining of the renal pelvis and calyces is diffusely inflamed. Infection of the renal substance is usually confined to one or more wedge-shaped areas, the apices being in the medulla. In this zone of acute inflammation there are micro-abscesses, some of which may bulge under the capsule of the kidney, but rarely they rupture into the perinephric area, producing *perinephric abscess*. Collections of polymorphonuclear leukocytes can be seen in and around the lumina of the tubules throughout their length. The glomeruli are usually spared structurally, but may become functionless because the tubular part of the nephron is destroyed. The infectious process tends to remain confined within the originally involved segment of renal tissue and to subside gradually over a period of one to three weeks. As healing takes place, the area contracts, polymorphonuclear leukocytes are replaced by mononuclear cells, and scar tissue is deposited. Eventually a linear scar involving a streak of medulla and corresponding cortical tissue is all that remains. Remnants of glomeruli and tubules filled with a colloid-like material lie in this fibrous matrix.

A considerable amount of work has been done on the pathogenesis of pyelonephritis in laboratory animals. The kidney can be infected either by the intravenous route or by introducing bacteria into the urinary tract; the lesion is the same regardless of the route of inoculation. In order to infect the kidney by way of the bloodstream it is necessary to inject large numbers of bacteria, probably because only a minute proportion of the inoculum is trapped by the kidney. As a general rule, coliform bacteria, although the most common cause of human pyelonephritis, are incapable of infecting a normal kidney, although pathogenic strains of Staphylococcus, enterococcus, occasional strains of Proteus, and rare strains of coliform organisms will do so. In the presence of an obstructive lesion, however, the susceptibility of the kidney to infection by all these bacteria, including the coliforms, is greatly increased. Obstruction has been produced by introducing artificial calculi into the bladder, by partial or complete ureteral ligation, or by mechanical injury of the kidney. Even small injuries of the medulla caused by needle puncture lead to obstruction of a few collecting tubules and localized susceptibility to infection. Experiments of this kind have demonstrated that bacterial multiplication begins in the medulla and then spreads into the corresponding area of cortex. It is thought, therefore, that infection spreads in retrograde manner from the obstructed collecting tubules in the medulla throughout the nephron. Characteristic wedge-shaped areas of acute pyelonephritis involving both medulla and cortex are also produced when small numbers of bacteria, e.g., 10 to 100 living organisms, are inoculated into the medulla. By contrast, as many as 100,000 coliform bacteria must be inoculated into the cortex in order to establish even local infection. A conspicuous feature of the areas of acute pyelonephritis produced in laboratory animals is lack of tendency for infection to invade neighboring, unobstructed areas of renal parenchyma. The process remains confined to the area of intrarenal hydronephrosis, eventually "burns out," and shrinks to a scar, leaving adjacent kidney unaffected. This seems compatible with acute pyelonephritis in man, wherein there is usually no measurable evidence of even temporary impairment of renal function despite evidence that both kidneys are acutely infected. It is reasonable to presume, therefore, that the disease in man is one of patchy renal involvement, leaving large segments of tissue unaffected. Evidence obtained in animals indicates that the medullary zone is the critical one from the standpoint of pathogenesis of acute bacterial infection. Factors that may be responsible include the following: (1) *Ammonia formation.* Evidence has been obtained that high local concentration of ammonia, as may be present when the body is dealing with an acid load, may be sufficient to inactivate complement, thus rendering ineffective a major defense mechanism against bacterial infection. (2) *Hypertonicity.* The unusual osmolarity in this area of the body may be sufficient to affect the activity of complement and phagocytes, as well as to permit survival of bacterial protoplasts. (3) *Differences in the blood supply.* The blood flow to the medulla is far less than that to the cortex.

Clinical Manifestations. Symptoms of cystitis and urethritis include frequency of urination, burning pain on urination, and passage of cloudy, occasionally blood-tinged urine. The patient may complain of a foul odor to the urine, lassitude, and suprapubic discomfort. Fever and leukocytosis are rarely evident in urinary tract infection confined to the bladder and urethra; as a general rule, their presence should be looked upon as evidence of infection of the upper part of the tract. Nevertheless, absence of fever and leukocytosis does not by any means exclude the possibility of kidney involvement.

The clinical picture of acute pyelonephritis may be characteristic: sudden rise of body temperature to 38.9 to 40.6° C, shaking chills, aching pain in one or both costovertebral areas or flanks, and symptoms of bladder inflammation. Physical examination reveals tenderness in the region of one or both kidneys; at times a tender kidney may be detected by palpation. Laboratory tests show polymorphonuclear leukocytosis, and the urine is laden with leukocytes. Stain of the sediment reveals numerous bacteria, usually gram-negative bacilli, and culture confirms this. In a small proportion of cases blood culture is also positive. There are no signs of impaired renal function or of acute hypertension as is sometimes seen in acute glomerulonephritis.

In the absence of an obstructive lesion of the urinary tract, such as stone or tumor, this illness is self-limited, rarely lasting more than a week or ten days.

The clinical picture just described is easy to recognize and is seldom confused with anything else. Yet there must also be subclinical forms, because typical evidence of previous attacks of acute pyelonephritis is encountered at autopsy in patients lacking a history of symptoms of urinary tract infection. Possibly the size of the area of renal tissue involved in an episode is the determining factor. In addition to the "classic" clinical picture and the subclinical form, acute pyelonephritis at times presents with symptoms that do not point to the urinary tract. Dysuria may be lacking, and there may be no fever. There may only be backache, without demonstrable tenderness in the kidney region. Some patients have pain in either the upper or the lower abdomen, together with symptoms of disturbed gastrointestinal function. Others complain only of general fatigue. Mild anemia may be caused by repeated episodes of acute pyelonephritis. The urine can be free of pus cells or bacteria for brief periods. Repeated urinalyses on succeeding days should, however, always reveal presence of pus cells and bacteria.

Acute urinary tract infection, complicated by pyelonephritis, frequently arises in debilitated patients in hospitals and nursing homes who have been subjected to urethral instrumentation, especially the indwelling catheter. In such people the infection may take a fulminating course, with bacteremia and shock, and can in fact be the terminal event of prolonged illness. Gramnegative sepsis and bacteremic shock are described in Ch. 214.

Course. The symptoms of inflammation of the urinary tract tend to disappear after several days even without bacteriologic cure. Recurrence of symptomatic infection is frequent in this group. Bacteriuria also tends to be highly recurrent. Persistence of fever and leukocytosis strongly suggest the presence of obstruction to flow of urine by stones or other mechanical means or a large renal or perinephric abscess. In the unobstructed female patient, recurrence is usually associated with reinfection with a new bacterial strain. Early recurrence, however, may be due to emergence of bacteria from a partially suppressed focus. Persistent infection with the same organisms should alert the physician to the presence of obstruction, calculus, or neurogenic lesions. Frequent follow-up examination of the patient's urine is essential to the management to be described below.

Concept of Significant Bacteriuria. Bacteriuria literally means the presence of bacteria in the urine. The concept of "significant bacteriuria" was introduced to distinguish between bacteria that are actually multiplying in the urine from contaminants in collection vessels, periurethral tissues, the urethra itself, and gross fecal or vaginal contamination. This separation can be accomplished by knowledge of the site and manner in which the urine is collected from the patient and enumeration of the number of organisms present in the sample. The criterion of 100,000 or more organisms per milliliter of urine for diagnosis of significant bacteriuria is an excellent *operational definition* when the clean voided method is used to collect specimens. It is based on the finding that contaminants will usually be present at numbers ranging from 1000 to 10,000 per milliliter. Organisms found in urinary tract infections grow well in urine; they usually achieve concentrations of greater than 100,000, and are often in the range of 1 to 10 million per milliliter. With proper instruction and cleansing, and prompt processing or refrigeration of specimens, it is usually not difficult to obtain reliable results by the clean voided method in both males and females. It is emphasized that, because the reliability of the method will differ with experience and care, it is often wise to avoid overdiagnosis by obtaining multiple specimens, particularly in the asymptomatic patient. Thus, survey and screening procedures for bacteriuria generally require two or three consecutive positive specimens, indicating that the patient has "persistent significant bacteriuria." Bacterial counts lower than 100,000 per milliliter may occur in patients with true bacteriuria, but when the clean voided method is used, these counts can only be established as valid when shown to be persistent and when the same species of bacteria and preferably the same serotype can be repeatedly isolated. Bacterial counts are higher when urine is allowed to incubate for some time in the bladder. A first morning specimen is preferred, but is not essential. Low or borderline counts may be due to dilution in a well-hydrated patient.

Aseptic methods of collection of urine such as from the renal pelvis or ureter, or by bladder puncture, *permit the diagnosis of significant bacteriuria regardless of the number of organisms found,* provided that the specimen is not contaminated prior to culture.

Bacteriologic Findings. The species of bacteria most likely to be recovered in individuals with bacteriuria depends, for the most part, upon previous history of infection, receipt of antimicrobial therapy, hospitalization, and instrumentation of the urinary tract. In this respect, the bacterial flora found in individuals with asymptomatic bacteriuria is no different from that in cases of clinically obvious pyelonephritis. Enterobacteriaceae are by far the most common organisms identified. *E. coli* generally accounts for more than 80 per cent of all species recovered in so-called uncomplicated cases, whereas Proteus, Klebsiella, Enterobacter, *Pseudomonas aeruginosa,* enterococci, and *Staphylococcus aureus* are more likely to be found in patients who have had previous infection or instrumentation (the so-called complicated group). Occasionally, organisms such as *Serratia marcescens,* Mima-Herellea, *Candida albicans,* and even *Cryptococcus neoformans* may be significant and produce disease in diabetics and in patients treated with corticosteroids and immunosuppressive agents. Diphtheroids, *Staphylococcus epidermidis,* and microaerophilic streptococci are highly suspect as contaminants. They usually will not be isolated on repeated culture. They should not, however, be dismissed if repeatedly recovered under optimal conditions of collection.

Despite the abundance of anaerobic flora in the gut, they are actually rare in urinary infections, presumably owing to the poor growth of these organisms in urine.

Microscopic Methods. Rapid diagnostic methods are available either by preparation of a Gram stain of unsedimented urine and examination with an oil immersion lens, or by study of the centrifuged urinary sediment for bacteria, employing the high dry objective under reduced light with or without the addition of methylene blue. The Gram stain has been the most widely used of these methods and correlates about 80 to 90 per cent with quantitative culture. Examination of the unstained sediment as prepared for search for formed elements in the urine is very helpful. It is much less time consuming than preparation of a stained slide, and can be done in conjunction with the routine examination for formed elements. This method lends itself particularly well in office practice to assessing the presence of a urinary tract infection. The criterion for a positive sediment is the presence of many (preferably more than 20) obvious bacteria. The presence of marked pyuria can mask bacteria in the sediment. Fresh urine is required, because crystals will also obscure the bacteria. If crystals do form, the urine should be warmed until they dissolve.

Ten or more leukocytes per high-powered field in the centrifuged specimen is usually accepted as representing pyuria. When inflammation of the bladder mucosa is intense, there may be some erythrocytes in the urine, and gross hematuria sometimes occurs. *Proteinuria* is not common in urinary infections.

Epidemiology and Natural History. Extensive epidemiologic studies have provided information of the frequency of bacteriuria in various populations. Bacteriuria in the newborn period has been difficult to define because of problems inherent in collection, but information is being obtained with the widespread use of the bladder puncture method. Infection of the urinary tract in this age group appears to be part of a generalized, life-threatening gram-negative sepsis, and is more common in boys than girls. Symptomatic urinary infections, particularly among girls, are prominent in the preschool years, and are frequently associated with important obstructive or neurogenic lesions. Urologic investigation is extremely valuable in this age group. *It is mandatory in males of any age because of the high frequency of important structural abnormalities* found (valves, malformations, obstructive and neurogenic lesions). The prevalence of bacteriuria among schoolgirls is 1.2 per cent; it is only 0.03 per cent in boys of the same age. The incidence rate in girls is 0.3 per cent per year; it is linear with time throughout the school years and is unaffected by menarche. The cumulative frequency or urinary infection in girls occurring at one time or another during the school years exceeds 5 per cent. Bacteriuria in schoolgirls is independent of socioeconomic status and race, and is not increased in diabetic girls. The prevalence of bacteriuria rises with age, and is increased in lower socioeconomic groups, probably because of limited antimicrobial therapy delivered to this population. Urinary infection is common after marriage. The "honeymoon cystitis" syndrome may be due to either infection or local irritation, and these should be clearly differentiated by culture. Bacteriuria in pregnancy varies from 2 to 6 per cent, depending upon age, parity, and socioeconomic groups. Early detection and treatment of bacteriuria in this age group will prevent the emergence of symptomatic infection. Elderly women may have frequencies of bacteriuria as high as 10 per cent; this rate may rise even higher in hospitalized patients, particularly diabetics. Bacteriuria in the male begins to appear in the "prostate" years, and is often initiated by instrumentation.

Role of Instrumentation. Persistent bacteriuria follows single catheterizations in relatively healthy individuals at a frequency of 1 to 2 per cent; the risk is much higher in the debilitated patient and in males with prostatic obstruction. With open indwelling catheter drainage bacterial colonization exceeds 90 per cent within three to four days. This may lead to life-threatening pyelonephritis and gram-negative sepsis. Fortunately, it is partially avoidable by (1) careful preselection of criteria for catheterization, and (2) use of aseptic closed drainage or antimicrobial bladder rinse during prolonged catheterization. The catheter should be removed as soon as it is no longer needed.

RENAL MEDULLARY NECROSIS
(Renal Papillary Necrosis, Necrotizing Papillitis)

Renal medullary necrosis is a severe complication of pyelonephritis—ischemic necrosis of the renal papilla and adjacent portions of the renal medulla. The lesion is most often, though not invariably, associated with severe acute and chronic pyelonephritis. It is especially common in patients with diabetes and pyelonephritis, about half the reported cases having involved such persons. Obstruction of the urinary tract is also regarded as a predisposing factor, but this may relate only to the aggravating effect of obstruction on infection in the kidney. European clinicians report fairly frequent occurrences of renal medullary necrosis in women who have habitually ingested large quantities of analgesic medicines containing phenacetin for headache. These patients also usually have infection of the urinary tract. The relative roles of infection and phenacetin in the pathogenesis of the lesion cannot be specified with certainty.

Although infection appears to be the most important factor in the pathogenesis of this lesion, there can be little doubt that the peculiarities of blood supply of the medulla must also be factors. This could help to explain the frequent occurrence of the lesion in patients with diabetes and generalized vascular disease, as well as the role of obstruction, which must impair the blood supply of this area.

The zone of necrosis may occur throughout the pyramid from the extreme tip as far proximally as the corticomedullary junction. Eventually this usually sloughs, so that chunks of necrotic tissue often migrate down through the urinary passages.

The clinical manifestations of renal medullary necrosis are intensification of symptoms of pre-existing pyelonephritis. There may be pain in the lumbar region, colicky pain along the ureteral radiation, and hematuria. Fever may be high. Manifestations of gram-negative bacteremia may supervene. This lesion should be considered always in elderly patients with diabetes who show rapid deterioration in clinical status with signs of active pyelonephritis and increasing renal decompensation.

The diagnosis can sometimes be made by finding pieces of renal medullary tissue in the urine sediment. Pyelography may also be of assistance: in addition to the scarring and asymmetry of chronic pyelonephritis, cavities and sinuses in the region of the papillae may be demonstrated.

Therapy is not notably effective, but should be directed toward control of infection and whatever measures can be employed to improve the status of patients who have diabetes mellitus or who are habitual abusers of analgesic medicines.

Management. The therapeutic principles are similar for all urinary infections, including bacteriuria, cystitis, or pyelonephritis. *Recognition and relief of obstruction* *are essential.* Therapy is then directed to sterilization of the urine and careful follow-up to detect recurrence, using significant bacteriuria as a guide. Infections uncomplicated by obstruction or many previous episodes will generally respond to oral therapy with sulfonamides, tetracycline, ampicillin, chloramphenicol, nalidixic acid, cephalexin, co-trimoxazole (trimethoprim plus sulfamethoxazole), or nitrofurantoin. The last-named drug is particularly useful in recurrent infections because of relatively less frequency of emergence of resistant strains. It should not be used to treat systemic infection and is contraindicated in the presence of any degree of azotemia, because adequate concentrations cannot be achieved in the urine under these conditions. Oral preparations of carbenicillin are reserved for Pseudomonas infection. Drugs are selected on the basis of relative cost, side effects, and antimicrobial susceptibility, all of which may be highly variable. Antimicrobial susceptibility tests should be used to guide therapy of recurrent episodes. The initial attack is usually due to *E. coli,* which is sensitive to most of the commonly used agents. It can be treated "blindly" with a sulfonamide, ampicillin, or tetracycline with about equal probability of success. Bacteria should disappear within 24 to 48 hours even if pyuria and symptoms continue. It is important to recognize bacteriologic failure early and change to another drug. Generally, short courses of treatment, from 10 to 14 days, are quite adequate; short-term high-dose therapy, sometimes with parenteral agents such as ampicillin, cephalothin, or gentamicin, may be required in some instances of failure with lower doses or when the patient is too ill to receive an oral agent. Recurrence within a few weeks after treatment is usually due to persistence of the same focus, whereas later recurrence, particularly in females, is more often the result of reinfection. Highly recurrent infections may be managed by either very close follow-up and treatment of each episode or by prophylaxis with nitrofurantoin, cotrimoxazole, or urinary antiseptics such as methenamine mandelate or hippurate. *The last-named agents require an acid urine,* preferably at pH 5.5. This may be achieved by addition of a high protein diet, ammonium chloride, ascorbic acid, or methionine. Methionine is an effective acidifier, but it may have to be given in doses as high as 10 grams per day. The dose can be titrated downward by measuring urinary pH. Prophylaxis should not be given for more than three to six months if at all possible. Cessation of prophylaxis permits reassessment of the patient. Prophylaxis can then be reinstituted if frequent infections recur. Some female patients require only a single dose of nitrofurantoin given at bedtime for effective prophylaxis. The drug must be changed if bacteriuria persists or recurs during treatment. This usually means that an organism insusceptible to the agent is now colonizing the urine.

The patient should be instructed to generously drink fluids and void frequently. Double voiding in patients with vesicoureteral reflux is recommended. Voiding after intercourse is felt to decrease the chance of recurrent infection. *Frequent follow-up to detect silent recurrence* is the key to good management. Quantitative urine cultures ideally should be done once monthly for the first three months after each infection and then at three-month intervals for at least two years. Recurrence even after several years of freedom from infection is not uncommon in females.

Complex urinary infections, that is, those in the presence of obstructive uropathy, neurogenic bladders, or catheters, are exceedingly difficult to eradicate and may be managed by suppressive therapy with urinary antiseptics *if shown effective,* or simply left alone unless systemic complications develop. Sepsis in these cases is usually precipitated by obstruction which should be promptly relieved. Antimicrobial therapy is discussed in Ch. 214. *Bacteriuria in the aged* is frequent, usually uncomplicated, and highly recurrent. It should not be over-zealously treated if simple measures fail, because toxicity and expense of therapy may outweigh the risk of disease.

Beeson, P. B.: Urinary tract infection and pyelonephritis. *In* Black, D. A. K. (ed.): Renal Disease. 2nd ed. Oxford, Blackwell Scientific Publications, 1967.

Bengtsson, U.: A comparative study of chronic non-obstructive pyelonephritis and renal papillary necrosis. Acta Med. Scandinav. (Suppl.), 388, 1962.

Kass, E. H. (ed.): Progress in Pyelonephritis. Philadelphia, F. A. Davis Company, 1965.

Kaye, D. (ed.): Urinary Tract Infection and Its Management. St. Louis, C. V. Mosby Company, 1972.

Kleeman, C. R., Hewitt, W. L., and Guze, L. B.: Pyelonephritis. Medicine, 39:3, 1960.

Kunin, C. M.: Detection, Prevention and Treatment of Urinary Tract Infections. 2nd ed. Philadelphia, Lea & Febiger, 1974.

O'Grady, F., and Brumfitt, W.: Urinary Tract Infection. London, Oxford University Press, 1968.

618. CHRONIC PYELONEPHRITIS

Solomon Papper

Definition. Chronic pyelonephritis is defined as a chronic disease of the kidney resulting from bacterial infection. It is characterized anatomically by an inflammatory reaction especially involving the interstitium (i.e., chronic interstitial nephritis). The interstitial tissue consists of elongated cells (interstitial cells) and their branching processes, fragments of basement membrane-like material, and collagen. The interstitium is found largely in the medulla and papillae surrounding blood vessels, loops of Henle, and collecting ducts. With time and progression, all elements of the kidney may become diseased: the vessels, the glomeruli, and the tubular structures. At the termination of its course, the anatomic features of chronic pyelonephritis may be indistinguishable from the various glomerulopathies, at which time the general term "end-stage" kidney is sometimes applied.

Chronic renal infection associated with urinary tract obstruction is common. However, there is some debate concerning the prevalence of chronic nonobstructive pyelonephritis. The diagnosis of chronic pyelonephritis without obstruction may have suffered twice from polarized excesses. At one time, the diagnosis was rarely made; most chronic renal diseases were labeled chronic glomerulonephritis. Subsequently, with greater interest in quantitative bacteriology of the urine, a tendency evolved equating chronic interstitial nephritis with pyelonephritis.

The following are some of the reasons suggesting that many, and perhaps most, instances of chronic interstitial nephritis may not be due to bacterial infection: (1) Chronic interstitial nephritis is also seen in other conditions: heavy metal nephropathy, papillary necrosis, analgesic abuse syndrome, Balkan nephropathy, nephrocalcinosis, hyperuricemia, and radiation nephritis, as well as when no cause is apparent; (2) most patients with chronic interstitial nephritis do not have a history of acute infection; (3) apparently few patients with acute pyelonephritis or chronic bacteriuria without obstruction progress to chronic renal disease; and (4) bacterial infection, when present, may not necessarily be a primary event, but rather may be superimposed on interstitial disease of other cause.

In any case, the dilemma of how often chronic, nonobstructive pyelonephritis occurs as a primary disease is still with us. Therefore we divide chronic pyelonephritis into two categories according to the presence or absence of structural and/or functional abnormalities of the urinary tract. This also serves to emphasize the importance of a search for such mechanical abnormalities in patients with bacteriuria, as well as in patients with renal disease of unknown nature.

Pathology. Grossly, the kidneys may appear irregular in outline, giving evidence of underlying scar formation, with normal areas between the scars. This emphasizes the fundamental focal, wedge-shaped nature of the condition. In some instances, the two kidneys differ considerably in size, a circumstance viewed by some authors as more consistent with pyelonephritis than with other forms of interstitial nephritis, but this is not established fact. On microscopic examination, one sees a chronic inflammatory reaction (lymphocytes and plasma cells) of the interstitial tissue with ultimate scar formation. The scarring results in distortion of the tubular structures—some small and some dilated tubules which may be filled with eosinophilic casts ("colloid casts"). The glomeruli, although frequently surrounded by a cuff of fibrosis, are spared until relatively late, when they, too, may sclerose. Vascular involvement is variable, but in patients with hypertension, afferent arteriolar sclerosis is found. In recent years, abnormalities of the papillae, including papillary sclerosis and deformity, have been found. Dilatation of one or several calyces with cortical scar formation directly over the dilated calyx is regarded by some as diagnostic of chronic pyelonephritis as distinguished from other forms of interstitial nephritis.

When structural or functional obstruction is present, there may also be diffuse dilatation of the pelvis and calyces.

As stated, if the lesion of interstitial nephritis is sufficiently advanced and uniform, it may be indistinguishable from glomerulonephritis.

Pathogenesis. The particular predilection of the renal medulla to infection is of interest. This may be a consequence of a relatively low blood flow and medullary hypertonicity. The latter has been shown to inactivate phagocytosis, as well as complement-mediated bactericidal activity. Obstruction of the urinary tract may add to medullary vulnerability to infection.

In patients with urinary tract obstruction, there may be virtually constant renal infection with consequent progressive tissue damage. Obstruction results in increased pressure in the conduit system which in and of itself may result in abnormal structure and function of the kidney.

The mechanism of progression in nonobstructive pyelonephritis is less evident. It is possible that as acutely infected areas heal, scar tissue is formed. The latter may cause destruction of adjacent renal structure, including the development of areas of intrarenal hydronephrosis.

The latter are more susceptible to new infection, and so the process of infection causing scar, which in turn predisposes to infection, may be self-perpetuating and may account for the heterogeneous anatomic appearance of scar tissue, chronic inflammatory reaction, and acute inflammation, as well. Another possible mechanism of continued renal damage with or without persistent bacterial infection has its basis in the observation that bacterial antigen persists in the kidney long after the disappearance of viable bacteria. It is therefore possible that previous asymptomatic renal infection initiates the disease, and persistent bacterial antigens lead to its progression by immunologic mechanisms.

There are some factors other than structural and functional abnormalities in the urinary tract that may predispose to chronic pyelonephritis. Some of these, such as pregnancy and diabetes mellitus, remain unproved, although highly suspect as predisposing features. However, instrumentation, sickle cell trait, and other underlying renal disease are well-established factors.

Clinical Manifestations. *Pyelonephritis with Mechanical Abnormalities of the Urinary Tract.* The major structural and functional alterations in the urinary tract predisposing to chronic pyelonephritis are (1) mechanical obstruction, (e.g., enlarged prostate, congenital malformations, renal calculi), (2) neurogenic bladder, and (3) vesicoureteral reflux (see Ch. 625). In some patients, obstructive symptoms are evident. In others, infection or the uremic syndrome is the only manifestation of obstructive uropathy. Because urinary tract infection is far less likely to be cured in the presence of obstruction and because obstruction itself is potentially destructive, it is critical that every patient with infection have radiographic examination of the urinary tract. In some instances, intravenous urography suffices; in others, special radiographic studies for vesicoureteral reflux and cystoscopy are needed.

Pyelonephritis without Mechanical Abnormalities of the Urinary Tract. It is in this group of patients that the problem of chronic pyelonephritis versus other forms of chronic interstitial nephritis presents itself. As previously stated, even the presence or absence of bacteriuria may not distinguish the nature of the underlying process. Chronic pyelonephritis may be associated with periods of "inactivity" without bacteriuria, whereas, on the other hand, bacterial infection may be superimposed on a renal disorder of different cause. In considering other causes of chronic interstitial nephritis, it is especially important to explore the more treatable ones, e.g., analgesic abuse syndrome, heavy metal nephropathy, and urate nephropathy.

When a patient has a long history of episodes of urinary tract infection, decreased renal function, pyuria, white blood cell casts, and bacteriuria and the pyelogram shows an irregular renal outline caused by cortical scars and caliectasis, the diagnosis of chronic pyelonephritis is established. However, this "classic" picture is present in relatively few patients.

Patients more often present as follows: (1) a urinalysis done for other reasons reveals white blood cells, bacteria, and little protein; (2) the blood urea nitrogen determined as a screening test for other purposes may be elevated in a patient previously not suspected of renal disease; (3) the manifestations of renal functional insufficiency may present insidiously when renal disease has not been suspected, i.e., anorexia, nausea, vomiting, fatigue, weight loss, nocturia, polyuria, and anemia.

Inadequately explained splenomegaly is a common accompaniment of chronic pyelonephritis.

The characteristics of the nephrotic syndrome, i.e., heavy proteinuira and edema, are not features of pyelonephritis.

The relation of hypertension to pyelonephritis remains incompletely resolved. It seems that there are patients with unilateral pyelonephritis whose hypertension is cured by nephrectomy. Whether the mechanism is the same as in renovascular hypertension is not known. It seems agreed that when renal failure develops in patients with chronic pyelonephritis, hypertension often occurs. However, it is conceivable that this is a feature of the renal failure rather than of the disease itself. On the other hand, many patients with chronic pyelonephritis never develop high blood pressure. The matter is further complicated by the higher incidence of urinary tract infection in patients with essential hypertension and nephrosclerosis.

Laboratory. *Urinalysis.* The urine generally has white blood cells, ranging from few to many. Red blood cells may be present, but generally in small numbers. White blood cell casts may be seen. More than a trace to one-plus proteinuria is uncommon, and 24-hour urinary protein is surely less than 3 grams and usually less than 1.5 grams. Bacteria may or may not be present. Glitter cells which are not diagnostic of chronic pyelonephritis may be seen with special stains; these are polymorphonuclear cells containing granules that exhibit brownian movement.

Renal Function. Early in the course of chronic pyelonephritis, even before azotemia develops, the medullary interstitial reaction may result in tubular dysfunction, especially of the loop of Henle and collecting ducts. This may result in (1) a defect in concentrating ability, sometimes with polyuria, (2) sodium wasting, and (3) disturbed urinary acidification. The latter may cause hyperchloremic acidosis.

Later in the course, there are the evidences of generalized functional deterioration, including reduction in glomerular filtration and renal plasma flow, as well as tubular functional impairment. When severe enough, renal failure ensues.

Pyelography. The renal size may be normal early in the course, whereas later small kidneys are characteristic, except when obstruction is present. Classically, the renal outlines are described as irregular because of cortical scar formation, and one or more calyces are blunted, dilated, and distorted. As stated, some authorities regard a dilated calyx with overlying cortical parenchymal scar as unique to chronic pyelonephritis, as distinguished from other varieties of interstitial nephritis. However, there appear to be instances of chronic pyelonephritis in which these features are absent, i.e., the pyelogram may be normal.

Renal Biopsy. Since the lesion of pyelonephritis is not uniformly distributed in the parenchyma, biopsy may be normal. If diseased tissue is obtained, it can only disclose interstitial nephritis, not its cause. However, early enough in the course, biopsy can exclude glomerulonephritis.

Course. If there is a remediable obstructing lesion treated surgically early enough in the course, the disease may not progress. In the absence of structural malformation, the course is extremely variable. The disease may progress very slowly and be asymptomatic for many years. Even when renal failure and azotemia ensue, appropriate care of the body fluids may be associated with a prolonged period of months to years of reasonably comfortable life.

In those patients who have hypertension, vascular complications, especially coronary artery disease and cerebral vascular disease, may determine an unfavorable course before renal failure does.

Treatment. If a remediable obstructing lesion is found, this should be corrected promptly with operative care. If successfully accomplished, antimicrobial agents are more likely to be effective in eradicating infection, and a stable or even improved state may result.

In the absence of obstruction, the approach to antimicrobial treatment described in Ch. 617 should be undertaken.

Hypertension should be treated to prevent vascular complications. If renal failure is already present, antihypertensive therapy must be undertaken with special care, because deterioration of renal function may follow the lowering of blood pressure.

The treatment of renal failure, including nondialytic measures, dialysis, and renal transplantation, is considered in Ch. 603 and Ch. 605 to 607.

Beeson, P. B.: Urinary tract infection and pyelonephritis. *In* Black, D. A. K. (ed.): Renal Disease. 2nd ed. Oxford, Blackwell Scientific Publications, 1967.

Braude, A. I.: Current concepts of pyelonephritis. Medicine, 52:257, 1973.

Freedman, L. R.: Urinary tract infection, pyelonephritis, and other forms of chronic interstitial nephritis. *In* Strauss, M. B., and Welt, L. G. (eds.): Diseases of the Kidney. Boston, Little, Brown & Company, 1971.

Heptinstall, R. H.: Pathology of the Kidney. Boston, Little, Brown & Company, 1966.

Hodson, C. J.: The radiological contribution toward the diagnosis of chronic pyelonephritis. Radiology, 88:857, 1967.

Kincaid-Smith, P., and Fairley, K. F. (eds.): Renal Infection and Renal Scanning. Melbourne, Australia, Mercedes Publishing Services, 1970.

Kleeman, C. R., Hewitt, W. L., and Guze, L. B.: Pyelonephritis. Medicine, 39:3, 1960.

Papper, S.: Clinical Nephrology. Boston, Little, Brown & Company, 1971.

OTHER SPECIFIC RENAL DISEASES

William B. Schwartz

619. THE NEPHROPATHY OF POTASSIUM DEPLETION

Potassium depletion often produces characteristic structural and functional disturbances in the kidney. The changes occur regardless of the cause of the depletion; primary aldosteronism, Cushing's syndrome, renal tubular disorders such as Fanconi's syndrome, and gastrointestinal losses from diarrhea or vomiting can all produce a deficit great enough to induce renal injury. It is not certain how long potassium deficiency must be present before renal abnormalities can occur. Occasionally, renal disease has been recognized in a patient who has been depleted for only several weeks, but in most instances depletion has been present for months or years.

The characteristic histologic changes in the kidney consist of multiple vacuoles in the tubular epithelium, usually most numerous in the proximal convolutions. These vacuoles (which do not contain fat or glycogen) are virtually pathognomonic of the disease. In most patients, however, the tubular abnormalities are less specific and are limited to mild degenerative changes or to diffuse foamy swelling. The glomeruli and blood vessels are usually not involved. Occasionally, despite striking functional abnormalities, the histologic appearance of the kidney is entirely normal.

The most frequent and striking functional abnormality is an inability to concentrate the urine even after prolonged restriction of water or after the administration of vasopressin. Diluting ability, on the other hand, is usually well preserved. The exact nature of the defect in concentrating power in man is not known, but it would appear from studies in animals that inability to establish a normal degree of medullary hypertonicity and reduced permeability of the collecting ducts to water are both important factors.

Many patients have no urinary symptoms, but in some, nocturia, polyuria, and polydipsia are prominent complaints. Occasionally these symptoms are of sufficient severity to suggest the diagnosis of diabetes insipidus. The polyuria and related symptoms probably result from impaired concentrating ability, although it has also been proposed that excessive fluid intake induced by a primary abnormality of the thirst mechanism may contribute.

Examination of the urine may reveal slight proteinuria and cylindruria, but often no abnormalities are found. Tubular excretion of phenolsulfonphthalein and para-aminohippurate is often reduced. Blood urea nitrogen and creatinine concentrations are ordinarily within normal limits or only slightly elevated, but frank azotemia may be induced by complications such as sodium depletion, hypotension, or pyelonephritis. Renal potassium wasting is *not* a feature of the disease; its presence indicates that an underlying disorder of adrenal or renal origin is responsible for the potassium depletion.

Pyelonephritis is said to occur with unusual frequency in patients with the nephropathy of potassium depletion, but, in view of the relative frequency with which pyelonephritis complicates virtually all types of renal disease, it is difficult to attach any special significance to this observation.

In some instances, urinary abnormalities, slight azotemia, and inability to concentrate the urine lead to an erroneous diagnosis of irreversible renal disease such as chronic glomerulonephritis. In other instances, kidney injury resulting from potassium depletion may complicate pre-existing renal disease and contribute to the development of serious renal failure.

Repair of potassium deficiency is usually followed within several months by improvement or correction of renal functional abnormalities. Serial renal biopsies indicate that in most instances the structural abnormalities can be completely reversed within a few months to a year.

Hollander, W., Jr., and Blythe, W. B.: Nephropathy of potassium depletion. *In* Strauss, M. B., and Welt, L. G. (eds.): Diseases of the Kidney. Boston, Little, Brown & Company, 1971.
Schwartz, W. B., and Relman, A. S.: Effects of electrolyte disorders on renal structure and function. N. Engl. J. Med., 276:383, 452, 1967.

620. THE NEPHROPATHY OF HYPERCALCEMIA

Hypercalcemic nephropathy is characterized in its early stages by tubular injury and polyuria, and in its late stages by progressive renal insufficiency. The changes in structure and function of the kidney are similar, regardless of the metabolic disturbance responsible for elevation of serum calcium concentration. The usual causes of hypercalcemic nephropathy are *hyperparathyroidism, sarcoidosis, vitamin D intoxication, excessive ingestion of milk and alkali (milk-alkali syndrome, Burnett syndrome), multiple myeloma, malignant disease,* and, less frequently, *immobilization* (particularly in *Paget's disease*) and *hyperthyroidism.*

The characteristic pathologic changes are in the collecting ducts and in the distal convoluted tubules, the epithelium in both areas showing degenerative changes and often necrosis and calcification. Calcified casts, which form in sites adjacent to tubular injury, lead to obstruction of nephrons with resultant dilatation of proximal segments. In longstanding hypercalcemia, calcification of the interstitium and occasionally of the glomeruli and vessels leads to progressive scarring and loss of renal mass. At this stage hypertension often develops, and the resultant nephrosclerotic changes may come to dominate the histologic picture.

Clinical findings vary with the duration and severity of the hypercalcemia. Moderate elevations of serum calcium concentration produce a clinical picture characterized initially by evidence of tubular dysfunction. Injury to the distal nephron impairs the countercurrent mechanism for concentrating the urine and leads to polyuria and polydipsia. Tubular secretory capacity is affected, as evidenced by impairment of phenolsulfonphthalein excretion. Azotemia develops only after a prolonged period and is a consequence of obstruction of nephrons rather than of primary glomerular injury. The urine frequently contains a small quantity of protein as well as casts, erythrocytes, and leukocytes. Roentgenographic examination of the abdomen may demonstrate *nephrocalcinosis,* which is usually seen chiefly in the area of the renal pyramids. Patients with hypercalcemia are likely to have hypercalciuria and therefore to develop *renal calculi,* often complicated by pyelonephritis.

It is worth emphasizing that, when an elevated serum calcium concentration is found in a patient with renal insufficiency, it should be assumed, at least initially, that the calcium disorder is primary since renal failure with secondary hyperparathyroidism rarely produces hypercalcemia. Hypercalcemia occurs with significant frequency, however, in patients with chronic renal failure who undergo successful renal transplantation; in these patients persistence of the parathyroid hyperplasia characteristic of secondary hyperparathyroidism may lead to a state of *autonomous hyperparathyroidism (tertiary hyperparathyroidism)* and to elevations in serum calcium concentration sufficient to threaten the integrity of a transplanted kidney. Transient hypercalcemia has also been noted as an uncommon finding during recovery from *acute renal failure.*

Hypercalcemic nephropathy is best treated by correcting the underlying metabolic disorder. Removal of a parathyroid adenoma, control of hyperthyroidism, discontinuance of excessive milk and alkali intake, or ambulation of the patient with Paget's disease usually leads to prompt reduction of the serum calcium concentration to normal. Reduction in serum calcium concentration after withdrawal of excessive vitamin D is generally slower, but can be hastened by administration of corticosteroids. Steroids may also be effective in the hypercalcemia of a sarcoidosis, metastatic bone disease, and multiple myeloma.

Severe hypercalcemia (15 to 20 mg per 100 ml) presents a special therapeutic problem because it may produce a syndrome characterized by rapidly progressive renal failure, oliguria, confusion, lethargy, and coma. This syndrome of so-called *hypercalcemic crisis* is seen most frequently in association with hyperparathyroidism and with malignant disease. It usually proves fatal within a short time unless a prompt reduction in serum calcium concentration is effected. As an initial approach to accomplishing such a reduction it is current practice to administer 2 to 3 liters of normal saline intravenously over a period of six to nine hours. The expansion of extracellular volume depresses the proximal reabsorption of calcium and thus increases calcium excretion. The concomitant administration of a diuretic such as furosemide serves to further enhance the excretion of calcium, and to accelerate the fall in serum calcium concentration. When diuretic therapy is employed, fluid balance must be followed closely and saline given in quantities sufficient to avoid contraction of the extracellular fluid; if contraction is allowed to occur, it will enhance calcium reabsorption and lower urinary calcium excretion. Still a further technique for lowering serum calcium concentration is the administration of mithramycin, which exerts its effect by diminishing skeletal resorption. Mithramycin usually produces a marked reduction in serum calcium concentration within one or two days. If hypercalcemia does not respond adequately to other measures, it can usually be quickly controlled by the intravenous administration of inorganic phosphate. Phosphate salts are thought to act both by increasing calcium deposition in bone and by diminishing bone resorption. The usual program of treatment consists of the infusion of 500 ml of a buffered 0.1 molar phosphate solution (1.5 grams of phosphorus) over eight or nine hours. The chief risk attendant on such treatment is that of producing severe hypocalcemia; but, with the regimen described above, such an occurrence is uncommon unless renal failure and a diminished ability to excrete phosphate lead to marked hyperphosphatemia. In the patient with renal insufficiency the period of infusion should generally be extended to 24 hours; serum calcium concentration should be measured several times during this interval.

Phosphate therapy may also be of use for the prolonged management of mild or moderate hypercalcemia that cannot be controlled by therapy directed toward the underlying disease state. For example, in certain patients with malignancies the daily oral administration of 1 to 3 grams of phosphorus (as sodium phosphate) may provide the only effective means of holding calcium concentration at or near normal levels. Whether or not such treatment entails an appreciable risk of producing clinically significant soft-tissue calcification has not as yet been clearly determined.

The prognosis in hypercalcemic nephropathy depends on the severity and chronicity of the renal disease. Renal failure of recent onset induced by acute hypercalcemia is often completely reversible. However, renal insufficiency that has developed gradually in association with chronic hypercalcemia is often little affected by restoration of a normal serum calcium concentration; when improvement occurs, it is likely to be slow, sometimes taking many months. The prognosis is particularly poor if severe hypertension and nephrosclerosis are present. Nevertheless, in every instance of hypercalcemia a vigorous effort should be made to restore the serum concentration to normal in the hope of preserving remaining renal function or of at least slowing the advance of renal insufficiency.

For additional discussion of hypercalcemia, see Ch. 872.

Epstein, F. H.: Calcium and the kidney. Am. J. Med., 45:700, 1968.
Goldsmith, R. S., and Ingbar, S. H.: Inorganic phosphate treatment of hypercalcemia of diverse etiologies. N. Engl. J. Med., 274:1, 1966.
Massry, S. G., Mueller, E., Silverman, A. G., and Kleeman, C. R.: Inorganic phosphate treatment of hypercalcemia. Arch. Intern. Med., 121:307, 1968.
Schwartz, W. B., and Relman, A. S.: Effects of electrolyte disorders on renal structure and function. N. Engl. J. Med., 276:383, 452, 1967.
Singer, F. R., Neer, R. M., Murray, T. M., Keutmann, H. T., Deftos, L. J., and Potts, J. T.: Mithramycin treatment of intractable hypercalcemia due to parathyroid carcinoma. N. Engl. J. Med., 283:634, 1970.
Suki, W. N., Yium, J. J., Von Minden, M., Saller-Hebert, C., Eknoyan, G., and Martinez-Maldonado, M.: Acute treatment of hypercalcemia with furosemide. N. Engl. J. Med., 283:836, 1970.

621. RENAL TUBULAR ACIDOSIS

Renal tubular acidosis (RTA) is an uncommon disease characterized by a defect either in urinary acidification ("distal" RTA) or in bicarbonate reabsorption ("proximal" RTA). The tubular abnormality in both forms of RTA may occur as either a *primary* or a *secondary disorder.*

DISTAL RENAL TUBULAR ACIDOSIS
(Type 1 RTA)

The characteristic abnormality in distal RTA is an inability of the tubule to establish a normally steep concentration gradient for hydrogen ion between blood and tubular fluid. The cardinal clinical finding is that urine pH, even in the face of severe metabolic acidosis, cannot be reduced to a value of less than 6.0.

Primary distal RTA is a disease of unknown origin that often becomes overt during infancy or early childhood but sometimes first manifests itself in early adult life. In some cases the disease is familial, occurring as an autosomal dominant with a variable degree of expression and greater penetrance in females. There are numerous clinical complications of primary distal RTA, the most notable of which are discussed here.

Osteomalacia: Hypophosphatemia and a high rate of phosphate excretion, i.e., increased phosphate clearance, are typical features of the disease and are often accompanied by roentgenologic evidence of rickets or osteomalacia. The clinical and roentgenologic manifestations are closely similar to those encountered with vitamin D deficiency or with resistance to vitamin D. In addition to the disturbance in phosphate metabolism, an important contributory factor to the development of osteomalacia appears to be the metabolic acidosis. In some patients, osteomalacia produces bone pain as its primary manifestation; in others, the initial clinical difficulty is a disturbance in gait resulting from abnormal skeletal growth.

Hypercalciuria and renal calculi: Hypercalciuria is an almost constant feature of the disease and frequently leads to the formation of renal calculi. A low urinary citrate excretion is thought by some investigators to contribute to the tendency to form stones. Symptoms of renal colic are frequent and may be the first manifestations of the underlying tubular disease. Complications of renal calculi, such as ureteral obstruction or pyelonephritis, are encountered commonly and are often responsible for both secondary renal damage and hypertension. Diffuse calcification of the renal medulla (*nephrocalcinosis*) is a characteristic, though not consistent, roentgenologic finding and at times is an important clue to diagnosis.

Hypokalemia and muscle weakness: Hypokalemia, accompanied by continued renal excretion of potassium (renal potassium wasting), is commonly present. The loss of potassium results from an impaired ability of the distal tubule to secrete hydrogen ion, with the result that a larger than normal fraction of sodium-cation exchange takes place by exchange with potassium. The major deleterious effects of potassium deficiency are on the musculoskeletal system and the kidneys. On occasion severe potasssium depletion may lead to quadriplegia and a clinical picture that closely mimics *familial periodic paralysis* (see Ch. 480). Longstanding potassium deficiency of the magnitude encountered in RTA is also prone to produce *hypokalemic nephropathy* (see Ch. 619).

Renal insufficiency: In the early stages of the disease, kidney function is typically normal or only slightly impaired; but over a period of many years there is usually a progressive loss of function which culminates in severe renal insufficiency. The major factors responsible for renal damage appear, as mentioned earlier, to be obstructive uropathy and pyelonephritis.

Secondary distal RTA is seen in a variety of disease states. It has been noted with particular frequency in *hyperglobulinemic states* (e.g., Sjögren's syndrome, cryoglobulinemia), in *amphotericin B nephropathy*, and after *renal transplantation*. It is also seen as a complication of certain *genetically transmitted systemic diseases* such as Fabry's disease. Few data are yet available on the natural history of secondary distal RTA.

PROXIMAL RENAL TUBULAR ACIDOSIS
(Type 2 RTA)

Proximal RTA is characterized by a defect in proximal bicarbonate reabsorption which increases the delivery of bicarbonate to the distal nephron and thus overwhelms the normal acidifying mechanism. The inherent acidifying capacity of the distal tubule is preserved, however, so that if plasma bicarbonate concentration (and thus filtered load of bicarbonate) is reduced sufficiently to allow nearly complete proximal reabsorption of bicarbonate, urinary pH falls to a level of less than 5.5.

Primary proximal RTA occurs chiefly in male infants and has as its sole clinical manifestations metabolic acidosis and growth retardation. Osteomalacia and nephrocalcinosis do not occur. Treatment with alkali and correction of the acidosis lead to a marked improvement in the rate of growth. Within a few years the defect in bicarbonate reabsorption usually disappears, and alkali therapy can then be safely discontinued.

Secondary proximal RTA is seen in association with multiple abnormalities of tubular function in such genetically transmitted disorders as cystinuria (see Ch. 820) and *Wilson's disease* (see Ch. 945), with the administration of *outdated tetracycline,* and in a variety of metabolic disorders, including *secondary hyperparathyroidism*.

The potassium deficiency in "proximal" RTA has a different cause from that seen in the "distal" form of the disease; in proximal RTA, potassium wasting results not from a defect in distal hydrogen ion secretion but from a flooding of distal exchange sites with sodium bicarbonate and consequent acceleration of sodium-cation exchange.

Treatment of Proximal and of Distal Renal Tubular Acidosis. The treatment of renal tubular acidosis consists of the administration of alkalinizing salts, such as sodium bicarbonate or sodium citrate, in quantities sufficient to restore plasma bicarbonate concentration to normal or nearly normal levels. In "proximal" RTA, in which there may be a gross defect in bicarbonate reabsorption, large quantities of alkali (as much as 5 to 10 mEq per kilogram of body weight per day) are sometimes required in order to achieve this purpose.

Correction of potassium deficiency is also an important therapeutic goal. In nearly all patients with "distal" RTA, correction of acidosis will in itself lead to retention of dietary potassium and repair of the potassium deficit; but in patients with "proximal" RTA, administration of supplemental potassium will usually be required to achieve repair.

If severe bone disease is present, treatment with large doses of vitamin D may be indicated; but if such therapy must be employed, serum calcium concentrations should be followed carefully because of the risk of hypercalcemia. In some patients, hypercalcemia will develop before the goal of restoring serum phosphorus to normal is achieved.

Gill, J. R., Bell, N. H., and Bartter, F. C.: Impaired conservation of sodium and potassium in renal tubular acidosis and its correction by buffer anions. Clin. Sci., 33:577, 1967.

Morris, R. C., Sebastian, A., and McSherry, E.: Renal acidosis. Kidney Int., 1:322, 1972.

Nash, M., Torrado, A. D., Greifer, I., Spitzer, A., and Edelmann, C.: Renal tubular acidosis in infants and children. J. Pediatr., 80:5, 1972.

Rodrigues-Sorianao, J.: The renal regulation of acid-base balance and the disturbance noted in renal tubular acidosis. Pediatr. Clin. North Am., 18:529, 1971.

622. THE NEPHROPATHY OF ACUTE HYPERURICEMIA

Acute uric acid nephropathy occurs as the result of a sudden, marked elevation of serum uric acid concentration in patients undergoing intensive treatment for leukemia or lymphoma. This disorder, though relatively infrequent, is a serious complication that can lead to progressive renal failure, anuria, and death. It can occur with any form of treatment, such as cortisone, radiation, or chemotherapy, that abruptly reduces the number of circulating white cells or diminishes the mass of splenic and lymphoid tissue. The increase in the size of the uric acid pool results primarily from the metabolism of nucleic acid released during the process of cellular destruction. With massive cellular destruction, uric acid concentration occasionally reaches a level as high as 50 to 75 mg per 100 ml.

Severe hyperuricemia is most likely to occur in patients with pre-existing hyperuricemia or in whom there is already some impairment of renal function that restricts the ability to excrete an abnormally large uric acid load. The untoward effects on kidney function result either from obstruction of ureters and pelvis by masses of uric acid or from intrarenal precipitation of uric acid within the collecting ducts and the distal tubules. Deposition in the proximal tubules ordinarily does not occur. The observed pattern of deposition can readily be understood if it is appreciated that at a pH above 7.0, uric acid (pK 5.5) is present almost entirely as the highly soluble urate anion, whereas at a pH of 5 to 6 a large fraction is present as the un-ionized and poorly soluble uric acid. Thus it is only in the distal tubule and collecting duct, where marked acidification of the filtrate takes place, that conversion of urates to uric acid creates a condition favorable to uric acid precipitation. Abstraction of water by the distal nephron and the resulting increase in uric acid concentration in the urine are undoubtedly additional factors favoring precipitation in the tubules and the pelvo-ureteral system.

The single most important consideration in uric acid nephropathy is *prophylaxis*. Until relatively recent years the most effective means of preventing renal injury was through the administration of alkalinizing agents in quantities sufficient to keep the urine pH above 7, the excess uric acid in both tubules and urinary tract thus being maintained in a soluble state. To achieve this goal sodium bicarbonate has to be administered at frequent intervals during the day and a carbonic anhydrase inhibitor (such as Diamox) at bedtime. Now, however, *allopurinol,* a potent inhibitor of xanthine oxidase, provides an even more reliable and physiologic approach to prophylaxis. Allopurinol, by blocking the conversion of hypoxanthine and xanthine to uric acid, prevents a rise in serum uric acid concentration (and in uric acid load delivered to the kidney), even in the face of extensive destruction of neoplastic tissue. When used in doses of 200 to 800 mg per day, it virtually eliminates the hazard of acute uric acid nephropathy.

When a patient presents with the problem of uric acid nephropathy and azotemia, cystoscopy and retrograde examination should be carried out in order to make certain that extrarenal obstruction is not present. If uric acid deposits are found to be blocking the pelvis and ureters, irrigation may serve to relieve the obstruction, but in some instances a pyelostomy will be necessary. In those instances in which obstruction is intrarenal rather than extrarenal, one should attempt to reduce plasma uric acid concentration and to alkalinize the urine in the same fashion as described above in the consideration of prophylaxis.

In some instances, osmotic diuresis with mannitol is helpful in initiating urine flow in the oliguric patient. If such efforts are ineffective, and if anuria or severe azotemia persists, some form of dialysis should be used for the purpose of removing uric acid and dealing with the clinical and chemical manifestations of the uremic state. Despite all these measures, there is a high mortality rate among patients who develop severe hyperuricemic nephropathy, and, as mentioned earlier, prevention of renal damage should always be the primary concern.

DeConti, R. C., and Calabresi, P.: Use of allopurinol for prevention and control of hyperuricemia in patients with neoplastic disease. N. Engl. J. Med., 274:481, 1966.

Frei, E., III, Bentzel, C. J., Rieselbach, R., and Block, J. B.: Renal complications of neoplastic disease. J. Chronic Dis., 16:757, 1963.

Muggia, F. M., Ball, T. J., and Ultmann, J. E.: Allopurinol in the treatment of neoplastic disease complicated by hyperuricemia. Arch. Intern. Med., 120:12, 1967.

623. BALKAN NEPHRITIS

During recent years a chronic and progressive nephritis of unknown cause has been noted in a large percentage of the population living in certain areas of Yugoslavia, Bulgaria, and Rumania. The disease occurs only in small villages located in valleys along river bottom land, and is not seen in neighboring cities or in adjacent foothills or mountains. Approximately one third of the population in the endemic areas has been found to have some evidence of renal disease, such as proteinuria, and between 5 and 10 per cent have been found to have significant azotemia. Several members of the same family are often affected by the disease. Proteinuria occurs in adolescents and in young adults, but azotemia is rarely encountered in patients under the age of 30 to 40 years.

The cause is unknown, and epidemiologic studies to date have not been fruitful. The renal lesion is apparently not the consequence of a previous streptococcal infection, of urinary tract infection, or of the excessive use of analgesics such as phenacetin. It is not related to exposure to toxic agents such as cadmium or lead, or to other factors such as the water supply, nutrition, alcohol intake, or economic status. A curious feature is that people who move out of the affected area in childhood almost never develop the disease, whereas those who move into the area frequently develop renal disease, usually in a period of about ten years. Further studies on various environmental factors are obviously required and are, in fact, in progress.

The kidneys in the patient with the advanced form of the disease are characteristically small, their weight averaging 40 to 60 grams. The most severe atrophy is noted at the outer portion of the cortex, the deeper portions of cortex being more or less spared. From both biopsy and postmortem examination it appears that the primary lesion involves the interstitium and the tubules rather than the glomeruli. Interstitial fibrosis is prominent and there is a minimal infiltration of round cells. Many tubules are atrophied, and the remaining tubules are often hyperplastic and show mitotic figures. The glomeruli are relatively uninvolved and appear to degenerate only late in the course of the disease, apparently as a consequence of the interstitial lesion.

The clinical picture in Balkan nephritis is characterized by an insidious onset, usually without a history of edema or hematuria. The urine is found to contain small quantities of protein, usually not exceeding 1 gram per day; and the sediment is scanty, containing only a few leukocytes and erythrocytes and an occasional cast. It is noteworthy that blood pressure is usually normal, though in a small percentage of cases hypertension has been noted. Diminished concentrating ability occurs early, a finding consistent with the histologic observation that tubular damage is a prominent feature of the disease. Hyperchloremic acidosis gives further evidence that injury to tubules is out of proportion to glomerular injury. Renal failure, once present, generally progresses slowly, usually over a five- or ten-year period, to a fatal termination. There is no specific treatment. The most pressing problem remains that of determining the cause of the disease.

Griggs, R. C., and Hall, P. W.: Investigations of chronic endemic nephropathy in Yugoslavia. *In* Metcoff, J. (ed.): Renal Metabolism and Epidemiology of Some Renal Diseases. York, Pennsylvania, The Maple Press Company, 1964, p. 312.

Hall, P. W., Dammin, G. J., Griggs, R. C., Fajgelj, A., Zimonjic, B., and Gaon, J.: Investigation of chronic endemic nephropathy in Yugoslavia. II. Renal Pathology. Am. J. Med., 39:210, 1965.

Wolstenholme, G. E. W., and Knight, J. (eds.): The Balkan Nephropathy. Boston, Little, Brown & Company, 1967.

624. ANALGESIC NEPHROPATHY

Studies over the last two decades have demonstrated a remarkably high incidence of renal disease among individuals who ingest large quantities of analgesics. Early reports laid the responsibility for analgesic-induced renal damage on phenacetin, but with continued observations it has become apparent that singling out phenacetin as the sole etiologic factor is not justified; phenacetin is typically given as part of pain-relieving compounds containing agents such as aspirin and caffeine, and available evidence suggests that such agents in combination are usually responsible for the development of renal damage.

The circumstantial evidence relating excessive ingestion of analgesics to the development of renal disease is impressive, but there are those who remain unconvinced that there is such an entity as analgesic nephropathy. The skeptics note that not all epidemiologic studies have demonstrated an increased incidence of renal damage among abusers of analgesics; they also note that most investigators have found it difficult to produce renal damage in animals given analgesics in doses equivalent to those consumed by patients. Nevertheless, the weight of the epidemiologic findings strongly supports the view that excessive analgesic intake often does produce kidney disease and, indeed, that it produces disease of a rather characteristic type.

Pathology. The characteristic pathologic findings of analgesic nephropathy consist of interstitial nephritis and extensive papillary necrosis. The interstitial lesion typically consists of round cell infiltration with associated severe tubular atrophy and mild glomerular sclerosis. The mechanism through which the renal lesions are produced remains undefined, but it has been suggested that the primary toxic effect of analgesics is on the papillae and that interstitial damage occurs secondarily. It should be emphasized that papillary necrosis, seen in the absence of pyelonephritis, urinary tract ob-

struction, or diabetes mellitus (see Ch. 617), should strongly raise the possibility of analgesic abuse.

Clinical Manifestations. The typical patient with analgesic nephropathy has taken ten or more analgesic tablets a day for eight to ten years or longer. However, some individuals who have taken as few as five tablets a day for only a few years have also been observed to develop renal injury.

Analgesic nephropathy occurs most commonly in women; in nearly all studies there is a three- to fivefold predominance of females over males. Most patients attribute their intake of medication to headaches or musculoskeletal discomfort, but a considerable number have no somatic complaints and have taken analgesics solely for the psychotropic effects. Even among patients with physical complaints there is a remarkably high incidence of psychoneurotic difficulties, notably depression and anxiety. Most observers believe that emotional problems are a near-constant feature in those who abuse analgesics.

It should be emphasized that some patients with analgesic nephropathy steadfastly deny the use of medications. Thus when the diagnosis is suspected, it may be necessary to speak with the family or local pharmacist in order to obtain accurate historical data regarding drug exposure.

A third or more of patients who abuse analgesics have a history of peptic ulceration or gastritis, and many of these also give a history of gastric surgery. The upper gastrointestinal difficulties are thought to be the consequence of injury to the gastric mucosa produced by continued exposure to analgesic compounds.

Patients with analgesic nephropathy often develop gross hematuria and renal colic, findings almost always accounted for by necrosis and sloughing of renal papillae. Occasionally a sloughed papilla will obstruct the ureter, and fulminant pyelonephritis may ensue; in the patient with pre-existing renal damage this sequence of events often produces a rapid and life-threatening deterioration of renal function.

The physical examination is usually unremarkable

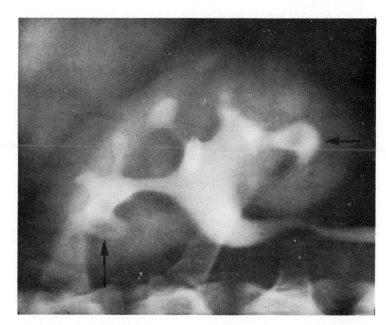

Tomogram of a kidney demonstrating renal papillary necrosis in a patient with analgesic nephropathy. Arrows indicate "ring shadows" in two calyces.

save for the frequent presence of hypertension. Laboratory studies ordinarily reveal mild to moderate anemia, small quantities of protein in the urine, and pyuria. The urine is often sterile even in the face of pyuria, but organisms in significant numbers are found in approximately one third of patients. The finding of pyuria without bacteriuria should itself raise the possibility of chronic interstitial nephritis. Renal function may be normal at the time that the patient is first seen, but in most instances it is already somewhat impaired.

In the patient with moderate or severe kidney disease, x-ray examination by intravenous pyelography almost always demonstrates small kidneys and calyceal clubbing. These findings are indistinguishable from those of chronic pyelonephritis, but when seen in association with evidence of papillary necrosis (such as a "ring sign"), they point strongly towards a diagnosis of analgesic nephropathy (see accompanying figure).

Treatment. Patients with renal dysfunction who continue to ingest analgesics usually develop progressive renal failure. However, those who discontinue the ingestion of drugs will often, for a period of years, show little further deterioration of function. The stability of function in the face of moderate or severe renal damage is almost unique for analgesic nephropathy. Remarkably, some patients who discontinue analgesics may even demonstrate a significant rise in filtration rate and concomitant striking reduction in plasma creatinine concentration. These prognostic considerations emphasize the importance of dissuading the patient from the continued ingestion of analgesic medications.

Gault, M. H., Rudwal, T. C., Engles, W. B., and Dossetor, J. B.: Syndrome associated with the abuse of analgesics. Ann. Intern. Med., 68:906, 1968.

Linton, A. L.: Renal disease due to analgesics. 1. Recognition of the problem of analgesic nephropathy. Can. Med. Assoc. J., 107:749, 1972.

Murray, R. M., Lawson, D. H., and Linton, A. L.: Analgesic nephropathy; clinical syndrome and prognosis. Br. Med. J., 27:479, 1971.

Nanra, R. S., and Kincaid-Smith, P.: Chronic effect of analgesics on the kidney. Prog. Biochem. Pharmacol., 7:285, 1972.

625. OBSTRUCTIVE NEPHROPATHY*

Francis P. Muldowney

Back pressure arising from urinary tract obstruction may result in important structural and functional derangements of the kidney, and obstructive uropathy is one of the most frequent etiologic factors in patients presenting with unexplained uremia. Clinical progress may be deceptively slow or viciously accelerated, depending on whether obstruction is incomplete or complete, and especially on whether infection is also present. Since obstruction is clearly a remediable cause of kidney damage, accurate diagnosis and appropriate management assume considerable importance for restoration and preservation of renal function.

Etiology (see accompanying figure). The many causes of obstruction may be considered under three headings: those inside the lumen of the urinary conduit

*The assistance of Mr. Daniel G. Kelly, F.R.C.S., in the preparation of this manuscript is gratefully acknowledged.

(intraluminal), those within the wall (intramural), and those causing pressure from outside. The accompanying table lists the major causes in each category. In unilateral (nonuremic) cases, the ureteropelvic junction is a common site of obstruction under all three etiologic headings. In bilateral (uremic) cases the most frequent causes are prostatic obstruction and urinary stone, comprising together some 55 per cent, with bladder tumor contributing a further 20 per cent. Retroperitoneal fibrosis is covered in detail in Ch. 107.

Incidence and Prevalence. Obstructive lesions of the urinary tract have been found in 3.8 per cent of a large series of routine autopsies. Corresponding figures from a population of uremic subjects at autopsy show a rise to fully 25 per cent, including those in whom obstructive uropathy was either a contributory or a major factor. A much higher relative incidence of obstructive versus other causes of renal disease is to be expected in particular at-risk age groups such as infants and children on the one hand (congenital strictures or ureteropelvic dysfunction) or elderly males (prostatic obstruction) on the other.

Pathogenesis and Pathology. In slowly developing or partial obstruction gross dilatation of the renal pelvis and calyces may occur, especially when the impedance is situated high up—for example, at the ureteropelvic junction. In such cases, the distended sac may accommodate 2 to 3 liters of fluid, with a greatly thinned renal cortex, but clinical manifestations may be few. When infection has supervened, pyonephrosis with total destruction of renal parenchyma is the end result, usually with correspondingly severe clinical manifestations. When obstruction develops rapidly or is complete, distention of the renal pelvis and calyces is much less but intraluminal pressure above the level of obstruction may be very high. Correspondingly severe symptoms of loin pain, caused by distention of the renal capsule, or ureteral colic, caused by repeated ureteric peristaltic waves, are usually present. Occasionally, however, complete obstruction of one ureter may occur with very little evidence of back pressure or dilatation, resulting nevertheless in gradual total loss of renal function on that side if not relieved within four to six months. In general, the degree of renal damage is related to the duration of obstruction. In either situation, the occurrence of infection behind the obstruction, either blood-borne or introduced during diagnostic instrumentation, transforms the clinical picture into an acute pyrexial illness with fever, accompanied by rapid destruction of renal tissue.

Infection is therefore an important determinant of the pathologic, functional, and prognostic picture. In lower urinary tract lesions, infection tends to occur early in the disease but is often relatively slow in progression. In upper urinary tract lesions, infection may not occur until much later but runs a more rapidly destructive course. In either case, the most important factor predisposing to infection is instrumentation of the urinary tract, by bladder catheter, cystoscope, or ureteral catheter.

Clinical Manifestations. Obstructive nephropathy is one of the most important causes of that ubiquitous nephrologic problem, "unexplained uremia," and, as mentioned above, is present at least as a contributory factor in 25 per cent of such cases at autopsy. All patients presenting with renal failure, or in whom there is abrupt deterioration of renal function unexplained by their primary renal problem, should be carefully screened to exclude onset of obstruction.

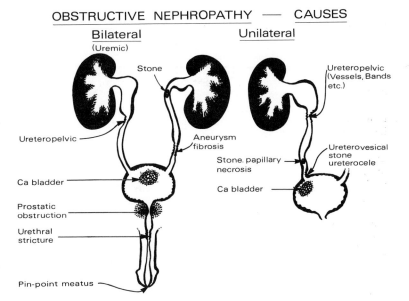

OBSTRUCTIVE NEPHROPATHY — CAUSES

Common sites of urinary tract obstruction.

Equally important is the mode of presentation in the form of recurrent urinary tract infection. Symptoms caused by complicating infection are commonly the presenting complaint with obstructive lesions at all levels. Persistent or recurrent urinary tract infection should always raise the suspicion of an obstructive lesion, even when specific localizing symptoms are absent.

In lower urinary tract lesions, the history of pattern of micturition provides an extremely useful guide to both diagnosis and treatment. Thus, for instance, a subject in whom rectal examination indicates apparently gross prostatic hypertrophy may nevertheless have minimal symptoms of urinary hesitancy or dribbling, and therefore does not merit further instrumentation or operation. On the other hand, a palpably normal prostate may give rise to severe obstructive symptoms by virtue of median lobe enlargement impinging inward on the prostatic urethra. In either case the history is of overriding importance.

Lower urinary tract obstruction — for example, in prostatic hypertrophy — is associated classically with hesitancy in commencing micturition, poor stream of urine, and inability to empty the bladder completely, with resulting stop-and-start urination and postmicturition dribbling. Sudden temporary urinary retention may result from vascular congestion of the prostate, e.g., after alcohol ingestion, with suprapubic pain caused by bladder distention. In chronic cases overflow incontinence from a distended bladder may produce deceptively large urinary volumes and thus cause suprapubic bladder enlargement to be overlooked. *Urine flow may be very large in such cases* owing to the associated defect in urinary concentrating ability producing hypotonicity.

Acute upper urinary tract obstruction of one or both ureters results in severe colicky pain referred to the groin, with associated symptoms of weakness and sweating. Chronic cases caused by gradually developing obstruction at the ureteropelvic junction present with dull pain in the renal angle but little or no severe colic. A minority of cases may obstruct one ureter without overt symptoms, with resulting silent loss of renal function on that side.

In some cases, development of high-renin hypertension or primary erythrocytosis may be the presenting features, leading to discovery of unsuspected unilateral hydronephrosis in, for example, pelviureteric obstruction.

Diagnosis and Differential Diagnosis. Background etiologic factors such as family history of stone (cystinuria), arthritis (primary gout), lymphoma (secondary gout), drug therapy (periureteral fibrosis), diabetes (papillary necrosis), or neurologic disorders such as multiple sclerosis must be considered. Microscopic examination of the urinary sediment may reveal red cells, cystine or uric acid crystals, or rarely fragments of a necrosed renal papilla. Frequently, however, no specific abnormality is found in the urine. Physical examination may disclose loin tenderness or palpable renal swelling; careful supra-

Causes of Obstructive Uropathy

Intraluminal	Intramural	Extramural
Stone	Congenital:	Prostatic obstruction
Bladder tumor	Ureteropelvic dysfunction (10% bilateral)	Ureteropelvic juncture — vessels, bands, etc.
Papillary necrosis (diabetes)	Ureterovesical stricture (simple or ureterocele)	Aortic aneurysm
Clot	Bladder neck obstruction	Periureteral fibrosis
Ureteral tumor	Pinpoint meatus	Retroperitoneal tumor or nodes
	Acquired:	Extraurinary growth (carcinoma of colon, diverticulitis)
	Urethral stricture	Pelvic tumor
	Ureteral stricture (tuberculosis, etc.)	Inadvertent ligature
	Neurogenic bladder dysfunction	

pubic palpation and percussion will show a distended bladder. Rectal or vaginal examination may point to extraurinary growth.

Further investigation may then proceed along two lines—the assessment of glomerular filtration rate; and the definition of anatomic outlines of kidneys, ureters, and bladder. If serum urea or creatinine is normal or only slightly raised, glomerular filtration rate (GFR) reduction even if present will not interfere with radiologic procedures such as intravenous pyelography, which may be pursued utilizing normal dosages of intravenous dye. If plasma urea or creatinine is significantly raised, a more exact measurement of GFR may be made by measuring the disappearance rate of ^{51}Cr labeled EDTA from venous blood. This method circumvents the difficulty of conventional clearance measurements in the presence of temporary anuria or oliguria. Values less than 50 per cent of normal are clearly indicative of *bilateral* renal dysfunction. A "double-dose" of intravenous dye (i.e., 35 to 70 grams of iodine rather than the normal 15 to 30 grams) is needed if GFR is in the range 70 to 25 ml per minute. Below this filtration level, doses of up to 70 grams may be given by slow intravenous infusion. In severely uremic cases, pyelography is best postponed until immediately after dialysis. Utilizing this method, good visualization of the renal tract can be expected in 90 per cent of cases no matter how low the GFR. Retrograde pyelography is therefore almost never necessary. Certain extra precautions must, however, be taken to ensure useful results from intravenous pyelography. In addition to the conventional 5-, 10-, and 20-minute films, repeated late exposures over a period of 24 hours may show delayed nephrotomograms or dilated ureteral outlines. Nephrotomography is particularly useful in the definition of renal size and outline. Postmicturition films when feasible may show incomplete bladder emptying (residual urine) or prostatic encroachment.

While preliminary GFR assessment is taking place, a simple straight roentgenogram of the kidney-ureter-bladder area may give important information. A radiopaque stone may be seen along the line of the ureter, especially at the ureterovesical junction. Nonopaque stone (uric acid) is more difficult to exclude. In either case unilateral renal enlargement may be visible.

In order to obtain the maximal information, it is helpful to study the pyelogram films in a definite sequence, as follows:

Are two kidneys present?

Is there a difference in size?

Is there a delay in appearance of dye on one or other side?

Is there evidence of calyceal or pelvic dilatation?

Is there thinning, deformity, or shrinkage of the renal cortex?

Is there dilatation of the ureter and down to what level?

Is there displacement of the ureter medially (periureteral fibrosis) or laterally (aortic aneurysm or tumor)?

Does the bladder outline show a filling defect or deformity?

Does complete emptying of bladder dye occur after micturition?

Adequate answers to most of these questions can be supplied in 90 per cent of cases. Rarely, resort to cystoscopy may be necessary with or without retrograde ureteral catheterization and pyelography. Owing to the danger of introducing infection, these procedures are performed only when absolutely necessary for establishment of the diagnosis or with a view to operative treatment. If, for instance, prostatectomy has been decided upon, preliminary cystoscopy is essential in order to exclude associated asymptomatic pathology such as bladder tumor, diverticulum, or stone which may be present in 10 per cent of cases.

Treatment. The principles of treatment are to (1) relieve obstruction, (2) prevent infection, and (3) treat infection if present, with antimicrobial choice and dosage according to the degree of reduction of GFR (see Ch. 617). Surgical correction of obstruction is aimed at achieving comfort and preventing further damage to the threatened kidney. Before definitive relief of obstruction is attempted, it may be necessary in severely ill or uremic patients to employ dialysis with or without temporary external diversion of urine. Temporary diversion is useful when some doubt exists as to the ultimate viability of the kidney and when immediate radical relief of obstruction may appear hazardous. In some cases also the exact nature of the obstructing lesion may be in doubt for some time, e.g., whether prostatic enlargement is benign or malignant.

The decision to attempt surgical relief of obstruction must therefore be tempered initially by consideration of the aforementioned factors, and subsequently by other important aspects of the obstructive lesion itself such as its nature, location, and duration. Formerly, nephrectomy was commonly advised for unilateral cases, especially when infected, but such an approach obviously fails to provide for possible partial recovery of function on the affected side. Nephrectomy can now be advised only when extensive renal damage or pyonephrosis indicates an irrecoverable situation, especially when the remaining kidney might become involved in the destructive or infective process.

Urgent surgical relief is indicated for high-level lesions such as ureteric stone which is impacted, i.e., not moving spontaneously over a period of days. An initial attempt at dislodgment by cystoscopy and retrograde ureteral catheterization should be quickly followed, if unsuccessful, by direct open ureterolithotomy, because complicating infection must then be expected. Any other cause of recent *total* ureteral obstruction likewise demands surgical relief in order to restore function. "Recent" in this connection implies within the past four to six weeks or at most within four months, because total obstruction of longer duration is likely to have permanently destroyed the kidney.

Postponement of surgical intervention may be preferable in noninfected patients when obstruction is only *partial,* or when there is reasonable expectation of spontaneous relief. Time thus gained will help the eventual decision, based on the nature of the primary lesion. Even when infection is present, time may be gained in this way during which the response to antimicrobial therapy may be assessed. Such caution is particularly advisable in *lower* urinary tract disease, such as prostatic enlargement, in which eradication of infection may relieve many symptoms originally thought to be obstructive in origin. If significant residual bladder urine volumes (more than 100 ml) persist at this stage, however, surgery is indicated. The presence of infection in *high* urinary tract obstruction is a more urgent indication for surgical relief, because the complication of gram-negative septicemia represents a very serious hazard.

After relief of obstruction, whether by temporary external diversion or by definitive surgery, diuresis follows with rapid return to normal of blood urea and creatinine. The subsequent urinary flow may in some cases achieve massive proportions with considerable loss of solute, suggesting a diuresis of proximal tubular origin. Such a postobstructive diuresis is encountered especially in relatively chronic cases with evidence of increase in body sodium and water stores. Usually the diuresis with negative salt balance is self-limited and represents merely a restoration to normal of the previously expanded extracellular fluid volume and as such it does not require treatment. In a small minority, however, intravenous saline replacement may be necessary in this phase. Falling blood pressure or serum sodium concentration, or the occurrence of a secondary rise in serum urea or creatinine, are indications for fluid replenishment.

Prognosis. Prognosis in obstructive nephropathy depends largely on whether treatment is instituted before irreversible damage has occurred. Without treatment, the subsequent natural history of the disorder is dependent on whether the obstructing lesion is complete or incomplete and unilateral or bilateral, and especially on whether infection is present. Complete blockage with infection can totally destroy the kidney(s) within days. Chronic partial blockage, as for example in congenital pelviureteral obstruction, may be consistent with many years without symptoms, but, if bilateral, is likely to present ultimately in the "unexplained uremia" category.

With treatment, much depends on the duration of obstruction prior to relief, and especially on whether infection has been present. Experimental data suggest that complete obstruction for one week results in a permanent 50 per cent reduction in GFR on the affected side. Obstruction of longer duration is associated with correspondingly more severe permanent damage. After three months gross GFR reduction is seen but with potential for partial recovery. Loss of maximal concentrating and acidifying ability may be a prominent residual tubular defect, but sodium excretion, although relatively high in the basal state, nevertheless responds normally to both volume expansion and mineralocorticoid administration, indicating preservation of tubular function. If the history suggests obstruction for longer than four to six months, recovery of function appears very unlikely. Operative interference is therefore not indicated unless complicating pyonephrosis, severe polycythemia, or developing high-renin hypertension supervenes.

Better, O. S., Arieff, A. I., Massry, S. G., Kleeman, C. R., and Maxwell, M. H.: Studies on renal function after relief of complete unilateral ureteral obstruction of three months' duration in man. Am. J. Med., 54:234, 1973.

Bricker, N. S., and Klahr, S.: Obstructive nephropathy. *In* Strauss, M. B., and Welt, L. G. (eds.): Diseases of the Kidney. 2nd ed. Edinburgh and London, Churchill/Livingstone, 1971.

Kerr, W. S.: Effects of complete ureteral obstruction in dogs on kidney function. Am. J. Physiol., 184:521, 1956.

Keuhnelian, J. G., Bartone, F., and Marshall, V. F.: Practical considerations from autopsies on azotemic patients. J. Urol., 91:467, 1964.

Legrain, M., Bitker, M., and Kuss, R.: Obstructive Nephropathy in Adults. Proc. 3rd Int. Cong. Nephrol. Washington, 2:336, 1966 (New York, Basel and Karger, 1967).

Muldowney, F. P., Duffy, G. T., Kelly, D. G., Duff, F. A., Harrington, C., and Freaney, R.: Sodium diuresis after relief of obstructive uropathy. N. Engl. J. Med., 274:1294, 1966.

Proca, E.: Errors and pitfalls in the management of acute urinary obstruction complicated by uraemia with special reference to stone. Br. J. Urol., 44:9, 1972.

626. TOXIC NEPHROPATHY

George E. Schreiner

Toxic nephropathy is a functional or structural change in the kidney caused by a chemical or biologic product. By extension, the concept is often applied to the renal effects of physiologic substances circulating in abnormal concentrations. This situation obtains in hypokalemic, hypercalcemic, and hyperuricemic nephropathies, which are considered in detail in Ch. 619, 620, and 622. The classification of toxic nephropathy is contained in Table 1, and a partial list of nephrotoxins is shown in Table 2.

The peculiar susceptibility of the kidney to an enormous range of drugs and biologically active materials stems from its huge blood supply relative to weight, its large endothelial vascular surface, its high oxygen consumption and glucose production, the fact that excreted compounds are concentrated along the luminal surface of the nephron, and the fact that many drugs occupy, at least transiently, an intracellular position if they are involved in secretory or reabsorptive transport processes. It is possible that some reabsorbed drugs may be concentrated along with sodium in the hypertonic interstitial tissues of the papillae.

Toxic nephropathy accounts for an appreciable fraction of all reported series of acute renal failure. In the past 15 years at Georgetown Hospital it represents 20 per cent of the total experience with acute renal failure. The most frequently encountered nephrotoxins in the series were carbon tetrachloride, mercury, sulfonamide drugs, radiographic contrast media, analgesics, ethylene glycol, and antimicrobials.

Toxic nephropathy may also account for a significant segment of so-called geographic renal diseases. The World Health Organization has cited some 25,000 cases of an interstitial nephritis that has been reported by various investigators as Yugoslavian, Bulgarian, and Balkan nephritis. This disease has a distribution conforming to specific altitudes and river valleys. Pathologically it resembles a toxic nephropathy, but the specific agent has not been identified. As more sophisticated renal diagnostic techniques are correlated with renal biopsy and histochemistry, it is likely that the number of

TABLE 1. Classification of Toxic Nephropathy

Class 1. Drugs, chemicals, or their metabolites with a reasonably *direct* effect, producing an identifiable morphologic or persisting functional change in the nephron. Model: bichloride of mercury.

Class 2. Compounds producing sensitivity disease identifiable as the *nephrotic* or *nephritic* syndrome in which the initial step may be subtle alteration in the renal cell or alteration of a protein, producing an immune reaction. Model: aminonucleoside nephrosis and nephroallergens producing the nephrotic syndrome.

Class 3. Compounds producing sensitivity reactions of the angiitis or vasculitis type involving the kidney as a vascular organ. Model: sulfa sensitivity.

Class 4. Compounds that may produce *chronic nephrotoxicity,* when the mechanism extends over a period of months or years and the evidence remains largely epidemiologic or circumstantial. Model: lead nephropathy.

Class 5. Compounds that aggravate pre-existing renal disease or predispose to secondary renal disease such as pyelonephritis. Model: diuretics and cathartics predisposing to pyelonephritis via potassium deficiency.

TABLE 2.   A Partial List of Nephrotoxins

Metals: Mercury (organic and inorganic), bismuth, uranium, cadmium, lead, gold, arsine and arsenic, iron, silver, antimony, copper, and thallium

Organic solvents: Carbon tetrachloride, tetrachlorethylene, methyl cellosolve, methanol, and miscellaneous solvents

Glycols: Ethylene glycol, ethylene glycol dinitrite, propylene glycol, ethylene dichloride, and diethylene glycol

Physical agents: Radiation, heat stroke, and electroshock

Diagnostic agents: Contrast agents in high concentration (pyelography and aortography) and bunamiodyl

Therapeutic agents: Antimicrobials: Sulfonamides, penicillin, streptomycin, kanamycin, vancomycin, bacitracin, polymyxin and colistin, neomycin, tetracycline, and amphotericin. *Analgesics:* Salicylates, para-aminosalicylate (PAS), ? phenacetin, phenylbutazone, zoxazolamine, phenindione, puromycin, tridione, paradione

Osmotic agents: Sucrose, mannitol

Insecticides: Biphenyl, chlorinated hydrocarbons

Miscellaneous chemicals: Carbon monoxide, snake venom, mushroom poison, spider venom, nephroallergens, cresol, beryllium, hemolysins, aniline, and other methemoglobin formers

Abnormal concentration of physiologic substances: Hypercalcemia, hyperuricemia, hypokalemia, hypomagnesemia, etc.

---

recognized nephrotoxins will increase during the next decade owing to both chemicals now in existence and substances still to be produced through the remarkable ingenuity and industry of the organic chemists.

SPECIFIC NEPHROTOXINS

Mercury and Other Heavy Metals

Mercury.   Mercury in various forms acts as a nephrotoxin. Acutely it produces tubular necrosis with renal failure. In organic form or with prolonged exposure it may produce the nephrotic syndrome or chronic renal damage. Frequently encountered mercuric compounds are chloride, iodide, oxide, cyanide, and salicylate. Mercurous compounds include the chloride (calomel), iodide, and oxide salts. Organic mercuric compounds associated with nephrotoxicity include merbromin (Mercurochrome) and the mercurial diuretics.

Epidemiology.   Inorganic mercury poisoning usually occurs by accident, in suicide attempts, or after its use as an abortive agent. Poisoning has occurred in a wide variety of industries, including the manufacture of paint, alloys, and scientific instruments. Agricultural exposures are due to disinfectants and pesticides. Medical poisoning stems from mercurial diuretics, ammoniated mercury ointments, and absorption from the skin of widespread dermatoses, such as psoriasis. Inhalation toxicity may occur. The urinary excretion of inorganic mercury normally ranges from 0.1 to 1 μg per liter. Patients with chronic industrial exposure often excrete amounts in excess of 300 μg per liter. Psoriatic patients have had mercuriuria demonstrated from 500 to 1000 μg per liter.

Clinical Manifestations.   Mercury produces a lingering, bitter, metallic taste that may be followed by a sensation of constriction in the throat, suffocation, substernal burning, esophagitis, gastritis, abdominal pain, nausea, and vomiting. Ulcerations occur on the palate or lips; diarrhea may be blood tinged. Circulatory collapse is signaled by feeble pulse, peripheral vasoconstriction, syncope, and shock with oliguria and anuria. It is important to obtain urine before oliguria sets in. The urine usually shows albumin, epithelial cell casts, erythrocytes, glycosuria, aminoaciduria, and increased mercury content, particularly in the precipitable fractions. Leukocytosis is the rule.

Pathology.   Mercurial vapor, dust, or liquid dissolves locally on moist surfaces of the mucous membranes. Mercuric salts are well absorbed by the gastrointestinal tract and vagina, and ammoniated mercury by the intact skin. Absorbed mercury is bound quickly to circulating protein, and appears in blood, kidney, liver, heart, brain, and some endocrine organs. Inorganic salts are excreted largely by the colon, kidneys, salivary glands, biliary system, and skin, and organic materials predominantly by the kidney. The most striking pathologic changes occur in the form of granular or vacuolar degeneration of the proximal tubules. Mitotic figures and basophilic cytoplasm may be seen in the early phases of healing. Early calcification of the site of necrosis may occur. In severe cases all segments of the tubule may be involved, and patchy tubulorrhexis may occur. Extrarenal autopsy findings include induration of surface membranes in pharynx, esophagus, and stomach, erosive gastritis, softening of the muscular coat of the intestine, severe colitis, congestion of liver and spleen, degeneration of myocardium, and focal hemorrhages in the cerebral cortex. It appears that mercury initiates cellular destruction by combining with the sulfhydryl groups of protein in the mitochrondrial membrane, leading to the disintegration of mitochondria and necrosis of nuclei and subsequent loss in enzyme activity.

Fourteen cases of acute renal failure caused by mercury have been studied at Georgetown Hospital. The dose expressed as inorganic mercury ranged from 0.4 to 10 grams. Oliguria occurred within the first 48 hours, and persisted for an average of 15 days (range 7 to 22). Tissue necrosis was a catabolic factor, and the BUN increased an average of 31 mg per 100 ml per day during the first week. Thirteen patients required hemodialysis, and three died. None of the patients died who underwent hemodialysis within 48 hours after the ingestion of mercury and the administration of BAL. Six cases of nephrotic syndrome secondary to mercury have been observed.

Treatment.   Prevention is exceptionally important. The use of mercuric salts for douching and surgical irrigation should be discouraged. Bottles should be labeled as poison and should be secured in a safe place. Acute ingestion is a medical emergency. Emesis usually occurs, but if not, the stomach should be emptied with a large lavage tube, and rinsed with egg white or concentrated albumin or medicinal charcoal. A useful lavage solution combines 1 pint of skim milk, 50 grams of glucose, 20 grams of sodium bicarbonate, and three eggs beaten into a mixture. One gram of medicinal charcoal can combine with 850 mg of mercuric chloride. After absorption, BAL (2,3-dimercapropanol) acts as an effective antidote because it appears to compete with biologically important sulfhydryl groups. Injections of 2.5 to 3 mg of BAL per kilogram of body weight should be given every four hours up to six injections, depending on the severity of poisoning. BAL may produce transient nausea, vomiting, diarrhea, burning stomatitis and excessive lacrimation. It is a mild hypoglycemic agent. In severe poisoning large doses of BAL are given immediately, and dialysis is carried out shortly thereafter to remove the mercury-BAL complex; the patient is then re-treated with BAL. Exchange transfusion may also be of value. Patients who remain oliguric should be given the same conservative management as other patients with acute renal failure (see Ch. 604).

Treatment of patients with nephrotic syndrome caused by mercury calls for immediate removal of the agent, administration of adrenocortical steroids, and a regimen similar to that recommended for other patients with the nephrotic syndrome. These patients may be subject to repeated renal damage by mercurial diuretics. Hypersensitivity reactions to mercurial diuretics have included generalized pruritus, urticaria, asthma, exfoliative dermatitis, and sudden death. Cystine, penicillamine, BAL, or other sources of sulfhydryl compounds may be used to augment the treatment of mercury sensitivity and especially ventricular fibrillation, which is the cause of sudden death.

Acrodynia (pink disease) occurs in children throughout the world, and is characterized by irritability, emaciation, stomatitis, and erythema of acral parts. The children have fever, leukocytosis, albuminuria, and mercuriuria from mercury used in teething powder or diaper rinses.

Bismuth. Bismuth toxicity arises chiefly from industrial poisons, antisyphilitic therapy, and soluble bismuth compounds such as the subcarbonate and the mixed thioglycolates. Bismuth may produce either acute renal failure or nephrotic syndrome. Sore mouth, diarrhea, peripheral neuritis, stomatitis, obstructive jaundice, and pigmentation of the gum margins may occur, together with evidence of acute renal failure with hyposthenuria, cylindruria, and the desquamation of renal tubular epithelial cells.

Uranium. Uranium causes proximal tubular necrosis in a distribution similar to that of mercury. Uranium nitrate may produce a central lobular lesion in the glomeruli. Uranium has been implicated in some cases of geographic nephritis.

Cadmium. Cadmium is widely used in the metal plating and industrial chemical industries. Interstitial nephritis may follow chronic exposure, and acute poisoning produces proteinuria and proximal renal damage. The most significant feature of cadmium nephrotoxicity is a peculiar proteinuria, ranging from 70 to 2600 mg per 24 hours. There is a low molecular weight protein (20,000 to 30,000) that precipitates with nitric acid but not with boiling, and migrates as an alpha globulin. Cadmium proteinuria is clinically significant and is best treated by removing the patient from the toxic environment. Cadmium is soluble in acid; acid foods and beverages placed in cadmium-plated containers such as ice cube trays may be a source of poisoning.

Lead. Lead nephrotoxicity has been implicated in severe renal disease produced from the drinking of whiskey made in stills improvised from automobile and truck radiators. In Queensland, Australia, the eating of paint or drinking of rain water from porches painted with lead paint has been found to result in a high incidence of chronic nephritis associated with increased skeletal lead content and increased lead in the urine. Unexposed subjects may excrete about 0.08 mg per liter of lead, and asymptomatic exposed subjects may excrete up to 0.15 mg per liter. Patients with lead poisoning may excrete from 0.15 to 0.30 mg per liter. Lead nephropathy is a predominantly tubular syndrome with renal glycosuria, aminoaciduria, albuminuria, casts, and increased excretion of lead, delta-aminolevulinic acid, coproporphyrin, urobilinogen, urobilin, and bile pigments. Roentgenograms show typically the increased density at the ends of the shafts of the long bones. Ziehl-Neelsen acid-fast, intranuclear inclusion bodies may be seen on renal biopsy.

Treatment of lead nephropathy lies in immediate removal of the subject from the source of exposure. Attempts may be made to increase excretion by such agents as sodium citrate, dimercaprol, and disodium calcium ethylenediamine tetraacetate.

Gold. Gold salts are used in rheumatoid arthritis in the form of gold sodium thiosulfate, sodium aurothiomalate, aurothioglucose, and aurothioglycanide. Cutaneous manifestations of hypersensitivity include urticaria, purpura, itching, maculopapular to exfoliative dermatitis, and polyneuritis. Bone marrow depression may be encountered. Nephrotoxicity is usually heralded by proteinuria and microscopic hematuria. The nephrotic syndrome may supervene. Brun et al. studied the localization of gold in renal biopsies of patients receiving gold therapy. Deposits of the metal were found in the proximal tubules shortly after injection. Subsequently (one to four years) they were localized in the distal tubules. In the interstitial tissues gold was stored in macrophages, and could be demonstrated up to 28 years after the last injection. At Georgetown Hospital four patients with the nephrotic syndrome after gold therapy have been observed. Three subsequently developed laboratory features of systemic lupus erythematosus.

Arsine. Arsine intoxication produces shock, hemoglobinuria, and acute tubular necrosis, which has been successfully treated by hemodialysis.

Arsenic. Arsenic may produce a toxic nephritis leading to oliguria and uremia, aggravated by the dehydration from associated diarrhea. The urine contains albumin, casts, erythrocytes, and leukocytes. Arsenic may be recovered in the dialysate of such patients treated with hemodialysis.

Silver. Silver may produce renal tubular degeneration, with sparing of the glomeruli, interstitial deposits of silver, and interstitial edema. It has been reported in persons who regularly handle photographic developers.

Iron. Acute tubular necrosis has been reported with a mortality rate of 50 per cent in children who accidentally ingest large doses of ferrous sulfate. It is presumably related to the mucosal damage in the gastrointestinal tract, metabolic acidosis, hepatic damage, and shock. Chronic renal failure, interstitial fibrosis, and iron deposition may be seen in hemochromatosis and severe transfusion hemosiderosis. In rabbits saccharated iron oxide produces a nephrotoxic lesion.

Antimony. As used therapeutically for leishmaniasis, antimony can lead to transient oliguric renal failure.

Copper. Copper sulfate ingestion can produce vomiting, dehydration, hypotension, sulfhemoglobinemia, and acute renal failure. Tubular degeneration and necrosis are seen, particularly in the ascending loop and distal convolution.

Thallium. Thallium is used in rat poisons, depilatories, and denaturing agents for alcohol. It causes albuminuria, tachycardia, colic, and a neurologic syndrome.

Solvents

Carbon tetrachloride is used as a cleaning agent, grease solvent and vermifuge, and in fire extinguishers. It is heavier than air. Nephrotoxicity may occur after either inhalation or ingestion. It is aggravated by the simultaneous ingestion of alcohol, even in small amounts. The initial symptoms are irritation at the exposure site, followed by headache, mental confusion, coma, and convulsions. Narcosis, encephalomyelitis, cerebellar degeneration, and optic and peripheral neuritis may occur. Gastrointestinal symptoms are prominent, particularly when the substance has been ingested, and include nausea, vomiting, and abdominal pain. The delayed manifestations are toxic hepatitis with jaundice, tender hepatomegaly with hepatic failure, and a toxic nephropathy with anuric acute tubular necrosis. Renal involvement may be insidious and delayed for as long as a week after exposure. The urine is typical of acute renal failure, with proteinuria, cylindruria, pyuria, hematuria, and desquamation of renal tubular epithelial cells. Bleeding manifestations, particularly scleral and periorbital hemorrhages, epistaxis, and hypoprothrombinemia may be seen. In the Georgetown Hospital experience, the most frequent signs and symptoms encountered were oliguria, nausea and vomiting, hepatomegaly, and abdominal pain. Half or less than half of the patients had bleeding, fever, hypertension, jaundice, rash, edema, ascites, and renal tenderness. Patients were azotemic, but the creatinine/BUN ratio averaged 16 per cent, considerably higher than the 11 per cent ratio in the entire group of acute renal failure. This may reflect some impairment of hepatic urea synthesis. The patients were usually hyperuricemic, hyponatremic, hypokalemic, hypochloremic, hypophosphatemic, and acidotic. Serum glutamic oxaloacetic transaminase was elevated. Hyperbilirubinemia, hyperglycemia, abnormal thymol turbidity, cephalin flocculation tests and elevated or high alkaline phosphatase levels were usual.

Treatment consists of removing the patient from the area of exposure and providing adequate ventilation, gastric lavage, and catharsis. The use of unsaturated oils by mouth has been suggested but not clinically proved to be helpful. People chronically exposed to carbon tetrachloride should be warned about the synergism with alcohol. After hepatic or renal failure has ensued, standard therapy for these complications should be employed. Hemorrhagic phenomena require the judicious use of blood transfusions.

Glycols

Ethylene glycol is commonly encountered in antifreeze solutions. Part of the compound is rapidly converted to oxalic acid, which may be deposited in the kidneys and other organs such as the meninges. In the kidney there is destruction of epithelial cells with preservation of the basement membrane, focal regeneration, and tubules filled with masses of calcium oxalate crystals that are birefringent on polarized light. Nephrons are dilated above the crystalline obstruction. Focal mononuclear cell infiltrates and interstitial edema are also seen.

The clinical events may be divided into three stages: During the first 12 hours central nervous system effects resemble those of ethanol intoxication. In severe poisoning this may include stupor, coma, convulsions, and death. During the second 12 hours the manifestations are predominantly cardiopulmonary, with tachypnea, cyanosis, pulmonary edema, and death in cardiac failure. After the first day the problem is mainly renal injury, with slight pain, tenderness over the kidneys, proteinuria, oliguria, and anuria; death may result from uremia.

Ethylene glycol poisoning is a medical emergency, and should be treated with immediate hemodialysis aimed at removal of the circulating alcohol to diminish the substrate for conversion to glycolic and oxalic acid. Gastric lavage and parenteral solutions of sodium bicarbonate may also be used. After anuria has supervened, the treatment is the same as for acute renal failure in general.

Physical Agents

Radiation nephritis is encountered clinically after radiation of tumors in or near the kidneys. The kidney is said to be the most radiosensitive of all major organs. The major syndromes include acute and chronic nephritis and benign and malignant hypertension. Clinically, radiation nephritis is characterized by proteinuria, hypertension, anemia, cardiomegaly, congestive heart failure, encephalopathy, and chronic uremia. In *acute* cases the mortality rate is about 50 per cent; survivors generally begin to improve within six months from the onset. In *chronic* radiation exposure the nephritis may be manifested only by proteinuria, anemia, hyposthenuria, and slowly progressive decline of renal function. These symptoms may occur as a continuum from the acute disease or may be discovered later in patients who have never presented with an acute syndrome.

Histologic study reveals marked thickening of the renal capsule, hyaline obliteration of the glomeruli, focal necrosis of the fibrinoid or hemorrhagic type, proliferation of Bowman's capsule, pericapsular fibrosis, tubular degeneration and atrophy, diffuse interstitial fibrosis, and fibrinoid necrosis of arterioles. There is a remarkable tendency to development of malignant hypertension and necrotizing arteriolitis.

The treatment is not essentially different from that for acute and chronic nephritis from other causes; the hypertension should be treated vigorously with antihypertensive drugs. When radiation nephritis is unilateral, the resulting hypertension may be benefited by nephrectomy.

Heat stroke may be encountered in hyperthermal industrial environments or military situations in the desert, and acute renal failure may be the dominant manifestation. Lack of acclimatization may be a primary factor in pathogenesis. Hemolysis, shock, hemoconcentration, volume depletion, and hypernatremia have been prominent clinical features. Acute renal failure ensues in up to 10 per cent of the patients who survive heat stroke.

Diagnostic Agents

Contrast media: Iodide is an essential component of all absorbable contrast media. A significant percentage of persons manifest iodine hypersensitivity in the form of urticaria, skin rashes, glottal edema, and occasionally anaphylactoid reactions with shock and acute tubular necrosis. Excluding hypersensitivity, organic iodides are, nevertheless, nephrotoxic. The highest incidence seems to be associated with an oral contrast medium, bunamiodyl (Orabilex), and with other double doses of dehydration techniques that have been used for attempted visualization of diseased gallbladders. Toxicity is also associated with abdominal aortography, especially when high concentrations of contrast material are used by direct rapid injection.

The numerous mechanisms suggested to explain the nephrotoxicity of contrast media have included renal vasoconstriction, erythrocyte agglutination and crenation from hyperosmolar injections, and loss of the dispersing effect of albumin, coagulation defect, and high concentration of the material in the tubular cell of a patient who has impaired hepatic excretion. Experimentally it has been shown that stasis with obstruction to urinary flow potentiates the toxicity.

Pathologic changes follow the particular route of pathogenesis: vasculitis in some cases of iodine hypersensitivity, proteinuria and glomerular damage from vasoconstriction and capillary thrombi, and acute tubular necrosis from shock or direct toxicity to the tubular cell. Recent reports suggest a specific reaction between the myeloma kidney and contrast material. Some may be due to dehydration incurred in preparation for pyelography. McAfee surveyed 13,207 abdominal aortograms and uncovered 12 fatal and 27 serious nonfatal instances of nephrotoxicity. Crawford noted reduced renal function in 50 per cent of patients receiving more than 40 ml of Urokon above the renal artery.

Intravenous pyelography, using less concentrated material, appears to produce fewer complications in even the presence of renal insufficiency. Retrograde pyelography carries the risk of infection from instrumentation and edema of the ureters, producing obstruction, and has been associated with papillary necrosis.

Cholecystography: It has been estimated that more than 100 cases of acute renal failure have been caused by bunamiodyl. The major pathologic finding is tubular necrosis, accompanied by deposition of birefringent green-brown crystals at the base of the tubular epithelial cell that are anisotropic with polarized light. Bunamiodyl is more completely absorbed from the intestine than other cholecystographic media and is therefore delivered in higher concentrations to the kidney, particularly in the presence of liver disease and an abnormal gallbladder. Wennberg recently demonstrated depression of glomerular filtration rate caused by bunamiodyl. Renal failure has also occurred in patients with underlying renal disease subjected to dehydration and specialized techniques of rapid intravenous or double-dose cholecystography.

Therapeutic Agents
(Antimicrobial Drugs)

In the presence of infectious disease and its circulatory consequences, recognition of nephrotoxicity from antimicrobial agents may be difficult. Dehydration, hypotension, vomiting, and allergic reactions may lead to renal failure that is not, properly speaking, direct nephrotoxicity. However, a number of antimicrobials do appear to produce direct renal damage.

Sulfonamide compounds may precipitate in the nephron or calyces, and may be excreted in high concentrations into a urine with a low pH. This can produce sulfonamide concretions, obstructive uropathy, and parenchymal damage from crystals. Occasionally direct tubular necrosis, interstitial nephritis, or necrotizing angiitis may also occur. Other lesions have been reported from acetazolamide.

Streptomycin may produce necrosis of the proximal tubular epithelium, cylindruria, and albuminuria. Since the excretion of streptomycin is predominantly renal, underlying kidney disease may be associated with higher and more toxic blood levels.

Kanamycin has been associated with proteinuria and microscopic hematuria in 10 and 20 per cent of the patients, respectively, at dosage levels of 25 to 50 mg per kilogram per day. Oliguria may develop, and tubular necrosis seems to be aggravated by prior therapy with streptomycin or viomycin.

Bacitracin produces renal tubular necrosis.

Polymyxins A, B, C, D, and E have nephrotic properties of varying severity. Only polymyxin B has received extensive clinical use. It may produce albuminuria, casts, epithelial cells in the urine, decrease in concentrating ability, and tubular degeneration. Polymyxin B accumulates if renal function is impaired or if the dose exceeds 3 mg per kilogram per day. Nephrotoxicity is dose related.

Colymycin (colistin) is chemically similar to polymyxin and has a similar nephrotoxicity.

Neomycin is not normally well absorbed from the gastrointestinal tract. It produces foamy vacuolization of the epithelial lining of the proximal convoluted tubules, and progressive renal failure has been reported after intraperitoneal administration.

Tetracycline accentuates azotemia by its catabolic effect in increasing nitrogen turnover. Deteriorated tetracycline, used after its expiration date, has produced a largely reversible Fanconi type of syndrome consisting of reduced renal function, polyuria, polydypsia, glycosuria, aminoaciduria, hyperphosphaturia, hypercalciuria, hypophosphatemia, hypokalemia, hyperuricemia, and severe metabolic acidosis with debilitating lethargy. Instances have also been demonstrated of heavy Bence Jones proteinuria, transient hyperglycemia, and a macular papular rash. The characteristic lesion is tubular degeneration with desquamation of epithelial cells, granular cytoplasm, vacuolization, hemosiderosis, evidence of reparative epithelial cell regeneration, and pale staining nuclei. Among the degradation products believed to account for the syndrome, two have been biochemically identified as epianhydrotetracycline and anhydrotetracycline. Clinical manifestations may appear in three or four days after ingestion of as little as 10 to 12 capsules.

Amphotericin B is dangerous chiefly because of renal damage. Cylindruria is the first manifestation, and may be accompanied by hematuria, pyuria, and proteinuria. The glomerular filtration rate and renal blood flow may decline by half or more. Maximal concentrating capacity decreases; serum urea and creatinine increase. Therapy may have to be terminated. Examination of kidney tissue shows necrosis and degeneration of proximal and distal tubules with flattened epithelium, regenerative foci, and calcification prominent in casts and interstitial tissue. Thickening of the glomerular basement has been noted in some patients.

Analgesic Abuse
(Phenacetin Nephropathy)

Mixed analgesic preparations are among the most frequently used drugs in medical therapy and self-medication. In 1953 Spuhler and Zollinger noted an increase in interstitial nephritis and a high incidence of medullary necrosis in patients who had abused analgesic therapy. Many such patients have now been reported from Switzerland, the Scandinavian countries, Australia, New Zealand, South Africa, Canada, and the United States. At Georgetown Hospital, nine patients with this

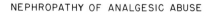

NEPHROPATHY OF ANALGESIC ABUSE

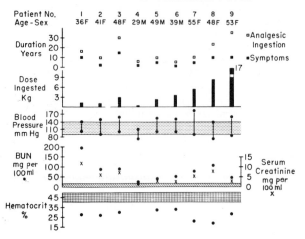

entity have been studied, and some of the findings are summarized in the accompanying figure.

Satisfactory understanding of the pathogenesis of analgesic nephropathy is lacking. Anti-inflammatory effects, salicylates as uncoupling agents, hypokalemia, manufacturing contaminants (acetic-4-chloranilid), methemoglobinemia and sulfhemoglobinemia, sensitivity reactions, and predisposition have all been suggested as playing a role in the disease. Direct toxicity has not been demonstrated in animals except when excessive amounts of phenacetin have been used; similar levels of aspirin ingestion are fatal. In general, clinical cases have occurred in which the cumulative ingestion calculated as phenacetin is in excess of 1 kg. Continuing investigation may add more epidemiologic and circumstantial evidence for an association between chronic interstitial nephritis, renal papillary necrosis, and/or a unique susceptibility to pyelonephritis of patients who chronically ingest analgesic mixtures.

Insecticides

Biphenyl is a citrus fungicide that produces polyuria and focal tubular dilatation resembling small cysts. Chronic exposure to *DDT* may produce fatty degeneration of the tubular epithelium, and anuria has been reported following exposure to *chlordane.*

Aye, R. C.: Renal papillary necrosis. Diabetes, 3:124, 1954.

Becker, C. G., Becker, E. L., Maher, J. F., and Schreiner, G. E.: Nephrotic syndrome after contact with mercury. A report of five cases, three after the use of ammoniated mercury ointment. Arch. Intern. Med., 110:178, 1962.

Brun, C., Olsen, S., Raaschou, F., and Sorensen, A. W. S.: The localization of gold in the human kidney following chrysotherapy. A biopsy study. Nephron, 1:265, 1964.

Crawford, E. S., Beall, A. C., Moyer, J. H., and De Bakey, M. E.: Complications of aortography. Surg. Gynec. Obstet., 104:129, 1957.

Doolan, P. D., Walsh, W. P., Kyle, L. H., and Wishinsky, H.: Acetylsalicylic acid intoxication. Proposed method of treatment. J.A.M.A., 146:105, 1951.

Freeman, R. B., Maher, J. F., Schreiner, G. E., and Mostofi, F. K.: Renal tubular necrosis due to nephrotoxicity of organic mercurial diuretics. Ann. Intern. Med., 57:34, 1962.

Frimpter, G. W., Timpanelli, A. E., Eisenmenger, W. J., Stein, H. S., and Ehrlich, L. I.: Reversible "Fanconi syndrome" caused by degraded tetracycline J.A.M.A., 184:111, 1963.

Goodman, L. S., and Gilman, A.: The Pharmacological Basis of Therapeutics. 3rd ed. New York, The Macmillan Company, 1965.

Lauler, D. P., Schreiner, G. E., and David, A.: Renal medullary necrosis. Am. J. Med., 29:132, 1960.

Longcope, W. T., and Leutscher, J. A.: The treatment of acute mercury bichloride poisoning with BAL (2,3-dimercaptopropanol). Med. Clin. North Am., 34:469, 1950.

Luessenhop, A. J., Gallimore, J. C., Sweet, W. H., Struxness, E. G., and Robinson, J.: The toxicity in man of hexavalent uranium following intravenous administration. Am. J. Roentgenol., 79:83, 1958.

Maher, J. F., and Schreiner, G. E.: Cause of death in acute renal failure. Arch. Intern. Med., 110:493, 1962.

Maher, J. F., and Schreiner, G. E.: The clinical dialysis of poisons. Trans. Amer. Soc. Artif. Intern. Organs, 9:390, 1963.

McAfee, J. G.: A survey of complications of abdominal aortography. Radiology, 68:825, 1957.

Pendergrass, E. P., Hodes, P. J., Tondreau, R. L., Powell, C. C., and Burdick, E. D.: Further consideration of deaths and unfavorable sequelae following the administration of contrast media in urography in the United States. Am. J. Roentgenol., 74:262, 1955.

Rich, A. R.: The role of hypersensitivity in periarteritis nodosa as indicated by 7 cases developing during serum sickness and sulfonamide therapy. Bull. Hopkins Hosp., 71:123, 1942.

Schreiner, G. E.: Dialysis of poisons and drugs: Annual review. Trans. Amer. Soc. Artif. Intern. Organs, 16:544, 1970.

Schreiner, G. E.: The nephrotoxicity of analgesic abuse. Ann. Intern. Med., 57:1047, 1962.

Schreiner, G. E., and Maher, J. F.: Toxic nephropathy. Am. J. Med., 38:409, 1965.

Schreiner, G. E., Maher, J. F., Marc-Aurele, J., Knowlan, D., and Alvo, M.: Ethylene glycol—two indications for hemodialysis. Trans. Amer. Soc. Artif. Intern. Organs, 5:81, 1959.

Schwartz, W. B., Hurwit, A., and Ettinger, A.: Intravenous urography in the patient with renal insufficiency. N. Engl. J. Med., 269:277, 1963.

Setter, J. G., Maher, J. F., and Schreiner, G. E.: Acute renal failure following cholecystography. J.A.M.A., 184:102, 1963.

Spuhler, O., and Zollinger, H. U.: Die chronischinterstitielle Nephritis. Z. Klin. Med., 151:1, 1953.

Strauss, M. B., and Welt, L. G.: Diseases of the Kidney. 2nd ed. Boston, Little, Brown & Company, 1971.

Wennberg, J. E., Okun, R., Hinman, E. J., Northcutt, R. C., Greip, R. J., and Walker, W. G.: Renal toxicity of oral cholecystographic media. J.A.M.A., 186:461, 1963.

Yow, E. M., Moyer, J. H., and Smith, C. P.: Toxicity of polymyxin B. II. Human studies with particular reference to evaluation of renal function. Arch. Intern. Med., 92:248, 1953.

627.   RENAL CALCULI

William C. Thomas, Jr.

Renal calculi are concretions consisting of crystals and a matrix of organic matter. Crystals usually constitute the predominant portion (> 90 per cent) of the mass of most calculi, but those occurring as a consequence of urinary tract infections have a higher proportion of matrix material. Occasionally this latter type of calculus may be almost devoid of crystals. Renal calculi are to be distinguished from calcific deposits within the renal parenchyma. Such deposits occurring at sites of previous inflammation or degenerative change are designated by the term "nephrocalcinosis." Elsewhere in the text are specific presentations of a number of disorders often complicated by nephrolithiasis; this chapter is largely limited to a discussion of broadly applicable principles in the cause and management of renal calculi.

Etiology. *General Factors.* Our knowledge of the cause of various types of calculi is incomplete, but from available evidence it appears that a combination of factors rather than any single event is most often responsible for calculus formation. The likelihood and type of calculous disease is modified by geographic factors, sex, race, and probably diet. In the United States the incidence is greatest in the Southeast, but there are other areas of the country where the incidence is also high. South Africa, portions of India, and Southeast Asia are regions where calculous disease occurs with unusual frequency. In the Southeastern United States "hard water" has been thought by some to be the important factor favoring calculus formation, but such a correlation fails to explain why calculi are infrequent in other "hard water" regions of the world. In India and Southeast Asia protein-poor, predominantly cereal diets have been considered to be of importance in the development of bladder calculi in children. Although these and other suggested explanations to account for the regional incidence of calculi have some attractiveness, none has sufficient investigative support to warrant complete acceptance.

Recurrent calculi composed of calcium oxalate and phosphate are relatively uncommon in women and rare in blacks of either sex. The disproportionate occurrence of such calculi in white males is unexplained, but holds true even in the high incidence areas of the Southeastern United States and South Africa. Women, however, are more susceptible than men to urinary tract infections. Thus women with magnesium-ammonium-phosphate or calcium-phosphate stones that develop as a complication of infection with urea-splitting organisms outnumber similarly affected men. Certain disorders predisposing to calculus formation, especially hyperparathyroidism, overcome the protective influence of sex or race, and this provides a diagnostic lead when searching for the cause of calculi in white women or blacks.

There is an increased incidence of calcareous renal calculi in patients with small bowel disease or in those subjected to ileal resection. Patients who have undergone jejunoileal anastomosis in an effort to control morbid obesity are especially prone to develop calculi. It is now known that such patients usually have a significant hyperoxaluria as probably the most important factor favoring stone formation. Frequently these patients also have some degree of acidosis, presumably from loss of intestinal bicarbonate, and a consequent decrease in urinary citrate.

Although there is disagreement as to the complete explanation of the hyperoxaluria in patients with small bowel disease, there is good evidence that such patients absorb a larger than usual proportion of dietary oxalate. Also, it has been suggested that malabsorption of bile salts may contribute to the hyperoxaluria in this syndrome through the action of colonic bacteria on glycocholic acid to provide absorbable precursors of oxalate.

Structure and Composition of Calculi. Although all calculi must initially be small, it is the aggregation of crystals and matrix into a dense mass with subsequent growth to macroscopic size that accounts for their medical significance. The crystalline components of calculi are formed from the less soluble crystalloids predominant in the urine. It has not been determined whether the matrix component of all calculi can be formed entirely from nonspecific proteinaceous material and cellular debris present in urine, or is dependent on the presence of specific compounds secreted by cells lining the urinary tract.

Examination of sectioned calculi usually reveals a distinct lamellar and sometimes radially striated organization. In most stones there is a small identifiable nidus around which the bulk of the calculus appears to have formed. In calcium oxalate renal stones, the most common variety, this nidus often consists of calcium phosphate, frequently in hydroxyapatite form. There is evidence that such a nidus may originate within the cells of the renal tubules or collecting ducts or beneath the papillary epithelium. As one means of stone formation, it has been suggested that extrusion of this type of nidus into the renal pelvis may promote apposition of crystals and matrix material from an appropriately constituted urine. There are other data, however, to indicate that the nidus of a stone need not be of specific composition. For example, calcium oxalate bladder stones of children in Southeast Asia regularly contain a core of uric acid crystals.

Crystalloids in Urine. Normal urine contains in solution a number of crystalloids, e.g., calcium, magnesium, phosphate, oxalate, and urate, at concentrations exceeding those achievable in water. The maintenance of this supersaturated state may be attributed to a number of factors. Urea, apparently by its interaction with water, increases the solubility of crystalloids, and the concentrations of sodium, potassium, chloride, and other soluble ions in urine also enhance the solution stability of the less soluble components. Organic acids, especially citrate, that form soluble chelates with calcium and magnesium are additional urinary constituents that promote the solubility of calcium or magnesium salts. One should be aware, however, that the potential of urinary organic acids to chelate metal ions is markedly decreased when urinary pH is low (< 5.0).

In addition to the aforementioned factors that may account in part for the supersaturation of urine, specific inhibitors to the crystallization of calcium salts have been detected in urine and also in serum. A deficiency of these biologic "water conditioners" may be important in determining susceptibility to calculus formation. One of these constituents, inorganic pyrophosphate, has been studied in considerable detail. It is a product of intermediary metabolism and is present in serum at concentrations of 75 to 160 μg per 100 ml. Urinary excretion of pyrophosphate by subjects receiving diets free of dairy products ranges from 4 to 10 mg per day, and, within limits, the amount in urine varies directly with orthophosphate excretion. Although urinary pyrophosphate may be a protective constituent, the amount excreted is the same in calculous and normal subjects and is insufficient to account for the solution stability of calcium salts.

A more potent inhibitor of crystal formation than inorganic pyrophosphate has now been identified in urine. This is a water-soluble, acidic compound of low molecular weight, but of undefined composition. Very small amounts of this compound, especially when acting in concert with citrate, prevent crystallization of calcium salts from highly supersaturated solutions. Observations to date indicate that there is a decreased excretion of this biologic "water conditioner" by patients with idiopathic calcareous calculi, but the data are too limited to assess the importance of this deficiency to the genesis of renal calculi. A number of investigators have observed that calcium-containing crystals form more readily in urine from patients with calcareous calculi than in that from normal subjects. This difference is consistent with a deficiency of inhibitors of crystal formation in the urine of stone formers.

The formation of renal calculi is thought to be dependent on the presence of metastable concentrations of crystalloids, but there must also be a component or nidus promoting the formation and aggregation of crystals. Whatever the initiating event, the growth of most calculi is dependent on the presence in urine of metastable concentrations of crystalloids. Such states of supersaturation may be achieved by various means: by increased excretion of specific crystalloids of limited solubility; decrease in urinary pH which converts urates to less soluble uric acid; or infection with urea-splitting bacteria to release ammonia, which causes an increase in urinary pH and provides a setting for crystallization of magnesium-ammonium-phosphate or calcium phosphate complexes. In addition to increased concentrations of crystalloids or alteration of urinary pH, reduced excretion of those urinary constituents that normally inhibit crystal formation would also induce a metastable state of crystalloids. This latter type of change is possibly of more importance to the development of idiopathic calcareous calculi than is increased excretion of calcium or oxalate.

Diagnosis. The medical history often provides important information. Infection as an etiologic or complicating factor is suggested by a history of fever preceding the initial episode of renal colic. Also, in postpartum women with calculi it is important to ascertain whether urinary tract infection occurred during pregnancy. Is there a family history of calculi? Genetic disorders such as renal tubular acidosis and cystinuria are expected in kindred, but idiopathic calcareous calculi may also occur in families. The occurrence of renal calculi in childhood may indicate the presence of a familial disorder, but infection or anatomic defects are more common causes in this age group. The contributory effect of intestinal disease to calculus formation was mentioned previously. A number of medications have been causally related to renal stone formation, and patients should be questioned about chronic use of medicines, particularly acetazolamide, absorbable alkali, silicates, allopurinol, or large amounts of ascorbic acid. The type of water used and unusual dietary habits are additional items of relevant information.

Clinical Manifestations. Many patients with renal calculi are asymptomatic. Inflammation or infection resulting from calculi may lead to symptoms, but passage of a calculus into the ureter with resulting renal colic is the classic manifestation of calculous disease. Passage of small, sandlike concretions with relatively little pain is not uncommon, particularly with uric acid lithiasis and sometimes in patients with calcium oxalate stones. Gross hematuria, especially in the absence of accompanying renal colic and a demonstrable ureteral calculus, should be regarded with suspicion as possibly indicative of infection or a coexistent neoplasm. Microscopic hematuria, however, is quite regularly present in patients with calculi. The malingerer, feigning renal colic in order to obtain narcotics, may demonstrate considerable ingenuity in developing a symptom complex.

Laboratory Findings. Careful examination of fresh urine provides immediate, valuable information. For example, an acid urine and urate crystals may be present in those with uric acid calculi, and octahedral crystals of calcium oxalate are frequent in patients with oxalate stones. A high urine pH (7.0 or higher) may signify infection or a renal tubular disorder. The presence of bacteria in fresh uncentrifuged urine usually indicates significant infection. As mentioned, microscopic hematuria is usual, and there may be few to many white blood cells. The pH of each freshly voided specimen of the patient's urine should be determined for 24 hours. Appropriately selected pH paper (pH range 4 to 9) is adequate for clinical purposes. If the pH is consistently high and infection is present (values between 8.5 and 9.0 always indicate infection), the pH determinations should be re-

peated after eradication of the infection. In normal persons receiving a regular diet, urine pH will be less than 6.0 at some time during the 24 hours. If this degree of acidity is not achieved, the presence of renal tubular acidosis is likely, and should be confirmed by definitive tests. The occasional patient with uric acid stones may excrete unusually acid urine (pH 4.5 to 5.5), but most uric acid stone-formers do not excrete urine of such acidity.

A qualitative test for cystine should be performed in every patient with radiopaque calculi, and freshly voided, concentrated urine is desired for this analysis. If positive, a quantitative analysis of the 24-hour excretion should be obtained. Although cystinuria is not a rare disorder, only a small proportion of cystinurics develop calculi.

A urine culture is indicated in the evaluation of patients with calculi. Of particular relevance to the problem of stone formation are infections with urea-splitting bacteria. It is pertinent to note that some strains of *E. coli* and staphylococci are capable of splitting urea.

Although of limited clinical value, it is sometimes desirable to know the amount of calcium excreted per 24 hours by patients with radiopaque stones. This is conveniently done by having the patient abstain from dairy products (milk, cheese, and ice cream) for one or two days and then, while continuing the diet restriction, collect urine for one or two 24-hour periods. The calcium ingested with this regimen will usually be less than 300 mg per day, and the amount excreted by normal subjects will be less than 175 mg per 24 hours. With unrestricted diets urinary calcium values may be as much as 300 mg per 24 hours in normal subjects. Urinary calcium is increased in the majority of patients with calcareous calculi, but will be normal in patients whose primary problem is infection. Reliable oxalate analyses are not generally available, but, when possible, urinary oxalate should be measured in patients with calcium oxalate stones. The amount of phosphorus in urine reflects dietary phosphorus, and is a useless measurement unless the amount ingested is accurately known.

In patients with calcareous calculi, serum analyses are required chiefly to establish the presence or absence of hypercalcemic states, particularly hyperparathyroidism or renal tubular acidosis. With the patient in a postabsorptive state, determinations of creatinine, carbon dioxide, chloride, uric acid, phosphorus, and calcium are sufficient. Abnormal values should be confirmed by repetition of the tests. The serum concentrations of bicarbonate and chloride may be normal in patients with mild renal tubular acidosis. Phosphorus concentrations in the sera of patients with idiopathic calcareous calculi are often slightly less than those of normal subjects, and uric acid values are frequently increased.

When the calculus is available, both its central and peripheral portions should be subjected to chemical or crystallographic (by x-ray diffraction) analysis. Much information as to cause and treatment may be gained from this.

Radiologic Findings. A plain film of the abdomen or renal tomography in a patient properly prepared with laxatives is often informative, but contrast urography can also be helpful. Roentgenographic visualization of the urinary tract should not be delayed if an infected patient is suspected of having ureteral obstruction. Uric acid and the rare xanthine calculi are radiolucent and may be large or small. It is not uncommon for a patient with idiopathic calcareous calculi to have stones of mixed composition—uric acid and oxalate, and a relatively small proportion as oxalate will induce radiopaqueness of a predominantly uric acid calculus. Also, it should be realized that patients with gout have an increased incidence of the radiopaque oxalate stones.

Large or staghorn-shaped radiopaque calculi are usually the result of infection and are composed of magnesium-ammonium-phosphate or calcium phosphate, but cystine stones may achieve a similar size and configuration. Detectable laminations are not uncommon in large calculi resulting from infection. Calcium oxalate calculi are usually small (2 to 5 mm in diameter), dense, and frequently multiple. Such calculi in children may indicate the presence of oxalosis. When large (diameter greater than 10 mm), extremely dense (more dense than adjacent bone) stones are present in children or adults, hyperoxaluria should be suspected. The coexistence of nephrocalcinosis and renal calculi is not uncommon as a sequel of infection, but may also indicate the presence of medullary sponge kidneys, renal tubular acidosis, hyperparathyroidism, sarcoidosis, and rarely oxalosis.

Stones are often of mixed composition, particularly when infection has supervened; for example, at the center of a large calculus there may be either a radiolucent area composed of urates or a radiologically dense oxalate stone. The rare calculus consisting largely of matrix material may be barely visible radiologically.

Finally, roentgenographic visualization of the urinary tract may reveal anatomic abnormalities conducive to calculus formation. Obstruction, localized deformity, or medullary sponge kidneys are probably the most common such abnormalities.

Treatment. *General.* Avoidance of dehydration is important in calculous disease of all types, but especially in patients with cystinuria, those with a susceptibility to uric acid concretions, and those with urinary tract infections. To maintain continuously dilute urine usually requires a daily intake of approximately 4 quarts of liquids, which should be distributed throughout the 24 hours. Although dairy products are frequently omitted during test procedures, there are no data to suggest that continued avoidance is beneficial in reducing the incidence or growth of calcareous calculi in man. In contrast to the poor absorption of oxalate from vegetables, many beverages (e.g., tea, beer, fruit juices, cola drinks) contain significant amounts of oxalate in absorbable form. In patients with oxalate stones it is probably wise to limit the intake of these particular liquids to no more than 1 pint daily until the specific role of diet in the pathogenesis of calculi is more fully delineated. In patients with small bowel disease and hyperoxaluria, more stringent reductions in dietary oxalate and correction of any existing acidosis are indicated. The possible usefulness of taurine and cholestyramine in reducing the hyperoxaluria of patients with intestinal disease has not been adequately defined.

Every effort should be made to eradicate infection promptly. In paraplegic patients in whom high incidence of calculi correlates with urinary tract infections, dramatic reduction in stone development has been achieved by prompt and effective treatment of incipient infections. The size of ureteral calculi that can be passed spontaneously is surprising. Therefore it is often wise to delay instrumental intervention until it is certain that the calculus will not be extruded.

Specific. Details regarding the rationale for treatment of patients with cystinuria, renal tubular acidosis, and uric acid calculi are recorded in other parts of the text. Suffice it to say here that if treatment with absorbable alkali is to be instituted, the amount required varies, depending on renal function, but for adults with normal glomerular filtration rates it is usually from 100 to 250 mEq of cation per day regardless of the salt used. For example, with sodium bicarbonate these amounts of cation are provided by 8.4 to 21.0 grams, respectively. Cystinurics to be treated in this manner require the larger amounts because of the need to maintain urinary pH in the range of 8.0. Dosage with alkali should be spaced equally throughout the 24 hours to ensure continuous control of urinary pH.

Patients with single or very infrequent calcareous calculi that are passed without undue difficulty should be advised to drink copious amounts of liquid, but usually need not be considered candidates for continuous medicinal treatment.

Several largely empiric modes of therapy are currently in widespread use for patients with recurrent calcareous calculi. Each of these programs was devised in an effort to modify urine in a way that enhanced the solubility of the least soluble salts. Administration of divided doses of orthophosphates, usually as a neutral mixture of monobasic and dibasic salts, in amounts sufficient to provide 1500 to 2100 mg of phosphorus per 24 hours has been remarkably effective in preventing stone formation in uninfected patients with calcareous calculi of various causes. Diarrhea is the major adverse symptom, but most males can tolerate the aforementioned doses. Amounts of phosphates providing less than 1500 mg of phosphorus are usually ineffective in preventing stone formation in males, but many females are adequately treated with 1200 mg of phosphorus per day. Potassium phosphates may be substituted for sodium salts in patients with hypertension. This form of therapy is contraindicated in patients whose renal function is impaired to the degree that there is inadequate excretion of a phosphate load. Phosphate administration induces an increased excretion of inorganic pyrophosphate, and possibly other phosphorylated inhibitors of crystal formation, and usually causes a modest reduction in urinary calcium. There is uncertainty, however, that these are the changes that account for the prevention of calculus formation by phosphates.

Hydrochlorothiazide administration, 50 mg twice daily, has proved effective in preventing stone formation in a large majority of patients so treated. Thiazides reduce urinary calcium and augment magnesium excretion, but frequently cause symptomatic hypokalemia. Complete replacement of the potassium deficiency may lessen the effectiveness of this form of therapy. In calculous patients with hypertension or in those with a hyperactive intestinal tract, hydrochlorothiazide is probably the therapy of choice. Magnesium oxide has been advocated for patients with oxalate stones on the basis that increased urinary magnesium promotes oxalate solubility, but published experiences with this form of therapy indicate it to be of limited effectiveness. In patients who form two types of stones, e.g., uric acid and calcium oxalate, it is often useful to use both allopurinol and phosphates or hydrochlorothiazide.

Patients with calculi caused by infection are the most difficult to manage. None of the regimens mentioned are effective in such patients. The infection should be treated, but it is difficult to prevent recurrence. In addition to control of infection, treatment directed to reducing the urinary phosphorus to several hundred milligrams per day has been used by a number of investigators. This program requires that the patient avoid dairy products and, to further decrease phosphate absorption, ingest 30 ml of aluminum carbonate gel after each meal and at bedtime. Caution must be exercised to guard against phosphate depletion with this regimen. When infection cannot be eradicated by antimicrobial drugs, surgical removal of calculi, especially if they are large, is advisable.

Boyce, W. H. (ed.): Symposium on renal lithiasis. Urol. Clin. North Am., 1:179, 1974.

Dent, C. E., and Sutor, D. J.: Presence or absence of inhibitor of calcium-oxalate crystal growth in urine of normals and stone-formers. Lancet, 2:775, 1971.

Smith, L. H., Jr. (ed.): Symposium on stones. Am. J. Med., 45:649, 1968.

Stauffer, J. Q., Humphreys, M. H. and Weir, G. J.: Acquired hyperoxaluria with regional enteritis after ileal resection. Ann. Intern. Med., 79:383, 1973.

628. CYSTS OF THE KIDNEY

George E. Schreiner

POLYCYSTIC DISEASE

Polycystic disease is the most prevalent renal cystic disease (Table 1). It is inherited as a dominant, non-sex-linked disease emerging at two prominent age peaks, in infancy and in adult life. Progressive dilatation of renal tubules leads to obstruction, infection, rupture of cysts, bleeding, hypertension, and progressive renal failure. There may be associated anomalies, such as cysts in the liver, pancreas, spleen, or lung, or berry aneurysm of the cerebral vessels. Sporadic cases are found without familial history and scattered through childhood. More often the adult disease emerges after the next generation has already been "planted." The infantile type may be autosomal recessive, but the adult disease is a hereditary dominant. Penetrance is high and rises with increasing age. Clinical surveys in large families usually reveal that half or more of the members are afflicted. In advanced age penetrance for cysts is almost total. However, once present, cysts may vary in signficance to mortality or health.

Embryology.   Nephrogenesis is usually complete by 35 weeks. Theories no longer accepted for the pathogenesis of polycystic disease include fetal papillitis with secondary fibrosis and obstruction, cyst formation as a neoplas-

TABLE 1.   Simple Classification of Cystic Disease

1. Polycystic disease
    Infantile (Potter, Type 1)
    Adult (Potter, Type 3)
2. Multicystic disease
3. Multilocular cysts   } (?Potter, Type 2)
4. Simple cysts
5. Medullary cystic disease
6. Medullary sponge kidney
7. Dysplasia
8. Miscellaneous cysts of renal origin
9. Miscellaneous cysts of nonrenal origin

TABLE 2.   Some Representative Incidence Figures

Year	Place	No. Polycystic Cases	Ratio to Autopsies
1897	Kiel	16	1:636
1928	Leningrad	192	1:261
1933	Mayo	9	1:1019
1934	New York	14	1:428
1935	Göttingen	38	1:222
1949	Great Britain	16	1:375
1950	Minnesota	70	1:779
1954	Copenhagen	143	1:773
1955	Mayo	35	1:323
1965	Georgetown	——	1:165

Total = 533 +   Avg. = 1:498

tic process, congenital syphilis, and fetal interstitial nephritis. Popular theories include (1) "nonunion" of ureteric bud and tubules, (2) noncanalization owing to lack of "organizer," and (3) persistence of primitive nephrons that fail to atrophy. A microdissection study subclassified four types: (1) hyperplasia of interstitial portion of collecting tubules, (2 inhibition of ampullary activity, (3) multiple developmental anomalies, and (4) urethral obstruction. Infantile cysts may be totally isolated; adult cortical cysts are younger, larger, and glomerular and do not connect. Juxtamedullary cysts are older and have entering and exiting tubules. In the medulla the cysts involve collecting ducts and may open to a calyx.

Physiology.   In studying polycystic patients with normal, medium, and low filtration rates, we have found progressive loss of concentrating ability and a salt-losing tendency. Bicarbonate wasting may contribute to systemic acidosis. In an excellent family study (M-M), 10 of 12 noncystic family members had U_{max} greater than 900 mOsm per kilogram (1060 ± 134). In 11 of 13 family members with cysts but without azotemia, U_{max} was less than 700 mOsm per kilogram (657 ± 169). Patients with renal failure have osmotic U/P ratios near unity. This is a pitressin-resistant concentrating defect. Dilution capability is preserved. Cyst fluid has variable concentrations of Na, K, H, Cr, PAH, and inulin, indicating entry of solutes into cysts and selective transport of water and solutes out of cysts. Cyst/plasma ratios of Cr are above 1.0 in deep cysts. Concentration of amino acids in cysts may add 50 to 100 mOsm per kilogram. Such osmols have the potential of drawing in water for expansion of cysts. Protein, red cells, bacteria, and cellular debris may be found. Enzymatic breakdown of protein could yield amino acid mOsm.

Incidence (Table 2).   Since early diagnosis is difficult, the clinical incidence varies with the vigor of the diagnostic pursuit. Isotopic scans, ultrasound studies, infusion nephrotomography, and other diagnostic techniques enhance the yield. Measurement of concentrating ability in absence of other causes may be the most sensitive screening test. Yet polycystic disease is still often a surprise diagnosis at autopsy.

Pathology.   The kidneys are enlarged and often asymmetrical. They have a nodular surface produced by projecting cysts that may be filled with watery, serous, hemorrhagic, pustular, or viscid fluid or clear urine. Cut surface reveals the entire parenchyma honeycombed by cysts protruding from various levels. About one fifth of polycystic patients have intracranial aneurysm, and 4 per cent of patients with clinical aneurysms have polycystic disease. Cysts may coexist in liver, spleen, lungs, and pancreas, but are rarely clinically significant. Mild renal cysts may occur in hepatic cystic disease and may be clinically subordinate. Histologically, cysts of various caliber, location, and content may be demonstrated. The internal lining may be flattened or cuboidal and rarely may have papillary projections or glomerular tufts. Recently, it has been shown that interruptions of the elastic laminae of small renal arteries, ruptured arteries, and microaneurysms can be demonstrated in the renal parenchyma. It is not clear whether vessel rupture is cause or effect. Degenerative changes from pressure, calculi and secondary infection may be seen. Many cases of renal carcinoma have been reported in polycystic kidneys. Earlier functional evaluation and renal biopsy studies are needed in polycystic families, because little is known of the natural history of cysts in the presymptomatic decades.

Diagnosis. The *infantile type* is usually diagnosed by palpation of bilateral renal masses, roentgenographic findings, or presentation with uremia. Nausea, vomiting, dehydration, and abdominal distention are the most prevalent. We have one such patient six years old. The small cyst variety is the most difficult to diagnose. The *adult type* may be totally asymptomatic for several decades, with a chance finding on roentgenographic examination or even at autopsy. Segmental disease has been described. Patients with large cysts (greater than 3 cm) have more severe disease, are more symptomatic, and die younger. With progressive enlargement, presenting symptoms include lumbar or abdominal pain (28 per cent), palpable mass (20 per cent), hypertension (17 per cent), bladder symptoms of frequency, urgency, and dysuria (17 per cent), painless hematuria (17 per cent), and painful hematuria (10 per cent). Other patients may present with any of the protean manifestations of uremia. Renal osteodystrophy and hyperparathyroidism are especially prevalent in younger patients. Hypertension and palpable kidneys are present in about three quarters of the patients at the time of diagnosis. Kidneys may grow to a size of 6 kg or more and produce weakness, a dragging sensation, increasing abdominal girth, and the displacement of other organs.

Complications. Many patients with polycystic disease present or die with complications such as vascular accidents from ruptured aneurysms or hypertensive disease, secondary pyelonephritis, infected cysts, perinephric abscess, obstruction, gross hematuria, calcification of cyst wall and formation of urinary calculi, and associated renal carcinoma. Both erythrocytosis and polycythemia have been noted. Dalgaard found calculus and/or colic in 18 per cent of 350 patients. Rarely dystocia has been reported owing to distended abdomen of the fetus from infantile cystic disease. We have seen subdiaphragmatic abscess from ruptured infected cysts and obstructive uropathy reversible by surgical decompression. A family history of polycystic kidneys can readily be obtained in the majority of cases by taking a detailed history and surveying causes of death in siblings with emphasis on cerebral aneurysm and kidney disease. Spurious histories are encountered in families with a pathetic desire to hide the trait. General problems we have encountered include psychologic "block" to family surveys; the problems of marriage, pregnancy, and contact sports; questions of elective surgery and medical procedures; economic problems generating from inability to get life, health, hospital, or disability insurance or to meet medical requirements of a job; and the emotional impact of watching other members of the family die from a known affliction of the observer.

Laboratory Findings. These include albuminuria, hematuria, pyuria, passage of epithelial cells, and all the progressive laboratory findings associated with renal failure. Hyperchloremic acidosis, bicarbonate wasting, and defect in excretion of an acid load may be seen. A salt-losing tendency with dehydration, increasing azotemia, and hyponatremia is much more frequent than in other renal diseases.

Roentgenography. Important roentgenographic findings include enlarged or displaced kidneys with varying densities, loculation, or calcification, elongated pelves, crescentic deformities of calyces (wine-glass sign), hydronephrosis and other obstructive phenomena, and "unfolding" of the calyceal system. The small cyst, infantile type, is best diagnosed by observation of nephrographic phenomena persisting up to 72 hours. This parenchymal opacification results from concentration of iodine in tubular cells and excretion into the lumina of dilated tubules. Less than 10 per cent of polycystic disease is unilateral. Most "unilateral" disease on x-ray is bilateral at autopsy or surgery. Recently infusion nephrotomography and renal angiography have been found useful in differentiating neoplasm from cyst. The renal scan may

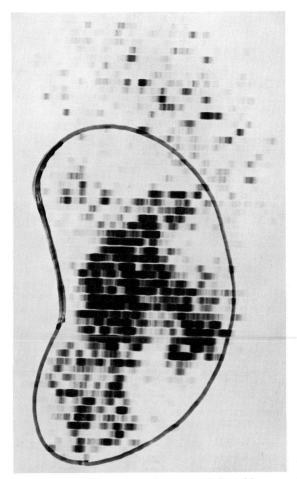

Isotope scan of a kidney; the cystic areas are indicated by areas of diminished or absent radioactivity.

give a characteristic appearance of "holes," as seen in the accompanying figure.

Prognosis. The infantile type is rapidly fatal from uremia or complications. The adult type may be latent and rarely may not interfere with longevity. Progressive cystic disease proceeds to hypertension, uremia, vascular accidents, infections, and death, with the peak mortality in the latter half of the fifth decade. Patients with small cysts (less than 3 cm), without cysts in other organs, or without hypertension tend to live longer. Prognosis can be improved by continuous medical care and treatment of infection and acute obstruction, management of chronic uremia, and avoidance of—or special care during—pregnancy. Polycystic patients often do not tolerate strict salt restriction. The age of diagnosis and the subsequent life expectancy are related. Under 50, one third of males are alive 12½ years later. Over 50, only 14 per cent are alive 2½ years later.

Treatment. The treatment is medical. Marsupialization, bivalving with unroofing, puncture and aspiration, and unilateral nephrectomy have all been tried and have failed. Decompression or heminephrectomy is justified only when extrarenal obstruction is demonstrated. Treatment for infection is as outlined in Ch. 617. Treatment of chronic renal failure and acute renal failure is detailed in Ch. 603 and 604. Bed rest is indicated for hematuria and transfusions for symptomatic anemia of blood loss. In patients suffering recurrent pain from enlarging cysts, we have had some success with the use of acetazolamide, 500 mg daily, as a single dose, or with combinations of acetazolamide and a thiazide diuretic. Strict control of hypertension is essential to halt progression.

Sympathetic understanding of the psychologic problem is important. The diagnosis of polycystic kidneys carries with it the responsibility to conduct a family survey and advise the patient and family members concerning the basic diagnosis, the management of possible complications, and the social concerns of marriage, pregnancy, and choice of occupation.

Hemodialysis has been successfully used for transient exacerbations of renal failure caused by infection, obstruction, dehydration, hyponatremia or hypotension. It may occasionally result in prolonged improvement even in apparently moribund patients. Recent history of a good urinary volume forms a reasonable guide in selection of patients for dialysis. Polycystic patients make good transplant candidates, because the graft does not acquire the disease of the recipient and because immunologic problems are absent. Bilateral nephrectomy is usually indicated before transplantation. Erythrocytosis may follow the relief of azotemia and may be reversed by removal of a cystic kidney, presumably indicating erythropoietin production.

Bialestock, D.: The morphogenesis of renal cysts in the stillborn: A study of microdissection technique. J. Pathol., 71:51, 1956.

Bricker, N. S., and Patton, J. F.: Cystic disease of the kidneys: A study of dynamics and chemical composition of cyst fluid. Am. J. Med., 18:207, 1955.

Dalgaard, O. Z.: Polycystic disease of the kidneys. In Strauss, M. B., and Welt, L. G. (eds.): Diseases of the Kidney. Boston, Little, Brown & Company, 1971, p. 1223.

Gardner, K. D., Jr.: Composition of fluid in twelve cysts of a polycystic kidney. N. Engl. J. Med., 281:985, 1969.

Hatfield, P. M., and Pfister, R. C.: Adult polycystic disease of the kidneys (Potter, type 3): J.A.M.A., 222:1527, 1972.

Martinez-Maldonado, M., Yium, J. J., Eknoyan, G., and Suki, W. N.: Adult polycystic disease: Studies of the defect in urine concentration. Kidney Int., 2:107, 1972.

Osathanondh, V., and Potter, E. L.: Development of human kidney as shown by microdissection. I. Preparation of tissues with reasons for possible misinterpretation of observations. Arch. Path., 76:271, 1963.

Osathanondh, V., and Potter, E. L.: Pathogenesis of polycystic kidneys. Historical survey. Arch. Path., 77:459, 1964. Type 1 due to hyperplasia of interstitial portions of collecting tubules. Arch. Path., 77:466, 1964. Type 2 due to inhibition of ampillary activity. Arch. Path., 77:474, 1964. Type 3 due to multiple abnormalities of development. Arch. Path., 77:485, 1964. Type 4 due to urethral obstruction. Arch. Path., 77:502, 1964.

Safouh, M., Crocker, J. F. S., and Vernier, R. L.: Experimental cystic disease of the kidney: Sequential, functional and morphologic studies. Lab. Invest., 23:392, 1970.

OTHER CYSTS

Serous or *solitary* cysts are thin sacs with flattened epithelium frequent in the lower pole and rarely communicating with a nephron. Congenital in origin, they may grow to 12 liters, produce backache, dragging sensation, palpable mass, obstruction, or urographic abnormality. They may contain blood and calcification. Solutes generally approximate those of plasma water. *Multilocular* cysts have septa or a honeycombed interior. When large they may resemble polycystic disease and may account for some older reports of unilateral polycysts. Comparative features are outlined in Table 3. A few cases of *segmental* cystic disease have been reported with histologic criteria for polycystic disease. *Lymphatic cysts* are found near the hilum and are associated with veins and vascular atresias. They begin 1 to 2 cm in diameter in the newborn but may enlarge. *Diverticula* of pelvis and calyces are associated with infection and obstruction, and they may appear as *cystic dilatations* of the parenchyma. They are suspected by their location. *Perirenal* cysts may follow traumatic extravasation or may be neoplastic. The latter originate in aberrant mesodermal tissue (wolffian or müllerian ducts, lymph channels), are varied in form, are usually unilateral, and are on the left side in females. *Renal hematomas* may liquefy and cavitate. *Angiomas* may produce profuse bleeding over long periods. *Mesenteric* cysts form below the kidney and simulate tumor or cause obstruction. *Dermoid* cysts contain all germ layers and may contain hair, bones, teeth, and other tissues. Infectious erosion of the renal parenchyma or dissolution of infected infarcts in *pyelonephritis* may produce cystlike areas, filled with fluid or pus. *Renal tuberculosis* may produce *caseocavernous abscesses* or ulcerations of the pelvis. Retention cysts of chronic glomerulonephritis are rarely of clinical importance. *Echinococcus cysts* occur from infestation by the larval stage of the dog tapeworm. This is prevalent in

TABLE 3.   Characteristics of Cystic Disease

	Polycystic	Multicystic
Hereditary	+	−
Bilateral	+	Rare
Unilateral	Rare	−
Progressive enlargement	+	−
Associated renal anomalies	−	+
In adults	+	−
In children	Rare	+
Functioning cysts	+	−
Communicating cysts	+	−
Measurable renal dysfunction	+	−
Dysplasia	−	+
Normal tissue between cysts	+	−
Thick capsule	−	+

certain sheep-raising countries. The manifestations include tumor, pain, dysuria, hematuria, eosinophilia, and excretion of ova, hooklets, and scolices in the urine. A complement-fixation test may be positive. *Toxoplasma* may produce microscopic pseudocysts in the kidney. *Renal aneurysm* may produce flank pain, hematuria, hypertension, and urographic filling defects. Renal cysts are associated with angiomatous tumors of the cerebellum in *Lindau's disease* and of the retina in *von Hippel-Lindau disease.*

Treatment of most cysts depends on type, location, and manifestation. Known serous and pustular cysts may be aspirated by needle. More often, because of the threat of malignancy, most cysts require surgical exploration and removal. Normal parenchyma should be preserved whenever possible. Erythrocytosis may be reversed by cyst removal, but cysts rarely contain granular cells or significant erythropoietin. They probably stimulate erythropoietin production in nearby tissue. Advances in renal plastic surgery now permit more frequent choices between partial and total nephrectomy. The latter should be avoided in benign conditions.

Boggs, L. K., and Kimmelstiel, P.: Benign multilocular cystic nephroma: Report of 2 cases of so-called multilocular cysts of the kidney. J. Urol., 76:530, 1956.

Hutchins, K. R., Mulholland, S. G., and Edson, M.: Segmental polycystic disease: N.Y. State J. Med., 72:1850, 1972.

Isaac, F., Schoen, I., and Walker, P.: An unusual case of Lindau's disease: Cystic disease of the kidneys and pancreas with renal and cerebral tumors. Am. J. Roentgenol., 75:912, 1956.

Moore, T.: Unilateral cystic kidneys. Br. J. Urol., 29:3, 1957.

Parkkulainen, K. V., Hjelt, L. V., and Sirola, K.: Congenital multicystic dysplasia of the kidney: Report of nineteen cases with discussion on the etiology, nomenclature, and classification of the cystic dysplasias of the kidney. Acta Chir. Scand., Suppl. 244, 1959.

Vertel, R. M., Morse, B. S., and Prince, J. E.: Remission of erythrocytosis after drainage of a solitary renal cyst. Arch. Intern. Med. 120:54, 1967.

UREMIC MEDULLARY CYSTIC DISEASE

Uremic medullary cystic disease, familial juvenile nephrophthisis, and some forms of salt-losing nephritis now appear to be facets of the same disease. There is definite hereditary predisposition exhibiting in various pedigrees as a recessive, a dominant, or an incomplete recessive affecting young children, older children, young adults, and a few rare survivors in the fifth and sixth decades. The majority are in the second and third decades. Male-to-male transmission (? X-linked) has been reported. There is a frequent association with red and blond hair. The disease may present insidiously with pallor, polyuria, anemia, or failure to thrive and grow. Hypotension, salt-wasting, and symptomatic bone disease are frequent. The normochromic anemia is refractory. The urine is deceptively benign, although modest proteinuria is frequent in older patients. Salt wasting is almost the rule. Hypertension is rare. The patients progress inexorably, but at varying rates, into uremia, with any or all of its features. Prominent are hyponatremia, hypochloremia, hypocalcemia, hyperphosphatemia, hyperphosphatasemia, metabolic acidosis and retarded growth. The osteodystrophy may be predominantly rachitic, osteomalacic, hyperparathyroid, or a mixture. Roentgenologic changes include widening of zone of calcification, metaphyseal fraying, decreased bone density, delayed maturation, pseudofractures and deformities, exostoses, localized osteosclerosis, subperiosteal cortical bone erosion, brown tumors, periosteal new bone, and extraosseous calcification—especially articular (hands, feet), periarticular, and soft-tissue, e.g., cornea, conjunctiva, and kidney. Parathyroid and adrenal hyperplasia and myelofibrosis occur. All tubular defects are distal with impaired concentrating ability, poor response to ADH, impaired acidification, impaired ammonium excretion, salt wasting, and a tendency to hyperkalemia. Infection is rare except after instrumentation. Notably absent are phosphaturia, glycosuria, aminoaciduria, or any disorder of proximal tubular function.

Pathologically, the kidneys are contracted (45 to 100 grams), granular, and lobulated. There are glomerulosclerosis, periglomerular fibrosis, diffuse, severe interstitial fibrosis, tubular atrophy and dilatation, colloid casts, localized lymphangiectasia, and cysts widespread in medulla, but often randomly distributed elsewhere. They vary from 50 mm to 2 cm in diameter. Cut sections from patients with nephronophthisis and medullary cystic disease are indistinguishable. Overemphasis on macroscopic cysts and their anatomy has confused the issue. Goldman et al. have traced 50 members of a family through five generations and found a dominant pattern. Eighteen of 25 persons in the first three generations had either overt renal failure or transmission to offspring. In other families it has been recessive. In some cases there is no family involvement. The cause and progression resemble human toxic nephropathy from a variety of agents, including heavy metals, and the lesions resemble early diphenylamine intoxication in rats. The disease could be an inborn error of metabolism that permits accumulation of a toxic substance, affecting distal tubular development in fetal life or early infancy.

Treatment consists in genetic counseling, management of abnormal physiology such as the salt depletion, treating the full range of defects seen in renal tubular disease, especially osteodystrophy and anemia, and ultimately resorting to the definitive therapy of terminal renal failure—dialysis or transplantation. Patients with renal transplants in place for more than two years have not acquired the defect, indicating that medullary cystic disease is purely renal in origin.

Fanconi, G., Hanhard, E., Albertini, A., von Uhlinger, E., Dolivo, G., and Prader, A.: Die familiare juvenile Nephronophthise (die idiopathische Schrumpfniere). Helv. Paediatr. Acta, 6:1, 1951.

Gielson, N., Heinegard, D., Holmberg, C. G., et al.: Renal medullary cystic disease or familial juvenile nephronophthisis: A renal tubular disease. Am. J. Med., 48:174, 1970.

Goldman, S. H., Walter, S. R., Merigan, T. C., Jr., Gardner, K. D., Jr., and Bull, J. M. C.: Hereditary occurrence of cystic disease of the renal medulla. N. Engl. J. Med., 274:984, 1966.

Herman, R. C., Good, R. A., and Vernier, R. L.: Medullary cystic disease in two siblings. Am. J. Med., 43:335, 1967.

Levin, N. W., Rosenberg, B., Zwi, S., and Reid, F. P.: Medullary cystic disease of the kidney, with some observations on ammonium excretion. Am. J. Med., 30:807, 1961.

Mongeau, J. G., and Worthen, H. G.: Nephronophthisis and medullary cystic disease. Am. J. Med., 43:345, 1967.

Rayfield, E. J., and McDonald, F. D.: Red and blonde hair in renal medullary cystic disease. Arch. Intern. Med., 130:72, 1972.

Strauss, M. B.: Clinical and pathological aspects of cystic disease of the renal medulla. Ann. Intern. Med., 57:373, 1962.

Strauss, M. B., and Sommers, S. C.: Medullary cystic disease and familial juvenile nephronophthisis. N. Engl. J. Med., 277:863, 1967.

SPONGE KIDNEY
(Nonuremic Medullary Cystic Disease)

Sponge kidney, first recognized in 1939, has now been recognized in several hundred patients. It is a congenital anomaly which can be manifested by pain, colic, calculi, recurrent infection, or hematuria; but more often it is asymptomatic and discovered as an incidental finding on roentgenography, biopsy, or autopsy. Branching, radial ducts and cysts are found ramifying from calyces along the pyramids. They may fill on intravenous pyelography, and may *not* fill on retrograde pyelography. Flow is slow, and contrast material hangs behind. They may be uni- or bilateral, segmental, or focal. The roentgenographic appearance has been likened to a sponge, grapes, flowers, and twigs. The cysts are filled with fluid, cellular debris, and concretions. Calcium apatite, carbonate, oxalate, and triple phosphate have been found. Nephrocalcinosis may occur. Hypercalciuria, pyelonephritis, and hypertension may supervene. Distal tubular defects have been noted, but so uncommonly that they may be related to the complications rather than the disease. Similar cysts have been noted in congenital hepatic fibrosis. Reported cases in Ehlers-Danlos syndrome, hemihypertrophy, and congenital pyloric stenosis may be special forms of sponge kidney. The roentgenographic pattern has been seen in two generations of one family and in two siblings, but is generally nonfamilial. The prognosis is related to infection, obstruction, and calculous disease. The asymptomatic form is benign and usually without any counterpart functional disorder. Instrumentation should be avoided.

Abeshouse, B. S., and Abeshouse, G. A.: Sponge kidney: A review of the literature and a report of five cases. J. Urol., 84:252, 1960.
Copping, G. A.: Medullary sponge kidney: Its occurrence in a father and daughter. Can. Med. Assoc. J., 96:608, 1967.
Lagergren, C., and Lindvall, N.: Medullary sponge kidney and polycystic diseases of the kidney: Distinct entities. Am. J. Roentgenol., 88:153, 1962.
MacDougall, J. A., and Prout, W. G.: Medullary sponge kidney: Clinical appraisal and report of twelve cases. Br. J. Surg., 55:130, 1968.
Morris, R. C., Yamauchi, H., Palubinskas, A. J., and Howenstine, J.: Medullary sponge kidney. Amer. J. Med., 38:883, 1965.

629. TUMORS OF THE KIDNEY

George E. Schreiner

Neoplasia of the genitourinary tract accounts for about one fifth of adult tumors and about one quarter of childhood tumors. About 7000 people annually in the United States develop renal cell carcinoma. Renal masses are considered malignant until proved otherwise. Our ignorance of the mechanisms of renal neoplasia parallels our general lack of knowledge of the pathogenesis of unrestrained cell growth. A classification of renal tumors is given in Table 4.

Unending subclassifications of tumors and morphologic grading have generally proved to be a sterile pathologic exercise. Older designations, such as hypernephroma, adenocarcinoma, alveolar carcinoma, and embryonic carcinoma have been dropped in favor of "renal carcinoma" or tumors of epithelial cell origin. Multiple sections often reveal more than one histologic type.

Pathology.   Tubular epithelium gives rise to adenocarcinoma. The epithelial lining of the pelvicalyceal system yields transitional cell carcinomas, and immature parenchymal tissue is the source of Wilms' tumor. Carcinoma accounts for 80 per cent of renal malignancy.

TABLE 4.   Classification of Renal Tumors

1. Neoplasms of renal parenchyma
    Benign tumors
       Fibroma
       Adenoma
       Papillary cystadenoma
       Endometriosis
    Epithelial neoplasms
       Renal carcinoma
       Embryonal nephroma (Wilms' tumor, nephroblastoma)
    Mesothelial neoplasms
       Sarcoma
       Neurogenic tumors
          Neuroblastoma
          Schwannoma
          Sympathicoblastoma
2. Neoplasms of the pelvis and calyces
    Papilloma
    Papillary carcinoma
    Squamous cell carcinoma
    Hemangioma
3. Tumors of the renal capsule
    Fibroma
    Fibrolipoma
    Malignant sarcoma
    Angiosarcoma
    Chondroma
4. Perirenal tumors and cysts
5. Tumors metastatic to the kidney

Cell types are *clear* and *granular*. Anatomic staging is as follows: IA—intracapsular tumor; IB—intrarenal but extracapsular (invasion through tumor capsule); II—perinephric microscopic III—perinephric gross; and IV—distant metastases. Renal carcinoma has a male preponderance, with a peak incidence at 45 to 60 years of age. Extension into the renal veins or through the renal capsule offers a bad prognosis (vein invaded—30 per cent five-year survival, versus 60 per cent when the vein is not invaded). Degeneration and calcification are a good prognostic feature. Renal carcinoma may spontaneously regress. A metastatic lesion may regress after removal of primary site, or may occur as late as 20 years after primary removal. Spread is by direct invasion or by vascular and lymphatic channels. Venous occlusion may result from spread of the tumor up the inferior vena cava. Favorite metastatic sites are lungs, liver, bones, and brain. They may be solitary.

Embryonal nephroma (Wilms' tumor) may occur in the fetus or rarely in later life. Seventy-five per cent appear before the age of five; about two thirds occur before two years of age. Eight per cent are bilateral. More than 50 confusing names have been applied to this tumor. It grows rapidly, may approach the weight of the rest of the body, and metastasizes most frequently through the veins to the lungs or through the lymphatics to the periaortic nodes. Widespread metastases in many organs may be seen.

Clinical Manifestations.   Since early renal tumors are asymptomatic, diagnoses are achieved by way of accidental or routine diagnostic studies. The classic triad of hematuria, mass, and pain must now be considered a later finding. Fever, leukocytosis, evidence of metastases, abdominal and flank pain, albuminuria, anorexia, weight loss, nausea, and vomiting are the most common symptoms. Even so, in less than half the children with Wilms' tumor is diagnosis achieved within one month of onset of symptoms. Demonstration of hematuria varies with the skill and persistence brought to the urinalysis. Erythrocytes in urine should never be considered a normal finding; suspicion of tumor should become greater during a systemic exclusion of other causes of hematuria. Because of venous extension and vascular spread, examination of patients with nephroma should be cautious, and treatment should be instituted as early as possible. Hypertension has been reported with widely varying incidence in embryonal nephroma; it may not revert on tumor removal. Presumably the tumor produces pressors directly or indirectly via ischemia. Nephroma may simulate or coexist with infantile polycystic disease.

In adult renal cell carcinoma the most prominent manifestations, in order, are hematuria, weight loss, lassitude, flank pain, fever, and abdominal pain. A firm spherical mass may be demonstrable by palpation, or roentgenographic studies may reveal it. Distant metastases may be observed before local signs appear. Notable are "cotton ball" metastases to the lung, osteolytic lesions in the long bones (femur, humerus), and involvement of lymph nodes, liver, adrenals, and contralateral kidney. No organ is exempt; unusual cases have been diagnosed by finding lesions in such places as the eye and vagina. Pelvic angiography and pulmonary fluoroscopy with an image intensifier have revealed asymptomatic metastases unrecognizable by other means.

Unusual Features. Renal carcinoma may present curious features and it has been called the "internist's tumor." These features include large tumor without distortion of the calyceal system, leukemoid reaction with leukocytes ranging up to 100,000 per cubic millimeter, polycythemia, eczematoid dermatitis, hypertension, hypercalcemia, peripheral neuropathy, plasmacytosis, and amyloid disease. Renal carcinoma has emerged as a major consideration in fevers of unknown origin. It may mimic a prolonged septic disease, or it may form an arteriovenous fistula to produce congestive heart failure. Both adult carcinoma and Wilms' tumor have been associated with erythema and polycythemia. Elevated blood and tumor levels or erythropoietin have been reported. Renal carcinomas have polycythemia in 2.3 per cent of cases, and should be considered in the differential diagnosis of polycythemia. We have seen secondary polycythemia, including granulocytosis and thrombocytosis, in a patient with a small renal carcinoma not demonstrable by x-ray. Parathormone-like activity has been reported, with hypercalcemia responding promptly to excision of renal carcinoma. Tumor patients may be hypertensive but are not inordinately so, and renin has not been isolated in a tumor.

Laboratory Findings. In addition to anemia or polycythemia, renal carcinoma characteristically brings about an unusually high sedimentation rate (up to 150 mm per hour). On electrophoresis, serum albumin is reduced, and alpha$_2$ globulin is elevated. A special form of tumor, the clear-cell PAS-positive renal carcinoma, has been associated with evidence of increased glucoprotein synthesis and abnormal serum glucoproteins.

Roentgenographic findings include irregularity of renal margin, multiple calcifications, deformity of infundibulum or calyces, and displacement of the kidney by outward growth. Infusion nephrotomography, mainstream and selective angiography, technetium radioscans, venography, and lymphangiography have vastly improved the early diagnosis. Neovasculature giving a "tumor blush" on arteriography is virtually diagnostic and can separate tumor from cyst. Perinephric insufflation has also been used.

Prognosis and Treatment. Embryonal nephroma was once 90 per cent fatal. The combination of early diagnosis, restriction of palpation, preoperative irradiation, prompt nephrectomy, and postoperative irradiation has dramatically reduced mortality, so that half or more of the patients can survive. Actinomycin D and vincristine have also been used postoperatively. Standard chemotherapy of recurrent disease has generally been ineffective save for sporadic success with progestational agents, androgenic hormones, and, more recently, Lomustine (C-C Nitrosurea). Immunotherapy may hold some promise. Earlier diagnosis and prompt nephrectomy have bettered the former 20 per cent survival in renal carcinoma, but the outlook is still grave. Statistics are confused by the delayed appearance of metastases. Renal carcinoma may stimulate fibrosis such as that seen in periureteral fibrosis. The resulting obstruction can falsely simulate metastases or contralateral spread. The physician who diagnoses or suspects a space-occupying lesion has an urgent obligation to achieve definitive diagnosis and surgery when indicated. There is no infallible way to distinguish clinically between a solitary cyst and a potential malignant disease. Papillary tumors of the renal pelvis yield positive exfoliative cytology in the urine.

Pelvic tumors derive from transitional epithelium and resemble tumors of the urinary bladder. Group I tumors are benign papilloma with excellent prognosis. Group II are noninvasive or focally invasive papillary carcinoma, also favorable. Group III are fully invasive but confined to the kidney and give good surgical results. Group IV spread outside the kidney and pelvis (lymph nodes, bone, liver, and lung) and carry an ominous prognosis. They may occasionally metastasize to unusual sites, including other tumors. About 80 per cent of patients have hematuria, half of it gross. Flank pain or frequency is also found. Pyelography is usually positive. Nephrectomy and ureterectomy are treatments of choice. Renal perfusion pumps used for kidney transplantation have been used for prolonged "open-kidney" surgery with subsequent autotransplant. Cytogenetic studies have revealed karyotypic abnormalities, marker chromosomes, and aneuploidy said to predict greater malignancy in early stages of noninvasive carcinoma of the bladder. The relative risk for coffee drinkers compared to that for nondrinkers is 1.24 for men and 2.58 for women. Transitional tumors occurred in 9 of 104 analgesic abusers and none of 88 pyelonephritic controls.

Bengtsson, U., Angervall, L., Ekman, H., and Lehman, L.: Transitional cell tumors of the renal pelvis in analgesic abusers. Scand. J. Nephrol., 2:145, 1968.

Bottiger, L. E.: Studies in renal carcinoma. I. Clinical and pathologic anatomical aspects. II. Biochemical investigations. Acta Med. Scand., 167:443, 1960.

Burns, W. A., and Kadar, A. T.: Unusual metastases from a transitional cell carcinoma of the renal pelvis and ureter. Med. Ann. D.C., 42:65, 1973.

Clarke, B. J., and Goade, W. J., Jr.: Fever and anemia in renal cancer. N. Engl. J. Med., 254:107, 1956.

Cole, P.: Coffee drinking and cancer of the lower urinary tract. Lancet, 1:1335, 1971.

Editorial: Analgesic abuse and tumors of the renal pelvis. Lancet, 2:1233, 1969.

Falor, W. H.: Chromosomes in noninvasive papillary carcinoma of the bladder, J.A.M.A., 216:791, 1971.

Foot, N. D., Humphreys, G. A., and Whitmore, W. F.: Renal tumors: Pathology and prognosis in 295 cases. J. Urol., 66:190, 1951.

Grabstald, H., Whitmore, W. F., and Melamed, M. R.: Renal pelvic tumors. J.A.M.A., 218:845, 1971.

Johnson, S. H., III, and Marshal, M., Jr.: Primary kidney tumors of childhood. J. Urol., 74:707, 1955.

Rubin, P.: Cancer of the urogenital tract. Kidney: Localized renal adenocarcinoma. J.A.M.A., 204:219, 1968.

Wagle, D. G.: Vagaries of renal cell carcinoma. J. Med. (Basel), 3:178, 1972.

630. MISCELLANEOUS RENAL DISORDERS

George E. Schreiner

Hoxie, H. J., and Coggin, C. B.: Renal infarction: Statistical study of 205 cases and detailed report of an unusual case. Arch. Intern. Med., 65:587, 1940.

Woods, J. W., and Williams, T. F.: Renal infarction. *In* Strauss, M. B., and Welt, L. G. (eds.): Diseases of the Kidney. Boston, Little, Brown & Company, 1971, pp. 789–794.

INFARCTION

Definition. Infarction is the ischemic death of tissue. Total ischemia of the cortical area is better termed *renal cortical necrosis* (see Ch. 604). Bland infarction without reaction is the same as *focal cortical necrosis* and may be seen in trauma, preeclampsia, infectious shock, and in most of the causes of cortical necrosis. The term *renal infarct* is usually applied to the segmental type. These are usually due to *arterial* obstruction such as *embolism* (mural thrombi, cholesterol plaque material, endocarditis), *thrombosis, trauma,* surgical injury, intrarenal *narrowing* (scleroderma, malignant nephrosclerosis), stasis (shock, diabetic acidosis), and sickle cell disease, or to *venous* thrombosis as seen in neoplastic states (hypernephroma, lymphoma), dehydration (infantile diarrhea), septicemia, and hypercoagulable states. In one study of 205 human infarctions, about 77 per cent accompanied a cardiac lesion. The early red lesion evolves rapidly into a central and peripheral dead zone and a marginal area which is presumably the source of the pressor materials that produce the often-accompanying hypertension.

Diagnosis. The diagnosis is suggested by history, flank pain, renal tenderness, transient hematuria and albuminuria, and a space-occupying lesion or change of size or nonfunctioning kidney on pyelography. Total renal infarction with recovery is followed by calcification of the necrotic tissue and hypertrophy of the contralateral kidney. Infarction may produce acute or accelerated hypertension, and should be suspected when that is coupled with history of trauma to the kidney or renal surgery. The hypertension usually peaks at two to three weeks after a single infarction, and may subside as the ischemic tissue progresses to scar formation. Renal infarcts presenting as space-occupying lesions have to be distinguished from cysts and tumors. Nephrograms with "black" areas, scintigrams with "cold" areas, or anomaly in the distribution of dye in the segmental arteriogram may be an aid to diagnosis. Identification of small renal infarcts as embolic phenomena may be the clue that leads to a primary diagnosis, e.g., asymptomatic myocardial infarction.

Heparin perfusion during selective arteriography may have therapeutic benefit.

Treatment. Embolectomy or endarterectomy should be considered as emergency treatment when the blood supply to one kidney is threatened. Aortic repair may be indicated when dissection involves the renal artery. Vascular prostheses with a side arm have also been used to bypass an irreparably damaged renal artery involved in the Leriche syndrome. Anticoagulant therapy may be indicated for a central source of embolization. When diagnostic studies indicate unilateral renal infarct as a cause for accelerated hypertension, surgical intervention may be indicated if the hypertension does not spontaneously ameliorate within two months.

Baum, S.: Renal ischemic lesions. Radiol. Clin. North Am., 5:543, 1967.

Halpern, M.: Acute renal artery embolus: A concept of diagnosis and treatment. J. Urol. 98:552, 1967.

CHYLURIA

Chyluria is lymph in the urine. The entity has been known since Hippocrates. Biochemically the urine contains a colloidal suspension of fat in molecular form, albumin, lecithin, cholesterin, fibrinogen, and soaps producing a milky or creamy appearance resembling lactescent serum. The major component is usually triglycerides. The proteinuria may be sufficient to meet criteria of the *nephrotic syndrome.*

Parasitic (tropical) chyluria is caused by *Filaria sanguinis-hominis (W. bancrofti). Nonparasitic chyluria* is due to a rupture of a lymphatic into the collecting system resulting from observation of lymphatics anywhere between the intestines and the thoracic duct. Specific causes include tumors, fibrosis, pregnancy, and trauma. Pyelonephritis may be associated.

Milky urine, intermittent (postural) or constant, is the major sign. It may be mistaken for pyuria. Milky urine is stable, containing 2 to 4 per cent fat, and does not exhibit fat droplets on microscopy. Retrograde pyelography may demonstrate pyelolymphatic backflow. Oral fats labeled with Sudan 3 or isotopic ^{131}I will appear in the urine. Ether will extract both chyle and the label.

Major items to be differentiated are lipiduria and pyuria. *Lipiduria* has fat droplets that rise to the top on centrifugation. It may be associated with fractures, eclampsia, diabetes, phosphorus, arsenic, and carbon monoxide poisoning.

Primary treatment is identification and removal of the obstruction. A low fat diet reduces chyluria.

Caserta, S. J.: Description of chyluria: Report of a case. N. Engl. J. Med., 255:1239, 1956.

Tuller, M. A., Feuer, M. M., Schapira, H. E., and Ho, Peh-Ping: Recumbent chyluria: Demonstration of unilateral renal-lymphatic communication. Am. J. Med., 33:951, 1962.

Yamauchi, S.: Chyluria: Clinical laboratory and statistical study of 45 personal cases observed in Hawaii. J. Urol., 54:318, 1945.

PNEUMATURIA

Pneumaturia is the passage of gas bubbles in the urine.

In noninfected patients, pneumaturia is usually due to a vesicovaginal or vesicoenteric fistula. Vegetable fibers and fecal contamination may be found in the urine. Such fistulas may be congenital in infants, may result from gross infections or neoplasms, or may follow radical pelvic surgery. Bubbles may also be caused by gas-forming bacteria proliferating in urine. *E. coli, A. aerogenes,* or yeast may be involved. The gas is carbon dioxide. Pneumaturia, although rare, is most frequent in elderly diabetic women.

Bubbling or frothing urine is noted by the patient at the end of micturition or by physician and nurse in the last drainage by catheterization. A gas shadow may be seen in the bladder on roentgenographic study.

Treatment consists of reassuring the patient; finding and repairing the fistula, if present; or treating a specific infection and eliminating glycosuria.

NEPHROPTOSIS

Definition. Nephroptosis is excessive mobility of the kidney. It is to be distinguished from *ectopia*, which is congenital or acquired permanent abnormal placement of the kidney, and *malrotation*, or pivoting of the kidney on its vertical axis, the pelvis and ureter deviating from the normal position. When observing the percutaneous biopsy needle during normal respiratory excursions, most physicians are amazed by the normal mobility of the kidney, which has a fascial attachment to the diaphragm. It is therefore difficult to say how much mobility is "excessive." On palpation the fingers should not be able to slide above the upper pole. On urography the ureteropelvic junction should not descend on standing more than one to one and a half vertebral spaces.

Nephroptosis occurs in about one fifth of adult women and much less frequently in men. There is a right-sided predominance. It is more common in thin, hyperkinetic people.

Pathogenesis. The kidney is held within its normal excursion by its vascular supply (pedicle), its fascia (Gerota) anchored to the diaphragmatic attachments, peritoneal adhesions, intra-abdominal pressure and support of other organs, and its form fit to the lumbar gutter. Nephroptotic kidneys usually have diminished renal fat and poorly developed fascia. A long, thin torso, shallow lumbar gutter, generalized visceroptosis, faulty posture, atrophy of abdominal muscles, and multiple pregnancies may all be contributing causes.

Clinical Manifestations. Nephroptosis is largely asymptomatic, but has been too often made the organic focus for neurotic or hypochondriacal personality. Other than a vague dropping or dragging sensation, specific symptom complexes come from torsion, kinking, ureteral obstruction, infection, and stretching of the vascular pedicle. Recently, orthostatic hypertension and postural hyperaldosteronism (via angiotensin) have been identified with nephroptosis, accounting for 7 of 47 operated patients in one series of renal hypertension. Fibromuscular hyperplasia may accompany the condition. The arteriogram, renin excretion, and aldosterone secretion may be abnormal *only* in the upright position. Recently, we have seen severe orthostatic hypotension (90 to 60/40 to 30 mm Hg) in bilateral nephroptosis. The mechanism could be reduced renin or increased prostaglandins. *Dietl's crisis* is an acute prostrating ureteral colic coming on shortly after assuming the upright posture or after postural fatigue, e.g., in a waitress. The severe pain can be accompanied by nausea, vomiting, hypotension, oliguria, swelling, and tenderness of the kidney. It is relieved by a short period in the Trendelenburg position, followed by horizontal resting, at which time the urine may increase in volume and may contain albumin and erythrocytes. It is thought by some that, in the absence of nephroptosis, Dietl's crisis may occur owing to spasm of the renal pelvis characterized by decreased intrapelvic volume and increased frequency and intensity of peristalsis, analogous to spastic colon.

Diagnosis. Diagnosis is usually made by relating symptoms to posture or occupation and relief by assumption of the horizontal position. Physical examination is performed with the patient in the supine and standing positions, the weight on the leg opposite the side being palpated. Intravenous pyelography in the conventional supine position followed by a view of the upright position is a valuable adjunct. Urinalysis may reveal hematuria and albuminuria from vascular distention or pyuria and bacteria from secondary infection.

Treatment. Reassurance and explanation are the major components of treatment. Weight-gain regimens and exercises to strengthen the abdominal wall may be helpful. Short rest periods in the horizontal position and sensible shoes may work wonders for women whose jobs cause standing fatigue. Often a change of occupation or prolonged rest may be necessary to establish the postural relationship. Patients with recurrent pyelonephritis related to postural fatigue accompanied by ureteral kinking may occasionally benefit from nephropexy. When fibromuscular hyperplasia is present, nephropexy should be combined with arterial repair. The uncomplicated nephroptotic kidney should not be subjected to surgery or used as a psychosomatic crutch.

Derrick, J. R., and Hanna, E.: Abdominal renal mobility and hypertension. Am. J. Surg., 106:673, 1963.
Ginn, H. E., Jr., and Parry, W. L.: Postural hypertension and edema caused by excessive mobility of the kidneys. South. Med. J., 57:735, 1964.

ANOMALIES OF THE GENITOURINARY TRACT

Because of the complex embryologic development of the various specialized structures in the genitourinary tract, developmental mishaps are more common than in any other organ system and affect more than 10 per cent of all humans. Anomalies of the kidney include deviation in number, size, structure, form, and location. In addition, anomalies of the pelvis, ureter, bladder, and urethra may lead to obstruction or infection secondarily involving the kidney.

Kidney. *Bilateral renal agenesis,* often associated with malformations of the ear, is incompatible with life. Toxic or environmental factors would be most damaging at the fourth week of pregnancy. *Unilateral agenesis (solitary kidney),* which has an incidence of about 0.16 per cent, results from failure of the renal bud, the nephrogenic blastema, or the vascular supply. Arrested development of the wolffian duct results in associated nondevelopment of the rest of the urinary tract on the involved side. No ureteral orifice or ridge is revealed on cystoscopy. Solitary kidney may give rise to anuria when it becomes involved in acute parenchymal disease. As a cardinal principle, the presence of two kidneys should be established before doing any instrumentation or surgical procedure. *Supernumerary kidney,* completely separated and free, is extremely rare. *Fused supernumerary kidney* has an incidence of about 0.025 per cent. *Renal aplasia* may consist of unorganized parenchyma surrounded by fat, and may produce hypertension. *Renal hypoplasia* is generally unilateral and medial in position. In the adult this must be distinguished from renal atrophy secondary to pyelonephritis. Hypoplastic kidneys frequently become infected, demonstrate constant albuminuria, are symmetrically reduced in size, and show small nephrons on biopsy together with atrophic blood vessels. *Renal hypertrophy* may exist congenitally contralateral to a hypoplastic kidney or may be acquired. Functional hypertrophy regularly occurs in transplanted kidneys. *Fetal lobulation* is normal in infants, but persists in about 5 per cent of adults. Fusion of the two kidneys, which is found in about 0.2 per cent of people, may occur at the lower poles, at the lower or upper pole tips *(horseshoe kidney),* at both poles *(doughnut kidney),* throughout *(cake kidney),* or at the contralateral upper and lower poles *(sigmoid kidney).* The common variety, the lower-pole horseshoe kidney, lies close to the spine, with anterior rotation of the pelves. The vascular supply is almost always anomalous. Surgical separation is sometimes feasible for intractable infection or stone. *Congenital ectopia* (incidence 1 per cent) usually results in a pelvic location for the kidney and has been mistaken for tumor. The position of congenital ectopia is defined by the length of the ureter and vascular supply. In acquired ectopia the ureter and blood vessels were originally of normal length, but upon loss of fascial support the vascular pedicle lengthened and the ureter became redundant. *Malrotation* is frequent in ectopic kidneys. In *crossed ectopia,* the kidney crosses the midline, and lies adjacent to or fused with its mate.

Renal Pelvis. The normal renal pelvis is flask shaped, with upper, middle, and lower major calyces branching into minor calyces. Increase in number of major calyces up to six has been observed. *"Double kidney"* is really double pelvis, and results from the reduplication of the ureteral bud. It is found in about 4 per cent of urograms. The duplication has varying degrees of completion, and may or may not be accompanied by double ureter. *"Spider pelvis"* is a congenitally long, thin pelvis simulating compression. *Congenital hydronephrosis* may result from a variety of conditions present in fetal life. *Extrarenal pelvis* should be considered a normal variant from *intrarenal pelvis.* It becomes important, however, in the pathophysiology of obstructive uropathy.

Blood Vessels. Anomalies of the blood vessels are receiving increased attention because of their possible role in unilateral renal disease with hypertension. They are being discovered with increasing frequency since the advent of the radiohippuran and other radioiodide renograms and increased use of transaortic or retrograde aortography and renal angiography. *Arterial anomalies* include *congenital atresia, tortuosity,* and *aberrant vessels.* Minor anomalies are present in about 25 per cent of people. Renal arteries and veins may derive from the pedicle, aorta, vena cava, adrenals, pancreas, and liver. Anomalous vessels usually involve either pole, and upon crossing the upper portion of the ureter or the ureteropelvic junction may produce obstruction. *Renal artery aneurysm* and intrarenal *arteriovenous fistula* are rare but do occur.

Ureter. Ureteral malformations include agenesis, duplication, triplication, ectopia, ureterocele, herniation, postcaval ureter, aplasia, congenital stricture, congenital valves or folds, hydroureter, diverticula, torsion, kinks, and involvement with aberrant vessels.

Bladder. Malformations of the bladder include agenesis, hypoplasia, reduplication, diverticula, hypertrophy, urachal cysts and fistulas, trigonal folds, and cloaca formation. Vesical neck anomalies are discussed in Ch. 625.

Related Congenital Anomalies. Congenital cysts are discussed in Ch. 628. Malformed ears, particularly asymmetrical, are associated with some genitourinary anomalies. Congenital deficiency of the abdominal musculature is regularly associated with genitourinary problems. Renal anomalies have been described in Marfan's syndrome. Nerve deafness is associated with hereditary nephritis.

Diagnosis. The diagnosis of congenital renal and urinary anomalies is usually made during the course of investigation for other anomalies, as an incidental urographic finding, or when symptoms develop because of infection or obstruction. Most malformed and malrotated kidneys have defects in drainage and are liable to ascending pyelonephritis. Anomalous structures can be mistaken for cysts or tumors and may become significant factors in the course of pregnancy or of surgical procedures on nearby structures. The longest recorded survival in renal agenesis is 39 days.

Benjamin, J. A., and Tobin, C. E.: Abnormalities of kidneys, ureters and perinephric fascia: Anatomic and clinical study. J. Urol. 65:715, 1951.

Campbell, M. F.: Principles of Urology. Philadelphia, W. B. Saunders Company, 1957, Chapter 6.

Smith, E. C., and Orkin, L. A.: Clinical and statistical study of 471 congenital anomalies of kidneys and ureter. J. Urol. 53:11, 1945.

Part XIV

DISEASES OF THE DIGESTIVE SYSTEM

631. INTRODUCTION

Marvin H. Sleisenger

In the chapters that follow, important new ideas and clinical advances in the major diseases and disorders of the gut and liver are presented, and subjects previously treated as isolated topics have been expanded to chapters or important subdivisions of chapters. Among these are an approach to the recognition and differential diagnosis of the acute abdomen (see Ch. 653), diagnosis and treatment of gastrointestinal bleeding (see Ch. 644), vascular diseases of the intestine (see Ch. 658 to 661), and a sizable number of other less common but important diseases of the colon and rectum (see Ch. 670 to 679).

Advances in the technical aspects of diagnosis and management of gastrointestinal disease have been carefully considered. The role of flexible endoscopy, particularly esophagogastroduodenoscopy and colonoscopy, is described. These instruments have greatly influenced the approach to a number of major diseases of the upper and lower intestine, in the areas of both diagnosis and treatment. Appropriately mentioned are the arteriographic techniques which are of immense aid in diagnosis, particularly of diseases which cause massive gastrointestinal bleeding. A description of the usefulness of isotopic scanning and sonographic techniques will also be found.

Therapy for gastrointestinal diseases continues to be nonspecific for many diseases and disorders; however, the number of entities for which specific therapy, replacement type therapy, or symptomatic therapy is effective is growing. For example, it now appears that prolonged therapy with steroids is beneficial for patients with chronic active hepatitis. Instillation of vasoconstrictive substances through arterial catheters or directly into the stomach appears to help in halting massive upper gastrointestinal bleeding; the efficacy of hourly or two-hourly administration of antacids, particularly active aluminum hydroxide gel preparations, although being questioned, seems to be established in therapy for peptic ulcer disease; likewise, administration of these substances to debilitated, postoperative, chronically ill, intubated, or recumbent individuals in prevention of so-called "stress ulceration" is indicated.

Surgical procedures for gastrointestinal disease are an important part of the therapy for complications of peptic ulcer and of chronic inflammatory disease, for cancer and other tumors of the gastrointestinal tract, for calculous biliary tract disease, for portal hypertension, and for complications of acute and chronic inflammation of the pancreas. Of these, peptic ulcer disease is clinically the most important cause for major surgical intervention in gastroenterology. Procedures are evolving which are less mutilative and perhaps more specific for diminishing the vagal influence on gastric secretion while not increasing the possibility of undue antral (gas-trin) influence. Thus the selective vagotomy and the "superselective" vagotomy will be watched very closely and evaluated in terms of a trade-off between reduction in postoperative complications of peptic ulcer surgery and a somewhat increased incidence of recurrence as compared with partial gastrectomy and vagotomy. There is no question that colectomy is a specific procedure for universal ulcerative colitis, especially in view of improved technique for construction of ileostomies, and now clinicians are less and less willing to treat universal colitis indefinitely. In addition, the hazard of carcinomatous degeneration of the bowel in this disease with passing decades is real and affords the physician further reason to intervene surgically. There is no substitute for eradicative surgery for gastrointestinal cancer; radiation and chemotherapeutic agents are relatively ineffective except for some types of squamous cell cancer of the upper gastrointestinal tract.

The usefulness of intensive replacement therapy for patients with malabsorption becomes increasingly evident. Parenteral hyperalimentation for appropriate periods (postoperatively, particularly), followed by frequent supplemental feedings of high calorie substances (medium-chain triglycerides, protein hydrolysates), adequate therapy with both water-soluble and fat-soluble vitamins, and supplementation with calcium and iron, all may maintain these patients in adequate nutritional balance. More specific therapy for this condition may be found in the use of broad-spectrum antimicrobial drugs for those who have bacterial overgrowth.

The newer information concerning the pathogenesis of gallstones is providing the basis for a long-term study of the medical treatment of this disease by administration of a conjugated bile salt, chenodeoxycholate. The rationale is that increasing the cholesterol solubility in bile will not only prevent further crystallization but will also gradually dissolve existing stones. It is too early to tell whether or not the therapy will be effective on a long-term basis, and if continuous therapy will be necessary. Also, the long-term side effects are not yet evaluated. Meanwhile, the mainstay for therapy of symptomatic calculous gallbladder disease is surgery. The question of operation for those with "silent" stones is moot; the majority of observers feel that those under age 60 who are otherwise in good health with asymptomatic stones should undergo cholecystectomy.

Although covered in great detail in Part VIII, the infectious diarrheas are worthy of brief note here. It appears that an increasing number of these infectious organisms cause diarrhea not by virtue of invasiveness or tissue damage but by the elaboration of an endotoxin which, by increasing the concentration of adenylcyclate, leads to the secretion of water and electrolytes into the lumen. This mechanism is also stimulated by the administration of a number of drugs, particularly xanthines, and by endogenously produced substances, particularly prostaglandins.

The clinical pharmacology of the gastrointestinal tract has not changed much since the last edition of this book. The mainstays of therapy for most diseases and disorders of motility and secretion remain antacids, anticholinergics, sedatives, and tranquilizers. Steroids are useful at times for chronic inflammatory disease and for chronic aggressive hepatitis; broad-spectrum antimicrobials are often effective in the bacterial overgrowth syndrome and for Whipple's disease. The clinical usefulness of gastrointestinal hormones or their antagonists is still in the experimental stage and is not yet practicable.

Section One. DISORDERS OF MOTILITY

Thomas P. Almy

632. INTRODUCTION

Most gastrointestinal symptoms have as their immediate cause some disturbance of the motility of the gut, and the most common intestinal disorders in clinical practice are those in which disturbed motility is unassociated with a recognizable morphologic or biochemical lesion, i.e., they are "functional" disorders. Much less commonly, the most impressive physiologic and clinical effects of a morphologically definable disease process are disturbances of gut motility, the understanding of which represents the key to effective therapy. These two kinds of disorders are considered together in this section.

Rhythmic contractility is an intrinsic property of the intestinal wall. In the absence of extrinsic nerves or humoral influences, peristalsis is maintained by local reflexes for which the afferents arise in the mucosa, and the efferents include the myenteric ganglia. Extrinsic neural and humoral mechanisms serve to regulate and adapt the intrinsic motility of the gut to the needs of the total organism. A purposeful alternation of propulsive and nonpropulsive patterns of activity, adapted to civilized habits of eating, working, sleeping, and defecating, is referred to as normal intestinal function. The most common and clinically important disorders of intestinal motility occur during periods of stress in persons with normally innervated intestines, when the aforementioned patterns are long sustained as bodily accompaniments of emotional tension.

By contrast certain disorders, such as achalasia, congenital megacolon, and the esophageal disorder in diabetic neuropathy, are based upon permanent defects in integrative mechanisms. The high pressures generated at the sites of colonic and esophageal diverticula appear to result from patterns of disordered motility, the neural basis of which is as yet unclear.

Our knowledge of these disorders has been extended rapidly in recent years through the improvement of methods for the observation and recording of intestinal motility in intact man. The comparison of electromanometric recordings of intraluminal pressure with cineradiographic images of the barium-filled intestine has contributed much to our understanding of mechanisms, and at times has directly aided the diagnosis. The true diagnostic limitations of these methods, however, have not been fully defined.

633. DISORDERS OF SWALLOWING

Normal deglutition is accomplished by peristaltic movements, triggered by reflexes arising from voluntary contractions of the muscles of the buccal and pharyngeal cavities. The elevation of the tongue and larynx thrusts the food bolus against the posterior wall, raises the pressure in the pharynx, and seals off the aditus of the larynx. A fall in the pressure follows immediately (see Fig. 1) in both the superior (cricopharyngeal) and inferior (vestibular) esophageal sphincters, and a gradient of pressure is established favorable to propulsion of the bolus. The wave of high pressure generated in the pharynx then sweeps progressively downward to the stomach. The reflex pathways subserving this mechanism lie in the fifth, seventh, ninth, tenth, and eleventh cranial nerves, and the effectors include both skeletal muscle (tongue, pharynx, larynx, upper one third of the esophagus) and smooth muscle (lower two thirds of the esophagus). In the latter region the efferent pathway is autonomic and cholinergic, the postganglionic neurons lying in the esophageal wall (Auerbach's plexus). The lower esophageal sphincter or esophagogastric sphincter, although anatomically indistinct, normally

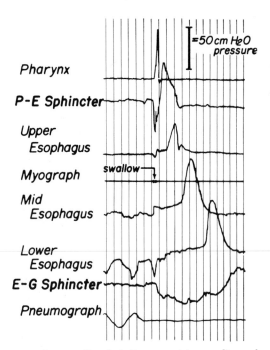

Figure 1. A composite of electromanometric recordings, showing simultaneous pressure changes throughout pharynx and esophagus during a single swallow. Read from left to right; interval between vertical lines = 1 second. P-E Sphincter = pharyngoesophageal sphincter. E-G Sphincter = esophagogastric sphincter or lower esophageal sphincter. (Adapted from Code, C. F.: An Atlas of Esophageal Motility in Health and Disease. Springfield, Ill., Charles C Thomas, 1958.)

presents a functionally important high pressure barrier to the reflux of gastric contents. It is under dual control—a neural mechanism (fast component), comprising cholinergic and alpha-adrenergic stimulatory fibers as well as beta-adrenergic and nonadrenergic inhibitory fibers; and a hormonal mechanism (slow component), which largely determines its tone but permits rapid relaxation and contraction in the act of swallowing. Both exogenous and endogenous gastrin have been shown to increase resting sphincter pressure, whereas secretin, cholecystokinin, and glucagon oppose the action of gastrin. These hormonal effects participate in the important adaptive reactions of the sphincter, which cause it normally to increase its strength of contraction when intra-abdominal or intragastric pressure rises, or when gastric acid secretion is increased.

Difficult swallowing, or *dysphagia,* may result from a defect or disorder in any part of the mechanism outlined above or from mechanical obstruction to the bolus propelled by this mechanism. In other patients a complaint of dysphagia will be found to relate entirely to difficulty in initiating the voluntary act of swallowing or to defects in the reflex coordination of oropharyngeal movements. When dysphagia is due to motor dysfunction, difficulty is experienced with both liquids and solids, whereas, in the presence of a mechanical obstruction or stenosis, the strong peristaltic movements above the lesion serve to propel through it any particle smaller than the stenotic lumen. Thus the patient with an obstructing carcinoma may experience the sudden onset of dysphagia on swallowing a bolus of meat or toast, and, as the lumen progressively narrows, may have to limit his diet to semiliquid and ultimately liquid foods.

Pain on swallowing, if mild, is likely to be incorporated in the experience of dysphagia. Its location often accurately reflects the level of the esophagus principally affected. At times esophageal pain is more severe, outlasts the normal duration of the deglutition, or is dissociated from it in time. Its location is usually substernal, beneath the xiphoid process, and in the episternal notch. It may radiate to the anterior neck and lower jaw, the dorsal spine, the sides of the chest, the shoulders and arms, and the epigastrium. Rarely it may originate in one of these sites. Its quality is most often either crushing or burning. The latter sensation, commonly called *heartburn,* characteristically radiates upward to the neck, and results from inflammation of the mucosa of the lower esophagus usually brought about by reflux of gastric juice.

Esophageal *regurgitation* is a common manifestation of obstructive disorders, and is to be distinguished from vomiting by the absence of nausea, the tendency to occur during or immediately after meals, the lack of digestion of regurgitated food, and the absence of bile or of a sour or bitter taste.

634. DISORDERS OF THE UPPER (PHARYNGOESOPHAGEAL) SEGMENT

The "lump in the throat" is a familiar transitory sensation accompanying fear or acute anxiety. Related is the "globus hystericus," in which a person suffering emotional conflict is incapable of initiating the voluntary movements of deglutition.

In any *disease of the brainstem,* the *cranial nerves,* or the *muscles* of this segment, the coordinated contraction of the pharyngeal musculature and relaxation of the pharyngoesophageal sphincter may fail to develop, with resultant gagging, coughing, and regurgitation of fluids through the nose. The specific cause is usually made obvious by associated symptoms and signs, and may be pseudobulbar palsy, bulbar poliomyelitis, myasthenia gravis, the oculopharyngeal syndrome, dermatomyositis, myotonic dystrophy, or sarcoidosis. This mechanism is important in the causation of the hypopharyngeal (Zenker's) diverticulum (see Ch. 639). The prognosis and treatment are those of the underlying disease.

SIDEROPENIC DYSPHAGIA
(Plummer-Vinson Syndrome, Paterson-Brown-Kelly Syndrome)

Sideropenic dysphagia is a disorder characterized by dysphagia referable to the upper segment, atrophy of the mucous membranes of mouth and pharynx, koilonychia, hypochromic microcytic anemia, hypoferremia, gastric achlorhydria, and stenoses or webs of the upper esophageal mucosa demonstrable by roentgenography or by endoscopy. It occurs mainly in women subsisting on low intakes of iron and vitamins, chiefly those of the B complex. The prognosis is excellent in most cases, but these patients should be observed for later development of carcinoma of the pharynx or esophagus, to which they are unusually susceptible. It is effectively treated with a good general diet, at first soft or semiliquid in consistency, with oral or parenteral iron in the amounts used for iron deficiency anemia and vitamin supplements. Occasionally the stenotic lesions require bouginage.

635. DISORDERS OF THE LOWER (ESOPHAGOGASTRIC) SEGMENT

The motility of the lower esophagus may be altered by diffuse disease of the muscular wall or by disturbances of intrinsic neural mechanisms. In systemic lupus erythematosus and other connective tissue diseases, disordered swallowing is strikingly associated with *Raynaud's phenomenon.* It is commonly seen in *scleroderma* (progressive systemic sclerosis), where it may antedate the appearance of cutaneous changes. In an advanced case the esophagogram reveals dilatation and absent peristalsis, a patulous vestibule allowing free regurgitation of barium from the stomach. In milder instances, and often in the absence of dysphagia, the patient with scleroderma will show defects in peristalsis only while swallowing barium in the recumbent position or when recorded electromanometrically (Fig. 2A). Esophagoscopy may reveal peptic esophagitis, to which acute or chronic blood loss may be due. The therapy is that for regurgitant esophagitis and other aspects of scleroderma.

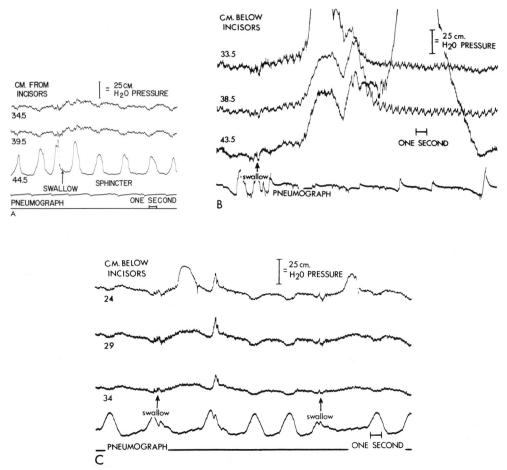

Figure 2. Electromanometric recordings from lower esophagus and lower esophageal sphincter. *A, Scleroderma.* Note absence of peristalsis; fluctuations in sphincter pressure coincide with inspiration. *B, Diffuse esophageal spasm.* Note extremely large, sustained or repetitive contractions beginning simultaneously at three levels. *C, Achalasia.* Note absence of peristalsis; pressure in the sphincter (here at 34 cm) does not fall on swallowing. (Reproduced from Kelley, M. L., Jr., by permission.)

Healthy persons may fail to generate a primary peristaltic wave, and instead exhibit incoordinate contraction of the lower esophagus after 1 to 10 per cent of swallows. These phenomena may occur after the majority of swallows in elderly persons (presbyesophagus) and in a number of disorders of the nervous system, including multiple sclerosis, amyotrophic lateral sclerosis, parkinsonism, pseudobulbar palsy, and both diabetic and alcoholic neuropathy. In many of these diseases, the esophagogastric sphincter may fail to relax. These defects of neuromuscular activity are seen in exaggerated form in three disorders apparently localized to the esophagus—diffuse spasm, hypertensive esophagogastric sphincter, and achalasia—which appear together or sequentially in the same patient with significant frequency, and hence may be pathogenically related.

DIFFUSE ESOPHAGEAL SPASM
(Corkscrew Esophagus, "Curling")

Particularly in some elderly persons, deglutition may evoke strong, uncoordinated, nonpropulsive contractions of the body of the esophagus (Fig. 2B). Although in most instances this condition is asymptomatic, it may induce dysphagia or substernal pain, at times simulating angina pectoris. On barium swallow, the esophageal lumen appears in the form of an irregular series of concentric narrowings, or a spiral coil (curling, Fig. 3). In some cases the esophagus is abnormally sensitive to methacholine (see Achalasia, below).

This disorder is usually chronic and nonprogressive. Rarely, it is followed by typical achalasia. When required, pain can be prevented or relieved by an anticholinergic agent, e.g., propantheline, 15 to 30 mg three times daily, or isopropamide, 5 to 10 mg twice daily orally. Severe cases may require a long esophagomyotomy for relief of symptoms.

HYPERTENSIVE ESOPHAGOGASTRIC SPHINCTER

In rare instances the resting pressure in the esophagogastric sphincter has been shown to exceed by far the normal upper limit of 40 cm of water. At times of spontaneous or induced emotional conflict, both roentgenographic and manometric studies indicate the occurrence of varying degrees of "spasm" of this sphincter, unassociated with disturbed peristalsis in the body of the esophagus, yet often giving rise to a sensation of obstruction at the xiphoid level. Long persistence

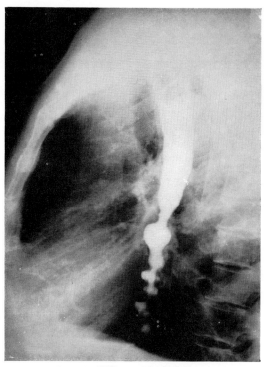

Figure 3. Diffuse esophageal spasm.

of the myenteric (Auerbach's) plexus or of the vagal motor nuclei. This varies greatly in degree, at times amounting to complete atrophy and at times being undetectable by ordinary histologic criteria, and appears to be proportional to the duration and severity of the motility disturbance.

Even in those patients without evident structural damage to the ganglia, physiologic abnormalities are demonstrable at any time. In manometric studies the total motor activity in the resting state varies widely; but, consistently on swallowing, a moving peristaltic wave fails to develop in the body, and the LES fails to relax normally (Fig. 2C). Whereas the motility of the normally innervated esophagus is altered by methacholine only when given in subcutaneous doses of 25 mg or more, injection of only 5 to 10 mg in a patient with achalasia is sufficient to induce a strong, sustained, incoordinated, often painful contraction of the body of the esophagus. In accordance with "Cannon's law," stating that a tissue deprived of its autonomic nerve supply is excessively sensitive to the chemical transmitter of the nerve impulse, this is held to be pharmacologic evidence of partial or complete aganglionosis. Recently, the LES in achalasia has been shown to be excessively sensitive to stimulation by gastrin.

With failure of relaxation of the LES on swallowing, food and liquid accumulate in the esophagus until, in the vertical position, the hydrostatic pressure exceeds the resistance of the sphincter, and the contents pass bit by bit into the stomach. The esophagus may be greatly dilated and elongated (Fig. 4), but, if the level of total motor activity is high, may long remain of normal caliber. The wall of the esophagus often becomes greatly thickened, although just above the LES conspicuous thinning or a pseudodiverticulum may appear. With severe retention, the mucosa and submucosa are often

of this phenomenon and more severe pain and dysphagia are seen when it is associated with diffuse spasm or hiatus hernia. Treatment is based largely on psychophysiologic principles (see Irritable Colon in Ch. 637) if other lesions have been excluded.

ACHALASIA OF THE ESOPHAGUS
(Cardiospasm, Aperistalsis, Megaesophagus)

Definition. Achalasia is a chronic disorder of motility that leads to obstruction at the level of the lower esophageal sphincter (LES). The previously accepted name, cardiospasm, is inappropriate, because the LES ("cardiac" sphincter) not only is contracted with moderately excessive force but also fails to relax normally (achalasia) on swallowing. Moreover, it is clear that peristalsis fails to progress normally through the lower two thirds of the esophagus.

Prevalence, Epidemiology, and Etiology. Although one of the more common causes of esophageal obstruction, achalasia is a relatively rare disease in medical practice in the United States, where no regional, ethnic, or familial predisposition has been recognized. It develops usually in the third to sixth decades, and is rare in children. No environmental factors of etiologic importance are known.

In Latin America, however, an identical disorder occurs endemically among the poor, chiefly in rural districts, in whom an association with Chagas' disease is suggested by epidemiologic and serologic evidence and by characteristic degenerative changes in the myenteric plexus. In such patients the esophageal disorder is often associated with disturbances elsewhere, such as megaureter or megacolon (see Ch. 273).

Pathology and Pathologic Physiology. The fundamental lesion in achalasia is degeneration of the ganglion cells

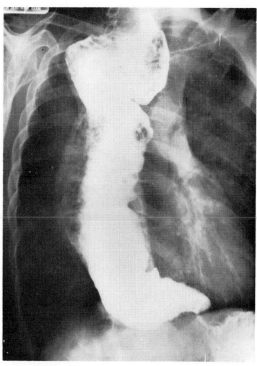

Figure 4. Achalasia. Far advanced changes.

inflamed. Rarely, carcinoma of the lower esophagus appears to be a complication of longstanding megaesophagus. Because patients often lie down before the esophagus empties itself, acute and chronic aspiration pneumonia is a moderately common complication.

Clinical Manifestations. The leading symptom, *dysphagia,* is usually insidious in onset; but in many instances it may begin suddenly and may be intermittent or of variable severity, despite the persistence of the morphologic and physiologic changes in the esophagus. From the beginning, some difficulty will be experienced in swallowing liquids as well as solids. Nevertheless, the patient often learns that he can obtain relief by drinking a liquid after a meal, presumably because the added fluid raises the hydrostatic pressure in the lower esophagus sufficiently to open the sphincter. Substernal *pain* after eating, lasting a few minutes, occurs variably in some patients, apparently because of spasm of the body of the esophagus.

In the more severe and chronic cases, there may be striking *loss of weight* or symptoms of *pneumonia* or lung abscess resulting from aspiration of esophageal contents.

Diagnosis. The symptom of dysphagia should lead promptly to the observation of a barium swallow; in a typical case of advanced achalasia the dilated, elongated, tortuous body of the esophagus, joined by a smooth conical tip to an elongated narrow sphincteric zone, permits easy recognition. Sometimes the disease is suspected because the esophagus produces the shadow of a large paramediastinal mass on plain film of the chest. Even when the esophagus is less strikingly enlarged, fluoroscopic study in the horizontal position will reveal defects in the primary peristaltic wave. Esophagoscopy usually reveals that the sphincter dilates to allow passage of the instrument into the stomach, and thus permits exclusion of an organic stricture. Manometric studies of swallowing and of the response to methacholine (see above) may be of great diagnostic value. In some cases of minimal dilatation of the esophagus, it is impossible to make a clear distinction between achalasia and diffuse esophageal spasm on the clinical and manometric findings.

By these means, achalasia can and must be differentiated from *carcinoma* of the fundus of the stomach or terminal esophagus. In such instances, during endoscopy direct biopsy of the lesion or (better) cytologic study of aspirated contents may reveal neoplastic cells. In *scleroderma* of the esophagus comparable defects in peristalsis are seen in the body of the esophagus, but the LES is most often patent and there is no abnormal sensitivity to methacholine. In *regurgitant esophagitis* the manometric findings are not typical of achalasia, and evidence of regurgitation, of mucosal inflammation, of stricture, or of hiatal hernia is usually obtained by fluoroscopic study, by esophagoscopy, and by measuring the pH of the lower esophageal contents.

Treatment and Prognosis. Initial conservative management is recommended because many patients are able to eat adequately and with minimal distress when freed from stress and emotional tension. The only medication frequently useful is a mild sedative. Anticholinergic drugs, such as atropine sulfate, 0.5 to 1.0 mg, or propantheline, 15 to 30 mg, can prevent or relieve painful spasms of the body of the esophagus, but do not relax the LES. Amyl nitrite inhalation (or glyceryl trinitrite, 0.4 mg sublingually) relaxes the sphincter, but only transiently.

The damage done to the innervation of the esophagus in this disease is, nevertheless, irreversible, and truly effective therapy requires that this be compensated by lasting damage to the sphincter, permitting drainage of the esophagus by gravity. Forcible stretching or rupture of the muscle fibers is accomplished by bougies and other dilators passed and positioned in the sphincter under fluoroscopic control. Although use of the pneumatic or hydrostatic dilators is attended by pain and a small risk of esophageal perforation, lasting relief of dysphagia is obtained in 60 to 80 per cent of patients after one or two treatments. These procedures are recommended for any case of achalasia in which severe dilatation and significant retention are regularly present and in which accurate placement of the dilator is technically feasible.

When adequate dilatation has not been possible or its results have been unsatisfactory, surgical division of the sphincter often becomes necessary. Yet the more radical and successful the destruction of the sphincter, the more likely is the postoperative occurrence of regurgitant esophagitis (discussed later) here worsened by the ineffective clearing of regurgitated material because of defective peristalsis. The most satisfactory compromise appears to be the Heller procedure, in which the muscle of the vestibule is sectioned longitudinally and the mucosa left intact. About 80 per cent of the patients may be expected to remain free from dysphagia, to gain weight, and to escape the symptoms of esophagitis.

Whether the sphincter has been damaged by dilation or by surgery, measures should be instituted to prevent regurgitant esophagitis. The patient should not lie down for one to two hours after eating, straining and chronic coughing should be controlled; and tight corsets should be discarded.

Cohen, S., Lipshutz, W., and Hughes, W.: Role of gastrin supersensitivity in the pathogenesis of lower esophageal sphincter hypertension in achalasia. J. Clin. Invest., 50:1241, 1971.

Ellis, F. H., Jr., and Olsen, A. M.: Achalasia of the Esophagus. Philadelphia, W. B. Saunders Company, 1969.

Kramer, P.: Progress in gastroenterology: The esophagus. Gastroenterology, 54:1171, 1968.

Leading Article: Esophageal dysfunction in diabetes. Br. Med. J., 2:466, 1969.

Pope, C. E., II: The esophagus, 1967–1969. Gastroenterology, 59:460, 1970.

DIAPHRAGMATIC HERNIA, HIATAL HERNIA, AND REFLUX ESOPHAGITIS
(Regurgitant Esophagitis, Peptic Esophagitis)

Definition. Gaps in the diaphragm resulting from congenital defects, relaxation of supporting tissues, or trauma may permit the stomach, colon, or other abdominal organs to herniate into the chest. *Traumatic hernia* may result in acute chest pain, dyspnea, hiccup, vomiting, and shock, usually in association with other internal injuries; on the other hand, large herniations may result but remain asymptomatic, later to be discovered on routine roentgenographic examinations. *Nontraumatic hernia* may be present at birth or delayed until adult life and may involve (1) the pleuroperitoneal hiatus (foramen of Bochdalek), (2) the gap (usually posterior) left by congenital absence of a portion of the diaphragm, and (3) an anterior substernal opening (foramen of Morgagni). By far the most common and clinically important, however, is (4) *herniation through the esophageal hiatus,* a slitlike opening, bounded by muscle bundles from the right crus of the diaphragm, in which the vestibule of the esophagus is normally located, bound in turn to the inferior surface of the diaphragm by the phrenoesophageal ligament. The clinical manifestations of esophageal hiatal hernia are due in large part to one of its complications, reflux esophagitis. Therefore, although the latter is often seen in the absence of a hernia, these conditions are here described together.

Prevalence and Pathology. The true prevalence of hiatal hernia is not known. Because it is essentially a dynamic process, estimates based on autopsies are too low. In roentgenographic surveys it is extremely common, especially in older women. Peptic esophagitis is the most common benign cause of persistent esophageal pain. In about 75 per cent of instances the hernia is of the *sliding* type, in which the esophagogastric junction lies inside the thorax at the apex of the herniated mass. In these a "short esophagus" exists—the result rather than the cause of the herniation; congenital primary short esophagus is exceedingly rare. In 25 per cent the hernia is *rolling* or *paraesophageal,* in which the apex of the herniated mass is some portion of the greater curvature of the stomach. This has rolled upward, medially and anterior to the sphincter, which may remain in its normal position or may be displaced above the diaphragm. (The latter hernia is often called the *mixed* type.) With the sliding and mixed types, mucosal inflammation may be found in the terminal 1 to 5 cm of the esophagus. Early lesions show edema and vascular engorgement and increased thickness of the basal layers of the stratified epithelium; with advancing disease mucosal erosions, hemorrhage, cellular infiltration, and fibrosis appear. In the end, an elongated, smoothly tapered stricture may be found.

Etiology and Pathogenesis. Normal closure of the esophagogastric sphincter in the face of increases in intra-abdominal pressure is maintained chiefly by the neural and hormonal adaptive mechanisms of the sphincter itself. Earlier emphasis upon the muscular sling provided by the right crus of the diaphragm and upon the short intra-abdominal segment of the esophagus as contributors to the closing mechanism has been offset by convincing evidence that the sphincter can remain competent when totally displaced into the thorax. *Thus the hiatal hernia is no longer considered essential to the production of reflux esophagitis.* The resting pressure and the adaptive increases in pressure in the LES may be reduced by a number of mechanisms which inhibit gastrin release (for example, acid in the pyloric antrum or anticholinergic drugs) or augment the release of secretin or cholecystokinin (for example, fatty meals). For other reasons, smoking and ingestion of alcohol also diminish sphincter tone. On the other hand, any sustained or recurrent influence which increases the intra-abdominal pressure (pregnancy, obesity, ascites, coughing, retching, weight lifting) may determine the frequency and severity of regurgitation and the probability of hiatal hernia formation. The pressures generated within a hernia and the probability of associated reflux esophagitis appear to be the greater, the *smaller* the hernia. Once inflammation occurs in the terminal esophagus, sustained contraction of its musculature raises the local pressure and reflexly diminishes the pressure within the (more distal) sphincter, thus accentuating the reflux.

Reflux esophagitis also occurs in other settings: (1) in prolonged use of intragastric tubes, especially postopera-

tively; (2) after operative disturbance of the diaphragmatic crura or the esophagogastric sphincter; (3) in scleroderma, in which the sphincter is immobilized by inflammation; and (4) in chalasia of infants, in which innervation of the sphincter is retarded. It can occur in the absence of hydrochloric acid or, indeed, of the stomach; it is likely that bile salts have a primary injurious effect. (See Gastroduodenal Syndromes in Ch. 636.)

Hemorrhage in cases of hiatal hernia is believed to arise either from the inflamed esophagus or from the hernial sac itself. Usually it is due to multiple erosions, but when severe it can often be traced to a discrete ulcer in the engorged mucosa of the herniated stomach.

Clinical Manifestations. The majority of hiatal hernias are virtually or wholly asymptomatic, and the most common problem for the physician is to judge whether this condition is in fact responsible for the complaints of the patient. There is no relation between the severity of symptoms and the size of the hernia unless, as some suggest, pain is *inversely* related to size.

In the absence of complications, *pain* usually is described as a dull, early postprandial, retrosternal fullness, disappearing spontaneously after a few minutes to one hour; it is often associated with belching or hiccup. It is often worse on lying down or on exertion after heavy meals; sometimes it radiates to the back, the jaws, the shoulders, and down the inner aspects of the arms, closely simulating angina pectoris. Particularly with large hernias, and with displacement of thoracic structures, there may be dyspnea, palpitation, or cough.

The earliest manifestation of esophageal reflux is usually *heartburn.* It is worse after heavy meals, on lying down, and on bending forward, as in tying a shoe; conversely, it is often improved by sitting or standing upright, by draughts of any liquid, and by ingestion of an effective antacid. With development of true esophagitis the pain becomes more severe, lasts longer, and is worsened by irritating food and drink of all kinds. Still later, dysphagia appears, worse for solid foods, and as it progresses the development of a severe stricture may be indicated by some amelioration of the heartburn.

Hemorrhage may take the form of acute hematemesis and melena or chronic blood loss. In the latter instance, the stools are usually not discolored and are only intermittently positive for occult blood, and the presenting manifestation may be a sideropenic anemia of unknown cause. Neither in acute nor in chronic hemorrhage should hiatal hernia or reflux esophagitis be accepted as the cause until a search has been made for other potential sources.

Diagnosis. The positive diagnosis of hiatal hernia rests usually upon roentgenographic findings or upon such findings considered together with clinical manifestations. With large hernias, the recognition above the diaphragm of a portion of the stomach, marked by its coarse rugae (Fig. 5), is usually simple. Diagnosis of the smaller sliding hernias depends upon precise location of the esophagogastric junction and the demonstration of reflux by fluoroscopy and cineradiography, and is aided by tilting the head downward and by the Valsalva maneuver. Rarely, the displacement of the sphincter upward into the chest may be recognized at esophagoscopy or by manometric techniques.

In the presence of a hiatal hernia or other predisposing cause, the existence of *reflux esophagitis* should be suspected when there is recurrent or persistent heartburn or otherwise unexplained, usually mild, upper gastroin-

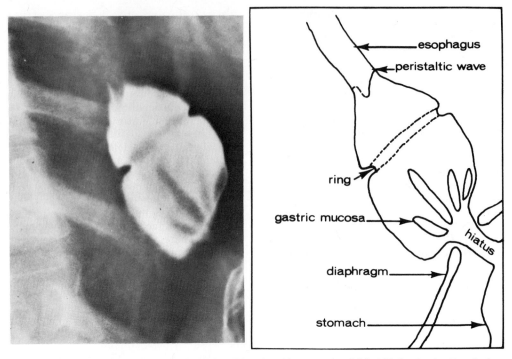

Figure 5. Roentgenogram of a small sliding hiatal hernia, with an associated Schatzki ring (contraction ring).

testinal bleeding. Esophagoscopy and biopsy may reveal epithelial thickening, deep rete pegs, and inflammation of the mucosa, but negative findings do not exclude the diagnosis. Esophagitis may rarely be due to *syphilis* or *tuberculosis,* or, more commonly, to *candidiasis,* particularly in children or debilitated adults with concomitant thrush (see Ch. 266). The regurgitation of gastric juice can be confirmed by aspiration of lower esophageal contents and measurement of its pH, with the patient supine. It may be helpful to infuse into the lower esophagus 0.1N HCl at the rate of 10 ml per minute for 30 to 60 minutes or until pain is experienced (Bernstein test). Reproduction of the pain by this means strongly supports the diagnosis of reflux esophagitis.

Strictures of the lower esophagus resulting from chronic peptic esophagitis must be differentiated from those due to lye or other corrosive poisons, to prolonged intubation, to foreign bodies, or to congenital stenosis or atresia, as well as from carcinoma or achalasia.

As it is capable of causing substernal pain radiating to the shoulders and arms, hiatal hernia may enter importantly into the differential diagnosis of angina pectoris, myocardial infarction, dissecting hematoma of the aorta, gallbladder disease, pancreatitis, and the "splenic flexure syndrome." Patients frequently exhibit two or more of these disorders simultaneously; management therefore requires thorough clinical and laboratory study and judgment based upon careful and repeated inquiry into the setting in which the attacks occur.

Treatment. In the conservative treatment of hiatal hernia, control of symptoms is attempted through the frequent feeding of small meals, the reduction of weight, and the removal of other causes of increased intra-abdominal pressure. Thus efforts are made to control chronic coughing, to reduce effort in defecation, and to eliminate bending forward, as in scrubbing floors or weeding gardens. No food should be taken for three hours before retiring, and the head of the bed should be elevated 10 inches on blocks. With symptoms of reflux esophagitis, the diet should be reduced in fat content, use of alcohol and tobacco should be interdicted or drastically reduced, and a nonabsorbable antacid such as Maalox or Aludrox should be given in dosage of 15 to 30 ml *immediately* after each feeding. The antacid is used in this instance not so much to buffer gastric acid as to heighten the endogenous release of gastrin. For the same reason, anticholinergics are held to be contraindicated. Except in the presence of esophageal stricture, no restriction of dietary residue is required.

The vast majority of symptomatic cases of hiatal hernia and early reflux esophagitis will be relieved by careful adherence to the aforementioned regimen. Frequent recurrence of substernal pain, heartburn, or dysphagia under these conditions is a clear indication for more radical measures. These are directed at repair of the hernia and the relief of lower esophageal obstruction.

In most instances, surgical reduction of the hernia and reconstruction of the hiatus, performed through either the abdomen or the posterior thorax, is the treatment of choice. If an early esophageal stricture exists, it may be necessary preoperatively to pass metal bougies of gradually increasing diameter over a previously swallowed string as a guide. Because the sacrifice of the esophagogastric sphincter is an invitation to postoperative recurrence of esophagitis, surgical resection of the strictured zone is regarded as a measure of last resort. In recent years the interposition of a loop of jejunum or descending colon between the resected esophagus and the fundus of the stomach has seemed to prevent or delay this complication, but the precise value of this procedure has not yet been determined.

The results of surgical repair are usually excellent in rolling hernias, but only about 80 per cent successful in controlling symptoms of the sliding hernia. With fundoplication and other procedures which firmly anchor the LES within the abdomen, despite present questions as to their rationale, recurrence rates as low as 7 per cent have been reported.

LOWER ESOPHAGEAL RING

In many elderly patients, roentgenographic study of the lower esophagus reveals a symmetrical, annular, shelflike constriction a few centimeters above the diaphragm (Fig. 5). The diameter of the ring may be as small as 5 to 10 mm; yet its detection requires careful fluoroscopy or cineradiography, with the esophagus well distended with barium. It usually lies below the esophagogastric sphincter, at the junction of esophageal and gastric mucosa; it is often associated with hiatus hernia.

In some such patients, attacks of severe lower substernal pain occur acutely on swallowing large and poorly chewed boluses that become lodged in the ring. Relief is afforded in some cases by bouginage and in others by actual cutting of the ring.

Edwards, D. A. W., et al.: Symposium on gastroesophageal reflux and its implications. Gut, 14:233, 1973.
Pope, C. E., II: Reflux esophagitis. *In* Sleisenger, M. H., and Fordtran, J. S. (eds.): Gastrointestinal Disease. Philadelphia, W. B. Saunders Company, 1973, pp. 430–449.
Schatzki, R., and Gary, J. E.: The lower esophageal ring. Am. J. Roentgenol. Radium Ther. Nucl. Med., 75:246, 1956.
Wilkins, E. W., Jr., and Skinner, D. B.: Medical progress: Surgery of the esophagus. N. Engl. J. Med., 278:824, 887, 1968.

636. DISORDERS OF GASTRODUODENAL MOTILITY

The motility of the stomach and the duodenum may logically be considered together, because these two organs have the common purpose of mixing the food with digestive juices and as the interaction of these two segments is considerable.

On the ingestion of food, initially a small amount is propelled through the stomach into the duodenum, after which the pylorus appears to close and the body of the stomach to dilate progressively as the remainder of the meal enters from the esophagus. After a period of nonpropulsive churning movements, a series of peristaltic waves appears, beginning at or slightly above the antrum and carrying through the pylorus to the second portion of the duodenum. Under normal conditions the stomach is emptied in this manner, after which peristalsis ceases.

The pyloric sphincter is stimulated to contract, and gastric emptying is retarded, by the instillation into the duodenum of fat, of solutions of hydrochloric acid, of hypertonic sodium chloride or glucose, or of amino acids. These effects are believed to be mediated by secretin and cholecystokinin, which stimulate the sphincter when injected intravenously, and the action of which is opposed by endogenous or exogenous gastrin. Thus a form of servomechanism exists, regulating the rate of gastric emptying and, under normal conditions, limiting the

regurgitation of duodenal contents into the stomach in the process of digestion.

GASTRODUODENAL SYNDROMES

Disturbances in this motor pattern have been correlated with a number of important digestive symptoms. Vigorous gastric peristalsis in the absence of food has long been associated with normal *hunger*. The sensation of *nausea*, on the other hand, is clearly accompanied by cessation of gastric phasic contractions and simultaneous sustained contraction or spasm of the descending portion of the duodenum. The resulting gradient of pressure and the open pylorus lead to duodenogastric regurgitation, with exposure of gastric and even esophageal mucosa (as the esophagogastric sphincter is often simultaneously relaxed) to the irritant action of bile acids as well as to pancreatic enzymes. This phenomenon can be totally asymptomatic, but in many instances can be correlated with the syndrome of *dyspepsia* (mild epigastric distress, early satiety, abdominal distention, belching, heartburn, and bitter regurgitation). Further, it has been demonstrated to occur with significantly increased frequency in patients with irritable colon, duodenal ulcer, gastric ulcer, and cholelithiasis; and it is considered of probable etiologic significance in chronic gastritis, gastric ulcer, and reflux esophagitis.

Vomiting. Whether or not preceded by nausea, the mechanism of vomiting involves close coordination of visceral and somatic movements. The gastric fundus and corpus are flaccid, the antrum and the proximal duodenum strongly contracted, and the esophageal vestibule (cardia) relaxed. The pharyngoesophageal sphincter is likewise relaxed, the glottis closed, and the larynx and soft palate elevated. At the moment of emesis the diaphragm forcibly descends and the abdominal wall contracts, squeezing the flaccid stomach and causing ejection of its contents. All this activity is triggered by the vomiting center in the floor of the fourth ventricle on chemical, humoral, reflex neural, or psychic stimulation. Persistent vomiting is most readily treated by drugs that depress this center or the vestibular apparatus, or both. The most effective short-term medication is a phenothiazine such as prochlorperazine, 5 to 10 mg (or promethazine, 12.5 to 25 mg) three times a day. For more prolonged use meclizine, 25 to 50 mg daily (or cyclizine, 50 mg), is safer and may be effective.

The Mallory-Weiss Syndrome. This signifies the hematemesis or melena that follows typically upon many hours or days of severe vomiting and retching, and that is traceable to one or several slitlike lacerations of the mucosa, longitudinally placed at or slightly below the esophagogastric junction. These lacerations may extend to or even through the muscularis, with rupture of blood vessels mainly in the submucosa. They are attributed to incoordination of the act of emesis, resulting from fatigue of the vomiting center and consequent forcible distention of the cardiac portion of the stomach while the vestibule remains contracted. Although usually recognized only at autopsy, the characteristic history of hematemesis that follows prolonged vomiting, usually after alcoholic indulgence, may often lead to the detection of these lesions by emergency esophagoscopy. Supportive medical treatment is indicated unless the threat of exsanguination makes emergency surgery mandatory.

Aerophagia. Aerophagia, or the swallowing of air, is

well nigh universal at meal times, though differing widely in degree. Its symptomatic results include belching, epigastric pain or fullness related to distention of the stomach, pain in the right lower quadrant, or in the right or left upper quadrant associated with distention of various parts of the colon, and the passage of flatus by rectum. All these symptoms, or any one of them, may be signified by the term *flatulence* or "gas." As aerophagia is for the most part a compulsive habit and a manifestation of emotional tension, it should be treated as such. The patient's consciousness of the habit can be increased by having him hold a tongue blade between his teeth, thus making swallowing much more difficult.

Acute Gastric Dilatation and Volvulus. Aerophagia may lead to serious overdistention of the stomach under two conditions: (1) during complete or partial *paralytic ileus* (see Ch. 637) after surgery, trauma, or acute medical conditions, when *acute gastric dilatation* may occur; and (2) in *torsion* or *volvulus* of the stomach, in which the most dependent portion of the greater curvature rotates forward, upward, and to the left. Under both conditions the rise in intragastric pressure may lead to increased gastric secretion and congestion of the gastric wall. The upper abdomen on examination is distended and tympanitic; a plain roentgenogram of the abdomen reveals the greatly enlarged gastric air bubble, which in volvulus characteristically presents a broad, smooth upward convexity beneath the left diaphragm.

Milder degrees of distention may give rise only to a feeling of pressure and pain in the epigastrium and left hypochondrium, relieved at times on change of position leading to escape of the gas by belching or, after traversing the intestines, on passage of flatus. In such cases decompression by stomach tube and constant suction of gastric contents should give prompt relief. Prevention of recurrences may demand effective treatment of aerophagia (see above).

In some instances of severe distention or torsion, a large volume of potassium-rich fluid is lost to the gastric lumen from the extracellular space, and the gastric circulation is impaired to the point of necrosis of the gastric wall, with resulting muscular weakness, severe shock, and death if the process is unchecked. In such cases, rapid parenteral repletion of extracellular water and electrolytes, followed by operative intervention, may be lifesaving.

PYLORIC STENOSIS

Definition. Pyloric stenosis, broadly defined, is any obstruction of the pyloric canal. What is commonly called pylorospasm is actually only the failure of relaxation of the sphincter in the absence or diminution of antral propulsive waves. True spasm of the pylorus, especially in adults, is usually associated with nearby duodenal or gastric ulcer or severe gastritis, and is to be differentiated from infiltration of the wall with inflammatory cells, fibrous tissue, or malignant cells.

Congenital hypertrophic pyloric stenosis is an obstructive narrowing caused by thickening of the pyloric muscle, possibly resulting from immaturity of enzymatic mechanisms in its intrinsic ganglion cells. It occurs in up to 3 per 1000 live births, four times more frequently in male than in female infants, and apparently as the expression of a single dominant gene. Never found before the fifth day of life, it is influenced also by multiple environmental factors affecting early infant feeding.

Clinical Manifestations. Typically, an infant between the ages of ten days and three months develops projectile vomiting, constipation, dehydration, and rapid loss of weight. Curiously, the appetite is well preserved, and feeding may be resumed immediately after vomiting. The vomitus may contain blood but no bile. Inspection after a feeding may reveal visible peristaltic waves passing from left to right across the upper abdomen. In many instances a firm tumor mass, 1 to 2 cm in diameter, is felt a few centimeters below the costal margin at the external margin of the right rectus muscle. Roentgenograms after a barium meal indicate gastric dilatation and a symmetrically narrowed, elongated pylorus.

In those patients not treated surgically (see below), attacks of nausea and vomiting occur at intervals for many years, sometimes throughout life. Rarely, such attacks begin in adult life and lead to the discovery of an identical hypertrophy of pyloric muscle.

Treatment. Initially an infant with this disorder is continued on breast milk or a formula yielding soft curds, supplemented with thick cereals. It may be necessary to make up deficits of water and electrolytes parenterally. Traditionally, atropine sulfate (0.06 mg) is given before each feeding, but the value of anticholinergics is not clearly documented. Phenobarbital (8 mg) may be combined to good effect with each dose of atropine. In most instances, as soon as dehydration has been corrected and acid-base balance restored, a Ramstedt operation (pyloromyotomy) should be performed. This requires a longitudinal incision that severs all the circular muscle fibers of the pylorus, leaving the mucosa intact. Although the mortality rate of this procedure is from 1 to 5 per cent, permanent cure is the rule.

In older children and adults, initial treatment of presumed pyloric stenosis should be the same as for peptic ulcer with obstruction (see below). Anticholinergics should not be used. During this interval the possible diagnosis of gastric cancer is studied by cytologic and gastroscopic means, and that of pyloric or duodenal ulcer by repeated roentgenographic examination. Unless the obstruction disappears completely within four to six weeks, it should be relieved surgically by pylorotomy or gastrojejunostomy.

MEGADUODENUM

The term *megaduodenum* is applied to gross dilatation of the duodenum from its upper end to the middle of the transverse portion. No point of true stenosis is to be found. The muscularis is hypertrophic, but the myenteric ganglion cells are damaged or absent. Although physiologic studies are so far lacking, the pathogenic mechanism is considered to be aperistalsis, comparable to the disorder in congenital megacolon, with which it is sometimes associated. A similar phenomenon has been observed in certain cases of South American trypanosomiasis (Chagas' disease), in which megacolon and megaesophagus may also be present.

This form of obstruction of the lower duodenum is to be differentiated from stenosis caused by malignant disease at the same site and from "superior mesenteric ileus," in which the transverse duodenum appears to be compressed between the lumbar vertebrae and the superior mesenteric artery near its origin from the aorta. Treatment is by duodenojejunostomy.

Barnett, W. O., and Wall, L.: Megaduodenum resulting from absence of the parasympathetic ganglion cells of Auerbach's plexus. Ann. Surg., 141:527, 1955.

Carter, C. O.: The inheritance of congenital pyloric stenosis. Br. Med. Bull., 17:251, 1961.
Jones, F. A., and Gummer, J. W. P.: Clinical Gastroenterology. Oxford, Blackwell Publications, Ltd., 1960, pp. 102–117.
Swenson, O.: Pediatric Surgery. 2nd ed. New York, Appleton-Century-Crofts, 1962, pp. 262–270.

637. DISORDERS OF INTESTINAL MOTILITY

Among the significant disorders of intestinal motility, some are adaptive mechanisms of general occurrence among persons under stress. Paralytic ileus and the irritable colon are both here interpreted in this light. These interrelated disorders are presented in the following pages, together with mechanical obstruction of the intestine, so often important in differential diagnosis.

Other disorders are thought to be due to excessive stimulation by humoral agents. These are the metastatic carcinoid syndrome and the diarrhea seen in patients with medullary carcinoma of the thyroid. Still others are known to be related to defects in the efferent cholinergic nerves regulating intestinal motility *(megacolon),* or thought to result from defects in the afferent limb of intestinal reflex arcs *(diabetic pseudotabes; tabes dorsalis).*

NORMAL COLONIC FUNCTION

The human colon has two main functions: (1) the absorption of water and crystalloids, and (2) the formation of a reservoir to permit the orderly and convenient evacuation of feces. The daily delivery from the ileum of 0.5 to 1.0 liter of liquid intestinal contents is regulated by the valvelike ileocecal sphincter, the tone of which is diminished by gastrin concurrently with its stimulation of ileal propulsive motility. In the colon the luminal contents are subjected over long periods to slow phasic contractions, kneading or accordion-like movements, which facilitate absorption. During this time the colon is sacculated or haustrated in outline. At long intervals, usually after the ingestion of food, this pattern of motility is replaced by one of *mass peristalsis,* in which haustra disappear, the proximal portions contract and the distal ones relax, and the entire colon undergoes shortening. In this manner feces are advanced rapidly.

The rectum is usually empty until part of the contents of the sigmoid is forced into it by mass peristalsis. This distends the rectal walls, produces discomfort in the sacral area, and initiates the defecation reflex by which the contraction of skeletal muscles of the abdominal wall and the coordinate relaxation of the anal sphincter assist in the emptying of the terminal colon. Voluntary inhibition of the reflex can be achieved by vigorous contraction of the external sphincter and a thoracic pattern of breathing. With time the walls of the rectum become adapted to the fecal mass; their tension decreases, and the stimulus to defecation subsides until renewed by further additions to the rectal contents.

DIARRHEA

Definition. Diarrhea signifies the passage of excessively liquid or excessively frequent stools. Never a com-

plete diagnosis in itself, its recognition demands careful study to determine its cause. Its duration and course vary widely, depending upon the natural history of the underlying disease.

Etiology. The causes of diarrhea are legion, and are best considered in relation to underlying pathogenetic mechanisms, briefly outlined as follows:

Excessive Intraluminal Volume. In these conditions excessive ingestion of food or fluid is only a minor factor, and fluid accumulations are due chiefly to one of the following:

1. *Decreased absorption of water and solute* (osmotic diarrhea), including that resulting from saline cathartics, lactase deficiency, sprue, postgastrectomy syndrome, and congenital chloridorrhea.

2. *Increased secretion into the lumen,* of which the classic model is cholera. Recent evidence makes clear that the same mechanism is active in infections with enteropathogenic *E. coli* and other gram-negative organisms, as well as with peptide hormone-producing tumors (medullary carcinoma of thyroid, islet cell tumors). It is mediated by or reproduced by the action of prostaglandins on the production of cyclic AMP by adenyl cyclase in the intestinal epithelium. Abnormal secretion into the *colonic* lumen is characteristic of diarrhea caused by ileal disease or ileal resection, resulting from the action of excess bile acids on colonic mucosa, as well as of the diarrhea of villous adenoma of the colon or rectum.

Exaggerated Propulsive Motility. Exaggerated propulsive motility, mediated by neurohumoral factors, including acetylcholine, serotonin (5-HT), and prostaglandins, may be an independent and important variable. The most common example is the irritable colon syndrome. Excessive 5-HT, as produced in the malignant carcinoid syndrome, produces hyperperistalsis of the small bowel, with often severe diarrhea (see below). Mild increases in stool frequency occur in thyrotoxicosis. Local increases in intraluminal pressure caused by partial obstruction of the intestine by tumors, strictures, or fecal impactions lead to exaggerated propulsive activity and to diarrhea.

In many inflammatory or neoplastic diseases of the bowel, more than one of these mechanisms are thought to be operative at one time. The main practical advantages in considering them lie in general orientation of differential diagnosis and in utilization of the oral route for repletion of body fluids in cholera-like syndromes.

Differential Diagnosis. The formidable task of identifying the one or the several causes of diarrhea in a given patient can be facilitated by efforts to estimate, in succession, the *location,* the *mechanism,* and the *nature* of the disease process. The location is suggested by the character of the stools and the zone of reference of pain. If each stool is *large* in volume, it may be presumed that the distal colon is reacting as it would to an enema and is itself not diseased, and therefore that the chief site of the disorder is in the proximal colon or small intestine. In such instances, any accompanying pain is usually referred to the periumbilical area or the right lower quadrant. On the contrary, if some stools, though attended by notable urgency, are of *small* size, the conclusion is justified that the distal colon does not tolerate accumulation of a normal amount of feces, and therefore that it is diseased. In such instances, the stool is more likely to contain visible mucus or flecks of blood, and pain is felt in the lower abdomen or the sacral region. With respect to the *mechanism,* osmotic diarrhea should cease if oral intake is interrupted for 24 hours or more. The *nature* of the disease process is estimated from its manner of onset and course over time; history of exposure to toxic, infectious, and allergenic agents; the extent of debility; and the personality and life situation of the patient. The diagnostic study of the patient usually includes sigmoidoscopy, gross and microscopic examination of the stools and cultures for pathogenic bacteria, barium enema, and small bowel x-rays, in the order named. Other useful laboratory tests are mentioned elsewhere under the specific diseases.

Treatment. It is frequently necessary to mitigate the diarrhea or its consequences before the recognition of the true cause permits specific therapy. In most acute infectious diarrheas, the disease is brief, and the diarrhea serves a useful purpose in ridding the body, at least subtotally, of the offending agent. Hence, the first indication is to replace the losses of fluid and electrolytes, usually with infusions of physiologic saline and 5 per cent glucose, guided by measurements of urinary output and plasma volume. Replacement of potassium and further adjustments of acid-base balance are guided by serial determinations of serum sodium, potassium, chloride, and bicarbonates. If oral administration is possible, water, sodium chloride, and glucose should be forced through dilute sweetened fruit juices, tea, and salty broths in sufficient quantity to maintain a urinary output of in excess of 1500 ml per day. Cold liquids and concentrated sweets are poorly tolerated.

Lying flat in bed, with constant use of heating pad or hot water bottle, is usually helpful. Most of the conventional binding agents, such as bismuth, pectins, and kaolin, are of a low order of effectiveness. Aluminum hydroxide gel in large doses (20 to 40 ml four times a day) is often useful. Codeine sulfate, 0.03 to 0.06 gram, or morphine sulfate, 0.008 to 0.015 gram, may be given every three to four hours during acute diarrhea, but will produce severe distention and cramps in most instances. The synthetic opiate, diphenoxylate hydrochloride, carries apparently less risk of addiction and is often effective in doses of 5 to 10 mg three times daily before meals and at bedtime. Camphorated tincture of opium (paregoric) is used in doses of 4 ml after each bowel movement until diarrhea is controlled. In prescribing any of these agents, the physician assumes the responsibility for eventually freeing the patient from dependence upon them.

Fordtran, J. S.: Diarrhea. *In* Sleisenger, M. H., and Fordtran, J. S. (eds.): Gastrointestinal Disease. Philadelphia, W. B. Saunders Company, 1973, p. 291.

Phillips, S. F.: Absorption and secretion by the colon. Gastroenterology, 56:966, 1969.

CONSTIPATION
(With Emphasis on Habitual Constipation or Rectal Constipation)

Definition. Constipation ordinarily signifies the passage of excessively dry stools or the evacuation of the bowels less often than every other day. By many patients, however, the same term is used to refer to a sense of incomplete emptying of the rectum or to the small size of their stools.

Pathogenesis. Inadequate propulsion of feces may result from mechanical obstruction (as in carcinoma of the sigmoid colon), from diminished contractions of the prox-

imal intestine, e.g., paralytic ileus, or from failure of the distal colon to relax, e.g., irritable colon and congenital megacolon. In most instances, however, constipation results chiefly from failure of the defecation reflex (habitual constipation, rectal constipation, or dyschezia).

Early in childhood, despite great variations in the intensity of "toilet training," the habits of defecation become subject to complex patterns of conditioned reflex behavior. Their disruption in adult life is usually associated with major changes in the pattern of living, e.g., travel or going away to school, with intercurrent illness, with emotional tension, or with willful neglect. The mechanical efficiency of defecation may be impaired by the use of high toilet seats, bedpans, or other departures from the primitive squatting position. Weakness of the muscles of the back or of the abdominal wall caused by neurologic disorders or by multiple pregnancies is occasionally an important factor. Failure of relaxation of the anal sphincter may be due to neighboring painful lesions such as anal ulcers or thrombosed hemorrhoids. These are, however, more often a result of the constipation than a cause.

Prolonged retention in the rectum (or rarely in the sigmoid colon) results in excessive dehydration or *impaction* of feces. This may lead to cramping lower abdominal pain and to paradoxical diarrhea, as watery brown stools are passed around the hardened mass. Many patients with constipation complain also of anorexia, bloating, belching, passage of flatus, headache, malaise, weakness, or faintness. Such symptoms are related in part to the attendant disturbances of intestinal motility and in part to the anxiety aroused by the constipation itself.

Diagnosis. In any constipated patient who has not recently been given an enema or a laxative, the finding of more than a few grams of feces on digital examination of the rectum indicates that habitual constipation is present. (Conversely, the usual finding in irritable colon or in megacolon is an empty rectum.) The search for localized anal and rectal lesions should be made carefully with both anoscope and sigmoidoscope. In most instances a barium enema, and in some an upper gastrointestinal roentgenographic series, is indicated to exclude intrinsic intestinal disease. Careful thought should be given to the possible etiologic importance of constipating medications such as opiates, anticholinergics, ganglionic blocking agents, tricyclic antidepressants, and nonabsorbable antacids. Search should be made for systemic diseases such as myxedema, hyperparathyroidism, lead poisoning, scleroderma, and mental depression, of which constipation may at times be the presenting symptom.

Management. The goal of treatment is an empty rectum, or the maximal possible restoration of normal habits of defecation, with minimal disturbance of normal intestinal motility. In bedridden patients, or in others whose daily habits are greatly disrupted, this must be postponed, and an effort is made to avoid fecal impaction by tapwater enemas or mild laxatives at one- or two-day intervals. Any painful anal lesion such as an ulcer or thrombosed hemorrhoid should be treated at once with sitz baths, local anesthesia by ointments or suppositories, and nightly mineral oil. Fecal impactions should be digitally broken, softened by a retention enema of cottonseed oil (150 ml) or dioctyl sodium sulfosuccinate (5 ml of a 1 per cent solution diluted to 90 ml in water), and evacuated by enemas of tapwater or soapsuds.

The cooperation of the patient is enlisted through explanation of the mechanisms of his constipation and of the goal of therapy. He must be persuaded that a daily bowel movement is desirable but not necessary. A large breakfast is prescribed, to contain fruit, cereal, toast or rolls, preserves, and coffee or milk. His diet should be high in vegetable fiber. He is required to sit on the toilet daily within the hour after breakfast, remaining ten minutes, and to distract his attention by a newspaper, magazine, or other device. All previous cathartics or enemas are forbidden; in their place a rounded teaspoon of a hydrophilic colloid (psyllium or agar) is taken with 400 ml of water at bedtime and again on arising. Mineral oil, 15 to 45 ml at bedtime only, may be substituted.

The patient is warned that one to four weeks are required for the achievement of desired results and that his bodily discomfort may in the meantime increase. When relief of this distress is needed, at intervals of two or three days, an enema of tapwater or of prepared hypertonic solutions (Travad, Clyserol, Fleet) is taken after the morning toilet visit. As normal habits are restored, the enemas and mild laxatives are cancelled; they may be recommended for future prophylactic use when the patient's habits of living are again disturbed.

Miner, R. W. (ed.): The colon: Its normal and abnormal physiology and therapeutics. Ann. N.Y. Acad. Sci., 58:293, 1954.

Rakatansky, H., and Kirsner, J. B.: Drugs for gastrointestinal diseases. *In* Modell, W. (ed.): Drugs of Choice, 1972–73. St. Louis, C. V. Mosby Company, p. 321.

IRRITABLE COLON
(Mucous Colitis, Spastic Colon, Unstable Colon, Adaptive Colitis)

Definition. Irritable colon signifies a variety of disturbances of colonic function that accompany emotional tension and participate in the general bodily adaptation to nonspecific stress.

This disorder is considered to account for more than 50 per cent of all gastrointestinal illness, and ranks with the common cold as one of the leading causes of recurrent minor disability.

Symptoms and Their Mechanisms. *Abdominal pain* of some degree occurs in most patients. It is usually located in the hypogastrium or left lower quadrant; it is commonly felt in the other quadrants of the abdomen but very rarely in the periumbilical region. In some instances severe pain is felt far laterally over the left costal margin and radiates to the precordium, the left shoulder, and the inner aspect of the left arm (the *splenic flexure syndrome*). In most instances, the pain of irritable colon is relieved by the passage of feces or gas. Hence it is believed to be due to distention or spasmodic contractions of the colon at various points (explaining its variable location). *Constipation* is probably related to heightened nonpropulsive activity (spasm), chiefly in the sigmoid colon, and *gaseous distention* of the proximal colon and *passage of flatus* are commonly associated. *Diarrhea* of varying severity may occur, together with urgency and tenesmus, usually in the morning before and after breakfast. Commonly the *stools are small,* whatever their consistency (hence the term "irritable colon"); they often contain visible *mucus,* or mucus alone may be evacuated with no fecal residues. Diarrhea and myxorrhea appear to represent the motor and secretory response of the colon to exaggerated cholinergic stimulation.

Extracolonic symptoms, often encountered in these patients, emphasize the generalized character of the body's adaptive response. Thus *anorexia, nausea, belching,* and *occasionally vomiting* indicate a concurrent disturbance of gastroduodenal motility. The syndrome of *neurocirculatory asthenia,* including palpitation, shortness of breath, precordial discomfort, and fatigue on mild exertion, is often present. *Headache* is common, and sweating, flushing, faintness, sighing respirations, and hyperventilation may be noted.

Natural History and Pathogenesis. This disorder may begin at any age, but usually in early adult life or in adolescence. Its course is extremely variable, but in most instances individual episodes of illness can be measured in terms of days, weeks, or months. In many persons the predominant symptoms are pain and constipation, in others painless diarrhea; but irregularly alternating constipation and diarrhea are not uncommon. There is rarely any significant dehydration or loss of weight.

The onset and recurrences of irritable colon usually coincide with periods of life stress and emotional conflict, and the symptoms often disappear spontaneously when these influences abate. Relevant disturbances of colonic function have been observed in the laboratory when emotional conflicts have been induced in patients through stressful interviews (Fig. 6) and have appeared

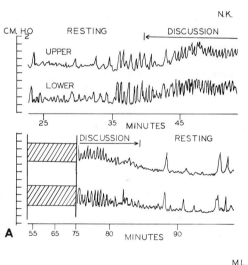

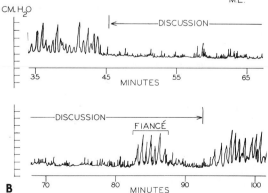

Figure 6. *A,* Heightened nonpropulsive contractions of sigmoid colon during stress interview in subject with spastic constipation. (Tandem balloons.) *B,* Reduced phasic activity of sigmoid colon during stress interview in a subject with functional diarrhea. (Single balloon.)

as normal bodily manifestations of emotion, not unlike blushing and weeping. The emotional state accompanying constipation has been described as one of assertive independence, defensiveness, or self-confident resistance to a noxious situation. The attitudes commonly observed with diarrhea are those of dependence, helplessness, and self-reproach. These impressions have been consistent in both clinical and laboratory studies. The pathways by which these reactions are mediated probably include the central and peripheral portions of the autonomic nervous system, as comparable disturbances have been produced transiently by administration of methacholine or neostigmine. It is probable that other chemical mediators, such as serotonin and cholecystokinin and other intestinal hormones, are involved.

Diagnosis. The diagnosis of irritable colon must be based upon (1) the recognition of characteristic symptoms, (2) the exclusion of other disease processes suggested by the symptoms, and (3) repeated and conscientious testing of the hypothesis that the symptoms are related to life and stress and emotional tension. On examination of the patient one commonly finds a palpable, tender sigmoid colon, enlarged areas of tympany over the proximal colon, and proctoscopic signs of mucosal engorgement, spasm, and excessive mucous secretion; yet none of these findings is specific for the disease or is a significant departure from the normal. The condition cannot be diagnosed, but may be suggested, by roentgenographic examination of the colon.

The syndrome of irritable colon may be mimicked very closely by *abuse of cathartics;* by *specific infections* of the colon such as amebiasis, shigellosis, or lymphogranuloma venereum; by *allergy* to ingested food or drugs; and by intolerance of *specific disaccharides,* particularly lactose. The differentiation from early *ulcerative colitis* or from *carcinoma of the colon* can usually be made by proctoscopy, biopsy, and barium enema. Differentiation from *diverticular disease* may be more difficult, because the symptoms and motor disturbances of the colon in this disease closely resemble those of irritable colon, and the two conditions may coexist or be interrelated (see Ch. 639).

Broadly, irritable colon must be differentiated from all the various causes of abdominal pain, constipation and diarrhea. Of particular note, the pain of *gallbladder disease* may be simulated by gaseous distention of the hepatic flexure, the pain and tenderness of acute or chronic *appendicitis* by distention of the cecum, and the migration of pain to the precordium in the "splenic flexure syndrome" may simulate *angina pectoris* or *myocardial infarction.*

Because of the ubiquity of stress and emotional tension, symptoms of irritable colon may be superimposed upon those of other and more serious diseases, or may reflect the anxiety occasioned by them. Careful consideration of the significance of each process is required, lest a carcinoma go undetected or the removal of a symptomless gallbladder prove useless in the relief of unrelated abdominal distress.

The establishment of a diagnosis of irritable colon on positive grounds depends upon a profound understanding of the social history and personality of the patient. As the process of acquiring this understanding is of both diagnostic and therapeutic value, it is described under the heading of Management.

Management. The recognition of irritable colon as a bodily reaction to stress calls for treatment directed to the patient as a whole rather than to his colon. As in the relief of blushing or weeping, both the environment and the attitudes of the patient must be considered.

At the first visit, the patient is called upon for a brief autobiography, including his relations with parents, marital partner, employers, and others. His speech and expression are observed for evidences of emotion, and topics of special meaning for him are thus usually easily recognized. The several visits required for adequate laboratory investigation and early symptomatic management provide opportunities for further discussion of these topics. Careful note is made of the dates of important events, so that a "life chart" may be constructed, correlating these with the course of bowel symptoms.

After several visits, such a procedure permits the reasonably certain acceptance or rejection of the diagnosis of irritable colon on the positive grounds of coincidence with life stress and correlation with emotional tension. A decision should then be made as to the prognosis and needs for future therapy. Those patients whose episodes of illness appear but *little related in time to easily recognizable stress situations* and who have made a uniformly inadequate adjustment to major personal problems may be considered the "more neurotic" group. The further efforts of the physician are best limited to reassurance regarding the benign character of the illness, manipulation of important environmental factors, explanations to responsible relatives, sympathetic listening, and the conscientious use of placebos.

On the other hand, the "less neurotic" patient who has made a satisfactory adjustment to most life situations, whose bowel symptoms are intermittent and closely related in time to specific difficulties, e.g., new job or marital problem, can often profit by relatively brief and simple psychotherapy in the hands of the general physician. This begins with *reassurance* as to the absence of serious disease and usually a simple explanation of his illness as an expression of emotional tension. He is urged to ventilate his feelings to the physician or members of his family or friends, or to sublimate them through more active and vigorous pursuit of sports, games, or hobbies. He is encouraged to make his own changes in ways of living as a result of the insight acquired.

A patient with irritable colon should be referred to a psychiatrist if his emotional tension is severe and out of proportion to his bowel disorder, if he seems psychotic, if he requires expert manipulation of psychotropic drugs, or if he declares his need of such help.

Concurrently, symptomatic management may be required. The most common problem is habitual *constipation,* which should be treated as outlined above. With *diarrhea* the usual binding agents are ineffective. The most rational therapy is an anticholinergic drug in sufficient dosage to dry the mouth, i.e., propantheline, 15 to 30 mg, or tridihexethide, 25 to 50 mg. This should not be given continuously but in anticipation of the hours of more severe diarrhea, usually in the early morning or just prior to social or business engagements. In some cases, diphenoxylate hydrochloride, 5 mg three times daily before meals and at bedtime, is indicated and is more effective. In view of the chronic and benign nature of the illness, use of opiates, even on a temporary basis, is rarely desirable. Severe abdominal *pain* is best relieved by a hot water bottle or a warm tapwater enema.

Sedatives, tranquilizers, and antidepressants may be required to deal with extreme degrees of anxiety and insomnia. Their use should be guided by the principles set forth in Ch. 321 and 336, and they should not be routinely prescribed for patients with irritable colon. The most convenient "placebo" is tincture of belladonna in doses of 10 to 15 drops in water three times daily before meals.

Prognosis. The "more neurotic" patients, as defined above, may be expected to have symptoms of varying severity, mitigated only temporarily by the solicitude of the physician or favorable life situations. The "less neurotic" should have symptoms at long intervals, reduced in frequency and severity, but rarely abolished, by a high degree of insight and alteration to their environment.

Almy, T. P.: Experimental studies on the irritable colon. Am. J. Med., 10:60, 1951.
Chaudhary, N. A., and Truelove, S. C.: The irritable colon syndrome. Quart. J. Med. (N.S.), 31:307, 1962.
Hislop, I. G.: Psychological significance of the irritable colon syndrome. Gut, 12:452, 1971.

INTESTINAL OBSTRUCTION
(Ileus)

Definition. Intestinal obstruction is broadly defined as any impairment, arrest, or reversal of the normal anad flow of intestinal contents. This concept thus includes obstruction caused by mechanical factors and that caused by failure of peristalsis for reasons of deficient neural stimulation (paralytic ileus) or vascular insufficiency.

Etiology. The majority of severe cases are due to *mechanical factors* that locally occlude the intestinal lumen. The most common of these are extramural, constricting the entire circumference of the gut, and include *hernias* (especially inguinal and femoral), peritoneal *adhesions* caused by previous operations or local inflammatory disease, and *volvulus* (usually of the sigmoid or ileocecal regions). *Mural thickening* resulting from disease or congenital defect of the intestinal wall may narrow or obliterate its lumen; examples are benign and malignant tumors; inflammatory strictures caused by diverticulitis, regional enteritis, or previous operative anastomoses; and congenital atresia or imperforate anus. Least common are *intraluminal* factors, including fecal impactions, meconium, foreign bodies, intussusception, gallstones, and large worms.

Another large group of cases is due to general or regional *failure of peristalsis (adynamic ileus)*. This may occur after any abdominal operation and in many severe, acute diseases such as pneumonia and myocardial infarction. It is an impressive feature of many painful conditions in the thoracolumbar area, such as renal and biliary colic, retroperitoneal hematoma, or spinal injuries, but is most severe in the presence of peritonitis. An initially identical picture may result from *ischemia* of the bowel wall caused by *vascular insufficiency*.

In many cases more than one of these mechanisms play a part. Thus, postoperative adynamic ileus may lead to volvulus and subsequent ischemia of the twisted loop. The possible combination of mechanical and physiologic factors calls for periodic reconsideration of the diagnosis in individual cases.

Pathogenesis. Whatever the etiologic mechanism, the immediate effect of ileus is to interrupt the normal pathways of intestinal propulsion and absorption of liquid and gas. *Even in the absence of oral intake,* 7 to 10 liters of water and contained solutes (net flux) enter the upper gastrointestinal tract each day, most of which is to be ab-

sorbed at lower levels. In intestinal obstruction, this cycle is interrupted. Even if vomiting does not occur, this liquid is withdrawn from the body fluid compartments to lie in the intestinal lumen. The result is dehydration, loss from extracellular fluid of sodium and chloride ions, alkalosis, and shift of potassium ion from intracellular to extracellular fluid to compensate for loss of potassium into the gut. Hypovolemia and hypokalemia may lead to acute renal insufficiency, even in the absence of arterial hypotension. Hypokalemia itself further inhibits peristalsis.

Stasis within the gut leads to multiplication of its bacteria, absorption of indoles and other of their metabolic products, and accumulation of gas produced by bacterial action and air swallowing. The resultant distention of the gut leads to dangerous increases in intraluminal pressure, especially in closed-loop obstructions caused by hernia or volvulus, or in complete occlusion of the colon, in which the contents are trapped proximally by the ileocecal valve. Mucosal blood flow is reduced by this increased pressure, as well as by torsion of, or extrinsic pressure upon, the mesenteric vessels. As the gut wall becomes necrotic, plasma proteins and blood exude into the lumen, and bacterial toxins gain access to the peritoneum and the circulating blood.

Mechanical obstruction of the small intestine is usually first indicated by epigastric or periumbilical colicky *pain* and *vomiting*. Early examination of the abdomen may reveal increased tympany but little distention, and the *bowel sounds* are characteristically hyperactive, high-pitched, and coincident with the episodes of pain; the higher the obstruction, the more frequent and severe the pain and the higher the expected pitch of the sounds. Loose stools and flatus may be passed before obstipation sets in. With lower sites of obstruction, distention is more prominent and vomiting may be delayed in appearance, and may resemble dilute feces in odor and appearance—the result of bacterial proliferation related to stasis in the small bowel lumen. In later stages the bowel sounds may become less active, and the development of continuous pain, increasing tenderness to direct pressure and rebound, rigidity of the abdomen, and signs of hypovolemia warn of strangulation of the bowel. Fever is a late and unimpressive feature.

In *paralytic ileus* distention and obstipation are the prominent symptoms, vomiting is less marked, and colicky pain is absent. Early auscultation of the abdomen often reveals absent bowel sounds (none in a period of three minutes or more).

In *colonic obstruction* distention is usually prominent, and pain, often delayed in onset, with less frequent paroxysms, is located either in the hypogastric area (with left colon lesions) or in the epigastrium and right upper quadrant (with disease of the right colon). Bowel sounds are low pitched and less frequent. Vomiting is delayed and often feculent. Rectal examination may reveal unchanged blood or a palpable mass. Previous pelvic surgery, as opposed to abdominal surgery, suggests a colonic rather than a small intestinal site of obstruction. The signs of strangulation (see above) may be evident in the initial examination.

Laboratory Findings. Early in the course, the fluid shifts are manifested by diminished urinary output, fall in serum chloride and potassium, and rise in plasma bicarbonate and pH and in the blood urea nitrogen. As these abnormalities worsen, the hematocrit may rise, and urinary specific gravity and osmolality may become fixed. With strangulation the peripheral leukocyte count rises, far out of proportion to the body temperature.

Early and repeated *roentgenographic examination* of the abdomen is essential. Films taken of the patient in the horizontal position aid in localization of the obstruction in the small or large intestine. Typically, marked gaseous distention of centrally located, horizontal small intestinal loops produces a "ladder" appearance, with no colonic gas. In closed loop obstruction of the colon with a competent ileocecal valve, only the laterally located, haustrated colonic segments are gas filled. With cecal or sigmoid volvulus, characteristically large distended sacs, without mucosal folds, are seen. In paralytic ileus, gas may be found anywhere in the gut, including the stomach and rectum. Films taken in the upright or lateral decubitus positions reveal fluid levels which indicate the degree of accumulation of fluid and gas; the latter is relatively *less* prominent as strangulation develops. Cautious performance of a barium enema, without preparatory cleansing of the bowel, is often indicated in localizing a point of colonic obstruction, but barium or other contrast media should never be given by mouth.

Treatment. The effective management of cases of intestinal obstruction calls for frequent re-evaluation of the status of the patient by clinical and laboratory methods and modification of the therapeutic plan to deal with the changing conditions thus discerned. The cardinal principles of therapy are *replacement* of metabolic losses, *decompression* of the intestine, and *removal of the cause* of obstruction.

Intake of fluid and food by mouth is suspended, and an infusion of equal parts of 0.9 per cent sodium chloride and 5 per cent dextrose in water is begun. As soon as the adequacy of renal function can be estimated or the serum potassium level has been reported, potassium chloride should be added to the infusion and delivered at a rate not exceeding 40 mEq of potassium per hour. An electrocardiogram should be taken before therapy; repeated observation of the T waves and S-T segments can serve, along with repeated determinations of serum potassium and chloride, to gauge the effectiveness of replacement. In the presence of severe dehydration, associated hemorrhage, or signs of strangulation, the central venous pressure, arterial pressure, urinary output, and hematocrit should be monitored, and administration of water, electrolytes, albumin, and whole blood should be adjusted accordingly. When strangulation is suspected, antimicrobial drugs are used in the manner recommended for cases of vascular occlusion.

Decompression of the mechanically obstructed intestine may be largely achieved by nasogastric intubation and constant suction. If this fails, and in all cases of paralytic ileus, the long balloon-tipped intestinal tube (Miller-Abbot or Cantor type) should be passed, with repeated roentgenographic verification of its position. Such a procedure will greatly diminish the symptoms of the patient, but will not benefit his fluid and electrolyte depletion, and may render less clear the signs of strangulation. For this reason, intubated patients must be carefully observed, and, if local tenderness and leukocytosis are not diminished after 24 to 36 hours, surgical intervention is required.

Removal of the cause of ileus requires *operation* in most cases of complete mechanical obstruction and in many cases of severe adynamic ileus. It must be postponed in all instances until dehydration, electrolyte loss,

and shock have been overcome; but, in the face of evident strangulation or closed loop obstruction of the colon, it must be accomplished as rapidly as possible. Just before operation, intensive antimicrobial therapy should be started; penicillin, 1 to 2 million units, and streptomycin, 1 gram, should be given in divided doses daily; or ampicillin, 0.5 to 1.0 gram every six hours. The surgical procedure depends upon the findings at laparotomy and the judgment of the surgeon, particularly as to the viability of the bowel.

Some cases of volvulus tend to right themselves on conservative management, permitting later surgery at a time of election, and rare cases of ileocolic intussusception in childhood are relieved by the intracolonic pressure exerted by a barium enema.

Prognosis. The outlook for recovery from intestinal obstruction depends chiefly upon the presence or absence of strangulation and its consequent toxemia, and the presence or absence of renal insufficiency resulting from excessive loss of fluid and electrolytes. These are in turn influenced by the type, location, and degree of obstruction, the existence of related primary disease (such as peritonitis leading to paralytic ileus), and the extent of delay in initiation of effective therapy. For persons recovering from ileus, the outlook for recurrence depends upon the underlying causes; with most patients with mechanical obstruction who recover without emergency operation, the probability of recurrence is so great as to dictate interval elective surgery.

Miller, L. D., Mackie, J. A., and Rhoads, J. E.: The pathophysiology and management of intestinal obstruction. Surg. Clin. North Am., 42:1285, 1962.

Neely, J., and Catchpole, B.: Ileus: The restoration of alimentary-tract motility by pharmacological means. Br. J. Surg., 58:21, 1971.

Silen, W., Hein, M. F., and Goldman, L.: Strangulation obstruction of the small intestine. Arch. Surg., 85:121, 1962.

PSEUDO-OBSTRUCTION OF THE COLON

Pseudo-obstruction is a rare disease of unknown etiology, manifested by episodes of ileus of both large and small bowel. Its usual onset is in early life. Its course is rarely acute, being more commonly a relapsing one over periods of 3 to 20 years. Histologic study of bowel wall reveals mild round-cell inflammation and fibrosis of the mucosa and submucosa, with normal ganglion cells. Motility of the colon and of the upper small bowel is reduced on manometric examination.

The symptoms include poorly localized abdominal cramps, distention, vomiting, mild diarrhea, and some signs of malabsorption. Bowel sounds are reduced, and plain x-rays of the abdomen reveal distended loops with air-fluid levels anywhere in the bowel, including the rectum. The disease is distinguished from scleroderma of the intestine by its earlier onset, absence of skin changes or Raynaud's phenomenon, and lack of striking therapeutic benefit from broad-spectrum antimicrobials.

During acute phases, supportive therapy is provided by nasogastric suction, parenteral fluid replacement, and ampicillin, 4.0 grams per day intravenously. The prognosis for the recurrent form of the disease is poor.

Maldonado, J. E., Gregg, J. A., Green, P. A., and Brown, A. L., Jr.: Chronic idiopathic intestinal pseudo-obstruction. Am. J. Med., 49:203, 1970.

MEGACOLON

The persistent enlargement of all or a long segment of the colon to a diameter greater than 5.5 cm is referred to as *megacolon.* This disorder may be acquired or congenital in origin, and may or may not involve permanent defects in intrinsic innervation of the bowel.

Psychogenic megacolon, or stool-holding, is a common disorder of children after the first year of life. The desire to avoid pain on defecation leads to retention of impacted feces and involuntary soiling. A similar process occurs in adult psychotic patients, mainly with depression, and is complicated by treatment with phenothiazines and tricyclic antidepressants. Treatment is by disimpaction, large and repeated doses of mineral oil, and, in the adult, repeated cleansing enemas.

Similar *acquired colonic dilatation* may accompany the severe constipation of myxedema or lead poisoning, the mural infiltration of scleroderma or amyloidosis, the neurologic deficits of diabetes or parkinsonism, or long-standing incomplete obstruction of the sigmoid or rectum. In *Chagas' disease* (South American trypanosomiasis) megacolon is found as a late complication, owing to destruction of the ganglia of Auerbach's plexus by the tissue reaction to the parasite. The mechanism of this colonic disorder, as well as of its sometimes associated megaesophagus, megaduodenum, or megalobladder, is similar to that of congenital megacolon, as described below.

CONGENITAL MEGACOLON
(Idiopathic Megacolon; Hirschsprung's Disease)

Definition. Congenital megacolon is a chronic disorder of intestinal motility, usually beginning in infancy, characterized by aganglionosis of the distal bowel, and resulting clinically in severe and unremitting constipation.

Etiology and Pathology. Congenital megacolon occurs once in 2000 births, more commonly in male children, and with significantly increased frequency in sibs. The basic lesion is a congenital absence of myenteric ganglion cells in a distal segment of the colon, with neighboring autonomic nerve fibers increased in number or size. The aganglionic segment may be located just inside the anal margin or may extend upward a variable distance into the rectum and sigmoid, or less often as high as the distal ileum. Because its muscle is persistently contracted, it presents a functional obstruction to the passage of feces. This narrow, usually empty segment connects by a short conical portion with a greatly dilated, more proximal segment. The dilated segment has normal myenteric ganglia, hypertrophic muscular coats, and normal propulsive activity; it is usually filled with putty-like feces. Several lines of evidence now suggest that the basic defect is a failure of development of intramural nonadrenergic inhibitory neurons, which migrate downward during embryonic life from a point of entry in the upper esophagus. Megaloureter, megalobladder, Down's syndrome, and cardiac septal defects may be associated congenital anomalies.

Clinical Manifestations. Many patients will have had an episode of intestinal obstruction in the first few days of life. After a remission of several weeks or months there is the gradual return of severe and continuous constipation, sometimes with occasional vomiting. The abdomen progressively enlarges, the costal margin flares, and colonic peristalsis may be plainly visible. Nutrition is poor and growth may be retarded. A mild anemia is common. Neonates and infants may develop pseudo-

membranous enterocolitis or perforation of the colon or the appendix.

Diagnosis. A plain roentgenogram of the abdomen may reveal the fecal retention as a large ovoid mass mottled by small irregular gas shadows. The diagnosis is supported, and differentiation made from acquired megacolon, by demonstration of a distal narrow segment of colon on barium enema, best seen in the lateral position. Pressure studies of the anal canal reveal a failure of the normal relaxation of the internal sphincter on distention of the rectum. Final diagnosis presently requires demonstration of absent ganglia on open biopsy of the wall of the narrowed rectum, performed per anum under general anesthesia. The diagnosis, however, can often be excluded by the finding of submucosal ganglion cells on suction biopsy of the rectum.

Treatment and Prognosis. Except in neonates, the much greater frequency of acquired than of congenital megacolon dictates a trial of therapy (see above) for the former condition before the aforementioned diagnostic measures are instituted.

In a small minority of cases of true megacolon with a very short aganglionic segment near the anus, the colon can be successfully emptied by the daily use of laxatives (magnesia magma, cascara, or senna) and enemas of physiologic saline or soap suds. Rarely, such a patient grows to early adulthood in a fair state of health, but with continuous dependence on these measures.

All the remainder of the cases require surgical relief. The procedure of choice is the resection of the aganglionic segment, with division of the internal anal sphincter and with end-to-end anastomosis of the normally innervated upper colon to the stump of the rectum just inside the anus (Swenson's "pull-through" procedure). Histologic study of the segment removed is necessary to ensure that the anastomosis has been made to normally innervated bowel. If this condition is satisfied, the results are lasting and almost uniformly excellent.

Davidson, M., Kugler, M. M., and Bauer, C. H.: Diagnosis and management in children with severe and protracted constipation and obstruction. J. Pediatr., 62:261, 1963.

Ehrenpreis, T.: Hirschsprung's Disease. Chicago, Year Book Medical Publishers, 1970.

Passarge, E.: The genetics of Hirschsprung's disease. N. Engl. J. Med., 276:138, 1967.

Schnaufer, L., et al.: Differential sphincteric studies in the diagnosis of anorectal disorders of childhood. J. Pediatr. Surg., 2:538, 1967.

Swenson, O.: Congenital megacolon. Pediatr. Clin. North Am., 14:187, 1967.

DIABETIC DIARRHEA

Definition. Persistent or episodic watery diarrhea in patients with diabetes represents a now well-defined functional disorder best referred to as diabetic diarrhea. It occurs infrequently, even among diabetics; its importance lies in the social disability imposed by the symptoms and in the availability at times of striking benefits from therapy.

Etiology and Pathogenesis. This disorder is most frequent among those whose diabetes has been poorly controlled by therapy and is complicated by neuropathy, particularly by other signs of visceral neuropathy, i.e., impotence, urinary incontinence, defects of sweating, pupillary abnormalities, gastric atony, and orthostatic hypotension. Degenerative changes in autonomic ganglia and in dorsal nerve roots have been occasionally observed at postmortem examination. The clinically evident disturbances in motility of the bowel are believed to be associated with defective innervation. The observation of dramatic improvement in some cases with the use of antimicrobial therapy (see below) has indicated that the diarrhea may be due to bacterial overgrowth in the small bowel.

Clinical Manifestations. The diarrhea in this disorder usually occurs in the form of severe and explosive attacks lasting one to a few days each, and separated by periods of either normal bowel function or constipation of variable severity. Less often, diarrhea is continuous. Movements characteristically are associated with great urgency, often waking the patient from sleep, and the penalty for sound sleep is often fecal incontinence. The stools are voluminous, watery, brown, and foul; they only rarely contain gross blood. The attacks are associated with little pain, and usually do not lead to serious dehydration or shock.

Physical examination reveals little except collateral evidence of peripheral or autonomic neuropathy (see above) or of the ocular or vascular complications of diabetes. Gastrointestinal roentgenograms may show atony and delayed emptying of the stomach; the small intestine appears normal in pattern, but passage time may be greatly accelerated or delayed. Chemical examination of the stools may or may not reveal an excess of fat, and the pancreatic juice is normal in volume and enzyme content.

The diagnosis should be suspected whenever explosive watery diarrhea recurs or persists, especially with nocturnal attacks of fecal incontinence. The probability is increased by the finding of neuropathy. The diabetes is not always clinically apparent or previously recognized.

Treatment. Control of the diabetes (maintenance of normal weight through adequate diet and insulin, freedom from ketosis, minimal glycosuria and hyperglycemia) is sufficient to eliminate or substantially diminish the symptoms in about half the cases. Standard medicaments for symptomatic control of diarrhea, including anticholinergics and opiates, are generally ineffective. The tetracyclines have been shown to terminate attacks in a few cases within an hour of the ingestion of a single dose, e.g., tetracycline, 250 mg. When diarrhea occurs frequently or continuously, the same dose may be given once daily or even once weekly (see Part XIV, Section Three).

Prognosis. Even without therapy, this disorder is not progressive in severity, but attacks may be expected to recur with variable frequency over many years or even decades. Severe electrolyte disturbances or dietary deficiencies seldom result. Health and survival are usually limited instead by the other complications of diabetes.

Malins, J. M., and Mayne, N.: Diabetic diarrhea. Diabetes, 18:858, 1969.
Whalen, G. E., et al.: Diabetic diarrhea. Gastroenterology, 56:1021, 1969.

638. GASTROINTESTINAL ALLERGY AND FOOD INTOLERANCE
(Food Idiosyncrasy)

Introduction. The gastrointestinal mucosa is rich in lymphocytes and plasma cells and is exposed to a myriad of potential antigens in food, in drugs and other chemicals, and in microorganisms, resulting in a great variety of antigen-antibody reactions. In addition, it apparently has the capacity to form and react with autoantibodies, as has been postulated in atrophic gastritis. Any and all clinical phenomena resulting from antigen-antibody reactions in the intestinal wall are connoted by the term *gastrointestinal allergy,* and these may include some aspects or some cases of established disease entities of uncertain or variable etiology, e.g., ulcerative colitis. The term *food allergy,* on the other hand, includes all manifestations of hypersensitive reactions to ingested foods, many of which, e.g., urticaria, are in tissues other than the intestine. *Food intolerance* or *food idiosyncrasy* connotes a variety of gastrointestinal disorders attributed in whole or in part to nonallergic mechanisms incited by specific foods or properties of foods.

Pathogenesis and Symptoms. The mucosa is slightly permeable throughout life to whole proteins, but markedly so in the neonatal period, when sensitization of its lymphatic tissue is most likely to occur. Probably as a result of this, many asymptomatic persons have circulating serum precipitins to proteins of cow's milk, hen's eggs, and other foods. Sensitization to chemicals and drugs may occur at any age and may be occult, as when milk from penicillin-treated cows is ingested. In a minority of those sensitized, later exposure to an antigen may give rise to reactions in the gut mucosa characterized pathologically by edema, vascular engorgement, ecchymoses, erosions, excessive mucous secretion, and often spasmodic muscular contractions. The resulting symptoms vary in nature and in time of onset with the segment of gut affected, but commonly include abdominal pain, nausea and vomiting, diarrhea, and mucoid stools. Urticarial eruptions and wheezing may be associated; and in severe cases hematemesis, melena, purpura, arthralgias and prostration may occur. In such acute cases recovery is usually prompt and complete, but in others of more insidious onset the course of symptoms is prolonged and highly variable.

Management. The presumptive diagnosis of intestinal allergy often can be made from a careful history, establishing a consistent temporal relationship between exposure to antigen and onset of symptoms. This impression, the more convincing if a single foodstuff is involved, can be confirmed prospectively by a food diary and notation of the time of symptoms, and then can be tested by elimination and reintroduction of the suspected allergen. The latter is best accomplished without the patient's knowledge, by stomach tube or by admixture with barium given for gastrointestinal roentgenograms, permitting (with suitable controls) observation of the motor effects of contact with the allergen. The gastric or colonic mucosa may be directly viewed by endoscopy after exposure to suspected antigens and to control materials. These methods can give valid information if practiced with great care. Skin tests, levels of serum antibodies, and changes in circulating leukocytes are of little value. According to present evidence, the levels of antibodies in the stool or in intestinal secretions (coproantibodies) more closely reflect antigen-antibody reactions in the gut mucosa, and may be diagnostically useful.

Once an offending antigen is recognized, its removal should constitute effective treatment, provided all sources of the antigen can be identified. Food additives, insecticides, and bread molds are examples of sources often difficult to eliminate. In some conditions, e.g., hypersensitivity to milk protein in ulcerative colitis, reaction to the exogenous antigen may constitute but one of many pathogenic factors in the disease, and the results of total exclusion are of doubtful value.

Differential Diagnosis. The symptoms of gastrointestinal allergy are nonspecific and may be mimicked by a wide range of gastrointestinal disorders, most commonly food poisoning and the irritable colon.

Many other reactions to ingestion of food are based on either nonallergic or questionably allergic mechanisms. The inconsistency in the clinical responses to exposure to the postulated food stimulus is based both on variations in the other influences on intestinal function and on the need for a threshold amount of the offending substance to evoke a clinically evident reaction. Some food idiosyncrasies are clearly *spurious* in that they are not, on repeated careful testing, consistently enough evoked by the suspected food. Intolerance of *roughage* is truly rare, and of probable significance only with marked stenosis of the esophagus, the large or small bowel, an abdominal stoma, or the anus. It should be remembered that food residues constitute only one third to one half of the bulk of the stool. Often certain foods are poorly tolerated because of previous *conditioning,* having been eaten under conditions of anxiety, depression, or disgust. In other instances, *motor disturbances* are brought about by physiologic mechanisms, such as the delayed emptying of the stomach (and feeling of fullness) after a fatty meal, and the osmotically induced distress of the postgastrectomy "dumping" syndrome (see Ch. 643).

Most clearly recognized nonallergic mechanisms of intolerance are related to defects of *digestion* and *absorption.* Gastric achylia may be manifested by a distaste for meat, and pancreatic achylia by steatorrhea on ingestion of fat. Intolerance of wheat, rye, and barley appears to be due to deficiency of a peptidase in the jejunal mucosa (*gluten enteropathy*—see Part XIV, Section Three), and intolerance of milk seems most often due to *deficiency of intestinal lactase* or, in some infants, *sensitivity to cow's milk proteins,* with resulting steatorrhea and severe electrolyte depletion. In the latter instance it is still not clear whether the intolerance is due to hypersensitivity or to defects in peptidase activity. Aside from lactase deficiency, bloating of the abdomen commonly attends the ingestion of beans and other legumes, apparently because of *bacterial fermentation of their nonabsorbable carbohydrates,* such as raffinose. Bloating that follows the eating of onions and cabbage appears to be due to their content of flavone compounds which directly inhibit intestinal motility. Considering the many unknowns in the chemistry of foods, many other nonallergic mechanisms must await discovery.

Sensitivity to cow's milk proteins occurs in about one of every 200 neonates, and is manifested chiefly by watery diarrhea, often with mucus and occasionally with rectal bleeding. There is often a family history of concurrent appearance of eczema, urticaria, or other allergic phenomena. The child fails to gain weight, has edema, and is found to have iron deficiency anemia, eosinophilia, hypoproteinemia, and positive tests for occult blood in the stool. In some infants an acute ulcerative colitis is found, with friable, bleeding, and acute inflamed rectal mucosa. The syndrome is dramatically relieved by elimination of milk and recurs with resumption of milk feedings.

Eosinophilic gastroenteritis is a rare but well defined clinicopathologic entity, in which one or several areas of the bowel, usually the stomach and small intestine, are the sites of infiltration with eosinophils, and in which the patient experiences intermittent nausea, vomiting, diarrhea, and abdominal pain after ingestion of specific foods. There is usually a history of hay fever, asthma, urticaria, or some other allergic disorder; eosinophilia of peripheral blood is common, and skin tests are often positive for suspected allergens. Protein-losing enteropathy, low serum immunoglobulins, and malabsorption are observed in many cases.

In patients with mainly mucosal involvement, upper gastrointestinal x-rays show nodular mucosal surfaces, and multiple suction biopsies of stomach and jejunum reveal a patchy eosinophilic infiltrate, sometimes with villous atrophy. This form must be distinguished from gluten enteropathy, connective tissue disorders, and protozoan or helminthic diseases of the bowel. In others, involvement chiefly of the muscular layers leads to polypoid or infiltrative thickening of the gut wall, the roentgenographic appearance of which resembles carcinoma, lymphoma, or Crohn's disease. *Eosinophilic granuloma* usually presents as an obstructing tumor mass at or near the pylorus in a patient lacking a clear-cut allergic history or a significant eosinophilia. Diagnosis prior to histopathologic examination is virtually impossible. Rarely, subserosal involvement gives rise to ascites with high eosinophil counts in the fluid.

Treatment is first attempted by elimination diet, but often requires temporary or chronic use of corticosteroids (e.g., prednisone, 20 to 30 mg daily for ten days, then tapered or discontinued). The eosinophilic granuloma is excised surgically.

Greenberger, N., and Gryboski, J. D.: Allergic disorders of the intestine and eosinophilic gastroenteritis. *In* Sleisenger, M. H., and Fordtran, J. S. (eds.): Gastrointestinal Disease. Philadelphia, W. B. Saunders Company, 1973, pp. 1066–1082.

Ingelfinger, F. J., Lowell, F. C., and Franklin, W.: Medical progress—gastrointestinal allergy. N. Engl. J. Med., 241:303, 1949.

Klein, N. C., Hargrove, M. D., Sleisenger, M. H., and Jeffries, G. H.: Eosinophilic gastroenteritis. Medicine, 49:299, 1970.

Taylor, K. B., and Truelove, S. C.: Immunological reactions in gastrointestinal disease: A review. Gut, 3:277, 1962.

Waldmann, T. A., Wochner, R. D., Laster, L., and Gordon, R. S.: Allergic gastroenteropathy. N. Engl. J. Med., 276:761, 1967.

639. DIVERTICULA OF THE INTESTINAL TRACT

Saccular outpouchings of the wall of the gut occur at all levels from the hypopharynx to the sigmoid colon and are known collectively as *diverticula.* With the single exception of Meckel's diverticulum, all appear to be acquired herniations of mucosa and submucosa through defects in the muscular layers, often clearly the result of excessive intraluminal pressure (pulsion diverticulum) and sometimes with clear-cut evidence of disordered or incoordinate motor activity in the adjacent bowel.

ESOPHAGEAL DIVERTICULA

Most diverticula of the esophagus occur at one of three locations, and at each of these the lesion has distinctive features.

Hypopharyngeal (or Zenker's) diverticulum is an evagination of the mucosa and submucosa directed posteriorly between the lower margin of the inferior constrictor muscle of the pharynx and the upper border of the cricopharyngeus muscle. It is considered a *pulsion* diverticulum, resulting from sharply localized increase in pressure at this point, when swallowing occurs without perfectly coordinated relaxation of the pharyngoesophageal sphincter. It is usually seen in men over 50 years of age, and enlarges progressively downward to the left of the cervical spine, eventually displacing and compressing the upper esophagus. Symptoms include dysphagia for both liquids and solids; regurgitation with aspiration of food and coughing, chiefly at night; and, ultimately, loss of weight. The sac may sometimes be felt as a mass in the left side of the neck, but is usually first identified on a lateral roentgenogram of the barium-filled pharynx and upper esophagus. Small diverticula usually require no treatment; when dysphagia and weight loss have been severe, the patient should be repleted by tube feeding and the diverticulum surgically resected in one stage, with myotomy of the pharyngoesophageal sphincter.

The *midesophageal* diverticulum is usually located at the level of the bifurcation of the trachea, and extends anteriorly and laterally from the esophagus; its orifice is wide. Its formation is often attributed to the contraction of adherent inflammatory tissue (usually tuberculous lymph nodes), but disordered esophageal motility may also be present. It usually causes no symptoms, and is recognized by its roentgenographic appearance.

The *epiphrenic* diverticulum, rarest of the three, is located a few centimeters above the vestibule and is thought to result from the high pressures of incoordinate contractions in achalasia, diffuse esophageal spasm, or reflux esophagitis. The symptoms and indicated management are usually pertinent to these associated conditions.

GASTRIC DIVERTICULA

Diverticula of the stomach are rare, and are chiefly of two types. The *juxtacardiac* diverticulum, accounting for three fourths of all cases, is found 2 cm below the cardia on the posterior wall of the stomach. Unassociated with any other gastric disease, it is usually asymptomatic but has been incriminated as a cause of recurrent epigastric pain and, rarely, of hemorrhage or perforation. Its identity can be verified on barium x-rays or on gastroscopy by its characteristic location and pliable wall. The *juxtapyloric* diverticulum, accounting for most of the remainder of cases, is the result of pressures resulting from ulceration, inflammation, surgical reconstruction, and the healing of these processes. Differentiation from active ulcer or carcinoma may require gastroscopy, biopsy, and cytologic examination of the gastric contents.

DIVERTICULA OF THE SMALL BOWEL

Diverticula of the small bowel are relatively common, especially in the elderly. Their frequency decreases from the pylorus to the ileocecal junction. Diverticula of the duodenum have been reported in 2 to 22 per cent of unselected cases at autopsy. In most instances they are found on the lesser curvature of the duodenum and the mesenteric border of the jejunum, at the sites of defects in the muscular wall through which major blood vessels (or the common bile duct) penetrate. In the duodenum they more often number but one or a few, whereas in the jejunum they are commonly multiple. Heterotopic gastric or pancreatic tissue is sometimes recognized in their walls. They are usually found as an unexpected and clinically silent abnormality on barium roentgenographic studies. In a minority of patients with duodenal diverticula, abdominal pain, nausea, vomiting, and weight loss may occur without other explanation. In a few, hemorrhage, obstructive jaundice, perforation, and peritonitis may be seen. The same complications may rarely be observed in jejunal diverticula, wherein bowel obstruction is sometimes due to inflammatory stricture or muscular thickening. Of particular interest is the association of a form of malabsorption syndrome (a variant of the "blind loop syndrome") with jejunal diverticula, in which stasis of intestinal contents has permitted massive bacterial overgrowth (see Part XIV, Section Three). Otherwise, in the absence of complications, no treatment is required; in severely symptomatic cases, surgical resection is warranted.

Meckel's diverticulum is a common developmental anomaly of the ileum, found in 0.3 to 2.0 per cent of the population, and represents the persistence of the stalk of the fetal yolk sac. It may remain attached to the umbilicus by a fibrous cord or (very rarely) by a patent sinus, and is almost always found 2 to 3 feet above the ileocecal junction on the antimesenteric border. Its wall includes all the layers of the intestine, including the muscularis; its mucosa often contains islands of heterotopic gastric, pancreatic, or colonic glands. Although the majority of these pouches are clinically silent, symptoms may arise in a number of ways: (1) intestinal obstruction, with periumbilical cramps and vomiting, may be caused by intussusception or by volvulus around the fibrous attachment to the umbilicus; (2) impaction of intestinal content may lead to inflammation and ischemic necrosis, both pathologic and clinical features closely resembling those of acute appendicitis; and (3) peptic ulceration may result from the secretion of heterotopic gastric glands, including parietal cells, with resulting pain and often perforation or severe hemorrhage in the form of brick red or mahogany stools. In 60 per cent of instances these symptoms occur before the age of ten; hence this anomaly figures importantly in the differential diagnosis of abdominal pain, the acute abdomen, intestinal obstruction, intestinal bleeding, and peritonitis in childhood.

DIVERTICULAR DISEASE OF THE COLON
(Diverticulosis)

The presence of multiple herniations of the mucosa and submucosa of the colon through the circular muscle layer is commonly referred to as *diverticulosis*. This condition, recognizable during life only at laparotomy or on barium roentgenographic studies, probably affects 20 per cent of the American population over the age of 40 years. Although the majority of those harboring diverticula suffer no ill effects or only moderate discomfort, about 20 per cent may develop inflammatory complications *(diverticulitis)* (see Ch. 654). The entire spectrum of disorders associated with these pouches is connoted by the term *diverticular disease of the colon.* These diverticula are easily distinguished from the "wide-mouthed diverticula" of the colon seen in progressive systemic sclerosis (scleroderma).

Prevalence. Both diverticulosis and diverticulitis vary greatly in prevalence in different countries. In North America and northern Europe, the frequency is extremely high, as indicated above; it is approximately 40 times more common than in certain native, nonwhite populations in developing tropical countries. The condition is exceedingly rare below the age of 35, and its prevalence rises steeply as age advances.

Morbid Anatomy and Pathogenesis. A typical diverticulum is a small pouch, the fundus of which measures 3 to 25 mm in diameter, lying beneath the serosa and connected by a narrow neck with the lumen of the colon. It passes through the muscularis at the points of penetration of blood vessels from serosa to submucosa; their close proximity to these vessels is probably a factor in the causation of major hemorrhage in otherwise uncomplicated diverticulosis. In some instances they appear uniformly distributed from cecum to sigmoid, in others virtually confined to the sigmoid and descending colon. Rarely, one or a few diverticula are found in the right colon alone; significantly the rectum, having an intact longitudinal muscle layer, is never involved. In many cases the wall of the distal colon is thrown into many thick, arcuate or concertina-like folds, each consisting of a double layer of thickened circular muscle (myochosis); the taeniae are conspicuously shortened. The diverticula appear at the apices of the small intervening haustra.

Their protrusion is attributed in part to the high intraluminal pressure observed in the affected segments of bowel. Further, the folding of the muscular wall converts the colon into a series of isolated chambers in which high pressures can be confined. In some instances, high pressure and myochosis have been apparently well developed before any significant formation of diverticula, and it is believed that the motility disturbance is the primary change, continuation of which brings about not only herniation of mucosa but also the impaction, vascular congestion, minor necrosis, and perforation which lead to diverticulitis and pericolonic abscess.

Etiology. The cause of the colonic hypermotility is unknown. Such a change is believed to occur in patients with the "irritable colon," and some clinical studies suggest that diverticular disease may be a sequela of that disorder. There appears to be a motor incoordination of the affected segments of bowel, but the neural basis for this has not been recognized by morphologic or physiologic means. The great international variations in prevalence are compatible with the hypothesis that diets high in content of vegetable fiber retard development of diverticula; this is confirmed by dietary experiments on diverticulosis in aged laboratory animals.

Clinical Features. Most commonly, patients experience one or several attacks of griping *pain* in the left lower quadrant or the hypogastrium, lasting one to ten days,

with exacerbation after eating. The sigmoid colon in such instances may be felt as a distinct, firm, tender mass. Unless true diverticulitis has developed, rebound tenderness, abdominal rigidity, fever, and leukocytosis are absent. In the intervals between attacks, moderate to severe constipation and a sense of abdominal fullness, relieved by passage of flatus, are commonly reported. Brief episodes of moderate or profuse *rectal bleeding* are not infrequently observed in patients with diverticular disease in the absence of inflammation. These usually cease spontaneously. Chronic low-grade blood loss more commonly arises from areas of diverticulitis, or from some unrelated lesion such as carcinoma or Crohn's disease.

The *diagnosis* of diverticular disease depends chiefly upon the barium enema, although the pockets are readily shown after barium by mouth. The deeply folded wall of the distal colon itself gives rise to the "sawtooth" pattern of the barium outline, and hence this does not constitute evidence for diverticulitis. In view of the high prevalence of diverticula in aged persons, caution must be exercised in attributing rectal bleeding to this source, lest a carcinoma or other more dangerous lesion go undetected.

The *treatment* of early symptomatic diverticular disease is essentially that of the irritable colon with mild constipation. A diet high in fruit and vegetable fiber is recommended, supplied in part by unprocessed bran, 2 teaspoonfuls three times a day with meals, increasing the dose as tolerated. This may be supplemented by the use of hydrophilic colloids, such as agar, psyllium seed, or methylcellulose. Relief of pain may be obtained with anticholinergics, such as propantheline, 15 mg four times daily, or with meperidine, 50 to 100 mg; but opiates are contraindicated because they dangerously elevate intracolonic pressures. Antimicrobial drugs should be reserved for clear-cut cases of diverticulitis.

Patients with demonstrated myochosis of the sigmoid whose painful episodes recur despite vigorous medical therapy may require surgical relief, either by resection of the most affected portion of the colon or by sigmoid myotomy. Both procedures are effective in two thirds or more of the cases.

Almy, T. P.: Diverticular disease of the colon: The new look. Gastroenterology, 49:109, 1965.

Cross, F. S.: Esophageal diverticula: Related neuromuscular problems. Ann. Otol. Rhinol. Laryngol., 77:914, 1968.

Ellis, F. H., Schlegel, J. F., Lynch, V. P., and Payne, W. S.: Cricopharyngeal myotomy for pharyngo-esophageal diverticulum. Ann. Surg., 170:340, 1969.

Horner, J. L.: Natural history of diverticulosis of the colon. Am. J. Dig. Dis., 3:343, 1958.

Nobles, E. R.: Jejunal diverticula. Arch. Surg., 102:172, 1971.

Noer, R. J.: Hemorrhage as a complication of diverticulitis. Ann. Surg., 141:674, 1955.

Painter, N. S., Almeida, A. Z., and Colebourne, K. W.: Unprocessed bran in treatment of diverticular disease of the colon. Br. Med. J., 1:137, 1972.

Reilly, M.: Sigmoid myotomy. Br. J. Surg., 53:859, 1966.

Section Two.   PEPTIC ULCER

640.   PATHOGENESIS AND PATHOPHYSIOLOGY

Morton I. Grossman

Definition.   Peptic ulcer is a sharply circumscribed loss of the tissue lining those parts of the digestive tract exposed to gastric juice containing acid and pepsin. These consist of the lower esophagus, the stomach, the upper intestine (usually only the first part of the duodenum), the small intestine adjacent to a surgically produced connection with the stomach, and those Meckel's diverticula that contain functioning gastric glands.

Pathology. *Acute Lesions.*   Acute lesions must be clearly distinguished from chronic ulcers because they are different diseases. Acute lesions are almost always multiple and they are superficial, rarely extending through the muscularis mucosae. Lesions that do not extend through the muscularis mucosae are called erosions, whereas those that do extend through this layer are called ulcers. Thus multiple acute lesions are mainly erosions, but chronic lesions are always ulcers (see accompanying figure).

Chronic Ulcers.   When the unqualified term ulcer is used, chronic ulcer is meant. In contrast to acute lesions, chronic ulcers are usually single (figure). About 4 per cent of patients with gastric ulcer and about 20 per cent of patients with duodenal ulcer have two ulcers at the same time. About 40 per cent of patients with gastric ulcer have evidence of past or present duodenal ulcer.

The margins of chronic ulcers are thickened, rounded, and overhanging because of the excavation beneath them. Askanazy was the first to describe the four histologic zones of the ulcer floor: a surface layer of fibrin and pus, a narrow zone of fibrinoid necrosis, a zone of granulation tissue, and a cicatricial or fibrous zone. Chronic ulcers usually destroy the entire muscular coat. During healing a single layer of epithelial cells covers the granulation tissue of the crater floor and then differentiates toward normal mucosa. There is no regeneration of muscle; a permanent scar in the muscular coat marks the site of a healed ulcer.

Gastritis.   Chronic gastritis is present in the stomach of almost all patients with chronic gastric or duodenal ulcer. The proximal 80 per cent of the stomach has acid-secreting oxyntic glands; the distal 20 per cent has pyloric glands that produce gastrin but no acid. In patients with duodenal ulcer the gastritis is limited to the pyloric gland area and is mild, seldom showing intestinal metaplasia. In patients with gastric ulcer the extent of the gastritis is correlated with the location of the ulcer. With ulcers near the pylorus the gastritis is usually confined to the pyloric gland area. Most gastric ulcers are located in pyloric gland mucosa at or near the boundary between pyloric and oxyntic glands. The higher the ulcer is located in the stomach, the larger is the extent of the pyloric glands, the more severe is the gastritis, and the more it extends into oxyntic mucosa. The severity and extent of the gastritis do not change with healing of the ulcer. Histologically, chronic atrophic gastritis accompanying gastric ulcer is indistinguishable from the sporadic form common with advancing age but differs from the form associated with pernicious anemia; in the latter the antrum is spared, and antibodies to parietal cells and to intrinsic factor are often present.

Intestinal metaplasia is a common feature of the gastritis associated with gastric ulcer. The converse heterotopia, gastric mucosa in the duodenum, is equally common in patients with duodenal ulcer. In both instances the incidence is related to acid secretion: the higher the level of acid secretion, the greater the incidence of gastric heterotopia in the duodenum; the lower the level of acid secretion, the greater the incidence of intestinal heterotopia in the stomach.

Pathogenesis.   Acid and pepsin are required for ulcer formation. Ulcers occur when there is an imbalance between acid-pepsin and mucosal resistance. Increased acid-pepsin secretion, decreased mucosal resistance, or the two acting together are ulcerogenic.

Epidemiology.   Peptic ulcer is a common disease, but there is much variation in frequency of occurrence from time to time and from place to place. In male Massachusetts physicians the lifetime prevalence of duodenal ulcer was 7.7 per cent and of gastric ulcer 0.9 per cent. The incidence rates peaked at 3.7 per thousand per year at age 55 to 64 for duodenal ulcer and at 1.4 per thousand per year at age 65 to 74 for gastric ulcer.

Based on the numbers of patients who went to physicians, the ratio of duodenal to gastric ulcers in one study was about 4 to 1 in men and 2 to 1 in women. The ratio of men to women was about 2 to 1 for gastric ulcers and 4 to 1 for duodenal ulcers.

The prevalence of peptic ulcer at autopsy is considerably higher than in clinical studies, probably because many ulcers never cause enough symptoms to lead to diagnosis. In an autopsy series from Leeds, England, the peak prevalence of ulcers plus scars was at ages 46 to 65

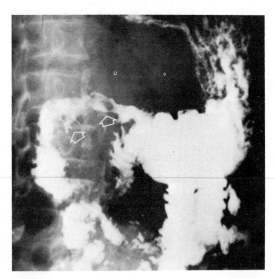

Enlarged gastric rugal folds, along with increased gastric secretions, have produced a mottled appearance of the barium in the stomach. Two duodenal ulcers are present (open arrows). Thickened mucosal folds are present in the second portion of the duodenum and in the jejunum. The patient had the Zollinger-Ellison syndrome. (From Goldberg, H. I., *In* Sleisenger, M. H., and Fordtran, J. S. [eds.]: Gastrointestinal Disease. Philadelphia, W. B. Saunders Company, 1973.)

with rates of 27 per cent in men and 15 per cent in women.

In almost all parts of the world morbidity from duodenal ulcer is reported as more common than from gastric ulcer, but deaths from gastric ulcer equal or exceed those from duodenal ulcer. In a few populations, for unknown reasons, gastric ulcer has been reported to be more frequent than duodenal ulcer; examples are fishermen of a village in Norway and Indian miners high in the Peruvian Andes. Mortality rates for gastric ulcer (in number per 100,000 deaths) range from 30 in Japan to 3 in Israel, and for duodenal ulcer from 10 in Scotland to 0.5 in France. Mortality, prevalence, and incidence of new cases all show a higher rate in town than in country. However, high rates have also been reported from areas that are not industrialized such as South India, Assam, South Nigeria, and Uganda.

Duodenal ulcer was a rare disease before 1900. By 1914 it had become common in Europe and North America. The sharp rise in duodenal ulcer was accompanied by a modest increase in gastric ulcer. From 1914 to about 1955 they remained at a relatively constant level and then began to decrease and are still decreasing. Cohort analysis, following all persons born in the same year, shows that death rates steadily increased for cohorts born up to the year 1890, whereas death rates for cohorts born after 1890 steadily decreased.

Environmental Factors. Of the many environmental factors that have been suspected as possible contributing causes of peptic ulcer, the only one that has been adequately studied is smoking. It is clear from all studies on this subject that smokers have more ulcers, both gastric and duodenal, and higher morbidity and mortality rates from their ulcers than nonsmokers. No relation between amount of smoking and ulcer incidence has been found; heavy smokers were not found to have more ulcers than light smokers. The nature of the relation between smoking and ulcer is not understood. Smoking neither stimulates nor inhibits gastric acid secretion but does inhibit pancreatic bicarbonate secretion, and some have suggested that this is related to its ulcerogenic action.

Although a role of diet in ulcer causation is often hypothesized, there is as yet no direct evidence to incriminate either particular diets or elements of diets such as hot spices.

Duodenal ulcer is equally common among all social classes, but ulcer of the body of the stomach is primarily a disease of the poorer economic grades. Despite the persistent myth of the hard-driving executive's proneness to ulcer, occupational differences are in fact small.

Genetic Factors. Genetic factors contribute to both gastric and duodenal ulcer. Gastric and duodenal ulcers are inherited independently. Close relatives of gastric ulcer patients have three times the expected number of gastric ulcers, and close relatives of duodenal ulcer patients have three times the expected number of duodenal ulcers. Concordance for ulcer, that is presence of ulcer in the second twin if one twin has ulcer, is more common in monozygous than in dizygous twin pairs. There is strong evidence that the increased familial incidence of ulcer is due to genetic factors and not simply to a shared environment. For both gastric and duodenal ulcer, the mode of inheritance is polygenic. None of the genes associated with ulcer of the body of the stomach have yet been identified. Duodenal ulcers, alone or with gastric ulcers, and ulcers of the prepyloric part of the stomach show abnormal frequencies of two genes: ABO blood groups and secretor status of blood group substances. Persons with blood group O are 1.4 times as liable to have duodenal or prepyloric ulcer as those with groups A, B, or AB, and persons who are nonsecretors are 1.5 times as liable to these ulcers as those who are secretors. Group O nonsecretors are 2.5 times more liable than secretors of groups A, B, and AB. The excess of group O and nonsecretion is greater in patients with recurrent ulcers after operations than in unoperated patients. The basis for the association of duodenal ulcer with group O and nonsecretion is not yet known.

The group O and nonsecretion factors explain only a small part of the variation in ulcer occurrence. Probably the most important genetic factor in peptic ulcer is the inheritance of acid-peptic glandular mass and the capacity to secrete acid and pepsin that is linked to it; the mode of this inheritance is not yet known.

Psychosomatic Factors. Popular wisdom holds that ulcers are caused by "nerves." At least two notions are implied: (1) that persons who have certain psychic traits are prone to develop ulcers, and (2) that situations that produce psychic tension are likely to bring on ulcers. These are hypotheses awaiting definitive testing. Since it is well established that emotional factors can alter gastric function, it is plausible to hypothesize a role for these factors in ulcerogenesis.

The most complete formulation of the interaction of psychic with other factors is that of Mirsky, whose postulates can be paraphrased as follows. The capacity to secrete acid and pepsin, of which serum pepsinogen level is an index, is genetically determined. Persons genetically endowed with high capacity to secrete acid-pepsin also tend to have a psychic conflict between persistent infantile wishes to be loved and cared for and repudiation of these wishes by their adult sense of shame and pride. Persons who have this combined physiologic and psychic pattern (high acid-pepsin secretory capacity and conflict over dependency wishes) are predisposed to develop duodenal ulcer. Ulcer is most likely to develop when a social event or a series of such events causes an exacerbation of the basic psychic conflict. The mechanism by which the exacerbation of the conflict leads to ulcer is not known, but it probably is not through further increase in acid-pepsin secretion.

Ulcers Caused by Drugs. If all the drugs that cause ulcers when given in massive doses to animals were withdrawn from human use, the pharmacopeia would be noticeably thinner. The drugs that are strongly suspected of being ulcerogenic in man are salicylates, indomethacin, phenylbutazone, and glucocorticoids. Salicylates and indomethacin applied topically break the mucosal barrier to hydrogen ions. This cannot be the sole mechanism by which they produce ulcer in lower animals, however, because they are also ulcerogenic by the parenteral route and do not break the barrier when so given. The mechanism of ulcerogenesis by these drugs is not understood; they do not stimulate acid secretion.

The only drug with a highly incriminating dossier for ulcerogenesis in man is aspirin. It is implicated in peptic disease in two ways. First, there is strong but not conclusive evidence that major bleeding episodes, probably mainly from acute diffuse hemorrhagic lesions, may be provoked by ingestion of aspirin. Second, there is mounting evidence that chronic ingestion of aspirin can cause gastric ulcer. Aspirin-induced gastric ulcers occur in stomachs that do not have the atrophic gastritis that is so characteristic of nonaspirin ulcers.

Peptic Lesions Caused by Stress. The acute diffuse lesions brought on by stress are pathologically and clinically distinct from chronic peptic ulcer. Many different kinds of stress can cause the lesions. Some prominent examples are sepsis, advanced carcinomatosis, shock, severe trauma, surgery, extensive burns (so-called Curling's ulcer), and acute respiratory insufficiency. One category of stress lesions deserves separate mention, namely, those associated with brain injury (so-called Cushing's ulcer). Any kind of acute brain injury, including surgical, traumatic, and cerebrovascular accidents, can cause the lesions. There is good evidence that hypersecretion of gastric acid and pepsin plays a role in stress lesions caused by brain injury, but hypersecretion has not been found in the other kinds of stress lesions. Although ischemia, breaking of the barrier to hydrogen ions, and mucus deficiency have been invoked in the pathogenesis of stress lesions, these are speculations without convincing supporting evidence. Hemorrhage is the main clinical manifestation of stress lesions; perforation occurs occasionally; pain is rare. Stress-related acute gastric lesions are a common life-threatening disease about which little is known.

Association with Other Diseases. The impression that two diseases appear together more frequently or less frequently than would be expected by chance must always be viewed skeptically, because it is easy to draw false conclusions about such associations from studies of nonrandom samples of broader populations. Duodenal ulcer is thought to be more common in patients with chronic obstructive lung disease, hepatic cirrhosis (especially after portacaval shunt), and gastric ulcer in those with rheumatoid arthritis. The evidence for these associations is contradictory, and in no instance is the mechanism for the possible association fully understood. In hepatic cirrhosis hypersecretion caused by a stimulant arising in intestinal mucosa and rendered more effective by bypassing the liver is postulated. In rheumatoid arthritis the ulcerogenic actions of the drugs used for treatment may well be involved.

Patients with hyperparathyroidism have a high incidence of duodenal ulcer. At least a part of this association is due to the occurrence of both parathyroid tumor and gastrinoma in some patients with multiple endocrine adenoma. Since the diagnosis of gastrinoma may not always be obvious, the question of whether patients with hyperparathyroidism without gastrinoma also have an increased incidence of duodenal ulcer must be regarded as unanswered.

Pathophysiology. *Mucosal Resistance.* Since most gastric ulcers and many duodenal ulcers occur in patients who do not have increased gastric secretion, a decrease in resistance of the mucosa to acid-peptic injury is presumably involved. Unfortunately, the factors that determine mucosal resistance have not yet been clearly identified. Some suggested contributory factors include mucosal blood flow, regeneration of epithelium, secretion of mucus, and integrity of the barrier to back-diffusion of hydrogen ions.

Gastric mucosa, like all tissue, requires adequate blood supply to remain intact. Reliable methods for measuring mucosal blood flow in patients with ulcer have not yet been devised. Although impaired blood supply is a theoretical possibility as a contributor to ulcerogenesis, there are no clues suggesting that it is so implicated. This same statement can be made for most factors that have been suggested as being involved in ulcerogenesis.

The epithelium of the entire gastrointestinal tract is rapidly replaced. It is estimated that the surface cells of the human stomach are replaced every four to six days. Good methods for measuring mucosal regeneration rate in man are available, but these have not yet been applied to the study of patients with peptic ulcer. Patients with atrophic gastritis have an increased rate of cell shedding from the gastric surface as measured by the rate of appearance of DNA in gastric washings; this also applies to the atrophic gastritis associated with gastric ulcer.

The notion that mucus somehow protects the mucosa against damage by acid-pepsin is very old and is still widely held, but there is no known biologic or physicochemical basis for such an action. Some sulfated mucosubstances inhibit peptic activity, but these do not occur in human gastric juice or gastric mucosa. The interstices of a gel of mucus are too large to offer significant resistance to diffusion of hydrogen ions or pepsin. The methods presently available have not shown any defects in secretion of mucus in patients with ulcer.

Back-Diffusion. Acid secreted into the gastric lumen diffuses back into the mucosa very slowly provided that the mucosa is normal; the leakback rate is only a few per cent of the maximal rate of acid secretion. This is spoken of as a "barrier" to back-diffusion. A variety of chemical agents, some arising in the body, others ingested, can break this barrier and allow markedly increased rates of back-diffusion of acid. Bile acids are endogenous barrier breakers. Exogenous barrier breakers that are likely to enter the human stomach include alcohol, salicylates, and oxethazaine. To break the barrier the chemical must enter the mucosa. If the agent is ionizable, it must be in its un-ionized lipid-soluble form to enter the mucosa; for example, aspirin must be in acid solution. Manifestations of a broken barrier include decrease in the electrical potential difference across the gastric mucosa and increased bidirectional permeability to sodium with increased accumulation of sodium in the gastric lumen. As acid diffuses through the broken barrier, it causes additional damage manifested by leakage of interstitial fluid and plasma into the gastric lumen and bleeding.

The locus of the barrier to back-diffusion of hydrogen ions is not known. Because Hollander used the term "mucous barrier" and Davenport used the term "mucosal barrier to hydrogen ions," it is commonly assumed that these two are the same barriers. There is no evidence that mucus has anything to do with the barrier to hydrogen ions.

Gastric Acid Secretion. CAPACITY TO SECRETE ACID. The capacity to secrete acid is determined mainly by the number of parietal cells in the gastric mucosa, and this is mainly genetically determined. The capacity to secrete acid can be estimated by measuring the response to a high dose (such that a higher dose would not give a greater response) of a stimulant such as gastrin, pentagastrin, histamine, or betazole, which all give about the same highest attainable response.

Secretory capacity is less in women than in men, a difference partially accounted for by difference in body size. Secretory capacity declines with age, presumably because of increasing incidence of gastritis that destroys acid-secreting cells. These sex and age differences are seen in patients with ulcer as well as in control subjects.

GASTRIC ACID SECRETION IN PATIENTS WITH ULCER.

Normal adults have on average about one billion parietal cells and can secrete about 22 mEq of acid per hour. The corresponding values for duodenal ulcer are 1.9 billion and 42 mEq and for gastric ulcer 0.8 billion and 18 mEq. The variations around the means are very large, so there is much overlap between these groups. However, on average, patients with chronic duodenal ulcer secrete more acid than normal subjects both at rest and in response to stimuli. At all times, day and night, in the fasted and fed states, the acidity of the gastric contents and of the first 5 to 10 cm of duodenum is greater than normal.

REGULATION OF GASTRIC SECRETION IN MAN. Two substances activate the parietal cell to secrete acid: the hormone *gastrin* which reaches the parietal cell by way of the blood, and the neurohumor *acetylcholine* which is released at the parietal cell by the postganglionic endings of the vagus nerves.

Gastrins: Scattered among the mucous cells of the pyloric glands are specialized cells, the G-cells, that produce gastrin and store it in granules.

Gastrin occurs in several molecular sizes. Gastrins with chain lengths of 13, 17, and 34 amino acid residues, designated G13, G17, and G34, have been isolated and chemically identified by Gregory. Each of these occurs in sulfated and nonsulfated forms. Pentagastrin, β-Ala-Trp-Met-Asp-Phe-NH$_2$, a synthetic peptide that contains the last four amino acids of gastrin, is widely used as a stimulant for gastric acid secretion in diagnostic testing.

In antral mucosa the predominant form of gastrin is G17, whereas in blood plasma after eating the most abundant form is G34. The greater abundance of G34 in plasma can be accounted for at least in part by its slower removal; the half-time of G34 is longer than that of G17. A higher blood level of G34 than of G17 is needed to give equal rates of acid secretion.

The richest source of gastrin is antral mucosa. The concentration of gastrin in the mucosa of the upper half of the duodenum is about half that in antral mucosa, and much lower concentrations are found in more distal intestine.

The concentration of gastrin in antral mucosa as measured by bioassay is normal in patients with duodenal ulcer and decreased in patients with gastric ulcer. In patients with duodenal ulcer serum gastrin concentration is normal in the fasting state and greater than normal after feeding.

Patients with gastric ulcer tend to have elevated concentrations of fasting serum gastrin. The increased blood gastrin level is correlated with decreased acid secretion. Dragstedt hypothesized that gastric stasis stimulated gastrin release that in turn caused hypersecretion leading to gastric ulcer. Since the elevated serum gastrin levels seen in some patients with gastric ulcer are associated with decreased acid secretion, Dragstedt's hypothesis is not supported.

All kinds of vagotomy (truncal, selective, proximal gastric) cause an increase in serum gastrin, both fasting and after feeding. Antrectomy causes a modest decrease in fasting serum gastrin level. The serum gastrin response to feeding is absent after Billroth II reconstruction and near normal after Billroth I, indicating that duodenal gastrin is releasable by feeding.

Until the distribution of the various molecular forms of gastrin has been studied in the serum of normal subjects and of patients with duodenal ulcer and gastric ulcer, no definitive conclusions can be drawn about correlation between gastrin and acid secretion and about differences between normal subjects and ulcer patients.

Acetylcholine: Cholinergic nerves supply both parietal cells and antral G cells. These cholinergic nerves are activated both by vagal impulses and by so-called short reflexes that are completed within the wall of the stomach. Vagal activation occurs as a result of stimuli acting in the head (the cephalic phase) and in the stomach (the gastric phase). Cephalic stimuli include chewing, tasting, and swallowing food (as in sham feeding), the sight, smell, or thought of food (conditioned reflex), hypoglycemia induced by insulin, and interference with glucose utilization by nonmetabolizable sugars such as 2-deoxyglucose. Gastric stimuli include distention of the stomach and the action of chemical agents, particularly partially digested protein, on the gastric mucosa. The gastric stimuli initiate both long vagovagal reflexes and short intramural reflexes; the long reflexes are more effective. All these mechanisms, cephalic vagal, gastric long vagovagal reflexes, and gastric short intramural reflexes, activate cholinergic fibers to both parietal cells and gastrin cells. Atropine does not inhibit release of gastrin in response to a meal, so either the cholinergic mechanisms for gastrin release are atropine resistant or there are additional noncholinergic (perhaps nonneural) mechanisms that can fully substitute. Atropine blocks direct vagal stimulation of the oxyntic glands and markedly inhibits the response to gastrin.

The vagus nerve influences gastric secretion in at least three ways: (1) direct cholinergic stimulation of parietal cells, (2) release of gastrin, and (3) sensitizing the parietal cell to stimulation by gastrin and other stimulants. Vagotomy removes that part of the tonic cholinergic background that is vagally dependent and thereby desensitizes the parietal cell to stimulation by gastrin. After vagotomy the highest attainable response to gastrin is reduced and the dose of gastrin needed to get that reduced response is increased. The magnitude and sensitivity of the response to gastrin can be restored to prevagotomy levels by giving a background of a cholinomimetic drug to replace vagal tone. *Thus vagotomy does not reduce the capacity of the stomach to secrete acid but takes away one of the stimulants required to fully activate that capacity.* Antrectomy, removal of the major source of gastrin, reduces the response to vagal stimulation and to other stimulants such as gastrin and histamine. The response cannot be restored to the preantrectomy level by giving a background of gastrin; the mechanism by which antrectomy reduces the capacity to secrete acid is not understood. Antrectomy and vagotomy have additive effects. For example, the highest attainable response to histamine is about 40 per cent of the preoperative level with vagotomy alone, about 50 per cent with antrectomy alone, and about 20 per cent with the two together.

Other factors: Partially digested protein bathing the intestinal mucosa stimulates gastric acid secretion, the intestinal phase. A part of this effect is mediated by antral-type gastrin that is mainly in the first part of the duodenum. Other unidentified humoral agents from the duodenum and jejunum are probably also involved.

Three mechanisms for inhibition of gastric acid secretion are recognized. The first is inhibition of gastrin release by acid bathing the antral mucosa. When antral pH is 1.5 or lower, all forms of gastrin release are almost totally suppressed. The other two inhibitory mechanisms operate from the intestine in response to acid and to fat. Secretin is one inhibitor of acid secretion released by acid, but it is likely that other unidentified hormones and nervous mechanisms are also involved. Fat inhibits acid secretion regardless of the stimulus. The cholecystokinin released by fat inhibits gastrin-stimulated secretion, but other unidentified inhibitors, enterogastrones, are also involved. Secretin and cholecystokinin are weak inhibitors of acid secretion, so they are unlikely to contribute significantly to regulation of acid secretion.

Caffeine and theophylline stimulate gastric acid secretion, an action that may be secondary to inhibition of breakdown of cyclic AMP.

POSTULATED ABNORMALITIES IN ULCER PATIENTS. The increased average rate of secretion in patients with duodenal ulcer could be due to one or more of these factors: (1) increased capacity to secrete, (2) increased responsiveness of acid-secreting cells, (3) increased drive to acid secretion, and (4) decreased inhibition of secretion. These factors are not entirely independent. For example, gastrin not only drives secretion but also stimulates growth of mucosa. Acetylcholine drives secretion and sensitizes to other stimuli; whether it also stimulates growth of mucosa is not known. Of these factors, increased capacity to secrete is the one most clearly involved in the hypersecretion seen in duodenal ulcer. Increased capacity to secrete acid is present long before the duodenal ulcer appears and stays relatively constant during exacerbations and remissions. There is some evidence that increased sensitivity to stimulation is also present, but this cannot be considered as fully established. There is also some evidence for increased drive in the form of greater than normal increments in serum gastrin after feeding, but the relative importance of this factor is not yet clear. Defective inhibitory mechanisms may contribute to hypersecretion. For example, acidification of a test meal causes less suppression of gastrin release and of acid secretion in duodenal ulcer patients than in controls.

Basal acid secretion rate divided by maximal rate can be used as an index of basal "drive." In both duodenal ulcer patients and controls, this fraction increases as basal rate increases, indicating that some unidentified factor other than maximal capacity is a major determinant of high basal rates.

A popular notion holds that the hypersecretion of duodenal ulcer is caused by excessive vagal activity. The only evidence in support of this idea is that the hypersecretion is eliminated by vagotomy. However, since vagotomy decreases the response to all forms of stimulation, the decrease in secretion that follows vagotomy cannot be accepted as proof that vagal overactivity caused the hypersecretion. There is no satisfactory method for measuring vagal "tone."

Impaired release of secretin or impaired capacity of the pancreas to secrete bicarbonate could contribute to the increased duodenal acidity seen in patients with duodenal ulcer. However, there is no convincing evidence for impaired secretin release, and capacity to secrete bicarbonate is actually increased, proportionately to the increased capacity to secrete acid.

In gastric ulcer associated with duodenal ulcer, the secretory pattern tends to be like that of duodenal ulcer. The higher in the stomach the gastric ulcer is located, the lower the secretory capacity; ulcers near the pylorus give secretory patterns like duodenal ulcer, whereas those near the cardia show marked hyposecretion. The decrease in acid secretion in gastric ulcer can be accounted for mainly by the associated gastritis that causes loss of parietal cells, but increased back-diffusion may also contribute.

Pepsins. Seven pepsinogens belonging to two immunochemical groups occur in human gastroduodenal mucosa. Group I pepsinogens are limited to mucous neck cells and zymogen cells of the oxyntic gland area, and Group II pepsinogens are present in these cells and also in the mucous cells of pyloric glands and Brunner's glands. Group I and II pepsinogens are present in blood plasma, but only Group I is found in normal urine.

There is a strong correlation between capacity to secrete acid and capacity to secrete pepsin and also between capacity to secrete acid and pepsin and concentration of pepsinogen in blood. Determination by radioimmunoassay of the concentration of Group I pepsinogens in blood serum is a convenient and accurate method of assessing the secretory capacity for acid and pepsin.

The major stimulants for acid secretion, gastrin and acetylcholine, are also the major regulators of pepsin secretion. The ratio of pepsin to acid is higher in cholinergically stimulated gastric juice (e.g., insulin hypoglycemia) than in that evoked by gastrin. The increase in gastric secretion in patients with duodenal ulcer and the decrease in patients with gastric ulcer involve both acid and pepsin.

Duodenogastric Reflux. Du Plessis (1965) hypothesized that reflux of bile from the duodenum into the stomach may be an important factor in the pathogenesis of gastric ulcer. Patients with gastric ulcer do reflux duodenal contents into the stomach more often and in larger amounts than controls, both in the fasting and fed states, but the overlap between controls and gastric ulcer patients is great. Over the short term this reflux leads to breaking of the gastric barrier to back-diffusion of hydrogen ion, and over the long term it is presumed to lead to gastric atrophy, factors that may make the mucosa less resistant to ulceration. Further studies are needed to assess fully the role of this factor.

Gastric Emptying. Since the stomach shows an exponential pattern of emptying, rate of emptying can best be expressed as a half-time. The half-time for gastric emptying shows wide variation in both ulcer patients and control subjects. There is a tendency for rapid emptying of a mixed meal in patients with duodenal ulcer, but the overlap with normal subjects is great. Some patients with duodenal ulcer or with gastric ulcer have markedly impaired gastric emptying. In most instances this impairment of emptying cannot be accounted for by anatomic narrowing of the gastric outlet, and its pathogenesis is not well understood.

641. DIAGNOSTIC STUDIES AND MEDICAL TREATMENT

Jon I. Isenberg

DIAGNOSTIC STUDIES

Radiography. Radiography is at present the most commonly used technique in the diagnosis of peptic ulcer disease. Ulcers may rarely be visualized on standard abdominal radiograms if air is trapped in the crater.

Barium sulfate suspension is usually used as the radiopaque contrast material for routine gastrointestinal radiography. An absorbable water-soluble contrast agent is used in patients with suspected perforated ulcers. Air contrast films help to define clearly the mucosal pattern of the upper gastrointestinal tract. Delayed films, taken about one hour after ingestion of barium, may demonstrate a collection of barium within an ulcer which was not seen on the initial fluoroscopic examination.

For certainty of diagnosis, the ulcer niche should be seen on more than one x-ray film. When an ulcer is viewed in profile, the niche appears as a collection of contrast material which extends beyond the confines of the gut wall. When the ulcer niche is seen en face, it appears as a puddle of barium, often surrounded by a halo and/or radiating folds to the ulcer. The halo is due to mucosal and submucosal edema surrounding the ulcer.

Ulcers of the esophagus usually occur within the lower half (Fig. 1). Ulcer and diverticulum of the esophagus may have similar radiographic appearances. Esophagoscopy (see below) can distinguish one from the other. The presence of an esophageal ulcer, particularly with an accompanying esophageal stricture, should suggest the possibility that the lower esophagus is lined with columnar epithelium (Barrett's syndrome). Almost all ulcers of the esophagus are visualized on radiography.

The great majority of gastric ulcers (approximately 85 per cent) occur in pyloric gland mucosa at or near the junction with oxyntic gland mucosa. Approximately 85 per cent of gastric ulcers occur on the lesser curvature of the stomach. About 90 per cent of endoscopically visualized gastric ulcers are seen on upper gastrointestinal series.

Gastric ulcers vary in diameter from less than 1 cm to

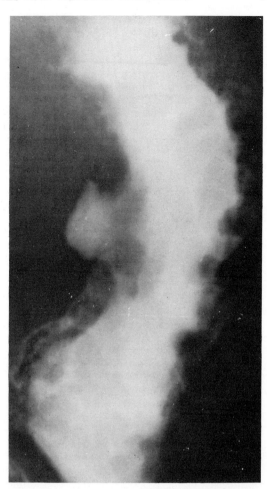

Figure 2. A benign ulcer of the lesser curvature is surrounded by an ulcer collar—the broad lucent band resulting from edema at the ulcer orifice. Gastric mucosal folds radiate from this mass of edema. (From Goldberg, H. I., *In* Sleisenger, M. H., and Fordtran, J. S. [eds.]: Gastrointestinal Disease. Philadelphia, W. B. Saunders Company, 1973.)

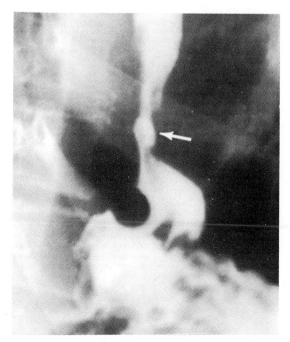

Figure 1. B. H., a 44-year-old housewife with intermittent dysphagia for four years and burning midepigastric pain, recurring after meals and during the night, for eight months. Esophagoscopy revealed chronic esophagitis with stricture; biopsies did not demonstrate neoplasia. The roentgenogram demonstrates an ulcer crater in the esophagus. Antacid therapy facilitated healing, and the dysphagia subsided.

greater than 10 cm. Nearly 80 per cent of gastric ulcers are less than 2 cm in widest diameter. When seen in profile, an apparent density surrounds the neck of the ulcer; this is due to an undermined margin of gastric mucosa which produces a narrow ring around part or all of the ulcer (Hampton's line), and often due to a thicker radiodense ulcer "collar" caused by edema and inflammation of the adjacent mucosa (Fig. 2). Although these radiographic changes tend to be more common with benign ulcers, they may rarely be seen in ulcerating gastric cancers.

Gastric ulcers may not be visualized because (1) the ulcer may be shallow and barium may not collect within it, (2) there may be mucus or blood within the ulcer crater, (3) the edematous margins around the ulcer may occlude the mouth of the ulcer, (4) the positions used may not throw it into profile, or (5) the patient may be too large or may be unable to permit adequate radiographic examination.

Approximately 4 per cent of all gastric ulcers seen on gastrointestinal radiograms are malignant. Radiographic features which tend to distinguish benign gastric ulcer from gastric cancer include the following: (1) most benign ulcers extend beyond the confines of the gastric wall, whereas gastric cancers tend to occur within the confines of the gastric wall; (2) benign ulcers tend to be round or ovoid, whereas cancers often are irregular in shape; (3) benign ulcers usually have a smooth base, whereas the base of a cancer may be nodular; (4) the gastric folds radiate to the lip of a benign ulcer, whereas there may be no radiating folds around a cancer, or the folds may be blunted and stop some distance from an ulcerating cancer; and (5) the stomach around a benign ulcer is usually pliable and has normal motility, whereas the wall around a cancer is rigid and has poor motility. Some ulcerating carcinomas may "heal" radiographically. Therefore other studies, such as endoscopy, biopsy, and cytology (see below), are needed to assist in distinguishing benign gastric ulcer from gastric cancer.

Benign gastric ulcers within the body of the stomach may produce infolding of the gastric wall opposite the ulcer. With healing of the ulcer, this cleft or incisura in the gastric contour may persist, producing an "hourglass stomach."

Most duodenal ulcers are located within the duodenal bulb (Fig. 3). However, ulcers may be located in the postbulbar area as well as the more distal duodenum and proximal jejunum. Approximately 85 per cent of endoscopically visualized duodenal ulcers (see below) are seen on upper gastrointestinal series (Fig. 4).

In the absence of a definite ulcer niche, radiographic findings which suggest duodenal ulcer disease include (1) spasm of the duodenal bulb; (2) eccentricity of the pyloric channel; (3) a persistent fold (i.e., incisura) extending across the duodenal bulb; (4) radiographic loss of the superior or inferior fornix of the duodenal bulb; (5) persistent spasm and/or fibrosis of the duodenal bulb, producing a "cloverleaf" deformity; and (6) distortion of the duodenal mucosa, suggesting edema, heterotopic gastric mucosa, or large duodenal folds. It is often difficult, if not impossible, to determine radiographically if there is an active ulcer in a scarred and deformed duodenal bulb. Giant duodenal ulcers (i.e., greater than 2 cm in diameter) may not be radiographically apparent, because they tend to simulate the normal superior or inferior fornix of the duodenal bulb (Fig. 5).

False-positive radiographic findings of duodenal ulcer may be due to ectopic pancreatic tissue with a minor pancreatic duct in the duodenal bulb, regional enteritis involving the duodenum, varicosities of the pancreaticoduodenal vein, carcinoma of the pancreas extending into the duodenum, and pancreatitis or cholecystitis producing inflammation of the adjacent duodenal mucosa.

Endoscopy. In the diagnosis of peptic ulcer disease, endoscopy is valuable in differentiating esophageal ulcer from diverticulum, in defining the bleeding site in upper gastrointestinal hemorrhage (see Ch. 644), in differentiating benign from malignant gastric ulcers, in differentiating recurrent ulcer from surgical deformity, and possibly in patients with x-ray-negative dyspepsia. In a scarred deformed duodenal bulb, duodenoscopy may demonstrate an ulcer not seen on radiographic study.

With the improved endoscopes, almost all ulcers of the esophagus and stomach are visualized, and approximately 85 per cent of radiographically demonstrated duodenal ulcers are seen. Conversely, about 10 to 15 per cent of duodenal ulcer craters seen endoscopically are not demonstrated radiographically. Mucosal lesions such as esophagitis, gastritis, and duodenitis are often not defined on radiographic study but can be diagnosed endoscopically, particularly with the addition of a directed endoscopic biopsy.

Endoscopically a benign gastric ulcer is usually round or ovoid and has a clear whitish base and a hyperemic border; the gastric folds radiate to the edge of the ulcer crater. Gastric cancers are often irregular in shape, have a necrotic hemorrhagic and nodular base, are surrounded by nodularity, and have clubbed folds radiating toward the cancer but stopping short of the ulcerated area. Multiple deep biopsies of the rim or direct brush cytology can often establish a histologic or cytologic diagnosis of cancer.

Secretory Studies. The following generalizations regarding both basal and stimulated acid secretion can

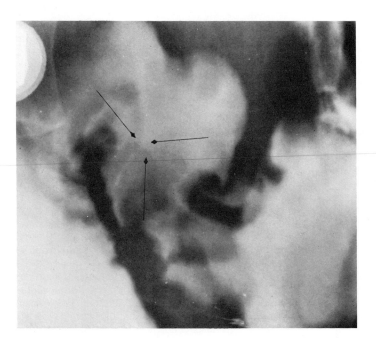

Figure 3. Edematous folds radiate from a pinpoint ulcer of the posterior duodenal wall (arrows). Compression of the duodenal bulb by the radiologist produced the best roentgenographic demonstration of this ulcer. (From Goldberg, H. I., *In* Sleisenger, M. H., and Fordtran, J. S. [eds.]: Gastrointestinal Disease. Philadelphia, W. B. Saunders Company, 1973.)

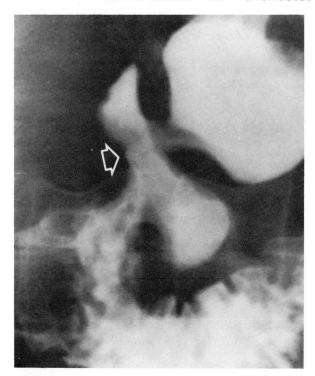

Figure 4. A small ulcer (arrow) has produced deformity of the duodenal bulb. Flattening of the superior surface of the bulb has resulted from edema and spasm. The superior and inferior recesses of the base of the bulb appear as diverticular outpouchings, so-called pseudodiverticula. (From Goldberg, H. I., *In* Sleisenger, M. H., and Fordtran, J. S. [eds.]: Gastrointestinal Disease. Philadelphia, W. B. Saunders Company, 1973.)

responses; that is, higher doses do not give higher responses.

Since ulcer disease does not occur in the absence of gastric acid—"no acid, no ulcer"—the finding of histamine-fast achlorhydria (i.e., all posthistamine determinations greater than 6) in a patient with radiographic evidence of gastric ulcer strongly suggests the diagnosis of gastric cancer. Unfortunately only about 20 per cent of patients with gastric cancer have histamine-fast achlorhydria. Thus for the differentiation of malignant from benign ulcer, achlorhydria is a highly *discriminative* test (a positive finding usually means cancer) but not a *sensitive* test (a positive finding is infrequent in patients with cancer).

Patients with duodenal ulcer disease tend to secrete more acid than control subjects in response to any stimulus. In about one third of male duodenal ulcer patients maximal acid output is greater than 42 mEq per hour, the upper limit of normal for control subjects. In addition, patients with duodenal ulcer almost always have a maximal acid output of at least 10 mEq per hour. If a lower rate is found, the diagnosis of duodenal ulcer disease becomes suspect. Maximal acid output of less than 10 mEq per hour is an insensitive criterion for absence of duodenal ulcer, because only about one sixth of normal subjects fall in this range.

There is evidence to suggest that duodenal ulcer patients with rates of stimulated acid secretion greater than approximately 45 mEq per hour may have a greater incidence of recurrent ulcer after vagotomy. No convinc-

be made: (1) patients with gastric ulcers of the body of the stomach tend to secrete subnormal amounts of acid; (2) patients with duodenal ulcer, prepyloric ulcer, or gastric plus duodenal ulcer tend to secrete more acid than normal subjects; and (3) patients with gastrin-secreting tumors of the pancreas (i.e., Zollinger-Ellison syndrome) tend to secrete more acid than most patients with duodenal ulcer. These generalizations refer to the "average patient." There is a great deal of overlap between groups.

Average basal gastric acid secretion in normal males and females is approximately 2.5 and 1.3 mEq per hour, respectively, but may range from 0 to 6 mEq per hour. Average basal secretion in patients with gastric ulcer is similar to normal, whereas average basal secretion for males and females with duodenal ulcer is approximately 5 and 3 mEq per hour, respectively. Some patients with duodenal ulcer disease may have no gastric acid at rest, whereas others may have greater than 10 mEq per hour. At rest only about one fourth of patients with duodenal ulcer secrete amounts of acid more than two standard deviations above the mean for normal subjects. Because of the wide overlap of basal secretion, it offers little assistance in the diagnosis of peptic ulcer disease. In most patients with gastrin-secreting tumors of the pancreas, basal secretion tends to be increased (i.e., greater than 10 mEq per hour in the intact stomach and greater than 5 mEq per hour in the postoperative stomach).

After subcutaneous injection of histamine acid phosphate (40 μg per kilogram), betazole (1.5 mg per kilogram), or pentagastrin (6 μg per kilogram), peak acid secretion is similar. These doses produce "maximal"

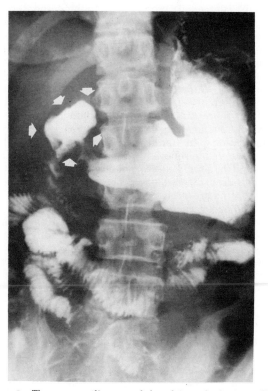

Figure 5. The arrows outline an oval-shaped, irregular barium collection at the site of the duodenal bulb. Serial roentgenograms demonstrated the same unchanging configuration. A giant duodenal ulcer occupied the entire bulb in the surgical abdomen. (From Goldberg, H. I., *In* Sleisenger, M. H., and Fordtran, J. S. [eds.]: Gastrointestinal Disease. Philadelphia, W. B. Saunders Company, 1973.)

ing correlation between degree of hypersecretion and severity of ulcer disease has been established in patients not operated on.

After vagal denervation of the stomach, insulin-induced hypoglycemia often fails to stimulate gastric acid secretion. The insulin test (0.2 U per kilogram intravenously) has been used to evaluate the effect of vagotomy on gastric acid secretion. If insulin-induced hypoglycemia produces an increase in gastric acid secretion after vagotomy, some vagal innervation to the stomach is assumed to persist but nonvagal mechanisms may also be involved. One year after vagotomy, approximately 50 per cent of patients have a secretory response to insulin. However, only about one of seven patients with an increase in acid secretion after insulin will develop recurrent ulcer disease. Therefore the vast majority of duodenal ulcer patients in whom vagotomy is performed do not develop ulcer recurrence regardless of whether they do or do not respond to insulin. There is a great deal of overlap in the insulin test responses in those with and without recurrence. The insulin test has so little predictive value as to which patients will develop recurrent ulcer that it is of limited practical clinical value.

MEDICAL THERAPY

The four goals of therapy of peptic ulcer disease are to relieve symptoms, to increase the rate of healing, to prevent complications, and to prevent recurrences. Unfortunately, in spite of the multitude of drugs used in the treatment of ulcer disease, there is a paucity of adequately controlled, prospective, double-blind trials in this common disease. The treatment of ulcer disease is therefore in large part empirical. Since the treatment of esophageal, gastric, and duodenal ulcer is similar, the following applies to all forms of acid-peptic disease except when stated otherwise.

Antacids. Antacids are widely used; approximately $110 million are spent on them each year. Surprisingly enough, there are no convincing data indicating that they improve healing, decrease recurrences, or decrease complications. In uncontrolled studies, antacids have been observed to relieve ulcer pain. However, in order to distinguish antacid effect from placebo effect in the therapy of ulcer disease, it is necessary that controlled double-blind prospective studies be conducted. Such clinical studies are currently in progress.

The rationale for the use of antacids in treating ulcer is as follows: (1) ulcer disease does not occur in the absence of gastric acid and pepsin; (2) peptic activity decreases markedly at pH greater than 3.5; (3) the incidence of experimental ulcers in animals can be decreased by antacids; and (4) ulcer disease usually resolves with surgical therapy which decreases gastric acid and pepsin secretion.

Most commercially available antacids consist of mixtures of magnesium, aluminum, or calcium salts. Factors that influence the in vivo efficacy of an antacid include the neutralizing capacity of the antacid, the rate of reaction with acid, the rate of gastric acid secretion, and the rate of gastric emptying.

Sodium Bicarbonate. Sodium bicarbonate is a potent, rapidly acting antacid. It is completely absorbed and so presents the body with a load of sodium and alkali. With normal renal function the body can tolerate the excess alkaline and sodium load. In patients with decreased renal function or salt retention, the alkaline and sodium load may lead to alkalosis and an increase in total body sodium and water. Because sodium bicarbonate is water soluble, it leaves the stomach rapidly, thus producing only transient intragastric alkalization, and therefore it is not used in the treatment of ulcer disease.

Calcium Carbonate. Calcium carbonate is a potent, rapidly acting antacid. In the duodenum most of the calcium is converted into poorly absorbed calcium carbonate, calcium phosphate, and calcium soaps. Less than 10 per cent of the calcium is absorbed from the gut. The advantages of calcium carbonate are that it is inexpensive and potent. Unfortunately calcium-containing antacids may cause hypersecretion or hypercalcemia. Oral calcium produces an increase in acid secretion in the fasting and fed state after a single or repeated dose, and in patients with and without ulcer disease. The increase in acid secretion is probably mediated in part by increased serum gastrin and occurs only after calcium-containing antacids, not with noncalcium antacids.

Repeated oral doses of calcium may produce an increase in serum calcium, phosphate, creatinine, and bicarbonate. Long-term ingestion of calcium carbonate plus sodium bicarbonate may result in the milk-alkali syndrome. This consists of an increase in serum calcium, blood urea nitrogen, serum creatinine, and serum phosphorus, plus systemic alkalosis. If recognized early in a patient with normal renal function, the milk-alkali syndrome may resolve on discontinuing calcium intake. If unrecognized, the milk-alkali syndrome may progress to renal calculi and permanent renal damage. Symptoms of the milk-alkali syndrome include anorexia, malaise, nausea, vomiting, weakness, muscle pain, polydipsia, and polyuria. The symptoms of milk-alkali syndrome are the same as those of hypercalcemia from other causes such as hyperparathyroidism, vitamin D intoxication or metastatic tumors.

Since there are many noncalcium antacids available which do not have the untoward effects of calcium but are effective antacids, some experts believe that calcium-containing antacids should not be used in the treatment of acid-peptic diseases.

Magnesium Hydroxide. Magnesium hydroxide is a potent antacid that reacts rapidly with hydrochloric acid. Magnesium trisilicate reacts with hydrochloric acid more slowly than magnesium hydroxide. Approximately 5 to 10 per cent of the ingested magnesium is absorbed from the gut and excreted by the kidneys. In patients with decreased renal function, serum magnesium level can increase and rarely may produce hypotension and respiratory arrest. Within the gut magnesium salts act as cathartics, so they can seldom be used as the sole antacid.

Aluminum Hydroxide. Aluminum hydroxide reacts with hydrochloric acid to form aluminum chloride. The neutralizing capacity of aluminum hydroxide preparations varies widely; some are ineffective antacids. In the gut aluminum hydroxide and aluminum chloride bind phosphate, producing nonabsorbable aluminum phosphate. Chronic ingestion of aluminum hydroxide can decrease serum and total body phosphate. It is therefore of therapeutic benefit in patients with chronic renal insufficiency and hyperphosphatemia. The adsorptive properties of aluminum hydroxide may decrease absorption of other drugs.

Fordtran found that in vitro buffering capacity correlated well with in vivo postprandial antacid activity. Patients with high levels of gastric acid secretion, "hypersecretors," tend to require larger amounts of antacid than low secretors to achieve a similar degree of neutralization. Because antacids rapidly leave the empty stomach, the effect of antacids in the fasting patient is transient, lasting about 10 to 20 minutes. However, when adequate amounts of antacids are administered one hour after a meal, their effect lasts up to three hours.

At present, antacids are the mainstay of therapy of acid-peptic disease, despite lack of carefully controlled prospective studies on their effect on rate of healing or recurrence rate. In the acutely ill symptomatic patient with ulcer disease, antacids should be given in doses of about 75 mEq (e.g., Maalox, 30 ml; Mylanta II, 18 ml) at hourly intervals during the day and evening, and about 150 mEq at bedtime. When symptoms resolve, antacids are given one and three hours after each meal and at bedtime. Hypersecretors should receive larger doses than those who are not. In patients with sodium retention or hypertension, low-sodium antacids should be given (e.g., Riopan).

Anticholinergic Drugs. Anticholinergics block the action of acetylcholine on postganglionic nerve sites. They are used in the treatment of ulcer to decrease acid and pepsin secretion. They also decrease salivary, bronchial, sweat, and pancreatic secretion and increase heart rate, produce mydriasis, decrease gastric and intestinal motility, and decrease urinary bladder tone and strength of contraction. There is no convincing evidence that any one anticholinergic has a selective action on a specific target.

Standard doses of anticholinergics (i.e., doses which produce dryness of the mouth) decrease basal and histamine or gastrin-stimulated gastric acid secretion by about 50 per cent. Because anticholinergics produce recognizable side effects in addition to decreasing gastric acid secretion, particularly dryness of the mouth, it is difficult to conduct double-blind studies comparing anticholinergic drugs with placebo. In gastric ulcer an anticholinergic (glycopyrronium) improved healing rate and decreased recurrence rate. Some studies suggest that anticholinergics are of value in duodenal ulcer for inducing pain relief and in prevention of recurrence. Other studies conclude that anticholinergics are of no therapeutic value in duodenal ulcer.

If anticholinergics are to be used in the therapy of ulcer disease, they should be prescribed in doses which produce a recognizable effect, such as dry mouth. They should not be used in patients in whom the anticholinergic effect may be harmful, as in patients with glaucoma, prostatism, gastroesophageal reflux, gastric retention, or chronic bronchitis. Anticholinergics probably have their greatest therapeutic effect in ulcer patients with nocturnal pain; a dose at bedtime may be effective in relieving nocturnal pain. Since the greatest amount of acid is secreted in response to a meal, anticholinergics are usually given about 30 minutes before eating.

Diet. Although bland diets have been used in the treatment of ulcer disease for the past 70 years, there is no evidence that a bland diet is more effective than a regular diet in ulcer healing, prevention of complications, or recurrence. During flare-ups of ulcer distress patients often restrict their diets to bland foods. There is no evidence that this reduces symptoms or shortens the attack.

In patients with ulcer disease, hourly milk and cream produced a lower intragastric pH than three regular meals. In addition, excessive milk and cream with antacid may be a factor in the pathogenesis of the milk-alkali syndrome and of atherosclerosis.

There is no evidence that spices in moderate amounts are ulcerogenic or alter the course of ulcer healing or frequency of recurrence. Also, the texture of the diet, soft versus rough, seems to be unimportant in ulcer pathogenesis or therapy. Since caffeine is a stimulant of acid secretion, caffeine-containing beverages (including cola drinks) should probably be excluded from the diet in ulcer patients. Alcohol, by its ability to damage mucosa, may be involved in the pathogenesis of erosions, and alcohol is therefore interdicted in the patient with ulcer disease.

In summary, at present there are no data to support altering the diet of patients with ulcer disease except to discontinue caffeine and alcohol, and to avoid substances which seem to produce symptoms. Also, bedtime snacks which will stimulate acid secretion while the patient is sleeping should be avoided. Food should not be used as an antacid, because the neutralization produced by food is always followed by increased secretion.

Hospitalization. In gastric ulcer hospitalization has been reported to increase the rate of ulcer healing when compared to outpatient management. The cost for prolonged hospitalization is often prohibitive, so it is recommended that patients with suspected or demonstrated gastric ulcer be hospitalized briefly to expedite careful evaluation of the ulcer by radiography, endoscopy with biopsy, and, if available, gastric cytology. Medical therapy can be initiated during hospitalization.

In hospitalized male veterans with gastric ulcer, the recurrence rate in two years was 60 per cent in those who healed slowly (less than 90 per cent in six weeks) and 40 per cent in those who healed more rapidly. Patients with large gastric ulcers, gastric ulcers plus duodenal ulcers, and black veterans tended to have a higher ulcer recurrence rate.

Serial radiograms of a gastric ulcer should be obtained at three- or four-week intervals for a maximum of 12 weeks. The ulcer should completely heal within this period. For those patients in whom the ulcer does not heal, surgery is indicated. Surgery is also recommended for the patient with second or third gastric ulcer recurrences.

The effect of hospitalization on duodenal ulcer has not been carefully studied.

Other Treatments. *Carbenoxolone Sodium.* Carbenoxolone sodium has been shown to increase healing in ambulatory patients with gastric ulcer to a rate comparable to that of inpatients. Carbenoxolone sodium increases the production and viscosity of gastric mucus, and also increases the life span of the gastric mucosal cells. These may be the mechanisms by which it increased gastric ulcer healing rate. Carbenoxolone sodium is structurally similar to aldosterone and therefore produces salt and water retention. The efficacy of carbenoxolone sodium can be maintained while avoiding salt retention with the administration of thiazide diuretics. Structurally similar aldosterone-blocking agents (e.g., aldactone) decrease the efficacy of carbenoxolone.

Sedation. Sedation has not been shown to be of value in the therapy of peptic ulcer disease. It is not recommended for routine use. Some physicians believe, however, that allaying anxiety in such patients may facilitate the recommended treatment program.

Estrogens. Estrogens have been demonstrated to be effective in increasing healing rate in duodenal ulcer, but not in gastric ulcer. Since they have untoward effects, particularly in males, they are not recommended.

Interdiction of Smoking. Discontinuing smoking has been shown to increase the healing rate in hospitalized patients with gastric ulcer. The incidence of gastric and duodenal ulcer is greater in smokers than in nonsmokers. Smoking should be discouraged in patients with peptic ulcer disease—not to the extent, however, that anxiety is produced.

Gastric Irradiation. Irradiation of the oxyntic gland portion of the stomach produces a decrease in acid secretion usually lasting less than one year. In some patients prolonged hypochlorhydria is produced. At present, gastric irradiation is employed only in those rare patients who are intractable to medical therapy and in whom surgery carries a prohibitive mortality.

642. CLINICAL AND ENDOCRINE ASPECTS

John H. Walsh

CLINICAL MANIFESTATIONS

Symptoms. In many patients the diagnosis of peptic ulcer disease may be made with reasonable certainty by history alone. Epigastric pain is the cardinal symptom. The location and character of the pain, its temporal pattern, and factors that aggravate or relieve it produce a characteristic clinical picture. It must be recognized, however, that patients may have peptic ulcer without typical symptoms and, conversely, that other patients may have typical symptoms without a demonstrable ulcer.

Location. Typical ulcer pain is epigastric, near the midline. Patients with gastric ulcer tend to localize the pain slightly to the left of midline, and those with duodenal ulcer, slightly to the right. Such subtle distinctions are rarely helpful in individual patients. The pain may be so sharply localized that the patient will indicate its site by pointing with one or two fingers.

Character. The pain may be described as burning, gnawing, cramping, boring, or aching, or as a sensation of pressure, heaviness, or hunger. It may be mild or severe. It may fluctuate in intensity, but, even when described as cramping, it usually comes in waves lasting at least several minutes. The pain is not aggravated by body motion. The difficulty which many patients have in describing the nature of the pain is probably due to its visceral origin.

Temporal Relationships and Pain Relief. The time course of the pain is the most useful feature which differentiates it from pain of other diseases. Usually, ulcer pain appears in clusters of days to weeks, interspersed with pain-free intervals of weeks to months. Thus chronicity and periodicity are typical of ulcer symptoms. The pattern of recurrent attacks may continue for many years without significant change; the pain may become more frequent or severe, or, in a minority of patients, it may diminish and finally disappear after a few years. The old adage "once an ulcer, always an ulcer" is true for the majority of patients with peptic ulcer.

The daily pain pattern roughly parallels the normal time course of gastric acidity. Thus pain is diminished in the early morning, when gastric acid secretion is low, and after meals, when acid is buffered by food. Pain is increased several hours after each meal, when acid secretion is high and is not buffered by food, and at bedtime. Likewise, measures which reduce intragastric acidity (oral antacids, food, nasogastric suction) typically relieve the pain. In some patients with gastric ulcer, a meal may produce transient worsening of the pain, followed by relief.

During the periods which are free of ulcer pain, the patient usually feels perfectly well.

Associated Symptoms. Nausea and/or excessive salivation may accompany peptic ulcer pain. Anorexia may occur in patients with gastric ulcer. Spontaneous vomiting is an occasional symptom, more commonly associated with gastric than with duodenal ulcers.

These features of ulcer pain are typical of patients with chronic uncomplicated peptic ulcer disease. Some patients may never experience pain and are found to have peptic ulcer disease only after they present with a complication of their disease (see below). Development of a complication may also lead to a change in the character of the pain (see below). Atypical symptoms are common in children and in elderly patients with peptic ulcer disease.

Physical Examination. Epigastric tenderness is frequently present, but is seldom marked, and is nonspecific. In fact, the general physical examination is of little help in establishing the diagnosis of uncomplicated peptic ulcer disease.

Differential Diagnosis. Any disease producing epigastric pain must be differentiated from peptic ulcer disease. Disease of only a few abdominal organs (stomach, liver, gallbladder, and pancreas) produces pain in this area; pain arising from the small intestine, large intestine, and bladder is felt lower in the abdomen. Pain arising in the gastroesophageal region and esophagus is usually felt in the subxiphoid area or retrosternally.

Pain from intrathoracic structures may also be referred to the epigastrium. Pain referred to the epigastric area may predominate in *pleuritis, myocardial infarction,* or *pericarditis.* These diseases are usually not confused with peptic ulcer disease. The pain they produce tends to be acute rather than chronic, constant rather than episodic, not related to meals or relieved by antacids, and usually associated with other pain or symptoms atypical of ulcer disease.

Pain arising from the esophagus (usually from *peptic esophagitis* or *peptic ulcer disease of the esophagus*) may exhibit some features typical of peptic ulcer pain such as temporal relation to meals and relief by antacids. However, lower esophageal pain, although occasionally epigastric, is usually felt as retrosternal "heartburn," and esophagitis is usually accompanied by symptoms of regurgitation of gastric contents which are accentuated by straining or by assuming a horizontal position.

Epigastric pain produced by intra-abdominal diseases not involving the stomach or duodenum can usually be distinguished easily from peptic ulcer disease. *Acute cholecystitis* may produce epigastric pain or pain in the right upper quadrant with rapid onset and duration of hours to days, and is frequently accompanied by tenderness over the gallbladder and fever. Patients will often have a history of previous attacks of biliary colic. *Acute pancreatitis* frequently produces epigastric pain, but the pain usually radiates to the back, and is aggravated by changes in position. Moreover, in either acute cholecystitis or pancreatitis, signs of acute abdominal inflammation (fever, direct and rebound tenderness, abdominal distention, or ileus) are typical and are not found in uncomplicated ulcer disease.

In the United States most gastric ulcers are benign, but the possibility of *malignant gastric ulcer* must be considered in every patient with gastric ulceration. Appropriate studies are discussed in Ch. 641.

Duodenitis. Duodenitis (inflammation of the duodenal mucosa) is frequently found in conjunction with active duodenal ulcer. It may also be found in patients with typical ulcer symptoms but without demonstrable ulcers. Such patients may have gastric hypersecretion, radiologic evidence of coarse duodenal folds, and histologic evidence of mononuclear infiltration and microscopic ulceration. Many patients with duodenitis later develop frank duodenal ulcer disease, and this condition may be a stage in the natural history of ulcer disease in some patients. Symptomatic duodenitis may also arise from eosinophilic or granulomatous infiltration of the duodenum.

Gastritis. In addition to gastritis associated with ulcer disease (see above), several forms of *chronic gastritis* may affect the stomach. Chronic superficial gastritis, atrophic gastritis, and gastric atrophy increase in frequency with age and sometimes are associated with epigastric symptoms but seldom produce any well defined pattern resembling peptic ulcer. Diseases infiltrating the wall of the stomach (carcinoma, lymphoma, granulomatous gastritis caused by Crohn's disease, eosinophilic granuloma, sarcoidosis, tuberculosis, or syphilis) may produce ulcer-like symptoms. Such symptoms are found in about a third of patients with adult hypertrophic pyloric stenosis and are relatively common in patients with Ménétrier's disease (hypertrophic gastropathy associated with protein loss into the gastrointestinal tract). Most of these diseases are rare. Their diagnosis depends on exclusion of peptic ulcer disease and demonstration of characteristic pathology by radiographic, endoscopic, and/or histologic examination.

Functional Dyspepsia. Functional dyspepsia is a syndrome with symptoms resembling many of those found in peptic ulcer disease but with no demonstrable pathologic lesion and with a prognosis free of complications of ulcer disease. Patients with functional dyspepsia have chronic and recurrent symptoms of epigastric distress. Pain-free intervals tend to be of short duration. Antacids frequently produce either partial or complete relief of epigastric pain, but food is likely to aggravate the distress. Often the pain is poorly localized, and the patients frequently complain of "gas." Nausea, vomiting, and pain may occur in the morning before breakfast. Nocturnal pain is encountered less frequently than in ulcer disease. The distinction between functional dyspepsia and peptic ulcer disease may be impossible to make by history alone. This is a diagnosis of exclusion, made only after careful radiographic and endoscopic examinations have excluded the diagnosis of peptic ulcer disease. As with duodenitis, a significant percentage of patients with "functional dyspepsia" will be found to have peptic ulcer disease when followed over a period of years.

ENDOCRINE HYPERFUNCTION AND ULCER DISEASE

Zollinger-Ellison Syndrome. One syndrome in which it has been established without doubt that ulcer disease is caused by hormonal excess is the Zollinger-Ellison syndrome. This syndrome is usually characterized by fulminant peptic ulcer diathesis or occasionally by diarrhea without ulcer, gastric acid hypersecretion, and a gastrin-secreting tumor, usually originating in the pancreas, which causes hypergastrinemia. The role of gastrin in the production of this syndrome was proved by chemical isolation of gastrin from such tumors and by bioassay of gastrin in serum and tumor extracts from patients with the syndrome. Gastrin radioimmunoassay has provided additional information about the pathogenesis of this disease and has permitted identification of many new patients.

The Zollinger-Ellison syndrome occurs in all age groups but is diagnosed most often between the third and fifth decades. The proportion of patients with ulcer disease who have the syndrome is unknown, but it is probably less than 1 per cent.

The predominant symptom is abdominal pain, which may be similar to that of ordinary ulcer disease or may be more severe. Intervals without pain tend to be shorter than in ordinary ulcer disease. Pain is present in more than 80 per cent of patients and usually has been present for a year or more before the diagnosis is established. Other prominent symptoms include diarrhea, vomiting, melena, and hematemesis. Recurrent ulceration after ulcer operation is unfortunately too often the first evidence of the disease. Some patients do not exhibit florid symptoms or may not have marked hypergastrinemia on a single determination and may be difficult to distinguish from those with ordinary ulcers.

In approximately three fourths of patients with the Zollinger-Ellison syndrome, there is an ulcer in the duodenal bulb or immediate postbulbar area. Ulcers in the distal duodenum or proximal jejunum are very suggestive but are found in less than one fourth of patients. Other radiologic features which are helpful in suggesting the diagnosis are hypertrophic gastric folds, increased quantities of gastric juice, dilatation of the duodenum and jejunum and mucosal edema, and irregularity in the small intestine. Occasionally there is a gastric ulcer (see figure in Ch. 640).

The diarrhea associated with the Zollinger-Ellison syndrome is due primarily to massive gastric hypersecretion and can be relieved by nasogastric aspiration or by total gastrectomy. The large amount of acid delivered into the upper intestine causes mucosal damage and increased intestinal motility. In addition, gastrin exerts an effect on the intestinal mucosa, decreasing absorption of salt and water, and also affects intestinal motility. The diarrhea is frequently accompanied by steatorrhea. Responsible factors include inactivation of pancreatic lipase and precipitation of conjugated bile salts at low intraluminal pH as well as direct damage of the mucosa by acid.

The gastrin-secreting tumors, or gastrinomas, responsible for the Zollinger-Ellison syndrome are usually small and may be difficult to find at operation or at postmortem examination. These tumors are most commonly located in the pancreas where they originate in the islets, but they may also originate in the duodenum. Metastasis and occurrence of multiple primary tumors are both common, so that the chances of locating a single benign operable tumor are probably less than one in four. Therefore treatment is total gastrectomy (see below).

Association with Other Endocrine Tumors. Individuals with the Zollinger-Ellison syndrome frequently have other endocrine abnormalities. The most common associated syndrome is hyperparathyroidism, which is found in about 20 per cent of patients with the disease. Hyperparathyroidism greatly affects the gastric secretory pattern in some of these patients. Hypercalcemia has been shown to release tumor gastrin and leads to increased acid secretion. Conversely, correction of hyperparathyroidism by parathyroidectomy may lead to transient or prolonged decreases in serum gastrin and acid secretion and may lead to periods of clinical remission. Other endocrine tumors found in the Zollinger-Ellison syndrome include pituitary, adrenal, ovarian, and thyroid. The abnormality may be carcinoma, single or multiple adenomas, or diffuse hyperplasia. The islet cell tumors may produce other substances such as insulin, glucagon, and ACTH.

A familial form of the Zollinger-Ellison syndrome was first described by Wermer. Several families have been described subsequently. There is autosomal dominant transmission with high but variable expressivity. The same pattern of glandular involvement and pathology is found as in the sporadic cases of multiple endocrine neoplasia.

Diagnosis. The diagnosis of the Zollinger-Ellison syndrome may be suggested by ulcer symptoms refractory to ordinary medical treatment, by radiologic findings, by gastric acid hypersecretion in the presence of ulcer symptoms, by recurrence of ulcer after an ulcer operation, or by the finding of an increased serum gastrin concentration. Gastric secretion is usually found to be excessive. Suspicion should be aroused when basal secretion is greater than 10mEq HCl per hour in an unoperated patient or greater than 5 mEq per hour in a patient with previous gastric surgery for ulcer. Confirmation of the diagnosis in most patients can be made by measurement of fasting serum gastrin concentration, with levels greater than 600 pg per milliliter in the presence of acid hypersecretion virtually diagnostic of the syndrome. In patients with hypersecretion in whom fasting serum gastrin level is equivocal (150 to 600 pg per milliliter), further evidence for the disease may be obtained by demonstration of minimal response of serum gastrin to a protein meal (normal subjects and duodenal ulcer patients show a twofold increase in serum gastrin concentrations after a protein meal) but an exaggerated increase in response to intravenous infusion of calcium and a paradoxical increase in response to intravenous secretin.

Patients with gastric ulcer tend to have moderately increased basal gastrin values, similar to those found in postprandial subjects. Gastric outlet obstruction leads to a moderate increase in basal gastrin which returns toward normal after a few days of gastric aspiration. Some patients with ordinary duodenal ulcer appear to have an exaggerated postprandial release of gastrin. Moderately to markedly increased fasting gastrin is found in many patients with achlorhydria who lack the normal inhibitory mechanism of antral acidification. The syndrome of *isolated retained antrum* after attempted antrectomy and gastrojejunostomy may produce gastric hypersecretion associated with hypergastrinemia. It is not clear whether there is a separate group of patients with hypergastrinemia caused by gastrin cell hyperplasia of the gastric antrum with autonomous release of gastrin not susceptible to acid inhibition.

Treatment. The usual treatment of the Zollinger-Ellison syndrome is total gastrectomy. Under some circumstances a period of medical treatment with anticholinergic drugs and antacids may be justified, especially for patients in whom the diagnosis is not certain and who have had no complications of ulcer disease. If operation is indicated, performance of less than total gastrectomy often leads to recurrent ulceration, frequently in the immediate postoperative period, and is often complicated by bleeding, perforation, and death. Occasionally it is possible to resect a single tumor and cure the disease.

643. COMPLICATIONS AND SURGICAL TREATMENT

James H. Meyer

COMPLICATIONS

Hemorrhage. Hemorrhage afflicts about 15 to 20 per cent of ulcer patients, being two to three times more common than perforation or obstruction. Duodenal ulcers bleed slightly more often than gastric ulcers; duodenal ulcers along the posterior duodenal wall or postbulbar ulcers bleed more frequently than anterior duodenal ulcers. Hemorrhage is usually from a major artery eroded by the ulcer and less commonly from smaller vessels in granulation tissue in the ulcer.

About 25 per cent of patients with bleeding ulcers have never recognized ulcer symptoms previously. In almost all patients hemorrhage is manifested by melena; but three patients in four (fewer with duodenal ulcer) experience hematemesis as well. Diaphoresis, pallor, palpitations, lightheadedness, mental confusion, or syncope are symptoms of associated hypotension which arises either as a direct result of blood volume loss or from a vasovagal reaction to sudden loss of blood.

Other than ulcer, the only common causes of upper gastrointestinal bleeding are acute gastric *mucosal lesions* (diffuse or localized, spontaneous or drug induced) and *esophageal varices*. Less common causes include *bleeding esophagitis, Mallory-Weiss tears, benign* (leiomyoma) or *malignant* (gastric carcinoma, lymphoma) *tumors, eosinophilic gastritis, milk allergy* (in children), and a variety of *rare vascular lesions* (hereditary hemorrhagic telangiectasia, phlebectasia of the jejunum, pseudoxanthoma elasticum, periarteritis, Ehlers-Danlos syndrome). Spontaneous upper gastrointestinal hemorrhage may accompany severe coagulation defects associated with underlying disease or anticoagulant therapy. As a diagnostic tool, the physical examination is helpful primarily in providing clues to bleeding lesions other than peptic ulcer, especially esophageal varices (e.g., hepatosplenomegaly, ascites, jaundice) and vascular abnormalities.

Upper gastrointestinal hemorrhage carries a significant mortality (about 10 per cent in ulcer disease). Therefore any patient experiencing melena, with or without hematemesis or associated symptoms or hypotension, should be hospitalized immediately for further evaluation and treatment. The over-all approach to the patient with upper gastrointestinal bleeding is discussed in Ch. 644.

Treatment. The program of immediate treatment consists of continued resuscitation as needed, reduction of gastric acidity, and continuous evaluation of the patient with the expectancy that surgical intervention may be required to save the patient's life. It is desirable that both physician and surgeon follow the patient's progress from the outset.

Many physicians prefer to treat the patient with continuous nasogastric aspiration as long as bleeding continues. When properly employed (proper tube placement, periodic venting), this procedure empties 90 to 95 per cent of secreted acid from the stomach and is therefore an adequate treatment. The appearance of blood in the gastric aspirate may also serve as an index of recurrent or continued bleeding. Alternatively, the patient may be treated with frequent antacids (see above) either from the outset or after the nasogastric tube is removed when bleeding has stopped. Most physicians prefer not to use anticholinergic drugs during hemorrhage, because these agents obscure signs of recurrent bleeding (they produce sustained tachycardia and diminish hyperactive bowel sounds which often indicate fresh blood in the gut).

If more than 3000 ml of blood is required for resuscitation, mortality increases significantly and is especially high if this quantity of blood is required in the first 48 hours. Emergency surgery is indicated in a patient who requires transfusion at a rate in excess of 3 units per day for the first 24 to 48 hours to maintain a stable circulation, once antecedent losses have been replenished. When bleeding has stopped under medical management but major hemorrhage subsequently reappears in spite of continued treatment, surgery should be undertaken, because it is likely that further medical treatment will not be successful and it is known that continued medical treatment in this situation carries a high mortality. Under these policies 15 to 30 per cent of bleeding ulcer patients will require emergency surgery.

Until recently, the traditional form of emergency surgery has been subtotal gastrectomy, usually with ligation or removal of the bleeding ulcer. Since the early 1960's, surgeons have favored the use of vagotomy plus pyloroplasty with ligation of bleeding vessels, citing lower mortality because of the speed and ease with which this operation can be performed. Retrospective analyses of mortality rates of these two operations in the bleeding patient are to date inadequate to substantiate the superiority of vagotomy plus pyloroplasty. Both operations effectively stop acute bleeding in 92 to 95 per cent of patients who are bleeding from a single, discrete ulcer, but are much less effective in stopping bleeding in patients with multiple stress ulcers.

Prognosis. Death from bleeding ulcer is more frequent in patients over 50 years of age. Bleeding gastric ulcers are more apt to be lethal than bleeding duodenal ulcers for two reasons: (1) patients with gastric ulcers are older than patients with duodenal ulcer, and (2) regardless of age, patients with gastric ulcer tend to bleed more profusely than patients with duodenal ulcer. Most forms of associated cardiovascular disease other than benign hypertension (ischemic or valvular heart disease, cor pulmonale) adversely affect the prognosis, as does any severe associated disease. It is not known whether earlier surgery in these higher risk patients would reduce mortality, because those patients are also the ones with higher operative mortality.

Thirty to 50 per cent of patients surviving the first hemorrhage without operative intervention will hemor-rhage again; the severity of the subsequent hemorrhage bears no relationship to the severity of the first episode. Continued morbidity (recurrent hemorrhage, intractable ulcer pain, subsequent perforation) is the rule in up to 70 per cent of ulcer patients who have bleeding. It is not clear whether surgery (emergent or elective) in the bleeding duodenal ulcer patient will significantly reduce recurrent bleeding. For the most part this is due to bleeding from recurrence of ulcer after surgery by either of the two procedures.

Impaired Gastric Emptying ("Outlet Obstruction"). This complication is seen in 5 to 10 per cent of ulcer patients. In the majority of cases (80 per cent), it appears as a complication of duodenal ulcer disease, usually of long duration. Gastric ulcers, most frequently prepyloric, are the second most common cause. Although pyloric channel ulcers may cause gastric outlet obstruction, ulcers at this site are infrequent.

In ulcer disease, impaired gastric emptying may develop as the result of narrowing of the lumen by fibrosis and/or inflammatory tumor around the ulcer. However, in many cases gastric motor dysfunction, associated with inflammation around the ulcer or with gradual dilatation of the stomach and stretching of gastric muscle beyond optimal force/length characteristics, plays a dominant role. Impaired gastric emptying is thus potentially reversible to the extent that gastric motor dysfunction can be corrected or that luminal narrowing by inflammation can be reduced with healing.

In the initial phases, mechanical outlet obstruction is usually not complete. However, ingested materials and gastric secretions gradually accumulate to produce gastric dilatation. With gastric dilatation, the patient begins to experience symptoms of constant epigastric fullness and discomfort, anorexia, sitophobia, and nausea. Vomiting (spontaneous or induced) may relieve these symptoms. The whole process tends to develop insidiously over days or weeks. The eventual development of protracted vomiting, usually of copious amounts of undigested food, brings the patient to the physician.

In the typical case the diagnosis is easily made by the history. However, about a fourth of patients with impaired gastric emptying never vomit before seeking medical attention, presumably because they have reduced oral intake to an amount that can be emptied by the partially obstructed stomach. In this minority the diagnosis is usually discovered during an upper gastrointestinal series which reveals a large, dilated stomach filled with solid and liquid material in spite of the customary overnight fast prior to the examination. In most patients physical examination confirms recent weight loss and evidence of dehydration. Abdominal distention and tenderness are rarely noted, and bowel sounds are normal. A gastric succussion splash may be elicited in about half the patients. Diagnosis suspected on the basis of historical and physical findings can be quickly confirmed by the placement of a large-bore orogastric (Ewald) tube; aspiration of 300 ml or more of gastric contents three or more hours after the last meal indicates gastric outlet obstruction.

Patients with gastric outlet obstruction must be hospitalized for treatment. The goals of hospitalization are fourfold: (1) correction of fluid and electrolyte deficits, (2) gastric decompression, (3) intensive ulcer treatment, and (4) surgery if obstruction persists.

In the face of protracted vomiting and no effective oral intake, fluid and electrolyte depletion may be profound.

Extracellular fluid and plasma volume deficits may be reflected by orthostatic hypotension, prerenal azotemia, elevated hematocrit, and abnormally low central venous pressure. Some degree of metabolic alkalosis and hypokalemia is common. The latter may accentuate gastric motor dysfunction. These deficits must be rapidly corrected; they contribute to continued morbidity and may be responsible for increased surgical mortality.

There are two sources of electrolyte losses in the patient with gastric outlet obstruction: (1) hydrochloric acid and lesser amounts of sodium and potassium chloride are lost with the gastric juice which is vomited or aspirated, and (2) considerable amounts of sodium and potassium are lost in the urine. For every H^+ ion lost in the gastric juice, one Cl^- ion is similarly lost and one HCO_3^- ion enters the circulation. During the early phases of obstruction, bicarbonate entering the bloodstream is cleared from the urine as $NaHCO_3$, and chloride losses are minimized by renal tubular reabsorption. At this stage the urine is characteristically alkaline and contains appreciable sodium, but is low in chloride. In effect, the kidney converts an HCl loss from the stomach to a net NaCl loss from the body (Na^+ lost in urine, Cl^- lost in gastric juice), and in this way metabolic alkalosis is minimized. However, as the body's deficit in NaCl mounts, secondary hyperaldosteronism intervenes. As a result, much more filtered Na^+ is reabsorbed by the renal tubules. Some is absorbed in exchange for K^+, and more is absorbed in exchange for H^+ secreted by the tubules. For every H^+ secreted by the renal tubules, one HCO_3^- enters the bloodstream. At this stage the urine is characteristically low in both sodium and chloride, but may contain significant amounts of potassium and may be paradoxically acidic. In effect, the kidney is no longer compensating for gastric losses; H^+ and Cl^- losses from the stomach are now aggravated by H^+ and Cl^- losses from the kidney. Sustained metabolic alkalosis, hypochloremia, and hypokalemia result.

Reversal of this sequence of events is accomplished by infusion of 0.15N NaCl intravenously. Potassium replacement as KCl may be started once an adequate urinary output has been established. Enough saline has to be given (1) to replenish continued gastric losses and (2) to replace antecedent sodium and chloride deficits. The adequacy of this replacement can be judged (1) by the disappearance of orthostatic hypotension and the return of venous pressure to normal, (2) by the reappearance of an alkaline urine with a rising sodium concentration, and (3) by rising chloride concentration in the urine. As these changes are observed, prerenal azotemia, metabolic alkalosis, and hypokalemia should disappear.

In the meantime gastric decompression is instituted to eliminate gastric dilatation and restore motor tone. This is accomplished by continuous nasogastric aspiration once the stomach has been lavaged free of solid debris through a large-bore orogastric tube. Usually a period of 72 hours is adequate to restore gastric tone. Continuous gastric aspiration, by removing secreted gastric acid, is also an effective treatment for active ulcer disease. This treatment thus serves to reduce inflammatory edema around the ulcer and thus may help to relieve the cause of the obstruction. With good management, fluid and electrolyte disturbances will have been corrected by 72 hours as well.

The end of the first 72 hours thus represents a point of reappraisal. If the nature of the obstructing lesion is in doubt at this time, an upper gastrointestinal series may be obtained to establish the diagnosis. This examination will also provide some indication as to how well the preceding treatment has restored gastric emptying. Some physicians assess gastric emptying by the saline load test. If more than 400 ml remains in the stomach 30 minutes after instilling 750 ml of isotonic saline, emptying is impaired. If the stomach does not empty, it is unlikely that further medical treatment will be effective, and surgery should be considered. If emptying is adequate, the patient may be begun on oral liquids and antacids. However, for the next several days continuous assessment of gastric emptying must be performed. If the patient has more than 300 ml of gastric residual at bedtime (four hours after the last intake) or more than 200 ml of residual after an overnight fast, or if the saline load test is abnormal, gastric emptying is still impaired and surgical treatment is indicated.

About 25 per cent of obstructed patients will require surgery by these criteria. Of those who escape surgery in a given episode, 15 per cent will have a recurrent episode of obstruction, frequently requiring surgery.

Perforation. Any peptic ulcer may eventually erode through the muscular and serosal walls of the viscus in which it is located. If such erosion establishes a communication between the lumen of the viscus and the surrounding body cavity, allowing spillage of luminal contents into this cavity, perforation has occurred. If, on the other hand, the transmural erosion is sealed by surrounding visceral structures or peritoneum before spillage of luminal contents supervenes, the ulcer is said to have penetrated.

Free perforation occurs in about 5 to 10 per cent of ulcer patients. About 90 per cent of these perforations arise from a duodenal ulcer, usually in the anterior duodenal wall. Nine per cent arise from gastric ulcers and the remainder from perforated malignant gastric ulcers or perforated marginal ulcers after subtotal gastric resection. Free perforation is almost always heralded by the sudden onset of intense, usually generalized and constant abdominal pain. Usually these dramatic symptoms follow years of intermittent ulcer-like pain, but in about 25 per cent of patients ulcer pain preceding the perforation will have been noted for less than three months, and 7 per cent of patients with perforation have never recognized ulcer symptoms previously. Perforation may arise at any age (peak incidence is in the fifth and sixth decades), and age-specific rates of perforation increase throughout life, even though ulcer disease generally remits in older life. Elderly patients who perforate frequently do not experience intense symptoms, so the diagnosis may not be appreciated. Ten per cent of patients who perforate hemorrhage simultaneously.

Physical examination usually confirms the diagnosis suspected on historical grounds. Generalized direct and rebound tenderness, boardlike rigidity of the abdominal musculature, and diminished or absent bowel sounds resulting from reflex ileus are signs of generalized peritonitis which accompanies perforation. Swallowed air escaping through the perforation into the abdominal cavity may result in loss of normal hepatic dullness on percussion; this air can be visualized radiographically under the diaphragm on upright or lateral abdominal films in 75 to 80 per cent of patients who have perforated. In the absence of a classic history, signs of generalized peritonitis from perforated ulcer could be ascribed to any abdominal catastrophe (e.g., rupture of a volvulus, diverticulum, gallbladder, or appendix; fulminant pancreatitis). Moreover, escaping luminal contents are occasionally confined to the upper abdomen or lesser sac or are spilled down the right gutter into the right lower quadrant; in these situations signs of peritonitis may be localized rather than generalized, so the condition may be misdiagnosed. In practice, however, the diagnosis of perforated ulcer is made correctly about 90 per cent of the time.

Peritonitis associated with perforation produces dehydration owing to fluid loss into the peritoneal cavity. Leukocytosis and fever also reflect peritonitis, but the latter is not a common sequel to perforation treated quickly. Serum amylase is often elevated as the result of perforation.

Three forms of treatment are available: (1) medical treatment, which consists of carefully monitored continuous nasogastric aspiration to allow the perforation to seal, (2) simple surgical closure of the perforation, and (3) surgical closure of the perforation combined with an operation for the ulcer disease. Medical treatment, *when properly managed,* is as safe and effective as surgical closure. However, surgical closure permits direct inspection of the abdominal cavity at laparotomy, minimizing errors in diagnosis. Consequently, surgical closure is the preferred treatment. Patients who perforate after longstanding ulcer symptoms continue to experience significant morbidity from ulcer disease after simple closure of the perforation. For this reason, most surgeons undertake definitive ulcer surgery at the time of closure of a perforation in patients with a longstanding ulcer history, provided that the patient's condition permits a more extensive procedure.

Penetration. Ulcers which penetrate are usually refractory to medical treatment. Posterior duodenal ulcers are most likely to penetrate. Penetration is heralded by a change in pain pattern. Classically visceral ulcer pain takes on somatic characteristics felt in the back, chest, or lateral abdomen. Often pain becomes constant and is no longer relieved by food or antacids. Some ulcers which penetrate into the head of the pancreas may result in localized pancreatitis and elevation of serum amylase. Definitive treatment for penetrating ulcer is surgical.

SURGICAL TREATMENT

Indications for Elective Surgery for Peptic Ulcer. It is uncertain whether sustained medical treatment can significantly alter the long-term course of ulcer disease. For the relapse-prone patient who experiences significant cumulative morbidity attended with economic loss and periods of absence from his life's pursuits, surgical treatment is an alternative, but unfortunately the operations available are all associated with continued postoperative morbidity in a significant number of patients (see accompanying table). Moreover, although surgery cures the ulcer in 90 per cent or more of patients, no guarantee can be made to the individual patient. For these reasons, the decision to operate electively for intractable ulcer disease must be carefully considered by patient, physician, and surgeon. The problem is to decide whether morbidity under medical management is likely to be greater than that which arises after surgery. Only a few guidelines can be offered to aid this decision.

Duodenal Ulcer. A period of observation under medical supervision is required to judge the virulence of duodenal ulcer disease in any individual patient. A significant number (probably about 25 per cent) of patients will experience only a single episode of duodenal ulceration which responds adequately to medical treatment; clearly these patients do not require surgery. Repeated recurrences more often than biannually indicate that the patient suffers from an unusually virulent form of the disease and that surgical treatment should be considered, but other factors must be taken into account as well. Among these factors is the disability produced by each recurrence. The personality of the patient must also be considered, for there is some evidence that a poorly motivated patient (as evidenced by poor work records antedating the ulcer disease or poor social adjustments) is more likely to experience postoperative morbidity. Only a minority of duodenal ulcer patients present with less equivocal indications for surgery: duodenal ulcers secondary to gastrinomas (see above), penetrating duodenal ulcers (see above), and giant duodenal ulcers. These are frequently refractory to medical treatment and are prone to complications, so surgical treatment is appropriate. Also, the development of one or more complications alters the prognosis; surgery may be required to treat these complications as they arise or may be subsequently elected because the patient has demonstrated, by the development of these complications, that he has virulent ulcer disease.

Gastric Ulcer. A similar line of reasoning applies to the patient with gastric ulcer. Recurrence is common (up to 40 per cent in two years), and morbidity from frequent recurrence is high. However, the problem of gastric ulcer differs from duodenal ulcer in two respects. (1) In gastric ulcer healing poorly under medical treatment, the possibility arises that the lesion is an ulcerated cancer which has escaped detection. Consequently, surgery may be undertaken even during the first occurrence if there is doubt about the nature of the lesion. (2) The patient with gastric ulcer tends to be older and may suffer from diseases associated with aging which alter operative risks and thus may influence the decision concerning surgery.

Outcome of Elective Operation for Duodenal Ulcer in Patients Followed Three to Eight Years*

Operation	Mortality (%)†	Ulcer Recurrence (%)	Postprandial Symptoms (%)‡	Weight Loss	Diarrhea (%)
Subtotal gastrectomy	0–2	2–5	36–40	++	7
Vagotomy and antrectomy	0–2	0–3	34–39	++	20–23
Vagotomy and drainage	0–2	7–9	21–40	+	25–26

*Results compiled from three randomized studies: Br. Med. J., 2:781, 1968; Ann. Surg., 172:547, 1970; and Surg. Gynecol. Obstet., 131:233, 1970.

†In these studies, high risk patients were not included; therefore mortality rates are lower than would be expected from the application of each procedure to all patients (see text).

‡Highest percentage of patients with any of several varieties of postprandial distress.

Types of Surgical Treatment. *Duodenal Ulcer.* Three types of operation are currently employed for duodenal ulcer: (1) *subtotal gastrectomy,* in which 75 to 80 per cent of distal stomach is removed and gastrointestinal continuity is restored by an anastomosis between the gastric remnant and the jejunum; (2) *vagotomy and "drainage,"* a procedure in which the vagus nerves are cut and the outlet of the stomach is widened by either a pyloroplasty or a gastroenterostomy; and (3) *vagotomy and antrectomy,* which consists of cutting the vagus nerves, removing the distal 50 per cent of the stomach, and re-establishing gastrointestinal continuity by gastroduodenostomy or gastrojejunostomy. "Drainage" is performed to obviate gastric stasis, which tends to occur after vagotomy. "Parietal cell vagotomy" is a promising new operation, not yet adequately evaluated, in which the surgeon cuts vagal fibers to only the part of the stomach proximal to antrum; no "drainage" procedure is required.

All three traditional operations are associated with some degree of postoperative morbidity (see table). The procedure of vagotomy and drainage does not require duodenal transection. This avoids postoperative leakage from a suture line through a badly diseased duodenum, a frequent source of postoperative mortality. This advantage of vagotomy and drainage, as opposed to the resective procedures, is not reflected by the table, because in studies presented there vagotomy and drainage was employed whenever operative conditions were not optimal. Nevertheless, it is apparent from the table that any reduced mortality from this procedure is offset by a significantly higher recurrence rate.

Gastric Ulcer. For gastric ulcer, the traditional surgical treatment is distal gastrectomy with gastroduodenostomy. In most instances this resection removes the ulcer; with high gastric ulcers it may be combined with a wedge resection of the ulcer or biopsies of the ulcer margins to ascertain the benignancy of the ulcer. Some have proposed that vagotomy and drainage be used for gastric ulcer. However, gastric ulcer recurrences are more frequent after this procedure than after distal resection.

Chronic Postoperative Morbidity. *Prandial and Postprandial Symptoms.* *Early satiety* (intense feeling of fullness before finishing a meal, experienced by 36 to 60 per cent of patients) and *bilious vomiting* (in 13 per cent) shortly after eating are complaints encountered after all three operations. The "dumping" syndrome, a symptom complex which includes any or all of the following: nausea, vomiting, abdominal cramps, borborygmi, flatulence, diarrhea, diaphoresis, palpitations, tachycardia, lightheadedness, and flushing, may be experienced while eating or immediately afterward, especially after meals high in sugar content. The syndrome is believed to arise from the rapid entry of hyperosmolar liquids into the gut. It is experienced in mild form by about 20 per cent of operated patients, but is troublesome in only about 7 per cent. Somewhat later postprandially (two to four hours), some patients (about 10 per cent) may experience *hypoglycemia* and symptoms thereof. Such patients exhibit abnormally rapid rises in both serum glucose and insulin concentrations which are thought to be related to rapid entry of glucose into the gut. All three operations accelerate the passage of liquid material into the gut.

These symptoms are usually more prominent in the first month after surgery and diminish as time passes. They may be ameliorated by the use of frequent small feedings taken without liquids and the avoidance of sugar in the diet (sugar is the most osmotically active dietary component).

Nutritional Problems. Some weight loss is common, particularly after resective procedures. Frequently weight loss is associated with reduced caloric intake as the result of early satiety or the desire to minimize postprandial symptoms. However, about a quarter of the patients have mild steatorrhea after these surgical procedures which may also contribute to malnutrition. Anemias occur in 20 to 50 per cent of patients, particularly after resection. Anemias usually appear more than five years after surgery; usually they reflect deficiency in iron, occasionally in folate or vitamin B_{12}. Osteomalacia may appear many years after subtotal gastrectomy.

Recurrent Ulceration. When the ulcer recurs in a duodenum left in continuity with the stomach, as after vagotomy and drainage, symptoms are typical of duodenal ulcer. However, when a recurrent ulcer arises at a gastrojejunal anastomosis ("marginal ulceration"), symptoms may be atypical. Pain frequently occurs in the left upper quadrant but may appear anywhere in the abdomen; marginal ulcers are refractory to medical treatment, frequently bleed, and occasionally perforate. Appropriate treatment is surgical. In patients who have had a subtotal gastrectomy, the treatment consists of a vagotomy. In patients who have had a prior vagotomy without resection, the treatment is antrectomy, often with attempts to cut more vagal fibers.

Postvagotomy Diarrhea. Although diarrhea may be associated with the dumping syndrome after any of the three procedures, a different form of diarrhea is seen in about one in four patients who have had a vagotomy (see table). This diarrhea tends to be episodic, lasting a day or two, and bears no relationship to dietary factors. In only a few patients is diarrhea disabling. For these few patients treatment with opiates or anticholinergics has been tried but has not been uniformly successful. The cause of postvagotomy diarrhea is unknown.

Rare Mechanical Problems. These problems arise almost exclusively in resected patients with gastrojejunal anastomoses. They include stomal obstruction, partial afferent loop obstruction, intermittent jejunal intussusception, gastro- or jejunocolic fistulas, and gastric bezoars.

644. GASTROINTESTINAL BLEEDING

David H. Law

Types of Bleeding. Bleeding may be manifested by *hematemesis* (vomiting of blood, either bright red or brown and precipitated, resembling coffee grounds), by *melena* (the passage of tarry black, sticky stool), or by *hematochezia* (the passage of fresh red blood per rectum). Bleeding, however, may be only occult, with normal-appearing stools which on chemical determination are shown to contain blood.

Degree and Effects of Bleeding. The pathophysiologic effects which result from gastrointestinal blood loss give rise to many of the symptoms and signs which have been shown to be of clinical importance in determining the presence and the severity of bleeding. In large part, however, this response to blood loss is unrelated to the site or cause of the bleeding, depending more upon the *rate* and *extent*.

After acute massive bleeding, typified by loss of greater than 1500 ml or 25 per cent of the circulating blood volume within a period of minutes to hours, cardiac output and systolic blood pressure decrease, followed by decrease in diastolic blood pressure and increased pulse. Blood pressure responses occur first in the form of orthostatic hypotension. Pulse rate seems to be a far less accurate parameter, even at a time when orthostatic hypotension is clearly evident, but it usually does rise. Compensatory vascular responses include constriction of the arterial bed with skin pallor, decreased splanchnic blood flow, and decreased renal blood flow with relative maintenance of cerebral and cardiopulmonary vascular systems. Vascular complications may include acute tubular necrosis, mesenteric vascular insufficiency with bowel infarction, and centrilobular necrosis of the liver. With continued acute blood loss, cerebral blood flow is embarrassed and there may be confusion, progressing to obtundation. Early electrocardiographic changes of T wave flattening or inversion and possibly S-T segment depression document insufficiency of coronary blood flow. Most of the early changes respond to correction of the diminished plasma volume, using blood transfusions or other plasma expanders such as electrolyte solutions or dextrans. If, however, blood loss continues unabated, the secondary effects of *shock*—increasing anoxia, cellular dysfunction, and acidosis—may lead to death. The mortality from massive gastrointestinal bleeding varies from 5 to 50 per cent, depending upon the cause of the hemorrhage and the age and condition of the patient.

More gradual compensatory physiologic mechanisms, including antidiuretic hormone and aldosterone release, act to re-establish intravascular volume, with a resultant drop in hematocrit and hemoglobin concentration. This plasma restoration begins rapidly, and up to one half the total compensation may occur within 8 to 12 hours. However, depending upon the patient's state of hydration, age, ability to resorb fluid lost into the gut, and rate of both oral and parenteral fluid repletion, this process may continue for 48 to 72 hours. For these reasons hematocrit and hemoglobin concentration values may be misleading during acute bleeding episodes. By recognizing these responses, the reduction in blood volume can be estimated and a logical sequence of diagnostic studies outlined to define the source of bleeding.

The degree of blood loss is the single most important parameter to be defined when a patient presents with gastrointestinal bleeding. This will establish the relative emergency of the problem and set the diagnostic and therapeutic pace to follow. Although the clinical history is often nondiagnostic, it will provide useful information in about one third of the cases and should be thoroughly evaluated.

Examination of the patient provides the best means of assessing blood loss based on the responses previously outlined. As a general rule, blood pressure less than 100 mm Hg or a pulse rate exceeding 100 per minute in an otherwise normotensive patient indicates a 20 per cent volume depletion. Associated pallor and/or postural hypotension lends support to this estimate. A pulse rate increase of 20 per minute or orthostatic blood pressure decreases of greater than 10 mm Hg further suggest acute blood loss in excess of 1000 ml.

Localization and Site. In the acute situation, several points of history may be useful in finding the site of bleeding. (1) Hematemesis indicates bleeding from above the duodenal-jejunal junction, whereas passage of red blood per rectum is most frequently associated with a bleeding site below the start of the jejunum and usually from the colon. (2) The onset of hematemesis after forceful vomiting suggests the Mallory-Weiss syndrome or esophageal rupture. (3) Typical abdominal pain may suggest peptic ulcer or reflux esophagitis. (4) Stress ulcers may occur hours to days after trauma, severe burns, or surgical procedures. (5) Associated diseases may suggest the source of gastrointestinal hemorrhage; i.e., alcoholism is associated with bleeding from gastritis and varices; arthritis is associated with salicylate and other drug ingestion which may cause gastritis; diverticulosis may bleed massively; emphysema carries an increased risk for development of peptic ulcer; and cirrhosis and peptic ulcer suggest sources of blood loss. (6) Past surgical procedures may suggest a bleeding site. (7) Medications and toxins (analgesics, adrenocortical steroids, antihypertensives, and alcohol) may be associated with bleeding. Qualitative characteristics of bleeding, such as the presence of clots or bright red, mahogany, or coffeeground material, have little quantitative significance but may help localize bleeding to a given area of the gastrointestinal tract.

The *physical examination,* in addition to demonstrating signs of blood loss, may show associated disease which is pertinent to gastrointestinal bleeding. One should focus particularly on the oral pharynx and skin changes of the upper trunk for the vascular lesions of Osler-Weber Rendu disease or the pigmentary spots of Peutz-Jeghers syndrome. Hepatosplenomegaly, adenopathy, the presence of a rectal mass, and overt congenital anomalies may be found.

Laboratory Studies. Immediate *laboratory* evaluation should include a white blood cell count, hematocrit, hemoglobin, blood urea nitrogen, and evaluation for bleeding diathesis. An abrupt leukocytosis up to 20,000 per cubic millimeter and an outpouring of platelets may be seen with acute hemorrhage. A nasogastric tube should be inserted to estimate the amount and character of blood present, and guaiac tests performed on gastric contents. A hemoglobin level of less than 11 grams per 100 ml and a blood urea nitrogen (BUN) greater than 40 mg per 100 ml, in an otherwise normal patient, indicates a blood loss greater than 1000 ml. Blood in the upper intestine is reflected in an increased level of BUN with essentially no effect on serum creatinine. With cessation of bleeding, the BUN returns to normal within two to three days.

Management. It is important to stress that management of the patient with massive bleeding frequently does not permit the luxury of a thorough diagnostic search. Immediate steps must be taken to minimize morbidity and mortality. The most important single aim in the management of *emergent* bleeding is the maintenance of an adequate blood volume. This requires adequate access to the venous system. With massive bleeding or shock, central venous pressure measurement may be a valuable guide in determining the need for increasing or decreasing subsequent plasma expansion. Simultaneously with typing and cross-matching of blood for transfusion, some form of *plasma expander* should be infused—normal saline, Ringer's lactate or even 5 per cent dextrose solution may be used initially, but dextran or plasma may be more effective while awaiting the arrival of whole blood. After establishment of intravenous access, an intragastric, large-bore tube should be passed. Blood in the gastric aspirate confirms a bleeding site proximal to the ligament of Treitz; however, failure to find blood does not exclude this possibility. If blood is present, one should continuously lavage the stomach with ice water or saline until it is free of clots and returns are clear. In addition to controlling hemorrhage, this may minimize vomiting and monitor the activity of bleeding. The patient with suspected esophageal variceal hemorrhage constitutes a special problem and will be discussed separately.

The use of vasoconstrictor drugs should be considered when bleeding is massive, but great care must be taken in the presence of hypertensive or arteriosclerotic cardiovascular disease. Intravenous infusion over 20 minutes of 20 units of vasopressin, diluted in 100 ml of 5 per cent dextrose in distilled water, may be effective. Direct selective arterial infusion of vasoactive agents (pitressin, epinephrine, or propranolol) may be directed at the bleeding lesion when arteriography identifies the lesion.

Specific Diagnostic Techniques. The clinical decision as to the diagnostic use of endoscopy or x-ray should be based on skills of the immediately available personnel. If peptic ulcer seems the most likely probability after considering all factors, a barium contrast study of the esophagus, stomach, and upper intestine would most likely yield a diagnosis, while minimizing diagnostic risks. Evidence suggesting the Mallory-Weiss syndrome, gastritis, or portal hypertension is an indication for *panendoscopy* as the *initial* diagnostic procedure if a trained physician is available. The availability of a wide selection of flexible fiberoptic instruments for direct visualization of the esophageal, gastric, and duodenal mucosa has greatly enhanced the detection of lesions responsible for gastrointestinal bleeding. It is the most reliable procedure for diagnosing mucosal disorders of the esophagus, stomach, and duodenum. Although skilled endoscopy in the emergent setting can be performed with minimal patient risk and provide vital diagnostic information, it should be emphasized that optimal visualization requires proper timing of the procedure, a clean stomach, and a relaxed, cooperative patient. These conditions are best accomplished when the patient's clinical situation is stable.

Radiologic evaluation must be performed with close cooperation between the primary care physician and a well-informed radiologist with a preplanned course of action and special handling to avoid delays or untoward risks while the patient is away from his room. Cinefluoroscopy and hypotonic duodenography have increased the sensitivity of this procedure, but the latter rarely offers anything in the management of the patient with emergent bleeding.

If routine studies are negative and the rate of blood loss is greater than 0.5 ml per minute, celiac and mesenteric angiography may be useful by showing puddling of contrast agent at the site of hemorrhage within a bowel. When a bleeding lesion is identified, the catheter may be left in place to infuse vasoactive drugs such as pitressin, propranolol, or epinephrine directly into the arterial system feeding the bleeding lesion. This approach, however, requires a skilled, trained angiographer and should be used only in a center equipped for the purpose.

When all the aforementioned studies are nondiagnostic and very active bleeding persists, small intestinal intubation with sequential aspirations of the intestinal content may localize the bleeding site. Barium contrast study may then be performed through the tube to document a lesion at the site of bleeding. This test is most useful for locating obscure bleeding sites between the ligament of Treitz and the ileocecal valve, such as small bowel tumors, ulcers, Meckel's diverticula, or vascular anomalies.

The terminal ileum is often seen during reflux from a barium enema and may show terminal ileitis, an infrequent cause of massive gastrointestinal bleeding. Colonic diverticula are increasingly frequent with age and therefore cannot necessarily be implicated as the cause of bleeding when they are visualized by x-rays. They are, however, a common cause of massive lower gastrointestinal bleeding. In such instances selective inferior mesenteric arteriography may reveal the precise site of hemorrhage.

On occasion emergency surgical intervention must be considered for the patient with shock caused by uncontrollable massive hemorrhage. In addition, certain patients with gastrointestinal bleeding have an increased mortality, suggesting the need for early surgery, such as those who rebleed while hospitalized with good medical management and those older than 60.

In the setting of nonemergent bleeding, a more deliberate plan, involving detailed history, physical examination, and selected special studies, including endoscopy and complete radiologic survey of the gastrointestinal tract, may be undertaken. Since bleeding may not be evident, laboratory data may be necessary to establish bleeding and to define its source. Inspection and chemical tests (i.e., guaiac) of fresh stool are important in assessing the presence and extent of nonemergent gastrointestinal bleeding. Vomitus and gastric and small bowel aspirates, in addition to stools, should be tested for the presence of occult blood in patients suspected of bleeding. When the aforementioned radiologic and endoscopic studies are nondiagnostic and persistent active bleeding is suspected, small intestinal intubation or passage of a weighted umbilical tape that will reach the small bowel may demonstrate the bleeding site.

Portal hypertension with gastrointestinal bleeding constitutes a special problem and is the most critical hazard to patients with portal hypertension. Approximately one third of cirrhotic patients die from this complication. When the patient with massive gastrointestinal bleeding also has portal hypertension, initial management should follow the guidelines noted above. Panendoscopy should be performed to establish that varices are, indeed, the site of blood loss, because up to one fourth of the patients with varices who present with gastrointestinal hemorrhage may be bleeding from another source. Treatment includes esophageal tamponade and initiation of intravenous pitressin, 20 units diluted in 100 ml of isotonic saline or dextrose, over a 20 to 30 minute period, repeated at two-hour intervals as indicated. Regardless of which tube is used for esophageal tamponade, ultimate survival with minimal morbidity depends on close supervision and strict attention to detail of the method. The immediate aim of therapy is to control hemorrhage, and this is possible in the vast majority of cases. Failure to control bleeding by tamponade may indicate that varices are not the source of bleeding. Ultimate therapy to prevent rebleeding is directed at elective surgical decompression of the portal system.

Operative mortality approaches 70 per cent when

emergent surgery is required to control variceal bleeding; therefore optimal prognosis necessitates surgical decompression of the portal bed as an elective procedure. The most important criteria for selecting a successful surgical candidate relate to the patient's age and hepatic function. A serum albumin above 3.0 grams per 100 ml, bilirubin less than 3.0 mg per 100 ml, sulfobromophthalein retention less than 20 per cent, prothrombin time less than four seconds elevated, absence of ascites, and a liver biopsy showing only minimal fatty metamorphosis and absence of alcoholic hepatitis in the presence of cirrhosis are the most important criteria to consider when selecting the ideal surgical candidate. Mortality and morbidity of shunt surgery seem related directly to abnormalities of these parameters reflecting hepatic reserve. Thus after the emergent gastrointestinal hemorrhage has been controlled, an intensive nutritional and rehabilitation program is essential to improve liver function in preparation for surgery. This may require up to three months to achieve maximal benefit.

Bleeding diathesis, although infrequently a cause of massive gastrointestinal hemorrhage, may be present in patients with blood dyscrasias, vascular abnormalities, or multiple systemic diseases which present with gastrointestinal bleeding. When the history, physical examination, or clinical course suggests such a possibility, the sequence of diagnostic studies should include expert hematologic consultation and the appropriate laboratory tests to detect these disorders.

Baum, S., and Nusbaum, M.: The control of gastrointestinal haemorrhage by selective mesenteric arterial infusion of vasopressin. Radiology, 98:497, 1971.

Brick, I. B., and Jeghers, H. J.: Gastrointestinal hemorrhage. N. Engl. J. Med., 253:458, 511, 555, 1955.

Isenberg, J. I., Walsh, J. H., and Grossman, M. I.: Zollinger-Ellison syndrome. Gastroenterology, 65:140, 1973.

Pitcher, J. L.: Safety and effectiveness of the modified Sengstaken-Blakemore tube: A prospective study. Gastroenterology, 61:291, 1971.

Schille, K. F. R., Truelove, S. C., and Williams, D. J.: Hematemesis and melena with special reference to factors influencing the outcome. Br. Med. J., 2:7, 1970.

Sleisenger, M. H., and Fordtran, J. S. (eds.): Gastrointestinal Disease. Philadelphia, W. B. Saunders Company, 1973, Chapters 12–16, 40–43, 50–63.

Section Three.   DISEASES OF MALABSORPTION

Marvin H. Sleisenger

The malabsorption syndrome is a constellation of symptoms and signs that are the result of abnormal fecal excretion of fat (steatorrhea) and of varying degrees of malabsorption of fat-soluble vitamins as well as carbohydrate, protein, minerals, other vitamins, and water.

MECHANISM OF NORMAL ABSORPTION

In view of the wide range of absorption defects that can be involved, each instance of the malabsorption syndrome must be analyzed against the background of the processes of *normal* absorption. Accordingly, a brief review of the processes of normal absorption is presented at this time.

During absorption, the end products of digestion must leave the intestinal lumen, traverse the mucosal cells, enter the terminal branches of the vascular and lymphatic vessels, and thus gain entrance into the general circulation. Two mechanisms, acting separately or together, are important in this process: *active transport* and *simple diffusion.* Both of these are presumed to take place in relationship to a hypothetical cell membrane.

Simple diffusion requires no energy, and is the passage of a molecule across a membrane barrier according to chemical concentration and electrical gradients. (Examples are the absorption of fatty acids, water, and bile salts in the jejunum. *Facilitated diffusion* is like simple diffusion, in that it requires no expenditure of energy, but a carrier mechanism permits a degree of effective transport exceeding that predictable on the basis of simple diffusion alone.) *Active transport* requires metabolic work with expenditure of energy that results in a net movement of substances against a chemical or electrical difference. An important mechanism of active transport systems is the "carrier," which makes possible penetration of the cell membrane. (Examples are the absorption of Ca^{++} and Fe^{++} in the jejunum and Na^+ and bile salts in the ileum.)

Fat Absorption. *Intraluminal Phase.* Sixty to 100 grams of fat are eaten daily by adults, principally as triglycerides containing long-chain fatty acids. This triglyceride must be digested (i.e., hydrolyzed) and solubilized intraluminally before absorption. Absorption, in turn, consists of uptake and transport, both processes requiring normally functioning mucosal cells.

The stomach plays a role in fat digestion. It reduces the size of particles and, by slowly emptying its acid chyme into the duodenum, ensures not only a normal rate of absorption but also an adequate stimulation for the flow of bile and pancreatic juice. *Gastric acid* may also be important in maintaining sterility of the upper small bowel. Heavy growth of the bacterial flora in this segment interferes with fat and vitamin B_{12} absorption (see below).

The initial intraluminal event in the jejunum is hydrolysis of triglyceride into two fatty acids and a residual β monoglyceride by *pancreatic lipase;* this enzyme, contained in high concentration in secreted pancreatic juice, is activated at the alkaline pH of the upper jejunum. Bile, by its emulsifying action, also facilitates hydrolysis.

At a critical concentration, conjugated bile salts, contained in bile provided by contraction of the gallbladder, form small spheres with detergent properties. These are amphipathic molecules with a portion polar and water soluble and a portion nonpolar and fat soluble. The latter resides at the center of the sphere and solubilizes monoglycerides and fatty acids and the fat-soluble vitamins, A, D, and K. This complex is known as a micelle. Di- and triglycerides remain in an oil phase until hydrolyzed to monoglycerides and fatty acids.

Micelle formation may be impaired in several ways: *inadequate hydrolysis* of triglyceride to monoglyceride and fatty acids (as in pancreatic insufficiency); *poor mixing* of pancreatic lipase and triglyceride (after subtotal gastrectomy); or *deficiency of conjugated bile salts* (as in bacterial overgrowth, cholestatic liver disease, or biliary tract obstruction, or after resection of distal ileum).

Cellular Phase. The monoglycerides and fatty acids of micelles cross the membrane, probably by passive diffusion, but the conjugated bile salts pass into the lower small intestine, where they are actively absorbed, and return to the liver for re-excretion into bile. Normally about 95 per cent of the total bile salt pool, 4.0 grams, is reabsorbed during each enterohepatic cycle, and each day the pool is circulated four to six times. Thus only 400 to 600 mg of bile salts are lost in the feces and are normally synthesized in the liver daily.

Although exact figures are not available, a considerable amount of fat may be absorbed in the absence of bile, indicating that the process is not entirely dependent upon micelles. The question of ileal absorption of fat has not been resolved. The rate of absorption of both free fatty acids and glycerides is determined mainly by both chain length and degree of saturation of the fatty acids involved.

The major site for fat absorption is the upper jejunum. For normal function, at least 90 cm of this segment must be free of bacterial overgrowth and must contain normal villi and patent lymphatics. These are the conditions for the uptake and transport of lipid which are phases of fat absorption. Triglycerides (neutral fat) after emulsification with fatty acids and bile salts *may* be absorbed unhydrolyzed, but apparently only in small quantity. Indeed, 80 to 90 per cent of neutral fat is either partly or completely hydrolyzed.

Conjugated bile salts also help to activate intracellular enzymes, which are required for resynthesis of fatty acids and monoglyceride into triglyceride, a necessary step in chylomicron formation; although unconjugated bile salts at high concentrations may appear to inhibit uptake of lipid as well as resynthesis of triglyceride intracellularly, decreased concentration of conjugated bile salts is responsible for diminished uptake and re-esterification. In the mucosal cells, molecules of triglyceride coalesce into large particles which are then coated with small amounts of protein, cholesterol, and phospholipid, thus becoming β-lipoproteins, called chylomicrons. These exit via the base of the cells, enter the lacteals whence they pass into the mesenteric lymphatic system, the thoracic duct, and, finally, the vena cava. Long-chain fatty acids (i.e., 10 or more C atoms) undergo this process. In the mucosal cells some fatty acids are incorporated into phospholipids.

Medium-chain triglycerides, with fatty acids of length C6 to C10, are more completely hydrolyzed than long-chain triglycerides, being split at two positions with release of three medium-chain fatty acids. Also, they form micelles more readily. Thus this lipid is more readily prepared for absorption than the long-chain triglycerides. Unsplit medium-chain triglyceride also appears to be taken up by cells (30 per cent of an oral dose) and is hydrolyzed by mucosal lipase, releasing fatty acids. Further, medium-chain fatty acids pass directly into the portal venous system without re-esterification. This independence of mucosal re-esterification and of the lymphatics is thought to be advantageous in patients with intestinal mucosal disease. Obviously, medium-chain triglyceride may be extremely useful in the therapy of patients with malabsorption syndrome, and its indications and usefulness will be discussed under Treatment (see below, Table 5).

Absorption of *cholesterol* appears to depend upon its separation from protein and release from fatty acid esters through hydrolysis by pancreatic esterase. The intestine also synthesizes cholesterol as well as very low density lipoproteins. Dietary vitamin A, largely in ester form, undergoes hydrolysis in the intestinal lumen to the free alcohol. The absorption of both cholesterol and vitamin A alcohol requires bile salts. Indeed, it now seems likely that absorption of cholesterol and all fat-soluble vitamins is more dependent upon micelle formation than are the hydrolytic products of neutral fat.

Protein and Amino Acid Absorption. Gastric pepsin may partially hydrolyze dietary protein; however, this action is almost entirely due to pancreatic proteolytic endopeptidases such as *trypsin, chymotrypsin,* and *elastase. Trypsinogen,* as well as precursors of the other endopeptidases, is activated by a mucosal enzyme, *enterokinase,* released by presence of food in the duodenum. *Trypsin* is liberated and, in turn, continues to activate trypsinogen as well as the other pancreatic endopeptidases. These substances attack the interior of the protein molecules, yielding oligopeptides which are further split by exopeptidases such as *carboxypeptidase.* Neutral and basic amino acids are released, as well as small peptides, di- to hexa-, in large quantities. These peptides enter the brush border where they are hydrolyzed by peptide hydrolases; some di- and tripeptides, however, enter the cells and are split into their constituent amino acids. Indeed, amino acid absorption is greater after administration of some dipeptides than with equimolar mixtures of amino acids.

Amino acids liberated intraluminally or within the brush border are transported across the cell membrane actively, i.e., by a process which consumes energy. It is Na^+ dependent to a varying degree. Thus neutral amino acids are more dependent and basic amino acids less so. Both types, however, are absorbed rapidly. Other active carriers operate for movement of glycine (which also is transported as a neutral amino acid), hydroxyproline, and proline; and for the dicarboxylic amino acids, aspartic and glutamic. Di- and tripeptides also enter the cells by one or more transport mechanisms. Resynthesis of protein from absorbed amino acids takes place to a limited extent in the mucosa; the liver, however, is the predominant site for such synthesis.

Most amino acids pass quickly into the blood, however, and enter the general "metabolic pool." The liver is the principal organ for their metabolism.

The rate of transport of amino acids is a function of their chemical configuration. Neutral amino acids are moved most rapidly; the principal component responsible for this rapidity is an intact carboxyl group attached to the α carbon, and affinity for an amino acid carrier is enhanced when the α NH$_2$ is intact and the side chain ("R" substituent) is nonpolar.

Carbohydrate Absorption. Dietary carbohydrate consists of starch and two disaccharides, sucrose and lactose. Amylose and amylopectin are the principal starches—long chains of connected (C_1-C_4) glucose molecules which are split in the duodenum by pancreatic amylase at these 1 to 4 α glucose-glucose linkages. Amylose is cleaved to yield maltose and maltotriose; amylopectin, however, yields molecules, α-limit dextrins, containing some branch points (C_6-C_1) present sequentially in amylopectin which are not split by the enzyme.

Maltose, maltotriose, α-limit dextrins, and other dietary disaccharides, sucrose and lactose, are split further by specific brush border *disaccharidases* into their component hexoses: glucose-glucose, glucose-fructose, and glucose-galactose, respectively.

The rate of absorption of hexoses in descending order is galactose, glucose, fructose. Glucose and galactose are actively transported, and fructose, whose absorption was thought to be "facilitated" by a poorly understood carrier, now appears also to be actively transported. Xylose shares the same transport system with glucose and galactose but not so avidly.

The exact mechanism of transport has not been elucidated. It is clear, however, that phosphorylation plays no role. Transport of glucose and galactose depends upon a process requiring both energy and Na^+. Possibly glucose and Na^+ bind to a carrier protein in the microvilli, and thus glucose moves into the cell. Na^+ then moves out of the cell via the so-called "Na^+ pump" mechanism. Na^+ also increases cellular permeability for glucose, although glucose may be transported at low concentrations of Na^+.

Vitamin B$_{12}$ Absorption. Vitamin B_{12} absorption is dependent upon the presence of intrinsic factor, a glycoprotein (50,000 to 60,000 m.w.) contained in gastric juice. Vitamin B_{12} is bound to intrinsic factor, and the complex in turn is bound to a specific ileal receptor. In some unknown manner, after several hours, vitamin B_{12} becomes "unbound" and passes into the blood. Whether uptake is energy dependent is not settled. Calcium ion is required for uptake of the vitamin B_{12}–intrinsic factor complex as well as a substance in pancreatic juice which somehow facilitates its absorption. Alterations in bacterial flora, such as are observed in the bacterial overgrowth syndrome (see below), lead to decreased absorption of vitamin B_{12} that, in most instances, can be reversed by the administration of broad-spectrum antimicrobial drugs. In some manner these bacteria bind the vitamin B_{12}.

Folic Acid Absorption. Dietary folic acid is in the form of polyglutamate conjugates of pteroylglutamic acid. About 1000 μg, as contained in yeast, liver, and green vegetables, is ingested daily in the Western world. The conjugated substance is water soluble and may be transported by *facilitated diffusion*. The glutamic acid residues are sequentially cleaved in the mucosal cell, yielding biologically active mono- and difolates. These forms of pteroylglutamic acid are then methylated within the mucosa, and the methylated folates, which are active forms, pass into the general circulation.

Water and Electrolyte Absorption. Water and electrolyte absorption takes place in the small intestine. *Water* moves across the membrane passively, i.e., secondary to osmotic gradients. However, under certain circumstances it can move against a gradient without requiring energy. The rate of water absorption in the small gut is five to ten times that in the stomach. To some extent, also, water follows the active transport of glucose and electrolytes, moving with them to maintain isotonicity of intraluminal contents. The small intestine usually absorbs over 7 liters of water per day.

Sodium absorption is an active process and is linked to an exchange with H^+ in both jejunum and ileum. A similar exchange mechanism for Cl' and HCO_3' exists only in the ileum. The sites of these exchanges in the cell are not known, but the exchanges are certainly mediated by carriers. It is also believed from in vitro studies that an Na^+ pump mechanism may be operative. In man, Na^+ transport is enhanced by absorption of glucose in the jejunum, either via this mechanism or by being "dragged" into the cell by the water in which glucose is carried. Some Na^+ also moves passively, i.e., down a gradient across the mucosa. Potassium movement seems to be passive, diffusing from the lumen proximally and into the lumen distally.

The amount of water and sodium absorbed represents the difference between influx from lumen to blood and efflux in the reverse direction. This net flux is diminished by hypertonicity of the intraluminal solution and is increased by hypotonicity. Changes in concentration of sodium in the lumen depend on relative rates of exchange of both sodium and water between blood and lumen.

During diarrhea, sodium concentration increases with increasing stool volume, and beyond 3 liters approaches values close to that of plasma. Conversely, potassium concentration progressively decreases.

Calcium and Iron Absorption. Calcium is absorbed actively in the duodenum. This transport is facilitated by *parathyroid hormone* and by *vitamin D,* and is inhibited by deprivation of this vitamin. The active form of vitamin D involved in the process is a kidney metabolite, *1,25-dihydroxycholecalciferol.* In vivo calcium absorption depends also upon pH and concentration of phosphates and fatty acids. Vitamin D absorption is necessary for calcium absorption, because 1,25-dihydroxycholecalciferol stimulates synthesis of a calcium-binding protein which is a key substance in the active transport of the cation. 1,25-dihydroxycholecalciferol also stimulates Na^+ dependent ATP-ase to release calcium from its binder in the cell.

Iron, 0.5 to 1.0 mg daily, is absorbed *actively,* in an amount sufficient for normal hematopoiesis and five to eight times this amount in people who are iron deficient. Absorption is a two-step process, principally in the duodenum, of uptake and transfer; the former is dependent upon oxidative metabolism. The latter, probably the rate-limit step, involves movement of Fe through the serosa to the circulation where it is bound to a globulin, *transferrin,* which transports it to tissues, particularly the liver. Iron absorption is diminished in chronic infection and by prior administration of large amounts of iron, and apparently is increased in pregnancy as well as iron deficiency. Animal hemoglobin is an important source of iron in the human, and is absorbed most rapidly, followed by Fe^{++}, then Fe^{+++}. After ingestion, hemoglobin is split in the upper gut; heme is readily absorbed, from which iron is split within the cell and passes thence into the circulation where it is bound by iron-binding protein. Some iron is released from heme intraluminally and is taken up directly by the cells.

In human subjects, absorption of inorganic iron depends upon its release from dietary compounds to which it is originally bound. Absorption of both Fe^{+++} and Fe^{++} is enhanced by chelation with ascorbic acid, carbohydrates, and amino acids at the pH of normal gastric juice.

These complexes remain soluble at the alkaline pH of the duodenum where iron is absorbed. Diminished iron absorption is associated with achlorhydria, because an acid pH is needed to solubilize ferric iron for chelation with ascorbic acid and other substances, in which form it is absorbed. Ferrous iron may also, however, be chelated at an alkaline pH. Over-all, iron absorption is regulated by the state of repletion, content of iron in absorbing cells, and factors affecting erythropoiesis. The influence of gastric and pancreatic juice proteins which bind iron is still uncertain.

CAUSES OF THE MALABSORPTION SYNDROME

The principal diseases and disorders that may give rise to the malabsorption syndrome are listed in Table 1. These conditions are discussed in detail in a subsequent portion of this section and are presented only in brief

TABLE 1.   Classification of Malabsorption Syndrome

I. Category 1: Defective Intraluminal Hydrolysis or Solubilization
  A. Primary pancreatic insufficiency
  B. Secondary pancreatic insufficiency
  C. Deficiency of conjugated bile salts
  D. Bacterial overgrowth (bile salt deconjugation)
    1. Blind loops
    2. Multiple strictures and jejunal diverticula
    3. Fistulas
    4. Postgastrectomy
    5. Scleroderma and pseudo-obstruction
II. Category 2: Mucosal Cell Abnormality and Inadequate Surface
  A. Primary mucosal cell disorders
    1. Disaccharidase deficiency and monosaccharide malabsorption
    2. A-beta-lipoproteinemia
    3. Vitamin B_{12} malabsorption
    4. Cystinuria and Hartnup disease
  B. Small bowel disease
    1. Celiac disease
    2. Whipple's disease
    3. Nongranulomatous ileojejunitis
    4. Allergic and eosinophilic gastroenteritis
    5. Amyloidosis
    6. Small bowel ischemia
    7. Crohn's disease (granulomatous enteritis)
  C. Inadequate surface
III. Category 3: Lymphatic Obstruction
  A. Lymphoma
  B. Tuberculosis and tuberculous lymphadenitis
  C. Lymphangiectasia
IV. Category 4: Infection
  A. Tropical sprue
  B. Acute infectious enteritis
  C. Parasitoses
V. Category 5: Multiple Defects
  A. Subtotal gastrectomy
  B. Distal ileal resection, disease, or bypass
  C. Radiation enteritis
VI. Category 6: Unexplained
  A. Hypogammaglobulinemia
  B. Carcinoid syndrome
  C. Hypothyroidism
  D. Diabetes mellitus
  E. Mastocytosis
  F. Hyperthyroidism and hypoadrenocorticism
VII. Category 7: Drug-Induced Malabsorption
  A. Cholestyramine
  B. Colchicine
  C. Irritant laxatives
  D. Neomycin
  E. p-Amino salicylic acid
  F. Phenindione

outline at this point. They can be divided conveniently into seven categories, based upon pathologic and pathophysiologic considerations.

CLINICAL MANIFESTATIONS

The signs and symptoms of the malabsorption syndrome include weight loss, anorexia, abdominal distention, borborygmi, muscle wasting, and passage of abnormal stools that are characteristically light yellow to gray, greasy, and soft. In many instances frequent movements are noted, but occasionally there is only one stool per day. In addition, edema, ascites, skeletal disorders, peripheral and circumoral paresthesias, tetany, and, rarely, convulsions may be observed.

The clinical features that result from deficiencies of fat-soluble vitamins include hyperkeratosis follicularis (vitamin A); bleeding, particularly ecchymoses and hematuria (vitamin K); and bone pain or fractures (vitamin D) (Table 2). Deficiencies of the vitamin B complex are manifested by glossitis, cheilosis, muscle tenderness, peripheral neuritis, and dermatitis (Table 2). The symptoms of the malabsorption syndrome may be intermittent or low grade, so that medical attention is not sought for a very long time—more than 35 years in some instances of adult celiac disease. Unfortunately, many of these patients whose malabsorption is mild escape diagnosis and suffer subtle changes for years. They do not exhibit obvious manifestations of malabsorption; they are chronically fatigued, lack drive, and may have symptoms of chronic depression. Further, they may lose weight only during the early months of illness and then will stabilize at a lower level.

In those with more severe malabsorption, the secondary manifestations may often overshadow the intestinal complaints. For example, about 20 per cent of patients with *adult celiac disease* will seek aid for bleeding or for skeletal pain or fractures. In many patients, weakness, fatigue, dyspnea, or dizziness, all caused by anemia, may be the presenting symptoms. Borborygmi and abdominal distention, which increase during the day and are often not relieved by defecation, are among the most common complaints. An extreme degree of such distress is frequently noted in patients with *scleroderma* of the small intestine.

Cramping lower abdominal pain is noted in a large number of diseases of malabsorption, usually preceding loose bowel movements, and thus does not distinguish between the various entities. Persistent or severe cramping pain, periumbilical or right lower quadrant, not relieved by movements is frequently seen in patients with *Crohn's disease* and, with stricturing and obstruction, may become chronic and associated with distention and emesis. Diffuse periumbilical pain is often suffered by patients with *nongranulomatous ileojejunitis, lymphoma, eosinophilic gastroenteritis, radiation enteritis, amyloidosis,* and, occasionally, *adult celiac disease.* Patients with *chronic pancreatitis* usually suffer recurrent deep epigastric pain that radiates to the midback; in patients with *lymphoma* of the small intestine and mesentery, the pain may be cramping (obstruction) or steady and intense (local invasion or spread).

Patients with malabsorption owing to *ischemia* of the small gut often also have periumbilical or midabdominal cramping pains 20 to 30 minutes after meals and often other evidence of widespread arteriosclerosis, or have

TABLE 2. Correlation of Laboratory Data with Absorptive Defects and Signs and Symptoms of the Malabsorption Syndrome

Clinical Features	Laboratory Evidence	Pathophysiology
Muscle wasting; small stature; edema	↓ Serum albumin	*Impaired protein metabolism* ↓ Absorption ↓ Intake
Skeletal deformity; pain fractures	X-ray: demineralization; collapsed vertebrae	↑ Enteric loss ?Impaired synthesis
Weight loss; pale, bulky stools	↑ Fecal fat ↓ Serum cholesterol, carotene	*Impaired absorption and excess loss of:* Fat
Paresthesias; tetany; + Chvostek; Trousseau; bone pain; fractures	↓ Serum Ca^{++}; ↓ or normal PO_4'''; ↑ alkaline phosphatase; x-ray: Looser's lines, Milkman's fractures; ↑ osteoid seams; ↓ serum Mg^{++}	Fat-soluble vitamins and calcium Vitamin D, calcium, magnesium
Bleeding: ecchymoses, hematuria	↑ Prothrombin time with response to vitamin K	Vitamin K
Hyperkeratosis follicularis	↓ Serum carotene, vitamin A tolerance	Vitamin A
A N E M I A / G L O S S I T I S G L — Paresthesias; neuropathy	Macrocytic anemia; megaloblastosis; ↓ serum B_{12} and ↓ absorption B_{12}	Vitamin B_{12}
A O / N S / E S / M I	Macrocytic anemia; megaloblastosis; ↓ serum folic acid	Folic acid
I A T I S — Koilonychia	Microcystosis, hypochromia; ↓ serum iron and ↓ saturation iron binding protein; ↓ iron in marrow	Iron
Dehydration; nocturia	↓ Plasma volume	Water
Muscle cramps, weakness	↓ Serum Na^+	Sodium
Muscle flaccidity, weakness; ↓ tendon reflexes, arrhythmias	↓ Serum K^+; EKG abnormalities	Potassium
Cheilosis; neuritis; dermatitis, glossitis; muscle weakness	↑ Urinary I3AA, Indican; ↓ serum B_{12}, folic acid	Vitamin B complex; folic acid vitamin B_{12}
Abdominal distention, flatulence; diarrhea	Low to flat oral glucose tolerance curve; ↓ absorption d-xylose; ↓ oral lactose tolerance; ↓ or absent rise of blood glucose after oral sucrose; ↓ or absent rise of blood reducing substances after oral galactose; fluid levels on x-ray; stools: acid pH, + Clinitest	Impaired hydrolysis of disaccharides, particularly lactose and sucrose, or ↓ absorption of monosaccharides and amino acids

chronic atrial fibrillation. Those with *hypogammaglobulinemia* may have other historic evidences of immunoglobulin deficiency (repeated infections, or even symptoms suggesting malignancy). *Eosinophilic gastroenteritis* may be highlighted by a specific "food allergy" or by a history of skin, nasopharyngeal, bronchial, or other allergy. Virulent peptic ulcer disease *(Zollinger-Ellison syndrome)* will usually highlight the history of malabsorption caused by gastric hypersecretion. Diarrhea associated with carbohydrate will be noted from childhood in those with *disaccharidase deficiency* or *monosaccharide malabsorption.* Surgical scars and associated histories will highlight cases of *massive resection, gastrectomy* and *ileal resection, bypass procedures,* and *blind loops.* Those with *enteroenteric* or *enterocolic fistulas* as well have a long history of inflammatory disease, usually Crohn's disease, or malignancy. Hepatobiliary tract disorders will have features of chronic obstruction of the common bile duct or of chronic intrahepatic disease.

Physical examination may reveal low blood pressure and evidences of malnutrition and multiple vitamin deficiencies: pallor, diffuse brownish pigmentation of the skin but not of the mucous membranes, hyperkeratosis, petechiae or ecchymoses, muscle wasting, edema, abdominal distention, skeletal deformity (particularly kyphosis), positive Chvostek and/or Trousseau signs, glossitis, cheilosis, impaired vibration sense, deep muscle pain, and clubbing of the fingers. In additions, signs of various underlying diseases may be noted: an abdominal mass *(lymphoma, regional enteritis);* fixation or severe limitation of joint movement and thickened skin *(scleroderma);* facial flush and hepatomegaly *(carcinoid syndrome);* puffed facies, bradycardia, and hair loss

(hypothyroidism); proptosis, thyromegaly, tachycardia, and tremor *(hyperthyroidism);* arthritis or skin rashes *(hypogammaglobulinemia);* nasopharyngeal congestion, skin rash, and wheezing *(eosinophilic gastroenteritis);* butterfly rash and splenomegaly (systemic lupus erythematosus); neurologic impairments *(abetalipoproteinemia);* diminished or absent peripheral arterial pulsations, skin lesions (particularly dermatitis herpetiformis), cataracts, and absent or diminished deep tendon reflexes or other evidences of diabetic neuropathy or retinopathy *(diabetes mellitus);* lymphadenopathy, arthritis, and signs of pulmonary disease *(Whipple's disease);* enlarged tongue and hepatosplenomegaly *(amyloidosis);* urticaria pigmentosa, flushing, pruritus *(mastocytosis).*

The malabsorption syndrome may be fatal, owing to the nature of the underlying disease *(lymphoma, pancreatic carcinoma, progressive scleroderma,* or *granulomatous enteritis)* or to the complications of malabsorption, which include superimposed infection, hypokalemia, or progressive inanition.

PATHOPHYSIOLOGIC BASIS FOR CLINICAL MANIFESTATIONS

In Table 2 may be seen the correlation between various absorptive defects and vitamin deficiencies, the clinical signs and symptoms, and the abnormalities of the routine laboratory tests in the malabsorption syndrome. Rarely does a patient manifest all the findings listed in Table 2, but many patients will exhibit many of them.

Impaired Protein Metabolism: Weight Loss, Edema. Protein metabolism, reflected by decreased muscle mass and lowered serum protein levels, is impaired for several reasons. Synthesis is below normal owing to defective protein absorption. Catabolism or breakdown is accelerated because of inadequate intake and absorption of carbohydrate. Decreased serum albumin may result also from abnormal loss of protein into the lumen of the gut, so-called *protein-losing enteropathy*. Such loss is usually associated with diseases that cause malabsorption by lymphatic obstruction or in which there is an inflammatory mucosal lesion, although it has also been reported in *adult celiac disease* (see below). *Hypogammaglobulinemia*, both congenital and acquired, has also been associated with steatorrhea, but the defective fat absorption cannot be related directly to low plasma globulins. In some instances, impaired hepatic function contributes to lowered serum protein levels.

The emaciation and weakness may be extreme (Fig. 1). The finding of hypotension and diffuse pigmentation makes the picture closely resemble severe *adrenal cortical insufficiency*. Hypokalemia as well as partial atrophy may underlie muscle weakness.

Clinical Effects of Steatorrhea. Excess loss of fat in the stool deprives the body of substantial numbers of calories and contributes greatly to weight loss and malnutrition. Perhaps the irritative effect of unabsorbed long-chain (C18) fatty acids which are hydroxylated contributes to the diarrhea with its severe losses of water, electrolytes, and other nutrients. In addition, binding of calcium by fatty acids contributes to hypocalcemia. Flatulence, fluid in loops of small intestine, and abdominal distention may be related to both diminished fat absorption and excessive carbohydrate fermentation. Failure to absorb fat-soluble vitamins A, D, and K also results in a variety of serious symptoms as recorded in Table 2.

Vitamin D Deficiency: Hypocalcemia and Skeletal Disease in Malabsorption Syndrome; Hypomagnesemia. Low serum calcium results from failure of normal absorption owing both to vitamin D deficiency and to chelation of calcium by unabsorbed fatty acids. Symptoms caused by depression of unbound or "ultrafilterable" calcium of the blood range from paresthesias of extremities and circumoral area to carpopedal and laryngeal spasms and muscle cramps. When levels are extremely low, the patient may even convulse. Clinically, hypocalcemia may be demonstrated by *Chvostek* or *Trousseau signs*. Obviously, the defect in calcium absorption involves more than deficiency of vitamin D, particularly its metabolite, 1,25-dihydroxycholecalciferol, active in calcium absorption, because the return of serum calcium to normal in

patients with adult celiac disease who are on a gluten-free diet is more rapid than may be attributed to the action of this vitamin.

Low levels of serum calcium stimulate parathyroid activity. Increased secretion of parathormone raises the level of blood calcium both by direct effect upon bone and by a renal mechanism. These processes lead to demineralization—*osteomalacia*. Osteomalacia principally affects the spine, rib cage, and long bones, with or without fractures (Milkman's fractures), and may cause extreme pain and disability.

In patients with poor protein nutrition, in part caused by malabsorption or protein-losing enteropathy (see below), particularly postmenopausal women and elderly men, the demineralization process is aggravated by *osteoporosis* or failure to deposit bone matrix.

Hypomagnesemia may also be noted in the malabsorption syndrome, causing symptoms that are identical with those of hypocalcemia. Differentiation is accomplished by the finding of lowered serum magnesium and by disappearance of symptoms only after administration of magnesium chloride or sulfate. Hypomagnesemia may also dramatically reduce the responsiveness of the parathyroids to hypocalcemia. Indeed, correction of magnesium deficiency may be essential to restoration of normal calcium by action of the parathyroid glands.

Vitamin K Deficiency: Bleeding Diathesis in Malabsorption Syndrome. As noted, *bleeding,* particularly subcutaneous, nasal, urinary, vaginal, and occasionally, gastrointestinal, is not uncommon in the malabsorption syndrome and may be the principal symptom. Defects in coagulation result from deficiency of plasma prothrombin owing to impaired absorption of fat-soluble vitamin K.

Vitamin A Deficiency. In the malabsorption syndrome *hyperkeratosis follicularis* may be noted, but *nyctalopia* is very rare.

Manifestations of Abnormal Carbohydrate Absorption. The abnormal carbohydrate absorption results in diminished glycogen stores in liver and muscle. Also, intraluminal fermentation of sugars contributes greatly to abdominal distention and flatulence. Failure to hydrolyze disaccharides, particularly lactose (*disaccharidase deficiency*), results in watery diarrhea as well as these local abdominal complaints (see below).

Anemia. Deficiency of vitamin B_{12} or folic acid may cause a macrocytic anemia with a megaloblastic bone marrow, whereas iron deficiency will cause a microcytic hypochromic anemia. With deficiency of vitamin B_{12}, folic acid, and iron, anemia with mixed features will be present. The former type is seen in *tropical sprue,* after *resection* of, or *disease* in, a large segment of the *terminal ileum;* rarely, in pancreatic insufficiency; in "primary" *malabsorption* of *vitamin B_{12}* (defective ileal receptor); and in conditions in which there is bacterial overgrowth in the upper small intestine—*"blind loops," jejunal diverticulosis, enteroenteric* or *enterocolic fistulas,* and *multiple small bowel strictures.* In contrast to pernicious anemia, in these conditions simultaneous feeding of intrinsic factor does not improve vitamin B_{12} absorption. In those cases caused by bacterial overgrowth as well as in tropical sprue, normal absorption of vitamin B_{12} may be restored by oral administration of a broad-spectrum antimicrobial drug—tetracycline, oxytetracycline, or ampicillin (1.0 gram daily) for 10 to 14 days (Table 3). Indeed, a brisk reticulocytosis may be noted in three to four days. Impaired absorption of vitamin B_{12} and mega-

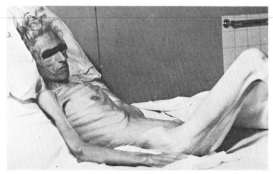

Figure 1. Extreme wasting in a patient with adult celiac disease (nontropical sprue).

TABLE 3. ^{60}Co-Vitamin B_{12} Absorption (Schilling)

Result after:	Pernicious Anemia and Total Gastrectomy	Megaloblastic Anemia Associated with:				
		Adult Celiac Disease*	Blind Loop Syndrome	Primary Malabsorption of Vitamin B_{12}	Tropical Sprue	Pancreatic Insufficiency*
		. . . Absorption . . .				
Vitamin B_{12}	Low	Low-normal or low	Low	Low	No change	Normal-low†
Vitamin B_{12} + intrinsic factor	Normal	No change	No change	No change	No change	No change
Vitamin B_{12} after antimicrobial therapy	Low	No change	Normal	No change	Normal or low	No change
Vitamin B_{12} after gluten-free diet	No change	Normal	No change	No change	No change	No change
Vitamin B_{12} + bicarbonate	No change	No change	No change	No change	No change	Normal‡
Vitamin B_{12} + pancreatic extract	No change	No change	No change	No change	No change	Normal‡

*Rare in adult celiac disease; very rare in pancreatic insufficiency.
†Rare to be low.
‡Very rare.

loblastosis may also be noted occasionally in patients with *adult celiac disease.*

Folic Acid Deficiency.   Folic acid deficiency may also underlie *megaloblastosis* and *anemia.* As there is often an associated deficiency of vitamin B_{12}, diagnosis may be established only by the finding of low serum folic acid levels (less than 5.0 ng), or of a reticulocytic response to administration of minimal daily effective dosage (0.05 to 0.5 mg parenterally). Usually, however, folic acid deficiency is corrected by adequate diet or oral supplementation.

Glossitis and Peripheral Neuropathy.   *Glossitis* and *peripheral neuropathy* can in part be attributed to deficiency of vitamin B_{12}. Since combined system disease may be induced or exacerbated by administration of folic acid, *vitamin B_{12} stores in tissues must be replenished before administration of folic acid alone for megaloblastic anemia.*

Impaired Iron Absorption.   Iron absorption may be subnormal except when the malabsorption syndrome is due to uncomplicated pancreatic insufficiency. Most often the iron deficiency is caused by poor absorption owing either to mucosal disease or to inability to release inorganic iron from organic compounds. However, occult blood loss may contribute to the anemia. Iron deficiency anemia is very common in *adult celiac disease* and may be noted also in the later stages of *tropical sprue.* When associated with deficiencies of folic acid and vitamin B_{12}, iron deficiency may not become apparent until these substances are repleted. Incorporation of iron into young marrow red blood cells requires both folic acid and vitamin B_{12}.

Diminished Absorption of Water and Electrolytes.   Common in the malabsorption syndrome are *dehydration, weakness,* and *hypotension.* Large amounts of water and electrolytes are lost if diarrhea is severe or if stools are very loose or bulky. Absorption of water in adult celiac disease is slower than normal, and diuresis after a water load is delayed. Thus patients with steatorrhea often have nocturia. *Hyponatremia* not caused by renal loss responds readily to administration of sodium, and symptoms of "low salt"—weakness, lethargy, nausea, cramps—rapidly disappear. *Hypokalemia,* if severe, causes muscle flaccidity and cardiac arrhythmias.

Vitamin B Complex Deficiency: Dermatitis, Neuritis, and Cheilosis.   Although *glossitis, neuritis* (peripheral neuropathy), and *dermatitis* in the malabsorption syndrome have been attributed to deficiency of B vitamins, proof of impaired absorption of these substances (vitamins B_1, B_2, and B_6) is not at hand. Perhaps deficiency results from metabolic action of abnormal bacterial flora that ordinarily do not inhabit the small bowel. However, conclusive demonstration of this mechanism also is lacking, particularly in *adult celiac disease.* Moreover, administration of vitamin B complex ($B_{1,\,2,\,6,\,12}$) does not always cure the glossitis, which may be partially due to iron deficiency.

DIAGNOSIS

Although the spectrum of clinical symptoms and signs of malabsorption syndrome is broad, those with mild chronic illness display one or more important clinical or laboratory abnormalities. A high index of suspicion of the diagnosis is essential for those with minimal complaints and seemingly normal-appearing stools. Unfortunately, there is no short cut to diagnosis of the syndrome and, equally important, of its underlying cause.

The clues to diagnosis of the malabsorption syndrome are the history, symptoms, signs, and laboratory abnormalities listed in Tables 2 and 3 that relate to malabsorption of fat and other substances, particularly fat-soluble vitamins, proteins, iron, and vitamin B_{12}. The average patient will complain of rather bulky, light-colored stools, often with increased frequency (but not necessarily so), abdominal distention, and variable weight loss, and will also show laboratory evidence of impaired absorption. However, special diagnostic attention must be tendered those with subtler histories and findings and especially those who complain principally of bleeding tendency or of some skeletal disability, chiefly pain. Other features commonly seen in many diseases of this syndrome include *hypotension, abdominal distention, diffuse brownish pigmentation,* and *clubbing* of the fingers and toes.

It is not usually difficult to establish solely by clinical examination that the malabsorption syndrome is present. Much more precise information as to *which* absorption defects are present is necessary, however, if the physician is to treat the illness successfully. In large measure, this essential information can be obtained only by the proper use of a number of laboratory procedures.

Laboratory Diagnosis

The pathophysiologic basis for the abnormal findings of the laboratory tests has been described and is presented in Table 2. The particular values of the individual tests in arriving at a diagnosis are considered in Table 4. The essential diagnostic tests, excluding routine blood studies (complete blood count, determination of Ca^{++}, K^+, and prothrombin time), include measurement of 72-hour stool fat and serum carotene, d-xylose absorption, tests of pancreatic function, tests for bacterial overgrowth, roentgenographic study of the small bowel, vitamin B_{12} absorption, and biopsy of the small intestine.

Measurement of Stool Fat: Serum Carotene. Because the most important feature in diagnosis of the malabsorption syndrome is steatorrhea, accurate measurement of fecal fat is extremely important. The only reliable method is the chemical analysis of a 72-hour stool collection, the patient ingesting 80 to 100 grams of fat per day. Normal excretion in these circumstances is 6.0 grams or less per 24 hours (Table 4).

This test is essential for diagnosis, because only in the so-called primary mucosal cell abnormalities (except for abetalipoproteinemia) is fat absorption normal (Table 1). Steatorrhea, however, does not indicate into which category of malabsorptive disorders the patient falls. If fecal fat is elevated, a roentgenographic study of the small intestine as well as a d-xylose test must be performed. Increasingly, small bowel biopsy is being done routinely if pancreatic disease is unlikely. Finally, determinations which reflect bacterial overgrowth (intestinal stasis) are required either when the roentgenographic

studies display a *blind loop, jejunal diverticula, strictures, enteroenteric* or *enterocolic fistula,* or the marked intestinal stasis of *scleroderma,* or when the biopsy is normal.

Depressed levels of serum carotene will usually be found in patients with steatorrhea. This test is useful in "screening" those in whom the malabsorption syndrome is suspected.

d-Xylose Absorption (Table 4). During recent years, absorption of d-xylose, a pentose, has been measured in the study of malabsorption. Twenty-five grams is given orally; if the patient does not vomit, has no delay in gastric emptying, is well hydrated, and has normal kidney function, 4.5 grams or more will be excreted in a five-hour collection of urine. It is absorbed actively like glucose, but its metabolism is not as rapid as that of glucose, and its renal excretion does not depend upon a threshold. As a measure of carbohydrate absorption, it is more reliable than an oral glucose tolerance test. In patients over 60, renal excretion diminishes; in such individuals, as well as in patients with delayed gastric emptying, liver disease with ascites, or renal disease, blood levels are measured and should reach 20 mg per 100 ml in two hours.

Although the fate of about half of the 50 per cent of the 25.0 gram oral load which is absorbed normally is unknown, it is clear that excretion in five hours is significantly diminished (less than 3.0 grams) with intestinal

TABLE 4.   Laboratory Tests Commonly Employed to Study Malabsorption

	Normal Values	Malabsorption Syndrome*
Serum:		
Albumin	4.0 to 5.2 grams/100 ml	Diminished
Carotene	0.06 to 0.4 mg/100 ml	Diminished, particularly in small bowel disease
Calcium	9.0 to 10.5 mg/100 ml	Diminished, particularly in small bowel disease
Cholesterol	150 to 250 mg/100 ml	Diminished
Potassium	3.5 to 4.7 mEq/L	Diminished
Magnesium	1.7 to 2.0 mEq/L	Diminished
Vitamin B_{12}	100 to 700 $\mu\mu$g/ml	Diminished, particularly in tropical sprue and bacterial overgrowth
Folic Acid	5 to 21 ng/ml	Diminished, particularly in small bowel disease
Plasma:		
Prothrombin time	Control value	Elevated
Tolerance tests:		
d-Xylose (25 grams orally)	Urinary excretion of 4.5 grams or greater per 5 hours	Diminished in diseases of the mucosa, particularly celiac disease, and in intestinal stasis (normal in pancreatic insufficiency)
Glucose (100 grams orally)	35 mg over fasting plasma level	"Flat curve" in celiac disease and diseases of intestinal wall and in monosaccharide malabsorption
Lactose (50 to 100 grams orally) (2.0 grams/kg in children)	Rise in blood glucose of 20 mg/100 ml	Low to flat curve in primary lactose deficiency, celiac disease, and diseases of the intestinal wall
Sucrose (100 grams orally)	Rise in blood glucose of 20 mg/100 ml	Low to flat in celiac disease and disease of intestinal wall
Vitamin B_{12} (μc ^{60}CO B_{12})	> 7% urine excretion/24 hours	Decreased with intestinal stasis, ileal dysfunction, or resection
Stool fat:		
Chemical determination (80–100 grams fat daily)	< 6 grams/24 hours	Increased
Miscellaneous:		
5-Hydroxyindolacetic acid (urinary excretion)	1.7 to 8.0 mg/24 hours	9 to 20 mg in adult celiac disease; 30 to 600 mg in metastatic carcinoid syndrome
Indole-3-acetic acid (urinary excretion)	Less than 18 mg/24 hours	
Indican (urinary excretion)	Minute amounts of $^{14}CO_2$/4 to 8 hours	Elevated in bacterial overgrowth and ileal dysfunction
Bile acid breath test		

*Usual findings. Some values for serum tests may be normal in some patients, e.g., carotene, calcium, and vitamin B_{12} in pancreatic insufficiency and calcium in tropical sprue.

disease affecting particularly the *jejunum,* after *massive resection,* and in marked *bacterial overgrowth,* presumably owing to bacterial action. The procedure thus serves to separate these patients from those with pancreatic insufficiency and from normal subjects. d-Xylose absorption has occasionally been found to be abnormal in *pancreatic carcinoma* with metastatic involvement of the small intestine.

Normal d-xylose absorption is strong evidence against the diagnosis of *adult celiac disease.* An abnormal result, however, casts strong doubt upon the diagnosis of *pancreatic insufficiency.* The test is also valuable in gauging the effect of therapy when pretreatment values have been low.

Pancreatic Function. Evaluation of pancreatic function by measurement of volume and bicarbonate concentration of duodenal aspirates after appropriate stimulation or concentration of enzymes after a test meal is in order if the d-xylose test is normal and roentgenographic study of the small intestine is normal or equivocally so. It is clearly indicated if biopsy is normal and there is no other apparent disease or disorder. Subnormal response strongly indicates pancreatic insufficiency or pancreatic ductal obstruction, although normal values do not exclude these possibilities.

Tests for Bacterial Overgrowth. The increasing clinical importance of bacterial overgrowth as a cause for malabsorption syndrome has stimulated development of tests which directly and indirectly indicate the presence of this condition. It may be present in a large number of diseases in which there is either small bowel stasis or contamination by lower gut organisms. These tests include the *bile salt breath test,* measurement of *urinary tryptophan metabolites,* and direct *culture* of jejunal aspirates.

Bile Salt Breath Test. The recent introduction of the so-called "bile salt breath test" promises to be enormously helpful in diagnosis of malabsorption caused by diseases or disorders in which bile salt deconjugation is abnormal. These include diseases of bacterial overgrowth and ileal dysfunction (diseased or absent long segment of terminal ileum). In either situation, bacteria (small intestinal in the former situation and colonic in the latter) will deconjugate a significant amount of orally administered ^{14}C glycine-cholate before it is absorbed; the released ^{14}C glycine will be further metabolized by bacterial enzymes to $^{14}CO_2$ which quickly diffuses into the circulation and is breathed out. Normally, only a minute quantity of $^{14}CO_2$ is detectable in four to six hours; however, when bacteria are present in the small gut or bile salt reabsorption by the terminal ileum is subnormal, $^{14}CO_2$ excretion in breath is elevated tenfold or more after ingestion of ^{14}C glycine-cholate.

Tryptophan Metabolites. The measurement of two urinary metabolites of L-tryptophan, indican and 5-hydroxyindolacetic acid (50HIAA), has been valuable in diagnosis of diseases of bacterial overgrowth and of ileal dysfunction (diseased, bypassed or absent terminal ileum) and of adult celiac disease. Elevated urinary levels of indoxylsulfate (indican) are found in virtually all diseases in which intestinal stasis is present or the terminal ileum is diseased or absent (greater than 100 mg per 24 hours). Return toward normal values may follow administration of broad-spectrum antimicrobials over a one- to two-week period.

The normal range of 5-hydroxyindolacetic acid is up to about 8.0 mg per 24 hours. In *adult celiac disease,* however-er, the urinary level is elevated—9.0 to 15.0 mg—reflecting perhaps an increased amount of circulating 5-hydroxytryptamine or serotonin. Treatment with a gluten-free diet restores normal excretion of this substance. Except for the metastatic *carcinoid* syndrome, in which levels are greatly elevated (300 to 500 mg per 24 hours), or *Whipple's disease,* in which an elevated level (15 mg per 24 hours) has been reported in several instances, excretion of this substance is usually normal in the various disorders which may cause the malabsorption syndrome.

The significance of these findings is not clear, but they indicate abnormal metabolism of tryptophan. Most likely this is related in some way to stasis and bacterial overgrowth, but also, as shown by appropriate loading tests with tryptophan, to a deficiency in vitamin B_6, which is necessary for its normal metabolism. The role of indolacetic acid in the pathophysiology of the malabsorption is not known, but there is evidence that it may have a suppressant effect upon the bone marrow.

Culture of Jejunal Aspirates. Techniques for culture of jejunal aspirates for fastidious anaerobic bacteria (clostridia, fusiforms, bacteroides) are increasingly available for diagnosis of intestinal stasis (bacterial overgrowth). Usually, the upper small intestine appears bacteria free in about one third of normal subjects; in the remainder, gram-positive or facultative anaerobes are present (lactobacilli and enterococci) in concentrations of 10^1 to 10^3 organisms per gram of content. Coliforms may be transiently present but rarely exceed 10^3. Normally, the terminal ileum has concentrations of organisms approaching 10^5 to 10^8 per gram, and these include gram-negative coliforms and bacteroides. In the colon enormous concentrations of anaerobes—bacteroides, lactobacilli, and clostridia—are usually present. When these organisms, particularly bacteroides and lactobacilli (but also clostridia and coliforms), luxuriate in the small intestine, the so-called bacterial overgrowth syndrome results (see Bacterial Overgrowth).

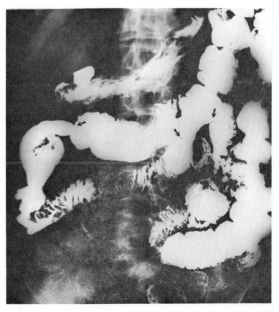

Figure 2. Small bowel series showing postoperative terminal ileum (arrow on left) and ileotransverse colostomy stoma (between arrows on right). Note the blind loop.

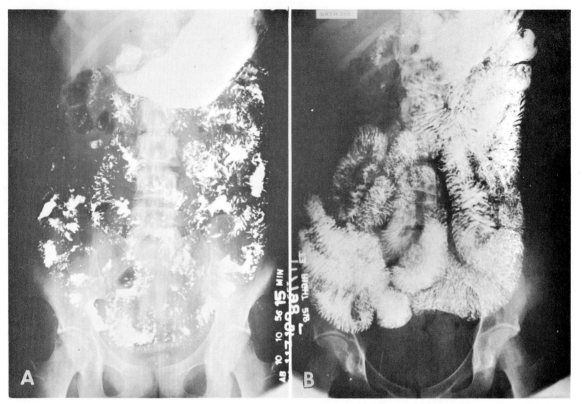

Figure 3. Small bowel roentgenographic series in patient (M.S.) with adult celiac disease. *A*, Before treatment. *B*, Six weeks after elimination of gluten from the diet. Note that the severely disordered pattern has improved.

Cultures of aspirates may now be obtained via sterile polyethylene tubes. Precise microbiologic technique for anaerobic organisms must, however, be practiced or the exercise will be futile.

Roentgenographic Studies. Diagnosis of the malabsorption syndrome may be facilitated by recognition of changes in the roentgenograms of the small bowel which point to bacterial overgrowth and include *strictures* or *fistulas, blind loops* usually from previous surgery (Fig. 2), or marked *stasis*, as in scleroderma. Dilatation of the proximal jejunum with "flocculation" and "scattering" of barium, slight coarsening of valvulae conniventes, and rather oddly shaped collections called "moulage," point strongly to *adult celiac disease* (Fig. 3). The factors underlying these changes are not completely understood but include some disturbance of motility or the effect of overproduction of mucus, caused perhaps in both instances by the collection in the gut of irritating substances such as fatty acids. Such changes, but particularly disordered transit and markedly thickened folds, may be noted in *Whipple's disease*. *Amyloidosis, radiation enteritis, hypoproteinemia, Zollinger-Ellison syndrome,* and *eosinophilic enteritis* may also be responsible. Differential diagnosis of various malabsorption states by roentgenographic examination of the small bowel, however, is often most difficult unless a characteristic finding for an underlying disease (e.g., tumor, stricture, or blind loop) is evident. Some roentgenographic changes associated with *chronic pancreatitis* or *cancer of the pan-*

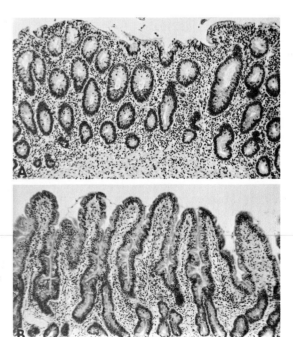

Figure 4. Jejunal mucosa of patient (F. G.) with adult celiac disease. *A*, Before treatment (60 ×). *B*, Twenty-eight months after elimination of gluten from the diet. Note the regeneration of the villi and the return toward normal of the columnar epithelium (60 ×).

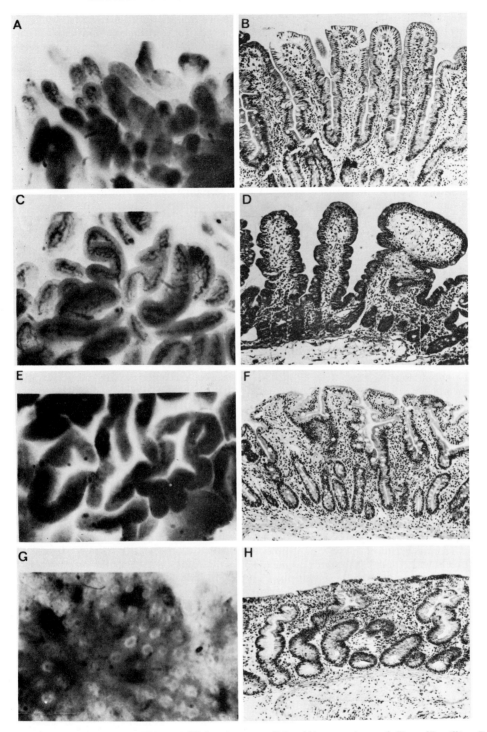

Figure 5.   Comparison of dissecting microscopy and light microscopy of jejunal biopsy specimens. *A*, Finger-like villi vs. *B*, normal villous pattern. *C*, Leaflike villi vs. *D*, normal villous pattern. *E*, Convolutions vs. *F*, partial villous atrophy. *G*, "Mosaics" vs. *H*, total villous atrophy. *E* through *H* are specimens from patients with adult celiac disease.

creas include diffuse calcification or displacement of the stomach by a pseudocyst in the former condition and widening of the duodenal loop or distortion or destruction of mucosal folds in the latter (see Ch. 646 and 648).

Vitamin B_{12} Absorption. Vitamin B_{12} absorption is tested after intramuscular administration of 1000 μg by oral administration of radioactive vitamin B_{12} and measurement of the excretion in the urine over a 24-hour period. Greater than 7 per cent of the administered dose should be excreted. The absolute values depend upon dose of labeled B_{12}.

Abnormal results are found after *resection* of the *terminal ileum*, extensive and severe *terminal ileal disease*, and *bacterial overgrowth*. It is also abnormal in *pernicious anemia*, after *total gastrectomy*, or in some patients with *pancreatic insufficiency*. Administration of tetracycline, 1 gram daily for two weeks, will usually restore vitamin B$_{12}$ absorption in bacterial overgrowth to normal. On the other hand, administration of the test substance with intrinsic factor will yield a normal result in patients with pernicious anemia and after total gastrectomy, but not after extensive resection of the terminal ileum or in pancreatic insufficiency. In the latter condition bicarbonate or pancreatic extract may be required (see Table 3).

Jejunal Histology. Histologic study of jejunal mucosa obtained by suction biopsy technique has further aided differential diagnosis of the malabsorption syndrome. The procedure is easily performed with one of several available tubes (Rubin tube or Crosby capsule). Prothrombin time must be normal. Characteristic findings have been associated with *celiac disease* in both children and adults and in *tropical sprue, Whipple's disease, amyloidosis,* and *eosinophilic gastroenteritis.* In some instances alterations may be noted in diffuse nongranulomatous *ileojejunitis,* in *lymphoma,* after *gastrectomy,* in *hypogammaglobulinemia* with steatorrhea, in patients with intestinal *lymphangiectasia* associated with protein-losing enteropathy who have dilated lacteals, and in individuals with *radiation enteritis, mastocytosis,* or severe *drug reactions.* Fat-laden epithelial cells are found in *abetalipoproteinemia.* Certain parasites, namely, *Giardia lamblia* and *Coccidioides immitis,* have also been found on biopsy.

A section of normal jejunal mucosa from a specimen obtained by suction biopsy is shown in Figures 4 and 5. The villi are long, delicate, and frondlike; the lining columnar epithelium is regular with basal orientation of nuclei. The crypts are normal, and cellular infiltration of the lamina propria is minimal. Proper interpretation of jejunal histology, it must be emphasized, depends upon correct (perpendicular) sectioning of the specimen, which, in turn, requires correct mounting before fixing.

The jejunal histology in *adult celiac disease and tropical sprue* is strikingly abnormal. In evaluation of small bowel biopsies from such patients, particular attention must be directed to configuration of the villi, morphology of the epithelial cells with their brush border, and the degree of the chronic inflammatory cell infiltration. The severity of changes may be graded from mild to moderate to severe. In the *severe* group (total villous atrophy) the changes consist of complete flattening of the mucosal surface without detectable villi or, at best, only very short and broad villi. Generally, there is a dense infiltration of chronic inflammatory cells and disorganization of the epithelial cells with a sparse brush border (Figs. 4 and 5). In the *mild* group (partial villous atrophy), the villi are formed but still are shorter and broader than normal. In some areas the villi approach normal in all respects. The epithelial cells with brush border generally may be nearly normal and the cellular infiltration is mild. In the *moderate* subdivision (subtotal villous atrophy), changes ranging between those of the mild and severe groups are noted (Fig. 5).

The degree of infiltration of the lamina propria and of alteration of the epithelial cells is proportional to the extent of villous atrophy. The brush border frequently appears intact in the crypts, although it is disorganized and sparse near the midportion and tip of the villus. Although the severity of the lesion varies considerably among patients, the variation within a limited region of the proximal jejunum in a single patient is minimal; however, definite differences between the samples from more distant locations in the same patient have been noted. Total villous atrophy, although characteristic of celiac disease, is not specific. Occasionally, it may be noted in *tropical sprue,* in *lymphoma,* or in *Whipple's disease,* and it has been reported in *diffuse nongranulomatous ileojejunitis* (often "ulcerative"), as well as in patients with *congenital hypogammaglobulinemia* in whom plasma cells are absent in the lamina propria. Some of the last-named will respond to a gluten-free diet and thus have adult celiac disease as well; the same coincidence may be noted in patients with *diabetes mellitus* after *gastrectomy,* and in *Sjögren's syndrome, mastocytosis, jejunal diverticulosis,* and even *cystic fibrosis.*

Changes of this nature have also been noted (but not responsive to gluten elimination) in patients with *eosinophilic gastroenteritis,* in some *parasitoses,* and in *intestinal ischemia, dermatitis herpetiformis, soy bean sensitivity, radiation enteritis, tuberculosis, viral enteritis,* and conditions caused by *colchicine* and *neomycin.* Recently, mild inflammatory cell infiltration of the lamina propria has been noted in biopsies from patients with bacterial overgrowth.

In *Whipple's disease* the diagnosis may be made by the demonstration of macrophages laden with periodic acid–Schiff staining material in lymph nodes or in the lamina propria of the intestinal wall. In addition, total villous atrophy may be noted (Fig. 6). Recent electromicroscopic studies during the active phase of the disease have revealed membranous structures, which may represent an infectious agent outside the macrophages. Deposits of amyloid have been found in the submucosa of the jejunum in patients with *amyloidosis,* particularly within the walls of arterioles.

In the past few years examination of fresh biopsy specimens under the dissecting microscope has yielded information about a number of diseases of the small intestine associated with malabsorption. The normal patterns of *finger-like villi* and *leaflike villi* are seen in Figure 5. The former are jejunal, and the latter are also normally present in the duodenum and upper jejunum. Epithelial convolutions usually indicate disease and, on histologic examination, correspond to *partial villous atrophy.* A most extreme change is noted with total villous atrophy, with *"mosaics"* or *"brain patterns"* as the picture under

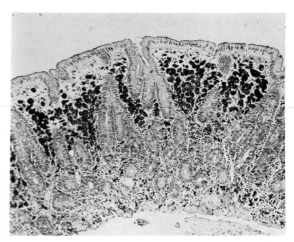

Figure 6. Jejunal biopsy from a patient with Whipple's disease. Periodic acid–Schiff stain. Note macrophages laden with stained material in the lamina propria.

the dissecting microscope. Examples of this classification are presented in Figure 5.

DIFFERENTIAL FEATURES AND TREATMENT OF INDIVIDUAL FORMS OF THE MALABSORPTION SYNDROME

Because the presenting clinical picture includes a wide range of symptoms — e.g., bulky stools, flatulence, distention anorexia, weight loss, weakness, glossitis, paresthesias, bleeding, bone pain — a careful history is of extreme importance in differential diagnosis. Particular atten-

tion must be paid to bowel habits in childhood, family history, previous illnesses and surgical operations, and dietary habits (including consumption of alcohol). A history of symptoms commonly associated with diseases that might underlie the malabsorption must be sought. Valuable clues may also be derived from a careful physical examination. In this way diagnosis of *tropical sprue, adult celiac disease, Whipple's disease, hypothyroidism, hyperthyroidism, hypoparathyroidism, scleroderma, lymphoma,* and other malabsorptive disorders may be facilitated.

The malabsorption syndrome must be differentiated from a wide variety of conditions characterized by a bleeding diathesis, by skeletal pain with or without frac-

TABLE 5. Representative Dosages for Agents Used in Management of Patients with the Malabsorption Syndrome

1. CALCIUM
   Oral: Calcium gluconate (91 mg Ca^{++}/gram), 1 to 5 grams three times daily
   Intravenous: Calcium gluconate injection. U.S.P. 10 per cent solution (9.1 mg Ca^{++}/ml), 10 to 30 ml administered slowly intravenously depending upon response
2. MAGNESIUM
   Oral: Magnesium sulfate (8 mEq/gram), 1.0 to 6.0 grams daily in divided dosage
   Intramuscular: (20% sol.) 10 ml two or three times daily
   Intravenous: Magnesium sulfate, 0.5 per cent solution, up to 1000 ml at a rate not faster than 1.0 mEq/minute
3. IRON
   Oral: Ferrous gluconate, 0.6 gram three times daily
   Intramuscular: (Imferon). Must be calculated according to severity of anemia. Detailed instructions accompany preparation.
4. FAT-SOLUBLE VITAMINS
   a. VITAMIN A
   Oleovitamin A capsules, U.S.P. (25,000 units per capsule), 100,000 to 200,000 units daily in severe deficiencies; maintenance, 25,000 to 50,000 units daily.
   b. VITAMIN D
   Synthetic oleovitamin D, U.S.P. (10,000 U.S.P. units vitamin D/gram), 30,000 units daily; increase dosage as necessary to raise serum calcium to normal. Dosage varies considerably depending on response as determined by level of serum calcium and urinary calcium.
   c. COMBINATION A AND D VITAMINS
   Concentrated oleovitamins A and D, U.S.P. (50,000 to 65,000 U.S.P. A units and 10,000 to 13,000 U.S.P. D units/gram) may be used rather than separate preparations.
   d. VITAMIN K
   Oral: Menadione, U.S.P., 4 to 12 mg daily. Vitamin K_1 tablets (Mephyton), 5 to 10 mg daily.
   Intravenous: (Bleeding episodes — acute situations.) Vitamin K_1 (Mephyton), 50 mg ampule. Administer 50 mg slowly over 10-minute period. Repeat in 8 to 12 hours if prothrombin time has not returned to normal.
5. FOLIC ACID, U.S.P. (5 mg tablets)
   Dose: Initial, 10 to 20 mg daily
   Maintenance, 5 to 10 mg daily
6. VITAMIN B_{12} INJECTION, U.S.P. (15 μg/ml)
   Dose: Initial, 30 to 60 μg daily for two to three weeks
   Maintenance, 100 μg monthly
   If combined system disease is present, a more intensive program is indicated.
7. VITAMIN B COMPLEX
   Any multivitamin preparation that contains daily requirements (thiamine 1.6 mg, riboflavin 1.8 mg, and niacin 20 mg). Use two or three tablets daily. Intramuscular preparations are available for severe deficiencies.
8. PANCREATIC SUPPLEMENTS, ORAL
   Recently these agents have been shown to be more effective when given at 6 to 12 regular intervals during the day rather than at meal times.
   a. *Pancreatin,* U.S.P. (0.3 gram tablet), 6 to 18 grams daily.
   b. *Viokase* (0.3 gram tablet), 4 to 12 grams daily in divided doses at meals or hourly per day.
   c. *Cotazym* (0.3 gram capsule), 4.0 to 12.0 grams daily, divided doses at meals or hourly per day.
9. BROAD-SPECTRUM ANTIMICROBIALS
   Oral: Chloramphenicol, tetracycline, or oxytetracycline (0.25 gram), 1.0 gram per day in divided doses for 10 to 14 days; ampicillin (0.25 gram), 2.0 to 4.0 grams per day in divided doses; kanamycin (0.5 gram), 2.0 to 4.0 grams per day in divided doses; sulfisoxazole (0.5 gram), 1.0 to 2.0 grams daily in divided doses; lincomycin (0.25 gram), 1.0 to 2.0 grams daily. Repeated courses often necessary or administration for three to four days each week indefinitely.
10. HUMAN ALBUMIN, SALT POOR (0.25 gram/ml)
    Intravenous administration of 50 to 100 grams each day for three to seven days to elevate a severely depressed serum albumin level
11. GLOBULIN, IMMUNE SERUM (0.165 gram/ml)
    Intramuscular injection of 0.05 ml/kg each three to four weeks in patients with hypogammaglobulinemia and recurrent infection.
12. CORTICOTROPHIN AND ADRENOCORTICOSTEROIDS
    a. Corticotrophin, 30 to 40 units intravenously each day, 10 to 21 days or longer for severely ill patients.
    b. Prednisolone or prednisone, 30 to 60 mg orally each day as needed; 5.0 to 15.0 mg maintenance dose.
13. ANTIDIARRHEAL AGENTS
    Oral: Diphenoxylate hydrochloride (2.5 mg), 5.0 mg twice or three times daily. Deodorized tincture opium, 10 drops twice to three times per day. Propantheline (15.0 mg), 30 mg twice or three times daily.
14. CHOLESTYRAMINE, ORAL RESIN
    4.0 gram dose, three to six times daily, before feedings.
15. CALORIC SUPPLEMENTATION
    Oral: (a) Medium-chain triglyceride (MCT). "Home or Hospital Mix" (MCT: 45 per cent calories; caseinate, 15 per cent; dextrose, 40 per cent). Ingredients homogenized with H_2O to one liter (MCT: 75 mg; caseinate, 60 grams; dextrose 160 grams). Keep at 20°C for one year. Defrost day's formula each morning; give three ounces at meals; gradually increase between-meal feedings to six ounces. Portagen (MCT: 45.0 grams fat/quart; 30 cal/oz; 10 per cent carbohydrate). Formula mix. Prepare according to instructions. Give 16 oz every day.
    (b) Vivonex, 80 grams = 300 cal: 90.8% CHO; 0.7% fat; 8.5% amino acids, plus minerals and electrolytes. Dissolve in 100 ml water. Feed up to 480 grams q.d.
    Intravenous: Prepare solution of approx. 0.9 cal/ml: 20% dextrose and 5% fibrin hydrolysate (w/v). Give 1500–3000 ml q.d. Increase amounts cautiously. Solution contains electrolytes, including Po_4'''
16. DRUGS FOR PARASITES
    Oral: Thiabendazole (25 mg/kg/day). Strongyloidiasis, two to three days; *Capillaria philippensis,* 30 days. *A. duodenale, N. Americanus,* 25 mg/kg/day twice daily for two days.
    Oral: Metronidazole (0.25 gram), 0.25 gram three times daily for 7 days for *Giardia lamblia.*
    Oral: Bephenium (5 gram packet). *A. duodenale,* one packet twice for one day; *N. Americanus,* one packet twice daily for three days.

ture, by evidence of vitamin B deficiency and extreme malnutrition, or by chronic diarrhea. Diagnosis of the malabsorption syndrome as a cause for these symptoms and signs must first, however, be based upon demonstration of abnormal fat absorption.

As the patient with the malabsorption syndrome may have extreme weight loss, weakness, hypotension, and diffuse pigmentation, differentiation from *Addison's disease* must be made. Abnormalities of serum calcium, carotene, or plasma prothrombin and impaired absorption of fat and xylose indicate the presence of the malabsorption syndrome (Table 4). Addison's disease may be excluded by the responsiveness of the adrenal gland to an intravenous infusion of corticotrophin. However, it must be stressed that patients very severely, acutely, and chronically ill with malabsorption syndrome, particularly *celiac disease,* may have evidence of hypoadrenocorticism and that administration of steroids is an indicated component of initial therapy.

The principal distinctive features of the individual forms of the malabsorption syndrome are discussed according to the seven categories of Table 1.

As there are numerous conditions that can produce the malabsorption syndrome, its treatment must be individualized. In contrast to the often gratifying response to dietotherapy shown by patients with *adult celiac disease,* or to antimicrobials by patients with *Whipple's disease, diseases with bacterial overgrowth,* and *tropical sprue,* successful management of malabsorption resulting from various other diseases or alterations of the gastrointestinal tract is often difficult. Dosage schedules for agents used in the treatment of malabsorption syndrome are listed in Table 5.

Category 1: Defective Intraluminal Hydrolysis or Solubilization

Primary Pancreatic Insufficiency. Pancreatic insufficiency results from *chronic relapsing pancreatitis, carcinoma of the pancreas,* or *cystic fibrosis,* or *after extensive resection* of the gland. In the first three instances, it is due to extensive parenchymal destruction and/or obstruction of the major ductal system. In chronic pancreatitis with malabsorption (see Ch. 646), the patient is frequently diabetic, the gland is noted to be calcified on flat film of the abdomen, and frequently, but not always, there is a history of recurrent attacks of inflammation. Occasionally the dominant symptoms of *carcinoma of the pancreas* are those of malabsorption rather than pain, anorexia, or jaundice. *Cystic fibrosis* is most often clinically apparent in early childhood; increasingly, however, the diagnosis is being made in young adults.

Whatever the cause of pancreatic insufficiency, failure of lipolysis results in moderate to severe steatorrhea, depending to some degree on the amount of gland remaining. Patients with this disease may show evidence of deficiency of either vitamin B_{12} or fat-soluble vitamins. In contrast to adult celiac disease, d-xylose absorption is normal in pancreatic insufficiency except in the unusual instance of carcinoma of the pancreas that has invaded the small intestine. As noted earlier, the diagnosis of pancreatic insufficiency is facilitated by analysis of duodenal fluid after stimulation of the pancreas. When lipolysis is markedly depressed, hydroxy fatty acids are not produced, providing a possible way of distinguishing pancreatic steatorrhea from steatorrhea of bacterial overgrowth and other nonpancreatogenous forms of malabsorption.

Secondary Pancreatic Insufficiency. Since pancreatic lipase is inactivated at an acid pH, conditions characterized by excessive gastric acid secretion, such as non-β islet cell tumor of the pancreas (Zollinger-Ellison syndrome) or massive small bowel resection, are associated with significant steatorrhea. As noted, defective lipolysis causes deficient formation of micelles. Although it is possible that a low pH in the upper small gut may also precipitate bile salts and cause mild histologic abnormalities, the importance of these factors as against inactivation of lipase remains to be determined.

Deficiency of Conjugated Bile Salts. Insufficient concentration of conjugated bile salt in the upper intestine, caused by severe liver disease or prolonged extrahepatic biliary tract obstruction, diminished bile salt pool, or significant reduction of conjugated bile salts resulting from bacterial overgrowth (see below), diminishes hydrolysis of neutral lipid and results in steatorrhea. The pathophysiologic mechanism is subnormal concentration (less than 2.5 mmoles per liter) of conjugated bile salts necessary for micelle formation.

Distal *ileectomy,* severely *diseased terminal ileum,* or *ileal bypass* (surgical or via cholecystocolonic fistula), by disrupting the enterohepatic circulation of conjugated bile salts, also causes steatorrhea, the degree proportional to the length of the resected, diseased, or bypassed segment (about 8 to 15 grams per 24 hours for distal 100 cm). Bile salt pool is diminished, the critical level of conjugated bile salts is not achieved in the jejunum, and micellar solubilization of lipid diminishes. Further, since bile salt absorption is subnormal, these substances make contact with colonic mucosa, inhibiting water and salt absorption, particularly in the ascending colon. Diarrhea—three to six loose to soft movements per day—results. When less than 100 cm of terminal ileum is involved, both the steatorrhea and diarrhea are mild. Patients with distal ileectomy generally lose from 15 to 30 grams of fat in stools per day. This large degree of steatorrhea may be due in small part to loss of absorptive function of the ileum, although it is likely that the diminished bile salt pool is responsible entirely.

Decreased conjugated bile salt pool is also notable in primary or *secondary biliary cirrhosis;* that the steatorrhea in these cases is due to liver disease is supported by disappearance of malabsorption with improvement of liver function. It is surprising, however, that the steatorrhea of complete obstruction is moderate, indicating other mechanisms for absorption in addition to proximal uptake of micellar lipid. Malabsorption of fat in *postnecrotic* (macronodular) or *portal* (micronodular) *cirrhosis* is usually mild unless *chronic pancreatitis* (usually caused by alcohol) is also present.

Bacterial Overgrowth (Increased Bile Salt Deconjugation). For many years, steatorrhea and vitamin B_{12} deficiency anemia have been clinically and experimentally associated with alterations in the anatomy of the small intestine, particularly surgically created *"blind" loops; enteroenteric, enterocolic,* or *gastrojejunocolic fistulas; afferent loop stasis* after subtotal gastrectomy and gastrojejunostomy; or *chronic obstruction* caused by adhesions or strictures, *jejunal diverticula,* or diseases with *motor abnormalities* such as scleroderma and pseudo-obstruction.

The common denominator in all conditions is bacterial overgrowth, which results from stasis in a segment of small bowel caused by anatomic factors, motor abnormalities, or contamination of small bowel by large bowel content. Concentration of anaerobic organisms greater than 10^7 per milliliter, particularly *bacteroides, clostridia,* and *lactobacilli,* is responsible for impairment of intraluminal solubilization of hydrolyzed lipid. Bacterial overgrowth may rarely play a role also in the malabsorption in *diabetes mellitus* with neuropathy (unclear), in *tropical sprue,* and after *subtotal gastrectomy* and Billroth II gastrojejunostomy. These patients may also have severe diarrhea as well as steatorrhea, possibly owing to impairment of Na^+ and water absorption by hydroxy fatty acids which result from bacterial action on unabsorbed fatty acids; also, short chain fatty acids, products of fermentation of sugars and amino acids, may cause diarrhea by increasing intraluminal osmolarity.

The mechanism of the malabsorption of vitamin B_{12} and fat caused by bacterial overgrowth is clear. Vitamin B_{12} is utilized by multiplying anaerobic organisms. Fat absorption is impaired by deconjugation of bile salts by bacterial enzymes. The decline in concentration of conjugated bile salts below a critical level (less than 2.5 mmoles per liter) impairs micelle formation, reducing uptake of lipid by the mucosa. Concentration of free bile acids is increased intraluminally; their absorption from the proximal small gut by passive diffusion is rapid, and their serum levels are elevated; these may also inhibit cellular resynthesis of triglycerides. Observations on patients with bacterial overgrowth indicate that less than 20 per cent of intraluminal fat is in a micellar phase 45 minutes after ingestion of a lipid meal (normal: more than 50 per cent). Since hydrolysis of fat is not impaired, steatorrhea is principally the result of impaired micelle formation.

Although the jejunal villi are not entirely normal in jejunal biopsy specimens of patients with bacterial overgrowth, demonstrating some infiltration of the lamina propria with lymphocytes, plasma cells, and occasionally polymorphonuclear cells, along with mild blunting, the appearance is strikingly different from the picture in adult celiac disease.

"Blind" Loops. A loop of intestine is "blind" either when it is disconnected from the main stream (rare) or when intestinal contents may gain access to it but not readily egress from it. An example would be a partly defunctionalized terminal ileal loop that has been partially excluded by either side-to-side or end-to-side ileotransverse colostomy (Fig. 2). Stasis and overgrowth of bacteria take place with subsequent invasion of the upper small intestine.

Multiple Strictures and Jejunal Diverticula. Strictures result from diffuse *granulomatous ileojejunitis, tuberculosis,* or *x-radiation* therapy. Frequently these patients have crampy abdominal pain, bloating, and other symptoms of progressive luminal narrowing, as well as other evidences of their underlying diseases. Most multiple jejunal diverticula are probably acquired. Stasis of intestinal content in these pockets of bowel leads to bacterial overgrowth.

Fistulas. Fistulas may complicate gastric or intestinal neoplasm or granulomatous enteritis, involving stomach, small gut and colon (gastrocolic), small gut and colon (enterocolic), or loops of small gut (enteroenteric). Malabsorption may also, of course, result from exclusion of significant lengths of absorbing surface from the main stream by large fistulas (gastroileostomy).

The diagnosis is greatly aided by a history of previous chronic enteric disease or of surgical procedure. Roentgenographic examination will often establish the diagnosis by the demonstration of one of these diseases or alterations. Frequently, however, the cause may not be demonstrated.

The megaloblastic anemia commonly associated with the "blind loop" syndrome will, unlike pernicious anemia, respond to the administration of broad-spectrum antimicrobial drugs. After 10 to 14 days of such therapy (tetracycline, 1.0 gram daily in divided dose), absorption of vitamin B_{12} is usually, but not always, restored to normal (Table 5). In contrast to those with pernicious anemia, these patients usually secrete hydrochloric acid.

Postgastrectomy. Afferent loop stasis after gastrectomy and gastrojejunostomy (Billroth II) is a cause for steatorrhea and malabsorption and may be due in part to bacterial contamination of the afferent loop (see Category 5).

Scleroderma and Pseudo-Obstruction. Although a disturbance of esophageal motor function is the most common gastrointestinal manifestation of scleroderma, severe involvement of the small bowel may cause malabsorption. Atrophy of the smooth muscle of the gut, submucosal fibrosis, and damage to the myenteric plexuses severely impair or abolish peristalsis. The resulting intermittent ileus may simulate closely the picture of complete intestinal obstruction. Severe involvement of the small intestine is usually associated with esophageal involvement, thickening of the skin, or other evidence of disseminated sclerosis, e.g., soft tissue calcification, telangiectasia, pulmonary diffusion defect, so that diagnosis is not difficult. Jejunal biopsy reveals normal villi, but there may be an increased number of inflammatory cells in the lamina propria.

Bacterial overgrowth is the principal factor in the steatorrhea and malabsorption of most patients with scleroderma involving the small intestine. As with the esophagus (see Ch. 634 and 635), small bowel smooth muscle is atrophic and is replaced with fibrous tissue. Motility is severely impaired; stasis and bacterial overgrowth result. Culture of small bowel content of such patients may yield a heavy growth of anaerobic organisms.

Pseudo-obstruction of the small and large intestine is a rare condition of unknown cause characterized by periodic episodes of prolonged ileus. It is chronic in some patients and may be associated with malabsorption resulting from bacterial overgrowth.

Treatment of Defective Intraluminal Hydrolysis

Primary Pancreatic Insufficiency. Replacement of digestive enzymes and insulin is important in the treatment of patients with primary pancreatic insufficiency. Among the available sources of enzymes are a commercial pancreatic extract, pancreatin, U.S.P.; a preparation containing whole raw pancreas, Viokase; and one containing hog pancreas extract, Cotazym. Doses of these preparations are listed in Table 5; occasionally, it may be necessary to increase the recommended amounts. Replacement therapy may be more effective when it is given in divided doses at regular intervals six times daily or even hourly during the day than when it is limited to mealtimes. Some patients with primary pancreatic insufficiency do not absorb vitamin B_{12} normally, a defect that may not be corrected by giving bicarbonate alone; pancreatic extracts, however, will increase absorption to normal. There is some indication that giving bicarbonate with pancreatic extracts may improve fat absorption, but this evidence is scanty.

Secondary Pancreatic Insufficiency. Hypersecretion of acid caused by *non-β islet cell tumor* is best treated by total gastrectomy (see Ch. 643); after *massive small bowel resection,* hypersecretion may appear and be relieved by vagotomy and pyloroplasty. In both conditions, large doses of anticholinergic drugs may be effective in reducing acidity.

Deficiency of Conjugated Bile Salts. Cases in which insufficient bile reaches the intestine pose a difficult problem in treatment. If possible, *cholecystocolonic fistulas* or chronic *obstruction* of the *biliary tree* should be corrected surgically. The keystone of medical management is a balanced diet without restriction of fat. For patients with chronic *cholestatic liver disease* it is important to provide calcium and fat-soluble vitamins A, K, and D in adequate amounts (Table 5). The demineralization of bone in patients with prolonged biliary obstruction results from osteoporosis and osteomalacia. Adequate supplements of vitamin D and calcium not only may prevent further osteomalacia but also may increase calcium deposition. The administration of a high protein diet and anabolic hormones, i.e., norethandrolone (Nilevar) or testosterone, and of estrogens intermittently, may help correct the osteoporosis. Because inactivity contributes to the skeletal demineralization, maximal ambulation must be encouraged.

Bacterial Overgrowth (Bile Salt Deconjugation). Absorption of vitamin B_{12} and of fat is impaired with *intestinal strictures, fistulas, blind loops,* and multiple *jejunal diverticula.* The surgical correction of the strictures, fistulas, or blind loops may effect a permanent cure and is therefore the therapy of choice.

In some patients with malabsorption syndrome associated with either *subtotal* (Billroth II) or *total gastrectomy* or *scleroderma,* long-term antimicrobial therapy should be undertaken. Tetracycline or oxytetracycline, 1.0 gram per day, or ampicillin, 2.0 to 4.0 grams per day, should be given for 10 to 14 days, and intermittently every other day for three days each week thereafter (Table 5). Chloramphenicol, also in a daily dosage of 1.0 gram, may be used in situations in which the risks of drug toxicity seem clearly to be outweighed by the potential dangers of the disease. Many of these patients, similar to those with bacterial overgrowth from other disorders, require continuous treatment. Rotation of antimicrobial drugs may be advisable in an effort to avoid the emergence of drug-resistant microbial populations. Aspiration of jejunal contents for cultures and periodic drug susceptibility determinations are necessary for therapeutic guidance. If organisms are not susceptible to the more usually employed drugs, courses of kanamycin (2.0 to 4.0 grams daily orally) may be given. All these drugs should be used in a rotational scheme. Occasionally, some patients with recurrent *regional enteritis* and strictures or fistulas, in whom the surgical approach is not feasible, will have to be managed in a similar fashion.

In addition to the assessment of clinical response, efficiency of antimicrobial therapy may be judged by the return of the bile salt breath test and urinary indican to normal or nearly normal levels.

Use of Medium-Chain Triglycerides (Table 5). Feeding preparations of medium-chain triglycerides, composed of fatty acids with six to ten carbons, appears to be valuable in a number of diseases that cause malabsorption, including those associated with defective intraluminal hydrolysis or solubilization of fat (see above).

Medium-chain triglycerides have been used in patients with defective intraluminal hydrolysis or solubilization and are most effective in those with pancreatic insufficiency who are also being given supplements of pancreatic enzymes (see above) and in patients with deficiency of conjugated bile salts (particularly biliary tract obstruction or bile fistulas).

Indication for medium-chain triglycerides is also strong in situations in which no specific therapy for malabsorption is available, such as after massive *small bowel resection* (short gut syndrome), *lymphatic obstruction,* and *biliary atresia.* Medium-chain triglycerides are a useful adjunct in malabsorption for which specific therapy is available (*celiac disease, bacterial overgrowth, Whipple's disease, parasitism,* and *tropical sprue* — all of which will be discussed in detail later in this section).

Category 2: Mucosal Cell Abnormality and Inadequate Surface

Primary Mucosal Cell Disorders

Disaccharidase Deficiency and Monosaccharide Malabsorption. Inability to split disaccharides because of disaccharidase deficiency (lactase or sucrase and isomaltase) may be primary or secondary. The primary type of *lactase deficiency* is either familial (very rare, fatal) or congenital with an autosomal dominant inheritance. Symptoms may appear during infancy, childhood, or adulthood. Primary lactase deficiency (as well as other primary disaccharidase deficiencies) is not associated with any discernible alteration of the villi or their brush borders which contain these enzymes. Bacterial fermentation of unsplit lactose produces lactic and other organic acids which increase osmotic load with water entering the lumen. Diarrhea, cramping abdominal pain, borborygmi, and flatulence result from ingestion of milk and milk products. Weight loss and steatorrhea are usually mild and appetite is good, although infants and children may not thrive well. This pathophysiologic concept applies equally to *sucrase deficiency.*

Lactase deficit is by far the most common, particularly in blacks, and is more common in Orientals than in whites. Dietary deficiency of lactose is not the cause. Adults diagnosed as having irritable colon syndrome (see Ch. 637) may be deficient in jejunal lactase. The reason for the clinical appearance of the disorder in adulthood is not clear; it is also occasionally unmasked after subtotal gastrectomy. Since no disease of the mucosal cells is evident, the deficiency is thought to be primary, but its clinical development is somehow acquired.

Diagnosis of lactase deficiency may be made by the measurement of blood glucose after the oral administration of lactose (Table 4). A rise of less than 20 mg per 100 ml is abnormal, and if the patient's blood glucose rises normally after he ingests a mixture of glucose-galactose of equal amount, lactase deficiency is extremely likely. Diagnosis may be confirmed only by the finding of low lactase activity in a jejunal biopsy specimen. Occasionally, these patients have lactosuria after administration of 50 grams of lactose during the lactose tolerance test.

Treatment of primary lactose deficiency is elimination of milk and milk products from the diet. It often dramatically relieves all symptoms. It may also be beneficial to patients with the secondary variety of deficiency.

Depression of lactase activity is also secondary to certain diseases affecting the brush borders of jejunal mucosal cells, such as *celiac disease*; but it is also found after *massive* small bowel *resection*, in *nonbacterial jejunitis, infectious diarrhea of childhood, Giardia lamblia infection, Whipple's disease, cystic fibrosis,* and *granulomatous* (regional) *enteritis.*

Deficiency of *sucrase* is rare; it is associated with deficiency of isomaltase. Recent studies indicate that it is a homozygotic deficiency affecting perhaps as many as 2 in 1000 individuals in the population. Symptoms include watery diarrhea and borborygmi, usually from infancy, and are caused by ingestion of sucrose and sucrose-containing foods. Secondary sucrase deficiency may often accompany secondary lactase deficiency.

Diagnosis of sucrase deficiency may be made by failure of blood glucose to rise at least 20 mg per 100 ml after ingestion of 100 grams of sucrose. Treatment may be either elimination or marked reduction of sucrose, dextrins, and starches from the diet.

Congenital *glucose-galactose malabsorption* is present from birth and is exacerbated by all sugars broken down to these hexoses. Diagnosis is made by failure of these children to absorb either of these substances. Treatment consists of feeding fructose or fructose precursor–containing foods.

Abetalipoproteinemia (Acanthocytosis). Abetalipoproteinemia is a disease characterized by a morphologic defect of erythrocytes, "spiny red cells," low to absent serum beta-lipoproteins, very low serum cholesterol, and, in some instances, mild steatorrhea, ataxia, nystagmus, motor incoordination, and retinitis pigmentosa. The cause of the disease is unknown, but it is related to an inability of the mucosal cells to invest lipid with a protein envelope necessary for entry to the lacteals. The severity varies—in milder cases, no steatorrhea or neurologic defects occur. Substitution of medium-chain triglycerides for ordinary triglycerides has led to weight gain in some patients, because the component fatty acids enter the portal, not the lacteal, system.

Vitamin B$_{12}$ Malabsorption. Very rarely, primary malabsorption of the vitamin B$_{12}$–intrinsic factor complex is noted, perhaps owing to absence of a specific but unidentified "receptor" in the ileal mucosa. These patients have been shown to have adequate intrinsic factor, normal ileal histology and calcium concentration, and alkaline pH. Treatment is monthly injections of vitamin B$_{12}$ intramuscularly (Table 5).

Cystinuria and Hartnup Disease. Rarely, patients may have genetic disorders of intestinal transport of amino acids. In *cystinuria* dibasic amino acids are involved—cystine, arginine, lysine, and ornithine; in *Hartnup disease,* neutral amino acids—e.g., phenylalanine and leucine. Tryptophan deficiency leads to nicotinamide deficiencies with rash, dementia, and ataxia. These patients are cured with adequate oral nicotinamide and protein, because they absorb small peptides normally.

Intraluminal Small Bowel Disease

These diseases include *adult celiac disease, Whipple's disease, nongranulomatous ileojejunitis, allergic* and *eosinophilic gastroenteritis, amyloidosis, small bowel ischemia,* and *Crohn's disease.*

Adult Celiac Disease. An important cause of chronic malabsorption in temperate climates is adult celiac disease (gluten enteropathy, celiac sprue, nontropical sprue). In some undemonstrated way, dietary gluten is related to this disease. Perhaps the intestinal mucosa of these patients is damaged by acidic peptides contained in the gliadin fraction of this substance, either because of a deficiency or absence of specific peptidases or by an immunologic reaction to them unrelated to enzyme activity. The process affects the mucosa principally with villous atrophy, columnar to cuboidal change of absorbing cells, and infiltration of the lamina propria with plasma cells and lymphocytes. Jejunum is more affected than ileum. The extent of this lesion may be roughly correlated with clinical severity.

Patients in this group have an abnormal incidence either of a history of childhood celiac disease or of evidence of the disease in relatives. The high incidence (80 per cent) of HLA-B in these patients suggests a genetic predisposition. Further, individuals with congenital IgA deficiency are predisposed to this disease.

Commonly, the symptoms of celiac disease disappear in later childhood and in adolescence, despite continued malabsorption. Although the clinical remission is sometimes permanent, the classic features of adult celiac disease may appear during the third to sixth decades. The patients then may present with a spectrum of disability, ranging from mild discomfort and diarrhea with perhaps some anemia to severe illness with an extreme degree of malabsorption, foul-smelling diarrheal stools, skeletal disorders, bleeding phenomena, and symptoms of hypocalcemia. There are no pathognomonic physical signs in this disease. There may be all degrees of malnutrition, as evidenced by muscle wasting and edema (Fig. 1). Hypotension and abdominal bloating are very common. Occasionally, there are clubbing of the fingers and pigmentation similar to that of Addison's disease. Signs and symptoms of celiac disease and their pathophysiologic bases are noted in Table 2.

Roentgenography of the small bowel gives findings that are characteristic but not specific. Frequently the only change is an altered pattern with some dilatation of proximal loops of small bowel and minimal coarsening of the jejunal folds. More severe impairment is manifested by marked dilatation of small bowel segments and clumping of the barium meal, with a waxy cast appearance of bowel segments (the *"moulage"* sign) (Fig. 3). As mentioned previously, the routine laboratory studies used in establishing the presence of the malabsorption syndrome are not specific.

Better techniques in diagnosis of adult celiac disease are measurement of d-xylose absorption and study of jejunal histology. Indeed, the diagnosis is untenable unless total or nearly total villous atrophy is found. Vitamin B$_{12}$ absorption is usually normal, but may be depressed if disease is extensive, involving the ileum. Other interesting findings, aside from those in Table 2, include frequent elevation of serum IgA and depression of IgM, along with reduced numbers of IgA-containing plasma cells in the biopsy.

A *trial of dietotherapy* may be important diagnostically in these patients. That the vast majority of adult celiac disease patients will respond favorably to an adequate gluten-free diet has been well established, and no other condition will respond so dramatically or so completely. Although clinical remission well within two months of institution of this therapy is the rule, nevertheless some patients may require six to twelve months or even longer.

Treatment of Celiac Disease. The basis for the use of the gluten-free diet in adult celiac disease lay in observations of its beneficial effects (in children initially) in celiac syndrome. Laboratory as well as clinical data strongly indicated that these patients cannot tolerate cereals with high gluten content. Thus when wheat, rye, oats, and barley are eliminated from the diet, diarrhea and steatorrhea cease, appetite improves, and rapid weight gain ensues. (Conversely, the introduction of gluten or gliadin into a histologically normal segment of small bowel causes mucosal inflammation with villous atrophy within 12 hours, associated with diarrhea and steatorrhea.)

The gluten-free diet excludes all cereal grains except rice and corn. To follow this diet, all labels must be carefully scrutinized to eliminate completely products that contain wheat, rye, barley, and oats as "fillers" (ice cream, salad dressings, canned foods, condiments, candy, etc.). As substitutes for the usual grains, rice, corn, and soy flours may be used. Recently, a wheat starch flour (Cellu Products Company) has become available. Beer and ale must be avoided, because they contain cereal residues; however, whiskies can be used, because the offending agent is not contained in the distillate. All other foods, except milk and milk products if they cause symptoms owing to lactase deficiency, are permitted, including fats. In general, the diet should be well balanced and high in protein. The complete diet is available in standard nutrition texts.

A substantial majority of the patients with adult celiac disease have responded to this diet, showing symptomatic improvement within a few days or a week, although a rare patient may require as long as 12 months. Weight gain has been so striking that patients have voluntarily restricted their caloric intake. The fact that a complete clinical remission with return to normal of pertinent blood components can be obtained in the majority of cases is significant, because previous treatment programs were usually only incompletely effective (Fig. 7). Follow-up biopsies demonstrate return to normal of mucosal histology in 50 per cent of patients who maintain that they adhere strictly to their diet, and marked improvement in most others. Complete restoration of villi and of the columnar epithelium in one patient is shown in Figure 4. Repeated biopsies in a minority of patients, however, reveal little or no improvement. It is difficult to ascertain whether they are ingesting some gluten; the physician should, however, also suspect other diseases which are associated with non-gluten-sensitive villous atrophy (*hypogammaglobulinemia,* particularly with *Giardia lamblia; lymphoma; dermatitis herpetiformis; collagenous sprue; Whipple's disease;* and *diffuse non-granulomatous ileojejunitis*). Absorption of d-xylose returns to normal, as does urinary excretion of 5-hydroxy-indolacetic acid, within a few weeks of elimination of gluten. Steatorrhea diminishes remarkably in all instances, but fat absorption returns completely to normal only in those patients who carefully eliminate all gluten.

Corticosteroids have been shown to produce significant improvement in adult celiac disease without entirely correcting the steatorrhea or biochemical abnor-

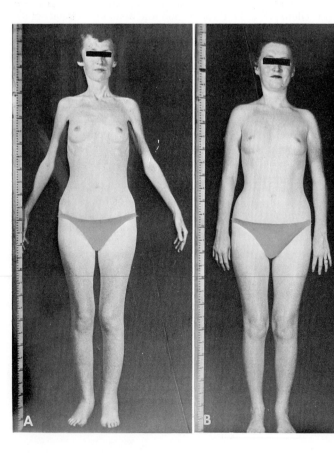

Figure 7. Appearance of patient (M. S.) with adult celiac disease. *A,* Before treatment. Note wasting and edema. *B,* Six weeks after elimination of gluten from the diet.

malities. These agents should be used for long-term therapy only in cases refractory to the gluten-free diet, for impaired protein metabolism and osteoporosis are troublesome features in this chronic condition.

Occasionally, a patient with adult celiac disease is critically ill, with severe diarrhea, wasting and anorexia, and serious protein and electrolyte depletion. There may also be bleeding, tetany, and edema. This situation demands a rigorous therapeutic regimen, employing intravenous vitamin K and calcium as well as infusions of salt-poor albumin (Table 5). It is in this clinical situation that corticosteroids may be lifesaving by greatly stimulating the appetite and perhaps by increasing absorption. Initially, corticotrophin, 30 units, should be given intravenously over an eight-hour period daily. After 10 to 14 days, either prednisolone or prednisone, 60 mg a day, may be substituted. Simultaneously, a gluten-free diet should be offered, and, as the patient's condition improves, drug therapy should be discontinued by gradual reduction in dosage over three to four weeks. These patients should remain on such dietotherapy permanently. Supplements (vitamin D and K, calcium, iron, folic acid, B-soluble vitamins, and vitamin B_{12}) are gradually withdrawn as clinical and chemical improvement proceeds; the program is set by results of reported essential laboratory determinations and personal observations.

Special Considerations and Complications of Adult Celiac Disease. LYMPHOMA AND CARCINOMA. The incidence of primary small bowel lymphoma and carcinoma in patients with adult celiac disease is high, about 13 per cent in a large collected series, with lymphoma contributing 10 per cent. Abdominal pain, weight loss, bleeding, obstruction, and perforation are the cardinal clinical features of this fatal complication. It is believed that lymphoma is more common in those not treated with a gluten-free diet. Relapse in those who have responded, associated with suggestive symptoms, should alert one to the possibility.

SMALL BOWEL ULCERATION. Nonmalignant ulcers of the jejunum and ileum may complicate celiac disease, and are manifested by exacerbation of severe diarrhea, abdominal pain, fever, and severe hypoproteinemia secondary to protein-losing enteropathy (see below). Perforation, bleeding, and/or obstruction are late manifestations.

NEUROLOGIC COMPLICATIONS. A syndrome similar to subacute combined degeneration of the spinal cord is noted early in celiac disease, despite remission with a gluten-free diet and no vitamin B_{12} deficiency (see Ch. 404 to 411 and Ch. 731).

CELIAC DISEASE AND THE SKIN. *Dermatitis herpetiformis* may be associated with patchy villous atrophy of the duodenum and upper jejunum; this abnormality does not extend beyond the proximal foot or so of the small gut, perhaps explaining why malabsorption in these patients is mild or even absent. Response to a gluten-free diet is poor, and instillation of gluten into the gut causes no inflammatory response as it does in gluten enteropathy. Partial and total villous atrophy have also been noted in *rosacea, atopic dermatitis,* and *psoriasis,* associated with varying degrees of steatorrhea and occasionally a dramatic response to a gluten-free diet. Conversely, a variety of skin disorders aside from hyperkeratosis have been reported in celiac disease, including *neurodermatitis* and *lichen planus.*

A rare patient with adult celiac disease who does not respond entirely to the diet may also have *pancreatic insufficiency* and will require oral pancreatic extract (Table 5).

COLLAGENOUS SPRUE. This disease resembles adult celiac disease in that it has the identical histologic picture, but it is not responsive to gluten elimination. Later, collagen is extensively deposited in the lamina propria beneath the epithelium.

HYPOSPLENISM. Recent studies indicate that an occasional patient will have splenic atrophy with hyposplenism and diminished immunologic response to antigens.

Whipple's Disease. In Whipple's disease, or lipophagic intestinal granulomatosis (intestinal "lipodystrophy"), there is a heavy infiltration of the intestinal wall and lymphatics by macrophages filled with glycoprotein. It is a generalized disease with steatorrhea as its principal feature, and it occurs predominantly in males in the fourth to seventh decades.

It may be difficult to differentiate this entity from other serious to fatal causes of malabsorption, particularly *lymphoma* and *tuberculosis.* Several manifestations such as polyserositis and postprandial pain are seen in all three diseases. However, nondeforming arthritis is most characteristic of Whipple's disease and is frequently the initial complaint. When gastrointestinal symptoms occur, the disease usually progresses rapidly with marked diarrhea, weight loss, weakness, and symptoms of anemia and deficiencies of fat- and water-soluble vitamins. Physical findings that suggest this disorder include lymphadenopathy, found in 40 per cent of the patients, and the various manifestations of polyserositis. Fever may be noted in about one third of the patients. Indefinite plastic or doughy abdominal masses have been described in approximately one quarter of the patients. The most consistent findings in the routine laboratory studies are anemia and an increased sedimentation rate; eosinophilia is occasionally present. Classically, steatorrhea is severe, with d-xylose absorption depressed and thickened folds. The roentgenographic findings in the small bowel are nonspecific, usually showing a "sprue-like pattern."

The diagnosis of Whipple's disease can be verified either by peripheral lymph node biopsy or, when this is normal, by biopsy of a mesenteric lymph node at laparotomy. Diagnosis may be established by identification of macrophages containing periodic acid–Schiff positive material in jejunal biopsy specimens obtained perorally (Fig. 6). Patchy villous atrophy may also be noted; thus identification of the engorged macrophages is crucial. Electron microscopic studies have revealed bacilliform bodies in and near these macrophages that may be infectious agents. Recent studies suggest that a pleomorphic organism is involved. Infiltration of the lamina propria also causes enlargement of villi and thickening of the submucosa.

Treatment of Whipple's Disease. Antimicrobial drugs by mouth are effective in treating Whipple's disease. Indeed, present information indicates that continuous treatment with penicillin G, 0.25 gram four times daily, or broad-spectrum antimicrobials, tetracycline or ampicillin, always brings about remission. The dose of tetracycline or ampicillin is 1.0 gram daily. The duration of therapy with antimicrobials is determined by the clinical response. Present data indicate that such treatment should be maintained indefinitely; otherwise, symptoms may return. Histologic as well as clinical improvement is noted after a period of weeks to months, with loss of diarrhea, reappearance of appetite, and tremendous gain of weight. The PAS-positive material slowly disappears from the mucosa, and the bacilliform bodies are no longer visible on electron microscopy. When remission has been sustained for nine months to one year, antimicrobial agents may be given intermittently, i.e., every other day or for three consecutive days each week (Table 5).

The symptoms of Whipple's disease may respond to corticosteroid therapy, as do those of other diseases characterized by arthritis and polyserositis, but the over-all result of such treatment is not satisfactory. Present evidence strongly indicates that only 40 per cent of patients achieve remission of the disease for two to six months while receiving corticotrophin or corticosteroids, and, in the majority, the disease relapses on cessation of such therapy. Many patients, particularly those whose illness is in a terminal phase, do not respond at all. The desperately ill patient should be given both corticotrophin intravenously, 40 units daily, *and* parenteral antimicrobial agents until the improvement of the patient permits withdrawal of the former agent.

Nongranulomatous Ileojejunitis. Steatorrhea and malabsorption may result not only from the complications of granulomatous enteritis (*strictures, fistulas,* or *massive resections*) (see Ch. 650), but also from nongranulomatous involvement of a large segment of the small intestine, particularly the jejunum. The small intestine is diffusely inflamed; mesenteric nodes are slightly enlarged, and serosal lymphatics are dilated. Although the mucosa is heavily infiltrated with inflammatory cells and has patchy ulcerations, the wall is not thickened as in Crohn's disease, nor are there strictures or fistulas.

The onset of this latter illness is abrupt, and signs and symptoms of malabsorption may predominate in a matter of one to two weeks. A daily remittent fever (39 to 40.5° C), abdominal cramping pain, usually periumbilical, and frequent watery stools are common complaints. Splenomegaly, occurring in 20 per cent of these patients with fever, may suggest an initial diagnosis of abdominal lymphoma. Usually, diffuse inflammatory changes are noted in roentgenograms of the small bowel. Stenotic segments and fistulas are not usually seen. The small bowel pattern may be indistinguishable from that of a wide variety of conditions associated with the malabsorption syndrome. One laboratory finding of help in the differential diagnosis is elevation of the leukocyte count, often with a substantial increase in the percentage of nonsegmented polymorphonuclear cells. Diagnosis may also be facilitated by a previous misdiagnosis of appendicitis. Often, however, diagnosis is made either by the response to treatment or by surgical exploration (see Ch. 650).

Treatment of Nongranulomatous Ileojejunitis. In diffuse ileojejunitis, corticosteroids may have a dramatic effect upon the clinical symptoms, including those that are due to malabsorption. Steatorrhea will diminish or cease; serum calcium, carotene, and plasma prothrombin concentration will return to normal. Serum albumin, often severely depressed to levels of 1.0 to 2.0 grams per 100 ml by "weeping" of serum protein into a large segment of inflamed gut, so-called protein-losing enteropathy (see below), likewise rises as the inflammation subsides. These improvements, as indicated by laboratory tests, accompany the disappearance of fever as well

as the increase in appetite, weight, and strength. Although such a therapeutic result is most salutary, it may not, unfortunately, be permanent. Recurrence is frequent, with progress of the disease in localized areas.

The consensus is that such patients, often acutely ill with fever and diarrhea, respond best to intravenous corticotrophin, 40 units daily, given over an eight-hour period for 10 to 14 days. The oral corticosteroid preparations are used after corticotrophin in the more serious cases and may be the principal therapeutic agents throughout the course of the less severe cases. The initial dose range in either instance is 40 to 60 mg of prednisone or prednisolone daily. The dose is gradually tapered over a week or longer to a maintenance level of 10 to 30 mg daily. The day-to-day clinical response best regulates the dose of drug at this stage of treatment. Broad-spectrum antimicrobials are not useful except in the presence of septic complications. Unfortunately, some of these patients have a relentless, refractory course and die of bowel perforation or intercurrent sepsis in two to three months, and the long-range outlook for permanent remission of this disease in those who initially respond is likewise not good.

Allergic and Eosinophilic Gastroenteritis. Increasingly, patients are seen with malabsorption, varying degrees of gastrointestinal bleeding, and protein-losing enteropathy; their small gut mucosa is infiltrated by eosinophils and is edematous but shows no vasculitis. The involvement in many instances is principally mucosal. In some patients, in whom the stomach is also involved, the deeper layers of the gut, including serosa, are infiltrated. In a minority of instances in adults, the disease is a response to a known allergen such as milk protein, meat, or even fruit. Even in the absence of an offending agent, these patients have histories of hay fever, eczema, and asthma, particularly in childhood, or other food idiosyncrasies.

The symptoms — cramping pain, diarrhea, weight loss, nausea, fever, and a degree of malabsorption — are related to the location and extent of the disease in the small bowel. Fat loss in stool is about 15 to 20 grams per day. If the stomach is also involved, epigastric pain, vomiting, and bleeding are common. Frequently, the patients have allergies, particularly hay fever and asthma, and many have urticaria as well as diarrhea after eating certain foods (milk, egg, cereal, meat). Marked eosinophilia is a constant finding and is greater than 20 per cent. The disease tends to be chronic with recurrent symptoms. Roentgenographic examination often reveals a nonspecific "malabsorption pattern" with coarsened folds of jejunum. Occasionally, narrowed segments may be seen. Hypoproteinemia caused by protein-losing enteropathy may be severe and may be associated with marked edema and ascites. Iron deficiency anemia resulting from occult gastrointestinal bleeding is common in children. Disease of the stomach, particularly antral, may cause hematemesis.

Another form of this disease is so-called *eosinophilic granuloma,* in which the process consists of localized nodular or pedunculated infiltrative eosinophilic lesions (involving the submucosa and muscle layer) without allergy or peripheral eosinophilia. *Eosinophilic gastroenteritis* may also involve the serosa of the bowel as well as peritoneum, with ascites the predominant manifestation.

Treatment of Eosinophilic Gastroenteritis. Effective therapy consists of withdrawal of offending foods, particularly milk for children. In more ill patients, prednisone, 20 to 40 mg daily orally with gradual tapering to a low maintenance dose, will bring remission of major symptoms and decrease of eosinophilia. With remission, edema and infiltrate of the jejunal mucosa also disappear in patients with no involvement of deeper layers. In patients with brisk bleeding from the stomach, surgery may have to be performed. Laparotomy, for severe pain or bleeding resulting from transmural small bowel disease, reveals thickened loops of jejunum, involved antrum, and enlarged mesenteric nodes. Biopsy differentiates this disease from granulomatous enteritis and tuberculosis. In the majority of patients the clinical picture, typical history, eosinophilia, obvious allergies, and response to treatment are sufficient to exclude *acute diffuse nongranulomatous ileojejunitis, lymphoma,* and *celiac disease.* Transoral jejunal biopsy will also be helpful.

Amyloidosis. Either the primary or the secondary form of the disorder may affect the gastrointestinal tract and cause malabsorption. Diffuse crampy pain and ileus are the most frequent abdominal symptoms. In the primary form of the disease, cardiac failure, macroglossia, and renal disease may be noted, but the Congo red test is negative. Roentgenographically, amyloidosis is characterized by dilated loops of bowel, occasionally with thickening of the jejuno-ileum and slow passage of the barium meal through the intestines. The diagnosis is made by tissue study. Gingival or tongue biopsies are frequently positive in *primary amyloidosis,* particularly when the disease is associated with myelomatosis; liver biopsy, although hazardous, may also establish the diagnosis. Biopsy of the liver or bowel at laparotomy may be necessary in some instances. Diagnosis may also be made from specimens of jejunal mucosa obtained by transoral suction biopsy.

In *secondary amyloidosis,* the presence of a chronic inflammatory illness and hepatosplenomegaly suggests the diagnosis. Congo red tests may show greater than 90 per cent retention of the injected material by the tissues.

Treatment is supportive, because the disease is too extensive for resection. If it is secondary to chronic infection or granulomatous disease, successful management of the underlying disorder may be helpful, although it is unlikely.

Small Bowel Ischemia. Chronic ischemia of the small bowel, caused by atherosclerosis of the celiac, superior, and inferior mesenteric arteries, may occasionally cause malabsorption, presumably because of impairment of mucosal cell function. No histologic damage, however, has been demonstrated in such instances (see Ch. 660).

The blood supply to the small intestine is occasionally severely compromised in patients with so-called collagen vascular disease, particularly *periarteritis nodosa* and *systemic lupus erythematosus.* Although malabsorption syndrome has been reported in these diseases, the documentation is unclear; *Degos' disease,* characterized by necrotic skin lesions and vasculitis of the small gut, may also cause malabsorption, although the far more serious and common clinical manifestation is infarction of the gut. A necrotizing type of arteriolitis leading to ulceration and perforation of the small gut is a serious form of vascular complication of the collagen vascular diseases.

Crohn's Disease. This important disease of the small bowel may cause malabsorption in a number of ways: by extensive damage to the mucosa; by multiple strictures (bacterial overgrowth); by fistulas between small bowel

and colon (bacterial overgrowth); or by necessitating ileectomy (defective solubilization and loss of absorptive surface) or massive resection (inadequate surface). Bacterial overgrowth and defective solubilization are discussed in Category 1 above; inadequate surface, a portion of Category 2, is discussed below. The clinical picture of diffuse Crohn's disease of the small intestine is discussed in Ch. 650. It is sufficient here to emphasize that an important part of this picture is the signs and symptoms of malabsorption, the range and severity of which are proportional to the extent (length of bowel involved), to severity (i.e., complications) of the disease, and to the type and extent of surgery which may have been performed.

Inadequate Surface

Most absorption takes place in the duodenum and first 90 cm of the jejunum. Clinical studies of patients who have had extensive resection of the small intestine indicate that survival is now reasonably certain with 90 to 120 cm of remaining normal small bowel, and is possible with shorter segments provided caloric intake is adequate. This length of jejunum is sufficient for normal carbohydrate absorption and, in most instances, for maintenance of positive nitrogen balance. The postoperative course is influenced by the site of resection—jejunum or ileum. Thus vitamin B_{12} absorption will be subnormal if a large length of ileum has been removed; conversely, sacrifice of a corresponding amount of jejunum will more seriously impair absorption of fat, calcium, and folic acid.

The three common causes for extensive resection of large segments of the small intestine are (1) *recurrent regional enteritis,* (2) *mesenteric vascular disease,* particularly thrombosis of the superior mesenteric artery, and (3) *malignant processes* involving the blood supply of the small bowel.

Treatment. Inadvertent surgical *jejunocolostomies* or *gastroileostomies,* which sidetrack large segments of small intestine, must be corrected surgically as soon as possible.

The patient who has had an *extensive resection of the small intestine,* nearly always right colon, ileum, and part of distal jejunum, requires continuous and meticulous medical care. For weeks or even for one or two months, nutrition may adequately be maintained by intravenous hyperalimentation which employs fluids containing adequate calories, protein, minerals, and vitamins. As little as 2 liters daily may satisfy nutritional requirements for an adult (Table 5). Certain complications may attend such therapy, and the physician must be aware of them. They are due to necessity for catheterizing the subclavian vein (sepsis, thrombosis, hemoor pneumothorax). Hyperosmolar, hyperglycemic dehydration, or hypophosphatemia may also ensue. The patient's fluid and electrolyte balance must, of course, be meticulously monitored on a daily basis.

Oral feedings should be initiated as soon as possible, preferably containing substances which require minimal hydrolysis and are easily absorbed. Such preparations as Vivonex have been useful, because they contain simple sugars and amino acids; however, as with all hypertonic preparations, diarrhea may be aggravated.

For periods of up to 12 months postoperatively, the remaining segment of intestine will show progressive improvement in absorptive capacity, associated with elongation and dilatation. It is important to remember that, since the amount of fat absorbed is proportional to the amount presented to the absorbing surface, the maximal intake of fat that does not cause symptoms is desirable. Regardless of which segment or its part—ileum or jejunum—remains, the diet should be high in protein, and frequent feeding (six times daily) should be recommended and may consist in part of protein and amino acids (Table 5). Vitamins A, D, and K and the B-complex vitamins as well as calcium, iron, and magnesium may be given orally, except in those instances in which adequate replacement is possible only by the parenteral route (Table 5). In general, a high protein intake will adequately maintain the serum albumin; however, occasionally, infusions of salt-poor albumin must be given.

Supplementation of the diet by medium-chain triglycerides (see above; Table 5) has been of distinct benefit to patients with massive small bowel resection, diminishing diarrhea and helping to stabilize weight by improving fat absorption; however, it must be noted that weight gain attributable principally to medium-chain triglycerides in these patients is slight. Drugs that decrease intestinal motility, such as diphenoxylate hydrochloride (5.0 mg twice or three times daily), anticholinergics (propantheline, 15 to 30 mg twice to three times daily), and/or small doses of tincture of opium (10 drops twice to three times daily) may help reduce diarrhea (Table 5).

Category 3: Lymphatic Obstruction

Lymphoma. The malabsorption syndrome secondary to lymphoma of the small bowel and mesentery may be clinically and roentgenographically identical to the classic picture of adult celiac disease. Several features, however, suggest the correct diagnosis. The symptoms of this disease are likely to be of much shorter duration and to include crampy abdominal pain and fever. Lymphadenopathy and hepatosplenomegaly do not appear until late in the course. Although intramural small bowel masses may be present in some cases, the roentgenographic study of the intestine generally does not reveal them. Unexpectedly, the usual therapeutic measures, such as diet, fat-soluble vitamins, and vitamin B_{12}, may lead to a temporary clinical and laboratory remission. The incidence of malabsorption syndrome caused by small bowel lymphoma is difficult to ascertain. It appears that as many as 10 per cent of patients with adult celiac disease may develop lymphoma. Although lymphatic obstruction is important in the pathophysiology of steatorrhea in lymphoma, widespread disease of the intestine will also contribute significantly to the malabsorption.

The diagnosis is usually established by laparotomy necessitated by some complication of the underlying disease, such as bleeding, perforation, or obstruction. In some patients, the diagnosis may be made from jejunal tissue obtained by peroral biopsy. The average duration of this illness after onset of symptoms is 13 months, despite resection and roentgen therapy.

Primary intestinal lymphoma, with malabsorption, may be a chronic condition in certain parts of the world, particularly in the Middle East in young Arabs and Sephardic Jews, and in Mexico. The clinical picture strongly resembles adult celiac disease in terms of chronicity and jejunal villous atrophy; however, most of these patients do not respond to elimination of gluten, and peroral biopsies will show evidence of lymphoma in the majority. In contrast to primary lymphoma of the small bowel with malabsorption in North America and Europe, which carries a prognosis of death one to two years after onset of symptoms (despite surgery, radiation, and chemotherapy), the young Middle Easterners may live with their disease for as long as ten years. Lymphoma also complicates *α-chain disease* in which heavy chains of IgA are produced excessively.

Treatment. Treatment of lymphoma of the small bowel and mesentery includes local resections as well as radiotherapy, and possibly therapy with chlorambucil and steroids or cyclophosphamide when the disease is disseminated. Despite this program, the course is frequently progressive, the average duration of life after onset of symptoms being one to two years. In these patients, continuous supportive therapy (high caloric diet, iron, vitamins, calcium, as needed) is frequently helpful and may result in successful maintenance of the patient's activity over a period of months. Indeed, these patients have also improved when given low-fat diets with vitamin and mineral supplementation.

Intestinal Tuberculosis and Tuberculous Lymphadenitis. Tuberculosis may result in a malabsorption syndrome through involvement of the mesenteric lymph nodes, although in some cases there may be associated disease of the intestinal wall. It is extremely rare in the United States, and it occurs almost always in persons with a history of severe pulmonary or lymph node tuberculosis.

Fever, palpable abdominal masses, a positive tuberculin skin test, evidence of old or recent disease on chest roentgenography, and calcification of mesenteric and pelvic lymph nodes on flat film all suggest the diagnosis, which may be confirmed by culture of sputum or gastric juice. Rarely, stool culture may be useful, but only if the other secretions are demonstrably free of tubercle bacilli. Roentgenographic studies, both barium enema and small bowel series, are particularly helpful when there is also deformity of the ileocecal segment resulting from hyperplastic lesions. Rarely, there may be diffuse small bowel abnormalities, such as coarsening of the folds, stricture formation, and edema, which suggest ileojejunitis. At times, exploratory laparotomy with node or bowel biopsy is necessary for diagnosis (see Ch. 234 and 240).

Treatment. Tuberculous involvement of the mesenteric lymph nodes should be treated by chemotherapy, as set forth in Ch. 240. A high caloric diet should be employed with calcium and vitamins as indicated. When there is an associated hyperplastic ileocecal tuberculosis with partial obstruction, appropriate local resection may be necessary.

Lymphangiectasia. In addition to the diseases just discussed, several other conditions may rarely cause the malabsorption syndrome by lymphatic blockade. These include *primary lymphangiectasia,* a genetically determined disease characterized by mild to moderate diarrhea, mild steatorrhea, and protein-losing enteropathy (see below), certain *protozoan diseases* (see Category 4), *the reticuloendothelioses, metastatic tumor* to the mesenteric nodes, and *neoplastic invasion of the main lymphatic channels* in the retroperitoneal tissues.

Category 4: Infection

Tropical Sprue. Tropical sprue can be differentiated from adult celiac disease. The disease occurs primarily in persons residing in certain areas of the Far East, India, and the Caribbean. Both nutritional deficiencies and bacterial contamination of the small gut appear to play causative roles. This disease responds to administration of broad-spectrum antimicrobial drugs, suggesting, but not proving, that infection is responsible. Histologic changes suggestive of tropical sprue may be noted in individuals newly arrived in the tropics; such changes may often be associated with an acute enteritis and a variable degree of malabsorption. Although the remarkable clinical improvement that follows folic acid therapy strongly suggests a vitamin deficiency, tropical sprue is not seen in some areas of the world where the population has a marginal or even inadequate diet; conversely, it has been noted in people with adequately "balanced" diets.

Clinically, three phases of the disease have been described. In the initial phase the patient complains only of fatigue, asthenia, and bulky stools. After weeks to months, the second phase of malnutrition is noted. Weight loss is prominent. Glossitis, stomatitis, cheilosis, and hyperkeratosis are observed in varying degrees. Moderate prothrombin depletion is present but is rarely associated with bleeding. Manifestations of impaired calcium absorption are not usually clinically apparent in patients with tropical sprue, in contrast to those with adult celiac disease. Iron deficiency anemia follows depletion of iron stores. Hypoalbuminemia with edema may be a late manifestation of this disease. Some laboratory criteria of impaired absorption are present (Table 4). The third stage is characterized by anemia and megaloblastosis and the symptoms of full-blown severe malabsorption described earlier in this section, although diarrhea may not be prominent. However, the clinical spectrum is wide—steatorrhea may be minimal, glossitis absent, and megaloblastosis inconstant. This inconsistent picture may indicate various causes.

Laboratory investigation reveals mainly steatorrhea and megaloblastic anemia. Small bowel roentgenographic findings and histologic changes of the jejunum are the same as those in adult celiac disease except that *total villous atrophy* is not as commonly encountered in tropical sprue. In many tropical areas, however, asymptomatic individuals often have histologic abnormalities suggestive of tropical sprue, making tissue diagnosis very difficult. Other routine laboratory studies, including d-xylose absorption, are also comparable in the two diseases. The gluten-free diet is ineffective.

Treatment for Tropical Sprue. The therapy for this disease is very effective. The similarity of tropical sprue to pernicious anemia, particularly in its hematologic aspects, prompted the use of liver extract, folic acid, and vitamin B_{12}, and remissions have also been noted with antimicrobial drugs, a low-fat, high-protein diet, and migration to a temperate climate. Administration of a broad-spectrum antimicrobial (tetracycline, 1.0 gram daily by mouth) along with 10 mg of folic acid daily is the best treatment and frequently brings remission, with disappearance of diarrhea and glossitis and gain in appetite and weight. However, response may be slow in some patients, and normal absorption and jejunal histology may not be noted for six months or longer. Parenteral vitamin B_{12} should be given for two months (Table 5). For those not responding completely within six months of treatment with antimicrobials and folic acid, therapy should be continued for as long as absorption continues to improve.

When remission has been achieved, 5.0 mg of folic acid daily is the maintenance therapy. In the presence of achlorhydria, addition of vitamin B_{12} to the regimen should be considered unless absorption of ^{60}Co B_{12} is normal (Table 5). If absorption of vitamin B_{12} remains subnormal after remission, monthly injections should be given.

Acute Infectious Enteritis. Bacterial and viral infections such as Salmonella, enteropathic *E. coli,* and a host of viruses may cause transient but severe malabsorption. Patients with this condition have steatorrhea and may have diminished xylose absorption. The serum calcium as well as the plasma prothrombin concentration may be depressed. Serum proteins may fall rapidly, largely owing to abnormal rate of loss into the inflamed gut. With recovery, absorption returns to normal.

Treatment. These patients may recover without specific antimicrobial therapy, provided that fluids and electrolytes have been rapidly and adequately replaced. Such infections are apt to attack patients who travel to tropical countries or are debilitated, or who have had abdominal surgery, particularly those also given broad-spectrum antimicrobials. Patients severely ill with salmonellosis (septicemia) may require treatment with broad-spectrum antimicrobials (see Ch. 213). The keystone of therapy for all infectious enteritis is rapid and complete replacement of fluid and electrolytes. Acidosis, hypokalemia, and hyponatremia are often severe (see Ch. 214).

Protozoan and Helminthic Diseases. Protozoan or helminthic diseases are a common cause of malabsorption in many tropical areas and are particularly associated with malnutrition. Because tropical sprue is also endemic in many of these countries, it is often difficult to assign a cause for malabsorption, especially in view of the histologic changes (blunting of villi, cellular infiltration of the lamina propria) which are present in many asymptomatic individuals who are malnourished with or without parasites. Some of these patients with mild to moderate steatorrhea (10 to 15 grams per 24 hours), however, have malabsorption syndrome caused by *hookworm, strongyloidiasis, Capillaria philippensis, coccidiosis,* and *giardiasis.* Parasites must be isolated and identified, and response to therapy, clinically, biochemically, and histologically, must be forthcoming before definite etiologic attribution of the malabsorption and malnutrition to parasitic infection can be made.

Patients with *Giardia lamblia* infection of the small bowel may suffer from malabsorption, particularly individuals with *subtotal gastrectomy; hypogammaglobulinemia* often associated with so-called "nodular lymphoid hyperplasia"; *tropical sprue;* or *severe malnutrition,* particularly in children. Thus the role played by the parasite is not completely clear despite demonstration of its invasion of the mucosa and report of some improvement in absorption after treatment with quinacrine (0.1 gram three times daily for one week). Recent evidence indicates that villous atrophy which is associated with the giardiasis of hypogammaglobulinemia is reversed with effective therapy for the parasite (see below, Category 6). In all doubtful cases it is wise to treat the patient (Table 5).

Category 5: Multiple Defects

Subtotal Gastrectomy. Steatorrhea and malabsorption after subtotal gastrectomy and gastrojejunostomy (Billroth II) or total gastrectomy are attributable to (1) loss of reservoir function with rapid emptying and dispersion of food through the small intestine, thereby diluting the normal output of pancreatic enzymes; or (2) stasis with bacterial contamination of the afferent loop of a Billroth II gastrojejunostomy. Deficiency of vitamin B_{12} will inevitably follow total gastrectomy, the lag period being determined by the liver store of the vitamin.

Treatment. Administration of ox bile extract is not helpful, probably because of its high content of unconjugated salts. As yet no preparation of pure conjugated bile salts is available for treatment. Pancreatic extracts may be tried in selected cases, although when given alone they have not produced consistent improvement. However, when pancreatic extract is combined with broad-spectrum antimicrobials (ampicillin or tetracycline, 1.0 gram per day in divided dosage, or lincomycin, 1.0 to 2.0 grams per day), in the treatment of patients after Billroth II operations, fat absorption may improve. These results indicate that in some patients bacterial contamination—probably originating in the afferent loop—plays an important etiologic role in the malabsorption syndrome that follows this procedure. Conversion of Billroth II to Billroth I has been reported to reduce steatorrhea in some patients.

Patients who have undergone Billroth II procedures should receive a high-calorie diet rich in protein, with frequent feedings containing as much fat as can be tolerated, in order to maintain good nutrition. After a total gastrectomy, 30 to 100 μg of vitamin B_{12} intramuscularly must be given monthly. Calcium, iron, and the fat-soluble vitamins may be added to this regimen as needed or when diarrhea or steatorrhea is so severe that deficient absorption of these substances may be anticipated (Table 5).

Distal Ileal Resection, Disease, or Bypass. As noted, resection, often required for granulomatous disease or vascular insufficiency, ileal bypass for obesity, or extensive ileal disease causes deficiencies of vitamin B_{12} and bile salts. Malabsorption is also in part due to loss of the reserve capacity of the ileum for absorbing fat, a function which would be carried on if proximal fat absorption were impaired by deficiency of bile salts.

Vitamin B_{12} should be replaced parenterally, as in pernicious anemia. If the megaloblastic anemia that appears does not respond entirely to vitamin B_{12}, folic acid should be added to the regimen (Table 5).

Treatment with cholestyramine, a bile salt–binding resin, is indicated and will often ameliorate the diarrhea caused by the effect of unabsorbed bile salts upon the colon. However, it may increase steatorrhea by further diminishing the bile salt pool. No replacement therapy for the bile salt deficiency is currently available clinically. Steatorrhea will be reduced, however, by feeding medium-chain triglycerides in place of dietary lipid (Table 5). Studies of the effect of potent pancreatic extracts and/or antimicrobials (broad-spectrum) are not available.

Radiation Enteritis. A few patients who receive high dosage x-ray therapy to the abdomen will develop a malabsorption syndrome on the basis of radiation injury to the bowel. It is difficult to assess how much of the defect in absorption is attributable to arterial damage, mucosal inflammation, or atrophy. Since the reaction to injury is slow, symptoms do not appear for weeks to months after exposure. In the usual patient, villous damage, mucosal and submucosal edema, and cellular infiltration are the main features and repair follows. However, larger doses cause ulceration of the mucosa and

endarteritis of submucosal vessels with transmural necrosis, followed by scarring with strictures and permanent loss of function. Thus malabsorption is principally due to disease of the small bowel wall; however, in some instances stasis caused by obstruction (bacterial overgrowth) contributes, and in others lymphatic obstruction (and perhaps ileal dysfunction) may contribute. Fibrosis and stricture are occasional sequelae of severe reaction, causing obstruction, usually chronic. Jejunal biopsy may reveal patchy villous atrophy.

Category 6: Unexplained

Hypogammaglobulinemia. The role of intraluminal immunoglobulins, particularly IgA, in maintaining the structure and function of the intestinal tract is not known, because their antibacterial activity as antibodies is minimal. Patients with hypogammaglobulinemia may, however, have steatorrhea and diminished d-xylose absorption, but the precise incidence is not known. Although the number of cases so documented is small, it is steadily growing. Evidence at hand indicates that most (if not all) of these patients have a deficiency of both plasma IgA and IgG and of intestinal IgA. Some patients have only plasma IgA ("selective") deficiency. IgM may be increased in serum and intestine in patients with selective IgA deficiency. The intestinal histology in diffuse hypogammaglobulinemia reveals normal histology or patchy villous atrophy, but *plasma cells are absent* and lymphocytes are reduced in all cases. Occasionally, it shows so-called "nodular lymphoid hyperplasia," and rarely it causes a granulomatous lesion. A high percentage of these patients with malabsorption will have *Giardia lamblia* infestation of their intestinal fluid, and in some the organism invades the mucosa. This infection is often associated with either villous atrophy or nodular lymphoid hyperplasia and appears to be present in a high percentage of these patients with steatorrhea. Although anaerobic bacteria may be present in the upper small bowel, their role in the pathogenesis of the steatorrhea is not proved. Other abnormalities include splenomegaly and gastric atrophy.

Treatment. Of those with villous atrophy, a rare patient will have a good to excellent response to the gluten-free diet. Antimicrobial drugs and injections of gamma globulin appear to be ineffective. The key to successful management appears to be eradication of giardiasis with atabrine or metronidazole (Table 5). Symptoms remit, absorption improves (including d-xylose), and villi regenerate. As noted above, patients with *celiac disease* have normal or elevated serum IgA, depressed IgM (one third), and normal IgG levels and have reduced IgA plasma cells and increased IgG and IgM plasma cells in the lamina propria.

Metastatic Malignant Carcinoid Syndrome. The presenting symptoms of this disease may be those of malabsorption. Steatorrhea may be caused by an increased production of 5-hydroxytryptamine (serotonin), which markedly increases gastrointestinal motility and thus impairs absorption. Other explanations for diarrhea and steatorrhea in this disease include lymphatic obstruction of the mesentery of the small bowel by tumor and ileal dysfunction. Treatment is that used for carcinoid syndrome in general. Methysergide (8.0 to 12.0 mg per day, orally) and cyproheptadine (80 mg per day in divided doses) have been reported to decrease diarrhea in this disease. Small doses of tincture of opium, however, seem most effective for the diarrhea. Parachlorphenylalanine, which inhibits hydroxylation of tryptophan to 5-HTP, has been effective in controlling diarrhea; however, side effects may preclude its general use. (see Ch. 869.)

Hypoparathyroidism and Pseudohypoparathyroidism. The association of steatorrhea and deficient parathyroid function has been recently confirmed. The mechanism by which parathormone is involved in fat absorption or transport is unknown. Symptoms of malabsorption may be the earliest manifestation of deficient parathyroid function. With vitamin D_2 therapy, diarrhea decreases, steatorrhea disappears, serum carotene and albumin levels rise, vitamin B_{12} absorption increases, and the roentgenographic appearance of the small bowel becomes normal. Diagnosis of hypoparathyroidism as a basis for malabsorption may be established by measuring hormone levels or by changes in urinary phosphate excretion after intravenous infusions of parathormone or calcium (see Ch. 839). Mild malabsorption (fecal fat about 10 grams per 24 hours) has been reported in pseudohypoparathyroidism. Parathormone in some way facilitates the effect of vitamin D upon calcium absorption by the intestinal tract. In pseudohypoparathyroidism the end organs, including the gut, are not responsive to parathormone. The effect of hypocalcemia per se upon intestinal absorption is not known.

Treatment. Administration of vitamin D and calcium will correct hypocalcemia and improve fat absorption as well as other manifestations of disease.

Diabetes Mellitus. Patients with longstanding diabetes mellitus may have severe diarrhea (see Ch. 637). Some with diarrhea will also have steatorrhea and malabsorption, and these patients are usually not well controlled by dietotherapy or insulin, or both, and a high percentage also have some evidence of neuropathy. In these patients, the intestinal difficulty may be due to involvement of the autonomic innervation of the small bowel, because they also have orthostatic hypotension, inability to perspire, and impotence. Possible changes in the microbial flora or mesenteric vascular insufficiency may also contribute to the malabsorptive state. Response to broad-spectrum antimicrobials supports the former hypothesis; however, careful bacteriologic studies of intestinal contents in a group of patients with diabetic neuropathy and diarrhea reveal that bacterial overgrowth is an uncommon cause for the steatorrhea of diabetic neuropathy. Although exocrine function is usually normal in diabetes, some patients have *pancreatic insufficiency* for which replacement therapy should also be given (Table 5) (see Ch. 646). Adrenal corticosteroids have been reported to benefit patients with this syndrome, but no satisfactory chemical documentation of such response has been presented. A disadvantage of such therapy would be the increased requirement for insulin. An increased incidence of *adult celiac disease* has also been reported in diabetics (see above).

Mastocytosis. Patients with overproduction of mast cells suffer not only from urticaria pigmentosa, but also from gastrointestinal symptoms. Perhaps the latter result from overproduction of histamine and perhaps of serotonin as well. Malabsorption is rare in these individuals. The lamina propria of the jejunal mucosa may or may not be infiltrated with mast cells; villi may be absent or stunted. Whether fat absorption is also impaired because of gastric hypersecretion or increased intestinal transit has not been determined.

Hyperthyroidism and Hypoadrenocorticism. Some patients with hyperthyroidism have steatorrhea. The pathogenesis is not understood. In one study of a group of patients with this disease, the possibility was raised that steatorrhea was due in part to excessive intake of fat in the diet (more than 120 grams per day). Successful therapy returns fat absorption to normal. Likewise, steatorrhea has been found in patients with Addison's disease in whom replacement therapy has corrected it.

Category 7: Drug-Induced Malabsorption

Some commonly used drugs may cause malabsorption. *Cholestyramine,* in doses of 12.0 or more grams per day, by binding bile salts renders them inactive in the process of fat solubilization and causes mild steatorrhea (7.0 to 15.0 grams of fat per day). *Colchicine* ingestion leads to mild malabsorption of fat (about 9.0 grams of fat per day), protein, and d-xylose by affecting epithelial cell replication and function. Certain *irritant laxatives,* presumably by markedly increasing transit, likewise may cause mild steatorrhea. *Neomycin,* frequently administered to patients with severe hepatic disease, causes steatorrhea, increased fecal loss of nitrogen, and impaired d-xylose absorption. The degree of malabsorption is dose related and may be noted with as little as 4.0 grams per day. It causes some blunting of villi and of their absorptive cells, reduces hydrolysis of fat, and precipitates bile salts. *Bacitracin, tetracycline, polymyxin,* and *kanamycin* may also cause malabsorption. Large doses (twice normal) of *p-aminosalicylic acid* lead to mild steatorrhea and decrease in absorption of d-xylose. *Phenindione,* an anticoagulant, may also cause steatorrhea. Anticonvulsants such as *diphenylhydantoin* in some way cause folic acid deficiency, as do *oral contraceptive* agents.

MALABSORPTION SYNDROME AND ENTERIC LOSS OF PROTEIN
(Protein-Losing Enteropathy)

Hypoalbuminemia without liver disease, inadequate protein intake, or albuminuria may be due to excessive loss of serum protein into the intestine. This loss has been noted in patients with mucosal ulceration of the stomach, small bowel, or colon; with mucosal disease without ulceration; or in lymphatic obstruction (Table 6). Intestinal lymphatic dilatation without obvious cause (lymphangiectasia, Fig. 8) is associated with abnormal enteric protein loss in some patients whose illness was previously termed "hypercatabolic hypoproteinemia." Many of these patients, regardless of the cause for plasma protein leakage, have some degree of malabsorption.

Edema or ascites, or both, secondary to hypoalbuminemia may overshadow enteric symptoms and, indeed, underlie presenting symptoms in patients with so-called *protein-losing enteropathy.* Most of these patients have specific diseases of the intestine. Thus the syndrome has been reported with gastric diseases such as *giant hypertrophic rugae* (Ménétrier's disease), *giant gastric ulcer, gastric cancer,* and *eosinophilic granuloma of the stomach.* A variety of inflammatory diseases of the small and large intestines are also associated with this syndrome: *granulomatous enteritis* and *enterocolitis; nongranulomatous ileojejunitis; acute infectious enteritis; ulcerative*

TABLE 6. Classification and Therapy of Diseases Associated with Enteric Loss of Plasma Protein

Disease	Therapy
A. Mucosal ulceration:	
Gastric carcinoma	
Gastric lymphoma	Surgical resection
Multiple gastric ulcers	
Colon cancer	
Granulomatous enteritis	
Diffuse nongranulomatous ileojejunitis	Corticosteroids
B. Mucosal disease without ulceration:	
Rugal hypertrophy (Menetrier's, etc.)	Resection, if local
Celiac disease	Gluten elimination
Tropical sprue	Antimicrobials; folic acid
Whipple's disease	Antimicrobials
Allergic gastroenteropathy	Elimination diet; steroids
Bacterial or parasitic enteritis	Antimicrobial drugs
Gastrocolic fistula	Resection
C. Lymphatic abnormalities:	
Capillaria philippensis	Thiabendazole
Primary lymphangiectasias	Low-fat diet or medium-chain triglycerides
Lymphenteric fistula	Resection
Lymphoma	Chemotherapy
Constrictive pericarditis	Pericardiectomy
Tricuspid valvular disease	Rx of heart failure

colitis; granuloma of the small bowel associated with *hypogammaglobulinemia, celiac disease, tropical sprue, lymphoma* of the small intestine, and *Whipple's disease;* and *lymphangiectasia* secondary to known causes such as *lymphoma* or *tuberculosis* or *Crohn's disease.*

Allergy to milk protein and, in rare cases, to cereals or even meat may underlie *protein-losing enteropathy* by affecting the small intestine. Biopsy is normal or shows mild infiltration of the lamina propria with eosinophils; the disorder usually begins in childhood; it is characterized by hypoproteinemia and edema; an iron deficiency anemia is common, as is diarrhea; eosinophilia is a permanent feature. This condition may well be a milder

form of *eosinophilic gastroenteritis* in which both protein-losing enteropathy and malabsorption may be more serious (see above). Infestation with a roundworm, *Capillaria philippensis,* has been described in the Philippines; it causes diarrhea, protein-losing enteropathy, and malabsorption, and proves fatal in two to four months unless vigorously treated (Table 6) (see Ch. 303).

Clinical Picture. As noted, the clinical picture may be dominated by signs and symptoms of hypoproteinemia. In most instances, the patient complains of some abdominal symptoms related to the underlying disease.

Diagnosis. The diagnosis of protein-losing enteropathy should be suspected in any patient with low serum albumin who has normal liver function and does not have an abnormal amount of protein in the urine. The abnormal loss may be confirmed by abnormal fecal excretion of ^{51}Cr after intravenous injection of ^{51}Cr albumin or by a rapid decay curve after intravenous ^{51}Cr chloride or ^{131}I-albumin.

Treatment (Table 6). Since therapy may be very successful, accurate diagnosis is extremely important. Resection of localized granuloma or ulcers of the stomach and bowel, or of localized giant gastric rugae, may lead to complete cessation of enteric protein loss. Patients with adult celiac disease and those with allergic gastroenteropathy who are sensitive to milk protein or other substances will respond to elimination of gluten or milk or other offending agents from the diet. Patients with intestinal lymphangiectasia of congenital origin respond to reduction of dietary fat to very low levels—5 grams or less—or to administration of medium-chain triglycerides in place of dietary fat. These regimens will usually reverse the abnormal protein loss in this disease, and may lessen it in any disease that obstructs lymphatics. Protein loss resulting from *acute, nongranulomatous ileojejunitis,* as well as *granulomatous enteritis* and *ulcerative colitis,* may disappear during therapy with corticosteroids, or, in the case of *viral enteritides,* with spontaneous recovery from the infection. *Acute bacterial enteritis* caused by Shigella or Salmonella, *Whipple's disease, enteric tuberculosis,* and instances of excessive protein loss associated with bacterial overgrowth in the small intestine *("blind loop syndrome")* all may respond to appropriate antimicrobial therapy. *Capillaria philippensis* is said to respond to thiabendazole, 25 mg per kilogram per day for 30 days (see Ch. 303). A similar effect has likewise been reported in enteric lymphoma after x-radiation and treatment with chlorambucil (Table 6).

Protein-losing enteropathy may be associated with *chronic constrictive pericarditis,* presumably caused by mediastinal lymphatic obstruction. Pericardiolysis or parietal pericardiectomy will alleviate or even completely reverse this enteric loss. Also, effective treatment of severe *right heart failure* may alleviate protein-losing enteropathy.

PROGNOSIS OF MALABSORPTION SYNDROME

The outlook for the patient with malabsorption syndrome depends upon both the nature of the underlying disease and the institution of appropriate therapy. (Proper treatment, of course, implies correct diagnosis.)

Specific therapy for patients with adult celiac disease (gluten-free diet) and effective agents for tropical sprue are available. Intelligent replacement therapy for those with deficient digestion (*gastrectomy, hepatobiliary dis-*

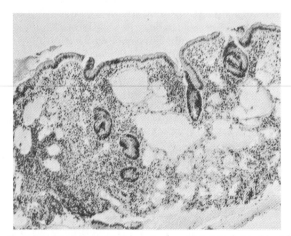

Figure 8. Jejunal biopsy demonstrating dilated lacteals of lymphangiectasia associated with protein-losing enteropathy.

ease, pancreatic insufficiency, massive resection of the small intestine, or *ileectomy)* often alleviates the major symptoms (Table 5).

Whipple's disease now appears entirely manageable, and perhaps even reversible, with the use of broad-spectrum antimicrobial agents and adrenal steroids. The malabsorption of diffuse *nongranulomatous ileojejunitis,* involving large segments of the small intestine, may be completely abolished by administration of adrenal steroids or corticotrophin. Likewise, isoniazid and streptomycin are similarly effective in *tuberculosis enteritis.* Elimination of an offender in the diet and use of corticosteroids are an effective combination against *eosinophilic gastroenteritis.*

The correction of conditions in which intestinal microbes play an important role may be accomplished by appropriate surgery, such as resection of fistulas or strictures, or by administration of broad-spectrum antimicrobial drugs. In either case, a normal or nearly normal state of health may be achieved.

The prognosis for patients with malabsorption associated with endocrine disorders is good. The patient with intestinal *scleroderma* or with *diabetes mellitus* who has neuropathy and bacterial overgrowth may be helped by the intermittent administration of antimicrobial drugs. Vitamin D and calcium will restore absorption toward normal in cases of *hypoparathyroidism.* Appropriate management of *hyperthyroidism* will reverse abnormal fat absorption, as will replacement therapy for *Addison's disease.* Specific treatment for *Giardia lamblia* will likely cure the patient with *hypogammaglobulinemia.* Broad-spectrum antimicrobial drugs are effective in treating tropical sprue. Resection of a non-insulin-secreting, *non-beta-cell tumor* of the pancreatic islets will diminish diarrhea and steatorrhea.

Because of the nature of the underlying disease, the outlook is bleak for a number of patients with malabsorption syndrome. These are the patients with advancing *biliary cirrhosis;* complicated *relapsing pancreatitis;* extensive *granulomatous enteritis* associated with recurrent fistulas, strictures, and mutilative surgery; progressive *scleroderma* of the intestine; *lymphoma* of the small bowel and mesenteric lymph nodes; and progressive *occlusive disease* of the *superior mesenteric artery.* Prognosis for those who have undergone *massive resection of the small intestine* – at once or in stages – is now vastly improved, however, because of intravenous hyperalimentation programs, improved feeding regimens of foods containing protein hydrolysates, and more potent antimicrobial drugs to treat infection. Therapy for *protein-losing enteropathy* is remarkably good if the correct diagnosis is made (Table 6).

On the whole, the prognosis for the malabsorption syndrome is optimistic, provided that the specific abnormality is identified and appropriate corrective measures are instituted.

Krone, C., and Sleisenger, M. H.: Studies on the pathogenesis of malabsorption: Lipid hydrolysis and micelle formation in the intestinal lumen. Medicine, 47:89, 1968.

Losowsky, M. S., Walker, B. E., and Kelleher, J.: Malabsorption in Clinical Practice. Edinburgh and London, Churchill, Livingstone, 1974.

Sleisenger, M. H., and Fordtran, J. S. (eds.): Gastrointestinal Disease. Philadelphia, W. B. Saunders Company, 1973, Chapters 4, 19–21, 66–67, 69–71, 73–76, 93, and 105.

Wilson, F. A., and Dietschy, J. M.: Differential diagnosis to clinical problems of malabsorption. Gastroenterology, 61:911, 1971.

Section Four. DISEASES OF THE PANCREAS

O. Dhodanand Kowlessar

645. ACUTE PANCREATITIS

GENERAL CONSIDERATIONS

During the past decade, rapid progress has been made in the understanding of basic pancreatic physiology and biochemistry. These advances have come from studies that have elucidated the factors controlling the secretion of pancreatic juice, the ultrastructure of the human pancreas by the use of the electron microscope, the sites of synthesis and discharge of pancreatic enzymes by the use of labeled amino acids and pulse chase radioautography, the precise electrolyte and enzyme contents of pancreatic juice, and the amino acid sequence and synthesis of potent pancreatic hormones. The information thus obtained, supplemented by contributions of clinicians, radiologists, and surgeons, has resulted in a better understanding of the pathogenesis of pancreatic inflammation, edema, and hemorrhage. It has further resulted in more exact and reliable diagnostic tests of pancreatic disease and, through utilization of therapeutic measures directed against specific etiologic mechanisms, in more rational and efficacious treatment. A brief review of pancreatic function will be helpful in understanding the etiology and pathogenesis of acute pancreatitis.

PANCREATIC PHYSIOLOGY, BIOCHEMISTRY, AND ANATOMY

Each day the human pancreas secretes between 1000 and 2500 ml of a clear, colorless fluid, of low viscosity containing 5 to 8 grams of protein, with a pH of 7.5 to 8.5. Pancreatic juice consists mainly of water, electrolytes, and approximately 24 proteins, of which the vast majority are enzymes. The main ions are Na^+, K^+, HCO_3^-, and, in lesser concentrations, Cl^-, Ca^{++}, Zn^{++}, $HPO_4^=$, and $SO_4^=$. Hydrochloric acid stimulates the release of *secretin,* which acts on the centroacinar cells to produce a watery secretion low in enzyme activity but high in bicarbonate. Secretin also acts in a feedback mechansim to inhibit *gastrin*-stimulated acid production and gastric motility. The augmentation of pancreatic secretion during digestion is the result of stimuli arising within the duodenum and a combination of integrated neurohumoral mechanisms acting on receptor sites on the acinar cells. Feeding stimulates vagal fibers originating in the hypothalamus to mediate the release of acetylcholine. Food distends the antrum, thereby releasing gastrin from "gastrin cells," and also causes the release of *cholecystokinin-pancreozymin* (CCK-PZ) from cells in the duodenal mucosa. Once released into the circulation, acetylcholine, gastrin, and CCK-PZ bind to receptor sites on the pancreatic acinar cell membrane where membrane-bound adenyl cyclase catalyzes the synthesis of cyclic 3-5′ AMP. A series of events is then activated which finally leads to the secretion of zymogen granules. At least two of the pancreatic proteins have been shown to be synthesized in attached ribosomes of the rough endoplasmic reticulum, whence they are transported into the intracisternal spaces to the Golgi complex for condensation, encapsulation, and formation of zymogen granules. The mature granules migrate toward the apex of the acinar cell, and under appropriate exogenous stimuli, a fusion of the zymogen granules and the external cell membrane occurs, allowing their contents to be ejected into the lumen by exocytosis.

Electrolytes are secreted by the human pancreas in a solution that is isotonic with the blood plasma. The concentrations of the cations Na^+, K^+, and Ca^{++} approximate the diffusible ionic content of the blood plasma. The Cl^- content varies inversely with the concentration of HCO_3^-, the latter increasing as the rate of secretion increases. The secretion of bicarbonate appears to be under the catalytic influence of carbonic anhydrase, which controls the formation of bicarbonate ion within the cell according to the following equation: $H_2O + CO_2 \rightleftharpoons H_2CO_3 \rightleftharpoons H^+ + HCO_3^-$. The main function of this balanced electrolyte pancreatic juice, apparently, is to adjust the duodenal contents to an optimal alkaline pH for the action of the pancreatic enzymes.

The proteolytic enzymes are synthesized and secreted as catalytically inert precursors or proenzymes and include trypsin(ogen), chymotrypsin(ogen) A and B, (pro)carboxypeptidases A and B, and (pro)elastase. (Pro)phospholipase A is also secreted in zymogen form. Enterokinase (secreted by the duodenal mucosa) in the presence of calcium catalyzes the transformation of trypsinogen to trypsin. In turn, trypsin catalyzes the formation of trypsinogen, chymotrypsinogen A and B, procarboxypeptidases A and B, proelastase, and prophospholipase A to their active forms.

The proteolytic enzymes hydrolyze dietary proteins to polypeptides of varying chain lengths and amino acids. The peptides undergo further hydrolysis by the brush border hydrolases followed by transport of the amino acids across the epithelial cell. α-Amylase splits starch to α-limit dextrins, maltose and maltotriose for further breakdown by brush border α-dextrinase and maltase. Lipase aided by conjugated bile salts acts on triglyceride to form monoglycerides and fatty acids. Once activated, phospholipase A in the presence of bile salts selectively removes the β-fatty acid from the lecithin molecule to form lysolecithin. The lysolecithin in human duodenal juice is an α-palmitoyl-lysolecithin.

ETIOLOGY OF ACUTE PANCREATITIS

A number of factors have been proposed for the etiology of pancreatitis. The three most important etiologic categories are gallstones, alcohol, and "idiopathic" processes, accounting for 90 to 95 per cent of all cases of acute pancreatitis; miscellaneous factors are implicated in the remaining 5 to 10 per cent of patients. The multiplicity of mechanisms for production of this disease demonstrates that this gland is capable of responding to a wide variety of stresses with a unitary reaction of varying degree.

Biliary Tract Disease. Biliary tract disease may be responsible for 10 to 95 per cent of various large series of pancreatitis. This wide range is related to the incidence of alcoholism in a given patient population.

The causative factors involved in the association of biliary tract disease and acute pancreatitis remain obscure. The importance of a mechanical factor in the pathogenesis of pancreatitis was stressed by Opie, who postulated his "common channel theory" from the observation of acute pancreatitis in a patient with a small stone impacted in the ampulla of Vater. This occurs in 8 per cent of the patients with gallstones and pancreatitis. In a recent study of patients with acute pancreatitis associated with gallbladder disease, there was a temporal relationship between an attack of pancreatitis and the appearance of gallstones in the feces, associated with transient jaundice and hyperamylasemia. Thus it would appear that the pancreatitis was due to an ephemeral mechanical blockage of the ampulla of Vater by migrating stones. It has also been suggested that duodenal contents, composed of unconjugated bile salts secondary to deconjugation of bile salts by microorganisms and lysolecithin secondary to the action of phospholipase A on bile lecithin, reflux into the pancreatic duct and initiate pancreatitis. It is equally possible that bacterial toxins derived from the biliary tree could reach the pancreas via anastomatic lymphatic channels, structurally altering the acinar cell membrane with release of pancreatic enzymes, which in turn initiates pancreatitis.

Alcohol. Alcoholism is responsible for 8 to 75 per cent of cases, depending upon the socioeconomic status of the patient population served by the hospital. The mechanisms whereby ethyl alcohol induces pancreatitis are not known. It is likely that after a large intake of alcohol, gastric acid secretion is stimulated by gastrin release and by direct stimulation of parietal cells. The acid in the duodenum promotes secretion of secretin and pancreozymin with an augmentation of pancreatic secretion by all three gastrointestinal hormones. Concomitantly, a direct effect of ethanol on the sphincter of Oddi would increase sphincteric resistance, with resultant increase in intrapancreatic ductal pressure. Another mechanism involves the reflux of bile into the pancreatic duct during vomiting and retching associated with heavy ethanol intake. Although the mechanical and reflux mechanisms appear cogent, it is possible, though not proved in man, that ethanol exerts a direct toxic effect on the pancreas. In long-term ethanol ingestion in rats, there are significant lipid droplets in the acinar cells, accompanied by mitochondrial swelling and reduction of their inner membranes, with associated degradation of acinar, centroacinar, and duct cells. There is also decreased protein synthesis in the pancreas, with inhibition of ^{32}P into pancreatic phospholipids. Although these experimental results are provocative, further work is needed to substantiate similar effects in man and to define the mechanism of the production of alcoholic pancreatitis.

Idiopathic Factors. Idiopathic factors consistently account for 20 to 50 per cent of large series and thus represent the third most common category; the precise etiology is unknown.

Miscellaneous Causes. A miscellaneous group of etiologic factors make up about 10 per cent of other causes of pancreatitis. Among these are the following: (1) *Metabolic-nutritional disturbances,* including hyperlipemia with genetically determined hyperlipoproteinemia (Types I and V), diabetic ketoacidosis, malnutrition (kwashiorkor), uremia, pregnancy (last trimester or early post partum), and *hypercalcemic states* (hyperparathyroidism, multiple myeloma, excessive doses of vitamin D, and sarcoidosis), which bring about excessive activation of trypsinogen by calcium ion, or by precipitation of calcium in an alkaline milieu in the ducts leading to obstruction. An increased incidence of parathyroid carcinoma causing hyperparathyroidism has been observed in those cases associated with severe pancreatitis. Of note also are the cases of severe pancreatitis occurring within the first 24 hours after the removal of a parathyroid adenoma. *Hereditary pancreatitis* appears to be transmitted as a non-sex-linked mendelian dominant trait modified by incomplete manifestation or sex-related expressivity. The attacks begin, in most cases, in childhood or early adult life, the average age of onset being 12 years, with approximately equal sex incidence. Cholelithiasis and alcoholism are infrequent concomitants. Pancreatic calcifications most often appear as discrete calculi in the larger pancreatic ducts. Aminoaciduria (increased lysine and cystine excretion and, to a lesser extent, arginine) has been observed in approximately 50 per cent of a small group of persons (with or without pancreatitis) so far studied in affected kindreds. However, aminoaciduria might be seen in some patients with nonfamilial pancreatitis. Carcinoma of the pancreas was a cause of death in a few members of kindreds with this entity. A particularly unique feature is the occurrence of portal vein thrombosis and splenic vein thrombosis complicating pancreatitis in a few cases. (2) *Infection* secondary to the reflux of infected material into the pancreatic duct, or from such systemic infections as scarlet fever, streptococcal food poisoning, typhoid fever, viral hepatitis, infectious mononucleosis, mumps, and coxsackievirus group B. (3) *Trauma:* Steering-wheel injuries, penetrating injuries from bullets or knife wounds, postoperative pancreatitis (after surgery in the area of the pancreas, as well as distant areas from the pancreas, e.g., transurethral resection), and electric shock. (4) *Vascular and autoimmune mechanisms:* Atheromatous embolization to intrapancreatic arteries, renal transplantation, extracorporeal circulation, polyarteritis nodosa, and systemic lupus erythematosus. (5) *Drugs:* Glucocorticoids, chlorothiazide, isoniazid, salicylates, sulfamethizole, indomethacin, salicylazosulfapyridine, L-asparaginase, immunosuppressive drugs (6-mercaptopurine and azathioprine), and oral contraceptives, especially in women who have Type 4 as well as Type 5 lipid patterns before therapy. (6) *Scorpion bite.* (7) *Pancreatic carcinoma.* (8) *Obstructive lesions* at the sphincter of Oddi secondary to benign polyps and regional enteritis of the duodenum.

PATHOGENESIS

The essential lesion in acute pancreatitis is necrosis of the acinar cells, and the clinical severity is determined by the extent of the damage to the exocrine pancreas. The underlying mechanism in the production of pancreatic inflammation is the escape of activated enzymes into the interstitial tissues, and the earliest responses to this chemical irritation are edema and vascular engorgement of the pancreas. Normally, the pancreatic proteases (trypsin, chymotrypsin, elastase, and carboxypeptidases) and phospholipase A are stored in the acinar cell as inactive precursors. The Golgi complex, ergastoplasm, zymogen granule, and the cell membrane segregate the exportable pancreatic enzymes in the acinar cell, as well as the lysosomal hydrolases. Two potent protease inhibitors which guard against intracellular activation of trypsinogen are also present in the exocrine cell. Theoretically, regardless of the etiology, a common denominator of the pathogenetic mechanism could be an increase in the permeability of the lipoprotein membranes which surround the exportable and lysosomal hydrolases with subsequent release of these enzymes with concomitant edema, coagulation necrosis, vascular injury, and hemorrhage.

Edema may occur anywhere in the gland, but is apt to be more severe in the head. The region affected becomes pale and indurated, with progressive engorgement of the blood vessels. In most instances the inflammatory edema subsides spontaneously, but in a small percentage of cases there is progression to hemorrhage, necrosis, and suppuration, or the inflammation becomes chronic. Progression of pancreatic edema to hemorrhagic necrosis is in part the result of enlargement of the pancreas within its capsule, which obstructs the pancreatic duct further and aggravates the vascular engorgement until ischemia supervenes. As elsewhere, ischemia superimposed on an inflammatory process results in infarction and hemorrhage. Activated elastase may bring about erosion of major blood vessels, with hemorrhage into the pancreas, the retroperitoneal tissues, and even the colon. Collections of blood, digested tissue, and pancreatic secretions may burrow along the tissue spaces into the gastrohepatic ligament and retroperitoneally into the lesser sac and flank, giving rise to the classic ascitic exudate of acute pancreatitis described as "beef broth," and to visible hemorrhagic areas in the costovertebral angle (Grey-Turner sign). The peritoneal effusion and peritoneal irritation during the early stages of acute pancreatitis are greatest in the lesser sac and at the base of the transverse mesocolon. This localized chemical peritonitis often results in a segmental paralytic ileus of the first jejunal loop, which has been described as a diagnostic sign, the "sentinel loop" of acute pancreatitis.

Thus the local pathology of pancreatitis at the inception is the result of edema, hemorrhage, and the onslaught of biochemical agents, i.e., the pancreatic enzymes. If the disease progresses without resolution, superimposed infection, especially by colonic bacteria, produces suppuration and results in pancreatic abscesses, as well as purulent collections in the various abdominal fossae, the lesser sac, the cul-de-sac, and the left subphrenic space.

Resolution may occur with fibrosis and calcification. The edema and other inflammatory changes subside during the first week of illness. Areas of necrosis are autolyzed and replaced by fibrous tissue. Cellular proliferation attempts to restore normal glandular architecture. By the end of the second week histologic repair may have proceeded to such a degree that the pancreas may appear normal. On the other hand, resolution is delayed in the more severe forms, with persistence of residual fibrosis, calcification, and acinar dysfunction.

DIAGNOSIS

Clinical Manifestations. *Pain* and *shock* are the outstanding symptoms of acute hemorrhagic pancreatitis; *pain* and *metabolic disturbances* dominate the clinical picture of acute edematous pancreatitis and chronic relapsing pancreatitis. However, all three—pain, shock, and metabolic disturbances—may be absent, as in painless pancreatitis.

The *pain* in acute pancreatitis results from distention of the pancreatic capsule, retroperitoneal extravasations, chemical peritonitis, and obstruction or spasm in the pancreatic ducts, extrahepatic biliary tract, and duodenum. Characteristically, the attack is sudden, and the pain is usually severe, constant, and widespread. It is frequently more intense when the patient is lying supine than when he is sitting or lying on the side with his spine flexed. Although usually originating in the epigastrium, the pain also may be experienced in other parts of the abdomen, and may radiate to the back, substernal area, and flanks. Physical examination discloses an acutely ill patient complaining of abdominal pain, with fever and tachycardia. The blood pressure may be slightly elevated in those in whom circulatory collapse has not supervened. *Cyanosis, cold* and *clammy skin, rapid* and *feeble pulse,* and *subnormal temperature* are present in the more severe attacks. The abdomen may be distended early as a result of paralytic ileus and the accumulation of peritoneal fluid. Peristalsis may be diminished or inaudible. *Tenderness* is invariably present in the epigastrium, and is associated with a moderate degree of muscular rigidity; it may be elicited elsewhere in the abdomen, depending on the sites of seepage of the pancreatic juice. Occasionally, a mass in the upper abdomen—an inflammatory *pseudocyst*—may be palpable. The systemic effects in acute pancreatitis are presumed to result from the absorption of activated pancreatic enzymes and the products of the activation of the bradykinin system.

Shock is the outstanding systemic phenomenon in *severe acute pancreatitis,* and may be so profound that death ensues within a few hours. The shock results from a combination of the following events: (1) presumed increase in serum proteolytic activity; (2) the release of the activated enzyme kallikrein, which in turn is responsible for the formation of kinins, whose main actions are stimulation of smooth muscle, dilatation of blood vessels, and lowering of blood pressure; (3) contraction of the blood volume, as great as 30 per cent, secondary to exudation of blood and plasma into the peritoneal cavity and possible protein leak; and (4) hyperlipasemia, which may then be related to hyperlipemia and to fat necrosis of the subcutaneous tissue and the bone marrow. Additional factors are (5) acute coronary insufficiency resulting from thrombosis and electrolyte disturbances (in turn, the lowered blood volume and shock contribute to the myocardial problem); (6) pulmonary embolus; (7) massive bleeding; and (8) intravascular coagulopathy.

In many cases, other metabolic disturbances can be uncovered. Serum calcium, potassium, and sodium are lowered. The depression of calcium is due partly to fixation by fatty acids in areas of fat necrosis and increased levels of circulating glucagon, which in turn stimulate the secretion of thyrocalcitonin with resultant inhibition of bone resorption. Glucagon can also directly inhibit bone resorption, induced either by parathyroid hormone or dibutyryl-3′-5′-adenosine monophosphate, indicating an additional glucagon action independent of thyrocalci-

tonin. Levels of calcium below 7 mg per 100 ml are usually accompanied by tetany.

Injury to the β-cells, as well as release of glucagon and glucocorticoids, secondary to pancreatic inflammation, are associated with *hyperglycemia, glycosuria,* and impaired glucose tolerance in about 50 per cent of the cases. These changes, although transient in the acute cases, may, with repeated attacks, progress to true "pancreatic" diabetes. *Coma* may be the presenting symptom of severe hemorrhagic pancreatitis; when associated with the commonly elevated blood sugar in acute pancreatitis, diabetic coma may be erroneously diagnosed. Likewise, confusion, restlessness, and disorientation have been observed during an acute attack ("pancreatic psychosis or encephalopathy").

Jaundice is seen in about 25 per cent of patients with acute pancreatitis, resulting primarily from obstruction of the terminal common duct as it traverses an edematous pancreas; in some patients, exacerbation of associated biliary tract disease may also be partly responsible. Intrahepatic cholestasis secondary to alcoholic liver disease may also contribute to the icterus.

Hyperlipemia with grossly opalescent serum has been observed in 3 to 8 per cent of patients with alcoholic pancreatitis and is due to a striking chylomicronemia or very low density lipoproteins. In follow-up studies of many of these patients, an underlying hyperlipidemia antedated the pancreatitis. Some authors have reported disseminated fat necrosis in the bone marrow and subcutaneous tissues. Acute and chronic bone lesions secondary to medullary necrosis have been described. *Pulmonary atelectasis, pneumonia,* and *pleural effusion,* particularly left-sided, are noted frequently. Significantly, pancreatic enzyme concentrations are higher in the pleural effusion than in simultaneously obtained serum. These enzymes are thought to reach the pleural fluid from the ascitic exudate by passage through the transdiaphragmatic lymphatic channels. Occasionally, *respiratory symptoms* may overshadow the abdominal complaints. Recently, mild to moderate degrees of respiratory insufficiency characterized by *arterial hypoxia* and *mild respiratory alkalosis* have been observed in a significant number of patients with acute pancreatitis.

The vascular phenomena in acute pancreatitis include peripheral *venous thromboses* and *thrombophlebitis* and mildly diffuse hemorrhage, widespread thrombosis, and disseminated intravascular coagulopathy.

Laboratory Diagnosis. *Serum Enzymes.* A diagnosis of acute pancreatitis may be made when an elevated serum amylase, usually greater than 300 Somogyi units, is found in a patient with acute, severe pain in the upper abdomen, tenderness, vomiting, fever, tachycardia, and leukocytosis. The serum amylase becomes elevated early in the course of the disease, usually within the first 24 to 48 hours. In most cases, values range from 300 to 800, but levels as high as 12,000 units have been reported. Apparently no constant relationship exists, however, between the severity of the disease and the height of the serum amylase values. Milder episodes may have considerable elevations. Conversely, in attacks with early fatality, the amylase values (as well as other enzyme levels) may be greatly decreased because of destruction of the pancreas. The serum *lipase* usually rises in parallel with the amylase activity, reaching its peak in 72 or 96 hours with a gradual fall; values greater than 2.0 ml of N/100 NaOH are significant. Elevations of the levels of glutamic oxaloacetic acid transaminase, alkaline phosphatase, and leucine aminopeptidase are usually secondary to obstruction of the common bile duct or associated liver disease.

A variety of diseases, intra-abdominal and extra-abdominal, may be accompanied by elevation of the serum enzymes, frequently posing a difficult diagnostic problem. Hyperamylasemia is encountered in *perforation of peptic ulcer, small bowel obstruction, salivary duct occlusion, parotitis,* and *uremia,* and after administration of opiates, notably codeine and morphine. Elevations of serum lipase have been reported in patients with *carcinoma of the pancreas; obstructive jaundice caused by stone, tumors,* and *cirrhosis of the liver; viral hepatitis; intestinal obstruction;* and *peritonitis.* It should be pointed out, however, that in these instances the serum enzyme elevations are not as high as in acute pancreatitis.

Urinary Amylase. Elevation of urinary amylase concentration has been used to diagnose acute pancreatitis in the absence of renal failure. Levels of urinary amylase higher than 6000 units per 24 hours or 300 units per hour are usually seen in patients with acute attacks of pancreatitis. A more precise method of diagnosing and following patients with acute pancreatitis is to determine concomitant concentrations of amylase (units per milliliter) and creatinine (milligrams per milliliter) in serum and in a simultaneously voided urine specimen. Thus C_{Am}/C_{Cr} can be determined by the following formula:

$$C_{Am}/C_{Cr} \, (\%) = \frac{(Am) \; urine}{(Am) \; serum} \times \frac{(Cr) \; serum}{(Cr) \; urine} \times 100$$

In normal subjects this ratio is 2.3 ± 0.1 per cent, whereas in renal insufficiency the ratio is 2.1 ± 0.2 per cent. In acute pancreatitis there is a significant increase in the ratio of 6.6 ± 0.3 per cent, with gradual fall to normal levels in 9 to 15 days. Acute exacerbations during the clinical course of pancreatitis are characterized by an increase in the ratio. In contrast to pancreatitis, patients with macroamylasemia (amylases with molecular weights of at least 160,000) were consistently associated with a low ratio of 0.34 ± 0.13 per cent. This low ratio can serve as a simple screening test for macroamylasemia.

Other Laboratory Data. Ancillary laboratory findings must be considered in making the diagnosis. The *leukocyte count* often ranges from 10,000 to 30,000 per cubic millimeter, with an increase in immature granulocytes. In mild cases, the leukocyte count may be normal. The hematocrit and erythrocyte count are usually not significantly lowered, except when there is hemorrhage into the gastrointestinal tract or peritoneal cavity. Elevation of *blood urea nitrogen* is not uncommon in the more severe cases, especially when shock and oliguria are present. *Glycosuria* appears in about 11 per cent of patients with acute pancreatitis, and disappears with resolution of the process. Transient *hyperglycemia* may be found more frequently than glycosuria. Bilirubin is usually slightly elevated—2.0 to 4.0 mg per 100 ml; higher levels may indicate that common duct obstruction underlies the pancreatitis.

A slight depression of serum *calcium* occurs in most patients between the third and fifteenth days of the disease, the lowest level occurring about the sixth day. Serum calcium below 7.0 mg per 100 ml portends a poor although not invariably fatal prognosis. Diminished serum albumin lowers the total serum calcium, so that hypoalbuminemia should be evaluated in the assessment of serum calcium and in replacement therapy. An unexpectedly normal serum calcium level in severe pancreatitis may be the first indication of hyperparathyroidism. *Hypokalemia* may be observed, and is most likely related to alkalosis, intravenous administration of saline solution, and loss of gastric juice because of continuous nasogastric suction. In severe cases, in which there is considerable tissue destruction, *shock* with oliguria causes hyperkalemia.

Electrocardiography. The electrocardiograms of some patients with acute pancreatitis may show depression of S-T segments in the limb leads and precordial leads as well as changes in the Q-T intervals. These changes may be due to the electrolyte imbalance or may be related to the shock in the more severe cases.

Roentgenographic Findings. Although in no way pathognomonic of acute pancreatitis, certain roentgenographic abnormalities are encountered with sufficient frequency to suggest the diagnosis. A survey film of the abdomen may reveal a localized paralytic ileus of jejunum ("sentinel loop"), usually in the left midportion of the abdomen, or calcification in the region of the pancreas (see accompanying figure) or the "colon cut-off" sign. The latter consists of an isolated gaseous distention of the colon and hepatic flexure owing to partial obstruction caused by spread of the inflammatory process from the head of the pancreas. Barium swallow may demonstrate displacement of the stomach, enlargement of the duodenal loop, or collection and stasis of barium in the dependent parts of the duodenum caused by an enlarged head of the pancreas or an inflammatory *pseudocyst.* *Pancreatic ultrasonography* (echography) will show pseudocysts as smoothly rounded transonic spaces, often with a distinct wall. This technique reliably estimates the size of even small pseudocysts. Also there may be an

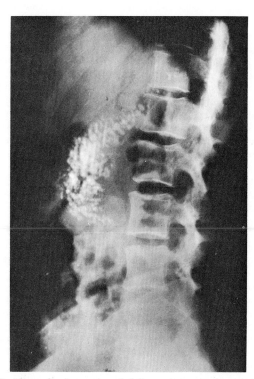

Left oblique roentgenogram of abdomen demonstrating pancreatic calcification.

enlarged edematous ampulla of Vater and irritability of the stomach and duodenum. In most instances the biliary tree may be adequately visualized by intravenous cholangiography, excluding bile duct obstruction as the precipitating event. Nonvisualization of the gallbladder after either oral or intravenous administration of dye, however, is a common finding during the acute episode, but does not necessarily indicate a disease of the gallbladder. Accordingly, the roentgenographic studies should be repeated several weeks after the attack has subsided, at which time, if the gallbladder is diseased, stones in the biliary tree and/or nonfilling of the gallbladder will be observed. The chest roentgenogram may show pleural effusion (usually on the left side), elevated left diaphragm, or linear focal atelectasis at the lung bases.

Other Diagnostic Procedures. Diagnostic tap of the peritoneum, performed under local anesthesia, in the left lower quadrant of the abdomen may reveal turbid yellow fluid in edematous pancreatitis or reddish-brown fluid in the hemorrhagic type. The peritoneal fluid amylase is considerably higher than serum amylase tested at the same time, and may remain elevated for two or three days after the serum amylase has fallen to normal levels. The determination of serum *methemalbumin* has been proposed as a diagnostic test for pancreatitis. Recent evidence suggests that elevated levels have occurred in other acute abdominal emergencies. However, if methemalbumin is detected within the first 24 hours in serum, pleural effusions, or ascitic fluid in a patient with clinical and biochemical evidence of pancreatitis, the diagnosis of necrotizing pancreatitis is justified.

Differential Diagnosis. The diagnosis of acute pancreatitis should be established as rapidly as clinical and laboratory facilities permit. However, the diagnosis is made difficult by the large number of abdominal catastrophes that may in many ways simulate this condition.

Perforated peptic ulcer, more than any other abdominal condition, may resemble acute pancreatitis. Usually a preceding history compatible with ulcer can be elicited, although occasionally perforation may be its first indication. Unlike pancreatitis, however, *boardlike rigidity of the abdomen* is the outstanding finding. A flat plate of the abdomen may show free air, usually under the right diaphragm. Hyperamylasemia, resulting from the escape of duodenal contents into the peritoneum or involvement of the pancreas in the process, may accompany perforation, but usually the values are not as high as in acute pancreatitis. (See Ch. 640 to 644.)

Biliary colic may resemble acute pancreatitis by virtue of pressure changes in the biliary tree and associated inflammation of the gallbladder. Pain, tenderness, and rigidity are frequently localized in the right upper quadrant of the abdomen. *Acute cholangitis,* caused by stones in the common bile duct, is usually associated with chills, fever, and jaundice. An elevated serum amylase is seen in about 20 per cent of cases of common duct stone, and differentiation may have to await the course of the disease.

The pain of *acute cholecystitis* is usually in the right upper quadrant and may radiate to the right scapula. Tenderness and guarding are present in the right upper quadrant. A striking feature is that, despite the pain, these patients do not usually look very ill, in contrast to patients with acute pancreatitis.

Acute *small bowel obstruction* may be a diagnostic problem in view of occasional associated hyperamylase-mia. The history of vomiting and the cramplike periumbilical pain with abdominal distention and visible peristalsis are helpful. In mechanical ileus, auscultation will reveal high-pitched notes, succussion splashes, and peristaltic rushes. Acute appendicitis involving a retrocecal appendix in close contact with the gallbladder may require differentiation. The amylase is usually normal in this condition.

Mesenteric thrombosis may present as intestinal obstruction with a less acute onset. This may be associated with bloody diarrhea, which is rare in pancreatitis. Shock is more acute, and diffuse tenderness and rigidity are more common. A flat plate of the abdomen may show a large, dilated, fluid-filled loop of bowel, the site of infarction.

Dissecting aneurysm usually presents with severe pain, shock, absent pulsations in the femoral vessels, and lowered blood pressure in the legs. A pulsating mass may be felt.

Nephrolithiasis on the left side may simulate acute pancreatitis. Hematuria and a flat plate of the abdomen revealing a stone will help in the differentiation.

Acute coronary occlusion may present with left upper quadrant or epigastric pain, nausea, and vomiting. Electrocardiographic changes and elevation of the serum glutamic oxaloacetic transaminase occur in pancreatitis, but Q waves are not ordinarily present in pancreatitis. Also, the lack of elevation of serum enzymes of pancreatic origin will help exclude acute pancreatitis.

Acute intermittent porphyria is usually associated with a history of vomiting at intervals, severe and frequent episodes of abdominal pain, and chronic constipation. The demonstration of porphobilinogen in the urine by the Watson-Schwartz test is helpful in establishing the diagnosis.

Acute systemic lupus erythematosus and *periarteritis nodosa* may present with an abdominal picture requiring differentiation from pancreatitis. The situation is further confused by the fact that pancreatitis may be a complication of these diseases. The history, coupled with other common findings in these diseases, will help in the differential diagnosis.

TREATMENT

Acute pancreatitis varies greatly in the degree of its severity. The milder attacks are presumably due to edema of the pancreas, and in this situation therapy is directed primarily to the relief of pain. In the more severe form with hemorrhage and necrosis and their concomitant physiologic and biochemical disturbances discussed previously, treatment may conveniently be divided into several distinct phases.

Control of Pain. The pain is usually severe, and should be treated promptly with adequate doses of analgesics. Meperidine (Demerol), with its minimal effect on the tone of the sphincter of Oddi, is probably the drug of choice and should be given parenterally in doses of 75 to 100 mg every four to six hours to assure prompt and adequate relief. Morphine and codeine should be avoided because of their spasmogenic effects. Sympathetic nerve blocks and continuous or fractional epidural anesthesia can be used to supplement the effects of meperidine in patients whose pain is persistent.

Treatment of Shock. Circulatory collapse is often the most immediate and major problem of the severe form of pancreatitis. Whole blood is probably the most effective treatment and, in view of the diminution of blood volume to approximately 70 per cent in severe cases, should be given promptly. Large volumes of fluid are often required; constant monitoring of central venous pressure and careful measurement of fluid intake and urinary output are necessary. Albumin and plasma are adequate temporary substitutes. Low molecular weight dextran may be highly effective and should be tried. It can decrease blood viscosity, expand plasma volume, and improve peripheral blood flow, and has antithrombotic activity. Patients with severe, unresponsive disease may be given an infusion of 1:500,000 isoproterenol hydrochloride (Isuprel), commencing with a dose rate of 0.5 to 4.0 μg per minute with careful electrocardiographic monitoring.

Inhibition of Pancreatic Secretory Activity. An important principle in the management of acute pancreatitis is the "splinting of the injured pancreas" by suppression of pancreatic secretion. Achievement of this goal is accomplished by cessation of oral intake of food, continuous nasogastric suction to minimize release of secretin through stimulation by gastric acid, and administration of drugs to inhibit pancreatic secretion. Propantheline (Pro-Banthine) bromide, 30 mg, or methantheline (Banthine) bromide, 50 mg, given parenterally every six to eight hours, have enjoyed wide popularity, although their efficacy remains in doubt. Their pharmacologic effects include suppression of gastric acidity, relaxation of the sphincter, and partial inhibition of pancreatic enzyme production. However, in the presence of *paralytic ileus* and *shock*, these drugs may be harmful and should be avoided.

Recently, *glucagon* in an initial dose of 1 mg intravenously, followed by 1.0 to 1.5 mg in 5 per cent dextrose or normal saline every four hours, has been reported to result in clinical improvement and relief of pain associated with a fall of serum amylase. It has been suggested that the beneficial effect observed was due to the inhibition of pancreatic secretion, thus suppressing the activity of the acutely inflamed gland. The serum calcium should be monitored if this form of therapy is used.

Antimicrobials. The prophylactic use of antimicrobials for the prevention of infection in severe cases of acute pancreatitis is purely empirical and without controlled studies. It has been proposed that the protein-rich exudate in edematous, poorly perfused tissues is favorable for bacterial growth. Appropriate cultures of blood, urine, sputum, and effusions are taken. Antimicrobial drugs should be withheld unless there is reason to suspect infection, evidenced by sustained or high spiking fevers (higher than 39° C) strongly suggesting either pancreatic abscess or cholangitis. Intramuscular ampicillin, 500 mg, and kanamycin, 250 mg, every six hours must then be initiated. Abscesses must be drained or obstruction of the common bile duct relieved along with cholecystectomy and cholecystostomy with continued appropriate antimicrobial therapy. An important clue to underlying cholangitis is persisting jaundice with bilirubin levels above 4.0 mg per 100 ml.

Fluids and Electrolytes. The continued gastric suction and the abstinence from any oral intake make it necessary to replace body fluids and electrolytes carefully. The amount of normal saline with supplemental potassium chloride to be administered may vary between 3 and 6 liters daily and should be estimated by considering the insensible loss, the amount of sweating, the elevation of temperature, the volume of gastric suction, and the anticipated urinary output. Glucose must be administered cautiously, for it may aggravate a diabetic state that has been precipitated by acute pancreatitis. When hyperglycemia and glycosuria are marked and diabetic acidosis is imminent, small doses of insulin must be given.

Hypocalcemia is fairly frequent, and calcium gluconate solution may be given intravenously as needed. *Hypokalemia* is combated by cautious intravenous administration of potassium chloride. Blood potassium determinations and electrocardiograms should be done frequently to avoid potassium toxicity.

Miscellaneous Measures. Abdominal distention and ileus are usually adequately managed by gastric suction, but occasionally it may be necessary to insert a long intestinal tube to deflate the small intestine. The adynamic nature of this ileus makes the passage of such a tube rather difficult.

Many drugs have been used in the treatment of acute pancreatitis, but since the disease is self-limiting in most instances, it is difficult to assess their efficacy. In recent years, the use of corticotrophin and cortisone has been advocated in acute fulminant pancreatitis, particularly when an abdominal exploration has been performed without previous knowledge of the existence of the disease. However, evidence has accumulated that steroids, when used in other diseases, have brought about lesions similar to those seen in pancreatitis. Thus caution should be exercised, and these drugs should be reserved for those patients in whom shock has developed that is unresponsive to the usual measures.

Peritoneal dialysis should be attempted in those patients whose symptoms fail to improve after a period of conservative therapy and who appear to be dying of their disease. The dialysate recently used with some success consists of sodium, 141 mEq per liter, calcium, 3.5 mEq per liter, magnesium, 1.5 mEq per liter, chloride, 101 mEq per liter, and lactate, 4.5 mEq per liter, given via a standard peritoneal dialysis catheter. After a half hour of delay, the fluid is removed by straight drainage, and the procedure is repeated. Dramatic improvement in shock, oliguria, and correction of electrolyte imbalance has occurred in many patients.

Surgical Measures. It has become accepted generally that immediate operation for pancreatitis can do no good and that elective surgery should await the subsidence of the acute attack. In cases in which it is impossible to make the diagnosis and in which there is evidence of progressively serious pancreatitis that has failed to respond to medical management, laparotomy and surgery are justified. If hemorrhagic, suppurative, or necrotic pancreatitis is found, aggressive drainage of the pancreatic bed may improve the prognosis. A major indication for surgery is infection in the biliary tree, especially cholangitis. Even if pancreatitis appears fulminant, relief of obstruction and drainage are mandatory. Surgical consultation should be obtained in all cases of pancreatitis, particularly in patients with serum amylase greater than 1000, because it appears that these patients are more likely to have acute or chronic cholecystitis and cholelithiasis. Likewise, patients with *pancreatic abscesses* and those with *pseudocysts* which do not decompress are clearly surgical candidates.

Management after Acute Attack. Management should be directed toward the prevention of future attacks. Patients should be given a low fat diet and small, frequent meals to minimize pancreatic secretion; they should be told to avoid alcohol. Anticholinergic and analgesic drugs to minimize pancreatic secretion and pain are useful adjuncts. Overeating, obesity, and alcoholic abuse seem to be important precipitating factors and should be interdicted.

PROGNOSIS

Recovery is universal for patients with acute edematous pancreatitis; however, the fatality rate among those with hemorrhagic or necrotic disease is high, approximating 50 per cent. It is difficult to state the percentage of patients with acute pancreatitis who develop the chronic relapsing form of the disease. Suffice it to say that continued alcoholism or neglected biliary tract disease is often associated with recurrent attacks. Another important determining factor is the degree of ductal obstruction that is the residue of the initial bout of inflammation. Correction or control of an underlying cause, e.g., an endocrine disturbance such as hyperparathyroidism, or the withdrawal of a potentially noxious drug may help to prevent further attacks.

Condon, J. R., Knight, M., and Day, J. L.: Glucagon therapy in acute pancreatitis. Br. J. Surg., 60:509, 1973.

Creutzfeldt, W., and Schmidt, H.: Aetiology and pathogenesis of pancreatitis (current concepts). Scand. J. Gastroenterol. (Suppl.), 6:47, 1970.

Dreiling, D. A., Janowitz, H. D., and Perrier, C. V.: Pancreatic Inflammatory Disease: A Physiologic Approach. New York, Harper & Row, 1964.

Geokas, M. C.: Acute pancreatitis (medical progress). Calif. Med., 117:25, 1972.

Levitt, M. D., Rapport, M., and Cooperband, S. R.: The renal clearance of amylase in renal insufficiency, acute pancreatitis and macroamylasemia. Ann. Intern. Med., 71:919, 1969.

Ranson, J. H. C., Roses, D. F., and Fink, S. D.: Early respiratory insufficiency in acute pancreatitis. Ann. Surg., 178:75, 1973.

Webster, P. D., III.: Pancreatic acinar cells and their clinical significance. Viewpoints on Digestive Diseases, 4:No. 5, 1972.

646. CHRONIC PANCREATITIS AND CHRONIC RELAPSING PANCREATITIS

The most common clinical form of chronic pancreatitis is *chronic relapsing pancreatitis,* suggesting exacerbations of acute disease superimposed upon a previously injured gland. Acute pancreatitis may recur frequently and not progress to chronic pancreatitis, but such attacks invariably damage the pancreas. The parenchyma of the gland, subjected to cycles of fat necrosis, edema, and calcification, is gradually and extensively replaced by fibrotic tissue with disappearance of acinar and islet tissue. During the early stages of relapsing pancreatitis, the functional reserve of the gland and its capacity for protein synthesis and recovery are so great that enzyme deficiencies are only transiently demonstrable during the acute attacks. Since the disease process is frequently more severe in the region of the head of the gland, and the islets of Langerhans are concentrated in the body and tail, disturbed carbohydrate metabolism appears relatively late. Calcium is deposited in the obstructed

main duct and intralobular ducts as well as in areas of fat necrosis in the parenchyma (see figure in Ch. 645). In the later stages, with extensive destruction of the parenchyma and islet tissue (probably greater than 90 per cent of the pancreas), the biochemical abnormalities of altered carbohydrate metabolism (diabetes), increased excretion of stool fat (steatorrhea), and increased excretion of stool nitrogen (azotorrhea) will follow.

Etiology. Chronic relapsing pancreatitis may be caused by a wide variety of etiologic factors, but the principal one is the toxic effect of *chronic alcohol ingestion.* A second cause, although less frequent, is *untreated biliary tract disease* (gallstones). *Trauma* may also be an important cause, because the initial event may leave residual damage to the ductal system. Recently, because of the recurrent nature of the disease, the possibility of an autoimmune mechanism or a hypersensitivity state has been suggested. Indeed, the serum of patients with pancreatitis contains one or more precipitating antibodies that react with homologous pancreatic homogenate. The inability to create experimental pancreatitis by the injection of antiserum, coupled with the incomplete understanding of the mechanism of antibody formation, makes these observations only of experimental interest at this time.

Clinical Manifestations. Chronic pancreatitis begins most often in the third or fourth decade of life, but may begin in early childhood or old age. It is more common in men than in women and, unlike gallbladder disease, has no predilection for obese persons.

The clinical syndrome is readily divided into two stages. In the earlier stage the outstanding feature is recurrent attacks of severe abdominal pain (relapsing pancreatitis); the later stage is characterized by metabolic disturbances, e.g., *diabetes, steatorrhea,* and *azotorrhea,* with concomitant weight loss (chronic pancreatitis). Pseudocyst formation and pancreatic calcification are also common complications.

The abdominal pain in both stages is the same as that described in Ch. 645, and it may persist for days to weeks. Between attacks the patient may be asymptomatic except for occasional complaints of fullness, abdominal distention, and dull epigastric ache. As the disease progresses, the intervals between attacks become shorter, and the pain may eventually be continuous, requiring constant therapy with narcotics, which in some cases may lead to addiction. *Nausea, vomiting, chills, jaundice,* and *tachycardia* may be associated with these painful episodes.

Physical examination of the abdomen during an acute exacerbation may reveal the signs of acute pancreatitis. In addition, an epigastric mass may be found, representing either an inflamed pseudocyst of the pancreas or an enlarged fatty liver. With repeated attacks, the parenchymal disturbances become irreversible, and cause *steatorrhea* and *diabetes mellitus.* Loss of weight, despite a good appetite and a satisfactory caloric intake, results from faulty digestion and absorption of fat. The stools become bulky, frothy, glistening, and foul smelling, and they may increase in frequency (see Part XIV, Section Three). Sometimes, diabetes and/or steatorrhea first attracts attention to the existence of a destructive inflammatory process in the pancreas.

Course and Diagnosis. *Dysfunction of Acinar Cells.* The degree of disruption of acinar cells as reflected by serum levels of amylase and lipase depends on the stage of the disease. During an acute attack, levels of serum amylase and lipase are increased (see above). These enzyme values tend to rise early and return to normal after the acute attack. Elevations may persist when the attacks occur in rapid succession, when activity is prolonged, or in the presence of pancreatic ductal obstruction by stone or perisphincteric fibrosis. With repeated attacks, more and more of the gland is destroyed; thus late in the disease, even though active pancreatitis is present, serum levels of amylase and lipase do not rise. At this stage, abnormal fat excretion, usually greater than 7 grams of fat, and nitrogen excretion, greater than 2.5 grams of nitrogen daily, will be found.

Deficient secretion of pancreatic juice is consistently encountered in chronic pancreatitis. The characteristic changes in pancreatic juice are subnormal volume and bicarbonate concentration after the intravenous injection of 1 clinical unit of *secretin* per kilogram of body weight. The normal volume response is 2 ml or more per kilogram in 80 minutes, and the maximal bicarbonate concentration should reach 90 mEq per liter in any 20-minute specimen. Volume response as well as enzyme concentrations may be normal in the face of diminished bicarbonate except when the disease is advanced. It has not been established whether this dissociation indicates a differentiation of function between the acinar and intralobular cells or a differential loss of function of the secretory cells.

Disturbance of Function of Islet Cells. In the early stages of relapsing pancreatitis, acute attacks may demonstrate temporary islet cell dysfunction, characterized by *glycosuria, hyperglycemia,* and even abnormal glucose tolerance curves. However, with advanced disease, there is further destruction of islet tissue, and frank *diabetes mellitus* is encountered.

Roentgenographic demonstration of calcification in the region of the pancreas furnishes additional evidence of chronic pancreatitis (see figure in Ch. 645).

Forward and upward displacement of the stomach by inflammatory masses or pseudocysts with lifting of the antrum may be seen along with indenting or flattening of the duodenal sweep. Endoscopic pancreatocholangiograms may demonstrate strictures, stones, dilatation, narrowing, and tortuosity of the pancreatic ducts.

In the *differential diagnosis* of the acute painful episodes of chronic relapsing pancreatitis, the same causes of abdominal pain that were discussed in Ch. 645 must be considered. In the later stage, when steatorrhea and malabsorption are present, *adult celiac disease, carcinoma of the pancreas, and Whipple's disease* should be excluded (see Part XIV, Section Three). *Primary atrophy of the pancreas* should be excluded. This is a disease of unknown cause, appearing in both sexes after the fifth decade. The fully developed clinical picture of pancreatic atrophy is that of a deficiency syndrome characterized by steatorrhea, weight loss, normal or increased appetite, occasionally edema, anasarca, and diabetes mellitus. Abdominal pain, pancreatic calcification, and increase of serum enzymes are absent. By the time the disease is recognized clinically, the pancreas has undergone nearly complete atrophy. This observation underscores the great reserve capacity of this gland. The predominant chronic symptom, steatorrhea, usually begins insidiously and is generally mild. Edema and anasarca are frequently the initial signs in this disease. When there is an associated decrease of islet cells, diabetes mellitus of varying degrees develops. Exploratory laparotomy may be necessary for exact diagnosis.

Pathologically, this entity is characterized by almost complete disappearance of the acinar cells and, to a lesser extent, of the islets of Langerhans. Fatty replacement of the atrophic tissue may be an accompanying finding.

Painless Pancreatitis. Although clinically the hallmark of chronic pancreatitis is recurrent bouts of severe upper abdominal pain lasting for days or weeks and followed by epigastric tenderness for even longer periods, the disease may be painless. The diagnosis is to be suspected when one encounters a patient who, without having experienced abdominal pain, has the sequelae of chronic pancreatitis, i.e., pancreatic calcification, diabetes mellitus, and steatorrhea. All of these may coexist, or they may occur in various combinations. Infrequently, at operation, painless jaundice may be found to have resulted from obstruction of the common bile duct by a chronically inflamed pancreas. Recent evidence suggests that acute or subacute edematous forms of pancreatitis may occur without abdominal pain. In one review of 25 cases of chronic pancreatitis at necropsy in a 35-year period, the pathologist was unable to discover any clinical record that abdominal pain had occurred in 15 patients (60 per cent). Such observations suggest that acute edematous pancreatitis may occur more frequently than is suspected and that it may undergo progression either to irreversible change or to complete resolution without recognition by either physician or patient.

Treatment. Palliation of acute symptoms and efforts to terminate the acute exacerbation have been discussed in Ch. 645. Management comprises bed rest, limiting the oral intake of fluids, nasogastric suction, adequate sedation and narcotics, and appropriate fluids and electrolytes.

Nonsurgical Treatment. Medical means for preventing attacks of chronic relapsing pancreatitis and halting the progression of the disease are few and of limited value. Adherence to a bland, low-fat diet, avoidance of overeating, abstinence from alcohol, and the use of anticholinergics (propantheline bromide [Pro-Banthine], 15 to 30 mg, or methantheline bromide [Banthine], 50 to 100 mg, given one half hour before meals and at bedtime) are the principal measures. Management of pancreatic insufficiency secondary to progressive pancreatic destruction requires control of diabetes and of excessive losses of fat and nitrogen, with their associated abdominal distention, cramps, borborygmi, increased flatus, passage of large, malodorous and frequent stools, and loss of weight. The dietary intake of fat is usually restricted to 70 grams a day, and 120 grams of protein and up to 450 grams of carbohydrate are offered to compensate for the calories lost by restriction of fat intake.

Six to 9.0 grams of potent pancreatic extracts (Pancreatin, Viokase, or Pancrelipase, 0.3 gram) should be given in divided doses with meals, plus 0.6 gram with "snacks." Alternatively, 0.6 gram may be given while the patient is awake, a program which may especially benefit the patient with severe steatorrhea. In patients with high basal acid output, it may be helpful to give 30 ml of an antacid before each meal, or 0.5 gram of sodium bicarbonate when the hourly program is used. Sodium bicarbonate therapy should be avoided in older patients. With a greater degree of effective digestion, the insulin requirement may be increased. Nutritional replacement should include folic acid, vitamin B_{12}, calcium, vitamin D, and vitamin K, if these deficiencies are established (see Part XIV, Section Three). In rare patients vitamin B_{12} malabsorption is associated with pancreatic insufficiency and may be corrected by giving these extracts, or, very rarely, bicarbonate alone. Replacement of dietary triglyceride with medium-chain triglyceride (MCT) is effective in patients with pancreatic insufficiency. Although MCT can be given in appetizing form, its use is not very convenient. It may be important in the management of some patients, especially in the hospital, when early weight gain is a desirable goal.

Surgical Treatment. The large number of surgical procedures employed in the treatment of pancreatitis reflect the continued efforts to relieve pain and to prevent progression of the disease. Cholecystectomy, common duct exploration, sphincterotomy, sympathectomy, ablation of the celiac ganglia, and vagotomy with either a gastric drainage procedure or antrectomy and gastrojejunostomy, as well as a number of types of resective or drainage procedures on the pancreas, have been used with varying success. The best results seem to follow procedures which have been individualized to each patient, dependent on the gross findings of the pancreas at surgery and on operative and endoscopic pancreatography.

Surgical drainage of pancreatic pseudocysts has been relatively successful. Internal drainage of such cysts is preferable to external drainage because of the difficulties and unpleasantness of prolonged drainage of material rich in enzymes. Ninety-five per cent resection of the pancreas, leaving a thin rim of pancreas, with suturing of the main pancreatic duct close to the duodenal surface, appears to be effective. Bilateral thoracolumbar sympathectomy in selected cases for relief of pain is sometimes helpful, but the relief lasts for only two or three years.

It is clear that several variables complicate appraisal of the results of surgical therapy. Such variables include the number of spontaneous remissions, the presence or absence of disease of the biliary tract, the effect of previous operations, continued use of or abstinence from alcohol ingestion, the stage of destruction and the activity of the disease in the pancreas, the presence or absence of diabetes, calcification, and pseudocysts, and the degree of pancreatic insufficiency. Even though the results of different surgical procedures vary, it appears that surgery should be offered to patients with documented, well established but early phase chronic pancreatitis in an attempt to prevent or modify the inexorable sequelae of this disease process.

Prognosis. Replacement therapy has made the outlook good for those patients with chronic pancreatitis and pancreatic insufficiency whose painful attacks have ceased or become infrequent. Recurrent painful attacks will usually not be prevented simply by diet and antacid medication. The best hope lies in the surgical removal of a stone in the common bile duct, sphincteroplasty with unroofing or retrograde dilatation of the duct of Wirsung for fibrosis of the ampulla of Vater, or direct procedures of ductal drainage or pancreatic excision. In all other instances, especially if the patient partakes of alcohol, the prognosis for health and comfort is guarded.

Dixon, J. A., and Englert, E.: Growing role of early surgery in chronic pancreatitis: A practical clinical approach. Gastroenterology, 61:375, 1971.

Fitzgerald, O., Fitzgerald, P., Fennelly, J., McMullin, J. P., and Boland, S. J.: A clinical study of chronic pancreatitis. Gut, 4:193, 1963.

Littman, A., and Hanscom, D. H.: Current concepts: Pancreatic extracts. N. Engl. J. Med., 281:201, 1969.

647. CYSTIC FIBROSIS OF THE PANCREAS
(Mucoviscidosis)

Cystic fibrosis of the pancreas is a generalized inheritable disease of unknown cause, associated with dysfunction of all exocrine glands, including those that are mucus producing. Although characteristically a disease of early childhood, cystic fibrosis is now recognized in adolescents and adults. The increased longevity has been attributed to earlier diagnosis, to increased use of antimicrobial drugs and other measures that control pulmonary infection, so frequently the cause of death, and to the effectiveness of potent pancreatic extracts and medium-chain triglycerides.

Etiology. The basic defect in cystic fibrosis is not known. The most commonly accepted theories for its pathogenesis are abnormal physicochemical secretions, autonomic dysfunction, humoral abnormality, and ion transport dysfunction. It appears that a humoral substance present in the body fluids of cystic fibrosis patients attaches to or acts upon the membrane surface of exocrine gland cells. This interaction results in a change in the metabolic activity within the cell with a concomitant alteration of cell membrane permeability with increased protein and mucopolysaccharide synthesis.

Whatever the nature of the basic defect in cystic fibrosis, it is an inherited disease expressed only in the homozygous state without X-linkage (autosomal recessive).

Incidence. The incidence of patients with the fully manifested disease (homozygotes) is estimated as 1 per 2000 live births, and that of heterozygotes as 2 to 5 per cent of the population. Approximately 5 per cent of all patients with cystic fibrosis survive past the age of 17, and the incidence in the white adult population is estimated to be 1 per 40,000. It affects equally all whites, is rare in blacks, and is very rare in Orientals.

Pathophysiology. The pancreas of patients with cystic fibrosis is characterized pathologically by obstruction of the large and small pancreatic ducts with amorphous eosinophilic concretions, followed by dilation of the acini, degeneration of the parenchyma, and fibrosis. The islets of Langerhans remain intact. The deficiency or absence of pancreatic enzymes, especially trypsin, lipase, and amylase, results in *steatorrhea* and *azotorrhea.* Carbohydrates are better utilized. *Diabetes mellitus* occurs in this disease, but ketosis is rare. The majority of these patients can tolerate protein better than fats, making a positive nitrogen balance possible with increased protein intake.

Generalized bronchial obstruction with secondary infection is a cardinal manifestation of the pulmonary involvement. The process leads to acute and chronic bronchitis, peribronchitis, patchy atelectasis, bronchiolectasis and bronchiectasis, poor alveolar aeration, hypoxia, hypercarbia, pulmonary hypertension, and cor pulmonale. In spite of their unusual susceptibility to respiratory infections, these patients are capable of developing good levels of circulating antibodies to many pathogenic bacteria to which they are exposed, and have adequate immunoglobulin responses to infections. Discovery of the constant presence of hemolytic *Staphylococcus aureus* and, more recently, of

Pseudomonas aeruginosa in their sputum and nasopharynx suggests a metabolic basis for the striking association of these organisms and cystic fibrosis.

Sweat and Salivary Electrolytes. The eccrine sweat defect is characteristic of cystic fibrosis in the pediatric age group, and is rarely seen in other pediatric disease except adrenal cortical insufficiency. A striking increase in the levels of sodium, chloride, and to a lesser extent potassium is present in virtually all homozygote patients with cystic fibrosis. A similar but less striking elevation of sodium and chloride has been found in the saliva, hair, and nails of patients with cystic fibrosis (see below).

Biochemistry of Secretions. The abnormal secretions which occur in this disease have been recognized as the basic pathologic lesion which results in bronchial and pancreatic obstruction. The increased viscosity of these secretions has been attributed to an increased fucose and decreased sialic levels of the glycoproteins and to a complex formed by the glycoprotein and calcium. To date, there has been no delineation of the underlying biochemical defect.

Recent Observations. Recent observations which may have some bearing on the disease include the following: (1) The isolation of a heat-labile, nondialyzable factor in serum of patients with cystic fibrosis which chromatographs with the macroglobulin fraction. This substance disorganizes the ciliary rhythm in explants of respiratory epithelium. It has also been detected in parents of children with cystic fibrosis, but in a lower concentration. It is present in only 1 of 25 control sera, the expected incidence of heterozygotes in the population. (2) Easily recognizable cytoplasmic intravesicular metachromasia, found in skin-fibroblast cultures derived from children affected with cystic fibrosis of the pancreas. A similar cytoplasmic metachromasia was seen in 13 of the 14 parents, obligatory heterozygotes. The exact reason for the accumulation of the mucopolysaccharides within the fibroblasts is not known.

Clinical Manifestations. *Chronic pulmonary disease* is characterized by chronic cough, wheezing, thick tenacious sputum, and repeated respiratory tract infections, which are the hallmarks of the disease in both children and adults. With irreversible damage to the bronchi, the pulmonary disease becomes progressive and leads to the distressing picture of pulmonary insufficiency and eventually death through such complications as *lobar atelectasis, lung abscesses, cor pulmonale, pulmonary hypertension,* mediastinal and subcutaneous *emphysema, pneumothorax, hemoptysis,* and *asphyxia.* The chest is usually hyperresonant, with depressed diaphragms and increased anteroposterior diameter. Clubbing of the fingers may be present. *Pancreatic insufficiency,* characterized by abdominal distention, large, bulky, foul-smelling stools, diarrhea, and abdominal cramps, may appear alone or in combination with respiratory disease. Malnutrition may be severe despite an exorbitant appetite and an apparently adequate caloric intake. This may lead to shortened stature and delayed puberty if the disease is first discovered during adolescence.

Fecal masses that may be so persistent and tenacious as to produce acute mechanical intestinal obstruction occur frequently in older children and adults and are known as the *meconium ileus equivalent.*

Chronic involvement of the paranasal sinuses is a regular finding; with progressive pneumatization it leads to a nasal voice, postnasal drip, and formation of polyps that often require surgical removal. Enlargement of sub-

maxillary salivary glands, hypertrophic osteoarthropathy, and ocular lesions (dilatation of the arteries and veins of the fundus with hemorrhage and papilledema) have been reported.

Diagnosis. The diagnosis of cystic fibrosis should be based on four criteria: (1) increase in electrolyte concentration in the sweat, (2) absence of pancreatic enzymes on assay of aspirated duodenal contents, (3) chronic lung disease, and (4) family history of the disorder. Usually two criteria are sufficient to establish the diagnosis.

An accurate *quantitative sweat test* performed by stimulation of the sweat glands by iontophoresis of a cholinergic substance (0.2 per cent pilocarpine nitrate) is mandatory. The sweat chlorides and sodium thus obtained will reveal mean values of 30 to 40 mEq and 60 mEq per liter, respectively, in normal children; in children with fibrocystic disease the means will be 105 to 125 mEq for chlorides and 120 mEq per liter for sodium, respectively. Values for sweat chloride greater than 60 mEq per liter and for sodium greater than 80 mEq per liter are considered diagnostic for children with cystic fibrosis.

Even though sweat tests have been used in the diagnosis of cystic fibrosis in adults, they are thought to be of limited value in this group. However, persistent elevated levels of sodium and chloride in the sweat of an adult or of an adolescent after strict salt deprivation constitute valid criteria for the diagnosis of cystic fibrosis of the pancreas. The clinical picture and duodenal aspiration appear to be more specific in the diagnosis of adult cystic fibrosis. A thick, viscid secretion with profound deficiency of amylase, lipase, and trypsin is obtained on duodenal drainage. Chest roentgenograms reveal generalized obstructive *emphysema* and *bilateral bronchopneumonia.* A family history of cystic fibrosis is of great diagnostic aid.

In patients with no lung involvement, but with symptoms and signs of *malabsorption,* the diagnosis of cystic fibrosis must be differentiated from that of *celiac disease,* with which it is most often confused, and from other causes of malabsorption. In celiac disease a jejunal biopsy will show virtual absence of villi, the d-xylose absorption test will be abnormal, urinary excretion of 5-hydroxyindolacetic acid will be elevated, and a clinical and biochemical response to a low gluten diet will be obtained (see Part XIV, Section Three).

Rectal biopsies in some patients with cystic fibrosis have shown widely dilated crypts packed with mucus, which can appear lamellated.

Treatment. Therapy of the chronic lung disease with various antimicrobials deserves major emphasis, because pulmonary involvement dominates the clinical picture and determines the fate of the patient. The choice of the antimicrobial regimen is the same as the treatment of chronic bronchitis and is discussed in Ch. 503.

Pulmonary physiotherapy in the form of postural drainage of each lobe three to four times daily often provides effective drainage of the involved lobe. In recent years, continuous nocturnal mist nebulization in a tent, with an appropriate small droplet nebulizer with a solution of 10 per cent propylene glycol, has been recommended. Agents such as deoxyribonuclease and N-acetyl cysteine have been recommended for daily nebulizations with the hope of diminishing the viscosity of pulmonary secretions. Pulmonary surgery is rarely indicated, because the pulmonary disease is usually bilateral and generalized.

The malabsorption seen in these patients can be ameliorated by a large intake of food with moderate restriction of fat intake and addition of pancreatic extracts to the diet. Concentrated pancreatic extract (Viokase or Pancrelipase) given hourly during the waking hours is satisfactory therapy (see Part XIV, Section Three). Medium-chain triglyceride preparations may aid in further decreasing steatorrhea and thereby help growth, development, and weight gain.

Prognosis. The prognosis in this disease is improving as early diagnosis and treatment become more effective. The pulmonary involvement usually determines the fate of the patient. Approximately 50 per cent of affected children die before the age of 10 years, more than 80 per cent before the age of 20 years, and most of the remaining survivors before 30 years of age.

Meconium ileus produces symptoms of intestinal obstruction shortly after birth and, unless surgically corrected, proves fatal. However, patients who survive the operation have essentially the same outlook as those without this complication.

Uncontrollable *gastrointestinal bleeding,* secondary to portal hypertension, and massive *salt depletion* in hot weather are additional hazards. In the older age group, *sinusitis* with its complications (notably polyps) has been a serious problem. Although pancreatic insufficiency is clearly present, digestive symptoms are minimal, and patients are able to tolerate an unrestricted diet. Sexual maturation proceeds normally, but with slight delay. A small number of women with this disease have given birth to healthy children. Only 2 to 3 per cent of males with cystic fibrosis who reach adulthood are fertile because of defective development of the wolffian duct derivatives.

Brusilow, S. W.: Cystic fibrosis in adults. Ann. Rev. Med., 21:99, 1970.
Danes, B. S., and Bearn, A. G.: A genetic marker in cystic fibrosis of the pancreas. Lancet, 1:106, 1968.
Lobeck, C. C.: Cystic fibrosis. *In* Stanbury, J. B., Wyngaarden, J. B., and Fredrickson, D. S. (eds.): The Metabolic Basis of Inherited Disease. New York, McGraw-Hill Book Company, 1972, pp. 1605–1626.
Spock, A.: Cystic Fibrosis. Current theories concerning pathogenesis. Minn. Med., 52:1429, 1969.

648. CARCINOMA OF THE PANCREAS

The diagnosis of malignant tumors of the pancreas and the periampullary region is a challenging and perplexing problem. The protean manifestations of this disease and retroperitoneal location of the gland make early diagnosis and treatment difficult. It is especially unfortunate that even the newer diagnostic techniques fail to establish an early diagnosis, because carcinoma of the pancreas is now the *fourth* leading cause of death among all sites of cancer in the United States.

Pancreatic carcinoma is predominantly a disease of males, with a sex ratio of 2 to 1. The mean age of onset of symptoms is 55 years. The most common tumors are adenocarcinomas, arising mostly from ductular epithelium. In two thirds of the cases, the head of the pancreas is the site; the body and tail contribute approximately 20 and 10 per cent, respectively. Extension of the tumor is by direct invasion of the remaining gland or duodenum and by adherence to adjacent structures. Extension via the perineural lymphatics and those accompanying the pancreaticoduodenal vessels is the rule. Metastases are most frequent to the regional lymph nodes and to the liver. Other sites of metastases, in their order of frequency, are lungs, intestines, adrenals, bone, and other organs.

Although not established, there are three frequently cited predisposing factors: chronic pancreatitis (especially calcific), heavy alcohol consumption, and diabetes mellitus.

Clinical Manifestations. *Symptoms.* Despite the still widely held opinion that carcinoma of the pancreas and ampulla of Vater is painless, *pain* is the most frequent first symptom. The pain is of three general types: (1) colicky, and frequently located in the right upper quadrant of the abdomen; (2) steady, dull, and midepigastric, radiating through to the low back; and (3) paroxysmal, near the umbilicus but felt over a wide area of the back, in the anterior chest, and over the abdomen. Other characteristic features of the pain are its severity, steady progression, and exacerbation at night, as well as its nonrelationship to normal events of the digestive cycle. This pain pattern may be due to the propensity of these tumors to infiltrate along nerve trunks and ducts with an accompanying desmoplastic response which tends to envelop and encase nerves, ducts, and blood vessels. The next most significant symptom is *jaundice,* which occurs in about 75 per cent of cases of carcinoma of the head of the pancreas, and is the symptom which causes most patients to seek therapy. It is almost always persistent and steadily progressive, and can become extremely deep, with accompanying pruritus. *Weight loss* occurs invariably and is usually extreme, frequently averaging more than 5 pounds per month. Gastrointestinal symptoms such as *anorexia, nausea,* and *vomiting,* although not specific for carcinoma of the pancreas, are very common complaints. An aversion for or complete rejection of food, rather than true anorexia, is considered distinctive of cancer of the pancreas. A feeling of *gastric fullness* and *flatulence* is common. Diarrhea, which may or may not be associated with steatorrhea, has been observed in 15 per cent of cases. *Constipation* is more common and may be related to the anorexia. *Bleeding* into the gastrointestinal tract, manifested by occult blood in the stool, is noted in about 50 per cent of cases, and is especially significant in lesions involving the stomach or duodenum and in carcinoma of the ampulla. *Thrombophlebitis* or phlebothrombosis, especially of the migrating type and resistant to anticoagulants, may be the first symptom in patients with carcinoma of the body and tail of the pancreas. *Emotional disturbances,* especially depression with crying spells, anxiety, intractable insomnia, and premonition of serious illness, are said to be unusually common with carcinoma of the pancreas, especially of the body and tail. Abnormal glucose tolerance or even frank *diabetes* is more common in carcinoma of the pancreas than in the general population. Uncommon manifestations of carcinoma of the pancreas include hypoglycemia, hypercalcemia, inappropriate antidiuretic hormone (ADH) secretion, excessive production of adrenocorticotrophic hormone (ACTH), and the carcinoid syndrome.

Physical Findings. Abnormal findings that may be noted on physical examination are evidence of weight loss, an enlarged, frequently hard liver, a distended gallbladder, jaundice, tenderness or resistance in the upper part of the abdomen, and a mass in the region of the pancreas. The gallbladder is visibly or palpably enlarged in about 50 per cent of patients with jaundice caused by carcinoma in contrast to patients with jaundice and chronic pancreatitis. Ascites and peripheral edema are noted in about 20 per cent of cases. Tumors arising in the tail of the pancreas may obstruct the splenic vein, leading to splenomegaly and hypersplenism; may obstruct the portal vein and produce esophageal varices; or may encase the splenic artery, resulting in an arterial bruit in the left upper quadrant. Subcutaneous fat necrosis, appearing as tender, subcutaneous nodules originating on the lower extremities and later involving other areas of the body, accompanied by polyarthralgia and eosinophilia, have been found only with the rarer *acinar cell carcinoma*. The high lipase content of these tumors may be responsible for this phenomenon.

Diagnosis. *Roentgenographic Findings.* Roentgenographic studies of the upper gastrointestinal tract may reveal a number of abnormalities owing to the tumor, such as changes in the mucosal pattern and rigidity of the duodenal wall, widening of the duodenal loop, "padding" of the gastric antrum, and disturbed motor activity of the small bowel. Occasionally, evidence of invasion of the duodenal wall—the "inverted 3" sign of Frostberg—will be noted. The ability to detect early changes is enhanced by *hypotonic duodenography,* performed with anticholinergic agents, glucagon or secretin. Spiculation (fine, sharply pointed serration along the inner aspect of the duodenal loop), flattening of folds, and nodular indentations along the inner aspect of the duodenal loop are the most reliable findings suggestive of pancreaticoduodenal cancer. Similar changes may occur in patients with chronic pancreatitis and collateral circulation secondary to portal hypertension. In the presence of obstructive jaundice, percutaneous transhepatic cholangiography will aid in the diagnosis of carcinoma of the head of the pancreas. These roentgenographic findings are invariably manifestations of progressive neoplastic change in the pancreas and surrounding structures.

Clinical Laboratory Findings. Early obstruction of the pancreatic duct will occasionally elevate the serum lipase and amylase. It is clear, however, that if the block has been prolonged, with resultant destruction of the acinar cells of the pancreas or replacement of the gland with tumor, these levels may be low. Unfortunately, significant change in either direction is infrequent. *Leucine aminopeptidase, nonspecific alkaline phosphatase,* and *5-nucleotidase* are elevated in carcinoma of the pancreas when there is an element of obstruction of the common bile duct or metastasis to the liver.

The *glucose tolerance test* is abnormal in 25 to 50 per cent of patients with carcinoma of the pancreas and is a more frequent abnormality than frank glycosuria or fasting hyperglycemia. Steatorrhea is found in approximately 10 per cent of the cases as judged by abnormal chemical fat excretion.

Pancreatic Drainage. Analysis of duodenal secretion after injection of *secretin* or *secretin followed by pancreozymin* is potentially of great diagnostic value. Precise localization of an obstructive lesion is possible. If both biliary and pancreatic secretions are absent, the obstruction must be in the head of the pancreas or in the ampulla of Vater. If the pancreatic and biliary flows are normal in volume, the lesion is not obstructive. If pancreatic secretions are ample despite absence of bile, the lesion must be in the extrahepatic biliary system, or duodenal obstruction is being bypassed by an anomalous pancreatic duct. With partial obstruction of the pancreatic duct, the quantity of bicarbonate and enzymes in the pancreatic secretion decreases, but the relative concentrations remain the same. Cytologic examination for malignant cells after secretin enhances the chance of positive diagnosis. The accompanying table presents a summary of the findings in carcinoma of the pancreas, chronic pancreatitis, and diseases of the biliary tract and liver after secretin stimulation. A significant rise in serum amylase or lipase, or both, after injection of secretin and pancreozymin strongly indicates pancreatic obstruction.

Radioactive Photoscanning. Radioactive photoscanning of the pancreas, utilizing ^{75}Se selenomethionine, results in decreased photoscan concentration in the area of tumors of the pancreas, as well as in pseudocysts. Uptake by the liver and inability to differentiate benign from malignant processes have limited the value of this technique.

Pancreatic Angiography. Pancreatic angiography, especially superselective angiography of vessels close to, or directly into, the pancreatic vessels, appears to help in establishing the diagnosis of carcinoma of the pancreas. The most reliable angiographic findings are irregular ar-

Significance of the Secretin* Test

	Total Volume Flow	Maximal HCO$_3^-$ Concentration	Total Enzyme Secretion	Biliary Pigment Response
Normal	2 ml or more/kg body weight/80 min	90 mEq/L in any 20-minute specimen	Normal	Normal
Pancreatic carcinoma				
Head	Greatly diminished	Normal to diminished	Normal to diminished	—
Body	Moderately diminished	Normal	Normal	—
Tail	Normal	Normal	Normal	—
With obstruction	Diminished	Normal to diminished	Normal to diminished	Obstructive (no bile)
Chronic pancreatitis				
Moderate	Normal	Diminished	Diminished to normal	Normal
Severe	Diminished	Diminished	Diminished	Normal
Biliary tract				
Common duct stone, stricture, or neoplasm	Normal	Normal	Normal	Obstructive (no bile)
Intrahepatic				
Hepatitis, cholangitis, and cancer	Normal	Normal	Normal	Normal (nonobstructive)
Cirrhosis and hemochromatosis	High	Normal	Normal	Normal

*With 1 clinical unit of secretin/kg of body weight.

terial or venous encasement, abrupt cut-off or occlusion of vessels, and occasional neovascular vessels. In the late phase of selective angiography the venous changes of occlusion or encasement of the splenic and superior mesenteric veins and their branches are best seen. Angiography also provides information regarding gallbladder size, liver metastases, and enlarged intrahepatic bile ducts.

Retrograde Cholangiopancreatography. Direct cannulation of the ampulla of Vater via fiberoptic duodenoscopy and retrograde cholangiopancreatography is a new and useful approach in experienced hands in evaluating patients with suspected pancreatic carcinoma. The abnormal features observed by these techniques are strictures, obstruction, dilatations, displacements, and nonvisualization of the pancreatic ducts.

Carcinoembryonic Antigen. Preliminary studies have shown that the carcinoembryonic antigen is positive in 90 per cent of patients with proved pancreatic carcinoma and 30 to 70 per cent positive in other digestive tract tumors. The significance of this finding awaits further evaluation.

Carcinoma of the pancreas can usually be diagnosed either grossly or by biopsy at operation, although such biopsy of the pancreas frequently reveals only inflammation. This finding is usually due to the fact that pancreatic carcinoma is surrounded by inflammatory tissue.

Treatment and Prognosis. The natural course of disease, whether it is primarily in the head or in the body and tail of the pancreas, is one of swift progression to death after onset of symptoms, regardless of whether metastases or contiguous extensions are present, and is uninfluenced by any surgical procedure except radical extirpation in suitable cases. Unfortunately, the over-all resectability rate is less than 25 per cent for adenocarcinoma of the head of the pancreas, and is far less for tumors of the body and tail. Surgical exploration should be performed on patients with suspected localized pancreatic carcinoma to determine the size and spread of the tumor, because resection of periampullary tumors has a five-year survival rate of 40 per cent. Palliative surgery for relief of vomiting, jaundice, and pruritus can be accomplished by cholecystojejunostomy and provides an average survival of 12 months. Recent evidence suggests that a combination of 5-fluorouracil (as a single weekly intravenous injection of 10 mg per kilogram of body weight) with 50 mg of testolactose (Teslac) three or four times daily with meals resulted in a significant prolongation of life of over a year. Medical therapy is usually directed at maintenance of good nutrition, with insulin, pancreatic enzyme replacement, and medium-chain triglycerides. The pain invariably requires narcotics. With increasing severity of the pain, serious consideration should be given to nerve blocks, rhizotomy, or cordotomy to ensure the patient's comfort. Carcinoma of the body and tail is almost never resectable, and five-year cures are extremely rare.

Cotton, B.: Cannulation of the papilla of Vater by endoscopy and retrograde cholangiopancreatography (ERCP). Gut, 13:104, 1972.

Ferrucci, J. R., Jr., and Eaton, S. B.: Radiology of the pancreas (current concepts). N. Engl. J. Med., 288:506, 1973.

Gullick, H. D.: Carcinoma of the pancreas: A review and critical study of 100 cases. Medicine, 38:47, 1959.

Waddell, W. R.: Chemotherapy for carcinoma of the pancreas. Surgery, 74:420, 1973.

Watson, D. W.: Pancreatic carcinoma (clinical seminar). Am. J. Dig. Dis., 15:767, 1970.

Section Five. INFLAMMATORY DISEASES OF THE INTESTINE

CHRONIC INFLAMMATORY DISEASES OF THE INTESTINE

Henry D. Janowitz

649. INTRODUCTION

Chronic inflammatory bowel disease includes a group of disorders characterized by acute and chronic inflammatory changes in all portions of the small and large intestines. The best and oldest known is *ulcerative colitis,* an inflammatory disease confined to the colonic mucosa and submucosa. Almost as well characterized is *regional ileitis* or *regional enteritis,* an inflammatory disease involving the entire wall of a portion of small gut. A more confusing group of inflammatory diseases involve both colon and ileum *(ileocolitis).* Furthermore, some disease which involves the colon but not the small bowel never-theless exhibits all the distinguishing features of regional enteritis of the small bowel, and thus differs from ulcerative colitis. Therefore some have designated this latter disease as *regional enteritis of the colon,* whereas many physicians simply designate regional enteritis, ileocolitis, and regional enteritis of the colon as Crohn's disease (after the man who precisely described regional enteritis) to avoid confusion without commitment to any etiologic theory.

650. REGIONAL ENTERITIS (Crohn's Disease of Small Bowel)

Definition. Regional enteritis is a chronic inflammatory disorder of the intestinal tract of unknown origin which may appear at any site but characteristically involves the terminal ileum (hence its original name, "terminal ileitis"). Clinically, regional enteritis is a diarrheal disease often associated with fever, abdominal pain, weight loss, abdominal masses, and anal or perianal lesions. The disease is also characterized by the frequent formation of enteric fistulas or sinus tracts. Characteristically the regional enteritis produces linear ulcers and deep fissures in the gut; inflammation (characterized by aggregations of inflammatory cells and sarcoid-like granulomas) may extend through the full thickness of the bowel wall.

Etiology. Forty years after its original description (in 1932), regional enteritis remains a disease of unknown origin, although considerable search has been made for causes. No infectious agent has been isolated, although the resemblance of its histopathology to that of noncaseating tuberculosis was noted early. The psychosomatic approach to this disorder has evoked little interest and very little supportive research and documentation. The recent heavy emphasis has been on investigations of the immunologic reactivity of patients with Crohn's disease. No characteristic or significant alterations in serum immunoglobulins have been described. Impaired cutaneous responses to tuberculin, stressed in the earlier literature, are not supported by recent studies. We have noted an absolute lymphopenia in some patients. With a widely accepted test of delayed hypersensitivity, most patients are not sensitized to dinitrochlorobenzene. Further evidence of depressed lymphocyte immunologic competence has been obtained by several groups who have shown that the circulating lymphocytes have a diminished response in vitro to phytohemagglutinin, suggesting impairment of thymic derived lymphocytes. This depressed responsiveness was present in an equal number (40 per cent) of patients with ulcerative colitis as well. Controversy exists regarding immunologic cross-reactivity between sarcoidosis and Crohn's disease. The active international standard Siltzbach-Chase Kveim antigen does not give a positive skin reaction in patients with Crohn's disease. More important is the observation that tissue from Crohn's disease patients introduced into the footpad of the mouse produces a local granulomatous reaction. Confirmation is required, but this evidence suggests that Crohn's disease may be due to a transmissible agent, with a long latent period, in a susceptible population.

Incidence, Prevalence, and Epidemiology. Epidemiologic studies tend to lump all forms of Crohn's disease into one, regardless of the location of the disease, and have the added difficulty of separating Crohn's disease of the colon from ulcerative colitis. It has its highest incidence in the United States, is thought to be infrequent in Central Europe, and is recorded frequently in Britain and the Scandinavian countries. It appears to be seen only infrequently in Africa, Asia, and South America.

Variable *incidence rates* (rate of occurrence of the disease per 100,000 persons at risk per year) have been reported. In the Baltimore study of patients over 20 years of age which utilized hospital cases only, the incidence in males was 2.5 and in females 1.2, for an average of 1.8. In the Oxford study of Evans and Acheson (1967), the incidence for both men and women was approximately 1.0.

Evidence regarding *prevalence* (all the patients affected with this disease at any one moment per 100,000 persons at risk) is difficult to obtain. Based on 36 reports, Mendeloff has estimated the range of prevalence as between 20 and 40 per 100,000 population. Fragmentary evidence suggests that the incidence of Crohn's disease may be rising in the western world.

There is no significant difference in regard to sex. In contrast to ulcerative colitis, Crohn's disease under age six appears to be extremely rare. The first incidence mode can be seen to occur between 15 and 20, with a second mode at age 55 to 60. In the United States, blacks and Indians are at low risk. Evidence has been accumulating that the incidence of inflammatory bowel disease in Jewish patients is strikingly higher than in the non-Jewish populations. In Baltimore, in Crohn's disease, the rate was six times higher for Jewish males and three times higher for Jewish females than the rates for non-Jews. Although these higher rates in Jews might be due to social, dietary, or genetic factors, current epidemiologic studies offer no explanation. There is a slight preponderance of urban over rural setting for Crohn's disease. Nevertheless, exhaustive study of socioeconomic status, for the United States, has demonstrated no significant difference for patient and control populations. Perhaps farmers are less vulnerable because of some occupational factor.

Genetics. Since the search for an exogenous (environmental) etiology in Crohn's disease has been fruitless, recent attention has been devoted to the problem of genetic susceptibility. No simple mendelian genetic mechanism has been forthcoming. A considerable number of family aggregations have been reported, the most frequent combination being two affected siblings, with parent (more often mother) and child combination a close second. This evidence may argue more for common environmental factors than for genetic influence. The literature contains no reference to a husband and wife both being affected, and studies on twins (concordance has been recorded in seven pairs of monozygotic twins) do not contribute to the solution of this problem. Family incidence of Crohn's disease is low; 1 in 15 to 1 in 50 patients have an affected first-degree relative. Although this incidence in first-degree relatives is higher than in the general population, lack of control data limits this interpretation. The association of Crohn's disease with other disorders of an inherited nature is pertinent. In one series eczema and hay fever were particularly common, possibly pointing to a genetically controlled immunologic mechanism. A stronger association exists with *ankylosing spondylitis,* which has some hereditary features, and which may appear before the clinical manifestations of the bowel disease. The association of Crohn's disease and ulcerative colitis within families is well recorded, but the uncertainties of this relationship do not advance our understanding. An interesting and curious feature in families with these diseases is that the index patient with Crohn's disease often has relatives with ulcerative colitis, whereas many series with families of ulcerative colitis patients have no relatives with Crohn's disease. One conclusion is that the genetic influence on etiology is likely to be polygenic, alleles at several different loci providing a genotype which determines susceptibility or resistance to environmental factors, although a virus-like maternal factor is a possibility.

Pathology. All areas of the gastrointestinal tract may be involved in regional enteritis, including rare lesions of the oral cavity and esophagus. Lesions of the stomach and duodenum occur more frequently, and the terminal ileum is the most common site of the disease. Although isolated regional jejunitis does occur, combined lesions of ileum and jejunum are more frequent. The lesion in the colon is discussed below (Crohn's disease of the colon). The *perirectal fistula* should be considered an integral part of Crohn's disease of the small bowel because of its frequency. All layers of the small intestine are involved, as are the regional lymph nodes. The bowel wall is remarkably thickened and rigid. Skip areas of disease are frequently seen with intervening normal bowel. Loops of affected small intestine may be adherent; frequently fistulas exist between these adherent loops. In addition, sinus tracts may extend into a thickened and inflamed mesentery, producing an inflammatory mass. Fistulas from the ileum to cecum and/or sigmoid are very common, but others may reach to the skin (often in old operative scars, occasionally to the navel), bladder, ureter, vagina, flank, and even the right hip joint. Frequently perianal inflammation arising in the crypts of Morgagni leads to anal and perirectal fistulas. An inflammatory mass may encase the ureter, producing ureteral obstruction and hydronephrosis. Superficial discrete ulcers which extend to form confluent linear ulcerations are characteristic of the macroscopic appearance of the intestinal mucosa, as are deep fissures which may extend through all coats and serve as the basis of fistulas. Microscopically, aggregations of inflammatory cells involving all layers predominate, with the sarcoid-granuloma most characteristic when present. Such granulomas are noncaseating collections of epithelioid cells (large mononuclear phagocytes) and multinucleated giant cells whose nuclei are arranged around the periphery or collected at the poles of the cell (Langerhans type) (Fig. 1). When a large number of sections are searched, granulomas have been found in the bowel wall in up to 75 to 85 per cent of patients.

The regional lymph nodes, often containing granulomas, are enlarged owing to nonspecific reactive changes. In one series, 38 per cent of lymph nodes contained granulomas, and in 63 per cent granulomas were present in the bowel wall. Further, 20 per cent of nodes may have this lesion without granulomas present in the bowel. Not all areas of the bowel and all regional nodes are equally affected in the same specimen.

A few available ultrastructural studies have not contributed to pathologic understanding or differential diagnosis but have confirmed the curious finding of neuronal hyperplasia in the mesenteric plexus.

Pathogenesis. An acute inflammatory reaction in the ileum has been well documented (albeit with little histologic confirmation), but most studies have demonstrated its disappearance without any of the sequelae of Crohn's disease, so that the transition from acute to chronic forms of regional enteritis is not recorded. Bacteriologic

and serologic evidence has associated some cases of acute ileitis with infection with the bacteria *Yersinia enterocolitica*, formerly known as *Pasteurella X*. (We need, however, to distinguish this situation from lymphoid hyperplasia of the ileum, frequently seen in the small bowel x-rays of youngsters studied for abdominal pain.)

Since all portions of the gastrointestinal tract from mouth to anus may participate in the pathologic process, an important question is the extent of dissemination. It is extremely rare to obtain characteristic pathologic changes in jejunal biopsies of patients with regional ileitis, and we have never had a positive rectal biopsy in patients with ileitis except when a local rectal or anal lesion was also present. Resected specimens show few lesions 6 cm beyond the edge. Although some scattered microscopic lesions have been noted in grossly normal colon adjacent to classic regional ileitis, in general the disease is localized and segmental rather than universal. Any scheme of pathogenesis must take into account other histologic features of this disease: hyperplastic reactive lymph nodes, the development of granulomas in regional nodes or in ectopic lymph follicles, inflammatory reactions in lymphatics and perilymphatics, ectasia of lymph channels, and the development of submucosal lymphedema secondary to obstructed lymphatics. Although the pathologic process may spread from ileum to adjacent large bowel by extension along sinus tracts with fistula formation, retrograde extension over any long segment does not occur in the absence of surgical intervention. Repeated surgical experience has demonstrated that in portions of the involved ileum excluded from the intestinal stream, completely diverting "bypass" operations lead quite regularly to subsidence of the inflammatory reaction and to recurrence of the pathologic process most frequently in the new "terminal ileum." One might postulate from this line of evidence that the exciting agent of the tissue reaction in Crohn's disease may be present in the intestinal stream, moving down and becoming more concentrated as it reaches the ileocecal area. Delay behind the ileocecal sphincter and above the anal sphincter favors its absorption and entry into submucosal lymphatics and lymphoid tissue with the characteristic tissue response in these loci.

Clinical Manifestations. The classic presentation of regional enteritis is that of a young person, in his or her late teens or early twenties, who has not been feeling well for an ill-defined time but whose indisposition has suddenly worsened. Whereas the past history may have included an occasional episode of cramps and diarrhea frequently ascribed to dietary indiscretions or "nerves," the patient now complains of more constant abdominal pain and more persistent diarrhea. The pain is most frequently cramping and periodic, and is often worse after eating; it is confined principally to the right lower quadrant; occasionally it radiates into the right upper thigh. At times it is more persistent, dull, and annoying. The stools become more frequent, small, loose to watery, often waking the patient at night as well, but are free of gross blood. Appetite clearly declines, and parents become alerted and alarmed by the obvious weight loss, which may be considerable. Often there is a low-grade fever, usually, however, not recorded at home. There may be a history of a recent appendectomy (performed for right lower quadrant pain and tenderness) or a slowly healing perirectal abscess.

Histories of some "allergic" phenomena, including pollen sensitivities and possibly intolerance to milk,

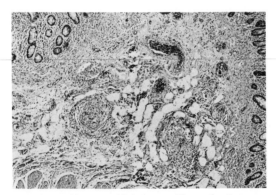

Figure 1. Regional enteritis. Submucosa of ileum, showing noncaseating granulomas with multinucleated giant cells. Hematoxylin and eosin stain, × 150.

seem to be present more frequently than by chance, but no obvious association with other so-called "immune" diseases exists. There may be a history of recurrent crops of aphthous ulcers of the mouth which may not only plague the patient but may also herald an acute exacerbation. Less frequently, persistent fever, malaise, and anorexia may overshadow the abdominal complaints, and the patient may be labeled as having "fever of unknown origin" or rheumatic fever (especially in the younger child). Failure of sexual and somatic development may be the sole clinical feature.

Less frequent is the patient who presents with fecal fistula in the unhealed scar of an appendectomy, or persistent mucopurulent drainage from the wound. Equally striking are the extraintestinal clinical manifestations of regional enteritis. These include joint symptoms, ranging from fleeting *arthralgias* to obvious *arthritis* and tender, swollen, hot joints, particularly knees and ankles. Backaches may also precede intestinal symptoms, later found to be due to *ankylosing spondylitis*. Skin manifestations include *erythema multiforme*, and especially the painful *erythema nodosum* of shins and feet and the rarer *pyoderma gangrenosum*. An intense *conjunctivitis* (often phlyctenular in nature) and uveitis and iritis with eye pain and visual disturbances may also accompany an underlying chronic intestinal inflammatory disorder. Except for ocular involvements, these extraintestinal manifestations parallel the intensity of the bowel symptoms. Less frequent concomitants include biliary colic caused by *cholelithiasis*, and renal colic associated with either showers of uric acid crystals in the urine or the presence of mixed, especially oxalate, *kidney stones*.

Although the presentation thus far appears to stress the youth of patients, the symptoms may begin at any age; indeed, there seems to be a bimodal distribution, with a second peak in the forties and fifties. A frequent and distressing clinical manifestation is delayed reappearance of general and intestinal symptoms after surgical intervention. Such clinical behavior heralds the discovery of recurrent enteritis, readily confirmed radiographically.

Physical Examination. Physical examination often reveals a well-developed young adult, with some evidence of recent weight loss, moderate pallor, and lassitude. Clubbing of the phalanges is usually not present unless there is extensive involvement of jejunum and ileum, or of ileum and colon. A large number of patients have either a palpable loop of thickened inflamed ileum or a clear-cut mass in the right lower quadrant. Pedal edema may be present. The cutaneous, joint, and eye manifestation cited above may be present. Examination of the rectal area may disclose nothing abnormal or may reveal a perianal or perirectal abscess; evidence of the prior surgical attempts to treat perirectal abscesses and fistulas; or, in patients with colonic involvement, the curious florid indolent ulcers of the anus which often make rectal examination difficult. Proctoscopy demonstrates a normal mucosa except in those with Crohn's disease of the rectum and anus. In children, evidence of retarded growth and delayed secondary sexual characteristics may be striking.

Laboratory Studies. Laboratory findings may include evidence of a mild to moderate anemia; the white cell count is usually normal except in the presence of suppuration. Absolute lymphopenia may be present. Albuminuria is rare and may indicate renal amyloidosis. The stools may reveal the existence of occult blood. The erythrocyte sedimentation rate, a crude but useful index of disease activity, is elevated. The serum albumin may be lowered, and often the gamma globulin fraction is elevated. Occasionally elevated blood uric acid levels in both females and males are present. Minor abnormalities in liver function tests may indicate the presence of fatty liver; more marked elevation in serum alkaline phosphatase or SGOT or SGPT determinations indicates the associated pericholangitis seen more frequently in ulcerative colitis and ileocolitis. Serum vitamin B_{12} levels and the Schilling test of vitamin B_{12} absorption may be abnormal, and variable amounts of unabsorbed fat can be detected by measuring fecal fat in a 72-hour collection (see Part XIV, Section Three); however, anorexia often precludes adequate fat intake, making this determination meaningless. The d-xylose test, a measure of carbohydrate absorption, is usually within normal limits.

Mechanisms of Disease Manifestations. The weight loss in regional enteritis is due in large part to failure of caloric intake, with a smaller contribution from failure of absorption. The reduced caloric intake derives mainly from loss of appetite but also from the generally restrictive diets that physicians recommend or patients adopt. The diarrhea of regional enteritis may arise from a multitude of causes: (1) failure of diseased ileum to resorb bile salts can result in excessive passage of bile salts into the colon where these products inhibit colonic fluid and electrolyte resorption; (2) loss of small bowel absorbing surface, as the result of disease or surgical resection, may produce general malabsorption with increased fecal output; (3) partial intestinal obstruction (caused by intestinal stenosis or mechanical obstruction from inflammatory masses or adherent loops of bowel) may produce diarrhea either as a result of excessive net secretion of fluid and electrolytes by dilated proximal bowel or as a result of intestinal stasis and bacterial overgrowth (see Part XIV, Section Three); and (4) lactase deficiency may be accentuated by the impaired nutritional status of these patients, because all brush border enzymes are decreased in the patients who are most ill (see below).

Absorptive Defects. Fat malabsorption is correlated with the length of inflamed or resected ileum, the incidence of steatorrhea increasing in those with more than 90 to 100 cm involved or resected. The mechanism is ascribed to the loss of bile salts (failure to be reabsorbed) in this portion of the gut, with resultant reduction of the bile salt pool and thus hepatic secretion of the bile salts needed for proper micelle formation and pancreatic lipase activity. Bacterial overgrowth in those with stenosis, stricture, fistulas, or surgically created blind loops may also contribute to steatorrhea. The bacterial overgrowth of colonic organisms is believed to deconjugate the bile salts needed for fat absorption. Carbohydrate absorption is usually quite normal (at least as measured by the d-xylose test) except in patients with jejunitis, or in those with stricture formation and consequent overgrowth of luminal bacteria which may metabolize this sugar. Lactose maldigestion secondary to intestinal lactase deficiency is seen in some patients, many of whom have themselves eliminated milk and milk products from their diets; the diarrhea of lactase deficiency in such patients arises from (1) the osmotic effects of unabsorbed lactose and (2) a lowered colonic pH (from bacterial breakdown products of lactose) which inhibits colonic water and electrolyte resorption. Vitamin

B_{12} malabsorption is related to the loss of normal ileal absorptive mechanism. When the length of involved or resected ileum exceeds 90 cm, the Schilling test is abnormal in all; thus malabsorption of vitamin B_{12} is correlated with fat malabsorption. The increased incidence of gallstones is ascribed to the alteration in bile salt pool and the secretion of "lithogenic" bile secondary to failure to reabsorb bile salts in the ileum (see Part XIV, Section Three).

Renal Calculi. Urinary uric acid crystals are more common in these patients. Several defects are believed responsible for this finding: (1) some patients have hyperuricemia, thought to result from increased catabolic rates; (2) the urine is more frequently acid, perhaps reflecting excessive loss of bicarbonate in the diarrheal stools; and (3) loss of excessive stool water results in the formation of a more concentrated urine. Some patients have in addition increased levels of blood uric acid, presumed to be associated with breakdown of tissue. Other types of renal calculi likewise appear to be correlated with fluid loss through the gut. The recognition of increased oxalate excretion in the urine and presence of oxalate stones has revealed a new metabolic complication. Ascribed at first to increased conversion of the glycine moiety of the deconjugated bile salts into the oxalate pathway, hyperoxaluria now appears to result from increased intestinal absorption of dietary oxalate.

Clinical Complications. Despite their frequency, certain manifestations of the disease are considered as complications. These include *local suppurative complications,* arising from extension of sinus tracts into the adjacent mesentery and giving rise to right lower quadrant abscess formation. These sinus tracts may also extend into the right psoas region, giving rise to a psoas syndrome of low backache, pain in the right upper thigh, and flexion deformity with limp. Healing takes place by a marked fibrotic reaction with narrowing of the intestinal lumen and *stricture formation,* accounting for the paradoxical increase in crampy abdominal pain with subsidence of systemic symptoms. The syndrome of incomplete intestinal obstruction rarely leads to complete obstruction unless there is a complicating local abscess or an impacted foreign body, usually of dietary origin (e.g., corn kernels, berries, peach pits). *Free perforation* of the ileum is reported with increasing frequency in recent years; usually, however, perforation of the bowel is confined by surrounding tissues and leads to sinus formation. *Massive hemorrhage* occurs in less than 5 per cent of patients with Crohn's disease of the small intestine, occasioned at times by stercorous ulceration proximal to a stenotic area. *Fistulization* may be considered an integral part of the basic disease; however, fistulas to the urinary bladder deserve some additional comment. Passage of frank feces through the urethra is quickly recognized by the patient. The passage of air or gas through the urethra, however, may require detailed specific inquiry by the physician. (This is also true of the passage of gas from the vagina.) Despite the frequently expressed fear of ascending urinary tract infections in the presence of an ileovesical fistula, patients tolerate this condition surprisingly well.

Renal Complications. *Uric acid* and *oxalate stones* have already been stressed. Right *hydronephrosis* and *hydroureter* from obstruction caused by a retroperitoneal inflammatory mass usually create few symptoms, and the urine is rarely infected. *Renal amyloidosis* is more common in Crohn's disease than in ulcerative colitis.

The writer has seen five instances in a series of 17 patients dying of ileitis in which the renal amyloid contributed to death.

Although *carcinoma* of the ileum or jejunum is rare, the 20 reported instances of adenocarcinoma in longstanding Crohn's disease of the small bowel, especially in excluded intestine, suggest that this is more than a matter of chance. Cancer in a "bypassed" loop is even more treacherous to diagnose, because these segments are almost always stenotic.

Neurologic Complications. Neurologic complications in the form of "startle reactions," tetany, and grand mal seizures, have been observed, usually on the basis of electrolyte and fluid disturbances, mainly hypocalcemia and hypomagnesemia. The clinical setting is one of a patient with profuse diarrhea, receiving steroids and intravenous fluids free of magnesium. We have seen a few patients with concurrent multiple sclerosis, one of whom had a diffuse vasculitis. Three of our younger patients suffered thrombosis of the middle cerebral artery without evidence of atherosclerosis.

Diagnosis. The history of malaise, anorexia with weight loss, and abdominal pain, especially in the right lower quadrant associated with increasing nonbloody diarrhea, together with the finding of thickened loops of intestine or a mass in the right lower quadrant, makes the diagnosis of Crohn's disease of the small bowel highly probable. The finding of an anal lesion or perirectal abscess or fistula or a cutaneous fistula increases the certainty of this diagnosis. Short of resection of bowel for histologic confirmation, characteristic x-ray findings in the small bowel (Fig. 2) confirm the diagnosis. Although the pathology of early regional enteritis may be insufficient to make the disease evident on barium contrast meal, patients with Crohn's disease should not be treated without x-ray confirmation. If the terminal ileum fails to visualize on barium enema examination because of failure of the barium to reflux from colon into ileum, an upper gastrointestinal series with small bowel follow-through is indicated. Failure to visualize ade-

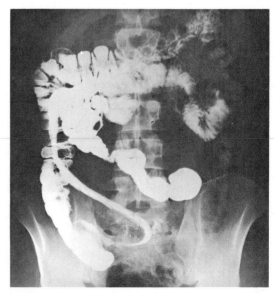

Figure 2. Involvement of terminal ileum in regional enteritis. Note narrowing of lumen with hoselike configuration of ileal contours.

quately the terminal ileum with barium by mouth is the most frequent reason for the failure to find radiographic confirmation of a strong clinical impression. The characteristic x-ray finding is segmental involvement of the bowel, most frequently the terminal ileum; at times, several segments of the ileum may be separated by "skip areas" of normal intervening bowel. Thickened, edematous mucosa with a "cobblestone" appearance reflects the submucosal cellular aggregates. Narrowing of the lumen, the so-called "string sign," represents a functionally contracted irritable segment or, in a later stage of the disease, fibrotic stenosis. Progressive thickening of the bowel wall stiffens the loops, which may be widely separated because of the thickened swollen mesentery, agglutinated by serosal inflammatory changes, or draped over a right lower quadrant inflammatory mass. The presence of sinus tracts and fistulas to adjacent loops of small or large bowel, especially the cecum or sigmoid colon, are classic findings. With the development of stenosis, dilatation of proximal loops of gut appears, together with pseudodiverticula. In the less common ileojejunitis, similar changes are found throughout contiguous loops of jejunum and ileum.

Rectal biopsy is rarely of use except when amyloidosis is suspected or an obvious anal lesion is present. Biopsy of the perirectal fistula may reveal the characteristic granuloma.

Differential Diagnosis. The differential diagnosis includes *acute appendicitis, appendiceal abscess, cecal diverticulitis* with localized perforation, *ovarian carcinoma, carcinoma* of the *cecum* invading the ileum, *lymphosarcoma, Hodgkin's disease, lymphoid hyperplasia, ileocecal tuberculosis, ileal carcinoid,* and the *"backwash" ileitis* of ulcerative colitis. In diagnosis of regional jejunitis, *nodular lymphoid hyperplasia* with dysgammaglobulinemia, the *erosive jejunitis* of *Zollinger-Ellison syndrome,* nonspecific *erosive jejunitis,* and *metastatic melanocarcinoma* must be considered. The differential diagnosis for *regional ileojejunitis* includes *nodular lymphoid hyperplasia* with dysgammaglobulinemia, *lymphosarcoma,* the *diffuse nonerosive ileojejunitis* reported on occasion in patients with *sprue, diffuse nongranulomatous ileojejunitis,* and prior *severe ischemia* of *small intestines.*

Of this list only a few diseases present real problems. *Acute appendicitis* may be extremely difficult to separate from an acute episode of regional ileitis in the absence of an antecedent history of bowel problems. Exploration is the method of choice if any doubt exists; current experience justifies removal of the normal appendix to prevent confusion in the future if the cause of the patient's syndrome is Crohn's disease of the ileum; fecal fistulas arise mainly from unsatisfactory surgical technique in manipulating the ileum, not the appendiceal stump. Extremely rarely, Crohn's disease may be confined to the appendix. Patients with known Crohn's disease of the ileum only rarely develop acute appendicitis.

Appendiceal abscess frequently cannot be distinguished from regional enteritis with right lower quadrant mass, and the roentgenographic findings in the ileum may mimic ileitis. Occasionally the disappearance of the abscess and clearing of ileal x-ray changes under the influence of antimicrobial drugs may resolve this clinical dilemma.

Lymphosarcoma usually occupies longer segments than the ileum, often extending across the ileocecal valve; although the appearances are similar in some respects, roentgenograms usually show no luminal narrowing as noted in regional ileitis. Further, and most important, the clinical picture is quite different.

Ileocecal tuberculosis is a rare disease in the United States and therefore is rarely considered in the differential diagnosis in patients without pulmonary tuberculosis. However, this diagnosis is important to consider in patients with pulmonary tuberculosis and ileocecal disease, or in areas of the globe where tuberculosis—especially milk-borne tuberculosis—is very common. At times the differential diagnosis cannot be made except at laparotomy. A negative tuberculin test in a patient with ileal disease is more likely found with Crohn's disease than with tuberculous enteritis. Moreover, tuberculous enteritis most often involves ileum and cecum; thus patients with disease confined to the ileum most often have Crohn's disease, but since ileocecal disease is found both in granulomatous colitis and in tuberculous enteritis, the distribution of the lesions is rarely helpful in distinguishing these two diseases.

Carcinoid of the ileum usually presents no problem, except when it is invasive, and the x-ray appearance may resemble regional enteritis. The innocuous *lymphoid hyperplasia* of the ileum seen in young patients is easily distinguished from the acute inflammatory changes seen in regional enteritis. This is true also of the roentgenographic changes of *nodular lymphoid hyperplasia* with dysgammaglobulinemia.

Some special problems arise in patients with known regional enteritis. The problem of right lower quadrant suppuration and appendicitis has been discussed. The coexistence of ileitis and cancer of the right ovary and/or cecum has tripped the unwary. One must be alert for the development of *adenocarcinoma* of the *ileum* in the stenotic phase of ileitis, or in patients who have had "bypass" operations in the past.

"Backwash ileitis" is a poor but widely used term to describe the changes in a short segment of terminal ileitis associated with universal ulcerative colitis, and diagnosed by barium enema. It should be distinguished from regional enteritis and does not represent clinically significant disease. It probably represents a direct extension of the associated ulcerative colitis through a patulous ileocecal valve, and is confined to the mucosal surface. It is easily separated from classic regional ileitis, but its distinction from ileocolitis of the Crohn variety may be difficult.

Eosinophilic gastroenteritis is also important in the differential diagnosis, especially of ileojejunitis. This illness, usually associated with a significant blood and tissue eosinophilia representing a response in some to a dietary allergy, may present with diarrhea, malabsorption, and protein-losing enteropathy. The stomach, duodenum, and entire small bowel may be involved alone or in various combinations. Although it is superficially similar to Crohn's disease, the intestinal films do not present with the characteristic infiltrated thickened loops of the latter disease; further, strictures and fistula are not present.

Treatment. There is no known specific therapy for this disorder. Accordingly, treatment is essentially supportive. It is empirical; its efficiency is still undetermined; and it involves review of the patient's activity, dietary intake, life style, and personal habits. It also requires consideration of a number of drugs currently employed in the management of ileitis and imposes important decisions regarding the necessity of surgical intervention. It also requires an awareness of the mortality rate, ranging from 5 to 18 per cent.

Medical Management. All approaches to the medical management of the patient with regional enteritis begin with an awareness of the high rate of recurrence (up to 50 per cent in some series) after surgery. Accordingly, the current therapeutic stance of most experienced clinicians in this field is one of surgical conservatism unless the patient cannot be managed medically in the presence of a continuously unfavorable course or some of the more dramatic complications.

Although it has yet to be shown that prolonged rest favorably affects this illness, management of the patient must begin with an evaluation of the patient's energy balance. Caloric intake usually being suboptimal, some restriction of energy expenditure is clearly in order. This is an individual matter, but all patients must establish and accept some limitations of activity. Although the physician must avoid being arbitrary, he will have to be firm in some situations.

Efforts to improve the patient's nutritional status are necessary and difficult. The victim of this illness needs to be encouraged to take a well-balanced, high caloric, high protein diet. Care must be taken to discourage food faddism and avoid arbitrarily conceived medical dietary advice. The patient's ability to tolerate milk and milk-containing products should be the criterion for lactose intake rather than a lactose tolerance test. Most patients have already established their tolerance by the time they see the physician. In the presence of profuse diarrhea or stenotic lesions, some reduction of the noncaloric residue of the diet is prudent. For patients with marked reduction in absorptive mucosal surface, medium-chain triglycerides are a reasonable supplement; however, they are often of limited use because of patient reluctance to ingest the oil (free from any lactose fillers) owing to the induction of diarrhea. Vitamin supplementation is rational in view of the restricted food intake of many patients (see Table 5 in Part XIV, Section Three).

The anemia of enteritis is rarely due only to vitamin B_{12} deficiency and iron deficiency from bleeding but rather to the effects of the chronic illness on bone marrow synthesis. When there is significant loss of the ileum vitamin B_{12} replacement is required. Oral iron preparations seem to be tolerated poorly by these sick individuals, and a parenteral form such as Imferon is useful.

The symptomatic treatment of abdominal pain, cramps, and diarrhea is an integral part of management. Judicious and temporary use of analgesics, anticholinergics, and opiates is very frequently required. The overuse of deodorized tincture of opium or the diphenoxylate and atropine combination (Lomotil) may lead to dependence and addiction.

Antimicrobial Therapy. Antimicrobial drugs modify the symptoms and course of ileitis very little. Local suppurative complications involving gram-negative organisms of the bowel require the appropriate drug; ampicillin, in doses up to 4 grams daily by mouth or 4 to 6 grams intravenously, provides an acceptable regimen. When stenosis, stricture, or surgical bypass with blind loops or small bowel to colon anastomoses leads to intestinal overgrowth with colonic organisms, tetracycline (0.25 gram every four to six hours) may be helpful in treating the attendant vitamin B_{12} deficiency and/or steatorrhea (see Part XIV, Section Three). Its use should be closely supervised, however, because of the risk of staphylococcal enterocolitis.

For a long time the relatively poorly absorbed sulfonamide derivatives, succinylsulfathiazole and phthalylsulfathiazole in doses of 1.0 to 3.0 grams every six hours were commonly prescribed. More recently, salicylazosulfapyridine (Azulfidine) in doses of 1.0 to 2.0 grams every six hours is the drug more widely used. This sulfonamide whose metabolites are concentrated in the intestinal tissues is a relatively poor antimicrobial agent. The mechanism of its limited usefulness in ulcerative colitis is not known, and its value in Crohn's disease is yet to be deomonstrated. This fact, however, has not prevented its therapeutic popularity, which may reflect a measure of physician desperation. Adverse reactions to this drug, which include nausea, headache and vomiting, skin rashes, high fever, leukopenia and agranulocytosis, hemolysis, and occasional jaundice, may occur in up to 15 to 20 per cent of patients. Recent studies relate the majority of toxic reactions to the serum levels of sulfapyridine achieved in those taking 4 or more grams daily. Since sulfapyridine is acetylated after absorption and conjugated as a glucuronide in the liver before being excreted in the urine, the majority of patients with adverse effects phenotypically acetylate slowly.

Anti-inflammatory Agents: Corticotrophin (ACTH and Adrenal Corticosteroids. Because these anti-inflammatory agents appear to affect the course of ulcerative colitis favorably, and because ileitis and ulcerative colitis have certain nonintestinal manifestations (arthritis, uveitis, erythema nodosum), adrenocorticosteroids, especially prednisone, are now also widely used in these diseases. They improve the patient's sense of well-being and often stimulate his capricious and depressed appetite. It is doubtful, however, that they have been shown to influence the long-term course of the illness for the better, and they do not affect the histopathology of the disease. Indeed, their hazards impose serious limitations for their long-term use, and until the National Cooperative trial in Crohn's disease gives its definitive answer one would do well to avoid their use if possible. Occasionally, in some desperately ill patients, especially those with diffuse ileojejunitis or recurrent enteritis after multiple resections, the use of corticotrophin intravenously (25 units every eight hours continuously) may be more helpful than the conventional doses of prednisone, 40 to 60 mg daily or on alternate-day schedules. However, enthusiasm for corticosteroids must be tempered by the realization that in at least one good recent study a higher than expected mortality for Crohn's disease was related in part to prolonged corticosteroid therapy; however, the series included many patients who were extremely ill.

Immunosuppressive Therapy. Azathioprine (Imuran) was introduced for the therapy of Crohn's disease with fistulas in 1969. It has been used sporadically since then, but convincing evidence of its value is yet to be presented. In daily doses of 2 mg per kilogram, this writer has observed no catastrophes when the white blood count remained above 3500. Immunosuppression requires at least three weeks' therapy, and the long-term undesirable effects of this therapy are unknown. Although only patients with renal transplants have thus far been reported to develop lymphomas while being treated with azathioprine, the possible risks of therapy when balanced with therapeutic effects do not justify using this agent except as part of a controlled study or as a measure of desperation.

Surgical Therapy. The early expectation that surgical excision would lead to a permanent cure in regional ileitis was soon followed by an era of disillusion based upon increasing evidence of recurrence. Recognition of the limited value of steroid therapy, however, has refocused attention on the effects of surgical therapy. Current evidence indicates that many recurrences develop during the first two to three years after operation, followed by a period of three or four years with little increase in rate of recurrence, only to be followed by a period of more frequent recurrences. Two to three years after resection and ileocolostomy, perhaps 30 per cent of patients have a recurrence; 40 to 50 per cent have a recurrence at five years, and perhaps as many as 60 per cent at ten years. The recurrences are usually on the ileal side of the ileocolonic anastomosis; in some the recurrences are solely radiographic; in others clinical severity parallels the original disease. Since as many as half of the surgically treated patients are faring well at the end of five years, this form of treatment should not be deprecated, especially in the young person when growth and education are critical.

If surgery is elected, the operation of choice is resection of the diseased ileum with an ileoascending colostomy to preserve the right colon for water absorption. These patients may have some period of watery diarrhea after resection with removal of the ileocecal valve. This often responds to bile salt binding therapy with cholestyramine (Questran, 1 to 4 grams daily in divided doses). The mortality and morbidity of this procedure is no higher than that from the older bypass operation (side tracking of the involved ileum with exclusion), and eliminates the risk of the late development of neoplasm in the excluded loop. When a suppurative complication in the right lower quadrant makes resection hazardous, especially an abscess or inflammatory mass encroaching on the right ureter, a bypass operation is to be preferred. Few factors are known to influence recurrence rate after surgery. The rate is higher in patients whose symptoms first appeared below the age of 40, and is higher the more extensive the involvement of the small bowel.

The indications for surgery are the obvious ones of intestinal obstruction, massive hemorrhage, and fistulization to the bladder. An internal fistula between adjacent loops of bowel or an intra-abdominal mass per se does not necessarily indicate surgery. A cutaneous fistula, often after exploratory laparotomy and appendectomy, may on occasion close under treatment with sulfonamides but usually requires surgery. The more difficult clinical problem is the patient who fails to improve or deteriorates under our current supportive management. This patient can be remarkably helped, albeit often temporarily, by resection. On occasion, severe or nonhealing perirectal fistulas are an indication for resection of proximal ileal disease.

Prognosis. Regional enteritis is a disease of quite variable course. It has the interesting characteristic of not spreading in a retrograde fashion in the absence of surgery. Extension to sigmoid or cecum by fistulization, however, is common. Over-all, mortality ranges from 5 to 18 per cent; however, it is from 4 to 12 per cent when related to the ileitis itself. In view of current unsatisfactory medical therapy, it is not surprising that the majority of patients ultimately come to operation, many of whom have multiple procedures. Thus in one surgical center, of 332 patients with Crohn's disease (large as well as small bowel), 295 sooner or later were submitted to surgical treatment, with an operative mortality of 5.8 per cent.

651. ULCERATIVE COLITIS

Ulcerative colitis is an inflammatory disease of unknown cause which involves the mucosa of the colon. Confined in some patients to the rectum, involving the left colon in many, it may also involve the entire colon. Its onset may be acute and fulminant, and its course often continues chronically in an intermittent or continuous form. Diarrhea is a common symptom and bleeding is an almost constant concomitant symptom, because friability in the mucosa is an integral feature of the illness. Although ulcerative colitis is capable of the most startling resolution and reversal, the more typical course is one of unpredictable recurrences. Thus like the more recently defined regional enteritis, ulcerative colitis constitutes an enigmatic clinical entity.

Incidence, Prevalence, and Epidemiology. Estimating the incidence and prevalence of ulcerative colitis is difficult. Most estimates are based on studies of hospitalized patients. Some patients—particularly those with disease confined to the rectosigmoid colon (ulcerative proctitis)—have such mild symptoms that they are not commonly hospitalized and hence are not accounted for in such surveys. Also, physicians are reluctant to examine and investigate thoroughly patients with mild chronic diarrhea or children with diarrheal disorders; thus some of these patients may have undiagnosed ulcerative colitis. Finally, granulomatous colitis cannot always be distinguished on clinical grounds from ulcerative colitis.

Incidence Rates (rate of occurrence of the disease per 100,000 persons at risk per year). In a study of the Oxford area, the incidence was 7.3 for females and 5.2 for males for an average of 6.5. In a Baltimore study of hospitalized patients over 20 years of age, the corresponding figures were 5.2 and 3.9, for an average of 4.6. To these figures should be added the incidence of ulcerative proctitis, which may range from 3 to 6.

Prevalence (all the patients affected with this disease per 100,000 persons at risk). In the United Kingdom, the data suggest that for each patient admitted to a hospital for the first time with ulcerative colitis, there were 12 patients at large in the population with the same disease. The range of prevalence for this disease has been estimated for proctitis as 40 to 80, and for ulcerative colitis as 35 to 70.

Although inflammatory bowel disease as a whole is being increasingly recognized, there is no evidence to support impressions of increasing incidence. In the United States, between 200,000 and 400,000 persons have been estimated to suffer from the disease, with between 25,000 and 30,000 new cases each year. In almost all series there is a preponderance of females over males. The first peak of incidence occurs between the ages of 20 and 25, as in Crohn's disease. Again, almost all series show a second rise in incidence in the decade from age 50 to 60. Kirsner and co-workers have suggested that this second peak may be related to mesenteric vascular disease. In the Baltimore study the urban black population was one third as likely to have ulcerative colitis as the white population. Among veterans of World War II in England and the United States, the incidence of ulcerative colitis among Jewish patients was two to four times greater than might be expected. In the Baltimore study the frequency of ulcerative colitis among Jews was 3.5 times the rate for non-Jews. Although impressions exist that the ulcerative colitis population has a higher socioeconomic and educational status than the general population, careful analysis does not confirm this.

Genetics. As with Crohn's disease, there is no simple mendelian genetic mechanism operative. Aggregation of families includes both ulcerative colitis and Crohn's disease; the incidence of familial disease is higher for Crohn's disease alone than for ulcerative colitis alone. In a recent study from Chicago, only 4 per cent of the control population had a family history of such bowel disease, whereas 11 per cent of those with chronic inflammatory disease had a family history of the same. Jews dominated this group and with onset at significantly lower age (less than age 20). Ulcerative colitis has been recorded in eight pairs of monozygotic twins with concordance in five. The association of *ankylosing spondylitis* with ulcerative colitis is similar to that of Crohn's disease. It may be that these two diseases have different environmental causes but occur in the same families because the genotypes determining susceptibility share genes in common.

Etiology. In the more than 100 years since Samuel Wilks separated nonspecific ulcerative colitis from epidemic forms of dysentery, many etiologic agents and concepts have been advanced. None has been convincingly demonstrated. No virus, bacterium, or protozoon has been shown to be specifically related to the disease. Occasionally after an epidemic of bacillary dysentery, a few individuals will be left with chronic ulcerative colitis, but this occurs in only a small minority. The disease occurring simultaneously in husband and wife is extremely rare, indicating that an environmental agent alone is not responsible. The relatively isolated dramatic response of the disease to withdrawal of milk from the diet has always raised the question of specific allergic factors.

Since all experienced clinicians have been impressed with exacerbation of ulcerative colitis in the setting of tensions, conflicts, and anxiety of their patients, much emphasis has been placed on the role of psychosomatic factors in initiating and perpetuating this disorder. George Engle, the most persuasive recent investigator of this aspect, has stressed the obsessive-compulsive immaturity of these patients and the dependency on parent or parent surrogate figures, and emphasized the "hopeless and helpless" reaction they experience at the loss of these figures by death, rejection, or removal. In similar approaches it is assumed that disturbances in secretory, vascular, and motor responses are mediated through the autonomic nervous system. Why only the colon should respond is obscure. More recently, these concepts have been both challenged and ignored by workers in the field. In the Baltimore study, in which the control population (patients with the irritable colon syndrome) and those with ulcerative colitis were meticulously interrogated for psychosomatic factors in their history, the results did not demonstrate that patients with inflammatory bowel disease had unusual health histories or significantly more of those factors which could be interpreted as evidence of life stresses and failure to adapt to them; indeed, there were more such factors in the patients with the irritable colon syndrome. Attention should also be paid to the failure of experienced clinicians to document the transition of the irritable colon syndrome into ulcerative colitis. However, the relatively crude investigative techniques used in these studies do not meet the criticism of more sophisticated psychiatrists. The inconclusive reports of the results of psychologic therapy cannot be interpreted in terms of etiology. Although the psychosomatic concept remains unproved, this does not gainsay the need to understand the emotional setting in which ulcerative colitis appears and exacerbates.

Immunologic mechanisms now occupy the forefront of investigations into the etiology, encouraged both by the concomitant presence of manifestations of hypersensitivity states such as *erythema nodosum, arthritis,* and *uveitis* and by the response to steroid therapy. More than 15 per cent of patients have high titers of circulating antibodies against colonic epithelial mucopolysaccharide antigens, and against certain cross-reacting bacterial lipopolysaccharide antigens, especially those of *E. coli* $01^.4$. These antibodies can bind to intestinal epithelial cells in vitro. But it has never been possible to demonstrate that these antibodies possess cytotoxic activity, or even that these antibodies are bound to colonic tissue in vivo. Anticolon antibodies also have been found in clinically healthy relatives of colitis patients, and classic ulcerative colitis has been reported in a patient with agammaglobulinemia. There is presently no evidence that anticolon or cross-reacting antibacterial antibodies in ulcerative colitis play any pathogenetic role in the disease. Individual patients with ulcerative colitis may have elevated serum levels of IgA and of secretory IgA in particular, in the presence of longstanding disease; but as a group, ulcerative colitis patients have no statistically different serum immunoglobulin levels or patterns from the general population, nor is there any consistent correlation between immunoglobulin patterns and disease severity. There is, however, some evidence to suggest that circulating immunoglobulins might be sequestered in diseased bowel, because a fall in concentration can be demonstrated across inferior mesenteric artery and vein during active disease. Moreover, serum IgM has been shown to rise acutely after bowel resection. Formation of antigen-antibody complexes in ulcerative colitis consumes the C1q component of complement. Pathologic processes might bind or catabolize immunoglobulins in diseased tissue in ulcerative colitis and initiate the formation of circulating immune complexes. Although no role has been identified for immunoglobulins in pathogenesis, circulating immune complexes could underlie such extracolonic manifestations as arthritis or erythema nodosum.

Lymphocytes from patients with ulcerative (and granulomatous) colitis are cytotoxic to intestinal epithelial cells in vivo and in vitro. There is also a cytophilic IgM antibody in the serum of patients with ulcerative colitis that confers this property upon normal lymphocytes. Neither lymphocyte cytotoxicity nor circulating cytophilic antibody reflects a basic underlying immune disorder in ulcerative colitis, because both disappear very rapidly when the inflamed colon is removed. The depressed responses of circulating lymphocytes to phytohemagglutinin in both Crohn's disease and ulcerative colitis in some patients appear also to be a secondary phenomenon.

Pathology and Pathogenesis. In contrast to the characteristic histopathologic features of Crohn's disease, the pathologic changes in ulcerative colitis are even more nonspecific. Throughout its course ulcerative colitis generally remains a disorder of the mucosa and submucosa of the colon. Under unusual circumstances the histopathologic process may extend through the muscular layer to reach the mucosa and may penetrate through the serosa.

The increasing use of rectal biopsy has made it possible to document the early pathologic features. The earliest lesion appears to involve the base of the crypts of Lieberkühn in the form of infiltration with polymorphonuclear leukocytes at the tip of the crypts with degenerative changes in the overlying epithelial cells. This is followed by the development of crypt abscesses with extension of the polymorphonuclear infiltrate into the crypts and necrosis of the crypt epithelium. A more heterogeneous cellular inflammatory reaction supervenes, involving lymphocytes, plasma cells, mast cells, and eosinophils, with vascular dilatation and engorgement. These so-called microabscesses of the crypts may next coalesce and separate the overlying mucosa from the lamina propria and its blood supply, producing ulceration of the mucosal surface and even its denudation. The extension of crypt abscess and ulceration results in the formation of residual islands of mucosa with undetermined edges. These fragments of epithelial tissue constitute the pathologic basis of *pseudopolyps*. Concurrent healing leads to some collagen deposition, but fibrosis is not prominent. Hypertrophy of the muscularis mucosae may also develop. Ineffective healing and regeneration lead to the presence of thin atrophic epithelium. These features are far from specific; similar changes have been described in a variety of infectious colitides, including *shigellosis* and *gonococcal infection,* and even in *amebic colitis.* However, the chronic recurrent nature of the changes, especially the crypt abscesses, and the development of either the atrophic mucosa or the multiple pseudopolypoid reactions are quite characteristic. Shortening of the bowel with narrowing of the lumen, loss of haustrations, and stricture formation in chronic cases appear to result infrequently from fixed fibrotic changes but more often from spasm and hypertrophy of the muscularis mucosae, which may account for their reversibility on occasion. Such reversals stand in marked contrast to the course of luminal narrowing in Crohn's disease.

In more severe forms the inflammatory necrotizing process may extend through all coats of the colon, leading to the clinical situation known as *toxic megacolon.* Here all elements are involved in the inflammatory reaction, and a vasculitis (swelling of the vascular endothelium, inflammatory changes in vessel walls, necrosis of blood vessels, and local thrombosis) is prominent. The inflammatory changes in the neural elements (especially ganglion cells) and musculature of the colon may account for the characteristic colonic dilatation in toxic megacolon. The extension of the pathologic process to the serosa, with deep ulceration through the muscular walls, together with loss of tone, sets the stage for free or walled-off perforations.

Grossly, the anatomic extent of the process differs widely. Perhaps as many as half the patients have the disease limited to the rectum alone, *ulcerative proctitis,* whose microscopic pathology in no way is different. Of the remainder, perhaps less than half involve the rectum and the left side of the colon from sigmoid to most of the descending colon. About one third of all patients have universal colitis. In about one fifth of the patients with involvement of the entire colon there is some superficial disease in the terminal ileum for a distance of 8 to 12 inches. The pathologic nature of "segmental colitis" involving portions of the right colon is more problematic; when significant ileal disease is present, patients are often found to suffer from Crohn's disease or regional (granulomatous) enterocolitis.

Clinical Manifestations. The wide diversity of clinical presentations is part of the highly variable course of this disease. Its onset may be most insidious or of catastrophic abruptness. In some patients (perhaps half) the initial symptoms of malaise, mild lower abdominal discomfort with slight increase in frequency, and softening of the stool with small amounts of blood are vaguely recalled. In another quarter of patients, the onset is more intense and more easily dated, often related by the patient to an upper respiratory infection, a "stomach virus," or a specific emotional trauma. More intense lower abdominal cramping pain, an increased number of loose to watery stools containing blood and often waking the patient at night, and mild systemic symptoms of easy fatigability and low-grade fever are characteristic of this moderately severe group. Perhaps in 15 per cent of patients there is an onset with profuse bloody diarrhea, high fever up to 39.5 to 40° C and severe abdominal diffuse pain. Such a sudden onset portends a grave illness.

Paralleling the diversity of the mode of presentation is the variability of the clinical course. A very small group will have but one attack and go into prolonged remission for years. The majority will have a chronic intermittent course with asymptomatic remissions between recurring attacks. The remainder (perhaps 5 to 15 per cent) will have a chronic, continuous, progressively relentless course. The outlook for survival after any episode is directly related to its severity. In an attack of mild disease the patient has few stools and lacks tachycardia, fever, and loss of appetite, whereas the patient with severe disease has severe bleeding, fever, anemia, and lowered serum albumin. Patients with mild disease rarely die, but as many as 35 per cent of those with severe attacks may die.

Those with mild colitis may also have vague lower abdominal distress, minor variations in the number and consistency of stools, and small amounts of rectal bleeding. This group of patients have few or no constitutional symptoms, except for perhaps a slight falling off of appetite. The patients usually continue their full activities, and if bleeding is not stressed, their symptoms may be interpreted as part of the irritable colon syndrome. Although in some the pathologic process is confined to the rectum or rectosigmoid, the mucosa of the entire colon may be involved. The group with the more limited distal disease, "ulcerative proctitis" or "idiopathic proctitis," may have all the attendant clinical features, both local and extraintestinal, as the more diffuse variants. Usually, however, the effects of illness are not striking, and reassuringly it tends to remain localized. Further, the immediate and long-term mortality in this variant is negligible and the risk of cancer is much reduced.

Intermediate in intensity, morbidity, and mortality between the "proctitis" variety and the severe form which may be fulminant and catastrophic is the group whose disease is moderate, about one quarter of patients. Diffuse lower abdominal pain, increasing number of stools both by day and — more troublesome — by night, tenesmus, more marked rectal bleeding than in the mild form, some anorexia, and low-grade fevers (37 to 37.5° C) are associated with disinclination to carry on usual activities.

The most dramatic and frightening presentation of ulcerative colitis is the severe disease which fulminates. Without any antecedent history, or in the first attack, or in the chronic course of mild and moderately severe ulcerative colitis, the illness begins explosively with high fever, profuse bleeding, marked diarrhea with profuse watery stools, associated with diffuse abdominal crampy pain, and prostration. With the extension of the pathologic process throughout all the coats of the colon, marked dilatation of the colon, "toxic dilatation," or "toxic megacolon," supervenes (Fig. 3). Death in an acute attack of ulcerative colitis is most frequent in this group.

In all forms of ulcerative colitis certain extracolonic manifestations may accompany the disease: they include *arthritis, uveitis,* and such skin manifestations as *erythema nodosum* and *pyoderma gangrenosum.* History-taking in the ulcerative colitis patient does not reveal any strikingly associated diseases except ankylosing spondylitis. In contrast to Crohn's disease, the extraintestinal manifestations (skin, eyes, joints) rarely precede the intestinal symptoms.

Physical Examination. In the mild forms, examination usually reveals no significant findings. In the more severe forms the physical examination reveals the ill, dehydrated, acutely or chronically sick and feverish patient. There may be diffuse abdominal tenderness, but except in patients with "toxic megacolon" or perforation, there is no evidence of peritonitis, localized or general. The spleen is rarely palpable. The skin, eye, and joint manifestations can at times all be present on physical examination. Clubbing of the fingers and toes is rare in the absence of concomitant small bowel involvement.

Laboratory Studies. Routine studies reveal a degree of blood loss which may be profound. Marked leukocytosis is usually present, as high, indeed, as 35,000 to 40,000. Remarkable increases in platelets may also be recorded in these same patients, and may play a role in thromboembolic phenomena. A hemolytic anemia may occur, usually in those receiving salicylazosulfapyridine (Azul-fidine), but a Coombs-positive autoimmune hemolytic anemia may be present unrelated to sulfonamides. A prolonged prothrombin time may result from associated liver damage, or from the effects of antimicrobial drugs on intestinal bacterial synthesis of vitamin K. A reduction in platelets and fibrinogen levels may document disseminated intravascular coagulation. Fluid, electrolyte, and serum losses lead to marked reduction in levels of serum potassium and albumin. The flat film of the abdomen usually reveals some gas in the colon, and allows visualization of the thickened edematous colonic wall.

Mechanisms of Disease Manifestations. Rectal bleeding arises from friability of the colonic mucosa and deeper ulceration. The cause of this friability (manifested by the elicitation of bleeding when the surface is gently stroked at sigmoidoscopy with a cotton swab, a pathognomonic feature of the disease) is undetermined, although some evidence suggests increased local concentration of fibrinolysins. The anemia is secondary to blood loss, usually grossly visible; on occasion, however, occult bleeding may continue from the friable mucosa. Chronic colonic bleeding may give rise to *iron deficiency anemia.* Azulfidine-related and rare idiopathic hemolytic anemias also contribute to the anemia. Hypoalbuminemia ensues as the result of colonic loss of serum albumin from altered, more permeable mucosa, although diminished protein intake (caused by loss of appetite) and, rarely, liver disease contribute to a limited extent. The diarrhea, which may be profound, results from the inability of the damaged colonic mucosa to reabsorb water and sodium and from the increased secretion of potassium.

Disturbances in Colonic Motility. The colon is primarily a storage or reservoir organ, and the motility waves ordinarily recorded from it (designated types I, II, and III) are of low amplitude and are believed to have a segmenting, restraining, or mixing function. The "mass movement" activity of the colon which results in evacuation and defecation is associated with the normal, rarely occurring, large amplitude type IV wave, which may reach 80 to 100 cm of water pressure. Colonic pain and frequency of rectal evacuation in ulcerative colitis have been associated with a marked increase in type IV activity; there is also some increase in type I and lack of type III (increase in tone superimposed on type I or II). The net effect is a reduction in segmenting but an increase in propulsive motility.

Diagnosis. Ulcerative colitis is a syndrome—a constellation of clinical features—an abnormal, inflamed colonic mucosa (demonstrated by sigmoidoscopy and barium enema), and a characteristic histologic substrate (demonstrated by rectal biopsy). Since the disease by definition is mucosal in location, the sigmoidoscopic examination is the single most important diagnostic tool, and will establish the diagnosis in 95 to 98 per cent of cases, because the rectosigmoid is almost universally involved. On occasion the lesion is patchy, and the rectum may not be clearly involved (possibly as a result of local steroid therapy); in these few instances colonoscopy may be useful. On sigmoidoscopy the earliest changes are edema and hyperemia of the mucosa, which give the granular appearance. This is followed by the development of such fragility that gentle wiping with cotton, or the pressure of the instrument alone, leads to bleeding. This finding is the most characteristic. The colon bleeds spontaneously as well. Discrete ulcerations are not seen frequently on sigmoidoscopy, but the mucopurulent, slightly foul exudate is characteristic. Pseudopolyps are also hallmarks

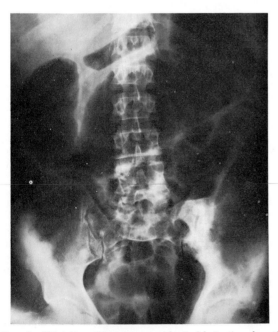

Figure 3. Dilatation of the transverse colon in fulminating ulcerative colitis.

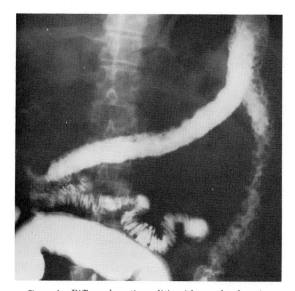

Figure 4. Diffuse ulcerative colitis with pseudopolyposis.

(Fig. 4). In most the diagnosis can be easily made by sigmoidoscopy; in some cases, however, the findings are extremely subtle, with friability the only positive finding. Here rectal biopsy may be helpful, with cellular infiltration, crypt abscesses, and atrophic epithelium (denudation of glands, evidence of previous mucosal ulceration). When the sigmoidoscopic examination is positive, there is little point in rectal biopsy except for serial study of the course of the patient; however, when the sigmoidoscopic lesion is equivocal, then biopsy may be helpful.

Radiologic Findings. Examination of the colon by barium enema is needed to determine the extent of disease beyond the sigmoidoscope, and to detect such complications as stricture, polyps, or cancer. Care must be used in the selection of patients for this examination. In the desperately ill patient, it is not only necessary but dangerous. The preparation of the colon for examination is also a serious concern. Cathartics and laxatives should not be used; rather, reliance is placed on several days of low-residue diet and gentle saline or tapwater enemas.

In the *acute stage* the roentgenographic findings are secondary to edema, ulceration, and alterations in motility. Spasm with narrowing and incomplete filling is associated with secretions within the lumen. Ulcerations are tiny and produce serrations along the contour of the filled bowel or small spicules in the film after evacuation. The bowel wall is fuzzy, and as ulceration proceeds "collar button"–like projections appear. In the *moderate* or *moderately severe stage,* the roentgenographic features are due to continued ulceration, beginning fibrosis, and epithelial regeneration, and pseudopolyps are the prominent features (Fig. 5). The results are shortening of the bowel, rigidity, and narrowing of the bowel lumen. The haustral markings, which are often missing in the normal left colon, disappear throughout. Some of the alterations in the shape of the colon are secondary to smooth muscle hypertrophy rather than collagen deposition. In this stage a patulous ileocecal valve allows visualization of the terminal ileum, which may (in 5 to 15 per cent of cases) have minimal involvement of the mucosa without narrowing of the lumen. In some patients early in the disease the barium enema may be entirely within normal limits. In others with "proctitis" the retrorectal space, which is increased owing to spasm and fibrosis of the rectal segment of the colon, may be the only evidence that this area has been involved in an inflammatory reaction.

Differential Diagnosis. Clinical presentation, the sigmoidoscopic findings, and the roentgenographic appearance usually establish the diagnosis with a high degree of accuracy. Yet certain other syndromes present real problems. Some acute *infectious colitides,* particularly shigellosis, may mimic the picture of acute fulminant colitis but usually are not chronic. The patient with the *irritable bowel syndrome* may have lower abdominal distress, intermittent cramps, and diarrhea. However, fever, the systemic symptoms, night stools, and bloody evacuations are absent, and a normal sigmoidoscopy establishes the difference authoritatively. *Amebic colitis* may be distinguished with some difficulty from acute ulcerative colitis, although the conventional teaching is that the ulcerations of amebic infection are larger and separated by islands of intact mucosa. If direct aspirates of the lesions fail to disclose the motile trophozoites, rectal biopsy may help by demonstrating them in the tissue. The patient with classic *ischemic colitis* is usually over 50 years of age, and has evidence of atherosclerotic vascular disease. However, *infarction of the colon* may be seen in young women taking oral contraceptive pills. The clinical picture of abrupt onset of lower abdominal pain, crampy in nature, fever, and rectal bleeding may mimic the acute onset of fulminant colitis, but the course with progression to gangrene or resolution with stricture formation helps to distinguish it. The typical x-ray features of intramural hemorrhage and edema with "thumbprinting" also help. But the occasional involvement of the rectosigmoid by ischemic colitis adds to the complexity of the differential diagnosis, because the proctoscopic features resemble nonspecific "proctitis." *Radiation colitis,* usually seen after radium treatment for carcinoma of the cervix, and occasionally seen in men after radiation and abdominal lymph node dissection for cancer of the testicle, presents with disturbances of bowel movements and bleeding at a variable time after the original exposure. Distinction from the other nonspe-

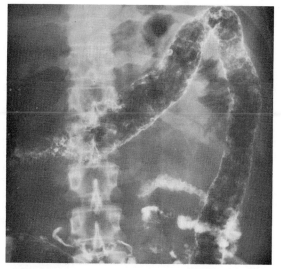

Figure 5. Evacuation film of colon of same patient as in Figure 4.

cific forms of colitis may be difficult, but the history is all important. *Acute proctitis* may occur after a large number of broad-spectrum antimicrobial agents; lincomycin has been especially stressed. *Gonococcal infection* of the rectum should also be considered. *Lymphogranuloma venereum* may simulate all the specific and nonspecific forms of proctitis. Positive Frei and complement fixation tests, together with presence or history of inguinal buboes, help to establish this diagnosis. *Cancer of the colon* and *diverticulitis of the sigmoid colon* may on occasion have a few clinical features in common with ulcerative colitis, but sigmoidoscopy and barium enema examination usually resolve the question. The interesting and important differential diagnosis of *ulcerative colitis* and *Crohn's disease of the colon* is discussed in Ch. 652.

Treatment.   *Medical Therapy.* It must be recognized that ulcerative colitis is a disease with an extremely variable course and with no known specific therapy. The aim of therapy is therefore supportive: in the acute episode to reduce the still significant mortality (up to 35 per cent in severe cases), and in the chronic forms to induce and maintain remissions and reduce the number, severity, and duration of exacerbations. Therapy thus includes the establishment of a good relationship between patient and physician in view of the disturbing nature of this illness to recur, correction of nutritional deficits, the restoration of fluid and electrolyte equilibrium, replacement of blood loss, and symptomatic relief of pain and diarrhea.

General Symptomatic Therapy. In all but the mildest forms, a period of restricted energy expenditure with appropriate rest periods is useful, especially if accomplished in a stable supporting environment. The diet should be adequate in total calories, contain enough protein to replace the losses caused by colonic leak and offset the effects of fever, and be palatable enough to appeal to the capricious appetite of these sick patients. Granted that no convincing evidence exists regarding the widely prescribed unpalatable low residue diet, it seems rational during episodes of marked rectal frequency to limit the amount of calorically insignificant cellulose residue of the diet proffered to the already irritated, inflamed colon. There is much anecdotal and a little scientific evidence that some patients dramatically improve on a diet from which cow's milk is excluded. This can be related only in part to intestinal lactase deficiency, but the patient's prior experience should guide the decision to withdraw milk and its products. Massive blood loss requires adequate blood replacement. The anemia of chronically ill patients is in part due to iron deficiency of chronic bleeding, to hemolysis, and to bone marrow failure to incorporate iron. The intolerance of a considerable number of patients to oral iron preparations is genuine, and the use of parenteral iron in the form of dextrose iron complex (Imferon) is justified. Although some apprehension is justified regarding the use of anticholinergics and opiates for the control of pain and diarrhea, because they may play a role in precipitating toxic dilatation of the colon, the judicious use of these agents is valuable on the basis of clinical experience. Tincture of belladonna (15 drops), codeine (15 to 30 mg), deodorized tincture of opium (6 to 10 drops), paregoric (4 to 8 ml), or Lomotil (2.5 to 5 mg) before meals and at bedtime gives the patient considerable comfort.

Antimicrobial   Therapy. Salicylazosulfapyridine (Azulfidine) has already been discussed in Ch. 650. This sulfonamide was introduced, however, for the treatment of ulcerative colitis, and in the opinion of most experienced clinicians it has a place in the management of milder forms of ulcerative colitis. The sulfonamide may be the sole drug used in treating patients who have mild disease and who are ambulatory. For those ill enough to be put to bed or hospitalized, however, it is inadequate. When used for those with mild disease, 2 to 8 grams in divided doses is prescribed; in view of the high percentage of patients developing nausea and anorexia or headache, it is wise to begin with smaller doses, or to add an antihistaminic to the regimen. Some clinicians are more comfortable with the use of other, non- or poorly absorbed sulfonamides in this group of patients.

In the sicker patients there is a place for maintenance therapy with the sulfonamide as well as for those who have gone into remission on corticosteroid therapy. In mild or moderately severe disease in remission, Azulfidine in doses of 2 grams per day is more effective in preventing relapses than are corticosteroids. Azulfidine has no place in the fulminatingly ill patient. Other antimicrobials also have no place in the management of ulcerative colitis except in the presence of toxic megacolon and suppurative complications.

Corticotrophin (ACTH) and Adrenocorticosteroids. Corticotrophin and corticosteroids were introduced into the therapy of ulcerative colitis on the assumption that their anti-inflammatory actions would be useful, especially because certain associated lesions of ulcerative colitis *(arthritis, uveitis, and erythema nodosum)* often responded to these compounds, and in the hope of reducing the colonic mucosal inflammatory reaction. Also, these agents stimulated appetite and elevated the patient's mood. Early studies revealed that a short course of cortisone induced an increased incidence of remission of this disease, but the effect was short lived and the long-term benefits have not been demonstrated. Yet the introduction of corticotrophin and steroid therapy with newer analogues of cortisone (prednisone or prednisolone) represents an advance in the management of the severe and the moderately severe attack.

In the mild forms, especially in those patients whose disease is confined to the rectosigmoid and distal colon, rectal instillations of steroids are of distinct use in inducing remissions, and their continued intermittent use may maintain remissions. Plastic disposable enema units containing 100 mg of hydrocortisone hemisuccinate or 20 to 40 mg of prednisolone phosphate are commercially available. This form of treatment may be used nightly as a retention enema until remission occurs, and maintained by instillation two to three times weekly. There is good evidence that these instillations may reach large sections of the colon (up to the hepatic flexure). The main effects are local, but some steroids are absorbed and the degree of adrenocortical suppression is minimal. In universal ulcerative colitis and in those sick enough to be hospitalized, rectal steroid therapy does not appear to be sufficient as the sole form of treatment.

In the moderately ill patient systemic oral steroids are the current drugs of choice. Forty to 60 mg of prednisone or its equivalent is a reasonable initial dose which should induce marked improvement and/or remission within two weeks, at which point it should be slowly tapered. In some patients the remission may be only partial and steroid therapy must be continued. Supplementation with Azulfidine at this point may be wise in the weaning period as well as for maintenance. Stepwise reduction in oral steroids should be continued while clinical well-being is maintained at a reasonably low dose. In view of the serious hazards of long-term corticosteroid therapy, which includes *profound suppression of endogenous adrenal activity, muscle weakness* and *wasting, osteoporosis* and *vertebral collapse, hypertension, diabetes, cosmetic deformities* with their attendant *psychologic disturbances, psychosis,* and *growth retardation* in children, doses above 15 to 20 mg should not be prescribed for longer than six to eight weeks. Although alternate-day therapy may minimize the incidence of undesirable side effects, the suppressive effect on symptoms is also lessened.

In the acutely ill patient with the fulminant presentation, intravenous therapy with corticotrophin or corticosteroids is the best current method of management. There is a general clinical impression that corticotrophin is superior to corticosteroids in this group; this judgment has, however, little supportive objective evidence. In these gravely ill patients corticotrophin should be given by continuous intravenous drip, 25 to 40 units per eight-hour period. If there is any question of adrenal responsiveness, intravenous hydrocortisone in doses of 100 mg given over each eight-hour period may be substituted. Fluid overload, sodium retention, and hypokalemia must be meticulously prevented. If a remission is to be achieved, it usually will be obvious within 7 to 10 days; it is hazardous to continue such therapy beyond 14 days. Failure of discernible response should lead to prompt colectomy at this point. If the expected clinical improvement occurs, the intravenous dose should be gradually reduced and supplemented by orally administered steroids. Dosage in turn is then gradually tapered until the patient can either be weaned or maintained on not more than 15 to 20 mg of prednisolone per day. The regimen may be supplemented in some by Azulfidine at this time.

Other complications of steroid therapy further limit the enthusiastic use of these compounds: *retinopathy, chemosis of lids, adrenocortical insufficiency* from too rapid withdrawal of the drug, or *inadequate adrenocortical reserve* which may persist for months after their use, and these agents may mask signs and symptoms of *sepsis* and *colonic perforation*. There is much discussion as to whether high-dose corticotrophin or prednisone therapy in the acutely ill patient increases the likelihood of perforation. Certainly in such circumstances the usual clinical signs and symptoms can be concealed. Demonstration of the preservation of liver dullness and measurement of abdominal girth should be part of the daily routine examination of this group of acutely ill patients. The activation of peptic ulcer and the precipitation of massive upper gastrointestinal hemorrhage are further reasons for close observation. Large doses of antacids, avoiding those containing magnesium which may aggravate the diarrhea, are widely and rationally used; their effectiveness in preventing ulceration and bleeding, however, is unproved. Cumulative experience supports the evidence that the mortality has been reduced considerably since the introduction of steroids, especially in the moderate to severe group in their acute attacks. It remains to be proved that the long-term outcome has been significantly altered. The earlier use of colectomy appears to be of major importance.

Immunosuppressive Therapy. Immunosuppressive therapy with azathioprine or 6-mercaptopurine has been used for a number of years for those patients not responsive to steroids or sulfonamides, or in an effort to reduce the dose of steroids needed to induce remission. There is little solid evidence to support this approach, although azathioprine (1.5 to 2.5 mg per kilogram of body weight daily) may be more effective than a placebo when given with steroids for exacerbations. Alertness for this drug's effect on the bone marrow as well as for possible intercurrent infections is essential. In view of its unproved nature and possible, albeit unknown, long-term effects, its use must be considered purely experimental and ethically should be confined to controlled clinical trials. This attitude is especially rational in view of the effectiveness of colectomy.

Psychotherapy. All who deal with patients with ulcerative colitis recognize the importance of the supportive role that the physician must play in this labile illness; indeed, most doctors act out their psychotherapeutic role intuitively. It is difficult to find convincing evidence that more formal psychotherapy by psychiatrists or lay analysts alters the long-term course of the illness. Despite this gap in knowledge, there is an obvious place for recommending psychotherapy for those patients and their families in whom personality problems and distorted interpersonal relationships exist. It is more difficult to decide whether all patients should have some exploration of possible psychic conflicts. If this is undertaken, the psychiatrist should be one who has experience with this illness and sensitivity to the often fragile psychic structures of these patients. There is little place for psychotherapy for the patient who is acutely ill. In general, psychotherapy should be reserved for the more quiescent interval phases of the disease.

Complications. *Local Complications.* These include the development of *anal fissures, rectal prolapse,* and *hemorrhoids* and are to be related to the intensity of the diarrhea. *Perianal abscess* and *fistulas* are rare in ulcerative colitis in contrast to Crohn's disease. *Rectovaginal fistulas,* however, may appear and do not heal with local surgical measures. The pseudopolyps carry with them no prognostic significance. They may disappear completely and have no relation to the development of cancer. *Massive hemorrhage* occurs in about 5 per cent of patients. Rapid replacement of blood and restoration of circulating blood volume are the initial factors in treatment. Hypoprothrombinemia should be corrected by ingestion of vitamin K. Although most patients will respond to medical management, an occasional patient may require colectomy, because the bleeding is from diffuse areas of the mucosa. At times inferior mesenteric arteriography may reveal a more discrete site of bleeding. The colectomy must be total to control bleeding; failure to remove the rectal stump usually requires further emergency surgery. *Strictures of the colon* occur in a little less than 10 per cent of patients, and are rarely of such magnitude as to compromise the intestinal lumen. They usually develop in the rectum or transverse colon, are of variable lengths, and may appear at any time in the course of the disease. They are not important symptomatically, because they only rarely cause abdominal cramping pain and obstipation. They require attention, because their differentiation from cancer is often difficult. *In fact, it is wise to consider every stricture in ulcerative colitis as carcinomatous until proved otherwise.* Exploratory laparotomy was the only method until recently, but colonoscopy and biopsy have been helpful when the strictured area can be thoroughly visualized and multiple biopsies taken.

Cancer of the Colon. The incidence of cancer of the colon is strikingly higher in patients with ulcerative colitis than in the control population, and contributes significantly to the colitis-related death rate. Current evidence relates this incidence to the duration of the colitis, rather than its activity, and to the extent of the colon involved. The risk of cancer rises regularly in all patients with the duration of the disease. After 20 years the cumulative risk of cancer in all patients is about 12 per cent, and at 25 years it is 25 per cent. In children it has been estimated that 3 per cent of those who develop the disease in childhood will have cancer of the colon after 10 years and 20 per cent per decade thereafter. The risk rises strikingly after the first decade of disease in children and after the second decade in adults.

The extent of colonic involvement with colitis plays an important role in determining the risk of subsequent cancer development. In proctitis it does not differ significantly from that in the control population. The incidence in left-sided colitis is much lower than in universal colitis. In this latter group the incidence may approach 13 per cent at 15 years, 25 per cent at 20 years, and 40 per cent at 25 years. Since childhood colitis is usually universal in type, this factor influences the high rate of malignancy. Most cancers of the colon are in the rectum, and this is true for ulcerative colitis, including universal colitis. Such cancers may, however, involve any segment of the colon, the transverse colon being the second most common location. The survival rate after surgery for cancer complicating ulcerative colitis is much lower than for cancer unrelated to ulcerative colitis. One reason is that cancer in ulcerative colitis is frequently multicentered (10 to 15 per cent). Clearly the population at greatest risk are those with universal colitis of more than 10 years' duration. Although prophylactic colectomy has been advocated for this group, no consensus exists at present on this point, although yearly sigmoidoscopy and barium enema examinations are widely proposed. The search for "precancerous" changes on biopsy may be more rewarding, particularly with the increasing use of colonoscopy as well as sigmoidoscopy. At present the value of serum carcinoembryonic antigen (CEA) levels in the diagnosis of malignancy in this disease remains to be established, because levels are elevated in 30 per cent of patients with inflammatory bowel disease.

Toxic Megacolon. At any time in the course of ulcerative colitis the patient may become gravely ill with the signs of systemic toxicity and marked dilatation of the colon. Although much ingenuity has been expended in establishing the criteria for defining this distention, usually the colon is more than 6 cm in width on the flat plate of the abdomen. This drastic episode coincides with extension of the previous mucosal inflammation through all coats of the colon, with evidence of involvement of neural and vascular components. Factors which decrease muscular tone or increase intraluminal pressure may be important in precipitating an episode of colonic dilatation: barium enema examination, injudicious use of opiates and anticholinergic drugs, or hypokalemia. In some patients no obvious triggering mechanism, except worsening of the pathologic process, can be found. Clinically, this is the most dramatic episode in all the variegated course of ulcerative colitis.

The patient is gravely ill, with high fever and rapid pulse, and dry. He complains of abdominal pain which may be continuous, and the abdomen is markedly distended. The previous diarrhea may cease abruptly. The abdomen is diffusely tender and ominously silent. Marked leukocytosis, hypokalemia, and a precipitous fall in serum albumin are usually present. The flat film reveals dilatation of all the colon or a segment, usually the transverse colon, and the edematous ragged colonic mucosa can be seen with the air contrast. If the colon has freely perforated, air may be seen under the diaphragm. Diffuse peritonitis and localized perforation are frequently overdiagnosed because of direct visceral tenderness elicited by pressure on the inflamed serosa of the dilated colon.

The diagnosis is made on the basis of the history of ulcerative colitis, acute worsening of the clinical picture, systemic toxicity, and dilatation of the colon on clinical and radiologic evidence. A few patients, however, will present initially with this condition. Barium enema examination should be avoided, and gentle proctoscopy in bed will make the diagnosis if the antecedent history of ulcerative colitis is not present.

Therapy of acute toxic dilatation of the colon should be intensive and meticulous. Correction of fluid and electrolyte deficits, especially of potassium, is needed. Anemia, hypoalbuminemia, and decreased circulatory blood volume require correction. Steroids are the therapy of choice, and if the patient has been on previous corticosteroids, corticotrophin or hydrocortisone in large doses is used as outlined above (25 to 40 units of corticotrophin or 100 mg of hydrocortisone, given over the course of each eight-hour period by intravenous drip). Since there is probably localized suppuration which has extended to the serosa, intravenous antimicrobial therapy is in order: ampicillin in doses of 8 to 12 grams daily intravenously is usually ordered. Daily flat film and physical examination two or three times a day are required. In view of the usual accompanying small bowel ileus, long-tube intubation should be promptly instituted along with cessation of feedings, anticholinergics, and opiates. The response to this vigorous form of therapy must be evaluated daily in terms of the patient's systemic improvement and regaining of colonic tone in terms of the distention of the colon clinically on flat film. The first 48 to 72 hours will usually indicate whether the hoped-for improvement is indeed beginning to take place. Failure to respond by the fourth or fifth day should lead to prompt subtotal colectomy (avoiding the trauma of the abdominoperineal resection in those desperately ill patients) and ileostomy. On occasion preliminary cecostomy or transverse colostomy has helped by decompressing the colon. The surgical difficulties in handling the thin, distended, often perforated colon should not be underestimated, even if performed by experienced surgeons, and the postoperative periods are often stormy, including localized or generalized peritonitis, walled-off abscesses, and the ominous iliofemoral thrombophlebitis. The mortality of toxic megacolon has been markedly reduced in recent years, in part because of steroid therapy and better systemic management, but probably in major part because of earlier surgical intervention. Of those who recover on current medical programs, the majority usually come to surgery during the next year because of persistent activity of the disease. An interesting clinical variant is the occasional patient who has a "subacute," perhaps a "chronic," megacolon, in contrast to the terribly sick "toxic" patient, and whose clinical course is more indolent, although similar.

Perforation of the Colon. Perforation of the colon is most likely to occur in the course of toxic dilatation, and is rare simply in the course of an acute attack. As noted, it is presumably the result of extension of the inflammatory ulcerative process through all layers of the bowel. Since the vast majority of these sick people are already receiving large doses of steroids, recognition is difficult, although sudden clinical worsening with increasing abdominal distention and tenderness of the colon may arouse suspicion. Obliteration of liver dullness must be sought for at all times, and the presence of free air under the diaphragm on x-ray examination makes the diagnosis. Surgical intervention is urgently required and colectomy indicated. Rarely, an episode of perforation may not be recognized and the patient survives; the perforation is documented later by an abdominal film showing free air in the peritoneal cavity.

Extracolonic Complications. As with Crohn's disease, a number of extracolonic complications or manifestations are part of the clinical syndrome. The *arthritis* may be severe, migratory, and accompanied by synovial swelling affecting knees, elbows, and ankles; however, the serologic factors of rheumatoid arthritis are missing, and there is no residual deformity. *Ankylosing spondylitis* and *sacroiliitis* occur with higher frequency than might be expected. *Iritis* and *uveitis,* unlike the arthritis, are not easily correlated with the degree of clinical colitis. Of the skin manifestations, *erythema nodosum* and *pyoderma gangrenosum* are the most common. The incidence of kidney stones is highest in those with ileostomies. The hepatic complications include *fatty infiltration, pericholangitis* and *chronic active hepatitis,* and, rarely, *sclerosing cholangitis* and its associated *carcinoma of the bile ducts.* It is not known at present whether colectomy improves liver function or structure. Massive peripheral or pelvic thrombophlebitis, especially *iliofemoral venous thrombosis,* is a grave complication, and may be related to marked thrombocytosis.

Surgical Therapy. Colectomy is curative in ulcerative colitis, at the cost of life with an ileostomy. The marked reduction in mortality from colectomy and the recent improvement in the quality of life with an ileostomy now makes colectomy an acceptable form of treatment for the patient with ulcerative colitis. Whether done in one or two stages, most experts agree that preservation of the rectum is not possible in this disease although ileoproctostomy (with or without active disease in the rectum) still has a few advocates. However, subsequent ileal dysfunction, intestinal obstruction, ileostomy prolapse or retraction, delayed healing of the perianal wound, and fear of psychogenic or neurogenic impotence present realistic limitations to the overenthusiastic use of surgery. The clearest indications for surgery are those complications for which no other therapy is available: massive uncontrollable hemorrhage, perforation of the colon, cancer of the colon, a stricture which cannot be distinguished from cancer, and medically unresponsive toxic dilatation. Close behind this group are the patients in a severe acute attack, which carries with it the highest mortality risk. This is the group which has until recently been usually treated with two to three weeks of intravenous steroids at high dosage plus massive antimicrobial therapy. Although continued disease activity, protein and electrolyte depletion, serious anemia, and localized suppuration make surgical intervention at this stage somewhat risky, it is the best choice. Some proponents of early surgery have advocated intervention after four to five days if the patient has not clinically shown remission in this period of time. Although this point of view

has yet to be unequivocably established, the trend of modern therapy is toward earlier intervention in the acutely ill patient. Moveover, there is probably little disagreement at present that the patient with intractable pyoderma gangrenosum and probably also persistent or serious uveitis should undergo colectomy. No solid evidence exists, however, that colectomy improves serious liver disease.

A decision for surgery in the patient with persistent symptomatic disease, sufficiently severe to prevent normal function, is indicated, especially for those who require unacceptably high levels of steroids (greater than 20 mg of prednisone daily) for suppression of symptoms. In others the decision for colectomy is more difficult, especially with childhood disease. These patients suffer a lower survival rate with or without malignancy, and growth and sexual maturation are retarded. Colectomy should be recommended for such children who are chronically ill, despite the reluctance and anxiety of both family and physician, but only after a period of medical trial, possibly not longer than two years.

The most difficult problem is the risk of cancer in the patient who has had the disease for ten years or more, either quiescent or with minimal medical therapy. Those with distal or only rectal involvement have little risk and can be followed with barium enema, proctosigmoidoscopy, and colonoscopy. It is those with universal colitis who raise the question of prophylactic colectomy. As indicated, no firm trend is visible at present. It should be pointed out that the development of the "continent" ileostomy of Kock of Sweden with its internal pouch and avoidance of an external mechanical appliance may simplify the decision in borderline patients.

652. CROHN'S DISEASE OF THE COLON
(Granulomatous Colitis)

Definition. Crohn's disease of the colon is a chronic inflammatory disease of the colon of unknown origin, characteristically of young adults, most frequently involving the proximal colon and its adjacent terminal ileum. Although any and all portions of the colon alone may be involved, it classically spares the rectum. A diarrheal disease of insidious onset and progressive course, it usually has little tendency to rectal bleeding, great tendency to fistulize both internally and externally, and, frequently, significant anal and perianal lesions. The characteristic pathology includes confluent linear ulceration, intramucosal fissuring, aggregates of mononuclear inflammatory cells, and epithelioid granulomas within the bowel wall or regional lymph nodes (hence the term granulomatous colitis). Because of similarities of clinical course, pathology, tendency to recur after resection, and coexistence with regional enteritis (Crohn's disease of the ileum), Crohn's disease of the colon is considered the same disease. The term "ileocolitis" is reserved for simultaneous involvement of the ileum and colon. The distinction from ulcerative colitis may be difficult on occasion, but this does not obliterate their differences and the therapeutic consequences of such differentiation.

Separation of Ulcerative Colitis and Crohn's Disease of the Colon. The year after the original description of regional enteritis, Colp described a patient with involvement of both ileum and cecum and demonstrated that the ileocecal valve is no barrier to the development of this process in the colon. Despite sporadic papers, it was not until 1960 that it became apparent that Crohn's disease could occur frequently in the colon as well as in the small bowel and could be differentiated from ulcerative colitis. The clinical and pathologic characters of Crohn's disease of the small bowel and ulcerative colitis have been presented in Ch. 650 and 651, respectively.

The features which distinguish ulcerative colitis and Crohn's disease of the colon should be emphasized: In Crohn's disease the small bowel is also involved in up to 80 per cent of cases; the lesion is segmental, sparing the rectum in perhaps more than half the patients; and fistulas are extremely frequent—all in marked contrast to ulcerative colitis. Clinically, in Crohn's disease rectal bleeding is a much less frequent occurrence, severe perianal and perirectal disease is often florid, free perforation and toxic dilatation are rarer, and, up to the present, development of cancer is extremely rare. In contrast to the mucosal pathology of ulcerative colitis, all coats are involved in Crohn's disease, with marked thickening and a high percentage of granulomas in the bowel wall and regional lymph nodes. Finally, in therapeutic contrast to ulcerative colitis, excision in Crohn's disease of the colon is often followed by recurrences in the small bowel. Our inability to differentiate these two entities even when adequate histologic material is present (in perhaps 15 per cent of cases) does not argue for their identity. The colon has a limited repertoire of disease, and other disorders are still to be separated from this group of inflammatory diseases, ischemic colitis being the most recently segregated entity.

Incidence and Distribution of Lesions.

The available data regarding the incidence and prevalence of Crohn's disease have been cited in Ch. 650. Despite the increasing recognition of this entity, the impression that the incidence of Crohn's disease of the colon rivals that of ulcerative colitis appears erroneous. Of over 600 patients with inflammatory colonic disease sick enough to require ileostomy and colectomy in the writer's series, less than 10 per cent had Crohn's disease of the colon.

The colon may be involved in Crohn's disease in one of several ways. The least significant is by way of fistula formation from a contiguous loop of small bowel which is the site of regional enteritis. This is relatively trivial, because the disease does not appear to spread, and the colonic area heals when the small bowel is resected and the fistula closed. Second, the colon may become involved only after an anastomotic operation for regional ileitis, and almost always directly adjacent to the anastomosis. More important, the colon alone may exhibit the disease. Finally, the colon and small bowel are simultaneously the seat of the pathologic process, with continuity of disease in the colon, and occasionally normal segment intervenes. When the colon is involved, less than 20 per cent of patients have the lesion confined to that organ; 80 per cent have disease in the ileum. Over-all, about two thirds of Crohn's disease involves the small bowel alone. The anal involvement in Crohn's disease of the colon is noteworthy. It may be in the form of edematous anal tags, chronic fissuring, anorectal fistulas, and indolent undermining ulceration. About 75 per cent of patients with Crohn's disease of the colon and 25 per cent of those with Crohn's disease of the small bowel have an anal lesion at some time in the course of this illness.

Pathology.

The pathology of Crohn's disease of the colon and rectum is fundamentally that of Crohn's disease of the small intestine. Because of the interest and difficulty at times of distinguishing colonic involvement from ulcerative colitis, some additional points should be mentioned. In contrast to ulcerative colitis, Crohn's disease is a discontinuous process, sparing the rectum generally in more than half the instances and involving the terminal ileum in a very high percentage of cases. Intense vascularity is characteristic of ulcerative colitis, not of Crohn's disease. Muscular shortening of the colon in ulcerative colitis contrasts with the fibrosis and stricturing of Crohn's disease. Pseudopolyp formation is characteristic of ulcerative colitis. External and internal fistulas are the hallmark of Crohn's disease, including such unusual sites as the stomach; the only fistula characteristic of ulcerative colitis is rectovaginal fistula.

The microscopic characteristics of both diseases have also been described under their respective categories. Ulcerative colitis is primarily a mucosal disease; Crohn's disease involves all layers. In Crohn's disease, in contrast to ulcerative colitis, fissuring is prominent, as well as aggregates of mononuclear inflammation and sarcoid granulomas in the bowel wall and regional lymph nodes. In biopsies of the rectum in Crohn's disease of the colon we have found about 10 per cent to have these granulomas when no gross lesion was visible on sigmoidoscopic or barium enema examination. Ultrastructural studies have disclosed no characteristic findings of these granulomas. Although crypt abscesses are not specific for ulcerative colitis, they are a prominent pattern in its histopathology, in contrast to Crohn's disease of the colon. The latter may also exist in a colon with sigmoid diverticular disease, and the clinical and radiographic features are as difficult to assign to each component as the pathologic findings.

Cancer as an important feature of the natural history of ulcerative colitis has already been emphasized; even in the small bowel in Crohn's disease, the incidence of adenocarcinoma is more frequent, especially in the bypassed ileum. Although some cancers have been observed in colons which are the seat of Crohn's disease, the data at present do not allow any firm statement regarding the risk of cancer development, for these patients have not been observed more than ten years, in part because the colons are usually removed before ten years of illness.

Clinical Manifestations.

Crohn's disease of the colon, like Crohn's disease of the small bowel, begins in young adult life. About a third of the writer's patients had their first manifestations between 16 and 20 years of age. In comparison with ulcerative colitis, an acute fulminant presentation is rare, toxic dilatation is rarer, and free perforation, rarest. Onset is usually slow and insidious, with diarrhea as the principal symptom in the majority of patients. The stools are small, frequent, and soft but not necessarily watery; some patients may be constipated, especially if they have anal lesions. Over three quarters of the patients lose weight. Crampy abdominal pain of a diffuse nature is prominent. Gross bleeding is noted only in less than half the patients; indeed, important rectal bleeding is most unusual except in the presence of rectal involvement. The history of a perirectal abscess or fistula often precedes the obvious clinical onset by years. *Aphthous stomatitis, arthralgias* and *arthritis, uveitis, pyoderma gangrenosum* and *erythema nodosum,* and backache caused by *ankylosing spondylitis* and *sacroiliitis* are secondary manifestations, as in other variants of inflammatory bowel diseases.

Physical Examination. In contrast to regional ileitis, patients with Crohn's disease of the colon rarely have a palpable right lower quadrant mass, even when the ileum is involved. Clubbing of the fingers and curvature of the nails may be present. Edematous perianal skin tags and perirectal fistulas may be noted.

Diagnosis. Confirmation of the clinical suspicion of Crohn's disease of the colon depends upon sigmoidoscopy and barium enema examination, and, on occasion, upon the small bowel series. In half the cases, the sigmoidoscopic examination is negative; in the others it may reveal an edematous mucosa, mucoid secretions, or a cobblestoned surface. Rarely a few discrete ulcers may be seen. In contrast to ulcerative colitis, however, bleeding from a friable mucosa is not present. Rarely, diagnosis may be made by biopsy findings.

The roentgenologic features are the same as in regional enteritis of the small bowel, i.e., segmental involvement with normal skip areas, longitudinal ulcerations, fissures, eccentric involvement, pseudodiverticula, strictures, internal fistulas, and sinus tracts (Fig. 6). In early cases nodular defects or irregularity of the contour of a short segment of colon may be the only findings, and may be obscured on the filled films. At times the evacuation films or examination of the colon from above may be the only way of documenting these changes. Strictures, as in ulcerative colitis, are difficult to distinguish from cancer; when the entire colon is diffusely involved in a symmetrical fashion, and when the ileum is normal, it may be impossible to distinguish Crohn's disease of the colon from ulcerative colitis by x-ray examination.

Differential Diagnosis. The important conditions which must be differentiated from Crohn's disease of the colon include *ulcerative colitis, cancer* of the *colon, tuberculosis* of the *ileocecal area, amebiasis,* and, rarely, *radiation enteritis* and *colitis.* When a left-sided colonic segment is the site of disease, *ischemic colitis* and *sigmoid diverticulitis* are the disorders which must be distinguished. The intramural abscess of diverticulitis and the longitudinal submucosal ulceration of Crohn's disease are similar on barium enema, but the very long tracts are characteristic of Crohn's disease.

Therapy. Current approaches to therapy of Crohn's disease of the colon reflect the perspective of experience with Crohn's disease of the small bowel. The unpredictable course of the disease, the significant reduction in longevity, and the high rate of recurrence of surgically treated ileitis have engendered a cautious and somewhat pessimistic view of all therapies available at present for Crohn's disease of the colon. All the modalities of medical treatment for ileitis are used in Crohn's colitis: general supportive measures, nutritional supplements, sulfonamides (especially Azulfidine), steroids (corticotrophin and adrenocorticosteroids), and immunosuppressives (azathioprine [Imuran]). Even more than in regional ileitis, the therapeutic value of all these methods remains to be demonstrated in sound controlled clinical trials. When multiple enteric and cutaneous fistulas lead to marked malnutrition and malabsorption, hyperalimentation with a central venous catheter may be effective.

Surgical intervention is clearly indicated for those complications for which no medical therapy exists: perforation, cancer, obstruction resulting from stricture, massive hemorrhage, and fistulization into stomach, duodenum, and bladder. The more difficult decisions concern those patients who are not able to carry out their usual daily activities and those who require more than 20 mg of prednisolone daily to suppress their symptoms over a period of months. Almost 75 per cent of patients ultimately come to surgery. Since considerable controversy exists at present regarding the fate of patients with total extirpation of the colon for Crohn's disease, the decision is by no means easy in sick patients. Diversionary ileostomy in the hope of resting an inflamed colon and possibly even subsequently utilizing this organ has become discredited. When the disease is segmental and especially since the left colon and rectosigmoid are free in at least half the patients, resection and anastomosis with sigmoid or rectum is the operation of choice. The rate of recurrence in these localized extirpations clearly resembles the rate of recurrence of Crohn's disease of the ileum alone (approaching 50 per cent). In the writer's experience, of 67 patients with Crohn's colitis, 31, or 46 per cent, had significant recurrences in the ileum after ileostomy and colectomy, 8 required multiple operations, and 6 had severe nutritional deficits. This experience is not paralleled by all observers. In some series recurrences have been observed in none or only 3 per cent. A review of the experience at St. Mark's Hospital in London indicated four recurrences in 56 patients (7 per cent), but others have reported as many as 16 recurrences in 37 patients treated similarly. These differences may relate in part to the extent to which the ileum is involved; in our group almost all had the ileal involvement. Accordingly,

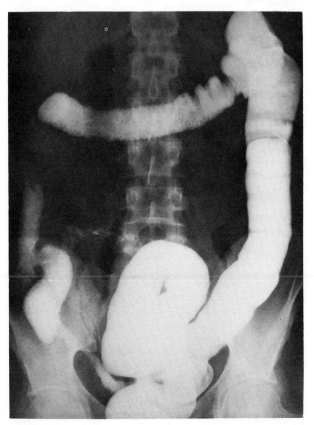

Figure 6. Crohn's colitis. Note involvement of terminal ileum as well as right side of colon.

some delay in deciding on colectomy seems warranted. Even the most vigorous proponents of ileostomy and total colectomy grant that the patients with Crohn's disease of the colon have a higher rate of stomal dysfunction and ileitis than patients with ulcerative colitis.

Regional Enteritis

Crohn, B. B., Ginzberg, L., and Oppenheimer, G. D.: Regional ileitis: A pathologic and clinical entity. J.A.M.A., 99:1323, 1932.
Gerson, C. D., Cohen, N., and Janowitz, H. D.: Small intestinal absorptive function in regional enteritis. Gastroenterology, 64:907, 1973.
Kayle, J.: Crohn's Disease. New York, Appleton-Century-Crofts, 1972.
Marshak, R. H., and Wolf, B. S.: Roentgen findings in regional enteritis. Am. J. Roentgenol. Radium Ther. Nucl. Med., 74:1000, 1955.
Monk, M., Mendeloff, A., Siegel, C., and Lilienfeld, A.: An epidemiological study of ulcerative colitis and regional enteritis among adults in Baltimore. I. Hospital incidence and prevalence, 1960 to 1963. Gastroenterology, 53:198, 1967. II. Social and demographic factors. Gastroenterology, 56:847, 1969.

Ulcerative Colitis

Edwards, F. C., and Truelove, S. C.: The course and prognosis of ulcerative colitis. I. Short term prognosis. Gut, 4:299, 1964. II. Long term prognosis. Gut, 4:309, 1964.
Engle, G. L.: Studies of ulcerative colitis. III. The nature of the psychological processes. Am. J. Med., 19:231, 1955.
Marshak, R. H., Korelitz, B. I., Klein, S. H., Wolf, B. S., and Janowitz, H. D.: Toxic dilatation of the colon in the course of ulcerative colitis. Gastroenterology, 38:165, 1960.
Sparberg, M., Genonessy, J., and Kirsner, J. B.: Ulcerative proctitis and mild ulcerative colitis: A study of 220 patients. Medicine, 45:391, 1966.
Wilks, S., and Moxon, W.: Lectures on Pathological Anatomy. London, Churchill, 1875.

Crohn's Disease of the Colon

Korelitz, B. I., Present, D. H., Alpert, L. I., Marshak, R. H., and Janowitz, H. D.: Recurrent regional ileitis after ileostomy and colectomy for granulomatous colitis. N. Engl. J. Med., 287:110, 1972.
Lindner, A. E., Marshak, R. H., Wolf, B. S., and Janowitz, H. D.: Granulomatous colitis, a clinical study. N. Engl. J. Med., 269:379, 1963.
Ritchie, J. K., and Lockhart-Mummery, H. E.: Nonrestorative surgery in the treatment of Crohn's disease of the large bowel. Gut, 14:263, 1973.

OTHER INFLAMMATORY DISEASES OF THE INTESTINE

Marvin H. Sleisenger

653. ACUTE APPENDICITIS (INCLUDING THE ACUTE ABDOMEN)

Definition. Appendicitis is acute inflammation of the vermiform appendix. It is rare before the age of two and reaches a peak incidence in the second and third decades. The vast majority of patients are between the ages of 5 and 30. Although incidence of the disease declines after the age of 40, the annual incidence is about 1.5 per thousand for males and 1.9 per thousand for females between the ages of 17 and 64. The disease is important because it is common and curable; it therefore constitutes the most important entity in the differential diagnosis of the acute abdomen.

Pathology. Usually, the appendix is swollen, hyperemic, warm, and covered with exudate. However, in the early stages it may appear only slightly discolored and, in the late stages, gangrenous with perforation. Microscopically, the picture ranges from some acute inflammatory cells in the lumen and mucosa to acute inflammatory changes transmurally with superficial mucosal ulcerations; in advanced stages, one or more perforations may be noted, particularly in patients over the age of 60.

Etiology and Pathogenesis. The initiating event in acute appendicitis appears to be obstruction, followed by increased intraluminal pressure, reduced venous drainage, thrombosis, hemorrhage, edema, and bacterial invasion of the wall. As the process proceeds, the appendiceal artery (an end artery) becomes occluded as a result of the inflammation, and venous stasis and perforation result.

Calculi are thought to be the most common cause of the initial obstruction. Indeed, about one third of inflamed appendices contain a radiologically demonstrable calculus, as compared with 2.7 per cent of normal ones. In turn, about a third of these are visible on plain films of the abdomen preoperatively, whereas they may be seen in only 1 per cent of a control population. The incidence of gangrene and perforation is significantly higher also in appendices which contain calculi. The nidus for these calculi is inspissated fecal material which is covered by a calcium phosphate–rich mucus; inorganic salts precipitate, hardening the calculus and increasing the likelihood for obstruction. It must be stressed, however, that two thirds to three quarters of patients with proved acute appendicitis do not have calculi. In these patients, obviously, an alternative pathogenetic mechanism must be responsible. Obstruction by parasites, lymphoid hyperplasia, and twisting of the appendix by adhesions have all been incriminated. An additional theory is malfunction of a valve system at the entrance of the appendix. Recently, mucosal ulceration has been considered by some to be the primary pathogenetic event rather than obstruction. Such ulceration may also result from viral infection.

Thus it is likely that the etiology of acute appendicitis is multiple. Regardless, increased intraluminal pressure, transmural swelling, and inflammation eventually compromise the appendiceal end artery and cause gangrene and perforation.

Clinical Picture and Diagnosis. The history of appendicitis is of short duration in the vast majority of cases—between 12 and 48 hours from onset to hospitalization. Over 95 per cent complain first of pain at onset, classically referred to the epigastric or periumbilical areas and later localizing in the right lower quadrant. This sequence, however, is found in only about half the patients. Further, a significant number will not localize clearly to the right lower quadrant, the pain being either diffuse or in the lower abdomen. When retrocecal, the pain may be referred to the thigh or right testicle and may even be felt as burning with urination.

Pain referred to the mid-epigastrium is due to stretching of the organ during early inflammation; later, when the process has reached the serosa and the peritoneum, it localizes over the site of disease. In some patients distress appears to be alleviated at the time of perforation; after perforation, localization of pain will depend on whether or not the process is quickly walled off locally. Thus if the spreading infection is not contained, generalized abdominal discomfort of variable severity will result. Anorexia and nausea (with or without vomiting) are the second and third most frequent symptoms. In almost all instances, pain precedes the appearance of these other complaints. About 10 per cent of patients will have constipation; diarrhea is relatively infrequent. Temperature usually ranges between 38 and 38.6° C; higher levels usually indicate perforation.

Physical Examination. The findings on physical examination differ widely and depend not only upon the stage of the inflammation but also upon the age of the patient. Tenderness to palpation is the most common and most reliable sign; indeed, without it, diagnosis is unlikely. It is usually confined to McBurney's point in the right lower quadrant, corresponding to the usual location of the organ. However, although rectal tenderness is present in about one third of patients, it may be so severe as to indicate pelvic peritonitis. On initial examination in a minority of patients, a mass may be felt in the right lower quadrant or in the pelvis or transrectally. Three quarters of patients will have unquestionable localized tenderness with localized rebound. Generalized rebound tenderness indicates diffuse peritonitis. Bowel sounds may be present or absent; absence associated with distention and generalized rebound tenderness is consistent with perforation and diffuse peritonitis.

On occasion, tenderness may be elicited in the case of retrocecal appendicitis by stretching the psoas by hip extension. Very rarely, because of the odd location of the appendix, tenderness may be in the right upper quadrant or even the left lower quadrant.

Laboratory studies consistently show a leukocytosis with an increase in polymorphonuclear cells — over 10,000 per cubic millimeter and greater than 75 per cent, respectively. Urinalysis is usually normal; however, about 15 per cent of patients have either a slight amount of protein or mild pyuria or hematuria. Presence of a calcified fecalith in the right lower quadrant on flat film of the abdomen is helpful, but its absence has no meaning in the diagnosis. Other findings on flat film include possible obliteration of the right psoas shadow, right lower quadrant sentinel loop ileus, and a right lower quadrant soft tissue mass with or without gas bubbles; with perforation and generalized peritonitis, fluid in the peritoneal cavity and obliteration of the peritoneal lines may be noted.

Differential Diagnosis of Appendicitis and of the Acute Abdomen. Appendicitis is first on the list of conditions causing acute abdominal pain which require surgery or immediate consultation with a surgeon. Here a few principles regarding the acute surgical abdomen in the setting of the differential diagnosis of acute appendicitis will be reviewed.

Pain Characteristics. Conditions associated with pain of sudden onset include perforated viscus or acute ischemia; occasionally, the onset of pain in acute small bowel obstruction is abrupt. The more gradual onset of pain usually indicates an inflammatory lesion, including appendicitis. However, the pain of diffuse inflammatory bowel disease is not localized as it is in appendicitis, except as a consequence of perforation or fistulization in granulomatous disease.

The type and radiation of the pain also help in differential diagnosis. For example, evidence of irritation of the diaphragm may be found on the right in *acute cholecystitis* and on the left in *acute pancreatitis;* sudden severe pain referred to the tips of the shoulders, associated with diffuse intra-abdominal pain and, later, distention, is more typical of perforated viscus, particularly

peptic ulcer. Ureteral obstruction causes pain which is frequently referred to the genitalia or groin. Steady continuous pain is more characteristic of inflammation, as in appendicitis; on the other hand, intermittent or crampy pain is more characteristic of *obstruction of a hollow viscus* such as the gallbladder or small bowel.

It is important again to stress that pain precedes nausea and vomiting in *appendicitis;* on the other hand, vomiting may be an earlier symptom of *acute cholecystitis* or *acute pancreatitis.* Bile-stained vomitus associated with acute cramping upper abdominal pain suggests *small bowel obstruction;* blood in the vomitus points toward a mucosal lesion proximal to the third portion of the duodenum. Relief of pain by vomiting suggests *gastric outlet obstruction.* Vomiting, of course, may accompany any intra-abdominal conditions, particularly if the patient has ileus or generalized peritonitis.

Physical Findings. Physical examination of the patient with an acute abdomen is of great importance, and the range of findings expected in acute appendicitis has been discussed. Localized tenderness and temperature elevation associated with continuing pain over a period of hours reflect either *localized peritonitis,* with or without perforation, or *vascular necrosis* of an ischemic organ. In such instances, the temperature is approximately 38.5 to 39.5° C. Higher temperatures are more often associated with urinary tract infections or bacterial pneumonias. A continuing rising pulse rate likewise indicates the possibility of gangrene or perforation of a viscus.

Careful examination of the abdomen is of extreme importance in differential diagnosis. *Diffuse peritonitis* is reflected by resistance of movement and change in position because of accentuation of pain; on the other hand, colic caused by *obstruction* of bile ducts, ureter, or small bowel early in its course is associated with restless movement. Later, in biliary tract and small bowel obstruction, infection and compromise of the blood supply may ensue and will cause the appearance of signs of localized tissue necrosis and peritonitis. The abdomen should be carefully examined for scars of previous surgery which may now underlie an *intestinal obstruction* caused by adhesions; hernias must be sought.

In examining the patient with an acute abdomen, the physician should palpate in that quadrant which is farthest removed from the site of distress. The important findings which indicate a surgical condition include persistent localized tenderness with unequivocal rebound, indicating localized peritonitis, and guarding. Guarding must be interpreted circumspectly, because it may be voluntary or involuntary. If it is the latter, underlying peritoneal irritation is likely. Generalized involuntary guarding is a classic finding for a perforated intra-abdominal viscus. The presence of an abdominal mass not previously noted, particularly when associated with other findings of inflammation, gangrene, or perforation, is very strong evidence for a surgical condition. Likewise, free air in the abdominal cavity, as evidenced by distention, absence of bowel sounds, and absence of liver dullness in the setting of acute abdominal pain, reflects a perforated viscus. Bowel sounds may be more active and high pitched in early obstruction or continuously active in diffuse acute inflammation (nonsurgical) of the small bowel. With increasing distention of small bowel loops, the sounds become less frequent and more high pitched. Bruits are an important finding, because they may reflect the presence of *arterial aneurysms*, the dissections of which may be the cause for the abdominal pain.

Rectal examination is crucial in differential diagnosis. Unequivocal tenderness indicates pelvic inflammation, and a mass usually reflects the presence of an abscess. As noted above, this examination often reveals positive findings in acute appendicitis. A glove specimen of stool must always be examined for occult blood. In females with acute abdominal pain, pelvic examination is essential to complement a careful gynecologic history.

Laboratory Aids in Diagnosis. The laboratory examination, consisting of urinalysis, complete blood count, serum electrolytes, BUN and creatinine, and x-ray examination of the abdomen and chest, is essential in differential diagnosis of the acute abdomen.

A *polymorphonuclear leukocytosis* strongly substantiates an acute intra-abdominal process with inflammation or necrosis; a low hematocrit reflects a disorder which is also capable of bleeding—*mucosal ulcerations, intestinal carcinoma,* or *ischemia* or *dissecting aneurysms.* An elevated hematocrit and BUN suggest dehydration, usually caused by vomiting and deficient fluid intake.

Urinalysis is vital in differential diagnosis, because the presence of pyuria, particularly white cell casts and bacteria on the smear of urinary sediment, is strong evidence for urinary tract infection and interdicts surgical exploration. Microscopic hematuria suggests stone or tumor of the genitourinary tract; red cell casts, on the other hand, suggest glomerulitis.

Important blood chemistries are *serum amylase,* elevation of which usually reflects acute pancreatitis; however, it may not be elevated in chronic relapsing pancreatitis, and it is elevated in other conditions such as *perforated peptic ulcer, strangulated obstruction* of the small bowel with perforation, and both *acute cholecystitis* and *acute common duct obstruction.*

Roentgenographic Studies in the Acute Abdomen. Roentgenologic examinations of importance include chest films, flat film of the abdomen, intravenous cholangiogram, and intravenous pyelogram. The flat and upright films of the abdomen may be specific for diagnosing free air in the peritoneal cavity, reflecting a perforation of a hollow viscus; in supporting the diagnosis of acute small bowel obstruction; in indicating the likelihood of calculus disease of either gallbladder or urogenital tract; of outlining a large obstructed stomach; and of revealing a variety of soft tissue masses which may reflect cysts or abscesses. Collections of extraintestinal gas often point to abscesses; occasionally, the biliary tree may be outlined by air, thus revealing a fistula to bowel. Diffuse calcification of the region of the pancreas indicates chronic pancreatitis. As noted, calculi in the right lower quadrant may help in the diagnosis of acute appendicitis. Flat film of the abdomen also may yield findings characteristic of acute pancreatitis, including "sentinel" loops and a "cut-off" of the colon. A routine chest x-ray is essential in order to reveal free intraperitoneal air under the diaphragm, to demonstrate pneumonia, or to show an elevated diaphragm on the left with or without pleural effusion and partial atelectasis as noted in acute pancreatitis, or on the right, reflecting subphrenic abscess.

The more special radiographic tests which may be of help in the differential diagnosis include an intravenous cholangiogram to evaluate the possibility of biliary tract obstruction and inflammation; cholangiographic demonstration of the gallbladder renders the diagnosis of acute cholecystitis highly unlikely. Intravenous pyelogram may establish the patency of the urinary tract or, conversely, establish ureteral obstruction or hydronephrosis unilaterally. Examination of the upper gastrointestinal tract with non-barium-containing radiopaque substances (Gastrografin) may help in the diagnosis of perforated ulcer.

Important in the differential diagnosis of acute appendicitis are those nonsurgical conditions which cause acute abdominal pain. These conditions may be excluded by appropriate attention to history, physical examination, and the laboratory studies enumerated in the preceding paragraphs. Chief among these are *pyelonephritis, pneumonia, pulmonary infarction, acute myocardial infarction,* and *pericarditis,* all of which may present with acute upper abdominal pain. Acute distention of the liver and its capsule resulting from acute right heart failure may simulate *acute cholecystitis; acute hepatitis,* viral or toxic (including alcohol), may closely simulate acute biliary tract disease. In these instances, however, an enlarged tender liver will be felt. Further, serum SGOT determinations will be markedly elevated (it is well to remember, however, that acute obstruction of the common duct with cholangitis may transiently raise SGOT to levels of a thousand units or more for 24 to 48 hours).

Systemic diseases, such as *sickle cell disease, acute intermittent porphyria, tabes dorsalis, heavy metal poisoning,* and *diabetic neuropathy,* all may present pictures simulating an acute surgical abdomen. Appropriate tests for sickling, for excretion of porphobilinogen (Watson-Schwartz test), for urinary lead, and for other evidences of syphilis or diabetes greatly aid in ruling out these conditions.

Acute pancreatitis, still considered a nonsurgical condition unless caused by common bile duct obstruction, usually presents with pain of many hours' to days' duration, associated with a history suggestive of biliary tract disease or indicative of acute and chronic alcoholism, and in its early stages abdominal tenderness is usually localized to the epigastrium. Markedly elevated plasma amylase (within 48 hours of onset) or urinary amylase (up to 5 days after onset) will help establish the diagnosis.

Special Considerations of Age in Differential Diagnosis of Acute Appendicitis. Great care must be extended to establish the diagnosis of this condition in the very young and very old. Children with diffuse abdominal pain which is preceded by anorexia, nausea, and vomiting and often associated with diarrhea are more likely to have *acute infectious gastroenteritis. Acute mesenteric adenitis,* presumably caused by viral illnesses and often associated with diffuse abdominal pain, is frequently confused with acute appendicitis in children. The difficulty is in those patients in whom there is some right lower quadrant tenderness and slight elevation of the white count. In such instances a diagnosis must be established at operation, because it is far safer to undertake a negative exploration than to neglect removal of an acutely inflamed appendix.

In young females diagnosis is confused by problems in the reproductive system, such as *ruptured graafian follicles, twisted ovarian cysts, ectopic pregnancies, dysmenorrhea, ruptured endometrioma,* and *acute pelvic inflammatory disease. Ruptured ectopic pregnancy* is usually of dramatic suddenness and is often associated with shock and massive blood loss; these findings in a pregnant woman make the diagnosis virtually certain. The *ruptured graafian follicle* is noted in midcycle; fever and leukocytosis are uncommon. Tenderness on moving of cervix on vaginal examination points toward a *twisted ovarian cyst,* the pain of which is out of proportion to the general well-being of the patient. *Gonococcal salpingitis* may be difficult to establish, because endocervical smears may be negative for the organism. Usually, however, the pain is more diffuse and tenderness not so well localized as in appendicitis. However, in questionable instances, exploration must be performed.

The differential diagnosis of appendicitis in the elderly may also be difficult. The classic picture is seldom noted, the history may be inadequate or misleading because of infirmity or the effects of medication, and the appendix perforates early. Findings on physical examination are usually not as dramatic, and, despite complications, fever may only be slightly elevated. Accuracy in diagnosis of patients over 60 years of age is below 70 per cent, and the incidence of perforation without a localized or generalized peritonitis at surgery is nearly 70 per cent—more than twice as high as all other age groups combined.

In elderly patients the principal problems in differential diagnosis are *cholecystitis, diverticulitis, mesenteric thrombosis, intestinal obstruction, incarcerated hernia,* and *perforated ulcer.* In these individuals it is well simply to recognize that one is dealing with a surgical abdomen, because, as stated, it is difficult to be clinically accurate in establishing acute appendicitis.

Right-sided acute diverticulitis may simulate acute appendicitis in every respect. In a few instances, *left-sided diverticulitis* may localize tenderness to the right lower quadrant, because the sigmoid is often more redundant in the elderly, and an excessively mobile loop may come to rest on the right side of the abdomen. In such instances, the patient also may have symptoms suggestive of diverticulitis, such as an episode of diarrhea associated with cramping or steady lower abdominal pain, slight temperature elevation, and, later, evidence of moderate to complete large bowel obstruction. When differential diagnosis is difficult, a cautious barium enema may help greatly in excluding acute diverticulitis as the cause of the problem.

Conversely, elderly patients must not be subjected to the risk of exploration falsely. Accordingly, all efforts should be extended to make certain that *acute myocardial* or *pulmonary infarction, pneumonia,* or other systemic disease or toxin is not responsible for acute abdominal pain simulating appendicitis.

Treatment. Unless strongly contraindicated, the only therapy for acute appendicitis is surgical removal of the appendix. Since mortality correlates with perforation and, except in elderly patients, perforation correlates with duration of symptoms, early diagnosis and appendectomy are essential for the lowest acceptable morbidity and mortality for the disease. When surgery is performed early in the disease in an otherwise healthy individual, mortality is only slightly above that for general anesthesia. In view of these facts and since the diagnosis is often difficult to make early in the course of disease, some normal appendices will inevitably have to be removed. To avoid the catastrophe of unoperated-upon acute appendicitis, normal appendices may have to be removed in 20 to 25 per cent of patients.

In patients in whom complications have already occurred prior to surgery, necessary measures to correct dehydration and combat infection must be instituted. If perforation is very likely or suspected, continuous nasogastric suction should be instituted. Those patients with temperatures higher than 39° C and with findings indicative of localized abscess or generalized peritonitis should be given broad-spectrum antimicrobials, usually high-dose penicillin and gentamicin or high-dose ampicillin.

The surgical approach, i.e., whether the usual transabdominal or other, to institute drainage of an established abscess is a decision for the surgeon to make. In those patients with obvious acute appendicitis for whom no surgeon is available, the patients may be treated with head-up position of the bed, intravenous fluids, broad-spectrum antimicrobial drugs, and nasogastric suction. The chance for recovery in otherwise healthy individuals with this program is surprisingly good.

Morbidity and Mortality of Surgery. Over-all, about 15 per cent of patients with acute appendicitis develop complications postoperatively; this figure is 35.6 per cent in those with perforation and localized peritonitis at the time of surgery and is 70 per cent in those with perforation and generalized peritonitis. The complications include *wound infection, intra-abdominal abscess,* mechanical *small bowel obstruction, fecal fistula,* and, much more rarely, *intraperitoneal hemorrhage. Pylephlebitis* is extremely rare (one in a thousand). In the elderly, of course, mortality is increased by the usual cardiovascular, pulmonary, renal, and cerebral complications.

The over-all mortality of acute appendicitis is now less than 1 per 100,000 population. It ranges from 0.18 to 1.6 per cent and is due principally to the interrelated factors of age and perforation. Indeed, mortality over the age of 60 ranges from 6.4 to 14 per cent. The cause of death in this group may be attributed equally to septic and nonseptic complications.

Special Considerations. *Incidental Appendectomy.* In view of the decreasing risk of appendicitis with advancing age and the extremely low risk of developing acute appendicitis, it is difficult to advocate elective appendectomy during laparotomy (for example, at age 37 years the risk is 0.0431 for males and 0.369 for females). Nevertheless, if the procedure should be performed, the patient, as in any other operation, should be fully informed of what was done.

Prophylactic Appendectomy. At present all data indicate that there is no place for prophylactic appendectomy. The one possible exception may be a move of indefinite duration to an area where neither adequate medical care nor surgical care is available on the part of an individual known to have a fecalith in the region of the appendix.

654. DIVERTICULITIS

Definition. Diverticulitis of the colon is a complication of diverticulosis defined as a micro- or macroperforation of a diverticulum. The etiology and pathogenesis of this complication are not clear; however, it is thought that increased segmental pressure causes a weakened area in the wall to perforate. There is no evidence for vascular occlusion or obstruction by stool as the cause.

Clinical Picture. The predominant clinical symptoms of diverticulitis are *pain* and *fever*. The pain is usually prominent and is frequently constant. Most commonly, it is localized in the left lower quadrant, because the sigmoid and descending colons are the sites of the largest number of diverticula. Occasionally, the patient will have a brief period of diarrhea or a few loose stools, and only rarely is rectal bleeding noted with diverticulitis. When the perforation and sepsis are of sufficient magnitude, the patient may also have chills with fever as high as 39 to 39.5° C. Usually, however, the fever is low grade, between 38 and 39° C.

Although the pain may be somewhat intermittent and even colicky at onset, it usually becomes steady and is of the same quality as noted in acute appendicitis. Indeed, acute diverticulitis has often been referred to as "left-sided appendicitis." The patient may present for examination after only a few hours or, when the situation is not so severe, after a few days of lingering but nagging left lower quadrant pain and low-grade fever.

Physical examination is extremely important in establishing the diagnosis. Since the process usually quickly involves the serosal surface and peritoneal cover, tenderness will be marked, and, as in acute appendicitis when the process has reached the peritoneal surface, will be both direct and rebound, though localized. Frequently, a tender mass may be discerned. When present for more than a few days, this mass may be astonishingly firm, even hard, and the distinction grossly from carcinoma is almost impossible. Rectal examination also will be painful, because inflamed bowel is often within reach of the finger; also, a mass may be palpable if a sizable abscess has formed.

In some instances the patient will present with complications of diverticulitis: *dysuria, pyuria,* and *pneumaturia,* all related to involvement of the urinary bladder. In extreme instances, the inflammatory process has perforated into the bladder; symptoms may be due to large collections of pus, not only adjacent to the colon, but also in the pelvis or under the diaphragm. Often the presenting symptom in these instances is simply septic fever. Rarely, the diverticulum perforates freely. In this instance the signs of free perforation are evident; that is, distention of the abdomen, generalized rebound tenderness, and absent bowel sounds.

Diagnosis. Diagnosis of diverticulitis should be suspected especially in patients with known diverticula who present with fever, leukocytosis, and signs of pericolic and peritoneal inflammation in the left lower quadrant. The diagnosis is even more likely if a mass is palpable. Fever between 38.5 and 39° C is also compatible with the diagnosis; when the process is more extensive and with formation of a *pericolic abscess* and its complications, the temperature is usually over 39° C, and the white count is proportionately higher. Urinalysis will reflect varying degrees of involvement of the urinary tract by this septic process; that is, with mild ureteral irritation a few red and white cells may be seen in the urinary sediment, but with direct involvement of the ureter or invasion of the ureter or the bladder by a pericolic abscess, the urine may be frankly septic and contain large numbers of red cells. Witnessing a patient pass gas on urination is also a sign, in the presence of other findings, that diverticulitis is the probable underlying diagnosis.

Some patients suffer much left flank pain owing to *hydronephrosis* resulting from obstruction of the ureter

by a *pericolic abscess.* An intravenous pyelogram shows no function or an obstructed kidney on the left.

The use of x-rays is of crucial importance in the diagnosis, especially flat film of the abdomen. Evidence of pericolic perforation and abscess formation may be suspected from collections of air and fluid in the left lower quadrant; free air may be seen under the diaphragm in instances of free perforation, and with complete sigmoid obstruction the dilatation of the proximal colon down to the point of the obstruction affords important information.

Sigmoidoscopy should be carefully performed. Air insufflation should not be used, and the importance of the examination is to exclude other conditions (see below). Usually, diverticulitis per se produces no abnormalities on sigmoidoscopy except an undue amount of spasm at the rectosigmoid junction.

Clinicians debate the advisability of using a barium enema in the diagnosis of diverticulitis, particularly in its acute phase. The concern is that the increased intraluminal pressure may produce further complications. The history, physical examination, and laboratory information are sufficient to make the clinical diagnosis in the vast majority of instances, and barium enema should await some subsidence of the acute phase of the illness. The single exception to this dictum is in those instances in which the clinical picture does not permit distinguishing between *acute ischemic colitis* of the left colon and sigmoid diverticulitis.

The roentgenographic features characteristic of diverticulitis are the presence of barium outside a diverticulum, the delineation of a pericolic mass, or the demonstration of a fistula originating in the colon. In some instances the distinction between diverticulitis and carcinoma may be difficult. The presence of irregularity, thickening, or even a sawtooth appearance of the bowel is not sufficient to make the diagnosis of diverticulitis, because these are typical for diverticula without perforation.

After diagnosis of diverticulitis has been established, intravenous pyelography should be done to ascertain whether or not obstructive involvement of the urinary tract is present, particularly on the left side. In some instances, as noted above, urinary symptoms may be the predominant feature, and radiographic examination of the urinary tract may have to be performed early.

Differential Diagnosis. *Diverticulosis.* For many years symptoms of *diverticulosis* have been attributed incorrectly to diverticulitis. *Diverticulosis* may periodically be associated with marked local tenderness, a palpable sigmoid loop, and some degree of large bowel obstruction, and thus the picture suggests diverticulitis. However, such patients usually do not have fever, the localized tenderness gradually recedes, the white count is not elevated, and there is no evidence of involvement of contiguous organs. Barium enema will reveal an irregular luminal contour with a narrowed sigmoid, possibly even a so-called sawtooth appearance of the mucosa. Barium must be noted outside the diverticulum, a fistula seen, or evidences of a pericolic or intramural mass detected before the diagnosis of diverticulitis is definitely made.

Carcinoma of the colon must be distinguished from diverticulitis because of similarity of age during which both diverticulitis and cancer of the colon appear. The differential diagnosis is especially difficult, because diverticulitis also often causes luminal narrowing with partial or complete bowel obstruction, may be associated with mild rectal bleeding, and may appear rather insidiously. Chronic obstruction, more persistent rectal bleeding, and weight loss are more characteristic of *cancer,* whereas localized tenderness with rebound, leukocytosis, and fever support the diagnosis of diverticulitis. In some cases, however, it may be impossible to distinguish the two conditions, especially when the barium enema has features common to both; that is, a mass, luminal irregularities, and partial obstruction. The matter can only be settled at exploratory laparotomy. In those instances in which the signs and symptoms of obstruction rather rapidly recede, repeat barium enema will reveal marked improvement only in the patient with diverticulitis. In the event that a suspicious defect remains, exploration will have to be done.

Granulomatous colitis may be difficult to exclude in the face of marked luminal narrowing or multiloculated channels parallel to the bowel wall on x-ray. Clinically, although both may exhibit pain, partial obstruction and lower abdominal mass, some rectal bleeding, fever, and leukocytosis, the history preceding the inflammatory event is usually markedly different. The patient with granulomatous colitis usually will have had previous episodes of lower abdominal pain, fever, and diarrhea, and it is unusual for such patients to present for the first time with advanced localized colonic disease.

Sigmoidoscopy may be crucial in making the differential diagnosis if the rectum is involved with granulomatous disease. Also, evidence elsewhere in the bowel of granulomatous disease, such as cobblestoning, long intramucosal sinus tracts, and skip areas, will help in the differential diagnosis (see Ch. 652).

Ischemic colitis of the left colon in elderly patients may present with signs and symptoms of bowel necrosis and localized peritonitis which are difficult to distinguish from diverticulitis. In these instances, gross rectal bleeding is prominent, and a barium enema is of crucial importance, because so-called "thumb printing" will be found in ischemic colitis, especially in the area of the splenic flexure and descending colon (see Ch. 659).

Treatment of Diverticulitis. The patient is given nothing by mouth, and continuous nasogastric suction is instituted if signs of obstruction are present or if the patient is nauseated. Appropriate intravenous fluid is administered. Broad-spectrum antimicrobials should be given to cover gram-positive cocci and anaerobic bacteroides; e.g., high-dose penicillin or gentamicin or ampicillin and kanamycin. Tetracycline or chloramphenicol should be added if sepsis is severe. Some favor clindamycin (against *B. fragilis*) in the latter situation.

As noted above, an intravenous pyelogram should be performed early if the clinical picture suggests urinary tract infection or left ureteral obstruction. Surgical consultation must be obtained early in all cases in which a mass is palpable or when there is suspicion of peritonitis or involvement of a contiguous organ.

Most patients respond well to this type of therapy with abatement of the fever, tenderness, and evidence of partial obstruction. Long-term therapy becomes identical with that for diverticulosis (see Ch. 639).

Indications for Surgery. Surgical intervention is necessary for generalized peritonitis or for failure of medical therapy as evidenced by enlargement of a mass, appearance of a mass during therapy, persisting intestinal obstruction, or the development of a fistula. Elective surgery is indicated for recurrent attacks of diverticulitis and for the inability to exclude a carcinoma as the cause for persisting deformity after recovery from the acute phase.

655. RADIATION ENTEROCOLITIS

Damage to the small intestine and colon may result from radiation therapy for abdominal and pelvic malignancy.

Incidence. Incidence of radiation injury varies between 2.5 and 25 per cent of patients treated with radiotherapy for pelvic and intra-abdominal malignancy. It is noted most commonly after the total dosage exceeds 5000 rads. Transient histologic inflammatory change may, however, be found in the rectal mucosa of nearly 75 per cent of individuals receiving such therapeutic irradiation.

Pathogenesis and Pathology. Radiation damage results from interference with cell replication. Further, damage to the mesothelial cells of the small submucosal arterioles results in varying degrees of occlusion and mucosal transmural necrosis. Accordingly, hyperemia and ulceration of the mucosa are frequent. With extreme damage, diffuse edema is followed by extensive fibrosis with multiple strictures and irreversible damage.

The pathologic changes range from diminution of crypt cell mitosis, shortening of the villi of the small intestine to varying degrees of hyperemia, edema, and inflammatory cell infiltration of the mucosa. Progress of damage is marked by crypt abscesses, sloughing of epithelial cells, and, later, mucosal ulcerations, diffuse or localized, are found. Two to 12 months after radiotherapy, the damage to the blood vessels becomes prominent. In these instances, repair of acute damage does not ensue. The mucosa and submucosa become progressively ischemic and fibrotic. *Abscesses* and *fistulas* may form with sinus tracts between loops of intestine and between intestine and neighboring organs.

Clinical Picture. Symptoms may appear early, that is, during the first or second week of therapy, or late, that is, six months or more after completion of therapy. Early, diarrhea and mild rectal bleeding may appear, resembling ulcerative colitis. Sigmoidoscopy reveals an edematous mucosa which may be friable; in more extreme instances, the acute changes also reveal a patchy or diffusely necrotic mucosa.

Later, symptoms of radiation include gross rectal bleeding, decrease in stool caliber, and progressive difficulty in defecation with marked constipation, all indicating severe rectal involvement. Small intestinal symptoms result from either fibrosis and obstruction or fistulization and abscess formation. If the damage is especially diffuse, malabsorption may be noted, as described in Part XIV, Section Three.

Diagnosis. Diagnosis of radiation enteritis is suspected with any of the aforementioned symptoms in patients who have received significant radiation. Sigmoidoscopy shows a picture which ranges from variable degrees of edema to a markedly inflamed and necrotic mucosa. Multiple telangiectases are common, as is rectal stricture. Since most cases are fairly clear cut, biopsy is usually not indicated.

Barium studies of the intestine are not specific and range from changes of diffuse edema and spasm to diffuse fibrosis with strictures, fistulas, and ulceration in more severe cases. Thus the picture may resemble localized malignancy in the colon or diffuse granulomatous disease in the small intestine. Long strictured areas may also be noted, however, in the colon.

Differential diagnostic usefulness of small vessel angiography to the intestine in radiation enteritis remains to be confirmed.

Treatment. Improving methods for monitoring radiotherapy will probably reduce the incidence of this complication; however, the increasing incidence of malignancy and of the efficacy of radiotherapy will probably increase the total number of such patients.

Symptoms caused by early reaction consist of mild diarrhea and perhaps some minimal bleeding which can be managed with the judicious use of tranquilizers, anticholinergic drugs, local analgesics, and warm sitz baths. If rectal bleeding is prominent, treatment with steroid retention enemas should be initiated as in ulcerative colitis (see Ch. 651). If the bleeding is more significant, transfusions may be required and even, possibly, surgery. Rectal strictures may be dilated, providing that it is early in their course and they are not extensive. Lubricants and stool softeners are often helpful; however, the progress to symptomatic occlusion of the lumen may necessitate proximal colostomy. Fistulas should be resected and abscesses drained. Resection of bowel and anastomoses are hazardous in view of the impaired blood supply.

In patients with malabsorption, treatment is as outlined in Part XIV, Section Three.

Prognosis. Prognosis depends on the extent and degree of damage, the age of the patient, the course of the underlying malignancy, and whether or not the patient has systemic vascular disease. Unfortunately, extensive disease of the colon usually means significant disease in the small intestine. The prognosis is guarded in those with ulceration, fibrosis, or fistulas in whom repeated resections or other major surgical procedures must be carried out. In such cases, age and cardiovascular status are also crucial determining factors.

656. PSEUDOMEMBRANOUS ENTEROCOLITIS

Pseudomembranous enterocolitis is an inflammatory disease of the small and large bowel; occasionally it involves either the small bowel or the large bowel exclusively.

Etiology and Pathogenesis. The cause for this disease is not known; however, it is usually seen in patients with underlying serious illness, in the postoperative period, with intestinal obstruction, and in individuals receiving antimicrobial therapy for a variety of infections. In some instances it is associated with recovery of *Staphylococcus aureus* from intestinal contents, but the exact relationship of the organism to the disease is not clearly defined. Shock or ischemia of the intestine may also play a role in the pathogenesis of this entity.

Pathology. The involved bowel is covered with yellowish-green membranous plaques which may become confluent. The changes in the mucosa range from mild edema to marked friability and ulceration. The "membrane" is made up of fibrin, mucus, and a variety of mononuclear and polymorphonuclear cells; staphylococci may also be seen in clusters. Mucosal ulcerations may be scattered, and the submucosal tissue is edematous and congested. In its advanced stage, the intestine is completely covered with the membrane, and the underlying bowel exhibits extensive necrosis and ulceration.

Clinical Picture. As noted above, the disease appears in the setting of other illness or disability. Its onset is abrupt, with fever from 38 to 40° C, associated with watery diarrhea containing mucus, pus, and, on occasion, blood. The amount of fluid lost may be extreme, and dehydration and metabolic acidosis may be prominent.

Diagnosis. The disease should be suspected when the symptoms described appear in particular settings. Stool may reveal clusters of gram-positive cocci, suggesting *S. aureus*. Sigmoidoscopy may reveal hyperemia, some friability, and whitish exudate. In more severe instances, scattered ulcers may be noted with marked hyperemia and edema. Roentgenographic examinations with barium yield nondiagnostic findings, some of which resemble ulcerative colitis. Culture of the stool may reveal an overgrowth of *Staphylococcus aureus*.

Treatment. Attention must be first paid to dehydration and electrolyte imbalance which includes hyponatremia and hypokalemia. As in enterotoxic diarrhea, enormous amounts of fluid may be required—10 to 15 liters in 24 to 36 hours. Potassium must be replaced before bicarbonate may be given for acidosis.

Shock must be combated with intravenous fluids, pressor agents, and 100 mg of prednisolone per 24 hours intravenously. If staphylococci are seen on fecal smear, then appropriate antimicrobial agents such as methicillin or cephalothin should be given; if the patient is sensitive to penicillin, erythromycin, 2 to 4 grams intravenously per day, should be administered. After the initial 48 hours of therapy, attention must be paid to replacement of protein which has been lost into the intestine by administration of salt-free albumin (50 to 100 grams per 24 hours).

Prognosis. Unfortunately, the mortality is extremely high in pseudomembranous enterocolitis, 50 to 75 per cent. The reason is that this disease is superimposed upon an already serious clinical situation. If fluid and electrolyte balance is quickly restored and blood pressure returns to normal with increasing urinary output and cessation of diarrhea, the prognosis is good. Such signs are usually noted within 72 hours.

657. PRIMARY NONSPECIFIC ULCERATION OF THE SMALL INTESTINE

This inflammatory disease of unknown etiology is rare, although in a majority of instances it is attributable to ingestion of enteric-coated potassium chloride. Such ulceration may also be associated with *vascular disease, central nervous system disease, infection, trauma,* and *malnutrition.*

The clinical picture consists of symptoms of small bowel obstruction and, more rarely, perforation or bleeding. Earlier, the patient reveals periumbilical colicky pain and perhaps nausea and vomiting.

If the patient has small bowel obstruction, the findings associated with this condition would be noted. Distention, diffuse tympany, absence of liver dullness, and generalized tenderness with rebound may be found on examination if the ulcer has perforated.

Laboratory investigation is normal unless the patient has been bleeding or has had protracted vomiting; plain films of the abdomen are of great value if small bowel obstruction is present. Barium contrast studies in the uncomplicated cases are most often unrevealing, although in rare instances ulceration and narrowing in the jejunum may be noted.

Treatment for the disease is surgical with resection of the involved segment. Potassium supplements (if prescribed) in such patients should always be given in liquid form.

NONGRANULOMATOUS DIFFUSE ILEOJEJUNITIS AND EOSINOPHILIC GASTROENTERITIS

Diffuse nongranulomatous ileojejunitis and *eosinophilic gastroenteritis* are described in Part XIV, Section Three. *Tuberculous enteritis* and *enterocolitis* are discussed in Ch. 234.

Acute Appendicitis (Including the Acute Abdomen)

Babcock, J. R., and McKinley, W. M.: Acute appendicitis: An analysis of 1662 consecutive cases. Ann. Surg., 150:131, 1959.

Deal, R. D.: Acute appendicitis. *In* Sleisenger, M. H., and Fordtran, J. S. (eds.): Gastrointestinal Disease. Philadelphia, W. B. Saunders Company, 1973, p. 1494.

Kazarian, K. K., Roeder, W. J., and Mersheimer, W. L.: Decreasing mortality and increasing morbidity from acute appendicitis. Am. J. Surg., 119:681, 1970.

Stone, H. H., Sanders, S. L., and Martin, J. D.: Perforated appendicitis in children. Surgery, 69:673, 1971.

Diverticulitis

Loeb, P. M., and Sleisenger, M. H.: Diverticular disease of the colon. *In* Sleisenger, M. H., and Fordtran, J. S. (eds.): Gastrointestinal Disease. Philadelphia, W. B. Saunders Company, 1973, p. 1415.

Reid, D. R. K.: Acute diverticulitis of the caecum and ascending colon. Br. J. Surg., 39:76, 1957.

Rodkey, G. V., and Welch, C. E.: Diverticulitis of the colon. Evolution in concept and therapy. Surg. Clin. North Am., 45:1231, 1965.

Radiation Enterocolitis

DeCosse, J. J., Rhodes, R. S., Wentz, W. B., Reagan, J. W., Dwarken, H. J., and Holden, W. D.: The natural history and management of radiation-induced injury of the gastrointestinal tract. Ann. Surg., 170:369, 1969.

Earnest, D. L., and Trier, J. S.: Radiation enteritis and colitis. *In* Sleisenger, M. H., and Fordtran, J. S. (eds.): Gastrointestinal Disease. Philadelphia. W. B. Saunders Company, 1973, p. 1406.

Pseudomembranous Enterocolitis

Birnbaum, D., Laufer, A., and Freund, M.: Pseudomembranous enterocolitis, a clinicopathologic study. Gastroenterology, 41:345, 1961.

Curtis, K. J., and Sleisenger, M. H.: Infectious and parasitic diseases. *In* Sleisenger, M. H., and Fordtran, J. S. (eds.): Gastrointestinal Disease. Philadelphia, W. B. Saunders Company, 1973, p. 1369.

Jeffries, G. H., Steinberg, H., and Sleisenger, M. H.: Chronic ulcerative (non-granulomatous) jejunitis. Am. J. Med., 44:47, 1968.

Karz, S., Guth, P. H., and Plonsky, L.: Chronic ulcerative jejuno-ileitis. Am. J. Gastroenterol., 56:61, 1971.

Lawrason, F. D., Alpert, G., Mohr, F. L., and McMahon, F. G.: Obstructive-ulcerative lesions of the small intestine. J.A.M.A., 191:641, 1965.

Watson, M. R.: Primary nonspecific ulceration of the small bowel. Arch. Surg., 87:600, 1963.

Eosinophilic Gastroenteritis

Greenberger, N., and Gryboski, J.: Allergic disorders of the intestine and eosinophilic gastroenteritis. *In* Sleisenger, M. H., and Fordtran, J. S. (eds.): Gastrointestinal Disease. Philadelphia, W. B. Saunders Company, 1973, p. 1066.

Gryboski, J. D., Burkle, F., and Hillman, R.: Milk-induced colitis in an infant. Pediatrics, 38:299, 1966.

Heiner, D. C., Wilson, J. F., and Lahey, M. E.: Sensitivity to cow's milk. J.A.M.A., 189:563, 1964.

Klein, N. C., Hargrove, M. D., Sleisenger, M. H., and Jeffries, G. H.: Eosinophilic gastroenteritis. Medicine, 49:299, 1970.

Leinbach, G. E., and Rubin, C. E.: Eosinophilic gastroenteritis: A simple reaction to food allergens. Gastroenterology, 59:874, 1970.

Ureles, A. L., Alschibaja, T., Lodico, D., and Stabins, S. J.: Idiopathic eosinophilic infiltration of the gastrointestinal tract, diffuse and circumscribed. Am. J. Med., 30:899, 1961.

Section Six. VASCULAR DISEASES OF THE INTESTINE

Robert K. Ockner

658. NORMAL ANATOMY AND PHYSIOLOGY OF THE SPLANCHNIC CIRCULATION

The supply of blood to the abdominal viscera depends upon three relatively large arteries which originate on the ventral aspect of the aorta. The most cephalad of these, the celiac axis, arises at the level of the twelfth thoracic or first lumbar vertebra, i.e., approximately at the insertion of the median arcuate ligament of the diaphragm (Fig. 1). Its subdivisions supply the liver and biliary structures (hepatic artery), spleen (splenic artery), and the stomach (left gastric and gastroepiploic, short gastrics, and branches of the gastroduodenal, including the right gastroepiploic). Important anastomotic connections between the hepatic branch of the celiac artery and the superior mesenteric artery (i.e., the pancreaticoduodenal arcades) are found in the region of the second portion of the duodenum, and branches of these also supply the pancreas and duodenum.

The second major splanchnic artery, the superior mesenteric, arises from the aorta just caudal to the celiac (Fig. 2). In addition to its pancreaticoduodenal anastomoses with the celiac arterial system, branches of the superior mesenteric artery supply those portions of the small and large intestines between the distal duodenum

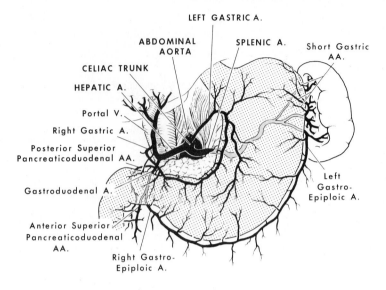

Figure 1. Arterial supply to the stomach and duodenum, showing major branches of the celiac axis and the superior portion of the pancreaticoduodenal arcades. (From Ockner, R. K., *In* Sleisenger, M. H., and Fordtran, J. S. [eds.]: Gastrointestinal Disease. Philadelphia, W. B. Saunders Company, 1973.)

and the distal transverse colon. The relatively large caliber of this vessel and its oblique take-off from the aorta render it particularly susceptible to entry by emboli originating in the heart and proximal aorta.

The third splanchnic arterial branch of the aorta is the inferior mesenteric. This vessel, the smallest of the three, arises at the level of the third lumbar vertebra and supplies the distal transverse and descending colon, sigmoid, and proximal rectum. Its branches connect with those of the superior mesenteric via the arc of Riolan ("meandering mesenteric artery") and the marginal artery (Fig. 2), and with the inferior and middle rectal branches of the hypogastric (internal iliac) arteries.

The system of abundant interconnections among the three major splanchnic arterial systems (i.e., the celiac, and the superior and inferior mesenterics) allows for the formation of collateral channels in the event that occlusive vascular disease develops. As a result, it is not uncommon for slowly developing complete or nearly complete occlusions of a single vessel to be associated with

little in the way of clinical sequelae. As with other systems, however, development of adequate collaterals requires time, and the sudden occlusion of even normal vessels (e.g., by emboli) usually results in infarction.

Blood flow in the splanchnic system depends not only on the patency of the large and medium-sized arteries described above, but also on systemic arterial pressure and the resistance at the arteriolar level. The latter is modulated not only in response to systemic arterial pressure itself (i.e., "autoregulation"), but also by a wide variety of other physiologic and pharmacologic factors. Thus resistance drops and flow increases during feeding and under certain neural and hormonal influences, including vagal stimulation, cholecystokinin, gastrin, secretin, and β-adrenergic stimulators, e.g., isoproterenol. Conversely, splanchnic vasoconstriction and decreased blood flow result from α-adrenergic stimuli, as occur in shock and other circumstances associated with endogenous catecholamine release. Digitalis glycosides also have been shown to cause splanchnic vasoconstriction. In the

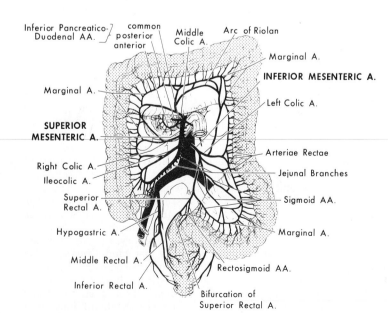

Figure 2. Arterial supply to the small and large intestines, showing the inferior portion of the pancreaticoduodenal arcades and the anastomoses between superior and inferior mesenteric arteries (arc of Riolan or "meandering mesenteric," and the marginal artery). (From Ockner, R. K., *In* Sleisenger, M. H., and Fordtran, J. S. [eds.]: Gastrointestinal Disease. Philadelphia, W. B. Saunders Company, 1973.)

final analysis, the adequacy of vascular perfusion is determined by the balance between tissue needs and local oxygen supply, and it is this balance, not merely the patency of any given vessel, that most often determines whether ischemia or infarction will occur.

659. ACUTE VISCERAL ISCHEMIC SYNDROMES

Acute Bowel Infarction: Mesenteric Artery Thrombosis. Thrombotic occlusion of the superior mesenteric artery may be asymptomatic if it evolves slowly enough to permit the formation of adequate collaterals, as noted above. More sudden occlusions, however, are associated with ischemic infarction of some or all of the supplied bowel. Most commonly, advanced atherosclerotic disease is responsible, but the syndrome may also occur in dissecting aneurysm, systemic vasculitis of all varieties, use of oral contraceptives, hypercoagulable states, and, rarely, without apparent explanation. Among causes of bowel infarction, the true incidence of arterial thrombosis is not certain, but it may be less common than previously thought in view of the increasingly recognized importance of *nonthrombotic* infarction (see below).

The clinical presentation of intestinal infarction (thrombotic or nonthrombotic) is often a misleading one. In its advanced stages, the associated abdominal pain, signs of intestinal obstruction, fever, leukocytosis, volume depletion, peritonitis with bloody abdominal fluid, hematemesis, and rectal bleeding are "classic" and render the diagnosis obvious. Earlier in the course, however, abdominal findings may be minimal, and the far less specific features of fever, leukocytosis, pain, and confusional state may dominate the clinical picture. Bowel sounds not only may be present, but may be hyperactive. The history is usually not helpful, but evidence of pre-existing "abdominal angina" (see below) or other conditions predisposing to thrombosis may aid in the evaluation of the problem.

The early diagnosis of bowel infarction depends upon a high index of suspicion, presumptive exclusion of other conditions likely to present as an acute abdomen, and, ultimately, surgical exploration. The demonstration of mesenteric vascular occlusion by abdominal angiography does not necessarily mean that the patient has an acute bowel infarction, because many patients with advanced occlusive disease are asymptomatic. On the other hand, the demonstration of *patent* vessels may serve to exclude *surgically correctable* vascular disease as a cause of bowel infarction (but will not exclude nonthrombotic infarction).

Initial therapeutic efforts should be supportive, i.e., correction of fluid and electrolyte imbalance (including administration of blood, plasma, or albumin as needed), cardiopulmonary support, and broad-spectrum antimicrobial drugs. Unoperated, acute bowel infarction carries essentially a 100 per cent mortality rate. Unfortunately, since many patients with this diagnosis are poor surgical risks because of age, advanced vascular disease affecting other vital organs, or poor general condition resulting from delay in diagnosis, surgery itself may contribute to

a fatal outcome. As a rule, however, operation should be undertaken as soon as the patient is in optimal condition, because time is of the essence. At surgery, infarcted bowel should be resected and, if large vessel thrombi are present and the patient's condition permits, corrective vascular surgery (bypass or endarterectomy) may be attempted. Because it is often difficult to define accurately the limits of viable bowel, many surgeons have recommended a "second look" operation after 24 hours, in order to resect any additional nonviable intestine. It should be recognized, however, that even under the best of circumstances, massive bowel infarction carries a mortality rate of at least 60 to 70 per cent, except in those cases caused by emboli (see below), in which a somewhat more favorable prognosis may be expected.

Nonthrombotic Intestinal Infarction. This syndrome presents clinically in a manner quite similar to that of thrombotic infarction, but only more recently has its frequency been appreciated. Characteristically but not invariably, it occurs in a setting in which systemic anoxia, hypotension, congestive cardiac failure, or severe dehydration impairs the delivery of adequately oxygenated blood to the bowel, even though the splanchnic vessels themselves are patent. The mucosa, being most sensitive to oxygen deprivation, undergoes hemorrhagic necrosis first, but necrosis of the entire bowel wall usually supervenes. Although experience is accumulating with the potential usefulness of administration of vasodilator substances as a means of restoring intestinal vascular perfusion, treatment of this extremely grave condition is essentially the same as that of thrombotic infarction, i.e., supportive therapy and, as soon as feasible, surgical resection of infarcted bowel.

Mesenteric Embolic Disease. As noted, arterial emboli to the splanchnic viscera most commonly lodge in the superior mesenteric artery. They usually arise from endocardial mural thrombi or vegetations, or from atherosclerotic plaques in the proximal aorta. The condition is associated with diseases (e.g., mitral stenosis) which occur in a somewhat younger population than that at risk for thrombotic or nonthrombotic infarction, and because of this and the fact that its dramatic clinical presentation often leads to earlier diagnosis, embolic disease carries a somewhat more favorable prognosis. Classically, a patient with mitral stenosis will experience the sudden onset of severe periumbilical pain, followed by vomiting and diarrhea. Initially bleeding may be absent and bowel sounds present, but ultimately the picture progresses, if untreated, to one identical with that of advanced thrombotic infarction. Treatment consists of urgent exploration, with embolectomy and, if necessary, resection of infarcted bowel, followed by a "second look" procedure. It is important to note that there are well-documented examples of cases in which early embolectomy has obviated the need for bowel resection, although a transient malabsorption syndrome may result.

Ischemic Colitis. The large bowel is subject to most of the same problems associated with impaired blood supply which affect the small intestine, and many of the same pathophysiologic, diagnostic, and therapeutic principles apply. Thus outright infarction of the colon (thrombotic or nonthrombotic) may lead to perforation and peritonitis, and may require surgical intervention. The clinical presentation of ischemic colonic disease takes on a broader aspect, however, in that patients may present with a self-limited episode characterized by left-sided abdominal pain, fever, leukocytosis, and passage of bloody stools. The potential confusion resulting from this superficial resemblance to acute ulcerative colitis may be compounded by sigmoidoscopic findings which also suggest ulcerative colitis. Sigmoidoscopy, however, may disclose a normal mucosa, or one which shows discrete ulcers or blue-black hemorrhagic submucosal blebs or nodules. All or part of the colon may be involved, but the process usually affects the region of the splenic flexure or rectosigmoid. For those patients in whom surgery is not indicated, barium contrast studies performed after subsidence of the acute phase disclose mucosal edema and hemorrhage, as reflected by a sawtooth irregularity or by so-called "thumbprinting." Eventually, the healing process is often associated with scar and stricture formation, possibly necessitating surgery at a later date because of partial obstruction.

The true incidence of ischemic colitis is difficult to estimate, but its presence should be suspected in any patient over 50 who first presents with what clinically resembles acute ulcerative colitis. Although reconstructive surgery of the inferior mesenteric artery is generally not feasible, the recognition of this entity may avert the use of potentially harmful corticosteroid therapy.

660. CHRONIC VISCERAL ISCHEMIC SYNDROMES

Abdominal Angina. This is an uncommon syndrome of postprandial epigastric or midabdominal pain resulting from relative bowel ischemia. It usually occurs 15 to 30 minutes after eating, i.e., at a time when intestinal blood flow and oxygen demand normally increase, and persists for one to two hours. The syndrome is almost invariably associated with extensive atherosclerosis affecting two or more of the major visceral arterial trunks. Clinically, in addition to the history of pain, patients exhibit marked weight loss. Although the over-all picture may suggest a diagnosis of advanced malignancy, careful questioning will usually elicit a fear of pain, which the patient has learned to associate with eating, resulting in diminished food intake. History and physical examination often provide evidence of atherosclerotic disease affecting other vessels, but the presence or absence of an abdominal bruit is of little help. Establishment of the diagnosis, which must be strongly suggested by the history, requires exclusion of other potentially confusing intra-abdominal pathology and the demonstration, by arteriography, of significant (i.e., more than 50 per cent) narrowing of at least two of the three major visceral arteries. If the occlusive lesions are close to their takeoff from the aorta, then surgical correction is possible in most patients, resulting in significant relief of symptoms.

Because a significant number of patients with bowel infarction give an antecedent history of abdominal angina, correct diagnosis and treatment of this disorder are essential. It must be emphasized, however, that in the absence of a convincing history, a positive arteriogram alone does not establish the diagnosis because of the relative frequency of advanced but asymptomatic occlusive disease. Furthermore, the long-term effect of surgery on the natural history of the disease has not been established conclusively.

Celiac Compression Syndrome. This more recently described syndrome is characterized by vague, intermittent epigastric pain, occasionally associated with other nonspecific gastrointestinal symptomatology. There is no clear relation to meals, but, as with abdominal angina, it is believed to represent visceral ischemia caused in this instance by isolated narrowing of the celiac axis. Most cases have been ascribed to celiac compression by the adjacent median arcuate ligament of the diaphragm, but excess neurofibrous tissue of the celiac ganglion has also been incriminated. The patients are for the most part relatively young women, who are otherwise healthy, without evidence of atherosclerotic disease or other significant abdominal pathology. An epigastric bruit, failing to radiate inferiorly, has been an almost invariable finding. Celiac arteriography will successfully demonstrate the narrowing, and in many cases reconstructive or bypass surgery has been effective in relief of symptoms. Despite these favorable reports, however, the diagnosis should be made only with caution, because similar degrees of celiac axis narrowing have been found incidentally (autopsy or angiography) in asymptomatic subjects, and because of persisting uncertainty as to why this lesion should be associated with pain in the presence of an adequate collateral circulation. It has been suggested that the pain is not ischemic, but rather arises in the celiac ganglion itself.

661. MISCELLANEOUS DISORDERS

Intramural Intestinal Hemorrhage. Bleeding into the wall of the intestine may occur as the result of spontaneous or iatrogenic hypocoagulable states (e.g., anticoagulant therapy), localized hemorrhagic infarction (e.g., vasculitis), or as the result of blunt abdominal trauma. Patients usually present with abdominal pain and exhibit variable findings suggestive of intestinal obstruction and bleeding. A significant obstructive picture is especially likely to be seen in those patients who sustain upper abdominal trauma, resulting in the formation of a large intramural hematoma in that portion of the duodenum which is fixed in position retroperitoneally. Barium studies show the "stacked coins" or "thumbprint" appearance typical of submucosal bleeding.

In most patients, intramural hemorrhage can be managed conservatively, including appropriate treatment of the underlying causative factors and nasogastric suction when indicated. In those patients with high-grade or unremitting intestinal obstruction, or in whom signs of peritonitis develop (suggesting perforation), surgery is necessary.

Abdominal Aortic Aneurysm. Pathologic dilatation of the abdominal aorta is usually due to advanced atherosclerosis, and most commonly affects that segment distal to the origin of the renal arteries. Mild degrees of dilatation (i.e., 4 to 5 cm or less) are rarely symptomatic and are almost never associated with significant morbidity or mortality. Aneurysms larger than 6 to 7 cm, however, and those of any size which are observed to be increasing in caliber or to be causing symptoms (usually because of erosion of adjacent vertebrae) constitute serious threats to life. Such aneurysms may lead to a rapid exsanguination, by rupturing into either the bowel, the free peritoneal cavity, or the retroperitoneal space. Since the operative mortality under these urgent conditions is unacceptably high, such high-risk aneurysms should be resected electively.

Superior Mesenteric Artery Syndrome. In certain persons with an "asthenic" habitus, it has been suggested that the third portion of the duodenum may be compressed between the superior mesenteric artery and the uncinate process of the pancreas, causing symptoms of postprandial obstruction. Some of these patients obtain relief by assuming the knee-chest position. The validity of this syndrome as a cause of significant gastrointestinal symptoms is questionable, and surgery is rarely if ever indicated.

Vascular Malformations. Hemangiomas of the small intestine are very uncommon vascular tumors found throughout the bowel, particularly the jejunum. They assume clinical importance as one cause of gastrointestinal bleeding of undetermined source. These lesions are most reliably diagnosed by abdominal angiography. Telangiectasias may also be causes of gastrointestinal bleeding, and may be associated with mucocutaneous telangiectasias (Osler-Weber-Rendu disease) or Turner's syndrome.

Boley, S. J. (ed.): Vascular Disorders of the Intestine. New York, Appleton-Century-Crofts, 1971.

Bynum, T. E., and Jacobson, E. D.: Blood flow and gastrointestinal function. Gastroenterology, 60:325, 1971.

Fagin, R. R., and Kirsner, J. B.: Ischemic diseases of the colon. Ad. Intern. Med., 17:343, 1971.

Williams, L. F., Jr.: Vascular insufficiency of the intestine. Gastroenterology, 61:757, 1971.

Section Seven.   DISEASES OF THE PERITONEUM, MESENTERY, AND OMENTUM

Robert K. Ockner

662.   DISEASES OF THE PERITONEUM

Anatomy and Physiology.   The abdominal cavity and viscera are lined by a continuous mesothelial membrane, the peritoneum. This structure forms a closed sac, except at the entry of the fimbriated ostia of the fallopian tubes, and consists of two anatomically distinct but contiguous portions. The *visceral* peritoneum encloses those organs which are entirely intraperitoneal, including the mesenteries by which they are suspended, whereas the *parietal* peritoneum lines the walls of the abdominal cavity (including the undersurface of the diaphragm and the pelvis) and the retroperitoneal organs (including the duodenum, ascending and descending colon, pancreas, kidneys, and adrenals). The two portions of the peritoneal membrane also differ in blood supply and innervation. The visceral peritoneum is supplied by the splanchnic arterial system, and its venous drainage enters the portal vein. In contrast, the parietal peritoneum receives branches of arteries which nourish the abdominal wall and diaphragm, and its venous drainage is by way of systemic veins. The visceral peritoneum does not contain pain receptors; afferent stimuli are transmitted via the visceral autonomics, whereas the parietal peritoneum is supplied by spinal nerves which also innervate the abdominal wall. As a result, irritation of the parietal peritoneum produces well-localized somatic pain (which may be referred to other sites in the same dermatome); in contrast, irritation of the visceral peritoneum produces a much less well-defined discomfort which is often poorly localized. The diaphragmatic portion of the peritoneum is supplied both by the phrenic nerve (spinal roots C3 to C5) and, in its more peripheral portions, by the intercostal nerves; as a result, pain resulting from diaphragmatic irritation may be referred either to the shoulder or to the thoracic or abdominal wall.

The peritoneal surface is a semipermeable membrane, and allows for the passive diffusion of water and solutes between the abdominal cavity and the subperitoneal vascular (blood and lymphatic) channels. In general, absorption of water and of solutes with a molecular weight of less than 2000 from the peritoneal cavity is accomplished via the blood vascular system; larger molecules and particulate substances enter the lymphatics. Movement of particles from the peritoneal cavity into the subdiaphragmatic lymphatics is facilitated by specialized areas of contact between the parietal peritoneum and the underlying lymphatics. In these areas, discontinuities exist between the peritoneal mesothelial cells and the lymphatic endothelial cells; basement membranes are scanty or absent. As a result, particles of substantial size (e.g., red blood cells) move freely from the abdominal cavity into the subdiaphragmatic lymphatics, a process which may be facilitated by respiratory motion of the diaphragm itself.

Water and electrolytes equilibrate rapidly (i.e., within two hours) between the blood vascular compartment and the free peritoneal cavity. *Net* fluid movement from the abdominal cavity into the plasma occurs at a maximal rate of approximately 30 to 35 ml per hour. This figure applies not only to the normal man, but also to patients with portal hypertension and ascites; this rate cannot be exceeded despite vigorous diuresis; rather, such diuresis only serves to remove fluid from other body compartments, and may cause hypovolemia.

Diagnosis.   Because of their wide diversity, few generalizations can be made regarding history and physical examination in diseases of the peritoneum. Abdominal pain and ascites may be present, as may other less specific complaints of fever, nausea, and vomiting, depending on the nature and localization of the process. Diagnosis of known or suspected peritoneal disease is therefore greatly dependent upon special techniques, including radiology, abdominal paracentesis, peritoneal biopsy, peritoneoscopy, and exploratory laparotomy.

Radiographically, ascites may be manifest by haziness and separation of bowel loops on plain abdominal films. Otherwise, peritoneal disease reflects itself only indirectly. For example, an inflammatory process resulting in scar formation may cause angulation, separation, or narrowing of intestinal loops or evidence of mucosal edema (owing to mesenteric lymphatic or venous obstruction) on barium contrast studies. If ascites is present, abdominal paracentesis is essential in order to establish its cause (see below). Peritoneal biopsy, particularly with the Cope needle, is a relatively simple and safe bedside technique which may yield a positive diagnosis of neoplastic or infectious causes in 50 to 60 per cent of cases. Peritoneoscopy, performed under the proper circumstances by a physician experienced in this technique, can be accomplished with little morbidity or mortality. A successful examination may obviate the need for exploratory surgery and may permit biopsy under direct vision of involved portions of the peritoneum or liver. If a diagnosis cannot be made in a patient with obvious peritoneal disease by means of the aforementioned procedures, exploratory laparotomy may be necessary.

ASCITES

The accumulation of fluid within the peritoneal cavity may result from any or all of three different pathophysiologic mechanisms. These include (1) increases in the permeability of the peritoneal capillaries (e.g., in neoplastic and inflammatory diseases of the peritoneum) and (2) diminished plasma colloid osmotic pressure (e.g., severe hypoalbuminemia of any cause). An elevation in portal venous pressure alone (i.e., in the absence of hypoalbuminemia) is ordinarily not adequate cause for ascites formation, as evidenced by its relative rarity in portal vein thrombosis not associated with liver disease. A third important mechanism for ascites formation is elevation of the hydrostatic pressure within the hepatic sinusoids. This may result from any of the conditions associated with *postsinusoidal portal hypertension*, including *cirrhosis, hepatic vein,* or *inferior vena cava obstruction,* and advanced *congestive heart failure* or *constrictive pericarditis.* In these conditions, elevated sinusoidal pressure increases the movement of protein-rich plasma filtrate from the sinusoid into the space of Disse and the hepatic lymphatics. Although the fluid may ultimately enter the thoracic duct, hepatic lymph may be lost directly from the surface of the liver into the free peritoneal cavity. This mechanism undoubtedly accounts for the not infrequent finding that patients with postsinusoidal portal hypertension of any cause, including cirrhosis and congestive failure, may have ascites with an unexpectedly high protein concentration, despite the fact that its formation may be considered to represent "transudation" rather than "exudation" in the usual sense.

Ascites formation in the cirrhotic, and in other situations in which plasma volume or renal vascular perfusion is abnormal, may be aggravated by renal retention of sodium and water. It seems unlikely, however, that these latter factors alone are sufficient for the formation of ascites, because neither primary hyperaldosteronism nor increased antidiuretic hormone secretion is associated with ascites formation in the absence of other contributing factors.

Evaluation of Ascites Fluid. Although laboratory analysis of fluid removed from the abdominal cavity may not provide a specific etiologic diagnosis, no patient with ascites can be considered to have been properly evaluated without this examination. Fluids with protein concentrations exceeding 2.5 grams are usually regarded as "exudates," whereas those with lower concentrations are designated "transudates." Although this classification is useful, exceptions in both directions occur not infrequently. Thus cases of neoplasm or infection of the peritoneum in association with "transudative" fluids and of cirrhosis and congestive heart failure in association with "exudative" protein levels are numerous and well documented. For this reason, ascites fluid protein concentrations must be interpreted only in the context of all other clinical and laboratory findings. Other chemical determinations may be helpful, including amylase (markedly elevated in pancreatic ascites), glucose (often less than 60 mg per 100 ml in neoplastic ascites), and triglyceride (in excess of plasma concentrations in chylous ascites). Bloody ascites strongly suggests neoplasm, especially hepatoma. Elevated leukocyte counts (in excess of 250 per cubic millimeter) indicate peritoneal irritation, e.g., neoplasm or infection. The differential leukocyte count is of help in that a very high percentage of lymphocytes strongly suggests tuberculous peritonitis. Cytology is an essential part of the examination and may be expected to yield accurate results in more than half the cases. Ascites fluid should be cultured for routine pathogens, acid-fast bacilli, and fungi.

Differential Diagnosis of Ascites. Although a wide variety of disease processes may be associated with the

TABLE 1.   Causes of Ascites Not Associated with Peritoneal Disease*

I. Portal hypertension
A. Cirrhosis
B. Hepatic congestion
1. Congestive heart failure
2. Constrictive pericarditis
3. Inferior vena cava obstruction
4. Hepatic vein obstruction (Budd-Chiari syndrome)
C. Portal vein occlusion
II. Hypoalbuminemia
A. Nephrotic syndrome
B. Protein-losing enteropathy
C. Malnutrition
III. Miscellaneous
A. Myxedema
B. Ovarian disease
1. Meigs' syndrome
2. Struma ovarii
3. Ovarian overstimulation syndrome
C. Pancreatic ascites
D. Bile ascites
E. Chylous ascites

*From Bender, M. D., and Ockner, R. K., *In* Sleisenger, M. H., and Fordtran, J. S. (eds.): Gastrointestinal Disease. Philadelphia, W. B. Saunders Company, 1973.

TABLE 2. Diseases of the Peritoneum

I. Infections
    A. Acute peritonitis
    B. Tuberculous peritonitis
    C. Fungal and parasitic diseases
        1. Candidiasis
        2. Histoplasmosis
        3. Schistosomiasis
        4. Enterobiasis
II. Neoplasms
    A. Secondary malignancy
    B. Primary mesothelioma
    C. Pseudomyxoma peritonei
III. Miscellaneous
    A. Vasculitis
    B. Granulomatous peritonitis
        1. Sarcoidosis
        2. Crohn's disease
        3. Starch peritonitis
    C. Familial paroxysmal peritonitis
    D. Eosinophilic gastroenteritis
    E. Whipple's disease
    F. Gynecologic disease
        1. Endometriosis
        2. Deciduosis
    G. Peritoneal lymphangiectasia
    H. Peritoneal loose bodies
    I. Peritoneal encapsulation

---

presence of ascites, more than 90 per cent of patients with this complication are found to have cirrhosis, neoplasm, congestive heart failure, or tuberculosis. For purposes of classification, causes of ascites may be divided into diseases not involving the peritoneum on the one hand (Table 1) and diseases of the peritoneum on the other (Table 2). Of those cases not associated with peritoneal disease, *cirrhosis* is by far the most common; it is considered in Ch. 709. *Portal hypertension* caused by disease of the heart and great veins accounts for a substantial number of patients with ascites of obscure origin. Included in this group are patients with *congestive heart failure* (especially right-sided), *constrictive pericarditis*, and *inferior vena cava* and *hepatic vein obstruction (Budd-Chiari syndrome)*. Clinically, patients with these conditions may not be readily distinguishable from those with hepatic cirrhosis; a high index of suspicion is necessary, and special diagnostic procedures may be required in order to establish or exclude the diagnosis. Hypoalbuminemia of any cause, including nephrotic syndrome and protein-losing enteropathy, may be associated with a classically "transudative" ascites.

Various endocrine conditions may be associated with ascites. These include *myxedema* and *diseases of the ovary*, among them *Meigs' syndrome*, in which transudative ascites is associated with ovarian fibroma or cystadenoma.

Ascites associated with pancreatic disease usually occurs in the presence of chronic *pancreatitis* and *pseudocyst*. The ascites fluid amylase concentration is elevated, often to very high levels, and drainage of the pseudocyst has usually been effective in managing this complication. Leakage of bile may be associated with the development of *bile ascites*. It is important to note that this situation is not necessarily associated with the fulminant clinical picture of fever, leukocytosis, and peritonitis which customarily is designated *bile peritonitis*. Rather, this latter, more ominous condition seems to occur primarily in those patients in whom the extravasated bile was infected originally.

Chylous ascites is due to the presence of lymph lipoproteins and chylomicrons in the peritoneal cavity. These lipid-rich particles impart a turbidity to the fluid which facilitates its diagnosis. It should be emphasized, however, that not all turbid abdominal fluids are "chylous." Establishment of the diagnosis requires direct evidence that the turbidity is indeed due to neutral lipid, a determination best made by analysis of the fluid for triglyceride concentration; alternatively, solvent extraction (ether or chloroform) which results in clearing of the fluid may be taken as presumptive evidence for the diagnosis. Other turbid abdominal fluids may be due to cellular debris, and are designated "*pseudochylous*" ascites, a condition occasionally associated with abdominal neoplasm or infection. The differential diagnosis of truly chylous ascites depends upon its chronicity and the age of the patient. *Chronic chylous ascites* in adults is caused in over 80 per cent of cases by abdominal neoplasm, usually *lymphoma*, with associated obstruction and disruption of the abdominal lymphatics resulting from extensive lymph node involvement. *Acute chylous ascites* ("chylous peritonitis") is associated with abrupt onset of abdominal pain. In some cases, this syndrome is due to *trauma, intestinal obstruction*, or *rupture* of a *chylous cyst*, but a specific etiologic diagnosis may not be possible even at laparotomy. In children, congenital malformations of the lymphatics, including intestinal *lymphangiectasia*, account for a higher proportion of the cases of chylous ascites.

INFECTIONS OF THE PERITONEUM

Acute Peritonitis

Although this syndrome may result from a chemical irritation or "burn" of the peritoneal surface (as in severe acute pancreatitis), most cases are due to *bacterial infection*. Most commonly, enteric organisms enter the peritoneal cavity through a necrotic defect in the wall of the intestine or other abdominal viscus resulting from *obstruction, infarction, neoplasm, foreign body*, or primary inflammatory disease such as *fulminant ulcerative colitis*. *Perforated peptic ulcer* and *ruptured appendix* are particularly frequent causes. If unchecked, bacterial contamination of the peritoneum results in a "spreading peritonitis," leading ultimately to marked exudation of protein-rich fluid into the abdominal cavity, paralytic ileus, and reflex spasm of the overlying abdominal musculature. The systemic consequences of this catastrophic event are predictable. Loss of fluid from the vascular compartment into both the free peritoneal cavity and the bowel lumen results in volume depletion and hemoconcentration; these factors, together with the possible systemic effects of the bacterial infection itself, may lead to shock and oliguria. The latter may progress to acute tubular necrosis.

Despite its often dramatic presentation, recognition of acute peritonitis may be difficult in those patients in whom the clinical manifestations are masked or suppressed. This applies particularly to the elderly and to those receiving corticosteroids, as, for example, in the treatment of acute ulcerative colitis. In these patients, a particularly high index of suspicion is necessary, and the only *early* manifestation may be a rise in pulse rate or unexplained hypotension. Diagnosis in such situations may depend upon the radiographic demonstration of free air in the peritoneal cavity and upon aspiration of abdominal contents to confirm the presence of polymorphonuclear leukocytes and bacteria. Fortunately, the peritoneum is often able to confine inflammatory processes of this type. As a result, acute peritonitis may be restricted to one portion of the abdomen and may not spread or become generalized.

Management of peritonitis includes restoration of fluid and electrolyte imbalance; the administration of fresh frozen plasma or albumin is often required. Antimicrobial therapy and nasogastric suction should be instituted. Analgesics are often necessary, but their premature use may hinder proper evaluation of the patient. The decision to operate must be individualized. In those patients who are seen early and who are good operative candidates, surgery should be undertaken as soon as feasible. However, in some patients (particularly those seen later in the course or who are poor operative risks), it may be desirable to attempt to control the process nonoperatively and to encourage its localization by means of antimicrobial drugs and other conservative measures. Localized abscesses so formed may be drained later, when circumstances are more favorable.

Subphrenic Abscess

Particularly challenging problems in diagnosis and treatment are posed by the collection of pus in one of the several more or less well-defined tissue spaces inferior to the diaphragm and adjacent to the liver, stomach, spleen, and lesser sac. Most often, subphrenic abscess develops secondary to other septic and inflammatory processes in the abdomen, especially *ruptured appendix* or *diverticulum, infected gallbladder, perforated ulcer* with bacterial contamination, *pancreatitis, penetrating abdominal wound,* or extension of an *intrahepatic abscess* beyond the liver capsule.

Clinically, the picture usually suggests a septic process, with malaise, fever, and leukocytosis. The subphrenic location is often not obvious, but may be suggested by a history of one of the aforementioned antecedent events, by direct clinical evidence such as pain, elevation, or impaired motion of the diaphragm, or by x-ray evidence of a pleural effusion associated with a subdiaphragmatic air-fluid level.

Antimicrobial therapy usually suppresses the process and helps to contain it, but may also obscure its recognition. Definitive therapy consists of surgical drainage.

Spontaneous ("Primary") Peritonitis

Bacterial peritonitis may also occur in the absence of an acute intra-abdominal precipitating factor. In this circumstance, the offending organism is often not enteric, and the syndrome is more likely to occur in patients who have pre-existing ascites, impaired immunologic defenses, or a cause for bacteremia such as localized infection elsewhere in the body or indwelling catheters. A well-recognized example of this circumstance is the child with nephrotic syndrome and ascites who develops *pneumococcal peritonitis* as a complication; the incidence of this entity has diminished considerably during recent decades because of the availability of antimicrobial drugs.

More common is spontaneous bacterial peritonitis in patients with advanced, decompensated *cirrhosis* and *as-*

cites. This syndrome may occur in up to 10 per cent of such patients, and although enteric organisms (particularly *E. coli*) are most often cultured, pneumococci and streptococci are frequent offenders. The cause of the syndrome is not known; perforated viscus, pneumonia, biliary tract infection, and other local sites of bacterial infection cannot be implicated. Possibly, the cirrhotic liver with spontaneous portal-systemic shunting is less effective in clearing bacteria from the portal blood, but this would not explain the occurrence of nonenteric organisms. The syndrome may be recognized by the sudden onset of abdominal pain, fever, and leukocytosis, occurring in the setting of decompensated cirrhosis and ascites. Blood cultures are positive in 75 per cent of cases; abdominal fluid usually yields a positive culture and contains an elevated number of polymorphonuclear leukocytes. Although appropriate antimicrobial therapy may afford a satisfactory bacteriologic response in the majority of patients, the over-all mortality exceeds 90 per cent.

Other Infections

Tuberculous peritonitis is discussed in detail in Ch. 239. It should be emphasized, however, that this disorder may present in a variety of ways, ranging from an acute abdomen to an insidiously developing, otherwise unexplained ascites resembling (or associated with) cirrhosis. Accordingly, its presence should be suspected in all patients with ascites, with or without an apparently adequate cause. Tuberculosis skin testing and appropriate cultures of ascites fluid for tubercle bacilli should be regarded as routine in the evaluation of ascites. The diagnosis is strongly suggested by a high percentage of lymphocytes in the abdominal fluid, and may be confirmed by means of a positive culture, peritoneal biopsy, laparoscopy, or, if necessary, exploratory laparotomy. The very satisfactory response of this condition to appropriate chemotherapy adds to the importance of early diagnosis.

Fungal and parasitic diseases may be associated with peritoneal involvement and, occasionally, with ascites. These disorders, including *histoplasmosis, candidiasis,* and *schistosomiasis,* are quite uncommon, but deserve consideration in otherwise unexplained cases of peritoneal disease with or without ascites.

TUMORS OF THE PERITONEUM

Secondary malignancy is the most common form of neoplastic involvement of the peritoneum. More than 75 per cent of such tumors are *adenocarcinomas,* but peritoneal involvement by *sarcomas, lymphomas, leukemias, carcinoids,* and *multiple myeloma* has been described. It is assumed that in these patients there is increased permeability of the mesenteric and peritoneal capillary bed, accounting for the formation of "exudative" ascites. The clinical picture is usually that associated with advancing malignancy, including weakness and weight loss, and variable complaints referable to the abdomen such as pain, distention, nausea, or vomiting. On abdominal paracentesis, the fluid obtained usually has a high protein content (more than 2.5 grams per 100 ml); cellular composition is variable, and occasionally the fluid is grossly bloody. The diagnosis is reliably made in most patients by means of cytology or peritoneal biopsy, but peritoneoscopy or surgical exploration may be necessary at times.

Treatment of this condition involves the intraperitoneal administration of antitumor agents, including alkylators, antimetabolites, or radioactive isotopes. Unfortunately, the prognosis of patients in this advanced stage of malignancy is poor. Intra-abdominal quinacrine has occasionally been successful in producing a fibrous serositis, thereby obliterating the free peritoneal space and reducing further fluid exudation. The usefulness of this approach is limited, however, by the frequent occurrence of fever, nausea, vomiting, and abdominal pain.

Primary Mesothelioma

This uncommon primary tumor of the peritoneum is associated with the gradual onset of abdominal pain and distention, nausea, vomiting, weight loss, and development of ascites. Cytology or peritoneal biopsy reveals a variable histopathology in which epithelial and mesenchymal elements are combined and because of which differentiation from other malignancies may be difficult. It has been suggested on epidemiologic grounds that exposure to asbestos fibers may play an etiologic role in the development of this tumor. This conclusion is based on the association, in most patients, with environmental exposure to asbestos fibers and evidence of pulmonary asbestosis, including "asbestos bodies" in the lungs. Because of more recent evidence suggesting that these so-called "asbestos bodies" are nonspecific and occur in up to 50 per cent of the general population, the importance of asbestos in the etiology of this tumor is at present uncertain (see Ch. 526). A significant number of patients with peritoneal mesothelioma have a similar process affecting the pleura. The prognosis of the disease is exceedingly poor, averaging one to two years' survival after diagnosis. Chemotherapy and radiation therapy have generally been unsuccessful.

Pseudomyxoma Peritonei

Classification of this rare disorder as a tumor is a matter of some uncertainty, because in many cases it appears to arise as a complication of certain relatively benign processes, including mucocele of the appendix. On the other hand, its neoplastic nature is suggested by a high incidence of cellular atypia in carefully examined pathologic specimens, as well as by evidence for low-grade malignancy in a high percentage of those patients in whom the syndrome develops subsequent to *mucinous cystadenomas* of the *ovaries*. The syndrome is characterized by abdominal distention resulting from the accumulation of a mucinous, gelatinous, translucent material. Most cases seem to originate as an outgrowth of pre-existing mucinous cystadenomas and cystadinocarcinomas of the ovary and mucocele of the appendix, but other tumors of the genitourinary tract or gastrointestinal tract may be associated with the process.

The condition usually presents as an increase in abdominal girth, with little in the way of other clinical signs of disease. At surgery, the abdominal cavity is found to contain gelatinous material existing in a variety of states, including cystic masses, lying freely without apparent attachment, or anchored to the peritoneal surface.

If the tumor is indeed malignant, it appears to be of low grade and rarely metastasizes. As a result, the course of the disease is prolonged and is characterized by recurrent episodes of intestinal obstruction and fistula formation. The most promising therapeutic approach at present appears to be one which combines surgical removal of the ovary, appendix, and as much mucin as possible, with intraperitoneal instillation of an alkylating agent.

Miscellaneous Diseases of the Peritoneum

The peritoneal membrane may be affected by a wide variety of systemic diseases, including *systemic lupus erythematosus* (see Ch. 81) and other "collagen vascular" diseases, *Whipple's disease* (see Part XIV, Section Three), and *sarcoidosis* (see Ch. 102).

Bender, M. D., and Ockner, R. K.: Diseases of the peritoneum, mesentery, and diaphragm. *In* Sleisenger, M. H., and Fordtran, J. S. (eds.): Gastrointestinal Disease. Philadelphia, W. B. Saunders Company, 1973, pp. 1578–1600.

Conn, H., and Fessel, M.: Spontaneous bacterial peritonitis in cirrhosis: Variations on a theme. Medicine, 50:161, 1971.

Levine, H.: Needle biopsy of the peritoneum in exudative ascites. Arch. Intern. Med., 120:542, 1967.

663. DISEASES OF THE MESENTERY AND OMENTUM

Mesenteric Inflammatory Disease. This syndrome includes a spectrum of conditions ranging from acute inflammation to a chronic fibrosing process associated with intestinal obstruction, ascites, and steatorrhea. Included are such conditions as "*mesenteric panniculitis*" and "*retractile mesenteritis*." The cause of this syndrome is not known, but it is believed to represent the sequel to some inciting event such as trauma, infection, or ischemia in the mesentery. Fat necrosis occurs, evoking an inflammatory reaction with subsequent scarring and granuloma formation.

Clinically, the acute syndrome ("mesenteric panniculitis") is characterized by recurrent abdominal pain, weight loss, nausea, vomiting, and fever. In most patients, a tender abdominal mass is palpable; leukocytosis may or may not be present. Radiographic examination is nonspecific, showing the effects of an abdominal mass and variable scarring, which include displacement and separation of intestinal loops, with angulation, stenosis, and extrinsic compression. In some patients the condition evolves into a more chronic process ("retractile mesenteritis"), characterized by continuing pain, fever, weight loss, and various signs of intestinal obstruction, ascites, and steatorrhea.

At surgery, the small bowel mesentery is found to be the principal site of involvement; it is thickened and fibrotic, particularly at the root. Microscopically in *mesenteric panniculitis,* there is infiltration of adipose tissue by foamy macrophages and lymphocytes, with fat necrosis, fibrosis, and calcification. In *retractile mesenteritis,* the thickening and fibrosis are more pronounced, and there is less evidence of acute necrosis and inflammation.

Although long-term experience with this syndrome is

limited, most patients seem to have a prolonged survival; many become asymptomatic after a period of months to years, whereas others exhibit the more chronic symptoms noted above. The role of corticosteroids is uncertain; although they may be effective in the management of those patients in whom acute symptoms predominate, there is no evidence that they affect the long-term prognosis or progression of the disease.

Mesenteric Cysts and Tumors.   Mesenteric cysts usually develop as the result of anomalies in the mesenteric lymphatic system, but may also consist of enteric or urogenital epithelium or celomic mesothelium. They may spontaneously wax and wane in size, and usually do not present symptomatically in patients less than 10 years of age. Symptoms are related to the size and position of the cyst, which on physical examination is nontender, round, and mobile. Spontaneous rupture, hemorrhage, or infection may occur, but these complications are unusual. Treatment consists of surgical excision.

Mesenteric tumors are rare and usually arise from the cellular elements normally present in the mesentery.

They include *fibromas, myxomas, lipomas,* and other less common neoplasms of mesenchymal or neural origin. Most are well differentiated, low-grade *fibrosarcomas* which produce symptoms such as pain, weight loss, abdominal mass, and compression of adjacent organs. They may be treated successfully by surgical excision. Others are more highly malignant and may metastasize distally. *Mesenteric lymphoid tumors* also occur, and certain of these have been associated with unexplained abnormalities in iron metabolism with hypochromic microcytic anemia.

Tumors of the omentum, unlike those of the mesentery, are chiefly muscular in origin (*leiomyomas, leiomyosarcomas*). About 40 per cent of these are malignant, and cause symptoms by virtue of local invasion and development of an abdominal mass; distant metastasis is unusual.

Bender, M. D., and Ockner, R. K.: Diseases of the peritoneum, mesentery, and diaphragm. *In* Sleisenger, M. H., and Fordtran, J. S. (eds.): Gastrointestinal Disease. Philadelphia, W. B. Saunders Company, 1973, pp. 1578–1600.

Section Eight.   NEOPLASTIC DISEASES OF THE ALIMENTARY TRACT

664.   INTRODUCTION

Lloyd L. Brandborg

Gastrointestinal cancer comprises 20 per cent of all cancers and accounts for 30 per cent of cancer deaths. In a single year in the United States there are about 133,000 new cancers and 97,000 deaths from cancers of the digestive organs. Cure rates of digestive organ cancer have remained constant for several decades. "Early" diagnosis and more effective treatment have not been achieved.

Striking geographic differences occur in the incidence of various gastrointestinal malignancies. There has been a marked decrease over the past several decades in carcinoma of the stomach in the United States. Carcinoma of the pancreas is increasing. Carcinoma of the colon has remained constant. Gastric carcinoma declines in migrants from countries with a high incidence to those with a low incidence, suggesting that environmental factors play a significant role in its causation. Carcinoma of the colon is virtually unknown in rural Africa, but the incidence in black people in the United States equals that in the white population. None of the factors identified in epidemiologic studies have been shown to cause any of the cancers of the gastrointestinal tract. Tantalizing clues are provided which require further intensive investigation.

Hereditary and genetic factors have been examined. There is an increase in gastric carcinoma in patients having blood group A, in pernicious anemia, and in patients having Lewis group specific substances, either Le^a or Le^b or both in saliva. Some families have been described with inordinately high incidences of carcinoma of the stomach or colon. Except for these patients and those with inherited multiple polyposis of the colon, gastrointestinal cancer does not have a familial distribution.

The symptoms of gastrointestinal cancer are not specific. Such phenomena as pain, bleeding, intestinal obstruction, weight loss, fever, or anemia should lead to a search for gastrointestinal malignancy. Most symptomatic gastrointestinal malignancies may be detected by roentgenographic, endoscopic, and cytologic techniques.

Specific chemical and serologic tests for gastrointestinal malignancy are not available. As the techniques become more sensitive, many of these tests become less specific. An example is the occurrence of carcinoembryonic antigen (CEA, see below) in many patients with nonmalignant disease.

Currently, surgery offers the main hope for cure of gastrointestinal cancer. It may also provide palliation. Preoperative irradiation therapy in gastrointestinal carcinomas may increase resectability and improve prognosis. Chemotherapy of gastrointestinal malignancy has been disappointing. Increased survival has not been shown. Occasional patients may enjoy striking remissions. Combination chemotherapy has not been widely studied in gastrointestinal malignancy. Hopefully, such an approach could improve survival as it has in leukemias, lymphomas, and other responsive cancers.

665.   NEOPLASMS OF THE ESOPHAGUS

Lloyd L. Brandborg

CARCINOMA OF THE ESOPHAGUS

Etiology.   Although the etiology of carcinoma of the esophagus is not known, a number of clinical conditions are associated with an increased incidence of the condition. Patients with *lye damage* of the esophagus have a

1000 times higher risk of developing carcinoma of the esophagus than the general population. Patients with *achalasia* have a reported incidence from 2 to up to 19 per cent. It is presumed that these lesions result from "irritation" caused by retention of esophageal contents. Whether successful brusk dilatation or myotomy, by virtue of eliminating stagnation, decreases the occurrence of carcinoma is not known. *Sideropenic dysphagia* is characterized by esophageal webs in the region of the cricopharyngeus, buccal mucosal atrophy, and a high incidence of carcinoma. This condition occurs most often in Scandinavia, particularly in northern Sweden, predominantly in elderly women. A strikingly high incidence of esophageal carcinoma occurs in some families with tylosis, an inherited disorder characterized by marked thickening of the skin of the hands and feet.

A statistical correlation exists between esophageal carcinoma and the use of cigarettes and alcohol. Atypical esophageal epithelium has been observed in the esophagus of smokers examined at autopsy. In view of the widespread use of cigarettes and alcohol, it is surprising that esophageal carcinoma is not more common.

Although it has been claimed that there is an association of esophageal carcinoma and hiatus hernia, prospective studies have failed to reveal such a relationship. Furthermore, most of the carcinomas associated with hiatus hernia are adenocarcinomas.

Incidence and Prevalence. The incidence of carcinoma of the esophagus is 5.8 per 100,000 in whites and 20.5 per 100,000 in nonwhites in the United States. Each year this amounts to 6800 new cases of esophageal cancer and 6400 deaths. Carcinoma of the esophagus is responsible for approximately 2 per cent of cancer deaths in the United States.

Epidemiology. The differences in geographic distribution of carcinoma of the esophagus are so striking throughout the world that it has been concluded that some environmental factors must have a role in etiology. The incidence in the United States in whites is 5.8 cases per 100,000 population per year, whereas in southern Rhodesia it is 157, in Transkei in South Africa it is 357, and in Kazakhstan in Asia it rises to 547 cases per 100,000 population. Statistical associations include long-term ingestion of very hot beverages, climate, vegetation, agriculture, trace metals in soils, and background irradiation. Genetic differences and chemicals in the diet may possibly contribute.

Pathology. Approximately one half of esophageal carcinomas occur at the level of the arch of the aorta, one third just above the esophagogastric junction, and the remainder in the hypopharynx and proximal esophagus.

If carcinomas arising in the cardia and fundus of the stomach are excluded, virtually all malignancies of the esophagus are squamous cell carcinomas. The gross appearance of carcinoma of the esophagus varies from hard, fibrotic infiltrative lesions to friable, exophytic papillary lesions. They are frequently ulcerated.

Esophageal carcinoma spreads by local invasion and lymphatic metastases. Microscopic lymphatic spread is common. These tumors frequently involve adjacent structures. The distal lesions invade the stomach and the left gastric and celiac lymph nodes. Extension into the diaphragm, vertebral bodies, pericardium, and heart is not rare. Lesions of the middle and upper third extend into the trachea and bronchi, and may involve the lungs and occasionally the recurrent laryngeal nerves.

Hematogenous metastases are less common than lymphatic extension and usually affect the liver, lungs, bones, and kidneys.

Clinical Manifestations. Carcinoma of the esophagus is unusual under the age of 40. The peak incidence occurs in the decade between the ages of 60 and 70. In most countries, males are afflicted approximately twice as often as females.

The most common symptom is progressive dysphagia. There is first difficulty in swallowing solid food, followed by inability to swallow semisolid foods and, finally, liquids. Occasionally, sudden esophageal obstruction occurs with a bolus of food that could have been easily swallowed a few days previously. Pain with swallowing, odynophagia, is due to extension of the tumor beyond the wall of the esophagus. It is located substernally, tends to be constant, is not always associated with swallowing, and is dull or burning. Occasionally, it may be felt in the back.

Other symptoms are due to chronic obstruction, extension of the tumor into adjacent organs, and hemorrhage. Brisk hemorrhage is uncommon (5 per cent of patients); however, occult bleeding is common.

Chronic obstruction leads to aspiration of secretions and undigested food, with severe coughing episodes and pneumonia; eating may become virtually intolerable. Food intake is reduced with ensuing weight loss. Regurgitation during the night, bad breath, bad taste, and thirst are frequent. Fever is common, usually because of pulmonary infection.

Symptoms of metastatic spread depend upon the organs involved. Involvement of the phrenic nerve or diaphragm may lead to unremitting hiccups. Extension into the trachea and bronchi produces coughing, infection, and tracheal or bronchoesophageal fistulas. Perforation into the mediastinum causes mediastinitis and empyema. Extension into the pericardium and heart causes pericardial effusions. A rare but dramatic symptom is exsanguinating hemorrhage caused by erosion into the aorta. Involvement of the recurrent laryngeal nerve will cause hoarseness. With distant metastases, patients may have jaundice, abdominal discomfort, ascites, cyanosis, dyspnea, and bone pain.

Diagnosis. *Every* patient with dysphagia should be investigated for carcinoma of the esophagus. The first procedure is a careful roentgenologic examination under fluoroscopic control (Fig. 1). Careful attention should be paid to the fundus of the stomach and cardia. Cineradiography is useful in detecting disordered motility. The most usual radiographic finding is a circumferential, irregular narrowing of the esophagus which is often ulcerated. There is slight or no dilatation proximal to the tumor. The mucosal folds are destroyed. In some smoothly tapering lesions, the differential diagnosis between benign stricture and carcinoma may be extraordinarily difficult.

Fiberoptic endoscopy permits direct visualization of the lesion. Directed biopsies give a diagnosis of malignancy in 50 to 75 per cent of patients. Directed cytology, either with lavage techniques or with the cytology brush, adds to the diagnostic accuracy. A benign biopsy cannot be relied upon, because in 25 to 50 per cent of patients biopsies taken out of obvious tumor reveal only "chronic inflammation."

Lavage cytology performed by skilled cytotechnicians and interpreted by skilled and interested physicians is

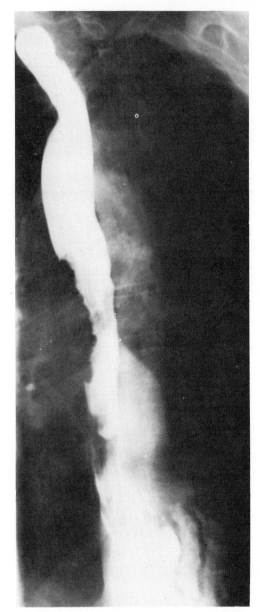

Figure 1. Extensive, sessile, ulcerated carcinoma of the esophagus.

Total obstruction is uncommon. The esophagus is dilated, often massively, and patients with achalasia may have symptoms of aspiration. The diagnosis may be made on a chest x-ray by finding a wide, mediastinal mass with a fluid level. The usual radiographic appearance is that of megaesophagus with a sharply tapering "beak" at the gastroesophageal junction. Test dilatation with a Hurst dilator has only a transient holdup at the cardioesophageal junction, whereas in malignancy the dilator usually cannot be passed. Manometric studies reveal absent peristaltic waves, a high pressure in the sphincter zone, and failure of the sphincter to relax in response to a swallow. The Mecholyl test is positive; however, a rare patient with carcinoma of the fundus or cardia which closely resembles achalasia radiographically may also have a positive Mecholyl test. Further, achalasia and carcinoma may coexist. (See Ch. 635.)

In *lye stricture,* the history of ingestion of caustic is usually clear; however, elderly patients may have ingested lye in childhood and not remember it. Because of the malignant potential of lye strictures, these patients should be followed periodically with roentgenologic examination, endoscopy, and exfoliative cytology.

Treatment and Prognosis. Treatment of esophageal carcinoma depends upon its location and whether it has spread. If distant metastases are absent, patients with distal esophageal carcinoma should have surgery. Lesions of the middle third are treated by either surgery or high voltage irradiation. Most patients with proximal esophageal carcinoma should receive irradiation therapy. Operative mortality for esophagectomy is between 15 and 20 per cent. Distal lesions are more favorable. Staged procedures, in selected patients, may improve the cure rate. A colon interposition, bypassing the cancer, is placed in the anterior mediastinum. The patient is then treated with therapeutic dosages of irradiation. Those patients surviving for six months then have an esophagectomy. Cure rates with irradiation alone or surgery alone are comparable and do not exceed 5 per cent.

Recent, uncontrolled observations suggest that preoperative irradiation in selected patients may improve resectability and perhaps even the incidence of cures. Irradiation, 4500 to 6000 rads tumor dose delivered to the entire esophagus, is followed in four to six weeks by resection. It is difficult to evaluate these observations, because only patients considered to be favorable candidates have received this treatment. However, a number of five-year cures have been reported.

Chemotherapy has not been shown to be of any value in esophageal carcinoma. Palliation is indicated in inoperable or incurable patients and consists of irradiation therapy, resectional surgery, or bypass surgery. Several prosthetic tubes are available which may be inserted through the tumor and which may relieve obstruction for some weeks or even months. Although nutrition may be improved, these devices may migrate through the tumor, erode into the mediastinum, or become occluded with tumor. Gastrostomy alone should not be done in patients with total obstruction caused by carcinoma of the esophagus, because this treatment only prolongs the patients' misery. They are unable to swallow their own secretions and suffer repeated pulmonary infections. If esophageal patency cannot be obtained with the aforementioned measures, these patients should be allowed to die with some dignity.

the most accurate means of diagnosing carcinoma when present and excluding it when suspected by other techniques. With an adequate test, carcinoma is diagnosed in 95 per cent or more of patients and false-positive diagnoses are exceedingly rare.

Differential Diagnosis. Only a few diseases may be confused with carcinoma of the esophagus. Most important is peptic *esophagitis* with *stricture* (see Ch. 635). Although most patients have a history of pyrosis, some have only a short history of dysphagia with little discomfort. The roentgenographic appearance may mimic malignant neoplasm. Eosphagoscopy with biopsy and cytology and lavage cytology will establish the benign nature of the stricture in virtually every patient.

The history of intermittent dysphagia in *achalasia* is much more characteristic than in carcinoma of the esophagus, which has a gradual increase in severity.

OTHER NEOPLASMS OF THE ESOPHAGUS

Carcinosarcomas

Carcinosarcomas are rare tumors of the esophagus. They tend to be polypoid and contain both carcinomatous and sarcomatous tissue. Exfoliative cytology may reveal both malignant sarcomatous and epithelial cells. Biopsy with histologic examination is probably more accurate. These tumors tend to be radiosensitive and should be treated with irradiation therapy if they are not resectable.

Malignant Lymphoma

Malignant lymphoma confined to the esophagus is extremely rare. The usual symptoms are either dysphagia or odynophagia. The roentgenographic appearance resembles monilial esophagitis. If the diagnosis can be established by exfoliative cytology or biopsy, irradiation therapy is the treatment of choice.

Leiomyomas

Leiomyomas are the most common benign neoplasms of the esophagus. Most often they cause no symptoms and are an incidental finding either at autopsy or surgery. They are usually less than 2 cm in diameter. They are intramural, extramucosal tumors and produce a smooth indentation in the esophagus on roentgenographic examination. Rarely, they may be "polyps" with a stalk. Even when they attain huge size, they may not produce symptoms. Rarely, patients have dysphagia and may even bleed. With large lesions, the diagnosis may be suspected by seeing a spherical mediastinal mass on chest x-ray. There is no evidence that leiomyomas undergo sarcomatous degeneration. The treatment of symptomatic esophageal leiomyomas is enucleation of the tumor. Resection is rarely necessary.

666. MALIGNANT NEOPLASMS OF THE STOMACH

Lloyd L. Brandborg

Ninety-five per cent of gastric neoplasms are malignant and 5 per cent benign. The most common benign neoplasm is the *leiomyoma*, which is usually an incidental finding at surgery or autopsy. The next most common is the *adenoma*. Other benign neoplasms of the stomach are exceedingly rare.

With the decreasing incidence of *adenocarcinoma* of the stomach in the United States and a constant incidence of gastric *lymphoma*, the proportion of malignant lymphomas has increased and possibly accounts for as many as 10 per cent of gastric malignancies. The other major malignant neoplasm of the stomach is the *leiomyosarcoma*, which accounts for about 1 per cent of gastric malignancies.

CARCINOMA OF THE STOMACH

Etiology. In spite of numerous experimental studies and epidemiologic investigations, a causative agent or agents responsible for carcinoma of the stomach remain elusive.

Genetic factors have been associated with an increased incidence of carcinoma of the stomach. Several families have been described with an unusually high occurrence. Studies of gastric carcinoma in twins have shown a higher frequency in monozygotic than in dizygotic twins. There is a 10 per cent increase in blood group A in gastric cancer patients when compared with suitable controls. Patients with pernicious anemia have been estimated to have a 10 per cent chance of developing gastric cancer. In these patients blood group A is also increased. Lewis group specific substances, either Le[a] or Le[b] or both, have been found in saliva in all patients with gastric carcinoma who have been examined. In the normal population 7 per cent of subjects are Lewis negative. These genetic factors are not etiologic, because the vast majority of subjects having them do not develop gastric carcinoma. They may be predisposing factors in response to other etiologic agents.

Adenomatous polyps have been considered to be "precancerous" in the past. Eight to 10 per cent of patients with adenocarcinoma of the stomach have one or more benign gastric polyps. However, many gastric adenomas observed over long periods of time have no growth, change in appearance, or malignant degeneration. Serial endoscopic observations have shown that some of these adenomatous polyps may even disappear. Benign adenomas may have small microscopic collections of cells that resemble carcinoma in situ. "Microinvasion" below the muscularis mucosae has been observed, but metastases have not been seen. Most often these cells have been found in proximity to areas of acute inflammation and granulation tissue and may not represent malignant change.

Atrophic gastritis, characterized by atrophy and intestinalization, is found in stomachs harboring carcinoma. In contrast to patients with adenomatous polyps, who are achlorhydric in 95 per cent of cases, 70 per cent of patients with gastric carcinoma secrete hydrochloric acid. It must be remembered also that decreased hydrochloric acid secretion is a feature of advancing age. Gastritis is probably not a predisposing factor, because histologic gastritis is very common in otherwise healthy individuals.

Patients with adult pernicious anemia have an increased incidence of gastric carcinoma. They are achlorhydric and achylic, and have intestinalization of their gastric mucosa and a high incidence of benign adenomas. Despite all these abnormalities, most of them do not develop carcinoma of the stomach.

Peptic ulcer of the stomach has been thought to be a precursor of carcinoma of the stomach. The finding of malignant cells in the margins of the ulcers has been offered as evidence. It is more likely, however, that ulcer in this circumstance develops as a result of peptic digestion of a small carcinoma. Further, virtually all such lesions have been described in patients secreting hydrochloric acid. Possibly neoplastic tissue is more susceptible to digestion than the surrounding mucosa. Although a benign gastric ulcer may degenerate into a malignant one, such an event must be extremely rare.

Previous surgery for benign peptic ulcer appears to be associated with an increase in carcinoma of the stomach. Several large reviews have shown that surgery for benign duodenal ulcer disease increases the risk of carcinoma in these patients. Carcinoma in association with duodenal ulcer is otherwise rare. The etiology and pathogenesis of gastric cancer in this situation are unknown. Possibly reflux of intestinal and pancreatic secretions into the gastric remnant may contribute. The interval between surgery for benign ulcer disease and the appearance of carcinoma of the stomach varies from 6 to up to 37 or more years. Any patient who develops gastric symptoms after several years of good health after surgery for benign peptic ulcer deserves a thorough investigation for malignancy.

Epidemiology. Striking geographic differences characterize the incidence and death rates from carcinoma of the stomach. The highest rates occur in Japan and Chile and the lowest in Egypt, Malaysia, and Nicaragua. Despite the marked differences, no environmental or dietary factor has been identified as being causative. Factors which have been found to be related to a high incidence include low socioeconomic status, urban dwelling, smoked fish in the diet, presence of carcinogens such as benzpyrene in barbecued meat or heated fats, background irradiation, trace metals in soil, types of soil, climate, and occupation.

Incidence and Prevalence. A striking and unexplained decrease in mortality from carcinoma of the stomach has occurred over the past four decades, from 33 per 100,000 population in 1930 to 7 to 8 per 100,000 population in the early 1970's. During the same interval, five-year cure rates have improved from 7 per cent to 9 per cent of all patients treated. These apparent small gains may be attributed to blood transfusion, better understanding of fluid and electrolyte therapy, better anesthesia, and the introduction of antimicrobial drugs.

Carcinoma of the stomach is twice as common in men as in women. This ratio tends to be maintained in all countries for which cancer statistics exist. In the United States the incidence in both men and women is approximately twice as high in blacks and Orientals as it is in whites. Carcinoma of the stomach has been observed in all age groups, but is most common in patients between the ages of 50 and 69.

Pathology. Carcinomas may be found at any site within the stomach. They may be divided into four gross classifications: polypoid, ulcerated noninfiltrating, ulcerated infiltrating, and the diffuse infiltrating varieties. (This classification corresponds to the Borrman classification.) The rare superficial spreading carcinoma is not included in the preceding classification. Most gastric carcinomas are adenocarcinomas of widely varying histology. The histology ranges from well-differentiated adenocarcinoma to mucoid carcinoma to undifferentiated carcinomas which may be difficult to differentiate from sarcomas.

Carcinoma of the stomach spreads by direct invasion and lymphatic channels. The pancreas, liver, and transverse colon are often invaded by tumor. Tumors in the proximal stomach often invade the esophagus for variable distances. The distensibility of the esophagus may be restricted. If the neural plexuses are invaded, these cancers may mimic achalasia. Extension across the pylorus from distal lesions is uncommon.

Probably lymph node metastases appear early. The local perigastric, preaortic, porta hepatis, and mediastinal nodes are frequently involved. Malignant deposits are frequently found in nodes in the hilum of the spleen and in the spleen itself. Occasionally metastases to the left supraclavicular space occur (Virchow's node), probably through the thoracic duct. Peritoneal implants are frequent, occurring in one third of patients coming to autopsy. In women the ovaries may have metastases, the so-called Krukenberg tumors.

Hematogenous metastases most often involve the liver, lungs, and bone. Pulmonary metastases may appear as a pneumonitis or as discrete masses, or may resemble miliary tuberculosis.

Clinical Manifestations. The mass survey studies in Japan have clearly shown that "early" gastric carcinoma confined to the mucosa does not produce symptoms. Most carcinomas of the stomach seen in the United States are already advanced. Symptoms are the result of ulceration, obstruction, necrosis, and disorders of gastric motility caused by tumor invasion.

Weight loss is the most common symptom and occurs in up to 96 per cent of patients. Approximately 70 per cent of patients have pain of variable intensity. Some patients have a mild and vague discomfort. Approximately 25 per cent of patients describe the pain as being similar to that of peptic ulcer. The pain may or may not be relieved by food or antacids. In a few patients it is of long duration. If the cancer has invaded the pancreas, pain may be referred to the back. The pain may be described as pressure sensations, fullness, aching, bloating, indigestion, dyspepsia, or gas pains. Some patients have pain immediately after eating. In others there is no apparent relationship to the ingestion of food.

Approximately 50 per cent of patients have vomiting. This usually implies pyloric obstruction, but occurs with carcinomas at any location within the stomach. Anorexia occurs in about 25 per cent of patients. The degree of weight loss often cannot be related to a reduction of food intake. Early satiety occurs in about 10 per cent of patients and is a fairly constant symptom in linitis plastica but may also occur with relatively small tumors.

Other gastrointestinal symptoms are changes in bowel habits such as constipation or diarrhea. Dysphagia is common with carcinoma of the fundus and cardia. A few patients may have odynophagia, and some have pyrosis. Gross hematemesis and melena are unusual, each occurring in 10 per cent of patients. Occult bleeding, on the other hand, is extremely common.

Other symptoms resulting from gastric carcinoma are unusual fatigability and symptoms of anemia such as dyspnea, dizziness and fainting, pallor, angina pectoris, and burning of the tongue. Some patients may have eructations, bad breath, and hiccups, and a few discover an abdominal mass. Peritoneal implants may cause ascites. Metastases in the liver or to the porta hepatis may produce jaundice. Bone pain may be the result of either pathologic fractures or invasion of the periosteum. Carcinomas may perforate and mimic perforated peptic ulcer.

Physical Examination. Only 45 to 50 per cent of patients with advanced gastric carcinoma have a palpable mass. Hepatomegaly is common but does not always indicate metastatic disease. Twenty per cent of patients will be emaciated or cachectic. Abdominal tenderness is noted in only 20 per cent of patients. Five per cent of patients have palpable peripheral lymph nodes caused by the metastases. Metastatic disease may also be manifest by hard nodular livers and palpable nodules on rectal examination. Rarely, a tumor nodule may be palpated or even seen in the umbilicus. Ascites is present in a few patients owing to hepatic or peritoneal metastases.

Jaundice may be seen with metastases to the porta hepatis or liver.

Differential Diagnosis. A number of other diseases may produce symptoms similar or identical to gastric carcinoma. The most important is benign *peptic ulcer. Cholelithiasis, pancreatitis, pancreatic neoplasm,* or *coronary artery disease* and other neoplasms of the stomach should be considered. Appropriate investigation will establish the correct diagnosis in most patients.

Laboratory Studies. The anemias of gastric carcinomas are of several varieties. Approximately two thirds of patients will have a hypochromic microcytic anemia. Macrocytic anemia caused by vitamin B_{12} or folate deficiency is not rare. A normochromic normocytic anemia may appear without bone marrow metastases. Occult blood is present in the stool in only about 45 per cent of patients on a single determination; when the stool is repeatedly tested, the percentage is much higher.

Gastric analysis is mandatory in every patient with a gastric ulcer. Ideally, the tube should be placed under fluoroscopic control with the tip in the middle of the antrum. If a fluoroscope is not readily available, the tube should be passed 55 to 60 cm from the nares. The secretagogue should be Histolog, 1.5 mg per kilogram subcutaneously or intramuscularly, or pentagastrin, 1 to 6 µg per kilogram intramuscularly. An ulcerating lesion in an achlorhydric patient is virtually pathognomonic of a malignant neoplasm. Presence of acid in no way excludes a diagnosis of cancer.

Roentgenologic Diagnosis. Roentgenologic examina-

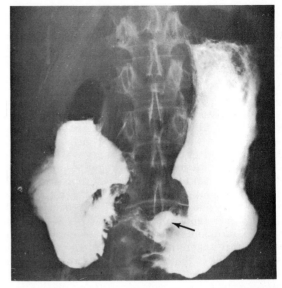

Figure 2. Carcinoma of the stomach. The tumor has involved the entire antrum and produced a characteristic filling defect and mucosal destruction. An ulcer within the mass is indicated by the arrow.

tion will detect 95 per cent of gastric lesions. The radiologist must procure good mucosal detail to avoid overlooking small lesions. One of the more difficult differential diagnoses is between malignant and benign

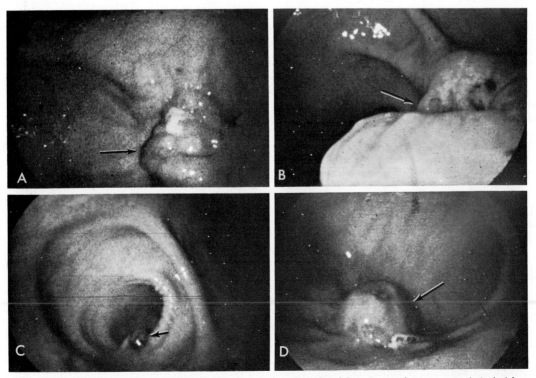

Figure 3. Four gastric lesions photographed with the gastrocamera (reproduced from 5 mm color transparencies). *A,* Adenocarcinoma (arrow) seen on the posterior aspect of the stomach near the incisura angularis. *B,* Benign gastric ulcer (arrow) from a tangential view, showing the incisura angularis with the antral region to the left and fundus to the right. The edematous rolled margins of the ulcer surround the typical necrotic center; there is no evidence of neoplasia. *C,* This adenomatous polyp (arrow) in the gastric antrum had bled persistently, causing the patient to become severely anemic. The 5 to 6 mm lesion was seen in only one of several carefully performed upper gastrointestinal series. Its size, shape, and smooth contours are consistent with the subsequently proved diagnosis of adenoma. *D,* Leiomyoma (arrow) on the posterior wall of the body of the stomach lying above the incisura angularis. Note the obviously submucosal character of this lesion and its typical umbilication by an apical ulcer.

ulcers. In some ulcers, this distinction may be impossible. Some features which favor malignant ulcer are effacement of folds and abnormal mucosal folds, a niche in a notch (an ulcer within an ulcer), an ulcer with a flat wavy base, and a triangular-shaped wide-based ulcer. Linitis plastica is characterized by loss of distensibility of the stomach and absent or marked reduction of motility. Other malignant lesions are characterized by rigidity, mucosal distortion, irregular and enlarged mucosal folds, and fixed filling defects. An ulcer within a mass is characteristic of carcinoma of the stomach (Fig. 2). Some ulcers have features of both benignancy and malignancy.

Gastroscopy. Fiberoptic endoscopy permits a more complete examination of the stomach than was possible with the previous semiflexible instruments. Still and motion picture photography provide a permanent record (Fig. 3). These endoscopes have biopsy and directed cytology instruments. If six to ten biopsies and cytology specimens are taken from every lesion, a positive diagnosis is possible in 85 to 95 per cent of patients. In some lesions it may be technically impossible to place the biopsy forceps or the cytology instrument on the lesion. With the end-viewing instruments it may be impossible to biopsy the proximal edge of an ulcer. It is also not possible to sample the entire stomach to detect an otherwise unrecognized carcinoma.

Exfoliative Cytology. Skillfully collected and expertly interpreted, exfoliative cytology is one of the most sensitive techniques for either diagnosing or excluding cancer of the stomach. As with all other procedures, there are limitations. The technique cannot detect submucosal malignancies which do not penetrate into the lumen of the stomach. Leiomyosarcomas, even when ulcerated, do not exfoliate diagnostic cells. Some large, necrotic tumors may have fibrin or necrotic membranes overlying them, preventing exfoliation of diagnostic cells. The diagnosis in these lesions is usually apparent by radiographic and gastroscopic appearance.

Lavage cytology is superior to abrasive instruments. The highest accuracy has resulted from the utilization of chymotrypsin as a mucolytic enzyme. Lavage cytology provides a total mucosal "biopsy." In laboratories regularly performing gastric exfoliative cytology, accuracy ranges from 90 to 95 per cent in patients with proved malignancy, and cancer is falsely diagnosed in less than 1 per cent of patients with benign disease. The diagnosis rendered by the responsible physician should include only three possible categories: (1) malignant cells present with an interpretation of cell type, (2) no malignant cells present, and (3) unsatisfactory test which must be repeated after appropriate cleansing of the stomach.

Use of All Techniques. All available techniques should be used in gastric cancer suspects. Overconfidence in one method to the exclusion of others is to be avoided. The application of roentgenologic, gastroscopic, and cytologic methods affords the greatest benefit to the patient under consideration. If all these techniques indicate a benign lesion, the patient with gastric ulcer warrants a trial of medical therapy. However, it is mandatory that these patients be repeatedly examined to ensure ulcer healing.

Treatment. The only curative therapy for gastric carcinoma is surgical excision. The type and extent of the procedure must be left to the discretion of the surgeon. Polypoid carcinoma may be treated with a limited gastrectomy if no evidence of metastasis is present. Antral lesions may be treated by a subtotal gastrectomy, including the regional lymph nodes in the vicinity of the tumor. Patients with cancer of the cardia and fundus should have a proximal gastrectomy. Super-radical gastrectomy, in which all areas of *predicted* metastases are removed, was advocated in the past, but these procedures double surgical mortality and actually decrease cure rates. Total gastrectomy is almost never indicated for treatment of gastric carcinoma. Palliative resection is indicated for patients with incurable disease. Even though survival may not be improved, these patients may derive considerable benefit from relief of obstruction and hemorrhage and from improved nutrition.

Chemotherapy may provide palliation for some patients. 5-Fluorouracil (5-FU) produces an objective response in 20 per cent of patients and subjective improvement in 40 per cent. A recommended regimen is 5-FU, 15 mg per kilogram given once weekly either intravenously or orally. The drug should be administered by physicians skilled in its use.

Systematic studies of radiation therapy of gastric carcinoma are not available. Such therapy should be considered if the patient is inoperable but has tumor largely confined to the vicinity of the stomach. It is impossible to predict whether this form of treatment will be effective without attempting it. Irradiation therapy is of some use in selected patients in controlling hemorrhage.

Prognosis. Advanced carcinoma of the stomach has a dismal prognosis. Sixty-five per cent of patients subjected to surgery are found to be incurable. Fewer than 10 per cent of all patients with the disease can be cured. Factors which favor a more favorable prognosis are a long history as opposed to a brief history. The gross appearance of the tumor is related to prognosis. The polypoid tumors and the ulcerating but noninfiltrating tumors have the best prognosis, and the ulcerated, infiltrating, and diffuse infiltrating varieties have extremely low cure rates. Superficial spreading carcinoma, which is usually diagnosed cytologically, and carcinoma of the stomach confined to the mucosa have cure rates in the order of 90 to 95 per cent.

OTHER NEOPLASMS OF THE STOMACH

Lymphoma

Malignant lymphoma may be confined to the stomach. With the decreasing incidence of carcinoma, it assumes an increasingly important proportion of gastric cancers. *Reticulum cell sarcoma* and *lymphosarcoma* are the most common types. *Hodgkin's disease, giant follicular lymphoma,* and *plasmacytoma* may also involve the stomach primarily. The symptoms of malignant lymphoma are similar to carcinoma except that some patients have a history similar to that of peptic ulcer, sometimes for as long as several years. Men and women are equally affected. The peak incidence is between the ages of 40 and 60. Anemia, overt bleeding, and marked weight loss are somewhat less frequent than with carcinoma of the stomach.

There are no distinctive roentgenographic or gastroscopic appearances to permit differentiation from carcinoma. Exfoliative cytology is diagnostic in up to 90 per cent of patients. It is possible to differentiate reticulum cell sarcoma, lymphosarcoma, and Hodgkin's disease by cytologic criteria.

Treatment consists of resection of the tumor followed by irradiation therapy. The surgeon should attempt to excise as much tumor tissue as possible even if it cannot be resected in toto. Some patients who have been deemed inoperable and treated with radiation alone have had long survival. Cure rates, as judged by five-year survival, are 50 per cent in patients treated with surgery followed by irradiation therapy.

Leiomyosarcoma

The history of patients with leiomyosarcoma is similar to that of patients with carcinoma of the stomach; however, bleeding is more common, particularly massive hemorrhage, because these tumors are frequently ulcerated. Metastatic spread tends to be confined to the abdomen. Treatment is wide surgical excision. Five-year survival after surgery is 40 per cent and is dependent upon the degree of anaplasia of the tumor rather than its size.

667. BENIGN NEOPLASMS OF THE STOMACH

Lloyd L. Brandborg

ADENOMA

Adenomas of the stomach are generally seen in patients over the age of 50. Ninety-five per cent of patients with adenomas have achlorhydria, and they occur in 2 per cent of patients with achlorhydria. The incidence in pernicious anemia varies widely from series to series and may be as high as 20 per cent in these patients.

Probably most adenomas of the stomach are asymptomatic. The most common symptom is a nondescript upper abdominal pain. It is not related to food, is described as a dull ache and occasionally gnawing sensation, and is not relieved by antacids or food. Rarely, nausea and vomiting may be present. Overt hemorrhage is unusual, but the tumor may bleed occultly.

The physical examination is usually normal. In a few patients the signs of iron deficiency anemia are present. A palpable abdominal mass caused by adenoma is virtually never found.

The roentgenographic appearance of gastric adenoma is that of a spherical filling defect often on a stalk of variable length. Fiberoptic endoscopy is more sensitive than radiology in detecting small polypoid lesions. It also assists in differentiating the nature of these lesions and permits biopsy and cytologic examination. Endoscopy frequently detects several gastric polyps when one is identified on roentgenologic examination.

If it is highly likely that a patient's symptoms are due to gastric adenoma, therapy is local excision, including the stalk. Because of the low potential of malignancy, polyps less than 2 cm in diameter may be followed annually with cytologic examination and endoscopy. Polyps larger than 2 cm in diameter, particularly if they are sessile, have a higher probability of being malignant. If surgical contraindications are not present, these lesions should be locally excised.

LEIOMYOMA

Although leiomyomas are the most common benign tumors found in the stomach at autopsy, they are rarely responsible for clinical symptoms. Intramural, extramucosal tumors, they occur with equal frequency in men and women and are seen most often in subjects between the ages of 40 and 60. Most are between 1 and 2 cm in diameter, but they can attain huge size. Evidence of previous ulceration of the mucosa overlying the tumor is found in as many as 60 per cent of cases.

The most important symptom of gastric leiomyoma is bleeding. Usually it is occult and leads to iron deficiency anemia, but on occasion it may be massive. Some patients may also complain of epigastric burning or gnawing pain and anorexia.

The roentgenographic features are those of an intramucosal, usually spherical, intramural mass projecting into the lumen of the stomach. An ulceration may be detected within the mass. Gastroscopically, the tumor is covered by a normal but somewhat stretched mucosa with flattened rugae. The central ulcer is visible if present.

Symptomatic leiomyomas should be treated by local excision or limited gastrectomy. Prognosis is excellent.

See references after Ch. 669.

668. NEOPLASMS OF THE SMALL INTESTINE

Thomas F. O'Brien, Jr.

Primary neoplasms of the small intestine which are of clinical importance arise from the epithelial, muscular, vascular, and lymphatic components of the small intestine. Thus *adenomas, adenocarcinomas, leiomyomas, leiomyosarcomas, hemangiomas,* and *lymphomas* represent the most frequently observed tumors of the small intestine.

MALIGNANT NEOPLASMS

Types. *Adenocarcinomas, lymphomas,* and *leiomyosarcomas* are the three most common primary malignancies of the small intestine. Adenocarcinoma occurs with the greatest frequency and leiomyosarcoma with the least.

Etiology. Very little is known or hypothesized about the etiology of small intestinal malignancy. Dietary factors do not appear to play an important role in the development of adenocarcinoma, and no major differences in incidence have been observed among population groups. Chronic small bowel disease, however, may represent a predisposing factor, because *celiac sprue* and chronic *regional enteritis* appear to be associated with a disproportionate number of primary small bowel malignancies. An hereditary factor is suggested by the unusual frequency of *primary small bowel lymphoma* in the Middle East, particularly Israel and southern Iran.

Incidence. Primary small intestinal malignancies are rare. Excluding carcinoids, they represent only 1 to 2 per cent of all malignant gastrointestinal neoplasms.

Pathology. More than 90 per cent of the *adenocarcinomas* of the small intestine are located in the duodenum, and most lie within 20 cm of the ligament of Treitz. The lesions are usually annular in configuration and reveal a moderate degree of differentiation under the microscope. More than half the patients will show extension to or beyond regional lymph nodes at the time of initial diagnosis.

All varieties of lymphoma may arise primarily in the small intestine, although *reticulum cell sarcoma* is by far the most common. *Lymphomas* tend to involve the more distal portions of the jejunum and ileum and rarely arise in the duodenum.

Leiomyosarcomas of the small intestine may arise in any portion of the small intestine; however, the jejunum and ileum are the usual sites. They tend to be bulky tumors, exceeding 5 cm in diameter. Central necrosis is a common feature. Metastatic spread occurs primarily by the blood-borne route or by direct extension, rather than lymphatically.

Clinical Manifestations. Malignant primary tumors of the small intestine are usually discovered in persons over 50 years of age. Lymphomas of the small intestine, however, tend to occur at a somewhat earlier age than adenocarcinomas or leiomyosarcomas. Men are afflicted with a frequency more than double that of women. Abdominal pain, malaise, anorexia, weight loss, and bleeding are common presenting symptoms. Although prodromal symptoms are usually present, sudden obstruction of the small intestine may be the first manifestation of a small bowel malignancy. A small bowel tumor, when palpable on physical examination, is almost invariably malignant. Free perforation is an important clinical manifestation of the sarcoma.

Diagnosis. Most primary small intestinal malignancies are identified by radiographic examination of the small bowel. Certain roentgenologic features characterize the various histologic types. Annular lesions of short length are typically found with an *adenocarcinoma* (Fig. 1). Longer, ulcerating lesions producing so-called aneurysmal dilatation of the lumen favor lymphoma. Diffuse small bowel involvement suggesting a malabsorption syndrome is a less common manifestation of lymphoma. *Leiomyosarcomas* are bulky tumors which displace adjacent bowel loops.

Visceral angiography has become a valuable tool in identification of malignant small bowel tumors. The source of blood supply is an important clue in the differential diagnosis of benign and malignant lesions. Benign tumors are invariably fed by a branch of the gastroduodenal or superior mesenteric artery. Blood supply from a renal or lumbar artery (parasitic blood supply) is characteristic of a malignant lesion.

Treatment. Surgery is required for the majority of patients with primary small bowel malignancies. Although in two thirds of the patients the disease will have spread at the time of surgical intervention, the procedure is usually indicated for relief of obstruction, control of hemorrhage, and alleviation of pain.

Radiation therapy, alkalating agents, and nitrogen mustard, together with corticosteroids, often prove effective for some patients with lymphoma. 5-Fluorouracil and its derivatives have not proved to be beneficial in most instances.

Prognosis. Prognosis in primary bowel malignancy is dependent to some extent upon location, histology, and duration of disease. Under favorable circumstances five-year survivals of 20 per cent have been reported with adenocarcinoma, 60 per cent with lymphoma, and up to 50 per cent with leiomyosarcomas.

BENIGN NEOPLASMS

The small intestine may give rise to a variety of benign small bowel tumors. Among these are *adenomas, leiomyomas, lipomas, fibromas,* and *hemangiomas.* Of these, the *leiomyoma* is the most important of the group to the clinician. They may arise at any level of the small intestine but favor the jejunum. Central necrosis with ulceration, resulting in severe hemorrhage, is a characteristic feature of the leiomyoma.

Hemangiomas are much less frequently found than adenomas or leiomyomas. They, too, are clinically important because of their propensity to bleed.

Clinical Manifestations. Benign small bowel tumors occur with equal frequency in men and women and are usually symptomatic in persons above 50 years of age. Colicky abdominal pain caused by luminal obstruction or intussusception is the predominant symptom. Massive gastrointestinal hemorrhage is suggestive of a leiomyoma. Benign small bowel tumors are rarely palpable.

Diagnosis. Barium contrast studies of the small intestine and visceral angiography represent the principal diagnostic methods. A small bowel series occasionally demonstrates localized intussusception, an important clue that the lesion is benign.

Treatment and Prognosis. Surgical excision is the treatment of choice for virtually all symptomatic primary benign small bowel tumors. Prognosis is excellent with resection.

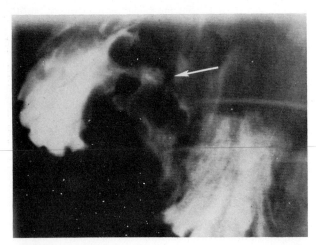

Figure 1. Adenocarcinoma of the duodenum, close-up view. The characteristic features of a small bowel adenocarcinoma are demonstrated here. Note the "shelving" edges at the proximal portion of the tumor. The central lumen shows destruction of the normal mucosal pattern with ulceration (arrow). (From O'Brien, T. F., Jr., *In* Sleisenger, M. H., and Fordtran, J. S. [eds.]: Gastrointestinal Disease. Philadelphia, W. B. Saunders Company, 1973.)

669. NEOPLASMS OF THE LARGE INTESTINE

Thomas F. O'Brien, Jr.

CARCINOMA OF THE LARGE INTESTINE

Incidence and Prevalence. Colorectal cancer is the second most common malignancy of the adult population in the United States (excluding skin cancer). It is exceeded only by lung cancer among males and breast cancer among females. Malignancies of the colon and rectum are responsible for approximately 15 per cent of all adult cancer deaths, resulting in an annual fatality rate of 16 to 18 patients per 100,000 population. A similar incidence has been noted in Great Britain, France, Germany, New Zealand, and a number of other countries which share an urbanized Western culture. In sharp contrast is a considerably reduced incidence in Japan, rural Africa, India, and a number of Latin American countries.

Etiology. The etiology of malignant tumors of the colon and rectum remains unknown. At least three factors must be considered in the development of large intestinal neoplasms, namely environmental factors, heredity, and pre-existing disease.

Environmental Factors. The contrasting prevalence of the disease among different cultures has led to increasing speculation that environmental factors, such as exposure to ingested carcinogens, play a primary role in pathogenesis. Considerable differences in dietary patterns exist between populations with high and low rates of large intestinal cancer. For example, those in cultures with a low incidence of large bowel cancer consume diets containing a large amount of plant fiber. Conversely, diets in areas where colon cancer is more prevalent tend to contain large amounts of highly refined carbohydrates and are generally low in fiber content. Perhaps related to these dissimilarities in diet are the significant differences in colonic bacterial flora which exist between the two groups. High fiber content diets produce bulky stools containing principally aerobic organisms (enterococci, streptococci), whereas the compact, small volume stools of low residue diets contain principally anaerobic organisms (bacteroides). Furthermore, it has been shown that some anaerobic organisms have the capacity metabolically to transform certain innocuous substances, such as bile acids, into potentially carcinogenic compounds. The latter phenomenon, together with the relatively prolonged colonic transit time of the small-volume stool, could lead to extended contact time between carcinogen and large bowel epithelium. Although unproved, this hypothesis is both popular and plausible.

In further support of the environmental theory is the observation that individuals from a "low-cancer" culture, such as native Japanese, develop large intestinal malignancies with an incidence similar to Americans when they establish residence in the United States and adopt Western dietary patterns.

Hereditary Factors. Genetic factors appear to play a primary role in several varieties of inherited colorectal neoplasms to be discussed.

FAMILIAL POLYPOSIS. Familial polyposis is inherited as an autosomal dominant trait. Multiple polypoid adenomas of the colon become apparent in patients between the ages of 10 and 15 years. In untreated cases, colorectal cancer will develop in 75 to 80 per cent of the patients. Unfortunately, some 40 per cent of index cases already have a malignancy at the time of original diagnosis. The identification of such an index case should prompt a thorough survey of all immediate family members with the usual diagnostic methods (see below). Subtotal colectomy with ileoproctectomy should be recommended to all asymptomatic patients in whom multiple polyps are present. The remaining rectal tissue, although subject to the development of polypoid adenomas and adenocarcin-

omas, can be inspected regularly with a proctoscope and suspicious lesions removed locally. The preservation of rectal function is desirable and more easily acceptable to asymptomatic patients.

GARDNER'S SYNDROME. Gardner's syndrome consists of multiple polyps of the small and large intestines associated with osteomas and soft tissue lesions. This disorder is also transmitted as an autosomal dominant trait. A variety of soft tissue lesions are seen, including sebaceous cysts, lipomas, fibromas, leiomyomas, and occasionally fibrosarcomas. These soft tissue tumors may occur in the skin, in subcutaneous tissues, or in a variety of mesenteric or retroperitoneal locations. Colorectal carcinoma occurs in these patients with a high frequency, similar to that observed in familial polyposis; however, the malignancies tend to develop at a later age in life. Prophylactic subtotal colectomy with ileorectal anastomosis is the treatment of choice.

FAMILY COLONIC CANCER WITHOUT POLYPS (THE CANCER FAMILY SYNDROME). Several kindreds have been described in which there is an unusual frequency of colonic cancer. The neoplasms tend to occur at an early age, and polyposis is *not* a feature. Pedigree studies suggest that the mode of inheritance is via an autosomal dominant trait.

PEUTZ-JEGHERS SYNDROME. Mucocutaneous pigmentation, primarily involving the buccal mucosa, perioral and periorbital skin, and distal extremities, characterizes this variety of gastrointestinal polyposis. The syndrome is transmitted by a single mendelian dominant trait responsible for both the melanin deposits and the polyps. Histologically, the latter are hamartomas rather than adenomas. In the great majority of cases the polyps are distributed primarily in the jejunum and ileum, although gastric polyps occur in approximately 25 per cent of cases, and colorectal polyps are seen in 30 to 50 per cent. The risk of associated gastrointestinal malignancy is small, of the order of 3 per cent of cases. In a recent review, it was reported that 15 of 125 female patients with Peutz-Jeghers syndrome had developed ovarian tumors. The wide distribution of the gastrointestinal polyps and the low incidence of associated malignancy make prophylactic bowel resection unrealistic.

TURCOT SYNDROME. This extremely rare condition features the association of malignant tumors of the central nervous system and familial polyposis. To date, only a single kindred has been described. No rational therapeutic management program has developed because of the insufficient case material.

CRONKHITE-CANADA SYNDROME. Diffuse gastrointestinal polyposis, alopecia, pigmentation, and onychotrophia characterize this syndrome. Diarrhea, hypoproteinemia, edema, and cachexia are important additional clinical manifestations. Patients with this syndrome have usually been in their fifth and sixth decades of life, and there is no predominant sex distribution. Although colorectal malignancy has not been associated with the polyposis, rapidly progressive cachexia and a fatal outcome are characteristic.

Predisposing Diseases. CANCER RISK AND POLYPOID ADENOMAS. Although formerly a subject of great controversy, there is general agreement that the polypoid adenoma of the colon is not a premalignant lesion. One or several such adenomas may be found in 15 per cent of the adult population (Fig. 2). One autopsy series in which meticulous inspection of the large bowel was

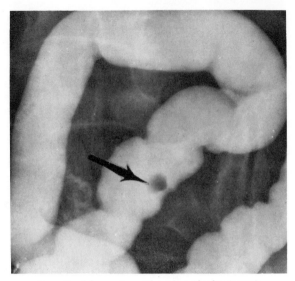

Figure 2. Adenomatous polyp, sigmoid colon (arrow).

carried out demonstrated adenomas in approximately three fourths of all those examined.

Most of the clinically detected polypoid adenomas are less than 1.5 cm in transverse diameter, and malignancy in lesions of this size is quite uncommon. Colorectal cancers, which assume a polypoid shape, are usually greater than 2.0 cm in transverse diameter at the time of discovery.

ULCERATIVE COLITIS. The development of colorectal carcinoma at a greatly increased rate in patients with chronic ulcerative colitis appears well established. Approximately 5 per cent of patients with prolonged disease develop this serious complication. At least three parameters appear important when considering the risk of malignancy in these patients: the duration of the disease, the age at initial onset of the disease, and the extent of colonic involvement with the disease. The majority of patients in whom ulcerative colitis is complicated by malignancy have usually had universal involvement of the colon by the inflammatory process, and their disease has been present in excess of 15 years on the average.

So-called childhood ulcerative colitis, with onset at less than 14 years of age, appears to have an unusual incidence of colonic carcinoma. An analysis of almost 400 cases from the Mayo Clinic places the cancer risk at 20 per cent for each 10 years of duration beyond the initial decade. This carcinogenic risk of longstanding ulcerative colitis makes duration of disease the most important single consideration in the decision for colectomy. To date there is insufficient evidence to establish a relationship between granulomatous-segmental colitis (Crohn's disease) and colorectal carcinoma.

Pathogenesis. *Normal and Abnormal Cellular Kinetics.* Radiothymidine-labeling studies of cellular proliferation in the colon have shown important differences between normal epithelium and areas of neoplasia. Mitosis of colonic epithelial cells is normally limited to a regeneration zone in the lower third of the base of the crypts of Lieberkühn. Newly formed epithelial cells then migrate to the mucosal surface over a period of approximately 72 hours, and are finally shed into the lumen in about 96 hours. No appreciable cellular division takes place once the cell has begun its journey out of the crypt. However, when surface epithelial cells of laboratory animals are exposed to chemical carcinogens, they begin to show considerable mitotic activity. Eventually polypoid adenomas develop which are histologically similar to those observed in humans. Parallel isotopic studies in humans with various hyperplastic colonic neoplasms have confirmed that increased cellular proliferation occurs within the superficial epithelium of such lesions. These studies support the theory that environmental carcinogens play an important role in colorectal neoplasms.

Pathology. The majority of rectal and colonic malignancies are adenocarcinomas. In a series of more than 50,000 cases of large intestinal malignancy, 86 per cent were adenocarcinoma in type. *Carcinoids, squamous cell carcinoma, leiomyosarcoma, adenoacanthoma,* and *lymphoma,* as a group, accounted for only 2 per cent of the total. The remainder were undifferentiated or poorly differentiated carcinomas. Multiple primary tumors within the colon are noted in approximately 5 per cent of patients at the time of initial diagnosis.

The distribution of large intestinal malignancies is similar in most large series. Approximately 15 per cent arise in the cecum and ascending colon, 10 per cent are distributed along the transverse colon, 5 per cent occur in the descending colon, 25 per cent occur in the sigmoid, and 45 per cent arise in the rectum. Metastatic spread may occur by direct invasion of surrounding tissues, by way of the regional lymphatics, or by multiple peritoneal implants. The liver is the principal site of major organ metastasis, with the lungs, brain, bones, and other viscera less frequently involved.

Microscopically, adenocarcinomas of the large intestine show a poorly formed acinar architecture, containing small amounts of mucus. A small number, perhaps 5 per cent, show considerable mucus production and have been assigned the term *mucoid adenocarcinoma.* Paradoxically, the well-differentiated mucoid carcinoma has a rather poor prognosis.

Clinical Manifestations. Carcinoma of the colon and rectum is primarily a disease of later life. Although sporadic cases may be observed in any age group, the disease occurs with increasing frequency above the age of 55 years and reaches its peak incidence beyond 65 years of age. Males and females develop tumors above the rectum with approximately equal frequency, whereas males predominate in rectal cancer.

The presenting clinical manifestations of colorectal cancer are primarily determined by the location of the tumor. Approximately 75 per cent of all large intestinal malignancies occur within, or distal to, the sigmoid colon. Characteristically, tumors in these locations grow circumferentially, producing some degree of bowel obstruction. For this reason a significant change in bowel pattern is reported by the majority of the patients. Common symptoms include increasing constipation or alternating constipation and diarrhea, usually accompanied by colicky lower abdominal pain.

Most tumors in this location have ulcerating surfaces, and because of their proximity to the rectum, visible blood is usually observed by the patient. When the tumors arise within or near the rectum, more severe obstipation, tenesmus, and visible blood are nearly always reported, and pencil-shaped stools are frequently observed.

In contrast, carcinomas arising in the cecum and ascending colon usually do not produce obstructive symptoms. Growths in this area often assume a polypoid configuration and may reach considerable size prior to discovery. Blood loss is typically occult, and is rarely observed by the patient. Frequently it is the symptoms of profound anemia which bring the patient to the physician. Quite often the tumor has metastasized to the liver at the time of initial examination, and jaundice, right upper quadrant pain, or a mass lesion may be noted.

Tumors arising in the middle third of the colon present with variable symptomatology. Vague discomfort, nonspecific dyspepsia, or colicky pain with gross or occult blood loss may be reported by the patient. Weight loss is variable, but when it exceeds 10 per cent or more of the patient's usual weight it usually indicates a poor prognosis.

Diagnosis. The diagnosis of a large intestinal malignancy is usually suggested by the patient's history. In addition, it must be strongly considered in all patients beyond the age of 45 years with unexplained anemia. A primary lesion in the large intestine must also be ruled out in those patients who present with evidence of metastatic liver disease such as jaundice and hepatic enlargement.

On physical examination, palpation of the abdomen may reveal a mass lesion, but this is highly variable and depends in large part upon the size of the tumor, degree of obesity, and location of the tumor in relationship to pelvic bony structures. Digital and proctoscopic examination of the rectosigmoid usually reveals two out of three lesions arising below the pelvic peritoneal reflection. The physician should be alert to those cutaneous manifestations suggestive of a familial syndrome associated with colorectal cancer. Superficial forceps biopsy of the lesion can usually be obtained safely by an experienced physician and will lead to rapid histologic confirmation of the diagnosis. Reluctance toward biopsy on the grounds of tumor dissemination is not justified. Comparative five-year survival studies of patients with and without circulating malignant cells after surgical manipulation have demonstrated that their presence is without prognostic significance.

Lesions beyond the reach of the proctoscope are best revealed by barium contrast radiographic examination. Typical lesions in the sigmoid colon produce a sharply demarcated narrowing of the lumen usually not exceeding 8 to 10 cm in length. The "napkin ring" or "apple core" appearance with shelving edges is a most characteristic radiographic feature (Fig. 3). Tumors arising in the cecum often assume polypoid rather than annular configuration and may be obscured by excessive barium filling of the cecum. In suspicious cases, when an annular lesion is not demonstrated, an air contrast barium enema can be diagnostic. A carcinoma lying within an area of massed diverticula can easily be overlooked, and repeat studies with special emphasis to the area of interest should be performed in suspicious cases.

Fiberoptic colonoscopy offers considerable promise for the visual inspection and biopsy of lesions beyond the reach of standard proctoscopes. Perhaps the greatest utility for this technique lies in the examination of pedunculated or sessile growths whose benignity or malignancy cannot be established on radiographic grounds. Techniques are rapidly developing for the complete excision of these lesions at the time of colonoscopy, thereby avoiding the necessity of laparotomy. Such techniques, however, require considerable skill on the part of the endoscopist and should only be performed by those with adequate training.

Exfoliative cytology, although advocated by Papanicolaou more than 20 years ago, has not gained wide acceptance in the diagnosis of colorectal cancer. Several series, however, have demonstrated a high degree of diagnostic accuracy for the method. A correct cytologic diagnosis is established in 80 to 95 per cent of patients with malignancy. The percentages of false-positive and false-negative reports are small in these series. Underutilization of the technique is probably accounted for by the belief that satisfactory specimens are difficult and unpleasant to obtain. In practice, however, quite satisfactory cytologic material may be obtained by a simple saline lavage of the colon preceded by several days of an elemental diet and a strong cathartic the night before the collection of the specimen.

Carcinoembryonic Antigen (CEA). A tumor-associated antigen, referred to as CEA, can be demonstrated in the serum of over 95 per cent of patients with disseminated colonic carcinoma and approximately 20 per cent of patients with localized disease. The CEA appears to be a glycoprotein with a molecular weight of approximately 200,000. In general, serum levels appear to be elevated in proportion to the mass of tumor tissue present. Serum levels of CEA below 2.5 ng per ml are clearly normal, whereas values which exceed 5.0 ng per ml are strongly suggestive of underlying disease (see below). Levels between 2.5 and 5.0 ng must be considered indeterminate, especially if underlying inflammatory disease is present.

The early promise of specific serologic diagnosis of large intestinal malignancy by means of the CEA has not been sustained.

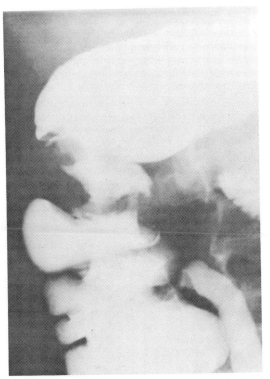

Figure 3. Carcinoma of the colon. This annular lesion in the ascending colon has produced a typical appearance of mucosal destruction and overhanging margins.

Positive tests can be obtained in a significant percentage of other gastrointestinal diseases, both malignant (hepatoma and gastric, pancreatic, and small bowel carcinomas), and nonmalignant (alcoholic cirrhosis, pancreatitis, and ulcerative colitis). Positive CEA tests have also been reported in lung cancer, breast cancer, prostatic cancer, neuroblastoma, and osteogenic sarcoma. These findings cast much doubt on the utility of the CEA as a screening test for colorectal cancer. The test may be useful in postoperative cases, because elevated levels tend to fall with successful resection. A return to elevated values is indicative of recurrent or disseminated disease.

Differential Diagnosis. Malignancies of the large intestine must be differentiated from other diseases which present with an abdominal mass, rectal bleeding, colicky abdominal pain, or a change in bowel habit. A number of diseases may produce these symptoms either singly or in combination. Included in the differential diagnosis are *diverticulosis coli,* with or without diverticulitis; inflammatory bowel diseases, including *ulcerative colitis* and *proctitis* and *ileocolitis* of the Crohn variety; and *benign tumors* (most frequently polypoid adenomas).

On rare occasions *pelvic endometriosis* may mimic a primary large bowel cancer. In this instance, usually the age, sex, and relationship of the rectal bleeding to menstrual flow are important differential diagnostic features in the history.

The finding of hemorrhoidal varices should not be accepted as sufficient explanation for rectal bleeding in any patient, especially in those over 45 years. Proctoscopy should be performed routinely in all patients with rectal bleeding, and radiographic studies should be obtained in most instances.

Treatment and Prognosis. *Surgical Resection.* Most patients with colorectal carcinoma require surgical resection of the primary tumor. The operation may be either curative or palliative in intent. A palliative resection is justified when lower bowel obstruction is imminent, even though known metastases are present. In a series of over 1800 cases from the University of Minnesota, the overall five-year survival of patients with colorectal carcinoma was approximately 30 per cent. Patients with rectal carcinoma generally showed a poorer prognosis than those with tumors of other segments of the colon. Patients without lymph node involvement, whose surgery took place between 1958 and 1963, showed a five-year survival of 43.5 per cent for carcinoma of the rectum and 62.5 per cent for other colonic cancers. The operative mortality for rectal carcinoma was more than twice that for higher lesions.

Rectal Fulguration and Radiotherapy. The higher operative mortality and poorer prognosis for rectal cancer has led to several innovations in therapy. Rectal fulguration and/or local radiation therapy have been successfully employed by some as an alternative mode of therapy for selected patients.

Chemotherapy. There has been disappointingly little progress in the development of effective chemotherapeutic agents for colorectal carcinoma. 5-Fluorouracil (5-FU) remains the most widely used agent. Objective tumor regression occurs in approximately 20 per cent of the treated patients. The rather slow cellular doubling time of colorectal cancers has been offered as an explanation for the general unresponsiveness to chemotherapeutic agents.

Some are cautiously optimistic that immunotherapy may play a role in future treatment. The identification of tumor-specific antigens within human neoplastic colon cells justifies the hope that specific antibodies can be developed and directed against the neoplastic tissues.

VILLOUS ADENOMAS

The villous adenoma is a special form of colonic neoplasm with interesting gross anatomic, histologic, physiologic, and clinical features. Villous adenomas occur with much less frequency than polypoid adenomas, and are usually seen in patients in the seventh decade of life. Grossly, the tumors are broad based, usually measuring more than 4 cm in transverse diameter, and consist of numerous frond-like projections. The majority are in the rectum and rectosigmoid portion of the colon. Those which can be reached by digital examination are very soft to palpation and appear velvety on proctoscopy. The epithelial cells of these tumors are abundant in mucin, and patients with villous adenomas often note considerable mucoid content in their stools. In rare instances a villous adenoma will secrete considerable volumes of fluid, rich in potassium, leading to severe hypokalemia.

In the microscopic evaluation of these tumors a clear distinction between atypical focal hyperplasia and carcinoma in situ can be very difficult for the pathologist. Such foci of cellular atypia can be found in up to 50 per cent of all villous adenomas upon careful serial sectioning. It is very unlikely, however, that 50 per cent of the lesions advance to infiltrating adenocarcinoma. The unpredictable course, together with frequently distressing clinical symptoms, dictates complete surgical excision whenever possible.

Castleman, B., and Krickstein, H.: Current approach to the polyp-cancer controversy. Gastroenterology, 51:108, 1966.

Devroede, G. J., Taylor, W. F., Sauer, W. G., Jackman, R. J., and Stickler, G. B.: Cancer risk and life expectancy of children with ulcerative colitis. N. Engl. J. Med., 285:17, 1971.

Griffiths, J. D., McKinna, J. A., Rowbotham, H. D., Tsolakidis, P., and Salsbury, A. J.: Carcinoma of the colon and rectum: Circulating malignant cells and five-year survival. Cancer, 31:226, 1973.

Margulis, A. R., and Burhenne, H. J.: Alimentary Tract Radiology. St. Louis, C. V. Mosby Company, 1973.

Morrissey, J. F.: Gastrointestinal endoscopy. Gastroenterology, 62:1241, 1972.

Sherlock, P., Erlich, A. N., and Winawer, S. J.: Diagnosis of gastrointestinal cancer: Current status and recent progress. Gastroenterology, 63:672, 1972.

Sleisenger, M. H., and Fordtran, J. S. (eds.): Gastrointestinal Disease. Philadelphia, W. B. Saunders Company, 1973.

Section Nine. OTHER DISEASES OF THE COLON, RECTUM, AND ANUS

David L. Earnest

670. INTRODUCTION

Certain diseases of the colon are not conveniently classified with other vascular, motor, malignant, or inflammatory conditions. In general, these miscellaneous colonic diseases are uncommon, often of uncertain etiology, and frequently perplexing to diagnose and treat. Properly taken and processed rectal biopsy specimens can significantly contribute to their diagnosis. A pedunculated or sessile mucosal mass may be biopsied with either punch or cutting forceps. Biopsy of an ulcerating lesion should be taken at its margin and should include some normal tissue. A suction biopsy tube can be used when there is diffuse mucosal disease. This instrument is especially useful if the abnormality is located above the peritoneal reflection. The use of conventional biopsy forceps for small mucosal lesions 12 to 14 cm or more above the pectinate line always carries the potential hazard of bowel perforation. Tissue specimens should be mounted on a piece of monofilament mesh with the mucosal side up and then placed in a fixative solution. Proper orientation of the tissue on the mesh may facilitate diagnostic interpretation by making it easier to section the specimen perpendicular to the mucosa.

671. COLITIS CYSTICA SUPERFICIALIS AND PROFUNDA

There are two types of benign, cystic, mucus-filled lesions of the colonic mucosa: *colitis cystica superficialis* and *colitis cystica profunda*. The superficialis type occurs predominantly in patients with pellagra and may develop at a time when typical skin lesions are absent. It has also been described in a few cases of adult celiac disease. Diarrhea is frequently the presenting symptom. The condition is characterized by very small mucus-filled cysts which lie superficial to the muscularis mucosae of the colon. Grossly, the cysts appear as thousands of minute gray blebs on the mucosal surface from which mucus can be expressed. Treatment with niacin or tryptophan for the underlying pellagra is curative.

In colitis cystica profunda the cysts are located below the muscularis mucosae and occasionally appear to "invade" the muscularis propria. They are filled with basophilic mucoid material and are lined by colonic epithelium, showing varying degrees of pressure atrophy. Pathologically, colitis cystica profunda must be differentiated from mucus-producing adenocarcinoma. Misdiagnosis has resulted in extensive cancer surgery for this benign condition.

The pathogenesis of cyst formation is uncertain. Congenitally ectopic mucosa may be responsible. However, communications between the cyst and the bowel lumen have been demonstrated, suggesting a weakness in the muscularis mucosae which allows herniation of mucosal epithelium into the submucosa. Another possibility is downgrowth of colonic epithelium during the healing process into areas of inflammatory ulceration. The frequently obtained history of preceding severe diarrhea or dysentery supports an inflammatory origin.

Cramping lower abdominal pain, rectal tenesmus, and mild diarrhea associated with blood and mucus in the stool are the most consistent symptoms. If palpated on rectal examination, the cystic lesion usually has a rubbery firm consistency and is not adherent to surrounding tissue. It may be sessile or polypoid and have either normal or ulcerated overlying mucosa. A nodular irregularity in the bowel wall may be the only radiologic abnormality on barium enema and may stimulate a large differential diagnosis. Biopsy of one of the cystic nodules should settle the diagnostic dilemma. Treatment consists of local surgical excision. There are no reports of recurrence in uninvolved intestine.

672. PNEUMATOSIS CYSTOIDES INTESTINALIS

Pneumatosis cystoides intestinalis is characterized by multiple gas-filled cysts in the submucosa or subserosa of both the small intestine and the colon. The majority of cases with involvement of the small intestine are in patients between ages 25 and 50 years who have either chronic obstructive pulmonary disease or peptic ulcer with some degree of pyloric obstruction. The exact cause of the gas-filled cysts is unknown.

The composition of the gas is similar to that of atmospheric air. It is postulated that air, forced into tissue spaces around an ulcer or from rupture of a pulmonary bleb, dissects along facial planes into the retroperitoneal space and out along blood vessels in the mesentery to the intestinal subserosa. Patients with pneumatosis in the wall of the rectum and sigmoid colon usually have undergone previous sigmoidoscopy. Presumably air entered the rectosigmoid wall through a small mucosal tear. Scleroderma of the intestine and inflammatory or ischemic bowel disease have also been complicated by intestinal pneumatosis.

The gas-filled cysts may vary in size from a few millimeters to several centimeters and look like multiple lymphangiomas or even multiple sessile polyps. Microscopically, the gas cysts are lined by a layer of endothelial cells which have a tendency to coalesce to form giant cells. A progressive fibrotic reaction may develop and ultimately obliterate the cyst. Because the cysts do not communicate with the bowel lumen, cyst rupture does not result in peritonitis except in ischemic bowel disease when pneumatosis of the intestinal wall is produced by invading bacteria.

Pneumatosis cystoides intestinalis produces no specific symptoms. It is usually an incidental finding during radiologic examination of the abdomen or intestine. Nevertheless, lower abdominal cramping pain, recurrent diarrhea, rectal bleeding, tenesmus, and partial bowel obstruction have all been described in patients with colonic pneumatosis. In addition, pneumatosis should be considered in the patient who presents with vague abdominal discomfort and free air under the diaphragm on x-ray examination, and who has no other evidence for a perforated viscus.

The most useful way of establishing the diagnosis is by barium x-ray examination of the small bowel and colon. Pneumatosis involving the rectosigmoid area can be recognized during sigmoidoscopy as pale bluish soft masses which protrude into the lumen and often collapse when biopsied.

When pneumatosis involves the small bowel, often no specific treatment is necessary except for the underlying or primary disease. The value of correct diagnosis is mainly in preventing unnecessary surgery. In contrast, surgery may be required for colonic pneumatosis if there is severe tenesmus, bleeding, pain, or partial obstruction of the lumen with no other apparent cause. Unfortunately, pneumatosis may recur and become more extensive after resection. If surgery is performed, the rectum should be spared, because pneumatosis in the rectum usually regresses after resection of more proximally involved colon.

pains in the rectum and occasionally mild tenesmus. Endometriosis of the more proximal colon is usually asymptomatic. Implants on the small intestine are often discovered incidentally during abdominal surgery. Bowel obstruction may develop from endometriosis at any level of the intestinal tract owing to fibrous adhesions, stenosis from fibrosis, or volvulus.

Clinical diagnosis of intestinal endometriosis primarily requires a high index of suspicion. The first diagnostic maneuver should be a thorough pelvic examination with combined rectovaginal palpation. Tender nodules with irregular induration in the cul-de-sac are suggestive of rectosigmoid endometriosis. Repeated pelvic examination later in the menstrual cycle should demonstrate some variation in character of the lesion. When a mass is palpable in the free portion of the sigmoid colon and none in the cul-de-sac, the diagnosis of endometriosis is much less certain. Radiologic, sigmoidoscopic, and mucosal biopsy findings may not significantly contribute to the diagnosis. Persisting uncertainty about a constricting rectosigmoid lesion, especially in an older woman, should prompt needle biopsy or surgical exploration to exclude adenocarcinoma.

The therapy of symptomatic intestinal endometriosis lies between watchful waiting, hormonal therapy, surgical excision, and castration. Treatment must be individualized and flexible during the course of the disease. Progestin therapy occasionally produces regression and even disappearance of symptomatic colonic endometriosis. However, this result is inconstant, and unless symptoms are promptly alleviated, obstructing lesions should be excised.

673. ENDOMETRIOSIS

Endometriosis refers to the presence of extrauterine endometrial tissue and the clinical sequelae produced by its normal function in an abnormal site. It is a disease of the reproductive period, with peak incidence between the ages of 30 and 40 years. It is uncommon in the 20's and, rarely, may produce symptoms after menopause. Intestinal involvement with endometriosis is usually greatest in those parts of the bowel that are pelvic in location, especially the rectosigmoid colon.

It is uncertain exactly how the heterotopic endometrium reaches the subserosa of the bowel wall. Nevertheless, under hormonal influence there is maturation, slough of the surface endometrial epithelium, and bleeding as occurs in the uterine cavity. Debris generated from this process may produce pressure necrosis of adjacent tissue, resulting in progressive dissection of the endometriosis through both subserosa and muscularis of the bowel wall. The mucosa is seldom penetrated, a fact which explains why periodic intraluminal intestinal bleeding infrequently occurs from endometriosis. A large bulky intramural lesion can develop which contains areas of fibrosis and marked smooth muscle hyperplasia. This firm mass, known as an endometrioma, may produce luminal obstruction, especially in the sigmoid colon.

Symptoms of endometriosis include dysmenorrhea, menometrorrhagia, intermenstrual pelvic pain, sterility, dyspareunia, and low backache. Involvement of the rectosigmoid colon is usually signaled by cyclic cramping

674. MALACOPLAKIA

Malacoplakia is a rare granulomatous disease of unknown cause which usually affects the urinary tract but which has also been reported in the colon. It is characterized pathologically by the presence of histiocytes containing peculiar intracytoplasmic dark, round laminated inclusions called Michaelis-Gutman bodies. These inclusions are PAS positive, stain for both calcium and iron, and appear to be a cellular reaction to breakdown products of bacteria. Colonic malacoplakia is most often noted as an incidental finding in elderly debilitated patients and is usually histologically associated with coexisting malignancy such as adenocarcinoma of the colon. An abnormal delayed immune response has also been found in these patients. Fever, diarrhea, hematochezia, and even death have occurred in patients with only intestinal malacoplakia. When visualized at sigmoidoscopy, areas of malacoplakia may vary from soft grayish-tan nodular lesions with serpiginous borders to confluent superficial ulcerations. Correct diagnosis is made from biopsy tissue. Its known high association with colonic adenocarcinoma should prompt evaluation for this possibility.

There is no specific pharmacologic treatment for intestinal malacoplakia. In the urinary bladder the disease has been successfully treated with streptomycin, para-aminosalicylic acid, and isoniazid. Excision or fulguration may be tried for localized disease.

675. MELANOSIS COLI, CATHARTIC COLON, AND SOAP COLITIS

The use of "irritant" purgatives has been associated with at least three colonic abnormalities: *melanosis coli, cathartic colon,* and *soap colitis.*

MELANOSIS COLI

Melanosis coli is an abnormal black or brown discoloration of the colonic mucosa which has been compared in appearance to tiger or crocodile skin or cross-section of nutmeg. The discoloration is due to brownish-black pigment in large mononuclear cells or macrophages in the lamina propria of the mucosa. The pigment granules have histochemical staining characteristics of both melanin and lipofuscin. Its exact origin, however, is uncertain.

Melanosis coli appears to result from chronic use of anthracin cathartics in the presence of fecal stasis. The pigment has been noted as soon as four months after the onset of taking cascara preparations and may disappear after the laxative is discontinued.

By itself, melanosis coli produces no specific symptoms and has no known unfavorable long-term prognostic significance. However, a few patients with carcinoma of the colon have also had melanosis coli. It is uncertain how many of them actually took laxatives. Without an accompanying history of anthracin laxative abuse or fecal stasis, the presence of melanosis coli probably warrants radiologic evaluation for an occult colonic neoplasm.

CATHARTIC COLON

Cathartic colon occurs predominantly in women who have taken irritant laxatives (cascara segrada, senna, aloe, podophyllin, castor oil, phenolphthalein, calomel) for a period of at least 15 years. It is a radiologic diagnosis characterized by loss of haustral markings, with lengthy inconstant areas of constriction having long tapering margins. At fluoroscopy, the distensibility of the narrowed segments can be demonstrated, excluding a stricture. The terminal ileum and ascending colon are most commonly involved. The radiologic differential diagnosis includes chronic ulcerative colitis, granulomatous colitis, and amebic colitis. An adequate medical history and examination of the stools for amebae will help exclude these differential possibilities. There should be no history of recent fever, recurrent diarrhea, or the passage of mucus or blood in stool. Treatment is cessation of use of the offending laxative. Bulk-forming and emollient laxatives should be considered if persistent constipation requires treatment.

SOAP COLITIS

The use of cleansing "soapsuds" enemas may produce a spectrum of symptoms from slight discomfort to severe prostration. The colonic mucosal reaction also varies from mild irritation to frank necrosis. Severe reactions have usually occurred in cases in which a concentrated soap solution was administered. Symptoms, which begin within a few hours after the enema, may include severe abdominal cramps, abdominal distention, mucorrhea, and serosanguineous diarrhea. Hypovolemia and acute hemoconcentration can result from rapid exudation of fluid into the colon. Hypokalemia may develop when exudation of colonic mucus is massive. Most patients recover with treatment consisting of close observation, careful replacement of fluid and electrolytes, and possibly administration of broad-spectrum antimicrobial drugs.

676. FECAL IMPACTION AND STERCORAL ULCER

Incomplete evacuation of feces for an extended time may lead to formation of a large firm mass of stool in the rectum and distal colon known as fecal impaction. The large irregular mass of feces cannot be expelled from the dilated rectosigmoid through the disproportionately small anal canal. Fecal impactions most often occur in children who have undiagnosed megacolon or psychiatric problems, in elderly, debilitated, or sedentary persons, and in patients with painful anal disease.

A sensation of rectal fullness, lower abdominal discomfort, headache, mild anorexia with weight loss, and a general sense of ill-being are the most commonly reported symptoms. Liquid stool above the fecal mass can expand the already distended colon and pass around the impaction, thus preventing complete obstruction. Unfortunately, this watery stool is occasionally interpreted as diarrhea, and the patient is improperly treated with constipating agents. The true diagnosis could be easily made by rectal examination.

Small pieces of a large impaction in the rectum should be removed digitally. Thereafter, warm water or saline enemas may then be given as well as mineral oil orally. More proximal sigmoid impactions can be broken up by advancing a large bore rubber tube through a sigmoidoscope into the fecal mass and gently flushing small amounts of water through the tube. Warm oil enemas are unnecessary and may produce burns of the heat-insensitive colonic mucosa. Enemas containing a dilute (5 to 10 per cent) solution of hydrogen peroxide have been used, but this technique risks rupture of an already distended colon by the liberated gas. Dilatation of the anus under anesthesia to allow removal of the impaction is occasionally necessary.

Complications of fecal impaction include urinary tract obstruction, spontaneous perforation of the colon, and stercoral ulcer. Progressive enlargement of the rectosigmoid by the impaction can compress the ureters near the ureterovesical junction or elevate the bladder, producing marked angulation of the urethra. The resulting obstruction may present as symptomatic urinary tract infection.

Spontaneous perforation of the colon in patients with fecal impaction usually occurs during attempts by the patient to pass the fecal mass. Unfortunately, vague lower abdominal pain often precedes physical findings of a perforated viscus by only a few hours. Treatment requires surgical closure of the perforation.

Stercoral ulcers in the rectum and colon likely result from pressure necrosis produced by a large fecal mass. The ulceration has a dark yellow-gray to greenish-purple irregular outline. Microscopically, there is little acute inflammatory reaction around the necrotic center. The ulcer usually heals rapidly after removal of the fecal mass. Chronic stercoral ulcers occasionally can be asymptomatic. Complications are bleeding and perforation. Perforation, occurring either spontaneously or during disimpaction, can result in a localized abscess or suppurative peritonitis.

677. NONSPECIFIC OR SOLITARY ULCER OF THE COLON

Discrete, usually single, ulcerations of unknown cause may develop in any segment of the colon or rectum. The cecum, ascending colon, and rectosigmoid colon are the most frequent locations. Symptoms and clinical course of the ulceration vary, depending on the segment of colon involved. Nonspecific ulceration in the cecum or ascending colon frequently presents with right lower abdominal pain. A tender mass may develop. Gross bleeding is uncommon. The usual initial differential diagnosis includes *appendicitis, pelvic inflammatory disease, ovarian disease,* and *tuberculous* or *idiopathic regional enteritis.* Perforation of the cecum with peritonitis is a frequent complication.

The sigmoid colon is the second most common site of nonspecific ulceration. The diagnosis is seldom made prior to surgery. Chronic lower abdominal pain, recurrent rectal bleeding, and a high incidence of perforation characterize the ulcer in this location. Misdiagnosis of *diverticulitis* is common. An inflammatory mass may develop, and surgery may eventually be required to exclude *carcinoma.*

In contrast to the acute symptoms of nonspecific ulceration elsewhere in the colon, solitary ulcer of the rectum is a more chronic condition which tends to be resistant to therapy. Dull pain in the rectum or left iliac fossa, which is increased during defecation, and the passage of small amounts of bloody mucus with stool are typical symptoms. Massive bleeding is unusual. The shallow rectal ulceration frequently occurs 7 to 10 cm above the anal margin and is usually demarcated from normal mucosa by a narrow area of hyperemia. The lesion may be round, have an irregular outline, or even be linear. A symptomatic preulcer, hyperemic, or "granular" phase can antedate the actual crater.

Multiple biopsies of the ulcer margin will exclude malignancy. Almost all forms of local and systemic therapy have not affected the chronic course of the ulceration. The only certain cure is total excision. However, since perforation is uncommon, treatment with stool softener, local anesthetics, and periodic re-examination is indicated unless symptoms become severe. Spontaneous healing may occur even after many years.

678. NONSPECIFIC ULCERATIVE PROCTITIS

Patients may present with rectal bleeding, tenesmus, and occasionally a mucosanguineous anal discharge and are found to have inflammation of the rectal mucosa with a clearly demarcated upper border above which the mucosa is normal. Histologic changes in tissue from rectal biopsy are usually compatible with ulcerative colitis, but barium enema demonstrates no abnormality of the colon above the rectum. This disease, ulcerative proctitis, appears to be a localized milder form of generalized ulcerative colitis, but with a better prognosis (see Ch. 651). In general, the disease runs a relapsing course without complications, except rectal stricture. Less than 15 per cent of patients with this disease will progress to develop diffuse ulcerative colitis.

679. DISEASES OF THE ANUS

GENERAL CONSIDERATIONS

Functionally, the most important parts of the anus are the neural innervation and muscular elements comprising the internal and external anal sphincters which maintain rectal continence. Anal sphincter dysfunction without perianal disease, a history of prior anal surgery, or evidence of more generalized neurologic disease should prompt evaluation for rectal carcinoma. Although various reconstructive techniques appear to improve some patients with anal incontinence, surgery should be considered only after the cause of sphincter dysfunction has been thoroughly investigated. In general, anal and perianal diseases produce disproportionately great symptoms when compared with the extent of tissue involved. In this chapter, a number of anal diseases are discussed briefly to acquaint the reader with diagnostic possibilities.

HEMORRHOIDS

Hemorrhoids or piles are varicosities of the hemorrhoidal venous plexuses. External hemorrhoids occur below the anorectal line and are covered by pain-sensitive anal skin. Thrombosis or rupture of the vein leads to a small, very tender, tense, bluish lump which can be seen on the outside anal surface. Conservative treatment is usually effective and consists of hot sitz baths, stool softeners, a recumbent position if possible, and avoidance of straining or strenuous work. Small anal skin tags may be left after resolution of the acute process. If the pile ruptures, the clot should be removed or the area excised.

Internal hemorrhoids are varicosities of the superior hemorrhoidal vein above the anorectal line and are covered by relatively pain-insensitive mucosa. These hemorrhoids tend to prolapse during defecation and usually become symptomatic by bleeding. A mucoid anal discharge is common with chronic prolapse and may lead to irritation of the anal skin. Bleeding from hemorrhoids is often noted by the patient as streaks of blood on the outside of stool or on toilet tissue. It is usually intermittent. Prolonged or excessive bleeding can result in iron deficiency and anemia. Use of an astringent suppository and the conservative treatment outlined above are often adequate. Surgical therapy may be indicated for recurrent bleeding, protrusion, thrombosis, ulceration, infection, or coexistent severe pruritus ani. Surgery should be avoided in patients with only moderately symptomatic hemorrhoids who have portal hypertension, incurable cancer, intractable heart disease, or persistent hemorrhoidal symptoms for less than six months post partum. Rectal bleeding should not be attributed to hemorrhoids without complete anorectal examination.

ANORECTAL ABSCESS AND FISTULA IN ANO

Patients with a rapidly developing painful anal mass may have an abscess in the perianal and perirectal tissue. After diagnosis, proper treatment requires surgical drainage. *Perianal abscess* occurs superficially, adjacent to the anal opening and below the anorectal ring. Severe throbbing pain is the major symptom. An *ischiorectal fossa abscess* involves deeper tissue of the buttocks and presents with perirectal discomfort and fever. Digital examination of the lower part of the rectum will demonstrate a tender mass bulging into the lumen. A *submucous abscess* extends upward in the submucous space above the anal valves. It may cause fever and dull rectal pain with no visible perianal abnormality except occasionally a purulent rectal discharge. A *pelvirectal abscess* arises from a primary infection elsewhere in the pelvis and usually presents with systemic toxic symptoms. An *anorectal abscess* may develop as a complication of acute hemorrhoids, an anal fissure, or injections into the anorectal area. A *tuberculous anorectal abscess* often presents as a gradually enlarging perianal or ischiorectal mass with less pain than that caused by a similar acute infection.

After an acute infection in the anorectal area, a chronic suppurative process may develop and form a *fistula in ano*. This fistula is a tract of chronic granulation tissue which connects two epithelial surfaces, either cutaneous or mucosal, and may have several external openings. The main symptom is persistent or intermittent drainage which soils the patient's clothing and leads to soreness and pruritus in the perianal area. Treatment requires complete surgical excision of the fistulous tract.

ANAL FISSURE

An anal fissure is a painful, usually elliptical ulceration of unknown cause which is commonly located posteriorly in the midline of the anal orifice and may extend into the anal canal as far as the pectinate line. Early, the fissure appears as a simple slit in the anal skin, but secondary changes soon develop, the most striking of which is a swelling at the lower end of the fissure known as a sentinel pile. If untreated, the ulceration can "erode" down to the internal sphincter muscle. Chronic spasm of the sphincter and postinflammatory fibrosis can produce a fibrotic, tightly contracted anal opening. Pain, especially with defecation, is the main symptom. Bleeding is usually only modest, but can be severe.

Most fissures heal spontaneously. Dilatation of the spastic sphincter, hot sitz baths, local analgesics, and stool softeners give good results in most cases. When the ulceration is deep enough to expose the sphincter muscle fibers, surgical therapy is usually required.

PRURITUS ANI

Pruritus ani refers to perianal itching which is frequently intense. In early cases, the primary rugae of the anus may be edematous and red. The skin is often moist and macerated. Multiple excoriations are evidence of frequent scratching. Later the perianal skin may become thickened or lichenified and have increased pigmentation. Superficial ulcers may be present, and with extreme chronicity leukoplakia may develop.

In evaluating the cause of pruritus ani, dermatologic abnormalities such as *seborrheic dermatitis, atopic eczema, psoriasis, lichen planus, neurodermatitis,* and *contact dermatitis* must be excluded. Involvement of the perianal skin with fungal or yeast infection, or parasitic infestation such as scabies or pinworm, may produce intense pruritus. Pruritus ani may also complicate many of the so-called surgical diseases of the anus such as *prolapsed hemorrhoids, prolapse of the rectum, benign* or *malignant tumors of the rectum,* or *chronic anal fissure* or *fistula.* An increase in perianal moisture from chronic diarrhea or vaginal discharge may also play a causative role. Finally, many patients with idiopathic pruritus ani have been shown to have an abnormally alkaline anal discharge. This may produce a chemical dermatitis and alter perianal skin resistance to normal bacterial flora.

Treatment of pruritus ani should begin with an exclusion of correctable underlying causes. A large number of idiopathic cases are cured by strict anal hygiene. Anesthetic ointments, abrasive toilet tissue and clothing, constipation or diarrhea, and gas-producing foods should be avoided. The use of bland soap, dusting powders (zinc, starch, or boric acid), and hydrocortisone or betamethasone cream is often helpful. In cases of idiopathic pruritus ani, oral administration of capsules of *Lactobacillus acidophilus* or malt soup extract (Maltsupex) has been shown to normalize the alkaline anal discharge and lead to improvement in symptoms.

ANAL MALIGNANCY

The most common malignant tumor of the anus is *squamous cell carcinoma.* Treatment of this widely metastasizing lesion requires radical surgical excision. *Intraepithelial squamous cell* carcinoma or Bowen's disease may present as an irregular reddish plaque. Wide local excision is usually adequate therapy. *Basal cell carcinoma* of the anus produces a superficial ulcerating lesion. *Paget's disease* may involve the perianal dermal apocrine sweat glands and present as an anal mass. Since both of these tumors do not metastasize widely, excisional biopsy is usually adequate.

Malignant melanomas of the anus are highly lethal, but fortunately rare. Initially, a small melanoma may be interpreted as a hemorrhoid by both patient and physician. Later the tumor becomes more polypoid and tends to ulcerate. Wide excision biopsy of a suspect lesion should be done immediately when the diagnosis is considered. Radical surgery for an advanced melanoma does not seem to improve survival.

PROCTALGIA

There are several conditions in which the main symptom is anorectal pain and for which there is no obvious cause, even after full proctologic examination.

Coccygodynia refers to pain in the coccyx area. This is thought to be due to tonic spasm of the levator ani, coccygeal, and pyriform muscles and to result from trauma to the coccyx. Diagnosis is made by eliciting pain during palpation of these muscles and movement of the coccyx. Treatment consists of improved sitting posture, warm sitz baths, massage of the spastic muscles, and systemic analgesics or tranquilizers which have a muscle relaxant property such as diazepam.

Proctalgia fugax is a rectal pain syndrome which frequently awakens the patient at night and most commonly occurs in young men. Most patients describe the discomfort as a severe cramping rectal pain unassociated with straining efforts. The pain usually lasts 30 to 45 minutes. Spasms of a segment of the levator ani muscle may be the source of the pain, but the true cause is unknown. Various recommended treatments have included hot sitz baths or warm water enemas, passing flatus or stool, sublingual nitroglycerin, and firm pressure upward against the anus. In many patients the symptoms respond to no treatment but resolve spontaneously after a period of months or years.

The *puborectalis syndrome* is characterized by chronic constipation, rectal tenesmus, and pain during and after defecation. This is thought to result from hypertrophy and spasm of the puborectalis muscle sling. Diagnosis is made on rectal examination by finding a constricting tender muscular ring at the upper end of the anus. Conservative treatment includes anal dilatation prior to defecation and the use of stool softeners. If this treatment is unsuccessful, surgical resection of a small segment of the puborectalis sling is usually curative without producing anal incontinence.

Tumors of the *cauda equina* of the spinal cord may also produce anal pain. Examination of the anus will demonstrate a weak sphincter and a small perianal area of diminished cutaneous sensation. Transient *sigmoidorectal intussusception* may also produce rectal pain which is difficult to diagnose.

Andrade, S., and Andrade, V. H.: Intestinal pneumatosis. Presentation of five cases. Am. J. Proctol., 19:39, 1968.

Epstein, S. E., Ascari, W. A., Ablow, R. C., Seaman, W. B., and Lattis, R.: Colitis cystica profunda. Am. J. Clin. Pathol., 5:186, 1966.

Folley, J. H.: Ulcerative proctitis. N. Engl. J. Med., 282:1362, 1970.

Gear, E. V., and Dobbins, W. O.: III. Rectal biopsy. A review of its diagnostic usefulness. Gastroenterology, 55:552, 1968.

Gray, L. A.: The management of endometriosis involving the bowel. Clin. Obstet. Gynecol., 9:309, 1966.

Lal, S., and Brown, G. N.: Some unusual complications of fecal impaction. Am. J. Proctol., 18:226, 1967.

Lewin, J., Harell, G. S., Lee, A. S., and Crowley, L. G.: Malacoplakia. An electron-microscopic study: Demonstration of bacilliform organisms in malacoplakic macrophages. Gastroenterology, 66:28, 1974.

Madigan, M. R., and Morson, B. C.: Solitary ulcer of the rectum. Gut, 10:871, 1969.

Nelson, S. W.: Extraluminal gas collections due to diseases of the gastrointestinal tract. Am. J. Roentgen., 115:225, 1972.

Pike, B. F., Phillippi, P. J., and Lawson, E. H.: Soap colitis. N. Engl. J. Med., 285:217, 1971.

Ziter, F. M.: Cathartic colon. New York State J. Med., 67:546, 1967.

Section Ten. DISEASES OF THE GALLBLADDER AND BILE DUCTS

Lawrence W. Way

680. INTRODUCTION

Biliary disease in adults includes congenital, metabolic, neoplastic, infectious, and parasitic conditions which cause considerable morbidity and pose challenging diagnostic problems to the clinician. Symptomatic cholelithiasis and its complications alone are responsible for over 300,000 operations in the United States annually, entailing great financial and emotional cost for the affected patients. Fortunately, improvements have recently been made in techniques of diagnosis and therapy, and preliminary findings suggest that even more dramatic advances may soon be made in the treatment of gallstone disease.

Physiology. Bile, an alkaline isotonic fluid (pH 7.8), is a mixture of the secretion of hepatocytes and the duct epithelial cells and has the composition given in Table 1. The volume of bile ranges from 500 to 1500 ml per day, depending on the amount and type of food ingested. The greatest fraction of the bile volume is produced by the hepatocytes and correlates directly with output of bile salts.

Bile salts are synthesized by hepatocytes from cholesterol by a process whose rate-limiting step involves the action of the enzyme 7α-hydroxylase. The two *primary bile salts*, cholate and chenodeoxycholate, are conjugated before secretion with either glycine or taurine to improve solubility. After entering the gut, bile salts aid in fat absorption, and then all but 5 per cent are reabsorbed in the ileum. Those that reach the colon are partially converted by bacteria to the *secondary bile salts*, deoxycholate and lithocholate. Deoxycholate is absorbed and re-excreted in bile; lithocholate, being insoluble, is mostly excreted in the feces. The actual composition of bile is 40 per cent cholate, 40 per cent chenodeoxycholate, 18 per cent deoxycholate, and 2 per cent lithocholate, each conjugated with glycine or taurine in a ratio of 3:1. Other than bile salt, the major solids in bile are cholesterol and phospholipid (mainly lecithin). The close correlation between the output of lecithin and that of bile salt suggests that the former may be leeched from the canalicular membrane by the traversing bile salt molecules. Cholesterol output is largely independent of bile salt.

Normally, only 10 to 20 per cent of the daily hepatic secretion of bile salt consists of newly synthesized molecules, because efficient ileal reabsorption and hepatic re-excretion allow repeated recycling through the *enterohepatic* circulation. In this way the bile salt pool, normally 1.5 to 3.0 grams, passes through the liver and gut more than twice during each meal, producing 6 to 8 cycles daily (i.e., each day about 20 grams of bile salt enters the duodenum). During an average day involving three meals, the bile salt pool is in continuous motion until at night the stomach and bowel are empty and the gallblad-

TABLE 1. Average Composition of Human Gallbladder Bile (Gram/100 ml)

			% Total Solids
Lipids	Bile acids	12.00	91
	Lecithin	3.00	
	Cholesterol	0.50	
	Bilirubin	0.15	9
	Protein	0.10	
	Potassium	0.05	
	Calcium and magnesium	0.06	
	Chloride	0.08	
	Bicarbonate and phosphate	0.04	

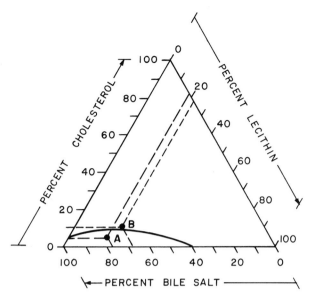

Figure 1. Phase diagram for plotting different mixtures of bile salt, lecithin, and cholesterol. The curved line represents the boundary of the micellar zone for aqueous solutions containing 4 to 10 per cent solids. Any mixture, such as A, falling within this area contains all its cholesterol in solution. Any mixture, such as B, falling outside this area has excess cholesterol as a precipitate or supersaturated solution. The points A and B actually depict the average composition of gallbladder bile obtained by Admirand and Small from normal persons and patients with cholesterol gallstones, respectively.

der fills. Reabsorption in the gut involves a mucosal active transport mechanism located in the terminal 100 cm of ileum. If the efficiency of the enterohepatic conservation is impaired by conditions such as a biliary fistula, Crohn's disease, or ileal resection, hepatic synthesis increases, but the maximal rate of 5 grams per day may be insufficient to restore intraluminal concentrations to normal if external losses exceed this amount.

The second component of bile, the ductular secretion, is generated by an active transport process which is stimulated by secretin, cholecystokinin, and gastrin, with vagal tone acting as a sensitizing influence. Ductular secretion results from active transport of Na^+ and HCO^- and seems to be useful in maintaining the alkalinity of bile.

Under basal conditions, tonic contraction of the sphincter diverts hepatic bile from the common duct into the gallbladder where it is concentrated by active absorption of Na^+, Cl^-, and HCO_3^- and passive return of H_3O. The absorptive mechanism is capable of concentrating gallbladder bile at a rate of 10 per cent of its volume per hour. Concentrations of bile salt may exceed 200 millimoles per liter, and since the gallbladder holds 40 ml, 8 millimoles (equivalent to 3 grams of cholic acid) or the entire bile salt pool can be sequestered here during prolonged fasting.

Cholecystokinin, released from the intestinal mucosa by fat, amino acids, and H^+, stimulates gallbladder contraction and simultaneous relaxation of the choledochal sphincter, emptying the gallbladder contents into the duodenum. Basal pressures in the biliary ducts and gallbladder are 10 to 15 cm H_2O. After eating, gallbladder pressure rises to 25 to 30 cm H_2O, slightly exceeding ductal pressure.

Bile salt molecules are amphophils possessing water-soluble and fat-soluble poles. In an aqueous medium, they are distributed randomly, until a critical concentration (about 2 millimolar) is reached, at which point spontaneous aggregation forms multimolecular structures called *micelles*. In micelles, the bile salt molecules line up with their hydrophilic portions facing the solvent (water) and their hydrophobic portions facing centrally. The hydrocarbon center of the micelle can incorporate biliary lecithin and cholesterol, and the entire aggregate remains water soluble. The addition of lecithin, a water-soluble compound, enhances the ability of bile salt micelles to incorporate other lipids. The ultimate cholesterol-carrying capacity of bile depends on the relative amounts of bile salt and lecithin (Fig. 1).

Pathogenesis of Cholesterol Gallstones. In Western cultures cholesterol is the principal ingredient (comprising over 50 per cent of total solids) of more than 90 per cent of gallstones, the remaining 10 per cent consisting mostly of bilirubin pigment stones in patients with hemolytic disease. In general terms an excess of cholesterol in bile seems to be a prerequisite, which in theory

could result either from diminished cholesterol holding capacity (bile salt and lecithin) or increased cholesterol concentrations.

Gallstones affect three times as many women as men, the differences beginning at puberty and declining somewhat in later years. This fact, combined with the higher incidence with multiparity and an apparently greater incidence in women who take birth control pills, suggests that female sex hormones may be partly responsible. In the United States the incidence in blacks, whites, and American Indians doubles in a stepwise fashion, so that at the upper extreme about 75 per cent of American Indian women over age 25 and 90 per cent of those over age 60 are affected.

Figure 1 is a phase diagram on which any aqueous mixture of bile salt, lecithin, and cholesterol can be represented by a point indicating the molar percentage each contributes to total solids. By in vitro testing, an area of the triangle (lower left) can be identified where cholesterol of the various combinations exists in stable micellar solution. Outside this area cholesterol forms a supersaturated solution or precipitates. The particular micellar zone depicted in Figure 1 pertains to solutions ranging from 4 to 10 per cent solids, which is comparable to bile.

Plotted on this diagram, bile from patients with gallstones tends to have relatively more cholesterol than that from normal persons, and simultaneous sampling from the gallbladder and hepatic ducts of patients with gallstones shows that bile is supersaturated as it emerges from the liver, implicating the hepatocytes rather than the gallbladder as the cause of the abnormality. Gallstone patients also have a total bile salt pool of 1.0 to 1.5 grams, about half the size of normal, and preliminary data indicate the presence of reduced amounts of the enzyme 7α-hydroxylase in their hepatocytes. These findings suggested the presence of diminished secretory rates of bile salts, but the few available measurements are conflicting; in one report, female American Indian patients had lower outputs, but in another (female whites) it was normal, presumably owing to more rapid recycling of the small pool.

The independence of cholesterol and bile salt output means that when bile salt secretion drops, the cholesterol:bile salt ratio climbs and the bile assumes greater lithogenicity. These observations appear to explain the shift in bile composition observed during fasting, a state that physiologically mimics interruption of the enterohepatic circulation. Instead of entering the gut, the bile salts during fasting become sequestered in the gallbladder, hepatic secretion drops, cholesterol secretion persists, and the bile becomes more lithogenic. Evidently supersaturation produced in this way is rather common in humans regardless of the presence of gallstones.

Therefore lowered micellar capacity caused by a scarcity of bile salt and lecithin has been demonstrated. One report on American Indian women also implicates abnormally high biliary cholesterol secretion, a consequence of obesity. So far neither men nor white women with gallstones, whether obese or not, seem to produce greater cholesterol than controls.

The aforementioned observations account for the production of lithogenic bile but do not explain why all persons with abnormal bile do not develop stones, why stone formation occurs mainly in the gallbladder, and why cholecystectomy is curative. Obviously, the gallbladder

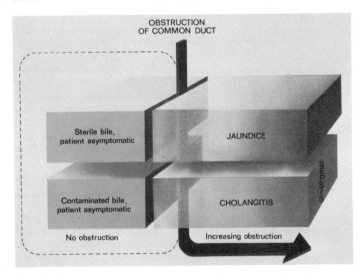

Figure 2. In the absence of obstruction there are no symptoms or active infection from bacterial contamination of bile. Obstruction, indicated by the arrow, produces either jaundice alone or cholangitis, depending on the original bacteriologic status of the duct.

possesses a critical role in the genesis of gallstones, possibly by supplying a nidus for crystallization (a small particle of bile pigment or mucoprotein can be found in the center of most stones), a mucoprotein lattice for further cholesterol deposition and stone growth, and an area of stasis to facilitate precipitation. Apparently the more supersaturated the bile, as in American Indian women, the more likely it is that gallstones will develop, but other initiating factors with quantitative importance must be postulated in any comprehensive theory on the pathogenesis of gallstones.

Dissolution of Gallstones by Chenodeoxycholic Acid. In preliminary experiments chenodeoxycholate given orally, 20 mg per kilogram per day, to patients with radiolucent gallbladder stones has partially or completely dissolved the stones within one to two years in a majority of cases. This treatment caused the bile to become unsaturated by lowering cholesterol output rather than by expanding the bile salt pool and increasing bile salt excretion (the expected mechanism). Other observations were that cholic acid had no beneficial effect, radiopaque gallstones were mostly resistant, and, after interruption of therapy gallstones returned in several patients. A nationwide clinical trial to determine the efficacy and safety of this treatment is in progress. Of concern is the possibility that lithocholate formed from chenodeoxycholate might damage the liver or that prolonged consumption of bile salts will interfere with endogenous cholesterol degradation. The potential impact of this or some analogous approach to curing cholesterol gallstones is certainly very great, but at this time treatment with chenodeoxycholic acid can only be justified within the framework of a clinical experiment.

Pathophysiology of Gallstone Disease. Obstruction caused by a stone is the primary cause of the manifestations of gallstone disease. By distending the gallbladder, blockage of the cystic duct produces biliary colic, and if the obstruction is unrelieved, acute cholecystitis may ensue. The intermediary steps leading from obstruction to acute inflammation are discussed later in more detail. The complications of empyema, perforation, and hydrops of the gallbladder develop, depending on whether a foothold is gained by secondarily invading bacteria. From the therapeutic standpoint, cholecystectomy cures cholecystitis, but it is important to appreciate that cholecys-

tostomy, which only relieves the obstruction, eliminates all the clinical manifestations of the disease.

An analogous situation holds for choledocholithiasis, in which obstruction is the key to all that follows. Pain, jaundice, pruritus, infection, and biliary cirrhosis are all dependent on the block to bile flow and, as with the gallbladder, surgical procedures which decompress the duct upstream from the stone allow acute symptoms to subside. The situation in the ductal system differs importantly from that in the gallbladder, because when ductal pressure exceeds about 25 cm per H_2O, bile is refluxed from the smallest ductules into hepatic venous blood. Pressures in this range and even higher are commonly produced by mechanical obstruction and are probably aggravated by infection. Regurgitation of ductal bacteria into the systemic circulation explains why the typical attack of cholangitis is accompanied by chills, positive blood cultures, and high fever. Fortunately, obstruction by calculus is rarely complete, because the combination of high-grade obstruction and infection (as in suppurative cholangitis) produces catastrophic sepsis (Fig. 2). It is also fortuitous that neoplasms, which uniformly give almost complete obstruction, occur most often in patients with sterile bile.

With unrelieved ductal obstruction, biliary cirrhosis gradually develops. About three months is the fastest that cirrhosis occurs; as might be expected, the earliest cases follow neoplastic (high-grade) obstruction. On the average, biliary cirrhosis from choledocholithiasis or biliary stricture takes five and seven years, respectively.

681. ROENTGENOLOGIC EXAMINATION

Because biliary disease usually results from obstructive lesions, radiologic techniques, if successful in outlining the system, are often diagnostic. Direct and indirect methods are available, and the diagnostic clinical strategy often revolves around the choice and timing of these procedures.

Plain roentgenograms can demonstrate the 10 to 15 per cent of gallstones which contain sufficient calcium to be radiopaque, but their relationship to the ductal system is not always obvious. Emphysematous cholecystitis, air in the bile ducts, and calcium in the wall of the gallbladder also have diagnostic appearances on plain films.

For *oral cholecystography,* the patient swallows tablets of iopanoic or tyropanoic acid, which are then absorbed from the gut, excreted in bile, and concentrated in the gallbladder. Films are exposed about 12 hours after the drug is taken. If the gallbladder is opacified, stones in its lumen are shown as radiolucent defects (Fig. 3). The gallbladder may not be visualized if the drug is not taken, if absorption by the gut or excretion by the liver is faulty, if the cystic duct is blocked, or if the diseased gallbladder mucosa cannot concentrate the bile. Oral cholecystography is the simplest and least expensive way of verifying gallstone disease in patients without acute symptoms. If hepatic and intestinal function are normal, nonvisualization is 95 per cent reliable in indicating gallbladder disease.

Intravenous cholangiography (IVC) relies on hepatic excretion of intravenously injected sodium or methylglucamine iodipamide in a concentration sufficient for ductal opacification. The procedure is used principally to identify common duct stones in patients who previously had a cholecystectomy and to verify acute cholecystitis when the findings of a normal duct and nonvisualized gallbladder are diagnostic. The disadvantage of intravenous cholangiography is that even with perfect liver function the concentration of contrast medium in bile is

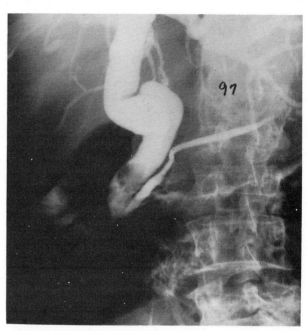

Figure 4. Retrograde cholangiopancreatogram, showing a large gallstone in a dilated common duct and a normal pancreatic duct. (Courtesy of Dr. Jack Vennes.)

barely above the threshold level; tomography must be used routinely, and, even so, false negative results are common in the search for choledocholithiasis. When the bilirubin exceeds 3.0 mg per 100 ml, the study is rarely successful and, because of its high cost and the occasional allergic reaction, should usually be deferred.

Transhepatic cholangiography is obtained by direct percutaneous puncture of an intrahepatic duct by a needle inserted through the eighth or ninth right intercostal space into the center of the liver. An abnormal clotting mechanism, ascites, and severe cholangitis are contraindications. If a duct is entered, water-soluble contrast medium is injected through the needle, and roentgenograms are obtained. Transhepatic cholangiography has proved particularly valuable in diagnosing biliary stricture and neoplastic obstruction of the bile ducts. A technically successful study is correlated with the size of the ducts, and only rarely can useful films be obtained in a condition such as sclerosing cholangitis.

Retrograde endoscopic cholangiography, involving cannulation of the ampulla of Vater via the duodenoscope, is a recently developed technique which will probably supplant transhepatic cholangiography in most instances, because it obviates the potential for bleeding from the hepatic puncture site (Fig. 4). With experience, the duct can be entered successfully in 90 per cent of attempts. Concomitant pancreatography is often possible, and in fact pancreatitis is a complication to be avoided by controlling the pressure of injection.

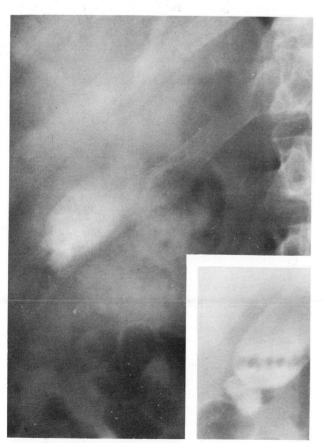

Figure 3. Oral cholecystogram, showing gallstones. In this case the stones are considerably less distinct on the supine than on the upright film (inset), where they float as a layer.

682. ASYMPTOMATIC GALLSTONES

In the absence of a population survey to determine the prevalence of gallstones, the exact percentage of asymp-

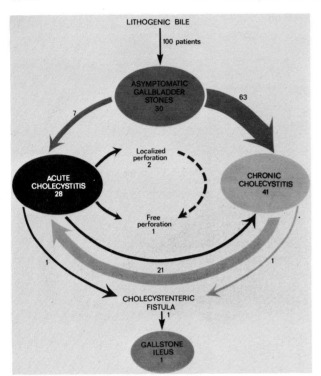

Figure 5. Natural history of cholecystolithiasis. The four ovals represent the major clinical syndromes, and the numbers represent the percentage of those operated on for each diagnosis. About 30 per cent remain asymptomatic.

tomatic stones, estimated now at 30 to 50 per cent of all cases, can only be guessed at (Fig. 5). Since the mortality of gallstone disease with the present plan of management, i.e., essentially treating only those patients with symptoms, is reasonably low, with a few exceptions asymptomatic patients should be followed expectantly and surgery advised only if symptoms develop. The asymptomatic patients for whom prophylactic cholecystectomy is recommended are (1) diabetics, because their mortality from acute cholecystitis is 10 to 15 per cent; (2) patients with nonfunctioning gallbladders or large (more than 2 cm diameter) stones, because their incidence of complications is considerably higher; and (3) patients with calcified gallbladders, because this change is so often associated with carcinoma of the gallbladder. Altogether these groups comprise less than half of the patients with asymptomatic gallstones. Confidence in the safety of expectant management is bolstered by knowing that at least three quarters of the asymptomatic patients who later develop symptoms will first experience episodes of biliary colic, and at that point cholecystectomy can still be performed electively.

683. CHRONIC CHOLECYSTITIS

The term chronic cholecystitis might be used to refer to any gallbladder, not acutely inflamed, which contains gallstones, or it might denote exclusively the presence of chronic inflammation. In actual practice,

chronic cholecystitis describes the *clinical* condition of symptomatic (nonacute) cholecystolithiasis. Chronic cholecystitis without gallstones is even less common than acute acalculous cholecystitis.

Two somewhat overlapping groups of patients are included in this category, depending on the occurrence of a previous attack of acute cholecystitis. In *primary chronic cholecystitis* the gallbladder appears grossly normal, the mucosa is slightly thinned, and the wall contains minor amounts of patchy scarring and cellular infiltration. Oral cholecystograms nearly always visualize the gallbladder and its stones. Symptoms tend to be vague, such as flatulence or food intolerance, and they sometimes persist after cholecystectomy.

In *secondary chronic cholecystitis* the gallbladder has been affected one or more times by acute cholecystitis. Signs of the resolved inflammatory disease consist of thickening of the wall by scar, adhesions to adjacent viscera, and patchy replacement of the mucosa by granulation tissue or collagen. In advanced cases the gallbladder may be so shrunken as to be almost unrecognizable. Nonvisualization is frequent on oral cholecystograms, biliary colic is the principal symptom, and relief is more predictable after cholecystectomy.

In about 5 per cent of patients with primary chronic cholecystitis, *cholesterolosis* gives the mucosal surface a streaked appearance, a condition which has been called "strawberry gallbladder." The changes are due to cholesterol located within clusters of large foamy macrophages in the submucosa. Cholesterolosis is seen occasionally without gallstones, but whether this situation gives symptoms is debated. That some patients become asymptomatic after removal of gallbladders which show only cholesterolosis is well documented, but it is also obvious that in most instances the condition is asymptomatic in the absence of gallstones.

Clinical Manifestations. The most specific symptom of chronic cholecystitis is biliary colic, a constant, severe, cramplike pain located in the epigastrium or right upper quadrant. It is caused by gallbladder contraction or obstruction of the cystic duct by a gallstone. Onset of pain takes only a few minutes; it quickly reaches a plateau in intensity and after an hour or two subsides more gradually. Even after the acute episode has resolved, a vague residual ache or soreness may remain. The absence of tenderness, muscular guarding, a palpable mass, fever, and leukocytosis distinguishes biliary colic from acute cholecystitis. Many patients have referred pain in the back at the level of the scapula. Vomiting may accompany the attack.

Considerably less reliable from the diagnostic standpoint are dyspepsia, fatty food intolerance, flatulence, and belching. Although these symptoms may be the result of chronic cholecystitis, they are often found in persons with normal gallbladders. The common occurrence of these complaints in the general population explains why cholecystectomy often fails to relieve them.

Hydrops, in which the lumen of the gallbladder contains mucus and gallstones, occasionally develops directly from chronic cholecystitis after cystic duct obstruction unaccompanied by acute inflammation. Hydrops produces constant discomfort in the right upper quadrant and a palpable mass without the clinical findings of acute cholecystitis.

Oral cholecystograms will demonstrate the gallstones in patients with primary chronic cholecystitis, but in secondary cholecystitis the gallbladder is often not visualized. In this case, a second examination should be performed; if nonvisualization persists and liver function and intestinal absorption are normal, significant gallbladder disease can be inferred. Because of the expense and risks of allergic reactions, an intravenous cholecystogram is not usually warranted for studying every patient with a nonvisualized gallbladder, but should be ordered selectively in puzzling cases.

Differential Diagnosis. The other common causes of chronic abdominal symptoms, such as *peptic ulcer* and *pancreatitis,* must be investigated in patients suspected of having chronic cholecystitis. Radicular pain from *spinal lesions* may mimic biliary colic, and vertebral films or, in some instances, myelograms of the T6-T8 segment may be indicated. *Angina pectoris* may cause pain thought to be abdominal, just as biliary colic may be felt in the precordial region. Postprandial pain or discomfort may result from the *irritable colon syndrome* or from *adenocarcinoma* of the *right colon.* Tragic delays in treatment have resulted from attributing pain from colonic carcinoma to gallstones.

Treatment. Dietary changes, anticholinergics, and antacids have no effect on the course of the disease but sometimes provide symptomatic relief for a while. Cholecystectomy is the treatment of choice. Cholecystolithotomy was tried at one time in patients whose gallbladders were normal in function and appearance, but gallstones recurred in most within a few years of surgery. At operation the common bile duct is inspected visually, operative cholangiograms are obtained, and the common duct is explored if there is evidence of choledocholithiasis.

Complications. *Choledocholithiasis* is the most common complication, affecting about 15 per cent of patients with cholecystolithiasis. The incidence of common duct stones increases with advancing age.

Mirizzi's syndrome results from gradual extrusion of a large gallstone from the gallbladder into the common duct. The cystic duct enlarges to accommodate the advancing stone, which eventually comes to reside in a common cavity comprising the residual gallbladder lumen, cystic duct, and common duct. Obstructive jaundice may develop.

About two thirds of patients with *acute cholecystitis* have previously had symptomatic chronic cholecystitis. The complication of acute cholecystitis is more common in the elderly and in patients with large gallstones.

Calcification of the *gallbladder,* relatively uncommon in acute and chronic cholecystitis, is of special significance because of its frequent association with carcinoma of the gallbladder. Whether it can be considered truly premalignant is not clear. The diagnosis is usually obvious when the abdominal x-ray shows an eggshell rim of calcium in the gallbladder wall.

Adenocarcinoma of the *gallbladder* is found mainly in elderly patients with cholelithiasis, most of whom have had biliary symptoms for many years. Since carcinoma of the gallbladder affects less than 1 per cent of patients with symptomatic cholelithiasis, it is hard to argue forcibly for early cholecystectomy just to prevent tumor.

Prognosis. Cholecystectomy predictably relieves biliary colic but is only 80 per cent successful in eradicating other types of preoperative complaints (e.g., dyspepsia or flatulence). Loss of the gallbladder does not impair gastrointestinal function.

The mortality of elective cholecystectomy is under 0.5 per cent, and most of the postoperative deaths follow cardiac and respiratory complications in elderly patients with pre-existing disease of these organs. The *postcholecystectomy syndrome* is discussed in Ch. 693.

684. ACUTE CHOLECYSTITIS

The patient with acute cholecystitis usually presents with acute right subcostal pain and tenderness. Obstruction of the cystic duct by a gallstone is usually the cause, and cholelithiasis is present in 95 per cent of patients. A variety of caustic agents produce cholecystitis when injected into gallbladders of animals, but the relation of this type of experiment to the human disease is obscure. More pertinent is the observation that when the gallbladder of dogs was filled with concentrated bile, obstruction of the cystic duct produced acute inflammation, presumably an effect of the bile salts. In control experiments, if the gallbladder was empty or distended with physiologic saline solution instead of bile, cystic duct obstruction was innocuous.

As in other biliary diseases, bacterial infection is secondary to the obstruction rather than a primary factor. Bacteria are present as contaminants in the gallbladders of about 25 per cent of patients with chronic cholecystitis. Early in acute cholecystitis the bile is positive in 50 per cent of the cases, but within a week after onset this figure reaches 90 per cent. Although infection is secondary, it is ultimately responsible for the most serious sequelae of acute cholecystitis—empyema and perforation.

Acalculous cholecystitis, accounting for 5 per cent of cases, is more common in men and in patients with unrelated sepsis. Many cases have been associated with prolonged fasting after major trauma, e.g., war injuries or surgical operations remote from the biliary system. At operation the bile is viscous and full of sludge. Perforation is more frequent, and the outcome is generally worse than in gallstone cholecystitis.

Primary gallbladder infection by *Salmonella typhosa* was responsible for cases of acalculous cholecystitis years ago when typhoid fever was more prevalent. *Polyarteritis nodosa* has occasionally been implicated.

Pathology. Subserosal edema, mucosal ulcerations, and submucosal hemorrhages are the earliest pathologic findings. The inflammatory process usually evolves slowly in contrast to that in appendicitis or diverticulitis, probably because the bacterial population within the gallbladder is relatively sparse at the moment of ductal obstruction. Cellular infiltration of the wall becomes prominent only after three to four days, reaching its greatest intensity at the end of the first week. During the second week, patchy mural gangrene and small intramural abscesses appear, the edema becomes organized, and the first signs of collagen deposition appear. Resolution of the acute changes takes another week or more.

The term *empyema* denotes a pus-filled gallbladder which clinically is characterized by a septic form of acute cholecystitis. On gross examination the condtion tends to be overdiagnosed, because gallbladder mucus containing precipitated calcium closely resembles pus. *Gangrene* and *perforation* are most common in the fundus where the blood supply is meager, or in the infundibulum where stones impact. With perforation, gallbladder contents may spill into the free abdominal cavity (bile peritonitis) or be confined by adhesions (pericholecystic abscess). Sometimes an adherent viscus is penetrated, making a *cholecystenteric fistula* through which the gallstones and pus may be discharged. If a large gallstone reaches the intestine and blocks its lumen, the presenting complaints are those of small bowel obstruction, i.e., *gallstone ileus.*

Chronic obstruction of the cystic duct causes *hydrops* (mucocele), a condition in which the gallbladder is distended with uninfected mucus (white bile). Hydrops may result either from resolved acute cholecystitis or from obstruction without inflammation.

Clinical Manifestations and Diagnosis. The attack begins with abdominal pain that mounts gradually in severity. The pain is usually located in the right subcostal region from the start, but sometimes begins in the epigastrium or left upper quadrant and then shifts to the region of the gallbladder as inflammation progresses. Two thirds or more of patients have had previous attacks of biliary colic. Early in the attack the patient may expect the symptoms to subside spontaneously as had happened before with similar pains, and medical aid is often not sought until 48 hours or more. Referred pain may be experienced in the back at the scapular level.

Anorexia, nausea, and vomiting are present in the average case, but the vomiting is rarely severe enough to be confused with bowel obstruction and is generally less than in acute pancreatitis. In the absence of complications, chills are rare; their presence should always suggest suppurative cholecystitis or associated cholangitis. Fever is also moderate, reaching an average temperature of 38° C in the absence of complications.

The right subcostal region is tender to palpation, and involuntary muscle spasm generally exists which limits the examination. If the patient takes a deep breath while the subhepatic area is being palpated, tenderness is suddenly worse and inspiratory arrest is produced *(Murphy's sign).*

In somewhat more than a third of the patients, a distended, tender gallbladder can be felt as a distinct mass, usually located farther to the right than the normal gallbladder. The presence of the palpable gallbladder is an important finding which clinches the diagnosis in an otherwise typical case. The gallbladder cannot be felt in the rest of the patients because of obesity, rigidity of the abdominal wall, or a deep subhepatic location, or because it is small and shrunken from previous inflammation. Other related conditions characterized by a tender mass in the same area are *pericholecystic abscess,* acute cholecystitis complicating *carcinoma* of the *gallbladder, torsion* of the *gallbladder,* or the rare case of gallbladder distention in *obstructive cholangitis* (e.g., suppurative cholangitis or Oriental cholangiohepatitis).

About 20 per cent of patients with acute cholecystitis are slightly jaundiced. This is sometimes due only to edema of the nearby common duct; however, two thirds of jaundiced patients will have a mechanical cause such as *common duct stones* or, less often, a *biliary tumor.*

After hospitalization, improvement is usually noticeable within the first 12 to 24 hours, and the signs and symptoms gradually subside over five to seven days.

Oral feedings can usually be resumed after a few days. Persistent severe pain after hospitalization, a rise in temperature or leukocyte count, development of shaking chills, or the appearance of more severe local or generalized abdominal tenderness all indicate progression of the disease and suggest the need for emergency operation.

Empyema can produce systemic toxicity and may herald perforation. After empyema develops, if the infection is subsequently controlled with antimicrobial drugs, the large tender gallbladder may remain palpable for several weeks, and return of well-being is similarly prolonged. The leukocyte count is 10,000 to 15,000 per μl or even higher with complications. Mild rises in bilirubin, alkaline phosphatase, and SGOT are frequent.

Roentgenograms of the abdomen may show calcified gallstones or an enlarged gallbladder. Oral cholecystograms will not visualize during an acute attack and are diagnostically unreliable because of unpredictable absorption and excretion of the contrast agent. Except in patients who become asymptomatic rapidly, oral cholecystograms should not be scheduled until four to six weeks after the attack; the rate of nonvisualization remains high even then.

Intravenous cholangiograms (IVC) may give useful information and should be ordered when diagnostic uncertainty remains, liver function is good, and more information would be useful for clinical management. This situation usually occurs in a patient for whom early operation would be appropriate, but an enlarged gallbladder is not palpable on physical examination. If on IVC the gallbladder fills, the diagnosis of acute cholecystitis is essentially excluded; if the ductal system is demonstrated but the gallbladder does not opacify, the diagnosis is confirmed. More difficult to interpret is the situation in which neither gallbladder nor ducts are shown. If the bilirubin level is normal and the upper abdominal pain and tenderness are typical, most such patients will turn out to have acute cholecystitis exactly as suspected.

Differential Diagnosis. *Acute pancreatitis, acute appendicitis,* and *perforated peptic ulcer* are the conditions which most often cause major diagnostic problems. Diagnosis is complicated by the fact that in acute cholecystitis the serum amylase may rise to 1000 per 100 ml or more. Acute cholecystitis and acute pancreatitis may coexist, and intravenous cholangiography can be quite helpful in these situations, because visualization of the gallbladder is expected in acute pancreatitis.

In women, gonococcal perihepatitis *(Fitz-Hugh-Curtis syndrome)* may be mistaken for acute cholecystitis, but adnexal tenderness is usually present on pelvic examination, a cervical smear usually reveals gonococci, and the patients are younger, often have higher fever, and are in less distress than would be expected in cholecystitis. Shoulder pain and a friction rub over the liver, common in the Fitz-Hugh–Curtis syndrome, are not found in uncomplicated acute cholecystitis.

Acute hepatitis, either *viral* or *alcoholic,* sometimes produces marked right upper quadrant pain and tenderness. A history of recent binge drinking, high SGOT levels, and liver biopsy aid differentiation. *Pneumonitis, pyelonephritis,* and *cardiac disease* have all on occasion produced acute pain suggestive of cholecystitis.

Treatment. Most patients with acute cholecystitis will improve with either expectant treatment or cholecystectomy performed during the acute attack. In general, the decision regarding the type of treatment should include

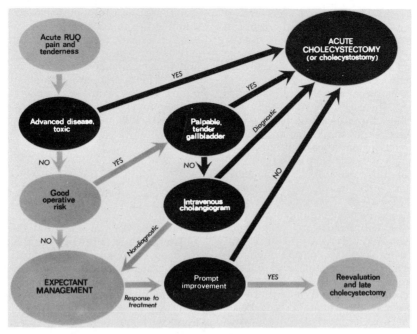

Figure 6. Algorithm for managing patients with acute right upper quadrant pain and tenderness, thought to have acute cholecystitis.

the following factors (Fig. 6): (1) whether the diagnosis is secure, (2) whether biliary complications have occurred or appear imminent, and (3) the over-all condition of the patient (operative risk).

Upon admission to the hospital, nasogastric suction should be started and fluid requirements given intravenously. Vomiting and fasting before hospitalization often cause dehydration which must be corrected. In many elderly patients, the acute biliary condition has aggravated pre-existing cardiac, pulmonary, or renal disease, and these systems must be evaluated and treated appropriately. Diabetes must be sought, because it is associated with a more ominous prognosis if surgery is delayed.

If the patient is first seen shortly after symptoms began, and if local signs and symptoms are mild, antimicrobial therapy need not be given. It is of more value later in the disease, especially for suppurative complications. Ampicillin, cephalosporin, or tetracycline is adequate, except in patients with empyema or perforation in whom cephalosporin plus gentamicin or kanamycin would be preferable.

Supported now by the results of controlled clinical trials, most experts advocate cholecystectomy during the acute attack, an approach which avoids the complications and prolonged morbidity of expectant treatment. This does not imply an emergency operation. The workup should proceed deliberately to confirm the diagnosis and to prepare the patient by procedures such as correcting fluid deficits. Cholecystectomy should then be scheduled for the next routine operating day.

In about 30 per cent of cases, the patient is a good surgical risk, the diagnosis is obvious within 12 to 24 hours, and cholecystectomy can be scheduled promptly. Another 30 per cent are good surgical candidates, but the gallbladder cannot be felt. In this situation the diagnosis should be regarded as tentative, because 10 to 15 per cent of patients whose only finding is tenderness will

have some other condition. An IVC should be performed preoperatively to verify the clinical impression.

Another third of patients will have serious coexistent cardiac, respiratory, or other disease whose treatment takes precedence. The cholecystitis should be treated expectantly while correcting the other problems. Progression of local abdominal findings requires continued reevaluation, balancing the risks of operation with the risks of continued delay.

About 10 per cent of patients require emergency surgery for complications present on admission or which appear later during observation and medical management. When emergency operation becomes necessary, *cholecystostomy* may be preferable to cholecystectomy in the seriously ill patient. In this procedure, the fundus is incised, stones and pus are removed from the lumen, and a catheter secured in the lumen is brought out through the abdominal wall and placed to gravity drainage. As in draining any abscess, this procedure allows the acute infection to resolve. Patients who recover should usually have a cholecystectomy six to eight weeks later. Those who continue to be poor surgical risks may be followed expectantly if postoperative cholecystography shows that the gallbladder and common duct contain no residual stones. If stones are present, surgery will be needed to avoid further acute attacks. In seriously ill patients, the cholecystostomy tube can be left in place indefinitely.

Recent experience suggests that postoperatively it is sometimes possible to extract residual gallbladder or common duct stones with flexible forceps or snares passed through the cholecystostomy fistula. The procedure is difficult to perform, and success is unpredictable.

After the cholecystostomy tube is removed from a patient whose biliary system contains no calculi, within the first year about 50 per cent of patients develop new stones and additional symptoms. Recurrent disease is less common after one year.

Complications. In *emphysematous cholecystitis,* a variant of acute cholecystitis, gas of bacterial origin can be seen in the gallbladder lumen and adjacent tissues. Clinically, emphysematous cholecystitis causes the same signs and symptoms as acute cholecystitis. Men are affected twice as frequently as women, about 30 per cent of patients have diabetes mellitus, and the gallbladder is acalculous in about half the cases. Gas does not occur until 24 to 48 hours after the attack begins, at which time a radiolucent halo outlines the lumen and an air-fluid level may be seen on upright films. Subserosal and then pericholecystic emphysema develop with time. Differential diagnosis of the x-ray findings includes *cholecystenteric fistula, appendiceal* or *subhepatic abscess,* and, rarely, *lipomatosis* of the *gallbladder.* In about half the cases the gas-forming organisms are clostridia, and the rest are *E. coli,* streptococci, and others. Treatment is the same as for acute cholecystitis in general, but the somewhat more aggressive nature of emphysematous cholecystitis and the association with diabetes mellitus mean that prompt surgery is usually required.

Empyema and *perforation* are usually manifested by greater sepsis and more marked abdominal signs. Perforation may take any of three forms: (1) free perforation into the abdominal cavity, (2) localized (contained) perforation with pericholecystic abscess, and (3) perforation into another viscus with fistula formation.

Free perforation, which has a 25 per cent mortality, is fortunately the least common type. It usually occurs early in the attack, often within the first three days, suggesting that when gangrene develops this quickly it cannot be walled off by adjacent viscera. Clinically, free perforation causes toxicity with high temperatures (greater than 39° C), leukocytosis over 15,000 per μl, and diffuse abdominal tenderness and rigidity. In more than half the cases, the correct diagnosis is unsuspected until laparotomy or autopsy, because a clear-cut history of preliminary right upper quadrant pain is often lacking. Treatment consists of intravenous antimicrobial therapy and emergency laparotomy with cholecystectomy.

Localized perforation most often appears in the second week of the attack at the peak of the inflammatory reaction. The diagnosis should be suspected with increasing local signs, especially when a mass suddenly appears. In most cases cholecystectomy can be performed; but in the severely ill patient, cholecystostomy and drainage of the abscess is the wiser procedure.

Fistula formation usually involves the nearby second portion of the duodenum or, less commonly, the colon, jejunum, stomach, or common bile duct. Rare fistulas have entered the renal pelvis or bronchus, or through the abdominal wall (empyema necessitatis). After intestinal fistulization the contents of the gallbladder are discharged into the gut, often aborting the acute attack. Clinically, the fistula itself may not be suspected, because it produces no unique findings; many are discovered incidentally during a later cholecystectomy. In the absence of biliary obstruction a cholecystenteric communication is not necessarily of pathophysiologic significance. Cholecystocolonic fistulas may cause malabsorption from diversion of bile, or from heavy bacterial contamination of the upper gut. If a particularly large gallstone enters through the fistula, it may obstruct the intestine, a condition called *gallstone ileus* (see Ch. 685).

Prognosis. The mortality of 5 to 10 per cent is almost confined to patients over 60 years of age with serious associated disease. Suppurative complications are more common in the elderly who can tolerate them least. In most instances, localized perforation can be managed satisfactorily at operation. Free perforation is considerably more ominous (25 per cent mortality), but is rare.

In patients who are treated expectantly, recurrent biliary symptoms are so common that an elective cholecystectomy should be planned in most cases. Another acute attack is not unusual during the month or two of waiting.

685. GALLSTONE ILEUS

Gallstone ileus is intestinal obstruction caused by a gallstone lodged in the intestinal lumen. The stone, passing through a cholecystenteric fistula, most often enters the gut in the duodenum, less commonly the jejunum, ileum, colon, or stomach. Although it is usually assumed that the initial event responsible for fistula formation is an attack of acute cholecystitis, only 30 per cent of patients with gallstone ileus give a history of recent right upper quadrant pain, and usually the clinical picture is that of bowel obstruction only.

After entering the gut, the gallstone moves downstream until is becomes too large for the intestinal lumen to accommodate. Obstruction is usually caused by gallstones over 2.5 cm in diameter, and because the lumen becomes progressively smaller aborally, the ileum is the final point of obturation in most cases. Typically, the patient's symptoms are intermittent at first as the stone transiently obstructs at various points and then dislodges, passing further along. This has been termed "tumbling obstruction," the brief periods of respite sometimes leading patient and physician to expect a spontaneous resolution of the symptoms. Eventually, however, vomiting, pain, and distention persist.

If the stone lodges in the duodenum, the diagnosis may be especially difficult in the absence of distention, hyperactive peristalsis, or x-ray findings of small bowel obstruction. Another uncommon variant is gallstone ileus of the large bowel. In these cases, the stone may have entered via a cholecystocolonic fistula or, less often, after traversing the entire small bowel. Obstruction of the colon, rare because its lumen is so wide, most often occurs when diverticulitis has narrowed the sigmoid.

Women are more often affected than men, and the average age is about 70 years. As a cause of intestinal obstruction, gallstone ileus is relatively uncommon but should always be high on the list in elderly patients, especially when incarceration in an external hernia is absent and there has been no previous laparotomy which might have produced adhesions.

On physical examination the findings are those of small bowel obstruction. Sometimes the large stone can be felt as a mass on abdominal, vaginal, or rectal examination, but it is rarely correctly identified as such.

Roentgenograms usually show air in the biliary tree if the films are carefully examined, and in some cases the radiopaque gallstone can be seen in its unusual location. Otherwise, the films are typical of bowel obstruction. Sometimes a gastrointestinal series is performed for the diagnosis of partial obstruction, revealing the cholecystoduodenal fistula.

Treatment consists of removing the obstructing gallstone through a small enterotomy and examining the proximal gut carefully to ensure that a second stone is not left which could produce an immediate recurrence. It is generally wise to leave the biliary disease undisturbed initially, because elderly patients tolerate long procedures poorly, and nothing much is gained by repairing the fistula primarily.

Postoperatively, if the patient has symptoms of biliary disease, an elective cholecystectomy may be scheduled several months later. Many patients become asymptomatic and the fistula closes spontaneously; for them, expectant management is best. About 50 per cent will require cholecystectomy.

The mortality rate, 15 to 20 per cent, remains high because of delay in diagnosis and the fragile state of cardiopulmonary function in elderly patients.

686. CHOLEDOCHOLITHIASIS AND CHOLANGITIS

In Western countries choledocholithiasis is usually the result of passage into the common duct of cholesterol gallstones formed in the gallbladder. Once there, they sometimes continue on into the duodenum, but the frequency of this event is not known and is rarely observed with certainty. The less common primary duct stone is usually associated with bile stasis caused by secondary dilatation of the duct from longstanding obstruction by stones, stricture, or ampullary stenosis. About 15 per cent of patients with gallbladder stones have concomitant choledocholithiasis. The incidence is even higher in elderly patients and in patients who seek medical care late. In rare instances choledocholithiasis is found in the absence of gallbladder stones; in such a case it is assumed that all the gallbladder stones escaped into the duct.

Clinical Manifestations. The natural history of choledocholithiasis is only vaguely known, because there is no solid information on the incidence and fate of asymptomatic patients. Available data suggest that 30 to 40 per cent of patients are asymptomatic at time of diagnosis, implying a relatively benign course in many cases. Obstruction by stones of the biliary or pancreatic ducts may produce any of the following syndromes: biliary colic, jaundice (without pain), cholangitis, pancreatitis, or a combination of these (Fig. 7). Secondary hepatic effects of persistent obstruction include biliary cirrhosis or hepatic abscesses.

Intermittent cholangitis, consisting of biliary colic, jaundice, and fever and chills *(Charcot's triad),* is the most common presenting symptom complex; in the absence of previous biliary surgery it is almost diagnostic in the Western Hemisphere of choledocholithiasis. Intermittency of symptoms is quite characteristic, a manifestation of intermittent partial obstruction. Whenever pain, chills with fever, and jaundice fluctuate together over a span of a few days or a week, cholangitis from biliary obstruction is almost certainly the cause. In a typical attack chills may precede the other symptoms, and dark urine from bilirubinuria may follow after a day or so. The pain, located in the epigastrium or right upper

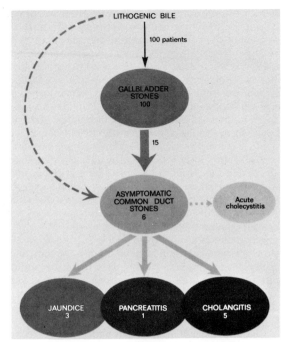

Figure 7. Natural history of choledocholithiasis, indicating that of 100 patients with gallbladder stones about 15 will develop this complication. Most acquire one of the syndromes in the bottom three ovals (with or without pain), but many probably remain asymptomatic.

quadrant, is indistinguishable from biliary colic caused by gallbladder stones and is steady, dull, and cramplike in quality. Pain may be referred to the upper back or even the precordium, occasionally suggesting coronary artery or esophageal disease.

The severity of the systemic reaction, i.e., fever and chills, varies widely from the usual mild transient illness to overwhelming sepsis with shock (see Suppurative Cholangitis, below). In the average case, the temperature rises to 38.5 to 40° C, preceded by chills and positive blood cultures. Localized tenderness in the subcostal region may be associated with extreme guarding and rigidity, but more often the local findings are minimal and are distinctly less severe than in acute cholecystitis. In most cases of common duct obstruction by stones, chronic inflammation and scarring of the gallbladder prevent it from becoming distended, as often occurs with periampullary malignancies. This serves as the basis for *Courvoisier's law:* a distended, nontender gallbladder in a jaundiced patient signifies neoplastic obstruction of the bile duct.

Laboratory Studies. In cholangitis the leukocyte count averages 15,000 μl but may go much higher in severe cases. Bilirubin values are usually in the range of 2 to 4 mg per 100 ml, and are uncommonly higher than 10 mg per 100 ml. Elevated serum alkaline phosphatase, leucine aminopeptidase, and 5'-nucleotidase levels indicate extrahepatic obstruction. The SGOT generally remains below 200 units, but values of 500 are not rare, and a few cases have been reported in which it has transiently exceeded 1000 units. In these instances the prompt drop within 48 hours and associated tenfold increase in LDH allows differentiation from serum hepatitis.

Differential Diagnosis. The same conditions considered for the patient with chronic cholecystitis must be excluded for biliary colic caused by ductal calculi. In patients who have had a cholecystectomy, differentiation between choledocholithiasis and biliary stricture as the cause of cholangitis usually depends on radiologic demonstration of the ducts. When the presenting syndrome is painless cholestatic jaundice, other causes, especially *periampullary* and *biliary neoplasms,* must be considered. With neoplastic obstruction the bilirubin averages about 18 mg per 100 ml and rarely fluctuates. Although jaundice from stones can certainly be as severe, the bilirubin is characteristically less than 10 mg per 100 ml and rises and falls episodically. The diagnosis of *intrahepatic cholestasis* from causes such as drugs, viral hepatitis, or pregnancy should in most cases be reached by exclusion only after visualization of normal bile ducts by direct or intravenous cholangiography.

Common duct stones may cause *acute pancreatitis* indistinguishable clinically from that resulting from alcohol or other causes and unaccompanied by specific signs of biliary disease. Pancreatitis caused by biliary calculi, despite numerous attacks, rarely progresses to pancreatic calcification, chronic pain, and pancreatic insufficiency, as so often occurs in the alcoholic variety. As a rule, gallstone disease should be searched for radiologically in every patient with acute pancreatitis, because further attacks can be avoided if the gallstones are removed.

Treatment. The potential seriousness of cholangitis warrants hospitalization for diagnosis and treatment in most cases. After blood cultures are drawn, antimicrobial drugs, chosen for their efficacy against enteric organisms, are given by the parenteral route. At present cephalosporin or ampicillin for mild attacks or either of these drugs plus gentamicin or kanamycin in severe infection has a good chance of controlling the infection. There is no strong rationale for choosing antimicrobial drugs based on their excretion in bile, because the block responsible for cholangitis also affects this process. Failure to obtain a rapid response may mean that the organisms were not susceptible to the initial drugs, justifying the addition of another drug or a shift from the initial regimen based upon the results of cultures and drug-susceptibility tests. The margin between mild and severe illness is small; antimicrobial therapy should be expected to control the acute attack within 48 to 72 hours, and if there is no improvement or worsening after this period, emergency surgery must be considered seriously.

Most acute cases respond satisfactorily to treatment and allow an orderly attempt at diagnosis. If oral cholecystography has already demonstrated gallbladder stones, laparotomy is indicated, and additional studies aimed at demonstrating the ductal pathology are usually not necessary. In patients with jaundice, acute pancreatitis, or upper abdominal pain who have had a cholecystectomy in the past, intravenous cholangiograms can be obtained if the bilirubin is below 3 or 4 mg per 100 ml, or direct opacification can be attempted by percutaneous transhepatic or, preferably, retrograde endoscopic cholangiography. Both these direct procedures are potentially hazardous in active cholangitis and should be postponed until infection is well controlled, proceeding then only under the protection of antimicrobial therapy.

Surgical exploration and choledochotomy should be scheduled after the diagnosis of choledocholithiasis has been made. If the gallbladder is present, cholecystectomy is done, and the common duct is opened and emptied of stones. A T tube is usually left in the duct to decompress biliary pressure in the postoperative period and to provide a route for additional cholangiograms a week or so later.

In patients with advanced disease, the common duct may be so packed with hundreds of stones that it is dilated to 3 cm or more in diameter. Rarely, the intrahepatic ducts become markedly dilated and contain innumerable stones, making complete extraction technically impossible. In either of these situations recurrent or persistent choledocholithiasis is almost certain unless a choledochoduodenostomy, sphincteroplasty, or Roux-en-Y choledochojejunostomy is performed to create a wide conduit between the duct and intestine through which residual stones can pass.

Retained Common Duct Stones. The methods for detecting duct stones at operation are about 95 per cent reliable, which means, unfortunately, that a few are overlooked only to be discovered on postoperative T tube cholangiograms. Two new approaches have recently made it possible to eliminate most residual stones without another laparotomy. One method depends on the ability of bile salt solutions to dissolve cholesterol gallstones. Several weeks after surgery a sterile solution of sodium cholate (100 mM) is infused into the T tube at 30 ml per hour continuously until the stone is gone. Oral cholestyramine must be given to prevent diarrhea from the large amount of bile salt delivered to the intestine. Disappearance of the retained stones occurs in about two thirds of patients within a two-week treatment period.

Instrumental extraction, an alternative technique, is somewhat simpler, faster, and about equally as successful. Under image intensification fluoroscopy the T tube is pulled out, a Dormia ureteral basket is passed into the duct, and the stone is grasped and withdrawn. If neither mechanical extraction nor chemical dissolution is successful, reoperation is usually necessary.

Prognosis. With accurate diagnosis and treatment, choledocholithiasis is cured by cholecystectomy and choledocholithotomy. Recurrent ductal stone formation is rare except as noted when the duct has become markedly dilated.

SUPPURATIVE CHOLANGITIS

The severest form of cholangitis, variously termed *suppurative* or *obstructive cholangitis,* involves the same causative factors as the "nonsuppurative" form but differs in that obstruction is complete, ductal contents become purulent, and clinically the manifestations of sepsis overshadow those of cholestasis. Hypotension and mental changes, such as lethargy or confusion, appear in addition to right upper quadrant pain, chills, fever, and jaundice. Because infection in the face of the high-grade obstruction progresses so rapidly, the serum bilirubin does not reach very high levels before the patient becomes moribund from sepsis. Costly delays in diagnosis are frequent, a consequence of failure to recognize the significance of mild icterus and abdominal pain in a patient with sepsis. All but a few cases are complications of choledocholithiasis, the others occurring with biliary stricture or neoplastic obstruction.

Laboratory tests reveal evidence of cholestasis with bilirubin values between 2 and 5 mg per 100 ml and elevated serum levels of alkaline phosphatase, 5'-nucleotidase, leucine aminopeptidase, and SGOT. The leukocyte count varies from normal to 40,000 per μl.

Tenderness is present to palpation in the right upper quadrant, but rigidity is rare. In some cases secondary cholecystitis develops, and an enlarged tender gallbladder may be found on abdominal examination.

There is no way to confirm the diagnosis by x-ray, because transhepatic or retrograde cholangiography would be extremely hazardous and intravenous cholangiograms are unsuccessful. Therefore diagnosis rests on recognizing the evidence of biliary obstruction and its relationship to the sepsis.

After initial resuscitation, consisting of intravenous infusions, antimicrobial drugs, and measures to restore cardiac, pulmonary, or renal function, emergency surgery offers the only hope of saving the patient. Hypoglycemia has been found in some patients whose depressed cerebral function seemed to improve with infusion of hypertonic glucose solutions.

At surgery when choledochotomy is performed, pus often squirts from the duct owing to the high pressure. If the patient's condition permits, thorough exploration can be performed to correct the obstruction by eliminating stones, repairing a stricture, or bypassing a tumor. Insertion of a T tube proximal to the obstruction is sufficient in patients who are unable to tolerate a longer operation, but sometime later it will be necessary to perform a second, more definitive procedure before the T tube can be removed.

The mortality is about 50 per cent, resulting from septic shock, renal failure, acute hepatic insufficiency, or a combination of these complications.

687. BILIARY STRICTURE

Biliary stricture, except in rare instances, results from surgical injury to the duct and usually follows cholecystectomy rather than procedures on the duct itself such as deliberate choledochotomy for common duct exploration. In some cases the surgeon may recognize the injury and attempt its repair. Often, however, it is not identified at the primary operation, and the first sign of trouble postoperatively might be excessive escape of bile along drains or the appearance of jaundice or cholangitis. A few noniatrogenic examples of biliary stricture stem from external trauma or scarring produced by choledocholithiasis.

Injury to the duct that is identified immediately or within a few days can sometimes be repaired without serious consequences. The patient who has signs of partial biliary obstruction and intermittent cholangitis weeks or months after cholecystectomy is the one who presents challenges for diagnosis and treatment. The symptoms closely resemble those of choledocholithiasis, the obvious clue being a history of previous cholecystectomy or attempt at repair of a stricture.

Leukocytosis and laboratory evidence of cholestasis parallel the clinical manifestations. The jaundice or cholangitis is generally mild and transient, and infection generally responds promptly to antimicrobial therapy.

Intravenous cholangiograms may be obtained if the bilirubin drops below 3 mg per 100 ml. Otherwise, transhepatic or retrograde cholangiograms will be necessary.

With persistent obstruction over several years, secondary biliary cirrhosis develops, and portal hypertension

may give rise to bleeding esophageal varices, or hepatic failure may ensue gradually. In other cases, uncontrolled sepsis results in multiple intrahepatic abscesses and death.

Differential diagnosis must include all the various causes of obstructive jaundice and cholangitis, but in most cases the major consideration is *choledocholithiasis.* A useful differential feature is that the initial symptoms of stricture nearly always begin within two years of the cholecystectomy, whereas a symptom-free interval longer than this is common with residual or recurrent common duct stones.

In all but a few cases an attempt should be made to repair the stricture surgically by creating a new unobstructed conduit between normal duct on the hepatic side of the lesion and the proximal intestine. This can sometimes be accomplished by a direct end-to-end anastomosis of the duct after excising the lesion or more often by choledochoduodenostomy or choledochojejunostomy to a Roux-en-Y jejunal segment. Loss of the duodenal end of the duct and choledochal sphincter with the last two operations is of no physiologic significance. By diverting alkaline bile from the duodenum, choledochojejunostomy predisposes slightly to peptic ulcer disease, but the problem is not of sufficient magnitude to weigh heavily in the choice of procedure unless the patient already has a peptic ulcer.

The over-all success rate of these operations is about 75 per cent, but it is important to note that even when there has been one or more previous failures, the odds still favor a good result after another try. For this reason, it is rarely wise to keep a patient with a known stricture indefinitely on a regimen of intermittent antimicrobial drugs for symptoms. The obstruction invariably produces cirrhosis or uncontrollable infection, and the opportunity to obtain a real cure is lost.

The mortality of 10 per cent is from the complications mentioned above.

688. UNCOMMON CAUSES OF BILE DUCT OBSTRUCTION

The following inventory briefly covers several uncommon causes of common duct obstruction manifested clinically by jaundice, colic, cholangitis, or a combination of these. *Pancreatic* and *duodenal tumors* are covered in Ch. 648 and 668, respectively. Other causes rarely encountered are compression by *neoplastic* or *inflammatory paraductal lymph nodes* and *duodenal Crohn's disease.*

Choledochal cysts occasionally produce their initial clinical manifestations in adults, presenting with jaundice, cholangitis, and, in some, a right upper quadrant mass consisting of the dilated duct full of stones. Diagnosis may require transhepatic cholangiography or may not be obvious until operation. The most definitive surgical procedure is excision of the abnormal duct, followed by Roux-en-Y jejunal anastomosis to the stump of the hepatic duct. The simpler cystenteric anastomosis may be preferable in some situations.

Caroli's disease consists of saccular intrahepatic bile duct dilatation which in most cases becomes symptomatic in patients between the ages of 20 and 50 owing to intrahepatic stone formation and cholangitis. Two forms are recognized: one a disease of the ducts only, and the more common type which is associated with hepatic fibrosis and medullary sponge kidney. The latter patients often have complications of portal hypertension before cholangitis or obstructive jaundice appears. Antimicrobial therapy may control attacks of cholangitis, and surgical procedures to facilitate ductal emptying or to extract stones may help in some cases, but the intrahepatic anomaly cannot be definitively corrected. Rarely the left lobe alone is involved, and lobectomy is curative.

Hemobilia presents with the triad of biliary colic, obstructive jaundice, and occult or gross intestinal bleeding. Most cases are caused by hepatic injury with secondary bleeding into the ductal system, usually beginning several weeks after the trauma. Hemobilia is occasionally caused by *biliary* or *hepatic neoplasms*, ductal rupture of an *hepatic artery aneurysm, hepatic abscess,* or *biliary calculus.* Inflammatory hemobilia has been reported mostly from the Orient, where it accompanies *biliary parasitism (Ascaris lumbricoides)* or *cholangiohepatitis.* The diagnosis can be verified preoperatively by selective hepatic arteriography. Treatment may require hepatic artery ligation for hemobilia secondary to trauma, but for the other types direct surgical management of the lesion is usually necessary.

Pancreatitis can produce transient jaundice by obstruction of the distal common duct where it is encased by pancreatic tissue. Prolonged obstruction can result from pressure by a pseudocyst or entrapment in severe pancreatic scarring from chronic pancreatitis. Diagnosis may be difficult in alcoholic patients in whom elevated bilirubin values are usually attributed to hepatic parenchymal disease.

Most *duodenal diverticula* arise within 1 to 2 cm of the hepatobiliary ampulla, and in some patients the common duct empties directly into a diverticulum. Duodenal diverticula may obstruct the common duct by anatomic distortion of its duodenal entry, by diverticulitis, or by an enterolith (of bile acids) in the sac. Even in jaundiced patients most duodenal diverticula are only incidental findings, but when definite proof implicates them in ductal obstruction, either choledochoduodenostomy or Roux-en-Y choledochojejunostomy is simpler treatment than attempting to excise the diverticulum or surgically to enlarge its entry into the duodenum.

Echinococcosis, by rupture of an hepatic cyst into the ducts, can give rise to biliary colic, jaundice, and cholangitis. Treatment involves surgical removal of the obstructing hydatid debris and daughter cysts from the ducts and excision of the parent cyst from the liver after its contents are sterilized by sodium hypochlorite (0.05 per cent) or hypertonic saline (30 per cent) solution. The practice of injecting formalin into the hepatic cysts is fortunately no longer used, because in patients with a biliary communication serious damage to the bile ducts and even death have occurred.

Ascariasis may produce colic, jaundice, and cholangitis by worms which invade the bile ducts through the choledochal sphincter from the duodenum. The worm eventually dies, but in some cases not until after depositing ova. Air is sometimes seen in the ducts, presumably entering through the sphincter with the ascarid. Treatment entails antimicrobial drugs and then piperazine after the acute symptoms are controlled. If progressive cholangitis occurs despite antimicrobial therapy, common duct exploration and extraction of the parasites may be necessary. After the nonsurgical regimen, follow-up intravenous cholangiograms should be obtained to verify that no worms remain in the duct; if residual defects are present, they should be surgically removed.

Throughout coastal regions of the Orient, from Japan to Malaysia, many persons of low socioeconomic status are affected by *Oriental cholangiohepatitis*, a form of chronic recurrent cholangitis caused by calcium bilirubinate stones formed primarily within the bile ducts. Among the various etiologic possibilities are the effects of parasites in the ducts (especially *Clonorchis sinensis* and *Ascaris lumbricoides),* diet (low in fat and animal protein), and excessive bilirubin excretion. In some regions, ova or fragments of adult parasites have been demonstrated within the center of the stones, but the disease has also been reported in populations without heavy parasitic infestation. Within the ducts, Clornorchis is especially capable of inciting ductal inflammation and scarring. Whatever the initial event, there is good evidence that β-glucuronidase, produced in the bile by secondarily invading *E. coli,* hydrolyzes bilirubin diglucuronide which then precipitates as sludge and stones of calcium bilirubinate.

Acute cholangitis is the usual presenting syndrome. Subcostal abdominal tenderness is present, and the gallbladder, which contains stones in only 20 to 30 per cent, is usually palpable, or even visible on abdominal inspection. Strictures sometimes develop in the hepatic ducts, leading to further stasis and intrahepatic stone formation. In advanced cases, one (usually the left) or both lobar ducts may become honeycombed with cysts or abscesses, producing atrophy of the hepatic parenchyma. Laboratory abnormalities consist of leukocytosis, elevated serum bilirubin (2 to 10 mg per 100 ml), and elevated serum alkaline phosphatase. During symptomatic episodes neither plain films nor oral or intravenous cholangiograms will demonstrate the pathology.

Most acute cases can be controlled with antimicrobials, but severe toxicity, fever (39 to 40° C), or septic shock mandates emergency laparotomy in as many as 30 per cent. If nonsurgical management is initially successful, transhepatic cholangiograms can be used later to outline the ducts.

The common duct stones should be removed through a generous choledochotomy. If it is impossible to empty the intrahepatic ducts, transhepatic lithotomy or even lobectomy may be required if there is unilateral lobar atrophy or abscess formation. Recurrence of choledocholithiasis is almost certain unless the junction between duct and intestine is surgically enlarged by sphincteroplasty, choledochoduodenostomy, or Roux-en-Y choledochojejunostomy.

Sclerosing cholangitis, a rare condition of unknown etiology, consists of benign nonbacterial chronic inflammatory narrowing of the bile ducts. The entire ductal system may be involved, or, less commonly, the process may be confined to the extrahepatic or intrahepatic portion. Males predominate in a ratio of 3:1, and the peak incidence occurs in the third and fourth decades. About one third of the cases are associated with *retroperitoneal fibrosis, Riedel's thyroiditis, regional enteritis,* or especially *ulcerative colitis.* When both are present, the severity of sclerosing cholangitis and ulcerative colitis is not correlated, and colectomy has an uncertain effect on the biliary disease.

The initial complaint may be jaundice or pruritus, although both eventually appear in most cases. There may be mild upper abdominal pain and sometimes fever, but a clinical picture resembling bacterial cholangitis is uncommon in the absence of previous surgical exploration of the ducts. Hepatomegaly is the only abdominal finding until late when secondary cirrhosis produces ascites or splenomegaly.

Jaundice may be constant or fluctuating, and bilirubin values are usually in the range of 2 to 10 mg per 100 ml. The alkaline phosphatase is quite high and remains elevated despite variations in clinical manifestations. Antimitochondrial antibodies are absent. Other liver function tests are normal until late in the illness when hepatic failure develops.

Preoperative diagnosis is difficult to establish except by exclusion. Transhepatic cholangiography will demonstrate the pathology if the intrahepatic branches are not affected, but retrograde cholangiography via endoscopy may eventually be a more reliable technique. The x-rays show diffuse irregular ductal narrowing with only a tiny residual lumen in the most severely involved areas. When considering the differential diagnosis, a short stenosis (1 to 2 cm) of the duct more likely represents a neoplasm or traumatic stricture than sclerosing cholangitis. Other causes of persistent cholestatic jaundice must be considered, especially *primary biliary cirrhosis, drug cholestasis,* and *neoplastic ductal obstruction.*

At operation the lumen is identified, often a tedious process, and then dilated with progressively larger probes. An operative cholangiogram should be obtained to show the extent and severity of involvement, and as large a T tube as possible should be placed in the duct and left there for several months. Since differentiation from scirrhous biliary malignancy may be difficult even at operation, biopsy of the duct should be obtained in all cases, and even then the pathologist may have trouble distinguishing sclerosing cholangitis from neoplasm.

Many experts favor postoperative administration of systemic corticosteroids for 6 to 12 months; but in the absence of conclusive proof of their value, others argue that on balance corticosteroids are too dangerous, because they foster suppurative complications. After surgery which introduces a few bacteria and a foreign body, episodic mild cholangitis occurs in most patients, and short courses of antimicrobial therapy can be given to hasten their resolution. Cholestyramine may be useful for pruritus at any stage of the disease.

Significant palliation follows surgery in most cases, but unfortunately is not often permanent. A few patients seem to recover completely; however, most have episodic remissions and exacerbations over five to ten years during which time secondary biliary cirrhosis develops. Death may follow uncontrollable biliary sepsis with hepatic abscesses, liver failure, or bleeding from esophageal varices.

689. CARCINOMA OF THE GALLBLADDER

About 6000 people in the United States die each year from carcinoma of the gallbladder, a number equal to the mortality from benign disease of the biliary tract. Gallbladder cancer accounts for 1 per cent of all cancer deaths and 3 per cent of gastrointestinal malignancies. Women outnumber men by 3 to 1, and the average age is 70. Because 85 per cent of cases occur in patients with gallstones, cholelithiasis is thought to be etiologically important; somewhat less than 1 per cent of patients with cholelithiasis will develop gallbladder malignancy.

All but a few gallbladder carcinomas are adenocarcinoma, the remainder being squamous cell carcinoma. The earliest spread is usually to the liver by direct extension and metastasis. Nodal metastases in the liver hilum are somewhat less common, and distant metastases appear only late.

The patients present clinically in one of the following ways: (1) unremitting deep jaundice from common duct and hepatic involvement; (2) acute cholecystitis, usually with a palpable mass; (3) chronic cholecystitis with intermittent right upper quadrant pain; and (4) advanced carcinoma. The diagnosis is rarely considered preoperatively, but in some instances clinical clues are present. In about two thirds of the patients a mass can be felt, and in one third there is local tenderness. Gallbladder symptoms in patients 70 years or older are associated with carcinoma in about 10 per cent. In all but a few cases, the oral cholecystogram does not opacify, and even when the gallbladder is visualized, the tumor can rarely be demonstrated. Because the tumor becomes surgically incurable before it has grown very large, there is a strong correlation between presence of a palpable mass and incurability. More than half the patients have had chronic biliary symptoms for several years, and presumably earlier cholecystectomy in these would have avoided the development of carcinoma.

Surgery is indicated in most patients if for no more than diagnosis. Resection is rarely possible for cure, but in some cases palliative procedures will relieve jaundice. If it appears curative, cholecystectomy and resection of adjacent involved liver should be performed if the general health of the patient permits, but most elderly patients cannot tolerate an hepatic lobectomy. Most cures have resulted from excision of the gallbladder with a tumor so small that it was unsuspected by the surgeon. Only scattered reports of five-year survivors have appeared. Most patients live for only a few months after the diagnosis.

690. BENIGN TUMORS AND PSEUDOTUMORS OF THE GALLBLADDER

This is a heterogenous group of uncommon lesions with uncertain clinical significance. The roentgenographic appearance may be distinctive, especially for adenomyomatous hyperplasia, but often is not. A pathologic classification is presented in Table 2.

Adenomatous hyperplasia, consisting of mucosal thickening, may be focal or diffuse. Gallstones are present in some cases. The diagnosis cannot be made by x-ray.

Adenomyomatous hyperplasia, the most common lesion, has sometimes been called *adenomyomatosis, diverticulosis, cholecystitis glandularis proliferans,* or *cholecystitis cystica.* Focal, segmental, and diffuse forms

TABLE 2.　Benign Tumors and Pseudotumors of Gallbladder—Classification

Benign pseudotumors:
1. Mucosal hyperplasia
   a. Adenomatous
   b. Adenomyomatous (adenomyoma)
2. Polyps
   a. Inflammatory
   b. Cholesterol
3. Mucosal heterotopia
4. Miscellaneous
   a. Fibroxanthogranulomatous inflammation
   b. Parasitic
   c. Other

Benign tumors:
1. Epithelial
   a. Adenoma, papillary
   b. Adenoma, nonpapillary
2. Supporting tissue
   a. Hemangioma
   b. Lipoma
   c. Leiomyoma
   d. Granular cell tumor

exist, but the first of these is by far the most common. Most pathologists agree that the lesion is not neoplastic; the absence of cases in children argues against a congenital origin. Located invariably in the fundus, the focal form consists of a thick button of smooth muscle invaded by cystic mucosal glands and punctuated by a central umbilication. Convincing cases have been reported in which patients were relieved of chronic abdominal complaints by cholecystectomy, but in most cases adenomyomatosis produces no symptoms.

Cholesterol polyps are a focal form of cholesterolosis consisting of submucosal histiocytes stuffed with cholesterol and located at a villous tip. Interestingly, diffuse cholesterolosis rarely gives rise to cholesterol polyps. The polyp is attached to the mucosa by a fragile stalk which can easily be broken. This has engendered speculation concerning a possible role for cholesterol polyps in the genesis of some cholesterol gallstones.

Papillary and *nonpapillary adenomas* are the only true benign neoplasms of the gallbladder seen with any frequency. Although the other lesions mentioned above clearly have no neoplastic potential, several cases of carcinoma have been reported in association with adenomas. It is doubtful, however, that many malignancies could arise in this way, because adenomas are rare compared with carcinoma of the gallbladder.

691. MALIGNANT BILE DUCT TUMORS

The main cause of early morbidity from tumors of the bile duct is biliary obstruction with gradual hepatocellular damage or secondary hepatobiliary infection. Except for a rare squamous cell tumor, bile duct malignancies consist of adenocarcinoma with either a scirrhous or a papillary pattern. Grossly, three types of pathologic presentations occur: focal stricture, diffuse thickening, and nodular mass. The first two varieties can easily be mistaken for a benign process, such as post-traumatic

stricture or sclerosing cholangitis. To further complicate differentiation, some tumors are so marked by desmoplasia that tumor cells may be hard to find in the extensive collagen stroma. In many cases, spread is confined to local lymph node metastases or hepatic invasion for months or years before there is more widespread abdominal or systemic involvement. The common hepatic duct or common bile duct is the site of origin in about two thirds of the cases. By contrast with carcinoma of the gallbladder, cholelithiasis is found in only one third of patients, and men slightly outnumber women. The average age at diagnosis is 70 years. A number of cases have been reported in younger patients with ulcerative colitis, and since some of these had previously undergone colectomy, it is thought that elimination of the ulcerated colon is not protective. Exposure to the chemical carcinogens benzidine, 3,3-dichlorobenzidine, and M-toluene-diamine has been etiologically implicated in some cases. Japanese- and Mexican-Americans are more often affected than whites in the United States. In the Orient, infestation with *Clonorchis sinensis* probably contributes to the higher incidence of *intrahepatic cholangiocarcinoma.*

Clinical Manifestations. The typical patient presents with unremitting deep jaundice, mild deep-seated upper abdominal pain, and weight loss. Pruritus is reported by many, usually after the jaundice, but preceding it in some cases. Diarrhea, presumably from steatorrhea, is reported by some. Pain, which affects over half the patients, is not of an intensity or character to be confused with biliary colic. In the absence of previous surgery, fever and chills are rarely present. Hepatomegaly without splenomegaly is found on abdominal examination. Tumors of the common duct sparing the cystic duct generally produce in addition to jaundice a distended nontender palpable gallbladder (*Courvoisier's law*). Otherwise, the abdomen is unremarkable, because palpation of the tumor itself is almost never possible. Most patients have occult blood in the stool.

The serum bilirubin exceeds 10 mg per 100 ml in most cases, with a mean value of around 18 mg per 100 ml. The alkaline phosphatase is raised and SGOT may be slightly elevated, although rarely higher than 200. Serum proteins are most often normal. The prothrombin time may be depressed but responds to parenteral vitamin K. Serum cholesterol averages about 400 mg per 100 ml.

Radiologic visualization of the biliary tree shows marked dilatation proximal to the obstruction. Excellent studies are usually obtained by transhepatic cholangiography, but retrograde cannulation of the duct, using fiberoptic endoscopy, may soon become the preferred technique. Only benign stricture of the duct is likely to create a similar radiographic picture, but if the patient has had no previous biliary surgery, benign stricture can be excluded.

Diagnostic confusion most often involves *primary biliary cirrhosis* and *jaundice* produced by *various drugs.* In neither of these does the bilirubin generally reach such high levels as with biliary tumors. Xanthelasma, found often with primary biliary cirrhosis, is only rarely seen with neoplastic obstruction. Antimitochondrial antibodies can be demonstrated in the serum of patients with primary biliary cirrhosis; how often they will be found with tumors is unclear, because the specificity of this test at present seems to vary between investigators, and there are reports of positive titers in some patients with longstanding extrahepatic obstruction.

Choledocholithiasis and *biliary stricture* are less likely to present with steady deep jaundice and weight loss. The clinical finding in these conditions is fluctuating, milder jaundice, usually associated with fever. Transhepatic cholangiograms can exclude calculous obstruction or stricture.

Treatment. Unfortunately, complete excision of the tumor is rarely possible, because unexpendable anatomic structures are involved early despite the slow growth of most biliary tumors. Nevertheless, a few cures can be expected when radical surgery is judiciously employed; and with new techniques for reestablishing bile flow, palliation is of increasing importance.

With proximal lesions, the findings at surgery consist of a collapsed gallbladder and small common duct, both grossly normal. That diagnostic pitfalls exist for the surgeon is underscored by the fact that many patients with tumors of the hepatic duct are subjected to at least one "negative" laparotomy before the problem is recognized. This could be largely obviated if operative cholangiograms that include the intrahepatic system were considered essential in diagnostic abdominal exploration for jaundice.

Distal lesions require radical pancreaticoduodenectomy (Whipple procedure) for complete removal. Because the operation has a 15 per cent mortality, it should rarely be performed if tumor would be left behind. Tumors of the supraduodenal duct are sometimes amenable to complete resection. Those of the left hepatic duct require a left hepatectomy, but secondary involvement of the right hepatic duct means this is rarely possible.

For most cases the goal is palliation. Distal tumors can be bypassed by cholecystojejunostomy or other types of biliary-enteric anastomosis. For proximal tumors a polyethylene tube is placed in the duct to maintain bile flow by spanning the tumor; the hepatic end is brought out directly through the liver substance, and the duodenal end is brought out through a choledochotomy. In this way the tube can be replaced later without reoperation when debris begins to plug the lumen, as usually happens after six months or so. Holes in the intraductal portion of the tube allow bile to reach the gut from the liver.

Prognosis. Cure is achieved in no more than 5 to 10 per cent, and survival is usually less than one year. If biliary drainage can be maintained, patients may survive for five to six years, even continuing their regular employment. Death eventually results from hepatic replacement with tumor or intrahepatic sepsis from recurrent ductal obstruction.

692. BENIGN TUMORS OF THE BILE DUCTS

The rare benign tumors of the bile ducts present with obstructive jaundice. *Papilloma,* the predominant morphologic type, is often multifocal and therefore difficult to cure. The next most common, *adenoma,* is more often localized. If the patient is an acceptable candidate, radical excision of the extrahepatic ducts is preferable to local curettement or limited resection.

693. POSTCHOLECYSTECTOMY SYNDROME

After cholecystectomy, a small percentage of patients continue to have significant abdominal symptoms. It was postulated by some that this postoperative disability resulted specifically from the absence of the gallbladder; hence the name postcholecystectomy syndrome. To avoid cholecystectomy, cholecystolithotomy was tried for chronic cholecystitis by several groups of surgeons, but an unacceptably high incidence of recurrent gallstones and persistent symptoms stimulated a return to cholecystectomy.

In many patients, the explanation for continued postoperative symptoms is that the gallstone disease was not the cause of their preoperative complaints. Patients with biliary colic, a symptom rather specific for chronic cholecystitis, are more often relieved than those with the vague symptoms of fatty food intolerance, dyspepsia, or flatulence. Success of cholecystectomy also correlates with the extent of pathologic change in the gallbladder wall; those with continued symptoms more often had minimal scarring and a functioning gallbladder.

In others, postcholecystectomy complaints can be attributed to overlooked organic disease, especially *choledocholithiasis, pancreatitis, peptic ulcer,* or *irritable colon syndrome.* These possibilities must be investigated by appropriate studies.

Last is a group of clinical entities whose clinical significance, incidence, or even existence in some instances remains in dispute. *Stenosis of the sphincter of Oddi, biliary dyskinesia, neuroma of the cystic duct stump,* and other cystic duct remnant lesions are the main examples. Perhaps it is fair to say that convincing evidence has been submitted to document the importance of each in specific cases, but as a group they are all quite rare. It should be appreciated in the management of patients with chronic abdominal pain that, in the absence of objective findings, exploratory laparotomy has a low rate of success for diagnosis and that surgical correction of minor variations in the gut anatomy usually fails to cure.

General

Kune, G. B.: Current Practice of Biliary Surgery. Boston, Little, Brown & Company, 1972.
Schein, C. J.: Acute Cholecystitis. New York, Harper & Row, 1972.
Sleisenger, M. H., and Fordtran, J. S. (eds.): Gastrointestinal Disease. Philadelphia, W. B. Saunders Company, 1973.

Specific

Adson, M. A.: Carcinoma of the gallbladder. Surg. Clin. North Am., 53:1203, 1973.
Dow, R. W., and Lindenauer, S. M.: Acute obstructive suppurative cholangitis. Ann. Surg., 169:272, 1969.
Dowling, R. H.: The enterohepatic circulation. Gastroenterology, 62:122, 1972.
Edlund, Y., and Olsson, O.: Acute cholecystitis: Its aetiology and course, with special reference to the timing of cholecystectomy. Acta Chir. Scand., 120:479, 1961.
Foulk, W. T.: Congenital malformations of the intrahepatic biliary tree in the adult. Gastroenterology, 58:253, 1970.
Grundy, S. M., Metzger, A. L., and Adler, R. D.: Mechanisms of lithogenic bile formation in American Indian women with cholesterol gallstones. J. Clin. Invest., 51:3026, 1972.
Longmire, W. P., Jr., McArthur, M. S., Bastounis, E. A., and Hiatt, J.: Carcinoma of the extrahepatic biliary tract. Ann. Surg., 178:333, 1973.
May, R. E., and Strong, R.: Acute emphysematous cholecystitis. Br. J. Surg., 58:454, 1971.
McSherry, C. K., and Glenn, F.: Biliary tract obstruction and duodenal diverticula. Surg. Gynecol. Obstet., 130:829, 1970.

Metzger, A. L., Adler, R., Heymsfield, S., and Grundy, S. M.: Diurnal variation in biliary lipid composition: Possible role in cholesterol gallstone formation. N. Engl. J. Med., 288:333, 1973.

Sandblom, P.: Hemobilia. Surg. Clin. North Am., 53:1191, 1973.

Schwartz, S. I.: Primary sclerosing cholangitis. Surg. Clin. North Am., 53:1161, 1973.

Small, D. M., and Rapo, S.: Source of abnormal bile in patients with cholesterol gallstones. N. Engl. J. Med., 283:53, 1970.

Thistle, J. L., and Hofmann, A. F.: Efficacy and specificity of chenodeoxycholic acid therapy for dissolving gallstones. N. Engl. J. Med., 289:655, 1973.

Thorpe, C. D., Olsen, W. H., Fischer, H., Doust, V. L., and Joseph, R. R.: Emergency intravenous cholangiography in patients with acute abdominal pain. Am. J. Surg., 125:46, 1973.

van der Linden, W., and Sunzel, H.: Early versus delayed operation for acute cholecystitis. Am. J. Surg., 120:7, 1970.

Way, L. W., Admirand, W. H., and Dunphy, J. E.: Management of choledocholithiasis. Ann. Surg., 176: 347, 1972.

Way, L. W., and Dunphy, J. E.: Biliary stricture. Am. J. Surg., 124:287, 1972.

Wenckert, A., and Robertson, B.: The natural course of gallstone disease. Gastroenterology, 50:376, 1966.

Section Eleven.   DISEASES OF THE LIVER

Graham H. Jeffries

694. MECHANISMS OF HEPATIC DISEASE

An understanding of the pathophysiology of liver disease provides the basis for a rational clinical approach to the patient. The chapters that follow will review selective aspects of the biochemical and regulatory functions of the liver, the pathophysiology of clinical manifestations of liver disease, and the differential diagnosis and treatment of diseases of the liver.

JAUNDICE

Jaundice or *icterus* refers to a yellow discoloration of the skin or sclerae by bilirubin. Jaundice is usually apparent when the serum concentration of bilirubin exceeds 2 to 3 mg per 100 ml. Mucous membranes, colored by capillary blood, usually appear icteric only when serum bilirubin levels are considerably elevated. In patients with longstanding jaundice of the obstructive type, the skin may assume a greenish hue that is due in part to melanin pigmentation.

Bilirubin Metabolism

Production. Bilirubin is a yellow tetrapyrrol pigment derived from heme-containing proteins. The hemoglobin of red blood cells is the major source of bilirubin (80 to 90 per cent). Normally, senescent red cells that have survived in the circulation for approximately 120 days are taken up by macrophages in the reticuloendothelial system (R-E system), and their hemoglobin is degraded to bilirubin. Biliverdin is an intermediate in the reactions that separate iron and protein (globin) from the molecule and open the tetrapyrrol ring at the α-methene bridge. The iron released from hemoglobin is stored in the R-E cells or is reutilized for heme synthesis.

When there is hemorrhage into tissues, the extravasated red cells are engulfed by macrophages which accumulate at the site of hemorrhage; the color changes of a subcutaneous hematoma reflect the conversion of hemoglobin to bilirubin.

Hemolytic disease states are usually accompanied by hyperplasia of the R-E system and an increased R-E cell production of bilirubin. When hemolysis is intravascular and hemoglobin is released into the blood, the pigment may be cleared by hepatic parenchymal cells or alternatively excreted by the renal glomeruli and reabsorbed by renal tubule cells; these parenchymal cells also have the capacity to degrade hemoglobin to bilirubin.

Small amounts of bilirubin are derived from the breakdown of hemoproteins other than hemoglobin—e.g., myoglobin and cytochromes. In studies on the incorporation of N^{15}-labeled glycine into the fecal pigment *stercobilin* (urobilin) that is derived from bilirubin, a small fraction (10 to 20 per cent) of labeled bile pigment was excreted within a few days of isotope administration. This "early-labeled" bile pigment is derived from the degradation of cytochromes, particularly in the liver, and from hemoglobin which escapes incorporation into peripheral red blood cells.

Transport and Distribution. Unconjugated bilirubin is a lipid-soluble molecule with minimal solubility in aqueous solution at the pH of plasma. The transport of bilirubin from the R-E cells and its subsequent distribution is determined by binding with plasma albumin; each albumin molecule has the capacity to bind two molecules of bilirubin. Unconjugated bilirubin, which is strongly albumin bound and thus nondialyzable, is not filtered by renal glomeruli and is not excreted in the urine. Conjugated bilirubin (see below) is water soluble and dialyzable from albumin solutions; in patients with obstructive jaundice and conjugated hyperbilirubinemia, the pigment is filtered and excreted in the urine. In patients with jaundice, bilirubin equlibrates between the intravascular and extravascular albumin pool. In the extravascular space, the pigment will distribute between tissue and plasma protein binding sites. Lipid-soluble, unconjugated bilirubin binds preferentially to albumin, and does not diffuse into cells other than the liver unless albumin binding sites are saturated (see Kernicterus in Ch. 696). The cerebrospinal and intraocular fluids do not become icteric in jaundiced patients.

Hepatic Uptake and Excretion. The transfer of bilirubin from plasma to bile can be divided into four steps: (1) passage from sinusoidal blood across the liver cell membrane, (2) concentration in the liver cell, (3) conjugation to diglucuronide, and (4) secretion into the bile canaliculus. The passage of bilirubin from albumin-bilirubin complexes in plasma across the plasma membrane into the liver cell is facilitated by low molecular weight binding proteins, designated Y and Z, in the liver cell cytoplasm. These intracellular binding proteins also bind other organic anions. In the liver cell, bilirubin is conjugated to form bilirubin diglucuronide. Conjugation with glucuronic acid is catalyzed by a microsomal enzyme, *glucuronyl transferase,* in the presence of uridine diphospho-glucuronic acid, and converts nonpolar, lipid-soluble, unconjugated bilirubin to a polar, water-soluble compound, which is excreted in bile.

The secretion of conjugated bilirubin from the liver cell across the membrane lining the bile canaliculi is an active process which is probably carrier mediated. *Conjugation of the pigment is a prerequisite for its secretion into the bile.* In the absence of bilirubin glucuronyl transferase (see Crigler-Najjar syndrome in Ch. 696), the bile is colorless, and bile pigment is excreted by unidentified metabolic pathways.

Intestinal Degradation.   Bacterial enzymes in the distal small intestine and colon convert conjugated bilirubin to colorless urobilinogens, which are excreted predominantly in the feces but are partly reabsorbed in the ileum and colon. Reabsorbed urobilinogen is either cleared by the liver and re-excreted in bile or excreted in the urine.

Pathophysiology of Jaundice

Hyperbilirubinemia with jaundice may be due to one or several mechanisms that include excessive pigment production, reduced hepatic uptake or conjugation of bilirubin, or decreased excretion of the conjugated pigment.

Excessive Bilirubin Production.   *Hemolysis,* an excessive rate of red blood cell destruction, is the most common mechanism of excessive bilirubin production. In the normal subject, the low serum bilirubin concentration predominantly in the unconjugated fraction reflects the efficient hepatic clearance of the pigment. Hepatic bilirubin excretion may increase to maximal levels when pigment production is increased by hemolysis, but the serum concentration of bilirubin (predominantly unconjugated) rarely exceeds 3 to 5 mg per 100 ml unless hepatic excretion is impaired by reduced blood flow, impaired hepatocellular function, or ductal obstruction.

In some patients with unconjugated hyperbilirubinemia, bile pigment may be excreted in excess of the amount derived from peripheral red cell destruction. This is typical of thalassemia and pernicious anemia, but is sometimes unassociated with hemolytic disease. *Ineffective erythropoiesis* may account for excessive bilirubin production and jaundice in these patients. Although the "early-labeled" pigment excreted in bile is partly derived from the metabolism of heme enzymes (cytochromes) in the liver, there is currently no evidence that jaundice may result from increased hepatic metabolism of cytochromes.

Reduced Hepatic Uptake of Bilirubin.   A defect in the transfer of plasma bilirubin to the liver cell may explain the unconjugated hyperbilirubinemia in *Gilbert's syndrome* (see Ch. 696), after recovery from acute *viral hepatitis,* in congestive heart failure and after portacaval shunt surgery. Certain drugs may also competitively interfere with bilirubin uptake (iodopanoic acid, novobiocin).

Reduced Hepatic Conjugation of Bilirubin.   Bilirubin conjugation with glucuronic acid is essential for normal bilirubin excretion. A deficiency or inhibition of glucuronyl transferase activity causes unconjugated hyperbilirubinemia. *Neonatal jaundice* is commonly due to immaturity of the hepatic excretory system, particularly in premature infants. In the *Crigler-Najjar syndrome* (see Ch. 696), glucuronyl transferase activity is congenitally absent, the serum concentration of unconjugated bilirubin reaches high levels, and brain damage caused by deposition of pigment in the basal ganglia (kernicterus) is usual. Rare patients have survived to adulthood.

Inhibition of glucuronyl transferase activity by a steroid excreted in maternal milk is an unusual cause for neonatal jaundice.

Reduced Excretion of Conjugated Bilirubin.   The excretion of conjugated bilirubin into the bile canaliculus is an active transport process which may be impaired by a variety of processes. In the *Dubin-Johnson* and *Rotor syndromes* there is a congenital defect in hepatic excretion of conjugated bilirubin and other organic anions including sulfobromophthalein (BSP); the normal excretion of conjugated bile salts in these patients suggests a separate transport pathway. Impaired excretion may result from hepatocellular injury as in *virus hepatitis,* or may be due to *drugs* that interfere with cell metabolism or increase the permeability of the biliary tree (methyl testosterone, estrogens), compete for excretion in bile, or damage bile ductules (chlorpromazine). Inflammatory, granulomatous, or neoplastic *infiltration* of the liver and extrahepatic *bile duct obstruction* by gallstone, stricture, or carcinoma commonly interfere with bile excretion. The mechanism by which water-soluble, conjugated bilirubin enters the plasma in patients with impaired hepatic excretion is uncertain. The pigment either may be transferred across the liver cell directly into sinusoidal blood or may diffuse from bile ductules or canaliculi when the permeability of the biliary system is modified by disease.

Classification of Jaundice

Patients with jaundice may be subdivided clinically into two groups in which the serum bilirubin is either predominantly unconjugated or conjugated. *Unconjugated hyperbilirubinemia* is due to excessive production, reduced uptake, or reduced conjugation of pigment, whereas *conjugated hyperbilirubinemia* may result from hepatocellular or biliary tract disease. The terms *hemolytic jaundice, hepatocellular jaundice,* and *obstructive jaundice* of intra- and extrahepatic types *(intra- and extrahepatic cholestasis)* are often used to describe these types of jaundice. *Cholestasis* refers to reduced bile flow and reduced excretion of bile constituents; pathologically, there is usually evidence of bile stasis with bile plugs in the canaliculi. Several of the mechanisms discussed previously may be responsible for jaundice in a particular patient. As an example, in acute viral hepatitis mild hemolysis may increase bilirubin production; parenchymal cell damage may impair uptake, conjugation, and excretion of pigment; and intrahepatic cholestasis resulting from disruption of bile canaliculi or inflammation may reduce bile excretion.

Fecal and Urinary Excretion of Bile Pigments

Unconjugated bilirubin, tightly bound to albumin and relatively nonpolar, cannot be dialyzed from plasma and does not pass the glomerular filter; jaundice with unconjugated hyperbilirubinemia is thus *acholuric.* Bilirubin diglucuronide, less avidly bound to plasma albumin, is partly dialyzable from plasma, and is excreted in the urine by glomerular filtration. In the presence of complete biliary obstruction, the urinary excretion of conjugated bilirubin will be equal to bilirubin production, and serum levels will stabilize at 15 to 25 mg per 100 ml.

The quantity of bile pigment excreted as urobilinogens in feces and urine is a reflection of the amount of bilirubin in the bile, the bacterial conversion of bilirubin to urobilinogens, and the capacity of the liver to excrete urobilinogen absorbed from the intestine. *Fecal urobilinogen* is increased by excessive bilirubin production, and is reduced when hepatobiliary disease impairs bilirubin excretion or when bacterial conversion of bilirubin to urobilinogens is inhibited by antimicrobial therapy. *Urinary urobilinogen* is increased when greater amounts of urobilinogen are absorbed from the intestine or when parenchymal liver disease impairs the hepatic excretion of this pigment. Reduced urinary levels suggest cholestasis or impaired renal function.

PHYSICAL CHANGES OF THE DISEASED LIVER

Liver enlargement is usually an indication of disease. A normal liver displaced by a depressed diaphragm or a Riedel lobe must be considered in the differential diagnosis. An increase in liver size may reflect changes in liver cells (infiltration with fat or glycogen, or an increase in the smooth endoplasmic reticulum), cholestasis (intrahepatic or extrahepatic), venous congestion, inflammation (hepatitis) or abscess formation, cellular infiltration (macrophages in Gaucher's disease, granuloma in sarcoidosis, hematopoietic cells in extramedullary hematopoiesis, tumor cells in primary or secondary neoplasms), or fibrosis with regeneration (cirrhosis in the alcoholic). A *small liver* is characteristic of acute and subacute hepatic necrosis and idiopathic cirrhosis. The *consistency* of the liver may indicate the nature of the underlying disease. Infiltration and fibrosis cause induration; palpable *nodules* may be neoplasm, cysts, abscesses, or regeneration nodules. *Tenderness* may be due to acute enlargement or inflammation, and may be elicited by direct palpation or by percussion over the right lower ribs. Expansile *pulsation* of the congested liver results from tricuspid regurgitation. Vascular *bruits* over the liver may be due to arteriovenous fistulas, vascular tumors, or pressure on the aorta by an enlarged liver. *Friction rubs* are usually associated with neoplastic infiltration of the liver capsule and peritoneum, but may be due to peritonitis.

PORTAL HYPERTENSION

The normal flow of blood through the liver approximates 1.5 liters per minute (25 per cent of the cardiac output); portal venous inflow from the splanchnic circulation contributes approximately 1 liter per minute, and the hepatic artery 0.5 liter per minute. Portal venous and hepatic arterial blood combine in the periphery of the hepatic sinusoids and flow centrally to the central vein and hepatic venous system. Hepatic blood flow is normally phasic with a pressure gradient between portal vein and inferior vena cava of 0 to 5 mm Hg.

Portal hypertension, an increased pressure gradient across the liver, may be due to an increased splanchnic blood flow, or to an increased resistance to blood flow through the liver.

An increase in splanchnic blood flow may be due to *arteriovenous fistulas,* either congenital or secondary to ruptured splenic or hepatic artery aneurysms. Massive *splenomegaly* in patients with *hematologic disorders* (polycythemia vera, agnogenic myeloid metaplasia, lymphoma, or leukemia) is sometimes associated with portal hypertension; both an increase in splenic blood flow and infiltration of hepatic sinusoids by hematopoietic cells or tumor cells contribute to the elevation of portal pressure. In patients with *tropical splenomegaly,* portal hypertension is also secondary to an increased splenic blood flow. *Cirrhosis of the liver* is often associated with an increased cardiac output and decreased peripheral vascular resistance. Spider angiomas and palmar erythema result from local arteriovenous shunts. It has been suggested that patients with cirrhosis and portal hypertension have a decreased splenic and splanchnic vascular resistance with increased blood flow that contributes to the portal hypertension. Splenic blood flow measured by injection of radioactive xenon into the splenic artery is increased in patients with cirrhosis, whereas portal blood flow measured after portacaval shunts was not increased. An increase in the vascular resistance within the liver is the major factor in the pathogenesis of portal hypertension in cirrhosis.

Portal hypertension secondary to an increase in vascular resistance across the liver is seen in patients with portal venous occlusion, in cirrhosis where blood flow from sinusoids is obstructed by fibrosis and nodular regeneration, and in patients with obstruction of the hepatic veins. *Presinusoidal obstruction* of the portal vein may be *intrahepatic* with occlusion of the distal branches of the portal system in portal triads as in *schistosomiasis* and *congenital hepatic fibrosis,* or may be *extrahepatic* when the portal vein is occluded by thrombosis or tumor. *Postsinusoidal obstruction* of the hepatic veins may be due to thrombus or tumor (Budd-Chiari syndrome). In *veno-occlusive disease* fibrosis around central veins and branches of the hepatic vein obstructs venous outflow. In patients with *acute alcoholic hepatitis,* acute sclerosing hyaline necrosis causes obstruction of central veins and adjacent sinusoids prior to the development of cirrhosis. With the progressive development of cirrhosis, scarring and nodular regeneration further obstruct blood flow. *Infiltrative disease* (secondary neoplasm or granuloma) sometimes leads to clinically significant portal hypertension.

Manifestations

The manifestations of portal hypertension are *splenomegaly,* the development of a *collateral circulation,* and *ascites.*

Splenomegaly. Splenic enlargement is commonly due to venous congestion, but may also result from lymphoid hyperplasia and cellular infiltration. The spleen is not always palpable in patients with portal hypertension, and, conversely, an enlarged spleen does not necessarily imply that a patient with liver disease has portal hypertension. Splenomegaly in cirrhotic patients is usually associated with an increased splenic artery blood flow.

Portal-Systemic Collateral Vessels. Collateral veins draining from the portal to the systemic venous system develop in response to an *increased pressure gradient* at sites of anastomosis between portal and systemic veins—in the esophagus and lower rectum, in the falciform ligament, in the retroperitoneal space, and in adhesions between the visceral and parietal peritoneum.

Esophageal collateral vessels between the left gastric and azygos veins develop as tortuous, dilated, thin-walled submucosal veins that may extend from the fundus of the stomach to the midesophagus (esophageal and gastric varices). Collateral vessels between the inferior mesenteric and internal iliac veins may form hemorrhoids. Collaterals from the left branch of the portal vein through patent umbilical or paraumbilical veins in the falciform ligament to the anterior abdominal wall may form a caput medusae—dilated, tortuous veins radiating from the umbilicus with centrifugal blood flow to epigastric, lateral thoracic, and saphenous vessels. A venous hum may be audible at the umbilicus (Cruveilhier-Baumgarten syndrome). These subcutaneous collaterals are most prominent when the patient is erect, and their origin from the portal system may be proved by showing that the glucose content of variceal blood exceeds that of peripheral venous blood during glucose absorption.

Acute upper gastrointestinal bleeding from esophageal varices is the major complication of portal hypertension.

Ascites. Ascites is an accumulation of lymph in the peritoneal cavity. Hepatic and intestinal lymph normally drains through the thoracic duct into the left subclavian vein. Ascitic fluid accumulates when hepatic and intestinal lymph is formed in amounts that exceed the capacity of the thoracic duct to drain lymph from the abdomen. Two factors, portal hypertension and a lowered plasma colloidal osmotic pressure, contribute to the increased transudation of fluid from hepatic sinusoids and splanchnic capillaries in patients with liver disease. A third factor, increased plasma aldosterone concentration, augments sodium and water retention by promoting distal renal tubular reabsorption of sodium.

Portal hypertension caused by hepatic venous outflow tract obstruction (hepatic vein occlusion or cirrhosis), with increased hepatic sinusoidal pressure, is the major factor that determines the selective accumulation of fluid in the peritoneal cavity of patients with liver disease. Large volumes of hepatic lymph drain from congested sinusoids through dilated hilar lymphatic vessels to the thoracic duct, or may leak from lymphatic vessels in the capsule and hilum of the liver into the peritoneal cavity. Ascites in patients with liver disease is not a stagnant pool. There is a rapid exchange of water and electrolytes between plasma and ascites across the visceral peritoneum, and an increased volume of lymph drains through the thoracic duct from the abdominal viscera and peritoneal cavity.

Portal hypertension without sinusoidal hypertension rarely causes ascites unless acute bleeding from esophageal varices precipitates hypoalbuminemia and stimulates aldosterone secretion. (See Hepatic Schistosomiasis in Ch. 702.)

Hypoalbuminemia with a lowered plasma colloidal osmotic pressure increases fluid transudation from hepatic sinusoids and splanchnic capillaries, and thus augments lymph flow from these congested vascular beds. Hypoalbuminemic patients without portal hypertension, however, develop ascites only as a manifestation of fluid accumulation in dependent parts, as in the nephrotic syndrome.

In cirrhotic patients with ascites there are increased urinary excretion and plasma concentration of aldosterone, owing in part to an increased adrenal secretion of aldosterone and in part to reduced hepatic metabolism of the hormone. Although it has been shown that inferior vena caval obstruction proximal to the hepatic veins in the dog stimulates aldosterone secretion, the exact mechanism of secondary hyperaldosteronism in patients with cirrhosis and portal hypertension has not been defined. A relative pooling of blood in the splanchnic bed with reduced renal blood flow may be the primary stimulus for the release of renin from the juxtaglomerular cells in the kidney and the subsequent secretion of salt-retaining hormone. Aldosterone secretion will be further augmented by hemorrhage, infection, and the administration of diuretic agents to these patients.

Ascites is sometimes precipitated by peritonitis (especially tuberculous) or tumor invasion of the peritoneal cavity. These complications must be considered in the differential diagnosis (see below).

The clinical manifestations of ascites are increasing abdominal distention with weight gain and an associated decrease in urine output. Distention of the abdominal wall may cause pain over the lower ribs at the insertion of the abdominal muscles, and may promote the formation of umbilical and inguinal hernias. On physical examination there may be shifting dullness, a fluid wave, and elevation of the diaphragms. Ascitic fluid may leak through the diaphragm to create a pleural effusion; this is more often seen on the right than on the left. The urinary excretion of sodium is considerably decreased and may be less than 1 mEq in 24 hours, whereas urinary potassium excretion is increased.

NEUROPSYCHIATRIC ABNORMALITIES ASSOCIATED WITH LIVER DISEASE

The neuropsychiatric manifestations of acute alcohol intoxication, prolonged excessive use of alcohol, alcohol withdrawal, vitamin deficiency in alcoholics, and head injury are often encountered in patients with cirrhosis. These are considered in Ch. 347. Wilson's disease (see Ch. 945) is important in the differential diagnosis of patients with juvenile cirrhosis.

Hepatic Coma and Precoma
(Hepatic Encephalopathy, Portal-Systemic Encephalopathy)

Patients with acute or chronic liver disease may develop a metabolic encephalopathy characterized by a variable disturbance of consciousness, psychiatric changes, a flapping tremor with hyperreflexia and increased muscle tone, hyperventilation with respiratory alkalosis, and a typical fetor.

Pathogenesis. Hepatic coma is associated either with severe impairment of liver function or with shunting of portal venous blood through collateral vessels into the peripheral circulation. There may be an accumulation of toxic substances which impair cerebral function or a lack of substances which are necessary for cerebral function. Of the several factors that may contribute to this metabolic encephalopathy, changes in ammonium metabolism have been studied most extensively. An increase in blood ammonium concentration parallels the severity of neuropsychiatric changes in cirrhotic patients with *chronic* encephalopathy after portacaval anastomosis. This increase in blood ammonium concentration resulting from enteric absorption of ammonia formed by bacterial deamination of amino acids or urea hydrolysis may be the major biochemical change that precipitates dysfunction of the central nervous system. In patients with *acute* hepatic coma, however, disturbances of ammonium metabolism may be of lesser importance, and blood ammonium levels may be normal.

Other agents which may impair central nervous system function in cirrhotic patients include *short chain fatty acids* (from the diet or from bacterial metabolism of carbohydrate) and bacterial metabolites of protein and amino acids, particularly biogenic amines which may function as false neurotransmitters.

The central nervous system of the patient with liver disease may be more susceptible to a variety of metabolic insults. Thus *hypoxia, electrolyte* and *acid-base imbalance, infection,* and *depressant drugs* may each contribute to metabolic encephalopathy in these patients. Although there may be changes in the serum concentration of electrolytes, elevation of blood ammonium concentration, and/or altered blood pH in patients with hepatic coma, these changes do not necessarily parallel electrolyte and pH changes and ammonium concentrations in the central nervous system. These changes *within the brain* are of primary importance in precipitating encephalopathy; alkalosis, which favors the diffusion of ammonia across the blood-brain barrier, increases ammonia toxicity. In patients with hepatic encephalopathy, there is a decrease in cerebral metabolism and oxygen utilization. There is some evidence that ammonia inhibits oxidative phosphorylation.

Clinical Features. The neuropsychiatric changes in hepatic encephalopathy are nonspecific. One of the more characteristic features of the metabolic encephalopathy associated with liver disease is its *rapid fluctuation. Disturbances of consciousness* may range from mild lethargy to deep coma. *Personality changes,* with depression or euphoria, irritability, anxiety, and paranoid features, together with a loss of concern for person or property, are evident. Intellectual function is variably impaired with *memory loss, inability to concentrate,* and a loss of the capacity for abstract thought. Speech may be slow and slurred, with a loss of modulation, and writing deteriorates; there may be dysphasia, perseveration, and apraxia. The common neurologic changes are asterixis, a "flapping" tremor of the outstretched hands, an increase in muscle tone, hyper-reflexia with clonus—often with flexor plantar responses—and ataxia. Hyperventilation causes repiratory alkalosis. The electroencephalogram shows the nonspecific changes of metabolic encephalopathy; high amplitude delta waves (2 to 3 per second) replace normal alpha waves.

Fetor hepaticus is a characteristic sweet, musty odor of the breath attributed to the excretion of mercaptans, particularly dimethylsulfide. Mercaptans produced by bacterial degradation of methionine escape hepatic detoxification and are excreted in excessive amounts in cirrhotic patients.

The *clinical course* of hepatic encephalopathy varies with its pathogenesis. In patients with *fulminant hepatitis* there is a rapid progression; mania and convulsions may precede the development of decerebrate rigidity and terminal deep coma. In patients with cirrhosis, encephalopathy may be acute or chronic and of varying severity.

Chronic encephalopathy usually improves with therapy (see below), but may progress to permanent neuropsychiatric syndromes (paraplegia, dementia) over a period of years.

CLINICAL MANIFESTATIONS RESULTING FROM IMPAIRED HEPATIC DETOXIFICATION

The liver cell is the major site of detoxification of many drugs and exogenous substances and of endogenous substances, including hormones. In general, by processes of oxidation, reduction, hydrolysis, or conjugation, mediated by enzymes in the smooth endoplasmic reticulum, relatively lipid-soluble substances are converted to water-soluble compounds that may be excreted in bile or urine.

Changes in Drug Metabolism. Several drugs (e.g., phenobarbital) stimulate the hepatic metabolism of drugs. Prolonged phenobarbital administration leads to hyperplasia of the smooth endoplasmic reticulum and an increase in the level of drug metabolizing enzymes. The concentration of hepatic binding proteins, Y and Z, which combine with drugs, also increases. The effects of alcohol (ethanol) on hepatic drug metabolism are of clinical importance. In the acutely intoxicated patient, drug metabolism is depressed; alcohol inhibits drug-metabolizing enzymes. The chronic alcoholic, withdrawn from alcohol, metabolizes drugs more rapidly than normal as a result of hyperplasia of the endoplasmic reticulum; this accelerated metabolism increases his tolerance to both alcohol and other drugs. When alcoholism causes alcoholic hepatitis or cirrhosis, drug metabolism is often depressed.

When hepatic detoxification is impaired in patients with liver disease, the pharmacologic action of some drugs may be augmented and prolonged as higher blood levels are maintained for longer periods of time than in normal subjects.

Endocrine Changes. The liver has a dual role in the metabolism of hormones. Several plasma proteins, alpha globulins, which bind hormones in the plasma, e.g., *thyroxin-binding protein, transcortin,* are synthesized by the liver; hormone activity may be influenced by protein binding in the plasma. Thyroxin and adrenal and gonadal steroid hormones are conjugated in the liver and partly excreted in bile. Conjugation forms polar, water-soluble molecules that have an enterohepatic circulation and are finally excreted in the urine.

Endocrine abnormalities in patients with liver disease may be due to malnutrition or chronic illness, to specific lesions of the endocrine glands (iron infiltration in hemochromatosis), or to altered hepatic metabolism, conjugation, and excretion of hormones by the diseased liver. Disturbances of gonadal function are particularly common in patients with cirrhosis. In males, there may be *hypogonadism,* with small testes, reduced libido and impotence, *gynecomastia,* and delayed development or regression of secondary sex characteristics. Depressed plasma levels of unbound 17β-hydroxy-androgens (particularly testosterone) with normal plasma levels of unbound estradiol have been documented in these patients with gynecomastia. In females there may be delayed menarche, oligomenorrhea, or amenorrhea with subnormal breast development. Normal cyclic hormonal activity is disturbed, and cessation of ovulation leads to sterility.

Cutaneous *striae, acne,* and *hirsutism* with truncal obesity and moon facies may suggest *Cushing's syndrome.* Although plasma cortisol levels may be slightly elevated in these patients, the urinary excretion of hydroxy- and ketosteroids is either normal or subnormal.

The appearance of some alcoholic patients with cirrhosis may suggest *hyperthyroidism.* There may be a tremor, peripheral vasodilatation with sweating, tachycardia, and a slight stare. Although the basal metabolic rate and the uptake and conversion of radioiodine by the thyroid may be increased (particularly if there is iodine deficiency), the serum protein-bound iodine concentration is normal.

NUTRITIONAL AND METABOLIC ABNORMALITIES IN LIVER DISEASE

Weight loss may be due to malabsorption, reduced caloric intake in patients with anorexia, or increased tissue catabolism in acutely ill febrile patients. The chronic alcoholic, deriving a major fraction of his calories from alcohol, consumes a diet that may be deficient in protein, folic acid, ascorbic acid, B vitamins, and minerals. Although body weight may be maintained by alcohol and carbohydrate, *muscle wasting* with progressive weakness is usual. *Hypokalemia,* magnesium deficiency, or alcoholic *myopathy* may accentuate muscle weakness in some patients.

Carbohydrate Metabolism. The liver has a central role in regulating blood sugar levels. During carbohydrate absorption, the monosaccharides glucose, fructose, and galactose are taken up from portal venous blood by liver cells, phosphorylated in the presence of specific hexokinases, and converted to glycogen or metabolized through pyruvate and Krebs cycle intermediates. During periods of fasting, or with secretion of epinephrine and glucagon, glycogenolysis or gluconeogenesis maintains or increases blood sugar levels.

Symptomatic *hypoglycemia* may occur in liver disease when hepatic glycogenolysis and gluconeogenesis are impaired. When liver glycogen stores are depleted by fasting, the ingestion of alcohol, which inhibits gluconeogenesis, may precipitate hypoglycemia *(alcoholic hypoglycemia).* Lowered blood sugar levels also result from massive hepatic necrosis (fulminant hepatitis) or a deficiency of enzymes necessary for glycogenolysis (glycogen storage diseases).

Diabetes mellitus in patients with cirrhosis is often due to associated pancreatic disease (chronic alcoholic pancreatitis, or hemochromatosis), or may be coincidental. Portal-systemic shunting is associated with a higher frequency of diabetes mellitus; plasma glucagon levels are significantly elevated in these patients. Cirrhotic patients often have an abnormal glucose tolerance curve owing to a reduced rate of glucose uptake and release from the diseased liver. Normal fasting blood sugar levels, with prolonged hyperglycemia and late hypoglycemia after a glucose load, are characteristic.

Triglyceride Metabolism. Postprandially, dietary triglyceride enters the circulation as a lipid emulsion (chyle) from the thoracic duct (fatty acids of chain length greater than C10), or passes directly as fatty acid into the portal venous blood (fatty acids of chain length less than C10). During periods of fasting, free fatty acid (FFA) is mobilized from peripheral fat depots and circulates as an albumin-FFA complex. Plasma FFA or triglyceride entering the liver cell is stored as triglyceride droplets, incorporated into plasma lipoproteins and thus transported to peripheral depots or catabolized to ketone bodies for peripheral utilization.

Triglyceride accumulates in the liver whenever there is excessive peripheral mobilization of fat or when liver cell injury prevents the normal metabolism of triglyceride. A fatty liver is commonly found in obese subjects, in diabetics, in normal subjects during starvation, and in alcoholics. The disturbances in triglyceride metabolism caused by acute and chronic alcohol ingestion are discussed in Ch. 709.

Cholesterol and Bile Acids. Cholesterol synthesized in the liver is either incorporated into plasma lipoproteins, excreted directly into bile, or converted to primary bile acids.

Plasma lipoproteins, containing varying amounts of cholesterol (both free and esterified), phospholipid, triglyceride, and specific proteins, are synthesized by the liver and intestinal epithelium. Cholestasis causes an increase in plasma cholesterol concentration; this is associated with an increase in high density lipoprotein with a high content of cholesterol and phospholipid. This does not cause a lipemic serum. Liver failure with impaired hepatic synthesis depresses serum concentrations of lipoprotein and cholesterol.

Cholesterol is excreted in bile as a micellar solution with conjugated bile salt and phospholipid. Changes in the concentration of these compounds may lead to the formation of gallstones (see Ch. 682 to 686).

The primary bile acids (cholic and chenodeoxycholic acids) are synthesized from cholesterol and are secreted in bile as their glycine and taurine conjugates (bile salts). These conjugated bile salts undergo an enterohepatic circulation with active reabsorption from the distal small intestine. Between 20 and 30 grams of conjugated bile salts are thus excreted in bile and reabsorbed daily; the daily fecal loss of bile acids (approximately 1 gram) is balanced by resynthesis from cholesterol.

The conjugated bile salts have important functions that depend on their detergent properties. In the bile they permit the formation of soluble micelles containing cholesterol; in the intestinal lumen they activate pancreatic lipase and form mixed micelles with monoglyceride and long-chain fatty acids, thus facilitating the absorption of fat and fat-soluble vitamins.

In patients with cirrhosis there is a greatly diminished total bile acid pool. This depressed bile acid pool does not lead to the formation of cholesterol gallstones, because decreased biliary bile acid secretion is accompanied by a parallel decrease in cholesterol excretion.

Liver disease may be complicated by *malabsorption* when biliary secretion of conjugated bile salts is insufficient to promote the formation of lipid micelles in the jejunum. The duration of malabsorption in patients with acute liver disease may be too short to cause deficiency states other than *hypoprothrombinemia* owing to malabsorption of vitamin K. In patients with chronic cholestasis (primary and secondary biliary cirrhosis, Ch. 709) steatorrhea may cause diarrhea and weight loss, whereas malabsorption of fat-soluble vitamins A, D, and K may lead to night blindness, bone demineralization, and hypoprothrombinemia.

Protein Metabolism. The liver cell contains enzyme systems that permit the synthesis of nonessential amino acids, synthesis of cellular and plasma proteins from amino acids, catabolism of plasma protein and amino acids, and conversion of ammonia to urea.

Amino acids derived from digested dietary proteins are absorbed in the upper small intestine, enter the portal venous blood, and are almost completely cleared by the liver to be catabolized or utilized in protein synthesis. During periods of fasting, amino acids are converted to pyruvate and phosphorylated hexose intermediates, which support gluconeogenesis and provide a source of glucose for brain metabolism.

Perfusion studies have shown that the liver is responsible for the synthesis of plasma proteins, with the exception of the immunoglobulins and antihemophiliac globulin (AHG). The factors which control protein synthesis are not well understood. Experimental studies suggest that the colloidal osmotic pressure of plasma has a regulatory function; albumin synthesis is depressed in laboratory animals or isolated liver preparations when the colloidal osmotic pressure of plasma is increased with dextran or gamma globulin. Adequate nutrition is essential for normal plasma protein synthesis; liver perfusion studies have shown that tryptophan exerts a specific role in activating albumin synthesis.

The sites of plasma protein degradation and the factors which regulate this are unknown. Studies with labeled albumin indicate that catabolism is in proportion to the total albumin pool. Catabolism by the liver, kidney, and gastrointestinal tract is well documented, but explains only a fraction of the total albumin catabolized daily.

Plasma proteins maintain the colloidal osmotic pressure of plasma, play a vital role in the transport of many substances (including iron, vitamin B_{12}, hormones, hemoglobin, bilirubin, and nonesterified fatty acids), and maintain normal blood clotting mechanisms.

Hepatic synthesis of plasma proteins may be impaired by hepatocellular failure. A reduced rate of plasma protein catabolism may partly compensate for reduced synthesis, which leads to *hypoproteinemia*. Severe *bleeding* may complicate a deficiency of blood-clotting factors. Excessive urinary excretion and elevated plasma levels of amino acids are manifestations of severe hepatocellular failure, particularly fulminant hepatitis. Although urea is synthesized by the liver, low blood urea levels are more often the result of dilution with fluid infused intravenously than of hepatocellular failure.

HEMATOLOGIC ABNORMALITIES

Anemia in patients with liver disease may be due to *blood loss* or *excessive destruction* and/or *reduced formation* of red cells. Changes in red cell morphology may reflect specific deficiency (iron or folic acid) or may result from changes in the lipid composition of the red cell membrane. Red blood cells from patients with cholestasis have an increased surface area related to the reversible accumulation of cholesterol from the plasma; these cells have a lowered osmotic fragility, and appear as target-cells on stained smears. Severe hemolysis in the alcoholic with liver disease may be associated with the appearance of poikilocytes (burr-cells) on peripheral smears.

Bleeding from the nose, upper gastrointestinal tract (esophageal varices, erosive gastritis, or peptic ulcer), or rectum (hemorrhoids) may precipitate acute anemia or chronic iron deficiency anemia. In the absence of blood loss, iron deficiency is uncommon in patients with liver disease; an increase in total body iron with hemosiderosis is more usual, particularly in alcoholic patients with pancreatic disease. The pathogenesis of this secondary hemosiderosis is not known.

Hemolysis is the most common cause of chronic anemia in patients with liver disease. Chronic, low-grade hemolysis in patients with splenomegaly is due to sequestration of red blood cells in the cortex of the congested spleen. Red cell production may fail to compensate for this increased destruction, particularly during periods of hepatic decompensation, so that the patient may exhibit a normochromic and sometimes macrocytic anemia with a normal reticulocyte count, reduced serum levels of haptoglobin, an increased serum level of unconjugated bilirubin, and a bone marrow showing cellular hyperplasia. Severe hemolytic anemia may be associated with hyperlipemia in alcoholic hepatitis *(Zieve's syndrome)* (see Ch. 709), but a causal relationship between the hyperlipemia and hemolysis has not been established. Acute viral hepatitis may precipitate hemolysis in patients with *glucose-6-phosphate dehydrogenase (G-6-PD) deficiency;* particularly high serum concentrations of bilirubin usually result.

A *deficiency of folic acid* may lead to a severe macrocytic anemia with *megaloblastic* bone marrow in alcoholic patients with liver disease. An inadequate vitamin intake, together with alcohol inhibition of folic acid utilization, contributes to the anemia. Treatment with a normal diet containing folic acid or with folic acid supplements corrects this deficiency. Rarely, a normochromic normocytic anemia may be due to *pyridoxine deficiency.*

Although *thrombocytopenia* (platelet counts less than 200,000 per cubic millimeter) and *granulocytopenia* (WBC counts < 4000 per cubic millimeter) may be associated with anemia in patients with liver disease and congestive splenomegaly, these abnormalities are rarely complicated by serious bleeding or infection. Severe thrombocytopenia and fatal aplastic anemia have been reported as complications of acute viral hepatitis.

Clotting abnormalities in patients with acute or chronic liver disease result from reduced synthesis of blood-clotting factors or their increased consumption. Many of the factors active in blood clotting—factors V, VII, IX, X, prothrombin, and fibrinogen—are synthesized by the liver. A lowered plasma concentration of these proteins, measured by blood-clotting tests (see Ch. 795), may be due to *malabsorption of vitamin K* which is required for the synthesis of prothrombin and factors VII, IX, and X, or may reflect *impaired hepatic protein synthesis.* Vitamin K malabsorption results from obstructive jaundice. Hepatic parenchymal disease, either acute or chronic, depresses the synthesis of clotting factors; the capacity of liver cells to produce fibrinogen appears to exceed that of other clotting factors, because fibrinogen levels are often maintained when other clotting factors are deficient. *Intravascular coagulation* with consumption of clotting factors, thrombocytopenia, and the appearance of fibrin split products in the plasma is a complication of fulminant hepatitis, decompensated cirrhosis, and metastatic cancer.

IMMUNE PHENOMENA IN LIVER DISEASE

Hypergammaglobulinemia is a common manifestation of *chronic active hepatitis, idiopathic cirrhosis,* and *primary biliary cirrhosis.* The gamma globulin increase is *polyclonal,* involving all classes of immunoglobulin (IgA, IgM, and IgG), although in primary biliary cirrhosis IgM may be increased selectively. Hypergammaglobulinemia is often associated with positive serologic tests for syphilis, heterophil antibody, antinuclear antibody, antimitochondrial antibody, and LE cell phenomena. Furthermore the titers of antibody against bacterial and viral antigens may be increased. An increase in circulating immunoglobulin in patients with liver disease usually reflects *infiltration of the liver* with plasma cells and lymphocytes, particularly in areas of parenchymal cell necrosis.

The role of *immunologic mechanisms* in the *pathogenesis* of chronic liver disease has not been established. The immune phenomena may be secondary to the release of antigens from damaged liver cells, or, alternatively, local immunologic processes may play an active role in destroying liver cells. The association between chronic liver disease, chronic thyroiditis, and Sjögren's syndrome suggests that autoimmune phenomena may indeed be important in pathogenesis (see Ch. 708 and 709). Depression of *serum complement* levels in patients with chronic liver disease cannot be correlated with immune phenomena, but appears to be related to impaired hepatic protein synthesis.

CARDIOVASCULAR CHANGES

Hepatocellular failure is often associated with an *increase* in *cardiac output* manifested by tachycardia, a precordial ejection systolic murmur, and peripheral vasodilatation. The cause for these circulatory changes is not known.

Some patients with cirrhosis exhibit central *cyanosis* with arterial oxygen unsaturation. In patients with portal hypertension, this may be due to portopulmonary venous shunts that bypass the pulmonary capillaries, or may result from pulmonary arteriovenous shunts or reduced aeration of basal lung segments in patients with tense ascites.

The plasma volume is usually normal or increased in cirrhotic patients prior to diuretic therapy. When patients with ascites are treated with diuretic agents, brisk diuresis is often accompanied by a fall in plasma volume which is particularly marked when fluid loss exceeds the volume of fluid mobilized from the ascitic pool. Hypovolemic shock may be a terminal complication of cirrhosis, precipitated by massive bleeding, by infection (especially gram-negative septicemia), or by paracentesis. Metabolic acidosis with hyperkalemia and hyponatremia are terminal events.

CHANGES IN RENAL FUNCTION

There are many causes for impairment of renal function in patients with liver disease. Many agents may cause acute cellular injury in both liver and kidneys; these include *hepatotoxins* (carbon tetrachloride, *Amanita phalloides*), *infectious agents* (leptospirosis, infectious hepatitis virus; see below), and *hypoxia* (shock). *Metabolic diseases* may damage both organs; in Wilson's disease the deposition of copper in the tissues is associated with cirrhosis and impaired tubular reabsorptive function with glycosuria, aminoaciduria, and hypouricemia.

In patients with cirrhosis and ascites several factors modify renal function. There may be a physiologic response to secondary hyperaldosteronism with sodium retention and potassium excretion, reversed by aldosterone-blocking drugs (see below). Abnormal excretion of a water load usually accompanies cirrhosis with ascites.

Hepatorenal Syndrome. This term refers to the functional renal failure which is a common terminal event in patients with cirrhosis and ascites, and a less common complication of obstructive jaundice after surgery. Progressive azotemia with hyperkalemia and hyponatremia, a reduced creatinine clearance, and progressive oliguria with a concentrated urine free of protein and formed elements and low in sodium are usually observed. Spontaneous recovery is rare. At postmortem examination, no significant pathologic changes are present in the kidneys.

The functional renal failure in patients with cirrhosis and ascites has been attributed to a decrease in renal blood flow resulting from hypovolemia after vigorous diuresis, abdominal paracentesis, or massive bleeding. Alternatively, increased renal vein pressure caused by increased intra-abdominal pressure was suggested as a mechanism. Although hypovolemia will contribute to renal failure, these mechanisms do not explain this syndrome. Studies of renal blood flow by isotope scanning and by renal arteriography have demonstrated an intrarenal shunting of blood with reduced cortical perfusion in cirrhotic patients with ascites and reduced creatinine clearance. Vasoconstriction of cortical vessels reduces glomerular perfusion, although total renal blood flow may remain normal. The agents which cause cortical vasoconstriction have not been identified, but it is known that sympathetic blocking agents do not restore cortical flow.

When a cirrhotic patient with ascites develops the hepatorenal syndrome, increasing jaundice results from decreased bilirubin excretion in the urine, and azotemia with increased blood ammonia levels usually precipitates hepatic coma.

CUTANEOUS MANIFESTATIONS OF LIVER DISEASE

Pruritus. Patients with obstructive jaundice (both intrahepatic and extrahepatic cholestasis) may suffer from generalized itching. This is probably caused by retained *bile acids.* The intensity of pruritus parallels the serum concentration of bile acids, and the oral administration of the resin cholestyramine lowers serum bile acid levels and relieves itching by binding bile salts in the intestine and preventing their reabsorption. *Itching is not related to the intensity of jaundice;* anicteric patients may itch because of retained bile salts, whereas deeply jaundiced patients may be free of pruritus when cholesterol and bile acid synthesis is impaired by hepatocellular failure.

Pigmentation. An increase in *melanin pigmentation* of the skin is typical of chronic obstructive jaundice (biliary cirrhosis) and in hemochromatosis. The pathogenesis is not known.

Spider Angiomas (Vascular Spiders). These cutaneous lesions, found in areas drained by the superior vena cava, have a central pulsating arteriole from which small vessels radiate over an area 1 to 10 mm in diameter. Multiple lesions may appear and disappear during the course of both acute and chronic liver disease, but are most numerous when liver disease is chronic and progressive. Small arterial spiders are also seen in normal subjects, and often appear during pregnancy. Their pathogenesis is not known.

Palmar Erythema. Cutaneous erythema, maximal over the thenar and hypothenar eminences and the pulp of the fingers and less often seen on the soles of the feet, is due to local vasodilatation with increased blood flow. The cardiac output is usually increased in patients with prominent palmar erythema.

Other changes in the hands include *Dupuytren's contractures* in patients with cirrhosis associated with alcohol ingestion, *clubbing* of the nails in patients with biliary cirrhosis, and white, opaque nails with loss of lunules in hypoalbuminemic patients.

Xanthomas. Prolonged obstructive jaundice with elevation of serum lipoprotein may be associated with deposits of lipid, predominantly cholesterol, in macrophages in the dermis or subcutaneous tissue. Flat lesions *(xanthelasma)* are common on the eyelids, on the neck, and in the palm creases, as yellow, slightly raised, soft deposits. Tuberous lesions, more common over areas exposed to pressure, are firm, nodular, and slightly yellow. These lesions may appear when serum cholesterol levels exceed 450 mg per 100 ml for several months, and may disappear when serum cholesterol levels fall below that value.

NONSPECIFIC SYMPTOMS IN PATIENTS WITH LIVER DISEASE

Many symptoms in patients with liver disease are also common manifestations of nonhepatic disorders. It is often impossible to determine whether these symptoms are primarily due to liver disease or whether they result from extrahepatic effects of the primary noxious agent. The prodromal symptoms of acute viral hepatitis—malaise, weakness, unusual fatigability, anorexia, fever, myalgia, and headache—are good examples. Although these symptoms are nonspecific, they are often helpful in differential diagnosis.

Fever. Fever is common in patients with acute liver disease and is usually due to tissue necrosis, infection, or drug hypersensitivity. In patients with acute metabolic encephalopathy, fever may be due to dysfunction of central thermoregulatory mechanisms. This usually occurs in fulminant hepatitis and in the alcoholic with a severe withdrawal reaction (delirium tremens).

Abdominal Pain. Abdominal pain may be localized to the right upper quadrant and may result from inflammation or stretching of the pain-sensitive capsule of the liver. Epigastric or midabdominal pain may be due to associated peptic ulcer disease, acute gastritis, or pancreatitis. Stretching of the abdominal wall by tense ascites may cause pain over the lower costal margin.

695. DIAGNOSTIC PROCEDURES

TESTS OF LIVER FUNCTION

Many biochemical tests have been used to estimate liver function. In interpreting tests of liver function one must remember that no test is diagnostic of specific liver lesion, that many tests may be normal in the presence of liver disease, and that factors other than liver disease may cause abnormal tests.

Serum Bilirubin. Spectrophotometric measurement of the amount of diazo-pigment formed by the van den Bergh reaction after one minute in the absence of alcohol gives an estimate of the *direct-reacting* serum bilirubin concentration; this is approximately equal to the serum concentration of *conjugated bilirubin*, which is diazotized in the absence of alcohol. When alcohol is added in the van den Bergh reaction, unconjugated bilirubin is able to react with the diazo reagent, and the total concentration of bilirubin (direct plus indirect reacting) in the serum is estimated. Normal serum contains less than 0.2 mg of direct-reacting pigment and less than 0.8 mg of indirect-reacting pigment per 100 ml. Measurements of serum bilirubin (direct-reacting and total) are helpful in separating diseases associated with unconjugated bilirubinemia from those causing predominantly conjugated hyperbilirubinemia, but are of no value in differentiating jaundice resulting from hepatocellular disease from extrahepatic cholestasis. Serial determinations of serum bilirubin concentration provide a more accurate measure of the impairment of bilirubin excretion during the course of liver disease than can be gained by a clinical assessment of the degree of jaundice.

Tests for *bilirubin in the urine* are helpful in differentiating jaundice caused by unconjugated hyperbilirubinemia; only conjugated bilirubin is excreted in the urine. Bilirubin may be excreted in the urine when the elevation of serum bilirubin is insufficient to cause jaundice.

Urinary and Fecal Urobilinogen. Urinary excretion of urobilinogen increases when the amount of urobilinogen absorbed from the intestine is increased by excessive pigment production or when hepatic excretion of urobilinogen is impaired by liver disease. Normally, urobilinogen can be detected in urine diluted to 1 in 16. *An increase in urinary urobilinogen excretion in the absence of increased fecal excretion of pigment is a very sensitive indicator of liver disease.* A quantitative measurement of the 24-hour fecal excretion of urobilinogen is of diagnostic value in hemolytic states and in patients with biliary tract disease. An increased fecal excretion of urobilinogen confirms that there is excessive bilirubin production, and a total absence of urobilinogen in the stool indicates complete biliary tract obstruction owing to atresia or neoplasm.

Sulfobromophthalein Sodium (Bromsulphalein, BSP) Clearance. The measurement of the hepatic clearance of this organic, anionic dye is the most sensitive test of liver function. Injected BSP, bound by plasma proteins (albumin and alpha globulin), is cleared by the liver and excreted in bile. BSP excretion by the liver depends on the selective uptake and concentration of dye by Y and Z binding proteins in the liver cell and the rate-limiting active transport of both unconjugated and glutathione-conjugated BSP into the bile canaliculi. BSP clearance varies with bile salt excretion, and can be increased experimentally by intravenous infusion of bile salt which augments excretion by increasing canalicular bile flow.

In the standard liver function test, the amount of BSP retained in the plasma is measured 30 or 45 minutes after an intravenous injection of the dye (5 mg per kilogram of body weight). The normal subject excretes more than 90 and 96 per cent of the injected BSP in 30 and 45 minutes, respectively. A reduced plasma clearance of BSP (increased retention of dye in the plasma) may result from changes in hepatic blood flow as in congestive heart failure or portal vein thrombosis, from reduced ability of liver cells to concentrate or excrete the dye as in hepatocellular injury and metabolic abnormalities, or from obstruction to bile flow in intrahepatic and extrahepatic cholestasis. Thus abnormal BSP excretion does not indicate a specific hepatic lesion. The dye should be injected with care, because leakage outside the vein causes severe pain and tissue necrosis.

Although the standard BSP test is a sensitive measure of liver function, the maximal capacity of the liver to excrete the dye is not measured. The maximal capacity of the liver to concentrate and to excrete BSP may be estimated by measuring plasma clearance when infusions of the dye are given. Either of these maxima may be reduced when all other tests of liver function remain normal. In some patients with liver disease, the maximal excretion rate of the dye may be reduced when hepatic storage is normal or increased.

Albumin. Normal levels of plasma albumin are maintained by an equilibrium between hepatic synthesis and degradation or loss. When synthesis is reduced in liver disease, the serum albumin concentration and the total body albumin pool decrease until a new equilibrium is established between synthesis and degradation. In view of the slow rate of albumin degradation (the half-time of plasma albumin degradation varies between 12 and 18 days), the serum concentration of albumin does not immediately reflect rapid changes in liver function, but decreases slowly when synthesis is impaired. In patients with cirrhosis, a depressed level of serum albumin reflects reduced synthesis and/or distribution of the albumin pool in an expanded extravascular space (ascitic fluid).

Globulins. Changes in the concentration of the serum globulins can be assessed by salt fractionation or by electrophoresis of serum. *Alpha and beta globulin* concentrations increase in patients with infection or obstructive jaundice and decrease when hepatocellular failure impairs their synthesis. The serum concentration of the *immunoglobulins* increases when antibody production is stimulated by exogenous or tissue antigen. Although immunoglobulin synthesis is not a function of the liver, measurements of serum gamma globulin concentrations are helpful in diagnosis. Extreme hypergammaglobulinemia suggests a diagnosis of chronic active hepatitis, or cirrhosis. Positive tests for antinuclear and smooth muscle antibody and LE cell reaction are frequent in patients with chronic active hepatitis, whereas antimitochondrial antibody tests are usually positive in patients with primary biliary cirrhosis (see Ch. 708 and Primary Biliary Cirrhosis in Ch. 709).

The serum *flocculation tests* are nonspecific tests in which the plasma proteins are precipitated or flocculated by a variety of agents. Positive tests depend on relative changes in the concentration of several plasma proteins and are not specific for liver disease.

Blood-Clotting Tests. Tests of blood coagulation provide a sensitive measure of hepatic synthetic function. The relatively short half-life (two to four days) of several of the blood-clotting factors leads to a rapid change in the one-stage prothrombin time when synthesis is depressed by acute parenchymal liver disease. In acute hepatitis, the prothrombin time is a valuable guide to the severity of parenchymal damage; marked prolongation of the prothrombin time (greater than 20 seconds) is an early reflection of massive necrosis. Whenever clotting tests are used to measure liver function, possible deficiency of vitamin K should be first excluded by parenteral therapy.

Cholesterol. Changes in serum cholesterol concentrations reflect changes in serum lipoprotein. In cholestasis, when cholesterol and bile acid excretion is impaired but cholesterol synthesis is normal, serum lipoprotein and cholesterol concentrations increase. When hepatic lipoprotein synthesis is impaired by hepatocellular disease, serum cholesterol concentrations fall.

Serum Enzymes. A large number of enzymes normally concentrated in the liver (and other tissues) are also present at low activity in the plasma. The level of enzyme activity in the plasma is determined by the rate of release from cells and the rate of clearance from plasma, in addition to the presence of activators or inhibitors in the plasma. Three patterns of abnormal plasma enzyme activity which depend on differences in enzyme synthesis and release are seen in patients with liver disease.

1. *Increased enzyme activity due to release from damaged liver cells.* Enzymes present in high concentration in the liver cell are released with damage to parenchymal cells. These enzymes include the *transaminases* and *dehydrogenases* which are measured routinely in clinical laboratories. The wide tissue distribution of these enzymes limits their specificity in localizing the site of cell damage unless other diagnostic criteria are used concomitantly or unless the elevation of serum enzyme is of such degree that liver cell damage could be the only source. In *acute hepatitis,* serum transaminase levels are usually elevated to levels in excess of 500 iu, but the degree of enzyme elevation correlates poorly with the extent of liver cell necrosis seen on liver biopsy. In patients with fulminant hepatitis, progressive clinical deterioration is often accompanied by a fall in serum enzyme activity (see Ch. 698). In *chronic active hepatitis,* the level of serum transaminase reflects the activity of the disease process and is a useful guide to therapy with corticosteroids (see Ch. 708).

2. *Increased enzyme activity due to de novo synthesis by liver cells and/or bile ducts with release into plasma.* The serum levels of alkaline phosphatase, 5'-nucleotidase, and leucine aminopeptidase are increased in patients with cholestasis—either intrahepatic or extrahepatic. Experimental studies have shown that the increase in serum alkaline phosphatase activity after bile duct ligation is due to the release of enzyme that is newly synthesized in the liver. The level of serum alkaline phosphatase is of no value in the differential diagnosis of obstructive jaundice. When the origin of the serum alkaline phosphatase is uncertain (serum enzyme activity may be derived from bone, intestine, or liver), the hepatic origin of the enzyme can be confirmed by measurement of serum 5'-nucleotidase or leucine amino-

peptidase activity; these enzymes are more specific for liver disease. Alternatively, differences in the heat stability of enzymes of hepatic and bony origin suggest the site of origin. Hepatic alkaline phosphatase is more heat stable than bone alkaline phosphatase. In the *absence of jaundice,* an elevated alkaline phosphatase suggests early cholestasis or hepatic infiltration by tumor or granuloma. A normal alkaline phosphatase in a jaundiced patient is usually indicative of parenchymal cell disease.

3. *Decreased serum enzyme activity due to impaired hepatic synthesis.* The serum level of some enzymes may decrease in patients with impaired synthesis. These enzymes include *ceruloplasmin,* a copper-containing oxidase, and lecithin-cholesterol acyltransferase, an enzyme which normally esterifies plasma cholesterol. These enzymes are not routinely measured as tests of liver function.

NEEDLE BIOPSY OF THE LIVER

Percutaneous needle biopsy of the liver by an intercostal approach under local anesthesia is a simple, safe bedside procedure that provides a tissue diagnosis of liver disease without subjecting the patient to the greater risk of general anesthesia and laparotomy with open surgical biopsy.

Indications. Needle biopsy of the liver is of proved value in the following situations:

1. In the differential diagnosis of jaundice, hepatic enlargement, and splenomegaly.

2. In the differential diagnosis of unexplained fever. A liver biopsy may suggest or establish the diagnosis of *miliary tuberculosis,* sarcoidosis, brucellosis, or neoplasm.

3. To assess the degree of hepatic fibrosis in chronic hepatitis and cirrhosis, to evaluate the course of hepatitis and acute liver disease, and to estimate hepatic stores of iron in hemochromatosis.

Contraindications. Liver biopsy is contraindicated in the following circumstances:

1. In patients who are uncooperative or who cannot control movements of the diaphragm, e.g., with severe recurrent cough.

2. In patients with bleeding disorders, with clotting defects (prothrombin time elevations greater than two to three seconds over control), or with vascular tumors in the liver.

3. In patients with severe cardiopulmonary disease that would be a contraindication to surgery should a biopsy complication ensue.

4. In patients with prolonged jaundice, probably extrahepatic in origin.

Complications. Needle biopsy of the liver is usually painless, but is occasionally followed by right pleuritic chest pain referred to the shoulder; a transient pleural friction rub may be audible at the site of biopsy. Serious complications include *hemorrhage* from the biopsy site and leakage of bile from dilated intrahepatic bile ducts or gallbladder, with *bile peritonitis;* this is usually a complication of extrahepatic obstruction. The incidence of these major complications should be less than 0.1 per cent.

PROCEDURES USED TO DIAGNOSE BILIARY TRACT DISEASE

The *radiographic procedures* used to visualize the biliary tree depend on the hepatic excretion of radiopaque dye *(oral cholecystography* and *intravenous cholangiography)* or on the direct injection of contrast agents into the bile ducts either at operation *(operative cholangiography)* or after cannulation of the ampulla via the duodenoscope *(retrograde duodenoscopic cholangiography)* or by needle (at *peritoneoscopy,* or by *percutaneous transhepatic* and *transvenous* transhepatic approaches). These techniques, as well as examination of duodenal bile *(biliary drainage)* and the *secretin test,* are of value in the differential diagnosis of obstructive jaundice. They are discussed in detail in Ch. 681.

The hepatic excretion of the most commonly used oral cholecystographic agent, *iopanoic acid,* involves a sequence that is similar to the excretion of bilirubin. In the plasma, iopanoic acid is albumin bound. Excretion depends on diffusion across the liver cell membrane, concentration in the liver cell by binding to Y and Z proteins, conjugation with glucuronide to form a water-soluble complex, and active transport of the glucuronyl conjugate into the bile canaliculi. Impaired excretion of iopanoic acid should thus be expected in patients with parenchymal liver disease or cholestasis.

DIAGNOSTIC PROCEDURES IN PORTAL HYPERTENSION

Esophageal varices may be demonstrated roentgenographically by a *barium swallow,* although *esophagoscopy* is a more accurate method for their identification.

Portal venous pressure can be measured indirectly by inserting a needle into the splenic pulp or by wedging a catheter in a branch of the hepatic vein. Comparative studies have shown that portal vein pressures measured directly through a catheter in the umbilical vein correspond to pressures recorded from wedged hepatic vein catheters in patients with cirrhosis. Measurement of wedged hepatic vein catheter pressure has the advantage of providing baseline inferior vena cava pressures. Portal pressure measurements are of value in establishing the presence of portal hypertension when this is in doubt in patients with splenomegaly or ascites. An elevated pressure is consistent with the diagnosis of chronic liver disease rather than presinusoidal portal vein obstruction. Repeated pressure measurements provide evidence of changes in portal pressure which may be of prognostic value; with recovery from acute alcoholic hepatitis, a fall in portal pressure suggests a better prognosis than a stable or rising pressure which reflects progressive fibrosis. The degree of pressure elevation does not appear to indicate the risk of hemorrhage from esophageal varices or the prognosis after portacaval shunt surgery.

The portal circulation can be visualized roentgenographically by *selective celiac arteriography* or by injection of contrast material into the spleen *(transsplenic venography)* or directly through the catheterized umbilical vein. The portal vein and collateral circulation should be demonstrated before portacaval shunt surgery is performed.

LIVER SCANNING

When compounds that are concentrated in the liver (either by parenchymal or Kupffer cells) are labeled with gamma-emitting isotopes and injected intravenously, their uptake by the liver can be assessed by surface scanning. ^{131}I-labeled rose bengal, ^{198}Au colloidal gold, and ^{99}technetium have been used. Space-occupying lesions (cysts, abscesses, or tumors) appear as filling defects. In patients with cirrhosis, hepatic uptake is decreased and irregular and splenic uptake may be increased. A liver scan is of value in providing evidence of a space-occupying lesion when this was not evident clinically. A liver biopsy should be performed to confirm the pathologic diagnosis; the biopsy needle may be directed to the site of infiltration demonstrated by the scan. Serial liver scans may be of value in documenting the response of a patient with metastatic neoplasm to therapy.

696. METABOLIC DISORDERS

Inborn errors of metabolism may cause chronic liver disease. In some of these conditions specific enzyme defects have been demonstrated (glycogen storage diseases [see Ch. 809], galactosemia [see Ch. 808]), whereas in others the underlying metabolic abnormality has not yet been defined (idiopathic hemochromatosis [see Part XVI, Section Four], Wilson's disease [see Ch. 945], Gaucher's disease [see Ch. 776]).

Disorders of Bilirubin Metabolism. Knowledge of several metabolic disorders has contributed greatly to an understanding of bilirubin metabolism and excretion.

Unconjugated Hyperbilirubinemia. Acholuric jaundice with unconjugated hyperbilirubinemia in the absence of other signs of anemia or liver disease may be due to one of the following conditions:

1. *Compensated hemolysis* in which increased red cell production masks excessive red cell destruction. This abnormality may be suggested by lowered serum haptoglobin concentrations and increased fecal urobilinogen and reticulocyte counts, but can be confirmed only by direct measurement of red cell survival using tagged erythrocytes. An increase in bilirubin production alone is insufficient to account for the unconjugated hyperbilirubinemia in patients with compensated hemolysis. Studies of bilirubin clearance using labeled bilirubin indicate that these patients also have a delayed clearance of pigment; the excessive bilirubin load unmasks this excretory defect (see Gilbert's syndrome, below).

2. *Excessive bilirubin production without hemolysis* ("shunt hyperbilirubinemia"). This is a rare condition in which abnormal catabolism of hemoglobin in red cell precursors in the bone marrow results in excessive pigment production (early-labeled bilirubin) and increased fecal urobilinogen excretion; peripheral red cell survival is normal.

3. *Idiopathic unconjugated hyperbilirubinemia (Gilbert's syndrome).* Mild unconjugated hyperbilirubinemia (usually less than 3 mg per 100 ml) without hemolysis or excessive bilirubin production is commonly recognized in healthy young subjects. Jaundice may be intermittent with exacerbations during intercurrent illness and particularly during periods of fasting. The absence of physical abnormalities, normal liver function tests, and normal liver histology exclude a diagnosis of viral hepatitis. This syndrome appears to have an autosomal dominant inheritance; unconjugated hyperbilirubinemia was detected in 16.1 per cent of parents and 27.5 per cent of siblings of patients with this disorder.

A defect in the hepatic uptake of unconjugated bilirubin from plasma has been documented by a depressed plasma clearance of labeled unconjugated bilirubin in patients with Gilbert's syndrome. In some patients, excessive bilirubin production from compensated hemolysis accentuates the excretory defect. Whereas fasting increases serum bilirubin levels in patients with Gilbert's syndrome, the administration of drugs which induce microsomal enzyme systems (e.g., phenobarbital) lowers the serum bilirubin, presumably by increasing the efficiency of hepatic pigment excretion.

4. *Parenchymal liver disease* may be associated with unconjugated hyperbilirubinemia. This has been recognized in patients during recovery from viral hepatitis. Other abnormal tests of liver function (positive flocculation tests, mildly abnormal BSP), and histologic changes on liver biopsy suggest hepatitis in these patients. Unconjugated hyperbilirubinemia in patients with congestive heart failure, or after portacaval shunt surgery for portal hypertension, reflects reduced hepatic blood flow and bilirubin clearance.

5. *Impaired bilirubin conjugation.* A defect in bilirubin conjugation is usually manifest during the neonatal period, and may be due to immaturity of the liver, inhibition of glucuronyl transferase, or deficiency of this enzyme.

a. *The immature liver* of the premature infant exhibits a reduced level of glucuronyl transferase activity. It has not been established, however, that this is the primary cause for physiologic jaundice; there may be other defects in the excretory mechanism.

b. *Prolonged neonatal jaundice in breast-fed infants* may be due to inhibition of glucuronyl transferase activity by an abnormal steroid (pregnane-3α-20β-diol) excreted in the mother's milk. Jaundice is maximal during the second to third week, and subsides rapidly if breast feeding is discontinued, or over a four- to eight-week period with continued breast feeding.

Transient neonatal hyperbilirubinemia, described in successive infants of several mothers, has been related to the presence of an inhibitor of glucuronyl transferase in the maternal plasma during pregnancy. Several of these infants developed kernicterus.

c. *The Crigler-Najjar syndrome* (congenital, nonhemolytic, unconjugated hyperbilirubinemia with glucuronyl transferase deficiency). This syndrome, characterized by severe jaundice, usually from birth, is transmitted in some patients as an autosomal recessive defect, and in others as an autosomal dominant. Patients with the autosomal recessive defect are deeply jaundiced (mean bilirubin levels 25 to 31 mg per 100 ml) and develop kernicterus. Their bile is colorless, and phenobarbital administration does not lower the serum level of unconjugated bilirubin. The autosomal dominant defect may cause less severe hyperbilirubinemia so that some patients survive to adulthood without kernicterus. When phenobarbital is given to these patients, the serum bilirubin concentration falls dramatically; this effect may be due to induction of glucuronyl transferase activity.

The homozygous *Gunn rat*, deficient in glucuronyl

transferase, provides a laboratory model of the Crigler-Najjar syndrome.

Kernicterus (Bilirubin Encephalopathy). This neurologic complication of severe unconjugated hyperbilirubinemia usually develops in the jaundiced infant during the first week of life with the appearance of spasticity, leading to head retraction, opisthotonos, muscle twitching, or convulsions. The infant may die during the neonatal period, whereas survivors exhibit mental retardation and spastic paraplegia with athetosis.

Normally, the binding of unconjugated bilirubin by albumin restricts pigment diffusion into tissue cells. However, when the concentration of unconjugated bilirubin exceeds the albumin-binding capacity (approximately 20 mg of bilirubin per 100 ml of plasma in the normal infant), unconjugated bilirubin is free to diffuse into tissues; the lipid solubility of the pigment enhances its diffusion across cell membranes and the blood-brain barrier. Depression of the plasma albumin level, the administration of drugs which bind albumin and thus displace bilirubin (sulfonamides and salicylate), and metabolic acidosis, all predispose to kernicterus. The biochemical mechanism for bilirubin encephalopathy has not been well defined.

Preventive therapy depends on the early recognition and treatment of conditions that may cause severe hemolysis in the newborn (ABO and Rh incompatibility or red cell enzyme defects). Infection and metabolic acidosis should be treated vigorously, and drugs which bind bilirubin should be avoided. Phototherapy (exposure to light of wavelength 440 mμ) may reduce the level of serum bilirubin by converting the tetrapyrrole pigment to colorless products with alternate pathways of excretion. Exchange transfusion is indicated when the serum bilirubin rises to dangerous levels; in sick premature infants with depressed albumin binding, serum bilirubin levels in excess of 10 mg per 100 ml plasma may be unsafe.

The Dubin-Johnson Syndrome. This is a familial metabolic disorder caused by impaired hepatic excretion of certain organic anions into the bile. Jaundice is associated with an increased serum level of conjugated bilirubin and bilirubinuria. The Dubin-Johnson syndrome is more common in females than in males, and often presents with jaundice during pregnancy when the hepatic excretory defect is accentuated by hormones. Jaundice is usually intermittent, and exacerbations are often associated with mild right upper quadrant abdominal pain. There is no hepatic enlargement. The excretion of oral cholecystographic agents is impaired so that the normal biliary system often cannot be visualized. Although BSP is concentrated and conjugated normally in the liver cell, biliary excretion of the dye is impaired, and large amounts of conjugated BSP passing back into the plasma may elevate the two-hour plasma BSP level above the 45-minute value. Patients with the Dubin-Johnson syndrome do not suffer from pruritus; there is no evidence for abnormal biliary secretion of the conjugated bile salts. In contrast to the retention of conjugated bilirubin and BSP, serum alkaline phosphatase levels are usually normal.

The diagnosis of the Dubin-Johnson syndrome is established by needle biopsy of the liver. Macroscopically the fresh liver tissue is black, and microscopically there are deposits of melanin-like pigment in the parenchymal cells, particularly in the centrilobular areas. The Kupffer cells do not contain pigment, the bile canaliculi are normal, and the liver is free of fibrosis or inflammatory infiltrate. Recent studies on mutant Corriedale sheep with a similar defect in organic anion transport and liver pigmentation suggest that the pigment may be an oxidation product of metanephrine glucuronide, an epinephrine metabolite normally excreted in bile but poorly excreted by these animals and by patients with the Dubin-Johnson syndrome. The hepatic pigment accumulates with increasing age in both conditions. The *Rotor syndrome* is a variant of the Dubin-Johnson syndrome, differing only in the absence of hepatic pigment.

The more important considerations in managing patients with this disorder of bilirubin metabolism are the reassurance that the abnormality is benign and leads to no disability or reduction in life expectancy and the avoidance of unnecessary biliary tract surgery.

697. ACUTE VIRAL HEPATITIS

Acute viral hepatitis is a common acute inflammatory disease of the liver caused by at least two strains of hepatotropic virus. *Hepatitis A* or *short incubation hepatitis* (formerly called *infectious hepatitis*) is due to hepatitis virus (or viruses) A, and *hepatitis B* or *long incubation hepatitis* (formerly called *serum hepatitis*) is due to hepatitis viruses B.

Etiology. Early information relating to the viral etiology of human hepatitis was based on indirect evidence derived from studies of epidemic hepatitis and from human transmission experiments. Hepatitis A and B were both shown to be caused by filterable agents that were relatively resistant to heat and chemical disinfectants. Epidemiologic and clinical studies suggested differences in the biologic properties of the two viral agents. Infectious hepatitis was believed to be transmitted by the fecal-oral route in the majority of patients in both endemic and epidemic outbreaks. Experimental studies suggested a short incubation period of two to six weeks, with the appearance of the infective agent in both blood and feces during the prodromal and early icteric phases of illness. Infection conferred immunity against further attacks of infectious hepatitis, but did not protect against serum hepatitis infection. Serum hepatitis was considered to be transmitted only by parenteral inoculation of infected blood or blood products with a long incubation period of six weeks to six months. The infective agent was thought to be confined to the circulation and not excreted in feces. The transmission of disease by transfusion of blood from healthy donors indicated a prolonged carrier state.

Early attempts to isolate the viruses of human hepatitis, to propagate them in tissue culture, or to transmit them to laboratory animals were unsuccessful, and knowledge of these agents was thus limited. The identification of a virus-like antigen in the serum of patients with *hepatitis B* has advanced knowledge of the epidemiology of this infection. Hepatitis B virus antigen (HBAg) was first called *Australia antigen* after its identification immunologically in the serum of an Australian aborigine. HBAg (also called serum hepatitis antigen and hepatitis-related antigen) can be identified by immunodiffusion, immunoelectrophoretic, complement fixation, and radioimmunoassay techniques, using serum which contains *hepatitis B antibody* (anti-HB). Electron microscopic studies of HBAg positive sera have demonstrated the presence of free particles with virus-like structure; larger Dane particles (42 nm) have a central core and surface capsid, whereas smaller particles (20 nm spheres or filaments) lack the central core. Immunologic studies have identified both core and surface antigens, designated HB_c-Ag and HB_s-Ag, respectively; these antigens promote the formation of corresponding antibodies—anti-HB_c and anti-HB_s. Two subtypes of HB_sAg (designated D and Y) have been identified.

Recent experimental studies indicate that marmosets can be infected with human hepatitis A; the use of this animal model should provide further knowledge of this virus.

Epidemiology. *Hepatitis A (Short-Incubation, Infectious Hepatitis).* Transmission of the hepatitis A virus is usually by the fecal-oral route, although infusion of infected blood obtained from viremic donors may cause sporadic infection. The occurrence of both sporadic and epidemic hepatitis depends on the distribution of infected material and the susceptibility of the exposed population. Thus poor sanitation, overcrowding, and exposure of a nonimmune population will contribute to an epidemic situation with a high frequency of infection in the young. Adults without previous exposure to hepatitis A infection are particularly at risk when traveling in or moving to an area of high endemic infection with poor sanitation. Explosive epidemics have been described after fecal contamination of drinking water and milk, and the concentration of virus by shellfish in polluted sea water has been a recent cause of several epidemics in the eastern United States. The common epidemics in institutions that house small children—orphanages, schools, and homes for the mentally retarded—reflect the exposure of a nonimmune population to many cases of anicteric or preicteric infection. The frequency of viral hepatitis (HBAg negative) in persons handling primates suggests that these animals transmit hepatitis A.

Hepatitis B (Long-Incubation, Serum Hepatitis). Transmission of hepatitis B virus by the parenteral route is well documented. This is a hazard among recipients of transfused blood (particularly blood from paid donors), pooled plasma, fibrinogen, antihemophilic globulin (AHG), and vaccines contaminated with human serum (e.g., yellow fever vaccine during World War II). Inoculation with minute amounts of infected blood may transmit hepatitis B virus infection; inadequately sterilized syringes, hypodermic needles, dental and surgical instruments, tattoo needles, and razors have all been implicated in the transmission of infection. Hospital personnel, particularly operating room staff, dialysis unit staff, and laboratory personnel, have an increased risk of accidental parenteral exposure. A high frequency of parenteral drug abuse is a major cause for infection in the young adult population.

The development of immunologic methods for the detection of hepatitis B antigen (HBAg) and antibody (anti-HB) has led to major advances in the understanding of hepatitis B infection and provides a means for reducing infection, particularly among recipients of transfused blood. Tests for HBAg identify many carriers of the hepatitis B virus; between 1 and 2 per cent of paid donors were found to be HBAg positive, whereas volunteer blood donors have a hepatitis carrier rate of between 1 and 2 per 1000. A majority of patients transfused with HBAg positive blood either develop HBAg positive hepatitis (either anicteric or icteric) or exhibit a rise in the titer of anti-HB in their serum. The frequency of posttransfusion hepatitis B infection is significantly decreased when transfused blood is derived from volunteer rather than paid donors and when HBAg positive blood is discarded.

Studies on the infants of mothers who suffered from hepatitis B infection during the last trimester of pregnancy or during the immediate postpartum period have shown a high frequency of neonatal infection. Although HBAg is sometimes present in cord blood, the relative importance of transplacental, perinatal, or postnatal transmission remains uncertain.

In epidemiologic studies, Krugman and co-workers have proved that hepatitis B infection can be transmitted by nonparenteral (fecal-oral) as well as by parenteral routes. Thus the terms infectious hepatitis (IH) and serum hepatitis (SH), which implied differences in the mode of virus transmission, are no longer accurate. The increased frequency of hepatitis B (HBAg positive), together with a higher frequency of detectable anti-HB in the relatives of HBAg positive blood donors or chronic renal dialysis patients, is best explained by nonparenteral transmission of the infective agent.

It is of interest to consider the factors which determined the spread of hepatitis B infection among populations that do not have parenteral exposure to blood or blood products. Under conditions of poor sanitation, nonparenteral transmission may be of greater epidemiologic importance; this may explain the high HBAg carrier rate in tropical Africa. Alternatively, it has been suggested that an insect vector may be important in the transmission of infection; HBAg has been recovered from several arthropods, particularly mosquitoes, captured from human dwellings in tropical West Africa.

The significance of the HBAg subtypes, D and Y, with respect to the severity or chronicity of infection in man is currently under investigation. The D subtype has a higher frequency than the Y subtype among healthy carriers (volunteer blood donors) and patients with chronic liver disease. In patients with HBAg positive hepatitis, the D subtype appears to be more frequent in patients with sporadic hepatitis without parenteral exposure or association with drug users; the Y subtype is more common in patients with needle-associated hepatitis.

Pathology. The hepatic lesion in uncomplicated viral hepatitis (both hepatitis A and B, whether anicteric or icteric) is characterized by parenchymal cell degeneration and necrosis, proliferation of Kupffer's cells, inflammatory cell infiltration, and cell regeneration. Parenchymal cells throughout the lobule, and particularly in centrilobular areas, undergo rapid necrosis so that the cell cords are disrupted. Degenerating liver cells either show *ballooning* of their cytoplasm or hyalinize to form *acidophilic bodies* that may exhibit pyknotic nuclei. Cell necrosis is closely followed by cell regeneration; this may be recognized by the appearance of cells in mitosis and by large cells with multiple hyperchromatic nuclei. An increased number of macrophages containing a yellow, acid-fast pigment (lipofuscin) accumulate at sites of cell necrosis. Numerous lymphocytes, plasma cells, and polymorphonuclear cells, both neutrophil and eosinophil, also accumulate focally at sites of cell necrosis in the lobules and in the portal areas.

Although necrosis disrupts the normal cell cords, the reticulum framework surrounding the hepatic sinusoids is preserved, and cell regeneration restores normal lobules. During the recovery phase an increased number of fibroblasts with collagen may appear in the portal areas, together with proliferating bile ductules; these changes, together with the inflammatory cell infiltrate, disappear with full recovery.

Intrahepatic cholestasis—dilated bile canaliculi containing bile plugs—particularly in centrilobular areas, is often seen in viral hepatitis when there is prominent clinical evidence of cholestasis. This may be due to a disruption of bile canaliculi by parenchymal cell necrosis, or it may result from a change in the composition of bile due to cell injury.

Rarely, viral hepatitis may cause more extensive zones of parenchymal cell necrosis bridging adjacent portal triads and/or central veins with collapse of the normal reticulum framework. This lesion has been termed *subacute hepatic necrosis. Massive hepatic necrosis,* usually associated with fulminant hepatitis, is associated with widespread necrosis. The term *acute yellow atrophy* refers to the shrunken, bile-stained liver in which zones of collapsed reticulum and sinusoids lie between islands of surviving cells.

Although complete recovery can be anticipated in patients with typical focal necrosis, the prognosis of patients with massive necrosis or subacute hepatic necrosis with respect to full recovery is poor. Massive necrosis in patients with fulminant hepatitis is usually fatal. In patients who survive, liver cell regeneration may restore normal liver structure and function or may result in a macronodular cirrhosis. Subacute hepatic necrosis has a variable clinical course. Of 52 patients who exhibited this lesion on liver biopsy, 4 died with fulminant hepatitis, 6 died after a subacute illness of several weeks, and the remainder survived the acute illness; of the survivors, 7 exhibited the clinical and histologic features of chronic active hepatitis, 5 had residual abnormalities of liver function with cirrhosis documented by biopsy in 2, and 28 recovered with normal liver function but with biopsy evidence of inactive cirrhosis in 9 of 19 subjected to repeat liver biopsy.

There is evidence from HBAg studies that *chronic active hepatitis* (see Ch. 708) may complicate viral hepatitis. This condition usually has an insidious onset, but may also follow subacute hepatic necrosis.

Extrahepatic lesions in infectious hepatitis appear in the gastrointestinal mucosa and the kidney. The mucosae are edematous and infiltrated with mononuclear cells; renal biopsies reveal interstitial edema without inflammation.

Currently, the relationship between the various lesions (hepatic and extrahepatic) of viral hepatitis and the distribution of the viruses is unclear. HBAg has been localized by immunofluorescence in liver cells, but the source of HBAg in healthy carriers is not known, and the relative importance of persisting infection or host responses (e.g., immunologic reactions) in the pathogenesis of severe or chronic lesions must still be defined. There is evidence that skin and joint lesions occurring during the prodromal period may relate to the formation of complexes between HBAg and anti-HB.

Clinical Manifestations. Acute viral hepatitis is commonly a mild disease without jaundice, particularly in those with relative immunity from previous infection, or in infants and children. Infection may be followed by a mild illness without clinical evidence of hepatitis; a rise in viral antibody titer or transiently positive test for

HBAg may be the only evidence of infection. In many subjects exposed to either of the viral agents, there is evidence of hepatitis without jaundice—*anicteric hepatitis. Icteric hepatitis* is usually a short, uncomplicated illness, but sometimes has a prolonged course *(chronic persisting hepatitis).* Acute exacerbations may follow partial recovery, or *recurrent hepatitis* may follow complete recovery. When a clinical picture of cholestasis is the dominant abnormality, the term *cholestatic hepatitis* is used. In jaundiced patients with hepatitis A infection, the risk of *fulminant hepatitis* with massive necrosis is less than 1 per cent. The risk of massive or subacute hepatic necrosis in patients with hepatitis B infection is increased in elderly patients, in diabetics, and in patients with severe illness, particularly neoplasms, which have required surgery and transfusion.

The clinical features of each of these variants of viral hepatitis will be discussed below. *Fulminant hepatitis* and *chronic active liver* disease are discussed in Ch. 698 and 708, respectively.

Anicteric Hepatitis. The symptoms of anicteric hepatitis are similar to those of many other viral infections; the onset of disease may resemble the prodromal (pre-icteric) period of icteric hepatitis. The diagnosis is suspected only in epidemic situations, in patients exposed to known infection, or in those who develop tender enlargement of the liver. A diagnosis is confirmed by liver function tests and liver biopsy. There is often slight hyperbilirubinemia with an increase in urinary urobilinogen and bilirubin and BSP retention. The serum enzyme changes are most helpful in diagnosis; serum transaminase and dehydrogenase levels are elevated, and serum alkaline phosphatase and 5'-nucleotidase may be slightly increased. On liver biopsy, the hepatic lesion is indistinguishable from that of icteric hepatitis except for the absence of bile stasis.

Icteric Hepatitis. THE PREICTERIC PHASE. The preicteric phase of nonspecific constitutional and gastrointestinal symptoms varies in duration from a few days to several weeks. It is usually abrupt in onset in patients with hepatitis A and often of insidious onset with hepatitis B; these symptoms may mimic those of other viral infections of the respiratory or gastrointestinal tract. *Fever* is usually most pronounced at the onset, and may be accompanied by a shaking chill; it is unusual, however, for shaking chills to be recurrent, although fever may persist until the early icteric phase. *Anorexia, weakness, headache,* and *myalgia* are common symptoms; there may be a striking loss of taste for cigarettes. Right upper quadrant pain with local tenderness and muscle spasm may simulate an acute abdominal emergency. Joint pains or acute migratory arthritis and urticarial or erythematous maculopapular rashes are sometimes seen, particularly in patients with hepatitis B infection. During this preicteric phase, the liver may become enlarged and tender, and the urine may become discolored with bilirubin.

THE ICTERIC PHASE. Gastrointestinal symptoms—anorexia, nausea, and vomiting with right upper abdominal discomfort—usually increase during the early period of increasing jaundice, the liver becomes more enlarged and tender, and the spleen may be palpable. Fever usually subsides a few days after the onset of jaundice. Within a few days of hospitalization and bed rest, nausea subsides, and the appetite improves in most patients. Typically, the patient is maximally jaundiced within two weeks, and thereafter clinical jaundice and serum bilirubin levels gradually return to normal within six weeks. Hepatic enlargement may subside with symptomatic improvement, but often persists during the icteric period. The maximal changes in urinary and fecal bilirubin excretion coincide with maximal serum bilirubin levels.

In patients with *cholestatic hepatitis* jaundice is usually more severe and prolonged and accompanied by *pruritus* secondary to bile salt retention. Liver enlargement usually persists during the period of jaundice, whereas hepatic tenderness is usually observed early in the acute illness. *Diarrhea* may be due to the cathartic action of nonabsorbed fatty acids.

Some patients with otherwise typical acute viral hepatitis may remain icteric with hepatic enlargement and abnormalities of liver function for a period of several months. A liver biopsy is indicated in such patients to confirm a diagnosis of *chronic persisting hepatitis;* the histologic features of typical viral hepatitis in spite of the prolonged clinical course indicate an excellent prognosis for full recovery.

Occasionally there may be acute exacerbations with anorexia, nausea, recurrent liver enlargement, and tenderness and jaundice after partial recovery from the initial icteric illness. Such exacerbations are sometimes precipitated by vigorous physical activity, and usually resolve promptly without long-term complications.

THE CONVALESCENT PHASE. The convalescent phase, leading to complete recovery and resumption of normal activity, may last for several weeks or months. During this period variable tiredness and malaise with mild hepatic tenderness may persist. These symptoms may be quite troublesome to the patient. They are often precipitated by unaccustomed activity and may be accompanied by mild elevation of serum transaminase levels and minimal BSP retention.

Laboratory Features. The hemoglobin and hematocrit are usually normal early in the illness, but mild hemolysis and repeated venipuncture for laboratory tests may cause anemia later in the course of the acute disease. A normal or reduced white cell count, with atypical mononuclear cells (virocytes) on smear, is usual during the preicteric and early icteric periods. The erythrocyte sedimentation rate is slightly increased. Aplastic anemia is an unusual complication of acute viral hepatitis. Thrombocytopenic purpura is occasionally seen, as in other viral illnesses. Evidence of acute hemolysis, usually with deep jaundice, may be secondary to a red cell defect, particularly G-6-PD deficiency.

The urine contains an increased amount of both urobilinogen and bilirubin in the early icteric period; bilirubinemia increases with increasing jaundice, whereas urinary urobilinogen excretion decreases to minimal levels when jaundice is maximal. Minimal proteinuria with microscopic hematuria, pyuria, and granular casts during the early icteric period may reflect the renal abnormalities that have been demonstrated on renal biopsy.

During the icteric period both direct- and indirect-reacting bilirubin are almost equally elevated in the serum, but during the convalescent period indirect bilirubinemia may persist (see Gilbert's syndrome in Ch. 696). Serum transaminase (glutamic-oxaloacetic or glutamic-pyruvic) levels, maximally elevated in the late prodromal or early icteric periods, may exceed 500 to 1000 IU. These increased enzyme levels may be sustained during the icteric period but usually fall toward normal during the icteric period. Serum elevations of alkaline phosphatase, 5'-nucleotidase, and leucine aminopeptidase are usually minimal and return to normal during the late icteric period. In patients with *cholestatic hepatitis* the increases in serum alkaline phosphatase, 5'-nucleotidase, and conjugated bilirubin are usually more prominent than the rise in serum transaminase levels. Serum cholesterol levels will increase in these patients. The typical changes in plasma proteins include a slight decrease in albumin and a late increase in gamma globulin, and the flocculation tests may be abnormal late in the prodromal period and return to normal during convalescence. The increase in gamma globulin levels in patients with acute hepatitis or in patients with *chronic persisting hepatitis* is considerably less than that seen in patients with *chronic active hepatitis* (see below). BSP retention decreases to normal levels during the convalescent period.

Diagnosis. During the prodromal period, symptoms may suggest some other viral infection—*influenza* or *gastroenteritis.* Abdominal pain may mimic *acute cholecystitis, pneumonia,* or *acute appendicitis.* In the icteric patient, other causes for jaundice must be considered; *drug-induced or toxic hepatitis* is usually indicated by a history of drug exposure, but cannot be clearly differentiated by the preicteric symptoms from viral hepatitis. Choledocholithiasis with obstruction is suggested by a history of calculous disease, biliary colic, predominant cholestasis with pruritus, high alkaline phosphatase levels with only slight increases in transaminase, and signs of bacterial infection—shaking chills and polymorphonuclear leukocytosis. *Infectious mononucleosis* with hepatic involvement is distinguished by lymphadenopathy, pharyngitis, and a positive *heterophil* test. *Leptospirosis* is usually accompanied by headache and photophobia, signs of meningeal irritation with abnormal cerebrospinal fluid, persisting fever, leukocytosis, and proteinuria or renal insufficiency. It is important to exclude an exacerbation of chronic liver disease with jaundice; *acute alcoholic hepatitis* or *chronic aggressive hepatitis* may present with jaundice (see below).

A percutaneous liver biopsy is of diagnostic value whenever the clinical picture is atypical. Lesions of extrahepatic obstruction, subacute hepatic necrosis, chronic active hepatitis, acute alcoholic hepatitis, or active cirrhosis can be distinguished from the changes of acute viral hepatitis.

Tests for HBAg are of value early in the course of hepatitis, or in patients with prolonged illness. The HBAg test usually becomes positive during the preicteric phase of hepatitis B infection, and the antigen test usually becomes negative with the appearance of anti-HB within two to three weeks of the onset of jaundice. When HBAg persists in the serum for periods in excess of four weeks, chronic active hepatitis must be considered as a diagnostic possibility.

Management of Acute Viral Hepatitis. Hospitalization of patients with acute viral hepatitis is indicated during the early icteric phase when symptoms are severe (e.g., severe vomiting) or when there is clinical evidence at the time of diagnosis of serious illness, particularly manifestations of subacute or massive hepatic necrosis (see below). High risk patients—pregnant, diabetic, elderly, or those with complicating disease—should also be observed in hospital. Patients treated at home should be advised with respect to diet, alcohol intake, physical activity, and measures to reduce their infectivity. The routine precautions to reduce cross-infection in hospital are those applicable to enteric diseases, plus careful disposal of needles and syringes. During the early symptomatic period frequent careful clinical observation and assessment of liver function are necessary for early recognition and treatment of massive or subacute hepatic necrosis. Liver function tests should be performed as often as is necessary to assess the patient's progress; a daily estimation of the prothrombin time after parenteral vitamin K_1 (10 mg intramuscularly) is valuable in detecting a sudden deterioration in liver function. A daily measurement of caloric intake is also helpful in assessing the patient's progress.

A liver biopsy should be performed if the diagnosis is not firmly established on the basis of clinical and biochemical findings, or if an atypical course suggests subacute hepatic necrosis.

Rest. The value of rest in acute viral hepatitis is suggested by the remission and exacerbation of symptoms that follow bed rest and physical activity, respectively. Nevertheless, the only controlled study on the effect of rest and activity in infectious hepatitis indicated that enforced rest was of no value in therapy and that activity did not cause complications, lengthen the course of the disease, or lead to chronic residual abnormalities. This controlled study was carried out on military personnel who were young and fit and who, irrespective of therapy, suffered no mortality or long-term sequelae that could be attributed to the viral hepatitis. In a civilian population of varied age, with other disease states complicating viral hepatitis infection, there are significant morbidity and mortality from subacute and massive hepatic necrosis. *Complete bed rest during the acute phase of viral hepatitis may protect some of these patients from these complications.* Until there is further information relating to a civilian population, it is recommended that all icteric patients rest in bed during the early symptomatic period when it may be difficult to assess the severity of illness, and that limited activity during the icteric period be permitted only for young, otherwise healthy patients. Elderly patients and patients with complicating disease should be ambulated when the serum bilirubin has fallen below 2 mg per 100 ml. It is important that ambulation to normal physical activity should be gradual for patients who have been confined to bed for long periods.

Diet. During the preicteric and early icteric periods, a poor appetite and nausea or vomiting may limit food intake. The patient should be served and encouraged to eat those foods that appeal to him. For some patients, it is possible to increase the caloric content of the breakfast when they have difficulty in eating other meals. If a total intake of 2000 calories daily is not maintained, intravenous glucose supplements should be given.

Corticosteroids. Although glucocorticoids effect a dramatic remission of symptoms and biochemical improvement in patients with viral hepatitis, it has not been established by controlled studies that these agents shorten the course of the acute disease or reduce the complications. Thus in mild, uncomplicated hepatitis there is no indication for their use. Corticosteroids are recommended, however, for acutely ill patients whose symptoms are severe and persist for several days in spite of bed rest. A daily dose of 30 to 60 mg of prednisolone, or equivalent doses of other steroids, maintained for a week and tapered slowly over a period of several weeks is suggested.

Sedatives. Sedatives and other drugs should be used with caution in patients with viral hepatitis. Smaller doses may be necessary to achieve a therapeutic effect. In acutely ill patients their side effects may complicate the clinical assessment of the patient.

Surgery. All surgical procedures should be deferred to the postconvalescent period if possible. There is evidence that abdominal surgery under general anesthesia increases the risk of subacute or massive hepatic necrosis.

Management of the Hepatitis (HBAg) Carrier. The routine screening of blood donors and patients with liver disease for HBAg has raised special problems in the management and education of subjects who may be otherwise perfectly healthy. When a person is found to be HBAg positive, it should be confirmed that a chronic carrier state exists by repeated tests. If tests of liver function are abnormal, a liver biopsy is advised to define the nature of the associated liver disease. If there are no clinical manifestations of liver disease and liver function tests are normal, liver disease is very unlikely. The healthy HBAg carrier should be excluded from donating blood and should be advised to maintain careful personal hygiene.

Prophylaxis. A single dose of pooled gamma globulin (0.02 to 0.04 ml of 16 per cent solution per kilogram of body weight, intramuscularly) protects against, or modifies, hepatitis A infection in exposed subjects. Susceptible persons probably develop anicteric rather than icteric hepatitis. Susceptible travelers to zones of known poor sanitation should receive a larger dose, 0.06 to 0.12 ml per kilogram, to give protection for five to six months.

Commercially available pooled gamma globulin does not confer protection against post-transfusion hepatitis B infection; these preparations do not contain significant hepatitis B antibody. In preliminary studies, however, there is evidence that commercial gamma globulin and gamma globulin containing anti-HB may both protect children against hepatitis B infection caused by nonparenteral exposure; the gamma globulin may also reduce the frequency of the chronic HBAg carrier state.

Although experimental evidence indicates that active immunization with heat-inactivated HBAg is effective in reducing infection, the development of commercially available vaccines requires further characterization of the viral agents and their cultivation in the laboratory.

698. FULMINANT HEPATITIS

Fulminant hepatitis resulting from massive hepatic necrosis may be due to *toxic liver injury* (e.g., carbon tetrachloride toxicity or acetaminophen overdosage), *hypersensitivity reactions* to therapeutic agents (e.g., halothane sensitivity), or *viral hepatitis*. In the case of toxic liver injury, the lesion is predictable and dose related; in the case of hypersensitivity reactions, the development of liver disease is unpredictable unless there has been a previous sensitivity reaction to the drug. Fulminant hepatitis may be caused by viruses A or B; predisposing factors have not been well documented, but the risk of infection during late pregnancy in malnourished patients is high.

Pathology. When a diagnosis of fulminant hepatitis is suspected by the clinical course, a percutaneous liver biopsy is usually precluded by the risk of bleeding caused by clotting abnormalities; the pathologic features are usually defined at postmortem examination. The liver is usually smaller than normal with a soft consistency and red-brown discoloration—thus the term *acute yellow atrophy*. Microscopically, there is confluent necrosis with disappearance of parenchymal cells, leaving a residual framework of collapsed reticulin, hepatic sinusoids, Kupffer cells, and inflammatory cells. Parenchymal cells surrounding portal tracts may be spared, or may exhibit evidence of degeneration or regeneration. The surviving Kupffer cells are usually hypertrophied and contain a yellow pigment—lipofuchsin. In portal areas, proliferation of bile ducts is commonly observed, and infiltration with inflammatory cells is usual. *Massive hepatic necrosis* usually leads to early death. *Subacute or submassive hepatic necrosis* represents a less extensive lesion in which areas of residual parenchyma are separated by zones of necrosis. Death may occur after a brief or protracted illness, or regeneration of parenchymal cells may permit survival. If the zones of parenchymal necrosis undergo fibrosis and surviving zones of parenchyma proliferate to form regeneration nodules, a macronodular cirrhosis will be the end result. Alternatively, prolonged survival may be accompanied by persisting piecemeal necrosis and the clinical picture of chronic active hepatitis (see below).

Pathologically, it is not possible to differentiate massive or submassive necrosis caused by toxic injury, drug hypersensitivity, or viral hepatitis.

Clinical Manifestations. In patients with fulminant hepatitis, the preicteric period is usually brief with severe symptoms, particularly abdominal pain, vomiting, and high fever. The clinical features which suggest a fulminant course are as follows: (1) High fever, severe abdominal pain, and vomiting which persist for several days after the initiation of bed rest. (2) A sudden decrease in the size of the liver. (3) Neuropsychiatric changes of early hepatic encephalopathy, including drowsiness, irritability, insomnia, and confusion. (4) Severe prolongation of the prothrombin time (more than 20 seconds with control of 12 seconds) with or without bleeding (uncorrected by parenteral vitamin K). (Serum bilirubin and transaminase levels do not reflect the severity of illness; patients may die in hepatic coma during the early icteric period, or may become deeply jaundiced, while serum transaminase levels often fall during the period of clinical deterioration.) (5) The appearance of ascites during the acute illness.

The complications of massive necrosis with acute liver failure include *hypoglycemia; bleeding* caused by deficient clotting factors; *disseminated intravascular coagulation,* which may accentuate liver cell necrosis; *acute hepatic encephalopathy* (described in Ch. 694) with terminal depression of medullary centers; *pneumonia* secondary to aspiration; *septicemia* with portals of entry at the sites of intravenous catheter lines, the gut, or urinary system; and terminal *renal failure* (hepatorenal syndrome).

Management. The patient with fulminant hepatitis requires intensive nursing care with monitoring and support of vital functions. In the comatose patient, a cuffed nasotracheal or tracheostomy tube should be inserted to ensure adequate ventilation, with respirator support if necessary, and to prevent aspiration. Continuous intravenous infusion of glucose solution is required to prevent hypoglycemia in a patient who has no hepatic glycogen stores and has depressed glyconeogenesis. Fluid and electrolyte balance should be achieved by accurate measurement of intake and output. In the absence of hepatic plasma protein synthesis, plasma albumin levels can be maintained by intravenous infusion of solutions of salt-poor albumin. Deficiency of clotting factors can be partially corrected by infusion of fresh-frozen plasma. The agitated, hyperactive patient should be restrained to prevent injury and should be sedated with small doses of diazepam (5 mg by intravenous injection); heavy sedation will deepen coma. General measures to treat hepatic coma are indicated (see Hepatic Coma in Ch. 709).

High doses of *corticosteroids* are usually given by intravenous infusion—e.g., prednisolone, 100 to 500 mg daily; the benefit of this therapy has not been established by controlled clinical trials, but is based on clinical impressions. Although there is evidence for disseminated intravascular coagulation in patients with fulminant hepatitis, treatment with heparin has not been of benefit in limited clinical trials.

A variety of measures designed to support the patient in acute liver failure have been described. These include *exchange transfusion, plasmapheresis, cross-perfusion* with a human volunteer or primate, or *extracorporeal perfusion* through a mammalian liver. Although isolated case reports suggest that exchange transfusion or plasmapheresis may restore consciousness in some patients and thus prolong life, it has not been established that these support measures actually improve survival. In one prospective controlled study, exchange transfusion was of no benefit in decreasing mortality. Studies in experimental canine hepatitis showed that infusion of immune serum improved the survival of infected animals. Treatment of patients with fulminant viral hepatitis, type B, with plasma containing hepatitis B antibody has been suggested; controlled trials are needed to establish the value of this therapy.

Recovery from fulminant hepatitis depends on liver cell regeneration; currently there are no measures known to potentiate liver regeneration in these patients. The better prognosis for recovery in children probably relates to a greater regenerative capacity; any measures which prolong survival and increase the chance of liver cell regeneration should be used in treatment.

699. HEPATITIS DUE TO OTHER VIRUSES

The viruses of yellow fever, rubella, cytomegalic inclusion disease, and herpes simplex may cause hepatitis. Yellow fever is discussed in Ch. 154. Infection with *rubella, cytomegalic inclusion virus,* and *herpes simplex* may cause *neonatal hepatitis* with jaundice and hepatosplenomegaly. Rubella and cytomegalic inclusion viruses are transmitted transplacentally, whereas herpes virus infects the infant during delivery. Hepatitis resulting from these viral agents may be part of a generalized disease. Although there may be complete recovery, with normal liver function and structure, these infections may be important but previously unrecognized causes for juvenile cirrhosis.

Many viral illnesses may be accompanied by minor, nonspecific changes in liver function (positive flocculation tests and slight transaminase elevation). There may be hyperplasia of Kupffer's cells and infiltration with mononuclear cells in portal areas—nonspecific reactive hepatitis.

INFECTIOUS MONONUCLEOSIS

Infectious mononucleosis is a systemic disease which is commonly associated with liver disease (see Part XVI, Section Nine). Jaundice is unusual, although hepatic enlargement with mild tenderness is often seen. The disturbances of liver function are those associated with hepatic infiltration: an elevation of the serum alkaline phosphatase, 5'-nucleotidase and leucine aminopeptidase, and BSP retention. Serum transaminase levels may be slightly elevated. Histologically, there is mononuclear infiltration predominantly in the portal areas with minimal evidence of cell necrosis.

No case of chronic liver disease has been proved to result from an attack of infectious mononucleosis.

This disease must be considered in the differential diagnosis of acute viral hepatitis. An atypical mononuclear cell reaction is common to these diseases, but tests for heterophil antibody, Epstein-Barr virus, and cytomegaloviruses differentiate them.

700. LIVER DISEASE ASSOCIATED WITH BACTERIAL INFECTIONS

In bacterial infection, liver disease may result from the effect of bacterial toxins on cell metabolism, changes in liver blood flow caused by endotoxin, shock or fever, localization and multiplication of bacteria in the liver, or the effect of antimicrobial agents.

Severe infections, particularly intraperitoneal, may cause obstructive jaundice with conjugated bilirubinemia, increased alkaline phosphatase, and minimal elevation of serum transaminase. In the absence of demonstrable lesions of the extrahepatic biliary system and normal operative cholangiograms, the jaundice in these patients is due to intrahepatic cholestasis resulting from unknown toxic factors.

Gram-negative septicemia with shock may cause acute hypoxic necrosis of the liver with jaundice as a terminal manifestation. The liver may be enlarged and tender. In *typhoid fever* there is focal necrosis of liver cells with acute and chronic inflammatory cell infiltration. An elevation of serum transaminases reflects parenchymal cell injury. In *leptospirosis,* jaundice is usually disproportionally greater than other evidence of liver involvement; the associated renal disease may impair urinary excretion of conjugated bilirubin.

Although the mucocutaneous lesions are most prominent features of *secondary syphilis,* liver disease is well documented. Hepatic enlargement with mild jaundice and elevated levels of alkaline phosphatase and transaminase in the serum are associated with polymorphonuclear infiltration of the portal tracts. Hepatic *tuberculosis* is discussed in Ch. 235.

701. ACUTE LIVER ABSCESS

Amebic abscesses are discussed in Ch. 279.

Pyogenic organisms which cause liver abscess may reach the liver by the biliary system (cholangitis), the portal venous system (portal pyemia in patients with appendicitis or umbilical sepsis), or arterial blood (staphylococcal septicemia or bacteremia from distant foci); by direct spread from contiguous structures (empyema of gallbladder or subphrenic abscess); or by penetrating wounds. Infection complicating biliary tract disease—*suppurative (ascending) cholangitis*—is now the most common cause for liver abscesses; the early diagnosis and treatment of acute appendicitis and umbilical sepsis in the newborn has decreased the frequency of abscess caused by pylephlebitis. The responsible organism for liver abscess reflects the source of infection; cholangitis is usually due to enteric organisms, particularly *E. coli,* anaerobic streptococci and Bacteroides species. Abscesses formerly regarded as being sterile probably harbored anaerobic organisms which were not isolated because of inadequate anaerobic transport and culture techniques. Abscesses are more often multiple than solitary and involve the right lobe more frequently than the left. A decreasing frequency in the young and increasing frequency in the elderly reflect the decreasing morbidity after appendicitis and the greater relative frequency of abscesses caused by biliary tract disease.

The *clinical manifestations* of liver abscess are the result of sepsis and the presence of a space-occupying lesion(s) in the liver. *Paroxysmal fever* with *chills* and a *polymorphonuclear leukocytosis* are usual; a liver abscess should be considered in the differential diagnosis of persistent unexplained fever (FUO). Blood cultures are positive in approximately 50 per cent of patients. Gastrointestinal symptoms and abdominal signs are often nonspecific and include anorexia, nausea, epigastric or right upper quadrant pain, and liver enlargement with tenderness. Jaundice may not be an early clinical finding unless there is associated biliary tract obstruction.

Abnormalities of liver function reflect associated biliary tract disease and focal inflammatory disease in relation to the lesion. In the absence of biliary tract obstruction, serum alkaline phosphatase levels are usually only mildly elevated, and transaminase levels are often normal. A decrease in synthesis and an increased catabolism of albumin cause hypoproteinemia in the majority of patients. An enlarging liver abscess may elevate the diaphragm or may be associated with a pleural effusion.

Diagnosis. The diagnosis of liver abscess is made too frequently at postmortem examination in patients who did not have the benefit of treatment. When symptoms and signs suggest the possibility of a liver abscess, the presence of a space-occupying lesion must be confirmed by *liver scanning.* Selective *celiac arteriography* is of value in differentiating avascular (cysts and abscesses) and vascular (primary or metastatic neoplasms) space-occupying lesions in the liver. Amebic liver abscesses should be diagnosed by appropriate serologic tests (see Ch. 279); the clinical manifestations of pyogenic and amebic liver abscesses are similar.

Treatment. *Surgical drainage* of pyogenic liver abscess is usually recommended as the treatment of choice. Preoperative *antimicrobial therapy* to cover gram-negative and anaerobic organisms should be continued postoperatively until bacteriologic studies have identified the causal organism and specific drug therapy can be provided. There have been no clinical trials to determine whether antimicrobial therapy alone without surgical drainage is as effective as the surgical approach in treating liver abscesses; multiple small abscesses may be less accessible to the surgeon.

Complications. The major complications of liver abscess are septicemia and rupture of the abscess into the pleural space or peritoneum to produce an *empyema, subphrenic abscess,* or *generalized peritonitis.*

702.   PROTOZOAN OR HELMINTHIC DISEASE OF THE LIVER

Parasites that commonly invade the liver include *amebae (E. histolytica* and malarial parasites*), schistosomes (S. mansoni), flukes (Clonorchis sinensis, Fasciola hepatica)* and *tapeworms (Echinococcus granulosus).* These diseases are discussed in Part IX.

Hepatic Schistosomiasis. Hepatic involvement in patients with *Schistosoma mansoni* results from portal seeding with ova that lodge in the portal areas and stimulate an inflammatory reaction with fibrosis. In acute schistosomiasis, the response to ova liberated two to eight weeks after infection is often associated with fever, diarrhea, hepatic and splenic enlargement, and intense eosinophilia. Transient abnormalities of liver function include increases in serum alkaline phosphatase and transaminase. In the later stage of hepatic parasitism, portal fibrosis interferes with hepatic blood flow and causes a presinusoidal portal hypertension, splenomegaly, and a collateral portal-systemic circulation. Bleeding from esophageal varices is a major complication. Liver function is usually good, so that patients may tolerate recurrent bleeding very well and do not usually develop ascites unless bleeding or malnutrition lowers serum albumin concentrations. Surgical decompression of the portal system by portacaval or splenorenal shunting is effective in preventing recurrent bleeding from esophageal varices, but it has not been established by prospectively controlled clinical trials that shunt surgery prolongs the life of these patients.

The diagnosis of hepatic schistosomiasis is established by demonstrating ova on liver biopsy; examination of "squash" preparations in glycerol is more helpful than routine histologic examination. The presence of ova in the stools or rectal biopsy of a patient with portal hypertension and splenomegaly suggests this diagnosis (see Ch. 296).

TOXIC AND DRUG-INDUCED LIVER DISEASE

703.   TOXIC HEPATITIS

A *hepatotoxin* is defined as an agent that causes liver injury in both man and animals in a predictable manner.

Liver injury is dose related and is usually manifest after a relatively short latent period. Hepatotoxins may cause liver cell necrosis or biochemical changes with necrosis; these changes may be manifest by impaired formation of bile, disturbances of lipid metabolism with fat accumulation, or altered enzyme activity. Some hepatotoxins may exert their effect indirectly by interfering with hepatic blood flow (Senecio alkaloids in veno-occlusive disease).

With elimination of a number of industrial hazards, exposure to hepatotoxins other than alcohol (ethanol) is now usually accidental or suicidal. Hepatotoxic agents are not often used pharmacologically unless the therapeutic dose is considerably less than the toxic dose, or unless therapy despite toxic side effects may still benefit the patient. Immunosuppressive agents and certain agents used in the chemotherapy of cancer may be hepatotoxic.

Poisoning by several hepatotoxic agents is discussed in Part III.

CARBON TETRACHLORIDE LIVER INJURY

The hepatotoxicity of carbon tetrachloride is believed to be due to the formation of toxic metabolites which bind to microsomal proteins. The increase in carbon tetrachloride toxicity after alcohol ingestion in man and laboratory animals has been related to an increase in the activity of drug metabolizing enzymes with increased formation of toxic metabolites; phenobarbital also increases carbon tetrachloride toxicity in laboratory animals.

The clinical features of carbon tetrachloride liver injury are similar to those of acute viral hepatitis, but with a shorter symptomatic preicteric period and with more rapid recovery, unless massive necrosis causes early death or renal tubular necrosis leads to irreversible or fatal renal failure.

The symptoms that follow inhalation or ingestion of the agent are predominantly gastrointestinal, with *anorexia, nausea* and *vomiting,* and right upper quadrant *pain* with *tender hepatomegaly* preceding the onset of jaundice. In many patients there may be hepatic enlargement with acute elevation of serum transaminase levels without jaundice. Acute renal failure is often a more prominent manifestation of poisoning.

Pathologically, there is centrilobular necrosis without inflammation during the period of maximal liver injury, followed rapidly by regeneration of parenchymal cells and hyperplasia of Kupffer's cells. Complete restoration of structure and function follows recovery from a single exposure. There is some evidence, however, that repeated exposure may sometimes lead to cirrhosis of the liver.

LIVER INJURY DUE TO ALCOHOL

Experimental studies in man and animals have shown that alcohol (ethanol) is a direct hepatotoxin. All the lesions of alcoholic liver disease in man have been produced by feeding alcohol to baboons for periods up to four years; these lesions included fatty infiltration, alcoholic hepatitis, fibrosis, and cirrhosis. A nutritious diet did not protect these animals from developing liver disease.

The clinical and pathologic manifestations of alcoholic liver disease are discussed in detail in Ch. 709.

SEX HORMONES AND THE LIVER

Methyl testosterone and C-17 alkyl substituted steroids (norethandronone) may cause intrahepatic cholestasis with conjugated hyperbilirubinemia, reduced clearance of BSP (with normal hepatic uptake and conjugation), and increased serum alkaline phosphatase and 5'-nucleotidase activity. This effect is dose related in man, causes no permanent liver damage or acute parenchymal cell necrosis, and is reversible. This type of cholestasis may be due to a change in the permeability of the biliary tree to bile salts.

During the third trimester of normal pregnancy there may be increases in serum cholesterol, alkaline phosphatase, and 5'-nucleotidase with reduced clearance of BSP. Occasionally, impaired hepatic excretory function may cause jaundice that recurs in subsequent pregnancies — *recurrent jaundice of pregnancy*. Recent studies have shown that natural estrogens reduce hepatic BSP clearance. It is probable that the physiologic changes in liver function during the third trimester of pregnancy are due to hormone effects on the liver. These observations are of particular interest in view of the recent reports that hormones given to suppress ovulation may occasionally cause hepatic dysfunction.

ACETAMINOPHEN LIVER INJURY

Self-poisoning with excessive doses of acetaminophen is now recognized as a relatively common cause for centrilobular liver necrosis with severe hepatitis in Great Britain. Therapeutic doses of acetaminophen cause no liver injury, because potentially toxic metabolites are rapidly conjugated with glutathione to nontoxic compounds. Excessive doses of acetaminophen (particularly with blood levels in excess of 300 μg per milliliter four hours after drug administration) exhaust the available glutathione, and toxic metabolites which bind covalently to microsomal protein accumulate and cause liver cell necrosis. Preliminary studies in laboratory animals and patients suggest that the early intravenous administration of a glutathione precursor such as *cysteine* or the sulfhydryl compound *cysteamine* protects against liver injury after excessive acetaminophen ingestion.

704. LIVER DISEASE DUE TO HYPERSENSITIVITY DRUG REACTIONS

Liver injury after drug therapy is more often due to a *hypersensitivity reaction* than to a hepatotoxic effect. In contrast to hepatotoxic reactions, the hypersensitivity reaction is quite unpredictable unless a previous reaction has been recorded, is not dose related, follows a variable latent period after drug exposure, cannot be reproduced in experimental animals, and may be associated with other manifestations of hypersensitivity (skin rash, fever, eosinophilia).

Drug hypersensitivity reactions involving the liver may be minor local manifestations of a generalized reaction, e.g., minor changes in liver function in patients with exfoliative dermatitis, or may be the predominant manifestation of the reaction. The common hepatic lesions are *intrahepatic cholestasis* and *parenchymal cell necrosis*. The former is illustrated by reactions to *chlorpromazine*, and the latter by reactions to *halothane*, *isoniazid*, or *alpha-methyldopa*.

CHLORPROMAZINE JAUNDICE

Approximately 1 per cent of patients treated with this phenothiazine develop a hypersensitivity reaction with intrahepatic cholestasis and jaundice. A greater number of patients develop changes in excretory function without jaundice. Early symptoms, beginning acutely usually within one to four weeks of initial drug exposure, or within a few days of repeated challenge, include *nausea, vomiting,* and *epigastric pain* often associated with *fever, lymphadenopathy, skin eruptions,* and *arthralgias.* The liver becomes enlarged and variably tender. Jaundice is obstructive in type with severe pruritus, dark urine, and pale stools, and tests of liver function reflect predominant *cholestasis* with conjugated hyperbilirubinemia and increased serum alkaline phosphatase, 5'-nucleotidase, and cholesterol levels. The serum transaminase levels may be elevated in the range of 100 to 200 IU. The white blood count may be normal or slightly elevated, with peripheral eosinophilia.

On liver biopsy, intrahepatic cholestasis, with bile plugs in dilated bile canaliculi and bile staining of parenchymal cells, and variable periportal infiltration with mononuclear and eosinophil cells are the predominant findings. There may be minimal centrilobular necrosis of liver cells.

Jaundice usually subsides within a few days or weeks of onset, with complete recovery, but occasionally chronic intrahepatic cholestasis may develop in spite of cessation of drug therapy. The clinical features in these patients may be similar to those in primary biliary cirrhosis, but periportal fibrosis is less severe, and eventual recovery without cirrhosis is usual.

Treatment. There is no specific therapy. The offending agent should be discontinued and avoided thereafter. Cholestyramine, 2 grams every four hours orally, may relieve pruritus by lowering serum bile acid levels. Vitamin K should be given parenterally if malabsorption causes an increase in prothrombin time. Corticosteroids are of little benefit either in relieving jaundice or in reducing pruritus.

HEPATITIS AFTER ANESTHESIA WITH FLUORINATED AGENTS

Acute liver disease, clinically and pathologically similar to viral hepatitis, is an uncommon complication of anesthesia with the fluorinated agents *halothane* and *methoxyflurane.* The mechanism of liver injury appears to be a *hypersensitivity reaction.* Liver disease is more common with repeated exposure to the anesthetic agent, and recurrent episodes have shorter latent periods between exposure and onset of symptoms; recurrent hepatitis has been well documented in several anesthetists after occupational exposure to halothane. Immunologic phenomena in patients with hepatitis after halothane exposure include peripheral eosinophilia, a transiently positive test for antimitochondrial antibodies in serum, and stimulation of cultured peripheral lymphocytes by halothane.

Several etiologic factors should be excluded before postoperative liver necrosis is attributed to an anesthetic agent; these include *hypoxia, hypotension, postoperative sepsis, biliary tract disease, viral hepatitis* (either coincidental or after transfusion), and *reactions to other drugs.* It is difficult to establish a diagnosis of hepatitis caused by anesthetic exposure with any degree of certainty unless there is a history of acute liver disease after previous exposure to the agent.

The treatment of patients with hepatitis caused by anesthetic agents is similar to that of acute viral hepatitis (see Ch. 697 and 698). When a patient has recovered from halothane or methoxyflurane hepatitis, further exposure to these anesthetic agents should be avoided.

ISONIAZID HEPATITIS

Severe hepatitis has been reported as a complication of *isoniazid* therapy for tuberculosis. Prospective studies in tuberculin-positive patients receiving isoniazid as a secondary chemoprophylactic agent have shown that approximately 10 per cent of patients exhibit transient elevation of serum transaminase levels (usually less than 100 IU). Overt hepatitis with jaundice is a rare complication which has usually been described during the first 12 weeks of treatment; jaundice is preceded by *fever, fatigue, weakness, myalgias and arthralgias,* and *anorexia.* Liver biopsies in jaundiced patients have shown focal necrosis, subacute necrosis (bridging), or multilobular necrosis with inflammation. Patients who continue drug therapy for longer periods after the onset of symptoms usually exhibit more severe liver lesions.

It is recommended that isoniazid therapy be discontinued in patients who develop symptoms associated with abnormal liver function tests; early cessation of therapy may prevent more serious and potentially fatal reactions.

705. FATTY LIVER

Fat accumulation in the liver (fatty liver) may be a physiologic response to an increase in lipid mobilization from peripheral fat, e.g., during early starvation, or may result from several disturbances of lipid transport and metabolism in a variety of disease states. Excessive lipid in parenchymal cells may arise from one or more of three sources: (1) the diet, (2) peripheral fat depots, and (3) hepatic synthesis. Lipid from any of these sources may accumulate when the supply is increased, or when a decrease in hepatic oxidation of fatty acids or reduced lipoprotein synthesis and release diminishes the clearance of lipid from the liver.

In *starvation,* free fatty acids are mobilized from adipose tissue, and are in part esterified in the liver to triglyceride. This physiologic response is probably the mechanism for the fatty infiltration of the liver observed in many patients after acute and chronic illnesses. In *protein malnutrition (kwashiorkor),* extreme fatty liver may be related in part to fat mobilization from depots (free fatty acid concentrations in serum are elevated), and in part to impaired lipoprotein synthesis. In *obese patients,* an excessive accumulation of fat in the liver may be a reflection of the general increase in the triglyceride stores. *Diabetic ketoacidosis,* with excessive mobil-

ization of depot fat, is usually accompanied by liver enlargement caused by fat. In each of these conditions the major clinical manifestation of fatty liver is hepatic enlargement; tenderness usually accompanies acute enlargement. *BSP retention* may be the only abnormality of liver function.

In several conditions fatty liver may be associated with severe derangement of liver function. This is particularly the case when fat accumulation is due to toxic injury causing decreased fatty acid oxidation or impaired lipoprotein synthesis. In *carbon tetrachloride* or *phosphorus* poisoning, fat accumulation is one manifestation of toxic liver injury. Large intravenous doses of *tetracycline* (usually more than 1 gram daily), particularly in pregnant women, have caused liver failure and death; a fine fatty vacuolization of the liver cells is the major pathologic change in the liver. In two syndromes, fatty liver is accompanied by severe encephalopathy with high mortality; the clinical picture is that of fulminant hepatitis. *Fatty liver of pregnancy* usually presents with vomiting, abdominal pain, and jaundice during the last month of pregnancy; bleeding, premature labor, renal failure, and coma with convulsions rapidly lead to death. The serum bilirubin and alkaline phosphatase elevations suggest severe cholestasis; disturbances of the clotting mechanism reflect impaired synthesis of clotting factors. *Reye's syndrome* is a rare disease described in children. Symptoms suggestive of an upper respiratory infection are followed by fever, progressive encephalopathy with delirium, convulsions, decerebrate posturing, coma, and death (see Ch. 397). Encephalopathy is associated with acute liver enlargement resulting from fatty infiltration; jaundice is unusual, probably because of the rapidly fatal outcome. Extremely high serum levels of transaminase, prolonged prothrombin time, and hypoglycemia indicate severe liver injury. The pathogenesis of this syndrome and the relationship between liver and brain injury are unknown; the suggestion that this syndrome may complicate viral infection has not been supported by virologic studies. *Small bowel bypass surgery* (particularly jejunocolic shunts) for the treatment of extreme obesity is often complicated by fatty infiltration of the liver with progressive impairment of liver function or the development of cirrhosis. Serial liver biopsies should be performed in these patients to monitor histologic changes.

The most common form of toxic liver injury leading to fatty infiltration of the liver is that due to *alcohol (ethanol) ingestion* (see Ch. 709).

Treatment of the underlying cause of fatty liver, e.g., correction or protein malnutrition, or withdrawal from alcohol, is usually effective in lowering the fat content of the liver. In patients with acute severe liver injury associated with encephalopathy, measures used in the management of patients with fulminant hepatitis have been applied with questionable success (see Ch. 698).

706. THE LIVER IN ACUTE HEART FAILURE AND SHOCK

Hypoxia secondary to reduced liver blood flow may cause centrilobular parenchymal cell necrosis. This often complicates *acute congestive heart failure* or *hypotension* of any cause. The liver may be enlarged and tender if the central venous pressure is raised. The predominant clinical manifestations are those of the underlying cardiovascular disease, which determines both therapy and prognosis. The biochemical changes in acute heart failure include slight hyperbilirubinemia with slight elevation of transaminases and alkaline phosphatase and BSP retention. In shock, the serum transaminase levels are sometimes markedly elevated but return quickly to normal levels with restoration of normal blood flow and parenchymal cell regeneration. Deep jaundice may be a terminal event in patients with prolonged shock.

707.   HEPATIC VEIN OCCLUSION
(Budd-Chiari Syndrome)

Occlusion of the hepatic veins is a rare condition usually caused by *tumor infiltration* (hepatoma, metastatic tumor) or *thrombosis* of the vessels. This may be a local lesion, or may extend from the inferior vena cava. *Polycythemia vera* is one of the more common causes of thrombosis of these veins. The major clinical manifestations of this condition are *hepatic enlargement,* with *pain* and *tenderness,* and *ascites.* In the acute form, hepatic vein occlusion is characterized pathologically by centrilobular congestion and necrosis of the adjacent parenchyma. A needle biopsy of the liver should establish the diagnosis when hepatic congestion resulting from an increase in central venous pressure has been excluded. The obstruction may be subacute or chronic when ascites and portal hypertension are the major clinical problems. *Hepatic venography* by direct injection of contrast material into a hepatic catheter is the most valuable technique for establishing the diagnosis.

Patients with chronic hepatic vein occlusion usually respond to a diuretic program (see treatment of ascites). Polycythemia vera should also be treated vigorously (see Ch. 758).

CHRONIC LIVER DISEASE

708.   CHRONIC ACTIVE (AGGRESSIVE) HEPATITIS

Chronic active hepatitis is characterized pathologically by a normal lobular architecture in which fibrous septa extend from enlarged portal tracts into the parenchyma, disrupting the liver cell plates adjacent to the portal zones and separating off rosettes of parenchymal cells. Piecemeal necrosis of liver cells adjacent to the expanding portal zones, infiltration of the portal areas with eosinophils, lymphocytes and plasma cells, and focal necrosis and inflammation within liver lobules are present in varying degrees and reflect the "activity" of the lesion. Progressive destruction of the normal lobular architecture with proliferation of fibroblasts in expanding portal areas and nodular regeneration of parenchymal cells may ultimately lead to cirrhosis in untreated patients.

Pathogenesis. It is now evident that the clinical and pathologic spectrum of *chronic active hepatitis* is a syndrome of diverse etiology. In a large percentage of patients the primary etiologic factor has not been identified. *Hepatitis B infection* is of importance in a significant number of patients; persistence of HBAg after acute hepatitis B is often associated with the development of chronic active hepatitis; chronic active hepatitis has been documented by liver biopsy in approximately 15 per cent of asymptomatic HBAg carriers without a past history of acute hepatitis; of patients diagnosed as suffering from chronic active hepatitis, between 10 and 30 per cent are HBAg positive. The clinical and pathologic features of chronic active hepatitis have been documented in patients with *drug-induced liver disease;* the laxative agent *oxyphenisatin* and *alpha-methyldopa* cause hypersensitivity reactions with typical clinical, biochemical, immunologic, and pathologic changes of chronic active hepatitis. *Wilson's disease* may present with features of chronic active hepatitis.

The factors which determine the chronicity of the disease process are poorly understood. In some patients chronic active hepatitis may be a host response to persisting viral (hepatitis B) infection, and in others it may be a reaction to toxic liver injury. *Immunologic phenomena* are a common feature; hypergammaglobulinemia parallels disease activity, and the patients' serum may contain a variety of antibodies which lack organ specificity, including antimitochondrial, smooth muscle, and antinuclear antibodies. The hypothesis that immunologic mechanisms relate to the pathogenesis of chronic active hepatitis is supported indirectly by the increased frequency of other diseases considered to have an immunopathologic basis in both patients and relatives of patients with chronic active hepatitis; Sjögren's syndrome, thyroiditis or thyrotoxicosis, and fibrosing alveolitis with pulmonary diffusion defects are commonly associated diseases. Studies on serum complement levels in patients with chronic active hepatitis have revealed that depressed complement levels are related to impaired hepatic protein synthesis and do not reflect immunologic activity.

Clinical Manifestations. Chronic active hepatitis is a disease with a wide clinical spectrum and insidious onset; it may be clinically silent for long periods, as in patients who present as asymptomatic blood donors and are found to be HBAg positive with elevated SGOT levels; patients with more active disease may present with symptoms suggestive of acute hepatitis with malaise, arthralgias, anorexia, and low-grade fever. Amenorrhea commonly results from disturbances of endocrine function. On physical examination, the patient may exhibit signs of both acute and chronic liver disease; these include jaundice, spider angiomas, liver enlargement with variable tenderness, and splenomegaly. The presence of ascites or manifestations of portal hypertension suggests that cirrhosis is already established. The important laboratory features of chronic active hepatitis are changes in *serum transaminase* levels and *hypergammaglobulinemia,* because it has been shown that these tests reflect the activity of the disease—the extent of liver cell necrosis and the degree of associated round cell infiltration in the liver. Patients who present with clinical manifestations of acute hepatitis and subsequently exhibit elevated levels of serum transaminase and gamma globulin for periods in excess of ten weeks are likely to be suffering from chronic active hepatitis or subacute hepatic necrosis. The prognosis of patients with extreme hyperglobulinemia (gamma globulin levels greater than twice normal) and with five- to tenfold elevations of serum transaminase (SGOT) persisting without improvement over a ten-week period is extremely poor without therapy; more than a third of these patients die within a period of six months. When disease activity is minimal, patients may remain well for long periods. Increases in the level of serum bilirubin and alkaline phosphatase caused by intrahepatic cholestasis and depression of plasma albumin and clotting factor levels caused by impaired hepatic plasma protein synthesis are variable features of advanced disease.

Diagnosis. The diagnosis of chronic active hepatitis should be confirmed by percutaneous *liver biopsy* whenever there is clinical or laboratory evidence of this disease. It is important to differentiate chronic active hepatitis from other liver diseases, particularly *chronic persisting hepatitis* which has a favorable prognosis for full recovery without therapy. The degree of irreversible liver damage—cirrhosis—can be determined only by morphologic studies. In all patients with chronic active hepatitis, potential etiologic factors should be fully evaluated, i.e., exposure to drugs and the presence of circulating HBAg or anti-HB. Wilson's disease must be excluded by slit lamp examination of the eyes for Kayser-Fleischer rings, and by measurements of serum ceruloplasmin levels and urinary copper excretion.

Treatment. It has been established by controlled clinical studies that corticosteroids increase the survival of patients with chronic active hepatitis. In the Mayo Clinic study, patients with biochemical and histologic evidence of severe disease (SGOT levels five- to tenfold elevated, and gamma globulin more than twofold increased for periods of ten weeks) were treated with prednisone (20 mg daily), a combination of prednisone (10 mg daily) with azathioprine (50 mg daily), azathioprine (100 mg) alone, or placebo; treatment with prednisone or prednisone with azathioprine was significantly more effective than azathioprine alone or placebo in inducing clinical remission and prolonging survival. The current indications for corticosteroid therapy in patients with biopsy-proved chronic active hepatitis are (1) biochemical evidence of severe disease as cited above, and (2) clinical deterioration with development of ascites or evidence of progressing liver failure. Patients with clinical features of chronic active hepatitis and pathologic evidence of subacute hepatic necrosis on biopsy should also be treated in view of the evidence that their disease is progressive. Patients with relative contraindications to steroid therapy—e.g., with diabetes mellitus—and those who develop complications of steroid therapy may benefit from a combined regimen of low-dose prednisone (10 mg daily) with azathioprine (50 to 100 mg daily). The value of alternate-day corticosteroid therapy has not been assessed.

The duration of corticosteroid therapy should be determined by the clinical, biochemical, and histologic response. The goal of therapy is to induce remission of active hepatitis; the patient should be asymptomatic, with normal or minimally elevated SGOT (less than twice normal) and normal gamma globulin levels, and with resolution of inflammation and liver cell necrosis on

liver biopsy; this end result can be anticipated in approximately two thirds of patients treated for one to three years. When complete remission is established, corticosteroids can be slowly withdrawn and discontinued; subsequent relapses usually occur within six months and require further therapy.

The decision whether to treat a patient with chronic active hepatitis of low-grade activity, e.g., a patient with mild symptoms and minimal elevation of SGOT and gamma globulin, may be a difficult one. Guidelines derived from controlled clinical trials are not available, and the potential benefit from corticosteroid therapy may be exceeded by the risks of long-term therapy.

Prognosis. With adequate therapy, remission of active disease with restoration of normal liver morphology or with residual inactive cirrhosis is achieved in approximately two thirds of patients. Approximately 20 per cent of patients with severe chronic active hepatitis fail to respond to steroid therapy and die with liver failure caused by progressive cirrhosis within a period of one to three years. The long-term prognosis of patients with chronic active hepatitis of low-grade activity has not been defined.

709. CIRRHOSIS OF THE LIVER

Definition and Classification. The cirrhotic liver is one in which the normal lobular architecture is destroyed by bands of fibrous tissue which separate nodules of regenerated liver cells (regeneration nodules). Clinically, patients with cirrhosis usually present with symptoms that relate to the primary etiology (e.g., chronic active hepatitis or manifestations of excessive alcohol intake) or with complications of cirrhosis (e.g., ascites, bleeding from esophageal varices, or hepatic coma). At the time of diagnosis, major etiologic factors causing chronic liver disease may be evident (e.g., documented hepatitis progressing to *chronic active hepatitis, excessive alcohol intake,* or *chronic biliary tract obstruction),* but in many patients the etiology will never be determined. Macroscopic and/or microscopic examination of liver tissue is necessary to establish the diagnosis of cirrhosis, but the pathologic changes in the liver may be the end-stage of several alternative processes which are not always evident at the time of autopsy examination.

In this chapter an *etiologic* classification is used; alternative terminology for cirrhosis will be referred to in the text.

1. Posthepatitic and idiopathic cirrhosis.
2. Cirrhosis in the alcoholic.
3. Metabolic cirrhosis (hemochromatosis and Wilson's disease).
4. Biliary cirrhosis (primary and secondary).
5. Schistosomal fibrosis.
6. Cardiac cirrhosis.

Hemochromatosis is discussed in Part XVI, Section Four, Wilson's disease in Ch. 945, and schistosomal fibrosis in Ch. 296.

POSTHEPATITIC AND IDIOPATHIC CIRRHOSIS (POSTNECROTIC CIRRHOSIS)

Pathogenesis. It has been shown by serial liver biopsy studies that acute viral hepatitis (usually type B, either icteric or anicteric) or toxic hepatitis complicated by subacute hepatic necrosis or chronic active hepatitis may lead to a macronodular cirrhosis. In many nonalcoholic patients there is no history to suggest previous viral or toxic hepatitis; i.e., the cirrhosis is idiopathic (cryptogenic). Idiopathic cirrhosis is sometimes associated with chronic ulcerative colitis; it has been suggested but not proved that chronic pericholangitis resulting from portal bacteremia may cause cirrhosis in these patients.

The association of hypergammaglobulinemia, positive antinuclear reactions, positive LE cell phenomena, and other positive serologic reactions with idiopathic cirrhosis has led to a theory that cirrhosis may be caused by immunologic destruction of parenchymal cells; this has not been proved (see Ch. 708). An increased formation of immunoglobulins with hyperglobulinemia may be stimulated by antigens released from necrotic cells, and may have no primary etiologic significance.

Pathology. The liver in posthepatitic or idiopathic cirrhosis is typically shrunken, with irregular large regeneration nodules and broad zones of fibrous tissue. Pathologically, this is referred to as *macronodular (postnecrotic) cirrhosis*. During the phase of *progressive (active) cirrhosis* after subacute hepatic necrosis or chronic active hepatitis, there may be microscopic evidence of cell degeneration and regeneration, and mononuclear infiltration (both lymphocytes and plasma cells) is prominent in the zones of fibrosis. Intrahepatic cholestasis with bile plugs in dilated bile canaliculi varies with the degree of jaundice, and bile duct proliferation is usual.

Clinical Manifestations. The progressive cirrhosis that follows subacute hepatic necrosis and chronic active hepatitis is often associated with malaise, weakness, anorexia, and jaundice. The patient often has a low-grade fever, and multiple spider angiomas may be seen. The liver is sometimes enlarged and tender, but is more typically shrunken and associated with increased percussion resonance over the right lower costal margin; the spleen may be slightly or massively enlarged. Ascites or peripheral edema may complicate portal hypertension or hypoalbuminemia, and increased bruising may be due to hypoprothrombinemia. Manifestations of disturbed endocrine function—acne, striae, gynecomastia, and amenorrhea—are particularly common in juvenile patients with active cirrhosis. Hypergammaglobulinemia parallels the degree of lymphocytic and plasma cell infiltration in the liver, and may be accompanied by serologic abnormalities. Chronic intrahepatic cholestasis with jaundice, hypercholesterolemia, and high alkaline phosphatase levels sometimes mimics primary biliary cirrhosis. It is not unusual for the biochemical evidence of hepatocellular failure to exceed the clinical evidence of this condition.

The only clinical manifestations of compensated idiopathic cirrhosis may be the cutaneous stigmata of chronic liver disease and splenic enlargement. In these patients, ascites, hepatic coma, and bleeding from esophageal varices may be late complications.

Treatment. Patients with chronic active hepatitis or subacute hepatic necrosis should be treated with corticosteroids to induce clinical remission. When cirrhosis is already established in these patients (confirmed by liver biopsy), corticosteroids will not reverse the existing cirrhosis, but by suppressing continued destructive activity they may prevent progression of the liver disease (see Ch. 708). Corticosteroid therapy is not indicated in patients with inactive posthepatitic cirrhosis.

The management of the complications of cirrhosis is discussed later in this chapter under treatment of portal hypertension, ascites, and hepatic coma.

CIRRHOSIS IN THE ALCOHOLIC

Pathogenesis and Epidemiology. The incidence of cirrhosis in the United States parallels the consumption of alcohol. Little is known, however, of the factors that determine individual susceptibility to cirrhosis; these would explain why many persons with a chronic heavy intake of alcohol do not develop liver disease; both genetic and dietary factors may be of importance. Some insight into the problem of liver disease in the alcoholic has been gained from experimental studies on the effect of alcohol (ethanol) on liver metabolism.

The Effects of Alcohol (Ethanol) on the Liver. Both in man and in laboratory animals, alcohol ingestion is associated with two prominent morphologic changes: the accumulation of fat (triglyceride) in parenchymal cells and degeneration of cell organelles (visible as *alcoholic hyaline*–eosinophilic cytoplasmic inclusions). These changes may result from a direct *hepatotoxic effect of alcohol* rather than a deficiency of dietary factors; they are seen when alcohol is substituted for carbohydrate in an adequate diet.

The pathogenesis of cirrhosis in the alcoholic was not clarified by earlier studies in laboratory animals; in the rat, prolonged administration of alcohol caused fatty infiltration and parenchymal cell degeneration, but these lesions did not progress to cirrhosis. Recent studies in baboons fed alcohol for periods of nine months to four years have reproduced all the pathologic lesions of human alcoholic liver disease.

Pathology. The liver in *acute alcoholic hepatitis* is enlarged and firm, and on microscopic examination the parenchymal cells are distended with droplets of fat, and may contain eosinophilic cytoplasmic inclusions (alcoholic hyaline). Central veins and centrilobular areas may be replaced by zones of *hyaline sclerosis*, a lesion which undergoes subsequent fibrosis and may contribute to the development of portal hypertension. There is variable inflammatory cell infiltration in portal areas and throughout the parenchyma, and bile stasis occurs in jaundiced patients.

Cirrhosis in the alcoholic is usually of the *Laennec* or *micronodular type*, with small uniform regeneration nodules separated by fibrous bands containing mononuclear cells and proliferating bile ductules. The pathologic changes of acute alcoholic hepatitis—inflammation, cell degeneration, and infiltration with fat—are often seen in the cirrhotic liver. Occasionally the liver is of the *macronodular type*, with coarse, irregular regeneration nodules and broad intervening bands of fibrous tissue.

Clinical Manifestations. A patient with *acute alcoholic hepatitis* may seek medical help because of *abdominal pain* caused by acute hepatic enlargement, gastritis, or pancreatitis; *vomiting*, with or without *hematemesis*, caused by gastritis, ulcer, or sometimes esophageal varices; *jaundice; abdominal swelling* with ascites; or because of symptoms caused by head injury, alcohol withdrawal, or thiamin deficiency.

On admission to hospital, the patient is usually *febrile*

and *dehydrated* and has an alcoholic fetor. An *enlarged, firm, tender liver,* abdominal distention with *ascites* and *jaundice,* with prominent spider angiomas and palmar erythema, are typically present. The early hospital course is often complicated by *delirium tremens.* Intense jaundice with *pruritus* in febrile patients may simulate extrahepatic biliary tract obstruction.

Liver function tests reveal conjugated hyperbilirubinemia, elevated serum transaminase levels (50 to 300 units), variable increases in alkaline phosphatase activity, and normal or depressed levels of albumin and clotting factors. The serum cholesterol concentration may be increased, normal, or depressed. *Hypokalemia* often results from increased urinary excretion of potassium. *Hyperuricemia* resulting from depressed urinary excretion of uric acid parallels lactic acidosis. Anemia may be due to bleeding or *hemolysis;* acute severe hemolysis is sometimes associated with *hyperlipemia* (Zieve's syndrome).

Cirrhosis in the alcoholic may present insidiously with anorexia, fatigue, and weakness, and a gradual onset of jaundice and ascites, or may present acutely with one or several major complications: acute upper gastrointestinal *bleeding,* sudden onset of *ascites,* liver failure with *jaundice* or *coma,* or symptoms of hepatic *carcinoma.* When the cirrhotic patient shows manifestations of acute alcoholic hepatitis, the term *florid cirrhosis* is often used. In the absence of these complications the only stigmata of cirrhosis may be a firm, enlarged, nontender liver with or without splenomegaly, and the cutaneous manifestations of chronic liver disease.

In *compensated cirrhosis* the only abnormalities of liver function may be mild BSP retention and an increased urinary excretion of urobilinogen. With progressive decompensation, serum protein concentrations fall, and hyperbilirubinemia and BSP retention increase. Serum enzyme levels are usually only slightly elevated.

Differential Diagnosis. In the differential diagnosis of acute alcoholic hepatitis other causes for acute jaundice must be considered, i.e., *viral hepatitis, extrahepatic obstruction,* and *drug reactions.* Infection should be considered in the febrile patient, although fever may be due to cell necrosis. In the compensated cirrhotic, an enlarged, firm liver may be suggestive of infiltrative disease. A needle biopsy of the liver usually resolves these differential diagnostic problems.

When cirrhosis is complicated by bleeding, ascites, or coma, other causes for these complications must be excluded. In cirrhotic patients, acute upper gastrointestinal *bleeding* may come from esophageal varices; but acute gastric erosions, peptic ulcer, and neoplasm must also be considered. Esophagoscopy, gastroscopy, and roentgenologic evaluation of the esophagus, stomach, and duodenum are necessary to establish the site of bleeding (see Ch. 644). Although *ascites* is usually due to portal hypertension with hypoalbuminemia, *constrictive pericarditis, bacterial peritonitis* (especially *tuberculous*), and *intra-abdominal neoplasm* must also be considered. Measurement of the venous pressure and a diagnostic paracentesis with analysis for protein, enzymes, bacteria, and cells are of value in differential diagnosis. In tuberculous peritonitis the protein concentration of ascitic fluid may exceed 2.5 grams per 100 ml and the ascitic fluid white cell count usually exceeds 250 per cubic millimeter, with lymphocytes predominant. Malignant effusions are often hemorrhagic, with a protein content greater than 2.5 grams per 100 ml and elevated lactic dehydrogenase activity; malignant cells may be found on cytologic examination.

Treatment. Long-term abstinence from alcohol is the single major factor that may modify the course of liver disease in the alcoholic. With abstinence, liver function may return to normal after an episode of acute alcoholic hepatitis, and minimal hepatic fibrosis may persist without progression. When cirrhosis is well established and portal hypertension with esophageal varices complicates the liver disease, abstinence from alcohol may not prolong the patient's survival.

Patients with *acute alcoholic hepatitis* should be treated with bed rest, alcohol withdrawal, and a diet containing adequate proteins, vitamins, minerals, and calories. Intravenous infusions of 5 per cent glucose, with potassium, magnesium and vitamin supplements, may be needed by the febrile, dehydrated patient. Oral supplements of ferrous sulfate (0.3 gram three times a day) or folic acid (5 mg daily) should be given to correct anemia caused by iron or folic acid deficiency. Salt intake should be restricted to 1 gram per 24 hours in patients with ascites, and fluid intake and output should be monitored with daily weights. On this regimen clinical and biochemical improvement is usual within two to three weeks, and is accompanied by a spontaneous diuresis and disappearance of ascites unless portal hypertension is already established by fibrosis.

Although corticosteroid therapy has been recommended for the treatment of severely ill patients, a recent controlled study indicated that prednisone was of no benefit.

TREATMENT OF THE COMPLICATIONS OF CIRRHOSIS

Portal Hypertension with Upper Gastrointestinal Bleeding. In the early management of bleeding, treatment is directed toward restoring blood volume and controlling the bleeding at the same time that diagnostic efforts are made to determine the site of bleeding. The alcoholic patient may bleed from *acute gastric erosions, peptic ulcer,* or *esophageal varices;* appropriate therapy depends on the site of bleeding. The several measures that may be used to control bleeding in cirrhotic patients include gastric lavage with ice water, local gastric hypothermia using an esophagogastric balloon, intravenous infusions of Pitressin, esophageal tamponade with an inflated balloon, or direct surgical procedures. *Lavage* with ice water is unlikely to control esophageal bleeding, but may be effective when bleeding is from gastric erosions. Infusions of Pitressin (20 units intravenously in 10 minutes) constrict the splanchnic arterioles, reduce splanchnic blood flow, and lower portal venous pressure. Bleeding from varices may thus be temporarily controlled. Similar results may be achieved without systemic side effects by continuous infusion of vasoconstrictor drugs into the superior mesenteric artery, selectively catheterized. *Esophageal tamponade* (with a Sengstaken esophageal tube) may be the only nonoperative procedure that will control massive bleeding from esophageal varices. The disadvantage of this procedure is the many complications that result from tamponade: asphyxia resulting from upward displacement of the balloon, aspiration, and esophageal erosion by pressure necrosis. These complications, however, will be minimized by using an additional smooth bore tube attached to the Sengstaken tube for aspiration of secretions proximal to the balloon and by tracheal intubation with a cuffed endotracheal tube.

Several surgical procedures have been recommended to control bleeding from esophageal varices. These include direct ligation of varices, transection of the esophagus with division of varices, esophagogastric resection, splenectomy, and splenorenal or portacaval anastomosis. Each procedure carries a high risk in the poor-risk patient with hepatic decompensation. The surgical procedure of choice is a *portacaval anastomosis,* which controls bleeding by lowering portal pressure; with the subsequent disappearance of esophageal varices, recurrent bleeding is unusual.

A portacaval anastomosis is recommended for the good-risk patient with documented bleeding from esophageal varices, unless bleeding has been precipitated by acute alcoholic hepatitis. In the latter instance, portal pressure may return to normal, and varices may disappear upon recovery from acute hepatic decompensation and resolution of hepatic inflammation and fatty infiltration. When esophageal bleeding complicates hepatocellular failure, surgery is contraindicated even when medical therapy is ineffective in controlling hemorrhage. There is no evidence that a prophylactic portacaval shunt is of value in prolonging the life of a patient with portal hypertension and esophageal varices that have not bled. Although prophylactic shunt surgery reduces the risk of subsequent variceal hemorrhage, the complications of surgery—hepatic encephalopathy and hepatic failure—result in considerable morbidity.

Ascites. When ascites complicates acute alcoholic hepatitis, therapy aimed at improving liver function usually leads to a spontaneous diuresis as the portal pressure falls toward normal and serum albumin levels rise. Sodium intake should be restricted to 1 gram daily, and diuretics should be used with caution.

When ascites is of longer duration and is associated with sustained portal hypertension and hypoalbuminemia, diuretic agents together with a restricted intake of sodium may be necessary to control sodium and water retention. Water intake may need to be restricted to a volume that equals insensible losses plus urine output in patients who fail to excrete a fluid load. The sole use of diuretic agents that act principally on the proximal tubule (mercurials and chlorothiazides) is contraindicated. These agents do not counteract the effect of aldosterone on the distal tubule; not only are they ineffective diuretics in cirrhotic patients with secondary hyperaldosteronism, but they also augment potassium loss and may precipitate *hypokalemic alkalosis* with hepatic coma in spite of oral potassium supplements.

To promote an *effective* and *safe* diuresis, an *aldosterone blocking agent* should be given in combination with one of the aforementioned diuretic agents. Spironolactone (50 to 200 mg daily) with hydrochlorothiazide (50 to 100 mg daily) is recommended. Oral potassium supplements (KCl in cherry syrup, 1 gram three times a day) may be necessary during the initial two to four days of combined drug therapy to prevent hypokalemia. Whereas edema fluid can be mobilized rapidly during diuresis, the maximal rate at which ascitic fluid can be removed by diuresis in the cirrhotic is approximately 900 ml per 24 hours. In patients free of peripheral edema, the rate of diuresis should not produce a daily weight loss in excess of 0.5 kg; if diuresis is more rapid, there will be a fall in plasma volume.

The complications of diuretic therapy include the following: (1) *Hyperkalemia* often results from the use of aldosterone-blocking drugs in patients with impaired renal function. (2) *Hyponatremia* may be associated with an abnormal distribution of sodium between the intracellular and extracellular fluid pools in patients with an increased total body sodium, with disproportionate water retention, or with sodium depletion after prolonged diuresis. (3) *Azotemia* may be due to contraction of the extracellular fluid pool or a decrease in glomerular blood flow owing to intrarenal shunting of blood. (4) *Hepatic encephalopathy* may follow rapid diuresis or disturbances of pH and electrolyte balance. These complications will be reduced if serum electrolyte concentrations and urinary electrolyte excretion are measured frequently during therapy. Diuretics should be discontinued when neuropsychiatric symptoms complicate rapid diuresis or electrolyte imbalance, and no attempt should be made to mobilize all ascitic fluid by prolonged therapy that increases the risk of complication without benefit to the patient. When long-term diuretic therapy is necessary to control ascites, diuretics should be given intermittently rather than continuously.

When ascites is associated with severe hypoalbuminemia, intravenous infusions of salt-poor albumin (50 to 100 grams daily) may potentiate a diuresis, but pulmonary edema caused by an expanded plasma volume must be avoided.

Paracentesis with removal of less than 1000 ml of ascitic fluid should be performed for diagnostic purposes, but is now rarely indicated for therapy of ascites except when impaired renal function prevents safe or effective diuretic therapy. Ascitic fluid should then be removed slowly through a small plastic catheter, and salt-poor human albumin (50 to 200 grams) should be infused intravenously over a period of 12 to 24 hours to prevent hypovolemia and shock that may result from a shift of fluid from the intravascular compartment into the peritoneal cavity.

Hepatic Coma. When a cirrhotic patient develops hepatic encephalopathy it is important to identify the precipitating cause. It may be due to gastrointestinal bleeding; fluid and electrolyte imbalances and pH disturbances, particularly during diuretic therapy; the administration of depressant drugs, both analgesic and sedative; intercurrent infection with fever; or increased dietary intake of protein. In the treatment of hepatic coma, gastrointestinal bleeding and infection must be controlled, depressant drugs withheld, and disturbances of fluid, electrolyte, and acid-base balance corrected. In all patients, measures that lower blood ammonium concentration by reducing enteric bacterial breakdown of amino acids and urea should be instituted. These measures include dietary *protein restriction* (complete in the comatose patient, or partial—20 to 40 grams—in patients with mild encephalopathy), *cathartics* (magnesium citrate, 240 ml twice daily), *enemas* to clear the intestine of its nitrogenous content, and *neomycin* (4 to 6 grams daily by mouth or by nasogastric tube) to reduce the bacterial flora.

Patients with chronic hepatic encephalopathy, who usually have extensive portal-systemic shunts, may be helped by long-term restriction of protein intake to 40 grams and the administration of neomycin, 2 to 3 grams daily. Lactulose, a disaccharide that is not absorbed but is metabolized by intestinal bacteria to organic acids, is effective in lowering the blood ammonia levels of patients with chronic encephalopathy; the unabsorbed sugar produces an osmotic diarrhea, and ammonia is retained in the fecal content at the acid pH.

A surgical approach to the management of the patient with chronic hepatic encephalopathy is excision or exclusion of the colon; the complications of surgery in chronically ill patients usually balance the potential benefit of removing a bacteria-laden gut.

BILIARY CIRRHOSIS

Primary biliary cirrhosis (chronic nonsuppurative destructive cholangitis) is a disease of unknown etiology. *Chronic intrahepatic cholestasis* is associated with progressive periportal fibrosis and chronic inflammation. Cirrhosis with nodular regeneration is a late pathologic finding. Although hypersensitivity reactions to drugs sometimes cause prolonged intrahepatic cholestasis, there is no evidence that acute intrahepatic cholestasis leads to primary biliary cirrhosis. It has been suggested that the primary lesion may be an injury to small bile ducts; these are often absent in liver biopsy specimens taken early in the course of the disease, but regenerate in the cirrhotic liver. Patients with primary biliary cirrhosis may exhibit hypergammaglobulinemia with circulating antibodies reactive against mitochondria (antimitochondrial antibody), but the significance of immunologic phenomena has not been established.

In *secondary biliary cirrhosis*, bile duct obstruction with or without infection causes periportal inflammation with progressive fibrosis, parenchymal cell destruction, and nodular regeneration.

Clinical Features. Primary biliary cirrhosis is most often diagnosed in women aged 40 to 60. The earliest symptom may be generalized *pruritus*. Jaundice with dark urine and pale stools and cutaneous xanthomas appear later with increasing intrahepatic cholestasis. At the time of onset of symptoms, the liver is usually firm and enlarged, and the spleen is palpable. Liver function tests at this time reflect cholestasis with good hepatocellular function; alkaline phosphatase, 5′-nucleotidase, and cholesterol levels may be markedly elevated, whereas serum albumin levels remain normal. During the period of maximal cholestasis the manifestations of malabsorption may become evident: *weight loss, diarrhea* with pale bulky stools, *bleeding* resulting from hypoprothrombinemia, and collapse of vertebrae and *pathologic fractures* with bone demineralization caused by malabsorption of vitamin D and calcium. *Xanthomas* usually appear when the serum cholesterol level exceeds 450 mg per 100 ml. Acute upper gastrointestinal bleeding is more often from a duodenal ulcer than from esophageal varices; a reduced flow of alkaline bile with normal gastric acid secretion may contribute to peptic ulcer.

The terminal stage of biliary cirrhosis is one of hepatocellular failure with rising serum bilirubin levels, a decrease in serum albumin and cholesterol with disappearance of xanthomas, and the onset of ascites.

Differential Diagnosis. The diagnosis of primary biliary cirrhosis must always be confirmed by exploratory laparotomy, with liver biopsy and operative cholangiography. Stenosing cholangitis, extrahepatic bile duct obstruction resulting from stone or stricture, and carcinoma involving the major extrahepatic or intrahepatic bile ducts should be excluded. The presence of antimitochondrial antibody is of diagnostic importance—patients with acute extrahepatic biliary obstruction do not exhibit this antibody.

Treatment. Supplements of fat-soluble vitamins should be given to prevent or correct deficiency caused by malabsorption. Vitamin K_1, 5 to 10 mg, and vitamins A and D, 10,000 units, should be given by mouth daily, together with calcium lactate or gluconate, 6 to 12 grams. *Pruritus* may be relieved by methyltestosterone or norethandrolone, 10 mg twice or three times daily, but these agents increase the jaundice. The bile acid sequestrant resin, *cholestyramine*, 8 to 12 grams daily in divided doses, is effective in relieving pruritus, lowering serum cholesterol levels, and reducing xanthomas when cholestasis is incomplete. Patients with duodenal ulcer or with complications of cirrhosis should be treated appropriately as outlined elsewhere.

Prognosis. The average life expectancy in primary biliary cirrhosis from the time of onset of symptoms is approximately five years. With supportive therapy the patient will be more comfortable and will suffer fewer complications during this period.

CARDIAC CIRRHOSIS

Chronic congestive heart failure with valvular heart disease and tricuspid incompetence or constrictive pericarditis may cause progressive fibrosis extending peripherally from centrilobular to portal areas. Regeneration nodules are not prominent. Fat may accumulate in hypoxic cells.

The liver is usually firm, with tenderness and an increase in size during more severe episodes of heart failure. Hepatic pulsation may be detected with tricuspid insufficiency. The changes in liver function are those of acute hepatic congestion, but hypoalbuminemia may be more severe when there is excessive enteric leakage of plasma protein. (See Part XIV, Section Three.) Although chronic congestive heart failure may raise the portal venous pressure, a portal-systemic collateral circulation, e.g., esophageal varices, does not develop in the absence of an increased pressure gradient between these systems.

710. CONGENITAL HEPATIC FIBROSIS

Congenital hepatic fibrosis is a variant of polycystic disease. Broad bands of fibrous tissue containing bile ducts surround the liver lobules and obstruct portal blood flow. Splenomegaly, portal hypertension, and bleeding from esophageal varices are the usual presenting manifestations in childhood or adolescence. With normal liver function these children usually tolerate recurrent bleeding and portacaval shunt surgery better than patients with cirrhosis. In adults, *polycystic disease of the liver* may cause massive liver enlargement without interfering with liver function. The complications include hemorrhage into a cyst with abdominal pain and bleeding from esophageal varices.

711. INFILTRATIVE DISEASE OF THE LIVER

HEPATIC GRANULOMAS

Hepatic granulomas are most commonly due to *sarcoidosis* and *tuberculosis,* but also occur in beryllium poisoning, brucellosis, fungal and parasitic infections, and Hodgkin's disease.

In sarcoidosis there are noncaseating granulomas, with mononuclear, epithelioid, and giant cells, and variable fibrosis. In patients with pulmonary tuberculosis or miliary tuberculosis, hepatic granulomas are particularly common. Small lesions may exhibit no caseation, and no organisms may be demonstrated; but larger lesions may have a central area of caseation.

Granulomatous disease of the liver may be associated with enlargement of the liver and BSP retention with elevation of alkaline phosphatase and 5'-nucleotidase without jaundice. A needle biopsy of the liver should be performed to establish the diagnosis of granulomatous disease. This is particularly helpful in the diagnosis of miliary tuberculosis in an ill, febrile patient without typical radiologic changes in the chest.

SECONDARY CARCINOMA OF THE LIVER

Primary carcinomas of the lung, gastrointestinal tract, and breast are the most common neoplasms that metastasize to the liver. Abdominal swelling or pain and jaundice are the presenting symptoms, but the liver is usually massively enlarged with multiple nodules before jaundice develops. The earlier biochemical manifestations of hepatic metastases are BSP retention and elevations of serum alkaline phosphatase and 5'-nucleotidase. Needle biopsy of the liver is helpful in providing a tissue diagnosis of secondary carcinoma, and may save the patient from the discomfort of an exploratory laparotomy. External radioisotopic scanning of the liver after the intravenous injection of a gamma-emitting radioisotope that is concentrated in the liver may be helpful in localizing large metastases that appear as "cold" areas in the surface scan. The presence of hepatic metastases from carcinomas of the colon and pancreas is usually associated with positive tests for carcinoembryonic antigen (CEA) in the serum; false positive tests have been reported in patients with decompensated alcoholic liver disease.

SARCOMAS OF THE LIVER

Hepatic infiltration with lymphoma, lymphosarcoma, or Hodgkin's disease is usually a manifestation of disseminated disease. Firm liver enlargement and biochemical evidence of intrahepatic cholestasis suggest, but are not necessarily diagnostic of, hepatic infiltration. Jaundice is more often the result of hepatic infiltration than invasion of the extrahepatic bile ducts by tumor; jaundice caused by intrahepatic cholestasis may develop, however, in the absence of liver infiltration. Splenomegaly is commonly associated with hepatic involvement in Hodgkin's disease. Percutaneous liver biopsy is less effective than biopsy through a peritoneoscopy in establishing the presence of liver involvement.

PRIMARY CARCINOMAS OF THE LIVER (HEPATOMA)

Hepatic carcinoma usually complicates cirrhosis of the liver; it has a higher incidence in postnecrotic cirrhosis and hemochromatosis than in Laennec's cirrhosis. This lesion should be suspected whenever a cirrhotic patient exhibits unexplained clinical deterioration with enlarging liver, right upper quadrant pain, or sudden onset of ascites. A vascular bruit may be heard over these tumors. Hypoglycemia is sometimes a prominent clinical manifestation. Changes in liver function include a rising alkaline phosphatase and elevated lactic dehydrogenase. A laboratory manifestation of hepatoma is the appearance of a fetal plasma protein, alpha-fetoprotein, in the plasma; sensitive radioimmunoassay techniques have recently detected this protein in the plasma of patients recovering from hepatitis. Hepatomas localized to one lobe of the liver have been excised successfully on several occasions, but usually cirrhosis and invasion of hepatic veins or local spread prevent surgical therapy.

Hepatoma can be produced with a high degree of regularity in several species of laboratory animals by injection of minute doses of the microtoxin known as *aflatoxin*. This substance is produced by Aspergillus growing on peanut (groundnut) meal that has been stored in appropriately hot, humid conditions. The incidence of hepatoma in man has long been known to show a marked geographic variation, and there is a correlation between the localities where hepatoma is the most frequently occurring carcinoma and the particular complex of circumstances that favors the production of aflatoxin. Obviously, it cannot be stated as yet that hepatoma in man is caused by aflatoxin, but this possibility that hepatoma is thus environmentally induced is being actively pursued in epidemiologic, clinical, and laboratory studies.

General

Davidson, C. S.: Liver pathophysiology. Its Relevance to Disease. Boston, Little, Brown & Company, 1970.

Scheuer, P. J.: Liver Biopsy Interpretation. London, Balliere, Tindall and Cassell, Ltd., 1968.

Schiff, L.: Diseases of the Liver. 3rd ed. Philadelphia, J. B. Lippincott Company, 1969.

Sherlock, S.: Diseases of the Liver. 4th ed. Oxford, Blackwell Scientific Publications, 1968.

Manifestations of Liver Disease

Berk, P. D., Bloomer, J. R., Howe, R. B., and Berlin, N. I.: Constitutional hepatic dysfunction (Gilbert's syndrome). A new definition based on kinetic studies with unconjugated radiobilirubin. Am. J. Med., 49:296, 1970.

Kaplan, M. M.: Alkaline phosphatase. N. Engl. J. Med., 286:200, 1972.

Reynolds, T. B., Ito, S., and Iwatsuki, S.: Measurement of portal pressure and its clinical application. Am. J. Med., 49:649, 1970.

Rothschild, M. A., Oratz, M., and Schreiber, S. S.: Albumin metabolism. Gastroenterology, 64:324, 1973.

Scheuer, P. J.: Liver biopsy in the diagnosis of cirrhosis. Gut, 11:275, 1970.

Schmid, R.: Bilirubin metabolism in man. N. Engl. J. Med., 287:703, 1972.

Acute Liver Disease

Chalmers, T. C., Eckhardt, R. D., Reynolds, W. E., Cigarroa, J. G., Jr., Deane, N., Reifenstein, R. W., Smith, C. W., and Davidson, C. S.: The treatment of acute infectious hepatitis. Controlled studies of the effect of diet, rest, and physical reconditioning on the acute course of the disease and on the incidence of relapses and residual abnormalities. J. Clin. Invest., 34:1136, 1955.

Chalmers, T. C., and Alter, H. J.: Management of the asymptomatic carrier of the hepatitis-associated (Australia) antigen. N. Engl. J. Med., 285:613, 1971.

Klatskin, G., and Kimberg, D. V.: Recurrent hepatitis attributable to halothane sensitization in an anesthetist. N. Engl. J. Med., 280:515, 1969.

Krugman, S., Giles, J. P., and Hammond, J.: Infectious hepatitis. Evidence for two distinctive clinical, epidemiological and immunological types of infection. J.A.M.A., 200:365, 1967.

Maddrey, W. C., and Boitnott, J. K.: Isoniazid hepatitis. Ann. Intern. Med., 79:1, 1973.

Redeker, A. G., and Yamahiro, H. S.: Controlled trial of exchange-transfusion therapy in fulminant hepatitis. Lancet, 1:3, 1973.

Sabbaj, J., Sutter, V. L., and Finegold, S. M.: Anaerobic pyogenic liver abscess. Ann. Intern. Med., 77:629, 1972.

Schweitzer, I. L., Dunn, A. E. G., Peters, R. L., and Spears, R. L.: Viral hepatitis B in neonates and infants. Am. J. Med., 55:762, 1973.

Sherlock, S.: Halothane hepatitis. Gut, 12:324, 1971.

Sherlock, S.: The course of long incubation (virus B) hepatitis. Br. Med. Bull., 28:109, 1972.

Shulman, N. R.: Hepatitis-associated antigen. Am. J. Med., 49:669, 1970.

Vittal, S. B. V., Thomas, W., Jr., and Clowdus, B. F.: Acute viral hepatitis. Course and incidence of progression to chronic hepatitis. Am. J. Med., 55:757, 1973.

Williams, R.: Problems of fulminant hepatic failure. Br. Med. Bull., 28:114, 1972.

Chronic Liver Disease

Boyer, J. L., and Klatskin, G.: Patterns of necrosis in acute viral hepatitis.

Prognostic value of bridging (subacute hepatic necrosis). N. Engl. J. Med., 283:1063, 1970.

Campra, J. L., Hamlin, E. M., Kirshbaum, R. L., Olivier, M., Redeker, A. G., and Reynolds, T. B.: Prednisone therapy in acute alcoholic hepatitis. Report of a controlled trial. Ann. Intern. Med., 79:625, 1973.

Conn, H. O.: A rational approach to the hepatorenal syndrome. Gastroenterology, 65:321, 1973.

Conn, H. O., Lindenmuth, W. W., May, C. J., and Ramsby, G. R.: Prophylactic portacaval anastomosis. Medicine, 51:27, 1972.

Gabuzda, G. J.: Cirrhosis, ascites and edema. Clinical course related to management. Gastroenterology, 58:546, 1970.

Golding, P. L., Smith, M., and Williams, R.: Multisystem involvement in chronic liver disease. Studies on the incidence and pathogenesis. Am. J. Med., 55:772, 1973.

Lieber, C. S.: Hepatic and metabolic effects of alcohol. Gastroenterology, 65:821, 1973.

Rubin, E., and Lieber, C. S.: Fatty liver, alcoholic hepatitis and cirrhosis produced by alcohol in primates. N. Engl. J. Med., 290:128, 1974.

Schenker, S., Breen, K. J., and Hoyumpa, A. M.: Hepatic encephalopathy; current status. Gastroenterology, 66:121, 1974.

Sherlock, S., and Scheuer, P. J.: The presentation and diagnosis of 100 patients with primary biliary cirrhosis. N. Engl. J. Med., 289:674, 1973.

Soloway, R. D., Summerskill, W. H. J., Baggenstoss, A. H., Geall, M. G., Gitnick, G. L., Elveback, L. R., and Schoenfield, L. J.: Clinical, biochemical and histological remission of severe chronic active liver disease. A controlled study of treatments and early prognosis. Gastroenterology, 63:820, 1972.

Soterakis, J., Resnick, R. H., and Iber, F. L.: Effect of alcohol abstinence on survival in cirrhotic portal hypertension. Lancet, 2:65, 1973.

Part XV
DISEASES OF NUTRITION

712. NUTRIENT REQUIREMENTS

Nevin S. Scrimshaw

GENERAL CONSIDERATIONS

The nutrient intakes recommended by most national and international organizations are defined as the amounts sufficient for the physiologic needs of virtually all healthy persons in a population. Conceptually, they are intended to cover the mean plus two standard deviations, although the data for actually calculating a standard deviation are rarely available. It is important for the physician to recognize that existing recommended dietary allowances for nutrients do not cover the additional needs that arise from microbial disease, trauma, advanced malignancies, disorders of the gastrointestinal tract, or metabolic diseases and abnormalities. Moreover, the intake recommended for any one nutrient presupposes that the requirements for energy and for all other nutrients are fully met.

Persons receiving less than the recommended allowance are not necessarily malnourished; it depends on their individual requirements, on the margin of safety inherent in the recommendation, and on whether other deficiencies are more limiting. On the other hand, persons consuming the recommended allowance are not necessarily adequately nourished. The presence of disease may interfere with absorption, increase utilization, or accelerate loss of an essential nutrient. This should be taken into account in prescribing diets for persons with acute or chronic disease. Moreover, imbalance among nutrients can render inadequate an intake which would otherwise be ample.

The 1974 Recommended Dietary Allowances of the Food and Nutrition Board (FNB) of the National Academy of Sciences are given in Table 1. They differ from those of the United Kingdom and FAO/WHO in their higher recommendations for calcium and ascorbic acid and slightly lower recommendations for calories.

The following nutrients have been established as necessary dietary constituents for man under physiologic or pathologic conditions, or both.

NECESSARY NUTRIENTS

Calories. The body requires a source of energy to maintain the normal processes of life and to meet the demands of activity and growth. Calorie requirements depend mainly on body size, basal metabolic rate, activity, age, sex, and environmental temperature. Clinical diseases associated with calorie deficiency are marasmus in children and cachexia in adults. A 70-kg male requires approximately 70 calories per hour under basal conditions and up to 600 calories per hour for very heavy muscular work, so that activity levels largely determine gain or loss of weight on a given diet. Carbohydrate and protein furnish about 4 calories per gram, alcohol about 7, and fat about 9. The report of the FAO Expert Committee on Calorie Requirements provides more detailed information.

Protein. Proteins in the diet vary in their usefulness, depending on the extent to which they contain those eight essential amino acids that cannot be synthesized within the body in the proportions needed for making new tissue. When protein is severely deficient relative to calories, kwashiorkor develops.

Protein requirements have two components: sufficient amounts and proportions of the essential amino acids, and adequate additional nitrogen from any utilizable source. The latter comes from both the dietarily dispensable amino acids and those essential amino acids present in excess of requirements. If the diet does not supply adequate calories, dietary protein will be utilized to meet energy needs at the expense of fulfilling requirements for protein. Protein requirements are greatly increased by microbial disease, trauma, and most other pathologic states.

Protein requirements are expressed in terms of reference protein which, in theory, is 100 per cent absorbed and utilized. Since only egg and milk approach this ideal, recommended dietary allowances for protein must be expressed in terms of the quality of the protein of the actual diet. In industrialized countries it can be assumed that the protein of the ordinary mixed diet is about 70 per cent utilized, but for cereal-based diets in most developing countries a figure of 60 per cent or less is more appropriate. Proteins of animal origin are generally the best utilized, followed by those from legumes, oilseeds, rice, oats, and Opaque-2 corn. Most other cereal proteins are of relatively poor quality.

Carbohydrates and Fats. Carbohydrates supply dietary energy and are necessary constituents of a balanced and palatable diet. There is no fixed requirement for carbohydrates, however, since they can be completely replaced as energy sources in the diet by protein and fats. Fats supply more than twice the energy of carbohydrate and protein per gram, and thus contribute a concentrated source of calories as well as palatability in the diet. The actual requirement for fat, however, is limited to a minute quantity of linoleic, linolenic, or arachidonic acid — all polyunsaturated fatty acids. Deficiency of these in young children leads to defective growth and scaly skin.

Fat-Soluble Vitamins

Vitamin A. Vitamin A (retinol) is essential for integrity of mucosal surfaces and is required in the form of its aldehyde for vision, particularly in dim light. Avitaminosis A results in skin and eye lesions and reduced resistance to infection (see Ch. 717), and hypervitaminosis A is equally serious (see Ch. 722).

Vitamin A is found preformed in animal tissue, and the beta-carotene of green and yellow vegetables is converted in the body to vitamin A with an efficiency of about 50 per cent. There are several other forms of carotene that have some activity but are still less efficiently

TABLE 1. Food and Nutrition Board, National Academy of Sciences–National Research Council Recommended Daily Dietary Allowances,* Revised 1974 Designed for the Maintenance of Good Nutrition of Practically All Healthy People in the U.S.A.

	Age (years) From Up to	Weight (kg)	Weight (lbs)	Height (cm)	Height (in)	Energy (kcal)†	Protein (grams)	Fat-Soluble Vitamins Vitamin A Activity (RE)‡	Vitamin A Activity (IU)	Vitamin D (IU)	Vitamin E Activity¶ (IU)	Water-Soluble Vitamins Ascorbic Acid (mg)	Folacin (µg)	Niacin†† (mg)	Riboflavin (mg)	Thiamin (mg)	Vitamin B₆ (mg)	Vitamin B₁₂ (µg)	Minerals Calcium (mg)	Phosphorus (mg)	Iodine (µg)	Iron (mg)	Magnesium (mg)	Zinc (mg)
Infants	0.0–0.5	6	14	60	24	kg × 117	kg × 2.2	420§	1400	400	4	35	50	5	0.4	0.3	0.3	0.3	360	240	35	10	60	3
	0.5–1.0	9	20	71	28	kg × 108	kg × 2.0	400	2000	400	5	35	50	8	0.6	0.5	0.4	0.3	540	400	45	15	70	5
Children	1–3	13	28	86	34	1300	23	400	2000	400	7	40	100	9	0.8	0.7	0.6	1.0	800	800	60	15	150	10
	4–6	20	44	110	44	1800	30	500	2500	400	9	40	200	12	1.1	0.9	0.9	1.5	800	800	80	10	200	10
	7–10	30	66	135	54	2400	36	700	3300	400	10	40	300	16	1.2	1.2	1.2	2.0	800	800	110	10	250	10
Males	11–14	44	97	158	63	2800	44	1000	5000	400	12	45	400	18	1.5	1.4	1.6	3.0	1200	1200	130	18	350	15
	15–18	61	134	172	69	3000	54	1000	5000	400	15	45	400	20	1.8	1.5	2.0	3.0	1200	1200	150	18	400	15
	19–22	67	147	172	69	3000	54	1000	5000	400	15	45	400	20	1.8	1.5	2.0	3.0	800	800	140	10	350	15
	23–50	70	154	172	69	2700	56	1000	5000		15	45	400	18	1.6	1.4	2.0	3.0	800	800	130	10	350	15
	51+	70	154	172	69	2400	56	1000	5000		15	45	400	16	1.5	1.2	2.0	3.0	800	800	110	10	350	15
Females	11–14	44	97	155	62	2400	44	800	4000	400	12	45	400	16	1.3	1.2	1.6	3.0	1200	1200	115	18	300	15
	15–18	54	119	162	65	2100	48	800	4000	400	12	45	400	14	1.4	1.1	2.0	3.0	1200	1200	115	18	300	15
	19–22	58	128	162	65	2100	46	800	4000	400	12	45	400	14	1.4	1.1	2.0	3.0	800	800	100	18	300	15
	23–50	58	128	162	65	2000	46	800	4000		12	45	400	13	1.2	1.0	2.0	3.0	800	800	100	18	300	15
	51+	58	128	162	65	1800	46	800	4000		12	45	400	12	1.1	1.0	2.0	3.0	800	800	80	10	300	15
Pregnant						+300	+30	1000	5000	400	15	60	800	+2	+0.3	+0.3	2.5	4.0	1200	1200	125	18‡‡	450	20
Lactating						+500	+20	1200	6000	400	15	80	600	+4	+0.5	+0.3	2.5	4.0	1200	1200	150	18	450	25

*Reprinted from Recommended Dietary Allowances. 8th revised edition. Washington, D.C., National Academy of Sciences, 1973. The allowances are intended to provide for individual variations among most normal persons as they live in the United States under usual environmental stresses. Diets should be based on a variety of common foods in order to provide other nutrients for which human requirements have been less well defined. See text for more detailed discussion of allowances and of nutrients not tabulated.

†Kilojoules (KJ) = 4.2 × kcal.

‡Retinol equivalents.

§Assumed to be all as retinol in milk during the first six months of life. All subsequent intakes are assumed to be one half as retinol and one half as β-carotene when calculated from international units. As retinol equivalents, three fourths are as retinol and one fourth as β-carotene.

¶Total vitamin E activity, estimated to be 80 per cent as α-tocopherol and 20 per cent other tocopherols. See text for variation in allowances.

**The folacin allowances refer to dietary sources as determined by *Lactobacillus casei* assay. Pure forms of folacin may be effective in doses less than one fourth of the RDA.

††Although allowances are expressed as niacin, it is recognized that on the average 1 mg of niacin is derived from each 60 mg of dietary tryptophan.

‡‡This increased requirement cannot be met by ordinary diets; therefore the use of supplemental iron is recommended.

utilized. One international unit (IU) is equivalent to 0.3 μg of retinol, or 6 μg of beta-carotene.

Vitamin D. Vitamin D is essential at all ages for maintenance of calcium homeostasis and skeletal integrity. It can be acquired by ingestion of vitamin D_2 (ergocalciferol) or D_3 (cholecalciferol) and by exposure to certain ultraviolet wavelengths of light that convert 7-dehydro-cholesterol in the skin to vitamin D_3.

One IU of vitamin D is 0.025 μg of pure vitamin D_3. Excessive amounts of vitamin D (of the order of 1000 to 3000 IU per kilogram per day) are potentially dangerous and may lead to hypercalcemia and attendant complications.

Most foods of animal origin have some vitamin D activity, and 1 quart of vitamin D–fortified milk supplies the daily requirement.

Vitamin E. The earliest evidence of vitamin E deficiency differs with the species, but eventually the hematopoietic, muscular, vascular, and central nervous systems are affected. The normal resistance of red blood cells to rupture by oxidizing agents is also markedly reduced in vitamin E deficiency. One IU of vitamin E is 1 mg of synthetic dl-alpha-tocopherol acetate. Recommendations are based on the formula, IU = 1.25 × body weight in kg.[0.75]

Abundant vitamin E is supplied by salad oils, shortening, margarine, fruits and vegetables, and whole-grain products. However, high intakes of polyunsaturated fatty acids may increase requirements sufficiently to induce a deficiency of this vitamin.

Vitamin K. The K family of vitamins occurs throughout nature and is required in microgram amounts by man and certain animals to maintain prothrombin and other clotting factors. The average diet apparently contains adequate amounts of vitamin K, and additional amounts are supplied by the gastrointestinal flora. Thus few malnourished human beings have presented findings indicating inadequate dietary vitamin K. Because of the lack of reliable information, a daily allowance for this vitamin has not been established. A group of older adults experimentally depleted of vitamin K were found to require slightly more than 0.03 mg per kilogram of body weight intravenously to obtain normal blood clotting.

(For the clinically important states in which deficiency of vitamin K develops, see Ch. 799.)

Water-Soluble Vitamins

Ascorbic Acid (Vitamin C). Ascorbic acid has many biochemical functions in the body and is essential for normal wound healing and resistance to infection. Man, higher apes, and the guinea pig lack the metabolic pathway to synthesize adequate amounts of ascorbic acid, and in these species a lack of sufficient dietary ascorbic acid leads to scurvy. The minimal daily intake of ascorbic acid to prevent scurvy in the adult is about 10 mg, but this does not allow tissue saturation. Ascorbic acid is furnished by fruits, particularly citrus fruits, as well as by most fresh vegetables. (For more information on ascorbic acid deficiency, see Ch. 721.)

Biotin. Biotin is essential for the activity of many enzyme systems in bacteria, animals, and, presumably, man. Biotin deficiency does not occur naturally in man because the vitamin is so widely distributed in all common foods. Experimental biotin deficiency in man, induced by feeding the metabolic antagonist avidin found in egg white, results in the development of serious clinical and pathologic changes. These include scaly dermatitis, pallor, extreme lassitude, anorexia, muscle pains, insomnia, precordial pain, and slight anemia.

Choline. Choline serves as a source of labile methyl groups in the body, and in addition is a constituent of several compounds necessary for nerve function and lipid metabolism. Choline is generally considered to be an essential nutrient in the diet, although human choline deficiency has not been demonstrated. The average mixed diet consumed by persons in industrialized countries has been estimated to contain 500 to 900 mg per day of choline, mostly from egg yolk, vegetables, and milk. Beef liver contains about 0.6 per cent choline.

Folacin. Folacin coenzymes function in the transfer of single carbon units in a number of intracellular metabolic processes, particularly in the synthesis of purine and pyrimidine ribotides and deoxyribotides and in amino acid interconversions. A folacin deficiency may arise from inadequate dietary intake, impaired absorption, excessive demands by tissues of the body, and metabolic derangements. Megaloblastic anemias resulting from folacin deficiency have been recognized with increasing frequency (see Ch. 731). The intake of food folacins depends on the highly variable amount destroyed by cooking. Folic acid (phenylmonoglutamic acid) and folacin (tetrahydropteroyl glutamic acid) occur in a wide variety of foods of animal and vegetable origin, particularly in glandular meats, yeasts, and green leafy vegetables.

Niacin. The term "niacin" is generic for both nicotinic acid and nicotinamide. Nicotinamide functions in the body as a component of two important coenzymes that are primarily concerned with glycolysis, tissue respiration, and fat synthesis. Tryptophan is a precursor of niacin in man, and the efficiency of conversion is such that an average of 60 mg of dietary tryptophan is equivalent to 1 mg of niacin. Good dietary sources of niacin are liver, other meats, fish, whole-grain cereals and enriched breads, dried peas, nuts, and peanut butter.

Pantothenic Acid. Pantothenic acid is of biologic importance because of its incorporation into CoA, on which acylation and acetylation and other interactions depend. Pantothenic acid deficiency induced in human volunteers by feeding the metabolic antagonist, omega-methylpantothenic acid, together with a deficient diet, resulted in serious clinical signs and symptoms within a few months. An important feature of the syndrome produced by pantothenic acid deficiency was reduced antibody formation. Neuropathy associated with low serum pantothenic acid has been observed in alcoholic patients habitually consuming extremely poor diets. A daily intake of 5 to 10 mg is probably adequate for children and adults. Ordinary cooking does not cause excessive losses of pantothenic acid, and the vitamin is so widely distributed in plant and animal tissues that deficiency does not occur spontaneously in human populations.

Food sources include organ meats, egg yolk, peanuts, plants of the cabbage family, and whole grains. Other meats, vegetables, milk, and fruits also contain moderate amounts of pantothenic acid.

Riboflavin. Riboflavin functions as a coenzyme or active prosthetic group of flavoproteins concerned with the oxidative processes. The requirement for riboflavin is related to body size, metabolic rate, and rate of growth. Deficiency of riboflavin produces lesions in mucous membranes, most easily seen in the tongue, lips, and cornea (see Ch. 718).

Riboflavin is soluble in water. It is widely distributed in all leafy vegetables, in the flesh of animals and fish, and in milk, but may be destroyed when food is exposed to sunlight or cooked.

Thiamin. Thiamin functions in carbohydrate metabolism as a coenzyme in the decarboxylation of alpha-keto acids and in the utilization of pentose in the hexose monophosphate shunt. Thiamin deficiency leads to beriberi, still seen among populations subsisting primarily on rice; but in the industrialized countries, signs of thiamin deficiency are limited almost entirely to chronic alcoholics (see Ch. 720).

Thiamin is widely distributed in foods and readily available. It is soluble in water, sensitive to oxidation, and destroyed rapidly by heat in neutral or alkaline solutions. Roasting and stewing of meat may reduce the thiamin content by 30 to 50 per cent, and vegetables may lose 25 to 40 per cent in cooking.

It has been generally assumed that thiamin need is related to caloric intake, particularly to those calories derived from carbohydrate. Although dietary fat does "spare" thiamin to some extent, the reduction in requirement appears to be small. Because it is possible that older persons use thiamin less efficiently, it is deemed advisable to recommend that a thiamin intake of 1 mg per day be maintained by older adults, even when they are consuming less than 2000 calories daily.

Vitamin B_6. Vitamin B_6 in the form pyridoxal phosphate or pyridoxamine phosphate has been shown to function in carbohydrate, fat, and protein metabolism. Vitamin B_6 is a collective term for a group of naturally occurring pyridines that are metabolically and functionally interrelated; namely, pyridoxine, pyridoxal, and pyridoxamine. The vitamin appears to be part of the molecular configuration of glycogen phosphorylase. Pyridoxine deficiency has occurred in children fed a proprietary formula in which the B_6 content was largely destroyed as a result of changes in the sterilization process. Symptoms were restlessness and irritability, and some developed convulsions. Pyridoxine deficiency may be responsible for anemia in adults.

Good dietary sources are liver, other meats, wholegrain cereals, soybeans, peanuts, corn, and many vegetables.

Vitamin B_{12}. Vitamin B_{12} is essential for the normal functioning of all cells, but particularly those of the bone marrow, nervous system, and gastrointestinal tract, because it facilitates reduction reactions and participates in the transfer of methyl groups. Its chief importance seems to be in nucleic and folic acid metabolism. Deficiency of vitamin B_{12} results in the development of megaloblastic anemia and signs of degeneration of the long tracts of the spinal cord. Sore tongue, paresthesias, and amenorrhea may also be present (see Ch. 411 and 731).

Cyanocobalamin is the principal one of several compounds with vitamin B_{12} activity. As little as 1.0 μg daily will cure most cases of megaloblastic anemia resulting from deficiency of this vitamin, but will not replenish liver stores. In a dose of 0.5 μg more than 70 per cent is absorbed, but as the dosage of vitamin B_{12} increases, absorption gradually decreases to 30 per cent in a dose of 5 μg. Vitamin B_{12} occurs predominantly in foods of animal origin, with very little present in vegetables. Nevertheless, except in vegetarians, deficiency states are likely to arise only as a result of superimposed infections, malabsorption, or lack of intrinsic factor (pernicious anemia).

Mineral Elements

Calcium. Calcium is a major mineral constituent of the body and makes up about 1.5 to 2.0 per cent of the body weight of the mature human, more than 99 per cent of it in bones and teeth. Active processes of bone formation and resorption constantly exchange calcium with body fluids. The small proportion of calcium distributed in body fluids and tissues contributes importantly to other functions, such as blood coagulation, neuromuscular irritability, muscle contractility, and myocardial function. Calcium is incompletely absorbed, and phytate, oxalate, and fatty acids of the diet form nonionized or poorly soluble calcium complexes, further interfering with intestinal absorption. Calcium requirements are increased during periods of growth, and in pregnancy and lactation, but intestinal absorption is more efficient as need increases.

Good sources of calcium include milk and most other dairy products, shellfish, egg yolk, canned sardines and salmon (with bones), soy beans, and many green vegetables. Adequate vitamin D is required for efficient absorption of calcium.

Copper. Copper-containing proteins in the body include ceruloplasmin, erythrocuprein, hepatocuprein, cerebrocuprein, cytochrome-C oxidase, tyrosinase, and monoamine oxidase. Copper depletion of a degree severe enough to cause hypocupremia has been observed in a few patients with iron deficiency anemia and edema, kwashiorkor, sprue, and the nephrotic syndrome. Anemia, neutropenia, and bone changes caused by copper depletion have been reported in Peruvian children.

A copper intake of 2 mg per day appears to maintain balance in adults, and an intake of 0.08 mg per kilogram per day is recommended.

Copper is widely distributed in foodstuffs, and a diet of even mediocre quality contains more than the recommended amount. The richest sources are liver, kidney, shellfish, nuts, raisins, and dried legumes. Milk is poor in both copper and iron.

Fluorine. Fluoride is incorporated into the structure of teeth and bone, and is necessary for maximal resistance to dental caries. In areas where natural water supplies do not contain this amount, the addition of fluoride to bring the concentration to 1 part per million has proved to be a safe, economical, and efficient way to reduce the incidence of dental decay. In communities where fluoridation has been introduced, the incidence of tooth decay in children has been decreased up to 50 per cent or more. The range of safety in fluoride intake is wide enough for safe accommodation to normal fluctuations in the fluoride content of foods among populations with fluoridated water supplies, without risk of inducing the first indication of an excess—slight mottling of the enamel. Some natural water supplies contain sufficient fluoride to induce mottling of the enamel, but no other associated adverse effects have been found (see Ch. 892).

Iodine. Iodine is an integral part of the thyroid hormones thyroxine and triiodothyronine, which have important metabolic roles. Dietary iodine deficiency leads to thyroid enlargement (goiter) as a result of increase in size and number of the epithelial cells in the gland (see Ch. 841).

Balance studies in adults indicate a daily requirement of 50 to 75 μg of iodine, approximately 1 μg per kilogram. Sources of iodine are food and water, but in large sections of the world, the amount of iodine in the water supply and locally produced foods is too low to meet human needs without hypertrophy and hyperplasia of the thyroid gland. Although today's wide diversification in the origin of foodstuffs has reduced the problem in many countries, iodization of salt is a desirable and effective measure of ensuring an adequate iodine intake for all segments of the population.

Iron. Iron is an essential constituent of hemoglobin and a variety of enzymes. An absolute deficiency owing to a low dietary intake, or a relative deficiency owing to high body losses of iron, results in the development of microcytic anemia and other clinical signs (see Ch. 737).

Iron is widely distributed in both animal and vegetable foods, but intake estimates based on food iron values in food composition tables are of limited value. Foods lose iron during preparation, gain iron from cooking vessels or from other contamination, or have much of the iron in poorly utilized bound forms.

Magnesium. Magnesium appears to activate the enzymes that catalyze the transfer of phosphate from ATP to a phosphate receptor, or from a phosphorylated compound to ADP. It appears to be associated with thermoregulation, neuromuscular contraction, and protein synthesis. Magnesium deficiency disease in man is similar to hypocalcemic tetany, and is reversed by administration of magnesium sulfate. Low serum magnesium levels have been observed in a variety of clinical conditions, including alcoholism, diabetes, malabsorption syndromes, kwashiorkor, neuromuscular conditions associated with parathyroid disease or without parathyroid disease, in surgical patients on restricted dietary regimens or parenteral feeding, and in patients receiving diuretic therapy.

Magnesium is widely distributed in ordinary foods. For example, cocoa, nuts and soy flour, barley, lima beans, corn, whole wheat flour, and oatmeal all contain over 100 mg per 100-gram edible portion.

Chromium, Cobalt, Manganese, Molybdenum, Selenium, and Zinc. Direct evidence for the essentiality of these trace or microelements in human nutrition is often difficult to obtain. Clear evidence that an element is required by mammals has provided a reliable index of a human requirement. Identification of elements in normal human enzyme systems has also afforded substantial evidence of a nutritional requirement.

There is evidence that *chromium* is a required nutrient. Continuing investigations of the relationship of this element to carbohydrate metabolism suggest its possible role in human nutrition.

Cobalt is an integral part of vitamin B_{12}. It is found in most common foods, and is readily absorbed from the gastrointestinal tract. Cobalt deficiency in man is unknown.

Manganese is an essential element, needed for normal bone structure, and is a part of enzyme systems that occur in man. A human deficiency has not been demonstrated, nor a recommended dietary allowance established.

Molybdenum and selenium have been shown to be essential in laboratory animals, and may also function nutritionally in man. There are insufficient data to establish a recommended dietary allowance. The close parallel of the functions of selenium and vitamin E in laboratory animals suggests a need for an evaluation of selenium in man.

Zinc has been recognized as an essential element in the nutrition of animals and humans, and there is some evidence for the occurrence of zinc deficiency in man under some circumstances. Patients exhibiting anemia, hepatosplenomegaly, short stature, hypogonadism, and geophagia have responded to zinc therapy when tissue levels of zinc and zinc intakes were low.

A mixed diet may be expected to supply adequate amounts of these microelements, and the risk of a deficiency in the United States is slight. Green leafy foods, fruit, whole grains, organ meats, and lean meats usually serve as generous sources of these elements.

At high levels of intake, all the elements are known to cause injury and to interfere with the utilization of other elements. Supplements should be used with caution and only with clear evidence of deficiency.

Beaton, G. H., and McHenry, E. W. (eds.): Nutrition: A Comprehensive Treatise, Vol. II: Vitamins, Nutrient Requirements, and Food Selection. New York, Academic Press, Inc., 1964.

Canadian Bulletin on Nutrition, Vol. 6, No. 1, Dietary Standard for Canada. Ottawa, Department of Public Printing and Stationery, March, 1964.

Department of Health and Social Security: Recommended Intakes of Nutrients for the United Kingdom (Report of the Panel on Recommended Allowances of Nutrients). Department of Health and Social Security Reports on Public Health and Medical Subjects No. 120. London, Her Majesty's Stationery Office, 1969.

Food and Agriculture Organization of the United Nations: Calorie Requirements: Report of the Second Committee on Calorie Requirements. FAO Nutritional Studies, No. 15. Rome, Italy, FAO, 1957. (Third printing, 1965.)

Food and Agriculture Organization of the United Nations/World Health Organization: Report of an FAO/WHO Expert Group, Rome, Italy, 23 to 30 May, 1961. Published jointly by FAO and WHO, FAO Nutrition Meetings Report Series No. 30 and World Health Organization Technical Report Series No. 230. Rome, FAO, 1962.

Food and Agriculture Organization of the United Nations/World Health Organization: Requirements of Vitamin A, Thiamin, Riboflavin and Niacin; Report of a Joint FAO/WHO Expert Group, Rome, Italy, 6–17 September, 1965. FAO Nutrition Meetings Report Series No. 41, World Health Organization Technical Report Series No. 362. Rome, FAO, 1967.

Food and Nutrition Board, National Research Council: Recommended Dietary Allowances, eighth revised edition, 1974. Publication 2216. National Academy of Sciences, 1974. Washington, D.C., Printing and Publishing Office, National Academy of Sciences.

World Health Organization: Energy and Protein Requirements. Report of a Joint FAO/WHO ad hoc Expert Committee. Rome, 22 March–2 April, 1971. WHO Technical Report Series No. 522 and FAO Nutrition Meetings Report Series No. 52. Geneva, World Health Organization, 1973.

713. ASSESSMENT OF NUTRITIONAL STATUS

Nevin S. Scrimshaw

The physician should always look for the clinical signs suggestive of nutritional disease in his patients. Inspection of those body areas in which signs of deficiency are most likely to be detected—the hair, eyes, lips, mouth, and skin of the face, neck, and arms—can be part of any examination, no matter how cursory, because neither formal examination facilities nor disrobing is essential. Suspicions aroused by clinical examination can then be verified by medical and dietary history and appropriate biochemical tests.

A manual of procedures developed primarily to guide

surveys of the assessment of nutritional status in populations has been developed by the U.S. Interdepartmental Committee on Nutrition for National Development (ICNND, 1963); a more concise document was prepared by a committee of experts convened in 1962 by the World Health Organization (WHO, 1963).

Clinical Examination: Inspection and Measurement. The over-all nutritional appearance of each patient should be appraised before examination of specific areas. This will indicate whether a person has excessive pallor, generalized skin lesions, or other indications of unsatisfactory health, possibly related to diet. Although simple inspection also reveals obvious overweight and underweight in individuals, weight for height is a more reliable means of discrimination. Similarly, a gross subjective estimate of subcutaneous fat can be obtained by pinching a double fold of skin over the outer surface of the upper arm (mid-triceps region), but skin calipers provide a more precise estimate.

Hair. Protein malnutrition causes the hair to change color and become fine, dry, and brittle. Characteristically, the hair of persons with severe protein deficiency can be pulled out of the scalp without discomfort; whole tufts of hair come out readily by the roots. Since the hair is brittle, the tips also break off easily. In whites, Indians, and Orientals who normally have brown or black hair, the change to a lighter color is readily detected, but without knowledge of prior hair color it might be thought to be genetic. The hair of blacks tends to become reddish in cases of protein deficiency before becoming lighter. In persons with naturally light and fine hair, the change is more difficult to detect.

Eyes. Both vitamin A and riboflavin deficiencies are known to affect the eyes. The xerophthalmia caused by avitaminosis A begins with a dryness of the bulbar conjunctiva, loss of the light reflex, lack of luster, and decreased lacrimation. It may proceed to keratomalacia, which is a softening of the cornea, and lead to ulceration, perforation, rupture, and destruction of the cornea. The final result is a scarred, opaque cornea and a sightless eye.

Bitot spots are often associated with vitamin A deficiency, although they cannot be regarded as specific to it. They appear as frothy, irregular, white or light yellow spots from one to several millimeters in diameter, most often on the conjunctiva lateral to the cornea. They look as if they could be wiped away, but are beneath the conjunctival epithelium. A small Bitot spot may consist of only a few tiny bubbles visible in the triangles, especially the outer ones. Both photophobia and the inability to see in dim light may be due to vitamin A deficiency.

The circumcorneal injection seen in riboflavin deficiency consists of penetration of the corneal limbus by the subconjunctival arterioles that normally terminate within 0.5 mm of the limbus. However, proliferation and congestion of the blood vessels in the sclerae and their extension into the clear corneal tissue is by no means pathognomonic of riboflavin deficiency. Excessive exposure to sunlight, smoke, dust, and other irritants is a recognized factor. Ariboflavinosis may also produce a moist, red lesion of the external angles of both eyes.

Skin. The areas of the skin most affected by nutritional deficiency usually are those most exposed to the environment. The skin of the face, neck, arms, and legs, and over pressure points such as the elbows, knees, and ankles is most likely to show positive findings in nutritional deficiencies.

Dyssebacea refers to a series of disturbances of the sebaceous glands characterized by increased oiliness, dermatitis, fissuring, and exfoliation. For positive identification, the lesion must be red and moist. In riboflavin deficiency, it occurs at the external angles of the eye, the nasolabial fold, and behind the ears, and may appear in other skin folds of the body. The nasolabial lesions should not be confused with acne in adolescents or with the irritation from nasal discharge in small children.

Xerosis, or generalized dryness of the skin, is thought to be characteristic of vitamin A deficiency, but difficult to evaluate in the individual because the appearance of the skin is influenced so much by bathing habits and exposure to dust and sunlight. The follicular hyperkeratosis widely ascribed to vitamin A deficiency consists of a "goose flesh" appearance which is not altered by temperature or brisk rubbing, and is most prominent on the skin of the outer forearm and thigh. Fully developed lesions consist of symmetrically distributed, rough, horny papules formed by keratotic plugs projecting from hypertrophied hair follicles; they make the skin look and feel like coarse sandpaper. Several well conducted therapeutic trials have failed to demonstrate any relationship between this hyperkeratosis and vitamin A deficiency, even when dietary fat is sufficient, and its specific etiology is not yet understood.

It is important to differentiate follicular hyperkeratosis from the perifolliculitis of ascorbic acid deficiency. The latter consists of perifollicular congestion, swelling, and, eventually, hypertrophy of the follicles. Only in this late stage is the skin rough to the touch. Other skin changes observed in severe ascorbic acid deficiency include petechiae, purpura, and hematomas. Because of increased capillary fragility, they are readily caused by a blood pressure cuff, shoes, or accidental bruising. Obviously, other factors increasing capillary fragility or interfering with blood clotting could cause these phenomena.

The cutaneous lesions of pellagra vary because of differences in the degree of deficiency, natural skin color, and conditioning factors, but they are sufficiently characteristic to be diagnostic in many instances. The most common chronic form is thickening, inelastic, fissured, and deeply pigmented areas of skin where exposed to sunlight or covering pressure points. Eventually, the skin in affected areas becomes dry, scaly, and atrophic. Erythema upon exposure to sunlight is an acute manifestation, with subsequent vascularization, crusting, and desquamation out of proportion to the precipitating exposure. In intertriginous areas a common, acute, but highly nonspecific reaction is redness, maceration, abrasion, and superimposed infection. Heat friction and poor personal hygiene contribute importantly to these signs. The symmetrical distribution of pellagrous lesions over skin exposed to sunlight and over pressure points is the most characteristic feature. Casal's necklace is a virtually diagnostic distribution of pellagrous dermatitis which sharply follows the neckline when a low-necked dress or an open shirt collar is habitually worn outdoors by persons on a niacin-tryptophan—deficient diet.

In severe protein deficiency, the skin of the legs, arms, and thighs shows marked pitting edema (which is a *sine qua non* of the diagnosis), and a dermatosis characterized by hyperkeratosis, hyperpigmentation, and desquamation. Although often similar in appearance to the lesions of pellagra, they are not limited to the exposed areas, and often extend to the thighs and lower trunk.

Neck. Endemic goiter resulting from a deficiency of iodine available to the thyroid gland usually can be detected by inspection and palpation (see Ch. 841).

Mouth. The mouth is one of the areas most sensitive to nutritional deficiencies, but the changes are nonspecific, confusing, and difficult to evaluate. Pallor of the lips and mucous membranes, like pallor of the skin and fingernails, may be a consequence of anemia, but its clinical appraisal is so subjective as to be of little value unless the anemia is severe. The stomatitis which may be a consequence of riboflavin deficiency has already been mentioned. Angular scars may be the result of past episodes of acute ariboflavinosis, but may also be wholly non-nutritional in origin. Poorly fitting dentures are a common cause.

The gums may reflect any of a variety of nutritional deficiencies, but the changes are difficult to differentiate from those resulting from local irritants and poor hygiene. This is especially true because neglect of both diet and oral hygiene are likely in the same individual. Marginal gingivitis and periodontal disease are reported to be common in persons whose diets are deficient in ascorbic acid, but attempts to prove such a relationship by ascorbic acid therapy have been failures. On the other hand, engorged, dark red, and bleeding gums are characteristic of scurvy.

Marginal and generalized gingivitis may also be found associated with deficiencies of vitamin A, niacin, and riboflavin. The problem is that many factors may play a causal role simultaneously so that the experimental correction of a single factor, even if contributory, does not necessarily effect a cure. General improvement of both diet and oral hygiene is usually required.

Marked hypertrophy of the filiform and fungiform papillae of the tongue is more frequently seen in populations in which vitamin B deficiencies, particularly of thiamin and riboflavin, are present. Papillary atrophy is also sometimes related to niacin or iron deficiency. Both nutritional megaloblastic anemia and the microcytic anemia of iron deficiency result in a smooth tongue. A markedly furrowed, so-called scrotal tongue is a possible manifestation of vitamin A deficiency.

Impression of the teeth on the borders of the tongue may be due to the edema resulting from protein deficiency as well as to defective dentures and a variety of other causes. When protein deficiency is the cause, evidence is likely to be present in the extremities as well.

Nutritional deficiencies may also cause changes in the color of the tongue, although they are usually difficult to evaluate. Reddening, either generalized or limited mainly to the distal third, may be associated with sprue. It affects first the tip and lateral margins, but may

---

TABLE 2.   Suggested Guide for Interpretation of Clinical Signs*

Dietary Obesity
Excessive weight
Excessive skin folds
Excessive abdominal girth

Undernutrition
Lethargy, mental and physical
Low weight in relation to height
Diminished skin folds
Exaggerated skeletal prominences
Loss of elasticity of skin

Protein-Calorie Deficiency Disease
Edema
Muscle wasting
Low body weight
Pyschomotor change
Dyspigmentation of the hair
Thin, sparse hair
Moon face
Flaky paint dermatosis
Areas of hyperpigmentation

Vitamin A Deficiency
Xerosis of skin
Follicular hyperkeratosis
Xerosis conjunctivae
Keratomalacia
Bitot's spots

Riboflavin Deficiency
Angular stomatitis
Cheilosis
Magenta tongue
Central atrophy of lingual papillae
Nasolabial dyssebacea
Angular palpebritis
Scrotal and vulval dermatosis
Corneal vascularization

Thiamin Deficiency
Loss of ankle jerks

Sensory loss and motor weakness
Calf-muscle tenderness
Cardiovascular dysfunction
Edema

Niacin Deficiency
Pellagrous dermatosis
Scarlet and raw tongue
Tongue fissuring
Atrophic lingual papillae
Malar and supraorbital pigmentation

Vitamin D Deficiency
Spongy and bleeding gums
Folliculosis
Petechiae
Ecchymoses
Intramuscular or subperiosteal hematoma
Epiphyseal enlargement (painful)

Vitamin D Deficiency
1. *Active rickets* (in children)
   Epiphyseal enlargement (over 6 months of age), painless
   Beading of ribs
   Craniotabes (under 1 year of age)
   Muscular hypotonia
2. *Healed rickets* (in children or adults)
   Frontal and parietal bossing
   Knock-knees or bow legs
   Deformities of thorax
3. *Osteomalacia* (in adults)
   Local or generalized skeletal deformities

Iron Deficiency
Pallor of mucous membranes
Koilonychia
Atrophic lingual papillae

Iodine Deficiency
Enlargement of the thyroid

Excess of Fluorine (Fluorosis)
Mottled dental enamel

---

*Adapted from World Health Organization Technical Report Series No. 258, Expert Committee on Medical Assessment of Nutritional Status. Geneva, WHO, 1963, pp. 59–61.

progress to include not only the entire tongue but all of the oral mucous membranes as well. A beefy red glossitis resembling raw beefsteak most frequently represents a deficiency of niacin, but other B vitamin deficiencies may be involved. Riboflavin deficiency is probably most often responsible for the purplish discoloration known as magenta tongue. Patchy areas of paler discoloration give rise to the name "geographic" tongue, which has no nutritional significance.

Teeth. The frequency and severity of dental caries is increased by a diet relatively high in soluble carbohydrates and decreased by adequate fluoride and phosphate intake. Any severe dietary deficiency in infancy and early childhood will delay tooth eruption and contribute to malposition of teeth. Malposition resulting from retarded mandibular development is a common sequela of early protein deficiency.

In children of many underdeveloped countries, a so-called hypoplastic line across the upper primary incisors has been described, in which a yellow or brown pigment becomes deposited. This is followed by the development of caries on the labial surface of the teeth. Subsequently, the teeth may break off along this line. A nutritional or febrile insult in the neonatal period is a probable cause.

Fluorosis, occurring in regions where the fluoride content of the water supplies is above about 2 to 6 parts per million of fluoride in drinking water, is characterized by mottled enamel and chalky white patches distributed over the surface of the teeth. In some cases, the entire tooth surface may be dull white and lusterless. Although cosmetically undesirable, the lesion is harmless, and such teeth are usually resistant to caries.

Edema. Edema of the lower extremities is characteristic of protein deficiency, and may also be seen in acute beriberi. In severe cases it becomes generalized.

Evaluation of Signs. The signs suggesting nutritional deficiency are easier to evaluate and more specific in children than in adults. In adults, lesions from other causes, such as aging and repeated trauma, and confusing signs such as pinguecula, pterygium, and geographic tongue, are more likely to be present. The clinical signs that suggest more or less strongly the possibility of a nutritional deficiency are summarized in Table 2.

It must be emphasized again that the aforementioned signs are largely nonspecific. Moreover, they are more reliable in the assessment of nutritional status of population groups than of single individuals. Excellent color illustrations will be found in several of the references listed at the end of this chapter.

It should be clear from the foregoing that clinical examination alone will rarely be sufficient to establish a definite diagnosis. Many of the signs are so nonspecific that they cannot be relied upon in a given individual even when appropriate for population surveys. A medical history and confirmatory dietary and biochemical data are required when clinical examination raises the question of nutritional deficiency in the individual.

Physical Methods Complementary to Clinical Examination. Although routine roentgenographic studies are rarely possible, or indeed required, it is valuable to carry out roentgenographic examinations if physical signs and other circumstances suggest that rickets, osteomalacia, infantile scurvy, beriberi, fluorosis, or protein-calorie malnutrition is present.

The test of dark adaptation is sometimes used as a measure of vitamin A deficiency. It is, however, difficult to perform, and is influenced by factors other than vitamin A. The same appears to be true of electroretinography.

Biochemical Tests. A single biochemical determination, if accurate, may decisively confirm or deny the nutritional origin of an uncertain complex of clinical signs. Here again, biochemical measures vary in their reliability and specificity. Serum levels of vitamin A and ascor-

TABLE 3. Tentative Guide to the Interpretation of Selected Biochemical Data Useful in the Appraisal of Nutritional Status of Adults*

	Deficient (High Risk)	Low (Medium Risk)	Acceptable (Low Risk)
Serum protein: gram/100 ml	<6.0	6.0–6.4	>6.5
Serum albumin (electrophoretic method): gram/100 ml	<2.8	2.8–3.4	>3.5
Nonessential/essential amino acid ratio (NE/E)†	<3.0	3.0–2.0	>2.0
Urea/creatinine ratio‡	<6.0	6.0–12.0	>12.0
Hemoglobin: gram/100 ml sea level			
Men	<12.0	12.0–13.9	>14.0
Women§	<10.0	10.0–11.9	>12.0
Hematocrit % (sea level)			
Men	<37	37–43	>44
Women§	<31	31–37	>38
Serum ascorbic acid: mg/100 ml	<0.20	0.20–0.29	>0.30
Plasma retinol: μg/100 ml	<10	10–19	>20
Thiamin, urinary excretion μg/gram creatinine	<27	27–65	>66–129
Riboflavin, urinary excretion μg/gram creatinine	<27	27–79	>80
N-methylnicotinamide, urinary excretion mg/gram creatinine	<0.5	0.5–1.59	>1.6–4.29
Pyridoxine, urinary excretion μg/gram creatinine¶	<20	–	>20
Serum folacin ng (mμg)/ml¶	<3.0	3.0–5.9	>6.0
Red cell folacin¶	<140	140–159	>160
Serum vitamin B$_{12}$ pg ($\mu\mu$g)/ml	<150	150–200	>200
Serum vitamin E (α-tocopherol) level, mg/100 ml (levels will vary according to method of analysis)	<0.50	0.50–0.70	>0.70

*Adapted from Sauberlich, H. E., Dowdy, R. P., and Skala, J. H.: Crit. Rev. Lab. Clin. Sci., 4:215, 1973.
†Value depends upon the analytical method employed and the procedure used to calculate the ratio.
‡These values are considered exceedingly tentative in view of the effect of age and the wide range of values reported in the literature.
§Nonpregnant, nonlactating.
¶Guidelines should be regarded as tentative and must be considered in terms of the microbiologic assay procedure employed. Values are based on the use of *Lactobacillus casei* as the test organism.

bic acid are quite useful, although very low levels may be present for some time before lesions appear.

For the B vitamins, blood serum levels are relatively insensitive, and measurement of thiamin, riboflavin, and niacin excretion in 24-hour urine samples is recommended.

Total serum protein and serum albumin are decreased markedly in protein deficiency, but only when the deficiency has progressed to the point at which it is beginning to be clinically evident. The ratio of urea to creatinine has been recommended recently as a measure of the loss of lean body mass in protein-calorie malnutrition. Anemia is also a laboratory-based diagnosis. A tentative guide to the interpretation of selected biochemical data is given in Table 3. It should be noted that most biochemical measures show only the current state of the patient, so that chronic nutritional lesions are possible even in those with normal serum levels of various nutrients.

Beaton, G. H., and McHenry, E. W. (eds.): Nutrition: A Comprehensive Treatise. Vol. III. New York, Academic Press, Inc., 1966.

Davidson, S., Passmore, R., and Brock, J. F.: Human Nutrition and Dietetics. 5th ed. Edinburgh, Churchill Livingstone, 1972.

Jelliffe, D. B.: The Assessment of the Nutritional Status of the Community. World Health Organization Monograph Series No. 53. Geneva, World Health Organization, 1966.

Jolliffe, N.: Clinical Nutrition. 2nd ed. New York, Hoeber Medical Book, Harper & Brothers, 1962.

Sauberlich, H. E., Dowdy, R. P., and Skala, J. H.: Laboratory tests for assessment of nutritional status. Crit. Rev. Lab. Clin. Sci., 4:215, 1973.

World Health Organization Technical Report Series No. 258: Expert Committee on Medical Assessment of Nutritional Status. Geneva, World Health Organization, 1963.

714. NUTRITION AND INFECTION

Nevin S. Scrimshaw

Malnutrition in man is inseparable from the occurrence and effects of microbial disease. Infection precipitates nutritional disease in the malnourished, and malnutrition worsens the consequences of infection. The interaction between the two is synergistic. Both are major health problems wherever poverty and ignorance result in poor dietary habits, as well as inferior environmental sanitation and personal hygiene. The World Health Organization monograph, *Interactions of Nutrition and Infection,* provides extensive documentation for the statements and conclusions of this chapter.

EFFECT OF INFECTION ON NUTRITIONAL STATUS

General. One of the earliest and most constant consequences of infection is loss of appetite and a decrease in the amount of food tolerated. Another is the almost universal tendency to change the diet to one that is more liquid and higher in carbohydrates at the expense of foods that are good sources of protein and other essential nutrients. This is a particularly common practice in the feeding of young children in less developed areas. Often milk as well as solid food is removed from the diet in favor of starchy gruels and cooking water from cereal grains or plant leaves when a child has diarrheal disease or other acute infections. In addition, therapeutic agents such as purgatives may reduce intestinal absorption, or antimicrobial drugs may interfere with intestinal synthesis of some nutrients. The direct influence of fever in increasing both basal metabolism and the loss of nutrients in sweat must also be taken into account. Sweat losses may amount to as much as 4 grams of nitrogen per day, together with significant quantities of electrolytes and iron.

Protein. Acute infections cause a stress response qualitatively the same as that observed in states of pain, anxiety, fear, and other psychologic stress. The stress reaction, mediated by cortisone and insulin, mobilizes amino acids from skeletal muscle and other tissues from which they can be spared for gluconeogenesis in the liver. This is necessary because in man the contribution of liver glycogen to maintain blood glucose is relatively limited. The stress reaction undoubtedly arose to enable individuals to fight, flee from sudden danger, or recover from wounds and infections, regardless of the timing of meals. However, it necessarily depletes the body of protein because the amino acids thus mobilized are deaminated to provide the carbons of glucose, and the nitrogen is excreted in the urine, largely as urea.

Nitrogen losses during severe infectious diseases have long been recognized and can be equivalent to the nitrogen of 2 or 3 kg of muscle during the acute phase of the illness. It is now clear that even such mild infections as vaccination against smallpox and immunization with the 17-D strain of yellow fever vaccine, as well as tonsillitis, otitis media, bronchitis, and localized abscesses, will also provoke this stress reaction.

The duration of the metabolic effect of stress depends upon the nature and extent of the precipitating cause. If the stress is of short duration, it may be balanced by an increase in nitrogen retention during the succeeding 24 hours. The catabolic period associated with an infectious disease episode, however, is likely to last for several days, and the anabolic period of increased nitrogen retention is generally at least twice as long. After the acute stress is over, dietary amino acids are returned to the depleted tissues; hence protein intakes above maintenance levels are required at this time. In individuals already depleted by low levels of protein intake, the urinary loss of nitrogen measured during stress is less than that observed in those who are well nourished. Nevertheless, increases in urinary loss of nitrogen during minor infections have been found even in experimental subjects receiving a nitrogen-free diet.

In infections associated with diarrhea, reduced absorption of nitrogen and other nutrients adds to the nutritional consequences. However, even in severe diarrheal disease the drop in nitrogen absorption may be only 10 to 15 per cent, and seldom exceeds 50 per cent. *Thus it is worthwhile to continue feeding persons with diarrhea even though stool volume may be increased.*

With so many factors adversely affecting protein nutritional status during infectious disease, it is not surprising that in underdeveloped countries the protein deficiency disease, kwashiorkor, is commonly precipitated by diarrheal disease, measles, or other infections in children who are already in a precarious nutritional state. Similarly, infections, especially of a chronic nature, are responsible for much of the protein deficiency seen in adults.

Vitamins. Blood levels of vitamin A are reduced in acute infections. Diarrheal and other infectious diseases, particularly measles, are frequently responsible for precipitating xerophthalmia and keratomalacia in children receiving diets deficient in vitamin A. It is probable that most clinical cases of avitaminosis A follow an acute infection. The absorption of vitamin A has been found to be reduced by severe *Giardia lamblia* infections. It is probable that other intestinal infections have this effect when sufficiently severe.

As was observed among prisoners of war of the Japanese during World War II, clinical beriberi is frequently precipitated in thiamin-deficient individuals by an infectious episode. The synthesis of thiamin and other B vitamins by intestinal bacterial flora may also be affected by both intestinal infections and chemotherapy.

Spontaneous respiratory infections have been found to induce megaloblastic anemia in monkeys maintained on a diet low in folic acid. Also, the dietary intake of hemopoietic B vitamins is not low enough to account for the megaloblastic anemia seen in many patients with complicating infections.

Well confirmed is the appetite of the fish tapeworm, *Diphyllobothrium latum,* for vitamin B_{12}. These tapeworms are a significant cause of anemia in people infected from eating raw fresh-water fish, a common custom in Scandinavia and among persons of Scandinavian descent in the United States.

The role of infections in lowering serum ascorbic acid and increasing urinary excretion of this vitamin has been demonstrated by many experimental studies in guinea pigs. In poorly nourished children, otitis media, pneumonia, pyelonephritis, and other infections have long been recognized as precipitators of scurvy. Malaria, typhoid fever, influenza, measles, tuberculosis, and vaccination against smallpox are among other specific infections reported responsible for the appearance of scurvy in vulnerable children.

Minerals. Early in an infectious episode there is a sharp decrease in blood levels of iron and zinc. It is well recognized that hookworm infection, if sufficiently severe, causes enough loss of blood to produce microcytic-hypochromic anemia even when dietary intakes of iron appear adequate. This may also occur with *Schistosoma haematobium* infections. Increased losses of calcium and phosphorus have been reported for tuberculosis in both guinea pigs and man. Losses of sodium, chloride, potassium, and phosphorus, which are sometimes severe enough to cause death, occur in diarrhea of infectious origin.

EFFECT OF MALNUTRITION ON INFECTION

There are large numbers of laboratory, clinical, and field observations which demonstrate that the severity and outcome of infection are frequently worsened by malnutrition. The prevalence of diarrheal disease, both upper and lower respiratory infections, and some other types of microbial disease is also influenced by malnutrition. Moreover, much of the high infant and preschool mortality in developing countries attributed to microbial disease would not occur in well nourished children. The relative influence of the various potential mechanisms whereby nutritional deficiencies influence resistance to infectious disease under field conditions is not really known. The following must be considered.

Antibody Formation. Although other mechanisms may be equally important in defense against infections, formation of antibodies specific for infectious agents or their toxins has received the most attention. This is because there are excellent techniques for detecting the presence of antibodies, and protective immunizations have been developed against many infections. Severe deficiencies of protein, vitamin A, ascorbic acid, riboflavin, thiamin, pantothenic acid, biotin, and niacin-tryptophan in laboratory animals are known to interfere with antibody formation. A number of studies confirm that protein deficiency in man can interfere with formation of antibodies. There have been several reports of false-negative tuberculin reactions in malnourished patients with tuberculosis. In human volunteers, antibody formation has been suppressed by inducing metabolic deficiencies of pantothenic acid or pyridoxine by feeding the corresponding antimetabolites, desoxypyridoxine and omega-methylpyridoxine. The same effect has been observed in cases of severe pellagra and moderately severe deficiency of several of the B vitamins.

Phagocytic Activity. The macrophages and microphages of the reticuloendothelial system are important protectors of the body against microbial diseases, particularly those caused by bacteria. Nutritional deficiency can reduce both the number and the phagocytic capacity of these cells. Children with kwashiorkor have little or no leukocyte response to superimposed infections. Macrophage activity is decreased in the presence of vitamin A, ascorbic acid, thiamin, and riboflavin deficiency in laboratory animals. Both animal studies and clinical observations of folic acid deficiency have shown production of phagocytes in mammalian bone marrow to be depressed to the extent of nullifying the effect of protective antibodies. Recently, relatively mild iron deficiency has been shown to reduce the killing power of leukocytes. Reduced cell-mediated immunity, as measured by delayed hypersensitivity skin tests, DNCB sensitivity, and lymphocyte transformation by PHA, has been demonstrated in children with protein-calorie malnutrition.

Tissue Integrity. The integrity of the skin, mucous membranes, and other epithelial tissues helps to prevent entry of the infectious agent. Various pathologic changes occur in tissues, depending on the type and severity of the nutritional deficiency. Mucous secretions may be reduced or absent, mucosal surfaces may become easily permeable, changes may take place in intercellular substance, or there may be epithelial metaplasia, edema in underlying tissues, and accumulation of cellular debris to form a favorable culture medium for the infectious agent. Deficiencies in vitamin A, ascorbic acid, thiamin, riboflavin, niacin, and protein are especially likely to cause tissue changes that lower resistance.

Wound Healing and Collagen Formation. How long an infection will be disabling depends on how rapidly it can be localized and contained. Nutritional deficiencies affect not only tissue integrity, but also wound healing, fibroblastic response to trauma, walling off of abscesses, and collagen formation. In protein-deficient rats, the walls of induced sterile subcutaneous abscesses were much thinner than those of spontaneous or induced abscesses in well nourished animals. The fibroblastic response in the deficient rats was markedly reduced, and as a result fatal septicemia frequently developed.

Ascorbic acid intake must be adequate for synthesis of the amino acids from which collagen is formed, particularly hydroxyproline and hydroxylysine, which are almost unique to collagen. The skin at the edges of wounds in scorbutic guinea pigs showed almost no hydroxyproline. Restoration of ascorbic acid to the diet induced rapid production of hydroxyproline and the onset of wound healing.

Nonspecific Resistance Factors. It is hard to assess the importance of various nonspecific mechanisms of resistance to infection such as those requiring properdin, interferon, or lysozymes. All would appear vulnerable to nutritional deficiencies, but there is no evidence of this occurring.

Destruction of Bacterial Toxins. Most of the destruction of bacterial toxins or resistance to them in the animal host occurs as the result of the toxins combining with specific antibodies. There is some evidence that other mechanisms may exist as well. For example, rats suffering from deficiencies of B vitamins or vitamin A are more susceptible than controls to diphtheria toxin, even though antitoxin titers and rate of disappearance of injected toxin are similar in the two groups. Probably because of the ethical difficulties of investigating the problem directly in man, there are no clinical observations of this phenomenon.

Intestinal Flora. There is evidence that changes in the intestinal flora induced by diet can influence susceptibility to some intestinal pathogens. In kwashiorkor, there is a tendency for the bacteria of the lower intestinal tract to appear at a higher level. In milder degrees of protein malnutrition it seems likely that intestinal organisms that are not normally pathogenic to the well nourished host may cause diarrhea. Not only is no known pathogen identified in most diarrheal episodes in malnourished children, but also the frequency and severity of these episodes are decreased when dietary supplements are provided. Changes in gastrointestinal motility secondary to malnutrition may also play a role in the severity of protozoal and helminthic infections.

Endocrine Balance. Prolonged adrenocorticotrophic hormone (ACTH) or cortisone therapy increases the spread of many infections, presumably by inhibiting local inflammatory reactions at the site of bacterial proliferation. These observations may have a bearing on the question of how malnutrition influences resistance to infection, since protein deficiency, caloric deprivation, and a number of other nutritional deficiencies influence endocrine balance.

Chung, A., and Viscorová, B.: The effect of early oral feeding versus early oral starvation on the course of infantile diarrhea. J. Pediatr., 33:14, 1948.

Gallin, J. I., Kaye, D., and O'Leary, W. M.: Serum lipids in infection. N. Engl. J. Med., 281:1081, 1969.

Law, D. K., Dudrick, S. J., and Abdou, N. I.: Immunocompetence of patients with protein-calorie malnutrition. Ann. Intern. Med., 79:545, 1973.

Scrimshaw, N. S.: Protein deficiency and infective disease, In Munro, H. N., and Allison, J. B., (eds.): Mammalian Protein Metabolism, Vol. II. New York, Academic Press, Inc., 1964, chap. 23, p. 569.

Scrimshaw, N. S., Taylor, C. E., and Gordon, J. E.: Interactions of Nutrition and Infection, World Health Organization Monograph Series No. 57. Geneva, World Health Organization, 1968.

Smythe, P. M., Brereton-Stiles, G. G., Grace, H. J., Mafoyane, A., Schonland, M., Coovadia, H. M., Loening, W. E. K., Parent, M. A., and Vos, G. H.: Thymolymphatic deficiency and depression of cell-mediated immunity in protein-calorie malnutrition. Lancet, 2:939, 1971.

Taylor, P. E., Tejada, C., and Sánchez, M.: The effect of malnutrition on the inflammatory response as exhibited by the granuloma pouch of the rat. J. Exp. Med., 126:539, 1967.

715. KWASHIORKOR, MARASMUS, AND INTERMEDIATE FORMS OF PROTEIN-CALORIE MALNUTRITION

Nevin S. Scrimshaw

Definition. The clinical spectrum of protein-calorie deficiency ranges from forms characterized only by growth retardation to the extremes of kwashiorkor and marasmus. Kwashiorkor results from a deficiency of protein relative to calories, is found in children whose caloric intake is adequate and even excessive, or may be superimposed on varying degrees of protein-calorie deficiency. When protein and calories are limited to about the same degree, the clinical condition that develops is marasmus.

Pathogenesis. The various forms of protein-calorie malnutrition are of major public health significance in most underdeveloped countries. They result from diets that are quantitatively and qualitatively inadequate in individuals with superimposed stress, usually episodes of infectious disease. A deficient diet results in turn from varying combinations of low food production, inadequate preservation and distribution of foods, restricted purchasing power, poor food habits, and deficient knowledge of the relation between diet and health. The excessive incidence of infectious disease is a consequence of poor environmental conditions, inadequate knowledge of epidemiologic factors, poor personal hygiene, and insufficient health services.

The clinical result depends on the severity and duration of the nutritional deficiencies of protein and calories, on the relative importance of the deficiency of protein to that of calories, on the nature and severity of other associated nutritional deficiencies, on the age of the person affected, and on the presence of other complications. The mild and moderate forms in children, frequently unrecognized or misinterpreted, are primarily characterized by inadequate growth and development. In adults they reduce work performance and resistance to infection.

Mild to Moderate Protein-Calorie Malnutrition in Children. Retarded growth is greatest in the first two years of life, when dietary inadequacy and frequency of infections are most pronounced. Insufficient or improper supplementation of breast feeding is usually a factor. After weaning, the usual diet is cereal grains, starchy roots, overdiluted milk, or even cornstarch. Often such a regimen not only fails to provide the needed calories but also is deficient in many essential nutrients, particularly proteins of high biologic value.

Not until the third to fifth year of life is the usual child in underdeveloped countries permitted an adult type of diet. The period of greatest dietary inadequacy coincides in general with increased exposure to an unsanitary environment and a greater frequency of diarrheal and parasitic diseases, measles, whooping cough, and other diseases of childhood. By the time children enter school this critical period of high morbidity from infection is largely past because of an acquired immunity and better nutrition.

The assumption that reduced growth of children in underdeveloped countries is due more to environmental than to genetic factors is supported by observations of children of different races living under similar adverse conditions. Conversely, well nourished children of the same genetic origins usually follow the growth pattern of well fed North American or European children in a healthy environment.

The shorter limb-to-trunk ratio often observed in poorly nourished populations is caused mainly by primary or secondary malnutrition during the period when growth, particularly of the long bones, is normally rapid in the young child. There is also x-ray evidence that such children have retarded ossification of centers in their wrists and hands. Children with early growth retardation experience a parallel impairment of psychomotor development that persists at least through the school years, although the latter stems partly from social deprivation.

Mild to Moderate Protein-Calorie Malnutrition in Adults. The consequences of the mild to moderate chronic protein-calorie malnutrition common among adult populations has been little studied. Adaptation to insufficient calories includes low weight for height and reduced caloric expenditure. Accordingly, it is probable that it seriously reduces work capacity and thereby contributes to the low social and economic development in these areas. The effects of such malnutrition on resistance to stress, particularly that resulting from infectious disease, also needs further attention. Pregnant and lactating women are a particularly vulnerable segment of adult populations of underdeveloped countries. Many women do not gain a normal amount of weight during pregnancy, and average weights of their children at birth are generally at least 200 to 300 grams lighter than those of well nourished mothers. Associated with this lower birth weight is higher neonatal and perinatal mortality as well as higher morbidity and poorer growth in infancy. The consequences of repeated pregnancy and lactation on poorly nourished mothers have received too little attention. It is noteworthy that such women look older than their chronologic age.

MARASMUS

The extremely low calorie diets responsible for the syndrome of marasmus are obviously also deficient in proteins and many other essential nutrients. Because calories are so inadequate, the child utilizes amino acids from the skeletal muscles and other less essential tissues for gluconeogenesis in addition to energy from fat deposits. Growth stops, but the amino acids and other nutrients liberated from the child's tissues permit a continuing synthesis of serum albumin, enzymes, and other essential metabolites, and no serious metabolic disturbances are observed.

The child with marasmus is emaciated owing to a loss of subcutaneous fat, extreme muscle wasting, and atrophy of most organs. Although the liver and other essential organs are much reduced in size, histologic changes are minimal. Despite the apt description of being reduced to "skin and bones," the child remains clinically alert, and maintains an appetite.

KWASHIORKOR

Clinical Characteristics. Clinically, the syndrome of kwashiorkor presents a pitting edema varying from a mild form localized in feet and ankles to severe, generalized edema, with eyelids swollen shut. Movement of the extremities may be limited, and fluid accumulates in the peritoneal cavity. Patients are usually extremely apathetic, with a weak, monotonous cry if disturbed. Anorexia is frequently severe; diarrhea is an almost constant finding. The characteristic alterations of the skin resemble the dermatosis of pellagra, with which they have been mistakenly identified. The lesions are pigmented, dry, hyperkeratotic, and sometimes desquamating, and vary in size from punctiform to large, confluent areas. They are most numerous where subject to irritation, especially in the perineal region. They frequently occur on the extremities and face, and may extend to the trunk.

Normally curly hair becomes dry, fine, brittle, and straight. It is easily pulled out or may even fall out. It may become reddish, yellowish, or even white. These pigmentation changes are often observed in stripes, indicating successive periods of normal and abnormal hair growth. The extremities are frequently cold and cyanotic. The abdomen may be distended owing to flaccid abdominal muscles and ascites. Hepatomegaly is sometimes found.

Biochemical Alterations. *Protein.* Low total serum protein is a diagnostic characteristic. It is due almost entirely to a low level of albumin, and is sometimes partially obscured by a relatively high level of gamma globulin resulting from a concurrent infectious process. There is a tendency for the beta globulin fraction to be both relatively and absolutely decreased; a relative increase in the alpha$_2$ globulin has also been found. Studies with I^{127}-labeled albumin indicate that the lowering of this fraction is due to a decrease in rate of synthesis and not to abnormal catabolism.

Total α-amino nitrogen in plasma is abnormally low because most amino acids are present in decreased amount. The greatest reductions are in tryptophan, cystine, valine, tyrosine, and methionine. Low levels of urea in both blood and urine indicate decreased protein metabolism. The synthesis of antibodies is also inhibited. A very marked increase in the proportion of urinary nitrogen excreted as purine derivatives has been taken as evidence of cellular breakdown in kwashiorkor. Other abnormal substances in the urine indicating impairment of important metabolic pathways are β-aminoisobutyric acid and ethanolamine.

Although the liver protein concentration in kwashiorkor is greatly reduced by fat, it is not decreased in absolute amount in relation to body size. However, a lowered ratio of nitrogen to deoxyribonucleic acid has been reported, suggesting a true loss of protoplasmic nitrogen. In any case, the level of nitrogen in the liver of children with kwashiorkor is markedly decreased over that for normal children of the same age. There is also a marked loss of muscle nitrogen in kwashiorkor, the degree depending largely upon the severity of pre-existing marasmus.

Lipids and Carbohydrates. All the lipid fractions that have been determined in the blood of children with kwashiorkor, including neutral fat, fatty acids, phospholipids, and cholesterol, have been found to be low, and levels of these substances rise rapidly in the course of treatment. An increase in fat content of the liver, found by gross and microscopic examination, is another diagnostic criterion. In true marasmus, on the other hand, the amount of liver fat is decreased. Blood glucose levels

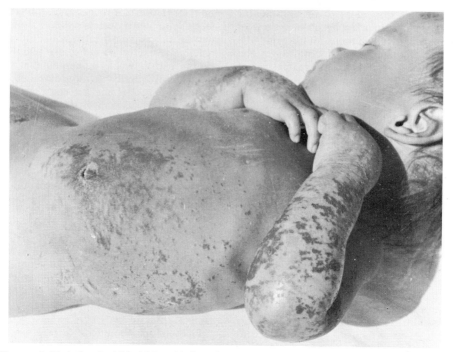

Figure 1. Edema and skin lesions in child with kwashiorkor. (Courtesy of Institute of Nutrition of Central America and Panama.)

are generally low. Although glucose tolerance is sometimes reduced, and a diabetic type of glucose tolerance curve is observed, this is not an invariable feature of the disease.

Enzymes. In acute kwashiorkor, lipase, trypsin, and amylase activities in the duodenal secretion are lowered almost to zero, and marked reductions in serum pseudocholinesterase, amylase, carbonic anhydrase, and alkaline phosphatase are recognized characteristics. The activity of these enzymes returns rapidly to normal with the administration of an adequate diet. Alkaline phosphatase levels, however, show a slight further drop before rising with therapy.

The activity of a number of enzymes has also been measured in liver obtained by needle biopsy from children with kwashiorkor. The outstanding finding is a decrease in xanthine oxidase activity per unit of protein, although cholinesterase and D-amino acid oxidase activity are also definitely lowered. Alkaline phosphatase activity in the liver is generally increased. These findings suggest that, although the activity of many key enzymes is maintained even in the presence of extreme protein deficiency, some are sufficiently affected to initiate the train of events culminating in death.

Vitamins. Levels of vitamin A and carotene in the serum of children with kwashiorkor are extremely low. It was assumed that this was due to low intake of vitamin A, until studies demonstrated that children with acute kwashiorkor upon admission to the hospital did not have an increase in serum vitamin A after a 75-mg oral dose of vitamin A palmitate. After three to five days of intensive protein therapy, however, a similar dose gave the same sharp increase in serum vitamin A that is found in normal children. It was also found that, in most cases, serum vitamin A levels rose with protein therapy, even when the diet contained no carotene or vitamin A. Analysis of liver biopsy material demonstrated that this

phenomenon occurred whenever there were adequate stores of vitamin A in the liver, and that in those few cases in which there was gross depletion of vitamin A, administration of protein alone produced no serum response. From this and similar studies, it appears probable that the *transport* of vitamin A and possibly of vitamin E, which also occurs in abnormally low amounts in blood plasma of children with kwashiorkor, is inadequate because of the lack of a protein carrier.

Blood levels of thiamin and riboflavin are within normal limits. Even though the pigmented skin lesions superficially resemble those of pellagra, there is no evidence of niacin deficiency. The urinary excretion of N-methylnicotinamide, in cases in Central America at least, is within normal limits. Levels of serum ascorbic acid are relatively low, but are not in the range commonly associated with clinical deficiency. No significant alterations of levels of vitamin B$_{12}$ in the blood have been found.

Electrolytes and Other Minerals. Potassium depletion is a major biochemical characteristic of kwashiorkor, and is a direct consequence of the protein deficiency. Other electrolyte changes are secondary to diarrhea (a symptom almost always present in kwashiorkor) or vomiting. Interpretation and correction of electrolyte changes in kwashiorkor are complicated by the abnormal distribution of water and the severe degree of potassium depletion. Magnesium deficiency may occur and lead to tetany.

Endocrine Function. On the basis of observed normal adrenal cortex function in marasmus and decreased glucocorticoid production in kwashiorkor, the hypothesis has been proposed that the severe restriction of calories in children in whom marasmus develops results in increased production of ACTH by the anterior pituitary gland which in turn stimulates the adrenal cortex to produce more corticosteroids. These hormones assure catabolism of muscle and other labile proteins sufficient to furnish amino acids to the liver for gluconeogenesis and likewise provide the liver with amino acids for synthesis of essential proteins. This mechanism does not operate when the child receives a diet with enough calories to meet minimal energy needs even though it is extremely deficient in proteins. Under these circumstances, children do not mobilize amino acids from their muscles, and instead present the serious metabolic disturbances of protein deficiency without further muscle wasting. The result is kwashiorkor.

Other Physiologic Changes. In the marasmic type of kwashiorkor seen in Central America, a relatively small heart, which rapidly increases in size with treatment, is found upon radiologic examination. Electrocardiographic findings have consisted of low voltage and minor abnormalities, including alterations in the T wave and changes in rhythm. To judge by the volume of feces excreted by children with kwashiorkor, these children suffer from a malabsorption syndrome which is not completely corrected even after some weeks of treatment. Good digestion and absorption of proteins still take place during the acute state, but fat is poorly handled at first. Although fat absorption improves very rapidly as the child recovers, some degree of steatorrhea persists even into late recovery. Despite the marked histologic alterations in the liver, the common tests for liver function have been found to give results within normal limits, with the possible exception of sulfobromophthalein retention, which is frequently high.

Electroencephalographic studies have shown diminished voltage and excessively slow rhythmic activity. Some authors have also reported abnormal focal activity and other alterations. These abnormalities tend to disappear as recovery progresses.

Pathology. The main pathologic alterations in kwashiorkor include fatty changes in the liver, of the large droplet type, beginning in periportal areas of the lobule and extending progressively to the central vein. The pancreas and other endocrine glands become atrophic, along with marked atrophy of the intestinal mucosa, to give changes like those in primary malabsorption. The skin shows atrophy of the epidermis, with varying degrees of hyperkeratosis and parakeratosis.

Coexisting Deficiencies. The clinical manifestations of protein-calorie malnutrition are further complicated by the presence of other nutritional deficiencies. Vitamin A deficiency with severe ocular lesions is frequent in both marasmus and kwashiorkor. Concurrent deficiencies of components of B vitamins, particularly riboflavin, are also common. The mild normocytic, normochromic anemia attributable to protein deficiency is often complicated and becomes much more severe because of simultaneous deficiencies of iron, vitamin E, folic acid, and other hematopoietic factors of the B vitamins. A recent report suggests that vitamin E deficiency is sometimes responsible. Dehydration and serious electrolyte imbalance are usual because of the coexisting diarrhea.

Treatment. The correction of dehydration and associated electrolyte imbalance and the treatment of infections are the immediate demands in management of protein-calorie malnutrition. The basic requirement, however, is a diet providing all essential nutrients. Three to 4 grams of protein of high biologic value and 100 to 140 calories per kilogram of body weight are useful in children with kwashiorkor, and up to 200 calories per kilogram in those with marasmus.

Prevention. The prevention of protein-calorie malnutrition depends upon teaching mothers the importance of feeding their young children properly. Efforts should be made to increase the availability of low-cost protein foods suitable for feeding to infants and young children, ensuring that the mother can obtain them through either commercial channels or welfare programs. There must also be effective public health measures for reducing the burden of microbial disease in vulnerable populations.

Béhar, M., Viteri, F., and Scrimshaw, N. S.: Treatment of severe protein deficiency in children (kwashiorkor). Am. J. Clin. Nutr., 5:506, 1957.

National Academy of Sciences–National Research Council: Pre-School Child Malnutrition: Primary Deterrent to Human Progress. An International Conference on Prevention of Malnutrition in the Pre-School Child, Washington, D.C., December 7-11, 1964. NAS–NRC Publication No. 1282, 1966.

Scrimshaw, N. S., and Béhar, M.: Protein malnutrition in young children. Science, 133:2039, 1961.

Scrimshaw, N. S., and Béhar, M.: Malnutrition in underdeveloped countries. N. Engl. J. Med., 272:137, 193, 1965.

Viteri, F., Béhar, M., Arroyave, G., and Scrimshaw, N. S.: Clinical aspects of protein malnutrition. In Munro, H. N., and Allison, J. B. (eds.): Mammalian Protein Metabolism. Vol. II. New York, Academic Press, 1964, Chap. 22, p. 523.

Waterlow, J. C., and Alleyne, G. A. O.: Protein malnutrition in children: Advances in knowledge in the last ten years. Adv. Protein Chem. 25:117, 1971.

Waterlow, J. C., Cravioto, J., and Stephen, J. M. L.: Protein malnutrition in man. Adv. Protein Chem., 15:131, 1960.

716. UNDERNUTRITION, STARVATION, AND HUNGER EDEMA

Nevin S. Scrimshaw

When a person's caloric intake is far below his daily energy expenditure, he must either bring the two into balance by reduced activity or draw upon his own tissues for energy. Initially, tissue fat is a major energy source, but protein is also required as a source of amino acids for gluconeogenesis. Cahill has shown that after several weeks of fasting, dependence on endogenous amino acids decreases, because even the central nervous system can then utilize fatty acids.

Once adipose tissue has been exhausted, lassitude, loss of ambition, hypotension, collapse, and death follow if the caloric intake deficit continues. The late stages of this syndrome are also observed in anorexia nervosa, terminal carcinoma, and other wasting diseases.

Keys provides the most comprehensive review of the world literature on starvation, and adds important experimental observations of his own. Others have described severe malnutrition in the prisons and concentration camps of World War II and famines in many parts of the world.

Dependent edema often accompanies severe, prolonged undernutrition (starvation). The edema is soft and pitting, and usually disappears when the person is recumbent for some time, as during sleep. The causes of the edema are not entirely clear. Hypoproteinemia (specifically hypoalbuminemia, thus lowering the colloid osmotic pressure) is frequent but by no means invariable. Loss of fat and muscle, leaving a "loose sack" of skin with fluid filling the empty spaces, has been thought of as a contributing phenomenon. Diminished renal blood flow and glomerular filtration resulting from diminished cardiac output would presumably lead to sodium retention and edema.

Treatment of starvation demands caution. *In all forms of severe undernutrition, refeeding must be instituted slowly.* Overeating was a cause of shock and death of concentration camp victims at the end of World War II. The same is true for nutritional treatment of patients severely undernourished because of non-nutritional disease, e.g., esophageal carcinoma. Sudden flooding of the intestine with rich food through a feeding jejunostomy or gastrostomy may produce shock and death.

Benedict, F. G.: A Study of Prolonged Fasting. Carnegie Institute of Washington, Publication No. 203, 1915.
Keys, A.: The Biology of Human Starvation. Minneapolis, University of Minnesota Press, 1950.
Mollison, P. L.: Observations on cases of starvation at Belsen. Br. Med. J., 1:4, 1946.
Owen, O. E., Morgan, A. P., Kemp, H. G., Sullivan, J. M., Herrera, M. G., and Cahill, G. F., Jr.: Brain metabolism during fasting. J. Clin. Invest., 46:1589, 1967.
Young, V. R., and Scrimshaw, N. S.: The physiology of starvation. Sci. Am., 225:14, 1971.

DEFICIENCIES OF INDIVIDUAL NUTRIENTS: VITAMIN DISEASES

Nevin S. Scrimshaw

717. HYPOVITAMINOSIS A (INCLUDING XEROPHTHALMIA AND KERATOMALACIA)

Etiology and Distribution.   The term vitamin A is used to include all compounds having vitamin A activity, but requirements are now expressed by the Food and Agriculture Organization and World Health Organization in terms of crystalline vitamin A_1 alcohol (retinol). The international unit, still used in many countries, is equivalent to 0.3 μg of retinol (or 0.344 μg of retinyl acetate) or to 0.6 μg of the provitamin beta-carotene. The recommended intake for adult males is 1000 μg of retinol per day, and for adult females, 800 μg, increasing to 1000 μg during pregnancy. During lactation 1200 μg of retinol per day is recommended. For children the recommendations are estimated from expected body weight for age, ranging from 420 μg per day at three to five months of age to the adult levels. Requirements are not influenced by physical activity or climate, but any pathologic condition that interferes with fat absorption is likely to impede vitamin A absorption, and infections can increase vitamin A needs.

Signs and symptoms of hypovitaminosis A are particularly common in Indonesia and most other countries of Southeast Asia and the Indian subcontinent, but are seen at least occasionally in nearly all economically underdeveloped countries. They are most often precipitated by infectious disease in infants and young children who already suffer from chronic malnutrition. Sporadic cases occur among particularly underprivileged infants in most of the industrialized areas of the world.

Clinical Manifestations; Pathology and Pathologic Physiology.   The best known and generally the earliest physiologic effect of hypovitaminosis A is the loss of night vision (nyctalopia). The retinal rods responsible for vision in dim light contain a light-sensitive pigment, rhodopsin, an aldehyde of vitamin A that breaks down to retinene when light strikes a rod. In vitamin A deficiency rhodopsin regeneration fails.

Xerophthalmia is a dryness of the only transparent epithelial structures of the body that are exposed to air and light. The conjunctiva is affected earlier and more constantly than the cornea. Typical is a fatty dryness, most pronounced at the thickened wrinkles of the corners; the eye loses its porcelain aspect and looks muddy-greasy, like oil paint.

Bitot spots are often present, ranging in severity from a few tiny air bubbles visible on the exposed conjunctiva between the corneal rim and limbus, to a frothy white coating that overflows onto the cornea. The meibomian glands sometimes enlarge to look like a string of beads along the margin of the eyelids. The cornea is more resistant, but becomes hazy, rough, and dry and insensitive to touch. Punctate superficial infiltrations or small erosions may be seen on the surface. As the disease progresses to *keratomalacia,* one of these erosions may enlarge rapidly, with protrusion and eventually prolapse of the iris and loss of the lens. Sometimes there is a rather sudden spongy swelling and melting down of the cornea, a colliquative necrosis, with subsequent shrinkage of the eyeball (Fig. 2).

The skin becomes dry as the sebaceous glands become covered with keratin, so that secretions are diminished. *Phrynoderma,* an elevated papular lesion caused by plugging of the mouth of the hair follicles with a dense keratotic mass together with hyperplasia of the epithelium lining the plugged follicles, has been mistakenly listed as a sign of vitamin A deficiency. This condition is not necessarily associated with low serum levels of vitamin A, and does not respond to prolonged vitamin A therapy. Moreover, it is different from the follicular lesion of vitamin A deficiency in laboratory animals, in which the upper third of the hair follicles contains loose keratin and becomes dilated.

The small intestine is the main site of the conversion of active forms of carotene to vitamin A and its absorption. Therefore, when the intestine is affected by diseases such as sprue, fibrocystic disease of the pancreas, lymphomas, or lipodystrophy (Whipple's disease), hypovitaminosis A is likely to result. The liver contains 90 per cent of vitamin A stores, but these may be markedly reduced in some hepatic diseases.

Lowered dietary intake of preformed vitamin A or of an active carotene precursor is the most obvious and common factor in hypovitaminosis A, but any condition interfering with the intestinal absorption and conversion of carotene to vitamin A and its transport to the liver will contribute to deficiency of this vitamin. Surgical removal of sections of the small bowel and excessive consumption of mineral oil are in this category. So are

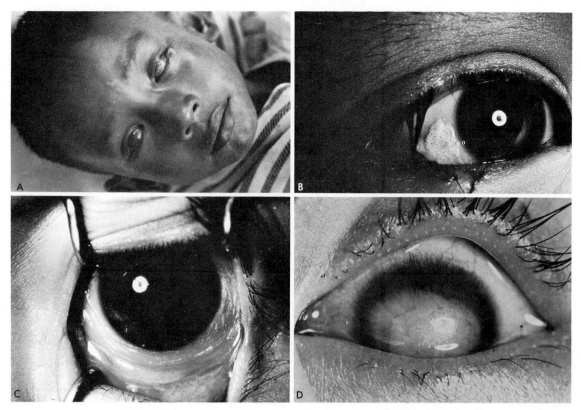

Figure 2. *A*, Keratomalacia in four year old boy. *Left eye:* Perforation of cornea, through which lens has escaped, with drop of vitreous substance visible on lower lid. *Right eye:* Necrosis of cornea with small ulcer. *B*, Bitot spot on transparent conjunctiva, nine year old child. *C*, Xerosis conjunctivae, showing Bitot spot and dryness of mucosal folds, four year old boy. *D*, Xerophthalmia with subtotal leukoma, after measles with perforating xerosis of cornea, in three year old child. (Courtesy of Dr. H. A. P. C. Oomen.)

massive intestinal infections with *Giardia lamblia* and probably also ascaris and hookworm. Severe protein deficiency (kwashiorkor) decreases the availability of transport protein. Dried skim milk fed to protein-deficient children in Indonesia increased the frequency of xerophthalmia, presumably by removing the limitation of protein and calories on growth and thereby increasing the need for vitamin A which the milk did not contain.

Treatment. Treatment consists of administration of therapeutic amounts of vitamin A, correction of the pattern of dietary intake, and, in cases of secondary deficiency, therapy of the underlying disease. In young children without serious eye involvement, the daily oral administration of 3000 µg of retinol is recommended. When there is reason to suspect that dietary fat, including the fat-soluble vitamin A, is not properly absorbed, the new water-miscible vitamin A preparations are indicated rather than fish liver oil. If no response is observed, or signs of keratomalacia are present, daily doses of 15,000 to 25,000 µg of retinol should be given intramuscularly for the first week in an attempt to prevent permanent impairment of vision. Improvement may be seen within a week, but maximal healing may take many weeks. If the lens is intact, residual corneal scarring can sometimes be treated by transplant.

When hypovitaminosis A is associated with protein deficiency, dietary protein alone will bring a prompt increase in serum vitamin A levels if the stores in the liver are adequate. Conversely, if protein deficiency is present, hypovitaminosis A will not respond to treatment with the vitamin alone owing to the lack of transport protein.

Prevention. Primary prevention depends upon assuring a diet with adequate vitamin A activity to meet all body needs and to maintain good stores of vitamin A in the liver. Foods of animal origin such as dairy products containing butter fat, egg yolk, liver, and fish liver oils are excellent sources. Sufficient quantities of the provitamin beta-carotene and other active carotenoids are also found in many vegetables and fruits. For populations in tropical and less developed countries, most of the vitamin A activity in the diet can come from fruits such as the mango and papaya. African palm oil, used in cooking in many parts of the world, is rich in vitamin A activity.

When processing has reduced the vitamin A activity of a food or when substitute foods of lower vitamin A content are introduced, fortification may be indicated. For example, margarine is routinely fortified with 10,000 IU of vitamin A per pound because it replaces butter, a good source of this vitamin. Similarly, skim milk for human consumption should be fortified with water-miscible vitamin A, because all vitamin A activity has been removed with the cream. Synthetic breakfast drinks replacing natural fruit juices can be made good sources of vitamin A.

Prevention of deficiency secondary to other disease requires measures to control the primary cause. Most important will be environmental sanitation and other public health measures to reduce the prevalence of infections.

Federation of American Societies for Experimental Biology: Nutritional Disease, Proceedings of a Conference on Beriberi, Endemic Goiter and Hypovitaminosis A, held at Princeton, New Jersey, June 1–5, 1958. Fed. Proc. 17:Part II, Supplement No. 2, 1958, pp. 103–143.

McLaren, D. S.: Malnutrition and the Eye. New York, Academic Press, Inc., 1963.

Scrimshaw, N. S., Taylor, C. E., and Gordon, J. E.: Interactions of Nutrition and Infection. World Health Organization, Monograph Series No. 57. Geneva, World Health Organization, 1968.

RICKETS AND OSTEOMALACIA

See Ch. 885 to 890.

ENDEMIC GOITER

See Ch. 841.

718. ARIBOFLAVINOSIS

Etiology and Distribution. The intake of riboflavin must be low for many months before symptoms become evident. Among persons whose diets contain limited riboflavin, the disease often appears during periods of physiologic stress such as pregnancy and lactation, and during the rapid growth of childhood. Ariboflavinosis is so commonly associated with diets deficient in niacin and protein that for years it was considered part of the pellagra syndrome.

Characteristic deficiency signs appear in persons on deficient diets for three to eight months, depending upon the exact level of riboflavin and individual variation.

Low urinary riboflavin excretion levels and mild clinical signs of ariboflavinosis are common among the low-income populations of developing countries. Moderate to severe ariboflavinosis is usually seen only in association with other deficiency diseases such as pellagra and kwashiorkor. In the industrialized countries it is likely to be one of the deficiencies seen in alcoholics and persons with long-standing infections, malignancies, and other chronic debilitating diseases.

Clinical Signs. Early symptoms of ariboflavinosis are soreness and burning of the lips, mouth, and tongue, and photophobia, lacrimation, burning, and itching of the eyes. The lesions of the lips may progress so that fissures extend from the angles of the mouth for a centimeter or more, and the lips themselves may appear dry and chapped. Shallow ulcerations and crusting sometimes develop. Neither the cheilosis nor the angular stomatitis is pathognomonic of riboflavin deficiency, because similar lesions may result from deficiency of niacin, iron, or pyridoxine.

The seborrheic type of dermatitis has a scaly, greasy appearance and is associated with erythema. Hard sebaceous plugs or fine filiform comedones may be seen over the bridge of the nose and on the malar prominences and chin. Dermatitis of the scrotum and vulva may also appear. In some instances, the redness, scaling, and desquamation of the skin of the scrotum extend to adjacent areas of the thigh which become raw and weeping.

The tongue in ariboflavinosis is characteristically purplish red or magenta and often has deep fissures. The papillae may be swollen, flattened, or mushroom-shaped, giving a pebbled appearance. In chronic deficiency the papillae may become atrophic. The glossitis of riboflavin deficiency cannot be clearly differentiated from that caused by lack of niacin, folic acid, or vitamin B_{12}.

Eye signs responding to administration of riboflavin include diffuse inflammation of the conjunctivae, and red, swollen eyelids with a sticky exudate. Photophobia may be intense. Injection and proliferation of the capillaries of the limbic plexus may develop.

Biochemical Function. Riboflavin functions as a coenzyme of the active prosthetic group of flavoproteins concerned with oxidative processes. Among these are cytochrome-c reductase, D- and L-amino oxidases, succinic dehydrogenase, diaphorase, and xanthine and aldehyde oxidases.

The concentrations of free riboflavin, flavin mononucleotide, and flavin dinucleotide in plasma can be readily measured, but are not reliable indicators of deficiency, nor are white or red blood cell levels of riboflavin any more specific. Either 24-hour urinary excretion of riboflavin or the excretion four hours after subcutaneous administration of 1.0 mg will be found reduced in those whose diets have been deficient in riboflavin for an extended period. Less than 50 mg in 24 hours or 20 μg in the four hours after the test dose indicate that prior intake has been inadequate.

Prevention and Treatment. Prevention requires a diet that includes foods that are rich sources of riboflavin such as milk, liver, other meats, eggs, and many green and yellow vegetables. For treatment, an adequate diet should be prescribed, and 5 mg of riboflavin given orally twice a day. Symptoms disappear in a few days, and the lesions clear up in a few weeks. In general, it is better to give a multivitamin preparation in treating ariboflavinosis because of the frequency of simultaneous deficiency of other B vitamins. When signs suggestive of such deficiencies are present, therapeutic doses of the appropriate vitamins should also be given.

Goldsmith, G. A.: The B vitamins: Thiamine, riboflavin, niacin. *In* Beaton, G. H., and McHenry, E. W. (eds.): Nutrition: A Comprehensive Treatise. Vol. II. New York. Academic Press, Inc., 1964, chap. 2, p. 145.

719. PELLAGRA

Etiology and Distribution. Although pellagra is caused by a primary dietary deficiency of niacin, the adequacy of dietary niacin is influenced by the quantity and quality of dietary protein, and particularly by the availability of tryptophan, which is a metabolic precursor of niacin. The term "niacin" is generic for both nicotinic acid and nicotinamide. One niacin equivalent is defined as 1 mg of niacin or 60 mg of tryptophan. The minimum required to prevent pellagra is 4.4 niacin equivalents per 1000 kcal per day, and a recommended allowance of 6.6 niacin equivalents per 1000 calories per day allows for individual variation.

Pellagra is traditionally associated with maize (corn) diets because this cereal grain has a low tryptophan as well as niacin content. It does not occur, however, where maize diets are supplemented with sufficient legume protein, as they are in Central America. It is still seen in the Yucatan peninsula of Mexico where the raising of henequen, maguey, hemp, or sisal takes most of the land, and in corn-eating populations of several Middle Eastern and African countries, notably in Egypt and Lesotho. In the 1930's it was still common in the southern United

States among low-income groups whose diets consisted mainly of pork fat and hominy grits made from degerminated corn, but the disease has now disappeared from the United States except in alcoholics. Until recently it was still seen among corn-eating populations of rural Yugoslavia, Rumania, and Greece.

The pellagra common in Indian populations subsisting on a diet of jowar (millet, *Sorghum vulgare*) is reported to be influenced by the relative excess of leucine as well as the low tryptophan and niacin of this cereal. Diets containing protein of animal origin or vegetable proteins of good quality contain enough tryptophan to prevent pellagra even when niacin intakes are low.

Experimental niacin-tryptophan deficiency in human subjects duplicates most but not all of the features of pellagra as it occurs in populations, because in the latter there are nearly always other complicating diseases and deficiencies. Pellagra in the industrialized countries at present is generally a result of the vitamin- and protein-deficient diets of chronic alcoholics.

Deficiency of folic acid probably accounts for the frequency of megaloblastic anemia in pellagra. The cheilosis, angular stomatitis, proctitis, scrotal dermatitis, and vaginitis may be more related to concomitant deficiency of riboflavin (vitamin B_2) or vitamin B_6 than to that of niacin. The neurologic and mental symptoms, especially the cord degeneration sometimes found, could possibly be caused by poor vitamin B_{12} absorption. Reversible achlorhydria often occurs. The peripheral neuropathy and occasional mental changes, suggesting Korsakoff's psychosis, are possibly due to concomitant deficiency of thiamin or pyridoxine. Because fatty liver may be present, deficiency of protein and especially of choline and methionine must also be considered.

Pellagra is encountered in patients with cirrhosis of the liver, chronic diarrheal disease, diabetes mellitus, and neoplasia. Prolonged infectious diseases, such as tuberculosis, or thyrotoxicosis may lead to deficiency owing to an increase in niacin requirement. Pellagrous dermatitis has also been reported in patients with malignant carcinoid, a rare tumor which may convert as much as 60 per cent of the body's tryptophan to serotonin instead of the usual 1 per cent. Decreased food intake and diarrhea presumably contribute to the development of pellagra in this condition.

Clinical Manifestations. The early signs of pellagra are nonspecific and include lassitude, anorexia, weakness, digestive disturbances, and often anxiety, irritability, and depression. As the deficiency progresses, soreness of the tongue gives way to severe inflammation of mucous membranes manifested by glossitis, stomatitis, esophagitis, diarrhea, urethritis, proctitis, and vaginitis. The mouth may be so painful that it is difficult to take even liquids, and the mucous membranes become bright red. The tongue is scarlet and swollen, with atrophy of the papillae. Not surprisingly, severe weight loss ensues.

The chronic dermatitis of pellagra may be difficult to distinguish from extensive exposure to dust and sunlight. It varies with the acuteness and severity of the deficiency state. At the earlier, acute stages it resembles sunburn. In chronic pellagra, which has developed more slowly, skin changes include thickening, scaling, hyperkeratinization, and pigmentation. Either type will usually be found on areas of skin exposed to sunlight—the backs of the hands and forearms, the anterior surfaces of the feet and lower legs, and the face and neck. Lesions following the sharp neckline of a dress or an open shirt are known as Casal's necklace. Other areas which may be involved are the axillae, groin, perineum, genitalia, elbows, knees, and skin under the breasts.

The early nonspecific psychic and emotional changes of early pellagra may, with increasing severity, progress to disorientation, delirium, and hallucination. The dementia may be hyperactive and manic or apathetic, lethargic, and stuporous. Other sensory and neurologic abnormalities and acute encephalopathy have been described in some cases. Anemia from associated deficiencies is common.

Biochemistry and Pathology. Nicotinamide functions in the body as the component of two important coenzymes, DPN (diphosphopyridine nucleotide) and TPN (triphosphopyridine nucleotide), which are functional groups in intracellular oxidation-reduction enzyme systems necessary for tissue respiration, glycolysis, and fat

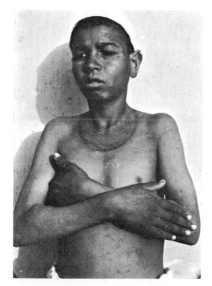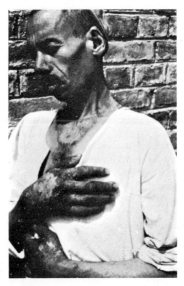

Figure 3. Modern pellagra. Egypt and the Balkans. (Courtesy of Dr. William J. Darby.)

synthesis. In endemic pellagra the combined excretion of the niacin metabolites, N^1-methylnicotinamide and pyridone, seldom exceeds 2 grams daily.

The skin lesions are hyperkeratotic, often with vesicles containing erythrocytes, fibrin, and melanin pigment. Microscopic examination reveals atrophy of the sebaceous glands and hair follicles and degeneration of the peripheral nerves of the skin. Pathologic changes have also been reported in the brain, spinal cord, and peripheral nerves. Mucous membranes show inflammation and atrophy.

Treatment and Prevention. The treatment of pellagra is a diet adequate in niacin and tryptophan and the administration of therapeutic doses of the vitamin. The best food sources of niacin are yeast, liver, lean meat, poultry, peanuts, and legumes. Potatoes, other vegetables, and whole wheat cereal and bread are fair sources. Most of these are also good sources of tryptophan as well. Although milk and eggs contain little niacin, they are also protective against pellagra because of their high tryptophan content. Enrichment of cereal flours with niacin and other B vitamins is a simple and inexpensive way of ensuring an ample intake of these nutrients.

In severe deficiency, niacinamide may be given in divided doses of 50 to 100 mg to a total of 300 to 500 mg for the first few days and then decreased to 150 mg daily. When circumstances make oral administration difficult, niacinamide can also be given intramuscularly in a dose of 100 mg three times daily. In advanced pellagra, bed rest is essential, and calorie intakes up to 3500 per day may be required. Acute symptoms improve within a few days, but several weeks of therapy may be required for complete recovery. Because concurrent deficiencies of other B vitamins are generally present, a multivitamin tablet containing 5.0 mg each of thiamin, riboflavin, and pyridoxine, should be given daily in the treatment of pellagra. Associated anemia may require either folic acid or iron therapy.

Goldsmith, G. A.: The B vitamins: Thiamine, riboflavin, niacin. *In* Beaton, G. H., and McHenry, E. W. (eds.): Nutrition: A Comprehensive Treatise. Vol. II. New York, Academic Press, Inc., 1964, chap. 2, p. 161.
Goldsmith, G. A., Sarett, H. P., Register, U. D., and Gibbens, J.: Studies of niacin requirements in man. I. Experimental pellagra in subjects on corn diets low in niacin and tryptophan. J. Clin. Invest., 31:533, 1952.
Spies, T. D.: Niacinamide malnutrition and pellagra. *In* Jolliffe, N. (ed.): Clinical Nutrition. 2nd ed. New York, Hoeber Medical Book, Harper & Brothers, 1962, chap. 18, p. 622.
Spies, T. D., Aring, C. D., Gelperin, J., and Bean, W. B.: The mental symptoms of pellagra. Their relief with nicotinic acid. Am. J. Med. Sci., 196:461, 1938.

720. BERIBERI

Etiology and Distribution. Beriberi occurs mainly in countries where polished rice provides a diet low in thiamin and high in carbohydrate. Among prisoners subsisting largely on polished rice in Japanese prison camps during World War II, beriberi developed when the thiamin supply was less than 0.3 mg per 1000 nonfat calories, with the acute episode usually precipitated by dysentery or other infectious disease. Deficiency signs may be anticipated when dietary intakes are less than 0.2 mg per 1000 calories, and intakes of 0.5 mg or more per 1000 calories are recommended. Because it is possible that older persons utilize thiamin less efficiently, they should maintain an intake of 1.0 mg per day, even when they are consuming less than 2000 kcal daily. The allowance of 0.5 mg per 1000 calories also applies to pregnant and lactating women and to children.

Beriberi is still seen occasionally in the rice-eating populations of Southeast Asia and the Indian subcontinent, and infantile beriberi has actually increased in some villages where newly introduced gasoline mills more completely separate the germ from the endosperm than does traditional hand-pounding. It has been described in some populations of Brazil and Africa among persons consuming cassava as the primary source of calories. It may also occur in association with pathologic states that interfere with the ingestion or absorption of food, and it is the most important of the B vitamin deficiencies common to alcoholism. Wernicke's syndrome is often associated with beriberi. Korsakoff's psychosis found among alcoholics is closely related to it (see Ch. 406).

Clinical Characteristics. The great majority of cases of beriberi are of the mild, subacute form, in which paresthesias and altered reflexes are the most characteristic findings. The muscle groups involved seem related to the length of the nerve controlling them, the amount of work they do, and possibly their blood supply. Laborers complain of disturbances of the lower legs, women more often of sensations in the fingers; other distributions can be related to the occupational use of muscle groups. Fullness or tightening of the muscles and fatigue pains resembling those of muscle ischemia are prominent, and, especially at night, muscle cramps occur.

In well developed cases, tachycardia is present, and the heart is enlarged. The edema may be generalized and massive or minimal without clear relation to the severity of the other symptoms. The most common characteristics of acute beriberi in prisoners of the Japanese in World War II were persistent tachycardia, symmetrical foot and wrist drop associated with muscle tenderness, mild disturbances of sensation over the outer aspects of the legs and thighs, and in patches over the abdomen, chest, and forearms. Most of these signs and symptoms have been reproduced experimentally in 30 to 120 days in adult subjects on thiamin intakes from 0.075 to 0.2 mg per 1000 calories.

The acute fulminating form of beriberi has been called Shoshin; it is dominated by circulatory insufficiency. The milder forms may develop into this often fatal type, but more often it is of sudden onset. When nerve lesions develop early, the heart is saved from extreme insufficiency because the patient is forced to rest. In terminal cases, severe dyspnea and violent palpitations of the heart allow the patient no rest, and precordial pain may be intense. The patient tosses and turns about violently and complains of heaviness, constriction, oppression, and sometimes actual pain over the epigastrium. The moans and shrieks of the patient are distorted by the coincident hoarseness and sometimes aphonia. Pupils are dilated, and respirations are frequent and superficial. The liver and heart are enlarged and the heart action tumultuous. Cyanosis is obvious, and the pulse is weak but regular.

The chronic, dry, atrophic type — with wrist drop and foot drop — is generally found only in older adults. They no longer show the biochemical changes characteristic of acute beriberi, nor do they respond satisfactorily to therapy.

The beriberi seen in *infants*, particularly from one to four months of age, is associated with poor thiamin content of, and possibly abnormal metabolites in, the breast milk of mothers subsisting on a rice diet. It begins with vomiting, restlessness, pallor, anorexia, and insomnia, and evolves variously. In acute infantile beriberi, the infant develops cyanosis, dyspnea, and running pulse with cardiac crises which are often fatal. If the process is more chronic, the symptoms are vomiting, inanition, anorexia, aphonia, opisthotonos, edema, oliguria, constipation, and meteorism. A subacute form that may evolve into either the acute or chronic type is also described. The infant develops puffiness, vomiting, oliguria, abdominal pain, dysphagia, aphonia, and even convulsions. These forms are not really distinct, and the signs and symptoms may be present in almost any combination. Case fatality is very high unless treatment is given.

Biochemistry and Pathology. Pyruvic acid tends to accumulate in the tissues in severe thiamin deficiency. Because thiamin pyrophosphate is a coenzyme in the reaction, reduced transketolase activity can be detected in the red blood cells of persons consuming diets low in thiamin. Urinary excretion of thiamin of 0 to 14 μg in 24 hours has been reported in beriberi, and early signs have been observed with excretions of less than 40 μg in 24 hours.

The pathology of thiamin-deficient states ranges from maximal disturbance of function with minimal histologic abnormalities in acute, severe deficiency to minimal biochemical changes and well defined peripheral nerve lesions in chronic deficiency. In fatal cases, hypertrophy of the heart is a constant finding.

Degeneration is found not only in peripheral, but also in cerebrospinal nerves, in terminal branches of the vagus and phrenic nerves, and sometimes in the spinal cord and fibers of the posterior root. In Wernicke's encephalopathy, histologic changes are found chiefly in the mamillary bodies, the related walls of the third ventricle, and the aqueduct and tegmentum of the medulla.

Treatment and Prevention. The treatment of beriberi consists of a balanced diet plus the administration of 5.0 to 10.0 mg of thiamin three times daily. In severe beriberi the thiamin should be given parenterally for the first few days, but oral administration is satisfactory for the treatment of most cases. Delay in the treatment of Wernicke's syndrome may result in cardiac death or in permanent cerebral damage with signs of Korsakoff's syndrome. Because other B vitamin deficiencies are often present in beriberi, a multivitamin preparation is also advisable.

The biochemical lesions are rapidly reversed, but structural defects require long recovery periods. Signs of heart failure disappear within a few days; within a few weeks the heart returns to normal size, and electrocardiographic abnormalities disappear. In longstanding cases of advanced neuropathy, complete restoration to normal may be impossible, although improvement may continue for many months.

Prevention requires an increase in the intake of thiamin for persons consuming rice diets. Parboiling causes the thiamin to pass into the grain so that it is not removed in the milling process. In practice, efforts to encourage parboiling or the use of home-pounded and undermilled rice have not been successful. Enrichment of rice at the mill with thiamin, riboflavin, and niacin has not been adopted by those countries needing it most. A generally improved diet, containing foods which are good sources of thiamin, and extensive distribution of synthetic thiamin are the measures that have been most effective in Asia.

Federation of American Societies for Experimental Biology: Nutritional Disease, Proceedings of a Conference on Beriberi, Endemic Goiter and Hypovitaminosis A, held at Princeton, New Jersey, June 1–5, 1958. Fed. Proc., 17: Part II, Supplement No. 2, September, 1958, pp. 3–56.

Goldsmith, G. A.: The B Vitamins: Thiamine, riboflavin, niacin, *In* Beaton, G. H., and McHenry, E. W. (eds.): A Comprehensive Treatise, Vol. II. New York, Academic Press, 1964, chap. 2, p. 109.

Spillane, J. D.: Nutritional Disorders of the Nervous System. Baltimore, Williams and Wilkins Company, 1947.

Weiss, S., and Wilkins, R. W.: The nature of the cardiovascular disturbances in nutritional deficiency states (beriberi). Ann. Intern. Med., 11:104, 1937.

721. SCURVY

Etiology and Distribution. Most mammals are able to synthesize ascorbic acid from glucose by way of glucuronic acid. Man, the primates, and the guinea pig lack the enzyme required for conversion of gluconate to ascorbate. If dietary intake of ascorbic acid ceases for several months, clinical scurvy develops. Scurvy has most commonly occurred in the spring in temperate climates or at the end of the dry season in tropical ones, because of the relative lack of fresh fruit and vegetables during the preceding months and because several months are required for the disease to become manifest. Although now rare, the disease is still seen in exceptional circumstances, and the treatment is specific and effective. The minimal daily requirement for ascorbic acid is controversial. A group of British volunteers remained in good health and had normal wound healing on a daily intake of 10 mg for almost a year, although plasma and leukocyte ascorbic acid contents were very low. In a notable human experiment by Crandon, under controlled conditions with complete deficiency of the vitamin, the plasma level of ascorbic acid fell to zero by the forty-first day, but abnormal hair and hair follicles appeared only after four months. Perifollicular hemorrhages were not evident until after five months on the experimental diet. Subjective symptoms of a less specific nature—fatigability and anorexia—preceded the appearance of objective signs.

Biochemistry and Pathology. The effect of ascorbic acid on enzymes depends on its properties as either a strong reducing agent or the source of peroxide from its oxidation with air. It is a reactant in such well defined enzyme systems as hydroxylation to form norepinephrine, 5-hydroxylation of tryptophan, tyrosine oxidase, and a number of others. In the oxidation of p-hydroxyphenylpyruvic acid, it protects the enzyme involved from inhibition by its substrate, a necessary function when large amounts of tyrosine are being metabolized. It is also a specific reductant of the ferric ion in its transfer from plasma transferrin to liver ferritin.

It is needed also for the conversion of proline to hydroxyproline and the synthesis of chondroitin sulfate in the ground substance of collagen; hydroxyproline is an amino acid found only in collagen. Ascorbic acid is a necessary component of the mucopolysaccharides of ground substance. In the vitamin's absence, defective ground substance is formed, and can be seen by electron microscopy to have lost its characteristic periodicity. At any rate, scar tissue does not form. Ascorbic acid is involved in the preservation of folinic acid, the reduced form of folic acid. Perhaps this contributes to the occasional macrocytic anemia seen in scurvy by diminishing the amount of folinic acid available. There is no good evidence that ascorbic acid is itself required for erythropoiesis.

The pathologic changes in scurvy are predominantly in the mesenchymal tissues of the body, especially in collagen, growing bones, teeth, and blood vessels. In growing bones the histopathology of scurvy is distinctive: a suppression of the orderly growth process and of the normal calcification of the cartilage matrix. In addition, hemorrhages may be found in the interior of the bone at the cartilage-shaft junction, together with fractures of the minute columns of cartilage matrix and, at times, dislocation, separation, or impaction of the epiphyses.

Subperiosteal hemorrhages are relatively uncommon in the adult but frequent in infantile scurvy. Loosening of the periosteal attachment leads to capillary bleeding, which may dissect the periosteum free over a large area. Most frequently these subperiosteal hemorrhages are found in the lower end of the femur, the upper end of the humerus, both ends of the tibia, and the costochondral junctions of the middle ribs.

Capillaries in the skin become fragile, and petechiae, ecchymoses, and hematomas result. Hemorrhages into the gums lead to swelling, tissue friability, and even gangrene.

The teeth become loose because of resorption of alveolar bone. In children the teeth also show abnormalities of development, with poorly formed matrix and porous dentine.

The laboratory detection of this deficiency or confirmation of the clinical diagnosis of scurvy requires measurement of the plasma or leukocyte concentration of ascorbic acid, or the urinary excretion of the vitamin with or without a "loading" test. With low levels of dietary ascorbic acid intake, plasma ascorbic acid levels fall sharply, but even levels below 0.2 mg may be associated with a wide range of tissue saturations, from 0 to approximately 50 per cent. At this level of nutriture, the white blood cell–platelet ascorbic acid level is most useful. It will average 20 to 30 mg per 100 ml in a well nourished subject, and on an ascorbic acid-free diet will decrease to 0 to 2 mg per 100 ml in three to five months. Clinical scurvy usually appears shortly thereafter.

Clinical Manifestations. Malaise, weakness, and lassitude are early and constant symptoms. Shortness of breath and aching in the bones and joints follow. The most distinctive physical sign and one of the earliest is perifollicular hemorrhage, usually in hyperkeratotic hair follicles, appearing particularly on the posterior thighs, anterior forearms, and abdomen. The hairs become fragmented, coiled, and buried in the follicles.

Petechiae are characteristic features of fully developed scurvy, and are usually most prominent in the same hair-bearing areas and in dependent parts of the body. Scorbutic petechiae are usually larger and more purplish than those in other forms of purpura, for example, in thrombocytopenia. Similarly, a tourniquet produces petechiae that are typically large and dark in color, appearing mostly on the hair-bearing areas of the forearm rather than on the flexor surface usually examined.

As scurvy becomes more advanced, ecchymoses appear, first at areas of irritation, pressure, or trauma. The "saddle area" and posterior thighs are the most frequent locations. Larger hemorrhages occur later in subcutaneous tissue, muscles, or joints, but are uncommon in the viscera, heart, or brain. Gums become swollen, inflamed, and "spongy," bleed easily, and are usually infected. Gum changes are less pronounced in edentulous subjects.

In untreated disease of long duration, postural hypotension and syncope are common. They may be part of the preterminal state in which vomiting and frank hypotension occur, resembling an Addisonian crisis.

Anemia, normocytic or macrocytic, with resultant pallor, is frequent. Two major causes of anemia must be considered. First, and most important, is the blood loss into the skin and deeper tissues or, uncommonly, into the gastrointestinal tract. Second is the possibility that dietary intake of folic acid may also be deficient. Many foods are important sources of both folic acid and ascorbic acid, and the two deficiencies may potentiate one another.

Most cases of scurvy seen in infancy *(Barlow's disease)* develop 6 to 12 months after the institution of artificial feeding. A few examples have been reported in infants considerably younger, but in these instances the mothers habitually subsisted on a diet inadequate in ascorbic acid. The concentration of ascorbic acid in human milk, invariably higher than that in maternal plasma, closely reflects the mother's intake.

Loss of appetite, listlessness, and irritability are early and insidious signs of infantile scurvy. The bony lesions and subperiosteal hemorrhages lead to tenderness, swelling, and evidence of pain on movement. Bleeding into the costochondral junctions of the ribs is noted externally as swellings—the "scorbutic rosary." Purpura and gum changes are similar to those in the adult except that pre-existing gum infection is less common.

Significance of Ascorbic Acid in Clinical Medicine. Although scurvy is now a rare disease, in several important clinical situations the state of ascorbic acid nutrition is a significant consideration. Resistance to infection is reduced in ascorbic acid deficiency, and microbial diseases have long been recognized to precipitate scurvy in individuals on borderline intakes of this vitamin.

Healing of wounds is defective in scurvy because of poor collagen formation. Experimentally deficient subjects fail to form new collagen in experimental wounds until the vitamin is administered. Delayed healing of wounds, postoperative breakdown of incisions, and delayed union of fractures may sometimes be at least partly the result of unrecognized but severe ascorbic acid deficiency. It is also known that extensive trauma and infectious diseases lower the plasma concentration of the vitamin. Ascorbic acid appears to be transported to wounds soon after injury, its concentration rising there as the plasma concentration falls, perhaps because the vitamin is needed for new ground substance and collagen formation.

Patients with thermal burns may develop ascorbic

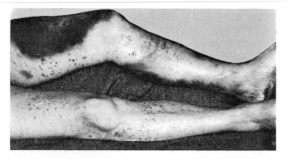

Figure 4. Ecchymoses, petechiae, and perifollicular hemorrhages on legs of patient with scurvy.

acid deficiency, especially when the burns are extensive and deep. Large doses of the vitamin may be necessary to maintain even low-normal plasma concentrations. Such deficiency leads to delayed healing of burns and impaired skin graft "takes."

Attention to nutrient intake, including that of ascorbic acid, is an essential part of the medical care of many illnesses. For example, the diet prescribed for peptic ulcer may be almost free of ascorbic acid, a situation which favors bleeding rather than healing.

Treatment and Prevention. Small amounts of ascorbic acid will promptly reverse the florid clinical manifestations of scurvy. Even in severe scurvy, 100 mg per day for several days, accompanied by a normal diet, usually produces rapid cure. Because retention is high in the deficient state, this is also sufficient to restore the normal 4- to 5-gram body content of the vitamin in a few weeks.

Prevention requires a diet containing adequate ascorbic acid. The vitamin is present in most fresh fruits and vegetables, and in liver. Citrus fruits are particularly good sources. Synthetic ascorbic acid is chemically identical, and is very cheap.

Attention must be paid to the prevention of infantile scurvy, for the disease continues to occur sporadically in the United States in spite of our knowledge of prevention. At least 2 ounces of orange juice or its ascorbic acid equivalent should be given to all infants after the first month.

When extensive wounds, fractures, or chronic infections are treated, supplementary ascorbic acid should be given if any reasonable doubt exists regarding previous nutrition with this vitamin. Patients with deep and extensive burns may require large amounts of ascorbic acid (200 to 500 mg daily) to maintain measurable blood concentrations.

Crandon, J. H., Lund, C. C., and Dill, D. B.: Experimental human scurvy. N. Engl. J. Med., 223:253, 1940.

Gupta, S. D., Chaudhuri, C. R., and Chatterjee, I. B.: Incapability of L-ascorbic acid synthesis by insects. Arch. Biochem. Biophys., 152:889, 1972.

Levenson, S. M., Green, R. W., Taylor, F. H. L., Robinson, P., Page, R. C., Johnson, R. E., and Lund, C. C.: Ascorbic acid, riboflavin, thiamin, and nicotinic acid in relation to severe injury, hemorrhage and infection in the human. Ann. Surg., 124:840, 1946.

Sebrell, W. H., Jr., and Harris, R. S. (eds.): The Vitamins: Chemistry, Physiology, Pathology, Methods. New York, Academic Press, Inc., 1967. (See Chapter 2, Ascorbic Acid, p. 305.)

Woodruff, C. W.: Ascorbic Acid, *In* Beaton, G. H., and McHenry, E. W. (eds.): Nutrition, a Comprehensive Treatise. Vol. 2. New York, Academic Press, Inc., 1964, p. 265.

722. HYPERVITAMINOSIS A AND D

Vitamin A is not normally excreted except during disease states. Therefore, massive doses may lead to increased storage in the liver and hepatomegaly. Toxicity from hypervitaminosis A brought on by eating polar bear liver has been reported since 1596 by Arctic explorers. A 500-gram polar bear liver may contain over nine million IU of vitamin A, more than twenty times the total normal liver reserves in man. Toxic symptoms are drowsiness, irritability, severe headache, and vomiting within a few hours after ingestion. Acute hypervitaminosis A was reported in an infant given a single dose of 300,000 IU. Drowsiness, hydrocephalus with protrusion of the fontanel, and vomiting ensued 12 hours after administration. Hepatosplenomegaly, hypoplastic anemia, leukopenia, precocious skeletal development, clubbing of the fingers, and coarse, sparse hair have been reported from long-continued high doses in children. Most symptoms, but not the hepatomegaly and abnormal bone growth, clear with discontinuation of the vitamin.

Overdosage of any form of vitamin D is dangerous. The syndrome of hypervitaminosis D is characterized by hypercalcemia and by generalized calcinosis (deposition of calcium phosphate in a matrix of mucoproteins) affecting joints, synovial membranes, kidneys, myocardium, pulmonary alveoli, parathyroid glands, pancreas, skin, lymph glands, arteries, conjunctivae and cornea of the eyes, and the acid-secreting portion of the stomach. In advanced stages, demineralization of the bones occurs.

The exact borderline between tolerable and noxious doses is not known. Certainly the continuous ingestion of 150,000 IU per day may result in symptoms. It is possible that some infants may show hypercalcemia on relatively small doses of 2500 to 4000 IU per day. Retardation of linear growth in children has been reported with 1800 IU per day. Complete recovery usually occurs when vitamin D is temporarily withdrawn. Treatment should include lowering of the calcium intake and a generous fluid intake.

Dam, H., and Søndergaard, E.: Fat-soluble vitamins. *In* Beaton, G. H., and McHenry, E. W. (eds.): Nutrition, A Comprehensive Treatise. Vol. II. New York, Academic Press, 1964, pp. 34–35.

Sebrell, W. H., Jr., and Harris, R. S. (eds.): The Vitamins: Chemistry, Physiology, Pathology, Methods. Vol. I. 2nd ed. New York and London, Academic Press, 1967.

Stimson, W. H.: Vitamin A intoxication in adults. Report of a case with summary of the literature. N. Engl. J. Med., 265:369, 1961.

723. OBESITY

Margaret J. Albrink

The differentiation of adipose tissue was a triumph of evolution. Phylogenetically the ability to store fat in true adipose tissue appeared first in the arthropods and became fully developed in birds and mammals; it was very likely an important factor in the liberation of life from the sea with its constant source of food. However, the ability to store fat in compact form, of great survival value when food was scarce, has become a handicap in affluent societies where overnutrition and underactivity have upset the ancient balance between caloric supply and demand. The consequence is obesity of epidemic proportions and the associated diseases of atherosclerosis, hypertension, and diabetes.

Definition. Obesity may be defined as excess adipose tissue. The dividing point between normal and excessive may be determined esthetically as fatness beyond the socially acceptable norms, or medically as adipose tissue in excess of that consistent with good health of mind and body. The latter definition includes the mild to moderate obesity characteristic of a large segment of our population, of paramount public health significance because of the associated toll of cardiovascular and other diseases.

Incidence. The exact incidence is uncertain because of difficulty in measuring degree of obesity. When compared to their desirable weight, 30 per cent of men and 40 per cent of women are 20 pounds or more overweight.

Etiology. Obesity results from the relative excess of caloric intake over caloric expenditure. Most cases of obesity seen in common clinical practice are due to the interaction of cultural forces that encourage excess intake with genetic factors that, other things being equal, favor the synthesis of fat.

Cultural Factors. First the agricultural, then the industrial, and finally the computer revolution have all served to make food increasingly available and life livable with a minimum of physical exertion. An important cause of widespread moderate obesity in the United States is the plethora of purified foods of high caloric content but low nutrient value.

Genetic Factors. Obesity, especially in its extreme form, tends to be familial. Obesity in children is much more common when both parents are obese than when neither parent is obese. Anabolic forces appear to be in operation from birth in very heavy people. (See below: Central Nervous System Regulation.) Heavy children usually become heavy adults, and differ constitutionally from lean persons in being statistically of shorter stature and greater breadth of trunk and in having small hands and feet. The localization of extreme deposits of fat, such as the massive adipose tissue over the buttocks of certain Bushmen, the so-called "Hottentot bustle," is an instance of genetically determined localized adiposity. This extreme example suggests that the number of adipose cells may be in part genetically determined and that the number and location of such cells or their precursors will determine in part the magnitude as well as the location of obesity.

Endocrine Factors. Many endocrine and metabolic abnormalities have been reported in very obese persons. Most are probably secondary to obesity (see below: Complications).

Sex. Women have a greater amount of subcutaneous fat than men. The relationship between parity and obesity and the frequent menopausal gain in weight, although difficult to document, suggest a possible role of female sex hormones in the regulation of fat metabolism. Administration of estrogens in rather high doses such as are present in birth control pills may cause obesity. The obesity of eunuchs suggests further that absence of male sex hormones also promotes adiposity. The hypogonad obesity that occurs in children just prior to adolescence disappears with puberty, at which time the adult fat distribution of each sex takes place. The effect of sex hormones could be explained by emotional factors and physical activity rather than by a direct effect on fat metabolism.

Age. The tendency to gain weight with advancing age is associated with increased mortality from cardiovascular and other diseases, and cannot be considered normal.

Central Nervous System Regulation of Food Intake. The role of the central nervous system in controlling food intake resides chiefly in the hypothalamus. A satiety center in the ventral medial hypothalamus exerts an inhibitory influence on a neighboring feeding center. Destruction of the inhibitory center releases the feeding center, with resultant massive overeating and hypothalamic obesity. Brain injury in man on occasion causes obesity, but the extent to which variation in the balance between these centers contributes to ordinary obesity is unknown. Very early overfeeding may "set" the regulatory centers in such a manner that obesity, manifest by an irreversibly increased number of adipose cells, persists in later life.

Behavioral and Emotional Aspects. Decreased activity rather than increased food intake is recognized in many obese persons, particularly obese women. Associated depression is a frequent concomitant of inactivity, and may be exaggerated by weight loss. The very obese person has a characteristic eating pattern in which the major caloric intake occurs at the evening meal or later.

Some distinctive behavioral traits have been described in obese persons, although whether they are causes or effects is uncertain. Unlike slender persons, the obese seem to depend on external rather than internal cues to initiate feeding. They eat in response to clock time, to the attractiveness and availability of food, and to other external cues rather than to internal signals of hunger and satiety. Correspondingly there is an inability to recognize and cope with inner needs and feelings. Behavior such as eating that should be dictated from inner needs is attached, rather, to external cues. Such lack of self-direction could result from lack of early life experiences which normally encourage development of ego identity. Another interpretation of dependence on external cues is that the obese are inwardly always hungry but outwardly always trying to exhibit socially acceptable behavior.

Like most of man's ills at one time or another, obesity has been blamed on the world's domineering mothers. The role of mothers in causing obesity in children can as well be attributed to their enforcement in early life of patterns of overeating as to the psychologic effects of overprotection.

Pathology. Two general types of distribution of obesity are described. Obesity in the male is most pronounced in the upper trunk and spares the extremities. In the female, distribution is predominantly in the lower trunk and involves also the extremities, particularly the lower extremities.

Excess adipose tissue is found subcutaneously, interspersed in muscle and about all organs. Extremely obese persons have generally enlarged organs; cardiac enlargement is mainly left ventricular, and may be due to the increased circulating blood volume and/or hypertension commonly present. The kidney, liver, and, indeed, the entire splanchnic area are of greater size than normal. Large fatty livers are frequently found in extreme obesity.

Cellularity. Hirsch, Salans, and Knittle and their colleagues, using a new method for estimating adipose cell size and number from adipose tissue sampled by needle biopsy, have studied the cellularity of adipose tissue. In man and in several other species the number of adipose cells increases until the onset of adult life. Thereafter the adipose mass is expanded only by increasing the size of existing cells. In man, probably no new adipose cells are laid down after age 20, although methodologic variability prevents exclusion of possible later addition of cells. Two periods of rapid adipose cell number expansion have been identified: very early in the first few years, and again between ages 9 and 13.

Two groups of obese persons can be identified: those with normal numbers of cells but increased cell size (hyperplastic) and those with increased numbers of cells which might or might not also be enlarged (hypercellular). The two types can best be separated by age of onset. Obesity of onset early in life is associated with increased numbers of adipose cells, whereas adult onset obesity is associated with normal cell number but increased size of cell. Extreme obesity is usually of the juvenile onset hypercellular type.

Sims and colleagues confirmed the hyperplastic nature of obesity of the adult onset type. Lean volunteers who purposely gain weight expand their existing adipose cells but do not add any new adipose cells. By the same token, weight loss in the obese is accomplished by shrinkage of existing adipose cells, not by loss of cells. Once laid down, the number of cells is immutable.

Hirsch et al. found behavioral differences between "adult onset" and "juvenile onset" diabetes. The lifelong hypercellular obese experience depression, fatigue, anxiety, and distortion in timing perception and body image during weight reduction. On both theoretic and practical grounds, therefore, weight reduction might seem more practical in adult onset obesity, where weight reduction and cell shrinkage should restore normal adipose cell size and number, than in the hypercellular obese, in whom no amount of dieting will reduce the number of adipose cells.

The cellularity of adipose tissue varies greatly from site to site so that information obtained by biopsy is of more statistical than diagnostic value in a single individual. There is some evidence that hypercellular obesity is distributed both on the trunk and on the extremities, whereas acquired hypertrophic obesity is more confined to the trunk. The finding of an obese trunk with thin arms and legs would thus suggest acquired obesity.

Pathogenesis. The balance between fat synthesis and fat mobilization depends on several key reactions in the adipose cell and the influence of various hormones, as well as state of nutrition, on these reactions. A shift in the adipose cell toward increased synthesis of fat or decreased mobilization of fat would operate to cause obesity.

Synthesis of Triglyceride. Triglycerides are synthesized within the adipose cell from one alpha-glycerol-phosphate molecule and three fatty acid molecules. The latter may be synthesized within the adipose cell from glucose, a reaction favored by reduced nicotinamide adenine dinucleotide phosphate (NADPH) (reduced triphosphopyridine nucleotide), or may be derived from circulating fatty acids of dietary or endogenous origin. By contrast, the alpha-glycerol-phosphate must be derived from glucose metabolized within the adipose cell. The glycerol liberated from triglyceride breakdown cannot serve this purpose since adipose tissue lacks appreciable glycerol kinase, the enzyme necessary for converting glycerol into alpha-glycerol-phosphate. The availability of glucose thus determines the availability of alpha-glycerol-phosphate, which in turn is obligatory for triglyceride synthesis in adipose tissue.

Circulating triglycerides such as those present in chylomicrons are evidently available to the adipose cell only if they are first broken down into glycerol and free fatty acids, a reaction taking place at or near the adipose cell wall under the influence of the enzyme lipoprotein lipase. This enzyme is increased in the carbohydrate-fed state, decreased in starvation. Since the enzyme appears in the circulation after heparin injection, it is also called post-heparin lipoprotein lipase. The free fatty acids liberated by the action of lipoprotein lipase enter the adipose cell, where they are re-esterified into triglyceride, provided alpha-glycerol-phosphate is present.

The latter must be derived from carbohydrate combustion. Carbohydrate combustion has the additional effect of generating NADPH via the pentose phosphate shunt, and NADPH favors the synthesis of fat from two-carbon precursors.

Insulin occupies a central role in the regulation of adipose cell metabolism. High insulin concentration inhibits lipolysis and favors fat synthesis. When insulin concentration is low, fat synthesis ceases and lipolysis proceeds. Insulin acts by stimulating the lipogenic actions of glucose metabolism noted above. In addition, insulin directly inhibits lipolysis.

In man and certain other species, the liver is an important site for new triglyceride synthesis. The triglycerides are packaged as very low density lipoproteins (VLDL) and secreted into the bloodstream. The VLDL triglyceride, just as with chylomicron triglyceride, is taken up by adipose tissue for storage under the influence of lipoprotein lipase when metabolic factors favor fat synthesis, that is, when carbohydrate metabolism is active and insulin is available.

Fat Mobilization. Fat is mobilized entirely in the form of free fatty acids. The release of fat from the adipose cell is accomplished by activation of an intracellular lipolytic system different from lipoprotein lipase. The activation is dependent upon generation of cyclic adenosine monophosphate (cyclic AMP). This system splits triglycerides into free fatty acids and glycerol. The liberated free fatty acids are either re-esterified into triglyceride, provided conditions favor fat synthesis, or are transported into the circulation bound to albumin as free fatty acids, either to be utilized by tissue or transported to the liver for re-esterification into triglyceride. A rise in concentration of circulating free fatty acids is evidence of fat mobilization.

Fat mobilization is favored by various hormones that activate the lytic system, of which epinephrine, norepinephrine, and growth hormone are probably of the greatest physiologic significance. Factors that stimulate epinephrine secretion such as exercise and trauma thus activate mobilization of fat. The absence of carbohydrate combustion as in starvation or diabetic acidosis also results in fat mobilization. Low concentration of circulating insulin characterizes both situations. The removal of the suppressing effect of insulin on lipolysis permits lipolysis to proceed. Alpha-glycerol-phosphate ceases to be synthesized from glucose in amounts sufficient for re-esterification of all the liberated fatty acids, and net loss of triglyceride from adipose tissue takes place. Through these systems the deposition or mobilization of fat is regulated by the presence or absence of food, especially carbohydrate, and by the presence or absence of emergencies that require fat as fuel for sudden bursts of energy.

Adipose Cell Metabolism in Obesity. Certain aspects of adipose tissue metabolism of obese persons are referable to the increased cell size of adult onset obesity. Hirsch and Salans and their colleagues have reported that the well known insulin resistance of obese persons is related to the oversized adipocytes and that normal insulin responsiveness is restored by weight loss and resulting cell size reduction. The large adipocyte is characterized by insensitivity to the stimulating effect of insulin on glucose oxidation and on synthesis of fatty acids from glucose and by increased basal and epinephrine-stimulated lipolysis. Similar abnormalities are found in the expanded adipocytes of lean individuals who have undergone forced weight gain. The abnormal findings are reversed by weight loss.

The decreased antilipolytic and lipogenic effect of insulin in large adipose cells has been proposed as a possible cause for the insulin resistance of the obese. Several theories have been advanced to account for the lack of insulin responsiveness. A lack of insulin binding sites on adipose cells or a defect in some aspect of intracellular glucose metabolism has been proposed, but no specific metabolic locus has been identified with certainty.

Prior diet exerts an important influence on adipose cell metabolism. The insulin insensitivity of both spontaneous and forced obesity can be overcome if sufficient carbohydrate is fed prior to biopsy. The large adipose cell thus appears to require more carbohydrate calories to maintain triglyceride storage than does the small adipose cell.

Several arguments can be made against the existence of a primary deficit in insulin responsiveness specific to large adipose cells. Similar insulin resistance is demonstrable in many, perhaps all, tissues of obese persons. The insulin resistance can be induced by forced weight gain and can be reversed by weight loss, and is therefore secondary. The resistance may, rather, be caused by a general lipolytic state which can be overcome by sufficient carbohydrate calories. The lipolytic state, in turn, perhaps through the known anti-insulin effects of increased intracellular free fatty acids, could be responsible for the insulin resistance at the tissue level. That increased lipolytic tendency and obesity coexist must mean that the weight-stable or weight-gaining obese person eats more than enough to overcome the lipolytic state.

Lipolysis is an adrenergic function. Its regulation and its modulation by nutrient intake may be controlled by the central nervous system, probably through certain hypothalamic centers. Such centers may also control the level of nutrient intake necessary to reverse the lipolytic state and may control the feeding behavior needed to ensure such intake. The observed lipolytic tendency of large adipocytes may merely reflect recent caloric deprivation relative to the requirements of the hypothalamic "set" for that individual. The nature of such a "set" if it exists, the signals to which it responds, and its potential for change are uncertain.

Manifestations and Complications. The sheer mechanical trauma of excessive body weight either aggravates or causes such troublesome ailments as osteoarthritis and flat feet, intertriginous dermatitis, varicose veins, and ventral and diaphragmatic hernias. Cholelithiasis and cholecystitis are more common in the obese than in the lean.

Obesity-Hypoventilation Syndrome. Dickens' graphic description of Fat Joe, a character in *Pickwick Papers* who fell asleep at the most inopportune moments, led to the eponym *pickwickian syndrome.* This condition, which appears in some very obese persons, is characterized by hypoventilation, somnolence, and carbon dioxide retention (Pco$_2$ values consistently elevated above 48 mm of mercury). Decreased compliance of the thoracic wall and consequent increased work of respiration are thus evidently penalties of extreme obesity. Failure to make the necessary increased respiratory effort to move the ponderous thoracic wall initiates the syndrome. Ventilation-perfusion disturbances also occur. Possible underlying pulmonary disease may be a factor in some pa-

tients. Hypoxia, pulmonary hypertension, secondary polycythemia, and, eventually, cardiopulmonary failure ensue. All symptoms are improved by weight loss.

Hemodynamic Complications. Very obese persons have a greater than normal total circulating blood volume and increased cardiac output, stroke volume, and cardiac work, probably because of the additional vascular bed of the excess adipose tissue. The blood volume per unit weight of adipose tissue, however, is less than that for lean tissue, with the result that the circulating blood volume per kilogram of body weight is less than for a lean person.

Hypertension. Studies around the world show a correlation between blood pressure and obesity. To a large extent the increased death rate of obese persons is due to hypertension. Increased stroke volume, a consequence of the increased cardiac output in the presence usually of a normal heart rate, may be in part responsible for the hypertension and left ventricular hypertrophy in obese persons. Peripheral resistance is normal or low. The hypertension and hemodynamic abnormalities are improved by weight loss.

Endocrine Complications. Sims and his colleagues, in studies of experimental obesity in man, have compared the metabolic abnormalities found in spontaneous obesity with those induced in normal subjects by forced overeating. Most of the abnormalities found in spontaneous obesity could be induced in the volunteers, and were reversed by weight loss in both spontaneous obesity and induced obesity. The abnormalities are therefore probably the result rather than the cause of the obesity. The picture in intact obese man, as in the large adipose cell, is that of decreased sensitivity to insulin. Increased concentrations of plasma glucose, amino acids, and insulin are the result. Since the induced obesity was achieved entirely by increasing cell size rather than number, the metabolic abnormalities were associated with adipose cell hypertrophy. The only metabolic difference between spontaneous and induced obesity was the greater number of calories required to maintain weight in induced obesity. The plasma free fatty acid concentration in induced obesity was found to be low, secondary to the high carbohydrate diet needed for weight gain. Free fatty acid concentration is elevated in spontaneous obesity only when there is associated diabetes, free fatty acids being normal in nondiabetic obese.

HYPERINSULINEMIA. Elevation of plasma insulin is a striking feature of obese nondiabetics. Fasting plasma insulin concentrations of 30 μU per milliliter or higher and postcibal concentrations in excess of 300 μU per milliliter are not uncommon in nondiabetic obese. In contrast, fasting and postcibal values for lean persons are usually well below 20 μU per milliliter and 150 μU per milliliter, respectively.

The insulin increase after a glucose challenge in the obese, when expressed relative to the basal insulin concentration, is appropriate for the degree of hyperglycemia. The basal insulin, however, is inappropriately high for the degree of fasting glycemia in obese persons. The increase in fasting insulin is thus the critical difference between thin and obese persons.

According to Felig and colleagues, the explanation for the elevated basal insulin may be the high fasting concentrations of those amino acids which stimulate the release of insulin and which are decreased in response to insulin. Insensitivity of the tissue to insulin accounts for the increase in insulin-sensitive substrates, such as certain amino acids as well as glucose and probably others. The fact of insulin insensitivity is communicated to the pancreas by increased concentrations of such substrates, but the resulting increased insulin concentration is less effective in restoring substrate levels to normal than is a similar concentration of insulin in slender persons. The reason for the insulin insensitivity of the obese is not known. In the case of obese adipose tissue, insulin insensitivity is related to increased cell size (see above). With weight reduction cell size returns to normal, and insulin sensitivity is restored.

THYROID FUNCTION IN OBESITY. Although the usual parameters of thyroid function are normal in obesity, Bray has reported an abnormality in the adipose tissue of obese persons which is corrected by administration of triiodothyronine. The defect is a deficiency in the mitochondrial oxidation of glycerol phosphate. Since this reaction may favor energy wastage and thus prevent weight gain in overfed persons, such a deficiency might cause obesity. However, in later studies similar deficiency was induced by forced weight gain in normal volunteers. Bray has also found an increase in the concentration of circulating triiodothyronine. The increase is probably secondary to tissue resistance to the action of triiodothyronine. Thus the demonstrated abnormalities in thyroid metabolism are the result of obesity, not the cause.

GROWTH HORMONE IN OBESITY. Several hormones of the anterior pituitary cause mobilization of fat from adipose tissue. The most important is growth hormone, which promotes mobilization and utilization of fat and conservation of protein and carbohydrate during caloric restriction. Growth hormone is secreted in response to hypoglycemia, hyperaminoacidemia, exercise, and other stimuli, and is spontaneously secreted during deep sleep. In both spontaneous and induced obesity the growth hormone response to hypoglycemia and to arginine infusion is reduced, as is the nocturnal rise. The normal increase in growth hormone in response to starvation is less marked in obese than in nonobese subjects. Obese persons respond to prolonged fasting with a less than normal rise in free fatty acids, a phenomenon probably reflecting the decreased secretion of growth hormone. The growth hormone hyposecretion is secondary to the obesity and is corrected by weight loss.

ADRENOCORTICAL FUNCTION IN OBESITY. Increased plasma cortisol concentration may occur in obesity. Increased cortisol secretory rate reported in spontaneous and induced obesity is related merely to increased body mass. The abnormalities are secondary to the obesity.

Diabetes. Diabetes is four times more common in obese than in lean adults, and with its toll of vascular disease accounts for some of the risk of obesity. The hyperinsulinemia of the obese may be a contributing factor to their increased susceptibility to diabetes. Over many years such increased insulin production may lead to pancreatic exhaustion and diabetes, accounting for the association between obesity and diabetes. When diabetes coincides with obesity, the rise of plasma insulin relative to plasma glucose after glucose ingestion is blunted, as in nonobese diabetics. The insulin increments, being superimposed on the increased basal levels, result in higher insulin values for each degree of glucose tolerance in the obese than in the nonobese. Weight loss greatly relieves the burden on the pancreas by decreasing both the basal and postcibal needs for insulin, with the result that glucose tolerance may become normal.

Atherosclerosis. The influence of obesity on atherosclerotic vascular disease and on serum lipids is discussed later in this chapter.

Diagnosis. Simple precise methods for measuring degree of obesity are lacking. The amount of body fat can be estimated from whole-body specific gravity or from the thickness of subcutaneous fat measured by skin-fold calipers or roentgenographically. The contribution of lean body mass to the total body mass can also be determined from whole-body radioactive potassium and the fat body mass indirectly calculated. The discussion of assessment of nutritional status (see Ch. 713) contains further information on methods for evaluating nutritional state.

The most commonly used method, however, remains the height-weight tables. In Table 1 may be seen the ranges of desirable weight, i.e., weight associated with lowest mortality according to insurance company data obtained from large numbers of policyholders. Desirable weight approximates that at age 25; this stresses the fact that weight gain during adult life is associated with increased mortality.

If a person weighs more than the upper limit of his ideal weight for his frame, he may be considered overweight, and if he is 20 pounds in excess of his ideal weight he is generally considered obese. Degree of obesity is often denoted as relative weight, the actual weight expressed as a percentage of desirable weight.

TABLE 1. Desirable Weights for Men and Women According to Height and Frame, Ages 25 and Over*

Height (in Shoes)†	Weight in Pounds (in Indoor Clothing)		
	Small Frame	Medium Frame	Large Frame
Men			
5 ft 2 in	112–120	118–129	126–141
5 ft 3 in	115–123	121–133	129–144
5 ft 4 in	118–126	124–136	132–148
5 ft 5 in	121–129	127–139	135–152
5 ft 6 in	124–133	130–143	138–156
5 ft 7 in	128–137	134–147	142–161
5 ft 8 in	132–141	138–152	147–166
5 ft 9 in	136–145	142–156	151–170
5 ft 10 in	140–150	146–160	155–174
5 ft 11 in	144–154	150–165	159–179
6 ft 0 in	148–158	154–170	164–184
6 ft 1 in	152–162	158–175	168–189
6 ft 2 in	156–167	162–180	173–194
6 ft 3 in	160–171	167–185	177–199
6 ft 4 in	164–175	172–190	182–204
Women			
4 ft 10 in	92–98	96–107	104–119
4 ft 11 in	94–101	98–110	106–122
5 ft 0 in	96–104	101–113	109–124
5 ft 1 in	99–107	104–116	112–128
5 ft 2 in	102–110	107–119	115–131
5 ft 3 in	105–113	110–122	118–134
5 ft 4 in	108–116	113–126	121–138
5 ft 5 in	111–119	116–130	125–142
5 ft 6 in	114–123	120–135	129–146
5 ft 7 in	118–127	124–139	133–150
5 ft 8 in	122–131	128–143	137–154
5 ft 9 in	126–135	132–147	141–158
5 ft 10 in	130–140	136–151	145–163
5 ft 11 in	134–144	140–155	149–168
6 ft 0 in	138–148	144–159	153–174

*Prepared by the Metropolitan Life Insurance Company. Derived primarily from data of the Build and Blood Pressure Study, 1959.
†1 inch heels for men and 2 inch heels for women.

Several height-weight indices are commonly used to express obesity, but, like other measures based on height and weight, actually measure body bulk rather than obesity. Of these indices the ponderal index, height/$\sqrt[3]{weight}$, and the body mass index, weight/height² × 100, are best, the latter being most independent of height.

The chief drawback of height-weight indices is their failure to take into account the variable contributions of lean and fat body mass to total body weight. The measurement of subcutaneous fat with skin-fold calipers avoids this difficulty. Skin-fold thickness, preferably measured at several sites, correlates rather well with total body fat estimated from specific gravity, and has the advantage of ease and simplicity of measurement. Special calipers have been designed for the purpose. The results of the community-wide study of Tecumseh, Michigan, although not necessarily representative of the world, provide guide lines for comparison of individual readings (Table 2). Ideal standards for skin-fold thickness are not yet available. As with weight, mean subscapular skin-fold thickness at age 25 (12.4 mm.) might be considered desirable.

Differential Diagnosis. *Hypothyroidism.* The weight gain in hypothyroidism is usually only moderate, and is due in part to accumulation of myxedematous fluid as well as to adipose tissue. The reduction in caloric expenditure contributes to the obesity. The usual measurements of thyroid function such as serum thyroxine concentration and I¹³¹ uptake are normal in ordinary obesity, and thus can be used to exclude hypothyroidism as a contributing cause of obesity. Hypothyroidism is rarely the cause of obesity.

Cushing's Disease. Hyperadrenocorticism causes moderate obesity that chiefly involves the face, causing the typical moon facies, the thorax, and abdomen, but spares the buttocks and extremities. The fat pad over the last cervical vertebra, the so-called buffalo hump, is characteristic, but may also occur in ordinary obesity, for example, the "dowager's hump" of the postmenopausal woman.

The presence of purple striae of the skin of the abdomen and elsewhere suggests Cushing's disease. However, striae are common in persons who gain weight rapidly. Obese adolescents frequently have striae of the upper arms, breasts, abdomen, hips, and thighs, although adrenal function is normal.

The differentiation of obesity with and without Cushing's disease may present difficulties because of the frequency with which the results of tests used to diagnose Cushing's disease are slightly abnormal in obesity. Elevated urinary 17-ketosteroids and 17-hydroxycorticosteroids as well as increased rate of cortisol secretion are common in obesity. The two most helpful tests for excluding Cushing's disease in obese patients are the diurnal variation in plasma cortisol conentration (usually lost in Cushing's disease but preserved in obesity) and the dexamethasone suppression test. Suppression is normal in the obese but impaired in Cushing's disease.

Stein-Leventhal Syndrome. In a woman, obesity, hirsutism, and infertility suggest this syndrome. The finding of large cystic ovaries on physical examination is confirmatory, although surgical exploration may be necessary for verification. Tests of adrenal cortical function are normal as a rule.

Insulinoma, Hyperinsulinism. The carbohydrate feeding necessary to counteract frequent hypoglycemic attacks may lead to obesity.

Treatment of Obesity. *General Considerations.* Reduction of excess weight in obese persons is associated with improvement in hypertension, in the hemodynamic abnormalities, and in diabetes, as well as with amelioration of the mechanical effects of the adipose mass. Weight reduction is highly desirable for a large segment of our population yet it is singularly difficult to achieve.

There is no satisfactory treatment for obesity. Once established, it is remarkably self-sustaining. Even if weight is temporarily lost, the former weight is regained with astonishing regularity—within months as a rule, within five years almost certainly. A patient who has successfully lost weight must be prepared for a lifetime of vigilance if he is to maintain his success. Nonetheless, the benefits to be expected from weight loss justify the utmost effort on the part of both physician and patient to bring about and maintain optimal weight. If successful, such measures correct or improve the hypertension, the diabetes, and the abnormal serum lipids associated with excess calories, and relieve the mechanical injuries resulting from the increased adipose mass.

Of the three main approaches to obesity—drugs, diet, and exercise—diet is the mainstay of treatment. An understanding of the physiologic changes that accompany caloric restriction is essential if the patient's progress is to be understood. Under dietary treatment, the outlook for the extremely obese patient who has as much as a hundred pounds or more to lose is dismal. Perhaps the most hopeful outlook can be expected for the slightly obese patient who has only a few pounds to lose. Because

TABLE 2. Subscapular and Triceps Skinfold by Age and Sex (Values in Millimeters)*

	Age (Yr)	Male Subjects, Percentiles			Female Subjects, Percentiles		
		20	50	80	20	50	80
Subscapular	20–24	8.0	12.1	19.2	8.6	13.2	21.7
	25–29	8.8	12.4	20.9	9.1	13.2	20.4
	30–34	9.1	15.1	24.3	9.0	13.6	21.2
	35–39	8.9	14.7	21.4	9.7	16.9	24.8
	40–44	10.9	16.3	23.5	11.4	17.6	28.2
	45–49	11.0	17.3	25.9	13.0	20.8	29.1
	50–54	9.9	17.3	24.6	13.4	21.0	33.2
	55–59	11.8	18.8	30.7	13.5	22.3	32.0
	60–64	9.3	16.8	24.8	15.5	22.4	33.6
	65–69	8.0	12.5	17.4	13.0	20.9	30.0
	70–74	8.7	14.3	23.1	14.0	22.6	29.9
	75–79	9.9	14.8	20.8	10.0	21.6	31.2
Triceps	20–24	7.2	11.0	17.8	12.5	17.5	23.4
	25–29	7.1	10.4	16.7	12.1	17.5	23.8
	30–34	7.9	12.3	17.8	13.0	18.1	25.0
	35–39	7.4	11.8	17.3	14.1	20.0	26.0
	40–44	8.0	12.4	17.6	15.2	20.7	27.3
	45–49	8.6	12.5	17.3	16.3	22.1	27.7
	50–54	8.7	12.0	18.7	18.1	22.7	26.9
	55–59	9.9	14.0	18.7	17.3	22.9	28.8
	60–64	8.6	11.7	17.8	18.3	24.7	31.5
	65–69	7.1	10.9	15.4	17.2	21.8	26.6
	70–74	8.1	11.8	15.3	16.0	21.2	26.0
	75–79	7.4	13.5	17.2	12.2	20.0	26.0

*From Montoye, H. J., Epstein, F. H., and Kjelsberg, M. O.: Am. J. Clin. Nutr., 16:417, 1965.

such patients account for the great majority of cardiovascular disease victims in this country, every effort should be made to reach them and to achieve weight reduction.

Diet. EFFECT OF CALORIC RESTRICTION. The seemingly simple and logical limitation of calories below caloric expenditure is often made difficult by the metabolic changes that occur in response to caloric restriction. After initial satisfactory weight loss of one to two or more pounds a week, a plateau is reached. The patient claims continued adherence to the diet, yet no further weight is lost. He finally yields to discouragement, abandons the diet altogether, and gains back all of the lost weight or even more.

One reason for this failure is that too much is expected of caloric restriction. Of the tissue lost, fat and protein tissue differ in their caloric density. Pure fat yields 9 calories per gram. Adipose tissue, consisting mainly of fat with little water, contains about 8 calories per gram of tissue. Protein, on the other hand, gives 4 calories per gram of protein, and carries with it about three or four times its weight in intracellular water. Protein tissue thus gives only about 0.8 calorie per gram, one tenth that of adipose tissue on a weight basis. If, for instance, a caloric deficit of 500 calories were derived only from protein tissue, it could be calculated that 620 grams of protein and water or more than a pound a day would be lost. If only fat tissue were lost, a mere 62-gram tissue loss a day, chiefly fat, would account for the 500 calories.

Actually a mixture of protein and fat tissue is lost. Some nitrogen loss is acceptable since the excess tissue of obese persons contains 10 to 30 grams of nitrogen per kilogram of excess weight. The tendency for negative nitrogen balance in the early days of caloric restriction favors loss largely of protein tissue and thus large weight loss. However, particularly in the very obese, with continued caloric restriction the body reacts by defense of its nitrogen reserves, and the nitrogen balance becomes less negative. If nitrogen balance is established, weight loss then results only from loss of adipose tissue, and occurs very slowly. The nitrogen-conserving defense is so great that positive nitrogen balance can occur on the same diet that initially caused nitrogen loss. Conceivably, protein synthesis taking place concomitantly with loss of calories from adipose tissue could create new protein-rich tissue that would more than equal in weight the adipose tissue lost, with resulting net weight gain despite continued caloric deficit. How long this state of affairs could last is not known, but the tendency toward positive nitrogen balance when undernourished persons are refed full diets may last for months.

The adaptation to caloric restriction includes a strong anabolic tendency that may be manifest not only as nitrogen retention but also as increased synthesis of fat from available carbohydrate. Adaptive hyperlipogenesis in laboratory animals is the greatly augmented synthesis of fat from carbohydrate on refeeding after a period of starvation. If this phenomenon occurs in humans, it would account further for the tendency to regain lost weight.

Not only do the logistics of weight loss from protein and fat tissue favor plateau and even weight gain in obese persons undergoing caloric restriction, but the tendency of such patients to retain sodium and extracellular water is further reason for weight gain. The resultant edema may be refractory to thiazide diuretics or salt restriction. The likelihood of depression, decreased activity, hunger, decreased metabolic rate, and weakness all

operate against the successful continuation of a calorically restricted diet.

SPECIFIC DIETS. Conservative nutritionists recommend a balanced diet, including 1 gram of protein per kilogram of ideal body weight and fat roughly equal in weight to the protein, the remainder of the calories to be made up from carbohydrate. From 800 to 1800 calories are commonly recommended, depending on activity, size, and desired speed of weight loss. However, the few available long-term studies show discouraging results on all diets. There is no basis for recommending any one diet over any other.

UNBALANCED DIETS. A variety of unbalanced diets have been proposed. Because they stimulate the patient's imagination, so-called "fad" diets, though the despair of dietitians, may elicit greater patient cooperation than conservative diets.

Two possibilities which might justify the various unbalanced diets are better patient acceptance or greater caloric loss for a given level of caloric intake. Some experimental evidence exists for both possibilities. Dietary imbalance of nutrients such as amino acids fed to laboratory animals may be recognized by the central nervous system and may lead to spontaneous decrease in food intake. Similar mechanisms interpreted as unpalatability or anorexia may limit intake of unbalanced diet in man and might facilitate adherence.

The second rationale, that certain foodstuffs are less efficiently used than others, has received some support from experiments in man and animals. The old concept of "luxuskonsumption," or the ability to maintain stable weight despite varying caloric intake, has been the subject of renewed interest and has been reviewed by Sims et al. Implicit in the concept is the assumption that calories fed in excess of those needed are less efficiently utilized and are in part lost as heat, with the result that less weight is gained than expected. The energy wastage of excess calories is explained in part by the greater number of energy-requiring metabolic steps required when fuel must first be converted to its storage forms than when it is utilized directly. The energy wastage of a high protein diet is well known and is attributed in part to the energy required for conversion of excess nitrogen to urea and its subsequent excretion by the kidneys. In hypocaloric diets the efficiency of protein, fat, and carbohydrate utilization is increased. This, together with a well-known decrease in metabolic rate with caloric deprivation, tends to minimize weight loss on weight reduction diets. Whether any particular hypocaloric diet will cause more rapid weight loss has not been demonstrated.

LOW PROTEIN DIET. On the assumption that a certain amount of excess tissue is nitrogen, and that the tendency of obese patients to retain nitrogen may defeat efforts at weight loss, some argument may be made for a low protein diet. The dangers of severe protein deficiency, especially liver disease, must be remembered. The classic concept that 1 gram of nitrogen per kilogram per day is needed for nitrogen balance has been revised downward by the World Health Organization to about 0.5 gram of nitrogen per kilogram per day.

LOW CARBOHYDRATE DIET. On theoretical grounds a low carbohydrate diet should be effective by discouraging lipogenesis and preventing reactive hypoglycemia with its attendant hunger. As noted under pathogenesis, dietary carbohydrate favors lipogenesis at several steps. It is also required for the manifestation of salt and water retention so commonly encountered during weight reduction. Limitation of carbohydrate to 50 or 60 grams a day but with *ad libitum* intake of protein and fat causes initial rapid weight loss (largely water), mild ketosis, and absence of hunger, and is usually well tolerated. Total calories are voluntarily limited to 1300 or so because of reduced palatability of fat without carbohydrate. More extreme, nearly total carbohydrate restriction may cause hypercholesterolemia. The safety of associated prolonged ketonemia and ketonuria has not been established. The complications of total carbohydrate restriction are similar to those of total starvation noted below.

STARVATION. The treatment of obesity by total starvation is usually well tolerated for repeated periods of 10 to 15 days each, sometimes much longer, and causes an average weight loss of a pound a day. Marked persistent ketosis occurs, but less than 100 calories a day are lost as ketones. Complications include decreased uric acid excretion, and hyperuricemia, sometimes manifested as clinical gout. Postural hypotension, anemia, and cardiac irregularities may also occur. Upon refeeding, excess excretion of uric acid may cause uric acid nephropathy. Intense retention of sodium and water causes edema and weight gain. Both the uric acid excretion and sodium retention are dependent on dietary carbohydrate, as little as 40 grams a day being sufficient. Unless dietary supervision is continued, the lost weight is readily regained. Starvation is best reserved for hospitalized patients in whom rapid weight loss is mandatory, for some reason such as planned surgery.

FORMULA DIETS. Prepared liquid diets of high satiety value have the advantage of simplicity but the drawback of monotony. Long-term studies indicate no greater success with these than with any other diets.

Drugs. Appetite-suppressant drugs are effective for only a few weeks, whereas treatment of obesity is lifelong. Dependence on the stimulatory effect of the amphetamine group makes withdrawal a problem. Such drugs have no demonstrated role in the long-term management of obesity. Although thyroid hormone is occasionally prescribed for obesity, weight loss occurs only with toxic doses. Negative nitrogen balance may occur. Such

treatment makes evaluation of thyroid function difficult because of suppression of endogenous thyroid secretion.

Exercise. The notoriously poor state of physical fitness of Americans undoubtedly contributes to their problem of obesity. Exercise, in addition to its obvious effect of expending calories, engenders a state of physical fitness with an accompanying sense of well-being. A program of gradually increasing exercise is an important part of the treatment of obesity. The caloric expenditure also varies with occupation (Table 3).

Jejunoileal Shunt. Bypass of all the small intestine except for a few inches of proximal jejunum and terminal ileum causes weight loss because of malabsorption. Severe nutritional cirrhosis and serious loss of water and electrolytes may occur unless patients are meticulously managed. The long-term results are not known.

Prevention. Prevention of weight gain after maturity is clearly more desirable than treatment of existing obesity. Once established, obesity seems to be self-perpetuating; the five-year cure rate is almost zero. Prevention means even further education of our already diet-conscious civilization. Such education might properly start with mothers who are responsible for establishing in their children life-long dietary patterns. Institutions, such as the army, that are responsible for feeding large segments of the population have an opportunity not only to establish restrained eating habits but to prevent weight gain in men during their tour of duty. Most important of all, and perhaps least achievable, would be the restraint by the food industry of its promotion of foodstuffs of high caloric but low nutritive value. The excess calories which contribute to mass obesity in the western world are derived mainly from products which the food industry has made too readily available. Purified fats and carbohydrates, either alone or combined in the form of rich pastries and other delicacies, are the worst offenders. Since an almost invariable result of food processing is the concentration of calories with loss of minerals and vitamins, a simple rule to apply would be to reduce the consumption of foodstuffs which require manufacturing at some stage of their preparation. The adoption in American homes of such simple diets with reservation of

TABLE 3.   Illustrations of How the Energy Expenditure May Be Distributed over 24 Hours and the Effect of Occupation*

| | Reference Man (65 kg, Age 20 to 39) | | | |
	Light Activity	Moderately Active	Very Active	Exceptionally Active
In bed (8 hours)	500	500	500	500
At work (8 hours)	1100	1400	1900	2400
Nonoccupational activities (8 hours)	700–1500	700–1500	700–1500	700–1500
Range of energy expenditure (24 hours)	2300–3100	2600–3400	3100–3900	3600–4400
Mean (24 hours)	2700	3000	3500	4000
	Reference Woman (55 kg, Age 20 to 39)			
	Light Activity	Moderately Active	Very Active	Exceptionally Active
In bed (8 hours)	420	420	420	420
At work (8 hours)	800	1000	1400	1800
Nonoccupational activities (8 hours)	580–980	580–980	580–980	580–980
Range of energy expenditure (24 hours)	1800–2200	2000–2400	2400–2700	2800–3200
Mean (24 hours)	2000	2200	2600	3000

*Adapted from "Energy and Protein Requirements." Report of a Joint FAO/WHO Ad Hoc Expert Committee. World Health Organization Technical Report Series, No. 522, Geneva, 1973, p. 29.

rich treats for special occasions would enhance appreciation of the special occasions and do much to eliminate obesity and its toll of vascular disease.

ATHEROSCLEROSIS AND OBESITY

The urgency of the problem of obesity is its role in the etiology of atherosclerosis and its most common lethal manifestation, ischemic heart disease.

Definition. Atherosclerosis is a type of arteriosclerosis in which the primary lesion is a thickening of the intimal layer of the aorta and large and medium-sized arteries.

Incidence. Most epidemiologic studies of atherosclerosis are concerned with coronary artery disease, which appears to have been increasing alarmingly in the United States during the current century. The annual incidence estimated from the Framingham study increased with age in males from less than 3.8 per 1000 at age 30 to 16 or more at age 55. Half of all deaths in men aged 50 are caused by ischemic heart disease. The incidence is much lower in females, but ten years postmenopausally approaches that of men. The annual death rate from atherosclerosis and degenerative heart disease in the United States for men aged 50 to 59 is the highest in the world. Sixty per cent or more of deaths from coronary artery disease are sudden deaths.

Etiology. Atherosclerosis is a multifactorial disease. Factors which have been most clearly implicated are serum cholesterol, smoking, and hypertension. Other important predisposing factors are serum triglycerides, diabetes, and obesity. Increased concentration of circulating serum insulin has been implicated by several studies. Although most epidemiologic studies have been concerned with ischemic heart disease, the same risk factors apply to other manifestations of atherosclerosis.

Obesity. Epidemiologic data show that members of ethnic groups with low incidence of ischemic heart disease, with a few unexplained exceptions, are leaner than Americans and do not gain significant weight after maturity. Among Americans, the prevalence of coronary artery disease is lowest in persons below normal weight, and increases proportionately with degree of overweight.

Considerable evidence suggests that adult onset obesity of mild degree, the type associated with increased size of adipose cells, is more closely related to atherosclerosis than is the juvenile onset hypercellular type. The Framingham study showed that certain manifestations of coronary heart disease, i.e., angina pectoris, preinfarction angina, and sudden death, were best predicted from subscapular skin-fold thickness. Triceps thickness, which when taken alone had no prognostic value, when taken in conjunction with other measurements was actually negatively associated with these manifestations. Unpublished studies by the author show, moreover, that skin-fold thickness is better correlated with serum triglycerides, glucose, and insulin concentrations when measured at the subscapular than at the triceps site, and that when adjustment is made for the former relationship, the correlations with triceps skin-fold are negative. There is no simple way to determine cell number and size in epidemiologic studies, but obesity which involves the trunk relatively more than the limbs is thought to be an indication of adult onset obesity and therefore of large adipose cells. The finding suggests that acquired obesity predisposes to electrical

abnormalities of the heart or to thromboembolic phenomena.

A large share of the effect of obesity on the atherosclerotic plaque may be explained by the fact that in the United States obesity is the single most important influence on virtually all other risk factors. The role of obesity in the etiology of hypertension, diabetes, and hyperinsulinemia has already been discussed. Obesity also has an influence on what could be the most important risk factor, the serum lipids. The status of glucose tolerance and serum lipids can best be ascertained after an overnight fast of 12 to 24 hours when the subject has been living and eating normally at least three months after an acute illness.

Serum Lipids. Two main groups of hyperlipoproteinemia are associated with increased incidence of atherosclerosis: hyperbetalipoproteinemia, in which lower density lipoproteins (LDL) are increased (Fredrickson Types IIA and IIB), and hyperprebetalipoproteinemia, in which very low density lipoproteins (VLDL) or endogenous triglycerides are increased (Type IV will constitute most of this group) (see Ch. 819). The predominant lipid in the first group is cholesterol; in the second, triglycerides. A classification based on lipid concentration is empirically useful: pure hypercholesterolemia (Type IIA) and hypertriglyceridemia. The latter in turn can be divided into mixed lipemia (cholesterol also elevated, Type IIB and some Type IV's) or pure hypertriglyceridemia (cholesterol normal, Type IV). Pure hypercholesterolemia may carry the greatest risk of coronary artery disease, but mixed lipemia and pure hypertriglyceridemia are more prevalent. Hypercholesterolemia and hypertriglyceridemia probably contribute about equally to the population of patients with ischemic heart disease. Recent investigations have shown that VLDL is the probable precursor of LDL. An increase in concentration of circulating VLDL as well as of LDL could be responsible for the LDL seen in the atherosclerotic plaque (see below).

HYPERCHOLESTEROLEMIA. According to the Framingham study, the incidence of coronary heart disease increases as serum cholesterol concentration increases. Between the ages of 45 and 54 the annual incidence of coronary artery disease is about six per 1000 among men with cholesterol concentrations below 200 mg per 100 ml; this increases to about 15 per 1000 among men with cholesterol over 260 mg per milliliter. There is no low concentration below which absence of myocardial infarction can be guaranteed and no upper limit above which it is inevitable. The overlap is great between normal persons and those with coronary artery disease; however, a cholesterol below 200 mg per 100 ml may be considered desirable and one above 260 undesirable. For laboratories which measure the cholesterol by an automated technique, which gives values a little higher than the true values, the aforementioned levels should be modified according to the criteria for the laboratory.

Comparison of different ethnic and geographic groups suggests that hypercholesterolemia is caused by the combined effects of obesity and of high intake of saturated fat and of cholesterol, acting on a genetic predisposition. Saturated fat intake constitutes nearly 20 per cent of calories in countries characterized by highest serum cholesterol concentrations.

The amount of cholesterol in the diet has an influence on serum cholesterol concentration which is most marked in the range between no intake and intake of 300 mg per day. Further increase in dietary cholesterol has only a small effect, if any, on serum cholesterol. The average dietary cholesterol intake of most Americans exceeds this and may be over 1000 mg per day. Weight gain and relative weight were the only factors measured in the Framingham study which were related to cholesterol concentration. Variations in diet had no discernible effect, probably because the intake of saturated fat and cholesterol was above the range in which a hypocholesterolemic effect of low intake of these components can be demonstrated. Obviously other as yet unidentified factors contribute to variation in serum cholesterol in the United States. Other dietary constituents such as pectins and cereal fiber may have a cholesterol-lowering effect.

HYPERTRIGLYCERIDEMIA. Epidemiologic data concerning the risk of elevated triglycerides are still rather meager but suggest that, as with cholesterol, the risk increases continuously throughout the range. The upper limit of normal is considered to be about 150 mg per 100 ml. Peripheral vascular disease may be a more common manifestation than in pure hypercholesterolemia. Endogenous hypertriglyceridemia is frequently associated with obesity of the adult onset type, and with impaired glucose tolerance, insulin resistance, and high basal insulin concentrations. In nondiabetics the postcibal rise in insulin, being superimposed on an elevated fasting level, may be high. In diabetics the insulin response is blunted. As in obesity, the high insulin output may eventually lead to pancreatic exhaustion and low insulin-output diabetes, thus accounting for the frequency of impaired glucose tolerance. Also as in obesity, the insulin-resistant state may be a fundamental aspect of endogenous lipemia.

The causal sequences among obesity, hypertriglyceridemia, hyperinsulinism, insulin resistance, impaired glucose tolerance, and ultimately atherosclerosis are not known.

Although it is not certain whether endogenous hypertriglyceridemia is caused by increased synthesis or impaired removal, it is exaggerated by factors which increase fat synthesis such as weight gain and very high carbohydrate diet. The latter causes so-called carbohydrate-induced lipemia, probably by increasing VLDL synthesis. Weight reduction or a low carbohydrate diet improves the lipemia. The amount of carbohydrate necessary to induce the lipemia is subject to marked individual variation. The triglyceride-lowering effect of a low calorie diet overrides the triglyceride-raising effect of a high carbohydrate diet.

Pathogenesis of Atherosclerosis. Of the three layers of an artery, atherosclerosis is a disease only of the intima. The characteristic lesion is the subendothelial atherosclerotic plaque. The earliest lesion is the "fatty streak," a subendothelial accumulation of fat which occurs in early childhood. This lesion is universal and is reversible. Its importance lies in the fact that during the third decade it progresses to the second stage, the raised subendothelial fibrous plaque in which fibrous connective tissue, collagen, and mucopolysaccharide appear and cause the lesion to encroach on the vessel lumen. Ischemia or necrosis of the organ supplied is the end result. The lesion progresses to ulceration, necrosis, calcification, and hemorrhage, the so-called complicated lesion. With each stage reversibility is lessened.

Progression of the universal innocuous fatty streak to the fibrous plaque is not inevitable but depends on dietary and other environmental factors. The single most important factor determining whether the fatty streak progresses to the atherosclerotic plaque is the lipid, particularly cholesterol, content of the lesion.

Study of the lipid components of the plaque show that cholesterol and triglycerides are probably derived from plasma, whereas phospholipids may be synthesized by the vessel wall. Little is known of the mechanism whereby lipids are transported across the endothelial barrier into the vessel wall. High density lipoproteins (HDL), low density lipoproteins (LDL), and possibly smaller very low density lipoproteins (VLDL) are small enough to enter by diffusion. The identification of LDL apoprotein within the plaque suggests that entire lipoproteins do enter the vessel wall from the serum. A certain amount of lipid exchange between intima and plasma is normal. The triglyceride can be metabolized by the vessel wall, and the remaining cholesterol-rich LDL disposed of in a manner unknown. Only when the rate of entry of LDL becomes greater than the rate of disposal does abnormal accumulation occur.

The localization of atherosclerotic plaques at sites of injury and at points of bifurcation of arteries and the greater incidence of atherosclerosis in hypertensive persons demonstrate that local injury and pressure relationships are important factors in plaque formation. Atherosclerosis is rare in pulmonary arteries unless pulmonary hypertension is present.

Recent work has focused on proliferation of the smooth muscle cell in the intima as the key event in the pathogenesis of the atherosclerotic plaque. The smooth muscle cells may proliferate from a few pre-existing intimal cells or may migrate from the media, the usual location of smooth muscle cells. Early in the atherosclerotic process the intimal smooth muscle cell accumulates LDL, thus becoming the well-known lipid-laden foam cell. Smooth muscle cells grown in tissue culture react to LDL accumulation by proliferation and by secretion of other constituents of the plaque: elastic fiber protein, collagen, and mucopolysaccharides. They later may secrete lipids into the extracellular space.

In summary, factors which increase endothelial permeability to lipoproteins, such as injury to the vessel wall, and factors which increase lipid concentration presented to the vessel wall in the circulation, would act to promote intimal smooth muscle cell proliferation which in turn leads to the atherosclerotic plaque.

An alternative theory attributes plaque formation to the intravascular coagulation initiated by increased platelet stickiness and platelet agglomeration or by a shift in the balance between fibrin formation and fibrinolysis in the direction of fibrin deposition, with secondary enmeshment of circulating lipids. Increased coagulability, superimposed on underlying atherosclerotic disease, may be of importance in the 50 per cent of myocardial infarctions in which thrombosis is a prominent part of the pathologic change.

Although atherosclerosis is a generalized disease, coronary artery disease may occur without atherosclerotic involvement elsewhere. Such isolated coronary artery disease is a common cause of morbidity and mortality among younger men and is associated, more than is generalized atherosclerosis, with overnutrition. Cerebral atherosclerosis occurs in taller, thinner persons about 20 years later than coronary atherosclerosis.

Treatment of Atherosclerosis. Specific treatment is directed toward individual organs. General treatment consists of identifying and correcting all the known risk factors (see above). The most important aspects of treatment are weight reduction, correction of hyperlipidemias, correction of hypertension, and cessation of smoking.

The general principles of weight reduction have been discussed above. Special attention to the diet is necessary when hyperlipidemias are not corrected by simple weight reduction. Whether such dietary intervention will reverse the atherosclerotic process is unknown, but optimism seems permissible on the basis of available knowledge.

Dietary Treatment of Hypercholesterolemia. In spite of lack of correlation between prevailing diet and serum cholesterol in the Framingham study, dietary *change* will have a small but definite effect on serum cholesterol concentration.

The National Diet Heart Study showed that reduction of total fat intake from 40 to 30 per cent of calories, reduction of saturated fat from 18 to 9 per cent of calories, reduction of dietary cholesterol intake from 700 to 400 mg per day, and an increase in the polyunsaturated to saturated fat (P/S) ratio from 0.4 to 1.5 effected an 8 per cent reduction of serum cholesterol in weight-stable persons. The effect was nearly doubled by weight loss, and weight loss in the control group caused a 5 per cent reduction. A further decrease of dietary cholesterol to 100 mg will be more effective, but such a diet is difficult to follow. The addition of polyunsaturated oils will have a cholesterol lowering effect which is about half the cholesterol raising effect of saturated fats. The safety of large amounts of unsaturated dietary fat is not certain. Most authorities now recommend only enough polyunsaturated fat to raise the P/S ratio to 1.0. Dietary cholesterol is derived entirely from animal sources. The important dietary sources of cholesterol may be seen in Table 4. Because one problem of cholesterol restriction is the maintenance of adequate protein intake, the protein values are also shown.

The elimination of eggs from the diet will do much to lower the cholesterol intake. Further reduction can readily be achieved by eliminating butter, organ meat, shrimp, and crab, and by substituting skimmed milk for whole milk. Recent studies have shown lower cholesterol in shellfish than previously thought. Protein can be supplied either by lean meat or by cheese, as preferred, as well as by vegetable sources. Although even lean meat contains substantial amounts of cholesterol, meat is the mainstay of the American diet, and its elimination will jeopardize patient cooperation. If meat is the only significant source of cholesterol in the diet, as much as 8 ounces a day can be permitted without exceeding 200 mg of dietary cholesterol.

The carbohydrate content of a very low fat diet may be sufficiently high to cause hypertriglyceridemia in susceptible persons (see below). In the average person moderate increases in dietary carbohydrate have little influence on triglycerides.

Treatment of Hypertriglyceridemia. The first step in the treatment of hypertriglyceridemia is weight reduction to or toward ideal weight (Table 1), or to weight at age 25. If simple weight loss does not lower serum triglycerides, restriction of carbohydrate to 40 or even 30 per cent of calories or more may be necessary. A decrease in serum triglyceride by as much as 50 per cent may be achieved.

Some evidence exists for the possibility that carbohydrate-induced lipemia is a response more to highly purified carbohydrates such as sucrose than to carbohydrate in general. For this reason it would be wise to eliminate sugar as such from the diet of obese or atherosclerotic patients, particularly if the triglycerides are elevated. Alcohol ingestion may raise the triglycerides and should be used only sparingly.

Prevention of Atherosclerosis. Preventive measures are the same as therapeutic measures except that they are directed toward patients of high risk who do not yet have atherosclerosis. Opinion is divided as to the advisability of drastic changes in the diet for children and young

TABLE 4. Approximate Cholesterol Content of Foods*

Item	Size Serving, Edible Portion as Purchased	Amount of Cholesterol (mg)	Amount of Protein (Grams)
Milk, whole	One glass (200 ml)	22	7
Milk, skim	One glass (200 ml)	6	7
Whole milk cheeses, as American, Cheddar, and cream	100 grams	85–100	21–36
Cheese, cottage	100 grams	15	13
Butter	1 tablespoon (15 grams)	38	0
Animal fat (lard)	1 tablespoon (15 grams)	14	0
Egg yolk	1 egg	300	3
Egg white	1 egg	0	5
Lean cuts of any poultry, meat except organs, fish except shrimp and crab	100 grams of meat only	30–90	16–32
Shrimp and crab	100 grams of meat only	100–150	16–24
Caviar	100 grams	>300	26–34
Organ meats	100 grams	150–375	16–26
Brain	100 grams	>2000	12

*Estimated from values listed in U.S. Department of Agriculture Handbook No. 8, Composition of Foods, 1963, and Feeley, R. M., Criner, P. E., and Watt, B. K.: J. Am. Dietet. Assoc., 61:134, 1972.

adults, not because of any doubt that prevention is desirable, but because of uncertainty regarding the best methods of prevention. Certain preventive measures can be recommended for the entire population: avoidance of cigarette smoking, of high intake of foods of high caloric density but low nutritive value such as sugar and fats, and of weight gain after maturity.

Albrink, M. J.: Overnutrition and the fat cell. *In* Bondy, P. K., and Rosenberg, L. (eds.): Duncan's Diseases of Metabolism. 7th ed. Philadelphia, W. B. Saunders Company, 1974.

Alexander, J. K., and Peterson, K. L.: Cardiovascular effects of weight reduction. Circulation, 45:310, 1972.

Bray, G. (ed.): Fogarty International Center Conference on Obesity. U. S. Government Printing Office, in press.

Damon, A., Damon, S. T., Harpending, H. C., and Kannel, W. B.: Predicting coronary heart disease from body measurements of Framingham males. J. Chronic Dis., 21:781, 1969.

Grinker, J., and Hirsch, J.: Metabolic and behavioral correlates of obesity. *In* Physiology of Emotion and Psychosomatic Illness. Ciba Foundation Symposium 8 (new series). Amsterdam, Elsevier Publishing Company, 1972.

Hatch, F. T.: Interactions between nutrition and heredity in coronary heart disease. Am. J. Clin. Nutr., 27:80, 1974.

Keys, A., Aravanis, C., Blackburn, H., Van Buchem, F., Buzina, R., Djordjevic, B. S., Fidanza, F., Karvonen, M. J., Menotti, A., Puddu, V., and Taylor, H.: Coronary heart disease: Overweight and obesity as risk factors. Ann. Intern. Med., 77:15, 1972.

Ross, R., and Glomset, J. A.: Atherosclerosis and the arterial smooth muscle cell. Science, 180:1332, 1973.

Sims, E. A. H., Danforth, E., Jr., Horton, E. S., Bray, G. A., Glennon, J. S., and Salans, L. B.: Endocrine and metabolic effects of experimental obesity in man. Recent Prog. Horm. Res., 29:457, 1973.

724. ANOREXIA NERVOSA

G. F. M. Russell

Definition. Anorexia nervosa is a chronic illness principally affecting young girls after puberty. It is characterized by severe weight loss which is self-induced, amenorrhea, and a specific psychopathology.

Historical Note. Sir William Gull described anorexia nervosa in 1868 and 1874 and concluded that "the want of appetite is due to a morbid mental state." This he attributed to the wiles of young women whom he considered "specially obnoxious to mental perversity." He advised that "the patients should be fed at regular intervals, and surrounded by persons who would have more control over them, relations and friends being generally the worst attendants." For a long time, confusion resulted from the concept of "Simmonds' cachexia," which embodied the mistaken view that panhypopituitarism usually caused loss of weight and wasting. Thus much needless effort was spent on the differential diagnosis of these two disorders which do not resemble each other.

Etiology. The cause of anorexia nervosa is unknown. Little is known about genetic aspects: morbidity is higher among sisters of patients (6.6 per cent), and concordance for the illness has been described in identical twins, but these observations are also explicable by the similarity of the home environment. Anorexia nervosa used to be considered a rare illness. However, a fivefold increase in incidence was reported in Malmö, Sweden, by Theander when he compared the 1950's with the 1930's. Similar observations in Britain have led to the hypothesis that culturally determined attitudes might lead to the illness. In recent years the upper social class bias for

anorexia nervosa has tended to disappear. The incidence of new cases ranges from 0.6 to 1.6 per 100,000 of the whole population, but the prevalence among schoolgirls around puberty may be as high as one in a hundred. The usual age of onset is 14 to 17 years, but it can be earlier (10 to 13 years) or later (up to 40 years). The illness is at least ten times more frequent in girls than in boys.

Psychopathology and Pathogenesis. Anorexia nervosa is usually thought to be a disorder of psychologic origin, especially from conflicts engendered by the experience of puberty and adolescence. The illness can also be viewed from a predominantly somatic perspective as a disorder of the feeding and endocrine functions normally controlled by the hypothalamus.

The psychologic basis of anorexia nervosa is supported by the observation that food refusal is often purposive. Psychodynamic formulations (not equivalent to causal explanations) emphasize the ambivalent emotional ties between the patient and her mother, conflicts caused by the advent of puberty, and the uncertainties that surround the search for a personal identity during adolescence. Psychologic explanations postulate an abnormal reaction to puberty (Thomä) or a disturbance of "body image" (Bruch). Some support has been given to the last hypothesis (Slade and Russell). Patients with anorexia nervosa have been shown to be abnormally responsive to their impressions of body size and weight. They eat less whenever they feel that their body is too large, instead of relying on the physiologic signals of hunger. Moreover, they tend to overestimate the width of their own body. They therefore see themselves as wider and fatter than normal girls, and further starvation ensues.

It has also been proposed that the pathogenesis of anorexia nervosa involves a disorder of hypothalamic function on the ground that destruction of the "feeding centers" in animals causes refusal of food and water. However, studies in anorexia nervosa have not revealed any primary disorder in the control of food intake, and there is often no true loss of appetite, so that the term "anorexia" is a misnomer. Emaciation has been described as a consequence of hypothalamic lesions in humans, but in such cases the clinical picture does not otherwise resemble anorexia nervosa.

The strongest evidence of a hypothalamic disorder in anorexia nervosa is specific failure in the function of the hypothalamic–anterior pituitary–gonadal axis: gonadotrophins are not released from the anterior pituitary, the ovarian production of estrogens drops, and ovulation fails to occur. These abnormalities often persist long after the malnutrition is corrected; gonadotrophins and estrogens rise again in the blood and urine, but cyclical variations in their levels and ovulation do not return for several months. These findings, together with the early onset of amenorrhea which may precede weight loss, indicate that the endocrine disorder is not simply the sequel of the malnutrition. The precise nature of the hypothalamic disorder is unknown. In male patients there is a corresponding endocrine disorder with reduction in gonadotrophin and testosterone levels in the blood and urine. There is also evidence of disordered thermoregulation in anorexia nervosa, but this can be corrected by restoring body weight to normal and is therefore probably secondary to malnutrition.

Clinical Manifestations. The illness usually begins in a girl aged 14 to 17 years. Her previous personality may have been normal. In some patients, however, there may be a preceding history of food fads or difficulty in making friendships; other signs of maladjustment are excessive tidiness or fears of meeting strangers or of taking school examinations. Loss of weight may be the first feature noticed by the parents, who draw the patient's attention to it. She is likely to explain the weight loss as the result of dieting for the purpose of improving her figure. Menstruation will have ceased by the time there has been a significant loss of weight, or this may happen as the first feature of the illness. There is often a change in the girl's temperament, consisting of impatience, irritability, and depression. She may become preoccupied with schoolwork or indulge in solitary exercises, thus withdrawing from her customary social life. The loss of weight can be very rapid, with a fall from 55 kg (121 pounds) to 35 kg (77 pounds) within two to three months. This is achieved mainly by avoiding carbohydrate-containing foods, but self-induced vomiting, the abuse of purgatives, and excessive exercising, in various combinations, may accelerate the loss of weight. The patient's life becomes unhappy and constricted. If she had a boyfriend, she loses interest in him and avoids any sexual contact. Relations with members of the family become strained. Parents may react to their daughter's food refusal by alternately pleading with her and trying to force her to eat. Food refusal leads to malnutrition which may persist for months or even years. The patient subsists on a diet of vegetables, fruit, and cheese, and avoids bread, potatoes, cakes, sugar, and other carbohydrate-containing foods. On some days she may take only black coffee. Sometimes, food avoidance alternates with orgiastic bouts of overeating, especially at night when the patient can no longer resist her cravings for food. These bouts are followed by vomiting. In severe cases the patient presents a pitiable sight of emaciation, apathy, weakness, and severe depression. There is a risk of death from suicide or complications of malnutrition – infections, potassium depletion, or hypothermia.

In spite of progressive malnutrition, the patient may reject her parents' entreaties to see a doctor, and she minimizes the extent of her dieting. When she does agree to seek help, she is likely to deny that she is unwell or admit only to insomnia, constipation, sensitivity to cold, or some depression of mood.

Mental Examination. Examination of the patient's mental state may reveal a variety of disturbances. There may be depression and agitation; compulsive features may be prominent, such as elaborate feeding rituals and the counting of calories eaten daily; hysterical mechanisms may account for her assertion that she is eating well, whereas at the same time she hides food surreptitiously or vomits in secret. In addition, however, more specific psychologic abnormalities will be present. Their central theme is the patient's fear of becoming fat as a result of "losing control over eating." To play safe she resolves to remain thin and sets herself a sharply defined weight threshold above which she is unwilling to rise, defending her chosen weight as "right" for her. She may betray an abnormal sensitivity about the shape and size of her body, saying that fat would go to her stomach (hips, thighs, or some other part of the body). She may overestimate her weight and maintain, with all sincerity, that she eats large amounts of food. In an extreme case she may deny that she is thin, or even state that she is fat in spite of obvious emaciation. The patient's distorted awareness of her size can be measured by getting her to estimate the width of her body at various levels

(e.g., face, bust, waist, and hips) by means of an apparatus which permits the separation of two lights until it corresponds to the selected body dimension. The patient's estimate is liable to exceed her actual measurements by as much as 50 per cent. Patients may offer a variety of other reasons for their reluctance to return to a normal weight, or they may conceal their abnormal attitudes which nonetheless become explicit by their behavior when they are under observation in hospital.

Physical Examination. Physical examination will reveal the signs of severe malnutrition in a young girl who has developed secondary sex characteristics. The malnutrition is of a calorie-deficiency type. The disappearance of subcutaneous fat leads to gaunt, hollow facial features; bony prominences stand out sharply, the limbs are reduced to sticks, the belly is flat, the breasts shrunken, and the buttocks wasted. The hands and feet remain cold and blue, even when the room temperature is warm. The central body temperature may be reduced by 1° C. The blood pressure is low (e.g., 90/60), and the heart rate is slow (50 to 60). The skin is dry, and there is an excessive growth of dry, downy hair over the nape of the neck and the cheeks, forearms, and legs (lanugo hair), changes attributed to a follicular keratosis. In older patients purpuric patches resembling senile purpura may appear over the dorsum of the hands, the forearms, and the legs after minor knocks.

In patients who vomit, dehydration ensues, together with a marked reduction in the levels of serum potassium (e.g., to 1.4 mEq per liter), which may lead to muscular weakness, tetany, and electrocardiographic abnormalities. There may also be a moderate fall in serum sodium and hypochloremic alkalosis. Serum cholesterol levels may be raised, especially in patients who overeat intermittently. Carotenemia may follow a high intake of carrots or spinach, and causes a yellow pigmentation of the palms and soles. Vitamin deficiencies occur only rarely.

Endocrine Changes. Patients who are wasted show a fall in the urinary output of gonadotrophins and estrogens; blood levels of luteinizing hormone (LH) are low. A course of clomiphene fails to raise the low serum LH levels. Specific measures of thyroid function fall within the normal range. Plasma levels of growth hormone and cortisol are normal or elevated, and can be raised further by the administration of insulin. Most of the physical abnormalities disappear when the malnutrition is corrected, and the patient's mental state is also likely to improve. An exception to this recovery is the disorder of gonadotrophin activity, as described above.

Side Effects of Refeeding. Peripheral edema may occur, especially when the diet has a high content of salt, water, and carbohydrates which cause water retention. A moderate normochromic normocytic anemia may result from hemodilution, or a more severe anemia may result from temporary hypoplasia of the bone marrow; occasionally, moderate iron deficiency anemia may occur. Acute dilatation of the stomach is a rare complication of too rapid refeeding.

Anorexia Nervosa in the Male. The illness in the male is rare, but resembles closely that in the female. The onset occurs around the time of puberty. The young boy rapidly loses weight as a result of avoiding carbohydrate-containing foods. Like the female, he expresses a fear of becoming fat, and resorts to a similar abnormal behavior of food refusal, possibly with vomiting, purgation, or exercising to excess. Because of the later age of physical maturation in the male, there is a greater risk of malnutrition causing retardation of growth and delayed puberty. The malnutrition is more likely to be of a type combining a deficiency of calories and proteins. The endocrine disorder in the male is analogous to that in the female. Urinary gonadotrophins and blood LH levels are low; the urinary output of testosterone is reduced. Questioning will elicit loss of recently acquired sexual interest and potency. As in the female, these hormonal abnormalities can be slowly reversed by treatment resulting in weight gain.

Treatment. There is no specific treatment; nevertheless the general management of patients can be rewarding. The approach is essentially empirical; the treatments used are those which have been found to be effective in practice. The immediate aim is to treat the patient's malnutrition, which can become severe and dangerous. Even during the early stages of treatment it is desirable to try altering abnormal attitudes, for the course of the illness is much affected by the psychologic state. Thus treatment is best administered in a psychiatric unit, but it is essential that there should be good nursing facilities. The long-term aim of treatment is to reduce the duration of the illness and prevent relapses.

Short-Term Treatment. SECURING THE PATIENT'S CO-OPERATION. The first need is to obtain as much cooperation from the patient as possible, notwithstanding her denial of illness. By the time there has been severe loss of weight, admission to hospital is the only certain way of restoring her nutrition to normal. The doctor's skills must therefore be focused on persuading the patient to come into hospital. Compulsory admission is best avoided whenever possible, because the patient's continued cooperation is essential throughout the course of the illness, which may last for a few years.

NURSING TREATMENT. The refeeding of the patient is best achieved by skilled nurses. After having assessed the severity of the feeding disorder, the nurse should try to establish a good relationship with her patient, one based on trust but not dependent on giving way to the patient's abnormal wishes to avoid food and weight gain. This is best achieved by the nurse asking the patient to look upon her as a person whom she can trust to decide on the amount of food to be eaten each day, and who will not allow her to become fat. The patient is told frankly that because of her illness she will be tempted to be deceitful about eating, vomiting, or taking purgatives. The nurse thus explains that close supervision will be necessary at first to reduce the strength of these temptations. The patient must be observed throughout every meal, and the nurse will cajole her into finishing all the food put on her plate. The avoidance of self-induced vomiting can be difficult. It requires round-the-clock nursing supervision, limiting the fluid intake to 1.5 liters daily, preventing access to the toilet for at least two hours after meals, and removal of vomit-bowls. The use of purgatives should also be stopped. As soon as the patient gains weight, she is complimented on her improved looks and is encouraged to use cosmetics and buy new clothes suitable for a person of normal weight.

The techniques of nursing are also important, but they will only succeed within the context of a good relationship with the patient. They consist of a close supervision and a positive encouragement to eat. Complete bed rest is seldom necessary for more than a few days, but it may facilitate a close watch being kept.

The nurse will decide on a judicious balance between restrictions and privileges, in collaboration with the doctor and psychologist. The balance is gradually altered in favor of added privileges which will be viewed by the patient as rewards for continuing progress. Thus the general management can also be fitted within a model of behavior therapy.

DIET. No special diets are needed. The patient is given her own choice of food so long as she does not exclude carbohydrate-containing foods. To begin with, the food intake should be 1500 calories daily; within seven to ten days she should be persuaded to accept full meals totaling 3000 to 5000 calories daily. Concentrated foods may be used to achieve this high intake (e.g., Complan, Metrecal, or Carnation breakfast food) by adding them to milk. Potassium supplements do not remedy the hypokalemia unless vomiting is controlled, and then they become unnecessary.

ADDITIONAL MEASURES. The nursing care described should be viewed as a form of *psychologic treatment* embodying the principles of psychotherapy and behavior therapy. Formal psychotherapy has only a limited place during the early stages of treatment.

Large doses of chlorpromazine are sometimes advocated to reduce the patient's resistance to eating, but they can be dangerous in undernourished patients, and are seldom necessary. In very agitated patients the nursing task can be facilitated by administering moderate, divided doses of chlorpromazine up to a total of 300 mg daily. There is no place for tube feeding. It is doubtful whether a modified leukotomy is ever justified. Weight gain can be achieved by conservative treatment, and the risk of suicide is increased after leukotomy.

ASSESSMENT OF PROGRESS. The patient is weighed daily before breakfast, and this provides the best check on her progress. A weight gain of up to 28 pounds (12.7 kg) in eight weeks should be possible. The patient should be seen to maintain a healthy weight for about two weeks before being discharged from hospital.

Long-Term Treatment. There is less known about the efficacy of long-term treatments. After discharge from hospital, it is necessary to provide outpatient supervision. Psychotherapy should be directed to whatever emotional problems have been identified in the patient and her family. Even when a normal weight is maintained, amenorrhea may persist for months or years. When the patient is eager to resume normal menstruation, one or two courses of clomiphene (50 to 100 mg daily for seven days) may be effective, but only when body weight has been restored to a normal level. In the event of a serious relapse, readmission to hospital will be necessary.

Prognosis. The short-term prognosis is usually excellent. Treatment should lead to a return to a normal weight; at the same time, the majority of patients show a marked improvement in their mental state. Deaths from malnutrition should not occur.

The long-term prognosis is more problematical. Relapses requiring readmissions occur in about half the patients. The illness often lasts two to three years or even longer. In a follow-up of severely ill patients who had been treated at least four years previously, 40 per cent had recovered, 27 per cent had menstrual irregularity or a moderately low body weight, 29 per cent had serious weight loss with amenorrhea, and 5 per cent had died. Poor prognostic signs are a later age of onset (early twenties as opposed to early teens), or an illness which has lasted more than five years. Even in these patients, however, good results can still be obtained from energetic treatment. In many patients the prognosis is good—their health returns to normal and they may marry and can bear children.

Bruch, H.: Eating Disorders: Obesity, Anorexia Nervosa and the Person Within. New York, Basic Books, 1972.

Gull, W. W.: Anorexia nervosa (apepsia hysterica, anorexia hysterica). Trans. Clin. Soc. London, 7:22, 1874.

Mecklenburg, R. S., Loriaux, D. L. Thompson, R. H., Andersen, A. E., and Lipsett, M. B.: Hypothalmic dysfunction in patients with anorexia nervosa. Medicine, 53:147, 1974.

Russell, G. F. M.: Anorexia nervosa: Its identity as an illness and its treatment. In Price, J. H. (ed.): Modern Trends in Psychological Medicine. 2d ed. London, Butterworth & Co. (Publishers) Ltd., 1970.

Russell, G. F. M.: The management of anorexia nervosa. In Robertson, R. F. (ed.): Symposium—Anorexia Nervosa and Obesity. Edinburgh, The Royal College of Physicians, 1973.

Slade, P. D., and Russell, G. F. M.: Awareness of body dimensions in anorexia nervosa: Cross-sectional and longitudinal studies. Psychol. Med., 3:188, 1973.

Theander, S.: Anorexia nervosa. A psychiatric investigation of 94 female patients. Acta Psychiatr. Scand., Supplement 211, 1970.

Thomä, H.: Anorexia Nervosa. Translated by G. Brydone. New York, International Universities Press, 1967.

NUTRITIONAL MAINTENANCE AND DIET THERAPY IN ACUTE AND CHRONIC DISEASE

Philip Felig

725. INTRODUCTION

Diseases resulting from deficiencies of specific nutrients in the diet are well recognized and have been covered in detail elsewhere (see Ch. 717 to 722). Except in underdeveloped areas of the world, problems of nutritional homeostasis in hospitalized patients are generally a secondary consequence rather than a cause of disease processes. The normal intake of nutrients may be interfered with in a variety of inflammatory, septic, or malignant disorders as a result of anorexia or vomiting, in association with primary disturbances of the gastrointestinal tract, and in the postoperative state. Nutritional maintenance also poses a problem in patients placed on therapeutic diets designed to limit the intake of calories, carbohydrate, protein, sodium, or potassium. Generally attention is focused on correcting the primary disorder, and little concern is attached to over-all nutritional requirements, since most patients are expected to tolerate limited periods of subnutrition without difficulty. Considerations of nutritional factors are often limited to providing vitamin supplements, with little attention to caloric and nitrogen balance. It is noteworthy, however, that sepsis secondary to debilitation, in the form of terminal bronchopneumonia, is a major cause of death in hospitalized patients. The sequence of events in

such patients is often as follows: primary disease (e.g., uremia, malignancy, ulcerative colitis) → poor nutrition and protein catabolism → depletion of body protein reserves (i.e., muscle) → weakness of respiratory muscles → atelectasis → pneumonia → death. In less severe circumstances, failure of adequate nutrition may prolong convalescence, predispose to infection, and interfere with wound healing.

An important goal in the medical management of disease is thus the maintenance of normal body composition in the face of reduced intake, increased metabolic requirements, or disordered metabolic machinery. From a practical standpoint nutritional considerations become an integral aspect of the therapeutic decision process in patients requiring short-term or long-term parenteral feeding, particularly when an anabolic response is necessary, and in patients on restrictive diets. To understand the principles underlying such nutritional interventions, it is first necessary to consider body composition in healthy subjects prior to the onset of illness, the metabolic response to nutritional deprivation in normal man, and the accelerated catabolism observed in disease states.

726. FUEL HOMEOSTASIS IN HEALTH AND DISEASE

Body Composition. Normal man may be considered not only in terms of his constituent organ systems, but also with respect to his underlying fuel reserves. The energy resources available in a 70-kg man are shown in Table 1. Body fat, comprising 15 to 25 per cent of body weight, constitutes the primary fuel depot, each gram providing 9 kcal. Smaller amounts of calories are available in the form of protein (4 kcal per gram), whereas carbohydrate stores (4 kcal per gram) are calorically insignificant. The enormity of fat stores relative to other nutrients is readily apparent. Furthermore, an increase in body weight, such as occurs in obesity, involves little change in the quantity of protein or carbohydrate but is associated primarily with an increase in fat. Thus a 25 per cent gain in weight is accompanied by a doubling in body fat. In contrast, weight loss, as observed in chronic debilitated states, involves a substantial reduction in body protein as well as fat. The ability to withstand a debilitating illness is accordingly reduced in the already wasted patient.

Short-Term Starvation. In individuals of normal weight or in those who are obese, even under circumstances of heavy exercise or the increased demands engendered by severe injury (Table 2), the magnitude of

TABLE 1. Body Composition and Fuel Reserves in a Normal 70-kg Man

Fuel	Tissue	kg	% Body Weight	Energy Value (kcal)
Fat	Adipose tissue	11–17	15–25	100,000–150,000
Protein	Primarily muscle	8–12	12–17	32,000– 48,000
Carbohydrate	Liver glycogen	0.070	<1	280
	Muscle glycogen	0.200	<1	800
	Blood glucose	0.020	<1	80

body fat stores is such that they might be expected to meet the total energy needs during periods of total starvation extending at least two months. However, it is not the depletion of fat which is the limiting factor in survival during food restriction. Death caused by starvation is a consequence of protein loss and generally occurs when one third to one half of total protein stores has been depleted. The continuous, obligate utilization of protein in the face of more plentiful fat reserves is a consequence of three factors: (1) protein constitutes the sole source of noncarbohydrate precursors which can be converted to glucose, inasmuch as net glucose synthesis from fatty acids does not occur in mammalian tissue; (2) certain tissues are obligate consumers of glucose; and (3) carbohydrate reserves (particularly liver glycogen) are extremely limited (Table 1) and are dissipated in less than 24 hours of starvation.

During short-term starvation the brain is the major site of glucose utilization. Glucose is consumed by the brain at a rate of 100 to 150 grams per day and undergoes terminal oxidation to CO_2 and water. Smaller amounts of glucose (50 to 75 grams) are converted to lactic acid by the formed elements of the blood, the renal medulla, and muscle tissue. The bulk of the energy requirements of muscle, heart, and visceral tissues are not dependent on glucose utilization (in either the fed state or starvation), but are met by the oxidation of free fatty acids mobilized from adipose tissue, and ketone acids formed in the liver in association with fat oxidation.

Since, as noted above, liver glycogen stores are limited to less than 100 grams, hepatic glycogenolysis can sustain brain glucose requirements for less than 24 hours. Synthesis of glucose from noncarbohydrate precursors (gluconeogenesis) consequently begins in the immediate postabsorptive state (10- to 12-hour fast). Amino acids, particularly large amounts of alanine, are released from muscle tissue and are taken up by the liver where they are converted to glucose. The rate of protein breakdown is approximately 60 to 75 grams per day, resulting in the appearance of 10 to 12 grams of nitrogen in the urine (6.25 grams N/gram of protein). Since muscle tissue is about 75 to 80 per cent water, this rate of protein catabolism results in a loss of approximately one half pound (200 to 300 grams) of lean body mass per day. A more rapid rate of weight loss reflects either a loss of body fluids (diuresis) or a catabolic state (see below).

The primary hormonal modulators of the gluconeogenic and ketogenic response to short-term starvation are insulin and glucagon. Fasting evokes a prompt decrease in serum insulin and a rise in circulating levels of glucagon. These hormonal changes, particularly the fall in insulin, provide the signal which stimulates lipolysis in adipose tissue and augmented gluconeogenesis by the liver. Insulin does not disappear entirely from the circulation; the small amounts remaining probably serve to prevent the massive ketogenesis and gluconeogenesis observed in diabetic ketoacidosis.

The catabolic processes precipitated by starvation may be dramatically altered by providing minimal amounts of carbohydrate. Administration of 100 grams of carbohydrate (400 calories) in the absence of other foodstuffs results in a marked diminution in urinary nitrogen losses to as little as 2 to 3 grams per day. This protein-sparing effect of calorically insignificant amounts of carbohydrate is of prime consideration in determining the composition of fluids administered to patients in whom food intake must be withheld for short periods (see below). Two points deserve emphasis regarding carbohydrate intake in otherwise fasted individuals: (1) increasing the carbohydrate content above 100 grams does not increase the protein-sparing effect; (2) positive nitrogen balance (anabolism) cannot be achieved unless an exogenous source of protein is provided as well.

Long-Term Starvation. As fasting continues beyond several days, a series of adaptations occurs designed to limit the rate and magnitude of protein breakdown. Total glucose utilization decreases as the brain consumes ketone bodies as an alternative oxidative fuel. Since less glucose is required, gluconeogenic processes are curtailed, and the outflow of alanine and other amino acids from muscle is greatly reduced. Urinary nitrogen excretion falls to as little as 3 grams per day, reflecting the catabolism of no more than 20 grams of protein and depletion of less than 100 grams of lean body mass. The expendable nature of fat as compared to protein is indicated by the fact that 95 per cent of caloric needs are met by combustion of free fatty acids and ketone bodies. The patient in this circumstance is on an "endogenous high-fat diet" in which protein breakdown continues, but at a greatly reduced rate. The precise signal (? hormonal) triggering this decrease in protein catabolism has not been identified.

Catabolic States: Inflammation, Sepsis, Trauma. The orderly adaptive processes directed at minimizing protein losses in prolonged or short-term starvation are predicated upon the absence of significant underlying disease. In association with acute or chronic inflammation, sepsis, or trauma (burns, injuries, or surgery), the response to nutritional deprivation is characterized by an accelerated rate of protein catabolism. The magnitude of the catabolic response is related in part to increases in energy expenditure. Oxygen consumption is increased by fever at a rate of 7 per cent per degree Fahrenheit. Thus a fever of 103° F results in a 25 to 30 per cent elevation in energy requirements (Table 2). In addition to the effects of fever, the nature of the underlying disease or injury will influence caloric expenditure. The trauma associated with elective surgery causes no increase in basal oxygen consumption. In contrast, compound fractures or severe infections (e.g., peritonitis) are associated with an increase of 50 per cent, whereas extensive body burns are followed by elevations of 100 per cent above normal (Table 2). These increased demands for energy are met by an accelerated rate of protein dissolution. Urinary nitrogen losses in the poorly fed patient with an extensive inflammatory process may amount to 25

TABLE 2.   Caloric Expenditure in Normal and Disease States

Normal Activity	Calories/kg Body Weight/Day	Disease States
Bed rest	25	Bed rest
Light exercise (light housework, office work)	30–35	Fever of 103° F
Moderate exercise (industrial work, heavy housework)	35–40	Peritonitis, sepsis
Heavy exercise (construction work, farm work)	40–45	Extensive burns

grams per day (more than twice the rate observed in uncomplicated starvation), reflecting the breakdown of over 150 grams of protein and resulting in a loss of more than 1 pound per day of lean body mass. The origin of the protein loss is primarily muscle, inasmuch as the integrity of visceral tissues (e.g., liver) is maintained. Although the fate of the amino acids mobilized from muscle has not been precisely defined, recent studies by Kinney suggest that this rapid loss of protein is coupled with an accelerated rate of gluconeogenesis. This increased production of glucose may serve to meet the needs of reparative tissues such as fibroblasts and phagocytes.

The over-all metabolic picture thus contrasts markedly with that which occurs in prolonged starvation in normal subjects. Oxygen consumption, protein dissolution, and gluconeogenesis are all accelerated. Even more striking is the dissimilarity in the response to glucose administration. In contrast to the protein-sparing effects of minimal amounts of carbohydrate in starvation, administration of 100 to 400 grams of glucose fails to influence substantially the course of protein breakdown. Positive nitrogen balance or even a substantial reduction in net nitrogen losses is achieved only by providing an exogenous source of amino acids as well as sufficient calories (in the form of carbohydrate and/or fat) to meet the increased energy demands of catabolic states.

Accelerated Starvation: Alcoholic Ketoacidosis and Alcohol-Induced Hypoglycemia. The response to nutritional deprivation in normal man not only is directed at minimizing protein losses but also involves a limitation of ketone acid (beta-hydroxybutyrate and acetoacetate) production so as to avoid metabolic acidosis. In addition, continuous production of glucose assures the maintenance of blood glucose concentrations above the hypoglycemic range. During periods of total starvation extending for several days to weeks in healthy subjects, ketone acid accumulation in blood does not exceed 8 mM per liter, serum bicarbonate remains above 14 mEq per liter, and blood glucose concentration remains above 50 mg per 100 ml. In contrast, in alcoholic patients, particularly after binge drinking and protracted vomiting, starvation-induced metabolic acidosis (caused by excessive ketone acid accumulation) and/or hypoglycemia may be observed. Clinically, patients with alcoholic ketoacidosis present in a comatose state or are alert but appear acutely ill and have rapid, deep respirations. Arterial pH is reduced to less than 7.2, and an increased anion gap is observed. In about 25 per cent of cases the blood glucose level is less than 50 mg per 100 ml. The nature of the metabolic acidosis is often not recognized or is mistakenly attributed to lactate, since the semiquantitative nitroprusside reaction for ketones (Acetest, Ketostix, Ames Co.) is often only faintly positive. The failure to detect the extent of ketonemia is due to the high ratio of betahydroxybutyrate (which is not detected in the nitroprusside test) to acetoacetate. The mechanism whereby alcohol accelerates the ketotic response to starvation involves augmented lipolysis and altered intramitochondrial oxidative pathways. In most instances a prompt clinical response follows the administration of parenteral fluids containing glucose.

Alcohol-induced hypoglycemia is observed in circumstances in which liver glycogen stores have been depleted by a period of one or more days of food abstinence or vomiting. Alcohol interferes with glucose homeostasis by inhibiting hepatic gluconeogenesis from lactate, pyruvate, and amino acids. This effect is mediated by changes in cytoplasmic redox (i.e., an increase in hepatic NADH) that accompany the metabolic degradation of alcohol. The hypoglycemic action of alcohol therefore does not become apparent until glycogen stores have been exhausted, and maintenance of the glucose supply to the brain is solely dependent on gluconeogenic processes. Consequently, this disorder is most likely to be encountered in the chronic alcoholic who has been eating poorly or has had protracted vomiting. In addition to the usual signs and symptoms of hypoglycemia, alcohol hypoglycemia is frequently accompanied by hypothermia. In contrast to insulin-induced hypoglycemia, glucagon is ineffective in raising the blood sugar level since glycogen reserves have already been depleted. As in the case of ketoacidosis, patients promptly respond to infusion of glucose.

727. PARENTERAL NUTRITION

The problem of assuring nutritional maintenance or minimizing losses in body composition in association with acute or chronic disease is particularly challenging in patients in whom feeding via the gastrointestinal route is precluded. Until recently the primary focus in parenteral nutrition has been mainly on water and electrolyte replacement with little emphasis on meeting total caloric and protein requirements. The development of new techniques involving the infusion of markedly hypertonic solutions containing glucose and amino acids (parenteral hyperalimentation) has revolutionized the field of parenteral nutrition. Weight gain and positive nitrogen balance are now attainable goals in patients fed intravenously. However, total parenteral nutrition is not without morbidity (as noted below, a variety of infectious and metabolic complications have been described), and consequently is not indicated for all patients in whom oral or tube feeding cannot be maintained. The factors determining the composition, tonicity, and volume of fluid to be administered will depend in large part on whether feeding via the intravenous route must be sustained for a relatively brief period of up to a week or whether one is dealing with a prolonged period of parenteral alimentation. In the former instance the goal is primarily to minimize losses in body composition, whereas in the long-term situation the objective is positive caloric and protein balance to facilitate repair and healing of inflamed or traumatized tissue and to hasten convalescence.

Short-Term Intravenous Nutrition. In the patient requiring intravenous feeding for a period of several days, treatment is directed at providing sufficient carbohydrate to meet cerebral glucose requirements without depleting liver glycogen stores. In this manner, the need for gluconeogenesis and its attendant dissolution of body protein is minimized. Simultaneously, the glucose infusion prevents the fall in serum insulin levels which would otherwise occur in a nonfed individual, thereby inhibiting the development of starvation ketosis. These protein-sparing and antiketogenic effects are achieved with as little as 100 grams of carbohydrate, which may be infused over 24 hours as 2 liters of a 5 per cent dextrose solution. The net effect of the conventional glucose infusion is not one of stimulation of glucose uptake by muscle or fat tissue, but inhibition of hepatic glycogenolysis and replacement of the liver (by the infusion) as the source of glucose for brain oxidative requirements. Such an infusion doubles circulating insulin levels (as compared to the five- to tenfold increase observed after a carbohydrate meal) and elevates blood glucose by 15 to 30 mg per 100 ml. Increasing the amount of glucose infused above 100 grams per day will not further reduce the small degree of protein catabolism which persists in nonfed patients, unless one achieves caloric balance by administering markedly hypertonic solutions (see below).

An alternative form of carbohydrate available in commercial parenteral fluids is fructose. There is no evidence, however, that fructose has any advantage over glucose. Furthermore, rapid administration of large amounts of fructose (0.5 gram per kilogram per hour) can result in the development of lactic acidosis.

In addition to meeting nutritional needs, the major goal in short-term intravenous therapy is the maintenance of fluid and electrolyte balance. Basal fluid requirements may be estimated at 2000 ml per day, which consists of (1) 800 ml to provide for insensible losses via the lungs and skin and sensible losses as sweat, and (2) 1200 ml to maintain a reasonable urine output. The electrolyte requirements are in the form of sodium and potassium. Although the urine will become free of sodium after five to eight days of total sodium restriction, negative sodium balance (and the possibility of plasma volume contraction) will prevail during this interval if exogenous sodium is not provided. The usual intake of sodium in the diet is 4 to 6 grams (174 to 261 mEq), which is ingested as 10 to 12 grams of NaCl. Sodium depletion can be readily prevented in normal man by infusing 500 ml of isotonic (0.9 per cent) sodium chloride containing 77 mEq of NaCl. Potassium supplementation is also necessary, because there is an obligatory daily loss of about 40 mEq per day.

The total carbohydrate, fluid, and electrolyte requirements during short-term intravenous therapy may thus be met with the following daily infusion regimen: 1500 ml of 5 per cent dextrose in water containing 40 mEq KCl; and 500 ml of 5 per cent dextrose in isotonic (0.9 per cent) saline.

It should be noted that this regimen is designed to meet basal fluid and electrolyte requirements in patients without cardiac or renal failure and does not take into account pre-existing deficits or abnormal losses. For the modifications necessary to meet problems of hydration and electrolyte imbalance, see Ch. 805.

Long-Term Intravenous Nutrition (Total Parenteral Nutrition, Parenteral Hyperalimentation). In circumstances requiring long-term intravenous nutrition, particularly in debilitated patients, the optimal goal is positive nitrogen balance and weight gain. The infusion program outlined above for short-term therapy is obviously nutritionally inadequate in that it provides only 400 calories and no amino acids. Although protein hydrolysates have been available for over 30 years, a major problem has been the provision by parenteral means of an adequate amount of calories (2500 or more calories per day) to promote anabolism. Fat emulsions providing 9 calories per gram are potentially the most efficient energy source; however, none are currently approved for clinical use in the United States. Ethyl alcohol (7 calories per gram) is also a relatively efficient source of calories, but the toxic effects associated with infusion of alcohol limit its usefulness. The achievement of caloric balance by infusion of carbohydrate (4 calories per gram) necessitates

the infusion of massive amounts of isotonic or moderately hypertonic fluid (6 liters of a 10 per cent solution), or, alternatively, the infusion of hypertonic solutions (20 to 25 per cent or four to five times the tonicity of plasma). The former regimen results in problems of fluid overload, whereas the latter approach leads to thrombosis of peripheral veins. These difficulties in providing adequate calories were solved by Dudrick and his colleagues with their introduction of parenteral hyperalimentation, a technique involving placement of a catheter in the superior vena cava followed by infusion of a hypertonic glucose–amino acid mixture.

Indications. Although total parenteral nutrition has been applied in a variety of clinical conditions, its usefulness has been documented in specific circumstances only. Furthermore, this technique involves a serious risk (in view of the complications enumerated below), and should be restricted to patients in whom a definite indication exists. The following disorders are likely to benefit from this form of therapy: (1) Gastrointestinal disorders, particularly chronic inflammatory bowel disease (regional enteritis, ulcerative colitis) complicated by fistula formation; the "short bowel syndrome" after extensive intestinal resection; and congenital lesions of the gastrointestinal tract amenable to surgical repair. (2) Extensive body burns and traumatic injuries in which caloric requirements are markedly increased. In such cases parenteral nutrition may be used as a supplement to oral feeding. (3) Acute renal failure. Over-all mortality and duration of azotemia have been demonstrated to decrease in patients with acute renal failure treated with a mixture of glucose and 1.8 per cent essential amino acids.

It should be emphasized that neither the presence of an acute focal, septic condition nor the requirement to "put the alimentary tract at rest" is a sufficient indication for this form of treatment.

Composition of Solutions. A variety of hypertonic glucose and amino acid mixtures are currently available in commercial form. The solution to be administered is generally prepared by mixing 500 to 600 ml of the commercial protein hydrolysate or synthetic amino acid mixture with 400 to 500 ml of 50 per cent dextrose. The resulting solution should provide 900 to 1200 calories per liter. The recommended concentrations of nutrients and electrolytes in the infusate are shown in Table 3. Inasmuch as commercial preparations vary markedly in their content of sodium, potassium, and phosphate, supplemental electrolytes may have to be added to the infusate to achieve desired concentrations. Particular attention should be focused on administration of adequate phosphate, inasmuch as the phosphate requirement in parenterally alimented patients may exceed the 40 mEq per day recommended in patients fed via the oral route. The concentrations of nutrients shown in Table 3 do not apply to patients in renal failure or with congestive heart failure. In the former circumstance, a sodium-free solution containing only essential amino acids (1.8 per cent) is employed. In cardiac failure the sodium content of the infusate is reduced to 20 mEq per liter or less.

Solution Administration and Patient Management. Because of the hypertonicity of the infusate, rapid dilution of the infusion mixture by high blood flow is necessary to prevent phlebitis or thrombosis. Consequently total parenteral nutrition necessitates administration of nutrient solutions through a catheter in the superior vena cava. The latter may be cannulated via an infra-

TABLE 3. Nutrient Concentration in Hypertonic Solutions Used in Total Parenteral Nutrition*

Glucose	200–250 grams
Protein hydrolyzate or synthetic amino acids	30–50 grams
Calories	920–1200 kcal
Sodium	40–50 mEq
Potassium	30–40 mEq
Calcium	5–10 mEq
Magnesium	4–8 mEq
Phosphate	15–20 mEq
Multivitamin concentrate†	2 ml

*Expressed per liter of infusate.
†Vitamin K and folic acid which are not present in the multivitamin concentrate are administered by intramuscular injection.

clavicular percutaneous subclavian vein puncture. Alternatively, a surgical cutdown may be performed with exposure of a peripheral vein through which the catheter is threaded to the superior vena cava. Strict asepsis must be used in inserting and maintaining catheters. The dressing over the puncture site should be changed every two to three days and an antibiotic ointment reapplied.

The solution is initially administered at a rate of 2 liters per day, and thereafter is gradually increased to 3 liters per day. In dealing with a markedly catabolic state, 4 to 5 liters may be administered. The solution should be infused at a constant rate over the entire 24-hour period.

While the patient is receiving total parenteral nutrition, a number of laboratory parameters should be followed so as to prevent or minimize metabolic complications. Fluid intake and output, body weight, and fractional urine glucose concentrations should be recorded daily. Blood sugar, blood urea nitrogen, electrolytes, and calcium and phosphate concentration should be determined at two- to three-day intervals. The importance of such monitoring is obvious from the complications reported in patients infused with hypertonic solutions.

Complications. Total parenteral nutrition is not without risk to the patient. The reported complications relate to either infection or metabolic disorders.

SEPSIS. This is the most frequently observed complication; it may occur in 25 per cent or more of patients. Fungemia caused by *Candida albicans* accounts for half the cases, with the remainder attributable to *Staphylococcus aureus* and *Klebsiella aerobacter.* In most instances the organism can be cultured from the catheter tip, implicating the catheter as the source of sepsis. Factors which may predispose to sepsis are prior antimicrobial use, the nutrient content of the infusate (which may serve as growth medium), and possible adverse effects of hypertonicity on phagocytic function. The incidence of septicemia may be reduced by placing an on-line membrane filter of 0.22 μ pore size in the infusion apparatus, frequent changing of the catheter, and meticulous care of the skin puncture site.

HYPERGLYCEMIA. In patients with normal pancreatic islet cell function, the dextrose-rich infusate invokes a hyperinsulinemic response which permits disposal of the administered glucose load without the development of hyperglycemia in excess of 200 mg per 100 ml. In patients with a predisposition to diabetes, the islet cell response is inadequate and hyperglycemia and glycosuria develop. In some instances this may take the form of *hyperglycemic nonketotic hyperosmolar coma* in which the blood glucose reaches levels of 1000 mg per 100 ml and is accompanied by dehydration, azotemia, obtundation, and occasionally seizures. Such patients should be treated with rapid-acting insulin intravenously and large volumes of water containing 2.5 per cent glucose. The development of a severe hyperosmolar state can generally be prevented by frequent monitoring of the urine and blood glucose levels and by administering insulin in doses of 10 to 20 units to patients with persistent hyperglycemia (above 200 mg per 100 ml) and glycosuria.

POSTINFUSION HYPOGLYCEMIA. If the intravenous infusion is suddenly dislodged or discontinued, a rapid fall in blood glucose occurs which may reach hypoglycemic levels. Presumably this is due to persistence of hyperinsulinemia and suppression of counter-regulatory hormones (glucagon, epinephrine, growth hormone, cortisol). This complication may be avoided by maintaining a constant infusion rate and by switching to a solution containing 5 per cent glucose several hours before terminating the infusion.

HYPOPHOSPHATEMIA. A decline in serum phosphate concentration to levels less than 1 mg per 100 ml is almost uniformly observed after hyperalimentation with phosphate-free solutions for periods of seven to ten days. Accompanying the hypophosphatemia is a decline in red cell levels of 2,3-diphosphoglycerate and an increase in red cell oxygen affinity as indicated by a left-shift in the oxygen dissociation curve. The clinical picture consists of circumoral paresthesias, obtundation, hyperventilation, and, in severe cases, seizures and coma. The hypophosphatemia is not due to urinary losses but is probably a consequence of shifts in body phosphate. Insulin-mediated glucose uptake in muscle and liver brought about by the hypertonic glucose infusion is accompanied by phosphate deposition in these tissues. This redistribution apparently occurs at the expense of plasma and red cell phosphate reserves. The syndrome may be prevented by adding phosphate supplements to the nutrient solution; in debilitated patients the requirement may be as high as 20 to 25 mEq per liter.

HYPERCHLOREMIC ACIDOSIS. In patients receiving synthetic amino acid mixtures rather than protein hydrolysates, the concentration of cationic amino acids (histidine, arginine, lysine) is substantially greater than that of metabolizable anions as reflected in a large cation gap. These cationic amino acids contribute hydrogen ions (thereby lowering blood pH) and chloride to body fluids upon conversion to urea or incorporation into peptide chains. The resulting effect is hyperchloremic metabolic acidosis. This syndrome may be prevented by adding a portion of the sodium supplements to the infusate in the form of bicarbonate rather than chloride when using synthetic amino acid mixtures.

HYPERAMMONEMIA. Abnormally elevated concentrations of blood ammonia have been reported in premature infants and in adults with liver disease receiving infusions containing casein or fibrin hydrolysates. It is probably due to an inability to metabolize preformed ammonia which may account for as much as 8 to 10 per cent of the total nitrogen content in protein hydrolysate solutions. This complication can be prevented or minimized by utilizing synthetic amino acid mixtures in patients with liver disease and in premature infants.

728. DIET THERAPY

Diets are employed in the care of the sick for the following purposes: (1) to regulate (either decrease or increase) the total caloric intake; (2) to restrict (or less frequently augment) the content of specific nutrients, such as protein, fat, sodium, or potassium; (3) to provide foods which are bland in flavor, as in patients with peptic ulcer disease; (4) to reduce fiber content, as in disorders characterized by chronic diarrhea; (5) to eliminate specific foods, as in allergic conditions; and (6) to modify the consistency of foods, as in "soft" or "liquid" diets. Here we will consider specific conditions (diabetes, obesity) and diets in which the treatment program is restrictive in total calories and/or specific nutrients (protein, carbohydrate, sodium, potassium). The use of bland or fiber-restricted diets is discussed in Ch. 637. The dietary treatment of hyperlipidemias is described in Ch. 723.

In prescribing a diet it is important to recognize not only the therapeutic goals but also the likelihood of patient acceptance. The patient's likes and dislikes as well as cultural, sociologic, and economic factors must all be considered. For example, the high protein, low carbohydrate diet advocated by some in the treatment of obesity has been referred to as a "rich man's diet," since the cost of a diet made up primarily of foods high in protein content (meat, fish) may be prohibitively expensive. On the other hand, diet treatment based on an extremely restrictive protein content (20 grams) may fail because the basic unpalatability and limited food selection result in noncompliance.

A second factor to be considered in the make-up of a diet is the influence of restriction of one nutrient on the availability of other dietary components. A diet which is extremely low in sodium (250 mg) requires restriction in protein intake inasmuch as unlimited ingestion of milk or meat will increase the sodium content of the diet. The use of such a diet for the patient with chronic congestive heart failure may contribute to mobilization of edema fluid, but at the expense of a depletion in lean body mass. Similarly, a diet low in protein (20 to 40 grams) as used in cirrhotic patients with portal-systemic shunting and in renal disease will generally be calorically inadequate. Caloric balance can only be achieved by means of a very high intake of carbohydrate in the form of concentrated sweets, which may cause difficulty if there is an associated diabetic tendency. Deficiencies in vitamins are also likely to occur on severely restrictive diets but are more readily corrected by giving a single multivitamin tablet daily.

A third principle requiring emphasis is the requirement for precision in nomenclature and the need for close communication between the physician and dietician. The term "diabetic diet" has no meaning as such. However, a prescription for a 1900-calorie, 200-gram carbohydrate, 80-gram protein, and 90-gram fat diet is readily interpretable. Similarly, a "low salt diet" does not specify the precise level of sodium restriction as indicated by a "500-mg sodium diet." Few physicians have adequate knowledge of nutrition to construct a palatable and effective diet. On the other hand, the dietician, even when given a precise diet order, may not be aware of the therapeutic priorities for a particular patient. Communication between the physician and dietician will permit the minor modifications which may transform an unpalatable regimen into an acceptable program. For ex-

ample, in the case of the patient in chronic renal failure on a restricted protein, sodium, and potassium intake, it is important for the dietician to know which nutrient may be most safely liberalized so as to improve patient acceptance without imposing serious difficulties in overall management.

The Normal Diet. In prescribing a therapeutic diet it is useful to begin by considering the normal diet. In an individual with a stable body weight and no marked shifts in body fluid, caloric intake equals caloric expenditure. As indicated in Table 2, the caloric requirements in a 70-kg man engaged in moderate activity are approximately 2500 to 2800 calories per day. In the "average" diet consumed in the United States, 15 per cent of these calories are derived from protein, 45 to 50 per cent are in the form of carbohydrate, and the remaining 35 to 40 per cent are derived from fat.

The normal diet can also be defined in terms of the relative contributions of six basic food groups (Table 4). Each of these basic food groups has a specific content of calories, protein, fat, and carbohydrate. In addition, for each of these groups an "exchange list" may be prepared, in which all of the specific food items of approximately equal carbohydrate, protein, and fat value are grouped. In this manner it becomes relatively simple to determine which foods are to be eliminated or reduced when intake of a specific nutrient is restricted. For example, it is clear that a diet low in protein entails a restriction in milk and meat. It is also obvious that a reduction in total calories can be achieved by substituting nonfat milk for whole milk and by restricting fat intake, while increasing vegetables (group A) as desired. It should be noted that certain vegetables such as potatoes, beans, peas, and corn are placed in the "bread group" because of their relatively high content of carbohydrate. The use of exchange lists, which is the fundamental tactic employed by the dietician in constructing a specific diet, is also extremely helpful to the patient in that it allows variety in food choices while maintaining specific nutritional guidelines.

Diabetes Mellitus. The fundamental role of diet in the management of diabetes is well recognized. Nevertheless, the specific principles involved in diet therapy have been poorly understood. The generally held notion is that carbohydrate is bad for people with diabetes and that a "diabetic diet" is a carbohydrate-restricted diet. In fact, the major emphasis in diet treatment in the diabetic should be directed at the following points in decreasing order of priority:

1. Regulation of total caloric intake so as to achieve an ideal body weight. For the maturity-onset diabetic in whom the incidence of obesity is 60 per cent or more, this generally entails a reduction in caloric intake. The importance of weight reduction in these patients is based upon the fact that obesity results in resistance to endogenous insulin; this is reversed by a return to ideal weight. With restoration to normal weight, the demand for endogenous insulin is reduced and an improvement in glucose tolerance will ensue. In contrast to the obese, maturity-onset diabetic, a hypercaloric intake is indicated in the thin, wasted insulin-dependent diabetic, particularly in childhood. Such patients require an increase in calories to restore body fat and protein and to permit normal growth.

2. The total carbohydrate content of the diet should not be disproportionately restricted, but the intake of concentrated sweets (candies, table sugar, pastries)

TABLE 4. Nutritive Values for Food Groups*

Food Group	Serving	Weight (grams)	Calories	Carbo-hydrate (grams)	Fat (grams)	Protein (grams)	Sodium (mg)	Potassium (mg)
1. Milk								
Whole milk	1 cup	240	170	12	10	8	120	335
Nonfat milk	1 cup	240	80	12	–	8	120	335
Low-sodium milk	1 cup	240	170	12	10	8	7	600
2. Meat								
Lean meat or fish	3 oz	90	219	–	15	21	75	300
Egg	1	50	73	–	5	7	60	65
3. Vegetables								
Group A†	1/2 cup	100	2-8	–	–	0.5-2.0	9	100-250
Group B‡	1/2 cup	100	35	7	–	2	9	100-200
4. Fruits	1/2 cup	100	40	10	–	0-1.0	2	75-250
5. Bread§								
Regular	1 slice	30	68	15	–	2	160	30
Low-sodium	1 slice	30	68	15	–	2	5	30
Low protein and low electrolyte	1 slice	30	68	17	–	0.1	9	3
Potatoes	1 small	100	68	15	–	2	4	407
Spaghetti	1/2 cup	100	68	15	–	2	1	61
6. Fat								
Butter, unsalted	1 tsp	5	45	–	5	–	–	–
Butter, salted	1 tsp	5	45	–	5	–	50	–

*Based on the Manual of Diets, Departments of Dietetics, Hospital of St. Raphael, Veterans Administration Hospital, and Yale–New Haven Hospital, New Haven, Connecticut, 1972.

†Includes all vegetables not listed in Group B or classified in "bread" group.

‡Beets, carrots, onions, green peas, turnips, squash.

§Includes high carbohydrate vegetables (potatoes, beans, and corn), cereals, and noodle products.

should be limited. There is no compelling evidence that isocaloric reduction in the carbohydrate content to 30 per cent results in improvement of the diabetic state. Such an approach may be deleterious in the long run, because the calories not taken as carbohydrate are generally made up in the form of a high fat intake which may have an adverse effect in accelerating atherosclerosis. Once the appropriate caloric intake has been determined, approximately 45 per cent of the calories should be provided in the form of carbohydrate. An exception is the diabetic with a carbohydrate-inducible (Type III or Type IV) form of hyperlipidemia, in whom a low carbohydrate, high fat intake is indicated (see Ch. 723). To avoid marked swings in the blood glucose concentration, particularly in insulin-dependent diabetics, simple sugars in the form of concentrated sweets should be avoided. Instead the carbohydrate in the diet should be primarily in the form of complex carbohydrates or starches (such as potatoes, beans, bread, and noodle products), because the glucose derived from these foods is released more slowly into the bloodstream.

3. Day-to-day regularity of food intake with respect to total consumption of calories and carbohydrates and with regard to the timing of meals is of importance in insulin-dependent diabetics so as to prevent insulin-induced hypoglycemia. An increase in the number and frequency of feedings in the form of a mid-morning, afternoon, and bedtime snack is also helpful in this regard. The regularity and frequency of feedings are predicated on the fact that, in contrast to the normal subject in whom insulin secretion is dictated by food ingestion, the insulin-dependent diabetic must match his food intake to the continuing action of injected insulin. The consistency in the pattern of food ingestion does not apply on those days in which there is a marked increase in caloric ex-

penditure as a consequence of moderate to severe exercise. In normal subjects exercise causes an inhibition in beta cell secretion, resulting in a fall in endogenous insulin levels which permits an increase in hepatic glucose output. In the diabetic subject receiving insulin injections such homeostatic changes in circulating insulin levels will not occur in response to exercise. Here, extra food should be taken so as to meet the needs of contracting muscles and to prevent hypoglycemia.

Dietary management in diabetes must be related to the two primary types of the disease. In the obese, adult-onset diabetic the primary goal is a hypocaloric intake and weight reduction. In the insulin-dependent diabetic the major dietary objective is regularity of food ingestion so as to prevent hypoglycemia. Despite the simplicity of these principles, less than 50 per cent of the diabetic population adheres to the recommended dietary regimen. Poor understanding on the part of the patient as well as the physician with respect to dietary goals and tactics is frequently responsible for failure. Often the basic prescription is clearly in error and unsuitable for the specific patient. For example, to many physicians a "diabetic diet" almost by definition means an 1800-calorie intake. Such a diet in a vigorous, nonobese 160 pound insulin-dependent diabetic is obviously too restrictive and is likely to have adverse consequences: (1) the patient will not follow the diet and will supplement his intake, generally with concentrated sweets, resulting in marked swings in the blood glucose; or (2) he may stick to the diet but will develop hypoglycemic episodes and/or lose weight. An 1800-calorie diet is equally inappropriate in the 180 pound, 5 foot 2 inch, 50-year-old, sedentary, noninsulin-dependent diabetic woman, in whom the major objective should be weight reduction by means of a more limited caloric intake.

Diet treatment is also useful in the prevention of diabetes. The most important nutritional factor contributing to the development of diabetes is obesity, irrespective of the ratio of individual foodstuffs in the diet. The notion that an increased intake of concentrated carbohydrate is in itself a major causative factor in diabetes has not been substantiated. Thus in patients with a predisposition to diabetes (e.g., strong family history; mothers with a history of large babies), the emphasis should be on *total caloric regulation* so as to prevent obesity rather than on disproportionate restriction in carbohydrate intake.

Obesity. The situation in which diets are most commonly used in the general population is in obesity (see Ch. 723). A wide variety of "fad" diets have been heralded in the lay press (water diet, grapefruit diet, the low carbohydrate "diet revolution," etc.). Unfortunately none of these provides more rapid weight loss or a greater likelihood for long-term success than is achieved by more conventional caloric restriction. To be particularly condemned is the practice of restricting carbohydrate intake to virtually zero while permitting unlimited ingestion of fat. Such a diet will cause ketosis and hyperuricemia and will result in weight loss only so long as total calories as well as carbohydrate are restricted. On the other hand, if fat intake is increased to high levels, weight loss will not occur, and the tendency toward hyperlipidemia may be exaggerated.

Generally, the most appropriate dietary approach to obesity is to restrict total caloric intake to 1000 to 1400 calories per day, while maintaining the protein contribution at 20 per cent or more. In this manner the amount of bulk in the diet is increased, thereby prolonging the amount of time spent on eating and providing the patient with more oral gratification.

A major cause for the failure of diet treatment in obesity is the patient's loss of motivation because of his expectation of totally unrealistic results (e.g., continued weight reduction at a rate of 4 pounds or more per week). It is therefore imperative that the following points be stressed to the patient: (1) Weight loss is most rapid in the first one to two weeks as a consequence of an initial (hypocaloric-induced) diuresis. (2) Subsequent weight loss will be dictated by the caloric value of the tissue lost (adipose tissue) and the extent of negative caloric balance. (3) Adipose tissue has a caloric value of 3500 calories per pound. (4) It is unlikely that on a long-term basis intake can be adequately restricted and/or activity substantially increased to achieve a negative caloric balance of greater than 500 calories per day. (5) The expected rate of weight loss should therefore be no greater than approximately 1 pound per week.

Protein-Restricted Diets. Protein, as noted above, contributes approximately 15 per cent of the total calories consumed in the American diet. The daily intake of protein by healthy adults in the United States varies between 70 and 125 grams, averaging about 100 grams. Diets in which protein content is restricted to 60 grams or less are frequently used in the treatment of chronic renal failure (see Ch. 603) and to a lesser extent in the management of patients with cirrhosis of the liver complicated by portal hypertension. In these conditions the concomitant requirement to limit the intake of sodium and (in patients with renal disease) restrict the ingestion of potassium complicates the over-all nutritional approach.

Since it has long been recognized that dietary protein contributes to the endogenous pool of urea, diets low in protein have been advocated in the treatment of acute or chronic renal disease for over 50 years. The nutritional management of renal disease gained impetus, however, after the classic observations by Giordano and Giovannetti in the early 1960's that patients with chronic renal failure achieved symptomatic relief, a decrease in blood urea nitrogen, and positive nitrogen balance when essential amino acid requirements were met by providing no more than 20 grams of dietary protein. This limited intake of nitrogen could be either in the form of natural foods containing proteins of high biologic value or as a synthetic mixture of essential amino acids. The principle is that with adequate calories and minimal requirements for essential amino acids, retained nitrogen, principally in the form of urea, can be used for the synthesis of nonessential amino acids which are then incorporated into tissue proteins. In this manner the accumulation of urea is reduced, and, to the extent that breakdown products of nitrogen metabolism contribute to the symptoms of uremia (nausea, vomiting, anorexia), clinical improvement is obtained. The extrarenal metabolism of urea and its incorporation into protein have subsequently been confirmed by a variety of techniques. In fact, recent data indicate that urea utilization can be further stimulated and dietary nitrogen requirements can be further reduced by feeding patients the alpha-keto analogues of the essential amino acids.

Despite its rational basis and initially enthusiastic reception, the over-all usefulness and frequency of implementation of the Giordano-Giovannetti diet are currently rather limited. It was early recognized that dietary manipulation provided symptomatic relief but in no way improved underlying renal function. Second, the increasing use of dialysis and renal transplantation programs lessened the need for purely symptomatic maneuvers. Third, implementation of the diet has proved to be extremely difficult with respect to food preparation and patient acceptance.

In addition to restricting total protein intake, the success of the Giordano-Giovannetti diet depends on two additional constraints: (1) the protein ingested must be of high biologic value; and (2) the caloric intake must be maintained at 2000 to 3000 calories per day. The biologic value or quality of food proteins is an index of the efficiency with which these foodstuffs can be used for anabolic processes and is dependent on the amounts and ratios of the constituent essential amino acids. Proteins such as eggs, meat, fish, and milk are of high biologic value since they can meet the essential amino acid requirements when supplied in minimal quantities. In contrast, bread, cereals, fruits, and vegetables contain significant amounts of protein (Table 4), but are lacking in one or more essential amino acids and consequently are of low biologic value. Formulation of a 20-gram protein diet thus involves the administration of one egg (or 1 ounce of meat, cheese, or fish) plus three fourths of a cup of milk (to provide 14 grams of high quality protein) plus one serving each of a fruit and vegetable. To provide the patient with an adequate amount of calories without increasing protein content, it is necessary to add to the diet low-protein bread, biscuits, and noodle products which are specially prepared from wheat starch (rather than wheat flour). A major problem is the lack of palatability and difficulty in preparation of such a diet. The result is poor compliance and often an angry, frustrated patient with a limited caloric intake and progressive wasting of lean body mass.

To meet the twin goals of symptomatic improvement plus maintenance of body protein reserves in chronic renal disease, a more moderate degree of protein restriction than that in the 20-gram protein diet is generally recommended. In *symptomatic* patients (i.e., patients with nausea, anorexia, or vomiting) in whom glomerular filtration rate (GFR) is between 5 and 10 ml per minute, dietary management consists of a 40-gram protein intake, composed primarily of high quality protein. In patients with a GFR below 5 ml per minute who fail to achieve relief with a 40-gram intake, the 20-gram protein diet is used while awaiting initiation of dialysis treatment or transplantation. The 20-gram protein diet should be used on a long-term basis only in circumstances in which dialysis is unavailable or impracticable. Institution of chronic dialysis treatment should not be delayed solely because a symptomatic response has been obtained while the patient is on a 20-gram protein intake. In patients on dialysis treatment, the recommendations regarding dietary protein content vary from 40 to 80 grams per day. The general trend at present is toward more liberalized protein intake so as to ensure adequate caloric ingestion and avoidance of wastage of lean body tissue.

In addition to reducing protein ingestion, a restriction in sodium (see below) and potassium content of the diet is generally necessary in patients with renal failure. The average intake of potassium in the normal diet is 3000 mg per day. In renal failure potassium ingestion is generally reduced to levels of 1000 to 2000 mg. Because potassium is so widely distributed in foods (Table 4), restriction in potassium becomes an important factor limiting the palatability and choice of foods. Since fruits and vegetables are quite variable with respect to their potassium content, diet planning is facilitated by grouping these foods on the basis of their potassium content (Table 5). It should be noted that the number of permissible foods can be increased by extracting their potassium content during preparation. For example, the potassium content of potatoes is 407 mg per serving when prepared in the usual manner, but is greatly reduced by cutting the potatoes into small pieces and boiling in a large volume of water. The caloric value of the protein-potassium restricted diet may be increased with such carbohydrate-rich foods as hard candies, honey, jams, jellies, and granulated sugar. However, chocolate candies should be avoided because of their potassium content.

Sodium Restriction. The intake of sodium in the normal diet ranges between 4 and 6 grams (174 to 261 mEq) per day, ingested primarily in the form of sodium chloride. The sources of sodium in the diet include naturally occurring sodium in foods (Table 4) and sodium added to foods. Among the foods rich in natural sodium are the milk, egg, and meat groups, particularly organ meats and shellfish. Bread is another important source of sodium (160 mg per slice) because of the baking soda and baking powder used in its preparation. Sodium is also added in the canning and freezing of vegetables, as a preservative in the form of sodium benzoate, and as a seasoning in the form of monosodium glutamate. An additional important source of sodium is table salt used at the time of cooking or eating. Each teaspoonful of table salt provides 2000 mg of sodium.

A restricted sodium intake is employed in the management of edematous states such as congestive heart failure, cirrhosis, and renal disease (nephrotic syndrome and oliguric renal failure), and in the treatment of hypertension. Since it is the sodium ion rather than chloride which must be limited in these conditions, and inasmuch as sodium may be present in the diet in a variety of forms (e.g., bicarbonate, glutamate, benzoate, propionate, or chloride), it is inappropriate to characterize diets in terms of *salt* intake. Instead the diet prescription should designate the precise number of *milligrams of sodium* to be provided each day. In general one of four categories of sodium restriction is employed: 2000 to 4000 mg, 1000 mg, 500 mg, and 250 mg.

The 2000 to 4000 mg (87 to 174 mEq) sodium diet represents a mild degree of sodium restriction which is attained by (1) elimination of table salt and sodium-rich seasonings added at meal times and (2) avoidance of salted foods such as pretzels, potato chips, processed meats (bacon, sausages, etc.), and salty fish (anchovies, sardines). Small amounts of salt may be used in cooking with this diet. This level of sodium restriction is useful as a maintenance diet in subjects in whom a diuresis has already been achieved.

A reduction in sodium intake to 1000 mg (43 mEq) requires, in addition to the measures outlined above, the elimination of salt in cooking and the avoidance of canned or frozen fruits and vegetables, unless specially

TABLE 5. Potassium Content of Fruits and Vegetables*

Fruits	Vegetables
Group I (less than 100 mg; average 75 mg) Applesauce, cranberries, pears (canned), pineapple (canned), blueberries (canned)	Group I (100–150 mg) Lettuce, cucumber, onions, cabbage, carrots (canned), corn (canned)
Group II (100–150 mg) Apples (raw or juice), grapefruit, cherries, tangerine, watermelon, pineapple juice, grape juice, peaches (canned)	Group II (150–200 mg) Carrots (raw or cooked), celery, beets, turnips, asparagus (canned), mushrooms (canned)
Group III (150–200 mg) Oranges (raw or juice), grapes, grapefruit juice, fruit cocktail	Group III (200–250) Tomatoes (fresh, canned, or juice), asparagus (fresh or frozen), broccoli, cauliflower, lima beans, spinach
Group IV (greater than 200 mg)† Apricots (canned), bananas, cantaloupe, dates, honeydew melon, prunes (raw or juice), raisins	Group IV (over 250 mg)† Potatoes, artichokes, Brussels sprouts

*Potassium content is given per serving (½ cup or small size for raw fruits such as apples, oranges and pears) and is based on the Manual of Diets, Department of Dietetics, Hospital of St. Raphael, Veterans Administration Hospital, and Yale–New Haven Hospital, New Haven, Connecticut, 1972.
†Fruits and vegetables in Group IV are generally omitted in potassium restricted diets.

processed as low-sodium dietetic foods. The ingestion of foods containing significant amounts of sodium such as regular bread and milk must be limited, generally to three slices and 1 pint per day, respectively. This level of sodium intake is often used when therapy is initiated in edematous patients.

In patients with severe refractory edema, it may be necessary to reduce the level of sodium intake to 500 mg (22 mEq) or less to effect a diuresis. This degree of restriction in sodium (500 mg) requires avoidance of all the foods omitted in the 1000 mg diet, substitution of low sodium bread for regular bread, and strict limitation in the intake of allowable foods (particularly meat, fish, eggs, and milk) to carefully measured amounts. A further reduction in sodium intake to 250 mg (11 mEq) is achieved by substituting low-sodium milk for regular milk. Because of the restriction in choices and amounts of food involved in such diets, it is difficult to maintain an adequate caloric or protein intake or to provide sufficient palatability to assure patient compliance. Con-

sequently, severe sodium restriction (250 or 500 mg diets), particularly on a long-term basis, should be employed only for patients who are clearly refractory to more moderate degrees of sodium restriction.

Cahill, G. F., Jr.: Starvation in man. N. Engl. J. Med., 282:668, 1970.
Cowan, G. S., and Scheetz, W. L.: Intravenous Hyperalimentation. Philadelphia, Lea & Febiger, 1972.
Dudrick, S. J., Macfadyen, B. V., Jr., Van Buren, C. T., Ruberg, R. L., and Maynard, A. T.: Parenteral hyperalimentation. Metabolic problems and solutions. Ann. Surg., 176:259, 1972.
Felig, P., Marliss, E., Owen, O. E., and Cahill, G. F., Jr.: Blood glucose and gluconeogenesis in fasting man. Arch. Intern. Med., 123:293, 1969.
Hyne, B. E. B., Fowell, E., and Lee, H. A.: The effect of caloric intake on nitrogen balance in chronic renal failure. Clin. Sci., 43:679, 1972.
Levy, L. J., Duga, J., Girgis, M., and Gordon, E. E.: Ketoacidosis associated with alcoholism in nondiabetic subjects. Ann. Intern. Med., 78:213, 1973.
Long, C. L., Spencer, J. L., Kinney, J. M., and Geiger, J. W.: Carbohydrate metabolism in man: Effect of elective operations and major surgery. J. Appl. Physiol., 31:110, 1971.
West, K. M.: Diet therapy of diabetes: An analysis of failure. Ann. Intern. Med., 79:425, 1973.

Part XVI
HEMATOLOGIC AND HEMATOPOIETIC DISEASES

729. INTRODUCTION

Ralph L. Nachman

This edition includes a number of new and exciting advances in the area of clinical hematology. Much of this new knowledge, which bears directly on the diagnosis and care of patients with hematologic disease, results from the direct application of the principles of molecular biology to clinical hematologic disorders. This is particularly appropriate since modern molecular biology stems in a real sense from the original observations made over a quarter of a century ago by Pauling on sickle cell hemoglobin. With this growing complexity and sophistication it has become obvious that many of the several areas within hematology have rapidly become the province of superspecialists such as red cell enzymologists, hemoglobinopathy experts, chemotherapists, and clotters. Despite this fragmentation, it is important to note that, although many primary hematologic disorders are relatively rare, hematologic symptoms, signs, and laboratory abnormalities are frequent secondary components of many common clinical disorders. A good history and physical examination still remain the essential prerequisites for adequate evaluation of a hematologic problem. It is true that many clinical hematologic disorders require complicated laboratory procedures before the final diagnosis is verified; it is clear, however, that these studies must be performed as part of an evaluation of the whole patient and not as a fragmented dissection of an isolated organ system.

In the chapters which follow, new information will be presented relating to several different areas which will have a long-range impact on the diagnosis and therapy of hematologic disease. Some of the most important new advances are noted here.

Red cell 2,3-diphosphoglycerate (DPG) plays an important role in the regulation of oxygen dissociation. DPG binds to the beta chains of deoxyhemoglobin and decreases oxygen affinity. As DPG rises, more oxygen is released to the tissue without a change in the tissue oxygen tension. Intraerythrocytic DPG levels thus play an important role in the physiologic adaptation to anoxia and anemia. Patients with severe chronic anemia tolerate very low hemoglobin levels owing to the elevated levels of red cell DPG.

Chronic granulomatous disease of childhood results from an inability of neutrophils to kill certain species of bacteria. The study of this disorder and similar related illnesses has greatly increased our knowledge of intracellular bactericidal mechanisms. Neutrophils generate H_2O_2 which in the presence of halide and the lysosomal enzyme myeloperoxidase kills phagocytized bacteria. Several new clinical disorders have been observed in which other qualitative defects in neutrophil function have been defined.

Viruses continue to play important roles in various hematologic disorders. Epstein-Barr (EB) virus causes infectious mononucleosis in man. The etiologic role of this virus in other lymphoproliferative states such as Burkitt's lymphoma remains to be determined. Considerable information has been accumulated concerning the etiologic role of RNA tumor viruses in a variety of animal cancers. Reverse transcriptase is a well-defined biochemical attribute of these tumor viruses. White cells from leukemic patients have been demonstrated to contain reverse transcriptase, which in the test tube synthesizes DNA homologous to certain tumor virus RNA. The story is inconclusive, but the evidence suggests that in the future viruses may be shown to be the causative agent of some forms of human leukemia.

Chemotherapy of leukemia and the lymphomas has made major strides in recent years. Combination chemotherapy and newer concepts of induction, consolidation, and maintenance have led to significant prolongation of survival in acute lymphocytic leukemia in childhood and in Hodgkin's disease in adults.

Some progress has been made in our understanding of hemorrhagic diseases. The role of the platelet as a first line of defense in hemostasis has been greatly clarified. It seems that this cell also significantly contributes to pathologic processes associated with arterial intimal disease. Much has been learned about the blood coagulation proteins and some of the control mechanisms which regulate the enzymatic conversion of fibrinogen to fibrin. Much interest and work have geen generated by clinical and molecular studies of the factor VIII diseases—hemophilia A and von Willebrand's disease.

These are only a few of the major advances which may well transform the face of clinical hematology in the coming years. It is certain that this is an area of medicine which is bound to substantially change in the next decade.

Section One.   THE ANEMIAS

730. INTRODUCTION

M. C. Brain

The function of the red blood cell is the transport of oxygen from the capillaries in the lungs to the systemic capillaries of the tissues and the facilitation of carbon dioxide transport from the tissues to the lungs. In physiologic terms, anemia can be regarded as a reduction in oxygen transporting capacity of the blood. The normal response to increased demand by the tissues for oxygen is met by an increase in cardiac output, and the symptoms of anemia first become apparent on exercise. Since oxygen is transported by the red blood cell in combination with hemoglobin, the principal protein constituent of the cell, anemia can be most simply and practically defined as a lowering of the hemoglobin concentration of the blood below the normal range for a population of comparable age and sex. However, the definition of anemia solely in terms of whole blood hemoglobin concentration makes several assumptions. First, the whole blood hemoglobin concentration does not take into account the influence of changes in plasma volume, nor does it provide information on the concentration of hemoglobin within the red blood cells, although the latter can be determined from knowledge of the cell count and the packed red cell volume or hematocrit. Second, and physiologically of greater importance, the definition of anemia in terms of hemoglobin concentration might be thought to imply that the hemoglobin concentration is the sole determinant of oxygen delivery by the red blood cells. Recent work on the regulation of the affinity of hemoglobin for oxygen has shown this not to be true. A number of factors are known to influence hemoglobin-oxygen affinity and hence both the amount and rate at which oxygen is released from red blood cells at the lowered partial pressure of oxygen in the systemic capillaries. These factors include blood pH, temperature, the concentration of hemoglobin within the red blood cell (the mean corpuscular hemoglobin concentration [MCHC]), the red blood cell concentration of organic phosphates (principally 2,3-diphosphoglycerate [DPG] and, to a lesser extent, adenosine triphosphate [ATP]) which are products of red cell metabolism, and the presence of genetically determined substitutions in key positions in the polypeptide chains of the hemoglobin molecule. All these factors may either increase or reduce hemoglobin-oxygen affinity and thereby enhance or diminish the amount and rate of oxygen release. Thus the physiologic consequences of anemia must reflect the hemoglobin concentration of the blood and the hemoglobin-oxygen affinity of red blood cells in the circulation. Whereas the hemoglobin concentration of the blood can be readily and rapidly determined, the measurement of hemoglobin-oxygen affinity is less simple. However, changes in hemoglobin-oxygen affinity caused by variations in pH and the MCHC can be readily calculated, as can the effects of DPG and ATP if the concentrations of these compounds in the red blood cell are known. Although changes in hemoglobin-oxygen affinity are rare and are therefore of less clinical importance than changes in hemoglobin concentration, it is important to be aware that they exist, because they may modify the physiologic effects of anemia.

An understanding of the pathologic and physiologic factors which give rise to anemia and its consequences requires an appreciation of the following: (1) the structure and function of the normal red blood cell, (2) the formation of red blood cells in the bone marrow and the factors which regulate erythropoiesis, (3) the disorders which influence the quantity and/or the normal constitution of red blood cells produced by the bone marrow, (4) the factors which influence the distribution and/or survival of red blood cells within the circulation, and (5) the disorders which result in loss of erythrocytes from the circulation.

The mammalian red blood cell is remarkable in that it carries out its function after loss of the nucleus which determined and controlled the synthesis of its constituents. The nucleus is normally extruded from the cell as it enters the circulation by passing into the venous sinuses of the bone marrow. For the first few days after entering the circulation the red blood cell retains cytoplasmic organelles, including mitochondria and ribosomes, and ribonucleic acids, and can be identified with supravital dyes which stain these constituents. The filamentous or reticulin-like pattern of the stained structures gave rise to the term *reticulocyte* for these cells. Once the mitochondria and ribosomes are lost, the cell's capability to synthesize proteins ceases. Thereafter the mature red blood cell has only a limited capacity to reconstitute membrane lipid and other nonlipid cytoplasmic constituents. As a consequence it has a finite life span of approximately 120 days. The maintenance of normal numbers of red blood cells in the circulation is thus dependent on continuous production from precursor cells in the bone marrow. In anemia the number of circulating red blood cells depends upon the capacity of the bone marrow to increase the number produced to compensate for the loss from the circulation—a response which may be ultimately restricted by the limitations imposed by the bony skeleton upon the expansion of the bone marrow within it.

The mature red blood cell is a highly deformable cell which in the resting state assumes the shape of a biconcave disc with an average diameter of 8.4 μ. The biconcave shape is primarily determined by the inherent physical strains within the membrane in relation to the ratio of membrane surface area to volume of the cell. The remarkable deformability of the red blood cell accounts for the low viscosity of blood at high flow rates despite the high proportion of red blood cells present in blood. Furthermore, the deformability enables the cell to pass repeatedly through the capillaries of the microcirculation, some of which have a diameter of 3 μ or less. Reduction in deformability resulting from a change in shape, or from a change in solubility or stability of hemoglobin with the formation of intracellular inclusions, predisposes the red blood cell to selective sequestration in the microcirculation, especially in the spleen, and can lead to shortened survival in the circulation.

Hemoglobin comprises approximately 95 per cent of the dry weight of the red blood cell and on average 34 per cent of the wet weight, the remainder being made up of water, anions, cations (principally potassium), glucose, phosphorylated glycolytic intermediates (principally 2,3-diphosphoglycerate which is present in the same molar concentration as hemoglobin), glutathione, adenosine and pyridine nucleotides, and the enzymes responsible for the metabolism of glucose to lactic acid. Glucose is metabolized by two linked metabolic pathways. The principal function of the Embden-Meyerhof pathway is the formation of ATP which is utilized in maintenance of the normal cation content of the red blood cells through ATP-dependent transport mechanisms, in maintenance of membrane lipid composition, and in cell shape. The hexose monophosphate shunt, the subsidiary pathway of glucose metabolism, is responsible for maintaining glutathione in a reduced state and thereby in protecting the cellular constituents (notably hemoglobin) from oxidative denaturation.

The hemoglobin within the red blood cell is formed of spheroidal molecules of a molecular weight of 64,458. Ninety-seven per cent of the molecule consists of the polypeptide chains of globin, and 3 per cent of the heme groups. Each molecule is formed from four subunits, comprising two pairs of identical polypeptide chains, to each of which is attached a heme group partially buried in the outer aspect of the molecule. In the red blood cells of adults, 97 per cent of the hemoglobin is made up of two α and two β chains and is designated *hemoglobin A. Hemoglobin A_2*, consisting of two α and two δ chains, forms 2 per cent, and *hemoglobin F*, formed from two α and two λ chains, provides the remaining 1 per cent. Hemoglobin F is the principal hemoglobin in the red blood cells of the fetus, and is gradually replaced by hemoglobin A with the onset of β chain synthesis in the last trimester of pregnancy. Hemoglobin F levels fall from birth and reach adult levels by the end of the first year of life. For the red blood cell to contain a normal concentration of hemoglobin requires balanced synthesis of both the α and β chains and of the heme groups by the erythroblasts in the bone marrow. Disorders of hemoglobin constitution and/or concentration within the red blood cell can arise through abnormalities of synthesis either of the globin (polypeptide chain) or of heme groups. Disorders of the constitution of the globin chains are not usually associated with major reductions in the amount of hemoglobin synthesized. Although many genetic variations in the primary amino acid structure of hemoglobin molecule have been recognized, they only become clinically important when such substitutions are at critical sites in the molecule, thereby influencing the function, solubility, or stability of the molecule. Deficient hemoglobin synthesis within the erythroblast can result from failure or imbalance of the synthesis of the polypeptide chains (the thalassemia syndrome), or through disturbances of heme synthesis, commonly caused by lack of iron, and more rarely caused by disorders in the porphyrin synthetic pathway.

The red blood cell formed in the bone marrow is the final stage in a sequence of cell divisions arising from a common multipotential hematopoietic stem cell. This common hematopoietic stem cell gives rise to a number of committed stem cells from which develop the erythroid, granulocyte, and megakaryocyte cell lines. The committed stem cells form a self-regenerating stem cell pool, as well as giving rise to differentiated erythroblasts which undergo three mitotic divisions during the course of maturation to the late normoblast and finally through extrusion of the nucleus to the reticulocyte. The time taken between an erythropoietic stimulus and the outpouring of reticulocytes from the bone marrow is approximately five days. It has long been recognized that anemia or hypoxia stimulates increased erythropoiesis. The response is mediated through the action of a specific erythropoiesis-stimulating hormone, *erythropoietin*. Erythropoietin is a relatively heat-stable glycoprotein with a molecular weight of between 40,000 and 70,000. It has been shown experimentally that erythropoietin stimulates the erythroid stem cell to undergo mitosis and accelerates the rate of cell division of the developing erythroblasts. Raised levels of erythropoietin have been demonstrated in the serum and urine of anemic patients. The primary stimulus to its release into the circulation has been shown to be hypoxia. There is much evidence to suggest that the kidneys are the principal site of erythropoietin formation or release. Destruction or removal of the kidneys is associated with diminished erythropoiesis; yet other organs and tissues must be responsible for erythropoietin formation, because erythropoiesis continues in anephric patients and erythropoietin has been detected in their serum. Although hypoxia is the principal stimulus to erythropoietin release, clinical evidence indicates a greater erythropoietic response to hemolytic anemia than to comparable anemia resulting from blood loss. Thus the products of red blood cell destruction may provide an additional stimulus to erythropoietin release.

The continuous formation of red blood cells from precursor cells within bone marrow is dependent upon both normal bone marrow function and the stimulus of erythropoietin. Disorders of red blood cell formation can arise from diminution of the number of pluripotent hematopoietic stem cells, as in aplastic or hypoplastic anemias, or from disturbances in maturation of the committed erythropoietic stem cell, as in isolated red cell aplasias. In acute and chronic leukemias the disorder of stem cell differentiation will adversely affect erythropoiesis. Similarly, infiltration of the bone marrow by malignant cells arising from other organs or the progressive sclerosis of the bone marrow in myelosclerosis will reduce erythropoiesis. In the latter circumstance, hematopoiesis, including erythropoiesis, may be undertaken at *extramedullary sites* in the body such as the liver and spleen. Erythropoiesis is quantitatively reduced in acute and chronic infections, by chronic inflammatory disorders such as rheumatoid arthritis, and by renal failure. It is influenced by the nutritional status of the individual, being particularly affected by deficiencies of vitamin B_{12}, folic acid, iron, and protein. Vitamin B_{12} and folic acid are essential cofactors in the synthesis of DNA. Deficiency of either one results in impairment of cell division with formation of megaloblasts, macroerythroblasts with defective nuclear maturation, and production of large red blood cells (*macrocytes*). Conversely, deficiency of iron through the impairment of hemoglobin synthesis results in the production of *hypochromic microcytic* (small) red blood cells. Defective hemoglobinization of the red blood cell is also a feature of the defective hemoglobin synthesis resulting from imbalanced globin synthesis of the thalassemia syndromes. Disorders of red blood cell maturation within the bone marrow, whether caused by disorders of cell division as in the megaloblastic anemias or by defective hemoglobin synthesis, are associated with *ineffective erythropoiesis*, a considerable proportion of the abnormal erythroblasts undergoing phagocytic destruction within the bone marrow and therefore failing to gain entry to the circulation. The extent of ineffective erythropoiesis can be assessed by measurement of the rate of clearance of radioactive iron from the plasma and of the proportion of the radioactive iron entering the circulation in labeled hemoglobin. In ineffective erythropoiesis there is rapid clearance of radioactive iron from the plasma, but only 20 to 40 per cent of the iron enters the blood compared with the 70 to 90 per cent in normal subjects. Ineffective erythropoiesis can also be assessed by the early excretion of C^{14}-carbon monoxide and C^{14}-stercobilin derived from the catabolism of newly synthesized heme after the administration of C^{14}-glycine. This latter method has shown that even in normal subjects a small proportion of the newly synthesized heme is catabolized to bilirubin, which may reflect the rapid turnover of nonhemoglobin heme proteins in the liver. In ineffective erythropoiesis the proportion of newly synthesized heme which is catabolized and the products excreted are greatly increased.

Red blood cells entering the circulation are normally uniformly distributed within the circulation, and the hematocrit of the venous blood corresponds closely to the whole-body hematocrit derived from simultaneous measurements of the red blood cell and plasma volumes. The distribution of red blood cells within the circulation is influenced by the spleen. Reticulocytes, until they mature, are preferentially sequestered within the spleen. In conditions which cause massive enlargement of the spleen, such as the congestive splenomegaly of portal hypertension, the proportion of red blood cells sequestered may be greatly increased. The sequestration of red blood cells in the spleen together with the associated increase in plasma volume can result in a lowering of the red blood cell count and hematocrit in the venous blood to produce an apparent anemia, although the red blood cell mass may be normal or only slightly below normal.

Red blood cells normally survive in the circulation for 120 days. The degree of anemia caused by shortened red blood cell survival is governed by the rate of the hemolysis and the ability of the bone marrow to compensate. Hemolytic anemia can usually be recognized by the association of an anemia, in the absence of evidence of blood loss, with an increase in the catabolism of hemoglobin as reflected by hyperbilirubinemia, and by reticulocytosis. Minor degrees of hemolysis accompany many disorders associated with ineffective erythropoiesis. Shortened red blood cell survival may be due to abnormalities inherent to the cell, such as congenital or familial disorders of the membrane, metabolism, or hemoglobin, or may be brought about by the action of extrinsic or environmental factors in the circulation. The latter include the effects of plasma factors (antibodies), the action of drugs or toxins, or changes in the vascular environment through which the red blood cells circulate. The extrinsic factors influencing red blood cell survival in general tend to be acquired rather than congenital or familial in etiology. But this distinction is not always valid, because congenital disorders of metabolism or of hemoglobin may predispose the cell to deleterious action of extrinsic agents such as oxidative drugs.

Loss of red blood cells from the circulation through frank or occult hemorrhage is a common cause of acute or chronic anemia, the degree of anemia reflecting the magnitude and duration of the blood loss and the reduction in body iron stores through loss of hemoglobin from the body. Thus chronic blood loss rapidly produces iron deficiency, with consequent impairment of erythropoiesis by the bone marrow.

The normal range of red blood cell values in adults is shown in Table 1.

The values of the red blood cell count, hemoglobin concentration, and packed cell volume in children between the ages of three months and puberty are approximately 10 to 20 per cent lower than the adult values, the difference being more marked in younger children. The differences between the sexes become apparent only at puberty. The lower values in children probably reflect the diminished affinity of hemoglobin for oxygen in children. Thus the lower red blood cell count and hemoglobin concentration meet the normal physiologic needs for oxygen transport.

CLASSIFICATION

Anemias can be classified according to the etiology of the disorder giving rise to anemia (Table 2) or in relation to the morphologic appearance and quantitative abnormality of red blood cell size (mean corpuscular volume [MCV]), hemoglobin content (MCH), and hemoglobin concentration (MCHC). Any attempt at classification is at best somewhat arbitrary, because in many disorders the degree of anemia and the morphologic appearance of the red blood cell are consequences of the effects of both the primary cause and the erythropoietic response by the bone marrow. Furthermore, it is difficult to combine a

TABLE 2. Anemias: Etiologic Classification

I. Principally caused by impaired production
  A. Disturbances of the proliferation and differentiation of stem cells
    1. Aplastic anemia: idiopathic; due to physical or chemical injury (radiation, benzol, lead, or cytotoxic and other drugs such as chloramphenicol, phenylbutazone, etc.)
    2. Pure red blood cell aplasia
    3. Anemia of chronic renal failure
    4. Endocrine deficiency (pituitary, thyroid, adrenal, or testicular hormones)
  B. Disturbances of proliferation and maturation of differentiated erythroblasts
    1. Defective DNA synthesis (vitamin B_{12}, folic acid, and metabolic defects in purine and pyrimidine metabolism)
    2. Defective hemoglobin synthesis
      a. Deficient globin synthesis (thalassemia)
      b. Deficient heme synthesis (iron deficiency)
      c. Sideroblastic anemia
    3. Protein malnutrition
    4. Anemia of chronic infections or inflammatory or neoplastic disease
    5. Myelophthisic anemias due to bone marrow infiltration or replacement (leukemias, myelofibrosis, Hodgkin's disease, multiple myeloma, metastatic carcinoma, etc.)
II. Principally caused by shortened red blood cell survival (increased rate of destruction)
  A. Intrinsic or red blood cell abnormalities
    1. Membrane disorders
      a. Inherited disorders of cell shape; spherocytosis, elliptocytosis, stomatocytosis
      b. Inherited disorders of membrane lipid synthesis
      c. Paroxysmal nocturnal hemoglobinuria
    2. Disorders of red blood cell metabolism
    3. Congenital or inherited enzyme deficiencies
    4. Disorders of hemoglobin (globin) structure, solubility, and stability (sickle cell anemia, hemoglobin C disease, unstable hemoglobins, etc.)
  B. Extrinsic or extraerythrocytic abnormalities
    1. Plasma factors
      a. Antibody mediated destruction
      b. Disturbance of cholesterol or plasma lipids (abetalipoproteinemia, liver disease)
    2. Physical factors (cardiac, microangiopathic, burns)
    3. Chemical or toxic agents (copper, lead, oxidative drugs: dapsone, phenacetin)
    4. Bacterial or other organisms: (Cl. welchii, malaria)
    5. Reticuloendothelial sequestration (splenomegaly)
III. Anemia of blood loss (acute or chronic)

TABLE 1. Red Cell Values in Adults: Normal Range

	Men	Women
Red blood cells	5.11 ± 0.38	$4.51 \pm 0.36 \times 10^6$ μl blood
Hemoglobin	15.5 ± 1.1	13.7 ± 1.0 gram/100 ml blood
Packed cell volume	46.0 ± 3.1	40.9 ± 3.0 ml/100 ml blood
Mean corpuscular volume	90.0 ± 4.8	90.4 ± 4.8 μm³/red blood cell
Mean corpuscular hemoglobin	30.2 ± 1.8	30.2 ± 1.9 pg/red blood cell
Mean corpuscular hemoglobin concentration	33.9 ± 1.2	33.6 ± 1.1 grams/100 ml red blood cells
Reticulocytes	0.2 to 2.0	0.2 to 2.0 per 100 red blood cells

logical pathophysiologic classification with the expected frequency with which the various etiologies may be encountered, the latter being influenced by the age, racial background, socioeconomic factors, and geographic location of the population encountered.

A classification of anemia on the basis of red blood cell morphology, as seen in the peripheral blood smear and supported by the quantitative measurements of cell size (MCV) and hemoglobin content and concentration (MCH and MCHC), can provide a valuable indication as to the possible etiologic mechanisms (Table 3). The introduction of automatic equipment for the rapid and accurate enumeration of red blood cells and determination of the MCV, MCH, and MCHC has greatly enhanced the diagnostic value of these measurements.

The classification shown in Table 3 fails to include much additional information which can be obtained from examination of stained blood smears. Quantitative data with the emphasis on mean values cannot reflect variations in cell shape, size, or hemoglobin content or cell staining, such as the polychromasia indicative of reticulocytosis. Only examination of the stained smear can lead to the recognition of intracellular inclusions such as *Howell-Jolly bodies* (nuclear remnants indicative of splenectomy or splenic dysfunction), *Pappenheimer bodies* (granules of hemosiderin), *punctate basophilia* (a feature of disorders of hemoglobin synthesis often seen in lead poisoning and in thalassemia), and malarial parasites. Disturbances of cell size *(anisocytosis)*, shape *(poikilocytosis)*, and staining can lead to the recognition of congenital or acquired causes of spherocytosis, of elliptocytosis, or of stomatocytosis. Poikilocytosis is a frequent accompaniment of disordered erythropoiesis, and is associated with disorders of hemoglobin synthesis as in iron deficiency or thalassemia. The abnormal shape of the *sickle cell* was recognized long before the molecular pathology of the sickle cell anemia was understood. Likewise, *target cells* in the absence of macrocytosis may suggest the presence of hemoglobin C. The presence of *red blood cell fragments* in the presence of hemolysis suggests a cardiac or microangiopathic mechanical hemolysis. Variation in hemoglobinization of erythrocytes can suggest partial response to iron therapy, be compatible with recent blood transfusion, or be a feature of the sideroblastic anemias. The recognition of megaloblastic anemia when associated with iron deficiency may not be accompanied by macrocytosis; however, the presence of multilobed polymorphonuclear leukocytes may provide the clue to an underlying vitamin B_{12} or folate deficiency. Likewise, knowledge of the differential white cell count and platelet count can lead to the recognition of hypoplastic anemias, myelophthisic anemias, and leuke-

mic disorders. Further information may be derived from examination of the reticulocyte preparation in the detection of *Heinz bodies* (precipitated denatured hemoglobin) and *hemoglobin H bodies* (β_4 inclusions). It may be helpful to examine a diluted wet preparation of blood in determining the nature of shape changes which can arise from the drying of conventional stained smears. Finally, the presence of intense rouleaux formation may indicate the presence of a paraprotein, whereas frank agglutination can point to the presence of cold-agglutinating antibodies.

Although knowledge of the red blood cell count, hemoglobin concentration, and MCV, MCH, and MCHC provides valuable information as to whether an anemia is macrocytic, normocytic, or microcytic, examination of the blood film can often give a more specific indication of the etiology of the disorder. This in turn can lead to further diagnostic investigations of erythropoiesis, such as a bone marrow biopsy, or of disorders of red blood cell membrane, metabolism, or hemoglobin, including the detection of antibodies on the membrane surface, or to evidence of frank or occult blood loss by appropriate inquiry or investigation.

PRINCIPLES OF THERAPY

As in all conditions, the principles of the treatment of anemia are primarily dependent on recognition of the cause of an anemia and, when possible, the correction of the cause with appropriate treatment. Consideration of the classification of the etiology of anemia provides a useful framework on which to base the principles of treatment. When a cause for aplastic or hypoplastic anemia can be identified, exposure to the agent or agents should cease and an incriminated drug should never again be given to the patient. Heavy metals may be excreted in response to appropriate chelating agents. In general the principal measures are supportive with blood transfusions. Erythropoiesis may be improved by androgenic steroids. Renal failure and endocrine deficiency states should be treated appropriately.

The cause of megaloblastic anemia should be sought and appropriate replacement therapy with either vitamin B_{12} or folic acid given. Neither of these vitamins should be prescribed without clear-cut indications. Among these indications is the folate deficiency associated with increased requirement for this vitamin in pregnancy and in the erythropoietic response to hemolytic anemia. Iron therapy should be given when anemia is recognized as being due to iron deficiency resulting either from inadequate intake or increased demand, as in pregnancy, or from blood loss. Patients with sideroblastic anemia may respond to treatment with pyridoxine. Iron therapy should be avoided in patients with anemia of other causes such as thalassemia or sideroblastic anemia, in both of which the hypochromic anemia may be mistaken for iron deficiency; nor should iron be given to patients with chronic hemolytic anemia. In all these disorders iron therapy can lead to tissue damage through iron overload. In the secondary anemias caused by infective or inflammatory disorders, the anemia only responds to the treatment of the underlying disease. The same is true for the myelophthisic anemias caused by marrow infiltrations. In hemolytic anemias treatment with corticosteroids may be indicated, depending upon the nature of the hemolysis, and splenectomy may be in-

TABLE 3. Anemias: Morphologic Classification

1. Macrocytic (MCV 93 cu mm)
    a. Megaloblastic erythropoiesis (deficiency of vitamin B_{12} or folic acid)
    b. Liver disease and obstructive jaundice
    c. Reticulocytosis
2. Normocytic
    a. Acute blood loss before reticulocytosis
    b. Hemolytic anemia when not associated with spherocytosis
    c. Anemia of chronic disease
3. Microcytic and hypochromic
    a. Iron deficiency
    b. Thalassemia
    c. Sideroblastic anemia

dicated when there is evidence that the spleen is playing a major role in red blood cell destruction. Anemia caused by acute blood loss and the anemias which fail to or cannot be expected to respond to specific hematinics may require blood transfusions. It must be recognized that blood transfusions are not without the risk of serious and sometimes fatal reactions, and that multiple transfusions increase the risk of both serum hepatitis and iron overload. Except for replacement of acute blood loss, the risk of circulatory overload and of transfusion reactions can be reduced by transfusing red blood cell concentrates from which the plasma has been removed. There is little cause to give blood transfusions if the hemoglobin is greater than 10 grams per 100 ml or to endeavor to maintain the hemoglobin above that level. Blood transfusions should be given after a full cross-match, including an indirect Coombs test, has established that the blood to be transfused is compatible. However, in patients with life-threatening autoimmune hemolytic anemia, the most compatible blood should be given despite the presence of a positive indirect Coombs test, because the survival of the transfused cells is likely to be no shorter than that of the patient's own red blood cells, and death from anemia can be prevented until more specific treatment with corticosteroids and/or splenectomy becomes effective.

Finch, C. A., and Lenfant, C.: Oxygen transport in man. N. Engl. J. Med., 286:407, 1972.

Gordon, A. S.: Regulation of Hematopoiesis. Vol. 1, Red Cell Production. New York, Appleton-Century-Crofts, 1970.

Harris, J. W., and Kellermyer, R. W.: The Red Cell Production, Metabolism, Destruction: Normal and Abnormal. 2nd ed. Cambridge, Mass., Harvard University Press, 1970.

Williams, W. J., Beutler, E., Erslev, A. J., and Rundles, R. W. (eds.): Hematology. New York, McGraw-Hill Book Company, 1972.

731. MEGALOBLASTIC ANEMIAS

Victor Herbert

Definition.   The megaloblastic (Greek: megas=large + blaste=germ) anemias are characterized by a common morphology of giantism of every proliferating cell and an underlying common biochemical defect of slowed DNA synthesis. Classically, the diagnosis of megaloblastic anemia is made when the first-visit evaluation of a new patient reveals anemia, often with pancytopenia, and the peripheral blood smear reveals the progeny of a megaloblastic bone marrow, namely, macro-ovalocytic red cells, granulocytes whose nuclei are hypersegmented ("hypersegmented polys"), and giant platelets. Although megaloblastic anemia is a single *morphologic* entity, the underlying slowed DNA synthesis may result from any of a wide variety of causes. Thus the *diagnosis* of megaloblastic anemia is usually very easy, but the *differential diagnosis* of underlying cause and therefore *proper therapy* rest on determination of the precise etiologic classification into which the patient fits.

Pernicious anemia is *not* a synonym for megaloblastic anemia. It is that etiologic subcategory of megaloblastic anemia which is due to inadequate intrinsic factor secretion of uncertain etiology (Table 1).

Etiologic Classification and Pathogenesis.   In about 95 per cent of cases, megaloblastic anemia proves to be a nutritional anemia (or, more broadly, a nutritional pancytopenia) caused by deficiency of vitamin B_{12}, folic acid, or, in some cases, both. Classification therefore usually falls in one of the six etiologic categories common to all nutritional deficiencies: inadequate ingestion, absorption, or utilization, and/or increased requirement, excretion, or destruction. Table 1 presents an etiologic classification of the causes of slowed DNA synthesis and therefore of the megaloblastic anemias, and Figures 1 and 2 present the flow charts of vitamin B_{12} and folate metabolism which provide the nutritional, physiologic, and biochemical underpinnings on which much of the etiologic classification rests.

As indicated in Figure 1, food vitamin B_{12} is liberated from its bonds by gastric acid and gastric and intestinal enzymes. The freed B_{12} (of which there is less when there is no gastric acid) attaches to the intrinsic factor (IF), a glycoprotein of molecular weight about 50,000 secreted by gastric parietal cells, and the B_{12}-IF complex dimerizes and passes into the ileum, where it is plastered onto specific brush border receptors for the IF-B_{12} complex in the presence of ionic calcium and a pH of more than 6. In the presence of trypsin and appropriate but unknown biochemical circumstances ("releasing factor"), the vitamin is absorbed and transported in the bloodstream, attached to the B_{12}-delivery protein, transcobalamin II (TC II, B_{12}-binding beta globulin), to be rapidly delivered to the liver, hematopoietic system, and other proliferative cells. Some B_{12} attaches in an apparently permanent fashion to granulocyte-related serum B_{12}-binding glycoproteins (TC I, a B_{12}-binding alpha globulin, and TC III, a B_{12}-binding globulin which moves with approximately the speed of transferrin on electrophoresis at pH 8.6). Normally, when a sample of blood is drawn, plasma B_{12}-binding protein is found to be approximately one third saturated with B_{12}, almost none of which is on TC II. Of the unsaturated B_{12}-binding protein, approximately 90 per cent is TC II. TC II delivers B_{12} to cells in an ionic calcium- and pH-dependent manner similar to the delivery of B_{12} to the brush border of the ileal cell by IF. The liver is the main storage organ for B_{12} in man, normally containing about 1 μg B_{12} per gram of liver, and there is a large enterohepatic circulation of the vitamin. It is this which explains why vitamin B_{12} deficiency occurs so slowly in vegetarians (whose enterohepatic circulation of B_{12} is usually intact) and relatively rapidly when B_{12} absorption (and therefore reabsorption) is shut off.

As indicated in Figure 2, food folates are predominantly in polyglutamate form. Prior to absorption, the excess glutamates must be split off by conjugases (gamma-glutamyl carboxypeptidases) present in bile and intestine; this process is variably inhibited by inappropriate pH (optimal pH for conjugase action is 4.6) and by conjugase inhibitors in beans, yeast, and some other foods. Once deconjugated, folate is absorbed primarily across the upper third of the small bowel, mainly as reduced monoglutamate, but partly as pteroylglutamic acid (PGA). The absorption of 5-methyl tetrahydrofolate (5-methyl THF) may be B_{12} dependent. Dilantin and certain other drugs inhibit folate absorption at step 2 in Figure 2. After absorption, folate is transported, mainly as 5-methyl THF, probably by a carrier protein, to cellular sites of utilization. Vitamin B_{12} appears necessary to get 5-methyl THF across cell walls (step 5 in Fig. 2), and this vitamin B_{12}-dependent cell uptake of folate helps explain why patients with uncomplicated vitamin B_{12} deficiency have a "pile-up" of folate in serum, resulting in a high serum folate and a low red cell folate. The "folate trap" in vitamin B_{12} deficiency consists in this folate "pile-up" compounded by inability to convert body folate stores (which are mainly methyl THF) to metabolically usable tetrahydrofolate (THF) because this conversion (step 6 in Fig. 2) is vitamin B_{12} dependent. Normal total body folate stores are in the range of 5 to 10 mg, about half of which is in the liver. There is an enterohepatic circulation of about 100 μg folate daily.

The defective DNA synthesis is due to inadequate thymidylate synthesis (step 11 in Fig. 2). Folate deficiency directly reduces the amount of 5,10-methylene THF available for thymidylate synthesis, and vitamin B_{12} deficiency reduces production of 5,10-methylene THF by blocking utilization of 5-methyl THF (at step 6 in Fig. 2) and possibly by directly reducing synthesis of thymidylate synthetase.

Incidence and Prevalence. Dietary vitamin B_{12} deficiency megaloblastic anemia is common among vegetarians because animal protein is the sole source of the vitamin. Conversely, it rarely occurs among meat eaters because the vitamin is almost indestructible by cooking or other processing. On the other hand, dietary folate deficiency megaloblastic anemia occurs in about one third of all the pregnant women in the world ("megaloblastic anemia of pregnancy") despite the fact that folate is found in nearly all natural foods, because folate is heat labile and is rapidly destroyed by extensive cooking, especially of finely divided foods such as beans and rice. Any pregnant women whose daily diet contains neither a fresh uncooked fruit nor a fresh lightly cooked vegetable, and all of whose food is heated at 100° C for periods in excess of 15 minutes, can be assumed to have folate deficiency until proved otherwise. Dietary folate deficiency is also present in over 90 per cent of hard-liquor alcoholics, a majority of wine and beer alcoholics, and about half of narcotic addicts, because these groups waste little money on solid food.

Pernicious anemia (megaloblastic anemia caused by inadequate secretion of gastric intrinsic factor) is age related, with an approximate incidence of 1 per million persons at ages 6 months to 1 year, 1 per 10,000 at ages 1 to 10, 1 per 5000 at ages 30 to 40, and a progressive increase in frequency thereafter so that the incidence is approximately 1 per 200 persons at ages 60 to 70. When statistics are corrected for age, there appears to be no specific sex or race predilection, and only a predilection for following by some years the incidence of gastric atrophy with its consequent histamine-refractory achlorhydria, which is present in about 15 per cent of people between ages 40 and 60, 25 per cent between ages 60 and 70, and 30 per cent over the age of 70.

Megaloblastosis caused by subnormal intestinal absorption of vitamin B_{12} (often with associated folate deficiency) is almost always present in active tropical sprue, which is endemic in the Caribbean and Southeast Asia, and has been most studied in Puerto Ricans, Haitians, Vietnamese, Pakistanis, and Indians, but is also found in other nationals from these two geographic regions. For unknown reasons, a person born in an endemic sprue region who gets sprue may have remissions and exacerbations of the disease throughout life; recurrences are seen in such persons even after they have been in a temperate zone and apparently symptom free for up to 20 years. For this reason, when a person born in Puerto Rico develops megaloblastic anemia in the continental United States, he should be considered to have tropical sprue until proved otherwise. Subnormal absorption of vitamin B_{12} is also present in the majority of patients with regional enteritis, and is also present in a majority with chronic pancreatic disease.

Hematologic and Other Pathology. The pathology of megaloblastic anemia is generated by slowed DNA synthesis per unit time, and this is observed in all proliferating cells. Normally, cells capable of reproducing themselves are in the resting state (i.e., 1 unit of DNA) most of the time. When they reproduce, they do so by rapidly doubling their DNA, dividing, and returning to the resting state. Thus at any instant 100 such normal cells may contain 101 units of DNA (99 cells with 1 unit each plus 1 cell which is about to divide and has rapidly doubled its DNA to do so). Unlike such normal cells, at any given instant few megaloblastic cells are resting, because nearly all are engaged in a slowed attempt to complete doubling their DNA, with frequent arrest in the S (synthesis) phase and lesser arrest in other phases. Thus the amount of DNA observed per cell may be almost 2 units, so that instead of the hypothetical 101 units of DNA per 100 normoblastic cells, there may be close to 200 units of DNA per 100 megaloblastic cells. This largely explains the apparent anomaly that megaloblastic cells are seen under the microscope to have larger than normal nuclei with *increased DNA content* and yet they have biochemically *defective DNA synthesis*. Megaloblasts have an even larger cytoplasm than nucleus, as compared with normal cells, because, although their synthesis of DNA is impaired, their ability to synthesize RNA is usually relatively unimpeded. This disparity or nuclear-cytoplasmic dissociation or asynchrony, as it is variously termed, is reflected in the finely particulate nuclear chromatin ("young nucleus," or nucleus with retarded maturation) of the erythroid megaloblasts at all stages of their development, even when hemoglobin is clearly visible in the cytoplasm ("old cytoplasm"), easily differentiating them from normoblasts with their coarsely clumped "old" nuclear chromatin.

Another striking feature of megaloblastic hematopoiesis is the megaloblastic myelopoiesis, manifested most dramatically by the presence of many giant metamyelocytes, whose increased DNA is eventually packaged in an increased number of mature neutrophil lobes.

The evolutionary biochemical and hematologic sequence in development of folate deficiency is indicated in Figure 3; the sequence in development of vitamin B_{12} deficiency is similar, but is measured in years rather than months.

When there is concomitant iron deficiency, as is often the case in pregnancy, various malabsorption syndromes, and alcoholism, and in about a third of cases of pernicious anemia, the erythroid megaloblastosis and macrocytic "overcolored" erythrocytes may be masked by the countervailing tendency of iron deficiency to produce microblasts and hypochromic microcytic erythrocytes. The result may be "intermediate megaloblasts" (cells halfway between megaloblasts and normoblasts) in the bone marrow, and in the peripheral blood both red cell forms may be present ("dimorphic anemia"), or one may dominate. The myeloid megaloblastosis in the bone marrow and the hypersegmented polymorphonuclear leukocytes ("hypersegmented polys") in the peripheral blood are not masked by iron deficiency, and they provide the

TABLE 1.   Etiologic Classification of Megaloblastic Anemias; A Tabular Lexicon

I. *Vitamin B_{12} Deficiency* (normal B_{12} body stores last 3 to 6 years after cessation of B_{12} absorption, but 20 to 30 years after cessation of only B_{12} ingestion, because of continuation of reabsorption of the 3 to 6 μg of B_{12} excreted daily in bile):
   A. Inadequate ingestion
      1. Poor diet (lacking microorganisms and animal foods, which are the sole B_{12} sources)
         a. Strict vegetarianism (eating no meat, fowl, seafood, eggs, milk, or any products thereof)
         b. Chronic alcoholism (no B_{12} or folate in hard liquor) (folate deficiency occurs first, and is more common, partly because body stores of B_{12} last much longer than those of folate)
         c. Poverty, religious tenets (Hinduism, Seventh-Day Adventism, certain Catholic orders), dietary faddism
   B. Inadequate absorption
      1. Gastric disorder, producing inadequate or absent secretion by gastric parietal cells of intrinsic factor
         a. Addisonian pernicious anemia (PA) (PA is that form of B_{12} deficiency disease due to inadequate intrinsic factor secretion of uncertain etiology)
            (1) Hereditary absence of normal intrinsic factor secretion; absent secretion at birth (circulating antibody to intrinsic factor never present) (supports theory that antibody only occurs when antigenic stimulus is produced by intrinsic factor which enters bloodstream from damaged parietal cells and is recognized as foreign by the immunologic surveillance system); rare
            (2) Congenital production of defective intrinsic factor molecule (one published case)
            (3) Autoimmunity-associated gastric atrophy. These patients almost always have nondiagnostic-for-PA circulating parietal cell antibody, which is index only of past or present gastric damage and *not* of amount of intrinsic factor secretion (circulating diagnostic-for-PA antibody to intrinsic factor is always present under age 21; there is a gradual decrease in measurable antibody, so that by age 65 only two thirds of cases present with measurable circulating antibody to intrinsic factor)
               (a) Juvenile pernicious anemia (usually presents between ages 3 and 14)
               (b) Hereditarily determined degenerative gastric atrophy (gradually progressing with increasing age) (almost half of all adult PA cases fall in this category)
               (c) Acquired gastric atrophy as the end result of superficial inflammatory gastritis; superficial gastritis with atrophy (almost half of all adult PA cases fall in this category, which includes acquired gastric damage related to iron deficiency, alcohol, etc.)
               (d) Endocrine disorders (hypothyroidism, polyendocrinopathy, etc.) associated with gastric damage
         b. Gastrectomy
            (1) Total
            (2) Subtotal (approximately 20% develop PA within ten years after surgery, associated with atrophy of remaining parietal cells)
               (a) Proximal
               (b) Distal
         c. Lesions which destroy the gastric mucosa (ingested corrosives, linitis plastica, etc.)
         d. Intrinsic factor inhibitor in gastric secretion
            (1) Antibody to intrinsic factor (in saliva or gastric juice)
               (a) "Blocking" antibody (attaches to intrinsic factor so as to block ability of intrinsic factor to take up B_{12})
               (b) "Binding" antibody (attaches to intrinsic factor at site distal to site of B_{12} attachment)
      2. Small intestinal disorder (affecting ileum, which is the main site of B_{12} absorption)
         a. Gluten-induced enteropathy (childhood and adult celiac disease); idiopathic steatorrhea; nontropical sprue
         b. Tropical sprue (B_{12} is often the first nutrient to be subnormally absorbed and the last to return to normal absorption)
         c. Regional enteritis
         d. Strictures or anastomoses of the small bowel
         e. Intestinal resection

         f. Malignancies and granulomatous lesions involving the small intestine
         g. Other conditions characterized by chronically disturbed intestinal function
         h. Drugs damaging B_{12} absorption
            (1) Para-aminosalicylic acid (PAS) (therapy of tuberculosis)
            (2) Colchicine (therapy of gout)
            (3) Neomycin (antimicrobial)
            (4) Ethanol (societal)
            (5) Metformin (and other biguanide oral antidiabetic agents?)
            (6) Oral contraceptive agents?
         i. Specific malabsorption for vitamin B_{12}
            (1) Due to long-term ingestion of calcium-chelating agents (ionic calcium required for B_{12} absorption)
            (2) Due to inadequately alkaline pH in ileum (Zollinger-Ellison syndrome, pancreatic disease, etc.) (pH > 6 required for B_{12} absorption)
            (3) Unknown causes (absence of intestinal receptors for B_{12}-intrinsic factor complex? absence of "releasing factor"?)
               (a) Congenital (Imerslund-Gräsbeck syndrome) (receptors probably functioning)
               (b) Acquired (forme fruste of sprue?) (receptors absent or nonfunctioning)
      3. Competition for vitamin B_{12} by intestinal parasites or bacteria
         a. Fish tapeworm (*Diphyllobothrium latum*) (decreasing in Finland because of pollution of fresh water killing the host fish)
         b. Bacteria: The blind loop syndrome (B_{12} adsorbing bacteria)
      4. Pancreatic disease (normal pancreatic exocrine secretion of trypsin and bicarbonate required for normal B_{12} absorption)
   C. Inadequate utilization
      1. Vitamin B_{12} antagonists
         a. Substituted B_{12} amides and anilides (experimental agents)
         b. Cobaloximes (experimental agents)
      2. Congenital or acquired enzyme deficiency or deletion
         a. Methylmalonyl-CoA mutase
         b. Methyltetrahydrofolate-homocysteine methyltransferase
         c. B_{12a} reductase
         d. B_{12r} reductase
         e. Deoxyadenosyltransferase
         f. Other enzyme reduction or deletion
      3. Abnormal B_{12}-binding protein in serum, irreversibly binding B_{12} and making it unavailable to tissues
         a. Increased TC I and/or TC III glycoprotein (myeloproliferative disorders) ("granulocyte-related" B_{12} binders)
         b. Increased TC II protein (liver disease) ("liver-related" B_{12} binders)
         c. Other abnormal B_{12} binding (a glycoprotein in some hepatoma cases, etc.)
      4. Inadequate serum B_{12}-binding protein (congenital or acquired)
         a. TC II protein (lack produces megaloblastic anemia) (it delivers B_{12} to blood cells, as transferrin delivers iron)
         b. TC I glycoprotein (lack not known to produce megaloblastic anemia) (it is mainly a storage protein for B_{12}, somewhat akin to ceruloplasmin for copper)
         c. TC III (lack not yet clearly established) (large amounts produced in vitro by granulocytes)
      5. Protein malnutrition?
      6. Malignancy?
      7. Liver disease?
      8. Renal disease?
      9. Thiocyanate intoxication?
   D. Increased requirement (normal adult daily requirement from exogenous sources is 0.1 μg)
      1. Hyperthyroidism
      2. Increased hematopoiesis?
      3. Infancy (increased requirement for growth)
      4. Parasitization
         a. By fetus
         b. By malignant tissue?
   E. Increased excretion
      1. Inadequate B_{12}-binding protein in serum (inadequate TC II particularly?)
      2. Liver disease (inadequate storage capacity for B_{12})
      3. Renal disease?

TABLE 1. Etiologic Classification of Megaloblastic Anemias; A Tabular Lexicon (*Continued*)

F. Increased destruction
   1. By pharmacologic doses of ascorbic acid
II. *Folic acid deficiency* (normal folate body stores will last only 3 to 6 months after cessation of folate ingestion or absorption):
  A. Inadequate ingestion
    1. Poor diet (lacking unprocessed fresh, uncooked, or slightly cooked food) (or fruit juices) (folates are heat labile)
     a. Nutritional megaloblastic anemia
      (1) Tropical
      (2) Nontropical
      (3) Scurvy (diets poor in vitamin C are also poor in folate)
     b. Chronic alcoholism with or without cirrhosis
  B. Inadequate absorption (affecting upper third of small intestine which is the main site of folate absorption) (since most food folates are in polyglutamate forms, biliary and intestinal gamma glutamyl conjugases are necessary to split off excess glutamates to make folates absorbable)
    1. Malabsorption syndromes
     a. Gluten-induced enteropathy (childhood and adult celiac disease) (idiopathic steatorrhea, nontropical sprue) (coincident B_{12} malabsorption rare)
     b. Any other chronic functional or structural disorder involving the upper small intestine
      (1) Tropical sprue (coincident B_{12} malabsorption almost invariably present)
      (2) Associated with herpetic and other skin disorders
     c. Drugs
      (1) Diphenylhydantoin (Dilantin) (anticonvulsant)
      (2) Primidone (anticonvulsant)
      (3) Barbiturates
      (4) Oral contraceptive agents (?)
      (5) Cycloserine (tuberculosis)
      (6) Ethanol (societal)
      (7) Metformin (diabetes therapy)
      (8) Dietary amino acid excess of glycine and/or methionine
      (9) Nitrofurantoin? (antimicrobial)
      (10) Glutethimide? (sedative)
    2. Specific malabsorption for folate
     a. Congenital nonconjugase defects (four cases published)
     b. Acquired nonconjugase defects
     c. Inadequate biliary or intestinal conjugase
     d. Conjugase inhibitors (such as are contained in some beans)
    3. Blind loop syndrome (folate-greedy bacteria) (more commonly, bacteria make folate and actually raise serum folate level of host)
  C. Inadequate utilization (metabolic block)
    1. Folic acid antagonists (dihydrofolate reductase inhibitors)
     a. 4-amino-4-deoxyfolates (Chemotherapy, immuno-(i.e., methotrexate) suppression, psoriasis)
     b. 2,4-Diaminopyrimidine (Malaria, toxoplasmosis) (i.e., pyrimethamine)
     c. Triamterene (Diuretic)
     d. Diamidine compounds (*Pneumocystis carinii*, (i.e., pentamidine protozoacidal) isethionate)
     e. Trimethoprim (Antibacterial)
    2. Diphenylhydantoin and possibly other anticonvulsants (possibly block cell uptake or use of folate)
    3. Enzyme deficiency
     a. Congenital
      (1) Formiminotransferase
      (2) Dihydrofolate reductase
      (3) Methyltetrahydrofolate transmethylase
      (4) Other enzymes
     b. Acquired
      (1) Liver disease
       (a) Formiminotransferase
       (b) Other enzymes
    4. Vitamin B_{12} deficiency (reduces methylfolate uptake by cells)
    5. Alcohol (both specific and nonspecific damage to folate metabolism)
    6. Ascorbic acid deficiency (increased hematopoiesis associated with bleeding reduces folate stores) (may also decrease ability of body to retain folates in their metabolically active reduced state)
    7. Dietary amino acid excess (glycine, methionine)
  D. Increased requirement (normal adult daily requirement from exogenous sources is 50 μg)

    1. Parasitization
     a. By fetus (especially in multiple and twin pregnancies)
     b. By malignant tissue (especially lymphoproliferative disorders, myeloproliferative disorders to a lesser extent, extensive carcinomatosis, etc.)
    2. Infancy (increased requirement for growth)
    3. Increased hematopoiesis (hemolytic anemias; chronic blood loss [including scurvy])
    4. Increased metabolic activity (hyperthyroidism, chronic temperature elevations)
  E. Increased excretion
    1. Vitamin B_{12} deficiency? (? of obligatory excretion of folate in urine and bile) (possible inability to reabsorb methylfolate excreted in bile, because B_{12} required for it)
    2. Liver disease?
    3. Kidney dialysis
    4. Chronic exfoliative dermatitis
  F. Increased destruction
    1. Oxidant in diet?
III. *Interference with purine ring synthesis and interconversion of purine bases:*
  A. Purine antagonists
    1. 6-Mercaptopurine (6-MP) Chemotherapy, immunosuppression
    2. Thioguanine Chemotherapy, immunosuppression
    3. Azathioprine Immunosuppression
  B. Enzymatic defects in ability to make purine nucleotide from preformed bases
    1. Lesch-Nyhan syndrome (there is an associated increased requirement for folate, which is needed at two steps in the increased de novo biosynthesis of purine)
IV. *Interference with pyrimidine synthesis:*
  A. Pyrimidine antagonists
    1. 5-Fluorouracil (5-FU) Chemotherapy (blocks thymidylate synthetase)
    2. 6-Azauridine Chemotherapy, psoriasis
  B. Enzymatic defects in ability to make pyrimidine
    1. Hereditary oroticaciduria (not responsive to therapy with vitamin B_{12} or folic acid, but responsive to yeast extract or its active ingredients, uridine or the pyrimidine nucleotides, cytidylic and uridylic acids)
V. *Inhibition of ribonucleotide reductase (cytidylic to deoxycytidylic acid):*
  A. Cytosine arabinoside (inhibits DNA polymerase also) Chemotherapy, antiviral
  B. Hydroxyurea Chemotherapy, psoriasis
  C. Iron deficiency: iron is required for ribonucleotide reductase, but it is not yet established that lack of iron can produce megaloblastosis; some workers have reported hypersegmented polys in iron deficiency which disappear with iron therapy, but coincident folate deficiency has not yet been excluded fully
  D. Procarbazine (depolymerizes DNA)
VI. *Inhibition of protein synthesis:*
  A. L-Asparaginase Chemotherapy
VII. *Mechanism unknown:*
  A. Benzene Solvent
  B. Azulfidine Ulcerative colitis
  C. Arsenic Poison
  D. Pyridoxine-responsive megaloblastic anemia (only about 10% of patients with pyridoxine-responsive sideroblastic anemia have megaloblastic morphology)
  E. Thiamine-responsive megaloblastic anemia (one case reported)
  F. Megaloblastoid anemias (differentiated from megaloblastic anemias by bizarre morphology, including marked polyploidy and few to no orthochromatic megaloblasts)
    1. Di Guglielmo's syndrome (erythremic myelosis) (a myeloproliferative disorder usually presenting as refractory anemia and eventuating in death from "erythroleukemia" or myelogenous leukemia); preleukemia
    2. Occasional cases of polycythemia vera and other myeloproliferative disorders
    3. Occasional cases of aplastic anemia (which cases may subsequently develop myeloproliferative disorders)
    4. Occasional cases of miliary tuberculosis (in such cases, the megaloblastoid marrow is often accompanied by monocytosis and leukopenia or leukocytosis)

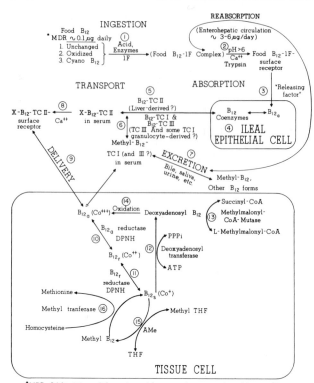

*MDR = Adult minimum daily requirement from exogenous sources to sustain normality

Figure 1.   Flow chart of vitamin B_{12} metabolism.

morphologic key to the existence of vitamin B_{12} or folate deficiency even in the presence of severe iron deficiency.

"Hypersegmented polys" are sought by either the simple "Rule of Fives" (i.e., if more than five of 100 neutrophils have five or more lobes, hypersegmentation is present) or the more elaborate "lobe average" (i.e., count the number of lobes in 100 "polys" and divide by 100; the normal lobe average is 3.17 ± 0.25; hypersegmentation is present if the lobe average is greater than 3.5; normally 20 to 40 per cent of "polys" have two lobes, 40 to 50 per cent have three lobes, and 15 to 25 per cent have four lobes; a substantial increase in percentage with four or more lobes means megaloblastosis, congenital hypersegmentation, or chronic renal disease). As Figure 3 indicates, in incipient megaloblastic anemia, hypersegmentation is present prior to the appearance of an obviously megaloblastic bone marrow or anemia. When the peripheral blood smears of all new patients are screened on a routine basis for hypersegmentation, one third of those found to have it are subsequently proved to have early vitamin B_{12} or folate deficiency, with low serum vitamin level but no anemia and no clinical suspicion of the diagnosis. The "Twenty Per Cent Rule" (i.e., if less than 20 per cent of 100 neutrophils have two or less lobes, hypersegmentation is present) is particularly useful when there are few or no "polys" with more than five lobes.

The megaloblastic anemias are due to ineffective erythropoiesis, and as such they have both a hemolytic component and an iron overload pathologic picture. The increased intramedullary "fetal" death rate of the erythroid cells is dramatically illustrated by the frequent finding of up to 25 per cent reticulocytes among

the bone marrow erythrons but 1 per cent or less in the peripheral blood, the high serum lactate dehydrogenase, and the modestly elevated serum bilirubin. Ineffective utilization of iron results in increased saturation of the iron-binding capacity and increased iron stores; this is so prominent that when a patient presents with megaloblastic anemia and normal rather than elevated serum and bone marrow iron, one should suspect iron deficiency, and should repeat the measurements of serum and bone marrow iron after vitamin therapy to determine whether overt iron deficiency has now been unmasked. Since megaloblastic anemia is usually associated with low normal total iron binding capacity, an elevated iron binding capacity is a clue to occult iron deficiency.

Megaloblastosis with underlying defective DNA synthesis is present in all proliferating cells; this is almost as striking in epithelial cells, particularly those of the alimentary tract and vagina, as in hematopoietic cells. Thus defective DNA synthesis results in a variable degree of secondary atrophy in epithelial cells of the tongue, stomach, and small intestine. It is this atrophy which produces secondary failure of gastric intrinsic factor secretion in one third of patients with tropical sprue, secondary failure of intestinal absorption of vitamin B_{12} in about half of patients with primary failure of intrinsic factor secretion, and the variety of other vicious cycles whereby vitamin B_{12} deficiency results in secondary decreased absorption of folate (and B_{12}) and folate deficiency results in secondary decreased absorption of vitamin B_{12} (and folate). These secondary malabsorption phenomena disappear after a variable period of vitamin therapy.

In addition to the defective DNA synthesis common to all megaloblastic anemias, a primary defect of unknown cause in ability to synthesize myelin is present only in vitamin B_{12} deficiency. This results in the insidious development of demyelinating vitamin B_{12} deficiency neuropathy, often beginning in peripheral nerves and progressing to involve the posterior and lateral columns of the spinal cord (variously called subacute combined degeneration, combined system disease, posterolateral sclerosis, and funicular degeneration) and the cerebrum ("megaloblastic madness"). (See Ch. 411.)

Clinical Manifestations.   Infrequently, the patient with megaloblastic anemia presents with bleeding caused by the thrombocytopenia, or infection caused by the leukopenia, but usually the presentation is with one or more of the symptoms of a gradually developing and slowly progressive anemia: easy fatigability, weakness, tiredness, shortness of breath, occasional faintness (particularly on suddenly arising from a recumbent or sitting position), headache, palpitations, and syncope. Before such symptoms are brushed off as "neurotic" (which they frequently prove to be), laboratory testing for anemia should be carried out, consisting at the least of determination of hematocrit (and/or hemoglobin) and examination of peripheral blood smear morphology.

If the patient has vitamin B_{12} deficiency and a good diet supplying adequate folate to substantially mask the hematologic picture, he may have no anemia and only slight morphologic evidence of megaloblastosis, and may present as a neurologic or neuropsychiatric problem, with paresthesias (especially numbness and tingling in the hands and feet) and diminished vibration and/or

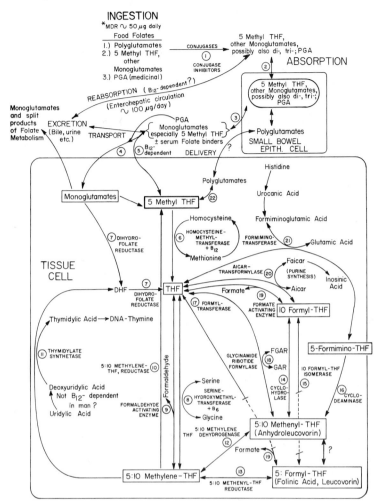

Figure 2. Flow chart of folate metabolism.

position sense (with loss of perception of 256 vps preceding by many months loss of perception of 128 vps, and loss of position sense in the index toes preceding by many months loss of position sense in the great toes). Examination with a "256" tuning fork may reveal complete loss of vibration sense from toes to iliac crest bilaterally before any loss of perception of vibration of a "128" tuning fork.

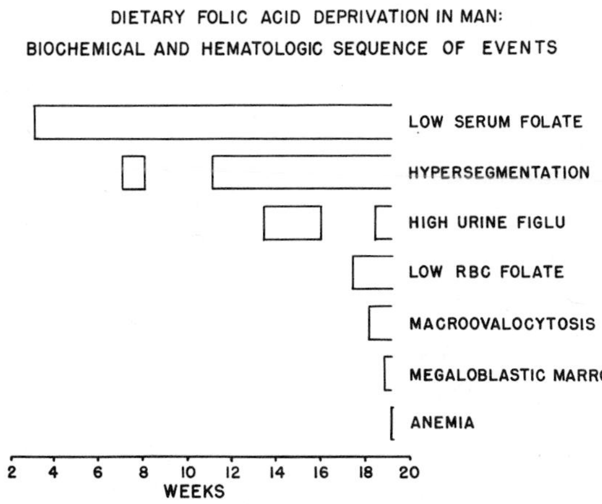

The classic neurologic disorder associated with vitamin B_{12} deficiency is combined system disease (subacute combined degeneration). Usually slow and insidious in onset, it is characterized by degeneration of the dorsal and lateral columns of the spinal cord, with paresthesias of the hands and feet, ataxia of the legs with variable spasticity and weakness, and eventual paraplegia. The classic symptoms are symmetrical paresthesias (numbness, tingling, burning) in feet and/or hands, followed by unsteadiness of gait associated with loss of position sense, manifested by inability to detect passive movements of the great toes. Prior to the appearance of deficits in the great toes, there may be inability to detect passive movements of the index toes. Knee and ankle jerks may be diminished or lost, or the knee jerks increased; extensor plantar responses, indicating damage to the spinal cord, commonly occur. Mental changes are variable, may include paranoid ideation and depression, and may be sufficiently severe to mimic paranoid schizophrenia or senility. (British workers have referred to this phenomenon as "megaloblastic madness"). Ataxic paraplegia similar to that resulting from vitamin B_{12} deficiency results from any kind of damage to the dorsal

DIETARY FOLIC ACID DEPRIVATION IN MAN:
BIOCHEMICAL AND HEMATOLOGIC SEQUENCE OF EVENTS

LOW SERUM FOLATE

HYPERSEGMENTATION

HIGH URINE FIGLU

LOW RBC FOLATE

MACROOVALOCYTOSIS

MEGALOBLASTIC MARROW

ANEMIA

2 4 6 8 10 12 14 16 18 20
WEEKS

Figure 3. Biochemical and hematologic sequence of events in folate deficiency.

or lateral columns of the spinal cord, as may occur with multiple sclerosis or chronic meningeal syphilis.

Subjective neurologic dysfunction, such as irritability, forgetfulness, and sleeplessness, occurs not only with vitamin B_{12} deficiency but even more frequently with folate deficiency. Such subjective stigmata are of limited differential diagnostic value in separating the two vitamin deficiency states; when caused by folate deficiency, these stigmata disappear dramatically within 24 hours of the start of folate therapy.

Occasionally, a chronic alcoholic with megaloblastic anemia caused by folate deficiency is erroneously diagnosed as having vitamin B_{12} deficiency because he has neurologic damage, including impaired position and vibration sense. However, associated thiamin deficiency in the alcoholic produces peripheral neuropathy mimicking that caused by vitamin B_{12} deficiency. Confusion may also arise in patients with folate deficiency and diabetes mellitus, because diabetic neuropathy may also mimic the neuropathy resulting from vitamin B_{12} deficiency.

The skin may have a lemon-yellow cast owing to the combination of pallor from anemia and low-grade icterus from the hemolytic component of the disorder. The "classic" pernicious anemia patient still appears as described by Addison in 1855:

> The countenance gets pale, the whites of the eyes become pearly, *the general frame flabby rather than wasted;* the pulse perhaps large but remarkably soft and compressible, and occasionally with a slight jerk, especially under the slightest excitement. There is an increasing indisposition to exertion with an uncomfortable feeling of faintness or breathlessness on attempting it; the heart is readily made to palpitate; the whole surface presents a blanched, smooth and waxy appearance: the lips, gums and tongue seem bloodless; *the flabbiness of the solids increases;* the appetite fails, extreme languor and faintness supervene, breathlessness and palpitation being produced by the most trifling exertion or emotion; some slight edema is probably perceived about the ankles. The debility becomes extreme; the patient can no longer arise from his bed; *the mind occasionally wanders;* he falls into a prostrate and half torpid state, and at length expires. *Nevertheless, to the very last, and after a sickness of perhaps several months' duration, the bulkiness of the general frame and the obesity often present a most striking contrast to the failure and exhaustion observable in every other respect.*

The parts of Addison's classic description which do not fit folic acid deficiency states as generally as those caused by vitamin B_{12} deficiency have been italicized. In folate deficiency, emaciation is more common than flabbiness, and diarrhea is more common than the constipation often seen in vitamin B_{12} deficiency.

About one third of patients with megaloblastic anemia have splenomegaly, but this may be observable only on abdominal radiography, because the spleen exceeds two to three times normal size in less than 10 per cent of cases. Moderate hepatomegaly may also be present.

A smooth or sore tongue is frequent, owing to megaloblastosis of the cells of the papillary surface. Almost 10 per cent of patients have hyperpigmentation, often most marked in the palmar creases, but occasionally in bizarre patterns such as occur with Addison's disease, sometimes with vitiligo. Occasionally low-grade fever is present.

Laboratory Findings and Differential Diagnosis. *Primary* laboratory findings include macro-ovalocytic anemia, leukopenia (with "hypersegmented polys"), thrombocytopenia (with giant platelets), and megaloblastic bone marrow. Reticulocyte count below 1 per cent is common with vitamin B_{12} deficiency, and that of 1.5 to 8 per cent is common with folate deficiency. *Secondary* findings include reduced haptoglobin, hyperbilirubinemia, increased fecal stercobilin, elevated serum lactate dehy-

TABLE 2. Separating Vitamin B_{12} Deficiency from Folate Deficiency: Laboratory Differential Diagnosis

Before therapy only:
1. Serum vitamin B_{12} (microbiologic: *Euglena gracilis, Ochromonas malhamensis; Escherichia coli, Lactobacillus leichmannii,* etc.) (radioassay using coated charcoal); normal: 200–900 pg/ml
2. Serum folate (*Lactobacillus casei*) (radioassay using coated charcoal); normal: 7–16 ng/ml
3. Erythrocyte vitamin B_{12}; normal: >100 pg/ml
4. Erythrocyte folate; normal: >150 ng/ml
5. Methylmalonate in urine; ↑ usually means B_{12} deficiency
6. Formiminoglutamate (FIGLU) (FGA) and urocanate in urine after oral histidine load; ↑ in B_{12} deficiency, folate deficiency, liver disease
7. "dU suppression" test (i.e., in vitro therapeutic trial)

Before or after therapy:
8. Gastric analysis: acid, pepsin, quality, quantity, intrinsic factor (IF) content
9. Tests of radio-B_{12} absorption (radioactivity in stool, plasma, liver, whole body, or urine) after physiologic dose (0.5–2 µg) of radio-B_{12} orally
   a. Urine (Schilling test)
      Stage 1: Radio-B_{12} orally + 1000 µg "cold" B_{12} IM, followed by 24-hour urine collection, another 1000 µg "cold" B_{12} IM, another 24-hour urine collection (normal result: >5% in 48-hour urine) (2 µg dose)
      Stage 2: Repeat Stage 1, but this time mix IF with radio-B_{12} before administering to patient (normal result: >5% in 48-hour urine) (2 µg dose)
      Stage 3: See text
10. Circulating antibody to human IF; normally absent

drogenase, formiminoglutamic aciduria (found not only in primary folate deficiency but also in primary vitamin B_{12} deficiency and primary liver disease), high serum iron and high saturation of transferrin, loss of gastric acid and abnormal liver function, and intestinal absorption tests. Megaloblasts are usually present in the buffy coat of centrifuged peripheral blood.

A serum B_{12} level below 100 pg per milliter is essentially diagnostic for primary vitamin B_{12} deficiency and *both* a serum folate of less than 3 ng per milliliter and a red cell folate below 150 ng per milliliter are diagnostic for primary folate deficiency. (Low serum folate alone may occur long before tissue folate depletion, and low red cell folate occurs also in primary vitamin B_{12} deficiency, because B_{12} is necessary to get methylfolate into red cells). One caveat: when the serum levels of both vitamins are low, the primary deficiency may be of just one, with resultant intestinal megaloblastosis producing malabsorption and therefore secondary deficiency of the other. For example, in megaloblastic anemia of pregnancy, both vitamin levels may be low, but treatment with only folic acid results in gradual rise to normal of the serum B_{12} level.

Methylmalonic aciduria occurs only in vitamin B_{12} deficiency and not in folate deficiency.

Absence of intrinsic factor in the gastric juice on in vitro assay is essentially diagnostic for pernicious anemia. One caveat: primary intestinal malabsorption of B_{12} or folate deficiency may produce secondary loss of intrinsic factor secretion; this will return to normal after vitamin therapy.

In vivo tests for detection of vitamin B_{12} malabsorption involve feeding 0.5 to 2 µg of the vitamin, labeled with ^{56}Co (half-life, 77 days), ^{57}Co (half-life, 270 days), ^{58}Co (half-life, 71 days), or ^{60}Co (half-life, 5.26 years), and measuring the amount absorbed by the amount of radioactivity in either stool, urine, blood, liver, or whole body. The test is divided into three stages: (1) Feed radio-B_{12} alone. Subnormal absorption means gastric or ileal dysfunction. It need not be done if in vitro radioassay for intrinsic factor is carried out. (2) Feed radio-B_{12} plus intrinsic factor concentrate. Subnormal absorption means ileal dysfunction, but does not rule out concomitant gastric dysfunction. (3) Only done if second stage is subnormal: Feed antimicrobial (or anthelmintic) for appropriate period, then feed radio-B_{12}. A normal result means that the patient had blind loop syndrome (or fish tapeworm). When pancreatic dysfunction is suspected, the third stage consists in feeding the radio-B_{12} with added bicarbonate or pancreatin, or both. When drug-induced B_{12} malabsorption is suspected, the third-stage test is carried out after withdrawal of the offending agent.

Every patient in whom tests reveal gastric or intestinal malabsorption of B_{12} that is not of a clear single cause should have the tests repeated after therapy with B_{12} (or after therapy with folic acid, if deficiency of folic acid is present). Vitamin B_{12} deficiency is a vicious-cycle disease (as is folic acid deficiency); severe deficiency of either B_{12} or folic acid may produce a variable degree of gastric and/or intestinal damage, and therefore may itself produce a variable degree of secondary reduction of gastric secretion of intrinsic factor and/or ileal ability to absorb B_{12} (and/or intestinal ability to absorb folate). This secondary malabsorption of B_{12} or folate is corrected by therapy.

Repetition of tests after therapy will establish which damage was secondary (i.e., a result of deficiency of B_{12} or folic acid) and which was primary (i.e., a lesion not produced by deficiency of B_{12} or folate). The B_{12} deficiency of a patient with regional enteritis may produce secondary gastric damage which may reduce intrinsic factor secretion; this secondary gastric damage may be corrected by B_{12} therapy. Conversely, the B_{12} deficiency of a patient with pernicious anemia may produce secondary ileal damage and resultant malabsorption of a test dose of B_{12} fed with intrinsic factor; this secondary ileal damage may be corrected by B_{12} therapy. Additionally, the B_{12} deficiency of either patient may make the malabsorption worse owing to his primary lesion.

Circulating antibody to intrinsic factor is present in two thirds of patients with pernicious anemia and, when found, is essentially diagnostic. Less than 10 per cent saturation of serum vitamin B_{12} binding capacity is also essentially diagnostic.

The dU suppression test on bone marrow cells aspirated from the patient is diagnostic for folate deficiency if a deficit in deoxyuridine suppression of radioactive iododeoxyuridine incorporation into DNA is found, and is corrected in vitro by pteroylglutamic acid (PGA) and methylfolate; it is diagnostic for vitamin B_{12} deficiency if corrected by B_{12} but not by methylfolate. This "therapeutic trial in the test tube" is the laboratory equivalent of the classic clinical trial discussed below.

Therapy. *Therapeutic trial* is diagnostic for vitamin B_{12} or folate deficiency. Such trial is carried out by giving the patient a diet devoid of foods high in vitamin B_{12} and folate, i.e., devoid of all fresh uncooked fruits and vegetables, fruit juices, nuts or other uncooked natural foods, and liver. After ten days on such a diet, and while continuing the diet, the patient is then treated with 1 µg of vitamin B_{12} parenterally daily if vitamin B_{12} deficiency is suspected, and with 50 to 100 µg of folic acid parenterally daily if folic acid deficiency is suspected. Unless

hematopoiesis is suppressed by infection, uremia, chloramphenicol, alcohol, or some other chronic systemic disease or drug, approximately three days after the start of therapy reticulocytosis will appear and will reach a peak at approximately seven days (range: five to twelve days) after the start of the daily vitamin therapy. The lower the initial red count, the higher the reticulocyte peak. The hemoglobin will gradually rise, and by approximately seven days after the start of therapy the white cell and platelet counts will rise to normal. The platelet count will usually, and the white count will in 10 per cent of cases, exceed normal before falling back into the normal range. It is important that the therapeutic trial vitamin dose not be larger than the aforementioned, to avoid "nonspecific" response (Fig. 4).

Immediate therapy is advisable in patients with megaloblastosis accompanied by anemia so severe as to be associated with dyspnea, congestive failure, and occasionally angina. Such symptoms, when found, usually occur in association with a hematocrit below 15 per cent. Rapid and dramatic relief of these symptoms may be obtained by administration of packed cells into one arm, accompanied by withdrawal of a slightly lesser quantity of whole blood from the contralateral arm. Venous pressure should be monitored, and only that amount of whole blood removed which is necessary to prevent elevation of the venous pressure. Packed cells may be given at the rate of 1 unit per five minutes by interposing a three-way stopcock and a 50-ml syringe between the bottle or bag of packed cells and the vein, drawing the packed cells from source into the syringe and then injecting into the vein. Using the three-way stopcock, venous pressure can be monitored and whole blood drawn off as required. In this procedure, packed cells with a hematocrit of approximately 80 are going into one arm while whole blood with a hematocrit of less than 15 is coming out the same or the other arm; there is therefore no dangerous sudden rise in circulating blood volume to induce the irreversi-

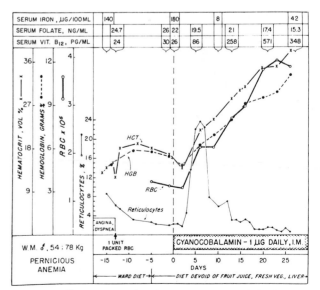

Figure 4. Therapeutic trial with 1µg of vitamin B_{12} daily. Note the "spontaneous" reticulocytosis present on admission (more frequent in folate deficiency), the termination of angina and dyspnea by a single unit of packed red blood cells (RBC), the initial high serum iron and folate, and their fall on vitamin B_{12} therapy.

ble congestive failure so dreaded when chronically anemic patients are given packed cells or whole blood in the conventional manner.

Immediate therapy with vitamin B_{12} and/or folate is advisable in patients with severe megaloblastic anemia and bleeding associated with platelet levels below 50,000 per cubic millimeter of blood or associated with infection accompanied by leukopenia with a white cell count below 2000 per cubic millimeter of blood. Immediate therapy with vitamin B_{12} and/or folate is also advisable in patients with severe infection, coma, severe disorientation, marked neurologic damage, severe liver disease, uremia, or other markedly debilitating illness complicating the deficiency of vitamin B_{12} and/or folate. When one of these reasons makes necessary immediate vitamin therapy before establishing the etiologic diagnosis, such therapy should be given intramuscularly with a minimum of 30 μg (1 ml) of vitamin B_{12} (cyanocobalamin) and 1 mg (1 ml) of folic (pteroylglutamic) acid, followed by 1 tablet (1 mg) of folic acid by mouth daily for a week and a minimum of 30 μg of vitamin B_{12} by intramuscular injection daily for a week. Some have recommended that potassium chloride be given at the onset of immediate vitamin B_{12} therapy to avoid the potential hazard of hypokalemia with subsequent arrhythmias.

After a week of therapy to carry the patient from the critical state to a state of well-being, all vitamin therapy should be stopped if necessary to make an etiologic diagnosis. However, with a combination of foresight and laboratory facilities, blood will have been obtained from the patient immediately on admission and prior to treatment, and diagnosis of vitamin B_{12} and/or folate deficiency will have been made from determination of the serum and erythrocyte levels of these vitamins, supplemented by the various tests which may be performed even when the patient is in a treated state. Initial therapy for inadequate absorption of vitamin B_{12} is 30 μg (or more) of cyanocobalamin daily for a week, or every other day for a total of five doses, to help replenish the body stores, followed by a minimum of 30 μg monthly. This quantity is not adequate to sustain complete normality and allows morphologic damage of moderate degree to persist; therefore a monthly injection of 100 μg of cyanocobalamin is preferable, because it will sustain in complete remission all patients with uncomplicated vitamin B_{12} deficiency.

Monthly maintenance therapy must be carried out for life in the patient whose inadequate absorption of B_{12} is due to lack of intrinsic factor secretion or to a noncorrectable structural or functional lesion of the ileum. Although there is no evidence that greater or more frequent therapy has any value, it has become general practice to give patients with neurologic damage 250 μg or more of vitamin B_{12} once or twice weekly for several months, followed by similar doses once or twice monthly for another year. Neurologic damage resulting from vitamin B_{12} deficiency, when of behavioral nature such as paranoia, may improve very rapidly (even within 24 hours) after the start of therapy. Objectively ascertainable neurologic damage, such as loss of position and/or vibration sense, improves more slowly, and there may be return of ability to perceive 128 vps before return of ability to perceive 256 vps, as well as return of ability to perceive passive motion of the great toes before return of ability to perceive passive motion of index toes. *Any neurologic damage which has not been corrected at the end of approximately 1 to 1 1/2 years may be considered to*

be irreversible. Neurologic damage caused by vitamin B_{12} deficiency begins as inability to make myelin, followed by gradual deterioration of the axon, followed by deterioration of the nerve head. This process occurs very slowly and is reversible until the nerve head deteriorates.

Oral therapy with large doses of vitamin B_{12} (500 to 1000 μg daily) should only be used when the patient with B_{12} malabsorption refuses parenteral therapy. Although there is usually sufficient diffusion-absorption from such doses to maintain patients in remission, this is not always reliable.

Oral therapy with vitamin B_{12}–intrinsic factor complexes should not be used, because such preparations are valueless to patients with structural or functional disorders of the small bowel and produce unreliable absorption of B_{12} in patients with pernicious anemia, many of whom become refractory owing to development in the gut wall of local antibody to intrinsic factor.

"Shotgun" antianemia preparations may actually harm the patient, because they may obscure the real nature of the anemia. For example, response to folic acid in a patient with megaloblastic anemia secondary to gastric carcinoma may obscure and delay the correct diagnosis.

The only recommended use of low (5 μg) daily dose oral B_{12} maintenance therapy is in the management of vegetarians who refuse to eat any animal matter.

Satisfactory clinical and hematologic remission may be obtained in any patient with uncomplicated vitamin B_{12} deficiency disease by daily parenteral administration of only 1 μg of vitamin B_{12} for ten days. Larger doses simply allow more rapid repletion of body stores. Initial therapy with doses of cyanocobalamin greater than 1 μg daily is desirable only when the vitamin B_{12} deficiency is complicated by other debilitating illness. Parenteral amounts of vitamin B_{12} greater than 30 μg daily have no proved therapeutic advantage, although it is possible that larger daily doses may result in slightly more rapid repletion of body stores. However, the percentage of the injected dose of vitamin B_{12} excreted in the urine rises logarithmically as the quantity of cyanocobalamin injected rises above 30 μg daily.

The most frequent complications of vitamin B_{12} deficiency, especially that caused by pernicious anemia, are infections, especially of the genitourinary tract, and variable degrees of congestive failure. These should be managed appropriately. Since the incidence of carcinoma of the stomach in patients with pernicious anemia is approximately threefold higher than chance, this entity should be looked for at yearly intervals.

In patients with chronic pancreatic disease, the intrinsic factor mechanism may not be operative and may be enhanced by feeding sodium bicarbonate, pancreatin, or trypsin.

Initial therapy with larger doses of pteroylglutamic acid than 0.1 mg daily is desirable when the folate deficiency state is complicated by conditions which may suppress hematopoiesis (infection, uremia, tumor; active inflammatory lesions such as rheumatoid arthritis, ulcerative colitis, or hepatitis; chloramphenicol or alcohol administration), or conditions which increase folate requirements (pregnancy; hypermetabolic states; states of increased hematopoiesis such as occur with hemolytic anemia or protracted blood loss). Therapy should then be 0.5 to 1 mg of pteroylglutamic acid daily.

There is no evidence that doses greater than 1 mg daily have greater efficacy than does 1 mg. Additionally, loss of folate in the urine becomes roughly logarithmic as quantities of administered pteroylglutamic acid exceed 1 mg. It is possible that the use of larger daily doses, especially if given in several spaced doses each day, may more rapidly replete the body folate stores, but the value of such rapid replenishment is uncertain.

When folate deficiency is due to malabsorption rather than inadequate ingestion, parenteral therapy is preferable initially, and maintenance therapy is preferably with 500 to 1000 μg (0.5 to 1.0 mg) of PGA daily rather than 100 μg (at least until further studies support the current impression that PGA is well absorbed even when the patient is only poorly capable of absorbing other nutrients [such as food folates]).

The best maintenance therapy for dietary folate deficiency is correction of the diet rather than permanent supplementation. Such correction often simply requires less prolonged cooking of the same foods the patient has always eaten, because prolonged cooking destroys folates. In other instances, such correction involves switching from canned to fresh fruits and vegetables, because the canning process may destroy 50 to 95 per cent of food folate.

Summary of Response to Therapy. Objective and subjective improvement occurs within a few days and a sense of well-being often within a day of the start of therapy with the lacking vitamin. Within 48 hours, the bone marrow returns sharply toward normoblastic. Reticulocytosis begins within two to five days after therapy is started and usually reaches its peak on about the fifth to twelfth day. The shape and height of the reticulocyte curve depend on the dose of vitamin B$_{12}$ or folic acid, the route of its administration, and the severity of the anemia. At approximately the time the reticulocytes reach their peak, the leukocytes and platelets will have risen to normal levels. Serum iron is usually elevated in untreated patients and falls abruptly within one to two days after starting therapy. This sequence of events should be followed by obtaining a blood count just prior to the start of therapy and a reticulocyte count at least once every two days from then until the reticulocyte peak has passed, plus a hemoglobin or hematocrit determination at weekly intervals for the first month and then every two weeks for the next month or two. If hematologic recovery does not follow the outlined response pattern, then either the diagnosis is wrong or complications suppressing hematopoiesis are present.

Arnstein, H. R. V., and Wrighton, R. J. (eds.): The Cobalamins. Edinburgh and London, Churchill Livingstone, 1971.

Beck, W. S.: Erythrocyte disorders—anemias related to disturbance of DNA synthesis (megaloblastic anemias). *In* Williams, W. J., Beutler, E., Erslev, A., and Rundles, R. W. (eds.): Hematology. New York, McGraw-Hill Book Company, 1972, pp. 249, 256, 278, 297.

Chanarin, I.: The Megaloblastic Anemias. Oxford, Blackwell; Philadelphia, F. A. Davis Company, 1969.

Herbert, V. (ed.): Symposium on vitamin B$_{12}$ and folate. Am. J. Med., 48:539, 541, 549, 555, 562, 570, 584, 594, 599, 602, 1970.

Herbert, V.: Detection of malabsorption of vitamin B$_{12}$ due to gastric or intestinal dysfunction. Semin. Nucl. Med., 2:220, 1972.

Herbert, V.: Drugs effective in megaloblastic anemias. *In* Goodman, L. S., and Gilman, A. (eds.): The Pharmacological Basis of Therapeutics, 5th ed. New York, Macmillan, 1975.

Herbert, V.: Folic acid and vitamin B$_{12}$. *In* Goodhart, R. S., and Shils, M. E. (eds.): Modern Nutrition in Health and Disease. Philadelphia, Lea & Febiger, 1973, p. 221.

Herbert, V., and Tisman, G.: Effects of deficiencies of folic acid and vitamin B$_{12}$ on central nervous system function and development. *In* Gaull, G. (ed.): Biology of Brain Dysfunction, Vol. 1. New York & London, Plenum Press, 1973, p. 373.

Herbert, V., Tisman, G., Go, L. T., and Brenner, L.: The dU suppression test using ^{125}I-UdR to define biochemical megaloblastosis. Br. J. Haematol., 24:713, 1973.

Jerzy Glass, G. B.: Gastric Intrinsic Factor and Other Vitamin B$_{12}$ Binders. Biochemistry, Physiology, Pathology and Relation to Vitamin B$_{12}$ Metabolism. Stuttgart and New York, Thieme Verlag and Intercontinental Medical Book Corporation, 1974.

Stebbins, R., Scott, J., and Herbert, V.: Drug-induced megaloblastic anemias. Semin. Hematol., 10:235, 1973.

Sullivan, L. W.: The megaloblastic anemias. *In* Mengel, C. E., Frei, E., and Nachman, R. (eds.): Hematology, Principles and Practice. Chicago, Year Book Medical Publishers, 1972.

Wellcome Trust Collaborative Study: Tropical Sprue and Megaloblastic Anemia. Edinburgh and London, Churchill Livingstone, 1971.

NORMOCHROMIC NORMOCYTIC ANEMIAS

732. ACUTE HEMORRHAGIC ANEMIA

Elmer B. Brown

Definition. Acute hemorrhagic anemia caused by loss of a large volume of blood may result from trauma, ulcerative lesions, abnormal blood vessels, or coagulation defects; it may occur from a severed blood vessel, from the gastrointestinal, respiratory, or genitourinary tracts, into a large muscle mass, or into various body cavities such as cysts or the pleural, peritoneal and retroperitoneal spaces. The hemorrhage is grossly evident except when blood is lost into the gastrointestinal tract, body cavities, or tissues. Clinical manifestations vary with the size, rate, and site of the hemorrhage, with the lesion responsible for the bleeding, and with the state of consciousness of the patient.

Clinical Manifestations. The manifestations of acute severe hemorrhage are remarkably consistent regardless of the underlying cause, because they depend on the volume of blood lost. As outlined in the accompanying table, the loss of as much as 500 ml of blood in five minutes usually produces only trivial effects on the circulation without changes in blood pressure or pulse rate. Withdrawal of a liter of blood often produces no fall in blood pressure in the recumbent subject, although if

Clinical Manifestations of Acute Blood Loss

Volume of Blood Lost		Clinical Manifestations
% of Blood Volume	*ml**	
10	500	Usually none; rarely vasovagal syncope
20	1000	Few changes supine; upright or with exercise, tachycardia and mild hypotension are often present
30–40	1500–2000	Marked postural hypotension and tachycardia; central venous pressure, cardiac output, and arterial blood pressure are reduced; pulse is thready; skin is cold and clammy; thirst, air hunger, headache, and syncope are frequent
50	2500	Severe shock, often leading to death

*Based on 5000 ml blood volume.

he sits up or attempts to walk, tachycardia occurs, the blood pressure often falls, and consciousness may be lost. When apprehension is added to the loss of even small amounts of blood, syncope caused by a vasovagal reaction may occur. Loss of 1500 to 2000 ml of blood leads to a fall in right atrial pressure, diminished cardiac output, hypotension, and a rapid, thready pulse. Additional symptoms are prostration, restlessness, thirst, tachypnea and air hunger, pallor with cold clammy skin, sweating, pounding headache, and frequent syncope. Rapid blood loss of greater than 40 per cent of the patient's blood volume leads to shock, the risk of renal tubular necrosis, myocardial infarction, and a high risk of death unless immediate replacement therapy is initiated. However, a previously healthy person may survive the gradual loss of as much as 50 per cent of his blood volume over a period of 24 hours. Hemorrhage into pleural, peritoneal, or retroperitoneal spaces usually causes pain, fever, and signs of serosal inflammation; bleeding into muscles may also produce marked limitation of motion.

Diagnosis. Initial assessment of the degree of hemorrhage may be difficult. When associated with multiple trauma, the amount of swelling surrounding the area of a wound correlates roughly with the amount of blood lost. Wounds of the thigh involving large muscles may be associated with a blood loss of 2500 ml or more. With gross disruption of tissues, as in gunshot or automobile injuries, the size of the wound correlates fairly well with the degree of blood loss — for an area of tissue damage the size of the patient's hand, loss of approximately 10 per cent of the patient's blood volume should be assumed. Upper gastrointestinal bleeding can be roughly quantitated by the fact that frank hematemesis indicates a large hemorrhage (usually more than 25 per cent of the blood volume), whereas melena alone indicates a much smaller blood loss. Generalizations of this type are important, because the initial hematocrit does not adequately reflect the size of the hemorrhage. Blood vessels of the skin and muscles constrict in an attempt to compensate for the decreased blood volume and to provide blood flow and adequate oxygen supply for vital organs. Replacement of plasma from endogenous sources is slow. The initial changes in blood counts after hemorrhage reflect the mobilization of platelets and leukocytes from marginated storage pools. Thrombocytosis to levels approaching 1 million per cubic millimeter may occur within an hour; a polymorphonuclear leukocytosis with white cell counts as high as 20,000 to 30,000 occurs within two to three hours. Metamyelocytes, myelocytes, and nucleated red blood cells often appear in the peripheral blood after severe hemorrhage. Replacement of plasma volume by fluid from the extravascular space is a relatively slow process, with the limiting factor being the rate at which albumin and other proteins are mobilized. After loss of 10 per cent of the blood volume, about half of the lost red cells and plasma are replaced by plasma alone after 24 hours. Loss of about 20 per cent of the blood volume requires 24 to 60 hours for restoration of the normal blood volume as reflected by a decreasing hematocrit for two or three days. Loss of red blood cell mass causes decreased tissue oxygenation only partially compensated for by adjustments in cardiovascular dynamics. Tissue hypoxia by a still unknown mechanism triggers erythropoietin production with measurable increases in plasma levels of this hormone within six hours. Increased levels of 2,3-diphosphoglycerate in circulating erythrocytes contribute to a shift of the hemoglobin oxygen dissociation curve for more efficient tissue oxygenation. Erythropoietin-stimulated erythropoiesis causes a fall of the plasma iron during the two to five days required for marrow stem cells to proliferate and mature into circulating reticulocytes to expand the red cell mass. Some reticulocytes are released prematurely from the marrow in response to hemorrhage, and their numbers increase to peak levels of 10 to 15 per cent after seven to ten days. Since reticulocytes are larger than mature erythrocytes, the mean corpuscular volume (MCV) rises (approximately 1 fl for each per cent of increase in reticulocyte count) and polychromatophilic macrocytes are seen in Wright-stained blood films. Depending on the size of the hemorrhage and the adequacy of iron stores, the red cell volume and hematocrit are restored to normal in about five or six weeks. Elevated platelet counts and leukocytosis have usually returned to the normal range within three to five days. Bleeding into the gastrointestinal tract produces an elevation of the blood urea nitrogen which may be accentuated if renal function is impaired. Resorption of blood from body cavities or tissues results in increased production of unconjugated bilirubin and may be associated with mild jaundice; iron released from hemoglobin bled into tissues is reutilized for new erythropoiesis.

Treatment. Treatment should be directed at stopping the hemorrhage, combating shock, and restoring blood volume. The patient should be kept warm and quiet; sedation and analgesics may be required. It is essential to begin an infusion through a needle or catheter of adequate bore to permit rapid fluid replacement, and this will sometimes require a surgical cutdown to find collapsed veins. The choice of solutions for initial replacement therapy depends on how critical the patient's condition is and what solutions are available. Most quickly available for rapid expansion of plasma volume are noncolloid electrolyte solutions (e.g., isotonic saline and Ringer's lactate) or dextran solutions, either a 10 per cent solution of low molecular weight dextran in isotonic saline (dextran 40, with an average molecular weight of 40,000) or a 6 per cent solution of high molecular weight dextran (dextran 70, with an average molecular weight of 70,000). Dextran 40 has the advantage of increasing the plasma volume by one to two times the amount infused, but is more rapidly cleared in the urine. Its effect is rapidly dissipated during the succeeding 12 hours, and in a few patients it may precipitate acute renal failure. Dextran 70 is cleared more slowly and sustains the plasma volume expansion for 24 to 48 hours. Both may produce circulatory overload, which can usually be avoided by administering the first 500 ml rapidly and the remainder more slowly with frequent monitoring of central venous pressure. When volumes of dextran solution in excess of 1000 ml are used, interference with platelet adhesiveness and coagulation mechanisms may accentuate bleeding. Plasma protein solutions and 5 per cent albumin in saline have the advantage of predictable volume expansion with physiologic materials, but carry the disadvantages of relatively high cost, slower time for reconstitution, and, with plasma solutions, the risk of hepatitis. Noncolloid electrolyte solutions such as isotonic saline or Ringer's lactate may be given quickly in acute emergencies for support of blood volume, but since they are rapidly distributed throughout the intravascular and extravascular compartments they must be supplemented with blood or colloid solutions. Use of fresh whole blood, packed erythrocytes, or saline-resuspended, concentrated red blood cells requires typing and cross-matching that cause too great a delay for routine use in the initial treatment of life-threatening hemorrhage. Use of uncross-matched universal donor blood cannot be condoned except in extreme emergencies. Rarely is red cell depletion so severe that blood transfusions cannot wait for careful cross-matching. Blood transfusions supplement initial volume expansion with dextran or other colloidal solutions and are the mainstay of the definitive treatment of acute hemorrhage. When bleeding is due to absence of platelets or coagulation factors, transfusion of fresh whole blood or concentrates of blood components is essential and may be lifesaving. With prolonged bleeding requiring replacement of more than 5000 ml of stored blood within 48 hours, thrombocytopenia caused by transfusion of nonviable platelets may cause bleeding. Anticipation of this complication as well as the risks of severe uncontrolled bleeding may favor early surgical attempts to identify and correct the cause of bleeding from gastrointestinal or other obscure sites. After the emergency is over, provision of a high protein diet and iron by mouth are indicated to replace the stores depleted by blood loss; no other supplements are needed.

Adamson, J., and Hillman, R. S.: Blood volume and plasma protein replacement following acute blood loss in normal man. J.A.M.A., 205:609, 1968.
Collins, J. A., and Ballinger, W. F.: The treatment of shock. *In* Ballinger, W. F., Rutherford, R. B., and Zuidema, G. D. (eds.): The Management of Trauma. Philadelphia, W. B. Saunders Company, 1973, Chapter 3.
Harris, J. W., and Kellermeyer, R. W.: The Red Cell. Production, Metabolism, Destruction: Normal and Abnormal, Revised ed. Cambridge, Harvard University Press, 1970, Chapter 4.
Mollison, P. L.: Blood Transfusion in Clinical Medicine. 5th ed. Oxford, Blackwell Scientific Publications, 1972.

733. ANEMIA ASSOCIATED WITH INFECTION AND CHRONIC SYSTEMIC DISEASES
(Simple Chronic Anemia, Anemia of Chronic Disorders)
Elmer B. Brown

Definition.   The anemia of infection and many chronic disorders is usually mild and nonprogressive in severity. It develops over a period of one to two months, is usually normochromic normocytic, and is characterized by decreased plasma iron, decreased transferrin iron-binding capacity, decreased bone marrow sideroblasts, increased reticuloendothelial iron deposits, mild hemolysis, and relative bone marrow failure. The occurrence of anemia in association with chronic disease of multiple etiologies makes the selection of an appropriate descriptive name difficult. The term "anemia of chronic disorders" may be the least restrictive for the anemia underlying cancer, lymphomas, connective tissue disorders, hepatic, renal and endocrine disorders, fractures and tissue injury, and chronic viral and suppurative infections. Other types of anemia, such as those related to blood loss, iron or vitamin deficiency, or hemolysis, may accentuate and complicate the underlying anemia of a chronic disorder. By its widespread association with many chronic diseases this anemia is the most common form seen in hos-

pital populations, and it is frequent in the population at large.

Etiology and Pathogenesis.   The mechanism can generally be framed in terms of three basic abnormalities: (1) moderate shortening of erythrocyte life span; (2) failure of the bone marrow to increase erythropoiesis sufficiently to compensate for the mild hemolytic anemia; and (3) an unexplained impairment of iron release from reticuloendothelial cells throughout the body. Examination of the interaction of these three basic abnormalities is essential before special features of anemias associated with specific diseases can be defined.

Decreased erythrocyte life span is of moderate degree and requires measurements with special erythrocyte labeling techniques; half-time survival of ^{51}Cr-tagged cells is reduced from a normal range of 30 ± 3 days to about 20 to 25 days. In absolute terms, erythrocyte survival is about 80 days instead of the normal 120 days. Cross-transfusion experiments have shown normal survival of red cells from anemic patients transfused into normal recipients, whereas cells from normal subjects transfused into the patient show decreased survival indicative of an extracorpuscular factor responsible for the decreased erythrocyte life span. Whether this unidentified factor acts in the plasma or adversely influences other portions of the erythrocyte's environment has never been defined.

Ordinarily, this mild degree of hemolysis would be compensated for by greater erythropoietic activity of the bone marrow which can increase red cell production six to eight times the normal rate. However, erythropoiesis in patients with chronic disorders rarely increases more than twofold; as a result, production of red cells falls behind destruction until a new balance is reached at mildly anemic levels. Normally the body responds to tissue hypoxia of anemia by increasing the output of erythropoietin which stimulates the differentiation of marrow stem cells into erythroblasts and speeds their maturation to circulating erythrocytes. One might suppose, under conditions of chronic disease, that either the stimulation of erythropoietin production is defective or the marrow is incapable of responding to this hormone. Experimental evidence indicates that erythropoietin levels are low and that the marrow is quite capable of responding to erythropoietin when injected in pure form or when stimulated by external hypoxia or cobalt administration. Thus the block to an appropriate erythropoietic response seems to be an insensitive "thermostat," failing to stimulate erythropoietin release in response to slowly developing anemia. The precise mechanism of this defect is unknown.

The third basic abnormality common to the anemias of chronic disorders is the impairment of iron release from reticuloendothelial cells. Normally, senescent erythrocytes are removed from the circulation by reticuloendothelial cells which digest hemoglobin, free its iron from the heme ring, and release it to plasma transferrin for transport to the marrow and reutilization in erythropoiesis. Within hours after infection or injury a block occurs to the normal release of iron by the reticuloendothelial cells, as evidenced by a precipitous fall in plasma iron concentrations. Further experimental evidence for this block was obtained by injecting ^{59}Fe-labeled, heat-damaged red cells that are rapidly cleared by reticuloendothelial cells and measuring the release and reutilization of ^{59}Fe into newly formed erythrocytes. Normal subjects reutilize 55 to 70 per cent of the ^{59}Fe for hemoglobin synthesis, whereas patients with the anemia of chronic disorders utilize less than 40 per cent. As a result of this block to normal iron flow, there is a buildup of ferritin and hemosiderin in reticuloendothelial cells in the bone marrow and throughout the body. The paucity or iron available for erythropoietic cells in turn leads to decreased numbers of marrow sideroblasts and other evidence of iron-deficient erythropoiesis. The three basic abnormalities are balanced so that the resultant anemia is mild and self-limiting. However, if blood loss, red cell fragmentation, or immune hemolysis increases the rate of red cell loss, if folate or vitamin B_{12} deficiency further decreases erythropoietic response, or if iron deficiency accentuates the block to iron flow, the anemia may be much more severe.

Various diseases have additional specific etiologic factors that might profitably be examined separately from the basic abnormalities that characterize the anemia of chronic disorders.

Renal failure is usually accompanied by anemia which may be quite severe. Anemia correlates roughly with the elevation of blood urea nitrogen, although a more nearly linear relationship exists between elevated BUN and decreased red cell life span. The factor or factors in uremic plasma that damage erythrocytes and cause anemia have not been identified, although many substances have been suggested. In some patients mechanical trauma and increased fragmentation of red cells lead to severe hemolytic anemia when renal failure is associated with malignant hypertension or various types of hemolytic-uremic syndrome. Other patients with renal failure have hemorrhagic tendencies caused by decreased numbers and function of platelets.

Deficiency of folate and iron aggravates the *anemia of patients undergoing dialysis;* folate is dialyzable and is lost into the dialysis bath, whereas iron is lost with blood in the dialysis coil. Since approximately 90 per cent of erythropoietin originates in the kidney, either directly or through a renal activating system, progressive renal disease leads to decreased erythropoietin production. In addition, the presence of uremia may blunt the bone marrow's response to the reduced amounts of erythropoietin released by damaged kidneys; dialysis may salvage some of the effectiveness of the available erythropoietin and cause amelioration of the anemia.

Rheumatoid arthritis in the active phase is frequently accompanied by the anemia of chronic disorders. A unique feature is the microscopic bleeding into the inflamed joints that leads to massive accumulation of iron in the hyperplastic synovial tissue. Sequestration of several hundred milligrams of iron in hypertrophied synovium may contribute to an iron deficiency state superimposed on the anemia of inflammation. Bleeding induced by the gastrointestinal irritation of aspirin, corticosteroids, and other anti-inflammatory therapeutic agents may further accentuate the iron deficiency.

Cancer in its later stages is almost always accompanied by the anemia of chronic disorders. Frequently there is no correlation between the degree of anemia and the extent of the tumor. Bone marrow invasion by cancer is often associated with the release of immature leukocytes and nucleated erythrocytes, but the extent of marrow metastases correlates poorly with the degree of anemia. Substances released from necrotic cancer cells and the red cell fragmentation from fibrin strands in vessels narrowed by tumor invasion have been postulated to explain the hemolytic anemia in cancer. Bleeding from tumors of the alimentary or genitourinary tracts or from vascular lesions of the skin causes hemorrhagic or iron deficiency anemia, and the inanition leading to calorie, protein, and vitamin deficiency accentuates the underlying simple chronic anemia.

Liver disease is associated with various complications in addition to the underlying anemia of chronic disorders. The increased plasma volume of cirrhosis may give an exaggerated impression of anemia when the concentration of erythrocytes is measured by hematocrit and hemoglobin determinations. Bleeding related to peptic ulcers, varices, and deficient coagulation factors may produce rapid blood loss anemia or slowly developing iron deficiency. Alcohol depresses erythropoiesis acutely and leads to folate deficiency anemia because of inadequate intake and defective absorption of the vitamin. Erythrocyte abnormalities—thin macrocytic target cells or burr cells—may contribute to the decreased red cell survival. Hypersplenism frequently associated with portal hypertension of liver disease also accentuates the hemolytic anemia of chronic disorders.

Endocrine disorders, including thyroid, pituitary, and adrenal insufficiency, are associated with a normochromic normocytic anemia most severe in hypothyroidism. Presumably these endocrine deficiencies lead to decreased erythropoietin production. In the case of *hypothyroidism* the diminished need of the tissues for oxygen leads to an adaptive partial atrophy of the erythron. Frequently, coexistent iron, folate, and especially vitamin B_{12} deficiencies are present with the anemia of hypothyroidism.

Clinical Manifestations.   The symptoms are primarily those of the underlying disease. As the anemia is mild and develops slowly, the patient can adjust to it with minimal accentuation of fatigue, dyspnea, and palpitations. When bleeding or hemolysis complicates the underlying anemia of chronic disorders in patients with leukemia, lymphoma, or chronic renal failure, symptoms of anemia may be disabling and lead to coronary insufficiency and congestive failure. Pallor, tachycardia, cardiac dilatation, and low-grade sustained fever are nonspecific signs common to many types of chronic anemia.

Diagnosis.   The anemia of chronic disorders is usually normocytic normochromic (MCV 87 to 103 fl and MCHC 32 to 36 grams per deciliter), but may be normocytic hypochromic or even microcytic hypochromic. When microcytosis or hypochromia is present, it is usually milder than that seen in well-developed iron deficiency anemia. The hematocrit usually remains constant in a range between 25 and 39 per cent at full development of the anemia after six to eight weeks. Erythrocyte morphology is unremarkable except for burr cells of uremia and some types of cancer and the thin, flat macrocyte of chronic liver disease. Reticulocytosis or polychromasia indicative of increased erythropoiesis is rare. Leukocytes and platelets are normal unless they reflect changes related to the underlying disease. Bone marrow morphology on Wright-stained specimens shows no specific abnormality; changes related to the underlying disease may include increased numbers of plasma cells in cirrhosis or rheumatoid arthritis and leukemic or tumor cell infiltration. Prussian blue stains for iron in bone marrow disclose decreased numbers of erythroid precursors with iron granules (sideroblasts), whereas reticuloendothelial cells show increased hemosiderin deposits. Plasma iron and total iron-binding capacity are both reduced; the per cent saturation of transferrin is normal or low. Differentiation from the plasma iron changes of iron deficiency anemia may be difficult; the major difference is a tendency toward increased transferrin concentration and absence of stainable marrow iron in iron deficiency. When iron deficiency and the anemia of chronic disorders occur together, the rise in transferrin usually seen in iron deficiency is blunted; absent marrow hemosiderin is the key diagnostic observation. Despite the underlying hemolysis, the serum bilirubin is usually normal unless there is associated liver dysfunction. Hemolysis is usually detectable only by special red cell survival measurements.

Treatment. The only effective therapy is that directed toward correction of the underlying disease. Since the anemia typically is mild and nonprogressive, no attempt at correction may be necessary. When symptoms of underlying heart disease are triggered by anemia, transfusions with packed erythrocytes to a hematocrit of 30 to 35 per cent may be temporarily beneficial. Attempts to stimulate erythropoiesis by administration of cobalt have been abandoned, because undesirable side effects outweigh the modest improvement of the anemia. Androgenic steroids may be effective in some patients with cancer or chronic renal disease. Purified erythropoietin is not yet available in sufficient amounts for adequate clinical trials. Corticosteroids frequently ameliorate the anemia of rheumatoid arthritis and other connective tissue diseases; they may also be beneficial in treatment of complicating immune hemolysis. No means has been found to bypass the block to iron flow in the anemia of chronic disorders. Since colloidal iron preparations given parenterally must be processed by the reticuloendothelial cells before iron is made available to transferrin, the colloidal iron is blocked as effectively as that from senescent erythrocytes. When bleeding causes superimposed iron deficiency, giving iron by mouth or parenterally will restore hemoglobin levels to those of the underlying chronic disorder, but not back to normal. Similarly, folate deficiency of alcoholic cirrhosis will respond to folate therapy by partial correction of anemia.

Cartwright, G. E.: The anemia of chronic disorders. Semin. Hematol., 3:351, 1966.

Harris, J. W., and Kellermeyer, R. W.: The Red Cell. Production, Metabolism, Destruction: Normal and Abnormal. Cambridge, Mass., Harvard University Press, 1970.

Kimber, C., Deller, D. J., Ibbotson, R. N., and Lander, H.: The mechanism of anaemia in chronic liver disease. Quart. J. Med., 34:33, 1965.

Strandberg, O.: Anemia in rheumatoid arthritis. Acta Med. Scand. [Suppl.], 454:1, 1966.

Williams, W. J., Beutler, E., Erslev, A. J., and Rundles, R. W. (eds.): Hematology. New York, McGraw-Hill Book Company, 1972.

734. APLASTIC ANEMIA

M. C. Brain

Definition. Aplastic or hypoplastic anemia is the term applied to a group of disorders characterized by reduction in all the cellular elements of the blood (pancytopenia), and associated with hypocellularity of the bone marrow. The degree of panctyopenia reflects the severity of the disorder and may vary during the course of the illness. Less marked reduction in cell counts may be encountered in hypoplastic anemia than in aplasia of the bone marrow. The bone marrow aspiration or biopsy may

on rare occasions yield a hypercellular or normocellular specimen. Such a finding probably reflects the chance sampling of a residual focus of marrow showing normal or increased cellularity. The distribution of active marrow by isotopic scanning techniques and the findings at necropsy usually reveal a diffusely hypocellular fatty marrow throughout the normally hematopoietic skeleton, although residual foci of hematopoietic marrow may be present. Reduced erythropoiesis may be confirmed by ferrokinetic studies with impaired clearance of iron from the plasma and greatly diminished, often negligible, incorporation of iron into red blood cells. Although the exact etiology of aplastic anemia is frequently unknown, the generalized failure of hematopoiesis, including erythropoiesis, granulopoiesis, and megakaryopoiesis, suggests that the primary defect is due to an absolute reduction in the numbers of pluripotent hematopoietic stem cells.

Although the term aplastic anemia is descriptive, it appears reasonable in the light of present knowledge to draw a distinction between the failure of bone marrow function associated with a hypoplastic or aplastic marrow and the failure of hematopoiesis that may be associated with hypercellular marrow, ineffective hematopoiesis. However, it must be recognized that certain bone marrow toxins which are known to produce aplastic anemia, such as benzol, may also give rise to pancytopenia with a hypercellular marrow exhibiting ineffective hematopoiesis. Furthermore, it seems reasonable to draw a distinction between the pancytopenia associated with aplastic anemia and the isolated reductions in red blood cells, granulocytes, or platelets through failure of formation of the differentiated cell lines. Disorders of formation of isolated cell lines probably reflect the action of toxic agents or the influence of immune mechanisms on the differentiation of committed rather than the pluripotent stem cell precursors in the bone marrow. Lack of fundamental knowledge of the precise etiologic mechanisms which can result in either aplastic anemia or isolated failures of formation of one of the hematopoietic cell lines may make the distinction between the disorders somewhat arbitrary. However, recent knowledge regarding the association of pure red cell aplasia with immunologic disorders and thymic tumors does suggest that different mechanisms may be operative and therefore validate the distinction. Aplastic anemia may develop without an apparent or recognized cause, or may follow exposure to ionizing radiation or a variety of chemical agents, including drugs, either known to be potentially toxic to hematopoiesis or recognized to only occasionally have this effect, or it may be familial or constitutional in etiology, becoming manifest in childhood or early adult life. The clinical course is influenced by the severity of the pancytopenia and especially by the degree of leukopenia or thrombocytopenia. If severe infective and hemorrhagic complications do not take place, or can be prevented, the patient may survive for a number of years, and occasionally complete or partial remissions may take place.

Etiology. A general classification of the etiology of aplastic anemia is given in Table 1. The exact cause of aplastic anemia is often obscure. In a considerable proportion of the cases no etiologic agent can be incriminated with certainty, and these are described as idiopathic. A small proportion of the idiopathic group occur in childhood or in early adult life, and when associated with other congenital abnormalities and a history of

TABLE 1. Etiologic Classification of Aplastic Anemia

Idiopathic
  Familial or constitutional (Fanconi's anemia)
  Acquired
Secondary
  Physical or chemical agents
    Ionizing radiation
    Drugs (cytotoxic; normally noncytotoxic)
    Nonpharmacological chemicals
  Infections
    Viral hepatitis
    Bacterial: miliary tuberculosis
  Metabolic
    Pancreatitis
    Pregnancy
  Immunologic
    Antibody mediated
    Graft versus host reaction
  Neoplastic
    Myelophthisic
    Paroxysmal nocturnal hemoglobinuria

aplastic anemia in other members of the family their separate designation as the constitutional type of aplastic anemia *(Fanconi's anemia)* is warranted. The majority of idiopathic cases are presumed to be acquired, and although no etiologic agent may be incriminated, this designation does not preclude exposure to some unrecalled or unrecognized environmental or ingested agent. In the secondary aplastic anemias in which a history can be obtained of exposure to chemical or physical agents, or when the onset was preceded by an event known to be associated with aplastic anemia, the exact causal relationship between the implicated agent or agents and the fundamental disturbance of hematopoiesis often remains obscure.

The agents which may give rise to aplastic anemia can be divided into two categories. First come agents that regularly produce bone marrow damage if the magnitude or the duration of the exposure is sufficient to produce cytotoxicity. These include exposure to ionizing radiations from x-rays, radioactive elements, or nuclear explosions; chemical agents such as benzol; and a variety of cytotoxic drugs used in the treatment of malignant disease, including nitrogen mustard, cytoxan, busulfan, the vinca alkaloids, and antimetabolites such as 6-mercaptopurine and methotrexate. The second category contains agents which have been recognized as being associated with aplastic anemia in only a small proportion of the population exposed to them. The incidence of aplastic anemia in this second category is so low that considerable periods of time have elapsed before the adverse reaction has been sufficiently widely recognized and reported for it to be appreciated as being a statistically significant risk. Drugs are the most common group in this second category. Chloramphenicol is now widely recognized as a potential cause of aplastic anemia. Inquiry as to exposure to drugs must include both drugs prescribed by physicians and drugs that can be purchased without prescription, including analgesics, hypnotics, and antihistamines. Inquiries should be made and evidence sought for the possibility of self-administration or abuse of mood-changing drugs, or the inhalation of organic solvents for the same purpose. When no history of drug ingestion can be established, the incrimination of possible etiologic agents may be exceedingly difficult, because many chemical compounds in common

daily use contain benzene derivatives or allied compounds which must be regarded with suspicion. Many such chemicals are used as solvents in common household cleaning agents, in dyes and paints, and in insecticides and fertilizers, and have been identified in animal feed supplements in which the manufacturing processes have resulted in toxic products derived from relatively nontoxic precursors. Thus the risks of exposure to potentially toxic compounds are well-nigh limitless. Despite frequent difficulty in establishing a definite etiologic agent, it is important that a full and detailed inquiry be made of the patient and relatives as to the possible exposure at work or in the home to potentially toxic chemicals, through a detailed history of daily activities and hobbies.

Since its introduction in 1948, *chloramphenicol* became recognized as the drug most commonly associated with aplastic anemia. It achieved rapid and widespread popularity with physicians by virtue of the range of its antimicrobial activity and the ease with which it could be administered. In 1952 a number of reports were published associating chloramphenicol with aplastic anemia, an association which was directly responsible for the establishment of a registry of drugs giving rise to aplastic anemia and other adverse hematologic drug reactions. The reports published in 1965 and 1967 by the Registry on Adverse Reactions showed that of 771 cases of pancytopenia 338 (44 per cent) followed the use of chloramphenicol, and that in 154 (23 per cent) chloramphenicol was the only drug taken in the preceding six months. Although the risk of developing pancytopenia and aplastic anemia after chloramphenicol is approximately 1 in 20,000 to 30,000, this is about 13 times greater than the risk of idiopathic aplastic anemia in the population as a whole. Awareness of the risk has resulted in a considerable and commendable reduction in the prescribing of chloramphenicol, partly through the increasing availability of other broad-spectrum antimicrobials of comparable activity and ease of administration. It is now generally accepted that chloramphenicol should only be prescribed in specific and serious infections in which it can be shown to be the *only* antimicrobial agent suitable on the basis of sensitivity testing. However, the awareness of the hazards of this serious complication of chloramphenicol differs in different countries, and there are still countries where it is widely prescribed or may, indeed, be obtained without prescription. The higher incidence of aplastic anemia in clinical practice in certain countries may reflect relative lack of control over the availability of this drug. Thus with increasing air travel the risks of exposure to chloramphenicol may persist despite the adverse publicity and the application of more stringent indications for its prescriptions in many nations.

It is now recognized that there are two independent types of bone marrow toxicity produced by chloramphenicol. It is well established that this drug induces a dose-related reversible bone marrow lesion characterized by maturation arrest and vacuolization in early erythroid cells, reticulocytopenia, and ferrokinetic changes indicative of suppressed erythropoiesis. This reversible effect of the drug results from inhibition of mitochondrial protein synthesis and consequent mitochondrial injury. It appears to be quite distinct from the much rarer and devastating complications of aplastic anemia, which may not be dose dependent or even directly temporally related to exposure to the drug. There is some evidence that the bone marrow aplasia may occur on the basis of a genetically determined biochemical predisposition to toxicity involving the DNA synthetic pathway. Although knowledge as to the mechanism of the reversible pharmacologic toxicity of chloramphenicol in the bone marrow may ultimately throw light onto the mechanism of marrow aplasia, it must be emphasized that currently these two mechanisms appear to be distinct and that the onset of aplasia cannot be predicted nor is it readily reversible. Thus the only way to avoid the calamitous consequence of aplastic anemia is to not expose the patient to chloramphenicol in any form.

Although the association of aplastic anemia with drugs other than chloramphenicol is well recognized, the low incidence of this complication and the fact that, as mentioned already, it is common for patients with aplastic anemia to give a history of exposure to a number of potentially toxic agents makes it difficult to calculate with any accuracy the possible risk of this complication. However, phenylbutazone was the second most frequently recorded drug in the A.M.A. Registry, having been administered alone or concomitantly with an apparently innocuous agent to 27 patients and having been associated with other potentially toxic agents in a total of 52 patients (6.3 per cent). Other drugs, including the hydantoin analogues used in treating epilepsy, sulfonamides, sulfonylureas, gold compounds, organic arsenicals, potassium perchlorate, and quinacrine, are known to be associated with aplastic anemia. At least 50 other drugs have been implicated, and many of them are chemically related to drugs established as being associated with aplastic anemia. Among those obtainable without prescription are a wide variety of antihistamine preparations. In addition, salicylamide, widely available as a sedative without prescription, has been reported in three patients as being associated with aplastic anemia.

Benzol and a wide variety of *aromatic hydrocarbons* derived from the refining of petroleum and coal products are included in many cleaning solvents and form the basis of many compounds used in the petrochemical and plastic industries. Aplastic anemia has been reported as following exposure to aromatic hydrocarbons by siphoning gasoline from gas tanks. The widespread use of these compounds in dyes, solvents, insecticides, cements, glues, and fingernail polish, and as diluents to paints, varnishes, and lacquers as thinners and paint removers, makes the risk of exposure of the general population very considerable. Furthermore, in many instances the relative purity of organic solvents is unknown and significant amounts of benzene may be present. Aplastic anemia is recognized to follow the ingestion of benzene trinitrotoluene or exposure to Stoddard solvent, widely used in the automobile industry as a cleaning agent.

Aplastic anemia is a recognized complication of "gluesniffing," and many of the glues and cements may contain benzene or benzene derivatives.

Insecticides such as gamma benzene hexachloride (Lindane), chlordane, and chlorophenothane (DDT) have been associated with aplastic anemia, and have been reported in the A.M.A. Registry. Many of these organic insecticides are used suspended in petroleum solvents which may contain benzene.

Aplastic anemia has occasionally been reported after exposure to hair dyes, tints, rinses, and sprays, but in view of the widespread use of these agents it appears that they represent a negligible risk.

Aplastic anemia has been associated with *hepatitis* in more than 50 patients. The onset of aplastic anemia is usually within two to six months after the hepatitis has resolved. The nature of the etiologic relationship between hepatitis and aplastic anemia is unclear. Viral etiology of the hepatitis has seldom been established. Furthermore, it is well recognized that many agents capable of producing aplastic anemia are also hepatotoxic; thus both the hepatitis and the aplastic anemia may have a common etiology. Even when the viral nature of the hepatitis is established, the possibility remains that hepatic dysfunction itself may increase the risk of aplastic anemia because of impaired or abnormal handling of potentially marrow-toxic agents.

The etiology of *pure red cell aplasia* can, like that of aplastic anemia, be divided into constitutional and acquired forms. More than 100 cases of chronic erythroid hypoplasia and aplasia have been described in childhood. The onset may be at birth but is more commonly recognized within the first two years of life. The occasional occurrence of the disorder in a sibling has suggested a genetic or inherited abnormality, although detailed family studies have not provided evidence to support this. A metabolic defect in the handling of tryptophan has been described in some of the affected children. The children may go into remission either spontaneously or in response to adrenal steroid administration. Acquired red cell aplasia may occur as an acute transient episode, particularly in children with congenital hemolytic anemia. This disorder, most frequently reported in hereditary spherocytosis, is thought to be due to suppression of erythropoiesis in association with viral illnesses and may reflect a direct action of viruses on erythropoiesis or be a consequence of an immunologic response to a viral infection. The recognition of this disorder in association with chronic hemolytic anemia probably reflects the dramatic onset of anemia caused by cessation of erythropoiesis and an increased rate of hemolysis, and may indicate increased susceptibility of an actively erythropoietic bone marrow to a variety of toxic factors. Pure red cell aplasia in the adult is associated with thymic tumors in about 30 to 50 per cent of patients. The presence of a thymoma and the response of these patients to either thymectomy or adrenal steroid or immunosuppressive treatment have suggested that the selective disturbance of erythropoiesis is due to an immunologic mechanism. Support for this has come from demonstration of antibodies in the patient's serum which react against erythroid precursor cells and from the selective suppression of erythropoiesis in laboratory animals given gamma globulin prepared from the patient's serum. Although anti-erythropoietin antibodies have also been demonstrated, the presence of high levels of erythropoietin in the serum of these patients makes it unlikely that this is the primary mode of action.

Incidence. Idiopathic aplastic anemia is rare and occurs predominantly in children and young adults of either sex. The incidence of secondary aplastic anemia will be directly related to the size of the population exposed to the causal agents. Increasing use of atomic energy and of radioactive isotopes and x-rays in both industry and medicine has increased the risks of exposure to ionizing irradiation. However, the widespread recognition of the hazard makes it unlikely that aplastic anemia will increase through this cause except by accidents or negligence. Nevertheless, numerous cases of aplastic anemia resulted from the two atomic bombs exploded over Japan in 1945, and the risk of aplastic anemia through atomic warfare and, indeed, other chemical agents under such conditions is ever present. The incidence of secondary aplastic anemia caused by drugs and other toxic chemical agents is difficult to estimate with accuracy. It has been calculated that 1 of every 20,000 to 30,000 patients receiving chloramphenicol develops pancytopenia. The incidence of secondary aplastic anemia will be dependent on the population exposed to known toxic agents. The increasing use of cytotoxic drugs in malignant disease, in order to produce suppression of immune system in a wide variety of disorders, and the use of methotrexate in the treatment of psoriasis have greatly increased the risk of the development of hypoplastic or aplastic anemia as a complication of treatment. In patients exposed to phenylbutazone, the incidence rises with age and reflects the relative preponderance of women receiving this and other related agents in the treatment of rheumatoid arthritis. The incidence of pure red cell aplasia depends on whether the disorder is constitutional or acquired. Both the constitutional and the acute acquired red cell aplasia seen in congenital hemolytic anemia are most commonly seen in childhood. Acquired pure red cell aplasia in the adult is mainly seen in middle age. There is a significant preponderance of females over males when pure red cell aplasia is associated with thymoma, whereas males exceed females in those patients in whom a thymoma cannot be demonstrated either radiologically or on exploration of the anterior mediastinum.

Pathology and Pathogenesis. The peripheral blood count reveals a reduction in all cellular elements, with lowering of the red cell count, packed red cell volume, and hemoglobin concentration, and reduction in the total circulating white cells, particularly those of the granulocyte series, although absolute monocytopenia is usually present. The platelet count is invariably reduced and may be very low. The anemia is usually normochromic but may be slightly macrocytic with red blood cells showing some slight changes in size and shape. The reticulocyte count varies from 0 to 5 per cent, but the absolute reticulocyte count is usually subnormal. The reticulocytes may be large and immature, possibly reflecting a response of the remaining erythroid cells to increased erythropoietin stimulation with a short bone marrow transit time. The presence of nucleated red blood cells in the peripheral blood is unusual and implies some other disorder of hematopoiesis. Absolute granulocytopenia is an invariable feature and is of importance in relation to the immediate prognosis, because an absolute granulocyte count of less than 200 per cubic millimeter puts a patient at great risk from infectious complications. The absolute monocyte count is usually reduced, and an absolute lymphocytopenia is a common finding. It is unusual to find immature cells of the granulocytic or lymphocytic cell lines in the peripheral blood.

These peripheral blood findings reflect the disordered hematopoiesis in the bone marrow. The specimens of bone marrow are usually aspirated without difficulty or pain and usually yield fragments which consist of fat spaces with few cellular elements. Occasionally bone marrow aspiration reveals a normocellular or hypercellular specimen, which may reflect the chance aspiration of a sample of bone marrow with residual normal activity, in which case aspiration should be carried out at other sites if the diagnosis is to be confirmed. Further information regarding over-all cellularity of the bone marrow can be obtained from the histology of needle or trephine biopsies. The relative proportions of the different cellular elements in the bone marrow seen on aspiration or on biopsy can vary from patient to patient. Both the degree of cellularity and the relative involvement of the different cell lines may reflect the nature and severity of the action of the toxic agent inducing disordered hematopoiesis. Although increases in precursor cells may be present, suggesting a "maturation arrest," or may be accompanied by changes in the chromatin pattern of the erythroid precursors with some megaloblastic-like features, an absolute increase in blast cells is uncommon. The presence of an increase in granulocyte precursors and a reduction in cytoplasmic granules within the maturing cells may make the distinction between aplastic anemia and subleukemic myelocytic leukemia difficult. However, the absence of blast cells in the peripheral blood and the presence of a hypoplastic or aplastic marrow at other sites usually distinguish between aplastic anemia and subleukemic leukemia. When the patient has received multiple blood transfusions, hemosiderosis of the bone marrow may be present and in due course will involve other organs, notably the liver, spleen, and heart. Enlargement of the liver and spleen may be due to hemosiderosis, because extramedullary hematopoiesis is uncommon. Other pathologic changes are related to infectious and hemorrhagic complications which are frequently encountered during the course of the illness and are the usual causes of death.

The mechanism by which exposure to irradiation or chemical agents induces the cellular damage which results in aplastic anemia is incompletely understood. Ionizing radiations and radiomimetic drugs are thought to inhibit mitosis, probably by causing disturbances of DNA replication or synthesis. The antimetabolites used in treatment of malignant disease either interfere with the formation of purines or nucleic acids or, in the case of the vinca alkaloids, inhibit chromatin separation through interaction with spindle proteins. Although exposure to radiation or cytotoxic drugs characteristically produces a transient depression of hematopoiesis, the persistent disorder of hematopoiesis characterizing aplastic anemia implies a more fundamental defect in stem cell proliferation and differentiation. A similar distinction must be drawn between the transient, reversible, and dose-related disturbance of hematopoiesis that follows ingestion of chloramphenicol and the more fundamental and probably unrelated disturbance of hematopoiesis characterizing aplastic anemia caused by this agent. Although the transient disorder of hematopoiesis caused by chloramphenicol can be regarded as a direct or metabolic effect on cell maturation, aplastic anemia would appear to imply some more fundamental derangement of the genetic information necessary for stem cell proliferation and differentiation. A variety of evidence supports the latter view.

Exposure to irradiation may be followed by persistent disorders of the chromosomal structure of lymphocytes which may be detected months or years after the radiation exposure. In aplastic anemia from any cause, the level of fetal hemoglobin in the erythrocytes produced by the bone marrow may be increased, suggesting some persistent derangement of the control of globin chain synthesis. Although initial results suggested that a high hemoglobin F might be a good prognostic sign, this interpretation has been questioned. In Fanconi's anemia, in which some as yet unknown inherited influence can result in the appearance of aplastic anemia in childhood or early adult life, chromatin breaks and other disturbances of the karyotype have been described. Furthermore, abnormalities of the red cell enzymes have also been described. The common association of Fanconi's anemia with developmental abnormalities affecting the structure or position of the kidneys and radiologic evidence of abnormalities of the bony skeleton suggests the presence of some fundamental derangement of genetic factors influencing development, although the causal relationship between these abnormalities and the subsequent development of aplastic anemia is as yet unexplained.

Still further support for the view that a fundamental disturbance of stem cell structure and function is the basis for aplastic anemia comes from the association between aplastic anemia and *paroxysmal nocturnal hemoglobinuria*. Hypoplastic or aplastic anemia may develop as a complication of paroxysmal nocturnal hemoglobinuria (PNH), or a small proportion of the red blood cells in aplastic anemia may show the increased susceptibility to complement lysis characteristic of PNH. The PNH red blood cells may be found at the onset or during recovery from aplastic anemia and be associated with frank hemolytic anemia. Since the membrane disorder characterizing PNH can be shown to be present in red blood cells, granulocytes, and platelets, it is probable that the lesion is due to proliferation of a modified stem cell line. In pure red cell aplasia there is an isolated failure of differentiation of the erythroid cell line which may reflect different susceptibilities of the various hematopoietic cell lines to agents capable of inducing aplastic anemia. A variety of drugs may induce transient erythroid hypoplasia and, in the case of chloramphenicol, be associated with morphologic changes in the erythroid precursors; however, the relationship of this response to pure red cell aplasia is ill understood and appears to be a fundamentally different reaction. As mentioned under Etiology, the association of pure red cell aplasia in adults with thymoma points strongly to an immunologic mechanism specifically directed against erythroid precursor cells.

Clinical Manifestations. The patient's symptoms are related to the rapidity of onset and the extent to which the different hematopoietic cell lines are affected. Acute aplasia induced by ionizing radiation or by cytotoxic drugs can develop rapidly, and in such circumstances the symptoms are predominantly due to the infective or hemorrhagic complications of severe granulocytopenia or thrombocytopenia. Anemia, unless it is due to some underlying disease, develops more insidiously, although gastrointestinal hemorrhage or increase in menstrual blood loss or uterine bleeding can rapidly exacerbate it. When the granulocyte and platelet counts are at levels which provide some protection against infection and spontaneous hemorrhage, the presenting symptoms are usually those of anemia: pallor, fatigue, dyspnea and tachycardia on exertion, and headache. Severe granulocytopenia may be accompanied by infections of the skin and oral and rectal mucosa, with the development of painful ulceration at these sites which may cause difficulties in swallowing and defecation, or by urinary tract infections. Thrombocytopenia is usually associated with bleeding into the skin from mucous membranes and spontaneous bleeding from the gums, nose, vagina, or rectum. Occasionally patients appear to tolerate severe thrombocytopenia without serious bleeding except at sites subjected to minor degrees of trauma. Intracerebral or subarachnoid hemorrhage may take place and is one of the causes of death. However, it is often remarkable how long patients survive with an increased hemorrhagic tendency caused by thrombocytopenia before this serious complication occurs.

The principal features on physical examination relate to the changes that result from anemia, the infective or hemorrhagic complications. At the onset of the illness physical examination may be unremarkable apart from petechiae of the skin at sites exposed to undue pressure and on the lower limbs. Larger bruises may be present at sites subjected to trauma, including venipuncture. Examination of the optic fundi often reveals flame-shaped hemorrhages and occasional Roth spots. The extent of the retinal changes is frequently related to the degree of anemia as well as to the severity of the thrombocytopenia. It is unusual for the spleen to be enlarged in the early stages of the disease; indeed, the finding of splenic enlargement usually suggests the presence of some other disorder causing pancytopenia. Severe anemia is accompanied by tachycardia, cardiac enlargement, a systolic hemic murmur, and signs of congestive cardiac failure. In the later stages of the disease, particularly when multiple transfusions have been given, increased pigmentation of the skin and enlargement of the liver and spleen may indicate development of hemosiderosis. Infective complications can be accompanied by chronic ulceration of the oral and rectal mucosa, and can give rise to fever. Hectic fever and rigors are usually due to widespread infections, which in the absence of a granulocyte response may be accompanied with few localizing symptoms or signs. Neurologic signs may be present when hemorrhagic or infective complications involve the brain, spinal cord, or peripheral nerves.

Diagnosis. Pancytopenia is a cardinal feature of aplastic anemia, and although the blood count may vary, it is unwise to make the diagnosis unless there is severe depression of all cellular elements at some stage in the disease.

The degree of anemia may vary, depending on when the patient is seen and the relationship of the blood count to previous blood transfusions. The morphology of the red blood cells in peripheral blood smears is usually normal, but slight macrocytosis and anisocytosis may be present. There is usually an absolute reticulocytopenia, although because of the degree of anemia the percentage of reticulocytes may be increased, and an absolute reticulocyte count should be calculated, because it is usually subnormal. The presence of an increased reticulocyte count should lead one to suspect the possibility of the development of paroxysmal nocturnal hemoglobinuria. It is unusual for nucleated red cells to be present in the peripheral blood, and, when found, some other disorder of hematopoiesis should be considered. The total white cell count is usually low, and an absolute granulocytopenia is a feature. The severity of the granulocytopenia is of considerable immediate prognostic significance, because a count of 200 per cubic millimeter or less suggests that the patient is in imminent danger of infective complications. The neutrophil granulocytes may be deficient in granules. Metamyelocytes, myelocytes, and blast cells are rarely found, and, if present, suggest the presence of leukemia rather than aplastic anemia. The absolute monocyte and lymphocyte counts are often depressed in severe cases. Thrombocytopenia is frequently present and may be severe. Large and bizarre-shaped platelets may be present in the blood smear. Severe thrombocytopenia is associated with prolonged bleeding time and positive tests for capillary fragility. Neither of these tests is of diagnostic value, and they do not warrant the discomfort they may produce for the patient. Coagulation tests are usually normal except for those dependent upon normal numbers of platelets. *Bone marrow* aspiration should be carried out and may be performed safely if attention is paid to aseptic techniques and to the prevention of subsequent hemorrhage by applying firm pressure to the site of aspiration for 15 to 20 minutes. Aspiration is achieved with little pain. The specimen often contains an adequate number of bone marrow fragments, although diluted with blood. A needle or trephine biopsy of the bone marrow may be helpful in the assessment of cellularity. Smears from the bone marrow aspirate usually reveal marked hypocellularity of the marrow fragments with a predominance of reticulum cells, mast cells, lymphocytoid cells, and plasma cells. Cells of the myeloid series are often grossly reduced in numbers, and those that are present are usually at the promyelocyte and myelocyte stages of maturation. Megakaryocytes may be absent or very infrequent. Erythroid precursors may be more numerous than those of the myeloid series and, although usually normoblastic, may show abnormal nuclear maturation with some megaloblastic features. Iron can usually be demonstrated in the reticulum cells and may be greatly increased if the patient has received blood transfusions. In view of the selective involvement of the bone marrow, a hypercellular specimen may be obtained, in which case aspiration at another site is advisable and a needle biopsy may be helpful.

The serum iron level is usually elevated, and the total iron binding capacity of the serum is reduced. Ferrokinetic studies may reveal a normal rate of plasma iron clearance and turnover but marked diminution of iron utilization. External scanning of the iron distribution into organs has shown that most of the iron is taken up by the liver rather than the bone marrow. The ferrokinetic studies are of little diagnostic value. The levels of erythropoietin in plasma and excreted in the urine are high and often exceed values found in patients with comparable degrees of anemia. The levels of fetal hemoglobin (hemoglobin F) may be increased. Except for the association with paroxysmal nocturnal hemoglobinuria, evidence for shortened red blood cell survival caused by hemolysis is usually absent and of little value in the presence of frank or occult hemorrhage.

The diseases most likely to be confused with aplastic or hypoplastic anemia are those which lead to pancytopenia by other mechanisms. They include subacute leukemia or preleukemia and other forms of myelophthisic anemia.

The greatest difficulty may be encountered in distinguishing between a hypoplastic anemia and subacute or subleukemic myelocytic leukemia. The presence of an increased number of blast cells and myelocytic precursors in the bone marrow can usually enable the distinction to be made, as can the finding of blast cells and other immature cells in the peripheral blood. The distinction usually becomes apparent during the course of the illness when a more obviously leukemic blood picture may develop. The distinction between a preleukemic state and a true aplastic anemia is sometimes rendered difficult by the development of acute myelocytic leukemia in a patient who has had aplastic anemia for many months or years. It is possible that the agent or agents

provoking aplasia, such as irradiation, are also leukemogenic. The finding of enlargement of the spleen or lymph nodes, generalized bone tenderness, or radiologic evidence of bone destruction should lead one to doubt the diagnosis. It is unusual for the level of immunoglobulins to be raised, and the finding of a monoclonal protein in the serum should arouse suspicion. Infiltration of the bone marrow by metastatic malignancy, metastasis, plasma cells, Hodgkin's disease, lymphosarcoma, or myelofibrosis, all of which can cause a myelophthisic anemia, can usually be recognized by the cellular infiltration seen in smears and histologic sections of biopsies.

Treatment. The principles underlying treatment are to recognize and, wherever possible, to prevent further exposure to any recognized or implicated causative agent, and then to endeavor to prevent hemorrhagic and infective complications, while correcting anemia by blood transfusion in the hope that the patient may go into spontaneous remission.

Whenever possible, all drug therapy should be discontinued unless specifically indicated, in which case drugs thought to have the least risk of marrow toxicity should be used. Only in the case of heavy metals, such as gold, are measures directed toward increasing excretion of the toxic agent from the body likely to be helpful. The patient should be advised against coming into contact with organic solvents in any form, and should only take those drugs specifically prescribed.

The general supportive measures required are determined by the severity of the pancytopenia. An ambulatory patient will often tolerate an anemia of 8 grams per 100 ml, and therefore a blood transfusion is only indicated when the anemia is more severe than this or when hemorrhage or intercurrent infections result in a fall in the hemoglobin concentration below this level. Blood should be given as packed cells which have been stored for less than seven days, and care should be taken in the cross-matching procedure, because it is not uncommon for the patient to develop group-specific antibodies after receiving multiple transfusions. The transfusion of platelet concentrates is indicated to control hemorrhagic complications when the platelet count falls to 10,000 to 20,000 per cubic millimeter. The platelets transfused should be blood group compatible and can be shown to have improved survival if they are drawn from an HL-A-compatible donor if this is feasible. The use of platelet transfusions is probably best reserved for the control of serious thrombocytopenic bleeding, because the development of antibodies to transfused platelets often limits their effectiveness when given on a regular or prophylactic basis. When severe granulocytopenia is accompanied by blood-borne bacterial infections, the transfusion of granulocytes prepared by using a cell separator or by filtration techniques may enable an infection which is not responding to appropriate antimicrobial therapy to be brought under control. The granulocytes so prepared have a very short survival and therefore can only be used to combat serious infective complications.

Apart from these specific measures, meticulous care should be given to the acutely ill pancytopenic patient with regard to the prevention of infection by scrupulous attention to aseptic techniques in setting up intravenous infusions, regular oral hygiene, and protection of the skin, particularly at pressure points. At no time should intramuscular injections be given, because the hematoma at the site of injection impedes the absorption of a drug and greatly increases the risk of infection at the injection site. The principal benefit of isolation procedures may be to constantly remind those looking after the patient of the risks of inappropriate procedures. Microbial cultures should be obtained on all infected lesions, and blood cultures should be performed whenever the patient's condition suggests systemic infection. Antimicrobial therapy should be given after cultures have been taken and should be modified in the light of the sensitivities of the organisms cultured. It is not uncommon for patients with granulocytopenia to have serious infections with bacteria which in other circumstances would not be regarded as pathogens. The prophylactic administration of antimicrobial drugs is of doubtful benefit and may predispose to infection with resistant organisms.

There is little evidence that adrenal steroids influence the degree of pancytopenia or the prognosis. Transient remissions have been documented, but these may reflect the natural history of the disease. Steroids may lessen the bleeding caused by thrombocytopenia and may occasionally reduce the fever in patients unresponsive to antimicrobial therapy. In view of the uncertainty as to the beneficial effects of adrenal steroids, it may be warranted to give prednisone or prednisolone in a dose of 20 mg per day for a trial period of one or two months. The possible benefits of adrenal steroid administration have to be weighed against the known side effects and the greater risk of bacterial infections. Likewise, there is no substantive evidence that splenectomy is beneficial; it should be considered only after multiple blood transfusions are associated with enlargement of the spleen and evidence that the survival of the transfused blood is significantly reduced. The immediate risks of hemorrhage at splenectomy have been reduced with the increasing availability of platelet transfusions, but any benefit must be balanced against the risk of increased susceptibility to bacterial infections that have followed splenectomy, particularly when associated with persistent hematopoietic disorders.

A variety of drugs have been used to enhance the hematopoietic activity of the bone marrow. There is no evidence that administration of vitamin B_{12} is of benefit; indeed, the fact that this has to be given as an intramuscular injection is a valid contraindication. Occasionally patients may become deficient in folic acid, but this is unlikely to take place if the patient is able to tolerate an adequate diet. Treatment with iron is contraindicated, because it will further add to the iron overload induced by multiple blood transfusions. There is evidence in childhood that the combined use of androgens and steroids in patients with constitutional aplastic anemia (Fanconi's anemia) or acquired aplastic anemia may be accompanied by partial or complete remission of the anemia, although the response of the granulocytes or platelets tends to be less satisfactory. Nevertheless, the reduction in blood transfusion requirements may be considerable and thereby both reduce symptoms and reduce the risks of iron overload and other complications of multiple transfusions. The experience of adult aplastic anemia with androgens has been far less encouraging, and although the anemia may improve, the over-all survival curve of adults with aplastic anemia has not been significantly influenced. Nevertheless, it is reasonable to try androgen therapy for a period of three to six months in the hope that a partial remission may be induced or that transfusion requirements may be reduced. The oral synthetic testosterone, oxymetholone (2 to 4 mg per kilo-

gram per day), is the drug of choice, because it has fewer side effects than intramuscular injections of testosterone enanthate (3 to 10 mg per kilogram once a week) or oral administration of testosterone propionate (0.25 mg per kilogram per day). Liver function tests should be performed regularly on all patients receiving androgen therapy, because cholestatic hepatitis may develop as a toxic manifestation of the treatment. In the absence of a remission in two to three months the drug should be discontinued, because the side effects of hepatotoxicity, fluid retention, and hirsutism, particularly in women, do not justify their continued use.

Bone marrow transplantation has been used successfully in a number of patients. This procedure should only be carried out in centers which have the ability to HL-A type the patient and potential donors, and must be accompanied by use of immunosuppressive drugs to prevent both graft rejection and the development of graft versus host disease. Although this approach is being actively explored in a number of centers and has been accompanied by dramatic success with recovery of hematopoiesis when the graft has taken, it is too early to assess its relative benefits and cost-effectiveness as against careful supportive therapy with the ultimate development of a spontaneous remission. It seems unlikely at present that this treatment will be applicable to more than a few highly selected patients for whom HL-A-compatible donors are readily available.

In patients with pure red cell aplasia and radiologic evidence of a thymoma, surgical excision of the thymic tumor has been associated with remission in approximately half the cases. These patients may benefit from use of adrenal steroids, although the dose required can maintain a sustained remission but may be too high to be tolerated by the patient without producing serious side effects. The evidence that pure red cell aplasia may have an autoimmune basis has led to the use of immunosuppressive drugs such as cyclophosphamide and 6-mercaptopurine, and a few patients seem to have successfully responded to such treatment. It is thus worthwhile giving a course of treatment with these drugs at a dosage which does not induce severe depression of the granulocyte or platelet counts. There is no evidence that splenectomy is of benefit in patients with pure red cell aplasia.

Prognosis. The immediate prognosis is related to the severity of pancytopenia and the degree of bone marrow aplasia. The initial prognosis of the severely pancytopenic patient is grave; approximately 30 per cent of them die within the first year. The initial survival may improve with the increased availability of platelet transfusions and of antimicrobial drugs in overcoming bacterial infections. Patients with less severe pancytopenia survive for a number of years despite persistent anemia, granulocytopenia, and thrombocytopenia. Spontaneous or drug-induced remissions may take place and are most likely to be seen in patients with mild pancytopenia and moderate hypocellularity of the bone marrow. Death usually results from infective or hemorrhagic complications. Hemosiderosis of the heart and liver may be a late sequel of patients requiring repeated blood transfusions.

Allen, D. M., Fine, M. H., Nechles, T. F., and Dameshek, W.: Oxymetha-
   lone therapy in aplastic anemia. Blood, 32:83, 1968.
Buckner, C. D., Clift, R. A., Fefer, A., Neiman, P., Storb, R., and Thomas,
   E. D.: Human marrow transplantation—current status. In Brown, E. B.
   (ed.): Progress in Hematology, Vol. 8. New York, Grune & Stratton,
   1973, p. 299.

Dacie, J. V., and Lewis, S. M.: Paroxysmal nocturnal haemoglobinuria: Clinical manifestations, haematology and nature of the disease. Ser. Haematol., 3:3, 1972.

Dameshek, W., Brown, S. M., and Rubin, A. D.: "Pure" red cell anemia (erythroblastic hypoplasia) and thymoma. Semin. Hematol., 4:222, 1967.

Erslev, A. J.: Aplastic anemia. In Williams, W. J., Beutler, E., Erslev, A. J., and Rundles, R. W. (eds.): Hematology. New York, McGraw-Hill Book Company, 1972, p. 207.

Erslev, A. J.: Pure red cell aplasia. In Williams, W. J., Beutler, E., Erslev, A. J., and Rundles, R. W. (eds.): Hematology. New York, McGraw-Hill Book Company, 1972, p. 227.

Harris, J. W., and Kellermyer, R. W.: The Red Cell. Production, Metabolism, Destruction: Normal and Abnormal. 2nd ed. Cambridge, Mass., Harvard University Press, l970.

Krantz, S. B., and Kao, V.: Studies on red cell aplasia. II. Report of a second patient with an antibody to erythroblast nuclei and a remission after immunosuppressive therapy. Blood, 34:1, 1969.

Registry on Adverse Drug Reactions, Panel on Hematology. Council on Drugs, American Medical Association. April-May 1965, June 1, 1967.

Sanchez-Medal, L., Gormez-Leal, A., Duarte, L., and Guadalupe, M. G.: Anabolic androgenic steroids in the treatment of acquired aplastic anemia. Blood, 34:283, 1969.

Williams, D. M., Lynch, R. E., and Cartwright, G. E.: Drug-induced aplastic anemia. Semin. Hematol., 10:195, 1973.

Yunis, A. A.: Chloramphenicol-induced bone marrow suppression. Semin. Hematol., 10:225, 1973.

735. SIDEROBLASTIC ANEMIA
M. C. Brain

The sideroblastic anemias are a heterogeneous group of disorders in which a normocytic or slightly macrocytic anemia is accompanied by ineffective erythropoiesis and defective hemoglobin synthesis, manifested by hypochromasia of a proportion of red cells in the peripheral blood, with the finding of *ringed sideroblasts* in the bone marrow. Ringed sideroblasts are nucleated red blood cell precursors, often showing defective hemoglobinization, which can be shown on iron staining to have a perinuclear ring distribution of iron-staining granules. The perinuclear distribution of the iron distinguishes this disorder from the increase in iron-staining granules which may be seen in megaloblastic anemias and in thalassemia. Electron microscopic studies have shown that the nonheme iron is located between the cristae of the perinuclear mitochondria, and may also be present as ferritin and ferritin aggregates in the cytoplasm. The presence of ringed sideroblasts may be suspected when basophilic granules are observed in hypochromic erythroblasts in Romanovsky-stained preparations. Studies of heme and globin synthesis have demonstrated that the defective hemoglobin synthesis is due to failure of incorporation of iron into protoporphyrin to form heme. Increased levels of erythrocyte protoporphyrin may be found, and the defective hemoglobin synthesis observed in vitro can be corrected by the provision of heme. The sideroblastic anemias may be classified as in Table 2.

Primary acquired sideroblastic anemia of adults is thought to be due to acquired disorder of the heme synthetic pathway. It has been thought by some to be a variant of erythroleukemia, and a proportion of patients subsequently develop either erythroleukemia or a chronic subacute myeloid leukemia. This type of sideroblastic anemia occurs most frequently in men and women late in life, and has no distinguishing clinical features. *Hereditary sex-linked* sideroblastic anemia is rare, but appears to be transmitted as a sex-linked recessive abnormality. The precise metabolic defect is still incompletely understood, and may involve different enzymatic steps in the protoporphyrin synthetic pathway in different subjects. Anemia occurs in early childhood and presents problems analogous to the chronic anemia caused by defective globin chain synthesis which characterizes thalassemic syndromes. However, it requires blood transfusions less commonly but, as in thalassemia, the chronic anemia and enhanced dietary iron absorption can lead to development of hemosiderosis of the liver and myocardium.

Pyridoxal phosphate functions as a coenzyme in the synthesis of delta amino levulinic acid, the product of the first synthetic step in porphyrin synthesis. Pyridoxal-responsive sideroblastic anemias may thus arise as an unexplained primary disorder; in alcoholism, in which the formation of pyridoxal phosphate from pyridoxine may be impaired; or as a consequence of isoniazid therapy, a drug which is a metabolic antagonist of pyridoxine. Sideroblastic anemia may also be due to pyridoxine deficiency as a complication of severe malabsorption syndromes. In patients in whom there is pyridoxal phosphate deficiency caused by ethanol ingestion, malabsorption, or drug antagonism, the anemia responds to the administration of physiologic concentrations of pyridoxal phosphate. Patients with acquired pyridoxine-responsive anemia not apparently caused by isoniazid ingestion or ethanol occasionally respond to pharmacologic doses of pyridoxine. The biochemical explanation for this is as yet unclear. Still other patients have been described who appear to respond to crude liver extract and may have a fundamental disorder of tryptophan metabolism. The sideroblastic anemia that results from lead poisoning is due to inhibition of delta levulinic acid dehydrase and ferrochetalase (heme synthetase), important steps in heme synthesis.

The degree of anemia may vary but is usually in the range of 7 to 8 grams of hemoglobin, with a lowered mean cell hemoglobin concentration. The red cells may show a varying degree of hypochromasia, and not uncommonly there may be a dimorphic blood picture with a varying proportion of normochromic normocytic cells with hypochromic microcytic red cells. Macrocytosis and a moderate degree of poikilocytosis may be present. The red cells may contain Pappenheimer bodies, demonstrable as iron-containing siderocytes on iron staining. Basophilic stippling is a feature of lead poisoning. The absolute reticulocyte count is usually reduced. The leukocyte

---

TABLE 2.   Sideroblastic Anemias: Classification

1. Primary
   a. Acquired sideroblastic anemia in adults (synonyms: chronic refractory anemia with sideroblastic bone marrow, refractory normoblastic anemia, sideroachrestic anemia, refractory sideroblastic anemia)
   b. Hereditary (sex-linked) sideroblastic anemia
2. Pyridoxine-responsive sideroblastic anemia
3. Secondary
   a. Sideroblastic anemia associated with rheumatoid arthritis, polyarthritis, carcinoma, myelofibrosis, leukemia, multiple myeloma, hereditary and acquired hemolytic anemias, malabsorption syndromes, or chronic alcoholism
   b. Drug-induced: isoniazid, cycloserine, and other antituberculous drugs
   c. Lead poisoning

and platelet counts are usually normal. The plasma iron and transferrin saturation are either normal or high. As mentioned earlier, the diagnosis is made on examination of the bone marrow which shows erythroid hyperplasia, defective hemoglobinization, and increased iron both in the marrow fragments and in the developing erythroblasts. The erythroblasts may show megaloblastic features and the associated defective maturation of white cell precursors. These changes are usually indicative of an accompanying folate deficiency, which can be confirmed by finding a low serum folate level. Myelopoiesis is usually normal, although an increase in blast cells and early precursor cells of the myeloid series may point to an associated subacute myeloid leukemia.

It is not uncommon for acquired sideroblastic anemia in the adult to be confused with iron deficiency anemia, although the high serum iron and the presence of iron in the bone marrow preclude this diagnosis.

Treatment should be directed toward correcting a folate deficiency when it is present and vitamin B_{12} deficiency has been excluded. A trial of pyridoxine of 50 mg a day for two to four weeks is indicated. A variable response may take place to either folate and/or pyridoxine treatment. Patients have been reported who only respond to pyridoxal phosphate given parenterally. Blood transfusions may be required when the hemoglobin level falls to below 8 grams per 100 ml and when symptoms or complications caused by anemia are present. The blood transfusion requirements may increase and will tend to exacerbate iron overload. Iron treatment by any route is absolutely contraindicated. When sideroblastic anemia is due to a drug, removal of the agent or treatment with pyridoxine can result in complete recovery. Except in those patients in whom the anemia is associated with a subacute leukemia, the prognosis in terms of survival is good, although chronic anemia usually persists.

Hines, J. D., and Cowan, D. H.: Studies on the pathogenesis of alcohol-induced sideroblastic bone marrow abnormalities. N. Engl. J. Med., 283:441, 1970.

Hines, J. D., and Grasso, J. A.: The sideroblastic anemias. Semin. Hematol., 7:86, 1970.

Moore, C. V.: Sideroblastic anemia. *In* Williams, W. J., Beutler, E., Erslev, A. J., and Rundles, R. W. (eds.): Hematology. New York, McGraw-Hill Book Company, 1972, p. 349.

736. MYELOPHTHISIC ANEMIA

M. C. Brain

The term myelophthisic anemia is applied to those anemias accompanied by the presence of nucleated red cell precursors and immature white cells in the peripheral blood resulting from a disturbance in the microarchitecture of the bone marrow brought about by infiltration of the bone marrow by abnormal cells or progressive fibrosis of the bone marrow, as in myelosclerosis. The disorder occurs when the bone marrow is extensively invaded or replaced with leukemic cells, the plasma cells of multiple myeloma, metastatic carcinoma or sarcoma, Hodgkin's disease and other malignant lymphomas, infectious or noninfectious granulomas, or lipid storage cells. Carcinomas of the breast, lung, prostate, stomach, kidney, and thyroid and neuroblastomas are most frequently associated with metastatic infiltration of the bone marrow. Extramedullary hematopoiesis can often be demonstrated at necropsy and can give rise to massive enlargement of the spleen and liver in a patient with a chronic myelophthisic anemia such as myelosclerosis.

The anemia may be moderate to severe; the white blood cell count may be elevated or depressed; and the platelet count may be normal or increased, but is more commonly reduced. A degree of anemia is often unrelated to the extent of bone marrow infiltration, suggesting that there is a more fundamental disturbance of hematopoiesis than can be accounted for by the extent of bone marrow infiltration. Survival of red cells may be reduced.

The clinical manifestations are usually those of the underlying disease, although not infrequently a myelophthisic anemia may be the presenting feature in a patient with widespread metastasis from a small primary tumor which may itself have given rise to few symptoms or signs. Bone pain may be severe, and may be either generalized or localized to the site of pathologic fractures. Symptoms may arise from the severity of the anemia, and bleeding may be associated with the thrombocytopenia. In patients with widespread metastatic adenocarcinoma, activation of coagulation within the blood can contribute to the thrombocytopenia and may rarely be associated with a microangiopathic hemolytic anemia. Enlargement of lymph nodes and the liver may be a manifestation of the underlying malignant disease; enlargement of spleen usually reflects the duration of the anemia and the extent of extramedullary hematopoiesis.

Myelophthisic anemia should be suspected whenever nucleated red blood cell precursors are found in the peripheral blood in association with a normocytic anemia and in the absence of other obvious disorders of hematopoiesis. In patients with known malignant diseases, the appearance of nucleated red cells in the blood is highly suggestive of bone marrow infiltration. In patients with moderate anemia the red blood cells show few morphologic changes. The presence of teardrop cells is suggestive of myelofibrosis, and when anemia is marked there may be greater degrees of poikilocytosis, polychromasia, and basophilic stippling. The blood picture may be complicated by a concomitant hypochromic anemia resulting from iron deficiency, by gastrointestinal blood loss, or by macrocytosis caused by folate deficiency in myelofibrosis. The reticulocyte count may be normal or increased. The total leukocyte count is often elevated, and usually exhibits a left shift with the presence of myelocytes and metamyelocytes. The platelet count will vary with the extent of the disease; large and bizarre platelets and occasionally megakaryocytic nuclei may be seen. The diagnosis of myelophthisic anemia is made by the finding of abnormal cells in the bone marrow. Aspiration of this may be difficult or, indeed, unsuccessful, or at best may yield a specimen containing few if any fragments diluted with blood. Owing to the focal nature of the infiltration, a normal actively hematopoietic bone marrow may be obtained. Nevertheless, all the slides should be surveyed extensively for presence of malignant cells; not infrequently these are found in small groups. A needle or trephined biopsy of the bone marrow is very helpful in the assessment of hematopoiesis, the recognition of bone marrow infiltration, and the demonstration of an increase in reticulin and fibrosis by silver stains characteristic of myelofibrosis. Bone marrow aspiration and biopsy may have to be carried out at more than one site before the diagnosis can be made with certainty. The diagnosis of the cause of myelophthisic anemia depends upon the identification of the underlying disease.

Treatment and prognosis depend on the cause of the disorder, and blood transfusions may be required to overcome the anemia.

Beutler, E.: Anemias associated with marrow infiltration. *In* Williams, W. J., Beutler, E., Erslev, A. J., and Rundles, R. W. (eds.): Hematology, New York, McGraw-Hill Book Company, 1972.

HYPOCHROMIC ANEMIAS

Elmer B. Brown

737.   IRON DEFICIENCY ANEMIA

Definition.   Iron deficiency anemia occurs when the supply of iron is inadequate to support optimal erythropoiesis. In its fully developed form it is characterized by hypochromia and microcytosis of the circulating erythrocytes, low plasma iron, low transferrin saturation, and marked depletion of bone marrow and other body iron stores.

Prevalence.   Throughout the world iron deficiency is almost certainly the most common cause of anemia. In parts of Africa and Asia, where marginal dietary intake and excessive iron loss owing to intestinal parasites occur together, more than 50 per cent of the population may suffer from iron deficiency anemia. Variable figures of the incidence of iron deficiency have been reported from surveys in temperate countries. Reasons for variation include the criteria used for detecting borderline iron deficiency as well as the nature of the population sampled in terms of age, sex, economic status, and local environmental factors. Fewer than 3 per cent of men are affected in most population surveys; 10 to 30 per cent of all women may show signs of iron deficiency; and 10 to 60 per cent of pregnant women and infants in the first year of life have iron deficiency anemia. Much more information is needed to define precisely the prevalence of iron deficiency in representative geographic and socioeconomic cross sections of the United States.

Iron Metabolism.   Iron is essential to human life because of its central role in the heme molecule that permits oxygen and electron transport. Every cell in the body contains some iron.

Distribution.   The body's iron can be divided into two main compartments: (1) an essential, functional component composed of hemoglobin, myoglobin, enzyme and cofactor iron, and plasma transport iron, and (2) a nonessential storage component made up predominantly of ferritin and hemosiderin, not required for health but providing a reserve of iron readily mobilizable into the essential functional compartment in time of need.

In the normal adult man there is about 50 mg of iron per kilogram of body weight, approximately 80 per cent of which is in the functional compartment and 20 per cent in a storage form. Women, with a reduction in red cell mass and hemoglobin concentration as well as

smaller iron stores, have a body iron concentration of about 40 mg per kilogram. Total body iron ranges between extremes of 2 and 6 grams in small women and large men. These differences are reflected in the amount and percentage distribution of iron in the body (Table 1). Approximately 85 per cent of the functional iron in the body is present in the red blood cells as hemoglobin, which contains 0.34 per cent iron by weight. Divalent iron in each of the four disc-shaped heme groups carefully positioned in the pocket of coiled globin chains binds oxygen reversibly for transport to all tissues. Oxidation of the iron to the ferric state (as in methemoglobin) causes hemoglobin to lose its capacity to carry oxygen. Myoglobin, one fourth the size of hemoglobin and with one iron atom per molecule, accounts for about 15 per cent of the functional iron. It is present in concentrations of 0.9 to 2.2 grams dry weight of human muscle; cardiac muscle contains consistently less myoglobin than skeletal muscle. Myoglobin functions as a reservoir of oxygen for muscle metabolism. A small but extremely important component of body iron is that bound to transferrin. Approximately half of the transferrin iron is in extravascular tissue fluids while a more easily measured fraction is circulating in the plasma in transit from sites of hemoglobin destruction, iron absorption, or storage depots to the bone marrow and other areas of utilization. Lactoferrin, an iron-binding protein of milk, mucosal tissues, and leukocytes, is similar to transferrin structurally but appears to function in the body's defense against bacterial infection by binding iron essential to bacterial growth. Iron present as an integral part of various enzymes or as a cofactor constitutes a small but important part of the functional iron compartment. Iron enzymes may be classified as heme-proteins (cytochromes a, b, c, c_1, a_3, cytochrome c oxidase, catalase, peroxidases, tryptophan pyrrolase, lipoxidase, and homogentisic oxidase) and iron-flavoproteins (cytochrome c reductase, NADH dehydrogenase, xanthine oxidase, succinate dehydrogenase, and acyl CoA dehydrogenase). Iron as an essential cofactor is required by aconitase and succinic dehydrogenase. Most of these enzymes function as reversible donors or acceptors of electrons and are critical to the metabolism of every cell in the body.

Nonessential storage compounds that account for the remaining body iron are ferritin and hemosiderin. Ferri-

TABLE 1.   Distribution of Iron in the Body

Compartment	Iron Content (grams)		Fraction of Total Body Fe (%)	
	Men	*Women*	*Men*	*Women*
Functional				
Hemoglobin	3.050	1.700	71.8	73.5
Myoglobin	0.430	0.300	10.1	13.0
Enzymes	(?) 0.010	0.010	0.2	0.4
Transferrin	0.008	0.006	0.2	0.2
Subtotal	3.498	2.016	82.3	87.1
Storage				
Ferritin-hemosiderin	0.750	0.300	17.7	12.9
Total	4.248	2.316	100.0	100.0

Values are based on data from various sources. Assumptions include a body weight for men of 80 kg, blood volume of 70 ml/kg, and Hgb of 16 grams/dl; for women the values used were a weight of 55 kg, blood volume of 65 ml/kg, and Hgb of 14 grams/dl.

tin, composed of a large, water-soluble, crystalline protein surrounding micelles of iron (up to 20 per cent by weight), is a ubiquitous compound found in many tissues of the body but predominantly in liver parenchymal cells and reticuloendoethelial cells of the liver, spleen, and bone marrow. Hemosiderin is a water-insoluble protein with higher concentrations of iron (up to 35 per cent by weight) that is readily identified by Prussian blue staining of tissues. Since the iron in these compounds is readily mobilizable for use by the essential functional iron compounds, there is wide variation in their amounts and percentage of total body iron.

Absorption. Iron absorption assumes great importance in human iron metabolism, because iron balance is regulated by controlled absorption rather than by excretion. Despite intensive investigation, many facets of the mechanism and control of iron absorption remain unexplained or controversial. Current information suggests that iron entering the stomach in various organic compounds of food is digested to soluble ferric salts that may be either reduced to ferrous ions or chelated in either the ferrous or ferric valence state to maintain stability and promote absorption. The presence of hydrochloric acid in the stomach is not essential for iron absorption, although an acid milieu prevents the formation of insoluble complexes of ionized iron. Other unidentified iron-stabilizing substances in gastric secretions – possibly mucoproteins – promote iron absorption. Entry of iron at the brush border of mucosal cells appears to be mainly by passive diffusion; exit from the cells to the plasma transferrin probably requires metabolic energy for active transport. Most of the iron destined to enter the bloodstream traverses the mucosal cell rapidly in the form of small molecules. Attempts to identify specific mucosal iron carrier substances have been unsuccessful. Likewise, efforts to identify subcellular fractions in the sequence of iron transfer across the mucosal cell have added little to our understanding of the precise process of iron absorption. Older theories implicating mucosal ferritin as a carrier of iron and the key to regulation of iron absorption through a "mucosal block" mechanism have been abandoned. The small quantities of ferritin in intestinal mucosal cells appear to function as a storage compound to accept a proportion of iron in excess of the rapid transport capacity. The ferritin is then lost when the cells are desquamated at the end of their three- to five-day life span. Luminal factors modifying the form in which iron is presented to the mucosal cell play an important role in the amount of iron that can be absorbed. Sugar, sorbitol, cysteine and other amino acids, ascorbic and succinic acids, mucoproteins, and various other components of the dietary constituents or intestinal secretions tend to stabilize iron in a soluble form and to promote iron absorption. Phytates, phosphates, carbonate, oxalate, pancreatic bicarbonate, and gastroferrin bind iron as relatively insoluble complexes and decrease iron absorption. The means by which the body's need for increased or decreased iron absorption is transmitted to the mucosal cell have not been completely defined. Multiple signals, including mucosal cell iron concentration, local hypoxia, tissue iron stores, rate of erythropoiesis, plasma transferrin saturation, plasma iron turnover, and humoral factors, have been suggested, but without compelling evidence for any precise mechanism.

Measurement of iron absorption has progressed from the tedious and cumbersome dietary iron balance studies to the use of radioactive iron with determination of unabsorbed iron in the feces, absorbed radioactivity in the circulating red blood cells, or total body radioiron using sensitive whole body counters. Studies of iron absorption can be divided conveniently into two groups: (1) those using simple iron salts such as ferrous sulfate or ferric chloride which give information applicable to the behavior of iron given therapeutically; and (2) those measuring the absorption of iron from foods.

Ferrous salts are better absorbed than ferric compounds, and various agents such as ascorbic and succinic acids and sorbitol enhance iron absorption. Other substances such as phytates, phosphates, and various antacid preparations bind iron and diminish its absorption. Maximal absorption occurs in the duodenum and upper jejunum where the villous surface is maximal and in which the luminal contents are acid or neutral; there is progressively less absorption distally from a more alkaline environment, although the potentiality for some iron absorption exists throughout the length of the gut from the stomach to the rectum. Iron absorption from mucosal cells is via intestinal capillaries with little lymphatic participation, and is virtually complete within several hours after ingestion. Uptake of iron is unidirectional without any back-flux except for iron lost into the gut lumen by desquamation of mucosal cells. There is no enterohepatic circulation. Small doses of iron are absorbed from the duodenum by an active process; with large doses of iron, passive diffusion occurs. Increasing the ingestion of simple iron salts results in increasing absorption of iron until toxicity becomes the limiting factor. Conditions associated with increased iron absorption include iron deficiency, hemolytic and sideroblastic anemias, hypoxia, cobalt and erythropoietin administration, hemochromatosis, cirrhosis and portacaval shunts, some types of pancreatic insufficiency, and the later stages of pregnancy. Decreased iron absorption is present in patients with iron overload, erythroid hypoplasia, generalized malabsorption states, malignant, infectious, and inflammatory diseases, and achlorhydria.

Less information is available about the absorption of food iron. Attempts have been made to classify the "availability" of iron in various foods by its release after incubation in digestion mixtures or by its ability to increase hemoglobin formation in anemic animals or human subjects. These efforts have been relatively unsuccessful. Radioactive iron biosynthetically incorporated into various foods or added as a simple salt to dietary food mixtures has allowed comparison of dietary iron absorption with that of simple iron salts. From these studies it was learned that heme iron is absorbed differently from various nonheme iron compounds in the diet. Heme is taken up by the mucosal cell where the porphyrin ring is split open to make iron available to the body. Heme iron absorption is not influenced by dietary composition (ascorbic acid, phytates, or phosphates) as is the case with nonheme iron compounds. Furthermore, the nonheme iron compounds of food behave as a single pool in their absorption characteristics and can be labeled with a single radioiron salt. ^{55}Fe labeling of heme (intrinsic tag) and ^{59}FeCl$_3$ for labeling of nonheme vegetable components (extrinsic tag) have allowed the precise measurement of the absorption of complex dietary iron mixtures. Results of this type of study indicate that iron in meat (primarily heme) is better absorbed (12 to 20 per cent) than iron from vegetable sources (primarily nonheme). Iron from vegetable sources is absorbed to a variable extent – about 1 to 7 per cent of usual doses in a meal—with substances such as phytates accounting for the diminished absorption. Rice and spinach are at the lower end of the absorption scale, whereas wheat and soybean iron are better absorbed. When mixtures of foods approximating those of usual diets are given, the percentage of iron absorption of the total mixture is similar to that of the least well-absorbed vegetable source, except for the heme component whose absorption is uninfluenced by other dietary components. Of importance in the consideration of food iron supplementation to prevent iron deficiency is the finding that diets containing foods with little heme (meat) and with a predominance of poorly absorbed vegetable iron sources, such as rice, impart their poor iron absorbability to the supplementary iron salt irrespective of the compound used.

Transport. Iron is transported in plasma bound to a specific carrier protein, transferrin. This β-globulin of about 75,000 molecular weight is synthesized in the liver and has an eight- to ten-day half-time in plasma; the 7 to 15 grams present in the body is almost equally distributed in the extravascular and intravascular spaces, with plasma concentrations varying from 215 to 350 mg per deciliter. At least 19 genetic variants have been described, but all that have been studied appear to be identical in their iron-binding properties. Transferrin can bind two atoms of ferric iron per molecule in the presence of bicarbonate. Binding of iron to transferrin receptor sites is a random process in vitro, and there is no exchange of iron from one molecule to another. Recent evidence suggests that release of iron to tissue receptor sites is a selective process, with one transferrin iron site being erythroblast oriented and the other site oriented toward receptors on liver parenchymal cells. If these functional differences in selective iron delivery are confirmed, the concept of transferrin as a passive plasma carrier of homogeneous iron atoms will be changed to one of actively controlling the distribution of iron in the body. Measurement of functional iron-binding capacity rather than direct determination of transferrin is employed clinically. Iron is present in equal amounts in plasma and serum; normal values range from 60 to 160 μg per deciliter, with a mean of 120 for men and 110 for women. Plasma transferrin is normally about one third saturated and the total plasma iron-binding capacity is 280

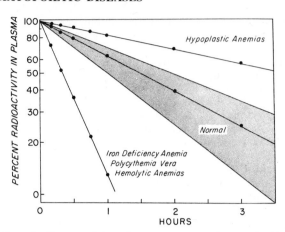

Figure 2. Plasma radioiron disappearance curves for normal subjects and for patients with increased and decreased erythropoiesis.

to 400 μg per deciliter. Plasma iron shows a diurnal variation, with morning values about 30 per cent higher than those in the evening. Menses, exercise, or normal meals have no appreciable effect on plasma iron concentrations. Highest concentrations are seen during reproductive years in both sexes, with a modest decline in old age. Variations in plasma iron and iron-binding capacity are seen in a variety of disorders, as illustrated in Figure 1.

Ferrokinetics. Since the pioneering studies of the kinetics of iron transfer were published by Huff and coworkers in 1950, there have been many refinements in technique that have added much to the precision of measurement and the complexity of mathematical analysis, but little to the clinical interpretation of ferrokinetic data. Measurement of plasma radioiron clearance and erythrocyte utilization are simple, useful tests available to any clinician with access to radioisotope facilities. If more sophisticated interpretation of deranged iron metabolism in a variety of diseases is desired, computer evaluation of prolonged plasma iron disappearance curves and external monitoring over liver, spleen, and sacrum are needed. By this type of analysis a number of compartments with various rates of iron interchange can be identified with analyses too complex for routine use. However, useful basic information is obtained by measuring the rate of disappearance of radioactive iron bound to plasma transferrin after intravenous injection and its subsequent incorporation into circulating erythrocytes 7 to 14 days later (Figs. 2 and 3). Plasma radioiron disappearance, measured at 10- to 15-minute intervals and plotted semilogarithmically, is linear with a half-time rate of disappearance normally between 60 and 120 minutes. More rapid disappearance rates (shorter half-time values) are found in iron deficiency and conditions with increased erythropoiesis such as polycythemia vera and hemolytic anemias. Slow rates of radioiron disappearance indicate erythroid hypoplasia from various causes. By extrapolating the plasma iron disappearance line back to zero time, one may obtain a close estimate of plasma volume by dividing the total count rate of the injected radioiron by the count rate at time zero. Calculation of the plasma iron turnover rate (PITR) requires only the additional measurement of plasma iron concentration. The formula for this calcula-

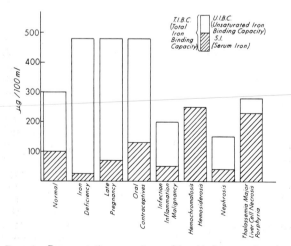

Figure 1. Representative serum iron and iron-binding capacity values in a variety of conditions.

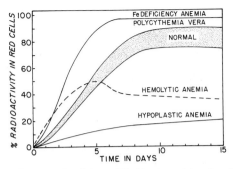

Figure 3. Patterns of radioiron utilization in peripheral erythrocytes for normal subjects and for patients with various disorders with increased or decreased erythropoiesis.

tion is shown at the bottom of this page. The PITR reflects changes in two variables, the size of the plasma iron pool and the rate of disappearance of ^{59}Fe from plasma. Normal values of PITR range from 25 to 40 mg per day. Increased PITR is observed in patients whose plasma radioiron disappearance is rapid and whose plasma iron values are normal or increased, e.g., hemolytic states and ineffective erythropoiesis with values four to ten times normal. Decreased PITR is seen in some patients with hypoplastic anemias, infection, or uremia or after irradiation when slow plasma radioiron disappearance rates are combined with normal or low plasma iron values. In iron deficiency anemia, in which there is rapid radioiron disappearance and low plasma iron values, the PITR is usually normal.

Measurement of the utilization of radioiron incorporated into hemoglobin of red cells during the one to two weeks after a plasma radioiron clearance study provides valuable information about the effective production of erythrocytes compared to total erythropoiesis reflected by the PITR. Iron utilization is calculated from the radioactivity in 1 ml of packed red cells multiplied by the red cell volume (calculated from the previously determined plasma volume and the hematocrit) divided by the count rate of injected radioiron, and is expressed in percentage terms. Normally 70 to 90 per cent of the injected radioiron can be accounted for in circulating cells two weeks after injection. Decreased radioiron utilization reflects decreased erythropoiesis with extreme reductions in aplastic anemia. Radioiron utilization to levels slightly above the normal range occurs sooner in iron deficiency or polycythemia. Complex intermediate curves reflecting rapid red cell production and destruction may be seen in various hemolytic anemias.

Storage. Iron in excess of the needs for hemoglobin, myoglobin, and essential intracellular enzymes is stored as ferritin and hemosiderin. Major sites of storage iron are hepatic parenchymal cells, reticuloendothelial cells of the bone marrow, liver, and spleen, and a poorly defined store in skeletal muscle. The immediate source of most reticuloendothelial iron stores is hemoglobin iron conserved from the breakdown of red cells at the end of

their life span. Hepatic parenchymal iron comes from plasma transferrin. Accurate measurement of diffusely distributed iron stores is difficult. Qualitative estimates are usually based on histochemical appraisal of bone marrow or liver hemosiderin deposits. More quantitative estimates can be obtained from measurement of iron excreted into the urine after injections of deferoxamine or other chelating agents; chelate iron mobilization correlates closely with the amount of iron mobilized by phlebotomy before iron deficiency anemia supervenes. Minute amounts of ferritin circulating in plasma are related to the amount of iron stores, and plasma ferritin measurement provides another means of determining body iron stores. Estimates of storage iron in normal adults have decreased in recent years to an average in men of 750 mg (range 200 to 1400 mg) and an average in women of 300 mg (range 60 to 500 mg). Approximately 65 per cent of storage iron is normally in the form of ferritin; the remainder is hemosiderin. In disorders of iron overload the proportion of hemosiderin increases progressively. Both storage forms are readily mobilized in response to need such as bleeding. Regulatory mechanisms controlling the buildup and mobilization of iron stores are poorly understood. Mobilization is frequently interfered with by infection, inflammation, and malignancy.

Excretion. The body has a limited capacity to excrete iron except by means of hemorrhage. Normally, excretion balances absorption, because most of the iron released from hemoglobin of senescent red blood cells is conserved and reutilized. Total daily excretion amounts to slightly less than 1 mg for men and postmenopausal women. Of this amount approximately 0.1 mg is excreted in the urine, and about 0.6 mg in the feces from mucosal cell desquamation, bile, and small amounts of blood loss; the remainder is lost from skin as desquamated cells and in sweat. Approximately 0.5 mg of iron is present per milliliter of blood. With normal menstrual blood losses of 25 to 60 ml monthly, this normal bleeding accounts for an additional 12 to 30 mg of iron lost monthly, or 0.4 to 1.0 mg per day, in women during their reproductive years. Iron loss occurs in pregnancy and delivery in amounts totaling more than 500 mg. Obligatory daily iron losses are about 50 per cent less than normal in patients with iron deficiency anemia.

Requirements. Since iron absorption must balance excretion for the body's iron stores to stay in balance, one may construct a table of iron requirements for different physiologic states (Table 2). In addition to the exceptional stresses on iron balance imposed by menstrual losses and pregnancy, one must also add the needs related to growth. These needs of iron to build hemoglobin, myoglobin, and other intracellular iron compounds are greatest at growth spurts of infancy and adolescence. An increment of 0.5 mg per day is an acceptable estimate in the absence of precise measurements.

These requirements of iron to meet special circumstances can be translated into terms of nutritional iron intake to prevent a negative balance from occurring. Assuming that absorption of iron from food mixtures nor-

$$\text{PITR (mg/day)} = \frac{0.693}{^{59}\text{Fe T/2 (hrs)}} \times \text{mg Fe/ml plasma} \times \text{plasma vol (ml)} \times 24 \text{ hrs}$$

TABLE 2. Estimated Dietary Iron Requirements

	Absorbed Iron Requirement, mg/Day	Daily Food Iron Requirement,* mg/Day
Normal men and nonmenstruating women	0.5–1.0	5–10
Menstruating women	0.7–2.0	7–20
Pregnant women	2.0–4.8	20–48†
Adolescents	1.0–2.0	10–20
Children	0.4–1.0	4–10
Infants	0.5–1.5	1.5 mg per kg‡

*Assuming 10 per cent absorption.

†This amount of iron cannot be derived from diet and should be met by iron supplementation in the latter half of pregnancy.

‡To a maximum of 15 mg.

mally averages about 10 per cent, the figures for dietary iron intake can be derived (Table 2). Iron concentrations of foods in most Western diets are related to calories, with about 6 mg of iron per 1000 calories. Although iron absorption may increase to about 20 per cent with the onset of iron deficiency, it is obvious that pregnant women can hardly eat enough food to provide for their markedly increased iron needs and that they, with many menstruating women and adolescent girls, are likely to fall behind in meeting dietary iron needs.

Pathogenesis. Iron deficiency develops because of one or a combination of the following factors: inadequate dietary iron intake, malabsorption, blood loss, or repeated pregnancies. Since excretion of iron is limited, assigning the cause of iron deficiency in adults to inadequate intake or malabsorption implies chronicity measured in years. More important are iron losses which occur most often from the gastrointestinal tract of men and from abnormal menstrual bleeding in women. A convenient way to consider these causes of iron deficiency is to divide them into two categories—low intake and high output.

Low Intake. Restrictions of dietary iron because of economic, religious, or cultural considerations lead to iron deficiency in many parts of the world. Economic and religious factors weigh heaviest in underdeveloped nations, whereas in the United States one might cite the inadequate meals of weight-conscious young women and mothers caught up in the harried pace of rearing children. In old age, absent or ill-fitting dentures combined with apathy, inactivity, and financial restrictions reduce the intake of foods with high iron nutritive value. Continual refinement and cleanliness of our food supplies combined with the use of noniron cooking vessels may have the undesired effect of reducing our iron intake. Assimilation of iron is often reduced owing to interaction of phytates from cereals, phosphates, and other substances in the foods we eat. Malabsorption of iron rarely if ever occurs as an isolated absorptive defect, but is present in sprue syndromes and is associated with iron deficiency. (Surprisingly, the steatorrhea of pancreatic insufficiency allows normal or even increased iron absorption.) Abnormal gastrointestinal motility secondary to gastrectomy or to a variety of causes for diarrhea is usually associated with decreased iron absorption. Patients with achlorhydria have inefficient absorption of food iron, and cannot increase iron uptake effectively when they become iron deficient.

High Output. Identification of the site of blood loss responsible for high output iron deficiency may be quite difficult. One reason for this difficulty is that increased menstrual blood loss, the single most common cause of iron deficiency in temperate countries, is often not recognized, and is difficult to quantitate. The best estimates of the frequency and extent of menorrhagia in randomly selected women indicate that the normal menstrual flow (25 to 60 ml) is exceeded in about 20 per cent of women, with occasional blood losses as high as 500 ml per month. Unfortunately, predictions of menstrual loss by the patient's account of the number and saturation of sanitary napkins and the number of days of flow are only partially successful. Contraceptive pills of the combined estrogen-progesterone type reduce menstrual blood loss by 50 to 60 per cent, whereas intrauterine devices tend to increase menstrual blood loss. Iron loss associated with pregnancy is easier to estimate and totals about 500 mg. Unless iron supplementation is provided, repeated pregnancies are almost invariably accompanied by iron deficiency.

Blood loss from the alimentary tract is frequently occult and intermittent, and may elude careful search with a battery of sophisticated techniques. In a recent study no demonstrable source of blood loss could be found in 16 per cent of patients with gastrointestinal bleeding. In those whose bleeding could be explained, the cause was hemorrhoidal bleeding in 10 per cent, salicylate ingestion in 8 per cent, peptic ulceration and hiatus hernia in 7 per cent each, diverticulosis in 4 per cent, neoplasm in 2 per cent, and a sprinkling of additional cases of esophageal varices, hemorrhagic gastritis, regional enteritis, ulcerative colitis, hemorrhagic telangiectasia, and intestinal polyps. Hookworm and other intestinal parasites are important causes of blood loss and iron deficiency in many countries. Blood donation—which must be specifically inquired about—doubles the amount of iron that must be absorbed when only three pints are removed per year. Blood removed for diagnostic studies from patients undergoing prolonged or repeated hospitalization is a cause for iron deficiency that can easily be overlooked. Rare causes of excess iron loss include the hemosiderinuria from chronic intravascular hemolysis of paroxysmal nocturnal hemoglobinuria and cardiac prostheses, and the iron that is trapped in the lungs of patients with pulmonary hemosiderosis. One cannot overemphasize the dictum that iron deficiency anemia in the adult man and the postmenopausal woman is due to blood loss until proved otherwise.

The sequence of changes in slowly developing iron deficiency is fairly predictable. Initially iron stores in reticuloendothelial and parenchymal cells are mobilized to provide the metal for functional iron needs. When demands for functional iron cannot be met from the stores, a signal of some sort is transmitted to the intestine to increase iron absorption. Transferrin concentration increases while the plasma iron concentration falls as demands of the bone marrow exceed the supply of iron released from senescent erythrocytes and intestinal absorption. Anemia appears when the supply of iron restricts erythropoiesis. Distorted cells reflecting skipped divisions and hypochromic cells reflecting insufficient iron for heme synthesis gradually replace the normal cells of the circulating blood. Later, increased cell division or more severe maturation defects lead to microcytosis and dyserythropoiesis of the fully developed iron deficiency anemia. The extent of the depletion of cell enzyme iron is variable in different tissues sampled in man, and little is known of the rate of these changes.

Clinical Manifestations. Iron deficiency anemia is accompanied by a wide diversity of symptoms. Some patients have no awareness of ill health despite marked anemia which may be recognized by chance examinations. Symptoms usually appear insidiously, and their onset is difficult to date. The gradual development of iron deficiency often allows remarkable adaptation, and may permit strenuous work with few symptoms. At the other extreme, marked tiredness, easy fatigability, dyspnea on exertion, palpitations, headache, irritability, paresthesias, lightheadedness, and other vague symptoms may trouble patients with borderline or mild anemia.

Examination usually discloses pallor, although on casual observation this finding may not be noticed. A peculiar greenish appearance of the skin of young girls, vividly described by careful observers before 1900 and termed chlorosis, has mysteriously disappeared. Vitiligo is a rare skin change in blacks. Angular stomatitis—most marked in edentulous patients—frequent papillary atrophy, and varying degrees of glossitis comprise the oral lesions associated with iron deficiency. Dysphagia resulting from postcricoid esophageal webs or strictures, associated with hypochromic anemia and achlorhydria, and most frequently seen in middle-aged women—the Paterson-Kelly or Plummer-Vinson syndrome—is rare in the United States, but is fairly common in the British Isles and Scandinavia. Whether this syndrome is due to iron deficiency or some associated disorder is not known. Multiple gastrointestinal complaints, such as anorexia, pyrosis, flatulence, nausea, eructation, and constipation, are common in association with iron deficiency. Occasionally bizarre cravings for cornstarch, ice, clay, and other substances may appear. These forms of pica are especially common in iron-deficient black women, but probably have a world-wide distribution. Gastritis, which is reversible after iron therapy, and permanent gastric atrophy have been described in numerous gastroscopic investigations of iron-deficient patients. Whether these gastric lesions are cause or effect of iron deficiency is debatable. Spoon nail (koilonychia) is the most advanced abnormality of the nails and is becoming very rare. Often, milder nail changes such as thinning, brittleness, lusterless appearance, longitudinal ridging, and flattening accompany prolonged iron deficiency, and are associated with depletion of cysteine in the nails. The frequent suggestion that these epithelial changes are related to the severity or chronicity of iron deficiency anemia may be questioned because of their virtual absence in patients with severe, lifelong iron deficiency owing to hookworm infestation. An attractive but unproved hypothesis is that the epithelial changes may reflect a chronically depressed intake of iron (and possibly other substances) rather than chronically increased loss of iron from bleeding.

Severe anemia often leads to cardiac dilatation, the occurrence of hemic murmurs, and, in older patients, the development of congestive heart failure. Enlargement of the spleen to slightly below the costal margin is observed in about 10 per cent of patients, and recedes after treatment. Claims of aggravation of menorrhagia by iron deficiency anemia and improvement after treatment are difficult to substantiate. Numbness and tingling without objective neurologic abnormalities are reported by about 25 per cent of patients. Extremely rare are the papilledema and increased pressure of cerebrospinal fluid that may be confused with intracranial tumors. Infants often show marked irritability and present difficulties in feeding.

Laboratory Findings. A number of laboratory procedures facilitate the identification of iron deficiency anemia. A well-stained blood film shows small erythrocytes (microcytosis) poorly filled with hemoglobin (hypochromia) with marked variation in size (anisocytosis) and shape (poikilocytosis). Mean corpuscular volume is less than 80 fl and mean corpuscular hemoglobin concentration is less than 30 per cent. Since the introduction of the Model S Coulter electronic counter into many hematology laboratories, the mean corpuscular hemoglobin concentration in iron deficiency anemia has been observed to be in the low normal range. The explanation for this seems to be that the volume of the erythrocytes, calculated from their number and degree of interference with the electrical field across the aperture through which they pass, is different from that measured by packing in a high speed centrifuge. Erroneous estimates of packed cell volume occur because of increased plasma trapping between distorted iron-deficient cells. Thus to identify iron deficiency, the key measurement to note in the printout of the Model S Coulter Counter is the mean cell volume. Plasma iron concentration is usually less than 80 μg per deciliter, associated with a total plasma iron-binding capacity of more than 400 μg per deciliter. Transferrin saturation (the product of plasma iron divided by total iron-binding capacity multiplied by 100) is 15 per cent or less. Examination of bone marrow particles shows normoblastic erythroid hyperplasia; sideroblasts and hemosiderin in macrophages are absent when the marrow particles are stained for iron. Defective heme synthesis is associated with elevated erythrocyte protoporphyrin concentration and decreased plasma bilirubin. Reticulocytes are present in normal numbers except for elevations secondary to recent hemorrhage. Erythrocyte osmotic fragility is decreased, reflecting the diminished hemoglobin concentration. The life span of erythrocytes is usually normal, although shortened survival has been reported. Thrombocytosis in the range of one million platelets per cubic millimeter, or, less often, thrombocytopenia, both of which return to normal after iron therapy, may be observed. Abnormalities of the leukocytes are rare and are usually confined to slight leukopenia and occasional hypersegmented neutrophils. Unfortunately there is no practical laboratory test to measure depletion of tissue enzyme iron.

Treatment. The two objects of treatment of iron deficiency anemia are (1) to replace the blood and tissue iron deficits, and (2) to recognize and, if possible, correct the underlying cause. Despite the vast array of therapeutic preparations containing iron, simple ferrous salts (ferrous sulfate, ferrous gluconate, and ferrous fumarate) given by mouth remain the mainstay of treatment for iron deficiency anemia. Large doses of ascorbic or succinic acid will increase iron absorption but only to a small extent that hardly warrants the extra expense. The addition of other substances found in "shotgun" mixtures such as copper, cobalt, molybdenum, intrinsic factor, and various B vitamins is of no benefit. The use of these shotgun hematinics must be condemned, because they may obscure the correct diagnosis as indicated by a response to iron alone; further, they encourage sloppiness in diagnosis, and they are unnecessarily expensive.

Enteric-coated and delayed-release iron preparations are poorly designed to exploit the fact of maximal absorption in the upper gastrointestinal tract. All too often their delay in iron release serves to dump the metal in the lower intestine, in which absorption is greatly diminished. When iron medication is prescribed in tablet form, the physician should warn the patient to keep the tablets out of reach of small children to reduce the danger of severe iron intoxication. Suitable warnings on the label and the use of child-proof containers will further reduce this risk.

A total daily dose of iron in the range of 180 to 240 mg provides for maximal rates of hemoglobin regeneration in adults. Three or four tablets of ferrous sulfate (60 mg of elemental iron) or ferrous fumarate (66 mg of iron) provide the requisite daily dose. Ferrous gluconate, with only 36 mg of elemental iron per tablet, requires a dosage of six tablets per day. These iron preparations are given in equal doses with or after meals and with a snack at bedtime. The advantage of increased absorption of iron salts taken on an empty stomach is often overweighed by the undesirable side effects of gastrointestinal irritation.

Approximately one patient in ten will experience unpleasant side effects such as nausea, epigastric pain, abdominal cramps, diarrhea, or vomiting of sufficient severity to require discontinuation of treatment. No effective iron preparation is free from causing gastric or intestinal irritation. Gastric symptomatology is dose dependent, and may be minimized by a gradual buildup of the iron dose during the first three days of treatment. A few patients are completely unable or unwilling to take iron by mouth; patience and understanding on the part of the physician can keep this group small. Treatment with iron should be continued for four to six months and even longer in the face of recurrent bleeding. Restoration of iron stores to provide a buffer against recurrent iron deficiency is a slow process.

Infants and toddlers are best treated with liquid iron preparations. Infants should receive a total of 60 to 90 mg of iron daily in water or fruit juices. Ferrous sulfate is available in concentrated drops containing 15 mg of iron per 0.6 ml, as a syrup with 30 mg of iron per 5 ml, or as an elixir with 44 mg of iron per 5 ml. Transient staining of the teeth by liquid iron preparations can be prevented by using a dropper or a straw. Most children weighing 35 to 75 pounds can satisfactorily take iron tablets in half the adult dosage; larger children usually receive adult doses of iron.

Response to adequate doses of iron given to a patient with iron deficiency anemia is quite predictable (Fig. 4). An initial sense of well-being is often observed within 48 hours. This improvement appears to be more than a psychologic effect from taking medications, as infants often lose their irritability and begin to eat better. Because this response occurs before any change in blood values is measurable, it has been attributed, without any real evidence, to replenishment of some vital cellular iron compound. The height of the reticulocyte peak and the rate of hemoglobin regeneration are proportional to the severity of the anemia; maximal daily rates of hemoglobin regeneration are 0.3 gram per deciliter.

Failure to respond to iron given by mouth should call forth the following considerations: (1) the patient failed to take the iron as prescribed; (2) the patient did not have iron deficiency anemia, and re-evaluation of the diagnosis is necessary; (3) blood loss exceeded new blood formation; (4) intercurrent infection, inflammation, or malignancy interfered with the response to iron; (5) the patient was unable to absorb the iron; and (6) an ineffective iron preparation was administered.

Parenteral administration of iron should be reserved for the following indications: (1) patients with malabsorption syndromes; (2) the relatively small group of patients who are unable or unwilling to take iron by mouth, including some people with ulcerative colitis, regional enteritis, and colostomies; (3) selected patients who prove unreliable in taking their prescribed iron; and (4) some patients with chronic uncorrectable bleeding with iron loss in excess of that which can be replaced by the oral route. Two satisfactory preparations are available for parenteral use. Both iron dextran (Imferon) and iron sorbitex (Jectofer) contain 50 mg of iron per milliliter. Iron sorbitex should be administered only by intramuscular injection, but iron dextran can be given by either the intramuscular or the intravenous route. The technique of deep intramuscular injections is important. The skin at the injection site (preferably the buttock) should first be displaced laterally before the needle is inserted into the muscle, so that reflux of the dark brown iron solution along the injection path, causing skin staining, can be prevented. After a test dose of 0.5 ml, 2 to 5 ml doses are given daily into alternate extremities until a calculated total dose is administered. Intravenous injection of iron dextran is reserved for patients in whom insufficient muscle mass or the discomfort of massive and prolonged intramuscular therapy precludes the intramuscular route. Usually iron dextran is injected undiluted in a dose of 2 to 5 ml per day, although the total dose may be diluted in 250 to 1000 ml of isotonic saline and infused during a two-hour period without untoward reactions. Dosage is calculated by the following formula: Normal Hgb (grams per deciliter) − patient's Hgb × 0.255 = iron dose in grams. This formula provides sufficient iron to replace the circulating hemoglobin deficit plus a 50 per cent excess for creation of tissue stores. Side effects such as local pain, lymphadenitis, headache, dizziness, fever, urticaria, arthralgias, myalgias, and hypotension occur in about 5 per cent of patients; rare fatal anaphylactic reactions have been reported. Urine that turns black on standing and urinary irritation may occur after injections of iron sorbitex, because one third of the dose is excreted into the urine, a fact that should be considered in total dose calculations.

Preventive iron therapy for groups prone to develop iron deficiency (infants, pregnant women, and blood donors) requires special consideration. Fortification of foods with iron salts seems a reasonable and fairly effective way to improve the iron intake of infants. Iron enrichment of bread remains a hotly debated subject both in terms of its efficacy in preventing iron deficiency of groups at special risk and in terms of risks of eventual iron overload in other groups. Pregnant women should be given iron during the last half of pregnancy, after the early period of "morning sickness" that might erroneously be attributed to the iron tablets and influence the patient's subsequent willingness to take this medication. One tablet of ferrous sulfate (60 mg of iron daily) is sufficient to provide for the extra iron needs of pregnancy. For repeated blood donors the dose of iron will depend on the rate of donation—one to three tablets daily may be required.

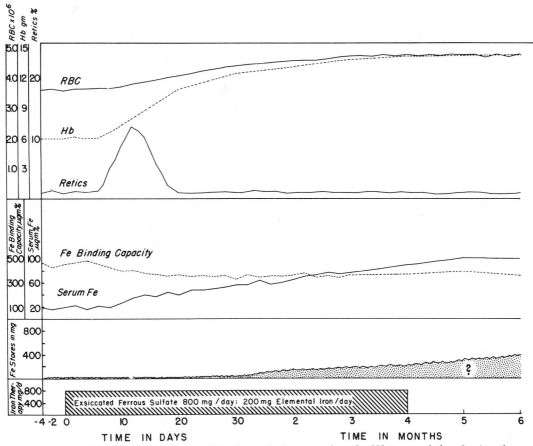

Figure 4. Schematized response to iron therapy. Reticulocytes begin to rise about the fifth to seventh day after iron therapy is started, reach a peak between the tenth and fourteenth days, and then fall to normal levels. Hemoglobin level begins to increase on about the seventh to tenth day. From four to eight weeks are required before normal values are attained. No accurate data are available to describe the reappearance of storage iron; its reaccumulation may be slower than shown; hence the question mark.

Prognosis. Prognosis in iron deficiency can only be applied to the underlying disorder causing the anemia. A vastly different prognosis is expected in a patient with a bleeding carcinoma of the alimentary tract and another with hemorrhoids. Patients rarely die of iron deficiency anemia itself, but they often die of the underlying cause. Recurrence of iron deficiency anemia after treatment is common; one third of women and one fourth of men have a recurrence in extended follow-up studies. These recurrence rates emphasize the importance of identifying and correcting the cause of iron deficiency.

Bothwell, T. H., and Finch, C. A.: Iron Metabolism. Boston, Little, Brown & Company, 1962.

Committee on Iron Deficiency: Iron deficiency in the United States. J.A.M.A., 203:407, 1968.

Fairbanks, V. F., Fahey, J. L., and Beutler, E.: Clinical Disorders of Iron Metabolism. New York, Grune & Stratton, 1971.

Gross, F. (ed.): Iron Metabolism—An International Symposium. Berlin, Springer-Verlag OHG, 1964.

Hallberg, L., Harwerth, H.-G., and Vanotti, A. (eds.): Iron Deficiency. Pathogenesis, Clinical Aspects, Therapy. New York, Academic Press, 1970.

Harris, J. W., and Kellermeyer, R. W.: The Red Cell. Production, Metabolism, Destruction: Normal and Abnormal. Cambridge, Mass., Harvard University Press, 1970.

Moore, C. V.: Iron nutrition and requirements. Scand. J. Haematol. (Series Haematologica), 6:1, 1965.

Williams, W. J., Beutler, E., Erslev, A. J., and Rundles, R. W. (eds.): Hematology. New York, McGraw-Hill Book Company, 1972.

Wintrobe, M. M.: Clinical Hematology. 6th ed. Philadelphia, Lea & Febiger, 1967.

738. HYPOCHROMIC ANEMIAS NOT CAUSED BY IRON DEFICIENCY

Hypochromic anemia occurs predominantly when hemoglobin synthesis is interfered with out of proportion to defects in erythrocyte proliferation. Biosynthetic abnormalities have been identified at one or more stages of protoporphyrin synthesis, iron incorporation into the heme ring—the prime defect in iron deficiency anemia—or globin synthesis. Compared to iron deficiency anemia, these disorders of hemoglobin synthesis are rare. As a group they can be differentiated from iron deficiency anemia by increased body iron stores with increased hemosiderin in marrow particles, the presence of sideroblasts and siderocytes, and increased plasma iron and transferrin saturation. Special distinguishing features are included with the following list of these disorders. (1) By far the most common of the hypochromic anemias not caused by iron deficiency are thalassemia and its variants resulting from interaction with abnormal hemoglobins. The basic defect is in the synthesis of globin chains. Thalassemia and its variants can be distinguished from iron deficiency by hemoglobin electrophoresis and detection of elevated levels of hemoglobins A_2 and F. (2) Homozygous Hgb-C disease and Hgb-

S-D are hypochromic anemias readily identified by appropriate hemoglobin electrophoresis. (3) Sideroblastic anemias can be subdivided into congenital, acquired, and pyridoxine-responsive categories. They share the common features of disordered heme synthesis with prominent ringed sideroblasts observable on iron staining of bone marrow particles. Electron microscopy discloses the siderotic granules to be diffuse iron aggregates in the intercristal spaces of mitochondria surrounding the nucleus of an erythrocyte precursor. Abnormalities in tryptophan metabolism and partial improvement of the anemia after pyridoxine or crude liver extract administration, as well as a high rate of leukemic transformation, have been reported in this group of disorders. (4) Chronic lead intoxication produces a hypochromic anemia resulting from defective hemoglobin synthesis. Stippling of erythrocytes and abnormal urinary excretion of coproporphyrin and aminolevulinic acid distinguish this disorder from iron deficiency, although in young children whose lead poisoning is due to pica of lead-based paint the two disorders may coexist. (5) Inadequate delivery of iron from plentiful stores to the marrow for hemoglobin synthesis has been observed in rare instances, such as in a child with congenital absence of transferrin, in pulmonary hemosiderosis, and in older people with an unexplained block in the release of iron from reticuloendothelial sites of hemoglobin catabolism.

Williams, W. J., Beutler, E., Erslev, A. J., and Rundles, R. W. (eds.): Hematology. New York, McGraw-Hill Book Company, 1972.

Wintrobe, M. M.: Clinical Hematology. 6th ed. Philadelphia, Lea & Febiger, 1967.

Section Two.   HEMOLYTIC DISORDERS

739.   INTRODUCTION

Lawrence E. Young

Definition. The essential feature of a hemolytic disorder is shortening of the life span of the red blood cells. The patient may have a compensated hemolytic state without anemia if the bone marrow responds adequately. As the marrow of adult man appears to be capable of increasing red blood cell production about eightfold, and as the normal life span of human red cells is about 120 days, anemia may not develop in some cases even if the average life span of the red cells is reduced to 15 to 20 days. The reserve capacity of the liver to excrete an increased quantity of bilirubin resulting from hemolysis may likewise result in maintenance of a normal concentration of bilirubin in the blood plasma. In a large proportion of the hemolytic states recognized clinically, however, patients are either anemic or mildly icteric, or both, so that the terms *hemolytic anemia* and *hemolytic icterus* are applicable.

Clinical Manifestations. In addition to pallor and mild icterus, the patient with a hemolytic disorder may present with fever, dyspnea, or shock if hemolysis is severe and anemia develops rapidly. The spleen is frequently enlarged but is by no means always palpable. In some instances, notably in hereditary spherocytosis, splenomegaly may be associated with accumulation of red cells in the splenic pulp; in others, enlargement may be due chiefly to proliferation of one or more cellular elements. The liver is also enlarged in many cases. Other clinical findings are related chiefly to the severity of the anemia and to the condition responsible for the hemolytic process. Chronic ulceration of the skin over or proximal to the malleoli may develop in sickle cell anemia, and rarely in hereditary spherocytosis and other chronic hemolytic disorders.

Gallstones containing chiefly bile pigment develop frequently in patients with chronic hemolytic disorders. Obstructive jaundice associated with choledocholithiasis or with cholestasis may develop rapidly and with extremely high concentrations of serum bilirubin because of the combination of excessive pigment production and biliary obstruction. Another major complication of chronic hemolytic disorders is rather sudden depression of erythropoiesis and fall in reticulocyte count, most often associated with acute infection. In such cases, the bone marrow may show hypoplasia or arrested maturation of erythroid cells. Folate deficiency may be demonstrable in some patients with chronic hemolytic anemia and may at times be associated with a megaloblastic marrow. Many of the "crises" in chronic hemolytic states are due chiefly to decrease in erythropoiesis for one reason or another. Anemia may suddenly become severe under these circumstances without significant increase in hemolysis above the patient's usual rate. Such episodes are often referred to as "hyporegenerative crises." Because folate requirement may be increased by persistent hemolysis, administration of 1 mg of folic acid by mouth daily may be justified in chronic hemolytic states of any type to prevent deficiency of this vitamin.

Diagnosis. Persistent reticulocytosis, with or without nucleated red blood cells in the peripheral blood, in the absence of blood loss should arouse suspicion of hemolysis. Large, diffusely basophilic red cells, which appear on supravital staining as prematurely released reticulocytes, are especially indicative of heightened bone marrow response. Estimates of compensatory increase in rate of erythropoiesis by use of reticulocyte counts require calculation of the number per cubic millimeter (normal is about 60,000) and recognition of the fact that maturation time of reticulocytes in the circulation may increase two- to threefold as anemia becomes severe. The rate of red cell destruction can be estimated most conveniently by measuring the survival time of the patient's cells after tagging with radioactive chromium (^{51}Cr). Rapid disappearance of similarly labeled normal donor cells from the patient's circulation points to an extracorpuscular hemolytic mechanism. Measurement of fecal urobilinogen excretion, usually in four-day collections of stool, also provides an estimate of the rate of red cell destruction, but such estimates may be falsely low in some cases. Fecal urobilinogen determinations have been made much less frequently in most centers since isotopic tagging of red cells became available. Since the amount

Classification of Hemolytic Disorders

I. Intracorpuscular abnormalities (sometimes combined with extrinsic challenge):
  A. Membrane defects
    Spherocytosis
    Elliptocytosis
    Stomatocytosis
    Chronic hemolytic anemia with paroxysmal nocturnal hemoglobinuria
  B. Enzyme deficiencies
    Defect in Embden-Meyerhof pathway of glycolysis
    Hexokinase
    Glucose phosphate isomerase
    Phosphofructokinase
    Fructosediphosphate aldolase
    Triosephosphate isomerase
    Diphosphoglyceromutase
    Phosphoglyerate kinase
    Pyruvate kinase
    Deficiency in enzyme activity related to the hexose monophosphate shunt pathway
    Glucose-6-phosphate dehydrogenase
    Phosphogluconate dehydrogenase
    Glutathione reductase
    γ-Glutamyl-cysteine synthetase
    Glutathione synthetase
    Glutathione peroxidase
  C. Hemoglobinopathies—qualitative defect in alpha or beta chains of globin
    Aggregating hemoglobins (S, C, D, I)
    Unstable hemoglobins (Zürich, Köln, etc.) with Heinz body formation
  D. Thalassemias—quantitative deficiency in synthesis of alpha or beta chains (may be combined with qualitative defect)
  E. Other types
    Low ATP concentration
    High ATP concentration
    ATPase deficiency
    Erythropoietic porphyria
    Increased red cell lecithin

II. Extracorpuscular causes (sometimes acting upon defective red cells):
  A. Immune mechanisms
    Warm-reacting antibodies
      Isoimmune
        Transfusion reactions
        Hemolytic disease of newborn
      Autoimmune
    Cold-reacting antibodies
      Cold agglutinin syndrome
      Paroxysmal cold hemoglobinuria
    Paroxysmal nocturnal hemoglobinuria (discussed in Ch. 740)
  B. Intravascular fragmentation
    Microangiopathic—intravascular clotting hemolysis
    Cardiac valvular hemolysis
    March hemoglobinuria
  C. Acquired membrane alterations
    Chemicals
      Drugs
        Nonimmune
        Immune
      Poisons
        Animal—spider bites, snake venoms
        Vegetable—castor beans, mushrooms
        Mineral—Cu^{++}
    Accumulated metabolites
      Due to kidney failure
      Due to liver failure
    Infectious agents
      Direct infestation
      Malaria
      Bartonella
    Indirect alteration
      Immunologically
      Nonimmunologically
  D. Hemolysis due to abnormal sequestration of normal red cells by the reticuloendothelial system
    Hypersplenism
    Eosinophilic granuloma syndromes (histiocytic reticuloendothelioses)

---

of urobilinogen excreted in the urine is affected by liver function, measurements of urinary urobilinogen are unreliable as indicators of the rate of red cell destruction. In the presence of modest hemolysis, urinary urobilinogen excretion may be normal if liver function is well preserved, or it may be greatly increased if liver function is impaired.

The concentration of bilirubin (predominantly unconjugated) seldom exceeds 8.0 mg per 100 ml of plasma. Hemolytic icterus has been recognized for many years as "acholuric"; little or no bilirubin is excreted in the urine unless liver function is impaired or the biliary tract becomes obstructed.

Since hemoglobinemia is largely the result of rapid intravascular hemolysis outside the microcirculation of the spleen, liver, and/or bone marrow, it is absent or minimal in many hemolytic states. The renal threshold for hemoglobin depends on the capacity of plasma haptoglobins to bind hemoglobin (normally 100 to 150 mg of hemoglobin per 100 ml of plasma) and on the ability of renal tubular cells to remove hemoglobin from glomerular filtrate. The haptoglobins, which are alpha-2 globulins with remarkable capacity to bind hemoglobin, are markedly reduced in the plasma in most of the clinically recognized hemolytic states, acute and chronic, including those with little or no hemoglobinemia. Reduction in haptoglobin concentration is due to rapid clearing of the hemoglobin-haptoglobin complex by the recticuloendothelial system.

Morphologic abnormalities of the red blood cells are best discussed in connection with the individual hemolytic disorders. In some examples of hemolytic disease, no abnormality of size or shape of the red cells is apparent. Fragmentation, best observed with phase microscopy or scanning electron microscopy, but also evident in customary examination of stained blood smears, is recognized increasingly as a final common pathway in many hemolytic states. Platelets and granulocytes are usually present in normal or increased numbers, but either or both may be decreased in some instances. The bone marrow typically shows normoblastic hyperplasia in response to hemolysis except during hyporegenerative periods which are most commonly associated with infection.

Splenectomy. Since the estimated benefits and hazards of splenectomy must be weighed in the management of many patients with hemolytic disorders, certain general considerations can be presented to advantage at this point. Often decision can be reached easily on the basis of precise diagnosis and abundant documentation in the literature of favorable or unfavorable results with a given disorder. In some of the disorders to be described, decision regarding splenectomy may be influenced by measurements of radioactivity over the body surface above the spleen in comparison with counts above the liver after transfusion of autogenous or normal donated red cells tagged with ^{51}Cr. Such measurements help to reveal the relative importance of the spleen in the hemolytic process. There are well-documented examples, however, of patients benefiting from splenectomy despite the fact that excessive splenic localization was not found in this type of preoperative study.

Immediate operative mortality from splenectomy performed primarily to relieve hemolytic disease is very low in the hands of experienced surgeons. Two possible sequelae of splenectomy deserve emphasis. The risk of sepsis with sudden onset and high mortality rate must be recognized in all asplenic persons regardless of the reason for splenectomy. The risk is greatest during infancy but persists throughout adulthood, especially with blood-borne inocula of pneumococcus, Meningococcus, *E. coli*, and *H. influenzae*. Splenectomized patients and their families as well as responsible nurses and physicians should be aware of the need for prompt diagnosis and treatment of infection in the absence of defense mechanisms normally provided by the spleen.

Another consequence of splenectomy is thromboembolism in patients with persistent thrombocytosis. Such patients are usually those who continue to have anemia and reticulocytosis as well as thrombocytosis for many years. The patient whose hemolytic anemia is not significantly relieved by splenectomy thus incurs the added risk of thrombophlebitis and embolic complications.

Classification. The classification in the accompanying table is based chiefly upon current concepts of pathogenic mechanisms. The disorders listed with intracorpuscular abnormalities of the red cell are hereditary except for that associated with nocturnal hemoglobinuria. Intrinsically defective red cells with shortened life span may be produced in patients with myeloid metaplasia, chronic myelocytic leukemia, deficiency of vitamin B_{12} folate, or iron, and in patients with lead intoxication. These conditions will not be discussed here because other features of the respective illnesses are usually more important than the hemolytic component of the anemia.

740. INTRACORPUSCULAR ABNORMALITIES

Lawrence E. Young

Erythrocytes from patients with certain types of intracorpuscular abnormality have been found to disappear rapidly from the circulation after transfusion to normal recipients. Normal donor cells, on the other hand, survive normally in the circulation of such patients unless there are complicating hemolytic mechanisms such as hypersplenism or the development of immune isoantibodies as a result of previous transfusions. Although there are unmistakable abnormalities of the red blood cells in this group of patients, hemolysis may be dependent upon or heightened by the presence of environmental factors that provide a critical challenge to the defective cells. The sequence of events by which most recognized types of abnormal red cells are destroyed in vivo becomes clearer each year. This group of disorders provides excellent material for studies in cellular biology.

MEMBRANE DEFECTS

Hereditary Spherocytosis (HS)

Definition. This condition is inherited as an autosomal dominant disorder and is characterized by the presence of spherocytes or abnormally thick red blood cells in the circulation. It has been found in many populations, but appears to be most common in northern European stocks. In such populations, the incidence has been estimated at from 200 to 300 per million.

Clinical Manifestations. Diagnosis may be made at birth if the condition is suspected, but in mild cases diagnosis may not be made until late in life. Moderate splenomegaly develops in nearly all cases. Leg ulcers are encountered infrequently. Roentgenographic examination reveals striation and thickening of the frontal and parietal bones in some cases. Anemia is rarely severe in the absence of hyporegenerative crises or other complications such as infection or hemorrhage.

Diagnosis. Spherocytosis is usually evident in blood smears or in wet preparations which show bizarre rouleau formation. The increase in osmotic fragility provides a reliable measure of the degree of spherocytosis. Mechanical fragility of the red cells is also increased. Both types of fragility are increased by sterile incubation of the blood at body temperature for 24 hours, a procedure that may cause changes in red cells similar to those produced during sequestration within the spleen. Autohemolysis, or spontaneous lysis of red cells in defibrinated blood incubated at body temperature, is best measured at 48 hours and is markedly increased in most cases of HS. The percentage of lysis after incubation is computed by measuring the concentration of hemoglobin in the serum in relation to the hemoglobin content of the blood sample prior to incubation. Autohemolysis is strikingly inhibited by addition of glucose or by slight acidification of the blood from HS patients. Such inhibition of autohemolysis is less evident in other types of chronic spherocytosis, and is sometimes not demonstrable in HS until after splenectomy. In order to establish the diagnosis, similar abnormalities should be sought in relatives of patients with spherocytosis, even when there is no history of anemia, jaundice, or splenomegaly. In some cases only the measurements of fragility with incubated red cells are clearly abnormal. In instances of suspected low gene manifestation or gene mutation, both parents of patients with suspected HS may be hematologically normal by all available criteria.

Pathogenesis. Spherocytes are readily trapped, probably for variable periods of time, within the splenic pulp. When washed from that site after splenectomy, they show much greater osmotic fragility than do spherocytes in the peripheral blood, although normal donor cells in the splenic pulp show little increase in fragility. Transfused spherocytes are readily trapped and destroyed in the spleen of hematologically normal recipients but survive normally in splenectomized normal recipients.

The red cell membrane in this disease is less deformable and more permeable to sodium than the membrane of normal red cells. Trapping of HS red cells within the cords of Billroth of the spleen is probably related to cellular rigidity, which depends both on the decreased surface area to volume ratio and on increased intrinsic rigidity of the cell membrane. Abnormality of contractile protein in the membrane is under continuing study. The relatively low pH and oxygen tension within the splenic pulp render ATP bound to deoxyhemoglobin less available than needed to maintain integrity of the red cell membrane. Hereditary spherocytosis cells lose lipid and protein from the membrane surface as they make their way through the cords, with the result that they become more nearly spherical and still more rigid. Eventually the cells are unable to escape through the small openings into the venous sinusoids. Fragmentation of the rigid cells to the point of ultimate destruction has been observed by phase microscopy and electron microscopy in the spleens of mice afflicted with a comparable disorder. Hemoglobinemia is not encountered in HS patients, but plasma haptoglobin concentration is consistently low.

Treatment. Splenectomy is invariably effective in lengthening the life span of the red cells to a nearly normal range. In most cases anemia is fully corrected and there is a decrease to normal in reticulocytes and serum bilirubin concentration. Spherocytosis and other demonstrable abnormalities of the red cells persist after splenectomy, but are of little or no consequence once the splenic trap is removed. Splenectomy can be recommended in most cases, even when well compensated, because of the threats of cholelithiasis and of severe anemia during periods of suppressed erythropoiesis. Splenectomy may prevent development of hemochromatosis, a recently reported complication in older patients. Operation is usually deferred to about age five to make minimal the risk of sepsis explained previously. Transfusion of normal red blood cells is seldom indicated except during the periods of severe anemia associated with hyporegenerative bone marrow.

Hereditary Elliptocytosis

Hereditary elliptocytosis is similar to hereditary spherocytosis in many respects. It has been found in many populations, and may be encountered more frequently than spherocytosis in some localities. It is inherited as an autosomal dominant abnormality with wide variations in gene manifestation both within and between families. In some families there is evidence for location of the gene or genes determining elliptocytosis on the chromosome bearing genes for the Rh blood group system. The degree of elliptocytosis varies from person to person and also among the red cells of any affected person. Many of the cells are usually abnormal in shape, some are greatly elongated, and others are slightly oval. There is no apparent relationship between the degree of elliptocytosis and the life span of the red cells. In the presence of active hemolysis, microspherocytes may be found in small numbers. Some affected persons have red cells with normal life span; others have a compensated hemolytic state; and a minority have overt hemolytic anemia. The very rare homozygous state is associated with severe hemolysis. Factors determining chronic hemolysis in the heterozygotes are unknown. Coexistence of elliptocytosis with hemoglobin S or hemoglobin C trait or with erythrocyte glyoxalase II deficiency does not appear to cause an additive, deleterious effect on the red cells. Coexistence of elliptocytosis with heterozygous beta thalassemia, on the other hand, may be associated with hemolysis.

Splenomegaly is common, and sequestration of red cells in the spleen is evident. Most patients splenectomized because of hemolysis associated with elliptocytosis have been benefited.

Stomatocytosis

Stomatocytosis is characterized by red cells with the appearance of a linear, mouthlike area of central pallor on stained films and with the appearance of bowls in wet preparations. There is marked increase in osmotic fragility, and in one form there is high concentration of calcium and sodium and low concentration of potassium with increased energy requirement for active cation transport. Reports to date suggest that this is an autosomal dominant character. Response to splenectomy is variable. Stomatocytosis may be produced in vitro by a variety of chemical agents, many of which are cationic detergent-like molecules.

Chronic Hemolytic Anemia with Paroxysmal Nocturnal Hemoglobinuria*

Definition. This rare disorder has been encountered in many parts of the world. It occurs in both sexes, with onset most common during the third or fourth decade. There is no report of familial incidence.

Clinical Manifestations. The disease is characterized by chronic hemolysis of a highly variable degree, with hemoglobinemia and usually, but not always, hemoglobinuria. Hemolysis is usually increased during sleep, regardless of the time when the patient sleeps. Episodes of increased hemolysis, sometimes lasting several days, occur irregularly, particularly after infections. During the period of hemolysis sufficient to cause hemoglobinuria, the urine passed on arising is usually brown or reddish brown. In severely affected patients, hemoglobinuria may be continuous, with further darkening of the urine after sleep. Hemosiderinuria, a regular feature of the disease, results in considerable loss of iron from the body. Renal function is usually unimpaired, but there may be complications such as pyelonephritis. Hemosiderin is not found in any significant quantity in the body outside the cells of the convoluted tubules and ascending loops of Henle in the kidney, unless the patient has had frequent transfusions. The liver and spleen may be slightly enlarged. No characteristic abnormality of the red cell is evident in blood smears or in tests of osmotic or mechanical fragility. Neutropenia and thrombocytopenia are commonly found. Alkaline phosphatase activity in the neutrophils is markedly decreased. Although erythroid hyperplasia of the bone marrow is usually present, marked hypoplasia of all elements is being found increasingly before or, rarely, after the hemolytic disorder becomes apparent. It has been suggested that in some cases the abnormal red cells may be derived from a mutant clone of precursors originating during a period of marrow aplasia, even when the aplasia seems related to drug usage. The recently recognized development of stem cell or acute myelocytic leukemia in patients with antecedent nocturnal hemoglobinuria has led to the suggestion that this hemolytic disorder may represent a somatic mutation which, at times, involves the stem cells. Thrombotic complications, particularly involving hepatic and cerebral veins, are frequently associated with greatly accelerated hemolysis. Dysphagia caused by increased esophageal pressure waves may occur, particularly during hemolytic crises. Severe abdominal pain of uncertain cause is also seen with such episodes.

Pathogenesis. The disease is characterized by the presence of a proportion of red cells which are more susceptible to the lytic action of complement than normal

---

*The author thanks Dr. Wendell F. Rosse for advice in the wording of this article.

cells. The proportion of abnormal cells may vary from 1 to over 90 per cent, and the severity of the disease roughly parallels this proportion. The activation of complement by unknown mechanisms results in the intravascular lysis of these abnormal cells, particularly during sleep. The nature of the membrane defect leading to increased lysis by complement is not known, but it appears to result in an increased binding of the later components (C3 and beyond) and an increased effectiveness of these components. Membrane-bound acetylcholinesterase is deficient on these cells, but the relationship of this to the increased lysis by complement is problematic.

Because of the membrane defect, the cells are lysed, no matter how the complement sequence is activated. In vitro activation by antibody is useful in demonstrating the presence of the lesion, but activation by the so-called alternate, or properdin, pathway which bypasses the initial steps of the classic antibody pathway in activating C3 is probably more important in initiating hemolysis in vivo.

The diagnosis is made by demonstrating increased lysis by complement in any of several systems. In the Ham test (acidified serum lysis test), complement is activated through the alternate pathway by the mild acidification of normal serum. It may be rendered more sensitive by augmentation of the magnesium concentration to 0.005 M. This test is specific for PNH if suitably controlled, including demonstration that the patient's serum lyses his own cells. The red cells of some patients with congenital dyserythropoietic anemia may be hemolyzed in normal serum because of the occurrence of naturally occurring antibodies against membrane antigens; these cells are not lysed by the patient's own serum nor by normal serum in any of the tests listed below.

Complement may also be activated by reduced ionic strength in an osmotic solution of sucrose. This provides a convenient method for diagnosis, but the test must be carefully performed. Lysis of PNH cells may also be induced by a factor from cobra venom and inulin, both of which activate the alternate pathway.

Treatment. Transfusion of washed, normal red blood cells is needed during periods of severe anemia. Transfusion of whole blood should be avoided in most cases, because constituents of normal plasma as well as leukocytes may accelerate hemolysis. Use of coumarin derivatives may be indicated in patients who have developed thrombosis, but it is difficult to justify for prevention of thrombosis. Their inhibitory effect on hemolysis is transient with tolerable doses. Use of heparin is controversial. Intravenous administration of 1000 ml of 6 per cent dextran daily or at longer intervals may inhibit hemolysis during critical periods of the disease but is not recommended for sustained use. All operative procedures, including splenectomy, are to be avoided if possible. Administration of iron, preferably by mouth, may be beneficial for patients who are not transfused and who develop evidence of iron deficiency. Administration of androgens, such as fluoxymesterone, 20 to 30 mg daily by mouth, may be beneficial by stimulating erythropoiesis and perhaps by reducing hemolysis. Prednisone, 20 to 30 mg every other day, may be useful in control of hemolysis in severely affected patients. Folic acid, 1 mg daily by mouth, is indicated to meet increased folate requirement.

Prognosis. This is a chronic disorder that terminates fatally in many cases. The patients may lead active lives between complicating episodes if suitably managed. In some instances, the abnormality of the red cells eventually disappears. A few women with this disease have borne normal children, but usually with complications during pregnancy or the puerperium.

ENZYME DEFICIENCIES

The accompanying figure shows the pathways of glycolysis in the mature human erythrocyte, with lines drawn under the names of enzymes thus far demonstrated to be deficient in certain individuals with hemolytic states. Although the hemolytic mechanisms are only partially understood, the relationship between enzyme deficiency and hemolysis is well documented in most instances. Under normal conditions about 90 per cent of glucose is metabolized anaerobically through the Embden-Meyerhof pathway with net increase in high energy adenosine triphosphate (ATP) serving multiple purposes. Another product of glycolysis is 2,3-diphosphoglycerate (2,3-DPG) which exerts major influence on the binding of oxygen to hemoglobin (see Ch. 730).

Defects in Embden-Meyerhof Pathway of Glycolysis

Hemolytic states associated with deficiencies of eight enzymes involved in the anaerobic pathway of glycolysis

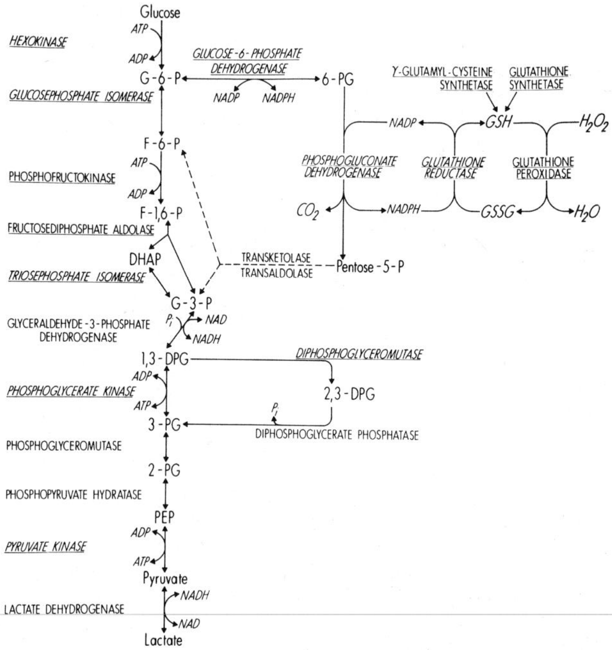

Pathways of glycolysis in mature human red cell (modified from Valentine).

Abbreviations: ATP = adenosine triphosphate; ADP = adenosine diphosphate; NADP = nicotinamide-adenine dinucleotide phosphate (TPN); NADPH = reduced nicotinamide-adenine dinucleotide phosphate (TPNH); G-6-P = glucose-6-phosphate; 6-PG = 6-phospho-3-ketogluconate; Pentose-5-P = pentose-5-phosphate; GSH = reduced glutathione; GSSG = oxidized glutathione; F-6-P = fructose-6-phosphate; F-1,6-P = fructose-1,6-phosphate; DHAP = dihydroxyacetonephosphate; G-3-P = glyceraldehyde-3-phosphate; P_i = inorganic phosphorus; 1,3-DPG = 1,3-diphosphoglycerate; 2,3-DPG = 2,3-diphosphoglycerate; 3-PG = 3-phosphoglycerate; 2-PG = 2-phosphoglycerate; PEP = phosphoenol pyruvate.

in red cells have been identified since 1962. Pyruvate kinase (PK) deficiency is the most frequently encountered example of this uncommon group of disorders and was the first to be described. The pattern of inheritance is autosomal recessive, except for phosphoglycerate kinase deficiency which is X-linked.

In PK deficiency, the prototype of this group, heterozygotes are phenotypically normal, but have measurable deficiency of enzyme activity in the red cells. Homozygotes have a lifelong hemolytic state of variable severity with splenomegaly and only partial relief from hemolysis after splenectomy. Spherocytosis is not prominent, but may be noted on close inspection of blood smears and wet preparations. Crenated red cells are frequently noted and are probably crenated spherocytes or irregularly contracted cells. Finding crenated spherocytes on the blood smear of a patient with splenomegaly and with a history suggesting hemolytic anemia since early childhood should stimulate the clinician to obtain enzyme assays on the patient's red cells.

Genetically determined heterogeneity of erythrocyte PK has been demonstrated, including evidence of kinetic abnormality of the enzyme. Most patients with PK deficiency develop anemia and jaundice in the neonatal period. Anemia is usually more severe than in hereditary spherocytosis. Osmotic fragility of the red cells is normal with fresh blood but is abnormally increased after the blood has been incubated for 24 hours at 37° C. Autohemolysis is moderately increased except in patients with a presumed variant of PK deficiency and usually is not diminished when glucose is added to the blood. In some cases of PK deficiency, however, glucose may inhibit autohemolysis. Use of the autohemolysis test for differential diagnosis must take into account these exceptional cases of PK deficiency along with the exceptional cases of hereditary spherocytosis in which glucose fails to inhibit autohemolysis until after splenectomy.

Hemolysis in PK deficiency generally is attributed to impaired glycolysis and consequent reduction in ATP generation, but further studies of the hemolytic mechanism are needed. PK-deficient reticulocytes may be spared to some extent from destruction in the general circulation, because their mitochondria provide ATP from aerobic metabolism. The PK-deficient reticulocytes, like normal reticulocytes, tend to be sequestered within the spleen. Within the hypoxic environment of the splenic pulp, aerobic metabolism, upon which the PK-deficient reticulocytes are dependent, is inhibited with consequent decrease in ATP content, increase in cellular rigidity, and irreversible sequestration of the reticulocytes. The partial relief of anemia and frequent reduction in transfusion requirement in this disorder after splenectomy may be attributable to removal of the hypoxic trap. Reticulocyte counts are frequently higher after splenectomy despite amelioration of anemia, thus reflecting the survival of reticulocytes which previously had been eliminated from the circulation by the spleen. Although splenectomy is much less effective than in hereditary spherocytosis, it can be recommended after infancy for patients requiring transfusions to maintain acceptable concentrations of hemoglobin.

In triosephosphate isomerase deficiency, enzyme activity is also low in leukocytes, muscle, and cerebrospinal fluid. A severe, progressive neurologic disorder develops in addition to hemolytic anemia. The hematologic picture is similar to that of PK deficiency except that autohemolysis is inhibited more constantly by glucose.

Glucosephosphate isomerase deficiency may be second in incidence to PK deficiency among the enzymes involved in the anaerobic pathway. Other examples of enzyme deficiency in the red cell related to anaerobic glycolysis are rare. In general, the clinical findings and course are similar to those of PK deficiency. Severe deficiency of lactate dehydrogenase, transmitted as an autosomal recessive trait, is not associated with overt hemolysis.

Deficiency in Enzyme Activity Related to the Hexose Monophosphate (HMP) Shunt Pathway

Glucose-6-Phosphate Dehydrogenase (G-6-PD)

The enzyme G-6-PD is involved at the beginning of the oxidative HMP shunt pathway, which under usual conditions accounts for about 10 per cent of glucose metabolism of the red cell. In normal red cells the proportion of total glucose metabolized through the shunt pathway may be increased many-fold if the cells are subjected to oxidants such as those derived from certain drugs. The resulting increase in generation of the reduced form of nicotinamide adenine dinucleotide phosphate (NADPH) and consequently of reduced glutathione (GSH) helps to resist oxidant stresses. Otherwise, these stresses may inactivate essential thiol (SH) groups on membrane proteins, and within the cell may cause formation of methemoglobin and degradation of hemoglobin to form Heinz bodies. Drugs such as phenylhydrazine may overwhelm this protective mechanism, especially in older red cells because there is a decline in G-6-PD activity with aging of red cells in the circulation. Red cells with a genetically determined deficiency of G-6-PD are unable to withstand lesser oxidative stresses. The outcome in any given red cell presumably is determined by the amount of stress and the severity of enzyme deficiency, but predictions based on estimates of enzyme activity by the usual methods may nevertheless be inaccurate.

Studies on hemolytic disorders related to the HMP shunt pathway constitute one of the most fascinating and clinically significant chapters in the history of hematology. G-6-PD deficiency in red cells has been shown to be due to a wide range of genetic variants, each of which is X-linked. The defect is fully expressed in male hemizygotes and female homozygotes. It is variably manifest in female heterozygotes because two populations of red cells are present, deficient cells and normal cells, in varying proportions. It is not known whether the heterogeneity in G-6-PD formation is produced by different mutations at a single locus on the X chromosome or whether mutations at different loci affect the production and function of the enzyme. There are two common types of G-6-PD. Type A, moving rapidly on starch-gel electrophoresis, is found in about 30 per cent of American blacks, including most of those who are enzyme deficient. Type B, moving more slowly on electrophoresis, is found in about 70 per cent of blacks and in nearly all Caucasians.

Manifestations in Blacks. The most common type of G-6-PD deficiency is found in blacks: about 10 per cent of American blacks, 8 to 20 per cent of blacks in West Africa, but only 2 per cent of South African Bantus. Activity of this enzyme in the red cells is reduced to 5 to 15 per cent of normal in hemizygous males and homozygous females. Enzyme activity in heterozygous females ranges from normal to figures nearly as low as those obtained from homozygotes. Red cell life span is only slightly reduced in G-6-PD-deficient blacks unless the cells are subjected to stress imposed by derivatives of certain drugs or by infection or possibly by diabetic ketoacidosis. More than 40 drugs have been found to produce hemolysis in G-6-PD-deficient persons. These include the antimalarial drugs primaquine and quinine (the latter also used in popular beverages), the antipyretics and analgesics acetylsalicylic acid and phenacetin in large doses, the nitrofurans, sulfones, many sulfonamides, para-aminosalicylic acid, probenecid, quinidine, phenylhydrazine, and water-soluble analogues of vitamin K. Naphthalene, of which moth balls are composed, is often ingested by children with effects similar to those of the drugs listed. Blacks whose G-6-PD-deficient red cells are challenged develop hemolytic anemia of varying severity, depending upon the dose and oxidative capacity of the derivatives of the chemical agent involved; in female heterozygotes the degree of enzyme deficiency appears also to influence the extent of hemolysis. Patients suffering from infection, acidosis, or impaired liver or kidney function, with consequent delay in drug excretion, may be more subject to hemolysis with a given dose of a potentially oxidant drug. Moreover, infection or acidosis may provoke hemolysis in the absence of an offending drug, and they may in fact be the most common precipitants of hemolytic anemia in these individuals. Infection may lead to hemolysis through increased production of hydrogen peroxide by leukocytes engaged in phagocytosis of organisms.

Hemoglobinemia and hemoglobinuria are usually of only moderate degree and short duration, and may not be observed. Plasma haptoglobin is usually reduced even in the cases of little or no hemoglobinemia. Many of the red cells may contain Heinz bodies during the first few days of hemolysis, but in typical cases most of the red cells containing Heinz bodies have been eliminated by the time the hematocrit reaches its lowest point. The red cells show fragmentation of widely varying degree from case to case prior to onset of the recovery phase. The cells may appear as though a portion had been torn away, but they do not as a rule show crenation or appear as irregularly contracted spherocytes. Careful inspection of the blood smear together with consideration of the patient's history and ethnic group helps to differentiate this type of hemolytic anemia from that caused by a defect in the Embden-Meyerhof pathway within the red cell. Typically hemolysis is limited in duration because of the more nearly normal G-6-PD activity in younger red cells which become more abundant in the circulation in response to hemolysis. Consequently, the erythrocyte level may return to normal even though administration of the offending drug is continued. Diagnosis by estimates of enzyme activity in the red cells may be difficult at the time of acute hemolysis and reticulocytosis. Confirmation of the clinical diagnosis by enzyme assay often must await the return to normal of the red cell age distribution unless special methods are used.

Manifestations in Other Populations. G-6-PD deficiency in populations other than blacks is usually more severe, with red cell enzyme activity in most cases in the range of 0 to 5 per cent of normal and with reduced G-6-PD activity in leukocytes and platelets as well as in red cells. At least 100 different forms of G-6-PD have been demonstrated among Caucasian and Oriental populations on the basis of biochemical characteristics of the enzyme. Among Caucasian populations G-6-PD Mediterranean is by far the most common variant enzyme, with a gene frequency of less than 0.1 per cent in Northern Europeans and of about 50 per cent among male Kurdish Jews. The frequency in Greeks is 2 to 9 per cent, in Italians 0.5 to 1.0 per cent, and in Sardinians 3 to 35 per cent. The distribution of variant enzyme types in other populations is less clearly determined; the incidence of G-6-PD deficiency is about 2 to 4 per cent in Chinese, 12 per cent in Thais, and 1 to 5 per cent in Indians.

Studies of Caucasians with G-6-PD activity in the range of 0 to 18 per cent of normal have shown that about 20 per cent of the circulating red cells are destroyed after ingestion of a single standard prophylactic antimalarial dose of primaquine (45 mg). The degree of hemolysis under these circumstances is not related to the estimated level of enzyme activity. G-6-PD-deficient Caucasians are generally more subject than are blacks to hemolysis after use of potentially oxidant drugs or as a complication of infection or of diabetic ketoacidosis.

Chronic hemolytic anemia in the absence of drugs or other extrinsic challenge is encountered in Caucasian and occasionally in Oriental males with marked deficiency of G-6-PD activity. Hemolysis appears to be continuous from infancy, but may be accelerated by the same types of challenges causing acute hemolysis in the much more common, nonanemic G-6-PD-deficient Caucasian or black. Most of the G-6-PD variants associated with a chronic hemolytic state are abnormally labile at temperatures of 40 to 46° C. Osmotic fragility of the red cells in the chronic state is normal or nearly so. Autohemolysis is increased only slightly and usually is inhibited by glucose. Ovalocytes are noted in some cases, but spherocytes are seen rarely. Data on spleen size and results of splenectomy are meager. Splenomegaly is not a regular feature as it is in hereditary spherocytosis and in PK deficiency. Studies with ^{51}Cr-tagged red cells show no unusual concentration of radioactivity over the spleen.

Favism is an acute hemolytic anemia occurring after ingestion of fava beans or after inhalation of pollen from the plant *Vicia faba* by persons with G-6-PD-deficient red cells. Several other plants may have a similar effect. Favism has been observed only in Caucasians and is most common among certain groups of Kurdish Jews, Sardinians, Greeks, and Italians. Since many Caucasians with G-6-PD deficiency suffer no hemolysis after challenge by bean or plant, an additional mechanism is suspected. Studies on isolated populations with high incidence of favism suggest that the additional determinant may be inherited. Anemia may be very severe and accompanied by hemoglobinemia. During the early phase of an attack the hemoglobin appears to be concentrated on one side of some of the red cells, leaving the cell envelope visible on the opposite side. Heinz bodies and spherocytes may be seen, and osmotic fragility may be increased transiently. There is marked leukocytosis, often with transient eosinophilia.

Neonatal Jaundice. Neonatal jaundice with development of kernicterus is a hazard for infants, especially males, with some types of G-6-PD deficiency. Hemolysis and hyperbilirubinemia can be induced in the newborn, particularly if premature, by use of drugs such as water-soluble, synthetic vitamin K preparations or by drugs given to the mother before delivery. Caucasian and Oriental infants may develop jaundice without exposure to drugs. In Hong Kong, for example, G-6-PD deficiency is claimed to be the most common cause of neonatal jaundice and kernicterus. Even in the presence of normal G-6-PD activity in the red cells, glutathione is unstable during the first few days of life. Since this instability can be corrected in vitro by addition of glucose, it is believed that hypoglycemia in the newborn may increase the risk of neonatal jaundice.

Use of Screening Tests. It is estimated from population surveys that at least 100 million persons in the world have red cells deficient in G-6-PD. Wide use of a simple screening test for this deficiency, such as that based on reduction of methemoglobin, is indicated as a part of comprehensive health care for populations known to be at relatively high risk. Tests done when the patient is well serve to forewarn both patient and physician. Tests performed during or immediately after a period of hemolysis are unreliable because some genetic variants, chiefly in blacks, have a high activity of G-6-PD in reticulocytes; i.e., the tests may yield "false negative" results.

Drug-Induced Hemolysis of Older Normal Red Cells. Since G-6-PD activity declines with aging of red cells in the circulation, even red cells with normal enzyme activity initially may become susceptible to hemolysis if challenged by large doses of a drug such as the commonly used phenacetin or by modest doses of a drug such as phenylhydrazine with high oxidizing potential. It seems likely that this type of drug-induced hemolysis of normal aging red cells would be accentuated in the presence of infection or of diabetic acidosis. This potential hazard should be kept in mind by the physician as he estimates the risk of contemplated therapy in many clinical situations.

Other Deficiencies Related to the HMP Pathway

Deficiency of 6-phosphogluconate dehydrogenase has been the subject of recent studies revealing genetic polymorphism with respect to this enzyme; relationship to hemolysis is not yet clear.

Glutathione reductase deficiency, inherited as an autosomal dominant trait, is found in leukocytes and platelets as well as in red cells, and is associated with hemolytic anemia, thrombocytopenia, and, in some cases, with leukopenia. A neurologic disorder characterized by spasticity may develop in these patients. Use of oxidant drugs may cause severe pancytopenia. The enzyme deficiency may be corrected by oral administration of 5 mg of riboflavin daily, at least in some cases.

Deficiency of red cell glutathione with an associated chronic hemolytic state may be caused by deficiency in either of the two enzymes involved in synthesis of glutathione, γ-glutamyl-cysteine synthetase or glutathione synthetase. Both types of enzyme deficiency probably are inherited as autosomal recessive traits. Use of potentially oxidant drugs causes acceleration of hemolysis in persons with deficiency of red cell glutathione synthetase; comparable observations are not yet reported in persons having deficiency of red cell γ-glutamyl-cysteine synthetase. Deficiency of the latter enzyme is associated with chronic neurologic disease in the cases reported, but relationship between the degenerative neurologic disorder and the enzyme deficiency is not established.

Deficiency of red cell glutathione peroxidase is associated with relatively mild hemolytic states. Since this enzyme normally helps to prevent peroxidative injury, increased susceptibility to hemolysis after use of oxidant drugs is anticipated and has been demonstrated in one presumably homozygously deficient patient. Available data suggest that this deficiency is most likely an autosomal recessive trait.

OTHER INTRACORPUSCULAR ABNORMALITIES

The hemoglobinopathies and thalassemias, some of which are associated with a hemolytic state, are considered in Ch. 746 to 751. It is noteworthy that the Heinz body anemias associated with unstable hemoglobins usually are detectable by the simple procedure of heating hemolysates at 50° C for one to two hours. The resulting turbidity owing to precipitation of unstable hemoglobin is not observed in the Heinz body anemias associated with deficiency in enzyme activity related to the HMP shunt pathway.

Patients have been described with hemolytic anemia associated with low ATP concentration in the red cells and very high glycolytic rate. The cause of increased ATP utilization by the cells is unknown. Several different types of red cells have been described with high ATP concentration but without an associated hemolytic state. In one patient with high ATP concentration and deficiency of ribosephosphate pyrophosphokinase, chronic hemolysis was documented. Examples of hemolytic anemia have been reported in association with ATPase deficiency in the red cells, probably as an autosomal dominant trait.

A large share of patients with erythropoietic porphyria have hemolytic anemia which is relieved to varying degree by splenectomy. Improvement both in the hemolytic state and in photosensitivity after splenectomy may be marked.

Other types of hereditary abnormalities of the red cell associated with hemolysis are not easily classified. An example is the hemolytic anemia associated with increased red cell content of lecithin (phosphatidyl choline) probably inherited by an autosomal dominant pattern.

General

Dacie, J. V.: The Haemolytic Anaemias: Congenital and Acquired. 2nd ed. Parts 1, 2, 3, and 4. London and New York, J. & A. Churchill, Ltd., and Grune & Stratton, 1960–1967.

Harris, J. W., and Kellermeyer, R. W.: The Red Cell. Production, Metabolism, Destruction: Normal and Abnormal. Revised ed. Cambridge, Mass., Harvard University Press, 1970, pp. 517–593.

Singer, D. B.: Postsplenectomy sepsis. In Rosenbert, H. S., and Bolande, R. P. (eds.): Perspectives in Pediatric Pathology. Chicago, Year Book Medical Publishers, 1:285, 1973.

Weed, R. I. (ed.): Hematology for Internists. Boston, Little, Brown & Company, 1971, pp. 49–127.

Williams, W. J., Beutler, E., Erslev, A. J., and Rundles, R. W. (eds.): Hematology. New York, McGraw-Hill Book Company, 1972. pp. 381–409, 460–474.

Specific Hemolytic States

Beutler, E.: Abnormalities of the hexose monophosphate shunt. Semin. Hematol., 8:311, 1971.

Konrad, P. N., Richards, F., II, Valentine, W. N., and Paglia, E. D.: γ-Glutamyl-cysteine synthetase deficiency: A cause of hereditary hemolytic anemias. N. Engl. J. Med., 286:557, 1972.

Rosse, W. F.: Variations in the red cells in paroxysmal nocturnal haemoglobinuria. Br. J. Haematol., 24:327, 1973.

Valentine, W. N.: Hereditary enzymatic deficiencies of erythrocytes. Introduction. Deficiencies associated with Embden-Meyerhof pathway and other metabolic pathways. Semin. Hematol., 8:307, 348, 1971.

EXTRACORPUSCULAR MECHANISMS

Wendell F. Rosse

741. INTRODUCTION

Hemolysis not resulting from intrinsic defects of the red cell itself may be caused by a variety of abnormalities. In some instances, this is the only manifestation of disease; more frequently it is secondary to some other pathologic process which adversely affects the ability of the red cell to survive. The general manifestations of the hemolytic anemia resulting from extracorporeal causes do not differ from those for hemolysis resulting from intracorpuscular lesions, which are discussed in Ch. 740.

742. HEMOLYSIS DUE TO IMMUNE MECHANISMS

Alteration of the red cell membrane by immunologic reactions is one of the more common mechanisms by which the life span of the red cell may be shortened. These immune processes are usually initiated by IgG or IgM immunoglobulins; the diagnosis often depends upon demonstration of an antibody on the cells or in the serum of the patient.

Antibodies may sometimes be demonstrated by ability to agglutinate the cells. This is effected by the fixation of one antigen binding site of the antibody molecule on one cell and the other on another cell. When several cells are thus bound together, an agglutinate forms. IgM molecules are able to do this readily, because they are large enough to bridge the distance imposed by forces responsible for mutual repulsion of the red cells (the "zeta potential"). Many IgG antibodies cannot directly agglutinate, because they are not able to bridge this distance. Their presence on the red cell surface is often detected by the addition of antibodies directed against antigens present on the antibody molecules (*antiglobulin reaction; Coombs' reaction*). These heterologous antibodies are able to react with IgG antibodies on two red cells, thus linking the cells and forming the agglutinate. This reaction has immeasurably increased our ability to define immunologic reactions involving red cells.

The mechanisms by which immune reactions effect hemolysis depend upon the nature of the antibody, its interaction with antigen, and its ability to fix complement. When most IgG antibodies interact with red cell antigens, an area changes in the heavy chain portion of the molecule which permits it to interact with receptor sites on phagocytic cells, neutrophils, and macrophages (monocytes). The red cell may thus be held in place, and the whole cell or a portion of the membrane may be ingested; the remaining membrane may reseal across the defect, and the resulting cell fragment is capable of escaping from the phagocyte. Since it has lost more membrane than contents, the red cell must assume the shape of a spherocyte.

The spleen plays an important role in hemolysis by this mechanism. Because of peculiarities of its circulation and the rich layer of phagocytic cells lining the sinusoids, it is the chief site of interaction between macrophages and red cells with IgG antibody on the surface. In addition, those spherocytes which survive the initial interaction are rigid and on subsequent circulation through the spleen may be trapped and destroyed in the fine interstices. However, even when the spleen is removed, if sufficient antibody is present, the cells may be destroyed in other parts of the reticuloendothelial system.

Red cells may be destroyed because of fixation of complement. The complement sequence is initiated when two IgG antibody molecules or one IgM antibody molecule react with two antigen sites in close proximity to one another. This fixes a molecule of the first component of complement (C1), which acts upon the fourth component (C4) which may be then firmly affixed to the red cell surface. The second component, also activated by C1, is affixed to the fourth component, and this combination is able to activate a third component (C3) which is also fixed to the membrane. The fixed, active C3 molecule may interact with membrane receptors on phagocytic cells different from those interacting with IgG. This allows the phagocytic cell to ingest either a portion of the membrane or, more commonly, the entire cell. Such phagocytosis may be prevented by an enzyme which cleaves the C3 molecule, leaving an inactive portion of the molecule on the red cell membrane; it is this fragment which is usually detected by anti-C3 antiserum in an antiglobulin (Coombs) reaction like that used to detect IgG antibodies.

The active C3 molecule on the red cell membrane is able to propagate the complement sequence; if the sequence is successfully completed, disruption of the membrane occurs and intravascular hemolysis follows. For reasons not clearly understood, the completion of the complement sequence is singularly inefficient on normal human red cells, and therefore intravascular hemolysis is uncommon in immune hemolytic anemia, except under unusual circumstances.

The hematologic manifestations and the mechanism of destruction depend in large part upon the nature of the antibody initiating the immune reaction. Although many classifications could be constructed according to the various properties of the antibodies, it has been found most convenient to classify the syndromes by whether the antibody is able to react with the cell at body temperature (*warm-reacting antibodies*) or only at reduced temperatures (*cold-reacting antibodies*).

Antibodies may also be classified as isoimmune and autoimmune. The former arise in response to antigens not present on the red cells of the patient. Autoimmune antibodies react with antigens of the patient's own red cells. This distinction is usually relatively simple to make in the untransfused patient, because the direct antiglobulin test will be negative if the antibodies are isoimmune and positive if the antibodies are autoimmune. In complex clinical situations in which transfusion has taken place, this distinction may be more difficult.

HEMOLYSIS DUE TO WARM-REACTING ANTIBODIES

Warm-reacting antibodies are those capable of reacting with the red cell antigens at 37° C. They may or may not fix complement, depending upon the spacing of the antigen sites with which they interact and the immunoglobulin subclass of the antibody. In some instances, the antibody is not readily detectable on the red cell membrane by the antiglobulin test, but fixed complement components indicate that the immune reaction has taken place.

Hemolysis Due to Isoimmune Antibodies

Transfusion Reactions

See Part XVI, Section Three.

Hemolytic Disease of the Newborn

Hemolytic disease of the newborn is due to the transplacental infusion of isoimmune antibodies from the mother to the infant when the infant's red cells contain an antigen against which they may react. The antibody is, in most instances, formed in the mother in response to the prior transplacental transfer of "incompatible" red cells from that infant or previous infants, with the resultant production of isoimmune antibodies; occasionally, prior transfusion may be the cause of maternal sensitization. Hemolytic anemia in the infant results from the interaction of the maternal antibody and the infant's red cells.

Clinical Manifestations. The clinical manifestations are dependent in part upon the degree of sensitization of the mother, the immunoglobulin class of the antibody, and the antigen with which the antibody is reacting. In its most severe manifestations, the infant is born with anasarca, marked anemia, and hepatosplenomegaly; such infants rarely survive. In other instances, marked hemolytic anemia with jaundice may result. The anemia may persist for days to weeks. If appropriate treatment is instituted quickly, the resultant outcome is usually good; in some instances of marked sensitization, the infant is delivered prematurely in order to institute treatment. Where there is lesser sensitization, the extent of hemolytic anemia may be minimal.

Diagnosis. Hemolytic disease of the newborn is usually diagnosed by finding a positive direct antiglobulin test on the cells of the infant. The antibody may be eluted and its specificity determined. Occurrence of the illness may be anticipated by demonstration of an isoantibody in the mother's serum before birth where a rising titer may be assumed to indicate increasing sensitization and therefore increased chance of severe hemolysis. In some instances, prenatal hemolytic anemia is diagnosed by examination of the amniotic fluid for bilirubin-like catabolic products.

Prevention and Treatment. The chief complications of hemolytic disease of the newborn are anemia and excessive bilirubinemia, leading to kernicterus. The standard treatment is exchange transfusion. More recently, exposure of the infant to ultraviolet light has been shown to lower the bilirubin level and reduce the number of exchange transfusions needed.

Since most of the transplacental infusion of fetal cells into the mother occurs at birth, it has been found possible to prevent sensitization of the Rh_0 (D) negative mother to the Rh_0 (D) antigen by injection of a large quantity of anti Rh_0 (anti-D) antibody shortly after parturition. Any cells that have leaked from the fetus to the mother are destroyed by the injected antibody, and sensitization of the mother does not occur. Clearly, this preventive treatment does not work if the mother has been previously sensitized by other pregnancies or by transfusion.

Hemolysis Due to Autoimmune Antibodies

When the antibody is directed against an antigen on the red cells of the host (autoimmune hemolytic anemia), the warm-reacting antibodies are usually IgG; although IgM and IgA antibodies have been described, their pathogenetic role is unclear. In approximately two thirds of the instances, the IgG antibodies will fix complement; when complement is not fixed, the antibody usually has specificity for the Rh locus of one of its antigens.

The hemolytic anemia which results may vary greatly in intensity. Usually the amount of hemolysis is related to the amount of antibody detectable on the red cell surface, but this is not clearly the case in some instances. In approximately one instance in fifty, immunoglobulin may not be detected on the red cell surface (*Coombsnegative immune hemolytic anemia*). In general, an antibody fixing complement probably causes a greater degree of hemolysis than one which does not.

Approximately one third of the time, there may be no other manifestation of disease, except perhaps for immune thrombocytopenia. In the remaining half to two thirds of the instances, an underlying disease may be defined at the time of the initial diagnosis or during the clinical course. The most common diseases associated with immune hemolytic anemia of the warm antibody type are *chronic lymphocytic leukemia* and *lymphoma* or *systemic lupus erythematosus*. It may be seen with other immune system diseases such as the *Wiskott-Aldrich syndrome, agammaglobulinemia,* and *malignant thymoma,* as well as a variety of other syndromes such as *rheumatoid arthritis, systemic sclerosis,* or *ulcerative colitis.*

Clinical Manifestations. The degree of hemolysis varies from patient to patient. In its classic presentation, immune hemolytic anemia is rapid in onset; well-documented instances of the development of severe anemia within a few days have been seen. The anemia can be so severe as to be fatal if not competently treated. The spleen is frequently enlarged and may vary in size according to the degree of hemolysis. The liver is less commonly enlarged. Jaundice and pallor may be present. The peripheral blood frequently shows spherocytosis and marked reticulocytosis; however, considerable hemolysis can take place in the absence of spherocytes. The white blood count may be elevated slightly. Hemoglobinemia may be chemically detectable, but hemoglobinuria is rare. There are few other manifestations associated with the anemia itself, although, if it is secondary to some underlying disease, symptoms of that disease may be manifest.

Diagnosis. The diagnosis usually depends upon the demonstration of immunoglobulins or components of complement on the red cells of the patient. This is usually done with specific antisera containing only antibodies against IgG or the inactive fragment of the third component of complement (C3). Tests with these reagents may reveal the presence of either or both on the surface. When complement alone is found, further efforts must be made to demonstrate the antibody. Cooling the cells to 4° C may reveal an IgG antibody on the surface *(cold-detectable antibody)* capable of reacting with the cell at 37° C but detectable only at reduced temperature. An antibody of low affinity may be detected in the serum, using papainized normal cells to increase the interaction of the antigen and antibody. The antibody may rarely be IgM or IgA, and specific anti-IgM or anti-IgA antisera may be needed to reveal its presence. The antibody may be cold reactive or drug related, and appropriate steps will be needed to reveal its presence, as described later in this chapter (Diagnosis) and in Ch. 744.

Treatment. The initial treatment of autoimmune hemolytic anemia caused by IgG warm-reacting antibodies is prednisone. In general, 1 mg per kilogram per day in divided doses is sufficient for initial therapy. If response to this dose of the drug is seen in elevation of the hematocrit, the amount of prednisone being administered can be rapidly tapered to approximately 0.3 mg per kilogram per day. Thereafter the dose may be tapered more slowly, at about the rate of 5 mg per day each month. In many instances of immune hemolytic anemia in childhood, remission occurs and prednisone may be omitted entirely; however, in adults, this is unusual, and great caution must be used in discontinuing prednisone completely. Many patients will maintain total remission on 2.5 to 10 mg per day; alternate-day dosage appears to be as good as daily dosage and may be attended by less severe side effects.

The mode of action of prednisone is not clear but appears to be multiple. Evidence has been adduced that it causes the removal of antibody from the red cell membrane when given in high doses. This effect appears to account for many of the instances of rapid remission obtained with the drug. In addition, it appears to suppress the production of antibody in two to three weeks in those patients achieving remission which can be maintained on small doses. Finally, it is thought that prednisone can interfere with sequestration of cells by the reticuloendothelial system. The basic mechanism of any of these actions is not known.

If prednisone is unsuccessful in initial therapy or if the dose of prednisone required to maintain remission is too high, other measures must be sought. In general, these consist of *immunosuppression* by other drugs (azathioprine, 100 to 150 mg per day; cyclophosphamide, 50 to 100 mg per day) or splenectomy. *Splenectomy* is generally preferred in younger patients, whereas in older patients immunosuppression may be wiser. If one of these treatments fails to bring about an adequate remission, the other method may be required. Seldom is a patient resistant to a combination of prednisone, immunosuppression, and splenectomy.

Transfusion may be necessary during the acute hemolytic phase of the disease. This is often attended by difficulty because of problems in obtaining an adequate cross-match; however, if it is clinically indicated, a transfusion that is not appropriately cross-matched is preferable to having the patient succumb to the anemia. The best chance of a proper cross-match is obtained if the antibody is isolated, either from eluates or from the serum, to determine whether specificity exists and, if it does, in selecting units of blood which are compatible. If the specificity cannot be identified, the blood bank is often obliged to test the patient's serum against all units of blood available of the appropriate type to determine which are optimal. When this procedure is carefully performed, few transfusion reactions will occur; however, one must be cautious about the simultaneous presence of isoantibody in addition to the autoimmune antibody.

HEMOLYSIS DUE TO COLD-REACTING ANTIBODIES

The term *"cold-reacting antibodies"* is probably a misnomer, because it has recently been shown that when the antigens against which these antibodies interact are isolated in vitro, interaction between antigen and antibody can occur at any temperature, including 37° C. Antigens against which these antibodies interact are located on a species of glycoprotein on the red cell surface; the placement of the antigen is probably temperature dependent such that in the warm, it is not available for interaction.

The fact that these antibodies are unable to interact with the red cell at 37° C means that the mode of destruction cannot be mediated by antibody (see above); since these antibodies are able to fix complement, complement is responsible for the hemolysis.

Cold Agglutinin Syndrome

The cold agglutinin syndrome is due to antibodies, usually IgM, which are able to act at reduced temperature and cause agglutination of the red cells. The presence of the antibody is readily demonstrable in the serum of the patient; the serum may on occasion be diluted several thousand fold and still be able to agglutinate red cells.

The antigens with which these antibodies interact are of three general sorts, called "I", "i," and "Pr." The *"I" antigens* are those which are most strongly expressed on adult cells; the *"i" antigens* are most strongly expressed on cells of newborn infants and of rare adults; the *"Pr" antigens* are equally well expressed on both cells and are destroyed by neuraminidase. The antigens are polysaccharide in nature, and some of them appear to be related to the polysaccharides of the ABH and Lewis groups.

The maximal temperature at which the antibody interacts with the red cell is variable. Since the interaction in vivo of antigen and antibody depends upon lowering the temperature of the blood below 37° C in the peripheral areas (arms, legs, and appendages), those antibodies which are able to interact at higher temperatures will, in general, have a greater opportunity to cause hemolysis than those which react only at lower temperatures.

Clinical Manifestations. The clinical manifestations of the cold agglutinin syndrome are due to two phenomena: (1) intravascular agglutination, which occurs when blood is cooled in peripheral parts of the body, and (2) hemolytic anemia, which occurs consequent upon the fixation of complement. Upon exposure to cold, patients with cold agglutinin syndrome may note that the hands, ears, nose, or feet may turn purple and become painful; this process is rapidly reversed upon rewarming and is distinguished from Raynaud's phenomenon in that there is no blanching phase and little evidence of hyperemia. If the symptoms of agglutination are sufficiently severe, pain may result upon breathing cold air or eating cold food, or from so small a stimulus as holding a glass of ice water.

The hemolytic anemia which accompanies cold agglutinin syndrome is rarely severe. Usually the patient has moderate hemolytic anemia which is exacerbated during the winter. The spleen may or may not be enlarged. Spherocytosis is usually absent. If the patient is exposed to severe chilling, he may have a sudden bout of hemolysis with consequent hemoglobinemia and hemoglobinuria. In some whose antibody has a high thermal amplitude, the anemia may be severe even when the patient is carefully protected from the cold; these people may require transfusion.

Cold agglutinin syndrome is seen in two major clinical settings: (1) *chronic cold agglutinin disease* of the elderly and (2) *postinfectious cold agglutinin syndrome.* Chronic cold agglutinin disease of the elderly is characterized by a gradual onset of symptoms and a chronic course. The antibody seen is usually monoclonal and is nearly always of the κ light chain type. Some patients with this syndrome have been found to have lymphoma; this is particularly true when the antibody is anti-i.

Postinfectious cold agglutinin syndrome usually follows infection with *Mycoplasma pneumoniae* (in which case the antibody is anti-I) or *infectious mononucleosis* (in which case the antibody is anti-i). Antibodies in these instances are not monoclonal, as in the chronic idiopathic type, but may be restricted in their molecular variation. The antibodies in infectious mononucleosis are highly variable; some may even be IgG. Although most patients with either Mycoplasma infection or mononucleosis may have a rise in the titer of the cold agglutinins in their serum, reaching a peak two to three weeks after onset of the illness, clinically manifest hemolytic anemia is uncommon, usually only when the amount of antibody is very great. The course of the illness is self-limited, and all manifestations usually disappear within two to three months.

Diagnosis. The presence of cold agglutinins is often suspected by casual observation of an anticoagulated sample of blood at room temperature. The sample may appear to be coagulated or show marked clumping, which disappears when warmed to 37° C. This is more rigorously tested by diluting the serum and testing it against normal adult and newborn cells; in some instances dilutions as high as 1 in 100,000 may cause agglutination.

The patient's cells invariably have on them relatively large amounts of the inactive fragment of the third component of complement which is detectable with antiglobulin reagents containing anti-C3. The reaction with anti-IgG is negative. The hemolytic ability of the antibody may also be tested by appropriate in vitro reactions.

Treatment. The treatment of chronic cold agglutinin disease is usually simplified if the patient is able to avoid cold exposure during the winter months. This may require near-incarceration in heated rooms and wearing heavy, warm clothes. Sometimes it may require traveling to warmer climates. If this is insufficient or not possible, treatment with chlorambucil (2 mg per day) has been suggested. In general, little benefit results from treatment with prednisone or splenectomy.

Paroxysmal Cold Hemoglobinuria

Paroxysmal cold hemoglobinuria was the first hemolytic disease to be specifically defined. It formerly was encountered in patients with syphilis; it now more commonly occurs as an autoimmune or postviral disease. The antibody is IgG in type and reacts with the P blood group antigen which is possessed by nearly all red cells. For reasons not clearly understood, the antibody is able to effect marked lysis by complement. This is detectable clinically by episodes of hemoglobinemia and hemoglobinuria after exposure to cold and is detected in vitro by

the *Donath-Landsteiner test,* by which the syndrome is frequently diagnosed. In some instances, the syndrome may be so severe as to threaten life; this usually occurs after viral infection in children. Paroxysmal cold hemoglobinuria is treated by protection from exposure to cold, by prednisone, and by cyclophosphamide, just as any other IgG antibody syndrome.

743. FRAGMENTATION HEMOLYTIC ANEMIA

The membrane of the normal red cell is readily deformable but with limits to its elasticity. When sufficient shear stress is placed upon the cell, it undergoes progressive deformation and, eventually, membrane rupture. The amount of shear stress required has been estimated at about 3000 dynes per square centimeter. Such stresses do not occur in the normal circulation, because the vessels of the circulatory system are designed to allow the smooth passage of the blood, and the turbulence of the blood passing through the normal heart does not generate forces of this magnitude. However, such shear stress forces may be generated when abnormalities occur in the circulatory system, and fragmentation of the red cells may result. The characteristic red cell fragments resulting from this phenomenon are called *schistocytes;* these usually have sharp points and have been called *"helmet" cells, "triangle" cells,* and other similar names.

Fragmentation within the circulation occurs in two general clinical situations: (1) when intravascular fibrinous coagulation or abnormalities of the vessel walls in small arterioles cause irregularities upon which red cells may be fragmented, much as cells may be fragmented by being pushed through a fine wire screen, and (2) when alterations in the heart and major vessels occur such that turbulence and other factors yield shear stress forces sufficient to fragment the red cells.

HEMOLYSIS DUE TO ABNORMALITIES OF THE MICROCIRCULATION
(Microangiopathic Hemolytic Anemia)

The first clear-cut description of fragmentation hemolytic anemia in patients in whom abnormalities of the arterioles could be demonstrated was in 1963 by Brain, Dacie, and Hourihane. They named the syndrome "microangiopathic hemolytic anemia." The mechanism of this hemolysis was elucidated by members of the same group, using an artificial circulatory system. They demonstrated that if blood were pumped through a bed of fibers of sufficiently small diameter so that the red cells could be looped over the fibers like clothes hung on a clothesline (without clothespins) and if sufficient force were applied as pressure, the cells would be severed by the strand much as a wire cheese knife cuts cheese. Since the opposite sides of the membrane were brought into apposition, they were sometimes able to reseal and the fragment was able to float away.

Fragmentation in vivo results when threads of sufficiently small size (usually fibrin) occur in the arteriolar side of the circulation where the blood pressure provides sufficient force to fragment the cells. The accompanying table lists some of the clinical states in which this occurs.

In many instances, there is a greater or lesser degree of intravascular coagulation. When the primary defect appears to be arteriolar damage, the amount of intravascular coagulation demonstrable by a diminution in procoagulants may be small or even absent. On the other hand, when intravascular coagulation is the major event and occurs on both the arteriolar and venous sides, marked diminution in procoagulants may be present with only minor amounts of fragmentation hemolysis.

Clinical Manifestations.   The degree of hemolysis may vary, depending upon the underlying process. Fragmentation hemolysis occurs in malignant hypertension, usually only when renal failure and papilledema are present; pathologically the kidneys usually show fibrinoid necrosis. The fragmentation hemolysis in carcinoma is usually seen only in adenocarcinoma and then only when widely metastatic; the degree of hemolysis may be considerable. The hemolysis in vasculitic lesions (e.g., Rocky Mountain spotted fever, periarteritis nodosa, Wegener's granulomatosis) is generally relatively minor, and the major manifestations are those of the underlying disease.

Diagnosis.   The diagnosis of fragmentation hemolysis is made by the demonstration of schistocytic forms in the peripheral blood. Evidences of intravascular hemolysis (increased plasma hemoglobin and lactic acid dehydrogenase, urine hemosiderin, and, perhaps, urine hemoglobin) are usually present. Ancillary evidence may include evidence of disseminated intravascular coagulation (see Ch. 801).

Treatment.   Treatment of fragmentation hemolysis depends in large part on the management of the underlying lesion. Reduction in blood pressure in malignant hypertension will reduce the rate of fragmentation hemolysis. Resolution of the septic shock or the Rocky Mountain spotted fever will also end the hemolytic episode. Irradiation or removal of vascular abnormalities (giant hemangioma, traumatic arteriovenous fistula) will usually end the hemolytic process. In those instances in which intravascular coagulation plays a major role, treatment with heparin may be of value. Heparin does not appear to be of value in widely metastatic carcinoma.

HEMOLYSIS DUE TO ABNORMALITY OF THE HEART AND GREAT VESSELS
(Traumatic Cardiac Hemolytic Anemia)

Abnormalities of the heart and great vessels may lead to such degrees of turbulence that fragmentation may occur. The resultant hemolytic anemia is in general mild. Instances of fragmentation hemolysis have been described in aortic stenosis, ruptured sinus of Valsalva, congenital stenosis of the aorta, traumatic arteriovenous fistula, marked aortic regurgitation, and marked tachycardia. In general, only lesions of the left side of the heart and general circulation lead to traumatic fragmentation hemolysis, because only on that side are the shear stress forces of sufficient strength.

When prosthetic devices are inserted into the heart or great vessels, fragmentation hemolysis is frequent. In one large series, 60 to 80 per cent of all patients with prosthetic aortic or mitral valves demonstrated clinically significant hemolysis. Patients with both aortic and mitral prostheses are more likely to have hemolysis than are those with only one.

Causes of "Microangiopathic" Fragmentation Hemolysis

Vascular abnormality predominant:
1. Thrombotic thrombocytopenic purpura (hemolytic-uremic syndrome)
2. Renal lesions
   a. Malignant hypertension
   b. Glomerulonephritis
   c. Transplant rejection
   d. Preeclampsia
3. Vasculitis
   a. Polyarteritis nodosa
   b. Rocky Mountain spotted fever
   c. Wegener's granulomatosis
4. Vascular anomalies
   a. Giant cavernous hemangioma (Kasabach-Merritt syndrome)
   b. Arteriovenous fistula
Intravascular coagulation predominant:
1. Septicemia with shock
2. Abruptio placentae

A frequent cause of severe hemolysis is regurgitation around the outside of the valve owing to poor seating; this is particularly common in prosthetic aortic valves. The material of which the valve is composed is of some importance; cloth-covered valves tend to give more hemolysis than others, and those with steel balls show less hemolysis than those with Silastic balls. When variance of the Silastic ball occurs, increased hemolysis may result. In general, increased hemolysis occurs in situations of increased turbulence, as when large quantities of blood are forced through small apertures by high pressure.

Fragmentation hemolysis may also occur after surgery for correction of the ostium primum defect with a patch. In certain instances, the defect in the mitral valve is insufficiently closed, and blood regurgitates forcefully against the patch. When this occurs, epithelialization of the patch may be prevented, and since the surface is relatively rougher than the endothelium, the forceful jet of blood may create forces sufficient to fragment the cells.

Clinical Manifestations.   The degree of hemolysis is variable from patient to patient, depending upon the underlying abnormality. In a given patient the amount of hemolysis tends to vary with the cardiac output. Hence patients tend to have more hemolysis during the daytime when active than at night. If the patient becomes markedly anemic, in compensation the cardiac output is raised and the degree of hemolysis may increase. This may be manifest to the patient as increasing hemoglobinuria.

As in all chronic intravascular hemolysis, considerable iron is lost into the urine as hemosiderin and hemoglobin. Hence the patients may become iron deficient, thus suppressing erythropoiesis. This will lead to more severe anemia which will lead to an increase in cardiac output and thus more severe hemolysis.

Treatment.   All patients with evidences of fragmentation hemolysis ought to be given iron supplementation (ferrous sulfate, 300 mg three times a day). When the degree of hemolysis is severe, parenteral iron therapy with iron-dextran may be needed. Transfusion may be required. However, if chronic transfusion is necessary, some consideration should be given to replacement of the valve if, as is usually the case, some defect in the valve placement is present. When hemolysis is due to a patch on an ostium primum defect, it may be necessary to replace the patch and further to replace the mitral valve so that regurgitation against the patch does not occur.

In those instances of traumatic fragmentation hemolysis in which no prosthesis has been inserted, the hemolysis is usually not severe enough to require treatment.

MARCH HEMOGLOBINURIA

March hemoglobinuria was first described in 1881 in an infantryman in the Prussian army who, after long marches, noted passage of dark urine. Since that time, many instances of hemoglobinuria occurring after running or after repeated trauma to some part of the body have been described. *Marathon runners* commonly demonstrate this syndrome, especially those with a stomping gait or those who run barefoot or in poorly cushioned shoes. *Karate experts* who practice their art by repeatedly striking their hand against hard surfaces, *pelota players, bongo drummers,* and *patients who strike their heads* repeatedly against the wall have all been found to have hemolysis as a result of their particular activity.

The red cells do not appear to be abnormal. The hemolysis apparently occurs because the red cells are forceably smashed within the microcirculation when the body part is struck against a hard surface or object. The cells may be popped like a balloon, and schistocytes are rarely if ever seen. The syndrome can be stopped by altering the activity so that forceable striking of a body part does not occur; e.g., marathon runners may be advised to use cushioned shoes or to alter their gait.

Clinical Manifestations. The patient commonly notes dark urine immediately after the activity; it generally clears by the second or third voiding. Anemia seldom occurs, and no other serious side effects, save for the fright of seeing dark urine, have been noted.

744. HEMOLYSIS DUE TO ALTERATIONS OF THE RED CELLS BY EXOGENOUS MATERIALS

During the normal circulation of red cells, the red cell membrane is not appreciably altered in such a way as to effect hemolysis until 120 days are reached. However, certain alterations in the environment have been defined which can alter the red cell membrane and shorten the life span of the red cells.

DRUGS

Drugs and other chemicals may diminish the life span of the red cell in several ways: (1) they may interact directly with the membrane of the normal cell, resulting in abnormalities which lead to hemolysis; (2) they may stimulate the formation of antibodies which then lead to the destruction of the red cell; or (3) they may effect certain reactions which are not usually toxic for the normal red cell but are injurious to red cells deficient in detoxifying mechanisms, usually related to deficiencies of the hexose monophosphate shunt. Since these deficiencies are usually on a congenital basis (e.g., glucose-6-phosphate dehydrogenase deficiency), this form of hemolysis is considered elsewhere (see Ch. 740).

Drugs which cause hemolysis directly are few in number, because this effect is readily detected and the drugs are not used. *Amphotericin* may do so by its ability to interact with lipids of the membrane. Certain lipid solvents may interact with the membrane and bring about its dissolution. This form of hemolysis is probably rare.

Immune hemolysis initiated by drugs is more common. There are basically two types: (1) "autoimmune" hemolytic anemia, in which the drug induces an antibody which reacts with antigens normally present in the red cell, and (2) "immune" hemolytic anemia, in which the antibody formed is directed against the drug and the red cell is lysed as a consequence of the interaction between antibody and drug. In this latter group, the drug may be firmly fixed to the red cell membrane *(haptene-like reaction)* or only loosely attached to the membrane *("innocent bystander" reaction).*

"Autoimmune" drug-induced hemolysis is almost exclusively due to a single drug, α-*methyldopa (Aldomet),* although L-dopa and mefanemic acid have been implicated as well. After taking the drug for at least two to three months, about 5 to 10 per cent of all patients will have a positive indirect antiglobulin (Coombs) test caused by the presence of IgG antibody directed against components of the Rh complex locus; complement is almost never fixed. Antibody may be detected in the serum without addition of the drug to the test. In most patients, little if any hemolysis will result, but in a small proportion of patients taking the drug, significant hemolysis occurs. The syndrome produced is that of warm-reacting IgG antibody with spherocytosis, splenomegaly, and response to prednisone therapy, if its use becomes necessary. When the drug is stopped, the antibody usually disappears within two to three months, and the direct antiglobulin test reverts to negative. The reason a drug should stimulate production of an antibody capable of reacting with autologous red cell antigens is not clear.

Many drugs serving as haptenes apparently stimulate the production of antibodies. These antibodies may be capable of destroying red cells as a result of their reaction with the drug. In some cases, the drug may be firmly attached to the red cell, as in the case of penicillin; in those instances, the IgG antibody will also be detectable on the red cell surface in the direct antiglobulin test. Since relatively small amounts of antibody are attached, complement is usually not fixed. In other instances, the drug is not firmly attached to the red cell. However, the interaction of drug and antibody results in the activation of complement at the red cell surface. If sufficient complement is fixed, hemolysis results, as outlined above. Since the initial steps of the immune reaction are not firmly associated with the red cell, antibody will not be detected on the direct antiglobulin test. In these reactions, the red cell has been called an "innocent bystander"; some doubt has been raised as to its complete innocence in this reaction.

Numerous drugs have been implicated in an "innocent bystander" reaction: *Fuadin* (an antischistosomal agent), *sulfonamides, quinidine, chlorpropamide,* and *thorazine,* to name a few. When the "innocent bystander" reaction is responsible for hemolysis, only complement will be present on the patients' cells (antibody having been washed away during the preparation of the cells for the test), and the indirect antiglobulin test will be positive only when the responsible drug is present in the reaction mixture.

MEMBRANE ALTERATION BY TOXIC SUBSTANCES

Toxins and Poisons

Toxic substances ("poisons") may bring about hemolysis by alteration of the membrane. These substances may be of animal origin, as in the case of hemolysis after snake bites or spider bites (see Ch. 57 and 59). In the former, phospholipases are thought to release the lipids of the membrane and destroy its integrity. Hemolysis, if present at all, is only a minor part of the complex clinical syndrome.

Some vegetable poisons such as *castor beans* and certain *mushrooms* may cause hemolysis. The mechanism of this has not been delineated. Certain minerals may also cause hemolysis, the best known of which is *copper*. This is thought to be the cause of the hemolysis which occasionally occurs in Wilson's disease. Its role has been very clearly demonstrated in patients undergoing dialysis in which the medium became so alkaline that copper salts were dissolved from the machine. The precise mechanism of its action is not clear; it may have to do with the fact that the copper ion is able to bind to the membrane sulfhydryl groups. Patients with *arsenical* intoxication sometimes have hemolytic anemia. Again, interference with the membrane structure is probably the cause, although the details have not been ascertained.

Failure of an Excretory Organ

The milieu in which the red cells circulate may be altered by failure of one of the excretory organs. When this occurs, some of the accumulated abnormal metabolites may alter the red cell membrane and result in hemolysis. With *liver failure,* commonly secondary to cirrhosis or alcoholic hepatitis, the red cells may become markedly overloaded with cholesterol. This at first leads to a spreading of the membrane, resulting in target cells which have a normal life span. However, if the process is further exaggerated and if the ratio of cholesterol to phospholipids is further altered, the membrane may become markedly abnormal, and a *spur cell,* a contracted, irregular cell fancifully resembling a spur for horses, may result. When this occurs, marked intravascular hemolysis may result.

Some patients with renal failure also exhibit hemolysis. The precise nature of the accumulated metabolite which is responsible for this phenomenon has not been demonstrated. In some instances, the defect may be demonstrated by an abnormal autohemolysis (sterile incubation) test.

Infectious Agents

Hemolysis is a frequent accompaniment of infections. This may be due to the fact that the infectious agent invades the red cell and directly effects its lysis. This most commonly occurs in malaria, particularly by *Plasmodium falciparum.* The sudden release of merozoites may result in sufficient hemolysis to cause hemoglobinuria *(blackwater fever).* The bacterial organism *Bartonella* may also invade the red cells and cause hemolysis.

Red cells may be altered indirectly by infections. In some instances, reactions may occur as the result of the infection which may result in immunologic damage to the cell. This is particularly true in cold agglutinin syndrome secondary to Mycoplasma or Epstein-Barr virus infections, but may also be found in bacterial and other viral infections as well. In these instances, the direct antiglobulin test will be positive.

Several infections with clostridial organisms causing gas gangrene may result in marked hemolysis; instances of hemolysis of all circulating red cells have been recorded. This is thought to be due to alteration of the membrane phospholipids by enzymes elaborated by the organisms, but this has not been proved. The red cells show marked spherocytosis, and readily apparent evidences of intravascular hemolysis are present. The occurrence of this complication usually indicates a very poor prognosis, although instances of recovery have been reported when the infection is adequately treated.

In other instances of infection of various sorts (e.g., *Salmonella, Neisseria, E. coli, D. pneumoniae*), hemolysis of a less dramatic degree may occur in the absence of evidence of immunologic reaction on the red cell membrane. This has been thought, as in the case of the clostridial infection, to be due to alteration of the membrane by the organism or some product elaborated by it; this theory remains to be proved.

745. HEMOLYSIS DUE TO OVERACTIVITY OF THE RETICULOENDOTHELIAL SYSTEM

Red cells are presumably destroyed normally in the reticuloendothelial system, although the causes and the details of this destruction are not known. In certain instances, overactivity of the reticuloendothelial system, resulting from either anatomic alteration or malignancy of its cells, has been thought to cause premature destruction of normal cells.

HYPERSPLENISM

See Ch. 788.

EOSINOPHILIC GRANULOMA SYNDROMES

See Part XVI, Section Ten.

Immune Hemolytic Anemia

Mollison, P. J.: Transfusion in Clinical Practice. 5th ed. Oxford, Blackwell Scientific Publications, 1973.

Pirofsky, S. M.: Autoimmunization and the Autoimmune Hemolytic Anemias. Baltimore, Williams & Wilkins Company, 1960.

Rosse, W. F., and Dacie, J. V.: Immune lysis of normal human and paroxysmal nocturnal hemoglobinuria (PNH) red blood cells. II. The role of complement components in the increased sensitivity of PNH red cells to immune lysis. J. Clin. Invest., 45:749, 1966.

Worlledge, S. M.: Immune drug-induced haemolytic anaemias. Semin. Hematol., 6:181, 1969.

Fragmentation Hemolysis

Brain, M. J.: Microangiopathic hemolytic anemia. Ann. Rev. Med., 21:133, 1970.

Bull, B. S., Rubenberg, M. L., Dacie, J. V., and Brain, M. C.: Microangiopathic haemolytic anaemia: Mechanisms of red-cell fragmentation. Br. J. Haematol., 14:643, 1968.

Davidson, R. J. L.: March or exertional hemoglobinuria. Semin. Hematol., 6:150, 1969.

Marsh, G. W., and Lewis, S. M.: Cardiac hemolytic anemia. Semin. Hematol., 6:133, 1969.

HEMOGLOBIN, THE HEMOGLOBINOPATHIES, AND THE THALASSEMIAS

C. Lockard Conley

746. INTRODUCTION

The primary role of the red cells is transport of oxygen, a function made possible by the hemoglobin within the erythrocytes. The amount of oxygen delivered by fully oxygenated blood is dependent not only on the hemoglobin content and rate of flow, but also on the affinity of the hemoglobin for oxygen at existing oxygen tensions. The effectiveness of hemoglobin in oxygen transport is the result of its variable oxygen affinity, a unique property dependent upon the tetrameric structure of the hemoglobin molecule.

The major hemoglobin component of the normal adult (Hb A) contains four polypeptide chains, two alpha chains each with 141 amino acid residues, and two beta chains each with 146 residues; it is designated $\alpha_2\beta_2$. A heme group containing an iron atom is affixed to each chain. A minor component comprising 2 to 3 per cent of the hemoglobin is designated Hb A_2, consisting of alpha and delta chains ($\alpha_2\delta_2$). The predominant hemoglobin of the fetus and newborn (Hb F) contains pairs of alpha and gamma chains ($\alpha_2\gamma_2$). There are multiple differences in amino acid sequences of beta, delta, and gamma chains, but the physiologic properties of the hemoglobins are similar. The fashion in which the globin chains and their heme groups are bonded together provides the iron atoms with precisely the environment necessary for reversible combination with oxygen. As oxygen is bound successively to each of the four iron atoms, stereochemical changes occur in the hemoglobin molecule that cause an increased affinity of the remaining iron atoms for oxygen. The sigmoid oxygen dissociation curve is the graphic representation of these relationships. Because of these allosteric effects, hemoglobin is fully oxygenated in the lungs even if the alveolar oxygen tension is appreciably less than normal; as oxygen is unloaded in the tissues, progressive reduction in the oxygen affinity of the hemoglobin provides for maximal delivery of oxygen with little change in oxygen tension.

OXYGEN AFFINITY OF THE RED CELLS

Pure hemoglobin has too high an affinity for oxygen to release appreciable amounts at normal tissue oxygen tensions. Within the red cell the oxygen affinity of the hemoglobin is modified by several mechanisms. Hydrogen ions stabilize the deoxy-state of hemoglobin, lessening oxygen affinity (Bohr effect). Carbon dioxide binds to hemoglobin and decreases its affinity for oxygen. Both these reactions facilitate release of oxygen in the tissue capillaries. Hemoglobin concentration in the erythrocyte influences oxygen affinity, with high values of the mean corpuscular hemoglobin concentration associated with lowered oxygen affinity. Certain phosphate compounds within the red cells significantly reduce the oxygen affinity of hemoglobin. Of these, 2,3-diphosphoglycerate (DPG) occurs in highest concentration (almost 1 mol per mol of hemoglobin), and is most important in regulation of oxygen dissociation. The deoxy-conformation of hemoglobin facilitates DPG binding to the beta chains, stabilizing this conformation and lessening oxygen affinity. Fetal hemoglobin binds less DPG than Hb A; therefore the oxygen affinity of red cells containing Hb F is higher than that of normal adult red cells, even though the oxygen dissociation curves of purified Hb A and Hb F are similar. The position of the oxygen dissociation curve is expressed as the P_{50}, the oxygen tension required to half-saturate the hemoglobin with oxygen. Because of its high concentration of Hb F, the blood of the fetus has a higher oxygen affinity than that of adult blood; the P_{50} is reduced and the oxygen dissociation curve is shifted to the left.

Each red cell produces its own DPG, an intermediate in glycolytic metabolism. The concentration of DPG within the red cell is markedly influenced by the environment of the erythrocyte. Anemia or anoxia causes the concentration of DPG within normal erythrocytes to rise. When normal red cells are transfused to anemic patients, the DPG level of the transfused red cells increases, demonstrating that the effect is initiated by extracellular mechanisms. In addition, alterations of DPG concentration may result from intrinsic disorders of the metabolism of the red cell; for example, in erythrocyte pyruvate kinase deficiency, DPG is usually elevated. The presence of DPG is largely responsible for reducing the oxygen affinity of the hemoglobin within normal red cells to a value appropriate for release of oxygen at tissue oxygen tensions. When the concentration of DPG rises, oxygen affinity is lessened, so that more oxygen is released in the tissues without a change in the tissue oxygen tension. This phenomenon is significant in adaptation to anoxia and anemia. In persons acclimatized to low oxygen tensions, as at high altitude, values for DPG are high, assuring that relatively large amounts of oxygen are released at tissue tensions even though the arterial blood is not fully saturated. The remarkable ability of patients with chronic severe anemia to tolerate extremely low concentrations of hemoglobin in the blood is largely attributable to the high values of DPG in the erythrocytes, permitting release of greatly increased amounts of oxygen per red cell at normal tissue oxygen tensions. These adaptive changes are promptly and effectively regulated, the oxygen affinity of red cells changing within hours after the onset of anemia or anoxia.

DEFINITIONS AND GENETIC CONSIDERATIONS

A *hemoglobinopathy* is an abnormality of hemoglobin synthesis manifested by the production of globin in which there is a structural abnormality. More than 180 genetically determined abnormalities of hemoglobin have been discovered. A separate gene determines the amino acid sequences of each of the globin chains. A single amino acid substitution in one type of polypeptide chain is accounted for by replacement of one nucleotide in an RNA codon. Thus the abnormality of sickle hemoglobin can be attributed to a change in a single purine base in the codon which specifies the sixth amino acid of the beta chain, with the result that glutamic acid is replaced by valine. Such a point mutation accounts for most of the inherited abnormalities of hemoglobin. Rarely two amino acid substitutions occur within a single polypeptide chain, as in Hb C Harlem. In certain abnormal hemoglobins, including Hb Gun Hill and Hb Freiburg, amino acid residues are missing from a globin chain, an abnormality that can be accounted for by loss of a segment of DNA ("deletion" of part of a gene) during nonhomologous crossing-over of genes. The hemoglobins Lepore contain the amino-terminal portion of the delta chain and the carboxy-terminal portion of the beta chain, an abnormal structure that can be explained by loss of DNA from portions of closely linked genes, with formation of a "fusion" gene. Hb Kenya contains the amino-terminal sequence of the gamma chain and the carboxy-terminal segment of the beta chain. Hb Constant Spring contains elongated alpha chains, an abnormality that may be explained by a mutation affecting a terminator codon. *Thalassemia* is an inherited impairment of hemoglobin synthesis caused by retarded production of a specific type of globin chain, not associated with a primary structural abnormality. The mechanism

is not clearly understood, but is related to insufficiency of messenger RNA. *Hereditary persistence of fetal hemoglobin* is an anomaly occurring in several forms. In the type occurring in blacks, beta and delta chains are not produced at all, perhaps because of deletion of closely linked genes. Complete compensation for the deficit is achieved by synthesis of gamma chains, and the homozygous carrier has exclusively Hb F but no anemia or other clinical manifestations.

The hemoglobinopathies are inherited as autosomal codominant traits; heterozygous carriers have both the normal and the abnormal hemoglobin in each red cell. The normal component almost always constitutes the larger fraction. The genes that determine the structure of one class of globin chains are alleles; thus a person heterozygous for Hb S and Hb C, both of which contain abnormalities of the beta chain, has no Hb A and transmits one or the other but never both of the abnormal hemoglobins to each child. Thalassemia is inherited as if closely linked to the structural gene for the same chain. The beta and delta chain genes are closely linked, but the alpha chain gene segregates independently; accordingly a person heterozygous for both Hb G Philadelphia (an

Clinical Disorders Associated with Some Abnormal Hemoglobins

Disorder	Abnormal Hb	Structural Change		Electrophoretic Mobility, Starch Alkaline pH*	Comments
Hemolytic anemia	S	beta 6	glu → val	−	Forms molecular aggregates when deoxygenated, producing sickle cell anemia in homozygotes
	C	beta 6	glu → lys	−	Low solubility lessens plasticity of red cells, causing hemolytic anemia in homozygotes
	D Punjab	beta 121	glu → gln	−	Mechanism unknown
	E	beta 26	glu → lys	−	
	Zürich	beta 63	his → arg	−	Unstable hemoglobin is precipitated by certain drugs, producing hemolytic anemia in heterozygotes
	Torino	alpha 43	phe → val	0	
	L Ferrarra	alpha 47	asp → gly	−	
	Hasharon	alpha 47	asp → his	−	
	Ann Arbor	alpha 80	leu → arg	−	
	Bibba	alpha 136	leu → pro	−	
	Leiden	beta 6 or 7	glu deleted	−	
	Savannah	beta 24	gly → val	−	
	Riverdale-Bronx	beta 24	gly → arg	−	
	Genova	beta 28	leu → pro	0	
	Abraham Lincoln	beta 32	leu → pro	0	
	Philly	beta 35	tyr → phe	0	
	Hammersmith	beta 42	phe → ser	0	
	Louisville	beta 42	phe → leu	0	Unstable hemoglobin causes chronic hemolytic anemia in heterozygotes; precipitated hemoglobin tends to form inclusion bodies within red cells, under certain conditions
	Toulouse	beta 66	lys → glu	−	
	Bristol	beta 67	val → asp	0	
	Sydney	beta 67	val → ala	−	
	Seattle	beta 70	ala → asp	0	
	Shepherd's Bush	beta 74	gly → asp	+	
	Santa Ana	beta 88	leu → pro	−	
	Borås	beta 88	leu → arg	−	
	Sabine	beta 91	leu → pro	−	
	Gun Hill	beta deletion of 5 residues between 91 and 97		−	
	Istanbul	beta 92	his → gln	−	
	Köln	beta 98	val → met	−	
	Casper	beta 106	leu → pro	0	

alpha chain variant) and Hb S (a beta chain variant) may transmit either, both, or neither of the abnormal hemoglobins to a child. The gamma chain gene appears to be duplicated, i.e., there are two gamma chain genes on one chromosome. The alpha chain gene also may be duplicated, at least in some individuals.

Hemoglobinopathies and thalassemias occur as a result of genetic mutations. Very high gene frequencies for harmful mutants are maintained in some areas of the world, presumably by strong selection pressures. Heterozygosity for Hb S appears to protect infants against the lethal effects of falciparum malaria, accounting for the maintenance of a high frequency of this deleterious abnormality in Africa. What selective advantage is conferred by Hb C in Africa, by Hb E in Southeast Asia, and by thalassemia in several parts of the world is unknown. New mutations account for a surprising number of the unstable hemoglobins; in these cases the abnormal hemoglobin is not detected in other members of the family.

Not all variations in hemoglobin are genetically determined. Increased levels of Hb F may occur in several acquired conditions, including pregnancy, aplastic anemia, leukemia, myeloproliferative disorders, and hemolytic anemias. Hemoglobin A_2 may be increased in pernicious anemia and decreased in iron deficiency and aplastic anemia. Hemoglobins with abnormal electrophoretic mobility have been encountered in lead poisoning and diabetes, presumably as a result of chemical alterations in Hb A induced by the metabolic disturbance.

CLINICAL SYNDROMES ASSOCIATED WITH HEMOGLOBINOPATHIES

Substitutions of amino acids in the globin chains do not necessarily cause untoward effects, and most of the known abnormal hemoglobins are not associated with disease. Two types of clinically important abnormalities have been identified: (1) Replacements on the surface of the molecule may cause abnormal *intermolecular* reactions, phenomena which explain the pathologic effects of Hb S and Hb C. Individual molecules function satisfactorily, and the peculiar interactions between molecules tend to occur only with the high intraerythrocytic concentrations of the abnormal hemoglobin found in homozygotes. Therefore the disease appears to be

Clinical Disorders Associated with Some Abnormal Hemoglobins (*Continued*)

Disorder	Abnormal Hb	Structural Change		Electrophoretic Mobility, Starch Alkaline pH*	Comments
	Peterborough	beta 111	val → phe	0	
	Wien	beta 130	tyr → asp	0	
	Olmstead	beta 141	leu → arg	−	
	H	alpha$_2$beta$_2$ → beta$_4$		+	Unstable hemoglobin occurring in some forms of alpha thalassemia; precipitation of hemoglobin and hemolysis are accelerated by certain drugs
Cyanosis due to methemoglobinemia	M Boston	alpha 58	his → tyr	0	Methemoglobin causes cyanosis in heterozygotes; some also have evidence of hemolytic anemia
	M Iwate	alpha 87	his → tyr	0	
	M Milwaukee	beta 67	val → glu	0	
	M Saskatoon	beta 63	his → tyr	0	
	M Hyde Park	beta 92	his → tyr	−	
	Freiburg	beta 23	val deleted	−	
Cyanosis due to increased deoxyhemoglobin	Kansas	beta 102	asn → thr	−	Decreased oxygen affinity of hemoglobin causes cyanosis in heterozygotes
Erythrocytosis (polycythemia)	Chesapeake	alpha 92	arg → leu	+	Increased oxygen affinity of hemoglobin hinders release of oxygen to tissues, causing compensatory erythrocytosis in heterozygotes
	J Cape Town	alpha 92	arg → gln	+	
	Olympia	beta 20	val → met	0	
	Malmö	beta 97	his → gln	0	
	Yakima	beta 99	asp → his	−	
	Kempsey	beta 99	asp → asn	−	
	Ypsi	beta 99	asp → tyr	−	
	Brigham	beta 100	pro → leu	0	
	San Diego	beta 109	val → met	0	
	Little Rock	beta 143	his → glu	0	
	Rainier	beta 145	tyr → cys	0	
	Bethesda	beta 145	tyr → his	0	
	Hiroshima	beta 146	his → asp	+	
Hydrops fetalis	Bart's	alpha$_2$gamma$_2$ → gamma$_4$		+	Unstable hemoglobin with high oxygen affinity occurring in high concentration in stillborn fetuses with homozygous alpha thalassemia

*Symbols indicate relative mobility as compared with Hb A, less rapid (−), more rapid (+).

recessively inherited. When a red cell contains two major hemoglobin components (for example, Hb S and Hb C), interactions may occur that importantly influence the pathologic effects. (2) Replacements in critical areas of the molecule may lead to *intramolecular* abnormalities with resultant alteration in oxygen binding or in molecular stability. These effects are manifested in heterozygotes, and in some the homozygous state presumably would be lethal.

Amino acid substitutions are likely to impair molecular function or stability when they occur in the area in which the heme group is attached, when they distort the conformation of the molecule, or when they occur at points of interaction between the polypeptide chains. The net result may be formation of methemoglobin, alteration of oxygen affinity, denaturation of the hemoglobin, or a combination of these effects.

Most of the known variant hemoglobins were discovered because of abnormal electrophoretic mobility under usual conditions of measurement. The electrophoretic method continues to be useful, but many amino acid substitutions do not alter net charge on the molecule and may be electrophoretically neutral. A number of abnormal hemoglobins have the same electrophoretic pattern. The method therefore has important limitations in the detection as well as in the recognition of mutant hemoglobins. Other types of investigation, including detailed analysis of the functional properties of the hemoglobin, may be required for identification.

747. SICKLING DISORDERS

The single amino acid substitution in the beta chain in Hb S, located on the surface of the molecule, has no significant effect on oxygen affinity or molecular stability. It causes a unique *intermolecular* reaction in which molecules of deoxygenated Hb S align in spirally arranged polymers, forming insoluble fiber-like structures which distort the erythrocyte, increase its rigidity, and thereby cause the sickling deformation. The attractive forces between molecules operate only at short distances, so that the sickling phenomenon is markedly influenced by the concentration of deoxygenated Hb S in the red cell. Conditions influencing the intracellular concentration of deoxyhemoglobin, in particular oxygen tension and pH, are critical determinants of the degree of sickling. Sickling may be enhanced by the low oxygen affinity of the red cells of patients with sickle cell anemia; the low affinity is attributable in part to elevated values of 2,3-DPG and in part to the high concentration of hemoglobin in irreversibly sickled cells. Sickling is not instantaneous when hemoglobin is deoxygenated, so that duration of exposure of red cells to low oxygen tension is also a conditioning factor. Whether intravascular sickling occurs depends on local conditions of blood flow, oxygen tension, and pH; on the concentration of Hb S in the red cell; and on the presence in the erythrocyte of another hemoglobin which may interact with Hb S to lessen or enhance sickling. Except for irreversibly sickled cells, the number of which seems to be correlated with severity of disease, erythrocytes quickly resume their normal shape when the hemoglobin is reoxygenated.

Manifestations of disease attributable to Hb S are caused by intravascular sickling of partially deoxygenated erythrocytes. The rigid sickle cells tend to be tangled, trapped, and fragmented in small vascular channels; in addition, the cell membrane may be damaged by the sickling distortion. Both factors shorten red cell survival with predominant destruction of erythrocytes within the RE system. The unyielding elongate and crescentic cells increase the viscosity of the blood, retard flow, occlude small blood vessels, and produce infarcts and other lesions as a result of local anoxia.

SICKLE CELL ANEMIA

Definition. Sickle cell anemia, the clinical expression of homozygosity for Hb S, is a serious disease characterized by unrelenting hemolytic anemia, recurrent episodes of pain and fever, and pathologic involvement of many organs. Affected persons are predominantly blacks who have obtained the mutant gene from both parents. Since sickle cell trait occurs in about 8 per cent of American blacks, about 16 per 10,000 are expected to be homozygous at the time of conception; the actual incidence of sickle cell anemia is lower because of its high mortality. First described by J. B. Herrick in 1910, the disease is of unique historic significance. Study of the sickling phenomenon led Hahn and Gillespie in 1927 to discover that the distortion of the red cells is related to the state of oxygenation of the hemoglobin. Pauling and his associates in 1949 demonstrated the existence of an abnormal hemoglobin and developed the concept of "molecular" disease. Subsequently the investigations of Ingram and others showed that the abnormality in Hb S is limited to a single amino acid substitution within a polypeptide chain of globin. These discoveries initiated an unprecedented era of scientific advancement, with rapid evolution of knowledge pertaining to molecular biology, genetics, and pathophysiology.

Clinical Manifestations. Manifestations of the disease appear after the newborn period, when Hb F is replaced by Hb S. Persistent hemolytic anemia, although usually severe, is remarkably well tolerated and is not often the cause of the presenting symptoms. Many patients lead reasonably normal lives, at least for long intervals, and may be capable of a surprising amount of physical exertion. Much of the havoc of the disease is related to the periodic occurrence of disabling "crises," acute self-limited episodes of pain and fever, usually incapacitating but often not associated with increase in the degree of anemia. Precipitating factors may not be apparent; but attacks tend to occur at night, on exposure to cold, or during infections, times at which erythrostasis may be enhanced. Pain frequently is experienced in the bones and large joints of the extremities and in the back. Agonizing pain of great severity may be localized to a single area, involve multiple sites, or have a migratory character. Episodes tend to subside within a few days, but some patients have more persistent grumbling discomfort. Dramatic episodes of severe abdominal pain and fever simulate acute appendicitis and other urgent intraabdominal disorders.

Most patients have a characteristic asthenic habitus with disproportionately long extremities and "spider" fingers, probably as a result of delayed closure of epiphyses. Sexual maturation tends to be delayed, and fertility is reduced. Pregnancies often are concluded successfully, although fetal loss and maternal morbidity and mortality are increased. Susceptibility to infection is enhanced. Pneumococcal infections, including meningitis, occur with increased frequency, probably because of decreased serum opsinizing activity related to an abnormality of the properdin pathway. A unique predisposition to salmonella osteomyelitis is a remarkable feature of the disease. Chronic ulcers of the legs, overlying the malleoli, tend to occur at puberty or later. Multisystemic involvement is caused principally by ischemia resulting from anemia, erythrostasis, and vascular occlusions. Segmentation of blood flow can be seen in conjunctival vessels, and the retinal vessels may be tortuous, sometimes with peripheral vascular occlusions. Many symptoms are referable to infarction of bones and bone marrow. In infancy the earliest manifestation may be the "hand-foot" syndrome, a painful swelling of the hands or feet, associated with appearance on roentgenograms of rectangular deformities of metacarpals, metatarsals, and phalanges. Later avascular necrosis of the femoral or humeral heads may cause permanent disability. Bone involvement is readily seen in dental films, which show radiolucency, abnormal trabeculation, and infarcts. Similar changes, with widening of marrow cavities and elevation of the periosteum, may be seen in other bones. Osteoporosis of the spine may be associated with a "fish" deformity of the vertebrae.

Repeated episodes of pneumonia tend to occur, sometimes in conjunction with painful crises. Infarction of the lung is responsible for many pneumonia-like illnesses. Pulmonary vessels are occluded by masses of sickled erythrocytes or by emboli arising in veins or in infarcted marrow. Rarely, repeated emboli lead to cor pulmonale. The heart is enlarged, and the dilated chambers and accelerated circulation give rise to impressive murmurs. These are most often systolic; they simulate the murmurs of valvular heart disease. Electrocardiographic abnormalities are not unusual. Congestive heart failure, uncommon in childhood, becomes more frequent as age advances. Vascular lesions in the nervous system may produce focal or multifocal neurologic manifestations, sometimes with convulsions. Hemolytic jaundice is persistent, and the chronic overproduction of bilirubin predisposes to formation of gallstones, cholecystitis, and obstruction of the biliary tract. The liver is usually enlarged. Erythrostasis in hepatic sinusoids may cause necrosis of liver cells, leading to episodes of marked jaundice with high levels of conjugated bilirubin and aberrations of liver function tests, suggesting both hepatocellular damage and intrahepatic biliary obstruction. Damage to the liver may cause chronic hepatic dysfunction, and the end result may be a peculiar form of cirrhosis. In addition to these disorders hepatitis may be acquired through blood transfusions. The spleen is enlarged in infancy, but infarctions lead to its shrinkage to a fibrous remnant, and splenomegaly is rare in adults. Even when enlarged the spleen does not function normally, probably a factor in the increased susceptibility to infection. Hyposthenuria is the most common evidence of renal dysfunction. Infarcts of the kidney or papillary necrosis may cause hematuria, and recurrent infarction may lead to progressive renal insufficiency. The nephrotic syndrome occurs more often than would be expected by chance and is sometimes associated with renal vein thrombosis. Priapism may lead to permanent deformity and impotence.

Anemia is normocytic, with hemoglobin concentrations ranging between 5 and 10 grams per 100 ml. The reticulocyte count persistently exceeds 10 per cent, and polychromatophilia, stippling, and target cells are usual;

siderocytes and Howell-Jolly bodies may be seen. Sickled erythrocytes may not be numerous in the blood smear, but in blood deoxygenated with sodium metabisulfite virtually all the red cells are sickled. Hemolytic jaundice is associated with a slight increase in the plasma hemoglobin. Thrombocytosis and leukocytosis tend to persist and increase during crises, when leukocyte counts of more than 20,000 per cubic millimeter are common. The bone marrow is hyperplastic with a predominance of erythroid precursors. At times necrotic marrow can be aspirated from areas of acute bone pain. Profound anemia may be the result of "aplastic crises," transient episodes of retarded erythropoiesis associated with reticulocytopenia; these occur most often in association with infections. Folate deficiency, attributable in part to the high folate requirement of chronic hemolytic anemia, may lead to a superimposed megaloblastic anemia.

Diagnosis. In typical cases the diagnosis is readily established by the demonstration of hemolytic anemia, positive sickling preparation with sodium metabisulfite, and the abnormal mobility of the hemoglobin on electrophoresis. Anemia may be overlooked in blacks, and the dramatic nonhematologic manifestations can be misleading. Recurrent joint pain and striking cardiac abnormalities often suggest rheumatic fever. Differentiation between the painful abdominal crises and other intra-abdominal disorders may be extremely difficult. Differential diagnosis of marked jaundice in patients with sickle cell anemia may require meticulous evaluation, including liver biopsy in appropriate cases. Limitations of the electrophoretic method should be recognized. Sickle cell anemia is clearly distinguished from sickle cell trait by this procedure in untreated patients, but after transfusions the patterns may be similar. The electrophoretic pattern of hemoglobin in untreated sickle cell anemia may be indistinguishable from that of other disorders, including sickle cell–thalassemia, sickle cell–hemoglobin D disease, sickle cell–hereditary persistence of fetal hemoglobin, and homozygous sickle cell anemia with heterozygosity for hemoglobin Memphis or alpha thalassemia, disorders which tend to be less severe. Accordingly, proof of diagnosis may require family studies and additional analysis of the hemoglobin. Special investigations are warranted when the clinical disorder is atypical, for example, when splenomegaly persists into adult life, when anemia is mild or absent, or when the disease is unusually benign.

Prognosis. The disease in the past has had a high mortality rate in early childhood, few patients reaching adult life. Recent decades have seen progressively increasing longevity, and increasing numbers of patients survive beyond the age of 50. This improvement in outlook is not attributable to advances in specific therapy, but is largely the result of better nutrition and more adequate prevention and treatment of infections. Infection remains the most common cause of death. Aplastic crises are a serious threat to life if not treated promptly. Death may result from renal or hepatic insufficiency, cardiac failure, or vascular occlusions in the nervous system. Widespread intravascular sickling is found in some patients dying suddenly or during a painful crisis. The clinical spectrum of the disease is broad, and mild cases of sickle cell anemia are increasingly recognized. Some older patients have chronic anemia but have not had the characteristic symptoms associated with the disease.

Treatment. Specific therapy is not available. The

painful episodes are self-limited; accordingly they appear to respond to a variety of therapeutic measures, but convincing evidence of efficacy is lacking. None of the drugs or agents reported to shorten a crisis has stood the test of a properly conducted controlled trial. A recent wave of enthusiasm for the therapeutic use of urea appears to be unjustified, and careful clinical trials have not demonstrated a beneficial effect of this drug. The lesions underlying the painful crisis are related to ischemia and infarction, and there is no proof that unsickling the red cells will relieve pain after the crisis has occurred. A more promising approach to treatment of sickle cell disease is the long-term use of an agent that modifies the hemoglobin molecule in such a way as to lessen the tendency to sickling. Sodium cyanate preferentially carbamylates the N-terminal residues of the hemoglobin polypeptides, increasing oxygen affinity and thereby lessening the tendency of the red cells to sickle. Clinical trials are in progress to determine whether therapeutic benefits of cyanate can be achieved at doses that are not excessively toxic; the preliminary results are not very encouraging, because neurotoxic and other untoward effects have occurred with doses of cyanate too low to improve anemia. Severe pain justifies the use of narcotics, with care to avoid respiratory depression. Narcotic addiction attributable to appropriate therapy is rare, because the painful episodes are too short to induce dependence. Hydration should be maintained by use of intravenous fluids as needed during the crisis. Careful attention should be given to oxygenation of the blood in patients with pulmonary lesions. Patients with sickle cell anemia should continuously receive supplemental folic acid (0.5 mg per day). Infections should be treated promptly. Transfusions may be lifesaving in aplastic crises and in the shock of abdominal crises, but their use in other situations should be carefully considered. Administration of usual volumes of blood raises the hematocrit value without markedly diluting the sickle cells, increasing the viscosity of deoxygenated blood and potentially enhancing the production of vascular occlusions. Partial exchange transfusions are effective in preventing crises when about 50 per cent of the red cells are replaced by normal erythrocytes. This procedure is particularly useful in preparing patients for surgical operations, and may be used in other critical situations. Leg ulcers tend to heal with conservative measures, particularly when anemia is corrected by transfusions and during bed rest; however, they often recur even after grafting procedures. When anesthesia is administered, good ventilation and high oxygen tensions in the inspired gas mixture should be maintained. Surgical procedures can be safely performed in patients in good general condition; nevertheless, major elective procedures such as removal of asymptomatic gallstones appear to be unjustified.

SICKLE CELL TRAIT

Persons heterozygous for hemoglobin S are said to have sickle cell trait, with rare exceptions innocuous and not associated with anemia. It occurs in Africa, the Mediterranean area, Arabia, and India. About 8 per cent of American blacks are affected. Each erythrocyte contains both Hb S and Hb A, and all the red cells sickle when deoxygenated; but the concentration of Hb S in the red cells is sufficiently low that intravascular sickling does not occur at physiologic oxygen tensions. Clinical manifestations may appear when unusual circumstances foster intravascular sickling. Hemolytic anemia simulating sickle cell anemia has been encountered in heterozygous carriers of Hb S with anoxemia owing to congenital heart disease. Infarction of the spleen has occurred during travel in unpressurized aircraft. Very rarely sudden death has been attributed to sicklemia, but documentation of the role of the sickle cells is not adequate. Hyposthenuria is relatively common. Unilateral renal hematuria may appear without demonstrable cause and may persist for weeks; it usually ceases without relation to therapeutic efforts, none of which are clearly effective. Recurrent gross bleeding from either kidney may occur, and nephrectomy is contraindicated. Infection of the urinary tract in pregnancy is reported to be increased in frequency in women with sickle cell trait. Diagnosis requires demonstration of the sickling phenomenon in addition to the electrophoretic abnormality of the hemoglobin.

OTHER HETEROZYGOUS SICKLING DISORDERS

Persons heterozygous for hemoglobin S and for another abnormality of either the alpha or beta chain may have no evidence of disease. Thus persons heterozygous for Hb S and J (an innocuous beta chain variant) have no Hb A in their red cell hemolysates, yet appear perfectly well. In certain other heterozygous states intravascular sickling of red cells is enhanced by the additional genetic abnormality.

Sickle cell–thalassemia resembles sickle cell anemia but is generally less severe, with atypical features including relatively mild anemia and persistent splenomegaly. It occurs predominantly in persons of black or Mediterranean ancestry. The beta thalassemia gene lessens production of Hb A, which occurs in low proportion. Electrophoresis of hemoglobin shows that the predominant hemoglobin is Hb S, with smaller fractions of Hb A and Hb F; sometimes Hb A cannot be detected and family studies are required to differentiate the disorder from sickle cell anemia.

Sickle cell–hemoglobin C disease occurs in American blacks with about one fourth the frequency of sickle cell anemia. Anemia tends to be mild, and some patients are asymptomatic. Splenomegaly is usual and may persist to old age; but atrophy of the spleen attributable to infarction occurs in some cases. The disease has special importance because of its predominantly nonhematologic manifestations. Symptoms may be referable to the eye, where peripheral vascular occlusions in the retina cause retinal avascularity and neovascular proliferations; these tend to bleed, producing vitreous hemorrhages with subsequent fibrosis and retinal detachment. Pain and dysfunction of the hip or shoulder are caused by avascular necrosis of capital epiphyses, especially the femoral head. Acute abdominal pain after anesthesia or during flight in unpressurized aircraft is the result of infarction of the spleen. Gross unilateral renal hematuria is not uncommon. Pregnancy may be complicated by severe anemia, infarcts of bone, and pulmonary emboli; but in many instances pregnancy is uncomplicated. Diagnosis is suggested by examination of the blood smear in which almost all the red cells are target forms. Electrophoresis of hemoglobin shows two major components, Hb S and Hb C; Hb A is absent.

Sickle cell–hemoglobin D Punjab disease has many of the features of sickle cell anemia and may be incapacitating because of vascular occlusive lesions, although anemia tends to be less severe. The rarity of the disease, its predominant occurrence in white persons, and the nonhematologic presenting manifestations obscure the diagnosis. Standard electrophoretic methods yield a pattern indistinguishable from that of sickle cell anemia, but Hb D separates from Hb S on agar gel at low pH.

748. DISORDERS ASSOCIATED WITH HEMOGLOBINS C, D, AND E

Homozygous hemoglobin C disease is an uncommon disorder occurring in blacks. Affected persons usually have few symptoms, but the spleen is enlarged. Chronic hemolytic anemia is rarely severe and is often discovered incidentally. Hb C is relatively insoluble, causing increased rigidity of the red cells with fragmentation and accelerated destruction. The blood film contains populations of target cells and microspherocytes, the latter representing older fragmented cells. *Hemoglobin C–thalassemia* causes a similar disorder. Heterozygosity for Hb C, *hemoglobin C trait,* occurs with high frequency in some areas of East Africa and in 2 to 3 per cent of American blacks. Some target cells are seen in the blood smear without anemia or other evidence of disease.

Homozygous hemoglobin D Punjab disease is a rare disorder causing mild or moderately severe anemia with numerous target cells in the blood smear. Hb D Punjab occurs in India but also in many other parts of the world, and several instances of the disease have been encountered in white families. Hemoglobin D–thalassemia resembles the homozygous disorder but can be differentiated by family studies. Persons heterozygous for Hb D alone have no hematologic abnormalities.

Homozygous hemoglobin E disease is manifested by mild microcytic and normochromic anemia, usually without splenomegaly. Large numbers of target cells are seen in the blood smear. The disease has been encountered with considerable frequency in Orientals. Persons heterozygous for Hb E and beta thalassemia have a more severe anemia, and the spleen is usually enlarged. The high frequency of the genes for Hb E and various types of thalassemia in Southeast Asia has led to the appearance of some complex genetic disorders, for example, hemoglobin E–alpha thalassemia disease, in which affected persons appear to have the characteristics of hemoglobin H disease in addition to hemoglobin E. Heterogeneity of the hemoglobin E diseases is related in part to the diversity of genetic factors.

749. HEMOLYTIC ANEMIAS CAUSED BY UNSTABLE HEMOGLOBINS

Congenital hemolytic disorders attributable to unstable hemoglobin molecules have been discovered in a few widely scattered cases. The patients present with anemia of varying severity, jaundice, and often splenomegaly. Affected persons are the heterozygous carriers of the abnormal hemoglobin, and homozygotes are unknown. Persons with *Hb Zürich* have a compensated mild hemolytic disorder without anemia except after administration of sulfonamides or during infections, when fulminant hemolytic anemia may occur. Drug-induced hemolytic episodes have been described in carriers of *Hb Torino* and *Hb Shepherd's Bush. Hb Köln* causes chronic hemolytic anemia, with recurring bouts of more severe anemia, jaundice, and dark urine; splenectomy has sometimes appeared to have a beneficial effect. Other unstable hemoglobins are not associated with distinguishing clinical features. Mild methemoglobinemia accompanies the hemolytic process in some instances, and the variant hemoglobin may have abnormal oxygen affinity. Increased oxygen affinity in Hb Zürich appears to have no clinical importance; reduced oxygen affinity in *Hb Seattle* is thought to increase anemia by lessening the stimulus for compensatory erythropoiesis. Diagnosis is suggested by demonstration of precipitates of denatured hemoglobin (Heinz bodies) in the red cells. In patients with Hb Zürich these may appear during hemolytic episodes as large globular inclusions. Heinz bodies are seen in many of the red cells of patients with Hb Köln after splenectomy. They can be demonstrated in other cases by incubating red cells with brilliant cresyl blue, a redox dye. The abnormal hemoglobin tends to precipitate when hemolysates are heated at 50° C. The dark urine contains a dipyrrole pigment thought to originate from heme groups dislodged from unstable hemoglobin molecules.

750. DISORDERS CAUSED BY HEMOGLOBINS WITH ABNORMAL OXYGEN AFFINITY

Cyanosis is caused by methemoglobinemia in the heterozygous carriers of the hemoglobins M and *Hb Freiburg.* The concentration of methemoglobin is not sufficiently high to cause major symptoms. In some instances there is an associated hemolytic disorder. Carriers of *Hb Kansas* also display cyanosis, in this instance caused by an increased concentration of deoxyhemoglobin in the blood in capillaries and venules. Hb Kansas has a low affinity for oxygen which facilitates the unloading of oxygen in the tissues, a phenomenon without apparent harmful effects.

Erythrocytosis (polycythemia) is the clinical expression of several abnormal hemoglobins with increased oxygen affinity. These variants have been discovered in scattered cases, and it is noteworthy that they cause one form of familial polycythemia without leukocytosis, thrombocytosis, or splenomegaly. Hematocrit values of heterozygotes have not exceeded 65 per cent, and homozygotes are unknown. Impaired release of oxygen activates the erythropoietin mechanism, producing the compensatory erythrocytosis. These hemoglobins should be sought by direct measurement of oxygen affinity in cases of unexplained erythrocytosis; electrophoretic mobility of the variant hemoglobin is not always abnormal. (See Ch. 754 to 758.)

751. THE THALASSEMIA SYNDROMES

The thalassemia syndromes are a heterogeneous group of inherited disorders manifested in the homozygote by profound anemia or death in utero, and in the heterozygote by red cell abnormalities of relatively trivial significance. Two major categories are recognized: *alpha thalassemia,* caused by retarded production of alpha chains of globin, and *beta thalassemia,* caused by retarded production of beta chains. Delta thalassemia has been described but is of no clinical significance. Impaired hemoglobin synthesis causes anemia and microcytosis. In addition, unbalanced production of globin chains leads secondarily to accumulation of uncombined alpha chains in beta thalassemia and to formation of the abnormal molecules γ_4 (Hb Bart's) and β_4 (Hb H) in alpha thalassemia; these tend to precipitate within red cells, hastening their destruction. In rare instances a thalassemic disorder is associated with one of the Lepore hemoglobins or Hb Constant Spring.

HOMOZYGOUS BETA THALASSEMIA

Definition. Homozygous beta thalassemia is the inherited disorder described by Cooley and Lee in 1925 and subsequently known as Cooley's anemia, Mediterranean anemia, target cell anemia, or thalassemia major. Occurring primarily in persons of Mediterranean ancestry, the disease is characterized by profound anemia, marked hepatosplenomegaly, and, typically, death in childhood.

Clinical Manifestations. Anemia appears after the newborn period and thereafter is severe, with marked pallor and mild to moderate hemolytic jaundice. The spleen and liver become tremendously enlarged. Deformation of the bones, particularly those of the head, contributes to the characteristic "Mongoloid" facies, and distorts the mouth and disturbs the alignment of the teeth. Roentgenograms show a "hair-on-end" appearance of the skull, enlargement of other marrow cavities with thinning of cortical bone, and abnormalities of trabeculation related to the marked hyperplasia of marrow. Cardiac enlargement and failure are explained by the anemia and by the deposition of large amounts of iron in the myocardium. Hemosiderosis is largely the result of the many transfusions required to maintain life. The hypochromic microcytic red cells are flattened, usually with numerous target and stippled forms and variable numbers of nucleated erythrocytes, polychromatic cells, and reticulocytes. Inclusion bodies can be demonstrated in many normoblasts and reticulocytes when stained with methyl violet. Leukocytosis may be marked and persistent. Much of the hemolytic activity appears to be intramedullary with resulting ineffective erythropoiesis. Serum iron is elevated with increased saturation of iron-binding protein. The proportion of Hb F is usually between 20 and 60 per cent, but values as high as 90 per cent may occur. Hemoglobin A_2 is not increased.

Treatment and Prognosis. With frequent transfusions and appropriate prevention and treatment of infections, life may be improved and prolonged. Massive deposition of iron is often the cause of cardiac failure and death. In selected cases splenectomy is beneficial when the spleen is actively sequestering red cells, but susceptibility to infection may be enhanced. Supplemental folic acid (0.5 mg per day) provides for the increased requirement. Chelating agents such as desferrioxamine have been used in an effort to reduce iron stores.

HETEROZYGOUS BETA THALASSEMIA

Heterozygous beta thalassemia (thalassemia minor) is manifested by mild anemia, usually with microcytosis, hypochromia, stippling, and target cells. Most frequent in Mediterranean populations, it is widely distributed throughout the world, occurring not rarely in blacks and less often in white persons from northern Europe. Symptoms are unusual, but some persons have anemia of moderate severity associated with jaundice and splenomegaly. Red cell abnormalities, which are variable and sometimes hardly detectable, are associated with resistance to osmotic lysis. Genetic heterogeneity is suggested not only by the clinical variability but also by differences in proportions of hemoglobins in hemolysates. Typically Hb A_2 is increased to about 5 per cent, sometimes with a slight increase in Hb F. But in some cases Hb F tends to be more elevated; in others Hb A_2 is reduced ($\delta\beta$ thalassemia). "Thalassemia intermedia," a term applied to instances of thalassemia which on clinical grounds appears to be intermediate between the typical heterozygous and homozygous disorders, has no specific meaning. Thalassemia minor is most often discovered during routine blood examination of blood smears or by detection of a low MCV using an electronic cell counter. It is often mistaken for iron deficiency anemia. Lead poisoning may be suggested by the numerous stippled cells, or other iron-refractory microcytic anemias may be considered. Diagnosis is suggested by demonstration of the same blood abnormality in other members of the family. An elevated level of Hb A_2 is confirmatory.

ALPHA THALASSEMIA

Homozygous alpha thalassemia is thought to be incompatible with life, and in a number of instances has appeared to be the cause of fetal death at about the thirtieth week. Most cases have been described in Orientals. The stillborn infant displays severe hydrops fetalis. Red cell hemolysates contain about 80 per cent Hb Bart's, a functionally inadequate hemoglobin with high oxygen affinity.

Heterozygous alpha thalassemia is manifested by very slight thalassemic abnormalities of the red cells with little or no anemia and by increased proportions of Hb Bart's (5 to 20 per cent) in cord blood. Identification is virtually impossible after the newborn period, although minor abnormalities of erythrocytes persist. It is widely distributed, occurring most frequently in Asiatic, African, and Mediterranean populations, and has been detected in almost 2 per cent of American blacks at birth. Rarely, heterozygous alpha thalassemia has occurred in persons who also had an alpha chain structural abnormality. Hemoglobin Q–alpha thalassemia, described in Orientals, is manifested by severe anemia. Hemoglobin I–alpha thalassemia was encountered in a black with mild anemia.

Hemoglobin H disease is a chronic hemolytic anemia associated with splenomegaly and intermediate levels of Hb H in erythrocytes. It has been found in persons of various ethnic backgrounds, including persons of apparently Northern European origin. Hemolytic episodes may be precipitated by sulfonamides. Red cells are hypochromic and microcytic. Intracellular inclusions of Hb H appear in erythrocytes after splenectomy, and may be induced before splenectomy by incubating blood with brilliant cresyl blue. The disease is thought to occur in persons heterozygous for alpha thalassemia and for a different alpha thalassemia gene with milder effects. The resulting deficiency of alpha chains is not so severe as in homozygous alpha thalassemia, and the disease is compatible with long life.

Charache, S., Weatherall, D. J., and Clegg, J. B.: Polycythemia associated with a hemoglobinopathy. J. Clin. Invest., 45:813, 1966.

Diggs, L. W.: Sickle cell crises. Am. J. Clin. Pathol., 44:1, 1965.

Herrick, J. B.: Peculiar elongated and sickle-shaped red corpuscles in a case of severe anemia. Arch. Intern. Med., 6:517, 1910.

Pauling, L.: Abnormality of hemoglobin molecules in hereditary hemolytic anemias. Harvey Lecture, 1953–1954, p. 216.

Weatherall, D. J. (ed.): The haemoglobinopathies. Clin. Haematol., 3:No. 1, 1974.

Weatherall, D. J., and Clegg, J. B.: The Thalassaemia Syndromes. 2nd ed. Oxford, Blackwell Scientific Publications, 1972.

White, J. M., and Dacie, J. V.: The unstable hemoglobins — molecular and clinical features. Prog. Hematol., 7:69, 1971.

752. METHEMOGLOBINEMIA AND SULFHEMOGLOBINEMIA

Ernst R. Jaffé

METHEMOGLOBINEMIA

Definition. Methemoglobinemia occurs when the concentration of methemoglobin within circulating erythrocytes is increased above the normal level of about 1 per cent. Since the abnormal pigment is intracellular, methemoglobinemia is perhaps a misnomer, but methemoglobincythemia and methemoglobinia are too clumsy, and convention dictates the use of the former term. Methemoglobin (ferrihemoglobin, hem*i*globin, ferric protoporphyrin IX-globin) is defined as an oxidation product of hemoglobin in which the sixth coordination position of ferric heme is bound to a water molecule (acid form) or to a hydroxyl group (alkaline form), each with its characteristic optical spectrum. Because of the additional positive charge, the sixth coordination position of iron is no longer available to bind molecular oxygen reversibly.

Etiology and Pathogenesis. The intracellular environment of hemoglobin is such that some oxidation of heme iron might be expected. Although the intrinsic structure of hemoglobin shields the iron against oxidation, metabolic processes are also normally active to protect hemoglobin against oxidation or irreversible denaturation and to reduce any methemoglobin which is formed to hemoglobin. An increase in the concentration of methemoglobin above the normal level can result from (1) the presence of a hemoglobin with an abnormal structure that makes it more susceptible to oxidation and/or unsuitable for reduction, (2) deficiency in the ability to reduce methemoglobin, and (3) exposure to drugs or chemicals which increase the rate of oxidation beyond the protective and reductive capacities of the cell. Whereas the first two mechanisms are associated with inherited disorders, the latter occurs in toxic or acquired methemoglobinemia.

Hereditary Methemoglobinemia Due to an Abnormal Hemoglobin (Hemoglobin M) (see Ch. 746 to 751). Substitution of tyrosine for histidine occurs at or across from the heme-binding site in the α chains of hemoglobin M Iwate and M Boston and in the β chains of hemoglobin M Hyde Park and M Saskatoon. Glutamic acid replaces valine in the β chain of hemoglobin M Milwaukee-1 one helical turn away from, but still facing, the heme iron. These alterations in the primary structure of hemoglobin increase the tendency of the heme iron to be oxidized and/or stabilize the methemoglobin form so that the normal mechanism for the reduction of methemoglobin is ineffective. Thus the methemoglobinemia does not respond significantly to conventional therapy (see below). As with other abnormal hemoglobins, hemoglobin M is transmitted as a codominant characteristic. Only heterozygotes for hemoglobin M have been identified, presumably because the homozygous state would be incompatible with life. Because only one pair of chains (either α or β) of a hemogloblin M is affected, and in the oxidized state, the concentration of methemoglobin does not exceed 25 to 30 per cent. Since α chains are already present in large amounts at birth, M hemoglobins with α chain substitutions are usually apparent immediately, whereas β chain abnormalities are often not manifest until later.

Hereditary Methemoglobinemia Due to a Deficiency in the Ability to Reduce Methemoglobin. The reduction of methemoglobin in human erythrocytes depends, primarily, on the activity of a reduced nicotinamide adenine dinucleotide (NADH or DPNH)-dependent methemoglobin reductase system. This system utilizes NADH generated by glyceraldehyde-3-phosphate dehydrogenase in the Embden-Meyerhof pathway of glycolysis to reduce methemoglobin to hemoglobin. Three other pathways capable of reducing methemoglobin are present in human erythrocytes, but are much less important: nonenzymatic reduction by ascorbic acid or reduced glutathione (GSH) and a reduced nicotinamide adenine dinucleotide phosphate (NADPH or TPNH)-methemoglobin reductase system, which requires an artificial electron carrier, such as methylene blue, to become effective in reducing methemoglobin. Significant methemoglobinemia is not observed in scurvy, glucose-6-phosphate dehydrogenase deficiency, marked GSH deficiency, or NADPH–methemoglobin reductase deficiency. Although other defects in the metabolic pathways of erythrocytes theoretically might lead to methemoglobinemia, they have not been identified.

The limited ability of erythrocytes from patients with hereditary methemoglobinemia not due to an abnormal hemoglobin to reduce methemoglobin in vitro has been demonstrated in numerous investigations. In most cases, this handicap has been traced to decreased activity of the NADH–methemoglobin reductase system. Methemoglobinemia as high as 40 to 50 per cent results from the accumulation of spontaneously formed methemoglobin in the absence of the normal mechanism for reduction. Data from family and biochemical studies are consistent with an autosomal codominant mode of inheritance. Marked deficiency in activity is seen in erythrocytes of affected homozygous patients, whereas approximately half normal activity is usually evident in cells from acyanotic, asymptomatic heterozygous subjects. At least eight different electrophoretic variants of NADH–methemoglobin reductase have been demonstrated. One variant is associated with only a slight decrease in activity. Thus, as is true for hemoglobin, glucose-6-phosphate dehydrogenase and other enzymes, multiple aberrations in the NADH–methemoglobin reductase system apparently exist, some with and some without functional consequences.

Toxic (Acquired) Methemoglobinemia. Methemoglobinemia occurs when oxidative stress overwhelms the protective capacities of erythrocytes and exceeds the ability of the cells to reduce methemoglobin. The heme iron may be oxidized directly by ferricyanide, ferric tartrate, bivalent copper, chromate, chlorate, certain quinones, alloxans, and some dyes with a high oxidation-reduction potential. Nitrite, a powerful reducing agent and one of the most common methemoglobin-forming compounds, produces methemoglobinemia by a reaction that is not completely understood, although the generation of hydrogen peroxide has been suggested. Nitrates, upon conversion to nitrites, especially in the gastrointestinal tract of infants, can lead to toxic methemoglobinemia. Erythrocytes of newborns also are less able than adults' cells to protect hemoglobin against oxidation and to reduce methemoglobin, owing to decreased activities of NADH–methemoglobin reductase and other enzymes. More complex reactions are postulated to explain the methemoglobin-forming properties of aromatic amino and nitro compounds (acetanilid, phenacetin, nitrosobenzene, phenazopyridine, primaquine, sulfonamides, prilocaine, benzocaine) and of aniline dyes in laundry marks and wax crayons. These compounds may be converted to metabolites which either act as direct oxidants or participate in a coupled oxidation with oxyhemoglobin. In the latter reaction, generation of hydrogen peroxide, peroxyhemoglobin, or free radicals is thought to cause the formation of methemoglobin. In addition to producing methemoglobinemia, some of these agents also can induce alterations which lead to hemolysis, especially in erythrocytes deficient in glucose-6-phosphate dehydrogenase activity.

Incidence and Prevalence. Although hereditary methemoglobinemia is rare, over 450 probable cases have been recorded. It is impossible to determine accurately how many are the result of a deficiency in NADH–methemoglobin reductase activity and how many are due to hemoglobin M. Patients in whom complete biochemical studies have not been performed, but whose chronic methemoglobinemia responds to therapy, presumably have had an abnormality in erythrocyte metabolism. Most of these patients probably have a deficiency in NADH-methemoglobin reductase activity; about 250 examples can be cited. The abnormality has a worldwide distribution, and is particularly prevalent in inbred populations.

The M hemoglobins also have a worldwide distribution with about 200 examples. Although many patients are of Northern European origin, a number have been reported from Japan, and the patient with hemoglobin M Hyde Park was a 77-year-old black man.

There have probably been thousands of instances of acquired methemoglobinemia, but most have been transient and either clinically insignificant or coincidental complications of another disease. The chronic methemoglobinemia ("enterogenous cyanosis") which is believed to result from the absorption of nitrites produced in a gastrointestinal (or urinary) tract persistently infected with nitrite-producing bacteria is extremely rare. More than 700 cases of toxic methemoglobinemia have been reported in infants fed formulas prepared with well-water containing high concentrations of nitrate; the mortality has been as high as 10 per cent. The anticipated increase in susceptibility to toxic methemoglobinemia of individuals heterozygous for NADH-methemoglobin reductase deficiency is seen in such subjects while receiving primaquine, chloroquine, or diaminodiphenylsulfone as malarial chemoprophylaxis.

Clinical Manifestations. The characteristic clinical picture of hereditary methemoglobinemia is presented by a patient with diffuse, persistent slate-gray cyanosis, often present from birth and not associated with clubbing of the fingers or evidence of cardiopulmonary disease. Concentrations of methemoglobin of 10 to 25 per cent are tolerated without apparent ill effect, but levels of 30 to 40 per cent may be associated with mild exertional dyspnea and headaches. These patients are really more blue than sick.

Toxic methemoglobinemia, especially if it develops rapidly, will produce symptoms of anoxia. Levels of 20 to 30 per cent methemoglobin are accompanied by dyspnea, tachycardia, headache, fatigue, fainting, nausea, anorexia, and vomiting. Some of these symptoms may reflect direct toxic effects of the causative agent. Lethargy and stupor may appear with methemoglobin concentrations above 55 or 60 per cent. The lethal concentration probably is greater than 70 per cent.

The decreased oxygen-carrying capacity resulting from untreated hereditary methemoglobinemia is sometimes associated with a mild compensatory erythrocytosis. This is often not as great as expected and is not observed with M hemoglobins. Segregation of methemoglobin in a population of older erythrocytes in NADH–methemoglobin reductase deficiency has been invoked to explain, in part, the absence of erythrocytosis. The heme groups of the normal hemoglobin chains in the M hemoglobins retain their capacity to bind oxygen, and normal oxygen affinities are observed with hemoglobin M Saskatoon and Hyde Park. The oxygen affinity, however, is decreased in hemoglobin M Boston, Iwate, and Milwaukee-1. This looser binding of oxygen may facilitate delivery to the tissues and may make an erythrocytosis unnecessary. In toxic methemoglobinemia, the methemoglobin not only decreases the available oxygen-carrying pigment, but also increases the affinity of the unaltered hemoglobin for oxygen, thereby further impairing the delivery of oxygen and enhancing symptoms.

Systemic effects usually do not occur in hereditary methemoglobinemia. The association of severe mental retardation has been noted in 21 children from 12 different families with NADH–methemoglobin reductase deficiency, perhaps caused by a generalized disorder not limited to the erythrocytes. Toxic methemoglobinemia may be associated with hemolysis, central nervous system depression, hepatic damage, or renal dysfunction, depending upon the causative agent or associated disease.

Diagnosis. Methemoglobinemia should be considered, even if only briefly, in the differential diagnosis of cyanosis. About 5 grams of deoxyhemoglobin per 100 ml of blood are required to produce visible cyanosis, but a comparable discoloration is produced by 1.5 to 2 grams per 100 ml of methemoglobin and by about 0.5 gram per 100 ml of sulfhemoglobin (see below). The greater visible effect of these abnormal pigments is due to the alterations in the absorption spectra. Blood which contains more than about 10 per cent methemoglobin (or sulfhemoglobin) appears unusually dark red or even brown, and does not change color upon vigorous shaking with air. Addition and mixing of a few drops of 10 per cent NaCN or KCN results in the rapid formation of bright red cyanmethemoglobin, but has no effect on the color of sulfhemoglobin.

Determination of the absorption spectrum is required to define the nature of the abnormal pigment. Acid methemoglobin has a characteristic spectrum with peaks at 502 and 632 mμ that disappear upon the addition of cyanide. Sulfhemoglobin has a peak at 620 mμ that is not altered by cyanide. The absorption spectra of methemoglobin M variants differ from those of normal methemoglobin with displacement of the peaks at 502 and 632 mμ toward lower wavelengths. Sulfhemoglobin, however, may be difficult to differentiate from methemoglobin M. The rate of formation of a complex with cyanide, the resulting absorption spectrum, and the electrophoretic migration of the methemoglobin form of hemoglobin M variants often differ from those of normal methemoglobin and help to establish the diagnosis.

NADH–methemoglobin reductase deficiency can be detected by a simple spot test, but confirmation of the diagnosis requires assay of this enzyme system in a hemolysate.

A careful history should provide clues to possible toxic methemoglobinemia. Parent-to-child transmission of congenital cyanosis should suggest the possibility of a hemoglobin M, whereas unexplained cyanosis in siblings but not in parents or offspring is more consistent with NADH–methemoglobin reductase deficiency.

Treatment. With toxic methemoglobinemia, concentrations of 20 to 30 per cent will disappear spontaneously in 24 to 72 hours after exposure to the offending agent terminates. More vigorous therapy is indicated if unconsciousness, stupor, or methemoglobinemia greater than 40 per cent supervenes. Oxygen administration and hemodialysis or exchange transfusion to remove the toxic agent may be helpful. Methylene blue, 1 to 2 mg per kilogram given intravenously during five minutes, will often correct the methemoglobinemia within 30 to 60 minutes. Repeated doses may be needed. Toxicity from methylene blue is uncommon, but doses over 15 mg per kilogram may cause hemolysis in infants. Individuals with glucose-6-phosphate dehydrogenase deficiency may respond suboptimally, and may develop hemolysis. Since neither methemoglobin M nor sulfhemoglobin will respond to methylene blue administration, failure to observe a significant change in color should alert the physician to the possibility of these abnormal pigments. Ascorbic acid has no place in the management of toxic methemoglobinemia because the rate at which it reduces methemoglobin is so much slower than that of the normal intrinsic mechanism.

Hereditary methemoglobinemia resulting from NADH–methemoglobin reductase deficiency usually does not require treatment except for cosmetic reasons. Intravenous methylene blue will reduce the methemoglobinemia rapidly, and daily oral administration of 100 to 300 mg will maintain the concentration below 10 per cent. Somewhat less effective is oral administration of ascorbic acid, 500 mg daily, to maintain the concentration of methemoglobin between 5 and 13 per cent. Despite good control of methemoglobinemia, therapy does not influence the mental retardation suffered by some patients.

Since the causal abnormality in the M hemoglobins resides in the structure of the hemoglobin, no effective form of therapy has been discovered.

Prognosis and Prevention. Methemoglobinemia, as an isolated alteration, does not have an adverse effect on the life expectancy of the patient or on the life span of the erythrocyte. The prognosis in toxic methemoglobinemia, once the acute episode is over, depends upon the precipitating circumstances. Toxic methemoglobinemia can be avoided by careful supervision of potential methemoglobin-producing drugs and chemicals, including thorough laundering of diapers to remove excess aniline dyes.

SULFHEMOGLOBINEMIA

Sulfhemoglobin, an incompletely characterized pigment not normally present, arises from the interaction of hemoglobin with soluble sulfides, especially hydrogen sulfide, in the presence of an oxidizing agent, usually hydrogen peroxide. Sulfhemoglobinemia is caused by the same aromatic amino drugs (acetanilid, phenacetin) that are associated with toxic methemoglobinemia. Why some patients develop methemoglobinemia and others have sulfhemoglobinemia is unknown. The concentration of GSH in the erythrocytes of some of the latter patients is elevated. Sulfhemoglobinemia may occur in patients with "enterogenous cyanosis," and has been attributed to the absorption of H_2S from the diseased gastrointestinal tract. The effect of sulfhemoglobin on the life span of human erythrocytes is uncertain, but many patients with sulfhemoglobinemia also have hemolysis. Since sulfhemoglobin cannot bind oxygen, the clinical effects are similar to those of methemoglobin. Sulfhemoglobin cannot be converted to hemoglobin, and there is no effective treatment. The pigment disappears when the erythrocytes containing sulfhemoglobin leave the circulation.

Cumming, R. L. C., and Pollock, A.: Drug-induced sulphaemoglobinaemia and Heinz body anaemia in pregnancy with involvement of the foetus. Scott. Med. J., 12:320, 1967.

Hsieh, H.-S., and Jaffé, E. R.: The metabolism of methemoglobin in human erythrocytes. *In* Surgenor, D. MacN. (ed.): The Red Blood Cell. 2nd ed. New York, Academic Press, 1975.

Jaffé, E. R., and Hsieh, H.-S.: DPNH-methemoglobin reductase deficiency and hereditary methemoglobinemia. Semin. Hematol., 8:417, 1971.

Kiese, M.: The biochemical production of ferrihemoglobin-forming derivatives from aromatic amines, and mechanisms of ferrihemoglobin formation. Pharmacol. Rev., 18:1091, 1966.

753. HEMOGLOBINURIA

Hugh Chaplin, Jr.

Definition and Mechanism. Hemoglobinuria (the presence of free hemoglobin in the urine) is a sign of variety of pathologic states and not a disease entity in itself. Hemoglobin generally finds its way into the urine by filtration from the plasma; uncommonly, it may be released from red cells which lyse within the kidney or urinary outflow tract. Normal human plasma contains an alpha$_2$ globulin, haptoglobin, present in amounts sufficient to bind 75 to 175 mg of hemoglobin per 100 ml of plasma. The tightly bound hemoglobin-haptoglobin complex, which has a molecular weight above 280,000, is not filtered by the normal glomerulus but is metabolized independent of the kidney at a linear rate of approximately 10 mg per 100 ml of plasma per hour. The total plasma hemoglobin binding capacity of the average normal adult, e.g., 3 liter plasma volume, is $125 \times 30 = 3750$ mg of hemoglobin, the amount contained in 11 ml of red blood cells. When hemoglobin entering the total plasma pool exceeds this relatively modest amount, the pigment exists free in the plasma, and is either metabolized or filtered into the urine and excreted. During metabolism of free plasma hemoglobin, some of the heme moiety is split from the parent molecule and binds to albumin, forming methemalbumin, which is readily distinguishable chemically and spectroscopically from free hemoglobin and hemoglobin-haptoglobin complex, and which is relatively slowly metabolized over 24 to 48 hours. Normal plasma also contains a beta globulin, hemopexin (50 to 100 mg per 100 ml), which selectively binds free heme in equimolar amounts.

It has been puzzling that free hemoglobin (molecular weight 66,000) should pass so readily into the glomerular filtrate when albumin (molecular weight 60,000) is filtered so poorly. It is known that under physiologic conditions oxyhemoglobin in dilute solution partially and reversibly dissociates into two alpha beta dimers each with a molecular weight of about 32,000. Recent studies by Bunn et al. suggest that it is this phenomenon occurring in the glomerulus that is responsible for the increased filtration of hemoglobin into the urine. The kidney has a limited capacity for tubular reabsorption of filtered hemoglobin; free hemoglobin will be excreted in the urine when the plasma free hemoglobin concentration exceeds 15 to 25 mg per 100 ml.

Occurrence. *Hemoglobinuria Following Intravascular Hemolysis.* Lysis of red cells within the circulation may occur under a variety of circumstances. The plasma will appear pink or red (free and haptoglobin-bound hemoglobin) or brown (methemalbumin). Isoimmune hemolysis occurs in relation to transfusion when the patient's plasma contains antibodies to donor red cell antigens. Hemolytic transfusion reactions usually involve incompatibility within the ABO system, but may occur within the other blood group systems, especially when complement-binding antibodies are involved, e.g., anti-Jk[a]. Repeated transfusion of group A, B, or AB recipients with group O "universal donor" blood may result in isoimmune hemolysis of the recipient's red cells owing to the cumulative effect of donor isoantibodies. Autoimmune hemolysis, particularly when complement components are part of the erythrocyte-autoantibody complex, may result in massive hemoglobinemia (as in "cold" autoimmune hemolytic anemia and in the rare condition of paroxysmal cold hemoglobinuria). It should be emphasized here that hemoglobinemia is not an inevitable accompaniment of severe iso- and autohemolysis; when red cell destruction occurs primarily extravascularly, i.e., by phagocytosis within the reticuloendothelial system (especially in the spleen), plasma hemoglobin levels will be low, and haptoglobin levels may be only minimally depressed. Severe hemoglobinemia has also occurred in relation to certain drug-antibody-erythrocyte complexes, as in patients sensitized to Fua-

din and quinidine. A number of intrinsic red cell defects may result in massive intravascular hemolysis under appropriate conditions. The most striking example is the poorly understood cell membrane defect in patients with paroxysmal nocturnal hemoglobinuria (PNH); also important are the enzyme-deficient cells, e.g., cells deficient in G-6-PD, which may lyse massively when exposed to sufficient concentrations of oxidant drugs or to components of the fava bean. Rarely, mechanical damage to red cells, as in severe microangiopathic hemolytic states or after extensive body surface burns, may cause gross hemoglobinemia; physical damage also accounts for the hemoglobinemia that accompanies many extracorporeal perfusion procedures. A number of snake and spider venoms contain enzymes that provoke rapid red cell lysis (lecithinase in the venom of the brown recluse spider, reported mainly in the south central United States). Massive destruction of red cells may result from direct erythrocyte parasitism in falciparum malaria. Hypotonic red cell lysis follows the intravenous infusion of distilled water, and may occur inadvertently when water is used to irrigate the bladder during exposure of the vascular prostatic bed in the course of transurethral resection procedures. A rare but interesting condition, "march (or exertional) hemoglobinuria," has been described, wherein hemoglobinuria follows prolonged exercise (usually, running) in susceptible individuals. Because of the variety of conditions under which this poorly understood phenomenon has been reported, it is likely that multiple factors may be responsible for its occurrence. The condition is clearly distinguishable from myoglobinuria.

Hemoglobinuria Originating in the Urinary Tract. Hemoglobinuria may accompany infarction of the kidney. Presumably, red cells lyse in the infarcted tissue, and the liberated hemoglobin "leaks" into the urinary outflow tract directly; cystoscopy reveals the unilateral origin of the pigmenturia. Rarely, when hematuria occurs coincident with a very dilute urine (specific gravity less than 1.006), hypotonic lysis of the cells occurs within the collecting system. In neither of the aforementioned conditions is hemoglobinemia found, and plasma haptoglobin levels are normal.

Clinical Manifestations and Implications. Hemoglobinemia and hemoglobinuria, when induced by the experimental infusion of hemoglobin, when occurring from nonimmune causes, and when unaccompanied by shock or dehydration, are generally asymptomatic and benign phenomena. Stroma-free hemoglobin administered intravenously has no demonstrable effect on renal function. Red cell stroma is known to have coagulant properties; signs of mild disseminated intravascular coagulation and mild transient impairment of inulin and creatinine clearances have been observed in monkeys receiving large amounts of hemoglobin-free autologous stroma intravenously. Nonetheless, massive hemoglobinuria occurring in patients with PNH and in human subjects mistakenly given distilled water intravenously has not been associated with renal impairment. Thus any symptoms occurring in association with hemoglobinuria are likely to be related to the cause of the hemolysis and not to the hemoglobinuria per se.

By contrast, hemoglobinuria can contribute importantly to severe renal damage when it occurs in association with a major antigen-antibody reaction, e.g., incompatible blood transfusion, and/or in association with markedly reduced renal blood flow, as in shock or severe dehydration. That hemoglobinuria per se is not necessarily the cause of renal shutdown after transfusion reaction has been demonstrated by Schmidt et al., who observed renal failure after the infusion of hemoglobin-free incompatible red cell stroma. Since hemoglobin and its breakdown products are relatively insoluble when in high concentration and at acid pH, the precipitation of hemoglobin products in the renal tubules will be favored by any condition that results in reduced urine volume and acid urine pH.

Diagnosis. Investigation of suspected hemoglobinuria should include studies of the plasma as well as of the urine. Plasma obtained at the time of active intravascular hemolysis will be pink or red; free hemoglobin and haptoglobin-bound hemoglobin (in acute hemolysis) will be demonstrable by electrophoretic, spectrophotometric, and gel filtration methods. If a blood sample is not obtained until 18 to 48 hours after intravascular hemolysis has ceased, the plasma will have a brown discoloration, and the only heme-containing pigment present will be methemalbumin, demonstrable spectroscopically by Schumm's test (appearance of a sharply defined band at 558 mμ after treatment with one tenth volume of concentrated ammonium sulfide).

During acute hemoglobinuria, the freshly voided urine will be pink, red, or deep port wine in color, depending on the hemoglobin concentration. Over a period of hours (whether in the bladder or during storage after voiding) the color turns brownish red or almost black owing to the formation of reduced hemoglobin, methemoglobin, acid hematin, and other breakdown products. Differential diagnosis should include hematuria, myoglobinuria, porphyrinuria, bilirubinuria, melanuria, betaninuria (beet pigment sometimes excreted in urine), and alcaptonuria (darkens only after storage and at alkaline pH). Hematuria can be quickly ruled out by centrifugation of the specimen. Several techniques employing benzidine reagents (which react with the iron-containing heme portion of the molecule) will help to rule out porphyrinuria, bilirubinuria, melanuria, and alcaptonuria, each of which can be separately identified by appropriate laboratory tests. Benzidine reagents will not, however, make the important distinction between hemoglobinuria and myoglobinuria, because they react with the heme groups of both molecules. The excretion of myoglobin in the urine should be suspected on clinical grounds when pigmenturia follows extreme excessive exercise (especially in the untrained individual who complains of severe postexercise muscle pain and weakness) and infarction of, or trauma to, a large muscle mass (crush syndrome). Although there are minor spectroscopic differences between hemoglobin and myoglobin, differentiation of these pigments is made easier by two physicochemical properties of myoglobin. Myoglobin does not bind to haptoglobin, and, because of its small molecular size (molecular weight 17,500), is rapidly excreted in the urine. Therefore during acute myoglobinuria, the plasma will be only slightly discolored or normal in appearance, and plasma haptoglobin levels will be normal. Second, hemoglobin is essentially insoluble at 80 per cent saturation with ammonium sulfate, whereas myoglobin remains in solution under these conditions. Thus the addition of 2.8 grams of ammonium sulfate to 5 ml of benzidine-positive red-brown urine will result in precipitation of the abnormal pigment if hemoglobinuria is present. Rarely, both pigments may occur together in the urine and may be identified by a variety of immunologic, electrophoretic, or gel filtration techniques.

Chronic hemoglobinuria, even at levels too low to discolor the urine, is always accompanied by *hemosiderin granules* in the urinary sediment. The hemosiderin is formed within tubular cells after reabsorption of hemoglobin, and is either released from the cells or appears within cells sloughed into the outflow tract. The brown granules are readily identified by the Prussian blue reaction with potassium ferrocyanide. Hemosiderinuria is a common accompaniment of many chronic hemolytic states, and is occasionally seen in patients with hemochromatosis. When hemolysis is sufficiently prolonged and severe (as in PNH), the cumulative loss of hemoglobin and hemosiderin in the urine may lead to frank iron deficiency.

Treatment. Therapy must be directed to the primary cause of the red cell lysis that is ultimately responsible for the hemoglobinuria. Assurance of adequate urine volume (by maintenance of adequate systolic blood pressure and good hydration) is essential. Special measures (including the use of mannitol and alkali) of importance in treating acute hemoglobinuria of isoimmune origin or under any circumstances, e.g., shock, in which acute renal shutdown is threatened are described in detail in Part XVI, Section Three.

Allison, A. C., and Rees, W.: The binding of hemoglobin by plasma proteins (haptoglobins). Br. Med. J., 2:1137, 1957.

Birndorf, N. I., Lopas, H., and Robboy, S. J.: Disseminated intravascular coagulation and renal failure. Production in the monkey with autologous red cell stroma. Lab. Invest., 25:314, 1971.

Blondheim, S. H., Margoliash, E., and Shafrir, E.: A simple test for myohaemoglobinuria (myoglobinuria). J.A.M.A., 167:453, 1957.

Bunn, H. F., Esham, W. T., and Bull, R. W.: The renal handling of hemoglobin. I. Glomerular filtration. J. Exp. Med., 129:909, 1969.

Ham, T. H.: Hemoglobinuria. Am. J. Med., 18:990, 1955.

Rabiner, S. F., Helbert, J. R., Lopas, H., and Friedman, L. H.: Evaluation of a stroma-free hemoglobin solution for use as a plasma expander. J. Exp. Med., 126:1127, 1967.

Schmidt, P. J., and Holland, P. V.: Pathogenesis of the acute renal failure associated with incompatible transfusions. Lancet, 2:1169, 1967.

Section Three. TRANSFUSION REACTIONS

Hugh Chaplin, Jr.

GENERAL CONSIDERATIONS

The true frequency of untoward reactions to transfusions of whole human blood is unknown. Incidences varying from 10 per cent to less than 0.2 per cent have been reported; the wide variation reflects principally the care with which the observer followed the recipients and the strictness of the criteria employed for defining reactions. A conservative estimate would be that 2 per cent of all transfusions are accompanied by some sort of unfavorable response. Thus with approximately 8 million units of whole blood administered annually in the United States, at least 160,000 recognizable reactions can be expected.

Caution must be exercised against erroneous diagnoses of transfusion reactions. Most of the symptoms of transfusion reactions are nonspecific (see accompanying table). Patients who receive transfusions are often seriously ill with disorders which themselves may be responsible for the acute onset of chills, fever, shock, or jaundice. The temporal association of the transfusion with the onset of symptoms certainly constitutes presumptive evidence of cause and effect, but important errors in patient care may result if wisdom and restraint are not exercised to assure a comprehensive consideration of possible causes other than transfusion.

Several complications of transfusions do not strictly qualify as transfusion "reactions," and thus are not included in the table. Among these are the development of *transfusion hemosiderosis* in the chronically anemic patient who receives a great many transfusions (usually more than 50) over a period of months or years, and the possible prejudicial effect of *sensitization to blood donor histocompatibility antigens* with respect to subsequent homograft survival. Another complication is the *transmission of diseases* such as syphilis, malaria, and hepatitis. The value of gamma globulin as prophylaxis against transmission of serum hepatitis has been controversial; a comprehensive evaluation of available evidence by the Public Health Service Advisory Committee on Immunization Practices has provided no justification for the prophylactic administration of conventional immune serum globulin. The possible value of hepatitis hyperimmune serum globulin for high-risk transfusion recipients is under investigation. An additional recognized complication of transfusion is the *"post-pump syndrome,"* an infectious mononucleosis–like illness occurring in 5 to 10 per cent of patients approximately one month after open-heart surgery. Possible causes include transmission of infectious mononucleosis or cytomegalovirus organisms via the transfusions, or transient host versus graft or graft versus host reactions involving recipient and donor leukocytes (principally lymphocytes).

There are several *complications of massive transfusion* (usually more than 3000 ml to an adult recipient within 12 hours). Citrate toxicity may occur, particularly during rapid intra-arterial transfusion or in patients with hepatic insufficiency or shunt bypass of the portal venous circulation. At citrate concentrations higher than 100 mg per 100 ml, skeletal muscle tremors may occur, along with prolongation of the QT segment of the electrocardiogram. Cardiac arrest may result if the citrate concentrations rise even higher. The manifestations of citrate intoxication can be prevented or eliminated by the simultaneous administration of calcium gluconate into another vein. Two other complications of massive transfusion are related to changes that take place in blood during storage in the blood bank. A hemorrhagic diathesis may develop, caused principally by the absence of viable donor platelets in blood stored more than 24 to 48 hours, even under ideal blood bank conditions. Depletion of the patient's own platelets by preceding massive blood loss is thus not compensated by the transfusion of viable donor platelets, and thrombocytopenia develops. Other

Categories of Transfusion Reactions

Cause of Reaction	Common Symptoms	Frequency	Shock	Prognosis
Contaminated blood	Chills, fever, headache, backache, delirium, bloody vomitus, and diarrhea	Rare	Yes ("red shock")	Serious
Bacterial pyrogens	Chills, fever, headache, malaise	Rare	No*	Good
Circulatory overload	Dyspnea, cough, hemoptysis, tachycardia	Rare	Rare*	Good
Air embolism	Sudden onset of cough, cyanosis, syncope, convulsions	Rare	Yes	Serious
Allergy	Itching, urticaria, fever, angioneurotic edema, bronchospasm	Common	No*	Good
Red cell incompatibility: intravascular hemolysis, extravascular hemolysis	Chills, fever, headache, backache, hemoglobinemia, hemoglobinuria, oliguria, jaundice	Moderate	Yes	Serious
Sensitivity to:				
Donor leukocytes	Chills, fever, headache, malaise, confusion	Common	Rare*	Good
Donor platelets	Chills, fever, headache, malaise, confusion	Rare	Rare*	Good
Donor plasma (IgA)	Anaphylaxis, collapse, chest pain	Rare	Yes	Serious
Unexplained (febrile)	Chills, fever, headache, malaise	Common	No*	Good

*Although shock is absent or rare as a general feature of these types of reactions, in the seriously ill or injured patient shock may be precipitated by the added stress of the transfusion reaction.

causes for hemorrhagic tendency are deficiencies of labile plasma coagulation factors in stored donor blood. Abnormal bleeding may occur on this basis in an adult who receives more than 8 to 10 successive units of stored blood in less than 24 hours; the complication can be largely prevented if every fourth unit of blood given within a 12- to 18-hour period is a "fresh" unit, i.e., drawn within three to four hours of administration. A unit of fresh-frozen plasma may be substituted at the same intervals if the patient's platelet count is adequate. A less frequent complication of massive transfusion of stored blood is the occurrence of clinically significant hyperkalemia in the recipient. During storage in ACD preservative solution at 4° C, donor red blood cells continuously lose potassium ion; thus the concentration of potassium in the suspending donor plasma will average 15 to 20 mEq per liter after two weeks of storage and 25 to 30 mEq per liter after three weeks. The danger of hyperkalemia is increased in the presence of impaired renal function. When renal insufficiency is known to exist, transfusion should employ blood stored less than five to seven days, and packed red cells should be used, whenever possible.

MECHANISMS OF REACTIONS

Contaminated Blood. The transfusion of banked blood contaminated by endotoxin-producing bacteria (usually gram-negative rods that grow well at refrigerator temperature) may give rise to extremely serious reactions in the recipient, with a fatal outcome likely in more than 50 per cent of the patients. Death usually results from profound and persistent vascular collapse. In addition to the symptoms listed in the table, a characteristic feature is the occurrence of "red shock"; i.e., unlike the more common hypovolemic shock in which peripheral vasoconstriction results in cold, gray, clammy skin, endotoxin shock may be accompanied by marked peripheral vasodilatation so that the skin is dry, warm, and pink. Thus it is essential that blood pressure be measured frequently in patients suspected of having reactions to contaminated blood, because dangerous hypotension may coexist with an outward appearance that belies the severity of the circulatory collapse.

Fortunately, with current blood banking procedures, contamination of stored blood rarely occurs. It is also fortunate that the diagnosis of significant bacterial contamination can be established within ten minutes. A small sample of residual donor blood from the container or tubing used for administration is centrifuged lightly (500 rpm for two to three minutes); a drop of the supernatant plasma is smeared, fixed by heating, and Gram stained. Unless most oil immersion fields contain several clearly definable organisms, contamination can be disregarded as the primary cause of the reaction. If the blood is cultured to confirm the diagnosis, incubation should be carried out at 30° C as well as at 37° C, because some contaminants will not grow at temperatures as high as 37° C.

Because of the extreme gravity of reactions owing to contaminated blood, rapid institution of comprehensive supportive therapy is essential. Intravenous therapy should include sufficient vasopressor drug to maintain the systolic pressure above 100 mm of mercury, corticosteroids (100 to 150 mg of hydrocortisone), broad-spectrum antimicrobials in high dosage, and additional whole blood if the estimated blood loss has not been corrected. Special measures to mitigate renal complications are discussed later.

Pyrogenic Reactions. The term "pyrogenic reactions" should be reserved for reactions related to the presence of demonstrable bacterial pyrogens (endotoxins) in the infused blood or in the transfusion equipment. Now that commercially manufactured pyrogen-tested disposable transfusion equipment is widely employed, the frequency of pyrogenic transfusion reactions has diminished strikingly. When parenteral therapy equipment does contain pyrogens, febrile reactions are "epidemic" among patients receiving intravenous infusions, and the aid of a specialized laboratory qualified to demonstrate the presence of bacterial pyrogens should be sought. Treatment is symptomatic.

Circulatory Overload. The onset of acute left-sided heart failure during transfusion may reflect actual hypervolemia caused by administration of excessive amounts of blood to a patient whose volume deficit has been seriously overestimated. Even in the absence of hypervolemia, pulmonary edema may be precipitated by the too rapid administration of blood to a patient who is profoundly anemic (hemoglobin concentration less than 4 to 5 grams per 100 ml) or in cardiac failure. A further cause for the symptoms of circulatory overload may be the presence of mechanical circulatory obstruction, e.g., mitral or aortic valve disease. Whatever the cause, treatment consists of slowing the rate of transfusion (cessation if necessary), changing to packed red blood cells, and digitalization. Rarely, a small phlebotomy is required. When there is reason to be concerned about possible circulatory overload in an elderly or severely anemic patient, or in one suffering from either cardiac or renal insufficiency, venous pressure should be monitored at frequent intervals during transfusion.

Air Embolism. Air embolism is rarely encountered as a life-threatening cause of transfusion reaction except when blood is being administered under air pressure after massive exsanguination. The accident occurs when all the blood in the container into which air has been pumped has been delivered and air is allowed to flow into the patient. This complication has been largely eliminated with the increasing use of plastic blood containers to which external pressure can be safely applied without the possibility of air infusion (provided that air has not inadvertently got into the bag, e.g., during prior component preparation). When air embolism has occurred, the administration tubing should be immediately clamped and the patient turned on his left side in the head-down, feet-up position so that air in the right ventricle floats away from the pulmonary outflow tract.

Allergy. Allergic reactions are relatively common and are generally mild (hives, bronchial wheezing, and congestion of mucous membranes). Treatment is symptomatic (antipyretics, antihistaminics). The drugs should be administered directly to the patient; under no circumstances should they be added to the container of blood. Marked angioneurotic edema or anaphylaxis may require prompt parenteral administration of epinephrine, vasopressor drugs, and corticosteroids.

Red Blood Cell Incompatibility. Incompatibility within the ABO system, with the resultant destruction of donor cells by alloantibodies in the recipient's circulation, is the most common cause of life-threatening reactions in contemporary transfusion practice. These preventable transfusion accidents almost always occur because of technical or logistic errors—the use of faulty techniques of blood typing and improper identification of blood samples, donor bottles, and patients. When the recipient's blood contains potent allohemolysins, acute intravascular hemolysis of the donor cells occurs. When the plasma hemoglobin concentration exceeds the hemoglobin binding capacity of the recipient's plasma (normally 75 to 175 mg of hemoglobin per 100 ml of plasma), *hemoglobinuria* occurs. Whereas many patients tolerate severe hemoglobinuria, e.g., paroxysmal nocturnal hemoglobinuria, without serious impairment of renal function, intravascular hemolytic reactions are potentially dangerous, especially when accompanied by shock, because of the possible development of oliguria, anuria, and uremia.

When donor red blood cell destruction occurs predominantly extravascularly, as for example in the presence of Rh antibodies demonstrable only by the indirect antiglobulin (Coombs) reaction, hemoglobinemia is generally much less severe, and jaundice is a more prominent feature, reflecting reticuloendothelial cell destruction of antibody-coated donor erythrocytes sequestered from the circulation predominantly in the spleen and/or liver.

Although the occurrence of an acute hemolytic transfusion reaction can generally be suspected on the basis of the symptoms and signs shown in the table, a special problem is presented by *anesthetized patients,* in whom the only sign of serious hemolytic reaction may be oozing of blood at the operative site. The bleeding tendency, which is often accompanied by severe transient thrombocytopenia, is generally thought to be the consequence of disseminated intravascular coagulation in response to thromboplastic substances liberated from the hemolyzing cells.

To determine quickly whether acute intravascular hemolysis has occurred, a blood sample is drawn from the patient into a clean, dry syringe or a syringe rinsed with physiologic saline. The blood is mixed with an anticoagulant by repeated gentle inversion (with care to avoid foaming, which causes in vitro hemolysis) and immediately centrifuged. If the plasma is obtained within two to eight hours of massive intravascular lysis, it will appear frankly pink or red. Plasma examined 12 to 48 hours after intravascular lysis is more apt to be brown, reflecting the presence of methemalbumin, which can be demonstrated spectroscopically by Schumm's test (appearance of a sharply defined band at 558 mμ after treatment with one tenth volume of concentrated ammonium sulfide). When donor red blood cell destruction has been largely extravascular, the plasma will show increased indirect-reacting (unconjugated) bilirubin; peak levels generally occur four to six hours after the transfusion.

To ascertain the basis for incompatibility, blood freshly drawn from the recipient should be sent immediately to the blood bank along with the donor blood container so that a thorough serologic review can be carried out. Along with the conventional retesting of the recipient's serum for the presence of antibodies against donor erythrocytes, such a review should include search for antibodies in the donor plasma that might cause destruction of the patient's cells, or cells of the other donors in the case of multiple transfusions.

In addition to general supportive measures, therapy of acute hemolytic transfusion reactions should be especially directed to minimizing possible renal complications (see below).

Delayed hemolysis of donor cells may occur (usually three to ten days after the transfusion) as a result of post-transfusion sensitization of the recipient. Red blood cell destruction generally occurs by an extravascular mechanism, and is manifested principally by jaundice and progressive anemia. The latter, if severe, may be treated safely by further transfusion, provided that serologic investigation has clarified the cause of the erythrocyte destruction so that repetition may be avoided.

Dangerous Universal Donor. A special instance of hemolytic transfusion reaction is the destruction of the group A, B, or AB patient's cells by high-titer alloantibodies in the plasma of a group O donor blood. In modern practice, every effort is made to screen group O donor bloods so as to detect those with dangerously high titers of alloantibodies. Except under emergency conditions, group O blood should be given to A, B, or AB recipients only if screening tests have defined the blood as "low titer." When a "dangerous universal donor" reaction does occur, its severity is usually tempered by the dilution effect of the recipient's plasma volume, the neutralizing effect of soluble group-specific A or B substance (or both) in the recipient plasma, and the large recipient red cell mass. Nonetheless, hypotension, hemoglobinemia, hemoglobinuria, and renal shutdown may result. Clinical management is similar to that described above for hemolytic reactions resulting from destruction of donor cells.

When an A, B, or AB recipient must be transfused with multiple units (4 or more) of low-titer group O whole blood, a cumulative effect of donor alloantibodies may result in relatively slow extravascular destruction of the patient's red blood cells. Jaundice and progressive anemia are the chief signs. If the patient requires further transfusion, it is advisable to continue with low-titer O blood and to resume type-specific blood only after two weeks have elapsed from the time of multiple Group O transfusions.

A special category of "dangerous donors" consists of those whose plasma contains alloantibodies (which may be of any blood group specificity) as a result of multiple prior transfusions or incompatible pregnancies, the latter usually associated with evidence of hemolytic disease of the newborn. In many blood banks, donor alloantibodies against red cells will be detected by routine screening of all donor sera against commercially available cells containing all the clinically important erythrocyte antigens. Even when such screening has not been performed, the donor alloantibodies will be detected if a sensitive technique is employed for the minor cross-match.

Sensitivity to Donor Leukocytes, Platelets, or Plasma. Transfusion reactions in this category are observed in patients who have had multiple previous exposures to the homologous antigens either by repeated transfusions or by pregnancies. The aid of an experienced serologic laboratory should be sought to demonstrate the presence in the patient's plasma of antibodies to donor leukocytes, platelets, and plasma proteins. The majority of such reactions are caused by recipient sensitization to donor *leukocytes;* symptoms appear within 30 to 90 minutes from the start of transfusion and subside over the succeeding four to eight hours. Treatment is symptomatic. The reactions can be prevented by several effective procedures for removing leukocytes from the blood prior to transfusion. In addition, there have been increasingly frequent reports that *donor* plasma containing antileukocyte antibodies active against recipient white cells may cause an anaphylaxis-like reaction with hypotension, tachycardia, prolonged fever (up to 48 hours), tachypnea, cyanosis, and x-ray findings of "allergic pneumonia." Eosinophilia is sometimes observed. Treatment is symptomatic. Although antibodies to donor *platelets* are commonly demonstrable in multitransfused recipients, symptomatic reactions to the platelets in a single unit of transfused blood rarely if ever occur. Reactions may be observed when a sensitized recipient receives multiple platelet concentrates in a single infusion. Shulman has described a rare form of delayed post-transfusion thrombocytopenia representing a complex immune response to incompatible donor platelets. The patients are generally multiparous women; profound thrombocytopenia develops five to seven days after transfusion and may persist for up to six weeks thereafter. Steroid therapy has been ineffective, but there are two reports of prompt termination of thrombocytopenia after exchange transfusions. An additional complication of platelet transfusion has been observed in severely leukopenic sensitized recipients; immediately after transfusion of multiple HLA-incompatible platelet concentrates, leukopenia becomes more profound and may not recover to pretransfusion values for 48 to 72 hours. Finally, dangerous acute post-transfusion thrombocytopenia may result when the plasma from multitransfused donors contains antibodies to recipient platelets. Rare but extremely serious anaphylactic reactions have been observed in recipients whose sera contain antibodies to donor *IgA globulin*. The patient's own serum lacks IgA globulin, and precipitating anti-IgA antibodies are demonstrable by agar immunodiffusion. Marked anxiety, collapse, and unconsciousness may occur immediately upon receipt of as little as 2 to 5 ml of donor plasma; measures to combat anaphylaxis must be undertaken immediately. Because the reactions may be provoked by such small amounts of IgA globulin, prevention requires extensive washing of donor red cells to accomplish virtual elimination of residual donor plasma.

Unexplained Febrile Reactions. These continue to make up a large proportion of the febrile reactions observed on a busy hospital service. Incompatibility between recipient's plasma and donor's red cells, white cells, platelets, and plasma cannot be demonstrated, nor can pyrogens be detected. There have been several well documented reports of symptomatic reactions associated with rapid destruction of donor red cells in the absence of any evidence of incompatibility by an elaborate battery of in vitro serologic tests. Therefore transfusion reactions that remain unexplained should not be comfortably dismissed as "idiopathic" but should stimulate persistent diagnostic investigation. Until the cause is found, the patient remains prey to recurring reactions with all subsequent transfusions.

MANAGEMENT OF RENAL COMPLICATIONS

A patient who has experienced severe hemorrhage with actual or impending hypovolemic shock, or who is suffering from bacteremia, may be precipitated into more severe circulatory collapse by any of the transfusion reactions described above. Under these circumstances the hazard of oliguric renal failure is ever present. The hazard is greatly increased when the reaction is of the acute hemolytic variety, in which the free hemoglobin that enters the urine may precipitate in the renal tubules.

The following recommendations for treatment of threatened or actual renal failure complicating transfusion reactions are based on a program developed by Barry and Crosby at the Walter Reed Medical Center. Urine flow, as a reliable indicator of renal function, is an important guide to management, and such measures as may be necessary should be taken to assure accurate measurement of urine volume at hourly intervals. The objective of treatment is to maintain a urine flow of at least 100 ml per hour until the effects of the reaction have subsided. Systolic blood pressure should be maintained at a sufficient level (above 100 mm of mercury) to assure adequate renal perfusion. Excessive elevation of blood pressure is to be avoided because of accompanying renal vasoconstriction. As soon as the reaction has occurred, 20 grams of mannitol as a 20 per cent aqueous solution should be infused intravenously during a five-minute interval. This dose should initiate diuresis in the patient capable of responding to mannitol. In the event of an acute hemolytic reaction, the infusion of 45 mEq of sodium bicarbonate subsequent to the test dose of mannitol may be indicated. Because some of the urine obtained at the end of the first hour may have been in the bladder before the reaction, an additional one-hour collection should be obtained to enable reliable evaluation of the patient's response to mannitol. If the urine flow is greater than 40 ml per hour, intravenous fluid containing approximately 50 mEq of sodium per liter as chloride or bicarbonate, e.g., 300 ml normal saline plus 700 ml 5 per cent dextrose in water, should be administered in sufficient volume to match the desired urine flow (100 to 150 ml per hour) until the possibility of renal injury is past and the patient is able to take oral fluids in sufficient volume to maintain satisfactory urine flow. The original dose of mannitol may be repeated whenever urine flow drops below 100 ml per hour for any two-hour period, but not more than 150 grams of mannitol should be administered in any 24-hour period.

If the patient does not respond to the aforementioned measures and renal shutdown has become established, Barry and Crosby recommend the following:

1. Restriction of fluid intake to 500 ml plus visible output per 24 hours.

2. Provision of 100 grams of carbohydrate per day at a constant rate to avoid periods of hypoglycemia and to decrease catabolism.

3. Control of hyperkalemia by the administration of 15 to 30 grams of sodium polystyrene sulfonate resin every six hours by mouth or by rectum.

4. Transfer of the patient within the first few days of oliguria to a renal center. Prior to transport, any EKG abnormality associated with hyperkalemia should be corrected by the infusion of 25 per cent glucose in distilled water containing 25 units of regular insulin and 200 ml of 10 per cent calcium gluconate per liter. An infusion rate of 3 ml per minute or more may be required during the first 30 minutes to return the electrocardiogram to normal. Thereafter, during transportation, rates of 0.25 to 1 ml per minute will usually protect the patient from cardiac arrest.

SUBSEQUENT TRANSFUSION OF THE REAC-TION-PRONE PATIENT

There is always an increased hazard in transfusing a recipient who has had a previous transfusion reaction. Therefore the indications for subsequent transfusions in these patients should be subjected to especially critical scrutiny, and transfusion should be avoided whenever possible. On the other hand, the added hazard should not engender indecision and delay, to the detriment of the patient. Informed of the possible causes for transfusion reactions, supported by the results of thorough investigation of previous reactions in the patient, and possessing a variety of sensitive cross-matching procedures as well as methods for separating donor blood to provide only the components actually needed by the patient, the physician can proceed with confidence to meet such a patient's transfusion needs. The transfusion should be administered slowly, and the patient should be watched especially carefully to detect the earliest signs of recurrent reaction so that the procedure can be discontinued if serious symptoms develop.

Barry, K. G., and Crosby, W. H.: The prevention and treatment of renal failure following transfusion reactions. Transfusion, 3:34, 1963.

Bjerrum, O. J., and Jersild, C.: Class-specific anti-IgA associated with severe anaphylactic transfusion reactions in a patient with pernicious anemia. Vox Sang., 21:411, 1971.

Cassell, M., Phillips, D. R., and Chaplin, H., Jr.: Transfusion of buffy coat-poor red cell suspensions prepared by dextran sedimentation. Transfusion, 2:216, 1962.

Chaplin, H., Jr., and Cassell, M.: The occasional fallibility of in vitro compatibility tests. Transfusion, 2:375, 1962.

Greenwalt, T. J., Finch, C. A., Pennell, R. B., et al.: General Principles of Blood Transfusion. 2nd ed. Chicago, American Medical Association, 1970.

Public Health Service Advisory Committee on Immunization Practices: Immune serum globulin for protection against viral hepatitis. Ann. Intern. Med., 77:427, 1972.

Shulman, N. R., Marder, V. S., Hiller, M. C., et al.: Platelet and leukocyte isoantigens and their antibodies: Serologic, physiologic and clinical studies. Prog. Hematol., 4:222, 1964.

Ward, H. N.: Pulmonary infiltrates associated with leukoagglutinin transfusion reactions. Ann. Intern. Med., 73:689, 1970.

Section Four.   HEMOCHROMATOSIS

(IRON STORAGE DISEASE)

Thomas H. Bothwell

Definition. The term hemochromatosis implies the presence of massive, generalized iron deposits in parenchymal tissues together with evidence of fibrotic changes and functional impairment in the most severely affected organs.

Pathogenesis. The amounts of iron normally absorbed and excreted daily are small, being between 0.5 and 1.0 mg in men and twice this figure in women. Any variations in absorption that do occur are directed toward maintaining a normal body iron content. There are three basic ways in which excessive amounts of iron can accumulate in the body.

First, there are conditions in which mucosal behavior is abnormal and amounts of iron are absorbed that are inappropriate to body needs. This occurs in idiopathic hemochromatosis, in which a daily absorptive rate of no more than 3 to 5 mg extending over half a lifetime leads eventually to massive iron overload with its attendant pathologic sequelae. The tendency to absorb iron excessively in the condition is inherited, being transmitted by a dominant or partially dominant autosomal gene. Inappropriate absorption of iron has also been noted in certain anemias, being a feature of thalassemia major and of other refractory anemias. The common denominator in such "iron-loading" anemias appears to be increased but ineffective erythropoietic activity. Excess iron absorption has also been noted sometimes in liver disease and in porphyria cutanea tarda, but why this should be so is not known.

A second cause of iron overload is too much iron in the diet. When large amounts of absorbable iron reach the lumen of the upper small intestine, the mucosal mechanism for excluding unwanted iron is overwhelmed, and excessive quantities are absorbed. This occurs most commonly in South African blacks who brew fermented drinks in iron containers. As a result, iron overload of varying degrees is found in the majority of adult men, and a small proportion exhibit fully developed hemochromatosis. Other potential sources of excessive iron in the diet are medicinal tonics and red wine.

Finally, there are situations in which iron is introduced into the body by another route. Multiple transfusions are used in the mangement of hypoplastic and other forms of refractory anemia. Each unit of blood contains approximately 200 mg of iron, and massive quantities of the metal can be introduced by this means. Since the body's capacity to excrete iron is very limited, subjects on regular transfusion therapy accumulate large amounts.

The eventual outcome in an individual patient can be modified by several factors. Caloric intake and hence iron intake tend to be greater in males, whereas menstruation and pregnancies increase iron losses in females. As a result, clinical manifestations of idiopathic hemochromatosis are four times more common in males than in females and occur at a younger age. Approximately a third of patients presenting clinically with the disease give a history of an excessive intake of alcohol. There are several reasons for the association. As mentioned previously, some alcoholic beverages, such as red wines, contain appreciable amounts of iron. Alcohol also stimulates iron absorption. Finally, the hepatoxicity of alcohol and iron are almost certainly additive. A similar interplay between genetic and environmental factors is seen in the hemochromatosis that occurs as a complication in thalassemia major. Such subjects have an inherent tendency to absorb increased amounts of iron. In addition, they receive multiple blood transfusions and are often subjected to misguided therapy with oral iron.

Pathology. Approximately one quarter of the 3 to 4

grams of iron normally present in the body is stored in the liver and reticuloendothelial system as a soluble complex, ferritin, and as a closely related but insoluble golden-brown compound, hemosiderin. In hemochromatosis the total body iron content is increased to between 20 and 40 grams, most of the extra iron being deposited as hemosiderin. Concentrations are greatest in the parenchymal cells of the liver and pancreas, but significant deposits are also present in other endocrine organs and in the heart. Varying degrees of fibrosis occur in affected organs, and in the liver cirrhosis is almost invariably present. Deposits in the reticuloendothelial system are relatively scanty in the genetic disorder idiopathic hemochromatosis, but are often heavy after multiple transfusions and are also prominent in the dietary iron overload that occurs in South African blacks. The degree to which the iron from transfused blood is redistributed from reticuloendothelial cells depends on the activity of the erythroid marrow and the plasma iron level. Redistribution, with offloading onto parenchymal cells, is particularly liable to occur when there is a hyperplastic marrow and when the transferrin of plasma is saturated with iron. Why reticuloendothelial deposits are so prominent in the dietary iron overload occurring in South African blacks is not known. A similar distribution has, however, been noted in animals given large amounts of oral iron. The cellular localization of the iron is important, because parenchymal deposits are noxious to tissues, whereas iron in reticuloendothelial cells seems to be harmless.

Clinical Features. Idiopathic hemochromatosis is usually regarded as a model of the effects of the slow accumulation of large amounts of iron in parenchymal tissues. Symptoms usually develop between the ages of 40 and 60 years, and presenting clinical features relate to one or more of a number of organs. The most prominent are skin pigmentation, diabetes mellitus, hepatomegaly with symptoms of hepatic dysfunction, cardiac failure, and evidence of panhypopituitarism.

In half the patients the skin is bronzed owing to the presence of excess quantities of melanin; hemosiderin is also present in the remaining half, and the skin has a slate-gray appearance. Pigmentation is most prominent on the exposed parts. Although a firm hepatomegaly is almost invariably present, liver function in the absence of associated alcoholism is often surprisingly good. Hepatic failure with coma can, however, be precipitated by intercurrent infections and other acute insults. The spleen is enlarged in about 50 per cent of patients, but complications as a result of portal hypertension are not common. Hepatoma may occur as a complication in older patients.

Diabetes occurs in the majority of subjects and may be mild or severe; insulin, occasionally in large doses, is usually needed for its control. Complications, such as nephropathy, neuropathy, and peripheral vascular disease, occur in about 20 per cent of patients. It has been customary to ascribe the diabetes to inadequate islet function as a result of iron deposits in the pancreas. There is, however, evidence that insulin levels are often normal. In addition, it has been shown that the incidence is high in the relatives of affected individuals, and that this is not related to the presence of iron overload.

Arrhythmias and refractory cardiac failure occur in a proportion of affected persons and are particularly troublesome in younger patients. Sexual impotence, testicular atrophy, and sparsity of body hair are commonly present. Although these are usually secondary to the liver dysfunction, the pituitary and other endocrine glands are sometimes directly affected. Recently, attention has been drawn to an arthropathy in some patients, affecting both small and large joints. It seems to result from chondrocalcinosis and iron deposits in the joints.

The symptom complex that is such a characteristic feature of idiopathic hemochromatosis is sometimes found in other forms of iron overload. For example, cirrhosis and diabetes have been reported both in South African blacks and in subjects who have had many transfusions; cardiac failure is also common in the hemochromatosis that occurs in thalassemia major. Other complications of excessive iron deposits have been recognized in South African blacks. Ascorbic acid deficiency and osteoporosis are both common in affected individuals, and there is some evidence that the iron overload is a causal factor in their occurrence.

Diagnosis. The diagnosis is not difficult when the classic tetrad of skin pigmentation, liver disease, diabetes, and heart failure is present. In fact, the combination of any two of these should alert the physician. Laboratory tests are required to confirm the diagnosis. The best screening test is the measurement of the plasma iron concentration and the plasma iron–binding capacity. In the absence of intercurrent infection or complicating hepatoma, the plasma iron is usually greater than 200 μg per 100 ml, and the transferrin is virtually completely saturated. It must be emphasized that this test does not define the degree of iron overload. The plasma is often saturated with iron both in affected relatives at a time prior to the development of significant stores and in patients with anemias resulting from ineffective erythropoiesis. Insight into the amount of parenchymal iron present can be gained in several ways. Injecting chelating agents such as deferoxamine (Desferal) and measuring the quantity of iron passed in the urine is helpful, because it has been established that this is positively correlated with the size of the iron stores. With an intramuscular dose of deferoxamine of 10 mg per kilogram, a normal person excretes less than 2 mg of iron over the next 24 hours, whereas subjects with idiopathic hemochromatosis usually excrete more than 10 mg. The test is particularly useful in distinguishing between idiopathic hemochromatosis and alcoholic cirrhosis with only moderate iron overload. Liver biopsy provides the final proof, with evidence of heavy parenchymal iron deposits together with a fibrous reaction. The amount of connective tissue varies from a fine portal-tract fibrosis to frank macronodular cirrhosis. Further useful information can be obtained by chemical estimation of the concentration of iron present in a needle biopsy specimen. In passing, it is important to emphasize that the physician's role extends beyond the diagnosis and treatment of affected patients. With up to one half of siblings showing a predisposition to develop the disease, it is important that they be defined and treated prior to the accumulation of massive quantities of iron.

Treatment and Prognosis. Apart from the management along conventional lines of complications, such as diabetes and heart failure, the specific treatment is to remove the iron as rapidly as possible. This objective is normally achieved by repeated phlebotomies. The 200 to 250 mg of iron removed in each pint of blood creates a deficit that leads to the mobilization of a similar quantity of iron from the body's stores. Weekly phlebotomies are tolerated well by most patients, and hemoglobin levels greater than 11.0 grams per 100 ml are often maintained with venesection programs that are even more vigorous. Once the stores are exhausted, venesections are continued at less frequent intervals to prevent reaccumulation of the iron. Successful removal of all the iron deposits, which is heralded by a drop in the plasma iron concentration, may occur only after weekly venesections have been carried out for two years or more. Provided the patient is eating a well balanced diet, no specific supplementation is required. When venesections are not feasible (e.g., in thalassemia), deferoxamine can be given on a daily basis. The amounts of iron excreted are, however, usually not more than 10 to 20 mg, and this method of treatment has not been widely applied.

Without therapy, idiopathic hemochromatosis is a fatal disease. Death usually results from cardiac failure in younger patients and from liver disease or its complications in older ones. Some subjects succumb to an acute abdominal crisis followed by shock. Although the cause has not been definitely established, it may result from gram-negative bacteremic shock. In one recent study only 33 per cent of untreated patients were alive at five years. In contrast, 89 per cent of those treated by repeated venesections survived. Such therapy is associated with a gain in weight, an increased sense of well-being, regression of skin pigmentation, and an improvement in hepatic and cardiac function; insulin requirements are also often reduced. Hepatoma can, however, still occur as a late complication.

Bothwell, T. H., and Finch, C. A.: Iron Metabolism. Boston, Little, Brown & Company, 1962.

Charlton, R. W., Bothwell, T. H., and Seftel, H. C.: Dietary iron overload, Clin. Haematol., 2:383, 1973.

Fairbanks, V. F., Fahey, J. I., and Beutler, E.: Clinical Disorders of Iron Metabolism. 2nd ed. New York, Grune & Stratton, 1971.

Section Five. POLYCYTHEMIA

Edward H. Reinhard

754. INTRODUCTION

Definition and Classification. Polycythemia is better defined as a sustained abnormal increase in red blood cell volume than as an increase in the number of red blood cells per cubic milliliter of blood; an abnormal increase in hemoglobin is invariably accompanied by an increase in erythrocytes, but the converse is not always so. Some writers apply the term *erythrocytosis* to polycythemias secondary to recognized causes, and the term *erythremia* to the idiopathic disorder otherwise known as *polycythemia (rubra) vera*. Polycythemic syndromes include polycythemia rubra vera, *"benign polycythemia," familial polycythemia,* and *polycythemia secondary to a variety of causes;* although relative polycythemia does not fit our definition of polycythemia in that there is no absolute increase in red blood cell mass, it will be discussed in Ch. 755, because this condition must always be considered in the differential diagnosis.

The polycythemic syndromes can be classified under the following headings: (1) *Relative polycythemia* includes polycythemia caused by fluid loss, fluid deprivation, or extravascular shift of fluid, and at least some cases of so-called benign or "stress" polycythemia. (2) *Familial polycythemia* is usually due to an inherited hemoglobinopathy (which will be discussed under secondary polycythemias), but there are rare reports of what appears to be familial polycythemia vera. (3) *Secondary polycythemias* can be divided into those that are due to an appropriate (or physiologic) increase in erythropoietin production, and those due to an inappropriate (or nonphysiologic) increase in erythropoietin production. (4) *Polycythemia vera* ("primary" polycythemia).

755. RELATIVE POLYCYTHEMIA

Relative polycythemia occurs when there is a decrease of plasma without comparable decrease of red blood cells so that the erythrocytes become more concentrated. Restricted fluid intake alone may lead within a few days to lowered plasma volume. More common mechanisms are increased loss of water and electrolytes because of diabetic acidosis, the postoperative state, diuretic therapy of congestive heart failure, vomiting, diarrhea, abnormal sweating, hyposthenuria, adrenal insufficiency, or excessive plasma loss owing to extensive burns or traumatic shock. The hemoconcentration accompanying dehydration rarely gives rise to more than a 25 per cent increase in hematocrit, but the leukocyte level may rise considerably more owing to mobilization from marrow and marginal leukocyte pools or stimulation of leukopoiesis by the disorder producing the dehydration. Restoration of fluid balance with appropriate amounts of water and electrolytes promptly abolishes the relative polycythemia. Release of erythrocytes from storage in the spleen in normal man is never sufficient to produce significant polycythemia.

GAISBÖCK'S SYNDROME, STRESS POLYCYTHEMIA, AND BENIGN POLYCYTHEMIA

Gaisböck in 1905 described 18 patients with hypertension associated with an elevated red blood cell count but without splenomegaly; subsequently this combination of findings became known as Gaisböck's syndrome. This term gradually fell into disuse, and some authors believed that these were patients in whom mild erythrocytosis and hypertension coexisted by coincidence.

In 1952 Lawrence and Berlin reported 18 patients with erythrocytosis in whom blood volume determinations revealed normal red blood cell mass and decreased plasma volume. It was thus apparent that these patients had relative polycythemia. Half of them had hypertension. The authors were so impressed by the anxiety-tension state of these patients that they attributed the relative polycythemia to "stress." Similar cases were described by other authors, and the diagnosis of "stress polycythemia" became popular. In 1964 Russell and Conley studied 25 patients with polycythemia who did not have the associated symptoms, the splenomegaly, the leukocytosis, and the thrombocytosis characteristic of polycythemia vera and in whom dehydration and arterial oxygen unsaturation were excluded. These patients formed a strikingly homogeneous group. They were predominantly white males with a mean age of 45 years, somewhat younger than that for patients with polycythemia vera. They tended to be moderately overweight and of stocky habitus. Slight plethora and suffusion of the eyes were common. Many of the patients were tense and nervous. Almost all smoked cigarettes. Twelve of the 25 had persistent hypertension. None of them had congenital heart disease, pulmonary disease, vascular shunts, clubbing of the fingers, or palpable spleen. The highest documented hematocrit values for the group ranged between 54.5 and 65 per cent. Blood volume determinations were done on ten of the patients. Some had a mild absolute polycythemia, whereas others had only relative polycythemia. Seven of these 25 patients had had significant vascular disease (myocardial infarction, intermittent claudication, cerebrovascular accident, Leriche syndrome, or thrombophlebitis). Russell and Conley believed that the recurring pattern of manifestations justified the concept of a unique syndrome that they called benign polycythemia. They emphasized that this is the same syndrome described by earlier authors under the designation Gaisböck's syndrome or stress polycythemia. They doubted, however, that stress played any part in the etiology of the erythrocytosis, and were of the opinion that multiple features of the syndrome are of constitutional pathogenesis and, at times, of familial occurrence. Some patients with high hematocrit values are undoubtedly normal persons whose hematocrit and red blood cell counts fall rather far from the mean on the normal curves of distribution. Patients with the Gaisböck or benign polycythemia syndrome do not require any specific treatment.

756. FAMILIAL POLYCYTHEMIA

It now appears clear that most instances of what were reported in the past as examples of familial polycythemia were, in fact, cases of genetically transmitted hemoglobin abnormalities, in which inheritance follows an autosomal dominant pattern. However, the incidence of polycythemia vera appears to be higher among American Jews and lower among American blacks even after correction for all biases which might lead to lower detection among blacks and higher detection among Jews. This different prevalence according to ethnic groups living in a somewhat similar environment suggests the influence of genetic factors. Furthermore, rare examples of what appear to be familial incidence of polycythemia vera have been reported in the literature. These findings, if valid, are best explained by polygenic inheritance (the operation of several genes often transmitted from both parents). There is an increased incidence of aneuploidy in polycythemia vera, but the chromosomal abnormalities are nonspecific and have been attributed by some authors to the abnormal and increased cellular proliferation of the marrow.

757. SECONDARY POLYCYTHEMIAS

SECONDARY POLYCYTHEMIAS ASSOCIATED WITH AN APPROPRIATE (PHYSIOLOGIC) INCREASE IN ERYTHROPOIETIN PRODUCTION

A variety of conditions associated with *tissue* hypoxia may lead to the development of this type of secondary polycythemia.

Pathologic Physiology. When there is prolonged lowering of the oxygen *tension* of the arterial blood despite a normal or elevated hemoglobin content, sustained secondary polycythemia often results. In this situation, the oxygen tension of the arterial blood is less than normal in spite of the increased oxygen carrying capacity. This, together with increased viscosity of the blood and the underlying circulatory burden imposed by the primary cardiac or pulmonary disease, results in decreased delivery of oxygen to the tissues. The plasma of hypoxic animals and of man has been shown to produce accelerated erythropoiesis in recipient animals. The mechanism by which erythropoietin-producing cells detect tissue hypoxia is not known, but the oxygen tension of arterial blood passing through the renal parenchyma somehow initiates a sequence of events in which the kidneys produce a *renal erythropoietic factor* (REF) which, in turn, may combine with or cleave an alpha-2 globulin in the plasma to form *erythropoietin*. This, when carried to the marrow, initiates the differentiation of erythroblast precursors into erythroid cells. Experimentally, erythropoietin also shortens the transit time of radioactive iron through the marrow compartment, which suggests that the maturation of the erythroid cells is speeded up. As the red blood cell mass is increased, the oxygen supply to the kidneys increases and the production of REF is reduced or shut off completely, thus slowing or stopping red cell production.

Some patients with significant arterial oxygen unsaturation caused by chronic obstructive pulmonary disease do not have erythrocytosis, or they may have considerably less erythrocytosis than comparable degrees of hypoxia resulting from high altitude or cyanotic heart disease would produce. The reason is not always clear. However, in some cases the red blood cell volume may actually be increased, but the hemoglobin and hematocrit values remain normal owing to a comparable increase in the plasma volume. Furthermore, acidosis makes more oxygen available to the tissues than would be predicted for a given degree of oxygen saturation (the *Bohr effect*), and many patients with chronic lung disease have respiratory acidosis. Lastly, the concentration of 2,3-DPG in the red cells influences the availability of oxygen to the tissues, and this may be increased in chronic lung disease. Thus many factors other than the arterial oxygen saturation may influence the P_{O_2} in and around the cells in the kidneys responsible for erythropoietin production.

Situations and Disorders Causing Secondary Polycythemia Associated with an Appropriate Increase in Erythropoietin Production

Polycythemia secondary to *cardiac or pulmonary disease* occurs when there is less than normal oxygen saturation of the blood entering the aorta because of short-circuiting of the pulmonary capillary bed by passage of part of the venous blood from the right directly into the left side of the heart or into the aorta, e.g., patent atrial or ventricular septum, dextroposition of the aorta, or pulmonary arteriovenous fistula; when the alveolar ventilation is restricted because of chronic pulmonary disease, e.g., emphysema or silicosis; or when there is thickening of the alveolar membranes, e.g., in mitral stenosis, or diffuse pulmonary fibrosis preventing normal transfer of oxygen from the alveoli to the blood. Tremendous obesity (pickwickian syndrome), massive abdominal tumor, or ascites may decrease pulmonary ventilation and thus contribute to the development of secondary polycythemia. Healthy persons living at high altitudes have polycythemia proportional to the diminution in oxygen tensions of the inspired air (and hence in the arterial blood).

Another important cause of secondary polycythemia associated with an appropriate increase in erythropoietin production is the presence in the red blood cells of an *abnormal hemoglobin* with an increased affinity for oxygen (approximately 50 per cent of the total hemoglobin). These patients are heterozygotes with mutant hemoglobin and normal hemoglobin. The abnormality is transmitted as an autosomal dominant. The first such report involved an 81-year-old man and 15 members of his family covering three generations, in all of whom a hemoglobin variant designated as hemoglobin Chesapeake comprised about 30 per cent of the total hemoglobin. Since the initial report, familial polycythemia has been found to be caused by many other hemoglobin variants, including J. Capetown, Yakima, Kempsey, Ypsilanti, Hiroshima, Rainier, Bethesda, and Malmö (see Ch. 746 to 751). In all these familial polycythemias, the affected members of the families have had hematocrits in the range of 45 to 58 per cent, with a proportionate elevation of the erythrocyte count and hemoglobin levels; none have had leukocytosis, thrombocytosis, or splenomegaly. There has been no significant associated disability.

All the hemoglobin variants associated with erythrocytosis have amino acid substitutions located at one of the structural sites involved in subunit rearrangement during oxygenation. These substitutions usually involve amino acids which play a direct part in chain-chain interactions, as a result of which the mutant hemoglobin has an abnormal or abolished interaction between subunits resulting in an increased affinity for oxygen. The affinity of hemoglobin for oxygen may be expressed as the partial pressure of oxygen at which hemoglobin is half saturated (P_{50}). At 37° C and pH 7.4, the P_{50} of normal blood is 26.5 mm Hg. All these hemoglobins associated with erythrocytosis have an increased affinity for oxygen, and the oxygen dissociation curve is shifted to the left. The P_{50} value for the blood of patients with Hb Chesapeake is 18 to 20 mm Hg, and for the blood of patients with Hb Rainier, Yakima, and Kempsey it is 12 to 14 mm Hg. This left shift of the oxygen dissociation curve has little effect on the uptake of oxygen in the lungs, but is associated with a significant decrease in oxygen release to the tissues, so that tissue oxygen tension is decreased at a normal hematocrit with resultant stimulation of erythropoietin production. Hence red blood cell production increases until tissue oxygen tension is restored to normal. Many abnormal hemoglobins have normal electrical charges and cannot be detected by electrophoretic mobility studies. In addition to screening hemoglobin electrophoresis, laboratory confirmation of the diagnosis is based on study of the oxygen dissociation curves of the whole blood and of dialyzed hemolysates from which 2,3-DPG has been removed.

A mild compensatory erythrocytosis may occur in patients with longstanding *methemoglobinemia* or *sulfhemoglobinemia,* particularly when the pigment abnormality is secondary to certain chemicals such as analine dyes or gum shellac. Methemoglobinemia associated with hemoglobin M is only rarely associated with erythrocytosis. Cobalt is thought to produce secondary polycythemia by indirect stimulation of erythropoietin production.

Polycythemia occurs in association with primary aldosteronism, and may be induced by the administration of large doses of androgens or vasopressin. Relative polycythemia is common in Cushing's syndrome, but a true polycythemia may occur if both corticosteroid and androgen production are increased.

Clinical Manifestations. The clinical symptoms associated with these secondary polycythemias vary widely. In contrast to the disabling acute symptoms that appear in normal individuals on ascent to an altitude of 10,000 feet or more, most permanent residents at such elevations make a satisfactory adjustment and are asymptomatic. By virtue of the increased oxygen-carrying power of the blood and an increase in erythrocyte 2,3-diphosphoglycerate, sufficient compensation for its lowered oxygen tension is achieved so that these people are able to carry on muscular work with comparative ease. However, Monge has described *chronic mountain sickness* in occasional persons living at such altitudes who presumably have chronic pulmonary disease as a superimposed additional cause of arterial anoxia. Recurrent bronchitis and laryngitis over a long period of time develop into an incapacitating illness characterized by headache, tinnitus, dyspnea, anorexia, vomiting, and lethargy. These symptoms are greatly aggravated by slight exertion. The chest is emphysematous, and the vital capacity is reduced. Cyanosis, clubbing of the digits, and congestion of the scleral capillaries are prominent. Examination of the blood reveals polycythemia greater than that of other residents at the same altitude. The blood volume is increased, and reticulocytosis, moderately increased bilirubinemia, and sometimes leukocytosis are found. Return to sea level promptly relieves the symptoms, and the polycythemia gradually subsides. *Brisket disease,* affecting 1 to 5 per cent of cattle grazing in certain areas at high altitudes in Utah and Colorado, is an interesting counterpart of chronic mountain sickness in man. Brisket disease affects young calves mainly and, unlike *Monge's disease,* is characterized by pulmonary hypertension followed by right heart failure. The animals do not have sustained arterial oxygen desaturation, and they do not develop significant polycythemia. All animals that have been studied show a thick muscular coat around the small pulmonary arteries; it has been postulated that excessive development of this muscular coat as well as excessive fluid and salt intake caused by grazing on marshy ground are factors that contribute to the pulmonary hypertension and cor pulmonale in the affected animals.

Polycythemias secondary to cardiac or pulmonary disease are accompanied by symptoms and signs characteristic of the primary disease. The patients are invariably cyanotic and often have clubbing of the digits. Cardiac failure is common. Slight splenomegaly may be due to congestive failure or chronic pulmonary infection. *Ayerza's syndrome* is a condition characterized by slowly developing symptoms of pulmonary insufficiency, cyanosis, and polycythemia owing to primary disease of the pulmonary artery and its branches (arterial and arteriolar sclerosis, syphilis, or congenital hypoplasia of the pulmonary artery), aggravated, in some cases, by emphysema and pulmonary fibrosis. In this condition right-sided heart failure eventually develops (see Ch. 546 to 550).

In some secondary forms of polycythemia the erythrocyte level may reach 8 million and occasionally 10 million cells per cubic millimeter, usually with somewhat less than corresponding hemoglobin and hematocrit values. Reticulocytosis and slight hyperbilirubinemia are characteristic. Leukocytosis is absent except when there is associated infection, which also seems in some cases to restrict the polycythemic response to the arterial unsaturation. The essential diagnostic criterion of secondary polycythemia of this type is decreased oxygen saturation of the blood, almost always less than 90 per cent. The arterial oxygen saturation should always be determined at rest and after standard exercise; under the latter circumstances the arterial oxygen saturation remains approximately 95 per cent in normal persons and in most patients with polycythemia vera, whereas in patients with polycythemia secondary to anoxemia the arterial oxygen saturation after exercise always falls to less than 80 per cent and usually to much less than this (occasionally as low as 30 per cent).

Treatment. The treatment of polycythemia secondary to heart or lung disease is chiefly that of the underlying cardiac or pulmonary disorder. Elimination of the offending drug or toxic exposure relieves the polycythemia caused by methemoglobinemia, sulfhemoglobinemia, or carboxyhemoglobinemia. In acute episodes of cyanosis, oxygen administration may be helpful. The polycythemia with resultant increased oxygen-carrying capacity of the blood is a useful compensatory physiologic response. However, if the hematocrit value rises to levels above 65 or 70 per cent, phlebotomies may result in temporary relief of symptoms, perhaps because the bleeding lowers blood volume and viscosity. When hematocrit values are plotted against blood viscosity, blood viscosity rises slowly with increasing hematocrit until the level exceeds 60 per cent, when the slope of the curve increases more rapidly.

SECONDARY POLYCYTHEMIAS ASSOCIATED WITH AN INAPPROPRIATE (NONPHYSIOLOGIC) INCREASE IN ERYTHROPOIETIN PRODUCTION

In all the types of secondary polycythemia discussed above, the increased production of erythropoietin appears to be appropriate in that normal animals or man exposed to similar hypoxia, cobalt, or androgens would respond in a similar fashion. However, there is another group of secondary polycythemias in which the mechanism for the elaboration of erythropoietin is nonphysiologic, because there is no hypoxia and only a small proportion of individuals with each of these disorders develop increased erythropoietin levels. Secondary polycythemia of this type has been reported in association with many types of *cancer* and a few *benign tumors*. The

tumors which produce secondary polycythemia most frequently are malignant renal tumors and brain tumors; the brain tumors have usually been vascular tumors most commonly located in the posterior fossa. Papilledema was present in most of them. In one series of 37 cases of brain tumor (usually hemangioblastoma) with associated polycythemia, the hemoglobin returned to normal after removal of the tumor in 21 instances. Polycythemia has also been observed in association with carcinomas of the liver, prostate, lung, rectum, and breast, as well as with melanosarcomas, multiple myeloma, and pheochromocytoma. Secondary polycythemia also occurs in association with many types of *renal disease* other than tumors, including medullary cystic disease, renal tuberculosis, hydronephrosis, and renal artery stenosis, as well as after renal transplantation. There is evidence that many tumors and even some benign cysts of the kidney elaborate a substance having erythropoietin-like activity that is responsible for the excessive erythropoiesis.

758. PRIMARY POLYCYTHEMIA
(Polycythemia Vera, Erythremia)

Primary polycythemia is a chronic disease of unknown cause characterized by hyperplasia of all the cellular elements of the bone marrow, nucleated red blood cells being most prominently involved, with resultant sustained elevation of the erythrocyte count and hemoglobin and usually, to a lesser extent, leukocytosis and thrombocytosis. It has been regarded by many persons as a malignant neoplastic disease of the erythropoietic tissue analogous to leukemia. The relationship of these two diseases is emphasized by the fact that in primary polycythemia the leukocytosis is sometimes so pronounced as to suggest a diagnosis of chronic granulocytic leukemia, and some patients with well-established polycythemia eventually have developed blood and bone marrow findings, and even pathologic changes at autopsy, suggestive of leukemia even when no radiation therapy has been given. Conversely, several patients with typical granulocytic leukemia have been observed to develop polycythemia. In patients with primary polycythemia treated with radioactive phosphorus, the incidence of acute leukemia as a late manifestation has varied in different series of cases from 0 to greater than 20 per cent.

Aneuploidy and several other nonspecific chromosomal aberrations have been reported in untreated patients with polycythemia vera. In P^{32}-treated patients, the frequency of these aberrations is somewhat higher. According to one study, the finding most typical of P^{32}-treated patients is dicentric chromosomes, and a dose response curve to the last P^{32} dose was demonstrated. A Philadelphia-like chromosome was observed in two patients with polycythemia vera and in one with benign erythrocytosis, all after P^{32} therapy. The authors speculated whether the development of leukemia complicating P^{32}-treated polycythemia might be dependent on the type and location of radiation-induced chromosomal damage, with subsequent establishment of a clone of cells with a selective developmental advantage. There is no evidence that tissue anoxia or excessive production of any known endocrine or humoral factor, including erythropoietin, constitutes the stimulus to excessive blood cell production in primary polycythemia. When marrow from patients with polycythemia vera is incubated in vitro with erythropoietin, the rate of heme synthesis increases over that of controls by only one tenth. Marrows from polycythemia vera patients in remission respond normally to erythropoietin. These data suggest that the disease is due to an abnormal cell line whose intrinsic stem cell defect does not allow normal control of erythrocytic production by the usual regulatory substance, erythropoietin. There is now considerable evidence for the existence of two different lines of primitive cells in the marrow of patients with polycythemia vera: an abnormal cell line which differentiates at an increased rate and is not responsive to erythropoietin, and a normal cell line which lies relatively dormant so long as the differentiated products of the abnormal cells are present in sufficient numbers to suppress erythropoietin production.

It is now well established that many types of fowl and animal leukemia are due to viruses. Likewise, it has been observed that a "polycythemic virus" (a variant of Friend virus, or a passenger virus present in spleen filtrate prepared originally from mice infected with Friend virus) when injected into normal mice results in polycythemia and splenomegaly. Furthermore, this virus can initiate erythropoiesis in hypertransfused-polycythemic mice. The only other substance known to initiate erythropoiesis in a hypertransfused-polycythemic state is erythropoietin. The fact that this polycythemia-inducing virus causes an increase in proerythroblasts, erythroblasts, and reticulocytes and an increase in Fe^{59} uptake in the bone marrow and spleen without detectable erythropoietin activity in the plasma and urine suggests that the virus acts directly on erythropoietic stem cells and not through the mediation of erythropoietin. It is not presently known whether these animal data are relevant to human polycythemia vera.

In untreated polycythemia vera, the erythropoietic cells in the bone marrow do not respond normally to erythropoietin. The erythropoietin activity of plasma and urine is not increased. However, when the hematocrits of patients with polycythemia vera are reduced to normal or anemic levels by bleeding, measurable amounts of erythropoietin appear in the urine. Patients with hypoxia-induced erythrocytosis usually have increased levels of urinary erythropoietin, but an occasional patient with polycythemia of this type may have a normal level of urinary erythropoietin. If this situation is suspected, it is helpful to measure urinary erythropoietin content before and after phlebotomy. In polycythemia vera, phlebotomy results in little or no increase in erythropoietin excretion, but in patients with polycythemia secondary to tissue hypoxia with normal urine erythropoietin content, phlebotomy results in a marked increase in erythropoietin excretion.

The *incidence* of polycythemia vera is high among Jews and low among blacks. Men are more commonly affected than women. The usual age of onset is in middle or later life, although, rarely, young adults or children are affected. Familial polycythemia has been reported, and in these families onset of the disease in childhood is more common; as previously stated, at least some familial polycythemias are due to inherited hemoglobin variants.

Pathologic Physiology. In uncomplicated primary polycythemia the cardiac output and work are normal, but the velocity of blood flow is slowed. Pulmonary functions are normal or nearly so. The arterial saturation of the blood is normal in most instances. Hypoxia has been demonstrated in some patients with polycythemia vera, but in such cases it has usually been attributed to unrelated coexisting cardiorespiratory disease. However, one study of 26 patients with polycythemia vera who had no evident heart or lung disease revealed that, although all of them had normal ventilatory function, 9 patients had an arterial oxygen saturation of less than 92 per cent, and 11 patients had a mean arterial oxygen tension that was significantly lowered (that is, less than 80 mm Hg). The diffusing capacity for carbon monoxide was significantly lower than normal in 10 of these patients, and the defect in diffusing capacity appeared to correlate well with the level of hypoxia. It was suggested that these abnormalities might be due to widespread thrombosis in small pulmonary arteries. Whether this is the correct explanation or not, it is important to emphasize that many studies have confirmed the fact that mild hypoxemia is not uncommon in patients with well established polycythemia vera, and the arterial oxygen saturation is of little value in distinguishing between primary and secondary polycythemia unless it is less than 88 per cent.

Many of the clinical manifestations, as well as intravascular thrombosis, the most common complication of untreated primary polycythemia, can be attributed directly or indirectly to three factors: (1) increased total blood volume, (2) increased viscosity of the blood, and (3) thrombocytosis. The feeling of fullness and aching in the head and the fatigability characteristic of this disease can be relieved by phlebotomies so promptly and consistently that the increased blood volume seems a major factor in their genesis. Some patients with this disease continue to have mild symptoms when the red blood cell level and hematocrit are in the upper normal range, and yet are completely asymptomatic when these values are reduced to the lower normal range. The extent to which the increased viscosity of the blood contributes to these symptoms and to the high incidence of intravascular thrombosis is not entirely clear, but the circulation time may be greatly prolonged with resultant visceral stasis; increased blood viscosity is at least an important contributory factor. As the hematocrit level rises above normal, there is a progressively more rapid increase in the blood viscosity; the higher the hematocrit rises above 60 per cent, the more imperative becomes the need to lower the hematocrit, and hence the viscosity, in order to relieve symptoms and minimize the danger of intravascular thrombosis. Paradoxically, when the hematocrit is greatly elevated, there is a tendency to bleed excessively from minor injuries; this may be caused, in part, by the distention of the capillaries and veins required to accommodate the huge blood volume. However, abnormal platelet function has been reported in patients with polycythemia vera who have thrombocytosis. The thrombocytosis may be pronounced, and undoubtedly contributes to the production of intravascular thromboses, because the incidence of thromboses is low in secondary polycythemia (high viscosity, normal platelet level).

In untreated polycythemia vera, the marrow iron stores are often depleted, and hypoferremia is not uncommon. Furthermore, as would be expected under these circumstances, the plasma iron disappearance time (T 1/2) is often markedly shortened. After repletion of iron stores by parenteral iron dextran administration, the plasma iron disappearance time approaches normal. In uncomplicated secondary polycythemia, the marrow iron stores are normal or increased, and the plasma iron disappearance time is more nearly normal than in polycythemia vera.

In polycythemia vera, there is very poor correlation between the hemoglobin value and the packed red blood cell volume on the one hand and the *total* red blood cell mass on the other. This is because the plasma volume in polycythemia vera may be normal, decreased, or increased.

The basal metabolic rate is frequently elevated. The increased production of blood cells results in an increased destruction of blood cells, and this increased cell turnover increases the metabolic rate. Since an end product of nucleic acid degradation is uric acid, it is not surprising that hyperuricemia or increased urate excretion occurs in 75 per cent of cases of untreated polycythemia vera and that at least 5 per cent of patients develop clinical gout.

Clinical Manifestations. Symptoms vary from none to so many that psychoneurosis is suspected. Common presenting complaints include headache or a feeling of fullness in the head, itching that is aggravated by a hot bath, paresthesias, dizziness, weakness, fatigability, dyspnea, and visual disturbances. A ruddy complexion usually of considerable duration, skin or mucous membrane hemorrhages, or awareness of a heavy sensation or fullness in the left side of the abdomen owing to enlargement of the spleen may be initial manifestations. The plethora is especially noticeable in the face, mouth, neck, hands, and feet. The veins of the scleras and retinas are distended and dark. Elevation of the systolic pressure occurs in more than half the cases, but diastolic hypertension is no more common than in the general population. Hepatomegaly occurs in about half the cases and splenomegaly in over three fourths.

The red blood cells frequently number from 7 to 10 million or more per cubic millimeter when patients are first seen. The erythrocytes usually appear normal, but the hemoglobin value may be increased less, in proportion, than the erythrocyte level because of a low mean corpuscular volume and mean corpuscular hemoglobin. Sometimes there is hypochromia (low mean corpuscular hemoglobin concentration) in addition to microcytosis, especially after large hemorrhages or repeated phlebotomies. The reticulocyte percentage is usually normal, but the absolute number is increased. Reticulocytosis occurs, and normoblasts may appear in the blood, especially after hemorrhage. The leukocyte count is greater than 10,000 per cubic millimeter in more than half the patients; it is frequently over 25,000, and rarely as high as 50,000. Metamyelocytes and occasional myelocytes are seen in the blood. The platelets are usually increased in number, and counts as high as 3 million and even 6 million have been reported (counts above 3 million are now rarely encountered when modern "direct" platelet counting techniques are employed). The serum bilirubin levels, urine urobilinogen, and stool urobilin values are commonly slightly increased. The bone marrow in polycythemia vera classically shows hyperplasia involving all the cellular elements, orderly maturation, and decreased or absent stainable iron. By contrast, in secondary polycythemia the marrow hyperplasia involves only the erythroid cells, and iron stores tend to be normal. There are many exceptions to these classic concepts and, in actual practice, bone marrow examination is of lim-

ited differential diagnostic value. Determination of the *absolute red blood cell volume* is the single most important procedure in establishing the diagnosis. Unless the red blood cell volume is greater than 38 ml per kilogram for males and 36 ml per kilogram for females, the diagnosis of polycythemia vera cannot be considered established. The serum uric acid concentration may be greatly elevated in either primary or secondary polycythemia.

Among the common complications of the disease are the vascular thromboses already referred to; the incidence of such thromboses can be greatly reduced by adequate therapy. Cirrhosis of the liver and occlusion of the hepatic veins *(Budd-Chiari syndrome)* have been observed. Hemorrhage from varices in the esophagus, stomach, bowel, or rectum may be massive, as may be bleeding from duodenal ulcers, which occurs in 8 to 16 per cent of cases. Many patients with polycythemia vera, after an extremely variable interval ranging from a few years to over 20 years, develop compensated myeloid metaplasia. During this phase they usually have severe splenomegaly and occasionally considerable leukocytosis with the appearance of increasing numbers of immature granulocytic leukocytes in the blood. The red blood cell count and hematocrit may remain perfectly normal without therapy. This phase may last from six months to several years, and is usually followed by the development of myelofibrosis, progressive myeloid metaplasia, often with a leukemoid blood picture, and progressive anemia.

Treatment. The treatment of primary polycythemia is directed toward maintenance of a reasonably normal blood volume, viscosity, and thrombocyte level. When the hematocrit rises above 55 per cent, blood should be withdrawn. Myelosuppressive therapy should be employed (1) whenever, in order to keep the hematocrit below 55 per cent, it is necessary to withdraw blood so frequently that iron deficiency of sufficient degree to produce symptoms develops, or (2) when the platelet count rises significantly above normal.

Radioactive phosphorus therapy is a very effective means of suppressing excessive hematopoiesis; 3.5 to 5 mc intravenously (or 4.5 to 6.5 mc by mouth) is a reasonable dose. If too much radioactive phosphorus is given, leukopenia, thrombocytopenia, anemia, or any combination of these may develop. Further treatment should not be given for at least two or three months, for this length of time is required before the red blood cell counts stabilize. An additional, somewhat smaller dose of P^{32} may then be necessary. Once the blood has been restored to normal by such treatment, it is desirable not to give further radiation therapy for at least one year and preferably several years, occasional phlebotomies being resorted to in the meantime as necessary. It seems likely that such conservative therapy will minimize the danger of a radiation-induced acute leukemia. Control of the manifestations of polycythemia vera by radioactive phosphorus is so smooth that patients so treated have a greater number of symptom-free days than from any other form of treatment available.

Nitrogen mustard, triethylene melamine, busulfan, chlorambucil, cyclophosphamide, phenylalanine mustard, procarbazine, cytosine arabinoside, and hydroxyurea have all been used successfully to reduce excessive hematopoiesis in this disease; the first two drugs are seldom employed for this purpose any longer, and there are only limited data concerning the long-term effectiveness of the last three drugs. If chemotherapy is being employed as the only form of therapy, busulfan should probably be avoided, because it produces the most persistent and prolonged platelet depression. However, if the red blood cell level is being controlled by phlebotomies and the only indication for drug treatment is control of marked thrombocytosis, busulfan may be the drug of choice. Any of these drugs may also be used as an adjunct to P^{32} therapy in the occasional patient who develops severe thrombocytosis or progressive leukocytosis refractory to P^{32}. During therapy with any alkylating agent, much closer supervision of the patient is necessary than when P^{32} is used.

It is apparent that at present there are many different ways of treating this disease. The author believes that phlebotomy should be used as the primary method of control of the hematocrit; busulfan, chlorambucil, cyclophosphamide, or phenylalanine mustard should be used as an adjunct to phlebotomies when needed to control a markedly elevated platelet count; and P^{32} should be reserved for treatment of elderly patients, patients who cannot be seen by the physician at frequent intervals, and those rare patients who are refractory to other forms of treatment. Irradiation of the spleen, if it becomes uncomfortably large, may relieve the discomfort. Splenec-

tomy is contraindicated, because an increase in the platelet level with resultant fatal thrombosis may result. Elective surgery of any sort should never be done until the platelet and hematocrit levels have been restored to normal. If emergency major surgery is unavoidable in a polycythemic patient with very high hematocrit and platelet levels, an immediate phlebotomy and P^{32} administration can be done within half an hour; rapid ambulation of the patient after surgery is imperative. Allopurinol should be given to control hyperuricemia.

It is paradoxic that after blood has been withdrawn repeatedly over a period of many years, in the late stages of the disease transfusions are often necessary, because myelofibrosis develops.

Adamson, J. W., and Finch, C. A.: Erythropoietin in the polycythemias. Ann. N. Y. Acad. Sci., 149:560, 1968.

Jepson, J. H.: Polycythemia: Diagnosis, pathophysiology and therapy. Can. Med. Assoc. J., 100:271, 1969.

Klein, H.: Polycythemia—Theory and Management. Springfield, Ill., Charles C Thomas, 1973.

Lertzman, M., Frome, B. M., and Israels, L. G.: Hypoxia in polycythemia vera. Ann. Intern. Med., 60:409, 1964.

Modan, B., and Lilienfeld, A. M.: Polycythemia vera and leukemia—the role of radiation treatment. Medicine, 44:305, 1965.

Reinhard, E. H., and Hahneman, B.: The treatment of polycythemia vera. J. Chronic Dis., 6:332, 1958.

Section Six.   DISEASES OF THE WHITE BLOOD CELLS

759. NEUTROPHIL FUNCTION

S. J. Klebanoff

The primary function of the neutrophilic polymorphonuclear leukocyte is the phagocytosis and destruction of microorganisms, and this functional specialization is reflected in its unique morphologic and biochemical characteristics. The neutrophil develops in the bone marrow in a continuous process, beginning with the pluripotential stem cell and continuing through the committed stem cell, myeloblast, promyelocyte, myelocyte, metamyelocyte, and band cell to the fully segmented mature cell. The most important morphologic feature of the mature neutrophil is the abundance of membrane-bound cytoplasmic granules. At least two granule populations exist. Dense, relatively large granules which stain reddish purple with azure dyes (azurophil or primary granules) develop in the promyelocyte. These granules, which contain myeloperoxidase, basic proteins, acid mucopolysaccharides, and a number of acid hydrolases, are primary lysosomes. During the myelocyte stage smaller, less dense granules are formed which contain alkaline phosphatase, lactoferrin, collagenase, and lysozyme. These specific or secondary granules are free of acid hydrolases and thus are not lysosomes in the strict sense of the term. No further granule formation occurs beyond the myelocyte stage. Approximately three fourths of the granules of the mature neutrophil are of the specific (secondary) variety, and the remainder are azurophil (primary) granules. Subpopulations with more limited enzyme composition

have been described. The mature neutrophil has a relatively short life span. It disappears from the circulation at an exponential rate with a mean half-life of 6.5 hours. Its extravascular life span is a day or two. Some of the cells which leave the circulation are removed by the fixed macrophages of the liver and spleen. The remainder pass into the tissues or migrate to areas of direct contact with the environment (oral cavity, bronchotracheal tree, cervical canal).

The neutrophil response to microbial invasion can be divided into several stages: (1) chemotaxis, (2) phagocytosis, (3) intracellular killing, and (4) digestion (Fig. 1). Neutrophils are discharged from the bone marrow in large numbers, producing a leukocytosis. The total blood granulocyte pool (TBGP) normally consists of a circulating granulocyte pool (CGP) of actively circulating cells and a marginated granulocyte pool (MGP) of cells which are sequestered or marginated along the walls of small blood vessels. This latter process is accentuated in areas of inflammation. The neutrophil extends pseudopods between the endothelial cells of small venules, opening up a passageway through which it passes. The channel immediately closes behind it, and the neutrophil migrates by ameboid movement along an increasing concentration gradient of a specific chemotactic agent or agents. Chemotactic agents are formed in a number of ways: (1) Bacteria elaborate low molecular weight (approximately 1000) factors which are directly chemotactic for neutrophils. (2) The components of the complement (C) system are activated sequentially with the release of chemotactic factors. Bacterial antigens combine with specific antibody to form complexes which activate complement either by the "classic" pathway involving the first three functional complement components, C1, 4, and 2, or by

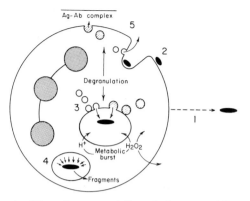

Figure 1. Schematic representation of the neutrophil response: (1) chemotaxis; (2) phagocytosis; (3) intracellular killing; (4) digestion; (5) extracellular enzyme release.

the "alternate" or properidin pathway which bypasses the early complement components. Activation by the "alternate" pathway also occurs when complement reacts with the endotoxic lipopolysaccharides of gram-negative bacteria. Three complement-derived components, C3a, C5a, and the trimolecular complex C567, have chemotactic activity. C5a is the predominant chemotactic factor in activated serum. (3) Proteinases released by bacteria, leukocytes, or damaged tissue act directly on complement components without activation of the entire complement sequence. C5 and C3 are cleaved to form the neutrophil chemotactic factors C5a and C3a. (4) Initiation of the kinin-generating and fibrinolytic pathways by Hageman factor activation results in the formation of kallikrein and plasminogen activator, respectively, which are chemotactic.

The chemotactic stimulus brings the neutrophil into direct contact with the microorganism, and phagocytosis rapidly follows. Cellular pseudopods surround the organism and isolate it from the extracellular environment in a vacuole lined by the invaginated cell membrane. A number of virulent organisms resist phagocytosis by virtue of the nature of their capsular material. These organisms are ingested when they can be trapped against a surface by the leukocyte (surface phagocytosis) or when the antiphagocytic nature of the capsular material is neutralized. Substances which react with particles to render them more susceptible to phagocytosis are termed opsonins. They may be heat stable or heat labile. Specific antibodies to surface antigens function as heat-stable opsonins. They attach to the bacterium through the antibody combining site on the F(ab')$_2$ portion and to the phagocyte through the Fc portion of the antibody molecule. The heat-labile opsonins are derived largely from complement, particularly C3. They are polyspecific and are not dependent on previous exposure to the organism. C3 when activated (C3b) attaches both to the bacterial cell wall and to receptor sites on the surface of the phagocyte. In general, antibody and complement combine to prepare the particle for ingestion, antibody serving both to identify the invading organism and to initiate adjacent complement activation.

Phagocytosis initiates a sequence of morphologic and biochemical events which result in the death of most ingested organisms. The granules adjacent to the phagocytic vacuole fuse with the vacuole, the common membrane ruptures, and the granular contents are discharged into the vacuolar space. All granular types

participate in the degranulation process. The metabolic machinery of the neutrophil is geared primarily to the production of energy (ATP) for chemotaxis and phagocytosis and to the production of H_2O_2 for microbicidal activity (Fig. 2). Energy production is dependent on glycolysis; it occurs in the absence of oxygen. H_2O_2 production, on the other hand, is dependent on the burst of metabolic activity which is associated with phagocytosis. There is an increase in glucose oxidation, particularly by the hexosemonophosphate (HMP) shunt. This is measured by the conversion of glucose carbon 1 to CO_2. There is a lesser increase in the conversion of glucose carbon 6 to CO_2 which measures the oxidation of glucose via the glycolytic pathway and Krebs cycle. Glycogen, which is present in large amounts in the neutrophil as particulate deposits, is broken down at an accelerated rate. Oxygen consumption is increased many fold and H_2O_2 is formed, possibly through a superoxide anion intermediate. Formate oxidation serves as a measure of H_2O_2 formation. Lactic acid production and phospholipid turnover also are increased.

Studies of the enzymic mechanisms responsible for the metabolic burst have focused on the oxidase responsible for the increased oxygen consumption and H_2O_2 production and on the link between this oxidase and the activation of the HMP shunt. The first two enzymes of the HMP shunt, glucose-6-phosphate dehydrogenase (G-6-PD) and 6-phosphogluconate dehydrogenase, reduce NADP to NADPH, and the continued activity of the shunt is dependent upon the reoxidation of NADPH. There are two prevalent views: (1) Oxygen is converted to H_2O_2 by NADH oxidase, a soluble enzyme which utilizes the NADH formed in the glycolytic pathway, and the H_2O_2 so formed activates the HMP shunt by a sequence of reactions, the oxidation of GSH by glutathione peroxidase and the reduction of GSSG by glutathione reductase, which result in the reoxidation of NADPH. (2) A granular NADPH oxidase is activated which meets the total requirements of the metabolic burst—increased oxygen consumption, H_2O_2 formation, and NADPH oxidation. The H_2O_2 formed by these or other mechanisms reacts with myeloperoxidase in the vacuolar space to form a microbicidal system (see below), whereas cytoplasmic components are protected from excess H_2O_2 by the glutathione system and by catalase.

A number of granular components released into the

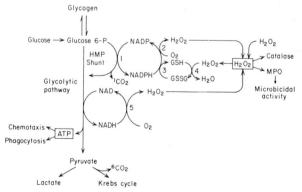

Figure 2. Leukocyte metabolism: (1) glucose-6-phosphate dehydrogenase and 6-phosphogluconate dehydrogenase; (2) NADPH oxidase; (3) glutathione reductase; (4) glutathione peroxidase; (5) NADH oxidase.

phagocytic vacuole during the degranulation process have antimicrobial properties. These include cationic proteins, lactoferrin, lysozyme, and myeloperoxidase. The pH in the vacuole falls, and H_2O_2 accumulates. Myeloperoxidase combines with H_2O_2 and a halide such as iodide or chloride to form a potent antimicrobial system which is effective against bacteria, fungi, viruses, and mycoplasma. Chloride ions are present in the leukocyte in excess, and small amounts of iodide are absorbed from the extracellular fluid or are released by the deiodination of the thyroid hormones. When iodide is the halide employed, iodination of the microorganisms occurs, and the extent of the iodination in intact leukocytes is a measure of the activity of this system in situ. H_2O_2 or other products of oxidative metabolism have some antimicrobial activity in the absence of myeloperoxidase. The ingested organisms vary in their sensitivity to the intravacuolar microbicidal systems. Some organisms (e.g., pneumococci) are susceptible to acid, whereas others (e.g., lactobacilli) are acidophilic; some are readily lysed by lysozyme, whereas most organisms resist the action of this enzyme; some organisms (e.g., streptococci, pneumococci) secrete H_2O_2 or acid into the vacuolar space, and this contributes to their own destruction, whereas others contain catalase and thus resist H_2O_2-dependent systems. The level and variety of the antimicrobial systems endow the neutrophil with an overkill capacity which allows it to function adequately despite a decrease in the activity of one of the systems. The death of the ingested organisms is followed by their digestion to low molecular weight fragments by acid hydrolases.

Although the neutrophil primarily serves a protective function, tissue damage may result from the release of granule components into the extracellular fluid because of cell disintegration, leakage during phagocytosis, or secretion when leukocytes are in contact with antigen-antibody complexes on a nonphagocytizable surface (Fig. 1). Neutrophil-mediated injury is seen in the Arthus and Shwartzman reactions and in experimental immune complex disease. In man, it may contribute to the tissue damage in acute glomerulonephritis, polyarteritis nodosa, rheumatoid or gouty arthritis, and transplantation rejection.

Karnovsky, M. L.: Chronic granulomatous disease—pieces of a cellular and molecular puzzle. Fed. Proc., 32:1527, 1973.

Klebanoff, S. J., and Hamon, C. B.: Role of myeloperoxidase-mediated antimicrobial systems in intact leukocytes. J. Reticuloendothel. Soc., 12:170, 1972.

Mayer, M. M.: The complement system. Sci. Am., November 1973, p. 54.

Stossel, T. P.: Phagocytosis. N. Engl. J. Med., 290, 717, 774, 833, 1974.

Ward, P. A.: Leukotactic factors in health and disease. Am. J. Pathol., 64:521, 1971.

760. NEUTROPHIL DYSFUNCTION SYNDROMES

S. J. Klebanoff

Metchnikoff over 70 years ago proposed that the destruction of microorganisms by "microphages" is essential to the host defense, and the increased incidence of infection in severe neutropenia or agranulocytosis fully

Neutrophil Dysfunction Syndromes

Defects of chemotaxis
Defects of phagocytosis
Defects of microbicidal activity
  H_2O_2 deficiency
    Hereditary
      Chronic granulomatous disease (CGD)
        X-linked
        Autosomal
      Familial lipochrome histiocytosis
      Severe leukocytic G-6-PD deficiency
    Acquired
  Myeloperoxidase deficiency
    Hereditary
    Acquired
Mixed defects
  Granule dysfunction
    Hereditary
      Chédiak-Higashi syndrome
    Acquired
      Toxic granulation

supports this thesis. What has become apparent within the past decade is that neutrophils may be present in adequate numbers in the bloodstream, yet still be unable to perform their function adequately. Defects have been described involving several aspects of the neutrophil response, namely, chemotaxis, phagocytosis, and microbicidal activity (see accompanying table).

DEFECTS OF CHEMOTAXIS

Decreased chemotaxis may result from a cellular defect in which the leukocytes are incapable of responding appropriately to a chemotactic factor, from a serum defect in which formation of chemotactic factors in the patient's serum is decreased, or from the presence of an inhibitor of chemotaxis in serum. A combined cellular and serum defect may exist. Chemotaxis is evaluated in vivo by the skin window technique and in vitro by the Boyden chamber technique. In the *skin window technique*, coverslips, applied to areas of abraded skin, are replaced at intervals, and the cells which have adhered to their undersurface are stained and counted. The cells which enter the lesion during the first six hours are predominantly neutrophils, after which mononuclear cells predominate. The *Boyden chamber* consists of two compartments separated by a membrane filter. The leukocytes present in one compartment migrate through pores in the filter under the influence of a chemotactic agent and are counted.

A cellular defect in chemotaxis has been described in the lazy leukocyte syndrome, congenital ichthyosis, the Chédiak-Higashi syndrome, newborn infants, diabetes mellitus, rheumatoid arthritis, some patients with acute infection, particularly those with toxic granulation, and in other isolated cases. A serum defect in the generation of chemotactic factors is seen in newborn infants, hereditary C2 deficiency, C3 hypercatabolism, C5 dysfunction, systemic lupus erythematosus, and diabetes mellitus. An inhibitor of chemotaxis is found in the serum of patients with cirrhosis and in the serum of isolated patients with multiple infections. Normal serum contains a chemotactic factor inactivator which is decreased in α1 antitrypsin deficiency.

The *lazy leukocyte syndrome* is characterized by low-grade fever, neutropenia, and recurrent gingivitis, stomatitis, and otitis media. The response of the patient's neutrophils to a chemotactic stimulus is decreased, as are random mobility (i.e., mobility in the absence of a specific chemotactic stimulus) and the release of granulocytes from the bone marrow. The formation of chemotactic factors in the patient's serum, however, is normal.

Job's syndrome is characterized by recurrent "cold" superficial staphylococcal abscesses, eczematous dermatitis, hyperkeratotic nails, and high IgE levels. Extensive neutrophil function studies failed to reveal a metabolic or microbicidal defect, suggesting that Job's syndrome should not be included as a variant of chronic granulomatous disease. A cellular defect in chemotaxis has recently been found in this condition as well as in some other patients with high IgE levels.

DEFECTS OF PHAGOCYTOSIS

Decreased phagocytosis may be due to a cellular defect or to a deficiency or dysfunction of either immunoglobulin or complement resulting in decreased opsonic activity. A cellular defect in phagocytosis has been described in some patients with diabetes mellitus, systemic lupus erythematosus, chronic myelocytic leukemia, myelofibrosis, and megaloblastic anemia. The sera of patients with hypo- or agammaglobulinemia have decreased levels of heat-stable opsonins resulting in an increased susceptibility to infection by encapsulated bacteria.

The opsonic activity of complement is dependent largely on C3. *C3 deficiency* with decreased opsonic activity is seen in systemic lupus erythematosus and progressive glomerulonephritis. Newborn infants, particularly with low birth weight, have decreased serum opsonic activity related either to C3 deficiency or to lack of transplacental transfer of IgM. Hereditary defects involving C3 include homozygous C3 deficiency and essential hypercatabolism of C3. The latter has been subdivided into Type I associated with a deficiency in the C3 inactivator KAF (conglutinogen activating factor), and Type II caused by the enhanced activity of a C3 inactivating enzyme. The patient's serum was deficient in a number of complement-mediated functions, namely, bactericidal activity and opsonic activity, and in the generation of chemotactic factors, resulting in an increased susceptibility to infection with pyogenic bacteria. The administration of normal serum or, in some instances, purified C3 produced a temporary increase in C3 levels with restoration of the complement-mediated functions. *C5 dysfunction* is found in infants with a syndrome consisting of generalized seborrheic dermatitis, intractable severe diarrhea, recurrent local and systemic infections, usually with gram-negative organisms, and marked wasting and dystrophy (*Leiner's syndrome*). Total hemolytic complement activity is normal, as is the level of the individual complement components. However, dysfunction of C5 is indicated by inability of the serum to opsonize particles dependent on C5 for optimal opsonization and reversal of this defect with purified C5. The generation of chemotactic factors in serum is defective in some patients.

The serum in *sickle cell disease* is deficient in heat-labile opsonins for pneumococci. It has normal levels of immunoglobulin, total complement, and the opsonic components of complement (C3, C5). A 5–6S pseudoglobulin of normal serum restores the opsonic activity of sickle cell serum. Decreased splenic clearance resulting from functional splenectomy also contributes to the decreased resistance to the pneumococcus in sickle cell disease.

CHRONIC GRANULOMATOUS DISEASE

Definition. Chronic granulomatous disease (CGD) is characterized by repeated and severe infection affecting lymph nodes, skin, lung, liver, bone, and many other tissues. *Staphylococcus aureus* and certain low-grade gram-negative organisms are the predominant pathogens. Tissue examination reveals multiple abscesses and granulomas and characteristic lipid-filled macrophages. The neutrophils (and monocytes) of these patients fail to kill certain ingested bacteria or fungi normally, and this is correlated with impaired leukocyte metabolic activity.

Incidence. CGD is a rare disease seen predominantly in males. Although generally found in infants and children, it is also seen in young adults.

Pathology. Miliary abscesses, varying in size from a few millimeters to several centimeters in diameter with occasional large abscesses, are seen on gross examination. Although any tissue may be involved, liver, spleen, lung, and lymph nodes are particularly susceptible. Patchy areas of hemorrhage and necrosis are common. Microscopic examination reveals evidence of an acute and a chronic inflammatory response; indeed, their coexistence is suggestive of CGD. An influx of polymorphonuclear leukocytes with abscess formation is seen, particularly in early lesions. Granulomas are a prominent feature, with areas of central necrosis surrounded by numerous plasma cells, lymphocytes, macrophages, and a few multinuclear giant cells. Tissue macrophages may be large with a foamy or vacuolated cytoplasm containing a characteristic yellow-brown lipid material. In some patients, the lipid-laden macrophages dominate the histologic picture, whereas, in others, only an occasional cell is seen. The organisms most commonly found in the lesions are staphylococci, enteric bacilli (Klebsiella-Aerobacter organisms, *Escherichia coli, Serratia marcescens,* Pseudomonas, Proteus, Salmonella, and Paracolon bacilli), and certain fungi (Candida, Aspergillus). Conspicuous by their rarity or absence from the lesions are β-hemolytic streptococci, pneumococci, and *Hemophilus influenzae*.

Pathogenesis. CGD is characterized by impaired host defense against certain microorganisms. Immunoglobulin levels are normal or elevated, and delayed hypersensitivity is unimpaired. Leukocytosis, with a high proportion of neutrophils, is characteristic of CGD as it is of infection in the general population. The peripheral neutrophils are morphologically indistinguishable from normal cells, although toxic granulation may be seen with longstanding infection. Chemotaxis and phagocytosis are unimpaired; however, the neutrophils do not kill normally those microorganisms generally found in the lesions. Other organisms (e.g. streptococci, lactobacilli, pneumococci) are readily killed by the patient's cells. This microbicidal defect is associated with a marked decrease in the phagocytosis-induced metabolic burst. The role of H_2O_2 deficiency in the microbicidal defect is emphasized by the improvement in microbicidal activity in vitro on the introduction of an H_2O_2-generating system into the cell. Indeed, those organisms which are killed well by CGD leukocytes generate H_2O_2, and their susceptibility to the intracellular microbicidal systems is due partly to the replacement of a defective leukocytic H_2O_2-generating system with H_2O_2 of microbial origin. The variability in the clinical course and in the mode of transmission suggests that different intraleukocytic molecular lesions can result in decreased H_2O_2 production and microbicidal activity. Several have been described. Leukocyte NADH oxidase activity was decreased in some patients, and two female patients were deficient in leukocyte glutathione peroxidase. Neutrophil dysfunction is also associated with a severe leukocytic deficiency of glucose-6-phosphate dehydrogenase, which is discussed later in this chapter.

A decrease in the intraleukocytic microbicidal activity results in the prolonged intracellular survival of ingested organisms. These sequestered organisms are protected from certain antimicrobials and from extracellular microbicidal systems, and multiplication and dissemination occurs. The organisms spread via the lymphatics and the bloodstream to the second line of defense, the fixed cells of the mononuclear phagocyte system. Lymphadenopathy and hepatosplenomegaly result. It is not known whether a defect exists in the fixed macrophage; however, its precursor, the blood monocyte, has decreased microbicidal activity. The fixed macrophages are unable to control the spread of infection, and miliary abscesses result.

Clinical Manifestations. CGD is characterized by repeated, severe, and widespread infections with staphylococci and certain gram-negative pathogens. Chronic suppurative lymphadenitis is the most common feature, with cervical lymphadenitis often its first manifestation. Enlargement of the inguinal, axillary, mesenteric, and mediastinal nodes also occurs regularly. The initial and most striking feature in some patients is a refractory eczematoid dermatitis, particularly around the eyes, nose, mouth, and other body orifices. Stomatitis, conjunctivitis, and persistent rhinitis occur with regularity. Wounds often are infected. Pneumonitis is seen in most patients, although it may be a late manifestation. The lesion progresses from a patchy bronchopneumonia with hilar node enlargement to massive consolidation, involving the entire lobe or lung. Lung abscesses are common, and pleural effusion and empyema may occur. A distinctive roentgenologic finding in some patients is discrete, usually round, homogeneous areas of consolidation ("encapsulating" pneumonia). The pulmonary lesions run a protracted course, leading in some instances to progressively increasing pulmonary insufficiency and death. Hepatosplenomegaly is a consistent feature of the disease. Liver scans may reveal focal lesions, either abscesses or sterile granulomas. Chronic subphrenic abscesses occur frequently. Osteomyelitis, often at multiple sites, is common. The metacarpal and metatarsal bones are particularly susceptible; however, the large bones may also be involved. A feature of the osteomyelitis of CGD is absence of sclerosis. Complete healing occurs with long-term antimicrobial therapy. Gastrointestinal manifestations include persistent, often bloody diarrhea, nausea, anorexia, and abdominal pain. Perianal and perineal abscesses with fistula formation occur frequently. Pigmented lipid histiocytes and granulomas with giant cells are seen in rectal biopsies. Pericarditis may occur, and anemia, either hypochromic microcytic or normochromic normocytic, is found in almost all patients.

Diagnosis. Any patient with severe staphylococcal or gram-negative infections since childhood who has normal or elevated immunoglobulin and WBC levels and normal delayed hypersensitivity should be suspected of having CGD. The diagnosis can be made with confidence by neutrophil function tests. A simple and commonly employed procedure is the nitroblue tetrazolium (NBT) reduction test. NBT is reduced to a blue-black substance (blue formazan) with low solubility by neutrophils activated by phagocytosis or exposure to endotoxin. Precipitation of formazan can be visualized microscopically or the dye extracted and measured spectrophotometrically (quantitative NBT reduction test). NBT is not reduced by CGD leukocytes. The leukocytes of many non-CGD patients with bacterial infection have increased spontaneous NBT reduction, i.e., NBT reduction in the absence of phagocytosis. A false negative result in this test should suggest the possibility of CGD. The diagnosis of CGD is confirmed by a decrease in leukocytic microbicidal activity, oxygen consumption, glucose C1 oxidation, formate oxidation, or iodination. The microorganism employed in the measurement of microbicidal activity is important, because the defect is selective, affecting staphylococci, gram-negative pathogens, and certain fungi.

Genetic Transmission. The most common form of CGD exhibits *X-linked* transmission. The affected children are males, and the mother and approximately 50 per cent of female siblings are carriers. The female carrier of the abnormal X chromosome has two populations of granulocytes, one with normal metabolic and microbicidal activity and a second with the same defect as affected children (Lyon hypothesis). When the leukocytes of carriers are treated as a single population, intermediate activity in the neutrophil function tests is observed. Two populations of cells are seen in procedures (slide NBT test, radioautographic iodination test) which measure the activity of individual cells. The presence of a variant or variants of CGD with *autosomal* inheritance is indicated by female patients, particularly female siblings with clinical and laboratory findings similar to those of the X-linked variety.

Clinical Manifestations in Female Carriers of X-Linked CGD. Unequal X inactivation may result in a preponderance of defective cells and in an increased incidence of infection. This, however, is rare in proved carriers, who are generally healthy. A chronic lupus-like illness, sometimes limited to the skin lesions of discoid lupus but on other occasions characterized by a more systemic disease, with arthralgia, cutaneous manifestations of lupus erythematosus, photosensitivity, fever, Raynaud's phenomenon, and recurrent stomatitis, has been noted in several CGD carriers. Tests for antinuclear antibodies are negative.

Therapy. The treatment of CGD remains the vigorous treatment of infection, namely antimicrobial administration and surgical drainage or excision. Both should be instituted promptly and antimicrobial administration maintained until healing is complete. Surgical excision of circumscribed suppurative lesions, e.g., lymph nodes, is preferable to incisional drainage, because the latter heals slowly with seeding at other sites. There are two considerations in the choice of antimicrobial agent: (1) sensitivity of the microorganism and (2) ability of the antimicrobial to reach and destroy the intracellular organisms. Viable microorganisms sequestered within intact leukocytes are protected from the lethal effects of many antimicrobials. The preferred antimicrobial based on sensitivity should be used despite poor penetrance, to combat extracellular organisms. Rifampin, which readily penetrates into leukocytes, is effective against sensitive intracellular staphylococci in vitro and in animal models, but has not yet been proved effective in man. It should be used in conjunction with other antimicrobials to minimize the development of resistance. Continuous antimicrobial therapy during periods of remission may be beneficial. Granulocyte transfusion has been advocated for life-threatening infections.

Whole blood transfusions may be required when the anemia is severe. The coexistence of CGD and the very rare Kell phenotypes, Kell null (K_0) or McLeod, has been observed in five patients, suggesting an association between the two genetic loci. Such patients are sensitized by transfusions with blood containing Kell antigens, making subsequent transfusions difficult. The Kell phenotype of patients with CGD should be determined, and those with either K_0 or McLeod phenotypes should not be transfused unless a compatible blood is available or the clinical situation warrants the risk of sensitization. Most patients with CGD have normal Kell antigens.

Prognosis. In some patients, the disease is apparent within the first year of life and progresses relentlessly, with remissions measured in weeks or months to death within the first decade. In others, there is a relatively late onset and long periods of remission measured in years.

Variants of Chronic Granulomatous Disease

Variants of CGD have been described which can be separated from "classic" CGD by clinical and/or laboratory findings but which have in common a leukocytic microbicidal defect caused by decreased oxidative metabolism.

Familial Lipochrome Histiocytosis. Three female siblings have been described with splenomegaly, pulmonary infiltration, hypergammaglobulinemia, arthritis, and an increased susceptibility to infection. The most striking histologic feature was the presence of numerous large, pigmented lipid-filled histiocytes. As in CGD, the patients' leukocytes were defective in microbicidal activity and in phagocytosis-induced oxygen consumption, glucose C1 oxidation, formate oxidation, NBT reduction, and iodination. This condition differed from "classic" CGD, not only in sex affected but also in the late onset of symptoms, absence of a chronic granulomatous response, and occurrence of arthritis.

Severe Leukocytic Glucose-6-Phosphate Dehydrogenase Deficiency. Patients with glucose-6-phosphate dehydrogenase (G-6-PD) levels which are 20 per cent of normal or greater do not have an increased incidence of infection and have leukocytes with normal metabolic and microbicidal activity. This includes all patients with the common African Gd A⁻ variant of G-6-PD who have normal leukocyte G-6-PD activity and most patients with the Mediterranean Gd B⁻ variant who have a partial deficiency of leukocyte G-6-PD. Patients with leukocyte G-6-PD levels of 5 per cent of normal or below, however, have neutrophil dysfunction and increased susceptibility to infection. The leukocyte abnormality differs from the more common variants of CGD in that the decrease in hexosemonophosphate shunt activity is not reversed by methylene blue. Further, the metabolic and microbicidal defect is not as severe, which correlates well with the milder clinical course. All the patients described have chronic nonspherocytic hemolytic anemia.

MYELOPEROXIDASE DEFICIENCY

Neutrophils in a normal human blood smear contain an abundance of peroxidase-positive granules. Myeloperoxidase (MPO) deficiency is indicated by a decrease in this peroxidase reaction. It may be hereditary or acquired.

Hereditary MPO Deficiency. Six patients from four families with a complete absence of MPO from neutrophils and monocytes have been described. The eosinophil peroxidase is present in normal amounts. The leukocytes are otherwise morphologically indistinguishable from normal cells. Genetic studies suggest autosomal recessive inheritance. Of these patients, four were reported to be in good health, the clinical history of one was not described, and one had severe disseminated candidiasis which began in adulthood and responded well to amphotericin B therapy. MPO-deficient leukocytes have decreased fungicidal and bactericidal activity despite normal phagocytosis, although the defect is not as severe as in CGD. Iodination also is impaired; however, in contrast to CGD, there is not a decrease in phagocytosis-induced NBT reduction, oxygen consumption, glucose C1 oxidation, or formate oxidation.

Acquired MPO Deficiency. Acquired MPO deficiency may involve all or a portion of the neutrophils; myeloperoxidase may be undetectable or decreased in amount, and the deficiency may be permanent or temporary. It has been observed in some patients with severe untreated bacterial infection, in acute encephalitis lethargica Economo, in a few patients with refractory megaloblastic anemia, and in some patients with acute myelogenous leukemia, chronic myelogenous leukemia with blast-cell transformation, or myelomonocytic leukemia. When tested, the microbicidal defect in the isolated leukocytes was comparable with that found in hereditary MPO deficiency.

THE CHÉDIAK-HIGASHI SYNDROME

The Chédiak-Higashi syndrome is a rare autosomal recessive disease characterized by the presence of giant lysosome-like granules in all granule-containing cells. It is seen in man, mink, cattle, and mice. Less than 100 cases have been described in man, with a roughly equal proportion of males and females. Its main clinical features are (1) partial oculocutaneous albinism with photophobia, rotatory nystagmus, and hair with a characteristic silken sheen when exposed to light; (2) repeated febrile episodes resulting chiefly from staphylococcal infections of the skin, lungs, and upper respiratory tract; and (3) a lymphoma-like "accelerated phase," with widespread tissue infiltration by lymphoid and histiocytic elements, characterized by lymphadenopathy, hepatosplenomegaly, neutropenia, hypogammaglobulinemia, hemolytic anemia, a bleeding tendency caused by thrombocytopenia and coagulation factor deficiencies, and peripheral neuropathy.

The diagnosis of the Chédiak-Higashi syndrome is made by demonstration of giant granules in circulating leukocytes. In the bone marrow, abnormally large, pleomorphic, azurophil (primary) granules are seen in promyelocytes which undergo a series of fusions to form giant granules containing myeloperoxidase and acid phosphatase. The specific (secondary) granules develop normally. The bone marrow neutrophil reserve is low, and neutropenia is common, particularly in the accelerated phase when lymphocytic infiltration of the bone marrow is apparent. The presence of giant granules in mature neutrophils is associated with some impairment in function. Chemotaxis, as measured by migration into a skin window in vivo or by the response to a preformed chemotactic agent in vitro, is decreased. Phagocytosis and the related metabolic burst are unimpaired; indeed, an increase in the initial rate of phagocytosis has been reported. However, degranulation with the release of the contents of the giant granules into the phagocytic vacuole is delayed or absent, and a delay in the killing of some bacterial species has been described. These abnormalities in neutrophil function combine to increase the susceptibility of the patients to pyogenic infections. The partial albinism is a consequence of the abnormal distribution of melanin in giant melanosomes, and the neurologic manifestations are associated with a lymphohistiocyte infiltration in the region of the degenerated peripheral nerves. Giant lysosomes are seen in both peripheral and central nervous system elements.

Treatment. The infections generally respond to conventional antimicrobial therapy, and the anemia and hemorrhagic tendency to multiple blood or platelet transfusions. The low serum folic acid levels and megaloblastic bone marrow changes can be corrected by folic acid therapy. Treatment of the accelerated phase with combined vincristine and prednisone administration has been advocated. Death usually occurs within the first two decades owing to infection but less commonly to hemorrhage or to the extensive lymphocytic infiltration of the accelerated phase.

Baehner, R. L.: Disorders of leukocytes leading to recurrent infection. Pediatr. Clin. North Am., 19:935, 1972.

Blume, R. S., and Wolff, S. M.: The Chédiak-Higashi syndrome: Studies in four patients and a review of the literature. Medicine, 51:247, 1972.

Dossett, J. H.: Microbial defenses of the child and man. Pediatr. Clin. North Am., 19:355, 1972.

Good, R. A., Quie, P. G., Windhorst, D. B., Page, A. R., Rodey, G. E., White, J., Wolfson, J. J., and Holmes, B. H.: Fatal (chronic) granulomatous disease of childhood: A hereditary defect of leukocyte function. Semin. Hematol., 5:215, 1968.

Johnston, R. B., Jr., Lawton, A. R., III, and Cooper, M. D.: Disorders of host defense against infection. Pathophysiologic and diagnostic considerations. Med. Clin. North Am., 57:421, 1973.

Klebanoff, S. J.: Intraleukocytic microbicidal defects. Ann. Rev. Med., 22:39, 1971.

Lehrer, R. I.: The role of phagocyte function in resistance to infection. Calif. Med., 114:17, 1971.

Nathan, D. G., and Baehner, R. L.: Disorders of phagocytic cell function. Prog. Hematol., 7:235, 1971.

Quie, P. G.: Infections due to neutrophil malfunction. Medicine, 52:411, 1973.

761. THE LEUKOPENIC STATE AND AGRANULOCYTOSIS

William N. Valentine

Leukopenia exists when a reduction below about 4000 per cubic millimeter occurs in the total blood leukocytes. Although the differential count may remain essentially normal, much more frequently the neutrophils are disproportionately low and the terms *neutropenia* or *granulocytopenia* are more accurately descriptive. *Lymphopenia* exists when the lymphocytes number below about 1400 per cubic millimeter in children or 1000 per cubic millimeter in adults. Although severe leukopenia merges into *agranulocytosis* with its frequently fulminant clinical manifestations, the more moderate and usual degrees of leukopenia are often well tolerated. No hard and fast rule exists, and host factors as well as the numbers of monocytes influence the incidence and severity of infections. In general, subjects with absolute granulocyte counts of 500 to 1000 per cubic millimeter have moderately increased risks, whereas below this the invasion of mucous membranes, skin, and blood by microorganisms becomes increasingly frequent and severe. With absolute counts below 200 per cubic millimeter, severe infectious complications become the rule.

Etiology and Pathogenesis. The kinetics of leukopoiesis have been more difficult to approach experimentally than those of erythropoiesis. In granulocytic leukopoiesis three compartments exist: the marrow, the circulating blood, and the body tissues in general. The marrow consists of a mitotic compartment containing cells capable of division and a postmitotic compartment composed of a reservoir of mature, nondividing cells in numbers perhaps 15 to 20 times as great as those present in the peripheral blood. This "ready reserve" can be rapidly mobilized, and its availability provides a source of additional granulocytes while granulopoiesis is increasing in response to sustained increases in demand. The total intravascular granulocytes are thought to be normally about twice those calculated from leukocyte counts and blood volume. Some are margined along vessel walls, but are in rapid equilibrium with actively circulating cells. The normal granulocyte circulating half-time in man appears to be about six to seven hours, and once granulocytes exit into the tissues there is little evidence of return to the intravascular compartment. The extravascular life span of leukocytes is difficult to ascertain, but in the steady state it has been estimated that there may be some 20 times as many tissue granulocytes as intravascular granulocytes. The numbers of circulating leukocytes are a result of their rate of production, rate of exodus from the blood to extravascular tissue, and rate of destruction. In the long term, supply and demand must be equal if normal balance is to be maintained; in the short term, excesses of demand may temporarily be met by drawing on the marrow reserve pool of mature granulocytes. The feedback mechanisms by which control is modulated are not fully understood. However, the techniques for in vitro culture of marrow in soft media have demonstrated that the formation of distinct colonies containing granulocytic and monocytic cells requires the presence of a "colony stimulation factor" (CSF). Variations in CSF presumably affect net granulopoiesis and may constitute one mechanism of control. However, there are probably multiple stimulatory and inhibitory controls modulating production rate, maturation, and release of granulocytes into the blood. At present, assessment of granulocytopenia depends upon evaluation of marrow cellularity, the marrow myeloid to erythroid cell ratios, the distribution of marrow granulocytes of different stages of maturation, the response of marrow cultures to various levels of CSF and to graded doses of bacterial endotoxin, and sophisticated granulocyte labeling procedures necessary in assessing leukocyte life span outside the marrow. The difficult availability and partial inadequacy of these procedures often render the peripheral leukocyte total and differential count the principal modality for evaluating granulocytopenia.

The granulocytopenic state may result, then, from (1) interference with normal marrow production of leukocytes and their delivery to the periphery, (2) increased utilization and destruction of granulocytes in the circulating blood and tissues other than marrow, or (3) combinations of the above. In addition, redistribution of leukocytes among the various body pools may result in relative or pseudogranulocytopenia when peripheral white cell counts form the basis of the evaluation.

Those disorders *interfering with normal granulopoiesis* can be subclassified. The marrow may be aplastic or hypoplastic on an idiopathic basis. There may be a similar lack of granulocyte precursors owing to exposure to ionizing radiation or certain drugs which predictably have cytolytic effects and interfere with marrow function on a dose-related basis. Such drugs include many of the chemotherapeutic agents used in the treatment of neoplasia or in producing immunosuppression: the alkylating agents such as nitrogen mustard, cyclophosphamide (Cytoxan), chlorambucil (Leukeran), and their congeners, busulfan (Myleran), procarbazine which interferes with deoxyribonucleic acid (DNA) polymerization, and the mitosis inhibitors such as vinblastine and vincristine sulfate (Velban and Oncovin). Chemotherapeutic agents which act as antimetabolites have similar effects. Among these are purine and pyrimidine antagonists such as cytosine arabinoside (Ara-C), 6-mercaptopurine, azathioprine (Imuran), thioguanine and 5-fluorouracil, and the folic acid antimetabolites such as methotrexate. The commonly employed phenothiazines have been intensively investigated, and appear to produce marrow aplasia or hypoplasia through inhibition of DNA synthesis, with resulting prolongation of marrow granulocyte generation time and reduction in cell division. Although adverse reactions are related to dose, there is considerable variation in host susceptibility. Mepazine and promazine have been relatively more frequently implicated than chlorpromazine. Other drugs whose administration carries a relatively or moderately high risk of causing either acute or chronic granulocytopenia and diminished granulopoiesis include the antithyroid drugs such as thiouracil, and to a lesser extent propylthiouracil and methimazole (Tapazole); the antimicrobials chloramphenicol, sulfonamides, and arsenobenzols; the anti-inflammatory agent phenylbutazone; and such therapeutic agents as gold preparations. Although adverse reactions to sulfonamides and the antithyroid drugs have some relationship to dose and duration of therapy, there are again wide variations in host susceptibility. For most of the other agents mentioned, idiosyncratic reactions appear to provoke granulocytopenia in certain sensitive individuals without much obvious relationship to dosage. This is particularly true of the severe aplasia produced by chloramphenicol, which, although rare, is chronic and often irreversible. This contrasts with the much more frequent occurrence of reversible and usually inconsequential leukopenia in many subjects receiving the drug. Other drugs at times producing granulocytopenia include the antidepressant dibenzazepine compounds such as imipramine; the antidiabetic drugs tolbutamide, chlorpropamide, and carbutamide; and the chinchona alkaloids such as quinidine. More rarely reported apparent offenders are procainamide, quinacrine (Atabrine), tripelennamine (Pyribenzamine), ethacrynic acid, thiazides, allopurinol, and various antimicrobial drugs. The list of offending or possibly offending agents is large and expanding. Exposure to environmental agents such as benzol, other solvents, insecticides, and sprays likewise carries the risk of quantitative granulopoietic depression. The hazards of exposure to benzol are particularly well documented.

In some disorders, *granulopoiesis is ineffective,* and there is increased intramarrow leukocyte death and inadequate delivery of granulocytes to the circulating blood despite normal or even increased cellularity of myeloid precursors. Ineffective granulopoiesis and granulocytopenia may be present at times in subjects with refractory anemia, leukemia, and other myeloproliferative disorders. They are classically present in folate and vitamin B_{12} deficiency states, and may be induced by drugs which impair absorption (diphenylhydantoin) or interfere with the metabolism (methotrexate) of substances such as folic acid. Certain other antimetabolites in large doses produce an aplasia and, in smaller doses, a hypercellular marrow characterized by a variety of morphologic abnormalities and degenerative changes. Alcohol ingestion in large amounts may at times produce a similar picture.

Granulocytopenia and/or agranulocytosis may also result from *replacement of normal marrow elements* by fibrous tissue, by leukemic blasts, by plasma cells in multiple myeloma, by lymphocytes in lymphosarcoma, and, more rarely, by carcinoma cells in large numbers.

Finally, there are certain *hereditary or familial disorders* characterized by impaired production of granulocytes. In *infantile genetic agranulocytosis,* there is a usually severe granulocytopenia, although the marrow contains abundant myeloid precursors. Late myeloid forms are conspicuously absent or severely reduced, however. Neutrophil survival has been reported as normal. *Familial benign chronic leukopenia* is a rare condition with little increased susceptibility to infection. Marrows are cellular, but late granulocytic precursor cells (bands and segmented forms) are reduced. *Cyclic neutropenia* is characterized by periodic, recurring episodes of severe granulocytopenia with intervening intervals of complete normality. Its familial nature has been sometimes demonstrable and sometimes not. Its cause is unclear. It has been suggested that there is mild marrow failure with the periodicity regulated by feedback mechanisms. During periods of granulocytopenia, the myeloid marrow elements are hypoplastic, and mature forms beyond the myelocyte are markedly reduced in number. In certain heritable conditions, granulocytopenia has coexisted with other abnormalities. In *pancreatic insufficiency with neutropenia,* a hyperplastic marrow, neutropenia, and deficient exocrine pancreatic secretion coexist. The disorder is not X chromosome linked. *Neutropenia with immunoglobulin abnormalities* is probably familial, and is associated with hypogammaglobulinemia and a cellular marrow. *Myelokathexis* is an unusual syndrome in which a high proportion of myeloid precursors in marrow have severe degenerative changes. The ineffective granulopoiesis and evidence of increased intramarrow death of granulocytes are also accompanied by shortened peripheral life span of granulocytes. In some cases of the *Chédiak-Higashi syndrome,* a disorder characterized by defective lysosomal membranes, ineffective granulopoiesis also appears to be present.

In contrast to defective production, granulocytopenia may also result from *increased utilization and destruction* of leukocytes, even in the presence of normal marrow function. *Infections* are common causes: bacterial (typhoid and paratyphoid fever, brucellosis, tuberculosis, and overwhelming infections even with microorganisms characteristically producing leukocytosis); viral (influenza, measles, infectious mononucleosis, infectious hepatitis, rubella); rickettsial, at times; protozoal (malaria, relapsing fever, kala-azar). *Splenic dysfunction* and almost any condition associated with splenomegaly may result in leukopenia alone or in combination with anemia or thrombocytopenia, or both. Thus leukopenia is frequently found in congestive splenomegaly caused by portal vein hypertension, in certain collagen vascular disorders such as lupus erythematosus and Felty's syndrome (rheumatoid arthritis, splenomegaly, and leukopenia), in Gaucher's disease, and in granulomatous disorders and lymphomas with splenic involvement. A nonhereditary, splenomegalic disorder of unknown cause, *primary splenic neutropenia,* has also been reported to be due to increased peripheral destruction of leukocytes. *Neonatal immunization neutropenia* is a somewhat controversial entity, thought by some to be secondary to fetomaternal leukocyte incompatibility and transplacental passage of a specific leukoagglutinin from mother to fetus. Others question its existence as an established entity.

Certain drugs (amidopyrine is the prime example, but sulfonamides, phenylbutazone, and gold have been implicated in rare instances) act as haptens and elicit antibodies leading to neutrophil destruction and severe agranulocytosis *(agranulocytic angina).* The initial administration of the drug does not cause agranulocytosis for at least 7 to 14 days, and sensitization may not develop for weeks or months. The experiments of Moeschlin convincingly support an immune mechanism of this type in the pathogenesis of amidopyrine-induced agranulocytosis. Blood from a sensitized subject receiving this drug and administered to a normal recipient promptly produced severe neutropenia in the latter. Further, agglutination of both homologous and heterologous leukocytes occurred when they were exposed to plasma from a sensitive subject receiving amidopyrine. The serum of a sensitized donor is totally inactive in the absence of the sensitizing drug. It is postulated that the agglutinated leukocytes are destroyed and lysed, perhaps mainly in the lungs. Although the explosive production of agranulocytosis by other drugs has often been attributed to a similar mechanism, this often is not the case, and the phenomenon is probably considerably rarer than originally believed. In this reaction to amidopyrine, not only is there profound destruction of granulocytes in the periphery, but granulocytic precursors in marrow are also temporarily eliminated.

Often the etiology of granulocytopenia is multifactorial. Thus infections may suppress marrow function by toxicity, by interference with metabolism of substances such as folic acid, and by causing accelerated leukocyte destruction. Nutritional deficiencies may interfere with leukocyte production and simultaneously result in production of defective cells with shortened life span. Antibodies may damage both marrow precursors and circulating granulocytes. Lymphomatous involvement of marrow and spleen may lead to the coexistence of diminished granulopoiesis and accelerated peripheral destruction of white cells.

Although the clinician most commonly equates the term leukopenia with granulocyte deficiency, certain lymphopenic states are also associated with profound susceptibility to infections. Thus lymphopenia is observed in hereditary thymic aplasia (hereditary lympho-

penia or Swiss type of agammaglobulinemia) commonly in conjunction with agammaglobulinemia. Affected children are liable to progressive viral infections and susceptibility to generalized vaccinia after vaccination; death usually occurs before the age of two years. Less severe or episodic lymphopenia has also been documented in other hereditary defects involving the thymus-dependent lymphocyte. These include the Wiskott-Aldrich syndrome, ataxia telangiectasia, and certain patients with "immunologic amnesia" in whom a complement-dependent lymphocytotoxic factor could be demonstrated in the serum during episodes of lymphopenia. In these situations, the lymphopenia is related to an underlying defect in the cellular immune mechanism which renders the patient extremely susceptible to bacterial, viral, protozoan, or fungal infections. In certain forms of Hodgkin's disease lymphopenia may be severe and anergy present.

Incidence. Agranulocytosis has become increasingly common with the proliferation of marrow-damaging chemotherapeutic agents utilized in the treatment of neoplasia and in immunosuppressive therapy, and by the more aggressive use of multi-drug therapy in malignancy. Indeed, with many protocols employed in the treatment of leukemia as one example, a period of agranulocytosis is accepted as the expected event to be endured prior to any evidence of remission. With other types of medication, agranulocytosis occurs in only a small number of patients exposed even to those drugs that cause the greatest number of cases. The gravity of complication rather than its frequency accounts for its great importance. Estimates of frequency have varied widely, but a recent estimate of phenothiazine-induced agranulocytosis has been 1 case in 1200 treated. Similarly, antithyroid drugs have been reported to cause this complication in about 4 of 1000, and chloramphenicol in as few as 0.01 per 1000 cases treated. The absolute frequency of agranulocytosis caused by each agent is a function of its rate of occurrence in those at risk and the frequency of its use in the general population. Although agranulocytosis occurs with a worldwide distribution, its induction by drugs or environmental factors parallels that of exposure of the population to offending agents.

Pathology. In granulocytopenias caused by underlying disease, the pathology of bone marrow and extramedullary tissues is that secondary to the disorder. Marrow may be replaced by fibrous tissue or by foreign or abnormal cells, or may be hypoplastic or aplastic. On the other hand, a hyperplastic but dysplastic marrow may accompany ineffective agranulopoiesis in certain leukemias, refractory anemias, and other myeloproliferative disorders. The myeloid precursors may exhibit vacuolization, asynchronous cytoplasmic-nuclear maturation, and other morphologic abnormalities. In vitamin B_{12} and folate deficiency, the marrow is hypercellular, and megaloblastic erythropoiesis is present, together with abnormal granulocytes such as giant metamyelocytes. In granulocytopenias in which peripheral leukocyte destruction is the predominant mechanism, the marrow granulocytes are most commonly increased, though with a paucity of mature forms owing to exhaustion of the marrow postmitotic reserve pool. In drug-induced agranulocytosis of the amidopyrine type, the marrow changes vary with the stage of the disease. Megakaryocytes and erythroid precursors are present in normal abundance. At the height of severe agranulocytosis, granulocytic elements, including myelocytes and metamyelocytes, are greatly reduced or absent. The prevalence of blast forms may erroneously arouse the suspicion of leukemia. In later stages, or in milder cases, there may be normal or hyperplastic granulocytopoiesis with a preponderance of less mature precursor cells. The marrow picture in agranulocytosis induced by the phenothiazines in its severe form is one of extreme aplasia. In the rare but exceedingly serious disorder sometimes induced by chloramphenicol, the chronic aplasia involves all cell series. In severe agranulocytosis, ulcerative lesions in the mouth, rectum, skin, and elsewhere are necrotic and contain large numbers of bacteria, but granulocytes are conspicuously absent. If death occurs as the granulocytic elements are returning to the blood, abscesses may make their appearance at affected sites. The localization of tissue reactions to invading microorganisms determines the remaining pathologic changes.

Clinical Manifestations. In leukopenia without infectious complications, the clinical manifestations either are nonexistent or are those of an underlying disorder. In acute, drug-induced agranulocytosis of the amidopyrine type (agranulocytic angina), the onset of the disease is sudden, usually with chills, high fever, and prostration. This pattern was initially regarded as being due to bacterial invasion, but since symptoms may follow within an hour of drug administration, the initial manifestations of this type of drug-hapten-antibody reaction are probably due to the period of rapid granulocyte lysis. Similar pyrogenic reactions occur in the absence of infection in patients developing antibodies and reactions against homologous leukocytes as a result of repeated transfusions. These prodromal symptoms, either mild or severe, are often followed by a brief but variable period in which fatigue, prostration, and neutropenia persist, but no new symptoms develop. This second stage is followed by return of fever, chills, and headache, frequently with ulceration of the oral pharynx and sometimes of the rectum and vagina, and manifestations of sepsis. This third stage is concomitant with bacterial invasion of the tissues, the most frequent lesions occurring at the sites where bacterial flora normally flourish in the absence of infection. In agranulocytosis not associated with an immunologic mechanism of the amidopyrine type, initial symptoms may represent invasive infection per se. In severe agranulocytosis of any etiology, fever is often as high as 40 or 40.5° C and prostration is extreme. In the absence of treatment or of spontaneous recovery, mental confusion, stupor, and death frequently supervene within the next few days. The ulcerated lesions are covered with a dirty gray membrane, but gross pus and abscesses are absent. Bacilluria may occur in the absence of pyuria. Regional lymph nodes become enlarged, pneumonitis may develop, and hypotension and hyperventilation may be prominent. Death is usually due to massive infection, often with gram-negative bacilli. The peripheral blood has few if any granulocytes, and these few, when present, usually show pyknotic nuclei, vacuolization, and toxic granulation. In acute, self-limited forms of agranulocytosis such as those often induced by amidopyrine, antithyroid drugs, phenothiazines, and sulfonamides, erythrocytes and platelets are usually normal. When hematopoiesis is widely depressed, other cytopenias coexist with lack of granulocytes. In amidopyrine-induced *agranulocytic angina* as well as in many other drug-caused agranulocytoses, if the offending agent is withdrawn, the granulocytopenia usually persists for five to ten days. Immature granulocyte precursors reappear in the marrow before return of mature

cells to the peripheral blood and tissues. A transient monocytosis and appearance of a few myelocytes often herald the beginning of recovery, the percentage of myelocytes sometimes being as high as 10 to 15 per cent. In a few days the white blood cell count rises rapidly to normal levels, or substantial leukocytosis may supplant the leukopenia.

In other circumstances in which severe neutropenia or agranulocytosis is slightly less severe, develops more slowly, or continues on a chronic basis, the onset of symptoms may be less explosive, and the course more indolent or fluctuating. In *cyclic neutropenia* the usual history is that at intervals of 15 to 35 days but most frequently at about 21 days, the patient experiences a few days of fever, oral ulceration, or skin infection corresponding with the development of profound neutropenia. The neutropenia usually lasts three to four days, during which time granulocytes may disappear from the blood. A compensatory monocytosis is sometimes present. Between the cyclic attacks, which most often develop in infancy or childhood, but which may have a later onset, affected subjects are completely well. Some of the hereditary disorders such as *infantile genetic agranulocytosis,* transmitted as an autosomal-recessive disorder, are very severe, with early onset, frequent infections, and usually early death. In some, such as *familial benign chronic leukopenia,* there is little increased susceptibility to infection and neutropenia is modest.

Differential Diagnosis. In the differential diagnosis of granulocytopenia and agranulocytosis, the history, physical examination, and marrow examination are crucial. Acute aleukemic leukemia and aplastic anemia are associated with characteristic marrow changes and usually with pancytopenia. Underlying disease in the form of neoplasia, collagen-vascular disorders, infections, and the presence of hepatosplenomegaly is defined by the history and physical examination and by laboratory studies. The history of drug ingestion or exposure to hazardous environmental agents is obviously of great importance. The familial or cyclic nature of certain granulocytopenias may also afford clues pointing to the correct diagnosis.

Prognosis. Prognosis depends upon the nature and severity of the underlying disorder and the granulocytopenia itself, upon the self-limited duration or chronic persistence of granulocytopenia, upon the initiation of proper antimicrobial and other therapy, upon the presence or absence of associated erythrocyte and platelet depression, and upon the potential reversibility of the lack of granulocytes. Before the advent of antimicrobial drugs, mortality in severe agranulocytosis, such as that associated with certain coal tar derivative drugs in Germany and the United States in the 1920's and early 1930's, was 50 to 90 per cent. This approached 100 per cent in patients over 60 years of age or with less than 1000 leukocytes per cubic millimeter. At present, with early and proper antimicrobial management most patients recover. Another factor clearly influencing prognosis is the recognition of offending drugs or environmental agents and their complete, immediate withdrawal.

Treatment. Patients with mild neutropenia without infection require only observation. Patients with sustained neutropenia are often managed on an ambulatory basis, sometimes with intermittent hospitalization for acute episodes of infection or for treatment of underlying disease. All patients with significant neutropenia should be carefully instructed on avoidance of crowds or undue exposure to infection in any form, on reporting promptly any untoward symptoms or febrility, and on the proper hygiene of skin, nails, and mucous membranes. Skin tests should be performed to provide information as to the patient's ability to express cellular immunity, and immunoglobulin levels of serum should be measured.

When agranulocytosis is detected, the patient should be hospitalized immediately even in the absence of signs of infection, because the earliest possible institution of antimicrobial therapy with the first indication of infection is important for survival. If infection or ulcerative mucous membrane lesions develop, early cultures of the lesions, the blood, the urine, and, if indicated, the cerebrospinal fluid are desirable, and should be repeated as indicated by the clinical course. Antimicrobial therapy should be directed toward broad coverage, and should not be withheld until the cultural results are known. However, therapy may require modification when the predominating organisms have been identified. It is, of course, important that all organisms cultured be tested for antimicrobial susceptibility. In many instances, the infecting organisms are those constituting "normal flora" rendered invasive by the presence of agranulocytosis in the patient. However, any microorganisms may be offending, and the possibility of sepsis with gram-negative organisms such as Pseudomonas and Proteus or with penicillin-resistant staphylococci must be recognized by the treatment regimen. For sepsis of unidentified type a satisfactory regimen includes gentamicin, 1.5 mg per kilogram of body weight every eight hours intravenously if the kidneys are functioning normally. The dosage should be reduced in subjects with uremia, but the drug may still be used with careful observation of renal function. In addition, 2 grams of cephalothin every four hours or 450 mg of 7-chlorolincomycin phosphate every six hours, both intravenously, should be administered. In patients with fulminant sepsis, 2 to 4 grams of carbenicillin every three hours intravenously may be used as a third drug. In many forms of acute agranulocytosis caused by drugs, the clinician can take some comfort that *if the offending agent is withdrawn,* agranulocytosis, and hence antimicrobial therapy, will be self-limited. In cases of doubtful etiology, *all* even remotely etiologic drugs should be withdrawn. The patient with agranulocytosis should be hospitalized in a single room, nurses or physicians with respiratory or other infections excluded, and visitors rigidly limited or excluded temporarily. The necessity for total "reverse isolation" with cap, gown, and mask precautions is advocated by some; but in the opinion of the writer, it is of doubtful efficacy if the regimen recommended above is employed. Nevertheless, in studies conducted in special facilities and dealing with severely neutropenic patients over prolonged periods (chiefly those being treated with extended chemotherapy), more stringent measures, employing "life islands" or laminar airflow rooms, vigorous measures to reduce skin and intestinal flora, and even sterilization of food, have probably further reduced intercurrent infections. Such facilities exist in only a few centers.

In patients in whom marrow function can be reasonably expected to return after agranulocytosis induced by therapy, every effort is required to support the patient during the critical period when granulocytes are absent. Neutrophil replacement by transfusion has proved to have some efficacy, but replacement of functional neutrophils in beneficial numbers is not feasible presently in most hospitals. However, in a few centers an increasing number of continuous-flow centrifuges designed to harvest leukocytes and platelets from large amounts of blood of compatible donors are being employed. Such harvesting techniques are becoming increasingly available, and may be a practical factor in the management of more cases of agranulocytosis in the not-too-distant future. The same can be said for currently experimental procedures such as marrow transplantation in subjects with leukemia and aplastic anemia. There is also increasing interest and, hopefully, potential for practical usefulness in techniques designed to bank or store patient's marrow for future use when it is expected that marrow function will be depressed or ablated by chemotherapy or radiation. These technical advancements, not yet available for most hospitals, are being increasingly evaluated for practicality and efficacy. In the meantime, transfusion of whole blood and separated platelets are of benefit when concomitant anemia and severe thrombocytopenia are present.

Granulocytopenia resulting from arsenic and gold may be treated by administration of BAL (British antilewisite; 2,3-dimercaptopropanol) in dosage of 1.5 ml of a 10 per cent solution in oil intramuscularly every four hours for two days, followed by similar dosage at 12-hour intervals for an additional eight to ten days. Of considerable importance in the treatment of agranulocytosis are attention to proper mouth care with frequent cleansing washes, avoidance of constipation and attendant anal abrasions by means of gentle enemas, and the maintenance of proper fluid balance by parenteral fluid administration when indicated. When the disorder is of short duration, maintenance of nutrition is usually not a major problem. Of great importance is the detection of an offending agent and its absolute prohibition at any future time.

Boggs, D. R.: The kinetics of neutrophilic leukocytes in health and disease. Semin. Hematol., 4:359, 1967.

Crosby, W. H.: How many "polys" are enough? Arch. Intern. Med., 123:722, 1969.

Finch, S. C.: Granulocyte disorders—benign, quantitative abnormalities of granulocytes. *In* Williams, W. J., Beutler, E., and Erslev, A. J. (eds.): Hematology. New York, McGraw-Hill Book Company, 1972, pp. 628–654.

Kostman, R.: Infantile genetic agranulocytosis. Acta Paediatr. Scand., 45 (Suppl. 105):6, 1956.

Kretschmer, R., August, C. S., Rosen, F. S., and Janeway, C. A.: Recurrent infections, episodic lymphopenia, and impaired cellular immunity. N. Engl. J. Med., 281:285, 1969.

Moeschlin, S.: Immunological granulocytopenia and agranulocytosis (clinical aspects). Sang, 26:32, 1955.

Morley, A. A., Carew, J. P., and Baikie, A. G.: Familial cyclical neutropenia. Br. J. Haematol., 13:719, 1967.

Pisciotta, A. V.: Immune and toxic mechanisms in drug-induced agranulocytosis. Semin. Hematol., 10:279, 1973.

Wiseman, B. K., and Doan, C. A.: Primary splenic neutropenia: A newly recognized syndrome, closely related to congenital hemolytic icterus and essential thrombocytopenic purpura. Ann. Intern. Med., 16:1097, 1942.

762. LEUKEMOID REACTIONS

Richard T. Silver

A leukemoid reaction is defined as a clinical syndrome in which changes are found in the peripheral blood suggesting leukemia. Usually, the white blood cell count is elevated, but a picture resembling leukemia may develop even when the white blood cell count is normal or reduced.

The most important distinction between a leukemoid reaction and leukemia is that the former is not an unregulated proliferation of leukocytes but an expression of a bone marrow response to some underlying cause. Thus the peripheral blood and bone marrow abnormalities return to normal when the cause has disappeared. Leukemoid reactions involve any of the white blood cells and can occur in a variety of diseases caused by bacterial and viral infections, allergy, poisonings, and malignancy, as well as in acute conditions such as hemolytic anemia, in hemorrhage, and after burns. It is unclear why certain leukemoid reactions are seen in some patients and some diseases and not in others. Leukocyte stimulatory and maturation factors and leukocyte kinetics are not well defined. Different types of leukemoid reactions occur with the same frequency as those cells which appear in the peripheral blood. Thus neutrophilic leukemoid reactions are most frequent; lymphocyte and then eosinophilic leukemoid reactions are next most common; and monocytic leukemoid reactions are relatively infrequent.

Neutrophilic leukemoid reactions are associated with neutrophilic granulocytic hyperplasia in the marrow. Such increases in neutrophilic leukocytes are seen, for example, in certain types of acute bacterial infections, acute hemolytic anemias, and metastatic disease of the bone marrow. Often, there is shift toward immaturity in both the marrow and the peripheral blood, for increased numbers of metamyelocytes and myelocytes are observed. Vacuoles and heavy, coarse granules may be seen in the cytoplasm of the granulocytes. Differentiation of a neutrophilic leukemoid reaction from chronic granulocytic leukemia is difficult if based only upon microscopic examination of the peripheral blood and bone marrow. Abnormalities suggestive but not diagnostic of chronic granulocytic leukemia include an increased platelet count (and correspondingly increased megakaryocytes in the marrow), increased numbers of circulating basophils and eosinophils, slight marrow fibrosis, and complete obliteration of marrow fat spaces. Anemia is less helpful in differentiating a benign from a malignant elevation of the white blood cell count, because it may be related either to the leukemia or to the disease causing the leukemoid reaction. Much more useful is the leukocyte alkaline phosphatase (LAP) score of the mature neutrophils in the peripheral blood. It is difficult to attribute an elevated white blood cell count to a leukemoid reaction unless there is a significant increase in the LAP score, whereas in the typical case of chronic granulocytic leukemia, the LAP score is low. Striking elevations of serum B_{12} and its binding proteins which are found in chronic granulocytic leukemia are rarely seen in neutrophilic leukemoid reactions, and this test can be helpful in differential diagnosis.

Leukemoid reactions should be readily distinguishable from acute granulocytic leukemia, even though in the latter disease the LAP score may also be increased. In a leukemoid reaction, the marrow shows relatively good preservation of erythropoiesis and granulocytes in all stages of maturation. There is no diffuse replacement of normal cellular elements by abnormal, immature cells as occurs in acute leukemia. *Auer rods,* usually considered strong morphologic evidence for acute granulocytic leukemia, have been seen in leukemoid reactions associated with disseminated tuberculosis.

Eosinophilic leukemoid reactions are often seen in parasitic and collagen-vascular diseases and in drug reactions. They are accompanied by eosinophilic proliferation in the marrow with a shift toward immaturity, and eosinophilic myelocytes and metamyelocytes may be observed. Eosinophilic (granulocytic) leukemia is indeed a rare clinical entity. Thus when a patient is observed with a high white blood cell count and a predominance of eosinophils, the condition is far more likely to represent a benign proliferation. It is noteworthy that eosinophils do not have alkaline phosphatase activity. Hence, in contrast to neutrophilic cells, eosinophilic leukemoid reactions and chronic eosinophilic leukemia cannot be distinguished by using the LAP determination.

Leukemoid reactions involving lymphocytes are seen, for example, in whooping cough, chickenpox, and infectious mononucleosis. In these conditions, the peripheral blood contains an increased number of lymphocytes, many of which are atypical and are known as "virocytes." There is considerable morphologic heterogeneity in contrast to the singular lymphocyte type seen in acute lymphocytic leukemia. The cytoplasm is vacuolated, and the cell border is serrated and wavy. Nuclear configuration and staining characteristics range from dark, clumped chromatin to lighter and more open or vesicular patterns. Most often, the bone marrow does not show a marked increase in lymphocytes or suppression of erythropoiesis or thrombopoiesis. Therefore marrow examination may be quite useful in excluding acute lymphocytic leukemia. Helpful distinction in diseases such as infectious mononucleosis, for example, may be made by utilizing serologic tests such as the heterophil reaction.

Striking increase in number of peripheral blood monocytes occurs infrequently, and rarely should cause difficulty in distinction from myelomonocytic or monocytic leukemia. Monocytosis has been seen in disseminated tuberculosis, in brucellosis, in other granulomatous diseases, and during marrow recovery after the vigorous use of chemotherapeutic drugs.

No therapy is required for a leukemoid reaction per se, although obviously the underlying condition should be appropriately treated. In those few but difficult instances in which it is initially impossible to distinguish a leukemoid reaction from leukemia, specific treatment must be deferred until the situation has clarified. The premature use of potent drugs in a patient without a primary hematologic malignancy is far more hazardous than deferring the onset of chemotherapy in a patient who subsequently proves to have leukemia.

763. THE ACUTE LEUKEMIAS

James F. Holland

Definition. The acute leukemias are a group of neoplasms which are manifest in the bone marrow. They are characterized by cells analogous to, and often individually indistinguishable by light microscopy from, normal immature hematopoietic cells. In the untreated state, acute leukemic cells enter the blood, where they usually become the predominant leukocyte, and invade other organs. The untreated disease leads to death after a brief and stormy illness, rarely lasting more than a year. Therapy has markedly altered prognosis, however, and the name "acute" as distinguished from "chronic" leukemia is no longer wholly descriptive.

Acute myelocytic leukemia arises from the marrow hematopoietic stem cell or its progeny; the term subsumes several subtypes of leukemia: *myeloblastic leukemia, promyelocytic leukemia, myelomonocytic leukemia, acute myelocytic leukemia* that is none of the foregoing, and *erythroleukemia*. Special forms of acute myelocytic leukemia often occur as the terminal events of chronic myelocytic leukemia, polycythemia vera, and myelofibrosis. Acute "pure" *monocytic leukemia* (Schilling) is characterized by monoblastic proliferation which can be distinguished cytochemically. Acute lekemias apparently derived from eosinophilic, megakaryoblastic, plasmablastic, and mast cells, although uncommon, display unique characteristics as well as some features in common with the other acute leukemias of marrow origin.

Acute lymphocytic leukemia arises in lymphoid tissue and is ordinarily first manifest by its presence in marrow. In some instances thymic infiltration precedes overt marrow disease, but it is not known whether the initial leukemogenic event in man is usually extramedullary. Many instances of lymphocytic lymphosarcoma and histiocytic lymphoma culminate in an acute leukemic phase which bears some resemblance to acute lymphocytic leukemia.

Acute leukemias and related lymphoreticular neoplasms occur throughout the vertebrate animals; examples are even known in some invertebrates. In the mouse, the species most extensively studied, a single transplanted leukemic cell can give rise to the full-blown disease. Removal of lymphoid target organs, such as thymus and spleen, causes a much higher frequency of acute myelocytic leukemia after leukemogenic viral infection than ordinarily would be the case. This indicates that host factors may in large part determine the type of leukemia which evolves.

Etiology.   The etiology of human leukemia has not been established. It is known that leukemias and related sarcomas of chicken, mouse, rat, hamster, guinea pig, cat, dog, cow, baboon, monkey, and gibbon are caused by RNA virus infection. In inbred laboratory mice the infection is not spread horizontally by contact, but transmission may occur through the germ line. Some selectively inbred strains such as AKR eventually develop leukemia in nearly every mouse. Mice may harbor and transmit the incorporated leukemic virus without manifestations of leukemia, allowing it to become apparent in progeny as if sui generis. In chickens, hamsters, and cats, horizontal leukemia or sarcoma *viral transmission* has been conclusively proved. The risk of neoplasm in healthy cats after known viral infection has been shown to be several hundredfold higher than in the general cat population.

When analyses are made of all cases of human acute leukemia, clusters in space and time cannot be shown. When analyses have been limited to children less than six years of age, however, significant clustering has been found in different parts of the world. Rare anecdotal instances of contact transmission are also provocative. Leukemic families have been reported in which several offspring have been affected. In one such family, fibroblasts from surviving members showed increased suscep-

tibility to transformation in vitro by SV 40 virus, a suggestive analogy to ease of induction of the neoplastic state in vivo.

Radiation leukemogenesis in man is well known. Radiologists sustained nearly tenfold the death rate from leukemia of other physicians before the widespread use of protective measures. Survivors of atomic bombings, patients who formerly were x-irradiated for spondylitis, and those who received therapeutic doses of ^{131}I for thyroid cancer all showed increased incidence of acute myelocytic leukemia. Patients with multiple myeloma, Hodgkin's disease, or other cancers, who were previously treated with alkylating agents, with or without x-irradiation, have increased frequency of acute myelocytic or acute histiocytic leukemia.

Chronic benzene exposure is leukemogenic in mice and can cause human acute myelocytic leukemia. Anecdotal data on other aromatic solvents suggest their possible human leukemogenicity, but less widespread use. Acute myelocytic leukemia has been reported after marrow aplasia induced by chloramphenicol and by phenylbutazone.

A few *constitutional diseases* lead to disproportionate frequency of acute leukemia. In trisomy 21 *(Down's syndrome)* both acute lymphocytic and acute myelocytic leukemia are increased. *Bloom's syndrome* characterized by chromosomal fragility and rearrangements, the pancytopenia of *Fanconi's syndrome*, and *idiopathic aplastic anemia* are sometimes followed by acute myelocytic leukemia. *Paroxysmal nocturnal hemoglobinuria* may represent a clonal stem cell disorder, first manifest by production of abnormal erythrocytes, culminating occasionally in acute myelocytic leukemia.

None of these data on family clusters, radiologic initiation, chemical induction, or constitutional predisposition are inconsistent with the possibility of underlying viral leukemogenesis in man. Available molecular biologic data from human experiments are essentially congruent with observations made in the known viral leukemias of mice. The discovery of an RNA-instructed DNA polymerase (reverse transcriptase) in the avian sarcoma and murine leukemia viruses was a monumental step. This enzymatic activity provides an explanation for the mechanism of transcribing oncogenic information from the RNA of an infecting virus into DNA polymers. Such heteropolymers can be incorporated into the host cell DNA, thereby introducing a heritable template for transcription in daughter cells. This provides information to maintain the neoplastic state and, under proper circumstances, to make new virus. The enzyme has been found in high concentration in every RNA oncogenic virus studied.

An RNA-instructed DNA polymerase has also been found in virtually every instance of fresh human acute leukemic cells. A DNA transcript prepared from the RNA of a murine leukemia virus underwent partial hybridization with RNA from human leukemic cells. This suggests that the human RNA had itself been transcribed from a DNA codon similar to the nucleic acid sequences of mouse leukemia.

An antibody to the purified reverse transcriptase of a known primate sarcoma virus cross-reacted with and inactivated the human enzyme, suggesting their near identity. In extracts of human acute leukemic cells, a virus-like particulate is found on centrifugation in a sucrose gradient, corresponding to the known density of murine leukemogenic viruses. On rupture of this particulate, reverse transcriptase activity is released. In the presence of labeled deoxynucleotide triphosphates, and using the RNA of the particulate as template, a DNA transcript is synthesized similar to the DNA transcribed from known primate sarcoma virus. In other experiments, the labeled transcribed DNA specifically hybridized with segments of DNA in human leukemic cells, but not in normal cells. This implies that nucleic acid sequences in the particular RNA template had been transcribed from sequences uniquely found in the DNA of the leukemic cell.

In two pairs of identical twins, each with one normal and one leukemic member, the patients' DNA's contained segments that hybridized with DNA transcribed from the 70s RNA recovered from particulates in the leukemic leukocytes. The normal twins had no such particle-related sequences in the DNA of their leukocytes. These data support the concept that the leukemia-associated DNA sequences were inserted after twinning, and not through the germ line.

These data, taken together, provide strong molecular biologic support for the viral etiology of human leukemia. Infectivity of the isolated particulate remains to be demonstrated. Since there is no proof of utility of laboratory animals or in vitro systems for this purpose, reservations must still be held until this investigative impasse is surmounted.

Pathogenesis. The recognizable leukemogenic event may precede clinical disease by many years. The time of appearance of the first leukemic cell and the interim behavior of the population of leukemic cells can only be inferred from data in man obtained during evident leukemia, or from animal models. Under the conditions of marrow crowding inherent in the fully developed leukemic state, the thymidine labeling index is substantially lower for leukemic blasts than for normal myeloblasts. This indicates that a large proportion of cells are not entering the DNA synthetic phase during the availability of labeled thymidine. It is clear evidence that many leukemic blasts are dividing slowly if at all. The largest leukemic myeloblasts or lymphoblasts are the cells which have the highest frequency of labeling. These large blasts mature, partially, to smaller blasts.

In some experimental murine leukemias, the doubling time progressively lengthens as the population density of cells becomes greater, thus deviating from exponential growth. This could be a result of lengthening of the cell cycle, cell death, and an increasing number of cells that do not divide. Some nondividing cells are sterile, whereas others may again be recruited into the mitotic cycle. Early in the pathogenesis of the human acute leukemic process, cells might divide more rapidly than normal cells, but this is usually not true when the disease has become advanced enough to measure.

Acute leukemic cells generally lack the appropriate metabolic programming for the physiologic aging that dictates leukocyte death or loss from the body across membrane surfaces. Such cells therefore accumulate, and, relatively insensitive to whatever humoral mechanisms control normal hematopoietic cell population size, they become an ever-increasing tumor that "spills over" into the blood. Normal immature hematopoietic cells are ordinarily excluded from the blood, perhaps because their nondeformability precludes traversing the interstices of the marrow sinusoids. Leukemia, in its literal sense, occurs late in the disease. The reason why immature acute leukemic cells eventually appear in the blood is not known; it probably depends on complex interactions with or invasion of the sinusoidal wall.

Myeloblasts demonstrate positive staining reactions for peroxidase and Sudan black which are negative in *lymphoblasts* and *monoblasts*. Myeloblasts do not stain, or at most have diffuse cytoplasmic periodic acid–Schiff (PAS) staining, whereas lymphoblasts often show large, coarse granules with this stain. Fluoride inhibits esterase activity of monoblasts for naphthol AS-D acetate, but not that of myeloblasts. Electron microscopic studies often show dissociation in nuclear and cytoplasmic age and other ultrastructural characteristics which distinguish leukemic blasts from other types of hematopoietic cells.

On direct preparations made from bone marrow, about half the patients with acute leukemia have a normal *karyotype*. This establishes that grossly visible chromosomal abnormalities are not essential in the pathogenesis. The half of patients with acute lymphocytic leukemia and half of those with acute myelocytic leukemia who have abnormal karyotypes (hyperdiploid for acute lymphocytic leukemia, hypo-, pseudo-, and hyperdiploid for acute myelocytic leukemia) are of great significance in studying pathogenesis. Indeed, in both major forms of acute leukemia, the aneuploid modal chromosome pattern disappears when a complete remission of the disease is achieved and is replaced by a normal karyotype. On relapse of the disease, the original leukemic karyotype reappears, almost without exception. This indicates that the acute leukemias are clones of abnormal cells, rather than abnormally functioning normal cells. This distinction has great importance when devising a therapeutic strategy.

The fact that cells are fundamentally abnormal does not preclude their demonstrating many normal characteristics, including maturation, albeit impaired. Leukemic cells form much smaller colonies of granulocytes and macrophages in agar cultures than do normal marrow cells, and then only in the presence of a glycoprotein colony-stimulating factor. Since the colony-stimulating factor(s) also enhance normal colony growth and are found in abundant quantity in the urine of some patients with acute myelocytic leukemia, a possible role of this bioregulatory substance in the evolution and pathogenesis of the leukemic state has been postulated.

The maturing granulocytes in acute myelocytic leukemia may have abnormal size and distribution of specific granules, sometimes appearing as a regional haze of eosinophilic dust. *Auer bodies* are highly refractile cytoplasmic rods derived from coalescence of azurophilic granules. They are seen in some of the myeloblasts or promyelocytes of about one third of patients with acute myelocytic leukemia. Rarely, these nearly pathognomonic markers are also seen in mature polymorphonuclear neutrophilic granulocytes of acute myelocytic leukemia, demonstrating that some maturation has occurred. The granulocytes of acute myelocytic leukemia show diminished migration across capillary membranes; this test also returns to normal during remission when granulocytes derive from the euploid stem cells.

In *acute lymphocytic leukemia*, it is commonplace to see different stages of lymphoid maturation in the marrow, up to and including lymphocytes morphologically indistinguishable from normal. The degree of immaturity of the predominant acute lymphocytic leukemic cell in the marrow is of prognostic importance. Patients with large primitive lymphoblasts do not respond so well as patients whose cells appear more mature.

The proliferation of acute leukemic cells in the marrow impairs normal hematopoiesis, even at population densities of leukemic cells when mechanical crowding alone cannot be responsible. One explanation relates this to inhibition of normal hematopoiesis by a hypothetical biochemical product of the leukemic cells. Alternatively, the affected cell in acute myelocytic leukemia may in fact be the early progenitor cell whose progeny are the stem cells for myeloblasts, erythroblasts, megakaryoblasts, and monoblasts. Leukemic proliferation of one cell might be associated with concomitant abnormalities of the other progeny, including hypoplasia. This interpretation would help explain the abnormalities in erythrocyte maturation commonly seen in acute myelocytic leukemia, which in the extreme are called *erythroleukemia*. In its end stages the natural evolution of erythroleukemia is for a clonal selection to myeloblastic proliferation. Megakaryocytes in acute myelocytic leukemia are also often bizarre in appearance and maturation, and their derived platelets may be abnormal.

Leukemic cells invade tissues; infiltration with enlargement of spleen, liver, and lymph nodes is common in all types of acute leukemia. Central nervous system leukemia, characterized by infiltration of the pia and arachnoid, occurs in about half the patients with acute lymphocytic leukemia and less frequently in acute myelocytic leukemia. It ordinarily becomes clinically manifest only in patients whose early death from hematologic manifestations of disease has been prevented by therapy. Leukostasis, infiltration of vascular walls, invasion into surrounding tissues, and hemorrhage occur particularly at high myeloblast counts, and may account for rapid death when the vessel is in the brain substance. Infiltrates of skin, testes, serosal membranes, and bone may be prominent. Enlargement of liver and kidney may also occur without infiltration by leukemic cells.

Acute myelocytic leukemic cells, particularly in promyelocytic leukemia, may secrete a vitamin B_{12}–binding protein in large quantity, accounting for high serum levels of B_{12}. Acute myelocytic leukemic cells, particularly those with monocytoid characteristics, may secrete *muramidase*. This low molecular weight lysosomal enzyme, also known as lysozyme, may appear in the urine, leading to tubular damage and renal insufficiency. In promyelocytic leukemia, and rarely in other types of acute myelocytic leukemia, secretion of thromboplastic substances accounts for the frequent (but not invariable) syndrome of disseminated intravascular coagulation, fibrinolysis, and major hemorrhage.

Epidemiology. The annual incidence per million of acute myelocytic leukemia is quite constant from birth throughout the first 10 years at about 10 cases. A slight peak in late adolescence occurs, and the incidence remains at a nearly constant 15 per million until age 55, after which the incidence progressively rises to 50 at age 75. This suggests some ubiquitous agent and cumulative injury.

The incidence of acute lymphocytic leukemia is sharply different. There is a peak incidence from 2 to 4 years reaching 50 per million annually, falling to 20 or less by age 8 until puberty, when the rate declines to about 10. The incidence remains below 10 until age 65, when it again climbs to about 15 per million at age 75.

These data are not inconsistent with an infectious disease with greatest susceptibility in childhood.

Numerous clusters of leukemia have been reported, although it has not been persuasively demonstrated that they occur more frequently than by chance. In three separate series, however, coincidences in time (within 60 to 75 days) and space (within 1 kilometer or 1 mile) have been seen in a total of 15 pairs of children less than six years old, sufficiently frequently to make their occurrence by chance highly improbable ($P \ll 0.01$). Of the 30 children involved, 27 were under four years. These occurrences, taken in conjunction with the virologic data aforementioned, are compatible with a contagious infectious origin of acute lymphocytic leukemia of young childhood. Further information about induction periods and periods of infectivity might provide additional clues that would bear on the appearance of leukemia in older patients.

Clinically, approximately 80 to 90 per cent of children with acute leukemia have acute lymphocytic leukemia, and 80 to 90 per cent of adults with acute leukemia have the acute myelocytic varieties.

Clinical Manifestations. The symptoms and signs of acute leukemia relate to decrease or disordered function of normal hematopoietic cells, and to tumefaction by leukemic cells.

Anemia. Asthenia, pallor, headache, tinnitus, dyspnea, angina, edema, and congestive heart failure may all indicate anemia. The anemia may result in part from diminished erythropoiesis; excessive hemolysis and blood loss are also often contributory. Evidence of specific antibody mediated hemolysis (positive Coombs test) is uncommon. Erythrocytes may show considerable variation in size and shape. Normoblasts and erythroblasts are common in the peripheral blood in erythroleukemia, but occasional nucleated red cells can also be seen in other types of acute leukemia.

Hemorrhage. Oozing gums, epistaxis, petechiae, ecchymosis, menorrhagia, melena, and excessive bleeding after tooth extraction are common initial manifestations of coagulation disorder in acute leukemia. Retinal hemorrhages, subarachnoid bleeding, and gross hematuria are rare initial manifestations, but may occur later. In nearly all instances the abnormal hemostasis can be correlated with decrease in circulating thrombocytes. Hemorrhagic manifestations are uncommon when circulating levels are above 50,000 per cubic millimeter; below this level, hemorrhage is inversely related to platelet count. Most thrombocytopenic bleeding occurs when platelets are 20,000 per cubic millimeter or less. Increased intravascular pressure (venous occlusion or dependency) augments the appearance of petechiae. Sepsis markedly accentuates thrombocytopenic bleeding, not only locally as in hemorrhagic pneumonia, but also systemically.

In promyelocytic leukemia, thromboplastic substances released from the cells can initiate disseminated intravascular coagulation which leads to activation of normal fibrinolytic systems and the appearance of fibrin split products in the blood. Massive ecchymosis and exsanguinating hemorrhage can occur if not promptly treated.

Infection. Acute leukemia is often first recognized by the occurrence of a respiratory infection from which the patient never fully recovers. Other bacterial infections are frequent before therapeutic control is attained: dental infections, sinusitis, bronchitis, pneumonia, perirectal abscess, urinary tract infections, paronychiae, and skin infections. Infections appear to be attributable to absolute granulocytopenia and, to some extent in acute myelocytic leukemia, to impaired function of the granulocytes present. Fever without recognizable infection is also common in acute leukemia, but this is always a diagnosis by exclusion. Every new fever in an acute leukemic patient could be the beginning of a bacterial infection with potential life-threatening consequences. Early, diligent, and repeated search is required before accepting an interpretation of "leukemic fever."

Infiltration. Lymphadenopathy, particularly of the cervical nodes in children, may be the first sign of the disease. It is often generalized. Splenomegaly is present in most patients with acute lymphocytic leukemia, and in about half of those with acute myelocytic leukemia. Hepatomegaly is usually present. Bulging interdental papillae are highly characteristic of acute monocytic or myelomonocytic leukemia. Tumefaction in bone may lead to bone or joint pain and tenderness. These are common in children, and the disease may present as a limp or protective restriction of motion. Confusion of acute leukemia with acute rheumatic fever was once common. Subepiphyseal decalcification in children and small areas of osteolysis may be recognized on x-ray films.

A diagnosis can be long delayed by failure to obtain a blood count. Pancytopenia without recognizably abnormal leukocytes is found in a small proportion of patients, the so-called aleukemic leukemia. Granulocytopenia with a normal number of circulating lymphocytes may occur in any kind of acute leukemia. Ordinarily, however, the peripheral blood contains immature myelocytic or lymphocytic cells, and the leukocyte count is elevated owing to the abnormal cells, sometimes in excess of 100,000 per cubic millimeter.

A suspicion or presumption of acute leukemia necessitates an examination of the bone marrow, because a diagnosis ordinarily cannot be established with certainty on peripheral blood findings alone. If cells are not obtained in adequate quantity (a circumstance that occurs from entrapment in reticulin fibers or cellular "packing"), a needle biopsy is also required. Other causes of hematologic disorders which mimic acute leukemia must be excluded. Among these are toxic cytopenias, isolated or multiple, and conditions such as infections, neoplasms, or marrow infiltrations that may lead to leukocytosis and to immature cells in the peripheral blood. The most commonly confused disorders are infectious mononucleosis, hematogenous tuberculosis, and drug-induced myelotoxicity. Drug-induced marrow aplasia may be succeeded by a marrow filled with myeloblasts. This normal cohort of repopulating cells matures in a few days, thus establishing the differential diagnosis.

Preleukemia is a term which has been applied to patients with symptoms and findings suggesting acute myelocytic leukemia but whose diagnosis cannot be established on the basis of the evidence then available. The marrow may be hypo-, normo-, or hypercellular. The change of marrow differential to a younger cell type, ordinarily with peripheral leukocytosis, may come suddenly after years of desultory mild illness. Adequate studies have not been performed to establish if karyotypic or other characteristics of neoplasia are present from the beginning.

Therapy. The treatment of acute leukemia is aimed at eradication or at least at marked destruction of the tumor, and at supporting the patient through manifestations of the disease per se, its complicating disorders, and the effects of therapy. The strategy of antileukemic treatment is conveniently divided into remission induction, sustaining or maintaining the remission, reinforcement of the remission, treatment of central nervous system disease, and, on an investigational basis, immunotherapy. Conversion of leukemic to normal or nonleukemic cells has not been achieved in vivo.

The possibility of cure of acute lymphocytic leukemia has become realistic. Although not yet at this level of accomplishment, chemotherapy of acute myelocytic leukemia is much better than a few years ago, and several long-term survivors without evident disease are known. Before undertaking the induction treatment of patients with acute leukemia, the conscientious physician should establish that he has the most current information, drugs, and professional resources available. Since the therapy has been progressively improving, much important information is embodied in current research undertakings. Several drugs of great usefulness have not yet been released from investigational status. Many supportive services are not available except in large centers participating in leukemia research. For these reasons, care of an acute leukemia patient should be carried out by a physician in cooperation with the closest leukemia center. Strategy can be planned and induction accomplished there, and the patient can be managed by his own physician during remission. This participation in ongoing research is also critical to continued progress toward universally curative therapy.

Single drug treatments of acute leukemia have largely given way to combinations of therapeutic procedures tailored to different body burdens of leukemic cells. Induction treatments are effective in abruptly lowering the leukemic population but are less effective in prolonging remissions. Drugs of value in maintaining remissions are somewhat less active in inducing them. Experimentally, immunotherapy is known to be ineffectual when leukemic populations are sizable.

Classification of Response. After therapeutic reduction of leukemic infiltration of the marrow, restitution of normal elements occurs. Clinical improvement and survival correlate well with disappearance or decrease of detectable leukemic infiltration and return of normal hematopoiesis. For convenience, codification systems have been devised for marrow (M), peripheral hematologic data (H), physical status (P), and symptomatic status (S).

In the best remission, the marrow is classified as M_0, indicating no recognizable abnormality in any constituent. When the blast cells are less than 5 per cent by Wright's stain, it is difficult if not impossible to be certain a blast cell is a leukemic blast and not a normal myeloblast. M_1 allows up to 5 per cent blasts and M_2 up to 25 per cent blasts; M_3 and M_4 are more abnormal. In similar fashion, the hematologic values in the peripheral blood can be classified as H_0, indicating no abnormalities whatever in erythrocytes, leukocytes, or platelets; H_1, for minor abnormalities within the range of normal; and H_2, H_3, and H_4, for more pronounced departures from normal. Similar rating scales exist for physical abnormalities (P) and symptomatic manifestations (S). These allow classification of individuals for clinical purposes into those with complete remission (M_1, H_1, P_1, S_1, or better), partial remission (all values 2 or better), improvement, no change, and progression.

Acute Lymphocytic Leukemia. Induction of remission is successfully accomplished in 85 per cent of children with vincristine and prednisone. The use of daunorubicin, methotrexate, 6-mercaptopurine, or asparaginase during this induction period has not significantly increased the induction frequency. The sequence of events includes a rapid fall in leukemic cells in the peripheral blood, often beginning within 48 hours. Leukopenia usually ensues, which is not ordinarily a cause for alteration in dose during vincristine and prednisone administration. In 7 or 14 days the population of leukemic cells in the bone marrow is noticeably decreased and the marrow cellularity is less. By 28 days half of children have less than 5 per cent leukemic cells remaining in their marrow, and a brisk erythroid hyperplasia is often present. Repopulation of the marrow with normal hematopoietic cells follows. The appearance of increasing platelet counts and granulocyte counts in the blood precedes return of marrow entirely to normal and is a favorable prognostic sign of an oncoming remission.

Administration of *E. coli* asparaginase immediately after the vincristine and prednisone administration significantly lengthens the subsequent remission duration without serious addition to the toxicity which simultaneous administration entails.

MAINTENANCE. Combined use of 6-mercaptopurine and methotrexate delays the emergence of resistant clones of cells. The probability of a single cell being or becoming refractory to both drugs simultaneously is much less than for a single drug, thereby accounting for some of the benefits which accrue to combination chemotherapy. Although immunosuppression exists during this drug regimen, attempts to change the dose and schedule of the combination, allowing for periods of immunologic recovery during the intermittency, have not yet proved superior to the uninterrupted administration of both drugs.

REINFORCEMENT. During remission maintenance, reinforcement with one or two doses of vincristine plus prednisone for one or two weeks has been applied every four to 12 weeks. Reinforcement has been proved of value when contrasted to maintenance chemotherapy alone.

CENTRAL NERVOUS SYSTEM TREATMENT. Central nervous system leukemia is rare early in the disease. CNS leukemia became clinically frequent only after systemic manifestations of the disease yielded to control, precluding early death. Without specific treatment to the central nervous system, nearly half of affected children develop infiltration of the meninges and brain substance, often as the first manifestation of relapse, giving rise to headaches, irritability, vomiting, personality change, meningismus, papilledema, cranial nerve palsies, and, in young children, separation of the cranial sutures. The failure of systemic treatment to control the central nervous system manifestations probably results from sanctuary of the leukemic cells beyond the blood-brain barrier where drug concentrations are substantially lower. Because of the high frequency of CNS manifestations, regional treatment for central nervous system leukemia with intrathecal methotrexate has been applied effectively before the clinical syndrome emerges. This therapy decreases the central nervous system manifestations and improves the duration of the hematologic remission as well.

The early administration of cranial radiation (2400 rads in 12 treatment days) to include the entire brain,

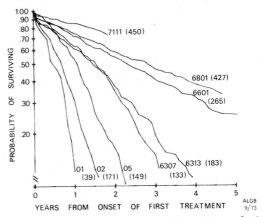

STUDIES IN ACUTE LYMPHOCYTIC LEUKEMIA (UNDER 20 YEARS OLD)

Successive improvement of survival in studies of Acute Leukemia Group B. Studies 01, 02, and 05 were begun between 1956 and 1962. The year when later studies began is given in the first two digits of subsequent numbers. The number of patients in each study is shown in parentheses. Each protocol contained several alternative therapeutic choices allocated at random.

retinas, and upper cervical cord has further reduced the appearance of CNS leukemia in patients treated with systemic chemotherapy at standard doses plus intrathecal methotrexate.

TREATMENT DURATION. The optimal duration of treatment for patients with acute lymphocytic leukemia is not well established. Some patients have sustained long-term remissions on particular regimens. Relapses in patients on these same regimens have almost always occurred within three years. Some investigators thus terminate chemotherapy after three years of treatment, whereas others are engaged in study programs which allocate patients at random to continue or terminate treatment after five years. Premature termination might, of course, lead to relapse, whereas adverse effects of unnecessary continuation would be cumulative toxicity and immunosuppression, leading to opportunistic infections or possibly to reinduction of leukemia through a repetition of the leukemogenic stimulus. Apparent freedom from disease has been produced in 50 per cent or more in recent protocols of at least four research centers.

Immunotherapy, using allogeneic leukemic myeloblasts and the BCG strain of tubercle bacilli, has been successful in reports by Mathe and colleagues. Seven of 20 patients repetitively treated with these immunologic stimuli after a short chemotherapeutic course have remained in remission for three to seven or more years. Unfortunately, this experience has not been duplicated elsewhere. This appears related in part to failure to reproduce the exact experimental design and in part to the progressive success of chemotherapy, which has preempted investigators' attention.

In children who fail to remain disease free, relapse of the leukemia can be detected in the marrow weeks or months before it is apparent in the peripheral blood. Reinduction into remission with vincristine and prednisone is ordinarily successful, but sustaining the remission with the drugs from which the child has just relapsed, or with new drugs, becomes progressively more difficult, and after a shorter remission florid leukemia reappears. Death usually comes during the florid uncontrolled leukemic state, although a small percentage of children die of intercurrent infection while in remission.

Acute Myelocytic Leukemia in Adults. The chemotherapy of acute myelocytic leukemia is more difficult than that of acute lymphocytic leukemia. Drugs known to affect the leukemic myeloblast also affect the normal myeloblast. Selective toxicity is heavily dependent on differences in kinetics of the leukemic and normal populations. Indeed, at the outset in florid leukemia, the population of normal myeloblasts is diminished if not absent; normal hematopoietic stem cells, through unknown mechanisms, are apparently in prolonged G_1 or in G_0 cell cycle status. The leukemic population is primarily in cell cycle, however. Because of this kinetic difference, maximal therapeutic advantage appears to derive from treatment programs of relatively short duration, five to ten days, which seriously injure the cycling leukemic population before substantial numbers of normal stem cells enter into the cycle. In the hiatus before a second course of treatment is administered, two to four weeks after the initiation of the first course, recovery of antibody synthesis and cellular immunologic functions is recognizable. It is presumed that the normal hematopoietic stem cell pool is similarly replenished, thus explaining the avoidance of irreversible marrow aplasia. Failure of remission induction or eventual relapse is ascribable to cells in the leukemic population which are, or become, relatively insusceptible to the drugs which can be given within the tolerance of nonlethal toxicity.

Age is a significant determinant of successful induction frequency in acute myelocytic leukemia; patients over 60 fare worse in virtually every study. This is not inherently a difference in the susceptibility of leukemic cells, but is rather due to a lesser recovery of normal stem cell functions and decreased resiliency in withstanding the nearly invariable complications of the induction phase.

Cytosine arabinoside, a highly specific inhibitor of the "S" or DNA synthetic phase of the cell cycle, can cause 20 to 35 per cent complete remissions of acute myelocytic leukemia. Given in combinations with other active antileukemic drugs, the remission rates reach 50 to 80 per cent. Cytosine arabinoside must be given frequently daily or by continuous infusion, to ensure that drug is present at some time during the S phase of each leukemic cell in cycle. Effective combinations of cytosine arabinoside with thioguanine, cyclophosphamide, CCNU, and, most successfully, the anthracycline antimicrobial drugs daunorubicin or adriamycin have been reported. Some investigators also add vincristine and prednisone. After induction, which can be accomplished in the majority of patients under 60 years of age with a single course of seven days of cytosine arabinoside and three days of daunorubicin (other regimens often require two or three repeated courses), efforts to sustain the remission are necessary.

The continuous drug administration regimens so useful in maintaining remission in acute lymphocytic leukemia of childhood are without equivalent impact in acute myelocytic leukemia of adults. Remissions can be sustained by intermittent courses resembling the induction treatment, or by rotating cycles of active agents in combinations. Median remission duration is 10 to 15 months on different programs, with second remissions, if they occur, of short duration. Central nervous system leukemia is substantially less common than in acute lymphocytic leukemia, in part because of earlier demise from

systemic disease. Intrathecal methotrexate or intrathecal cytosine arabinoside given in combination with cranial irradiation is temporarily effective in controlling central nervous system manifestations. Efforts to prevent clinical emergence of central nervous system leukemia will become more appropriate as increasing numbers of longer remissions are achieved.

The majority of patients with acute myelocytic leukemia show blastogenesis when their lymphocytes are incubated in vitro with their autologous leukemic cells. This is a manifestation of immune cellular recognition. Competence of the efferent immunologic arm is demonstrable by delayed skin hypersensitivity to leukemic cell membranes. Complete immunologic responses are detectable in animal leukemias, and are subject to augmentation with immunotherapy. First attempts to immunize patients with acute myelocytic leukemia in remission, using repeated BCG and allogeneic leukemic cell inoculations, have appreciably prolonged remission duration.

Less Common Acute Leukemias. Acute lymphocytic leukemia in adults can be effectively treated with nearly as good induction results as in children, using the programs for this disease outlined previously. Vincristine and prednisone induction, asparaginase intensification, 6-mercaptopurine and methotrexate maintenance with vincristine and prednisone reinforcement, and intrathecal methotrexate therapy with cranial irradiation have produced 70 per cent remission rates lasting two years in 40 per cent. Investigators whose programs for acute myelocytic leukemia of adults include vincristine and prednisone have treated adults with acute lymphocytic leukemia similarly, and have reported equally good induction results.

Acute myelocytic leukemia in children is even more responsive than the adult disease to the identical treatments.

The subvarieties of acute myelocytic leukemia have rates of response which are not importantly different from unclassified acute myelocytic leukemia, except for promyelocytic leukemia, which is particularly sensitive to daunorubicin. No in vitro or in vivo tests are sufficiently developed to predict reliably which drugs will be best for which tumor.

Supportive Measures. Massive leukemic cellular destruction releases a sudden load of purines to be oxidized to urate. This can lead to hyperuricemia and to urate nephropathy with uremia. If this possibility appears likely, short-term prophylaxis with a xanthine oxidase inhibitor such as allopurinol is appropriate.

Anemia is common and erythrocyte replacement is necessary to keep levels of hemoglobin above the threshold of physiologic dysfunction, at least above 7 grams per 100 ml. Thrombocytopenic bleeding should be prevented. The value of prophylactic platelet administration to preclude hemorrhage has been clearly demonstrated. Optimal platelet survival occurs when the genetic mismatch between donor and recipient is minimal. A sibling, particularly one who is HLA identical, is the best repetitive donor. Random donors are also of value, however, and enough platelets should be administered to protect against hemorrhage during the critical hypoplastic phase before remission ensues if the platelet count is less than 30,000 per microliter. Platelets which have been separated by flotation centrifugation suvive longer and are required less frequently than those which are precipitated and resuspended.

Prevention of infection is of great significance. Barrier

isolation with sterile filtered air circulating in a laminar flow pattern essentially eliminates exposure to exogenous airborne infection, and the likelihood of serious and fatal infections should thereby be decreased. Although most investigators have combined this isolation with oral nonabsorbable or systemic antimicrobial administration, equivalent effects have also been reported in patients isolated without prophylactic antimicrobial administration.

The nature of many serious infections depends upon the prevalence of particular organisms selected by the prior use of antimicrobial drugs in the hospital environment. In hospitals where extensive use has been made of antimicrobial drugs, Pseudomonas and Enterobacter infections outnumber infections caused by staphylococci and *E. coli*, the ordinary organisms in hospitals where extensive antimicrobial use has not been practiced. Opportunistic infections from fungi, *Pneumocystis carinii*, or cytomegalovirus may occur in granulocytopenic or immunodepressed patients who are protected against bacterial infection by early use of antibacterial drugs.

In the presence of granulocytopenia, new symptoms, signs, or unexplained fever require vigorous and immediate action. If infection is suspected, appropriate cultures and other diagnostic tests should be made and treatment started before results are returned. Evolving insusceptibilities in hospital organisms dictate the antimicrobials to be used which provide broad and effective coverage for gram-positive organisms and the likely spectrum of gram-negatives. Cephalothin or clindamycin has largely superseded ampicillin or methicillin, and Gentamicin has largely superseded kanamycin or polymyxin. Carbenicillin may be added if the suspicion of Pseudomonas is particularly strong. The antimicrobial regimen can be discontinued or changed early, if the initial clinical impression proves incorrect.

When visceral infection occurs in the presence of granulocytopenia, mortality is high despite treatment with antimicrobials, unless marrow recovery occurs nearly simultaneously, with the consequent return of granulocytes. Transfusion of allogeneic normal donor granulocytes, collected by differential centrifugation or by filtration leukophoresis on nylon filters, with subsequent elution, has proved a component of major effectiveness in the treatment of sepsis during granulocytopenia. Recovery of transfused granulocytes is best when donated by histocompatible sibling donors, but even granulocytes from random donors in adequate quantity, more than 10^{10} daily for several days, can cause significant improvement in survival from serious infections.

Baxt, J., et al.: Leukemic-specific DNA sequences in leukocytes of the leukemic member of identical twins. Proc. Natl. Acad. Sci. U.S.A., 70:2629, 1973.

Clarkson, B. D.: Acute myelocytic leukemia in adults. Cancer, 30:1572, 1972.

Cronkite, E. P.: Kinetics of leukemic cell proliferation. *In* Dameshek, W., and Dutcher, R. (eds.): Perspectives in Leukemia. New York, Grune & Stratton, pp. 158–186.

Doll, R.: The Epidemiology of Leukemia. Seventh Annual Guest Lecture, Leukemia Research Fund, 61 Great Ormond Street, London, WC1N3JJ.

Ellison, R. R.: Acute myelocytic leukemia. *In* Holland, J. F., and Frei, E., III (eds.): Cancer Medicine. Philadelphia, Lea & Febiger, 1973, pp. 1199–1234.

Henderson, E.: Acute lymphoblastic leukemia. *In* Holland, J. F., and Frei, E., III (eds.): Cancer Medicine. Philadelphia, Lea & Febiger, 1973, pp. 1173–1199.

Holland, J. F., and Glidewell, O.: Chemotherapy of acute lymphocytic leukemia of childhood. Cancer, 26:1480, 1972.

Holland, J. F., and Glidewell, O.: Survival expectancy in acute lymphocytic leukemia. N. Engl. J. Med., 287:769, 1972.

Todaro, G. J., and Gallo, R. C.: Immunological relationship of DNA polymerase from human acute leukaemia cells and primate and mouse leukaemia virus reverse transcriptase. Nature, 244:206, 1973.

Yates, J. W., and Holland, J. F.: A controlled study of isolation and endogenous microbial suppression in acute myelocytic leukemia patients. Cancer, 32:1490, 1973.

Yates, J. W., Wallace, H. J., Jr., Ellison, R. R., and Holland, J. F.: Cytosine arabinoside and daunorubicin therapy in acute myelocytic leukemia. Cancer Chemother. Rep., 57:485, 1973.

THE CHRONIC LEUKEMIAS

Charles M. Huguley, Jr.

764. CHRONIC GRANULOCYTIC LEUKEMIA
(Chronic Myelocytic Leukemia [CML], Chronic Myeloid Leukemia, Chronic Myelogenous Leukemia)

Definition. Chronic granulocytic leukemia (CGL) is characterized by abnormal proliferation of immature granulocytes—neutrophils, eosinophils, and basophils—in the bone marrow, the spleen, the liver, and sometimes other tissues.

Etiology. Except in a small percentage of patients, the etiology of chronic granulocytic leukemia remains obscure. Epidemiologic studies have been essentially negative with the exception of two well-established factors: exposure to ionizing radiation and chronic exposure to benzene. Evidence for a viral etiology has not been forthcoming. Genetic factors have seldom seemed to play a role.

The relationship to ionizing radiation was first demonstrated through the increased incidence of chronic granulocytic leukemia among radiologists who practiced in the era when careful shielding was not generally used. Later an increased frequency of the disease was found in patients with ankylosing spondylitis treated by radiation to the entire spine and in the Japanese population exposed to a single massive dose of radiation from atomic bomb explosions. There is also a clearly demonstrated increase in CGL among workers with chronic occupational exposure to benzene, mostly among those who had acute hematologic damage from the chemical. A relationship to other chemicals and drugs such as chloramphenicol and phenylbutazone is not established. There is no association with other cancer.

Incidence and Prevalence. Chronic granulocytic leukemia accounts for 15 to 20 per cent of all leukemia and has an over-all incidence of about 12 cases per million population per year. The disease is unusual below age 35 and thereafter increases steadily. It is slightly more common in males than in females.

Pathology. The essential feature of chronic granulocytic leukemia is accumulation of granulocytic precursors in the marrow, spleen, and blood. The marrow is usually devoid of fat, and 80 to 90 per cent of the cells are granulocytes. The distribution of granulocytes shows only a slight shift toward immaturity. In the early stages megakaryocytes are nearly always strikingly increased. Needle biopsy of the marrow will reveal some degree of fibrosis with positive stain for reticulin in about 25 per cent of cases. This fibrosis tends to become progressively more severe, and many patients end with a marrow picture similar to that of myelofibrosis. The spleen is usually very much enlarged. Its normal architecture is replaced by extramedullary myelopoiesis, including not only granulocytes but also erythroblasts and megakaryocytes. Infarcts are common. The liver is usually enlarged, although not massively. There are infiltrations with myeloid cells but usually not much damage to the liver cells. Other tissues are usually not involved early.

Although the numbers of granulocytes in the marrow, blood, and spleen are greatly increased, the mitotic index is usually lower than normal, because the mean generation time of immature cells is longer. There is an exchange of cells between the blood, the spleen, and the marrow.

About 90 per cent of patients with chronic granulocytic leukemia exhibit an abnormal chromosome called the Philadelphia chromosome (Ph[1]). This abnormality results from the deletion of a short arm from a chromosome of group 22. When present the Ph[1] chromosome is found in virtually all metaphases observed in the marrow, including erythroid precursors and megakaryocytes as well as granulocytes. It is not found in lymphocytes, skin, or connective tissue, indicating that the Ph[1] chromosome is an acquired abnormality of a common stem cell for granulocytes, red cells, and megakaryocytes. Since it nearly always persists despite vigorous treatment, there has been pessimism as to the possibility of ridding the body of the abnormal cell in order to permit repopulation by normal cells. Recently it has been possible, after vigorous therapy, to replace Philadelphia chromosome cells with normal cells. Whether this will alter the course of the disease remains to be seen, but it offers a basis for optimism.

Eventually 60 to 80 per cent of patients will develop a transformation into a pattern virtually indistinguishable from acute granulocytic leukemia. This change is called the *"blast crisis."* The pathologic manifestations are those of acute granulocytic leukemia. Occasionally a blast transformation will occur in extramedullary sites, particularly in lymph nodes, producing a histologic pattern resembling sarcoma. The demonstration that such cellular infiltrations contain the Ph[1] chromosome proves that the cells are immature granulocytes rather than other cells. Such tumors have been called *chloromas* or *granulocytic sarcomas.*

Patients who do not have the Ph[1] chromosome generally pursue an atypical course; e.g., the response to therapy is less predictable than it is in a typical patient with the Ph[1] chromosome, and prognosis is poorer.

Clinical Manifestations. Sometimes the disease may be diagnosed at an early stage by an incidental blood count. More commonly the patient experiences insidious onset of fatigue, sometimes accompanied by anorexia and weight loss. There may be fullness or heaviness in the left upper quadrant, or the discovery of a mass may bring the patient to the doctor. More rarely, the physician is consulted because of the manifestations of anemia, pain in the splenic region secondary to a splenic infarct, hemorrhagic or thrombotic manifestations, or an attack of gout.

The spleen is palpable in nearly all patients at the time of diagnosis and is usually quite large, frequently extending beyond the umbilicus. If there has been a recent splenic infarct, the organ may be tender and a rub may be heard over the area of infarction. The liver is also palpable. Less commonly it is possible to elicit sternal tenderness. Lymphadenopathy is rare. In short, the typical patient has relatively minor symptoms, and the usual physical finding is splenomegaly.

The essential laboratory abnormality is leukocytosis. The patient who presents with symptoms will characteristically have more than 75,000 WBC per cubic millimeter, and the count may exceed 500,000. The differential white cell count shows a spectrum of immature granulocytes similar to that seen in normal bone marrow. Myeloblasts rarely exceed 5 per cent of the count. Eosinophils and basophils are increased in percentage, which means a striking absolute increase. Monocytes may also be increased.

Anemia of varying degree may be present, but usually not until the white cell count exceeds 50,000 per cubic millimeter. About half of all patients at the time of diagnosis will have thrombocytosis which may be associated with bleeding as well as thrombotic manifestations. Some patients present initially with thrombocytopenia, and as the disease progresses thrombocytopenia becomes increasingly frequent.

The bone marrow is as described under Pathology.

Alkaline phosphatase activity in the mature neutrophils is strikingly decreased. Uric acid is elevated. The serum vitamin B_{12} level is high, as is the B_{12} binding protein transcobalamin I. The level of serum lactate dehydrogenase is considerably elevated in CGL.

Diagnosis. Leukocytosis with the characteristic shift to immaturity of the granulocytes and the increase in eosinophils and basophils suggests the diagnosis of chronic granulocytic leukemia. The presence of splenomegaly in most cases will serve to distinguish CGL from leukemoid reactions, although not from other myeloproliferative syndromes. The cellular marrow with granulocytic and megakaryocytic hyperplasia is characteristic. A bone marrow biopsy should be done to help distinguish CGL from myelofibrosis and also to search for some degree of fibrosis which is commonly present.

A cytogenetic study should be made on the marrow to establish the presence of the Ph[1] chromosome. If present, this abnormality corroborates the diagnosis of chronic granulocytic leukemia and indicates the probability of a rather typical course. Determination of leukocyte alkaline phosphatase activity of mature neutrophils in the peripheral blood, which is very low in chronic granulocytic leukemia and high in leukemoid reactions and in the other myeloproliferative syndromes, is an important test.

In the unusual case identified by a routine blood count, the diagnosis may at first be difficult. Sometimes patients are seen who have a persistent leukocytosis of 15 to 20,000 WBC per cubic millimeter with a mild shift toward immature forms. At this point the neutrophil alkaline phosphatase may not be much reduced. Many months may elapse before the more characteristic findings of the disease appear. In such cases the demonstration of the Philadelphia chromosome is especially helpful.

Treatment. Chronic granulocytic leukemia is remarkably easy to control until complications develop. Benzene was first used a century ago. Later, arsenic in the form of Fowler's solution was found to be effective. With the advent of radiotherapy, it was shown that the disease was readily responsive to radiotherapy directed to the spleen or to the whole body. Later radiophosphorus ^{32}P also proved effective. More recently it has been demonstrated that extracorporeal irradiation of the blood will control the disease.

With the advent of chemotherapy it was readily shown that most of the agents which produce leukopenia and are effective against any tumor are also effective against CGL. Busulfan has been found to be the drug which combines effectiveness with ease of use and is the standby of treatment. More recently dibromomannitol has proved equally effective.

Standard treatment consists of oral administration of busulfan (Myleran). It is available in 2 mg tablets, and the dose is 6 mg daily. The blood count must be monitored at weekly intervals and the dose adjusted as indicated. The fall in the white count is usually exponential after about two weeks. A safe rule is to reduce the dose of busulfan by half as the white count is reduced by half. However, if the white count falls more gradually and smoothly, the original dose may be maintained until the count is in the neighborhood of 15,000 per cubic millimeter. In any event therapy should cease when the count reaches this level, because there is a tendency for the decline to continue for a week or two after the busulfan is discontinued. Once the white cell count plateaus, it is advisable to resume busulfan in a reduced dose (2 to 4 mg daily) in order to bring the count down somewhat below 10,000 per cubic millimeter. The dose will then have to be titrated, ordinarily between 2 mg every other day and 4 mg daily and maintained until the spleen is no longer palpable and the platelet count has been reduced to normal. Both of these usually take longer than the return of the leukocyte count to normal. Control of the leukocyte count is achievable in over 90 per cent of patients. In perhaps 60 to 70 per cent it is possible to eradicate splenomegaly and have the platelet count, the hemoglobin, and the white cell differential return to normal, thus eradicating diagnostic features of the disease. At this point the leukocyte alkaline phosphatase may return to normal but the Ph¹ chromosome will persist.

Once control has been established, it is possible to continue treatment with a small dose of busulfan. Experienced hematologists, more commonly, will discontinue treatment and observe the patient. Relapse may occur within a few weeks or may require many months. In the latter case, the ordinary approach is to reinduce a remission and again stop treatment just as with the initial episode. Successive remissions become increasingly more difficult to achieve, and their duration will be shorter. If relapse occurs promptly after discontinuing busulfan, it will be easier to maintain the patient on regular dosage once a second remission has been obtained. Maintenance requires careful monitoring not only of the leukocytes but also of the platelets at intervals not to exceed two weeks because of the sometimes unexpected appearance of hematologic toxicity.

Other manifestations of busulfan toxicity usually occur with prolonged treatment and include the development of amenorrhea in females or aspermia in males and a dark pigmentation of the skin. These patients may develop a rare syndrome resembling Addison's disease but not accompanied by evidence of adrenal insufficiency. In addition, the so-called *"busulfan lung,"* a fibrosing process, is only partially relieved by steroid therapy.

Complications. Anemia, when present, is attributable primarily to crowding of the marrow and responds to control of the leukemia. Thrombocytosis may be accompanied by thrombotic complications. Bleeding may be associated with either thrombocytosis or thrombocytopenia which may be due to disease or to treatment. The mature neutrophils of CGL have been shown to be effective in control of infection when transfused into granulocytopenic recipients. Infection is not a usual complication of CGL. The patient in remission ordinarily leads a normal life until the resultant phase of the disease develops. Sixty to 80 per cent of patients will develop the "blast crisis," which occurs fairly suddenly and presents the picture of acute granulocytic leukemia. It is treated with various chemotherapeutic agents effective against acute granulocytic leukemia but less successfully. Remissions seldom last long.

About 25 per cent of patients with CGL will have some degree of fibrosis of the marrow at the time of diagnosis. This tends to progress and occasionally develops into a picture indistinguishable from myelofibrosis. At this point the hypocellularity of the marrow makes continued chemotherapy difficult, and the prognosis is poor. Another unusual outcome is development of a refractory state to chemotherapy. It becomes no longer possible to control the white cell count without producing unacceptable degrees of thrombocytopenia. Hydroxyurea or 6-mercaptopurine may be somewhat more effective than busulfan at this stage.

The untreated patient, or one in florid relapse with high leukocyte count and large spleen, has an elevated uric acid and greatly elevated uric acid excretion. This will be exaggerated by the destruction of leukocytes after treatment, which occasionally causes precipitation of uric acid in the renal tubules and anuria. Therefore it is advisable to administer allopurinol, 100 mg three times a day, during the initial weeks of treatment.

Prognosis. Recent reports of survival of patients with chronic granulocytic leukemia do not indicate an improved survival over the series of untreated patients reported by Minot in the 1920's. The median survival is between 2 1/2 and 3 1/2 years, and the range is ordinarily between one and ten years. It is somewhat paradoxical that the most easily controlled of all malignant conditions treated with chemotherapy has been so refractory to efforts at improving survival. Nevertheless, the quality of life is strikingly improved by treatment and is approximately normal until the appearance of the blast crisis. No means of preventing this complication is yet known. There is no clear evidence that any treatment accelerates or delays its onset. This failure has cast a pall of pessimism over all attempts at controlling chronic granulocytic leukemia. However, a recent clinical study has succeeded in eliminating the Ph¹ chromosome and repopulating the marrow with normal cells. The demonstration that there is indeed a clone of normal cells in the marrow suggests the possibility that the abnormal clone can indeed be destroyed and that some cases of chronic granulocytic leukemia may be curable.

The blast crisis often appears suddenly and is marked

by more than 30 per cent myeloblasts and promyelo-cytes in the peripheral blood and/or marrow. Some cases develop more insidiously and may be preceded by a rise in white count on a dose of busulfan which formerly controlled the white count, or by anemia, or thrombocytopenia or sustained unexplained fever. Another bad prognostic sign is rising percentage of basophils. Once the blast crisis develops, the duration of life is in weeks or months.

The immediate outlook for patients with chronic granulocytic leukemia is excellent. The major manifestations of the disease can be controlled in nearly all patients, and in the majority the blood counts and splenomegaly can be reverted to normal. However, within one to ten years, usually two to four years, complications will develop as described which lead to death within a few months.

Dowling, M., Jr., Haghbin, M., Gee, T. J., Wakonig-Vaar Tara, T., and Clarkson, B.: Attempt to induce true remissions in chronic myelocytic leukemia (CML). Am. Soc. Clin. Oncol., April 1973 (Abst. No. 50).

Ezdinli, E. Z., Sokal, J. E., Crosswhite, L., and Sandberg, A. A.: Philadelphia-chromosome-positive and -negative chronic myelocytic leukemia. Ann. Intern. Med., 7:175, 1970.

Galton, D. A. G.: Chemotherapy of chronic myelocytic leukemia. Semin. Hematol., 6:323, 1969.

Gralnick, H. R., Harbor, J., and Vogel, C.: Myelofibrosis in chronic granulocytic leukemia. Blood, 37:152, 1971.

Haut, A., Abbott, W. S., Wintrobe, M. M., and Cartwright, G. E.: Busulfan in the treatment of chronic myelocytic leukemia. The effect of long-term intermittent therapy. Blood, 37:152, 1971.

Medical Research Council's Working Party for Therapeutic Trials in Leukaemia: Chronic granulocytic leukaemia: Comparison of radiotherapy and busulfan therapy. Br. Med. J., 1:201, 1968.

Tjio, J. H., Carbone, P. P., Whang, J., and Frei, E., III: The Philadelphia chromosome and chronic myelogenous leukemia. J. Natl. Cancer Inst., 36:567, 1966.

765. CHRONIC LYMPHOCYTIC LEUKEMIA

(Chronic Lymphatic Leukemia)

Definition. Chronic lymphocytic leukemia (CLL) is characterized by accumulation in the lymphoid organs, bone marrow, and blood of long-lived cells with uniform appearance similar to that of the small lymphocyte. There is mild to severe immunologic deficiency characterized by hypogammaglobulinemia. Conversely, phenomena such as autoimmune hemolytic anemia and increased delayed hypersensitivity reaction to stimuli such as insect bites are common.

At present the whole subject of the lymphoproliferative diseases, including chronic lymphocytic leukemia, is in process of re-evaluation, stimulated by two developments: (1) our increasing sophistication in the morphologic separation of the various lymphoproliferative disorders and (2) the recognition of the important differences between T lymphocytes and B lymphocytes (see Ch. 60). The cells in nearly all cases of CLL tested have had the features of B cells.

Etiology. Epidemiologic studies have given very little insight into the etiology of chronic lymphocytic leukemia. It is clear that exposure to ionizing radiation is not a factor. It is also clear that genetic factors play some role, as evidenced by the appearance of multiple cases of CLL in some families. CLL is comparatively rare in Japanese, even among Japanese living in the United States. There has been no evidence of a relationship to any chemical carcinogen or to oncogenic viruses.

Incidence and Prevalence. Chronic lymphocytic leukemia is the most common type of leukemia and represents about 30 per cent of all cases. The annual incidence has been given as 15 per million. It is predominantly a disease of older people, being unusual below the age of 40. It is more common in males, in a ratio of about 3:2.

Pathology. Chronic lymphocytic leukemia must be considered as a leukemic form of well-differentiated lymphocytic lymphoma. It is not possible to distinguish between the lymph node pathology in the two diseases. The normal architecture is replaced by a sea of small lymphocytes. Lymph nodes are characteristically enlarged. The spleen is also nearly always enlarged but usually not to a conspicuous degree. Infarction is uncommon. Its architecture is similarly replaced by monotonous infiltration of small lymphocytes. The liver is often enlarged and demonstrates a lymphocytic infiltration which may be minimal or may consist of nodular masses. The bone marrow is involved. In early cases this may be patchy, and a bone marrow aspirate may be hypocellular without a particularly large number of lymphocytes, whereas a biopsy will show nodules of lymphocytes interspersed in normal marrow. Later the marrow becomes almost completely replaced with lymphocytes to the detriment of granulocytes, erythrocytes, and megakaryocytes, yielding a so-called "packed marrow" syndrome. Other organs may be involved, in particular the gastrointestinal tract and the skin.

Clinical Manifestations. In at least a quarter of patients with CLL, symptoms are absent and the diagnosis is suggested by a blood count obtained as part of a routine examination or for the diagnosis of some other illness. In other patients there is insidious onset of noncharacteristic symptoms, and in some the first sign of the disease is a complicating infection. There may be a vague feeling of malaise with easy fatigability. Sometimes there is loss of appetite and weight or a low-grade unexplained fever associated with night sweats. In an appreciable percentage of patients, with or without other symptoms, the physician will be consulted because enlarged lymph nodes or spleen have been observed by the patient. More rarely, bleeding manifestations bring the patient to the physician. Although generalized leukemia cutis may occur, it is rare. Nevertheless, skin manifestations are common. They may take the form of nonspecific leukemids represented by scattered papular or vesicular lesions, often intensely pruritic. These must be distinguished from hyperreactivity to insect bites or a generalized herpes simplex infection. Herpes zoster occurs frequently and may become generalized. Smallpox vaccination may produce a very severe local lesion, and it may go on to generalized vaccinia. The expanding lesions in the marrow encroach upon the bone, leading to demineralization and sometimes to collapse of vertebrae. (The use of steroids in treatment will aggravate demineralization.)

The blood picture is characterized by an absolute lymphocytosis composed mostly of uniform, small, mature-appearing lymphocytes. There will be some large lymphocytes, perhaps with a cleaved nucleus or nucleoli. Smudge cells are common. Early in the disease the absolute number of granulocytes is normal. There is often no thrombocytopenia or anemia at the time of diagnosis. The total white count is usually more than 20,000 but not usually more than 100,000. An occasional patient will have a normal or low white cell count consisting of the same type of abnormal lymphocytes. Most authorities would include such patients within the group of CLL. Examination of the marrow reveals an infiltration with small lymphocytes similar to those in the blood. The marrow may be difficult to aspirate, and a needle biopsy will demonstrate the infiltration of lymphocytes which may be patchy, In more advanced disease, the marrow will be packed with lymphocytes at the expense of the normal myeloid cells. At this point there will be neutropenia, thrombocytopenia, and anemia.

In chronic lymphocytic leukemia there is an accumulation of long-lived lymphocytes; the rate of cell production appears to be little if any above normal. These cells, predominantly of the B cell type, are characterized by an immunoglobulin coating of a monoclonal type. The percentage of T cells which react to antigen or phytohemagglutinin stimulation is reduced, and their absolute number is reduced. T cells may return to normal with treatment.

B cells are necessary for antibody formation. In CLL they appear to be abnormal so that the antibody response to antigens is diminished. Hypogammaglobulinemia is characteristic of the disease, and it increases in severity as the disease progresses. This leads to an increased susceptibility to infection which is the major cause of morbidity in patients with CLL. In advanced disease all patients will have hypogammaglobulinemia with a reduction in normal immunoglobulins. A monoclonal spike may be present, usually of IgM type. There is often a positive Coombs test, which may be accompanied by autoimmune hemolytic anemia. However, excessive hemolysis may occur in the absence of a positive Coombs test, and, in addition, anemia is caused by marrow replacement.

Although the serum uric acid concentration is usually normal, it may be elevated in rapidly progressive cases or after treatment.

Diagnosis. The diagnosis of CLL depends upon examination of the blood and marrow, as described under Pathology. Lymph node biopsy will show a diffuse, well-differentiated lymphocytic lymphoma. Lymphadenopathy and splenomegaly are usually present. Either may be massive but usually is not. Studies at the time of diagnosis should include careful history with an attempt to identify the earliest manifestations of the disease. There should be special examination of the skin, lymph nodes, liver, and spleen. The patient must have a complete blood count, including reticulocytes and platelet count, and a bone marrow examination. A needle biopsy of the marrow as well as the aspirate is desirable.

Other studies should include chest film, bilirubin, direct Coombs test, and studies of liver and kidney function. Determination of total protein and serum electrophoresis is important, and it is helpful to monitor the immunoglobulins. An abnormal electrophoretic pattern should be studied by immunoelectrophoresis to identify a monoclonal peak.

Treatment. Many forms of treatment have been effective, but in the past all have been of somewhat limited value, and there is therefore a considerable opinion that only the symptomatic patient should be treated.

As discussed under Clinical Manifestations, many patients (up to half) have the diagnosis of CLL made incidental to examinations carried out for other reasons. These patients may exhibit no morbidity from the disease and may show no progression for many years. Patients with "active" disease, by contrast, may be defined as those who have one or more of the following: unexplained weight loss, unexplained fever of more than two weeks' duration, rapidly enlarging or painful lymph nodes or spleen, anemia, thrombocytopenia, or such complications as hemolytic anemia, recurrent infections, or skin involvement.

Present experience suggests that the asymptomatic patient has little to gain from treatment and may be harmed. Active disease is an indication for treatment.

Radiation therapy can reduce the size of the spleen and lymph nodes. Whole body radiation has been particularly effective in controlling all manifestations of the disease. Of the various chemotherapeutic agents available, chlorambucil has been the most effective. It is usually administered daily, beginning with an oral dose of 12 mg and reducing the dose as the white cell count comes under control. More general improvement will be observed if treatment is maintained after the white cell count has been brought to normal for at least 12 weeks. Administered in this way, chlorambucil will lead to some improvement in all measurable parameters of disease in about two thirds of patients. About 10 per cent will obtain a return to normal status, including a normal blood differential and a reduction in marrow lymphocytes below 30 per cent, qualifying for a rating of "complete remission."

Since the abnormal lymphocytes of CLL proliferate slowly, they will not replenish themselves after treatment as rapidly as the normal cells of the marrow. Therefore it is logical to use chlorambucil in a single dose every two weeks, thus permitting time for recovery of normal cells between doses. This schedule has about the same effectiveness as daily chlorambucil, although response is slower, but with much less toxicity to the granulocytes and platelets. The dose is 0.8 mg per kilogram given at bedtime once every two weeks (this differs from the manufacturer's recommendations).

The addition of prednisone to chlorambucil has been shown to be associated with a much higher percentage of complete remissions. It has usually been given in a dose of 20 to 30 mg daily, but is also effective if given in a dose of 60 to 80 mg for four to five days every two weeks. The intermittent schedule may possibly protect the patient against some of the side effects of steroid therapy. Prednisone is mandatory for the treatment of autoimmune hemolytic anemia and other autoimmune phenomena. It is particularly effective in reducing the size of lymph nodes and may be helpful for thrombocytopenia.

Treatment should be maintained in an individualized dose for at least three months and certainly until maximal effect appears to have been achieved. This may require as long as a year. During this time careful monitoring of blood counts for hematopoietic toxicity will necessitate counts weekly until stability is achieved and then every two weeks. Treatment can then be stopped until the evidences of active disease return. A majority of patients will require constant treatment. It has not been shown that continued regularly spaced titrated therapy is more effective than the regimen described.

Complications. Most complications have already been mentioned. About 20 per cent of patients will develop an autoimmune hemolytic anemia which is usually responsive to prednisone. Not infrequently hemolysis may be precipitated by treatment. If the disease is controlled with chlorambucil, the hemolytic anemia may not recur. The anemia and sometimes the thrombocytopenia and neutropenia of advanced disease may be helped by the administration of an androgen on a daily basis. Fluoxymesterone in a dose of 10 mg three times daily has often been quite effective.

Infections require specific and vigorous treatment. The regular administration of gamma globulin has not been shown to be effective in preventing infections.

Monoclonal immunoglobulinopathy is present in 5 per cent or more of patients. It is usually of the IgM type and may be associated with a hyperviscosity syndrome.

Prognosis. Extensive tumor registry data indicate that patients diagnosed since 1955 have fared better than those diagnosed previously in the same hospitals. Although these data correspond to the introduction of chlorambucil, it may be that longer survival should be attributed to wider availability of blood banks, introduction of better antimicrobial drugs, and use of prednisone for treatment of hemolytic anemia and thrombocytopenia. Series reported from centers particularly interested in the care of patients with chronic lymphocytic leukemia seem to show a much better median survival (on the order of five to six years) than do series of patients derived from tumor registry data which indicate a median survival of less than four years. The difference may be artifactual in that referral centers tend to attract patients whose disease was discovered in the indolent phase because of routine yearly examinations, whereas district hospitals may handle a higher proportion of patients who have only sought help when symptoms had interfered with ability to work.

Have we been too impressed with the long, "benign" course of some patients? Has our pessimism about the past failure to prolong survival by treatment led us to be too conservative and nihilistic in our approach? Although many patients do survive for ten years or more before any treatment is deemed necessary, and some have lived longer than 25 years, we must not lose sight of the poor survival of the average patient. Patients with "indolent" disease have a median survival of only about two years longer than patients with "active" disease.

A number of "complete remissions" have been reported. A review indicates that such remissions have usually lasted many months and that the survival of such patients is considerably lengthened. Recent reports indicate a frequency of 10 to 50 per cent "complete remissions" after use of chlorambucil, chlorambucil plus prednisone, whole body irradiation, and a combination of cytosine arabinoside and cyclophosphamide. These reports should give us hope that a more aggressive attack upon the disease may lead to better survival than we have achieved in the past. Remissions have corrected all complications, and in some of those tested the normal immunoglobulins have returned to normal.

Boggs, D. R., Sofferman, S. A., Wintrobe, M. M., and Cartwright, G. E.: Factors influencing the duration of survival of patients with chronic lymphocytic leukemia. Am. J. Med., 40:243, 1966.

Cutler, S. J., Axtell, L., and Heise, H.: Ten thousand cases of leukemia: 1940–62. J. Natl. Cancer Inst., 39:993, 1967.

Han, T., Ezdinli, E. Z., Shimaoka, K., and Desai, D. V.: Chlorambucil vs. combined chlorambucil-corticosteroid therapy in chronic lymphocytic leukemia. Cancer, 31:502, 1973.

Huguley, C. M., Jr.: Survey of current therapy and problems in chronic leukemia. *In* Leukemia-Lymphoma, A Collection of Papers Presented at the 14th Annual Clinical Conference on Cancer, 1969, at The University of Texas M.D. Anderson Hospital and Tumor Institute at Houston. Chicago, Year Book Medical Publishers, 1970.

Johnson, R. E., Kagan, A. R., Gralnick, H. R., and Foss, L.: Radiation-induced remissions in chronic lymphocytic leukemia. Cancer, 20:1382, 1967.

Silver, R. T.: The treatment of chronic lymphocytic leukemia. Semin. Hematol., 6:344, 1969.

Zimmerman, T. S., Godwin, H. A., and Perry, S.: Studies of leukocyte kinetics in chronic lymphocytic leukemia. Blood, 31:277, 1968.

MYELOPROLIFERATIVE DISORDERS

Richard T. Silver

766. INTRODUCTION

The bone marrow, an organ diffusely spread throughout the bones of the body, consists of several different cell types that are strikingly different with regard to their physiologic roles. Depending upon the stimulus, a normal marrow response is unique and selective, occurring, for example, with an elevated white blood cell count after a pyogenic infection or with an elevated platelet count after hemorrhage. These reactions are self-limited, for the marrow reverts to its normal status once the provocative stimulus subsides. The myeloproliferative disorders refer to certain diseases in which the marrow proliferates more or less en masse. This proliferation is self-perpetuating, thus resembling a neoplastic disease, and results in common clinical, hematologic, biochemical, and morphologic characteristics. The concept of the myeloproliferative syndrome as a spectrum of disease with transitions from one form to another has achieved a certain popularity. There is a wide difference of opinion, however, as to which diseases should be included in the "myeloproliferative disorders," and a few hematologists find the term neither precise nor productive. Most would include in this group of diseases chronic granulocytic leukemia, polycythemia vera, myelofibrosis with myeloid metaplasia, and essential (idiopathic) thrombocythemia. At the onset of these illnesses, despite predominant proliferation of one cell type, there is evidence that the marrow *is* reacting en masse. Thus, for example, patients with chronic granulocytic leukemia initially may have an increased platelet count or even an increased red cell count in addition to an elevated white blood cell count. When first diagnosed, patients with polycythemia usually have, in addition to an increased red cell mass, elevations of white blood cell and platelet counts. Most patients with chronic myeloproliferative disorders have increased reticulin fibers in the bone marrow, presumably reflecting mesenchymal cell proliferation which reaches its greatest expression in the disease myelofibrosis with myeloid metaplasia (agnogenic myeloid metaplasia). All these illnesses involve the spleen as well as marrow. In some cases at diagnosis the bone marrow biopsy in the four conditions may be indistinguishable. Alterations are also seen in the levels of serum uric acid, vitamin B_{12} and its binding proteins, and leukocyte alkaline phosphatase activity. The terminal episode in many of these patients is often a disease resembling acute granulocytic leukemia.

The caveat regarding the myeloproliferative concept clearly relates to causation. The *Philadelphia chromosome,* the hallmark of about 90 per cent of the cases of chronic granulocytic leukemia, has not been found in the other diseases of the myeloproliferative group. Moreover, there is no current reason to indicate a common cause for these diseases. Although myelofibrosis may be seen in end-stage patients with polycythemia vera and chronic granulocytic leukemia, it is unlikely that this is the same disease as the idiopathic form. The similarities seen in these disorders may be explained on the basis of the limited manner in which the marrow can express itself in different disease states. Finally, transitions of chronic granulocytic leukemia and agnogenic myeloid metaplasia to polycythemia vera or idiopathic thrombocythemia are difficult to document.

In summary, whereas the term "myeloproliferative disorder" in a restricted sense is useful to refer to certain chronic proliferative diseases of the marrow which share certain characteristics, it should not embrace all the malignant hematologic disorders known to man.

Dameshek, W.: Some speculations on the myeloproliferative syndrome. Blood, 6:372, 1951.
Glasser, R. M., and Walker, R. I.: Transitions among the myeloproliferative disorders. Ann. Intern. Med., 71:284, 1969.
Myeloproliferative Disorders of Animals and Man. Proceedings of the Eighth Annual Hanford Biology Symposium at Richland, Washington, May 20–23, 1968, edited by W. J. Clarke, E. B. Howard, and P. L. Hackett. U.S. Atomic Energy Commission, published June 1970.

767. AGNOGENIC MYELOID METAPLASIA

Definition and Pathogenesis. The degree of confusion and controversy regarding the etiology, pathogenesis, and treatment of agnogenic myeloid metaplasia (*myelofibrosis with myeloid metaplasia* or *myelofibrosis with extramedullary hematopoiesis*) has been proportional to its polysyllabic length. No wonder this entity has been described in the hematologic literature under at least 35 additional names, ranging from *leukoerythroblastic anemia* to *pseudoleukemic-pseudoerythremic myelosis*. In order to understand this disease it is helpful to review the meaning of some terms constituting the name of this disorder. *Agnogenic* is derived from the Greek *agnostos* meaning unknown. *Myeloid,* as a general hematologic term, refers either to myeloid (or granulocytic) cells or to the marrow as a whole. In this sense it should be interpreted as referring to the marrow. *Metaplasia* is characterized by the proliferation of cells which are not usually histologically or functionally important in an organ or tissue. Therefore the term agnogenic myeloid metaplasia can be redefined as the causally unknown proliferation of cells which normally arise from the bone marrow in organs and tissues which are not usually involved in

blood cell formation. What is *extramedullary hematopoiesis?* In the early developmental stages of the human embryo, hematopoiesis is a function of embryonic connective tissue or mesenchyme. Erythrocytes are first formed in the blood islands of the yolk sac, followed by active hematopoiesis in the liver, spleen, and lymph nodes. Intramedullary blood formation within the bone marrow cavity has its onset at about the fifth month of gestation, and by the eighth month the marrow is the principal site of hematopoiesis as extramedullary (outside the marrow) hematopoiesis gradually subsides. At birth, significant extramedullary blood cell formation no longer exists. Nevertheless, the mesenchymal cells originally responsible for hematopoiesis persist throughout life. Normally inactive, they nevertheless retain their embryonic potential, and under a variety of stimuli they are capable of resuming active hematopoiesis. When the mesenchymal cells of the spleen and liver resume blood formation, once again there is extramedullary hematopoiesis (or myeloid metaplasia), for now there is production of marrow cells by organs not usually concerned with hematopoiesis. Such formation of blood outside the marrow cavity may occur secondary to a variety of clinical conditions, including, for example, severe hemolytic anemias, Hodgkin's disease, metastatic neoplasms to the marrow, irradiation, and infections such as tuberculosis, or may occur after poisoning of the bone marrow by fluorine, phosphorus, benzol, or strontium. In some patients with chronic granulocytic leukemia or polycythemia vera, myeloid metaplasia or extramedullary hematopoiesis occurs in association with fibrosis of the marrow during the course of the illness and/or as a consequence of therapy. In a certain number of patients the cause of the myeloid metaplasia is unknown; thus the term *agnogenic* myeloid metaplasia. This occurrence is most commonly (but not always) associated with fibrosis of the marrow; thus the term *myelofibrosis.*

Clinical Manifestations. Agnogenic myeloid metaplasia (AMM) occurs primarily in the older age groups. Nearly two thirds of the cases occur between the ages of 50 and 70 years, about equally in men and women. Symptoms may be of several years' duration, are usually insidious in onset, and are referable to anemia or to abdominal discomfort owing to splenic enlargement. Deafness caused by otosclerosis has been reported in 10 per cent of cases. Less often, migratory bone pain and symptoms of gouty arthritis may occur. The spleen is almost always enlarged when the patient is first seen, and without this physical finding the diagnosis on clinical grounds must be held suspect. On the other hand, the liver is palpable in only one third of the cases, and this finding may be associated with mild liver function test abnormalities. Hepatomegaly without splenomegaly does not occur in AMM. When an enlarged liver without splenomegaly is found in a patient with proved extramedullary hematopoiesis, a diagnosis of *secondary* myeloid metaplasia is almost certain.

Laboratory Findings. Severe degrees of anemia are uncommon when the patient is first seen. Usually the hemoglobin ranges between 9 and 13 grams per 100 ml. The white blood cell count is elevated in about half the patients, normal in one third, and low in the remainder. The leukocyte alkaline phosphatase score is variable, but usually it is normal or increased. The Philadelphia chromosome, the hallmark for the typical case of chronic granulocytic leukemia, is absent. Karyotypic abnormalities have occasionally been reported in AMM, although the majority of studies have been negative. A peripheral blood smear shows striking changes; typically there is a shift toward granulocyte immaturity, even with the appearance of a few myeloblasts and progranulocytes. The presence of these immature cells does not imply a shortened survival time. Marked changes in the red cells include variations in size and shape and teardrop forms. Polychromatophilia and nucleated red cells are characteristic. The reticulocyte count is usually elevated and reflects either dyspoiesis or hemolysis. The platelets may appear large and bizarre and may be increased, normal, or low in number. Megakaryocyte fragments may be seen. Normal or slightly elevated serum levels of vitamin B_{12} and its binding proteins have been reported in AMM, but a clear separation between the extremely high values in chronic granulocytic leukemia (CGL) and AMM is usually apparent. Radioactive iron studies reflect ineffective erythropoiesis and decreased red cell formation in medullary and extramedullary sites. Radioactive chromium-51 studies demonstrate shortened red cell survival in the majority of cases. Most likely this is due to hypersplenism, because the Coombs test is rarely positive and tests for red cell enzyme deficiencies are inconclusive.

The frequency of radiographic evidence of *osteosclerosis* in patients with AMM has ranged from 30 to 70 per cent and may be severe enough to be recognized on a routine chest x-ray in about one third of the cases. The distribution of osteosclerosis is primarily in the axial skeleton where changes are most apparent in the vertebrae, ribs, clavicles, pelvis, scapulae, and metaphyseal ends of the femur and humerus. Bones distal to the elbow and knee are rarely involved. Osteosclerosis of the skull may occur. The most frequent radiographic finding is a "ground-glass appearance" of the bones with loss of definition of individual trabeculae.

In almost every case (even when the marrow is very cellular) the bone marrow aspiration yields a "dry tap," but this finding must not be used as sole evidence for diagnosis. A closed needle biopsy can be readily obtained from the posterior iliac crest. If not, then an open surgical biopsy should be performed. In more than 90 per cent of the cases, the marrow shows fibrosis, and in some, osteosclerosis which is marked by the formation of broad irregular bone lamellae. Islands and clumps of megakaryocytes may remain. In a small but significant percentage of cases, the marrow at the time of diagnosis may be hypercellular, although the architecture in these instances is disorganized. When panhyperplasia occurs, the marrow findings may not be distinguishable from the histologic changes seen in polycythemia vera. Granulocytic hyperplasia is never found to the degree that occurs in chronic granulocytic leukemia. Striking increase in the amount of reticulin fibers is demonstrated by silver impregnation stain and may be found even before the classic increase in collagenous tissue is observed. Although the sine qua non for the diagnosis rests on the demonstration of myeloid metaplasia in the liver or spleen, the risks involved in biopsying these organs are rarely justified.

Course. As the disease progresses, the spleen gradually enlarges, and so may the liver. Anemia becomes more severe in degree and may be complicated by iron deficiency owing to blood loss or to folic acid deficiency. Bacterial infections occur more frequently and can be a major contributing factor leading to death. Of particular importance is the association of tuberculosis with myelofibrosis, and particular efforts should be made to exclude this infectious disease. Nearly all patients have elevated levels of serum uric acid, and attacks of gouty arthritis may develop. Within the past decade, the association of portal hypertension and ascites has been reported in a significant percentage of patients with AMM. Thrombosis of the hepatic vein and the development of the Budd-Chiari syndrome have been recognized. It has been suggested that portal hypertension is a manifestation of both high portal blood flow and a relative obstruction of portal flow at the hepatic sinusoidal level.

Treatment and Prognosis. No treatment affects the basic fibrosis of the marrow, and no form of therapy has been shown to prolong life. Survival time in AMM is difficult to state with assurance because of the problem of accurately determining the onset of the illness. Suggested estimated median survival times are approximately ten years from onset of disease and five years from diagnosis, although there is considerable heterogeneity with both shorter- and longer-lived survivors. Insofar as AMM can thus be a disease of long duration, presently no specific treatment should be undertaken unless the patient becomes symptomatic. All patients should receive at least 200 to 400 mg of *allopurinol* daily in order to avoid the complications of elevated serum uric acid levels. If a patient becomes symptomatic from anemia, *androgens* may be employed, although the high doses used to stimulate erythropoiesis lead to excess fluid accumulation and to masculinizing effects in women. Doses of testosterone enanthate, 600 mg weekly intramuscularly, or oxymetholone, 50 to 100 mg daily by mouth, can be used. Treatment must be continued for 6 to 12 weeks to evaluate its efficacy. It seems most effective in women whose spleen had been removed prior to the onset of therapy or in whom it had not been massively enlarged. Treatment becomes less impressive in patients with more advanced disease. The hemolytic anemia which is most often due to hypersplenism rarely responds to *corticosteroids*. In those patients who initially present with markedly elevated platelet counts, *busulfan* in a dose of 4 mg per day, followed by lower doses as the platelet count falls, may be instituted. In most cases, busulfan cannot be used for definitive reduction in spleen size, because prohibitive degrees of suppression of erythropoiesis and thrombopoiesis result. *Radiation therapy* to the spleen rarely produces meaningful reduction in spleen size, and the dose required often causes severe leukopenia, anemia, and thrombocytopenia. Although *splenectomy* is not automatically interdicted in patients with AMM, it should be reserved for those individuals with severe hemolytic anemia, thrombocytopenia and clinical bleeding, portal hypertension, or mechanical symptoms secondary to splenomegaly. Nevertheless, the postoperative morbidity of splenectomy is significant. Striking thrombocythemia after splenectomy, with thrombosis and hemorrhage, may develop. Often there is further gradual enlargement of the liver, and recurrent hemolysis and thrombocytopenia may occur owing to sequestration by the liver.

In summary, one cannot be categorical about the therapy of AMM, and each treatment modality has its significant attendant risks. On the other hand, future studies may show that earlier treatment, including splenectomy, of the relatively asymptomatic patient may alter the heretofore slow but nevertheless inexorable course of the illness.

Gardner, F., and Nathan, D.: Androgens and erythropoiesis. Further evaluation of testosterone treatment of myelofibrosis. N. Engl. J. Med., 274:420, 1966.

Silver, R. T., Jenkins, D., and Engle, R. L.: Use of testosterone and busulfan in the treatment of myelofibrosis with myeloid metaplasia. Blood, 23:341, 1964.

Silverstein, W. M., Gomes, M. R., ReMine, W. H., and Elveback, L. R.: Agnogenic myeloid metaplasia: Natural history and treatment. Arch. Intern. Med., 120:546, 1967.

Ward, H. P., and Block, M. H.: The natural history of agnogenic myeloid metaplasia (AMM) and a critical evaluation of its relationship with the myeloproliferative syndrome. Medicine, 50:357, 1971.

Section Seven. LYMPHORETICULAR NEOPLASMS

768.   INTRODUCTION

Paul P. Carbone

Neoplasms of the reticuloendothelial system are characterized as myeloproliferative or lymphoreticular. The myeloproliferative disorders include erythroid, myeloid, and megakaryocytic neoplasms that start in the bone marrow and only secondarily invade other tissues of the reticuloendothelial system (lymph nodes, spleen). Lymphoreticular neoplasms arise in lymphocytic cells, reticulum cells, or primitive precursor cells. The lymphocytic cells, primarily involved in immune reactions, are either T cells (thymus derived) or B cells (bone marrow derived). Malignant diseases of lymphoid cells, referred to as lymphoproliferative disorders, may be associated with immune disturbances or monoclonal gammopathies. Reticulum cells, referred to as histiocytic or macrophage cells, form the background population of all lymphoreticular tissues. The lymphoreticular cells are located primarily in lymph nodes, thymus, spleen, and liver, but components of the lymphoreticular system are also found in the submucosal areas of the respiratory and gastrointestinal tracts as well as in the marrow.

Lymphoreticular tumors may become clinically apparent as single or multiple tumors in the lymph nodes, spleen, or gastrointestinal tract and may or may not involve the bone marrow. Since lymphocytes and macrophages also normally occur in the peripheral blood, lymphoreticular tumor cells may circulate. Much confusion can be avoided by understanding these concepts. The term malignant lymphoma commonly refers to patients who present predominantly with solid tumors and must be further classified as to cell type, i.e., histiocytic, lymphocytic, or Hodgkin's. Since the tumor cells may exhibit different degrees of differentiation, i.e., well differentiated or poorly differentiated, that affect prognosis and response to therapy, subclassification for differentiation also is important. Occasional patients have such primitive cells that the terms stem cell and Burkitt's tumor are applied to indicate less differentiated populations. In the lymph node or tissue section, two populations of malignant cells may occur simultaneously with neoplastic lymphocytic and histiocytic components, and the term mixed lymphomas is used. When the marrow and peripheral blood manifestations are prominent, as contrasted to tumor or nodal enlargement, the term leukemia or leukemic phase is applied. Thus in patients with lymphoreticular neoplasms, one sees a complete spectrum from localized tumors only to

multiple tumors, leukemia, and mixtures. The presentation at the time of diagnosis reflects only a point in time, and the natural progression—untreated or after ineffective therapy—is toward dissemination.

Two other points deserve mention in understanding these disease processes. First, the cell type and disease progression may change with time to a less differentiated state. Patients with relatively well differentiated tumors may have subsequent biopsies that indicate less differentiation and even a stem cell–like picture. Clinically, this is important to appreciate, because therapy may need to be changed drastically in form or intensity. A second point relates to the identification of the pattern of lymph node involvement. The term giant follicle lymphoma, originally proposed by Brill and Symmers, referred to a *benign* form of involvement. Subsequent investigators recognized the fact that these patients did indeed die of cancer and that nodular involvement (follicular) occurred in patients with Hodgkin's disease, lymphocytic lymphoma, and, rarely, histiocytic lymphoma. Data from several centers indicate that the involvement pattern of follicular or diffuse can be applied to most histologic subtypes except Burkitt's tumor. In general, the prognoses of nodular forms are better than those of corresponding histologic varieties with diffuse patterns.

The current approach to classification of lymphoreticular neoplasms, as well as the previously applied terms, is shown in Table 1. The use of this classification and the appreciation of chronologic changes in cell type should clear up many of the previous difficulties with confusing names that encompassed grossly different prognostic categories.

The diagnosis of lymphoreticular neoplasms must always be based on an adequate tissue biopsy. Occasionally, multiple biopsies may be needed before the decision as to pathologic classification can be definitively made. Imprint preparations as well as cytochemical studies will help clarify the specific cell type and degree of differentiation. More recently, specific markers of the cell surface such as immunoglobulin receptors, complement receptors, immunoglobulin fluorescence, or rosette cell formation have classified cell variants that heretofore were difficult or impossible to categorize. Current histologic variants may in fact be lymphocytic cells but with cytologic variations. Electron microscopy studies may also be helpful in identifying the nature of the cell involved in the malignant process.

Besides insisting on adequate tissue for diagnosis, the physician responsible for the patient's care must work

TABLE 1. Classification of
Lymphoreticular Neoplasms*

Proposed Name	Old Name
Lymphoma, lymphocytic type, well differentiated	Lymphosarcoma
Lymphoma, lymphocytic type, poorly differentiated	
Lymphoma, histiocytic type	Reticulum cell sarcoma
Lymphoma, mixed lymphocytic-histiocytic type	Mixed lymphoma
Lymphoma, undifferentiated pleomorphic type	Stem cell lymphoma
Lymphoma, undifferentiated Burkitt type	Stem cell lymphoma

*From Berard, 1972. All varieties except Burkitt's may be classified as nodular or diffuse.

in concert with the clinical pathologist, nuclear medicine specialist, radiologist, and surgeon to establish the extent of disease. This process is known as staging. The complete extent of staging procedures has not been determined. One must do a careful history and physical examination, asking for symptoms, examining all nodal areas, determining liver and spleen involvement, and searching for abdominal or testicular masses. Careful examination of the oropharynx is a necessity, because much lymphoid tissue is located in those regions. In addition to routine laboratory studies, radioisotope scans (particularly bone and ^{67}Ga studies), bone marrow biopsy, x-rays of chest and abdomen, intravenous pyelogram, and lymphograms are all helpful in evaluating the extent of disease. Further emphasis on evaluating liver involvement has shown that liver function tests and even closed hepatic biopsies can be misleading. To achieve a greater degree of accuracy, laparoscopy with several direct biopsies of the liver and laparotomy have been used. Diagnostic laparotomy has been adopted by many centers because of the opportunity to do biopsies of other suspicious abdominal areas and to perform a splenectomy. In patients with Hodgkin's disease and non-Hodgkin's lymphoma, the spleen if involved seems to predict liver spread. The more extended procedures also aid in the shaping of radiotherapy fields to fit the specific pattern of involvement. Moreover, Kaplan and his colleagues have utilized these extended staging procedures to map out the natural history and pattern of spread so useful to modern approaches to treatment. Since patients with lymphoreticular disorders tend to be older than patients with Hodgkin's disease and generalized disease is more common, these additional staging procedures must be justified on the basis of risk and morbidity in relation to possible therapeutic benefit. The therapeutic benefit should be realized as leading to significant changes in approach or intensity of treatment.

769. LYMPHOCYTIC AND HISTIOCYTIC LYMPHOMAS

Paul P. Carbone

The non-Hodgkin's lymphomas include lymphocytic, histiocytic, mixed lymphocytic and histiocytic, pleomorphic (or stem cell type), and Burkitt's tumor. (Burkitt's

tumor is described in Ch. 769a.) As described in Ch. 768, each of the major cell types of lymphocytic and histiocytic lymphomas can be further classified by the degree of differentiation of the cell and by the presence or absence of a nodular histologic pattern. The pathologist identifies the cell type, but the designation of leukemia or lymphoma (solid tumors) must be integrated by the physician from all the information learned by physical examination, laboratory study, and further biopsies.

Epidemiology. Many animal lymphoid tumors have been associated with viruses, radiation, and genetic factors. Although virus-like particles have been reported in tissues from patients, no direct causal agent has been identified with certainty. Some animal viruses infect human tissues, but no increased incidence of lymphoid tumors has been seen in owners of sick animals. Using biochemical markers of viral information such as reverse transcriptase, tissue from patients has yielded positive results. An increased incidence of lymphocytic lymphoma and Hodgkin's disease has been reported in survivors of the atomic bomb explosions in Japan. Genetic and acquired immune deficiency disorders predispose to the development of lymphoid malignancies. Patients with ataxia telangiectasia, Wiskott-Aldrich syndrome, congenital sex-linked agammaglobulinemia, and Chédiak-Higashi syndrome all have associated increased risks of developing lymphoid tumors presumably related to immune deficiencies. Patients with acquired hypogammaglobulinemia, autoimmune disorders, and Sjögren's disease likewise seem to have increased risks of developing malignant lymphomas. Patients with kidney grafts and those on long-term immunosuppression have an increased incidence of secondary malignancies. More than half of such malignancies are primary lymphomas, particularly involving the central nervous system, an unlikely site for spontaneous occurrences.

Pathology. Misinterpretations as to histologic type as well as differentiating benign from malignant disorders are common problems. The lymph node biopsy result must be related to bone marrow, peripheral blood, and ancillary laboratory studies, particularly serum or urine immunoelectrophoresis. The classification of non-Hodgkin's lymphoma and the characteristic histopathologic sections are shown in Table 1 and the accompanying figure.

Lymphocytic, Well Differentiated Type. The pattern of lymph node involvement is usually diffuse, replaced by small, normal-appearing lymphocytes. The cytoplasm cannot be seen in most of the cells. The bone marrow is usually involved focally or diffusely. The disease most often occurs in elderly individuals, may be asymptomatic, and may present with small scattered lymph nodes. Bulky lymph node enlargement and splenomegaly also occur. Examination of the peripheral blood may reveal lymphocytosis, and with marrow invasion the diagnosis of chronic lymphocytic leukemia can be made. In young persons, the diagnosis of reactive hyperplasia or Hodgkin's disease, lymphocyte predominant type, should be entertained in the differential diagnosis. Occasionally admixtures of plasma cells occur that are associated with immunoglobulin paraproteins, particularly IgM, in the serum or urine.

Lymphocytic, Poorly Differentiated. The range of lymphocyte size and differentiation seen in the node is more heterogeneous. In children, mediastinal or abdominal tumors with a progression to leukemia are commonly seen with this pattern. This is called "convoluted cell" lymphocytic leukemia by Lukes (1973). Adults are more likely to show peripheral node enlargement and less often manifest frank leukemia. In the node, the cells are variable in size and often have clefted nuclei. Sometimes these abnormal cells in adults enter the peripheral blood and have been characterized as lymphosarcoma cell leukemia. Nodular varieties rarely occur in children.

Histiocytic Type. A wide spectrum of cell sizes and morphology occur, indicating various degrees of differentiation. Some cells may be multinucleate and confused with Reed-Sternberg cells. Phagocytosis and fibroblastic differentiation with marked sclerosis may be seen. The term malignant histiocytosis refers to a relatively benign-looking proliferation of histiocytes that exhibit phagocytosis. Erythrophagocytosis and progressive pancytopenia may be seen that lead to the patient's death. Other variants include leukemic reticuloendotheliosis and histiocytic medullary reticulosis. The former is relatively benign, with "hair cells" in the peripheral blood. The latter is a more fulminant disease, with fever, erythrophagocytosis, jaundice, pancytopenia, and hepatosplenomegaly.

Mixed Histiocytic-Lymphocytic Type. The pattern of involvement is usually nodular, but characteristically malignant histiocytic and lymphocytic cells occur. The histologic pattern of the disease may progress to a more malignant histiocytic type with time. Newer approaches to histologic identification by immunoglobulin markers have recognized the two populations as variants of B lymphocytes.

Undifferentiated or Pleomorphic Type. These tumors usually lack histiocytic or lymphocytic differentiation. The cells are pleomorphic and include bizarre giant forms. Subsequent evidence of cytologic differentiation to lymphocytic or histiocytic forms may occur. Unlike Burkitt's lymphoma, in which uniformity of cell size occurs, these tumors show striking variation on touch preparations.

Clinical Manifestations. The major clinical manifestation of lymphoreticular neoplasms is painless enlargement of one or more peripheral lymph nodes. The glands characteristically are firm and symmetrical, and tend to enlarge progressively. Systemic manifestations of fever, night sweats, or weight loss usually are not prominent features, occurring in only 20 per cent of the patients. In about 20 per cent, lymphoid structures of

the oropharynx, nasopharynx, or tonsils are involved. Palpable *splenomegaly* occurs in about 20 per cent of the patients and is more common in the lymphocytic than in the histiocytic varieties. *Gastrointestinal signs and symptoms* include obstruction, and malabsorption syndromes as a consequence of involvement of the intestinal tract occur in 15 per cent of patients. Diffuse patterns are more often associated with gastrointestinal involvement than nodular forms. The stomach and small intestine are the common gastrointestinal sites of disease. Primary lymphomas of the stomach may be confused with gastric cancer. Large mediastinal nodes are seen in about 20 per cent of the patients with non-Hodgkin's lymphomas as compared with 50 to 70 per cent of patients with Hodgkin's disease. Secondary findings related to intrathoracic tumor include superior vena caval obstruction and pleural effusions. Primary lymphomas of the lung are rare, whereas secondary spread to the lungs occurs commonly.

Hepatic enlargement and jaundice are relatively rare findings, but percutaneous biopsy evidence of liver involvement occurs in about 20 per cent. Further diagnostic procedures to evaluate the liver, including laparotomy, laparoscopy, and open biopsies, increase the yield of positives to about 50 per cent. The histologic subtypes of nodular or diffuse poorly differentiated lymphocytic forms are most likely to have liver spread.

Abnormalities in renal function may be secondary to parenchymal infiltration, obstruction of the outflow system, uric acid precipitation, anomalous protein excretion, or amyloid. Primary lymphomas of the *bone*, particularly histiocytic tumors, have been reported. The most frequent sites are the femur, pelvis, tibia, scapula, and humerus. They present as lytic lesions. Secondary lesions of the bone can be seen in advanced stages.

Primary lymphoreticular tumors of the *nervous system* are rare, but secondary compressions of the spinal cord or nerves may occur when large tumors impinge upon or invade the vertebral axis. The occurrence of free-floating cells or meningeal disease seems to be a late manifestation. Small cell glioblastoma (probably a lymphocytic tumor) with monoclonal gammopathy and primary histiocytic central nervous system tumors are seen.

Skin tumors, described as nodular infiltrations, dusky or blue colored, may be seen in few or many areas. The tumors occasionally ulcerate and become painful. Diffuse skin infiltration and exfoliative lesions may be a dramatic clinical presentation described as the "red

---

A, Normal lymph node (×11). Nodal architecture clearly shows nodules, germinal centers, and sinuses, particularly under capsule.

B, Diffuse lymphoma (×7). The normal nodal architecture is completely obliterated by a diffuse infiltrate of lymphoid malignant cells. The capsule, although intact here, can be disrupted with tumor cells extending outside the lymph node.

C, Nodular lymphoma (×7). The nodal structure is replaced by large nodules of malignant cells. The subcapsular area reveals fibrosis characteristic of an inguinal lymph node.

D, Well-differentiated lymphocytic lymphoma (×600). The malignant cells are small and uniform, with minimal cytoplasm, compact nuclear chromatin, and absence of mitoses.

E, Poorly differentiated lymphocytic lymphoma (×600). The cell size varies, particularly nuclear size with occasional mitoses. The nuclei are often irregular in shape. The nuclear chromatin is finely dispersed.

F, Mixed lymphocytic-histiocytic lymphoma (×600). Two morphologic populations of cells are clearly seen, small irregular lymphoid cells and large histiocytic cells with prominent nuclei.

G, Histiocytic lymphoma (×600). The cells are large and irregular, with clearly evident cytoplasm and large nucleoli.

H, Undifferentiated, non-Burkitt (×600). The pleomorphic cells are large and lack clear histologic differentiation with primitive nuclear pattern. A large multinucleate cell is also seen.

(Illustrations were kindly supplied by Dr. Costan Berard, Head, Hematopathology Section, Laboratory of Pathology, National Cancer Institute.)

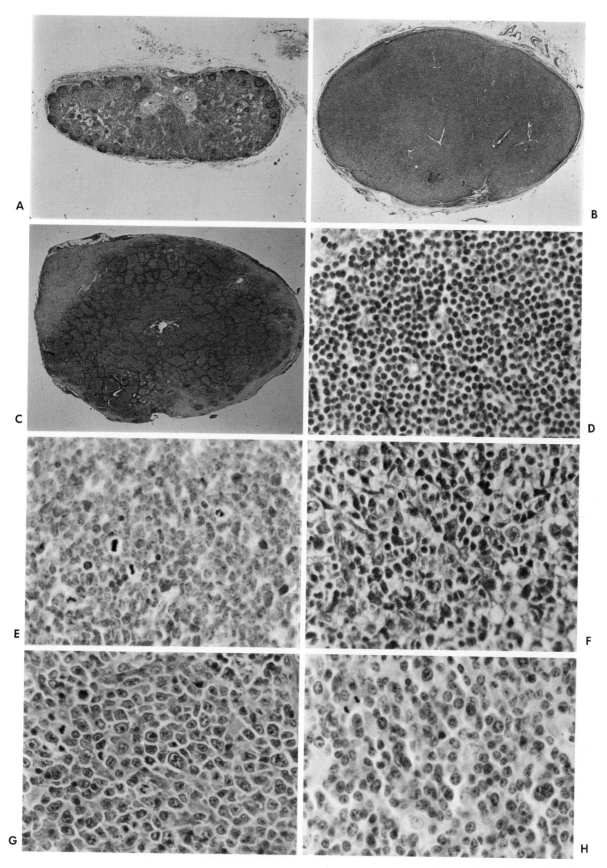

See opposite page for legend.

man's syndrome." Patients with B cell variant of *Sézary's syndrome* may have peripheral blood involvement without much marrow invasion.

In 10 per cent of the patients *anemia* may be present at the onset, but it occurs more often as the disease progresses. A brisk or chromic hemolytic anemia, often Coombs positive, may complicate the onset of more aggressive disease. Peripheral white blood counts are usually normal, but lymphocytosis occurs particularly in association with the well differentiated lymphocytic variety of lymphoma. Immature circulating cells occur in most children with poorly differentiated or stem cell lymphomas at some time during the clinical course. Leukemic transformation approaches 50 to 70 per cent during the first 12 months even if the initial bone marrow is not involved. Poorly differentiated lymphocytic cells occasionally invade the peripheral blood, appearing as moderate to large lymphocytes with notched nuclei. This manifestation has been called *"lymphosarcoma cell leukemia."*

Initial involvement of the marrow is seen in about 20 per cent of the patients with non-Hodgkin's lymphoma; however, the incidence is much higher, 40 per cent, in lymphocytic varieties as compared to histiocytic types. The finding of bone marrow involvement is usually associated with clinical Stage III disease (90 per cent) and rarely with Stage I disease.

Differential Diagnosis. The major considerations in the differential diagnosis of lymph node enlargement include infections, reactive lymphadenopathy, and other neoplastic illnesses. Principal among the infectious causes are diseases such as infectious mononucleosis, tuberculosis, syphilis, toxoplasmosis, cytomegalovirus infection, and many pediatric viral illnesses. Reactive hyperplasias of the lymph nodes may accompany acute or chronic infections of the extremities or throat, particularly after vaccinations. Lymphadenopathy has also been associated with diphenylhydantoin administration. Nonlymphoreticular neoplasms characteristically spread to local lymph nodes only. A careful search of the oropharynx and mucosal surfaces may reveal a primary cancer that should be biopsied rather than the neck nodes. Breast cancer may present as lymph node enlargement in the axilla with a small primary tumor in the breast that may escape initial evaluation. Occasionally, diffuse adenopathy with histologic features of a lymphoma can be seen in association with immunoglobulin abnormalities characteristic of Waldenström's macroglobulinemia. Differentiation between a primary macroglobulinemia and a lymphoma with paraproteinemia may be difficult. Immunoglobulin M paraproteinemia with lymphoma occurs in the diffuse varieties more often than in the nodular forms. Examination of the marrow may reveal the characteristic lymphoid plasma cell along with the hyperviscosity, purpura, and bleeding tendency in patients with macroglobulinemia.

Staging. After establishing the diagnosis, evaluating the extent of disease is the most important responsibility of the attending physician. The staging procedures currently recommended are shown in Table 2. More recent data with ^{67}Ga scan indicate that this is an important adjunct in finding disease sites for further evaluation, because inflammatory lesions and other tumors also take up ^{67}Ga. The staging originally applied to Hodgkin's disease appears to be most widely used

TABLE 2. Staging Procedures

1. History and physical examinations
2. Chest x-rays and tomograms as indicated
3. Complete blood counts
4. Liver function tests, serum electrophoresis, BUN, and creatinine
5. Bone marrow biopsy
6. Lower extremity lymphograms
7. Intravenous pyelogram
8. Bone and liver scans
9. Laparoscopy
10. Laparotomy when indicated

(Table 3). In it, extranodal sites are designated E. A clinical stage is based on the initial biopsy evidence of lymphoma and on the history, physical examination, and radiographic studies. A pathologic stage as a result of information derived from further special surgical procedures, such as liver biopsy or laparotomy, is included in the definition. The pathologic staging evaluation tends to result in an advance in the clinical stage in about 50 per cent. In one large series the distribution by stage for nodular and diffuse lymphomas is shown in Table 4.

A major tool in the evaluation of patients with lymphoreticular neoplasms is the *retroperitoneal lymphogram*. A radiopaque dye is injected into the small lymphatics of the foot under pressure. The dye is taken up by the abdominal lymph nodes and can be seen on the abdominal x-ray. In two thirds of patients with neck node enlargement, despite clinical evidence of localized disease, the lymphograms are abnormal. Since the dye persists in the nodes, the lymphogram findings may be used to follow the results of treatment. Repeat studies can be used to confirm disease activity.

The role of *laparotomy and laparoscopy* in the staging of patients with non-Hodgkin's lymphoma has become increasingly important, particularly in determining evidence of liver and extranodal involvement. The usual plan of staging is to do closed liver biopsies and bone marrow biopsy first in all patients. If the biopsy does not indicate disease in liver or marrow and the clinical evaluation of the patients does not reveal other evidence of Stage IV disease, then laparoscopy or laparotomy is indicated. The laparoscopic examination increases the yield of liver positives, precluding further exploration. Some institutions prefer to go directly to the laparotomy for wedge and needle biopsies of the liver, splenectomy, and thorough examination of abdominal lymph nodes and extranodal sites. Laparotomy

TABLE 3. Ann Arbor Staging Classification

Stage I:	Involvement of a single lymph node region (I) or a single extralymphatic site (IE)
Stage II:	Involvement of two or more lymph node regions on the same side of the diaphragm (II) or a solitary extralymphatic site and one or more of lymph node areas on the same side of the diaphragm (IIE)
Stage III:	Involvement of lymph node regions on both sides of the diaphragm (III), accompanied by spleen involvement (IIIS), or by solitary involvement of an extralymphatic organ or site (IIIE) or both (IIISE)
Stage IV:	Diffuse involvement of extralymphatic sites with or without lymph node enlargement

Clinical stage and pathologic stage defined for each patient; extranodal sites are designated by specific denominators; presence or absence of symptoms is designated B or A, respectively

TABLE 4. Distribution of Stage and Histology*

Clinical Stage	Histiocytic		Mixed		Lymphocytic, Poorly Differentiated		Lymphocytic, Well Differentiated		Pleomorphic		Total
	D†	N†	D	N	D	N	D	N	D	N	
I	9	3	5	5	6	9	3	1	3	—	44
IE	4	—	1	1	—	—	—	—	—	—	6
II	20	8	4	15	7	9	—	1	2	—	66
IIE	18	1	5	2	4	3	1	—	—	—	34
II	18	6	8	29	8	20	1	2	—	—	92
IIIE	2	1	1	1	—	1	—	—	—	—	6
IV	45	10	19	21	19	27	5	2	9	—	157
Total	116	29	43	74	44	69	10	6	14	0	405

*Modified from Jones, S. E., et al.: Cancer, 31:806, 1973.
†D = Diffuse.   N = Nodular.

has indicated evidence of liver involvement in at least 25 per cent of patients with prior negative percutaneous and laparoscopy biopsies. Mesenteric nodes are often found to be involved and must be considered in shaping radiation fields. The complications of laparotomy include occasional mortality, left side pleural effusions, infarction, pulmonary emboli, pancreatitis, gastrointestinal bleeding, and increased liability to subsequent infection. Because of these risks the indication for laparotomy must take into account the associated medical illnesses and the treatment program. If the treatment planned will not be influenced by laparotomy regardless of the result, the surgical exploration is not justified.

Treatment. The major modalities are irradiation, antineoplastic chemotherapeutic agents, and surgery. Historically, surgery was used for diagnosis, but also to remove obvious localized disease. This approach rarely resulted in long-term control unless the diagnosis was wrong or the histology extremely favorable (well differentiated lymphocytic, nodular). Therefore radiotherapy and/or chemotherapy form the basis of modern treatment.

Radiotherapy was recognized more than 30 years ago as an effective modality if administered in sufficiently high doses to forestall recurrences in the irradiated site. The usual dose for curative intent is 3500 to 4500 rads in patients with lymphoreticular neoplasms, administered at a rate of 1000 rads per week. The problem remains to define how much of the lymphoreticular system to radiate. In general, adequate radiotherapy should be administered to all involved sites in Stages I and II. Since more than half the patients have noncontiguous sites of involvement, more recent clinical trials have proposed extended radiotherapy to include all nodal areas and the spleen. With use of megavoltage equipment, total nodal irradiation appears to be well tolerated and capable of sterilizing disease. At some centers, experimental approaches to irradiate the entire body, the liver, and/or the lung are being tried, but the total dose administered has to be cut considerably. Radiotherapy may be used in combination with chemotherapy. Since we know that local disease may be controlled directly by radiotherapy, chemotherapy is used to treat occult disease in other sites.

Two additional points about radiotherapy must be emphasized. Since the abdomen is a major site of extranodal disease and mesenteric nodes are frequently involved, therapy techniques are available to permit total abdominal radiation. This includes spray radiation of the entire abdomen, with shielding of the liver and kidneys as the dose exceeds 1500 to 2000 rads. Another approach is the strip technique, in which the abdomen is radiated in a piecemeal fashion. The other use of radiotherapy is for special clinical problems. Obstruction of ureters, biliary system, bowel, and the respiratory airway, as well as compression of the nervous system, are medical emergencies. Radiotherapy to specific sites is very effective in relieving severe symptoms and signs quickly to prevent irreversible damage. Radiotherapy of the cranium combined with intrathecal chemotherapy is an accepted approach to meningeal disease.

The use of *chemotherapeutic* agents in the treatment of lymphoreticular neoplasms began in the 1940's, and their clinical usefulness spawned the search for many other new agents. Several have been used to treat patients with non-Hodgkin's lymphoma. The major categories of drugs and toxicities are shown in Table 5. The early trials indicated a relatively high proportion of responses as measured by tumor shrinkage in 30 to 50 per cent of patients using single drugs, but these responses were short-lived and clinical resistance followed. Following the lead of successful drug treatment programs in patients with acute leukemia, effective combination chemotherapy regimens were developed whereby tumor regressions were regularly achieved in most patients with non-Hodgkin's lymphoma. Most importantly, complete disappearances of tumor occurred in 50 per cent of the patients. Drugs with independent effectiveness and nonoverlapping toxicities were able to be combined at almost full doses, and the resultant effect against the tumor was additive or even synergistic. Most of the combinations employ an alkylating agent, a vinca alkaloid (usually vincristine) and a corticosteroid, and procarbazine. Some of the more common combinations are shown in Table 6.

The management of any patient should take into account the histologic type, the pattern of node involvement, the stage of the disease, and the associated medical condition of the patient. The initial approach should include a planned intent to achieve curative therapy or palliation. The decision must be firmly supported by what can be done under optimal circumstances with the best therapeutic modalities. For example, the physician must decide whether the x-ray equipment, expertise in treating with drugs, or management of complications is within the scope of his abilities and facilities. Respectable cure rates can be achieved by modern therapy. After frank discussion with the patient, the physician must advise on optimal therapy and where it

TABLE 5.   Doses and Toxicities of Drugs Used in Non-Hodgkin's Lymphoma

Drug	Dose and Schedule	Limiting Toxicities
1. Nitrogen mustard	0.4 mg/kg IV repeated q 3–4 weeks	Bone marrow suppression; nausea and vomiting
2. Cyclophosphamide	40 mg/kg q 3 weeks IV 15 mg/kg weekly IV 1–4 mg/kg/day PO	Bone marrow suppression; nausea and vomiting; cystitis; alopecia
3. Vincristine	0.025 mg/kg weekly IV	Neuromuscular; alopecia
4. Prednisone	1 mg/kg/day PO	Osteoporosis; diabetes
5. Asparaginase	200 units/kg/day IV	Allergic reactions; pancreatitis; renal failure
6. Bleomycin	5 to 30 mg twice a week or weekly IV (limited to 300 mg total)	Pulmonary fibrosis; skin ulcerations
7. Adriamycin	60 mg/m² q 3 weeks IV (maximum dose 500 mg/m²)	Cardiac toxicity; bone marrow suppression; alopecia
8. Bis-chloroethyl nitrosourea	3.4 mg/kg q 6–8 weeks IV	Bone marrow depression

should be given, either locally or by referral to special treatment centers. These decisions are often difficult, but they must be considered carefully before embarking on a therapeutic course. Since the answers to many questions are not yet settled or merely reflect personal opinion rather than scientific fact, the physician must be well informed or ask for help.

Although the therapy of patients with lymphoreticular neoplasms is changing rapidly, certain general statements appear valid. For patients with localized disease Stage I or II, the optimal therapy involves radiotherapy to the tumor-bearing areas, including the adjacent normal lymph nodes. The dose to be administered should be at least 4000 rads given over four weeks. Since disease extent is hard to determine with certainty, many oncologists are extending the treatment fields to include all lymph node areas and the splenic area, or bed, if splenectomy has been performed. The upper half of the body is treated en bloc, followed by a short rest and then treatment of the lower half. The anatomic sequence varies if disease exists only below the diaphragm. For patients with localized Stage IE or IIE in the abdomen, consideration should be given to the special abdominal radiation approaches mentioned above. Since the volume of tissue and potential damage to the normal tissues such as marrow, lung, and kidney are great, care must be taken to have well calibrated machines and expertly shaped fields. Therapists prefer megavoltage (linear accelerator) machines

that markedly restrict the amount of scatter to adjacent normal tissues. The ill effects of therapy of this intensity have been pulmonary or cardiac fibrosis, myelitis, pericarditis, bowel ulcerations, and marrow insufficiency.

The approach to patients with Stage III disease is not agreed upon by experts in the field. Even with the most aggressive total nodal radiotherapy, x-ray only produces median survivals of less than three years. Investigators tend to use a combination of chemotherapy and x-ray. The approach may be with chemotherapy first, followed by radiotherapy, or the alternate sequence.

For patients with Stage IV disease, which represents about 40 to 50 per cent of patients, most oncologists prefer combination chemotherapy programs attempting to achieve complete tumor regressions. The one possible exception relates to nodular or diffuse well differentiated lymphocytic lymphomas, in which less aggressive and even single agent chemotherapy may prove to be highly effective. Here one can choose one of several alkylating agents and add corticosteroids for certain clinical indications such as thrombocytopenia and hemolytic anemia. These patients often have marrow involvement and peripheral blood abnormal cells characteristic of chronic lymphocytic leukemia and immunoglobulin deficiencies of immunoglobulin G.

The characteristic effect of combination chemotherapy is rapid resolution of tumor with any of several combinations, but varying proportions will show re-

TABLE 6.   Combination Chemotherapies*

Hoogstraten (1969)	Cyclophosphamide Vincristine Prednisone	15 mg/kg weekly IV × 6 0.025 mg/kg weekly IV × 6 1.0 mg/kg daily PO × 42 days	
Luce (1971)	Cyclophosphamide Vincristine Prednisone	800 mg/M² day 1 2.0 mg/M² day 1 60 mg/M² daily × 5	} repeat q 15–21 days
Bagley (1972)	Cyclophosphamide Vincristine Prednisone	400 mg/M² daily × 5 1.4 mg/M² day 1 100 mg/M² days 1–5	} repeat q 21 days
Lowenbraun (1970)	Cyclophosphamide Vincristine Procarbazine Prednisone	600 mg/M² day 1 + 8 IV 1.4 mg/M² day 1 + 8 IV 100 mg/M² days 1–10 PO 40 mg/M² days 1–14	} repeat q 28 days
Bonadonna (1973)	Adriamycin Bleomycin Prednisone	75 mg/M² day 1 15 mg/M² day 1 + 8 100 mg/M² daily × 5	} repeat q 21 days

*From Carbone, P. P.: Cancer, 30:1511, 1972, and Bonadonna, personal communication.

bound tumor growth during rest periods or after cessation of therapy. To avoid this, other combinations are being evaluated and the use of maintenance treatment added. No single regimen has been agreed on for any single disease category. Moreover, some of the drugs still in the stage of investigation require special permission to use as part of an exploratory approach.

The *complications of chemotherapy* reflect the fact that the drugs injure all rapidly dividing cells, including the normal marrow and gastrointestinal tract, with resultant increased risks of infection, hemorrhage, and ulcerations. *Alopecia* appears common to many of the drugs, because the hair follicle is also dividing its germinal cells rapidly. It is usually reversible, as are most of the other side effects. Modification of the dose may be necessary to make the toxicity manageable.

Some of the newer agents have other toxicities, such as *pulmonary fibrosis* and *cardiac myopathy,* that restrict total dosages. Consideration must be given to the fact that drugs interact with each other or even synergize the effect of x-ray therapy. This is particularly true of adriamycin, a new agent. Some long-term toxicities have been uncovered, including hemorrhagic cystitis, azoospermia or anovulation, cytologic dysplasia, and even pulmonary or hepatic fibrosis; these must be explained carefully to the patient and his family. More recently, information is accumulating that, as patients do better and treatment becomes prolonged, *second cancers* develop, substantiating the effects seen in animals of the carcinogenic potential of x-ray and antineoplastic drugs. However, despite these hazards and risks, under optimal conditions more effective therapies are being devised, and patients are doing better for extended periods of time.

Several *special therapy problems* should be mentioned. First, the rapid turnover of tumor cells results in the production of excessive amounts of uric acid. Treatment itself may result in marked destruction of tumor, and *hyperuricemia* may ensue. Allopurinol, a metabolic inhibitor of xanthine oxidase, should be administered routinely at the start of therapy as a prophylactic measure, along with fluids to ensure adequate urinary output to prevent precipitation of uric acid in the renal tubules. *Hypercalcemia,* an uncommon complication of bone marrow involvement or the production of parathormone-like activity, can be managed with corticosteroids, oral phosphates, or mithramycin, a new antimicrobial that affects bone resorption. *Immune disturbances,* induced by the disease or occurring after treatment, result in an increased *risk of infections,* sometimes with exotic organisms. Accurate diagnosis must be attempted to institute effective therapy. These include fungus infections, viral illnesses, toxoplasmosis, and pneumocystis, whose treatment demands accurate elucidation. Platelet and white cell transfusions, particularly the former, should be available to treat acute problems that arise during the therapy. Pleural effusions and ascites caused by tumor cells on the parietal surfaces can be treated by using a variety of sclerosing agents or chemotherapeutic drugs.

Prognosis. Over-all survival figures for lymphoreticular neoplasms are meaningless, because survival is dependent on histologic subtype, presence or absence of nodularity, stage, sex, age, and treatment program. Such uncorrelated information is available from the End Results Studies of the National Cancer Institute.

Median survivals for localized lymphocytic and histiocytic lymphomas were three and six years, respectively. In disseminated disease the corresponding figures are twelve and six months, respectively. Few investigators report data based on the breakdown mentioned above. The best prognosis is associated with well differentiated lymphocytic lymphoma group, with median survivals of five or more years. In other cell types, nodular varieties do better than corresponding histiocytic forms. Nodular lymphocytic poorly differentiated and nodular mixed lymphomas have the next best prognosis (approximately four to five years). The diffuse poorly differentiated lymphocytic, diffuse histiocytic, and pleomorphic groups fare poorly, with median survivals in the order of one to two years. In most categories, females fare better than males. Age does not consistently affect survival but varies with subtypes. Unlike Hodgkin's disease, symptoms or absence of symptoms does not seem to affect the survival figures corrected for stages.

Data on survival by stage indicate that again histologic pattern influences the outcome. In Stage I patient survivals of five years or more range from 50 to 100 per cent, probably related to histologic differences between series. Stage II and III patients with nodular lymphocytic poorly differentiated and mixed lymphomas have a median survival of three to five years, whereas survival in the diffuse forms ranges from three to four years. Patients with the Stage II and III histiocytic lymphomas, rarely nodular, have a median survival of one to two years. For Stage IV patients, those with the nodular mixed and poorly differentiated variety have an estimated survival of three to four years. Patients with the same cell types and stage but diffuse forms have a median survival of one to two years. Poorest end results are reported in patients with histiocytic Stage IV disease, in which the median survival is six to twelve months. The figures quoted are to be reinterpreted as estimates based on retrospective reviews and analysis when therapy was not systematically controlled. More recent data with more aggressive radiotherapy and chemotherapy indicate that survivals may become considerably better as more attention is paid to staging evaluation and intensive treatment programs are applied.

Berard, C. W.: Lymphoreticular disorders; malignant proliferative responses; lymphoma: Histopathology of the lymphomas. *In* Williams, W. J. (ed.): Hematology. New York, McGraw-Hill Book Company, 1972, p. 901.

Carbone, P. P.: Non-Hodgkin's lymphoma: Recent observations on natural history and intensive treatment. Cancer, 30:1511, 1972.

Carbone, P. P., and DeVita, V. T.: Malignant lymphoma. *In* Holland, J. F., and Frei, E., III (eds.): Cancer Medicine. Philadelphia, Lea & Febiger, 1973, p. 1302.

Carbone, P. P., and Spurr, C.: Management of patients with malignant lymphoma: A comparative study with cyclophosphamide and vinca alkaloids. Cancer Res., 28:811, 1968.

Jones, S. E., Fuks, Z., Bull, M., Kadin, M. E., Dorfman, R. F., Kaplan, H., Rosenberg, S. A., and Kim, H.: Non-Hodgkin's lymphomas. IV. Clinicopathologic correlation in 405 cases. Cancer, 31:806, 1973.

769a. BURKITT'S LYMPHOMA

Paul P. Carbone

Burkitt's lymphoma has attracted a great deal of interest because of its unique geographical distribution, response to treatment, and epidemiologic features highly suggestive of an infectious origin. The clinical and pathologic features were originally described by Dennis Burkitt, a British surgeon, in East Africa in 1958. Burkitt's lymphoma also occurs in the United States, South America, and New Guinea. In Africa, Burkitt's lymphoma accounts for over 50 per cent of all childhood tumors; the incidence in the United States is not known, but more than 100 cases have been reported. The features of the disease and response to treatment are quite similar in Africa and in the United States.

Etiology and Pathogenesis. Burkitt's observations suggested that there were climatic restrictions for expression of this disease in Africa. These were weather and terrain conditions conducive to malaria, i.e., adequate rainfall and lack of freezing temperatures. Epidemiologic studies have confirmed these initial observations as well as time-space clustering of cases, further suggesting a viral etiology. Serologic and virologic studies have indicated that the Epstein-Barr virus (EBV) was associated with many cases. More recently, EBV has been proposed as the cause of infectious mononucleosis and possibly as a passenger virus in Burkitt's lymphoma. Malaria has also been associated with Burkitt's lymphoma, because those places that have eliminated malaria do not have a high incidence of this tumor. Malaria has been implicated as a possible co-carcinogen, i.e., priming the reticuloendothelial system, or as an immunosuppressive agent. Recently reverse transcriptase (RNA-dependent DNA polymerase) and Rauscher virus material have been found in some tumors. Despite all these associations, the cause of Burkitt's lymphoma and the causes of its peculiar distribution have not been uncovered.

Pathology. Burkitt's lymphoma, histologically, contains undifferentiated lymphoid cells of uniform size. The nuclei are round and vesicular with prominent nucleoli. The cytoplasm is basophilic with small vacuoles shown to contain fat by special stains. Large histiocytes ingesting tumor debris are scattered throughout the section. The cells can be differentiated from other lymphomas by their characteristic large size and lack of differentiation.

Clinical Features. The tumor affects primarily children (median age 7, range 3 to 60). Males are slightly more prone to develop the disease than are females. The clinical history of illness is short. In Africa, the most common presenting features relate to facial tumors (60 per cent). Abdominal masses occur in 30 per cent, usually as a result of ovarian, mesenteric, or retroperitoneal tumors. Peripheral adenopathy, splenomegaly, and/or hepatomegaly are rarely the main presenting features. Neurologic manifestations, such as paraplegia, cranial nerve paresis, and/or meningeal involvement, occur less frequently (10 per cent). In American patients abdominal manifestations predominate (75 per cent), and less than 25 per cent present with primary localized involvement elsewhere. Hematologic manifestations, such as marrow involvement and/or frank leukemia, are rare in contrast to other childhood lymphomas.

Because these tumors grow rapidly and because they involve the kidneys or obstruct the ureters, hyperuricemia and azotemia are common. The serum LDH may be extremely elevated and is of prognostic value; generally, high abnormal values that do not fall are associated with the poorest results. Metabolically, the tumor produces large amounts of lactic acid, and lactic

acidosis may be an added complication. After chemotherapy, tumor lysis may be so rapid that hyperkalemia may be fatal unless treated prophylactically by maintaining high fluid volumes and frequent serum K^+ determinations.

Diagnosis. The diagnosis can be established only by biopsy, because many of the clinical features, even in endemic areas, can be mimicked by other lymphomas, acute granulocytic leukemia (chloromas), and pediatric solid tumors such as Wilms' tumor, retinoblastomas, embryonal rhabdomyosarcomas, and neuroblastoma. Cytologic material should be prepared by touching a freshly cut surface of the tumor to the glass slides and then staining with standard hematologic techniques.

In the absence of the classic jaw tumor, Burkitt's lymphoma may not be suspected. The surgeon may first encounter the disease in the abdomen at laparotomy because of an expanding mass or intestinal obstruction. Attempts should be made to debulk the tumor as much as possible, because this may improve the over-all prognosis. Additional staging procedures include intravenous pyelogram, bone survey, bone marrow biopsy, lumbar puncture, lymphograms, and [67]gallium scans. It must be emphasized, however, that the tumor grows so fast that undue delay may be deleterious to the patient's eventual prognosis. Clinical staging schemes have generally acknowledged the good prognosis of facial tumors and limited abdominal disease. Conversely, central nervous system and bone marrow involvement convey a poor prognosis.

Management and Prognosis. Even in the localized cases, chemotherapy plays a major role in management. Cyclophosphamide, 40 mg per kilogram every three weeks intravenously for two to six courses, is the major therapeutic regimen. Patients who suffer a relapse quickly or fail to respond may receive vincristine, 1.4 mg per square meter, on day 1 and methotrexate, 15 mg per square meter, on days 1 to 4, alternating with cytosine arabinoside, 250 mg per square meter per day given in six-hour doses for three days.

When complete remission has been achieved, maintenance treatment has not been shown to be of value. X-ray therapy has not been a major modality in this disease except for treatment of obstructive symptoms. Ninety per cent of all patients achieve complete disappearance of tumor. About 30 per cent of these patients never relapse. The disease in one third of the remaining patients recurs early or produces central nervous system manifestations. These patients have a poor prognosis and will die usually in six months. The remainder have late recurrence (after six months) after a complete response. Characteristically, they respond to the same initial treatment. As mentioned above, care must be taken to prevent or manage the metabolic complications, particularly hyperuricemia, lactic acidosis, and hyperkalemia.

The long-term survival with Burkitt's lymphoma both in the United States and in Africa is extremely good, about 50 to 60 per cent. Best results are obtained in those patients with localized disease. Extensive abdominal disease or liver, central nervous system, or bone marrow involvement carries the poorest prognosis. Despite the strong evidence for tumor-associated antigens and spontaneous regressions in some patients, immunotherapy with BCG and/or allogenic tumor cells has not been shown to be better than chemotherapy alone.

Burkitt, D., and O'Conor, G. T.: Malignant lymphoma in African children: Clinical syndrome. Cancer, 14:256, 1966.

Cohen, M. H., et al.: Burkitt's tumor in the United States. Cancer, 23:1259, 1969.

Ziegler, J. L., et al.: Intensive chemotherapy in patients with Burkitt's lymphoma. Int. J. Cancer, 10:254, 1972.

Ziegler, J. L., and Magrath, I. T.: Burkitt's lymphoma. Pathobiology Annual 129. New York, Appleton-Century-Crofts, 1974.

770. HODGKIN'S DISEASE

Saul A. Rosenberg

Definition and History. Hodgkin's disease can be defined as a malignant disease, usually arising in the lymph nodes, with a histopathologic appearance which includes characteristic giant cells in an appropriate cellular background. The affliction has challenged clinicians and investigators because of its unknown etiology, its clinical and histopathologic features suggesting a granulomatous infection as well as neoplasia, the extreme variability of its microscopic and clinical picture, its peculiar associated immunologic abnormalities, and its frequent responsiveness to modern therapeutic approaches, which can result in cure of the disease.

In the absence of a known etiology or satisfactory animal model, it is being increasingly challenged that the characteristic giant cell of Hodgkin's disease, the so-called Reed-Sternberg cell, identifies a single disease entity. Nonetheless, considerable information and literature have supported the clinical value of considering Hodgkin's disease as a disease which can be variable yet reasonably predictable in its expression.

Thomas Hodgkin's name has been immortalized for his description, in 1832, of seven patients with a fatal illness in a report entitled *On Some Morbid Appearances of the Absorbent Glands and Spleen.* On later histopathologic review, Fox confirmed only two of Hodgkin's cases, and on clinical grounds suggested that a third patient of the original seven belonged to the entity now bearing Hodgkin's name.

Although numerous names have been given to this disease, such as *lymphogranuloma, lymphogranulomatosis, lymphadenoma,* and *malignant granuloma,* the name of Hodgkin's disease, initially suggested by Sir Samuel Wilks, has now received international recognition. Many pathologists have contributed to the characterization of this disease, but Dorothy Reed and Carl Sternberg are given credit for the clearest description of the virtually pathognomonic giant cell which bears their names.

Etiology and Pathogenesis. The cause of Hodgkin's disease is unknown. Although various etiologic agents, including bacteria, protozoa, and viruses, have been proposed, none have withstood the tests of time and confirmation. The problem of secondary invaders in the infection-susceptible patient with late-stage Hodgkin's disease has plagued the efforts of investigators for almost a century. The very nature of Hodgkin's disease, whether infectious in the usual sense or neoplastic, has long been a controversy and remains unsettled. The finding of aneuploidy and marker chromsomes in cells from Hodgkin's disease tissue is preliminary evidence that Hodgkin's disease is a true neoplasm. Whether this holds for all clinical and histologic types of Hodgkin's disease remains to be determined.

Any view of the cause of Hodgkin's disease must take into account the wide variety of histopathologic and clinical pictures, the usual rarity of neoplastic-appearing giant cells, the signs of an inflammatory reaction, the frequent infection-like symptoms, its anatomic predilections, its characteristic immunologic deficiencies, and its peculiar epidemiologic characteristics.

Epidemiology. In the United States the annual incidence of Hodgkin's disease is 35 per million for white males and 26 per million for white females, with an annual death rate of 23 per million and 13 per million, respectively. Nonwhites have a somewhat lower reported incidence than whites in all age groups, although the rates approach each other in the age range between 35 and 59 years. Hodgkin's disease has an unusual bimodal age-specific incidence curve, with one mode at ages 15 to 34 and another after the age of 50. The disease is distributed throughout the world, but the incidence peaks differ somewhat for various regions, e.g., absence of the first age mode in Japan.

Approximately 60 to 65 per cent of reported patients are male; 85 per cent of children with disease at age ten or younger are male, but between ages 15 and 35 the sex incidence is about the same.

Occurrence of the disease in two or more members of the same family has been documented in numerous reports and studies. Although the data are inadequate, it is likely that close relatives of patients with Hodgkin's disease experience a slightly increased risk of developing the disease. Observations suggesting a higher incidence of Hodgkin's disease among close unrelated contacts of those with the disease have been made recently. These provocative reports require confirmation and are difficult to establish statistically.

Pathology. The minimal requirement for the pathologic diagnosis of Hodgkin's disease is the presence of characteristic giant cells of the Reed-Sternberg type in an appropriate histologic setting. The morphologic findings, however, can be very diverse.

The most reliable characteristics of the Reed-Sternberg cell are the large inclusion-like nucleoli and the double or multiple nuclei of large size. Mononuclear forms are also found in typical lesions of Hodgkin's disease, but cannot be considered as reliably diagnostic. The Reed-Sternberg cells may vary considerably in appearance, depending on the type of histologic response and category. The distinctive multinucleated giant cells associated with the nodular sclerosis variety are presumed to be variants of the Reed-Sternberg cell, with abundant pale eosinophilic cytoplasm, well-defined cellular borders in lacuna-like spaces (in formalin-fixed tissue) with small to medium-sized nucleoli, and an unusual hyperlobation.

Recent reports have emphasized that cells indistinguishable from, or closely resembling, Reed-Sternberg cells may be found in conditions other than Hodgkin's disease. The appropriate cellular and architectural environment for these cells is required to permit the diagnosis of Hodgkin's disease.

There have been two major histopathologic classifications for Hodgkin's disease: that proposed by Jackson and Parker, and the Rye classification proposed in 1965. The relative frequency of the subgroups of these clas-

TABLE 1. Histopathologic Classification of Hodgkin's Disease

Relative Frequency (%)	Jackson and Parker	Rye, 1965	Relative Frequency (%)
5–10	Paragranuloma →	Lymphocyte predominance	10–15
80–90	Granuloma	Nodular sclerosis	30–70
		Mixed cellularity	20–40
5–10	Sarcoma →	Lymphocyte depletion	5–15

sifications is shown in Table 1. The major advantage of the Rye classification lies in recognition of the important subgroup of nodular sclerosis described by Lukes and his colleagues.

Clinical Manifestations. The presenting and subsequent clinical manifestations of patients with Hodgkin's disease can be extremely varied and considerably influenced by therapy.

A typical onset is in the observation, usually by the patient, of a painless, enlarging mass, most commonly in the neck, but occasionally in the axilla or inguinal-femoral region. Upon examination this is found to be a discrete, rubbery, painless lymphadenopathy, frequently with surrounding enlarged lymph nodes. In other instances, a chest roentgenogram, taken for a routine purpose, demonstrates mediastinal node enlargement; examination may then disclose lower cervical lymphadenopathy, which had not been noticed by the patient. Although these typical presentations may occur at any age with any histopathologic type, these patients are usually between 15 and 35 years of age and have the histologic variety of nodular sclerosis.

As the typical asymptomatic patient is evaluated more thoroughly with available diagnostic methods, the anatomic extent of disease is usually more widespread than was apparent on physical examination. In particular, mediastinal enlargement is found on routine or detailed radiologic examination, para-aortic involvement is noted on lower extremity lymphography, or splenic involvement is found at exploratory laparotomy in significant numbers of such patients.

Occasionally the lymphadenopathy makes itself known to the patient or his physician by producing local symptoms of pain, lymphatic or venous obstruction of an extremity, vena caval obstruction, or airway narrowing. The duration of lymphadenopathy prior to diagnosis is extremely variable. Some patients report that a particular mass had been present for several years, even waxing and waning in size. Typically several weeks to several months elapse between the time of the patient's first observation and the diagnostic biopsy.

Another group of patients with Hodgkin's disease have unexplained and persistent fever and/or night sweats as initial symptoms. Fatigue and weight loss may be associated complaints as these symptoms become more severe and prolonged. These patients tend to be in the older age group, are more often male than female, and, when evaluated, are found to have more widespread disease than the typical patient presenting without symptoms. Occasionally, in older patients, usually past the age of 40, the systemic symptoms are severe, often with associated anemia, but the lymphadenopathy is minimal. Extensive diagnostic efforts may be required to uncover the cause of the symptoms, including lymphography, bone marrow and liver biopsies, or even exploratory laparotomy. In rare cases, the diagnosis is not made before a postmortem examination. These older patients, with predominant systemic symptoms at the onset, usually show the histologic varieties of mixed cellularity or lymphocyte depletion.

Occasional patients with Hodgkin's disease have intermittent evening fever lasting several days, alternating with afebrile periods lasting days or weeks. Usually, the fever gradually becomes more severe and more continuous. This *cyclic fever* has been labeled as the *Pel-Ebstein* or *Murchison* type and is rarely a presenting manifestation of the disease.

Pruritus, usually generalized and severe, is another characteristic systemic symptom of Hodgkin's disease. It may appear as a mild localized symptom, but, if caused by Hodgkin's disease, it usually progresses and becomes generalized. The pruritus may be the only systemic symptom in the otherwise typical presentation of a young person, especially in women. Generalized severe pruritus may occur in patients with lymphoma other than Hodgkin's disease and in other medical and dermatologic conditions, but its presence should always suggest Hodgkin's disease. Its cause is unknown.

Rarely, patients complain of *pain* in the region of enlarged lymph nodes within a few minutes *after drinking alcoholic beverages*. Although this is suggestive of Hodgkin's disease, it is not diagnostic. Its mechanism is not known.

A wide variety of other symptoms may initially call the attention of the patient and his physician to the disease. These same problems occur more commonly as the course of the disease progresses.

The *clinical course* of the disease can be extremely variable. In addition, almost all patients receive treatment that may profoundly affect the course, sometimes resulting in apparent cure, and in many instances resulting in complications that become difficult to separate from the disease itself.

In the typical young patient with Hodgkin's disease, the disease progresses at a variable rate, over a period of months or years, to involve lymph nodes adjacent to those initially involved. In time, if not adequately controlled, typical extensions beyond the lymph nodes occur. There may be intrathoracic problems with compression of the airway or great veins, involvement of the pleura and/or pericardium with resultant effusions, increasing pulmonary parenchymal involvement, or local osseous involvement of sternum, clavicle, ribs, or vertebrae.

It is not uncommon for patients with early disease, apparently localized to the neck, to develop disease in the lymph nodes in the upper para-aortic region and/or spleen. Later, even the young patient with an initially favorable prognosis may develop widespread problems, as if there has been a loss of defense mechanisms. At this stage the *bone marrow* may become focally and then diffusely involved, with eventual marrow failure. Multiple *osseous lesions* may occur, usually of an osteoblastic or mixed osteoblastic and osteolytic radiologic appearance. These often produce pain, but rarely fractures. The *liver* may become progressively involved, diffuse infiltration of the portal spaces causing serious and even fatal hepatic dysfunction and laboratory features of intrahepatic biliary obstruction. Liver involvement in Hodgkin's disease has been noted to be closely, if not uniformly, associated with involvement of the spleen. Peripheral *neuropathies* as a direct result of tumor growth and epidural cord compression are seen increasingly as the disease progresses.

In time, virtually all patients with Hodgkin's disease develop increasingly severe systemic symptoms as their disease progresses beyond control. High continuous fever, drenching night sweats, malaise, fatigue, anorexia, and weight loss are all characteristic of the terminal picture of patients with Hodgkin's disease. Generalized pruritus is seen in a proportion of patients during their course but is not uniform in its appearance. Selected aspects of some of the clinical problems of patients with Hodgkin's disease require emphasis.

Hematologic Abnormalities. It is especially difficult to separate the effects of therapy for Hodgkin's disease from the effects of the disease itself on hematologic parameters. Anemia of a moderate degree may be found in patients who present with widespread disease, often associated with systemic symptoms. This is usually with normal indices, normal or low reticulocyte count, and a negative Coombs test. When analyzed in detail, there may be shortened red blood cell survival with inadequate marrow response, as is also seen in patients with advanced cancer or chronic infection. Excluding effects of therapy, which can greatly aggravate the situation, some patients develop profound anemia occasionally at the onset, but more commonly during the course of the disease. This may be due to extensive bone marrow involvement with the disease, hypersplenism, or, rarely, a Coombs-positive hemolytic picture. Often, combinations of these factors are responsible for the most severe anemias.

Bone marrow involvement by Hodgkin's disease can only rarely be demonstrated by the usual marrow aspirate technique and examination of marrow smears. The involvement is focal, is often associated with fibrosis, and can be discovered more readily by a marrow biopsy performed with a large-bore needle or open surgical technique.

The erythrocyte sedimentation is commonly elevated in patients with active disease, and sometimes it may be the only evidence that the disease has been inadequately treated or that clinical recurrence is imminent. Numerous other laboratory abnormalities have been reported to be correlated with disease activity. These include elevations of serum alpha-2-globulin, fibrinogen, haptoglobin, copper, zinc, and ceruloplasmin; depression of serum iron and iron-binding capacity; elevation of leukocyte alkaline phosphatase; and increase in urinary hydroxyproline and muramidase.

In the untreated patient, or if therapy has been minimal, moderate to marked neutrophilic leukocytosis and thrombocytosis are characteristic of active, symptomatic Hodgkin's disease. Occasionally, the granulocytosis may be so marked as to suggest chronic granulocytic leukemia. More careful study, however, usually demonstrates that this is a "leukemoid" reaction. Eosinophilia of a mild degree is not uncommon, but occasionally it is moderate or marked, tending to occur in patients with severe and longstanding pruritus. Absolute lymphopenia, even in untreated patients, is seen in a small percentage of cases and, when present, is a poor

prognostic sign. Absolute lymphocytosis rarely if ever is seen in Hodgkin's disease and should always suggest an error in diagnosis. Reed-Sternberg cells have been described in the peripheral blood in studies employing special techniques, but they are seldom seen with usual hematologic techniques. Rarely, leukemia of the acute myelomonocytic type occurs in patients with longstanding Hodgkin's disease.

Immunologic Abnormalities. The observation that patients with Hodgkin's disease frequently fail to develop a delayed type of skin reaction to tuberculin, even in the presence of active tuberculosis, has stimulated considerable study and speculation. Patients with Hodgkin's disease, even when apparently well, have a higher frequency of cutaneous anergy than does a control population.

Numerous studies have confirmed that patients with Hodgkin's disease have a defect in delayed hypersensitivity. In general, the more widespread and advanced the clinical extent of the Hodgkin's disease, the more complete is the loss of this immunologic reaction. The therapy used for Hodgkin's disease almost certainly contributes to the immunologic deficiencies observed. However, despite the immunosuppressive effects of therapy, recovery of parameters of delayed hypersensitivity has been observed as disease activity has been controlled.

It remains to be determined whether the defect in cellular immunity is uniformly observed in Hodgkin's disease, and thus may be of etiologic importance, or is a result of the disease and its therapy. Techniques of measuring cellular immunity are not yet sufficiently precise to be certain. It appears that the more sensitive the test, the more frequently it is abnormal, even in limited disease and prior to therapy.

The relatively well patient with Hodgkin's disease cannot be shown to be more susceptible to infections of any kind, even though he may be anergic to the usual skin tests. As the disease progresses with greater use of radiotherapy, chemotherapy, corticosteroids, and antimicrobials, bacterial, viral, and mycotic infections become more frequent. However, this is not substantially different from other hematologic and immunologic diseases in the late stages.

Selected Clinical Problems. *Epidural tumors* occur in Hodgkin's disease and other lymphomas. These may be seen in patients with otherwise favorable prognosis and must be recognized and managed as a medical emergency. Any patient who complains of back or neck pain, numbness, tingling or weakness of an extremity, or bladder or bowel dysfunction should be carefully examined for a transverse *spinal cord* or *cauda equina lesion.* This will require the cooperative efforts of neurologic, neurosurgical, radiologic, and radiotherapeutic consultants.

The problem of the *pulmonary infiltrate* in Hodgkin's disease is especially challenging. Involvement of the lungs is common, but its appearance is variable and must be distinguished from radiation effects, partial lung collapse, drug reactions, and especially the wide variety of pulmonary infections which occur in these patients. In some situations the therapeutic significance of these lesions is so great that a diagnostic thoracotomy is justified.

Virtually all patients with uncontrolled Hodgkin's disease who succumb to their disease will have episodes of serious infections. These occur most frequently during the later stages of the disease and are associated with the more intensive use of therapy, especially of myelosuppressive drugs and corticosteroids.

At the turn of the century, tuberculosis was so prevalent in patients with Hodgkin's disease that a causal relationship was proposed. Since tuberculosis has come under relative control in the United States and elsewhere, this infection is only rarely observed to coexist with Hodgkin's disease and is only rarely a cause of death in these patients. Although bacterial infections are commonly identified and respond to the modern use of antimicrobials, other infections complicate the later clinical course.

Fungal infections, especially of the lungs and meninges, with almost any species but especially Cryptococcus, are encountered in most series of patients with hematologic neoplasms, especially when corticosteroids are employed. *Pneumocystis carinii* and toxoplasmosis are being recognized with increasing frequency and must be sought, because effective therapy is now available. Viral infections, especially herpes zoster and cytomegalovirus infection, have frequently been described.

Diagnostic Evaluation. The progress being made in the treatment of Hodgkin's disease has paralleled the improvement in techniques for identifying the extent of the disease in the untreated patient. In view of the current choices of therapy, it is essential that all patients with Hodgkin's disease be evaluated completely by physicians experienced with the disease before therapeutic decisions are made.

A careful history and physical examination are essential to uncover characteristic systemic symptoms and to describe all the lymph node areas of the body. Not all palpable lymph nodes are pathologic in the sense that they contain Hodgkin's disease. However, if there are suspicious lymph nodes which, if involved, would change the therapeutic approach, biopsy should be done for confirmation. The lymphoid tissues in the oropharynx and nasopharynx should be evaluated by a skillful examiner. The size of the liver and spleen must be determined as carefully as possible. The bones should be examined for areas of tenderness.

Radiologic examinations should include routine chest films and whole lung tomography to identify mediastinal and hilar lymphadenopathy and pulmonary involvement. Lower extremity lymphography is essential in all patients, unless pulmonary function is seriously limited or bone marrow or other disseminated extralymphatic involvement has been documented. A skeletal survey complemented by bone scans is desirable to detect osseous lesions, most often first seen in the vertebrae and pelvis. Routine blood cell counts and determination of sedimentation rate, serum alkaline phosphatase, and urinalysis and evaluation of renal function are the minimal laboratory studies required for evaluation. Bone marrow biopsy, using a needle or an open technique, should be performed in all patients with advanced lymph node involvement.

In recent years, exploratory laparotomy and splenectomy have been employed to identify and confirm the presence of Hodgkin's disease in the abdomen and pelvis. Studies have demonstrated that approximately half the patients with clinical enlargement of the spleen do not have histologic involvement of that organ; conversely, in approximately one patient in four, spleens of normal size have demonstrable foci of Hodgkin's disease. The identification of involvement of the liver by Hodgkin's disease is especially difficult. It is unusual for marked and obvious liver involvement to occur early in the course of the disease. Abnormalities of liver function tests, including the Bromsulphalein excretion, serum alkaline phosphatase, and other enzymes, modest hepatomegaly, and nonspecific hepatic scan abnormalities may all be misleading. These abnormalities may occur nonspecifically, especially in patients with systemic symptoms, and histologic verification of hepatic involvement should be sought. Conversely, liver involvement can be demonstrated, although rarely, at laparotomy, with no laboratory abnormalities thought to be characteristic of that condition.

The advances in diagnostic ability and the results of detailed study of patients early in their course provide strong evidence that Hodgkin's disease presents in relatively orderly patterns of involvement, suggesting a unifocal origin. Before the distribution of disease has been altered by treatment, the lymph node involvement is not a random affair, but nodal disease occurs in contiguous regions (or those directly connected by lymphatic channels, such as the low neck and upper paraaortic lymph nodes) in 90 per cent or more of the cases when a second node group is involved.

Staging in Hodgkin's Disease. There have been several attempts to classify the extent of the disease, in previously untreated patients, to provide useful prognostic and therapeutic indicators. All the proposals acknowledge the poor prognostic significance of widespread disease and of systemic symptoms. The importance of an accepted staging classification in any disease is to facilitate the selection of appropriate treatment programs, to give an estimate of prognosis, and to permit a valid comparison among medical centers for evaluation of their therapeutic results and investigative programs. The disease stage of classification in current use is shown in Table 3 of Ch. 769.

Treatment. The treatment of Hodgkin's disease has undergone radical changes since 1940. These have resulted from advances in the availability and techniques of supervoltage radiotherapy, effectiveness of chemotherapeutic agents, and the realization that patients can be cured.

The advances and enthusiasm for aggressive treatment since 1960 have appeared and evolved rapidly. It is not yet possible to make an accurate assessment of the true curative potential of modern treatment. Nonetheless, there can be no doubt that considerable improvement in over-all survival rates is being observed, and a significant number of patients are being cured by appropriate evaluation and staging and the application of concepts of tolerable aggressive therapy.

Radiotherapy. The basic concepts of modern radiotherapy for Hodgkin's disease were enunciated years ago by the Swiss radiotherapist René Gilbert and were effectively put into practice during the kilovoltage era by Vera Peters, utilizing megavoltage apparatus by Kaplan, Johnson, and others.

The major considerations which determine the success of radiation therapy are the radiation dose per field, the extent of the fields employed, and the beam energy. It is inappropriate to employ kilovoltage x-rays in a curative attempt for a patient with Hodgkin's disease. Doses of 3500 to 4500 rads are required to relatively large fields to effect permanent eradication of any given site. Because of the limitations of present diagnostic methods in determining the true extent of the disease, lymphoid regions adjacent to known disease or contiguous via lymphatic channels are usually treated to full dose to achieve the best results. Modern equipment and methods permit the treatment of most of the commonly involved lymphoid tissues in two or three large single fields, the "mantle" or supradiaphragmatic field and the "inverted-Y" below the diaphragm.

Data are accumulating which support this philosophy of therapy for all carefully studied patients with Stage I, II, and III disease in providing relapse-free survival and probably increased cure rates as well. Extended field, so-called total lymphoid or total nodal radiotherapy should not be attempted by radiologists who do not devote their entire time to radiation therapy.

Chemotherapy. Chemotherapy has developed significantly since the initial experience with nitrogen mustard during World War II. Successful palliation now can be obtained in the majority of patients. Not infrequently, treatment with one agent will eliminate all evidence of Hodgkin's disease, but inevitably the disease recurs. No documented instance of apparent cure by single drug chemotherapy is on record. It is therefore not justifiable to utilize chemotherapy as initial treatment for patients with localized disease who have a chance for cure by intensive radiotherapy.

The alkylating agents vinblastine and procarbazine are valuable drugs for palliation of patients with Hodgkin's disease. In addition, vincristine and the corticosteroids are utilized in intensive combination approaches.

The principal alkylating agents are mechlorethamine (nitrogen mustard, HN-2), chlorambucil (Leukeran), cyclophosphamide (Cytoxan), and thiotriethylenephosphoramide (thio-tepa). *Nitrogen mustard* has the advantage of rapid action, but it must be given intravenously and causes brief but occasionally severe nausea and vomiting. The average duration of benefit is two to three months after a single dose. The advantage of *chlorambucil* is that it may be given orally, and its effect may be titrated more readily against both tumor and bone marrow response.

Cyclophosphamide is a good drug for Hodgkin's disease. Its gastrointestinal toxicity is mild, and it may be used intravenously or orally. An advantage is its lesser toxicity for blood platelet formation. However, it causes alopecia in many patients in whom administration of the drug is carried to the point of marrow toxicity, and hemorrhagic cystitis occurs in 10 to 20 per cent of patients with long-term administration.

Vinblastine provides significant objective improvement for the majority of patients with Hodgkin's disease. Although oral preparations have been tested, the clinically available form of the drug must be given intravenously. It is well tolerated, granulocytopenia being its major toxic effect. There is little or no depression of the platelet count when usual doses are used. The drug is usually given at weekly intervals. Although pronounced leukopenia may develop, rapid recovery is the rule. In some patients, injections may be spaced at two- to four-week intervals after the initial response is obtained. With maintenance therapy, the disease may be kept in remission for many months, occasionally for several years.

Procarbazine represents another class of drug which has definite activity against Hodgkin's disease. A high proportion of patients experience objective benefit for at least a short time. Its bone marrow toxicity is similar to that of nitrogen mustard, affecting all the formed elements. When used as the third sequential drug for Hodgkin's disease, the responses have been relatively short in duration, averaging two or three months, and marrow suppression may be prolonged.

There is no doubt that objective regression of Hodgkin's disease is observed in some patients treated with *corticosteroids.* However, the general experience is that the responses are brief in duration and overshadowed by the serious toxic effects of steroids, which are particularly distressing in leukopenic patients. The corticosteroids have been employed in combination drug programs, because they are not myelosuppressive.

Combination Chemotherapy. In recent years there has been great interest in the use of combinations of chemotherapeutic agents. It is possible to achieve greater cell destruction when drugs that do not have overlapping toxicity can be combined at relatively full dosage. The most successful and widely tested combination has been developed at the National Cancer Institute and consists of six two-week cycles of therapy with nitrogen mustard, vincristine, procarbazine, and prednisone – the so-called MOPP program. Since two-week rest periods intervene between successive cycles, the entire course requires six months. Although this is a prolonged and occasionally difficult therapeutic program, complete suppression of evidence of Hodgkin's disease can be obtained in 70 to 80 per cent of previously untreated patients. The value of this approach has been the high percentage of complete regression of disease and of long disease-free intervals without maintenance therapy.

In some series, the median duration of remissions is two to three years, with some patients in their first continuous unmaintained remissions approaching ten years in duration. This raises the realistic possibility that clinical cure of Hodgkin's disease can be achieved with combination chemotherapy, a result which had not been observed with effective but only palliative single-drug therapy.

Combination Radiotherapy and Chemotherapy. There have been numerous attempts to improve the results of radiotherapy by combining chemotherapy with it. To date, however, there are no convincing reports that such combined therapy has been beneficial. Moreover, the routine supplementation of radiotherapy with concurrent single-drug chemotherapy in localized Hodgkin's disease seems distinctly unwise, because the drug, by depressing hematopoiesis, may jeopardize completion of a potentially curative course of radiotherapy.

Recently there have been studies of the possibility of administering the MOPP cyclic combination chemotherapy after total lymphoid radiotherapy. This is an area of active clinical investigation at this time. Carefully controlled therapeutic trials will be required to prove if there is an advantage in terms of prolonged high quality survival of programs which of necessity are associated with greater morbidity and prolonged inconvenience to the patient.

TABLE 2. The Treatment of Hodgkin's Disease (November 1973)

Ann Arbor Pathologic Stage	Recommended Therapy	Estimated Five-Year Disease-Free Survival (%)	Experimental Therapy
IA, IEA, IIA, IIEA	Total lymphoid radiotherapy	90	Limited radiotherapy ± combination chemotherapy
IB, IEB, IIB, IIEB	Total lymphoid radiotherapy	75	Total lymphoid radiotherapy + combination chemotherapy
IIIA, IIIEA, IIISA	Total lymphoid radiotherapy	60	Combination chemotherapy ± total lymphoid radiotherapy
IIIB, IIIEB, IIISB	Total lymphoid radiotherapy or combination chemotherapy	40	Total lymphoid radiotherapy + combination chemotherapy
IVA, IVB	Combination chemotherapy	25	Total lymphoid radiotherapy + combination chemotherapy

Recommended Therapy. The recommended therapy for a patient with Hodgkin's disease must be individualized. Considerations of age, extent of disease, prior therapy, and availability of modern skills in radiotherapy and chemotherapy are important in making therapeutic decisions. However, the improving results of aggressive therapy after accurate clinical evaluation and staging in the untreated patient must be acknowledged. Although the value of some therapeutic regimens remains to be established, in terms of survival the recommended therapeutic approaches for the previously untreated patient with various stages of Hodgkin's disease are listed in Table 2. Estimated results are expressed as the percentage of patients likely to achieve a disease-free interval of five years. Careful evaluation and observation of a high proportion of patients, perhaps 90 or 95 per cent, who have survived disease-free for five years show them to be clinically cured of their disease. Trials are being conducted to further improve these results or to reduce the morbidity of their therapy. These newer approaches are also listed in Table 2.

Prognosis. Hodgkin's disease can no longer be accepted as a uniformly fatal disease. The advances in histopathologic classification and diagnostic evaluation and the selection of appropriate aggressive therapy are resulting in a continuous improvement in over-all survival.

Survival figures and prognostic factors which were accepted twenty or even ten years ago are not acceptable today. This is dramatically demonstrated by comparing over-all survival figures for all patients seen, not only from individual institutions, but from Public Health reports. The five-year survival rate has increased from approximately 25 to 50 per cent over the past twenty years. In some institutions the five-year survival rate is exceeding 75 per cent for all patients seen with the disease.

Even prognostic variables are being obscured by modern aggressive therapy. Such important factors as histology, stage of the disease, and presence of systemic symptoms, for example, are becoming less significant as the therapy has become more successful.

Within the context of the foregoing considerations, certain prognostic indicators can be re-emphasized. In general, the more widespread the disease, the poorer the prognosis. Patients with systemic symptoms as defined by the Ann Arbor Conference have a poorer prognosis than those without symptoms, independent of the extent of disease. Patients with the histologic varieties of mixed cellularity and lymphocyte depletion have a much shorter survival, on the average, than those with lymphocyte predominance and nodular sclerosis. All series show that female patients survive longer than males. Patients over the age of 40 have a poorer prognosis than children and younger adults. An important observation is that limited involvement of nonlymphoid structures does not indicate a poor prognosis.

The prognostic variables described above are not completely independent of each other. For example, systemic symptoms are correlated with the extent of disease, and the histologic type is correlated with the sex of the patient. Nonetheless, these prognostic variables are of practical value in considering the management of each patient and in evaluating the relative success of various therapeutic approaches.

Table 2 presents a reasonable estimate of prognosis, recommended therapy, and current appropriate investigative approaches for the various stages of Hodgkin's disease, as of November 1973. That such estimates and recommendations must be dated is testimony to the fact that the understanding and management of patients with Hodgkin's disease are dynamic and gratifying endeavors.

DeVita, V. T., Serpick, A., and Carbone, P. P.: Combination chemotherapy in the treatment of advanced Hodgkin's disease. Ann. Intern. Med., 73:881, 1970.

Easson, E. C., and Russell, M. H.: The cure of Hodgkin's disease. Br. Med. J., 1:1704, 1963.

International Symposium on Hodgkin's Disease, N.C.I. Monograph No. 36, May, 1973.

Jackson, H., Jr., and Parker, F. Jr.: Hodgkin's Disease and Allied Disorders. New York, Oxford University Press, 1947, p. 177.

Kaplan, H. S.: Hodgkin's Disease. Cambridge, Mass., Harvard University Press, 1972.

Rosenberg, S. A., and Kaplan, H. S.: Hodgkin's disease and other malignant lymphomas. Calif. Med., 113:23, 1970.

Symposium: Obstacles to the Control of Hodgkin's Disease, Rye, N.Y. Cancer Res., 26, 1966.

Symposium: Staging in Hodgkin's Disease, Ann Arbor, Mich. Cancer Res., 31, 1971.

Section Eight. CYTOTOXIC AND IMMUNOSUPPRESSIVE AGENTS

Paul Calabresi

771. INTRODUCTION

Although all active drugs exert a certain degree of toxicity on some cells in the body, the term *cytotoxic agents* usually denotes those compounds that affect the proliferative capacity of cells by their inhibitory action on DNA, RNA, or protein biosynthesis. Accordingly, they are sometimes also called *antiproliferative agents.* The desired result is selective cell death, with destruction of malignant·neoplastic cells and relative sparing of viability and function of normal cells. From the large number of compounds studied in experimental systems, only a few have demonstrated sufficient clinical antineoplastic activity, at acceptable levels of toxicity, to deserve the designation of *chemotherapeutic agents.*

Because these drugs inhibit biochemical sites that are not unique to cancer cells, they have also proved valuable in the management of several non-neoplastic disorders. Among these are certain conditions characterized by altered immune reactivity, including those observed in recipients of organ transplantations and in patients afflicted with connective tissue or autoimmune diseases. The term *immunosuppressive agents* has been used properly to describe drugs capable of suppressing measurable immune responses. It is an oversimplification, however, to attribute all beneficial effects of these drugs to suppression of the immune responses, because this does not take into consideration their anti-inflammatory action or selective enhancement and alterations of complex cellular and humoral immunologic interactions that are probably involved in these disorders.

Other non-neoplastic conditions that have been markedly improved by drugs originally developed for *cancer chemotherapy* include metabolic disorders, such as hyperuricemia and gout, dermatologic diseases, such as psoriasis, and infections caused by DNA viruses and other microorganisms. For these reasons, antiproliferative agents are attracting increasing interest, and their practical importance has expanded beyond the treatment of neoplastic disorders into many other areas of medicine.

772. PRINCIPLES OF CHEMOTHERAPY AND RATIONALE

THE CHEMOTHERAPEUTIC TRIANGLE

When using cytotoxic agents, the physician should always keep in mind the three principal entities involved in the chemotherapeutic triangle: (1) the host, (2) the drug, and (3) the tumor (see accompanying figure).

A series of primary effects and secondary responses involving these factors are illustrated in the figure. The relative preponderance or effectiveness of these interactions determines the final outcome for patients receiving chemotherapy. The effect of the tumor on the host is recognized as the "disease." The effects of the drug on the tumor are called "therapy," and those on the host are designated as "toxicity." The tumor may escape from the effects of the drug by one or more mechanisms of resistance. Although the mechanisms for natural and acquired resistance to drugs are not completely established, increased levels of target enzyme, deficiency of enzymes required for "lethal synthesis" of the active agent, impaired transport into cells, and increased catabolism of the drug have all been implicated. These and other mechanisms are usually exerted through selection by the drug of resistant cells, as a result of elimination of the susceptible population. The host responds to the toxic effects of the drug by metabolizing and eliminating the compound from the body. It is necessary therefore to be familiar with the mechanisms of detoxification and route of elimination of the drugs administered, as well as with the functional status of the organs involved. This is particularly true for cytotoxic agents, because the therapeutic:toxic ratio is small and the margin for error is slight.

Least understood are the defenses of the host against the tumor, although some degree of natural resistance and considerable variation between different individuals and types of tumors have been recognized for a long time. Recently, specific immunologic mechanisms have received considerable attention, and the importance of

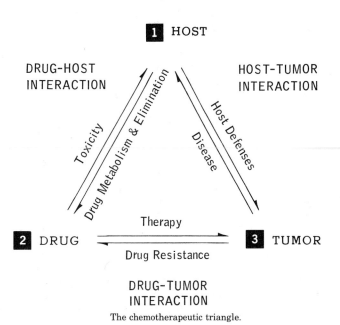

The chemotherapeutic triangle.

cell-mediated immunity through the lymphocyte has been clearly established. The role of humoral antibodies, on the other hand, may be beneficial to the host, when "cytotoxic antibodies" are present, or protective for the tumor when "blocking factors" are involved. Even more nebulous are nonspecific host defense mechanisms, including interferon, local inflammatory responses, phagocytic activity, reticuloendothelial system function, and others yet to be explored. Administration of cytotoxic agents to the host may have profound effects on host defenses, thereby altering a delicate balance that may exist between host and tumor. It is important to remember that these relationships also apply to other parasitic infestations in the body, including viruses, fungi, and bacterial microorganisms. Accordingly, suppression of host defenses may not only facilitate tumor growth, but may render the host more susceptible to infectious complications by pathogenic bacteria or opportunistic organisms.

CONCEPT OF TOTAL CELL-KILL

In order to achieve complete cure of a neoplastic process, every last clonogenic cell, i.e., one capable of giving rise to malignant proliferating daughter cells, must be eradicated. This may be attained surgically when the entire cancer can be excised or it may be accomplished by x-irradiation if sufficient mean lethal doses can be delivered without irreversible damage to normal tissues, so that less than one tumor cell remains. Although the same principles are applicable to chemotherapy, the result has been more difficult to achieve. This is both due to the limitations of currently available cytotoxic agents and because medical oncologists are usually asked to treat patients when the neoplastic process is large, widely disseminated, and not amenable to surgery or radiotherapy.

A number of fundamental principles established by Skipper and his colleagues, using the experimental leukemia L1210 model, offer an excellent basis for understanding the problems involved, and appear to have valid clinical implications. Briefly condensed, they are as follows: (1) A single clonogenic leukemia cell is capable, through its progeny, of producing enough cells eventually to kill the host; (2) the life span of the host is inversely related to either the number of leukemia cells inoculated or the number remaining at the end of therapy; (3) first-order kinetics obtain with respect to leukemic cell-kill by chemotherapy, i.e., a given dose of a given drug kills a constant percentage of cells, not a constant number, regardless of the cell numbers present at the time of therapy (fractional kill hypothesis); (4) it is possible to calculate the chances of killing the last cell in populations that are homogeneous with respect to drug sensitivity; and (5) host immune defenses can be augmented, but are detectable only when small numbers of leukemic cells remain.

It is clear that a reliable assay for determining surviving tumor cells would be a highly desirable guide for effective chemotherapy. Unfortunately, this has been available only for trophoblastic tumors of women. In patients with choriocarcinoma and related disorders, it is possible to measure quantitatively chorionic gonadotrophins in the urine. This enables assessment of the amount of tumor remaining after each course of treatment and continuation of chemotherapy until the assay indicates that all tumor cells have been killed. In certain leukemias and lymphomas, rough approximations of cell-kill can be made by counting the number of abnormal cells in the peripheral blood and the marrow or measuring changes in size of visible tumors. These neoplasms have responded most successfully to chemotherapy, not only because we are able to monitor the presence of residual tumor cells, but more important, because they are characterized by rapid growth and are more susceptible to cytotoxic drugs. In order to begin to understand the reasons underlying the results obtained with cytotoxic agents, it is essential to have a basic knowledge of cell-cycle kinetics.

CELL-CYCLE KINETICS

The percentage of cells in a tumor or a normal organ undergoing division at any given time represents the *growth fraction* or *proliferating pool*. The larger the growth fraction, the more rapid the growth. Since our most effective cytotoxic agents kill cells that are undergoing DNA synthesis and mitosis, the tumors with larger growth fractions are more susceptible to currently available drugs. These include choriocarcinoma in women, acute lymphocytic leukemia, lymphocytic lymphosarcoma, Burkitt's lymphoma, reticulum cell sarcoma (histiocytic lymphoma), Hodgkin's disease, testicular neoplasms, Wilms' tumor and Ewing's sarcoma. Other tumors characterized by a small growth fraction, including carcinoma of the lung and various types of adenocarcinomas, are less responsive to, or not inhibited by, cytotoxic drugs. Several normal rapidly proliferating tissues, particularly the bone marrow, the epidermal appendages (hair follicles and nails), and the epithelium of the alimentary tract, are extremely sensitive to cytotoxic drugs, and often constitute the limiting factor to the amount of chemotherapy that can be administered.

The intermitotic time of proliferating cells, i.e., the average time from one mitosis to the next, can be determined by using ^{3}H-thymidine. This interval can be divided into three phases: (1) the presynthetic phase (G_1), (2) the phase of DNA synthesis (S) and (3) the postsynthetic phase (G_2). At this point in the cycle, mitosis (M) transforms one G_2-cell into two G_1-cells, and the cycle may begin again. Implicit in the discussion of growth fraction is the concept that some cells in a tumor, or a normal organ, may be resting and nonproliferating. Some may be permanently incapable of reproduction, and others may be recruited into the proliferating compartment upon receiving an appropriate, but as yet unidentified, stimulus. These recruitable cells are considered to be in a fourth phase, designated as G_0.

Cells that are in cycle are the most vulnerable to cytotoxic drugs, particularly those that are S-phase specific, such as arabinosylcytosine (ara-C) and hydroxyurea. Other drugs, including methotrexate (MTX), 5-fluorouracil (FU), and 6-mercaptopurine (6-MP), exert their major effects during S-phase but, because of their inhibitory effects on RNA and protein synthesis, are self-limiting because they also produce delay of entry into S-phase. The vinca alkaloids are considered cell-cycle specific agents because they interfere with the process of mitosis.

Cells that are not in cycle (G_0) are almost completely insensitive to S-phase specific drugs but may still be affected by cycle-phase nonspecific agents. Alkylating agents, such as cyclophosphamide and 1,3-bis(2-chloroethyl)-1-nitrosourea (BCNU), are called cycle-phase nonspecific, because they react with DNA during any phase of the cell cycle, leading directly to the cell death or to a delayed lethal effect at mitosis. Actinomycin D and the anthracycline antibiotics, daunorubicin and adriamycin, bind to DNA and interfere with transcription, and are also cycle-phase nonspecific.

Normal tissues with large growth fractions, such as the bone marrow, may have fewer resting cells in G_0 than a slow-growing tumor with a small growth fraction. In this situation, chemotherapy with inhibitors of DNA biosynthesis (S-phase specific drugs) probably would be ineffective, because life-threatening marrow suppression would occur before significant antineoplastic effects. By contrast, the tumors that have responded best to our present generation of cytotoxic agents probably have a larger growth fraction of clonogenic cells than the marrow stem cells of the host. In these patients, judicious administration and scheduling of selected cytotoxic agents can progressively destroy the neoplastic cells while sparing significant numbers of marrow stem cells in G_0, which subsequently could reconstitute the host hematologically.

773. CLASSIFICATION OF DRUGS

ALKYLATING AGENTS

Alkylating agents were studied extensively during World War II in programs concerned with chemical warfare research. They became generally available in 1946, when secrecy restrictions were removed. Hundreds of biologically active compounds have been synthesized, using modifications of the basic chemical structure. A number of substances occurring naturally, including certain antimicrobial drugs with antineoplas-

tic activity, such as mitomycin C, porfiromycin, and streptozotocin, probably function as alkylating agents.

Five major types of alkylating agents have established clinical usefulness: (1) the nitrogen mustards, (2) the ethylenimines, (3) the alkyl sulfonates, (4) the nitrosoureas, and (5) the triazenes. The mechanism of cytotoxic action is thought to be similar for most of the agents in this class.

Mechanism of Cytotoxic Action

Most alkylating agents, except busulfan, generate highly reactive electrophilic carbonium ions that alkylate, by forming convalent linkages, with various nucleophilic substances. Although many biologically important groups may be targets for the reaction, it is thought that one of the most significant sites is the strongly nucleophilic 7 nitrogen of the purine base, guanine. This could lead to miscoding errors or depurination and, in the case of bifunctional alkylating agents, to cross-linking of adjacent macromolecules, which would interfere with normal mitosis by preventing separation of the strands of DNA. Polyfunctional alkylating agents are more cytotoxic than monofunctional alkylators, although the latter may cause mutagenic and carcinogenic damage that is not lethal to the cell and can therefore be reproduced indefinitely as an inherited mutation. Cells are most susceptible to cytotoxic action of nitrogen mustards or alkyl sulfonates when they are in G_1 or in mitosis (M). Progression from G_1 and S phases to mitosis is impaired after exposure to nitrosoureas, nitrogen mustards, and ethylenimine derivatives. Inhibition of mitosis with double complement of DNA and continuing synthesis of RNA and protein can lead to unbalanced growth, giant cells, and lethal cytotoxicity. Nonproliferating cells in G_0 can also be destroyed by alkylating agents. Cell death may occur during interphase, when many sites, including RNA and protein, are damaged, or may be delayed until mitosis when only cross-linking of DNA has occurred. Lymphocytes appear to be most sensitive to rapid cellular disintegration and lysis by highly reactive nitrogen mustards, whereas busulfan is more toxic to granulocytes. Suppression of the immune response may be pronounced, and depression of erythropoiesis and of platelet production also occur. The intestinal mucosa, the hair follicles, and the reproductive system can be damaged to varying degrees by different drugs in this class.

Nitrogen Mustards. *Mechlorethamine (Mustargen, HN₂).* The first of the nitrogen mustards to be used clinically, this compound is often abbreviated as HN_2, its chemical warfare code name. Mechlorethamine is a highly reactive agent and a powerful vesicant. For this reason, it is usually administered intravenously (0.4 mg per kilogram)* into the tubing of a rapidly flowing intravenous infusion. Since thrombosis and thrombophlebitis may occur when relatively high concentrations of the drug are in prolonged and direct contact with the intima of the injected vein, its administration into areas of elevated venous pressure, such as superior vena caval obstruction resulting from mediastinal tumors, must be avoided. The use of surgical gloves is advised to protect

Cytotoxic and Immunosuppressive Agents

I. Alkylating agents:	II. Antimetabolites:	III. Natural products:
Nitrogen mustards	Folic acid analogue	Vinca alkaloids
Mechlorethamine	Methotrexate	Vinblastine
Cyclophosphamide		Vincristine
Melphalan	Pyrimidine analogues	
Uracil mustard	Fluorouracil	Enzyme
Chlorambucil	Fluorodeoxyuridine	Asparaginase
	Fluorocytosine	
	Trifluorothymidine	Antibiotics
Ethylenimine	Cytaribine	Dactinomycin
derivatives	Azaribine	Daunorubicin
TEM	Idoxuridine	Adriamycin
Thiotepa		Mithramycin
		Bleomycin
Alkyl sulfonate	Purine analogues	IV. Miscellaneous
Busulfan	Mercaptopurine	agents:
	Azathioprine	Hydroxyurea
Nitrosoureas	Thioguanine	Procarbazine
BCNU	Adenine	Mitotane
Streptozotocin	arabinoside	Dacarbazine

*For conversion of milligrams per kilogram of body weight to milligrams per square meter of body surface, a ratio of 1:30 may be used. The conversion factor varies between 1:20 and 1:40, depending on age and body build.

the hands of the physician preparing and administering the solution. The drug must be dissolved and administered in a few minutes, because it decomposes on standing. Within a few minutes after administration, the drug is no longer detectable in active form and is bound to proteins or intracellular macromolecules. Less than 0.01 per cent is excreted in the urine. HN_2 has been administered intra-arterially, using techniques involving isolation and perfusion of a tumor-bearing area. The intracavitary use of mechlorethamine (0.2 to 0.4 mg per kilogram) after drainage of malignant pleural effusions can be an effective palliative measure. Intraperitoneal administration is often accompanied by severe gastrointestinal toxicity and is not recommended. Very dilute solutions (0.25 per cent) can be painted on the skin of patients with generalized mycosis fungoides with good results.

The major indications for HN_2 are in the treatment of generalized (Stage III and IV) Hodgkin's disease and other lymphomas, alone or in combination with other agents. The usual dose is 0.4 mg per kilogram administered as a single intravenous dose, because divided consecutive daily doses merely prolong the duration of nausea and vomiting, a direct central nervous system side effect which regularly follows administration of the drug. Premedication with a short-acting barbiturate and an antiemetic is recommended. When extensive neoplastic infiltration of the marrow is supected, as in malignant lymphoma, lymphocytic type, a reduced dose of 0.2 or 0.3 mg per kilogram is recommended. Beneficial palliative results have also been observed in carcinomas of the lung, breast, and ovary and, occasionally, in less common tumors.

The most serious toxic effect of nitrogen mustard is bone marrow depression, with resulting leukopenia and thrombocytopenia. After four weeks, recovery is usually adequate to permit administration of another course. Dermatologic complications include an idiosyncratic nonrecurring maculopapular skin eruption, overt clinical manifestations of herpes zoster, and local reactions caused by extravasation and vesicant action. The last-named complication may produce a painful, tender, brawny induration, which, in severe cases, may slough. If accidental extravasation occurs, the area should be promptly infiltrated with a sterile isotonic solution of sodium thiosulfate (1/6 molar), or normal saline if this is not immediately available, and an ice compress should be applied intermittently for six to twelve hours.

Cyclophosphamide (Cytoxan, Endoxan). Originally devised as a carrier or transport form of nitrogen mustard, cyclophosphamide is activated by enzymatic cleavage of the phosphorus-nitrogen linkage within the molecule. Although levels of phosphatases and phosphamidases capable of accomplishing this cleavage may be relatively high in some tumors, no evidence for this type of selective activity has been observed and the drug is mainly activated in the liver. Since this occurs through the drug-metabolizing microsomal oxidase system, it is subject to the influence of other compounds that affect these systems. Barbiturates stimulate these enzymes and would increase the activation and toxicity of cyclophosphamide, whereas corticosteroid and sex hormones appear to inhibit the effect. Since cyclophosphamide is frequently used in patients also receiving corticosteroid therapy, special caution is necessary, be-

cause a reduction in steroid dosage may increase the toxicity of a previously well-tolerated dose of the alkylating agent. After oral administration, maximal plasma levels are achieved in approximately one hour. Disappearance from the plasma is rapid, with a half-life of about four hours; urinary recovery of unchanged drug is less than 14 per cent.

The major advantage of cyclophosphamide is its versatility which permits a wide, intermediate range of activity, extending from that of the highly reactive intravenous mechlorethamine to that of the slow-acting oral chlorambucil. It can be administered intravenously at usual initial loading doses of 40 to 50 mg per kilogram, given at the rate of 10 to 20 mg per kilogram over two to five days. In patients with compromised bone marrow function, a reduction of one third to one half is recommended. Oral doses usually range between 1 and 5 mg per kilogram daily. The drug can also be administered intramuscularly or into body cavities, and is not associated with vesicant action. A good objective guide for prolonged regulation of maintenance therapy is the total leukocyte count, which should be kept between 2500 and 4000 cells per cubic millimeter.

The major clinical indications for cyclophosphamide are in the lymphoproliferative and myeloproliferative disorders. It is highly effective and has produced cures in Burkitt's lymphoma and is very beneficial in acute lymphoblastic leukemia of childhood, Hodgkin's disease, and other lymphomas. It is active in multiple myeloma, chronic lymphocytic leukemia, ovarian carcinoma, neuroblastoma, and retinoblastoma. Temporary beneficial results have also been observed in carcinoma of the breast, bronchogenic carcinoma, and other neoplasms. Because of its potent immunosuppressive action, it has been used clinically in Wegener's granulomatosis, rheumatoid arthritis, nephrotic syndrome in children, and other conditions associated with altered immune reactivity.

The most important toxic effects are on the bone marrow, but severe thrombocytopenia is probably less common than with other nitrogen mustards. By contrast, alopecia is more frequent and often more severe, though usually reversible. Nausea and vomiting are common, and mucosal ulcerations, hepatic toxicity, increased skin pigmentation, and interstitial pulmonary fibrosis have been reported. Sterile hemorrhagic cystitis, probably caused by accumulation of active metabolites in concentrated urine, has been reported in about 5 per cent of cases. Ample fluid intake and frequent voiding are helpful measures in the prevention of this complication. Because gonadal suppression resulting in sterility has been observed and the mutagenic and carcinogenic potential is high, the use of the drug in patients with reproductive capacity should be carefully considered with respect to possible benefits and risks.

Melphalan (Alkeran). This compound is a phenylalanine derivative of nitrogen mustard. It has the general pharmacologic properties of an alkylating agent of intermediate strength, demonstrating activity in the blood for about six hours. The drug can be administered orally, usually in daily divided doses of 6 mg for two to three weeks; then, after interrupting therapy for four weeks, a daily maintenance dose of 2 to 4 mg is instituted. It is particularly useful in multiple myeloma, alone or in combination with other agents. As with other alkylating agents, the clinical toxicity is mainly hematologic. Nausea and vomiting are infrequent, and alopecia does not occur.

Uracil Mustard. Although synthesized in an attempt to obtain more specificity for the alkylating moiety in pyrimidine biosynthesis, this agent behaves like other nitrogen mustards of intermediate activity. Plasma disappearance is rapid, with no detectable drug after two hours, and less than 1 per cent is recovered intact in the urine. The usual oral daily dose is 1 to 2 mg for three weeks or 3 to 5 mg for one week, with maintenance doses of 1 mg daily. The spectrum of clinical activity is similar to that of other nitrogen mustards. Bone marrow depression is the major toxic manifestation; nausea, vomiting, diarrhea, and dermatitis have been reported, but frank alopecia has not been observed.

Chlorambucil (Leukeran). An aromatic derivative of mechlorethamine, chlorambucil is the slowest-acting and least toxic nitrogen mustard in clinical use. Absorption after oral administration is good, but information on biologic persistence and elimination is inadequate. The usual oral dose is 0.1 to 0.2 mg per kilogram daily for at least three to six weeks. The total daily dose, usually 4 to 10 mg, is given at one time. The dosage is adjusted according to the clinical response, and when maintenance therapy is required, 2 mg daily is recommended. Chlorambucil is the treatment of choice in chronic lymphocytic leukemia. It is effective in Hodgkin's disease, malignant lymphoma, lymphocytic type, polycythemia vera, multiple myeloma, and, particularly, primary macroglobulinemia. It is useful in carcinoma of the ovary, breast, and testes, usually in combination with other agents. Good responses have been reported in the treatment of vasculitis as a complication of rheumatoid arthritis, and in autoimmune hemolytic anemias associated with cold agglutinins. Toxicity to the bone marrow is usually moderate, gradual, and readily reversible. Gastrointestinal and dermatologic toxicity are seldom encountered.

Ethylenimines. Triethylenemelamine (TEM) and triethylenethiophosphoramide (thiotepa) have been largely replaced by the nitrogen mustards, and have similar clinical indications and toxic manifestations.

Alkyl Sulfonate. *Busulfan (Myleran).* The cytotoxic action of this drug is quite selective, affecting primarily granulocyte production, and, to some extent, platelets. More than 90 per cent disappears from the blood within three minutes and is almost entirely excreted in the urine as methanesulfonic acid and other metabolites. The initial oral dose is 4 to 12 mg daily, and maintenance doses of 1 to 3 mg daily are recommended. It is the treatment of choice in chronic granulocytic leukemia and may be useful in polycythemia vera and myelofibrosis with myeloid metaplasia. It is of no value in acute leukemia or in the "blastic crisis" of chronic granulocytic leukemia. Gastrointestinal toxicity is rare. Occasionally, unusual complications have been reported, including generalized hyperpigmentation of the skin, gynecomastia, cheilosis, glossitis, anhidrosis, and pulmonary fibrosis, but their relation to the drug is poorly understood.

Nitrosoureas. *BCNU.* This abbreviation is used for 1,3-bis(2-chloroethyl)-1-nitrosourea; a related cyclohexyl compound is called CCNU. Disappearance of BCNU from the plasma occurs within five minutes. The usual intravenous dose is 1 to 2 mg per kilogram monthly. Bone marrow depression is the principal toxicity, with delayed onset and the nadir occurring after four or five weeks. Although useful in Hodgkin's disease and occasionally in malignant melanomas, the unique property of the nitrosoureas is that they cross the blood-brain barrier, probably because they are lipid soluble, and have demonstrated some promise in the treatment of primary and metastatic brain tumors.

Streptozotocin. This naturally occurring glucosamine nitrosourea is diabetogenic in animals and has been effective in patients with islet cell carcinoma of the pancreas and malignant carcinoid tumors. The usual dose is 1 gram per square meter intravenously for four weeks. Bone marrow toxicity is not significant, but nephrotoxicity may be severe.

ANTIMETABOLITES

Antimetabolites of nucleic acid biosynthesis are structural analogues of normally occurring substances, metabolites. They interfere with normal biosynthesis by competing with purines, pyrimidines, and their precursors for important enzymatic reactions. They may also be incorporated into nucleic acids in place of the corresponding normal nucleotides. Although the site of action for most of them has been defined, the mechanisms of cell death are incompletely understood. Cytotoxicity may be related to unbalanced growth of cells capable of synthesizing RNA and protein, but not DNA, or to coding, transcription, or translation errors after incorporation of the analogue into DNA or RNA.

The agents with recognized clinical value may be classified as follows: (1) folic acid analogues, (2) pyrimidine analogues, and (3) purine analogues.

Folic Acid Analogues. *Methotrexate (Amethopterin).* The folic acid analogues, aminopterin and subsequently methotrexate, were the first class of antimetabolites to demonstrate effective antineoplastic activity. Other "small-molecule" folate antagonists, pyrimethamine and cycloguanil, have been effective against malaria, and more recently trimethoprim has been useful in bacterial infections of the urinary and respiratory tracts. The primary site of action of methotrexate is the enzyme dihydrofolate reductase which catalyzes the reduction of folate and dihydrofolate to tetrahydrofolate. The kinetics of this inhibition are often referred to as "pseudo-irreversible," because the binding of the inhibitor to the enzyme is tight. This interferes with the transfer of single carbon fragments and blocks the conversion of deoxyuridylate to thymidylate, blocking DNA synthesis. Although RNA and protein synthesis are also inhibited by lack of tetrahydrofolate coenzymes, the thymidylate block is considered to be the most important site of cytotoxic action leading to "thymineless death."

Methotrexate is readily absorbed after oral administration. The mean plasma half-life is approximately two hours, and about 50 per cent of the drug is bound to plasma proteins. Transport across the blood-brain barrier is very poor, and intrathecal administration (0.2. to 0.4 mg per kilogram) is necessary to obtain high concentrations in the cerebrospinal fluid. The major route of elimination is through the kidney, with 50 to 90 per cent of the drug excreted unchanged in the urine, usually within eight hours. Impaired renal function can produce marked increase in toxicity.

The usual daily oral dose is 2.5 to 10.0 mg. Intravenous doses of 25 to 50 mg can be given once or twice weekly. Constant daily infusions of much higher doses have been administered but only when using the technique of leucovorin "rescue."

Methotrexate has produced cures in women with choriocarcinoma and related trophoblastic tumors in approximately 75 per cent of the cases. It is capable of inducing complete remissions in acute lymphoblastic leukemia of childhood, but is of more value for maintenance therapy. It can be useful in Burkitt's lymphoma, mycosis fungoides, and carcinomas of the breast, testes, and oropharynx. It is also effective in severe, recalcitrant psoriasis and as an immunosuppressive agent. In addition to bone marrow depression, it causes ulcerative stomatitis and gastrointestinal toxicity. These adverse reactions can reach serious proportions and even cause death, particularly in the presence of pre-existing folate deficiency or renal insufficiency. Other complications include dermatitis, alopecia, and hepatic dysfunction, sometimes leading to cirrhosis.

Pyrimidine Analogues. *Fluorouracil (FU) and Fluorodeoxyuridine (FUdR).* Both the fluorinated pyrimidine base (5-FU) and its corresponding nucleoside (FUdR) are converted in vivo to 5-fluoro-2′-deoxyuridine-5′-phosphate (F-dUMP). This fraudulent nucleotide has great affinity for thymidylate synthetase, the enzyme involved in transfer of a methyl group from N^5,N^{10}-methylenetetrahydrofolic acid to deoxyuridylic acid (dUMP) in the synthesis of thymidylate. This site of action is responsible for the major cytotoxic effects by blocking DNA synthesis. Inhibition of RNA synthesis and incorporation into RNA also occur and may explain why these compounds are cycle-specific but not phase-specific agents.

These drugs are usually administered intravenously; three hours after injection, no FU can be detected in the plasma. Metabolic degradation occurs primarily in the liver, and special caution must be observed in patients with impaired liver function or extensive hepatic metastases. Approximately 15 per cent of an injected dose of FU appears intact in the urine, most of it within one hour.

The recommended dosage schedule of FU is 12 mg per kilogram intravenously daily for four days and, after toxicity has subsided, 12 mg per kilogram (not to exceed 1 gram) as a single intravenous weekly maintenance dose. FUdR can be administered either at twice the daily dose of FU intravenously or by continuous intra-arterial infusion at doses of 0.1 to 0.4 mg per kilogram daily.

FU and FUdR have been most useful in the palliative treatment of carcinomas of the breast, colon, and rectum. Occasional responses have been noted in carcinomas of the stomach, pancreas, ovary, urinary bladder, and oropharynx. Topical FU (Efudex) as a 2 or 5 per cent solution of propylene glycol or in a hydrophilic cream base has been successful in eradicating premalignant actinic keratoses, as well as superficial basal cell carcinomas.

The major toxic manifestations are bone marrow depression and ulceration of the epithelium of the alimentary tract, with stomatitis, esophagopharyngitis, nausea, vomiting, and diarrhea. The nadir of the leukopenia is between 9 and 14 days. Dermatitis, hyperpigmentation of the skin, hair loss, and nail changes have been observed.

Other Fluorinated Pyrimidines. 5-Fluorocytosine (FC) is converted to the deoxyribonucleoside (FCdR), an active antimetabolite, by fungi such as *Candida albicans*. It is administered in oral doses of 50 to 150 mg per kilogram daily for one to three months, and is useful in fungal and cryptococcal infections.

Trifluorothymidine (F_3TdR) is beneficial as an antiviral agent when applied topically to the eyes of patients with herpes simplex keratitis. It is active also against vaccinia, another DNA virus.

Cytarabine (Cytosine Arabinoside, Ara-C, Cytosar). This analogue of 2′-deoxycytidine has a structural alteration in the sugar moiety instead of the base. Although the most important site of action has not been completely established, inhibition of DNA polymerase appears to be a primary locus, a concept supported by its cytotoxic effects as an S-phase specific inhibitor. The drug is also incorporated into DNA and RNA, and blocks ribonucleotide reductase. The drug is rapidly deaminated in the blood to an inactive metabolite, uracil arabinoside, which accounts for about 90 per cent of the material in the urine. Ara-C disappears from the blood in approximately 20 minutes, but after intrathecal injection may persist for several hours because of low levels of deaminase in the CSF. The drug is administered intravenously daily for 10 to 20 days, either by rapid injection, 2 to 4 mg per kilogram, or by continuous infusion, 0.1 to 1.0 mg per kilogram. Ara-C is a potent immunosuppressive agent and, depending on the dosage schedules used, can suppress either humoral or cellular responses, or both. It is effective against DNA viruses and has been used topically with beneficial results in patients with herpes simplex keratitis. In contrast to IUdR, systemic ara-C may have greater immunosuppressive than antiviral action, with detrimental effects in disseminated herpes zoster. Although it has not proved successful against solid tumors, it is the most active drug available in acute myelogenous leukemia, and is particularly effective in combination with thioguanine. Myelosuppressive toxicity can be severe, with leukopenia, thrombocytopenia, and anemia characterized by striking megaloblastic changes. Gastrointestinal disturbances, stomatitis, thrombophlebitis, hepatic dysfunction, dermatitis, and fever have been reported.

Azaribine (Triacetyl-6-Azauridine, Triazur). This triacetyl derivative of 6-azauridine blocks orotidylate decarboxylase and, thereby, the de novo synthesis of uridylate. Azaribine is well absorbed after oral administration, and provides good levels of 6-azauridine in the blood for approximately six to eight hours, almost 100 per cent of which is recovered intact in the urine. Occasionally, further metabolism to 6-azauracil, probably by gastrointestinal microorganisms, may produce reversible neurologic disturbances. The recommended oral dose is 125 mg per kilogram daily. It is extremely effective in the treatment of psoriasis and psoriatic arthritis. Recent evidence indicates that increased occurrence of thromboembolic disease in psoriasis is reduced by azaribine therapy. Relative absence of toxic manifestations makes it a safe and desirable agent, although at higher doses (270 mg per kilogram daily), it can produce reversible suppression of erythropoiesis. In this dosage it has been beneficial in patients with polycythemia vera and mycosis fungoides.

Idoxuridine (5-Iododeoxyuridine, IUdR, IDU, Stoxil, Herplex, Dendrid). Because the iodine atom in the 5-position of the pyrimidine ring is larger than hydrogen or fluorine and of similar size to the methyl group of thymine, IUdR behaves as an analogue of thymidylate, competitively inhibiting its utilization, and even replacing it in DNA. After parenteral administration, it disappears from the blood within two hours and is metabolized to, and excreted in, the urine as 5-iodouracil, uracil, and iodide. Topical therapy of herpes simplex keratitis is highly effective. Intravenous eight-hour infusions of 60 to 100 mg per kilogram daily for five days are used for systemic DNA virus infections. Beneficial results have been observed in patients with disseminated herpes zoster, vaccinia gangrenosum, and herpes simplex encephalitis. Immunosuppression has not been detected. Major toxic manifestations include bone marrow depression, stomatitis, and alopecia. Gastrointestinal toxicity is less frequent than with FU or FUdR. Transverse ridging of the nails and sensitivity to iodine are sometimes encountered.

Purine Analogues. *Mercaptopurine (6-MP, Purinethol).* This antimetabolite, after formation of the 5'-phosphate ribonucleotide, blocks by "pseudo-feedback inhibition" the formation of ribosylamine-5-phosphate catalyzed by PRPP-amidotransferase, the first committed step in the de novo pathway of purine biosynthesis. It can also block the synthesis of adenylate and guanylate from the "bridgehead" nucleotide, inosinate. The drug is well absorbed after oral ingestion, and about 50 per cent of the dose is recovered in the urine in 24 hours, largely metabolized to 6-thiouric acid and inorganic sulfate. Attempts to inhibit this degradation led to the development of allopurinol (Zyloprim), a xanthine oxidase inhibitor capable of blocking the catabolism of 6-MP, as well as the formation of uric acid from hypoxanthine and xanthine. Allopurinol has become an important agent in the management of hyperuricemia and gout. The usual oral daily dose of 6-MP is 2.5 per kilogram, but *this must be reduced to 25 per cent when allopurinol is being administered concomitantly* at doses of 200 to 600 mg daily to reduce or prevent hyperuricemia. The major clinical indication for 6-MP is acute lymphoblastic leukemia in children. It may be useful in adults with acute leukemia or in chronic granulocytic leukemia. It is not effective in chronic lymphocytic leukemia, Hodgkin's disease, malignant lymphoma, lymphocytic type, or solid tumors. Although active as an immunosuppressive agent, 6-MP has been superseded by its imidazolyl derivative, azathioprine (Imuran). The primary toxic effect is bone marrow depression. Stomatitis and gastrointestinal symptoms are uncommon. Cholestatic jaundice has been reported in as many as one third of adult patients; this is usually reversible upon discontinuation of therapy.

Azathioprine (Imuran). This imidazolyl derivative of 6-MP is probably the most widely used immunosuppressive agent in organ transplantation and disorders with altered immune reactivity. It is cleaved slowly to 6-MP and has similar actions, catabolism, and toxicity. The usual oral dose is 3 to 5 mg per kilogram daily, but this must also be reduced to 25 per cent if allopurinol is administered simultaneously.

Thioguanine (TG, Tabloid). In addition to being a potent "pseudofeedback inhibitor" and blocking interconversion of purines in a manner analogous to 6-MP, it is more significantly incorporated into DNA and RNA. After oral administration, peak blood levels are reached in six to eight hours, and approximately 40 per cent of the dose is excreted in the urine in 24 hours, mainly as inorganic sulfate and 2-amino-6-methylthiopurine, instead of 6-thiouric acid. Because of this, unlike 6-MP and azathioprine, no reduction in dose of TG is necessary when used together with allopurinol. The usual daily oral dose is 2 mg per kilogram. Clinically, it has a spectrum of antileukemic and immunosuppressive activity similar to that of 6-MP, and similar toxicity. It is particularly useful, together with ara-C, in acute myelogenous leukemia.

Adenine Arabinoside (Ara-A). This investigational compound appears to inhibit DNA polymerase and perhaps ribonucleotide reductase, with little effect on RNA or protein. It has demonstrated activity against several DNA viruses.

NATURAL PRODUCTS

An increasing number of naturally occurring substances have attracted attention because of their cytotoxic action. Some are derived from plants that were known for their toxic manifestations many centuries ago, such as the colchicine derivatives of the autumn crocus (*Colchicum autumnale*), and some are of more recent vintage, including the vinca alkaloids from the periwinkle (*Vinca rosea*). The enzyme asparaginase represents an interesting and unique approach to antineoplastic therapy. Finally, countless antimicrobial drugs have been isolated and tested for antitumor activity. Of these, only a few with special clinical pertinence will be discussed.

Vinca Alkaloids. The mechanism of action of these compounds is not clearly defined. Inhibition of the cell cycle occurs at metaphase as a result of spindle protein damage. Despite their structural similarity, remarkable differences in cytotoxic action and lack of cross-resistance have been noted among these agents. Oral absorption is unpredictable. Extravasation during intravenous injection may cause considerable irritation and should be treated with local injection of hyaluronidase and heat. The compounds are cleared in less than one hour from the blood and are excreted primarily through the biliary system. Increased toxicity may be encountered in obstructive jaundice. The drugs penetrate the blood-brain barrier poorly.

Vinblastine (Velban, VLB). This drug is administered at weekly intervals, intravenously. The initial recommended dose is 0.1 mg per kilogram, increased by weekly increments of 0.05 mg per kilogram until either moderate leukopenia or the desired beneficial effects are attained, up to a maximum of 0.5 mg per kilogram. Vinblastine is effective in the treatment of lymphomas, particularly Hodgkin's disease. Objective responses have been observed in neuroblastomas, Letterer-Siwe disease, choriocarcinoma, and carcinomas of the breast and testes. The major toxicity is bone marrow depression, usually leukopenia. Gastrointestinal manifestations may be encountered. Neurologic toxicity and alopecia occur less frequently than with vincristine.

Vincristine (Oncovin, VCR). This agent is administered intravenously, at weekly intervals. The initial recommended dose is 0.05 mg per kilogram, increased by weekly increments of 0.025 mg per kilogram to a maximum of 0.15 mg per kilogram, or until the desired response or toxicity is encountered. Vincristine is particularly effective in the induction of remission in children with acute lymphoblastic leukemia. Vincristine (2 mg per square meter) used together with prednisone (40 to 150 mg per square meter) daily can induce complete remissions in 90 per cent of cases, and with a third drug, such as daunorubicin (25 mg per square meter), this rate approaches 100 per cent. It is also very effective in Hodgkin's disease, malignant lymphoma, lymphocytic type, Wilms' tumor, and rhabdomyosarcoma. Responses have been described in choriocarcinoma and carcinomas of the breast, prostate, cervix, and kidney. In contrast to vinblastine, it does not produce bone marrow depression, which makes it particularly useful in combination with other myelosuppressive agents. The combination of nitrogen mustard, Oncovin, procarbazine, and prednisone, the so-called MOPP regimen, is considered the treatment of choice in advanced Hodgkin's disease. The dose-limiting toxicity is neurologic, with paresthesias, loss of deep-tendon reflexes, paresis manifested by footdrop, hoarseness, ptosis, and double vision. Neurogenic constipation may be severe and should be anticipated with an appropriate prophylactic regimen. Alopecia occurs in about 20 per cent of patients. The syndrome of inappropriate antidiuretic hormone (ADH) secretion has been observed in patients treated with vincristine.

Asparaginase. This enzyme, naturally present in guinea pig serum and currently prepared from *E. coli* as an investigational agent, catalyzes the hydrolysis of plasma asparagine to aspartic acid and ammonia. Because, in contrast to normal cells, certain neoplastic cells lack asparagine synthetase and are dependent on exogenous asparagine, a selective nutritional deficiency is produced. The resulting antineoplastic effect has stimulated considerable hope that exploitable biochemical differences may exist between normal and neoplastic cells. Unfortunately, this expectation has been somewhat tempered by the briefness of the remissions, by rapid development of resistance, and by allergic reactions after repeated administrations of foreign protein. Recommended intravenous doses range from 200 IU per kilogram daily for 28 days to 1000 IU per kilogram for periods not exceeding ten days. Asparaginase can produce complete remissions in up to 60 per cent of children with acute lymphoblastic leukemia; it is sometimes beneficial in other leukemias and lymphomas, and occasionally in malignant melanoma. Despite its notable immunosuppressive properties, hypersensitivity reactions occur in 5 to 20 per cent of patients, ranging from urticaria to anaphylactic shock. Inhibition of protein synthesis often results in mild impairment of hepatic, renal, pancreatic, central nervous, or clotting functions. Although usually expressed only as reversible aberrations of laboratory values, toxicity may occasionally be more severe.

Antibiotics. Antitumor antibiotics may (1) inhibit DNA synthesis, (2) impair RNA synthesis, or (3) block protein synthesis. Most of those with established clinical usefulness appear to belong to the second category and, after binding with DNA, inhibit DNA-dependent RNA biosynthesis. Bleomycin, however, inhibits DNA synthesis and reacts with DNA, causing strand scission. Most of these agents are rapidly cleared from the blood and are excreted mainly in the bile. They do not penetrate the blood-brain barrier significantly.

Dactinomycin (Actinomycin D, Cosmegen). This agent is administered intravenously in doses of 0.015 mg per kilogram daily for five days, to be repeated after two to four weeks if no toxicity persists. Dactinomycin is highly effective in gestational trophoblastic tumors and, in combination with radiotherapy and surgery, in Wilms' tumor. It is active in testicular tumors and rhabdomyosarcomas. It has an immunosuppressive effect and has been used in renal transplantation. Toxicity includes primarily bone marrow depression, stomatitis, and gastrointestinal reactions. Dermatologic manifestations include alopecia, as well as erythema, desquamation, and hyperpigmentation in areas subjected to radiotherapy. Extravasation can produce severe local injury.

Daunorubicin (Daunomycin, Rubidomycin, Daunoblastin). This anthracycline antibiotic is administered intravenously at doses of 0.8 to 1.0 mg per kilogram daily for three to six days. It is particularly effective in induction of remissions in children with acute lymphoblastic leukemia, usually in combination with vincristine and prednisone, and has some activity in lymphomas. The drug frequently causes bone marrow depression, stomatitis, alopecia, and gastrointestinal disturbances. A peculiar cardiac toxicity has been observed with arrhythmias and congestive failure, not relieved by digitalis. Vesicant action can occur if extravasated.

Adriamycin (Doxorubicin, Adriablastina). This 14-hydroxy-derivative of daunorubicin is also effective in acute leukemias but differs markedly in its strong activity in solid tumors. The currently recommended dose is 60 to 75 mg per square meter administered intravenously every three weeks. Vesicant action can occur if extravasated. Adriamycin is effective in the treatment of osteogenic, Ewing's, and soft tissue sarcomas. It is particularly beneficial in carcinomas of the thyroid and breast, and is active against neuroblastoma, lymphomas, and carcinomas of the bronchus and genitourinary systems in males and females. Myelotoxicity is a major complication, and alopecia, stomatitis, and gastrointestinal manifestations are common. Cardiomyopathy frequently occurs at total doses above 550 mg per square meter, and this level should generally not be exceeded. The structural similarities of the anthracycline antibiotics to the cardiac glycosides and their avid binding to cardiac DNA have been invoked as possible explanations for the arrhythmias and rapidly progressive congestive heart failure, unresponsive to digitalis. Since the drug is metabolized and excreted primarily by the liver, reduced dosages must be administered in the presence of impaired hepatic function.

Mithramycin (Mithracin). The usual daily dose is 0.025 mg per kilogram, administered during four to six hours intravenously for eight to ten days, as indicated for the treatment of patients with testicular tumors. The drug has an interesting and unique capacity for lowering the serum calcium level, possibly by interfering with calcium resorption from bone. Prompt reversal of dangerous hypercalcemia and hypercalciuria associated with metastatic disease has been observed with daily intravenous doses of 0.025 mg per kilogram for three to four days. The major toxic manifestation is a dangerous hemorrhagic diathesis, usually beginning with epistaxis. This is probably due to a combination of thrombocytopenia, abnormalities in multiple clotting factors, and capillary damage. Other myelosuppressive effects, gastrointestinal disturbances, and hepatic and renal abnormalities also occur.

Bleomycin (Blenoxane). The recommended dose is 10 to 20 mg per square meter, administered intravenously or intramuscularly once or twice weekly to a total dose of 400 mg. Preferential localization of drug occurs in the skin and the lung; other tissues inactivate the compound by removing 1 mole of ammonia. This probably accounts for the selectivity of therapeutic and toxic effects. It is of palliative value in patients with squamous cell carcinoma of the head, neck, and skin, lymphomas, and testicular tumors. Bleomycin alone does not produce bone marrow depression. The most serious toxicity is pulmonary. This begins with a picture indistinguishable from pneumonitis and may, in 2 to 15 per cent of cases, progress to pulmonary fibrosis, which has been fatal in about 1 per cent of patients. Stomatitis, alopecia, and marked dermatologic manifestations frequently occur, including hyperkeratosis, ulceration, and hyperpigmentation. Because anaphylactic reactions have been observed in patients with lymphomas, administration of a 1 mg test dose, followed by a 24-hour observation period, is recommended.

MISCELLANEOUS AGENTS

There are several substances, active as antineoplastic or immunosuppressive agents, that cannot be conveniently categorized under the aforementioned classification of cytotoxic drugs. Some of these are discussed elsewhere, including the steroid hormones—androgens, estrogens, progestins, and adrenocorticosteroids—and radioactive isotopes. Four other clinically useful compounds are listed below.

Hydroxyurea (Hydrea). This structurally simple compound inhibits DNA synthesis, probably by interfering with the enzymatic reduction of ribonucleotides to deoxyribonucleotides. It is an S-phase specific agent and does not block RNA or protein synthesis. It is well absorbed orally, peak plasma concentrations are reached in two hours, and it is undetectable in the blood within 24 hours. About 80 per cent is recovered in the urine; the rest is probably metabolized in the liver. The usual oral dose is 20 to 30 mg per kilogram daily, or 80 mg per kilogram every third day. Hydroxyurea is useful in patients with chronic granulocytic leukemia, who are refractory to busulfan and mercaptopurine. It has produced temporary remissions in malignant melanoma and is beneficial in psoriasis. Toxicity includes bone marrow depression, stomatitis, gastrointestinal disturbances, and, more rarely, alopecia, dermatitis, and neurologic manifestations.

Procarbazine (Matulane). The mechanism of action of this methyl hydrazine derivative is unknown, but it is capable of inhibiting DNA, RNA, and protein synthesis. It is rapidly absorbed from the gastrointestinal tract and readily equilibrates between the plasma and cerebrospinal fluid. Because of rapid metabolism, its half-life in the blood is approximately seven minutes, and in 24 hours 25 to 40 per cent is excreted as a metabolite in the urine. The recommended oral daily dose is 50 to 300 mg. It is effective in Hodgkin's disease, particularly in combination with nitrogen mustard, Oncovin, and

prednisone (the so-called MOPP regimen), and apparently lacks cross-resistance to other agents. Notable immunosuppressive activity has been reported. Major toxicity includes bone marrow depression and gastrointestinal manifestations. Neurologic, psychic, and dermatologic disturbances have been noted. Augmentation of sedative effects may accompany the concomitant use of CNS depressants. Ethyl alcohol may cause a reaction resembling the acetaldehyde syndrome produced by disulfiram (Antabuse). Because it is a weak monoamine oxidase inhibitor, sympathomimetics, tricyclic antidepressants, and other drugs or foods with high tyramine contents, such as bananas and ripe cheese, should be avoided.

Mitotane (o,p'-DDD, Lysodren). This derivative of the insecticides DDD and DDT causes selective destruction of normal or neoplastic adrenocortical cells. It also modifies the peripheral metabolism of corticosteroids. Approximately 40 per cent of the drug is absorbed after oral administration, and about 10 to 25 per cent is recovered as a metabolite in the urine. Blood levels are measurable for six to nine weeks after cessation of therapy. The drug is distributed in all tissues, fat being the primary site of storage. The initial daily dose is 8 to 10 grams, usually given in three or four portions. Maximal tolerated doses vary from 2 to 16 grams per day. Treatment should be continued for at least three months. Beneficial effects have been observed in 35 to 40 per cent of patients with unresectable adrenocortical carcinoma. Gastrointestinal disturbances are common. Somnolence, lethargy, vertigo, and dermatitis also occur. Adverse reactions are usually reversible with reduction in dosage, and do not contraindicate continuation of therapy. Discontinuation of drug and administration of exogenous corticosteroids are indicated if shock or severe trauma supervenes.

Dacarbazine (Dimethyltriazeno-imidazole Carboxamide, DTIC). The mechanism of action of this drug is uncertain. Originally considered an antimetabolite, it has demonstrated alkylating activity. It is not cell-cycle phase specific. After intravenous injection, plasma half-life is about 35 minutes, with 43 per cent excreted intact in the urine in six hours. Elevated urinary levels of 5-aminoimidazole-4-carboxamide (AIC) result from catabolism of DTIC and not inhibition of de novo purine biosynthesis. Intravenous daily doses of 4.5 mg per kilogram for five days every month are recommended. It is currently the most popular drug in disseminated malignant melanoma, used alone or in combination. Bone marrow depression and gastrointestinal manifestations are the major toxic effects. Fever, myalgias, malaise, alopecia, facial flushing, and paresthesias have been reported.

774. SELECTION OF PATIENTS

Proper use of cytotoxic agents requires more than a knowledge of their pharmacology. The physician must be thoroughly familiar with the natural history and pathophysiology of the disease before undertaking therapy. Most important is a careful evaluation of each patient in order to determine the benefit : risk ratio. Special attention must be directed toward factors that may potentiate acute toxicity. Among these, the presence of overt or occult infections, bleeding dyscrasias, poor nutritional status, and severe metabolic disturbances are important considerations. The functional condition of the major organs involved in metabolism and elimination of drugs, usually the liver and kidneys, must be determined. Of cardinal importance is the status of the bone marrow, which may be compromised by the disease process, earlier chemotherapy, or previous irradiation, particularly to the spine or pelvis. Cytotoxic agents have a potential risk for teratogenesis, mutagenesis, and carcinogenesis. Their use during pregnancy or during the reproductive years should be undertaken only after thoughtful consideration and appropriate precautions. Predictive tests for tumor sensitivity or selective immunosuppression are still research endeavors, but rational selection of patients for chemotherapy is feasible with the judicious application of available clinical and pharmacologic information.

775. SUPPORTIVE CARE

Notwithstanding careful precautions, moderate or severe toxicity may be encountered. The physician must be prepared to provide vigorous supportive therapy. Component blood therapy is often required, particularly platelet transfusions. Granulocyte transfusions are more difficult to obtain, unless access to a continuous flow cell separator is available. Accordingly, infectious complications in leukopenic and immunosuppressed patients are common. Although fever may be a manifestation of neoplastic disease, it generally indicates infection. Specific antimicrobial therapy requires prompt

identification of the responsible organism. Bacterial pathogens and opportunistic fungal, viral, or protozoal organisms may be causative agents. Some of these respond to the newer drugs described in Ch. 773. Cytotoxic drugs may produce metabolic complications. Hyperuricemia can be prevented by allopurinol; hypercalcemia can be controlled by corticosteroids and mithramycin; and inappropriate ADH secretion can be corrected by fluid deprivation. Other specific measures are discussed above in reference to individual agents. Finally, the importance of psychologic support cannot be overemphasized. Frank discussion of expected but unpleasant complications, such as gastrointestinal disturbances, paresthesias, and alopecia, should include appropriate reassurance of their reversibility. Because palliation is more frequent than cure, the physician's attitude is most important and should combine honesty with compassion.

Brodsky, I., Kahn, S. B., and Moyer, J. H.: Cancer Chemotherapy II. New York, Grune & Stratton, 1972.

Calabresi, P., and Parks, R. E., Jr.: Chemotherapy of neoplastic disease. *In* Goodman, L. S., and Gilman, A. (eds.): The Pharmacological Basis of Therapeutics. 5th ed. New York, Macmillan, 1975, in press.

DeVita, V. T., and Schein, P. A.: The use of drugs in combination for the treatment of cancer. N. Engl. J. Med., 288:998, 1973.

Greenwald, E. S.: Cancer Chemotherapy. Flushing, N.Y., Medical Examination Publishing Company, 1973.

Holland, J. F., and Frei, E.: Cancer Medicine. Philadelphia, Lea & Febiger, 1973.

Kaplan, S. R., and Calabresi, P.: Immunosuppressive agents. N. Engl. J. Med., 289:952, 1234, 1973.

Krakoff, I. H. (ed.): Medical Aspects of Cancer. Med. Clin. North Am., May 1971.

Proceedings of the National Conference on Cancer Chemotherapy. Cancer, 30:1473, 1972.

Sartorelli, A. C., and Johns, D. G.: Antineoplastic and Immunosuppressive Agents. Berlin–Heidelberg–New York, Springer-Verlag, 1974.

Skinner, M. D., and Schwartz, R. S.: Immunosuppressive therapy. N. Engl. J. Med., 287:221, 281, 1972.

Steinberg, A. D., Plotz, P. H., Wolff, S. M., Wong, V. G., Agus, S. G., and Decker, J. L.: Cytotoxic drugs in treatment of nonmalignant disease. Ann. Intern. Med., 76:619, 1972.

Young, C. W., and Burchenal, J. H.: Cancer chemotherapy. Ann. Rev. Pharmacol., 11:369, 1971.

Section Nine. INFECTIOUS MONONUCLEOSIS

William N. Valentine

Definition. Infectious mononucleosis is characterized typically by irregular fever, pharyngitis, lymph node enlargement, splenomegaly, absolute lymphocytosis with variably numerous morphologically atypical lymphocytes, the development in the patient's serum of heterophil antibodies against sheep, horse, and ox erythrocytes, and the development of antibodies to the herpes-like Epstein-Barr virus (EBV) present in certain Burkitt-lymphoma cell lines. It appears probable that EBV is the causative agent.

History. Although the first account of the disease is generally credited to Emil Pfeiffer, who in 1889 described an epidemic in children that he termed "glandular fever," substantial clinical differences from the typical syndrome and absence of serologic or hematologic

data render this assumption highly doubtful. Sprunt and Evans in 1920 first applied the name "infectious mononucleosis" to the disorder recognized as such today, and directed attention to the abnormal blood leukocytes. The latter were described in detail in 1923 by Downey and McKinlay. Paul and Bunnell in 1932 discovered the unusual concentrations of sheep cell agglutinins in the serum of subjects with the disease. In 1968, Gertrude and Werner Henle reported that patients with infectious mononucleosis acquired antibodies to EBV.

Etiology. The evidence supporting EBV as the etiologic agent of infectious mononucleosis is increasingly strong. Seroepidemiologic data have indicated that students entering college whose sera contains antibodies to

EBV subsequently fail to develop infectious mononucleosis. In contrast, the attack rate in EBV antibody-negative individuals ranges up to 15 per cent during the college years. EBV antibodies are regularly demonstrated in typical, heterophil-antibody-positive mononucleosis. Anti-EBV antibody has been shown to be absent in preillness sera, and to appear and rise in titer during the course of the disease. Unlike the transiently present heterophil antibodies, those directed against EBV persist for years. EBV has the capacity to "transform" lymphoid cells of subjects lacking antibody to it or lymphoid cells derived from umbilical cord blood or fetal lymphoid organs into lymphoblasts capable of long-term survival in tissue culture. Such transformation of cord blood lymphocytes by a factor convincingly identified as EBV has now been demonstrated when filtered throat washings from patients with classic mononucleosis (but not washings from healthy donors) are added to cultures. Moreover, the initial antibodies developing against EBV during acute mononucleosis have now been shown to be IgM in type. These are initially present in high titer, but subsequently become unmeasurable and are succeeded by IgG antibodies. This is precisely the expected course of events if EBV is the causative immunogen and the disease follows initial exposure to it. Nonetheless, there are some reservations, and it has been suggested that EBV could be a "fellow traveler" or latent virus emerging during the lymphoproliferative events of infectious mononucleosis. EBV has also been implicated in such diverse conditions as Burkitt's lymphoma, sarcoidosis, and viral hepatitis, and lymphoblastic cell lines containing EBV have been derived from other lymphoproliferative disorders and even on occasion from normal persons. Although the evidence for an etiologic relationship of EBV to infectious mononucleosis is very compelling, the transmission of EBV to a susceptible host with resultant unequivocal development of the disease is required if the last of Koch's postulates is to be fulfilled.

Incidence and Prevalence. Infectious mononucleosis is widely distributed, having been recognized in Europe, Asia, Australia, America, and elsewhere. Sporadic cases occur mainly, but not exclusively, between the ages of 15 and 30 years, with a slightly greater incidence in males. Epidemics have been reported chiefly in younger children, although in World War II a number of epidemics were observed in young adults. Unfortunately, in many reported epidemics clinical data fail to preclude other diagnoses, and hematologic and serologic data are inadequate or not convincingly confirmatory. Infectious mononucleosis has a low order of contagiousness, is rare in the endemic form among children, and most probably is largely, if not entirely, a sporadic disease. Large series of sporadic cases have been reported from college health dispensaries. Although earlier experience suggested the comparative rarity of the disease in blacks, it is now clear that it is not uncommon in this race. A high incidence has been found among hospital personnel, nurses, and medical students, but it must be recognized that hematologic studies are more frequent with mild illnesses in this group. In Connecticut from 1948 to 1967, the reported incidence of the disease increased some 25-fold. Although the increase was in part undoubtedly related to better recognition and reporting, similar upward trends in various parts of the world suggest that a true increase in incidence may

have occurred. At Yale University, about 75 per cent of entering students lacked EBV antibodies, and the annual student attack rate from 1962 to 1967 was 1.3 to 2.2 per cent.

Epidemiology. In the sporadic form of the disease, cases seldom appear in roommates, families, or other close contacts of patients with the disease. Evidence suggests that kissing may be one important mode of transmission. In epidemics reported before the development of the heterophil antibody test in 1932, serologic confirmation was unattainable, and those before about 1920 (and often later) were not substantiated by adequate hematologic studies. Variability in hematologic and serologic criteria for diagnosis in different reports, an unusual prevalence of atypical and subclinical cases in certain epidemics, and the handicap of the inability to demonstrate a specific etiologic agent combine to cast doubt upon whether reported epidemic and sporadic cases are necessarily the same disorder.

Pathology. The wide variety of clinical manifestations in infectious mononucleosis reflects the diffuse distribution of tissue lesions observed histologically. However, gross changes are confined almost exclusively to lymphoid tissues. Hyperplasia of nasopharyngeal lymphoid tissue is constant, and lymph node enlargement is present in varying degree. Histologically, lymph node reactions vary from a predominantly follicular hyperplasia to a blurred pattern, owing to proliferation of lymphocytic and reticuloendothelial elements in the medullary cords, and resemble malignant lymphoma in some instances. In properly prepared sections, the abnormal lymphocytes seen in the blood are also observed in nodal tissue. The spleen may be tense and swollen, the capsule and trabeculae being thinned and sometimes dissolved by lymphocytic infiltration. The normal splenic histologic pattern is usually partially effaced, with widely spaced follicles and with accumulations of normal and abnormal lymphocytes about the intratrabecular arteries, beneath the intima of veins, and in the blood sinuses. The changes in the spleen render it susceptible to rupture.

Other gross changes include hepatic enlargement and, occasionally, icterus and a skin rash. However, histologic lesions may be observed in virtually every body tissue, varying in distribution from case to case. These generalized lesions consist predominantly of perivascular aggregates of normal and abnormal lymphocytes, and resemble those of certain known viral diseases. Focal lesions are described in the myocardium, kidneys, lungs, skin, central nervous system, and elsewhere. The liver usually contains periportal lymphoid collars, and these occasionally attain the proportions seen in leukemia. Changes similar to those noted in the spleen are found in the capsule of the liver. Meningoencephalitis of mild to severe degree may be observed. In patients with severe nervous system involvement the meninges may be congested and edematous, and may contain increased numbers of mononuclear cells; perivascular cuffing with round cells may be found in brain tissue. Swelling and disruption of myelin sheaths and cellular infiltration of anterior nerve roots have been observed in patients with the Guillain-Barré syndrome associated with infectious mononucleosis. Custer and Smith are of the opinion that the widespread "infiltrates" of connective tissue and the cells composing the perivascular collars arise in situ from cells of the reticuloendothelial system rather than as cell migrations from distant locations. Particle sections of bone marrow fail to show lymphocytic infiltration, although smears of aspirates may contain increased mononuclear elements owing to dilution with peripheral blood. Granulomatous lesions have been described in particle sections on occasion.

Clinical Manifestations. The incubation period is uncertain, but in young adults it is usually in the range of 30 to 50 days. Initial symptoms are nonspecific; malaise followed by fever, sore throat, and headache frequently appears with increasing intensity during the first five or more days of illness. Nearly all patients seeking medical advice experience fever, most commonly from 37.5 to 39.5° C, although sometimes higher. A variably severe pharyngitis is commonly present in the first week of illness, but onset may be delayed to the second week or very occasionally later. Fusospirochetal organisms and hemolytic streptococci are frequently secondary invaders. In some patients (with the so-called "typhoidal" type of the disease) sore throat is absent, although pharyngeal injection and lymphoid hyperplasia are almost invariably present. The throat may be diffusely injected, or membranous pharyngitis may be observed. A palatal enanthem consisting of sharply circumscribed red spots, probably petechial, appearing in crops of usually 6 to 20 lesions, is commonly seen between the fifth and twelfth days of illness.

Lymph node enlargement is present in virtually all cases, but it may be relatively transient in some. The cervical lymph nodes are almost always involved, and posterior cervical nodal enlargement is of value in differentiation from other forms of pharyngitis. Cervical adenopathy is generally moderate but may be massive, and there is little correlation with the severity of pharyngitis. Axillary and inguinal adenopathy are common but not invariable, and enlarged mediastinal nodes may be detected roentgenographically in rare instances. There is no correlation between degree of lymph node enlargement and severity of illness. The enlarged nodes are normally discrete, nontender or slightly tender (unless they drain a secondarily infected area), firm, elastic, and nonsuppurating. Local heat and redness are not present. The spleen is variably enlarged in about 75 per cent of cases. Most commonly the enlarged spleen extends 2 to 3 cm below the costal margin, but more severe enlargement has been recorded.

The liver is palpable less frequently, but jaundice with or without hepatomegaly may occur, most commonly between the fourth and fourteenth days of illness. It is usually mild to moderate and is associated with bilirubinemia, but only rarely with acholic stools. Anicteric hepatitis occurs in most cases.

Although this constellation of signs and symptoms usually predominates in varying degree, giving rise to classification into pharyngeal, typhoidal, and icteric types, involvement by the offending agent is diffuse, and may result in symptoms involving almost every body system. Skin rashes—most commonly transient maculopapular or faintly erythematous eruptions—have been described in different proportions of cases in different series. Their incidence and importance as a physical finding are in dispute, and evaluation is complicated by possible confusion of infectious mononucleosis with other diseases producing exanthems. The most frequently observed lesions are small (2 to 5 mm),

usually pinkish or pinkish-brown, and involve mainly the trunk and upper arms. In Hoagland's extensive experience, skin rashes attributable to infectious mononucleosis itself occurred at the most in 3 to 4 per cent of cases. Neurologic manifestations indicative of involvement of the central and peripheral nervous systems may occur. Headache is common and frequently severe. Instances of isolated cranial and peripheral nerve palsies, nystagmus, papilledema, ataxia, skin hyperesthesia, paresis of an extremity, and toxic psychoses are recorded. Death from the Guillain-Barré syndrome, with ascending paralysis, involvement of multiple peripheral nerves, and high cerebrospinal fluid protein, has occurred.

Electrocardiographic and pathologic evidence of focal cardiac or pericardial involvement may be noted, but clinically significant cardiac involvement or permanent cardiac damage appears to be very rare. Likewise, pulmonary symptoms in the form of cough, sputum, and parenchymal infiltrates demonstrable by roentgenographic examination are uncommon, but have been described. Clinically significant renal disease does not ordinarily occur, but red blood cells, leukocytes, and albumin are sometimes found in the urine. In this regard, however, it must be remembered that hemolytic streptococcal infections are common complications of the pharyngitis. In somewhat less than half the cases, edema of the eyelids and a consequently narrowed ocular aperture are present. It should be emphasized, in addition, that, as with many illnesses, asymptomatic or subclinical cases occur and that the severity of the illness is extremely variable.

The characteristic "mononucleosis" most commonly appears by the fourth or fifth day of illness and persists two to eight weeks, occasionally for several months. Normal small lymphocytes and monocytes are found in abundance. A common, abnormal lymphocyte (Type I of Downey) has an oval, kidney-shaped, or lobulated nucleus with vacuolated, foamy, and usually nongranular cytoplasm. Others are larger with less condensation of nuclear chromatin and a nonvacuolated, more homogeneous cytoplasm (Type II of Downey), or may possess a finer chromatin pattern and one or two nucleoli, and may resemble lymphoblasts (Type III of Downey). Other forms of abnormal lymphocytes are also noted; the "Downey" cells individually are not specific for the disease. Their abundance in typical cases is characteristic, however. In the first two weeks of the disease, isotopic labeling evidence suggests that a high proportion of circulating lymphocytes are synthesizing DNA. The atypical lymphocyte in infectious mononucleosis is not only capable of in vivo proliferation, but has an increased potential for long-term in vitro proliferation as well. Thus long-term cultures derived from peripheral blood may be established, whereas in normal persons such cultures usually fail to thrive. Although cytochemical studies indicate some differences from normal lymphocytes or monocytes, differences observed by electron microscopy are insufficient to classify three types of "Downey" cells by this modality. The total leukocyte count is usually 10,000 to 20,000 per cubic millimeter at some point in the disease, but may be normal or appreciably higher. In the fully developed disease, mononuclear cells usually comprise 60 per cent or more of the leukocytes, and values of more than 90 per cent have been reported. At the outset, counts in the normal or leukopenic range without lymphocytosis are often present. Anemia and clinically significant thrombocytopenia are normally absent, although both acute hemolytic anemia and thrombocytopenic purpura are observed in rare instances; in the former the Coombs test may or may not be positive.

Heterophil antibodies agglutinating sheep and horse cells and hemolyzing ox cells almost always appear in the first two weeks of illness, and persist from four to eight weeks up to several months. Highest titers are usually observed in the second and third weeks of illness. The characteristic heterophil agglutinins are absorbed by beef erythrocyte antigen, but not completely by guinea pig kidney. Differential absorption studies are imperative in atypical cases, and serve in most instances to differentiate infectious mononucleosis from other conditions in which occasionally increased heterophil antibodies are observed. In most of the latter the antibody present is of the Forssman type, and is absorbable by guinea pig kidney. In serum sickness, the heterophil agglutinins are absorbed by both guinea pig kidney and beef antigen. However, a positive test for properly absorbed heterophil antibodies requires the presence also of appropriate clinical and hematologic manifestations if acute infectious mononucleosis is to be diagnosed. Purely serologic evidence may indicate persisting antibodies from a recent attack of the disease, or, rarely, a nonspecific anamnestic resurgence of heterophil antibodies during an unrelated illness.

In addition to heterophil antibodies, several other antibodies obviously not directed specifically at the original immunogen may be noted. Most common of these is a cold-reacting antibody against the human erythrocyte antigen i, most abundantly present in fetal red cells. When this is of sufficient titer and has a wide thermal range, hemolytic anemia in rare instances is the result. Sera from subjects with infectious mononucleosis may also react against Rhesus monkey erythrocytes, may possess cryoglobulins, and may have low titers of antinuclear antibodies. Early reports of frequent occurrence of a false positive VDRL test for syphilis now appear probably to be in error, and this serologic manifestation is probably rare. Its true incidence is currently controversial. In view of the rich serology, it is not surprising that immunoglobulin levels are elevated, usually returning to normal within three months. Although both heterophil and cold agglutinin antibodies are of the IgM class, their absorption from even high-titered sera removes less than 5 per cent of the increase in IgM.

Hepatitis with or without icterus occurs in most patients. Transaminase, alkaline phosphatase, and sulfobromophthalein retention tests for liver function are abnormal in a high proportion of cases. Elevations in SGOT and SGPT enzyme levels have been reported to be the most consistent abnormality. In one study the levels of both enzymes usually increased in the first week of illness, peaked in the second week, and returned to normal in about five weeks. Electrocardiographic changes such as abnormal T waves and prolonged P-R intervals are not uncommon. The cerebrospinal fluid may exhibit pleocytosis up to several hundred cells (chiefly lymphocytes). Moderate elevations in cerebrospinal fluid pressure have been observed.

Diagnosis. Diagnosis until recently rested on the triad of (1) clinical features of fever, pharyngotonsillitis,

lymph node enlargement, and splenomegaly; (2) absolute lymphocytosis persisting over a period of several days or longer and characterized by the presence of atypical lymphocytes, usually constituting 20 per cent or more of the leukocytes at some time during the acute stages; and (3) a positive heterophil agglutination test, with specific absorption studies when indicated. The time-consuming titrations and absorptions characterizing earlier serologic tests have largely been supplanted by a reliable, simple, quite specific and rapid screening slide test. This incorporates absorption with the classic combination of guinea pig kidney and boiled ox erythrocytes. It requires only a drop of serum, and sensitivity has been increased by substituting horse for sheep erythrocytes. Since antibody to EBV can be demonstrated with great consistency in infectious mononucleosis, the immunofluorescence, complement fixation, and membrane fluorescence tests for its presence may be extremely valuable, particularly in atypical or heterophil antibody negative cases. Antibodies to EBV are lacking in preillness serum where this is available; are present, often in high titer, early in the illness; and in any event develop within two to three weeks after the onset of symptoms. However, no single titer is diagnostic, because high titers may be present in other disorders. Although the absence of antibody would preclude the diagnosis, the usefulness of its presence is unfortunately limited by its lack of specificity, by the fact that high titers are often present when the patient is first seen and hence a rise may be difficult to demonstrate, and by inability to obtain anti-EBV titers except in comparatively few laboratories.

Typical cases are readily recognized. Atypical cases present substantial diagnostic problems. It must be remembered that transient lymphocytosis with a few atypical lymphocytes occurs in a number of febrile illnesses. A persisting negative heterophil antibody test does not exclude the diagnosis completely, but a firm diagnosis in its absence throughout the entire course of the disease is dangerous and unconvincing. However, heterophil antibody-negative cases, otherwise typical, have been shown to develop EBV antibody during the course of illness. Conversely, for reasons previously discussed, a positive slide test is not grounds for diagnosis in the absence of "mononucleosis" and appropriate clinical features. In the past, reliance on incomplete criteria for diagnosis or, indeed, at times on a single criterion has resulted in diagnostic confusion and frequent inclusion of questionable illnesses as instances of the disease.

Differential Diagnosis. Infectious mononucleosis may be confused with a variety of febrile illnesses, particularly viral, accompanied by some degree of lymphocytosis and atypical cells. The prominent *pharyngotonsillitis* requires differentiation from streptococcal infections, Vincent's angina, diphtheria, aphthous stomatitis, and other causes of acute sore throat. Generalized infections may be considered in the differential diagnosis in some cases. Constitutional symptoms associated with a skin rash may suggest a variety of exanthems. Adult *toxoplasmosis* may mimic the clinical syndrome of infectious mononucleosis, including the findings of pharyngitis, cervical lymphadenopathy, splenomegaly, fever, and lymphocytosis with atypical lymphocytes. No cross-reaction has been found, however, between heterophil and Toxoplasma dye test antibodies. A syndrome resembling infectious mononucleosis may accompany infection with cytomegalovirus. CMV mononucleosis and infectious mononucleosis both may be characterized by indistinguishable hematologic abnormalities, protracted fever, hepatitis and abnormal liver function tests, splenomegaly, and a variety of nonspecific immunologic aberrations. CMV mononucleosis occurs occasionally in healthy individuals, or some 21 to 34 days after massive transfusion therapy for nonsurgical conditions, or after open-heart surgery with extracorporeal circulation. In CMV mononucleosis the heterophil test is negative, pharyngitis is ordinarily absent, and lymphadenopathy is often not present. With special studies the virus may sometimes be isolated and specific CMV antibodies demonstrated. Syndromes simulating infectious mononucleosis in many respects have also been reported in infection with adenovirus. The hepatitis of infectious mononucleosis may simulate *infectious hepatitis* or homologous serum jaundice, and, indeed, lymphocytosis may also be observed in these disorders. Prominent neurologic features may simulate *encephalitis, poliomyelitis, Guillain-Barré syndrome,* or *lymphocytic choriomeningitis.* The abnormal blood picture may raise the question of *leukemia* or *infectious lymphocytosis.* The latter disorder is not accompanied by splenomegaly or lymph node enlargement, nor are the characteristic atypical lymphocytes or serologic features of infectious mononucleosis present. Hemolytic anemia and thrombocytopenia, when present, must be differentiated from similar findings in a variety of disorders.

Treatment. No specific therapy is available. Secondary bacterial invasion with streptococcal pharyngitis or Vincent's angina should be sought and treated with appropriate antimicrobial drugs and perborate mouth washes. In view of the peculiar liability of patients with infectious mononucleosis to allergic reactions to ampicillin, that antimicrobial should be avoided. Symptomatic treatment of the fever and pharyngitis with salicylates and sedation for pain is indicated when necessary. Splenic rupture occasionally occurs and may be heralded by abdominal pain and shock. This complication calls for prompt surgical intervention. Corticotrophin and 17-hydroxycorticosteroids have been reported to produce dramatic clinical improvements, but do not specifically influence the disease. They are not indicated, except possibly for very ill patients in extreme degrees of pharyngeal lymphoid hyperplasia or edema of the glottis threatening occlusion of the respiratory tract, and in rare instances of acute hemolytic anemia and thrombocytopenic purpura. They may be given to adults as a six-day course: prednisone, 80 mg the first day, and 40 mg a day for three additional days, followed by gradual reduction over the final two days of therapy. Although chloroquine has been advocated, there is little evidence of any significant effect on the basic disease. Very rarely, tracheostomy has been required for edema of the glottis or tracheal occlusion. The hepatitis is usually mild, and permanent sequelae are rare. However, it is probably wise to treat severely icteric patients with bed rest and close observation of liver function tests, as in other forms of hepatitis. Adequate rest and avoidance of activities in which splenic rupture may occur are important in the acute and convalescent period. The friability of the spleen is such that repeated or heavy-handed attempts at splenic palpation are to be avoided. The low order of contagiousness in sporadic cases precludes the necessity for strict isolation.

Prognosis. Infectious mononucleosis is essentially a benign disorder, although rare fatalities have occurred because of rupture of the spleen or severe neurologic involvement, particularly ascending paralysis with the Guillain-Barré syndrome. Very rarely myocarditis has been reported as a cause of death; also very rarely, edema of the glottis or secondary sepsis may be life threatening.

In terms of morbidity, the prognosis is extremely variable. As with other disorders, some patients have clinically inapparent disease or mild, transient illnesses that may or may not be diagnosed. In the more severely ill patients, the febrile period is usually of one to three weeks' duration, and there is a variable but definite period of postconvalescent asthenia. Brief recrudescences are sometimes seen. Serologic and hematologic abnormalities can persist for some time after convalescence. Although longstanding "chronic" infectious mononucleosis has been reported, most observers are of the opinion that a true chronic form of the disease has not been definitely recognized. Clinically significant sequelae of hepatic or cardiac involvement are ordinarily not observed. Occasional focal neurologic residuals are reported, but complete recovery is the general rule.

Carter, R. L., and Penman, H. G. (eds.): Infectious Mononucleosis. Oxford and Edinburgh, Blackwell Scientific Publications, 1969.

Evans, A. S., Niederman, J. C., and McCollum, R. W.: Sero-epidemiologic studies of infectious mononucleosis with EB virus. N. Engl. J. Med., 279:1121, 1968.

Henle, G., Henle, W., and Diehl, V.: Relation of Burkitt's tumor-associated herpes-type virus to infectious mononucleosis. Proc. Natl. Acad. Sci. USA, 59:94, 1968.

Klemola, E., von Essen, R., Wager, O., Haltia, K., Koivuniemi, A., and Salmi, I.: Cytomegalovirus mononucleosis in previously healthy individuals. Ann. Intern. Med., 71:11, 1969.

Remington, J. S., Barnett, C. G., Meikel, M., and Lunde, M. N.: Toxoplasmosis and infectious mononucleosis. Arch. Intern. Med., 110:744, 1962.

Stites, D. P., and Leikola, J.: Infectious mononucleosis. Semin. Hematol., 8:243, 1971.

Section Ten. EOSINOPHILIC GRANULOMA AND RELATED SYNDROMES

Philip H. Lieberman

Eosinophilic granuloma is a benign disorder characterized by infiltrates of eosinophils and mononuclear cells which have been considered to be histiocytes. This disease is complicated by a complex terminology which has its origin in the empiricism of yesteryear. "Histiocytosis X" is an old concept which refers to a spectrum of disease encompassing both the benign disorder eosinophilic granuloma and malignant lymphomatous diseases. The concept of "histiocytosis X" has been challenged recently on both historical and clinical grounds. The "Hand-Schüller-Christian syndrome" has been redefined over the years and is probably synonymous with the more exact designation "multifocal eosinophilic granuloma."

EOSINOPHILIC GRANULOMA

Eosinophilic granuloma occurs most frequently in children and young adults but is occasionally seen in the sixth and seventh decades of life. Approximately twice as many males as females are affected. Of particular importance is whether it is *unifocal* or *multifocal,* for if dissemination is present, one must expect a chronic disease state with generalized manifestations. If a unifocal bone lesion is found (verified by skeletal x-ray survey) and no secondary lesions develop within six months, one can be reasonably certain that the process is limited and that no further defects will develop. Unifocal bone lesions are found in long or flat bones, frequently in the calvarium or femur in children and not infrequently in ribs in adults. Multifocal lesions may involve any site, but are less frequent in the hands and feet. Bone pain and swelling are common presenting complaints, and pathologic fractures may occur.

In addition to orthopedic problems, patients with multifocal lesions frequently manifest fever, malaise, irritability, anorexia, pallor, and malnutrition. Many of the patients have recurrent bouts of otitis media, mastoiditis, and gum ulcerations and infiltrates. Careful history often reveals an allergic background. The periodicity of disease with attacks of hepatosplenomegaly, adenopathy, and debility is impressive. The patient may have transient or permanent diabetes insipidus at the onset of the disease, or it may develop at a later date. Despite the chronicity of the disease with periodic bouts of frequently severe illness, these patients almost all recover; some will have residual orthopedic defects or persistent diabetes insipidus. Much has been written about skin lesions in this disorder, with attempts to classify benign versus malignant forms on the basis of skin or mucous membrane histology. In general, skin biopsies are not helpful. Many patients develop dermatologic lesions which clinically and morphologically can best be described as seborrheic dermatitis. Laboratory studies have been disappointing. The blood counts are generally within normal range, except for occasional slight normochromic normocytic anemia in very ill patients or a slight shift to the left in differential counts when the patient develops secondary infections. Eosinophilia is not uncommon. Serum lipid and cholesterol studies have not been helpful. Immunoglobulin levels and tests of cellular immunity (dinitrochlorobenzene and tuberculin skin tests) have been within normal limits. Almost invariably studies of stools for ova and parasites have not been helpful. Occasional cases of infection by uncommon mycobacteria have been reported, but these are most unusual.

The basic lesion of eosinophilic granuloma of bone consists of aggregates of mature eosinophils and mononuclear cells; the latter have been considered to be benign histiocytes. Varying degrees of necrosis are encountered as well as the multinucleated giant cells common in many bone lesions. In areas of suppuration, foamy histiocytes can be seen. There may be some fibrosis, especially when the lesion is healing. Serial biopsies do *not* show a progression of the typical eosinophilic and histiocytic mixtures to a lipid phase followed by healing fibrosis, as was originally thought. More commonly, the lesion heals by direct fibrosis. Aside from skin there have been very few tissue studies of nonosseous lesions, presumably because of the benign course. However, lymph node biopsies are sometimes performed which show either nonspecific hyperplastic changes or large collections of eosinophils and benign histiocytes. The term "eosinophilic granuloma" has been used for apparently unrelated disorders such as diffuse or polypoid eosinophilic enteritis or cystitis. Nevertheless, it is believed that soft tissue lesions may also be present in the classic cases. Many of the children with multifocal eosinophilic granuloma have had episodes of pneumonitis, documented by roentgenograms, some of which may show diffuse pulmonary infiltration. Some of these attacks of pneumonitis probably represent secondary bacterial infections, for they respond to appropriate antimicrobial therapy. Occasionally typical morphologic lesions of eosinophilic granuloma may involve the mandible, maxilla, or orbital bones. Such patients present with ulcerative lesions of gums or classic proptosis. Although the classic triad of the Hand-Schüller-Christian syndrome, namely unilateral or bilateral exophthalmos, diabetes insipidus, and unifocal or multifocal areas of bone destruction, may be found in multifocal eosinophilic granuloma, they are also seen in other disorders such as malignant lymphoma or carcinoma.

Recent observations have indicated that the mononuclear cells involved in eosinophilic granuloma have an unusual type of membrane configuration similar to that seen in the Langerhans cell of the skin. These mononuclear cells thus may not be conventional histiocytes.

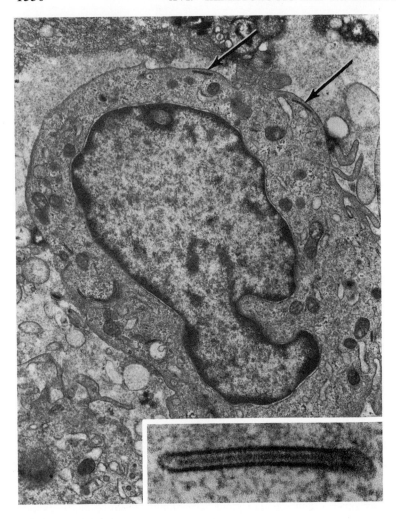

Electron micrograph showing a mononuclear cell characteristically found in eosinophilic granuloma. Arrows indicate two of the numerous Langerhans-type granules found in these cells. ($\times$ 10,800.) Inset: Langerhans granule. ($\times$ 128,000.)

The membranous "bodies" found in these cells result from an inversion of the plasmalemma. The pathogenesis of the peculiar membrane structures and the role the eosinophil plays, if any, in these changes is as yet unknown, but the suggestion that eosinophilic granuloma is an immunologic reaction is intriguing. Recent studies have shed much light upon the mechanisms of eosinophilia and its suppression by agents known to modify immune responses. Some of these latter agents have proved very effective in the clinical management of multifocal eosinophilic granuloma.

LETTERER-SIWE SYNDROME

The Letterer-Siwe syndrome, as formally defined by Abt and Denenholz, consists of (1) marked splenomegaly with moderate to considerable enlargement of the liver; (2) hemorrhagic diathesis; (3) lymphadenopathy; (4) localized tumefactions over bones (may be diagnosed radiologically); (5) secondary anemia with normal or somewhat diminished leukocyte count, normal differential count, and unremarkable platelet count; (6) splenic aspirates, containing increased numbers of nonlipid-containing macrophages; (7) no familial or hereditary disposition; (8) occurrence exclusively in infants; (9) acute onset unrelated to infection;

downhill course with duration from a few weeks to several years; (10) unknown etiology; and (11) generalized hyperplasia of nonlipid-storing macrophages in various organs. These criteria have been variously altered by authors throughout the years, but they are *nonspecific* and have included both benign and malignant disorders, causing much confusion. After eliminating various infectious diseases and nonspecific case reports, one is left with a group of malignant neoplasms principally characterized by the presence of histiocytic elements. On purely morphologic grounds, these disorders probably represent unusual forms of malignant lymphoma. It is probable that the Letterer-Siwe syndrome or disease and eosinophilic granuloma are independent entities. If it is true that eosinophilic granuloma may represent an immunologic response to an unknown etiologic agent, one would expect that rare overlapping of disease entities might take place and that the picture of eosinophilic granuloma might occur not only in rare lymphomatous disorders but also in other disorders, as, indeed, has been the case.

FURTHER NOTES ON TERMINOLOGY

It should be pointed out that, in addition to the inadvisability of using expressions such as "Hand-Schüller-

Christian syndrome," "histiocytosis X," and the "histiocytoses," the terms "reticuloendotheliosis" and "reticulosis" likewise do not belong in the lexicon of the modern clinician. The term "reticuloendotheliosis" was intended to describe proliferation of reticuloendothelial cells giving rise to circulating monocytes, thus being analogous to the terms "myelosis" and "lymphadenosis" used to describe disorders of the bone marrow and lymph nodes, respectively. The term "reticulosis" was introduced by Letterer as a synonym for reticuloendotheliosis. The use of these terms has caused confusion. "Reticulosis" has unfortunately become synonymous with malignant lymphoma in some parts of the world, and "reticuloendotheliosis" (and later "histiocytosis") has been used to describe not only the disorders under discussion in this section but also various lipid storage diseases and infectious granulomas.

TREATMENT

Management of Unifocal (Solitary) Eosinophilic Granuloma of Bone

1. Open biopsy for exact diagnosis.
2. Curettage (with or without bone chip packing).
3. Supervoltage radiation therapy to local "hazardous" sites such as cervical vertebrae or weight-bearing bones (300 to 600 r TD fractionated). Such noncancericidal dosages arrest progression of lesions and stimulate repair. High dosage radiotherapy can lead to tissue damage with resultant poor healing.
4. Supportive therapy, e.g., bed rest as indicated, a brace or cast to protect collapsed vertebra. (See below for diabetes insipidus.)
5. Surgery: (a) to relieve cord compression; (b) partial mastoidectomy if indicated; (c) skin grafts if necessary.
6. Observe for development of other lesions, which usually occur within the first six months after diagnosis. Incidence of solitary bone lesions increases with age. Patients with lesions in the mandible, mastoid, or facial or orbital bones are more likely to develop further disease. (a) Monthly history and physical examination. (b) Skeletal survey six months after biopsy if indicated. If necessary, repeat surveys every six months for one to two years.

Management of Multifocal Eosinophilic Granuloma of Bone

1. Open biopsy for exact diagnosis.
2. Curettage (with or without bone chip packing).
3. Chemotherapy is essential in management in order to prevent prolonged disease and to lessen morbidity and permanent deformity. This probably nonneoplastic disorder can best be treated with drugs used in cancer chemotherapy. Bone marrow depression is *not* necessary to achieve desired effect. Vinblastine, prednisone, and methotrexate used judiciously by experienced physicians can lead to marked suppression of the disease process. *Acute phase* (repeat every 4 to 6 months if new lesions develop): (a) Vinblastine, 0.1 mg per kilogram intravenously every week for three to five weeks. (b) Prednisone, 2 mg per kilogram by mouth three days each week for three to five weeks, with each cycle starting on days vinblastine is given. Total dosage should never exceed 80 mg per day. *Maintenance phase:* Methotrexate, 0.025 to 2.5 mg by mouth for three days, then without medication for 4 days.
4. Supervoltage radiation therapy to local "hazardous" sites, 300 to 600 r TD fractionated. There should be a prompt response, especially if radiation is administered after vinblastine-prednisone therapy is initiated.
5. Antimicrobial agents—used to treat otitis externa, mastoiditis, and sinusitis.
6. Surgery—for cord decompression, to relieve mastoid problems, and to excise calvarial lesions eroding through skin.
7. Supportive therapy: (a) maintain good nutrition; (b) whole blood transfusion when indicated; (c) bed rest, casts, braces, as indicated; (d) physical therapy as indicated; (e) *Reassurance* that the process is not neoplastic and that the patient will be able to regain normal life.
8. Diabetes insipidus: Pitressin tannate in oil and/or Diapid insufflation in conventional dosages (see Ch. 834).

Management of the Letterer-Siwe Syndrome (When Presenting as Histiocytic Lymphoma)

See Ch. 769.

Abt, A. F., and Denenholz, E. J.: Letterer-Siwe's disease. Splenohepatomegaly associated with widespread hyperplasia of nonlipoid-storing macrophages; discussion of the so-called reticuloendothelioses. Am. J. Dis. Child., 51:499, 1936.

Boyer, M. H. Basten, A., and Beeson, P. B.: Mechanism of eosinophilia. III. Suppression of eosinophilia by agents known to modify immune responses. Blood, 36:458, 1970.

Jones, C. R., and Lieberman, P. H.: Unpublished data.

Lichtenstein, L.: Histiocytosis X. Integration of eosinophilic granuloma of bone, "Letterer-Siwe disease," and "Schüller-Christian disease" as related manifestations of a single nosologic entity. Arch. Pathol., 56:84, 1953.

Lieberman, P. H., Jones, C. R., Dargeon, H. W. K., and Begg, C. F.: A reappraisal of eosinophilic granuloma of bone, Hand-Schüller-Christian syndrome and Letterer-Siwe syndrome. Medicine, 48:375, 1969.

Nyholm, K.: Eosinophilic xanthomatous granulomatosis and Letterer-Siwe's disease. Acta Pathol. Microbiol. Scand., Supp. 216, 1971.

Symmers, W. St. C.: The lymphoreticular system. *In* Wright, G. P., and Symmers, W. St. C. (eds.): Systemic Pathology, Vol. 1. London, Longmans, Green & Co., 1966, Chapter 5.

Tusques, J., and Pradal, G.: Analyse tridimensionnelle des inclusions rencontrées dans les histiocytes de l'histiocytose "X," en microscopie électronique. Comparaison avec les inclusions des cellules de Langerhans. J. Microscopie, 8:113, 1969.

Section Eleven.   LIPID STORAGE DISORDERS

Donald S. Fredrickson

776. GAUCHER'S DISEASE

Definition. Gaucher's disease is a relatively common familial disorder characterized by abnormal accumulation of glucocerebrosides in reticuloendothelial (RE) cells; the accumulation occurs because an enzyme necessary for the degradation of these glycolipids is deficient. The increasing mass of the storage cells accounts for most of the clinical manifestations of the disease, including hepatosplenomegaly, lymph node enlargement, and bone lesions owing to expansion of the involved marrow. At least three syndromes have been recognized: (1) a chronic non-neuronopathic or "adult" form, which is by far the most common, becoming evident at any age and associated with hypersplenism, bone lesions, skin pigmentation and pinguéculae, and preponderance among Ashkenazic Jews; (2) an acute neuronopathic form, which is manifest in infancy, is associated with severe neurologic abnormalities, and is usually fatal by three years of age; and (3) a "juvenile" form, which may begin at any time in childhood, combining the features of the chronic form with slowly progressive neurologic dysfunction. At least three different mutations are represented by the different forms of Gaucher's disease. No specific treatment is available.

Pathologic Physiology and Pathogenesis. Cerebrosides are compounds that contain equimolar amounts of sphingosine, fatty acid, and hexose. In the brain the hexose component is galactose, and the galactocerebrosides form an essential part of the myelin in the white matter. In tissues outside the brain, except for the kidney, practically all the small amounts of cerebroside present contain only glucose. These glucocerebrosides arise mainly from the degradation of more complex sphingoglycolipids, the most important source probably being the normal breakdown of both white and red blood cells. In Gaucher's disease there is a specific deficiency in the activity of glucosylceramide-β-glucosidase (glucocerebrosidase), one of the acid hydrolases found in the lysosomes. Glucocerebroside, a *relatively* insoluble compound, then accumulates in RE cells.

The morphologic hallmark of Gaucher's disease is the *Gaucher cell,* a round or polyhedral pale reticulum cell 20 to 80 μ in diameter, with a small eccentrically placed nucleus and a wrinkled ("crumpled silk") cytoplasm that contains an irregular network of fibrils. With electron microscopy the fibrils are shown to represent tubules or strands of glucocerebroside contained within secondary lysosomes having a single limiting membrane. Evidence of active phagocytosis or pinocytosis is present at the cell border, and fragments of erythrocytes are often visible. A few cells may have two or more nuclei. The cytoplasm does not stain with fat stains, but numerous wavy fibrillae are stained deeply with the periodic acid–Schiff reaction or with Mallory's

trichrome connective tissue stain. The cytoplasm also demonstrates strong acid phosphatase activity. Examination of unstained smears of aspirated bone marrow by phase microscopy affords the best visualization of the cells (see accompanying figure, part A).

Proliferation and expansion of the Gaucher cells are responsible for the enlargement of spleen, liver, and intrathoracic and intra-abdominal lymph nodes. The concentration of glucocerebrosides may be increased 50 to 100 times normal in these organs. The spleen may become tremendous in size. Hemosiderin may be increased in the skin and other organs. Gaucher cells are also scattered diffusely throughout the marrow, and in some areas form tumor-like accumulations that may expand, erode the cortex, and lead to pathologic fractures. Infiltration of the lungs, kidneys, thymus, tonsils, thyroid, adrenals, and lymphatic tissue of the intestinal tract also occurs. Functional impairment of these

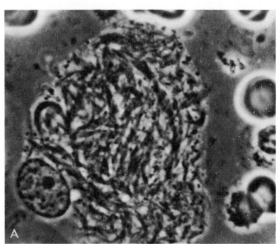
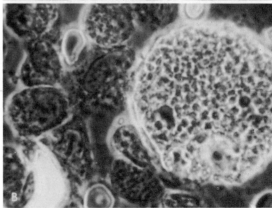

Appearance of the typical Gaucher cell (*A*) and a foam cell seen in Niemann-Pick disease (*B*). Both are viewed under phase microscopy in unstained smears of aspirated bone marrow. Magnification can be estimated from adjacent red cells.

organs is unusual, except for the lungs. Serious pulmonary infections are common in children, and pulmonary hypertension may occur in adults. Pathologic changes in the brains of adults are restricted to the presence of perivascular adventitial cells swollen in the typical Gaucher configuration. In children with the acute neuronopathic type of disease, such "perivascular cuffing" is accompanied by acute nerve cell degeneration with active phagocytosis of the cellular remains by histiocytes and microglia, and cytoplasmic storage of periodic acid–Schiff positive lipid in either neurons or glial cells. These changes are distributed focally in the cerebrum, cerebellum, brainstem, and spinal cord. In the juvenile form the ballooning of neurons is accentuated. An accumulation of both glucocerebrosides and gangliosides has been reported in the brains of infants with the acute neuronopathic type. It is not known why the severity of the effect on the brain is so different in the several forms of the disease.

Acid phosphatase activity, not inhibited by L-tartrate (in contrast to the prostatic enzyme), is characteristically elevated in plasma and has diagnostic value. The enzyme is apparently spilled into plasma from the Gaucher cells. Plasma cerebroside concentrations are elevated after splenectomy.

Clinical Manifestations. *Chronic Non-neuronopathic Type.* The disease affects both sexes equally. It has been reported in Caucasians, Negroes, and Orientals; but a very high proportion of cases occurs among Ashkenazic Jews. Manifestations may appear at any age; the diagnosis has been made in the first month of life and past the age of 80 years. The course is extremely variable and tends to be more severe in affected children. Often, particularly in adults, the patient has no symptoms for a long time except awareness of a progressively enlarging mass in the left upper abdomen. The spleen may become very large; the liver is usually palpable. The second most common presenting abnormality is related to bone lesions. From 50 to 75 per cent of patients have roentgenographic changes, mostly asymptomatic. A common change is expansion of the cortex of the lower end of the femur, producing a characteristic radiolucent area with the configuration of an Erlenmeyer flask. The phalanges, long bones, vertebrae, ribs, and pelvis are more commonly involved than the skull. Bone pain or aching and pathologic fractures may appear at sites of skeletal lesions. With destruction of the head and neck of the femur, walking may become progressively more difficult. The hip abnormalities are sometimes confused with Legg-Perthes disease. In younger patients episodic attacks of bone pain simulating acute osteomyelitis are common. The long bones are usually affected; fever, joint tenderness, and redness occur, and draining sinus tracts may form. The cause is believed to be interference with the blood supply of the highly vascular metaphysis. Attacks usually last several weeks and no longer recur when growth is complete.

A high percentage of patients with Gaucher's disease develop hematologic changes of hypersplenism at some time during the course of their disease: hemolytic anemia, leukopenia, thrombocytopenia, or any combination of the three. The peripheral cytopenia is accompanied by a normal or increased number of the progenitors of the involved formed element in the bone marrow. Chronic Gaucher's disease usually involves only a single generation, but it has been observed in two generations. Otherwise normal parents, siblings, and other close relatives of patients sometimes have slight splenomegaly or small Gaucher cells in the marrow. Although the disease sometimes appears to behave like a dominant trait, most patients probably are homozygous for an autosomal recessive allele or alleles.

Acute Neuronopathic Type. This "infantile" form of the disease is usually evident by three months of age but may become so any time between birth and 18 months. Among the earliest signs are splenomegaly, chronic cough, and psychomotor retardation. Other neurologic signs indicative of brainstem and cranial nerve involvement usually appear by the age of six months. The children have a stereotyped appearance: hepatosplenomegaly, strabismus, head retroflexed, lips retracted, and often spastic extremities held in flexion. The disease is fatal within three years; the average life span is about one year, respiratory infection and distress being the principal cause of death. Sex distribution is about equal. If one child in a family is afflicted, all other affected sibs will have the same form of disease. The disease appears to be transmitted as an autosomal recessive gene and is expressed only in the homozygote. The mutant gene is present in low frequency in many ethnic groups. Four of about 70 reported cases have occurred in Jews.

Juvenile Type. About 25 examples of subacute neuronopathic Gaucher's disease have been described. Hepatosplenomegaly, hypersplenism, bone lesions, and other features of the chronic type appear from infancy onward. These are combined with mental retardation, behavioral problems, seizures, choreoathetoid movements, and sometimes strabismus, trismus, and other evidence of brainstem involvement. In several related Swedish families, glucocerebrosidase deficiency was demonstrated. Glycolipids other than glucocerebrosides may be stored in the spleen and liver, and a clear-cut phenotype has not been established.

Diagnosis. Gaucher's disease should be ruled out in any patient with unexplained splenomegaly, especially with elevated plasma acid phosphatase activity (not inhibited by L-tartrate). A presumptive diagnosis is made from detection of Gaucher cells, usually in marrow aspirates. Diagnosis should be confirmed by demonstration of absence or severe deficiency in activity of glucosylceramide β-glucosidase. The enzyme activity can be measured most accurately in fibroblasts cultured from skin, bone marrow, or amniotic fluid (for prenatal diagnosis). Circulating white cells have also been used for this purpose. If there is any doubt, liver biopsy will permit confirmation of both specific enzyme deficiency and accumulation of glucocerebrosides, provided that the tissue is stored in the absence of fixatives.

Treatment and Prognosis. No specific therapy exists. X-ray therapy to bone lesions may alleviate pain, but usually does not arrest the destructive process. Bone pain may also respond well to corticosteroid therapy. Splenectomy corrects the manifestations of hypersplenism but does not otherwise influence the course of the disease. Because of the possibility that bone involvement may be accelerated by splenectomy, the indication for the procedure should be clear cut. The course is protracted, often extending over many years. Most older patients die of intercurrent diseases rather than Gaucher's disease per se.

Brady, R. O., and King, F.: Gaucher's disease. In Hers, H. G., and Van Hoof, F. (eds.): Lysosomes and Storage Diseases. New York, Academic Press, 1973, pp. 381–394.

Fredrickson, D. S., and Sloan, H. R.: Glucosylceramide lipidoses: Gaucher's disease. In Stanbury, J. B., Wyngaarden, J. B., and Fredrickson, D. S. (eds.): The Metabolic Basis of Inherited Disease. 3rd ed. New York, McGraw-Hill Book Company, 1972, pp. 730–759.

Reich, C., Seife, M., and Kessler, B. J.: Gaucher's disease: A review and discussion of twenty cases. Medicine, 30:1, 1951.

Schettler, G., and Kahlke, W.: Gaucher's disease. In Schettler, G. (ed.): Lipids and Lipidoses. New York, Springer-Verlag, 1967, pp. 260–287.

777. NIEMANN-PICK DISEASE

Definition. The eponym Niemann-Pick disease refers to several rare disorders characterized by extensive tissue storage of sphingomyelin. All patients have hepatosplenomegaly and large macrophages filled with lipid droplets in the bone marrow (see figure in Ch. 776, part B); some also have severe neurologic abnormalities. The "sphingomyelin lipidoses" fall into two major groups. In the first, there is clear-cut inheritable deficiency of activity of sphingomyelinase, a lysosomal enzyme that catalyzes the hydrolysis of phosphorylcholine from sphingomyelin. Sphingomyelin concentrations in tissues are 10 to 100 times normal. The second includes a heterogeneous group of disorders with clinical manifestations similar to the first. The tissue activity of sphingomyelinase is normal or only slightly deficient, however, and increases in sphingomyelin concentrations of liver or spleen are relatively small.

The sphingomyelinase-deficient disorders usually occur in either an acute neuronopathic form (type A) or a chronic, non-neuronopathic form (type B). All affected members of the same family are phenotypically the same, and the two disorders are presumably "allelic," i.e., they represent different mutations at or near the same locus governing the activity of sphingomyelinase.

Clinical Manifestations. *Type A.* Type A is usually manifested by six months of age by abdominal enlargement and evidence of physical and mental retardation. Hepatosplenomegaly and roentgenographic evidence of diffuse pulmonary infiltration may be present as early as one month of age. Throughout the nervous system the neurons and glial cells are ballooned with lipid, the nuclei are pushed to one side, and Nissl substance disappears. Neuronal loss, gliosis, and demyelination are severe. Retinal degeneration in the macular area usually causes a cherry-red spot to appear. The disease progresses to a vegetative state, and death nearly always occurs by the fourth year of life. There are a few exceptional patients, perhaps representing different mutations, who early have retinal changes and other central nervous system signs and who have a much more prolonged course. Both sexes are affected. The disease occurs in all races; it is disproportionately frequent in Ashkenazic Jews.

Type B. Children with type B may develop evidence of visceral involvement as severe and as early as those with type A, but the central nervous system apparently is spared, and mental development is normal. Chronic pulmonary infections and hypersplenism are sometimes life-threatening, but a reasonably normal life span may be possible. Types A and B are inherited as autosomal recessives.

Diagnosis. The typical presentation of Niemann-Pick disease is a very young child with hepatosplenomegaly in whose bone marrow foam cells (see figure in Ch. 776, part B) are present. From the appearance of the cells Gaucher's disease can be excluded but the diagnosis of Niemann-Pick disease cannot be made. Indistinguishable foam cells occur with severe hyperglyceridemia and many other lysosomal enzyme deficiencies. The next diagnostic step should be the culture of skin or marrow fibroblasts for assay of sphingomyelinase. When the assay is appropriately controlled, sphingomyelinase activity between 0 and 20 per cent of normal permits a presumptive diagnosis. Distinction between type A and type B rests on frequent observation for development of neurologic abnormalities. Niemann-Pick disease is also detectable prenatally by enzyme assays of fetal cells grown from amniotic fluid. Separation of types A and B in utero can only be presumed from phenotype of a previously affected sib. No certain test exists for diagnosis of the heterozygotes.

Indeterminate Forms of Sphingomyelin Storage. When the patient has unexplained hepatosplenomegaly and marrow foam cells and the tissue assay for sphingomyelinase is normal or slightly deficient, open liver biopsy is advisable. Tissue must be kept frozen without fixatives for chemical and enzymatic analyses. Careful morphologic examination is also advisable, but neither light nor electron microscopy is capable of distinguishing between most of the lipid storage diseases. Exhaustive analyses of the concentrations of phospholipids, neutral lipids, and glycolipids, in combination with assay of various lysosomal hydrolases and other appropriate enzymes, must be carried out.

In a number of patients an increase of only one- to twofold in sphingomyelin and cholesterol has been detected. These are usually children who have appeared normal for one or more years before moderate hepatosplenomegaly is noted. Later neurologic abnormalities appear; these may include seizures, behavioral disorders, and mental retardation. Frequently such abnormalities are familial and have been referred to as chronic neuronopathic forms of Niemann-Pick disease. If the sphingomyelinase activity is modestly decreased, such patients have been referred to as Niemann-Pick disease, Type C, or as Type D for a similar disorder occurring in related patients of Nova Scotian ancestry. They may possibly represent other mutations affecting sphingomyelinase, but probably they and other similar phenotypes in which the enzyme activity is unequivocally normal represent other undetermined lysosomal enzyme deficiencies in which sphingomyelin metabolism is only incidentally affected.

Treatment. There is no specific treatment for any of the sphingomyelin storage disorders. Chronic administration of sphingomyelinase has not been attempted. Because phospholipid storage leads to excessive lipid peroxidation and ceroid pigment deposition in tissues, long-term administration of an antioxidant, such as vitamin E, has been empirically recommended.

Brady, R. O., and King, F.: Niemann-Pick Disease. In Hers, H. G., and Van Hoof, F. (eds.): Lysosomes and Storage Diseases. New York, Academic Press, 1973, pp. 439–452.

Crocker, A. C., and Farber, S.: Niemann-Pick disease: A review of 18 patients. Medicine, 37:1, 1958.

Fredrickson, D. S., and Sloan, H. R.: Phosphorylcholine ceramidoses: Niemann-Pick disease. In Stanbury, J. B., Wyngaarden, J. B., and Fredrickson, D. S. (eds.): The Metabolic Basis of Inherited Disease. 3rd ed. New York, McGraw-Hill Book Company, 1972, pp. 783–807.

Section Twelve. PLASMA CELL DYSCRASIAS

Elliott F. Osserman

778. INTRODUCTION

Definition and Terminology. The term "plasma cell dyscrasia" is employed to encompass the wide range of pathologic conditions and biochemical abnormalities considered to represent unbalanced proliferative disorders of the cells that normally synthesize gamma (immuno-) globulins. The extent of the proliferative abnormality in the various plasma cell dyscrasias ranges from apparently autonomous, malignant proliferation (neoplasia) in typical multiple myeloma to apparently benign and stable dyscrasias manifested principally by their associated gamma globulin abnormalities. The plasma cell dyscrasias are characterized by (1) the proliferation of plasma cells in the absence of an identifiable antigenic stimulus; (2) elaboration of electrophoretically and structurally homogeneous, monoclonal, "M-type" (myeloma, macroglobulinemia) gamma globulins and/or excessive quantities of comparably homogeneous polypeptide subunits of these proteins, i.e., Bence Jones proteins, H-chains; and (3) commonly, an associated deficiency in the synthesis of normal immunoglobulins.

The major clinical patterns associated with plasma cell dyscrasia are listed in Table 1. Certain of these categories, such as myeloma, macroglobulinemia, amyloidosis, and heavy chain diseases, have sufficiently well defined clinical patterns to permit precise diagnostic classification. With increasing use of electrophoresis, however, many cases of M-type gamma globulin abnormalities are being found that apparently do not represent typical plasma cell myeloma or primary Waldenström's macroglobulinemia at the time of initial study. The fact that some of these patients ultimately develop

TABLE 1. Plasma Cell Dyscrasias

Clinically overt forms, with distinctive clinical and pathologic features:
    Plasma cell myeloma (multiple myeloma, myelomatosis, "solitary" and multiple plasmocytomas, plasma cell leukemia)
    Waldenström's (primary) macroglobulinemia
    γ Heavy chain (Franklin's) disease
    α Heavy chain (Seligmann's) disease (abdominal "lymphoma")
    μ Heavy chain disease
    Amyloidosis (Pattern I and Mixed Pattern I and II amyloidosis)
    Lichen myxedematosus (papular mucinosis, lichen amyloidosus)

Clinically occult (asymptomatic or presymptomatic) forms
    Plasma cell dyscrasia of unknown significance (PCDUS)
        Associated with chronic inflammatory and infectious processes, e.g., osteomyelitis, tuberculosis, chronic biliary tract disease, pyelonephritis, rheumatoid arthritis, chronic pyoderma, etc.
        Associated with nonreticular neoplasms, particularly cancers of the bowel, biliary tract and breast
        Associated with lipodystrophies, particularly Gaucher's disease, familial hypercholesteremia, and xanthomatosis
    Transient plasma cell dyscrasias
        Associated with drug hypersensitivity, sulfonamides
        Associated with (presumed) viral infections
        Associated with cardiac surgery: valve prosthesis

clinically typical myeloma or macroglobulinemia is well documented, but there are many cases (of the order of 20 to 30 per cent of patients with M-type gamma globulin abnormalities) that almost certainly do not belong in the diagnostic categories of myeloma or primary macroglobulinemia. Various designations have been given to these cases, including premyeloma, essential hyperglobulinemia, essential benign hyperglobulinemia, essential macroglobulinemia, idiopathic or essential cryoglobulinemia, the dysgammaglobulinemic syndromes, idiopathic or essential monoclonal gammopathy, paraimmunonoglobulinopathy, and others. The probable inaccuracies of all these terms are evident.

It is recommended that the inclusive term "plasma cell dyscrasia" be used, modified by the clinical pattern, e.g., myeloma, Waldenström's macroglobulinemia, or amyloidosis, when this is overt and evident. When no recognizable clinical pattern is associated with the finding of an M-type protein, the condition is classified as a plasma cell dyscrasia of unknown significance, because the ultimate course is not presently predictable. However, many, if not all, of the diagnostic categories listed in Table 1 overlap. Thus either amyloidosis can be the predominant feature of a plasma cell dyscrasia, in which case the diagnosis of "primary amyloidosis" is commonly, although inappropriately, applied, or the amyloid infiltrates can occur in association with otherwise typical myeloma. Also, a given case can progress from an asymptomatic status, i.e., plasma cell dyscrasia of unknown significance, to symptomatic myeloma, macroglobulinemia, amyloidosis, and so forth. Accordingly, the categories listed in Table 1 are tentative and somewhat indefinite diagnostic groupings in many instances.

In a significant percentage of cases the finding of an M-type protein abnormality is associated with another chronic disease such as recurrent cholecystitis and cholelithiasis, a chronic infection (particularly tuberculosis), or a nonreticular neoplasm (particularly rectosigmoid and biliary carcinoma). *These associations may not be coincidental,* but may represent plasma cell dyscrasias related to and possibly induced by these diverse chronic reticuloendothelial stimuli. For this reason, it is considered useful to document the associations by designations such as "plasma cell dyscrasia associated with chronic biliary tract disease" or "plasma cell dyscrasia associated with adenocarcinoma of the rectosigmoid."

Pathogenesis of Plasma Cell Dyscrasias. Although the etiologic factors responsible for production of plasma cell dyscrasias in man are still unknown, it is possible that some clues may have been provided by studies of experimental plasma cell tumors in mice. These studies have established the importance of genetic factors with the demonstration of the particular susceptibility of the inbred C_3H mouse strain and the F^1 hybrids of CBA $\times$ DBA/2 mice to develop plasma cell tumors spontaneously. In an effort to document genetic factors, chromosome studies have been carried out in several of these murine tumors as well as in human myeloma and macroglobulinemia, but thus far no consistent karyotypic abnormalities have been documented.

The *interdependence of genetic and carcinogenic mechanisms* is apparent in the interesting group of experimental *plasma cell tumors* that have been induced in BALB/c strain mice. A variety of plasma cell neoplasms can be induced in this strain by the intraperitoneal implantation of plastics, mineral oil–adjuvant mixtures, and mineral oil alone. The importance of genetic mechanisms is evident from the particular susceptibility of the BALB/c strain to develop plasma cell tumors in response to these forms of chronic peritoneal (reticuloendothelial) irritation. Significantly, strain C_3H mice, which develop spontaneous plasma cell tumors, are *not susceptible* to the induction of these tumors by intraperitoneal adjuvants and the like. With many other experimental tumors the intimate interaction of genetic factors, oncogenic viruses, and chemical and physical carcinogens has been established.

Cytology. The synthesis of specific proteins is the principal and probably the sole function of plasma cells. The abundant cytoplasmic RNA is responsible for the characteristic basophilia and pyroninophilia of plasma cells, and the highly developed Golgi apparatus is responsible for the typical paranuclear "halo" or clear zone. Electron microscopy of plasma cells has shown that the cytoplasmic RNA is organized in the form of granules (ribosomes) attached to a highly developed network of endoplasmic reticulum. All these structural features have now been related to the complex functions of protein synthesis and secretion. The nucleus of the plasma cell with its characteristically clumped chromatin (DNA) contains the genetic information that determines the structure of the protein to be synthesized. The synthesis of ribosomal RNA is carried out on DNA localized in the nucleolus. Messenger RNA's, which determine the structure of the specific proteins to be synthesized on these ribosomes, are derived from the nonnucleolar DNA's.

The different classes of immunoglobulins are probably synthesized by different cells. The possibility that a single cell may under certain conditions synthesize two types of immunoglobulins (e.g., IgG and IgM) either simultaneously or sequentially has not been excluded, but most studies have indicated the synthesis of only one type of immunoglobulin by a single cell. Immunohistochemical studies, using fluorescein-labeled antisera specific for each of the immunoglobulin groups, have generally shown IgG globulin synthesis in typical, mature, Marshalko-type plasma cells. IgA globulin has been localized in cells with relatively more abundant and vacuolated cytoplasm but still having the major features of plasma cells; IgM synthesis has been related to a population of somewhat smaller cells with proportionately less cytoplasm. These cells have been variously classified as lymphocytoid-plasma cells, plasmacytoid-lymphocytes, atypical plasma cells, and atypical lymphocytes.

Typical, ovoid plasma cells with eccentric nuclei, clumped chromatin, prominent nucleoli, paranuclear halo, and basophilic cytoplasm are widely distributed in lymph nodes, spleen, marrow, intestinal wall, and other tissues and organs. They constitute less than 5 per cent of the normal bone marrow population but increase significantly in association with infection, sensitivity reactions (particularly serum sickness), collagen diseases,

cirrhosis, parasitism, and certain neoplasms. In these conditions, the increase in plasma cells includes both "typical" and "atypical" forms (including multinucleated cells and cells with prominent nucleoli), and there are *no reliable morphologic criteria to distinguish these reactive plasmacytic populations from the cells that are found in the plasma cell dyscrasias.*

Normal Immunoglobulins and the Paraproteins of the Plasma Cell Dyscrasias. Figure 1 is a schematic summary of the present working hypothesis relating the synthesis of individual gamma globulin molecules (1, 2, 3, 4 . . . n) to specific plasmacytic clones. The normally broad, polydispersed serum gamma globulin peak represents the balanced synthesis of small quantities of a very large and presently indeterminate number (n) of individual and specific gamma globulin molecules by specific plasma cell populations. Normally, most of the proteins synthesized by these cells are complete immunoglobulin molecules, and there is only a small quantity of incomplete polypeptide subunits elaborated. These incomplete proteins, designated "gamma-u," are low molecular weight constituents (M.W. 20,000 to 25,000) and closely resemble Bence Jones proteins. Because of their small molecular size, gamma-u polypeptides are rapidly excreted by the kidney. Normally, 20 to 40 mg of gamma-u is excreted per 24 hours.

A plasma cell dyscrasia is considered to represent the excessive proliferation of a single clone of plasma cells, resulting in the synthesis of large quantities of a single protein related to one of the major classes of immunoglobulins and/or the synthesis of excessive quantities of a constituent polypeptide subunit of one of these proteins, usually of the Bence Jones type.

The proteins elaborated in the plasma cell dyscrasias have been shown to be very closely related and structurally similar to the normal immunoglobulins. As large quantities of these single proteins are synthesized in the plasma cell dyscrasias, they are more suitable for structural studies than the heterogeneous and polydispersed normal immunoglobulins. Significantly, much of our present knowledge regarding the structure and properties of normal immunoglobulins has been obtained from studies of the M-type paraproteins.

The biochemical and physiologic properties of the presently recognized immunoglobulins, IgG, IgA, IgD, IgE and IgM globulins, are presented in Ch. 60. In typical multiple myeloma, approximately 70 per cent of the serum "spikes" are IgG, 28 per cent are IgA, and 2 per cent are IgD. There have been only three cases of IgE myeloma reported to date. Bence Jones proteins, which represent free light chains, are elaborated in large quantities and excreted in the urine in approximately 50 per cent of cases of myeloma. Bence Jones proteins have molecular weights in the range of 20,000 to 25,000 but are commonly excreted as disulfide-bonded dimers. In any given case of plasma cell dyscrasia with Bence Jones proteinuria, the Bence Jones protein is *either* Type κ *or* Type λ, in contrast to excretion of small quantities of *both* Type κ and Type λ constituents in normal urine. In those cases of plasma cell dyscrasia in which there is a synthesis of both an M-type serum paraprotein and a Bence Jones–type protein, the Bence Jones protein is apparently identical to the constituent light chains of the corresponding serum paraprotein. This evidence is interpreted as indicating that a portion of the abnormal cells has retained the capacity to elaborate

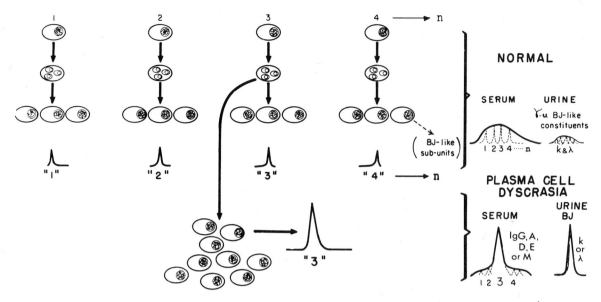

Figure 1. Schematic representation of the clonal hypothesis of immunoglobulin synthesis and the derangements in protein synthesis associated with plasma cell dyscrasias.

complete molecules with light and heavy chains, whereas others are capable of synthesizing only one of the constituent polypeptide subunits, i.e., light chains.

A fundamental question that remains unanswered is whether the proteins elaborated in the plasma cell dyscrasias are truly abnormal or whether they are, in fact, functional antibodies elaborated in great quantitative excess as a consequence of the proliferative abnormality. An increasing body of evidence obtained in recent years lends support to the latter hypothesis. Thus many human and mouse myeloma proteins and macroglobulins have been found to interact with a variety of synthetic haptens, polysaccharides, lipids, and bacterial antigens. The present consensus is that some of these reactions are probably cross-reactions between these proteins and antigens which are structurally related but not identical to the true antigens. Investigations are presently underway to identify the true antigens to which the myeloma proteins are directed, and this will unquestionably shed light on the pathogenic mechanisms responsible for plasma cell dyscrasias in man.

Electrophoretic Patterns of Serum and Urinary Proteins in the Plasma Cell Dyscrasias. As a result of the more general use of electrophoresis, increasing numbers of cases of plasma cell dyscrasia are being documented by the electrophoretic demonstration of M-type serum or urinary protein abnormalities, or both. These M-type abnormalities (see Figs. 3 and 4) are best appreciated by comparison with the patterns of normal serum and urine and the serum in certain disease states affecting the reticuloendothelial system generally (Fig. 2). The electrophoretic analyses illustrated were performed by the Spinco cellulose acetate method, which has certain advantages over filter paper techniques. For diagnostic purposes, the *contours of electrophoretic patterns are more significant* than the precise quantitation of individual peaks. A careful appraisal of the contours of each peak, particularly distinguishing a diffuse gamma elevation from an M-type spike, in conjunction with a rough

quantitative comparison of the patient's serum albumin, alpha-1, alpha-2, beta, and gamma globulins with a normal serum pattern will yield most of the clinically important information offered by this method.

In Figure 2, the normal serum pattern shows the characteristically broad contour of the major slow gamma peak, sometimes referred to as gamma-2, and a small secondary peak in the fast gamma region (between gamma and beta), which at times is designated gamma-1. The gamma-1 peak is detectable by cellulose acetate electrophoresis in most but not all normal sera. It is not resolved as a distinct peak by filter paper electrophoresis. The gamma-1 peak has been related to the faster migrating IgA and IgM globulins.

The electrophoretic pattern of the normal urinary proteins in Figure 2 shows albumin to be the major constituent, with lesser quantities of alpha, beta, and gamma globulins. Because of the extremely low concentration of protein in normal urine, the sample must be concentrated 50- to 100-fold by dialysis against 25 per cent dextran or polyvinylpyrrolidone (PVP) prior to electrophoresis. As in the case of serum proteins, the clinically important abnormal urinary proteins are detected as changes in the contours of the pattern and the relative concentrations of albumin and proteins of alpha, beta, and gamma mobility. Serial quantitation of 24-hour urinary protein excretion is useful for evaluating therapy but is not of particular importance diagnostically.

As illustrated in the lower patterns in Figure 2, the general suppression of plasmacytic function associated with the congenital and acquired forms of hypogammaglobulinemia is reflected in a *broad decrease* in gamma globulin, and, conversely, the generalized hyperactivity of the reticulendothelial system associated with certain chronic infections, cirrhosis, collagen diseases, etc., is reflected in a *broad elevation* of gamma globulin. The pattern illustrating a diffuse hypergammaglobulinemia shows an elevation of the slow, major gamma (gamma-2) peak owing to an increase in IgG

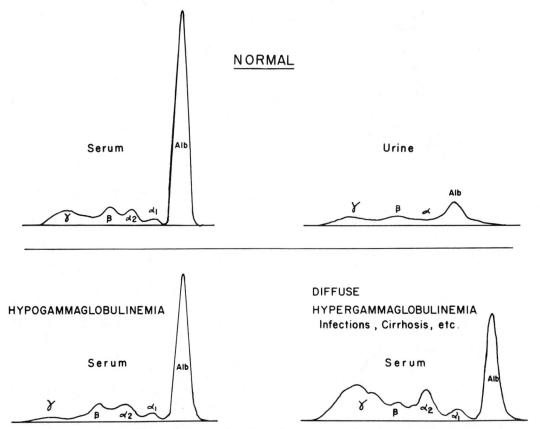

Figure 2. Representative electrophoretic patterns (Spinco, cellulose acetate system). *Top,* Normal serum and normal urinary proteins (concentrated 50×). *Bottom left,* Hypogammaglobulinemia (adult, idiopathic). *Bottom right,* Diffuse hypergammaglobulinemia.

globulins, and also an increase in the fast gamma (gamma-1) peak, reflecting an increase in IgA and IgM globulins.

The M-type serum and urinary protein abnormalities observed in myeloma, macroglobulinemia, and the other plasma cell dyscrasias are illustrated in Figures 3 and 4. In Figure 3, three sets of serum and urinary patterns from three cases of myeloma illustrate different combinations of abnormalities. Bence Jones proteinuria was present in all three cases of myeloma and was confirmed by the classic heat precipitation and re-solution at 90 to 100° C. Because of their small molecular size, the Bence Jones proteins are rapidly excreted, and their serum concentration is usually too low to be detected by conventional electrophoretic methods. Urine electrophoresis, however, demonstrates the Bence Jones proteins to have the same relative homogeneity as the myeloma serum globulins and electrophoretic mobilities, ranging from slow gamma through beta and into the alpha-2 mobility range. Urine electrophoresis is a more reliable method for the detection of Bence Jones proteins than the usual heat-precipitation procedure. *The finding in the urine of an electrophoretically homogeneous M-type component of gamma, beta, or alpha-2 mobility present in a concentration exceeding that of albumin indicates that the protein has a molecular size smaller than albumin (M.W. 70,000).* This is strong evidence in favor of Bence Jones proteinuria and can generally be confirmed by precipitation at 55 to 60° C and re-solution at 90 to 100° C *if the pH is carefully ad-*

justed to 4.5 to 5.0. False negative reactions will be obtained if inadequate attention is given to pH adjustment.

In the case of myeloma illustrated in Figure 3A the serum pattern shows a large, electrophoretically homogeneous peak of slow gamma mobility, and the urine pattern shows a large, abnormal M-type peak with a somewhat faster (more anodally positioned) mobility than the serum M-type peak. The lack of correspondence in mobilities of the serum and urinary proteins establishes their *nonidentity.* Immunoelectrophoretically, the serum protein was identified as an IgG globulin and the urinary protein as a Type κ Bence Jones constituent.

In Figure *3B,* the serum shows a small abnormal peak of slow gamma mobility and an obvious decrease in normal gamma globulin. The urine shows a very large abnormal peak of slow gamma mobility and a minimal amount of albumin. The serum and urinary proteins were both identified immunoelectrophoretically as Type λ Bence Jones protein. Bence Jones protein*emia* is usually not detectable by conventional electrophoresis, although it is almost always demonstrable by the more sensitive technique of immunoelectrophoresis when Bence Jones proteinuria is present.

In Figure 3C, the serum pattern shows two overlapping abnormal peaks of fast gamma (gamma-1) and beta mobility. The urine pattern has an abnormal beta peak along with significant quantities of albumin. In occasional cases of myeloma and other plasma cell dyscrasias, double peaks are found in serum patterns. Most frequently these have been shown to be due to an unusually high concentration of Bence Jones protein in the serum along with an M-type IgG or IgA globulin. Rarely, two distinct globulins or an IgG *and* an IgA or IgM globulin are found in the serum of a patient with a plasma cell dyscrasia. It is presumed that these double peaks indicate the simultaneous proliferation of more than one plasmacytic clone. In Figure 3C, the two serum peaks were immunoelectrophoretically identified, respectively, as IgA globulin and a Type λ Bence Jones protein. The abnormal urinary protein was identified as the same Type λ Bence Jones constituent present in the serum. There was no detectable IgA globulin in the urine.

In Figure 3D the serum and urinary patterns from a case of primary (Waldenström's) macroglobulinemia are illustrated. The serum has an M-type peak of slow gamma mobility indistinguishable from the IgG abnor-

mality illustrated in Figure 3A. Definitive identification of the abnormal protein as an IgM globulin in this as in all cases of macroglobulinemia was accomplished only by immunoelectrophoretic and ultracentrifugal analyses. The urinary protein pattern revealed nonspecific proteinuria with albumin as the predominant constituent. The virtual absence of the IgM globulin from the urine is noteworthy. Bence Jones proteinuria occurs in a smaller percentage (10 to 20 per cent) of cases of macroglobulinemia than of myeloma (50 to 60 per cent).

Serum and urinary electrophoretic patterns from plasma cell dyscrasias other than typical myeloma and macroglobulinemia are illustrated in Figure 4. The patterns in Figure 4A are from a case of generalized amyloidosis with predominant involvement of the tongue, heart, and gastrointestinal tract, classified as "Pattern I amyloidosis." There were no detectable skeletal lesions, but plasma cell dyscrasia was indicated by the finding of Bence Jones proteinuria,

Figure 3. Serum and urinary protein patterns in three cases of multiple myeloma (A, B, and C), each with an M-type protein abnormality in the serum and Bence Jones proteinuria. D, Macroglobulinemia with nonspecific proteinuria.

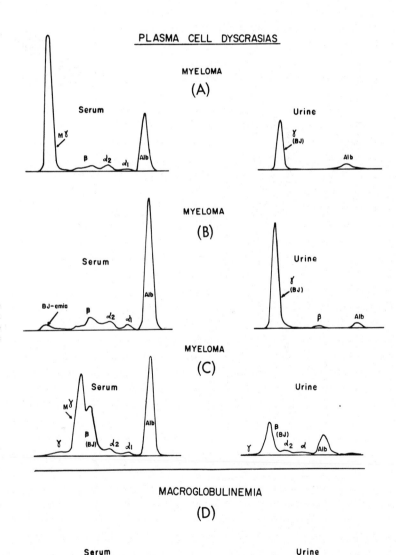

PLASMA CELL DYSCRASIAS

MYELOMA
(A)

MYELOMA
(B)

MYELOMA
(C)

MACROGLOBULINEMIA
(D)

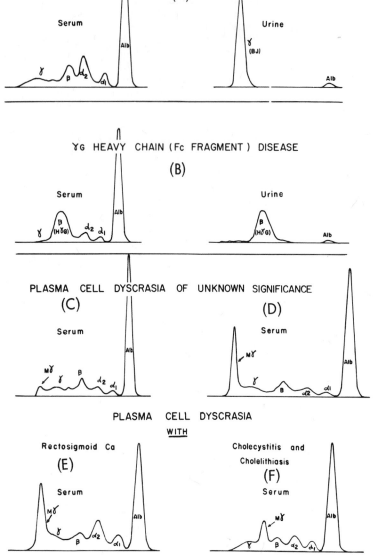

Figure 4. Representative electrophoretic patterns in plasma cell dyscrasias. *A*, Plasma cell dyscrasia and amyloidosis of "Pattern I" distribution with a characteristic Bence Jones–type abnormality in the urine pattern. *B*, γ Heavy chain (Fc fragment) disease with corresponding serum and urinary M-type peaks of β mobility. *C* and *D*, Asymptomatic plasma cell dyscrasias with a small (*C*) and a large (*D*) M-type serum peak. *E*, Plasma cell dyscrasia associated with an adenocarcinoma of the rectosigmoid colon. *F*, Plasma cell dyscrasia associated with chronic and recurrent cholecystitis and cholelithiasis.

and was confirmed by the finding on marrow aspiration of abnormal numbers of plasma cells. The abnormal urinary protein was immunoelectrophoretically identified as a Type λ Bence Jones constituent. The serum pattern shows an elevated alpha-2 globulin and a decreased gamma globulin, without an M-type peak.

In Figure 4*B*, the serum and urinary proteins from a case of γ heavy chain (Fc fragment) disease are shown. The protein elaborated in this conditon has been characterized as representing the major portion (Fc fragment) of the IgG H-chain with a molecular weight in the range of 50,000 to 55,000. Because these proteins are relatively larger than Bence Jones proteins, their renal clearance rate is relatively lower, and they are retained in the serum in sufficiently high concentrations to be detectable by conventional electrophoretic analysis. The abnormal serum and urinary protein peaks are of identical mobility and electrophoretically somewhat more polydispersed than the abnormal peaks in the

other plasma cell dyscrasias. The urinary protein pattern, however, is indistinguishable from the patterns observed with Bence Jones proteinuria, and identification of the abnormal protein as related to the IgG heavy chain and unrelated to Bence Jones proteins and light chains must be accomplished by appropriate immunochemical and physicochemical studies.

The serum electrophoretic patterns illustrated in Figures 4*C* and 4*D* are from two cases in which M-type protein abnormalities were discovered in the absence of overt signs or symptoms of myeloma, macroglobulinemia, or any other recognizable disease. These cases are classified as "plasma cell dyscrasia of unknown significance." As will be noted subsequently, the clinical and pathologic significance of protein abnormalities of this type are presently still obscure. In some cases, progression to overt forms of plasma cell dyscrasia, such as myeloma, has been documented, but in many cases the protein abonormality has been found to persist for as long as 20 years without the development of clinically recognizable disease. Rarely, protein abnormalities of this type have been found on subsequent analyses to have disappeared—i.e., transient paraproteinemias—and these almost certainly represent examples of the synthesis of excessively large quantities of functional antibodies.

The M-type gamma globulin abnormalities illustrated in Figures 4*E* and 4*F* were found in association with clinical conditions that may have been related to the development of plasma cell dyscrasias, notably an adenocarcinoma of the rectosigmoid with an intense plasmacytic infiltration surrounding the tumor and in the resected nodes (Fig. 4*E*), and chronic and recurrent cholecystitis and cholelithiasis with extensive plasmacytosis in the gallbladder wall and along the biliary tract (Fig. 4*F*). Until a direct relationship is established between these conditions and the plasma cell dyscrasias, their association must be considered coincidental, but the relative frequency of these associations warrants the search for an occult neoplasm or biliary tract disease in patients found to have asymptomatic M-type gamma globulin abnormalities.

Edelman, G. M.: The antibody problem. Ann. Rev. Biochem., 38:415, 1969.

Metzger, H. M.: Editorial. Myeloma proteins and antibodies. Am. J. Med., 47:837, 1969.

Osserman, E. F., and Takatsuki, K.: Considerations regarding the pathogenesis of the plasmacytic dyscrasias. Scand. J. Haemat., 4 (Suppl.): 28, 1964.

Potter, M.: Antigen binding M-components in man and mouse. *In* Azar, H. A., and Potter, M. (eds.): Multiple Myeloma and Related Disorders. Vol. I. Hagerstown, Md., Harper & Row, 1973, p. 195.

Potter, M.: The developmental history of the neoplastic plasma cells in mice. Semin. Hematol., 10:19, 1973.

Putnam, F. W.: Immunoglobulin structure: Variability and homology. Science, 163:633, 1969.

Seligmann, M., and Brouet, J. C.: Antibody activity of human myeloma globulins. Semin. Hematol., 10:163, 1973.

Solomon, A., and McLaughlin, C. O.: Immunoglobulin structure determined from products of plasma cell neoplasms. Semin. Hematol., 10:3, 1973.

CLINICAL PATTERNS OF THE PLASMA CELL DYSCRASIAS

779. MULTIPLE MYELOMA
(Plasma Cell Myeloma, Myelomatosis)

Multiple myeloma is generally defined as a neoplasm of plasma cells manifested primarily by widespread skeletal destruction and frequently associated with anemia, hypercalcemia, renal functional impairment, and increased susceptibility to infections. Amyloidosis, coagulation defects, and symptoms and signs related to cryoglobulins or increased serum viscosity are less commonly associated manifestations. Diagnosis depends upon the roentgenographic demonstration of diffuse osteolytic lesions and/or osteoporosis, documentation of

increased numbers of plasma cells in the marrow, and the finding of M-type serum or urinary proteins.

The frequency of myeloma has apparently increased in recent years and now is comparable to that of Hodgkin's disease in many large clinics. Improved diagnostic techniques are unquestionably partly responsible for the apparent increase. Males and females are approximately equally affected. The age of onset of symptoms ranges from young adulthood to advanced years, the peak incidence being in the mid-fifties.

The symptomatic stage of myeloma is preceded by a significant asymptomatic or presymptomatic period in most, and perhaps all, cases. In this presymptomatic period, M-type serum and/or urinary proteins are demonstrable and are usually first suggested by the finding on routine examination of an increased erythrocyte sedimentation rate or unexplained and persistent proteinuria. Because intravenous pyelography may precipitate renal shutdown in the presence of Bence Jones proteinuria, the increased hazard of the procedure should be considered in planning the investigation of a case with unexplained proteinuria The duration of the presymptomatic period in myeloma is impossible to define, but apparently can range up to 20 years. Repeated bacterial infections, particularly pneumonias, can occur during this period, presumably as a consequence of impaired immunologic mechanisms.

When myeloma becomes symptomatic, skeletal pains are the presenting and predominant manifestations in most cases. These may at first be mild and transient, or their onset may be sudden with severe back, rib, or extremity pain after an abrupt movement or effort. The abrupt onset of pain frequently indicates a pathologic fracture. With progression of the disease, more and more areas of bone destruction develop, frequently resulting in marked skeletal deformities, particularly of the sternum and rib cage, and shortening of the spine with as much as 5 or more inches decrease in stature. With earlier diagnosis and more effective chemotherapy and general management, these extreme degrees of skeletal deformity have become less common.

In most cases, multiple osteolytic ("punched-out") lesions are apparent on initial roentgenographic examination (Fig. 5). The skull, spine, ribs, clavicles, sternum, pelvis, and proximal long bones exhibit the greatest destruction, but any part of the skeleton, including the phalanges, may be involved.

In many cases, the initial roentgenographic appearance of the skeleton is that of diffuse osteoporosis without discrete osteolytic lesions. Histologic studies demonstrate a diffuse infiltration of the marrow spaces by myeloma cells, with generalized thinning of trabeculae not detectable by standard roentgenographic techniques. Virtually all patients with this initial pattern of diffuse osteoporosis eventually develop osteolytic lesions as the disease progresses. Possibly the rarest finding in myeloma is an osteoblastic reaction in the absence of a pathologic fracture; there are now several reported examples of this.

In occasional cases, myeloma presents as an *apparently single* skeletal lesion. Although these lesions are commonly designated as solitary plasmacytomas, most patients ultimately develop disseminated disease even if the original lesion is radically excised or irradiated. In cases of apparently solitary plasmacytomas, M-type protein abnormalities are almost invariably demonstrable.

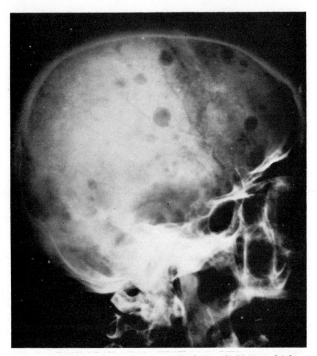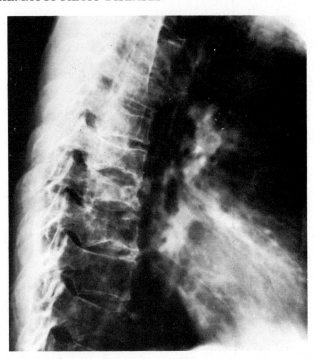

Figure 5. Characteristic x-ray abnormalities in multiple myeloma. Skull (left) shows multiple osteolytic ("punched-out") lesions. Thoracic spine (right) shows extensive osteoporosis and partial collapse of several vertebral bodies.

Skeletal destruction results in the release of bone salts, negative calcium balance, and hypercalciuria in virtually all cases. This is generally well tolerated if adequate hydration is maintained. Hypercalcemia ensues, however, if the renal excretory capacity for calcium is exceeded, usually as a consequence of inadequate hydration and diminished urine output. All too frequently, there develops a menacing sequence of hypercalciuria → osmotic diuresis + impairment of renal tubular reabsorption → dehydration → diminished urine output → hypercalcemia + azotemia → anorexia, nausea, vomiting, and further dehydration. This set of circumstances constitutes a major threat requiring prompt therapeutic intervention with rehydration as the primary goal. Prednisone is a useful adjunct in the management of hypercalcemia, but other chemotherapy is contraindicated until hydration is accomplished and renal function restored.

In occasional cases, particularly those of diffuse osteoporosis rather than local skeletal destruction, the initial symptoms are the nonspecific gastrointestinal complaints related to hypercalcemia and the polyuria and polydipsia secondary to hypercalciuria.

Anemia of variable severity is present in virtually all cases, either at the time of diagnosis or developing subsequently as the disease progresses. It may remain moderate (hemoglobin in the range of 7 to 10 grams) and be well tolerated or become severe enough to require repeated transfusions. The anemia is usually normocytic and normochromic, but may be macrocytic. It is characteristically refractory to iron, vitamin B_{12}, folic acid, and liver therapy. In occasional cases a hypochromic anemia may be related to blood loss from the gastrointestinal tract, to a defect in coagulation, or to plasmacytic or amyloid infiltrates of the intestinal wall. Several factors participate in the production of

anemia in myeloma, including marrow replacement, accelerated erythrocyte destruction, blood loss, renal insufficiency, the effects of radiotherapy and chemotherapy, associated infections, and nutritional factors.

Erythrocyte rouleau formation is observed in peripheral blood and marrow films, and in vivo erythrocyte aggregation ("sludged blood") is often demonstrable. This aggregation is probably due to erythrocyte coating by M-type proteins and may contribute to shortened red cell life span. Coombs reactions, however, are usually negative.

Leukocyte and platelet counts are usually within normal limits prior to cytotoxic therapy. Occasionally, however, moderate to severe leukopenia or thrombocytopenia may be observed prior to treatment and, indeed, with therapy, the white cell and platelet counts may rise toward normal. Thrombocytopenia may contribute to a bleeding diathesis and leukopenia to an increased susceptibility to infection. The precise mechanisms responsible for leukopenia and thrombocytopenia in the plasma cell dyscrasias are unknown. The differential white cell count frequently reveals a relative lymphocytosis (40 to 55 per cent) with a variable proportion of immature lymphocytic and plasmacytic forms. Plasma cells in the peripheral blood have been reported in up to 70 per cent of cases. An outpouring of plasma cells into the peripheral blood is occasionally seen in the later stages of disease, and is considered to represent a displacement phenomenon.

A clinical pattern consistent with a diagnosis of plasma cell leukemia, with hepatosplenomegaly and white cell counts in excess of 15,000 and over 50 per cent plasma cells, is occasionally observed, with weakness, anemia, and bleeding manifestations. In the peripheral blood the cells range from typical plasmacytes to immature and atypical forms. Bence Jones proteinuria and abnormal serum globulins occur with the same frequency as in myeloma. The majority of these cases pursue an acute or subacute clinical course. It is of interest that two known cases of IgE myeloma exhibited the clinical pattern of plasma cell leukemia.

Eosinophilia, with eosinophil counts as high as 15 to 25 per cent, is observed in occasional cases of myeloma and somewhat more commonly in macroglobulinemia and γ heavy chain disease. The significance of eosinophilia in these diseases is unknown.

Marked elevation of the erythrocyte sedimentation rate (ESR) is found in most cases of myeloma. When the M-type serum proteins are cold precipitable (cryoglobulins), the ESR may be markedly temperature dependent, i.e., slower at room temperature or in the cold and accelerated when performed at 37° C.

Pathologic Effects of M-type Serum Globulins and Bence Jones Proteins. Each M-type protein must be recognized to be individually specific and to possess specific physiochemical properties, such as solubility, intrinsic viscosity, thermostability, and reactivity with other proteins. Certain of these properties can be correlated with specific clinical and pathologic manifestations. Thus coagulation defects are related in certain cases to the interaction (protein:protein complexing) of specific M-type IgG or IgA globulins with specific coagulation factors, including fibrinogen, factors V, VII, prothrombin, and the antihemophilic globulin. Another group of protein-related symptoms are those produced by M-type IgG globulins which are cold precipitable, i.e., cryoglobulins. These include a Raynaud-type phenomenon, circulatory impairment, and, at times, occlusion and gangrene after relatively mild exposure to cold. Circulatory impairment, particularly in the central nervous system and retina, can also be related in certain cases to IgA and IgG globulins with a high intrinsic viscosity.

An association between Bence Jones proteinuria and renal functional impairment has long been implied, and is generally ascribed to the tubular precipitation of these proteins and blockage owing to cast formation. More recently, it has been found that Bence Jones proteinuria is occasionally associated with specific defects in renal tubular reabsorption mechanisms, including the adult Fanconi syndrome, indicating that certain Bence Jones proteins have the capacity to interfere with specific tubular transport mechanisms through direct (protein:protein) interaction with tubular cytoplasmic constituents. There is no evident correlation between the antigenic type of a Bence Jones protein and its nephrotoxic potential. The fact that a nephrotoxic potential is *not* common to *all* Bence Jones proteins is indicated by the persistence of apparently normal renal function in many cases with protracted and profound Bence Jones proteinuria. This is further evidence that several factors in addition to Bence Jones proteinuria, particularly hypercalciuria and dehydration, contribute to renal dysfunction in myeloma.

Bence Jones proteins have also been implicated in the pathogenesis of amyloidosis. It is postulated that Bence Jones proteins traverse capillary beds because of their small molecular size and polymerize and/or coprecipitate with as yet unidentified tissue proteins or polysaccharides to yield the complex proteinaceous tissue infiltrates designated amyloid (see Ch. 781).

Additional Clinical Manifestations. Hyperuricemia and hyperuricosuria are observed in most cases as a result of increased turnover of nucleic acids in the proliferating cell population. Hyperuricosuria is not infrequently associated with renal functional impairment resulting from precipitation of urate crystals or stone formation, or both. The danger of increased urate excretion is particularly great in the initial stages of cytotoxic chemotherapy, and warrants special attention to the maintenance of adequate hydration and possibly therapy with allopurinol. Gouty arthropathy is a rare complication.

Neurologic manifestations may develop from direct pressure on the spinal cord, nerve roots, or cranial or peripheral nerves, or as a result of a pathologic fracture of a vertebral body or long bone. Spinal cord compression leading to weakness and ultimately paraplegia is an especially serious complication because the osteoporosis and negative calcium balance produced by the myeloma are compounded by the osteoporosis of immobilization. Again, this complication of myeloma has become less common with improved therapeutic management.

Infiltration of peripheral nerves and nerve roots by amyloid can cause peripheral neuropathies or root symptoms that are usually symmetrical and are associated with other evidence of amyloidosis such as macroglossia, cardiac manifestations, and the carpal tunnel syndrome. Rarely, polyneuropathies develop in myeloma and the other plasma cell dyscrasias without demonstrable tumor or amyloid infiltration. The pattern of these polyneuropathies is nonspecific; apparently they are similar to the polyneuropathies of obscure origin occasionally associated with other neoplastic diseases.

Myopathies involving principally proximal muscle groups are also rarely associated with myeloma and other plasma cell dyscrasias and, again, the pathogenic mechanisms are completely unknown.

An apparent increase in the incidence of nonreticular neoplasms, particularly of bowel, breast, and biliary tract carcinomas, has been noted in association with myeloma in one comprehensive postmortem study (19 per cent) and in the author's series (22 per cent).

Immunologic Deficiency. Increased susceptibility to bacterial infections, particularly pneumococcal pneumonia, exists in many cases of myeloma and is at least partially the result of an impaired capacity for antibody formation. This is generally reflected in a decrease in the serum concentration of normal IgG, IgA, and IgM immunoglobulins irrespective of the type of M-protein elaborated. The basis for these deficiencies is presently unknown, but available studies indicate that diminished production is a more significant factor than increased catabolism or loss. Herpes zoster and generalized varicella infections occur with increased frequency in myeloma and other plasma cell dyscrasias, but apparently no more so than in Hodgkin's disease and lymphosarcoma. Susceptibility to other viral infections apparently is not increased. Studies of the homograft rejection reaction have demonstrated a significant prolongation of rejection time, indicating that the immunologic deficiencies in myeloma may include cell-mediated immune mechanisms.

Treatment. Both the comfort and useful life of patients with myeloma can unquestionably be extended by proper management. The importance of *ambulation and adequate hydration* cannot be overemphasized. The constant threats of hypercalcemia, hypercalciuria, and hyperuricemia necessitate continual attention to these cardinal aspects of general care. Many patients are immobilized and bedridden with pain when first seen. In these circumstances, all effort should be made to achieve ambulation by a combination of analgesics, orthopedic supports (particularly Taylor spine bracing), and local radiotherapy, as indicated. Plasma cell tumors are characteristically radiosensitive, and x-ray therapy is of established value in the control of localized symptomatic lesions. The field of irradiation and the dosage should be limited in order to spare the marrow as much as possible. A total dose of 1200 to 1500 roentgens is usually adequate for symptomatic control and for the facilitation of ambulation. Pain relief is frequently noted after as little as 200 to 400 r. Salicylates and codeine are usually more effective analgesics for the pain of myeloma than meperidine (Demerol) or propoxyphene (Darvon). Prednisone, as previously indicated, is a useful agent in the management of hypercalcemia, but hydration sufficient to achieve a 24-hour urine output of over 1500 ml is the principal need. Unless mobilization and hydration are accomplished by these measures, it is usually impossible to maintain a patient for the time required to accomplish a remission with chemotherapy.

Of the chemotherapeutic agents presently available, melphalan (1-phenylalanine mustard, Alkeran) and cytoxan (cyclophosphamide) are the two drugs most useful in the long-term management of myeloma. When properly administered, both agents can achieve significant objective and subjective remissions in approximately 80 per cent of cases. Although both melphalan and cytoxan are alkylating agents, their precise mechanisms of action must be different, because sensitivity or resistance to one agent does not necessarily imply the corresponding sensitivity or resistance to the other. Thus the two agents can be used sequentially with an increased possibility of achieving a remission. As yet it is not known whether there is a preferential order, but melphalan is generally the first agent employed in the author's clinic. Therapy is usually initiated with an eight- to ten-day course of 8 to 10 mg per day, i.e., an initial course of 64 to 100 mg, depending upon the patient's size, hematologic status, and general condition. After this initial course, continuous maintenance therapy at a dose of 2 mg a day is instituted. It is no longer considered necessary to interrupt therapy between the initial loading dose and institution of maintenance therapy. With this dosage regimen, it may be anticipated that the peripheral leukocyte count will fall to the range of 3000 to 4000 and be maintained in this range with continued therapy. This degree of marrow suppression is tolerated without complications and provides an index of the adequacy of dosage. In some cases, a decrease in white count below 3000 necessitates reducing the maintenance dose to 1 mg per day. With cytoxan, therapy is initiated at a dosage level of 200 mg a day for seven to ten days, after which the dose is reduced to 100 mg a day for maintenance. Again, in some cases it is necessary to reduce the maintenance dose to 50 mg a day because of leukopenia or thrombocytopenia, or both. With both melphalan and cytoxan, present evidence indicates that continuous drug administration is preferable to interrupted therapy.

With chemotherapy, the objective signs of improvement include a decrease in the concentration of abnormal M-type serum globulins, decreased Bence Jones proteinuria, hematologic improvement, cessation of further skeletal destruction, and occasionally recalcification of osteolytic lesions. In some cases, it has also been found that the concentrations of normal immunoglobulins increase, and this is associated with improved resistance to bacterial infections. It should be recognized, however, that several weeks may elapse between the institution of therapy and the first signs of improvement. Because of the rapid turnover of Bence Jones proteins, a decrease in Bence Jones proteinuria is the earliest objective sign of chemotherapeutic effect, and this has been noted within one week of initiating chemotherapy. A decrease in myeloma serum globulins is usually not observed until the fourth or fifth week. The duration of the remissions which can be achieved with chemotherapy has steadily increased in the past several years; there are now many patients who have been maintained in excellent clinical and functional remission for periods of six years or more. Thus the prognosis in myeloma has greatly improved in the past several years with the introduction of these agents.

An attempt to increase skeletal density by inducing fluorosis with sodium fluoride has been made in some cases with generally equivocal results. At present, this therapy is not recommended. The maintenance of ambulation and the encouragement of exercise are equally as important in the long-term management of myeloma as in the initial phase of therapy. Patients should be encouraged to walk, swim, or engage in other forms of exercise to the extent of their ability, avoiding only those activities which involve excessive lifting and straining.

Azar, H. A., and Potter, M.: Multiple Myeloma and Related Disorders. Vol. I. Hagerstown, Md., Harper & Row, 1973.

Farhangi, M., and Osserman, E. F.: The treatment of multiple myeloma. Semin. Hematol., 10:149, 1973.

Korst, D. R., Clifford, G. O., Fowler, W. M., Louis, J., Will, J., and Wilson, H. E.: Multiple myeloma. II. Analysis of cyclophosphamide therapy in 165 patients. J.A.M.A., 189:758, 1964.

Osserman, E. F.: Plasma-cell myeloma: II. Clinical aspects. N. Engl. J. Med., 261:952, 1006, 1959.

Snapper, I., and Kahn, A.: Myelomatosis: Fundamental and Clinical Features. Basel, S. Karger, 1971.

Waldenström, J.: Diagnosis and Treatment of Multiple Myeloma. New York, Grune & Stratton, 1970.

780. MACROGLOBULINEMIA
(Primary or Waldenström's Macroglobulinemia)

Macroglobulinemia is presently classified as a plasma cell dyscrasia involving those cell populations normally responsible for the synthesis of IgM globulins. The excessive proliferation of these cells results in the elaboration of large quantities of electrophoretically homogeneous (M-type) IgM globulins and a variable clinical pattern with anemia, bleeding manifestations, and symptoms related to the serum macroglobulins as the predominant features. Males and females are approximately equally affected. Symptoms generally begin in the fifth or sixth decade. As the disease slowly evolves, lymphadenopathy, splenomegaly, and hepatomegaly develop in a variable percentage of cases, producing a clinical pattern resembling a malignant lymphoma or lymphatic leukemia. Skeletal lesions of the type seen in myeloma are exceptionally rare.

Histologic studies of lymph nodes demonstrate a proliferation of lymphocytic-plasmacytic forms often arranged in a pattern of follicular hyperplasia. Immunofluorescent studies have confirmed the synthesis of IgM globulin in these cells, as well as in the corresponding lymphocytic-plasmacytic forms demonstrable in peripheral blood and bone marrow preparations. It is generally impossible to ascertain whether the cellular proliferations observed in macroglobulinemia represent reactive responses or autonomous neoplasia. The possibility that initially benign and reactive proliferations may undergo transformation to neoplastic proliferations is suggested in many cases of macroglobulinemia as in other forms of plasma cell dyscrasia.

When macroglobulinemia becomes symptomatic, anemia is the most common presenting manifestation, and is frequently profound, with hemoglobin levels in the range of 4 to 6 grams per 100 ml. Usually the anemia is due to a combination of factors, including accelerated red cell destruction, blood loss, and decreased erythropoiesis. Coating of erythrocytes with IgM globulin is apparently responsible for the marked rouleaux formation, positive Coombs reactions, and cross-matching difficulties encountered in many cases.

As previously noted, a large percentage of IgM globulins have specific physicochemical properties that are responsible for specific symptom patterns in certain cases. These properties include cold-insolubility (cryoglobulins), high intrinsic viscosity, and the capacity to form complexes with coagulation factors and other plasma proteins. *Cryoglobulin-related symptoms* include Raynaud's phenomenon, cold sensitivity, cold urticaria, and vascular occlusion with gangrene after exposure to cold. *Viscosity-related manifestations* are most evident in the retinal vasculature, in which a pattern of patchy venous bulging and localized narrowing ("sausage-effect" or "fundus paraproteinemicus") develops, frequently associated with hemorrhages, exudates, and visual impairment. Circulatory impairment in the central nervous system caused by increased plasma viscosity produces changing patterns of neurologic signs and symptoms, e.g., transient paresis, reflex abnormalities, deafness, impairment of consciousness ("coma paraproteinemicum"), frequently terminating with cerebral vascular hemorrhage. Cardiac decompensation and pulmonary symptoms may also develop secondary to increased viscosity in the systemic and pulmonary vascular beds. *Protein:protein interactions* with formation of complexes between IgM globulins and coagulation factors (fibrinogen, prothrombin, factors V, VII, etc.) are an important contributing factor to the bleeding diatheses (particularly epistaxes, oral mucosal bleeding, and purpura) exhibited in many cases. Interference with platelet function (platelet agglutination) and capillary damage secondary to increased serum viscosity are additional factors contributing to bleeding manifestations. It must be recognized that all these symptom patterns are also observed in occasional cases of myeloma with M-type IgG and IgA globulins possessing similar physicochemical properties.

Bence Jones proteinuria is present in approximately 10 per cent of cases of macroglobulinemia, but renal functional impairment is much less common than in myeloma, presumably because of the absence of the contributing factors of hypercalcemia and hypercalciuria. Amyloidosis has been observed in only a few cases of macroglobulinemia, and in all of these, the liver, spleen, and parenchymal organs have been the major areas of involvement (Pattern II) in contrast to the primary, atypical mesenchymal distribution (Pattern I) of amyloid usually observed in myeloma.

Peripheral neuropathies *(Bing-Neel syndrome)* and myelopathy may be progressive and incapacitating. Circulatory impairment in vasa nervorum is a postulated but still unsubstantiated mechanism. Myopathies and rheumatoid-like arthropathies have also been observed.

In the author's series of 57 cases, 15 had clinical or postmortem evidence of an associated nonreticular neoplasm, and an additional 12 had a background of longstanding infection, particularly tuberculosis.

Many of the laboratory findings in macroglobulinemia have already been considered. The presymptomatic cases are usually detected initially as a result of finding an unexplained elevation of erythrocyte sedimentation rate on routine examination, followed by electrophoretic demonstration of an M-type serum protein (Fig. 3) and, finally, its characterization as an IgM globulin by ultracentrifugation or immunoelectrophoresis, or both. The majority of IgM globulins are euglobulins and give a positive Sia water-dilution reaction, but this is not specific for macroglobulins because certain IgG globulins are also Sia-positive euglobulins. Approximately one third of IgM globulins are cryoglobulins, yielding a white precipitate or a thick clear gel on cooling. The temperature and duration of cooling needed for precipitation varies with individual cryoglobulins. With some cryoglobulins, precipitation or gel-formation occurs almost immediately after venipuncture, and a prewarmed syringe is necessary for blood sampling. Others require several hours at 10° C for precipitation. Similarly, the increased viscosity of serum containing a viscous M-type macroglobulin may be readily apparent when a tube of serum at room temperature is inverted, or viscosimetric determinations at different temperatures may be required.

Hematologic abnormalities, in addition to anemia, include an absolute lymphocytosis with "atypical, immature, and plasmacytic" forms in many cases, occasionally reaching leukemic proportions. Polymorphonuclear leukopenia, thrombopenia, and eosinophilia are also observed. Bone marrow aspirations characteristically reveal an increase in lymphocytic-plasmacytic forms, accompanied by eosinophils and mast cells in many cases. The small lymphocyte, with a dense pyknotic nucleus, which has been considered most typical for macroglobulinemia, probably represents a degenerating cell undergoing cytoplasmic shedding (so-called "clasmatosis").

Additional laboratory abnormalities in certain cases of macroglobulinemia include positive flocculation reactions, false positive serologic reactions, and positive rheumatoid factors. The latter are occasionally associated with rheumatic symptoms and arthropathy.

Treatment. The principal indications for therapy in macroglobulinemia are anemia, bleeding manifestations, and symptoms related to increased plasma viscosity. When the latter symptoms are severe and threaten central nervous system function and vision, plasmapheresis is indicated as a temporary measure. Sufficient plasma should be removed to effect a lowering of viscosity, and the red cells should be returned. In certain cases, a prompt and dramatic improvement in clinical status follows the removal of as little as 500 ml of plasma. Repeated plasmapheresis for a period of several weeks may be required until effective chemotherapy can be instituted.

Chlorambucil (Leukeran) is presently regarded as the chemotherapeutic agent of choice in macroglobulinemia. This should be administered continuously at a dosage level of 8 to 10 mg daily. Although this dosage level is significantly higher than the average employed in most cases of lymphatic leukemia or lymphosarcoma, it is usually well tolerated in macroglobulinemia. A large number of patients have been maintained in objective and subjective remission for periods up to nine years with continuous chlorambucil therapy. More limited studies with melphalan indicate it to be less effective in macroglobulinemia than chlorambucil. Prednisone may be of some value in the control of capillary bleeding.

MacKenzie, M. R., and Fudenberg, H. H.: Macroglobulinemia: An analysis of 40 patients. Blood, 39:874, 1972.
McCallister, B. D., Bayrd, E. D., Harrison, E. G., Jr., and McGuckin, W. F.: Primary macroglobulinemia. Review with a report on 31 cases and notes on the value of continuous chlorambucil therapy. Am. J. Med., 43:394, 1967.
Waldenström, J.: Studies on conditions associated with disturbed gamma globulin formation (gammapathies). Harvey Lect., Series 56:211, 1961.

781. AMYLOIDOSIS

Amyloidosis is a term applied to a variety of conditions associated with tissue infiltrates comprised of insoluble proteins and/or protein-polysaccharide complexes. With the relatively recent development of methods for the isolation and chemical and immunologic analysis of amyloids, it has become evident that there are *at least* two chemical types of amyloid. In one (Ig-type), immunoglobulin light chains appear to be the principal protein component; in the other (protein A-type), an apparently nonimmunoglobulin constituent (protein A) is the major protein. It must be stressed that other chemical types of amyloid will probably be defined by further studies, but the Ig-type and protein A-type probably comprise the majority of amyloidosis cases encountered clinically. In both types, the tissue infiltrates apparently represent noncovalently bonded polymers of the basic protein subunit, either alone or in combination with other proteins or polysaccharides. The polymers are sufficiently large to yield a characteristic fibrillar structure which can be visualized by electron microscopy and a distinctive green-yellow dichroic birefringence seen by polarization microscopy after Congo red staining.

As outlined in Table 2, there is some correlation between the chemical type of amyloid and the clinical pattern of amyloid distribution. Thus IgG-type amyloid has been mainly found in cases with either occult plasma cell dyscrasia or overt multiple myeloma. The pattern of distribution of amyloid in these cases is most frequently that previously referred to as primary-type, i.e., principal involvement of the tongue, heart, gastrointestinal tract, skeletal and smooth muscles, carpal ligaments, nerves, and skin. This distribution pattern, referred to as Pattern I, was manifested in 50 per cent of the cases in the author's series.

Protein A-type amyloid has thus far been mainly found in cases of amyloidosis associated with chronic infections (e.g., tuberculosis), rheumatoid arthritis, Hodgkin's disease, and familial Mediterranean fever. The pattern of distribution of amyloid in these cases most frequently is that previously referred to as secondary-type, i.e., principal involvement of the liver, spleen, kidneys, and adrenals. This distribution pattern, now designated Pattern II, was displayed by 17 per cent of the author's cases.

In a significant proportion of cases (30 per cent of the author's series), amyloid involves both Pattern I and II sites to varying degrees, and these cases are now referred to as Mixed Pattern I and II. Monoclonal IgG, A, D, and M globulins, indicative of associated plasma cell dyscrasias, are demonstrable in the majority (82 per cent) of Mixed Pattern I and II cases, but the specific role of these proteins in the amyloid deposits has not been determined. In a small percentage of cases (3 per cent in the author's series) amyloid is apparently localized to one tissue or organ. In all our cases of localized amyloidosis, abnormal collections of plasma cells were found in immediate juxtaposition to the amyloid deposits, and monoclonal immunoglobulins were also demonstrated in all three cases.

Ideally, disease classifications should be based on etiologic factors, and this should eventually be possible

TABLE 2. Patterns of Amyloidosis

	Previous Designations	Distribution	Associated Conditions	Type of Amyloid Protein
Pattern I	Primary-type, atypical, para-amyloid, pericollagen, mesenchymal	Tongue, heart, GI tract, muscles, ligaments, skin	Plasma cell dyscrasia, usually with Bence Jones only; overt myeloma	Ig-light chain
Pattern II	Secondary-type, typical, perireticular, parenchymal	Liver, spleen, kidney, adrenal	Chronic infections, rheumatoid arthritis, familial Mediterranean fever	Protein A
Mixed Pattern I and II	—	Various combinations of I and II sites	Plasma cell dyscrasia with complete IgG, A, D, and M globulins	Not known
Localized	Tumor-forming	Lung, GI tract, bladder, eye	Plasma cell dyscrasia	Not known

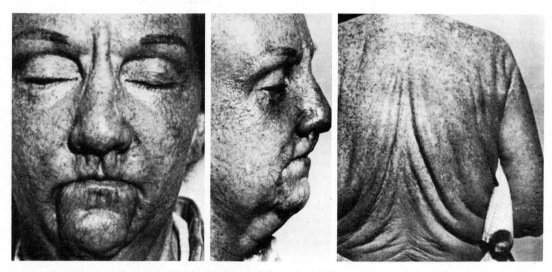

Figure 6. Lichen myxedematosus (papular mucinosis). A form of amyloidosis with extensive involvement of the dermis.

with amyloidosis. Until this is achieved, however, the presently suggested classification based on the predominant clinical patterns of amyloid distribution is considered preferable to previously employed designations such as primary, secondary, typical, and atypical. The terms primary and secondary have been particularly confusing, because in usage they have referred either to *presumed* etiologic factors or to particular patterns of amyloid distribution. Because of the prevalence of chronic infections and suppuration in the preantibiotic era, Pattern II amyloid was relatively more common and "typical" than Pattern I ("atypical"). In more recent series, however, Pattern I cases predominate.

The clinical manifestations of amyloidosis are variable and depend on the distribution and extent of the tissue infiltrates. In Pattern I amyloidosis the clinical manifestations may be any one or a combination of the following: cardiac involvement with decompensation (low output failure) characteristically refractory to digitalis and associated with decreased pulse pressure, low EKG voltage, conduction defects, and arrhythmias; tongue and salivary gland involvement with progressive macroglossia, change in taste sensation, xerostomia, and dysphagia; gastrointestinal manifestations, particularly anorexia, alternating diarrhea and constipation, abdominal cramps, borborygmi, spruelike manifestations with malabsorption, and gastrointestinal bleeding; carpal tunnel syndrome with median nerve involvement and arterial insufficiency caused by infiltration of the carpal ligaments; joint and muscle stiffness and limitation of motion, usually not painful or tender and readily distinguishable from rheumatoid arthritis; neuropathies and radiculopathies with varying sensory and motor deficits; or skin and subcutaneous tissue involvement evidenced by subcutaneous hemorrhages and purpura after minimal trauma, particularly in the eyelids and periorbital tissues. Monoclonal immunoglobulins, particularly Bence Jones proteins, and abnormal marrow plasmacytosis can be demonstrated in virtually all Pattern I cases, and overt skeletal lesions consistent with multiple myeloma develop in approximately 50 per cent of these cases.

In Pattern II amyloidosis, the process is usually manifested by the insidious onset of hepatosplenomegaly and progressive hepatic failure, proteinuria, and renal functional impairment, culminating in the nephrotic syndrome. Peripheral edema and anasarca frequently develop as a consequence of the combined effects of hypoalbuminemia (decreased albumin synthesis caused by hepatic dysfunction plus urinary loss) and abnormal arteriolar capillary permeability secondary to amyloid infiltration.

As would be expected, the clinical manifestations in Mixed Pattern I and II amyloidosis also reflect the extent of involvement of specific tissues and organs. Six of 30 cases of Mixed Pattern I and II amyloidosis in our series were associated with overt myeloma.

Lichen myxedematosus (lichen amyloidosus, papular mucinosis) is a rare form of amyloidosis or tissue proteinosis characterized by the progressive deposition of amyloid in the dermis of the face, trunk, and extremities (Fig. 6). Recent studies have established that this form of amyloidosis is apparently consistently associated with the elaboration of unusually basic (cationic) M-type IgG globulins. It has further been demonstrated in one case that the amyloid infiltrates of the skin were comprised, at least in part, by this specific protein, presumably deposited in combination with the mucopolysaccharides of the dermis. The possibility that lichen myxedematosus may be an autoimmune disease in which a monoclonal antibody is directed against antigenic constituents of the dermis has been suggested.

Diagnosis. The diagnosis of amyloidosis depends on biopsy documentation. If possible, an accessible site with apparent involvement should be biopsied (e.g., skin, muscle), but tongue biopsy should be avoided because of pain and the risk of infection. Liver and kidney biopsy are possibly associated with a risk of bleeding, but this has not been a significant problem in most series. Because amyloidosis of Pattern I and Pattern II frequently involves the arterioles of the rectal submucosa, rectal biopsy is a relatively safe and useful diagnostic procedure. All biopsy material should be stained with Congo red and examined by polarization microscopy. This technique not infrequently discloses amyloid deposits not revealed by the usual staining procedures.

In all cases of amyloidosis, detailed examination of the serum and urinary proteins by electrophoresis and immunoelectrophoresis is indicated, along with bone marrow studies, to document a plasma cell dyscrasia. In a case of amyloidosis with proteinuria, the finding of a negative Bence Jones reaction on heat-testing does not exclude the presence of an abnormal constituent of the Bence Jones type, because albumin and other serum proteins in the urine may mask a Bence Jones reaction.

Treatment. There is no known method to reverse the deposition of amyloid infiltrates except the identification and control of associated conditions, particularly osteomyelitis, pulmonary abscess, and tuberculosis. Several cases have been reported in which effective antimicrobial therapy or surgery or both for a chronic suppurative process have resulted in cessation of amyloid deposition and reabsorption of existing infiltrates. Unfortunately, this is rare; in most cases the amyloidosis continues despite apparently effective control of associated conditions.

Experience with melphalan therapy in cases of amyloidosis with overt myeloma or occult plasma cell dyscrasia is limited, but results have been generally discouraging. Most patients have continued to pursue a downhill course, succumbing to cardiac decompensation or complications related to tongue and gastrointestinal involvement. Corticosteroids occasionally provide slight symptomatic benefit. In cases of macroglossia, careful attention to oral hygiene is important to avoid irritation and ulceration of the tongue.

Cohen, A. S.: Amyloidosis. N. Engl. J. Med., 277:522, 574, 628, 1967.

Franklin, E. C., and Zucker-Franklin, D.: Current concepts of amyloid. *In* Dixon, F. J., and Kunkel, H. G. (eds.): Advances in Immunology. Vol. 15. New York, Academic Press, 1972, p. 249.

Glenner, G. G., Terry, W. D., and Isersky, C.: Amyloidosis: Its nature and pathogenesis. Semin. Hematol., 10:65, 1973.

Isobe, T., and Osserman, E. F.: Patterns of amyloidosis and their associations with plasma cell dyscrasia, monoclonal immunoglobulins and Bence Jones proteins. N. Engl. J. Med., 290:473, 1974.

Osserman, E. F., Takatsuki, K., and Talal, N.: The pathogenesis of "amyloidosis." Studies on the role of abnormal gamma globulins and gamma globulin fragments of the Bence Jones (L-polypeptide) type in the pathogenesis of "primary" and "secondary amyloidosis," and the "amyloidosis" associated wilh plasma cell myeloma. Semin. Hematol., 1:3, 1964.

782. γ HEAVY CHAIN DISEASE

γ heavy chain disease is a relatively rare form of plasma cell dyscrasia characterized by the elaboration of excessive quantities of polypeptide related to the heavy chains and, more specifically, to the Fc fragment of IgG globulin. The clinical pattern resembles a lymphoma with lymphadenopathy, splenomegaly, and hepatomegaly as the predominant manifestations associated with the nonspecific symptoms of weakness, fever, weight loss, and marked susceptibility to bacterial infections. Several patients have exhibited transient palatal erythema and edema resembling that of infectious mononucleosis, and in some there was transient spontaneous regression of the lymphadenopathy after an initially rapid onset. None have had clinical or roentgenographic evidence of skeletal destruction. Most have shown anemia, leukopenia, and thrombopenia, presumably owing to hypersplenism, and moderate to marked eosinophilia. Bone marrow aspirations and lymph node biopsies demonstrated proliferation of plasmacytic and lymphocytic forms along with eosinophils and large reticulum or reticuloendothelial cells.

Persistent proteinuria (4 to 15 grams per 24 hours) was generally the initial indication of an abnormality of protein metabolism. The characteristic serum and urinary protein electrophoretic patterns are illustrated in Figure 4B and have been described in Ch. 778. Total serum protein concentrations were generally within normal limits. The serum concentration of the abnormal protein ranged from 2 to 4 grams per 100 ml associated with marked decrease in the concentration of normal gamma globulin. Identification of the abnormal protein as related to the γ heavy chain (Fc fragment) and unrelated to Bence Jones and light chain polypeptides must be accomplished by immunochemical and physicochemical analyses.

In contrast to myeloma, erythrocyte sedimentation rates have been normal or only slightly elevated. Additional laboratory findings have included hyperuricemia with normal or only slightly elevated blood urea nitrogen levels and no other evidence of renal functional impairment.

Survival from the time of onset of symptoms has ranged from four months to over five years. Bacterial pneumonia and sepsis caused death in all cases.

Splenic radiation has produced temporary remissions with hematologic improvement. Limited trials of cyclophosphamide, melphalan, and steroids gave little or no benefit.

783. IgA HEAVY CHAIN (α-CHAIN) DISEASE

IgA heavy chain (α-chain) disease is the most recently identified plasma cell dyscrasia. As defined by Seligmann and his associates, the clinical pattern is that previously referred to as "Mediterranean-type abdominal lymphoma." The predominant features are a diffuse lymphoma-like proliferation in the small intestine and mesentery, chronic diarrhea, and malabsorption unresponsive to gluten withdrawal. Although all of Seligmann's cases were either non-Ashkenazi Jews or Israeli Arabs, we have recently documented the syndrome, with the specific α-chain abnormality, in a South American (Colombia) male of Spanish and Indian (Mestizo) descent. Thus, although genetic factors were considered to be of major importance, the disease is not exclusively restricted to the Mediterranean population.

Chronic diarrhea, malabsorption, and progressive wasting are the major clinical features. Small intestinal biopsies demonstrate a profound infiltration of the lamina propria with abnormal plasma cells. Intestinal absorption studies demonstrate impaired absorption of vitamin B_{12}, glucose, lactose, and fat. Roentgenograms of the small intestines show thickened mucosal folds, segmentation, and dilated intestinal loops. Bone marrow aspiration reveals moderate increases in plasma cells, and skeletal roentgenograms show moderate diffuse osteoporosis but no destructive lesions.

On electrophoretic analysis of serum, the distinctive increase in IgA heavy chains (α chains) has been evidenced by a markedly elevated, broad peak traversing the beta and alpha-2 mobility range. The electrophoretic polydispersity has been shown to be due to polymeric heterogeneity of the alpha chains. This tendency to polymerize also explains the relatively low concentration of alpha chains in the urine as compared with the excretion of gamma chains in IgG heavy chain disease. Confirmation of the identity of the abnormal serum protein as free α-chains is accomplished by demonstrating the absence of associated light chains by appropriate immunologic and chemical analyses.

The association of this particular form of plasma cell dyscrasia with the small intestine is of particular interest in view of the known preponderance of IgA-producing plasma cells in the intestinal tract. The possible role of antecedent chronic infection or irritation of the intestines in the pathogenesis of IgA heavy chain disease cannot be presently defined.

Frangione, B., and Franklin, E. C.: Heavy chain diseases: Clinical features and molecular significance of the disordered immunoglobulin structure. Semin. Hematol., 10:53, 1973.

Franklin, E. C., Lowenstein, J., Bigelow, B., and Meltzer, M.: Heavy chain disease. A new disorder of serum γ-globulins. Am. J. Med., 37:332, 1964.

Osserman, E. F., and Takatsuki, K.: Clinical and immunochemical studies of four cases of heavy (Hγ₂) chain disease. Am. J. Med., 37:351, 1964.

Seligmann, M., Danon, F., Hurez, D., Mihesco, E., and Preud'homme, J. L.: Alpha-chain disease: A new immunoglobulin abnormality. Science, 162:1396, 1968.

784. PLASMA CELL DYSCRASIA OF UNKNOWN SIGNIFICANCE AND PLASMA CELL DYSCRASIA ASSOCIATED WITH CHRONIC INFECTIONS, BILIARY DISEASE, AND NONRETICULAR NEOPLASMS

Use of serum electrophoresis as a routine clinical laboratory procedure has resulted in the detection of M-type protein abnormalities, such as are illustrated in Figure 4C and D, in otherwise asymptomatic persons. As previously noted, certain of these later develop signs and symptoms of myeloma, macroglobulinemia, or amyloidosis after many months or years. A fundamental question is whether M-type protein abnormalities are invariably manifestations of plasma cell dyscrasia that will produce clinical symptoms if the patient survives "long enough" (possibly several decades), or whether certain M-type abnormalities are truly benign and "essential." Since this question is presently unanswerable, the term "plasma cell dyscrasia of unknown significance" is considered preferable to "premyeloma" or "essential or benign monoclonal gammopathy."

In general, asymptomatic M-type protein abnormalities are more commonly observed in older subjects. In many cases there is a background of tuberculosis, syphilis or other chronic infection, chronic biliary tract disease, or a nonreticular neoplasm, particularly large bowel, breast, oropharyngeal, and biliary tract carcinomas. Although a coincidental association cannot be excluded, particularly in older subjects, there is increasing evidence that certain plasma cell dyscrasias in man may be induced by diverse forms of protracted reticuloendothelial stimuli comparable to those described in

mice. Because of the frequency of these associations, a careful search for an occult infection or neoplasm should be periodically carried out in all patients with asymptomatic M-type protein abnormalities, with particular attention to the bowel and biliary tracts.

To date, chemotherapy with melphalan or any other agent has not been deemed warranted in asymptomatic subjects, despite the knowledge that a certain percentage of them will later develop overt myeloma. Although there are obvious theoretical advantages to earlier chemotherapy, the unpredictability of the course in any one case and the significant toxicities of presently available agents are strong arguments against the institution of chemotherapy before a distinct clinical pattern is evident.

785. ASSOCIATION BETWEEN PLASMACYTIC AND MONOCYTIC DYSCRASIAS

A close functional relationship is known to exist between the monocyte-histiocyte-macrophage system and plasma cells in the processing of antigens and the synthesis of antibodies. As an apparently related phenomenon, there is a significant association between plasmacytic and monocytic dyscrasias in man. Thus monocytic leukemia develops late in the course of a small but significant number of cases of longstanding plasma cell myeloma, generally after several years of effective chemotherapeutic control of the myeloma. In all cases, the monocytic leukemia is associated with markedly elevated serum and urine lysozyme levels. The onset of monocytic leukemia is usually abrupt, although in some cases transient episodes of peripheral monocytosis and fever precede the development of the terminal leukemic phase.

Additional evidence linking monocytic and plasmacytic dyscrasias has been the finding of M-type gamma globulin abnormalities or diffuse hypergammaglobulinemia, or both, in several cases of monocytic leukemia not associated with overt myeloma. Significantly, many of these latter patients have had protracted chronic illnesses, particularly chronic pulmonary infections, tuberculosis, and osteomyelitis, similar to those associated with plasma cell dyscrasia. Thus comparable pathogenic mechanisms may be operative, and may constitute a proliferative stimulus to both plasma cells and monocytes, either simultaneously or sequentially.

Hallen, J.: Discrete gamma globulin (M−) components in serum. Clinical study of 150 subjects without myelomatosis. Acta Med. Scand. (suppl.) 462, 127 pp., 1966.

Isobe, T., and Osserman, E. F.: Pathologic conditions associated with plasma cell dyscrasia: A study of 806 cases. Ann. N. Y. Acad. Sci., 190:507, 1971.

Osserman, E. F.: Clinical and biochemical studies of plasmacytic and monocytic dyscrasias and their interrelationships. Trans. Studies, Coll. Physicians, Phila., 36:134, 1969.

Osserman, E. F., and Lawlor, D. P.: Serum and urinary lysozyme (muramidase) in monocytic and mono-myelocytic leukemia. J. Exp. Med., 124:921, 1966.

Waldenström, J. G.: Benign monoclonal gammapathies. In Azar, H. A., and Potter, M. (eds.): Multiple Myeloma and Related Disorders. Vol. I. Hagerstown, Md., Harper & Row, 1973, p. 247.

Young, V. H.: Transient paraproteins. Proc. R. Soc. Med., 62:778, 1969.

Zawadzki, Z. A., and Edwards, G. A.: Dysimmunoglobulinemia associated with hepatobiliary disorders. Am. J. Med., 48:196, 1970.

Section Thirteen.   DISEASES OF THE SPLEEN

Robert I. Weed

786.   INTRODUCTION

Aristotle may have been one of the first to suggest that the spleen was not necessary for the maintenance of life. In fact, there are references in ancient writings to removal of the spleen, in the belief that it would improve the wind of runners (perhaps, especially in runners who might have had splenomegaly because of malaria or another parasitic disease). Although today we are beginning to understand the functions of the normal spleen, it is an impressive fact that normal individuals can tolerate splenectomy, e.g., after trauma, with little evident ill effect. Indeed, we know far more about pathologic function than we do about normal function of the spleen, although much remains to be learned about the pathophysiology in disease states. The discussion in this section will include mention of splenic hypofunction as well as splenic diseases. Splenic diseases can be divided into primary hypersplenism, in which the abnormality appears confined to the spleen with no apparent associated systemic illness; secondary hypersplenism associated with a systemic disease, either malignant or nonmalignant; and a third group of miscellaneous disorders associated with splenomegaly, with or without hypersplenism.

Anatomy and Normal Functions.   There is considerable variation in ultrastructure as well as function of the spleen from one species to another, e.g., the spleens of sheep, cats, and dogs appear to act as erythrocyte reservoirs, whereas the human spleen normally contains only 20 to 30 ml of red cells. As illustrated in the accompanying figure, the spleen can be considered to contain three regions, structurally and functionally distinct, along the course of each branch of the splenic artery. The entire organ is encased in a capsule with supporting trabeculae, which extend into the splenic pulp. The splenic artery divides into trabecular branches which first enter the white pulp (on right in figure). This is made up primarily of periarterial collections of lymphocytes with germinal centers that contain variable numbers of monocytes, macrophages, and plasma cells. The location of the white pulp along branches of the artery proximal to the red pulp may be related to the relative rigidity of lymphoid cells compared to erythrocytes. Thus, as terminal arterioles branch out within the white pulp, the efficient filtering mechanism of the spleen may remove the lymphoid cells that arrive via the general circulation, permitting the erythrocytes to pass on into the red pulp.

Encircling the white pulp and interposed between it and the red pulp is a marginal zone that communicates with the periphery of the lymphoid follicles and contains lymphatic vessels that represent the efferent limb of the lymphatic circulation through the spleen. The arterioles that traverse the white pulp may terminate directly in splenic sinuses, or the terminal arterioles may simply end within the red pulp (on left in figure).

The red pulp consists of cords made up of fixed macrophages, a finger-like network of reticulin extending throughout the cords, and a basement membrane separating the cords from sinuses, with overlying endothelial cells lining the interior of the sinuses. Normally, less than 5 per cent of the blood passing through the spleen traverses the splenic cords in the red pulp, the rest being shunted directly through the sinuses without traversing the cords. However, for those cells that do traverse the cords, the challenge is formidable. Those that pass must be deformable and able to squeeze between the high endothelial cells at the terminal end of

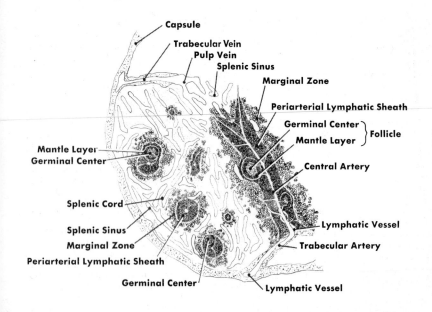

Diagrammatic representation of the structure of the spleen. (From Weiss, L.: Semin. Hematol., October 1970, p. 373.)

the arteriole, then between the macrophages lining the potential spaces which represent the normal circulatory pathways through the cords, and then to pass through 0.5 to 3 μ diameter slitlike openings or potential openings in the basement membrane which separates the cords from sinuses. After re-entering the sinuses, the cells then pass back into trabecular veins and into the general circulation. Under normal circumstances, erythrocytes make approximately 500 passages through the splenic circulation each day.

787. HYPOSPLENISM

Definition. As mentioned in Ch. 786, absence of the spleen is generally tolerated without evidence of clinical illness. There are, however, certain clinical and laboratory features which characterize "hyposplenism," whether it follows splenectomy or is associated with agenesis of the spleen or splenic atrophy secondary to multiple infarction.

Mechanisms. One of the functions of the normal spleen is to remove various inclusions from erythrocytes. Consequently, functional or genuine absence of the spleen is invariably associated with the persistence of such inclusions as *Howell-Jolly bodies.* The presence of Howell-Jolly bodies after splenectomy, or their disappearance at some interval after splenectomy, is an excellent illustration of how the peripheral blood may be used to evaluate splenic function (see next paragraph).

Diagnosis. Absence of splenic function is invariably associated with the appearance and persistence of these inclusions, and their subsequent disappearance after splenectomy may be taken as an indication of hypertrophy of an accessory spleen or spleens. Additional changes seen in erythrocytes after splenectomy include the appearance of target cells and acanthocytes (irregularly spiculated cells). Acanthocytes are noted regularly in the blood of all postsplenectomy patients, and after splenectomy their number often reaches a steady level between 10 and 20 per cent, although in some cases, up to 90 per cent of the cells may be acanthocytes. After splenectomy, *nucleated red cells* are found in the peripheral blood, especially when the spleen is removed for the treatment of hemolytic disease and also when the stimulus for increased erythroid production and release from the marrow persists after splenectomy. When the spleen is present and functioning normally, *siderocytes* (cells with iron-containing inclusions that are normally present in the bone marrow) are not seen in the peripheral blood, because the siderosomes are "culled" from the cells. After splenectomy, however, siderocytes are present in abundance in the peripheral blood, although it is necessary to use Prussian blue (PB) stain to identify them.

In *Heinz body anemias,* presplenectomy blood smears may show no evidence of the Heinz bodies, because the Heinz bodies have been pitted from the pathologic red cells. However, postsplenectomy, there is often an abundance of Heinz body–containing cells in the peripheral blood.

Leukocytosis, up to 20,000 per cubic millimeter or higher, if the patient is being treated with corticosteroids, and *thrombocythemia* to values of 500,000 to 800,000 per cubic millimeter are features that regularly characterize the peripheral blood of patients who have had their spleens removed. In evaluating leukocytosis in these individuals, it is important to recognize the predisposition of the splenectomized patient to develop leukocytosis. Potentially more important, however, is the thrombocytosis which normally rises to a maximum between the fourth and thirteenth postoperative day, and usually disappears within a month after surgery.

Treatment. If the platelet count exceeds values of 1,000,000 per cubic millimeter, there may be danger of thrombosis, including such serious complications as thrombosis of the portal vein. If the platelet count does rise above 1,000,000 per cubic millimeter, anticoagulation is indicated. Current investigations may establish that postoperative administration of aspirin interferes with platelet function sufficiently to justify the administration of aspirin in order to tide a patient over a period of thrombocytosis.

Prognosis. Potentially, the most significant consequence of absence of the spleen relates to the predisposition to develop serious infections, particularly those produced by *Diplococcus pneumoniae* and *Hemophilus influenzae,* although this is a controversial subject. There is general agreement regarding the increased risk of infection in children who undergo splenectomy under the age of four years. In older children and adults with hematologic disorders that require splenectomy, the increased incidence of infection associated with the diseases themselves makes it difficult to assess whether this risk is enhanced by splenectomy. There is no clear evidence that splenectomy in normal adults, e.g., after trauma, predisposes to infectious complications. Nevertheless, this potential complication of splenectomy, which is perhaps related to the role of the spleen as a large lymph node responsible for filtering and processing foreign antigenic material, as well as removal of foreign matter or injured cells by phagocytosis, requires further investigation to determine whether there is a significant predisposition of adults to infection after splenectomy.

788. HYPERSPLENISM

Definition. Hypersplenism, as a descriptive term, was first used by Chauffard in the last century to describe the role of the spleen in hereditary spherocytosis. The concept of hypersplenism which is generally accepted, however, was probably best defined by Dameshek during the period beween 1941 and 1955. This definition includes (1) splenomegaly, (2) pathologically low levels of one or more of the formed elements in the peripheral blood, (3) hypercellularity of the marrow precursors of those elements which are low in the peripheral blood, and (4) correction of the cytopenia by splenectomy. This definition of hypersplenism covers a variety of disorders, although it may exclude certain hematologic disorders that are improved by splenomegaly. Idiopathic thrombocytopenic purpura is an example, and even hereditary spherocytosis may satisfy all the criteria except for cytopenia, because in some cases there may be a compensated hemolysis without anemia.

Disorders which satisfy all the criteria of hypersplenism may be divided into primary disorders that have no apparent underlying cause and those states in which hypersplenism is clearly secondary to an underlying systemic illness.

PRIMARY HYPERSPLENISM

As with many disorders, the term primary or idiopathic represents a confession of ignorance, although ultimately an underlying diagnosis of lymphoma or collagen disease may become apparent months to years later. Nontropical splenomegaly has been suggested as a designation to describe this syndrome if one cannot establish a specific diagnosis based on pathologic findings or other distinctive clinical features. Nontropical splenomegaly, however, should be distinguished from the tropical splenomegaly syndrome (see below).

Pathogenesis. By definition, the pathogenesis remains poorly understood, and although it has been suggested that the splenic enlargement may represent an unusual or exaggerated response to an exogenous infection or insult, there is no conclusive evidence for this suggestion.

Pathology. Commonly, there is a wide separation of the fibrous trabeculae, although this is a feature common to all enlarged spleens. In some patients, lymphoid tissue constitutes an increased percentage of the total splenic tissue. In some cases, the sinuses in the red pulp are dilated and the hemosiderin within macrophages may be increased. Even in patients who may later prove to have an underlying lymphoma, the splenic histology is often nondiagnostic.

Clinical Manifestations. The clinical manifestations are those that one might anticipate with the classic picture of hypersplenism, and their extent depends on the degree of anemia, granulocytopenia, and/or thrombocytopenia.

Diagnosis. Evaluation of splenic size and abnormal function has become simpler in recent years by virtue of radioisotope techniques. In addition to careful palpation for splenic enlargement as part of the physical examination and examination of a roentgenogram of the abdomen for the size of the splenic shadow, more precise estimation can be obtained by a splenic scan after injection of damaged erythrocytes tagged with [197]Hg-labeled mercurihydroxypropane or [99]technetium, or [113]indium-tagged colloids. Removal of these labeled particles from the circulation by the spleen permits visualization and estimation of its size. Splenic scan may also identify defects suggestive of tumors or abscesses, although precise evaluation of tumors may require angiography. Evaluation of the destructive role of the spleen depends on the specific labeling of red cells or platelets with subsequent characterization of splenic radioactivity, compared to hepatic and precordial counts. In general, evaluation of splenic function in a hemolytic state may be helpful in predicting the possible benefit of splenectomy. Contribution of the spleen to hemolysis can be appraised by labeling of red cells with ^{51}Cr sodium chromate, reinjection, and following the cell survival, in conjunction with surface counting over the liver and spleen. In patients with hereditary or acquired anemias and enlarged spleens, the patients' own cells should be used. In other patients with splenomegaly who seem to be destroying transfused cells at an increased rate,

fresh cells from a normal donor should be used to evaluate whether splenectomy may decrease the transfusion requirement. Although there is considerable variation in the techniques employed and evidence of sequestration will not invariably predict benefit from splenectomy, an increasing splenic count in relation to the liver at the half-time (T/2) for red cell survival is evidence of significant splenic sequestration which supports a decision for splenectomy. Finally, it should be emphasized that "hypersplenic anemia" may represent (1) hemolysis, (2) splenic pooling, or (3) compensatory increase in plasma volume. These possibilities should be evaluated in each case.

Platelet sequestration can also be characterized with ^{51}Cr sodium chromate–labeled platelets. Studies of platelet survival are technically difficult and therefore are best done by those with experience in the technique. Careful studies of platelet distribution and survival have demonstrated that even in a normal-sized spleen, approximately one third of the total platelet mass in the peripheral circulation is sequestered there, and in splenomegaly the proportion of the total platelet mass may be even greater in the spleen. Studies of splenic platelet sequestration must therefore be evaluated in the light of this splenic pool both in normal and in pathologic spleens.

Treatment. Although by definition a preoperative diagnosis cannot be established in any patient with splenic enlargement, the condition is indicated by hypercellularity of normal bone marrow elements and peripheral blood cytopenia in one or more cell lines. Splenectomy is advisable when the hypersplenic syndrome becomes life-threatening as indicated by platelet counts of less than 20,000 per cubic millimeter or granulocyte counts less than 500 per cubic millimeter. Platelet counts of between 20,000 and 50,000 per cubic millimeter and/or granulocyte counts between 500 and 1000 per cubic millimeter constitute relative indications for splenectomy which may otherwise be called for because of mechanical or pressure symptoms.

Prognosis. The outcome of splenectomy in primary hypersplenism is generally satisfactory, provided that the criteria, as defined above, are satisfied. The long-term prognosis, however, depends upon the underlying disease, and, in fact, the establishment of idiopathic hypersplenism as the diagnosis is based on exclusion of specific causes of hypersplenism as demonstrated by splenic pathology, portal hypertension, or demonstration of systemic disease elsewhere.

HYPERSPLENISM SECONDARY TO AN UNDERLYING SYSTEMIC DISORDER

The accompanying table lists a wide variety of disorders which may be associated with hypersplenism. The reader is referred to specific chapters elsewhere within the book for discussion of the individual disorders. Nevertheless, it is important to recognize that the hypersplenic syndrome, including splenomegaly, hypercellular marrow, and cytopenia of one or more of the formed elements of the peripheral blood, may all be associated with a wide variety of underlying disease states that can be benefited by splenectomy.

Collagen Diseases. *Lupus erythematosus* is commonly associated with splenomegaly, and thrombocytopenia is

Secondary Hypersplenism

Collagen diseases:
  Lupus erythematosus, Felty's syndrome
Hematologic diseases:
  Hemolytic anemias: hereditary spherocytosis, hereditary ellipto-
    cytosis, thalassemia, sickle cell disease (in children), S-C, S-T dis-
    ease at all ages, autoimmune hemolytic anemia, unstable hemo-
    globin syndromes, pyruvate kinase deficiency, hereditary stomato-
    cytosis
  Myeloproliferative disorders: myeloid metaplasia, chronic granulo-
    cytic leukemia
  Lymphomas: Hodgkin's disease, non-Hodgkin's lymphomas (histio-
    cytic and lymphocytic)
Infections:
  Subacute bacterial endocarditis, malaria (tropical splenomegaly),
    kala-azar
Portal hypertension:
  Cirrhosis of the liver, portal vein thrombosis, myeloid metaplasia
Miscellaneous:
  Aneurysm of splenic artery, cavernous hemangioma

a clinical feature in approximately 15 per cent of patients with this disease. Leukopenia characterized by
both granulocytopenia and lymphopenia is also a
frequent clinical feature. Ten to 15 per cent of lupus patients have a hemolytic anemia, often with a positive
antiglobulin test. Thrombocytopenia may also be associated (see Ch. 81).

Felty's syndrome is a form of hypersplenism which
may occur in association with rheumatoid arthritis (see
Ch. 88). In Felty's syndrome, leukopenia may occasionally be severe enough to be life-threatening, and in
these cases splenectomy may be genuinely beneficial.

Hematologic Diseases. Several hematologic diseases
are associated with some type of hypersplenism. These
include congenital hemolytic anemia such as hereditary
spherocytosis and hereditary elliptocytosis, in which
splenectomy is clinically curative. In other congenital
hemolytic anemias such as thalassemia, sickle cell disease, unstable hemoglobin syndromes, pyruvate kinase
deficiency, and hereditary stomatocytosis, splenectomy
ameliorates the severity of the disorder. In autoimmune
hemolytic anemia, splenectomy may be clinically curative in some cases, and in other cases may fail to alter
the course of the disease. Patients who respond to
steroid therapy generally are benefited by splenectomy,
but some may benefit even though steroids are not effective.

In myeloproliferative disorders, particularly myeloid
metaplasia, splenomegaly is common. Although hematopoiesis can be demonstrated within the spleen, it is
not clear whether these marrow precursor cells have
arisen de novo within the spleen itself, or may represent marrow precursors that escaped from a pathologic
marrow, are trapped in the spleen, and continue to mature. Frequently, the enlarged spleen is a site for increased destruction of erythrocytes and platelets, so that
consideration of splenectomy becomes a major clinical
problem. In myeloid metaplasia, in particular, splenectomy should not be undertaken unless bone marrow
biopsy reveals an active bone marrow. Otherwise, although splenectomy may decrease transfusion requirements, no significant long-term benefit can be anticipated. The same applies to malignant lymphomas
associated with splenomegaly. Pancytopenia associated
with splenomegaly in malignant lymphoma should not
be interpreted as hypersplenism unless careful examination of the bone marrow reveals the latter to be active.

Infectious Etiologies. The hypersplenic syndrome is a
common feature of subacute bacterial endocarditis.
Splenomegaly is also a common accompaniment of malaria and of kala-azar. It may also be a feature of
tuberculosis and histoplasmosis.

Some patients who live in malarial areas develop a
syndrome that is characterized by marked splenomegaly and elevated levels of macroglobulin (IgM). This
has been called the *tropical splenomegaly syndrome*. An
important feature is that one finds normal transformation of the lymphocytes from affected individuals after
stimulation with phytohemagglutinin (PHA). These patients may have moderate lymphocytosis in the peripheral blood and lymphocytosis in the hepatic sinusoids as
well. Although the etiology is not clearly established,
patients with the tropical splenomegaly syndrome come
from malarial zones, many have positive trypanosomal
agglutination tests, and one of the hallmarks of the
disorder is a clinical response to antimalarial therapy
with proguanil. Thus it appears likely that this is a
complication of malaria associated with an exaggerated
response on the part of the lymphatic system, particularly the spleen. The red cell destruction is often characterized by splenic fragmentation of erythrocytes with
resultant spherocytosis but a negative antiglobulin test.

Portal Hypertension. Portal hypertension secondary to
cirrhosis of the liver, portal vein thrombosis, or disorders such as myeloid metaplasia in which there may
be major arteriovenous shunting occurring within the
pathologic spleen itself often leads to clinical hypersplenism. It is clear, however, that in many such patients the size of the spleen correlates rather poorly
with the severity of the cytopenias observed.

Miscellaneous. A variety of vascular anomalies, including aneurysm of the splenic artery or cavernous
hemangioma of the spleen, may be associated with
hypersplenism. In splenic artery aneurysm, the syndrome may exist for a long time and may even represent a lifelong disease state. In these vascular anomalies, in addition to splenomegaly, there may be
thrombocytopenia and also evidence of chronic intravascular coagulation with or without red cell fragmentation and destruction in the spleen. Physical examination may reveal a bruit over the splenic bed.

Diagnosis and Treatment. In all disorders in which
the hypersplenic syndrome is secondary to another
disease, attention must be paid to establishing the nature of the systemic illness, and primary treatment
should be directed toward that illness. However, if the
cytopenia(s) is severe enough and constitutes a clinical
problem, and if the bone marrow is demonstrated to be
hyperactive, splenectomy should be considered.
Frequently, the diagnostic work-up should include
liver biopsy except when thrombocytopenia is present,
and at the time of surgery portal vein pressures should
be measured. If elevated, a portacaval or a splenorenal
shunt should be considered at that time. Removal of a
large spleen in which there was significant shunting
may cause decrease in portal hypertension.

MISCELLANEOUS SPLENIC DISEASES WHICH MAY OR MAY NOT BE ASSOCIATED WITH HYPERSPLENISM

Splenic Abscess. Splenic abscesses are uncommon.
Most are secondary to metastatic spread of infection

from some remote site. About 10 per cent result from extension of contiguous infections, e.g., a perforated peptic ulcer, and 15 per cent develop secondary to some other splenic disorder or trauma, such as a hematoma. When small, they may be difficult to recognize. They may or may not cause left upper quadrant pain, but commonly cause fever, and, if large enough, splenomegaly. Rupture of a splenic abscess may lead to subdiaphragmatic abscess and, ultimately, pain in the left chest. A difficult diagnostic problem arises when the abscess is small and splenic enlargement is nil or minimal and the clinical problem is of septic fever without evidence of localization.

Splenic Infarcts. Splenic infarcts are encountered principally in hematologic disorders associated with vascular occlusive phenomena as in sickle cell disease or in disorders with marked and/or rapid hypertrophy, such as myeloid metaplasia. In sickle cell disease, the repeated infarctions ultimately result in splenic atrophy and "autosplenectomy." Sharp pain, splinting of the left diaphragm, and referred pain to the left shoulder, with or without friction rub, are the diagnostic features of a splenic infarct. Splenic infarction is generally managed conservatively, and the treatment should be based primarily on the underlying disorder.

Splenic Cysts. Splenic cysts are rare causes for splenomegaly. These may be divided into *true cysts,* which are formed from embryonal rests and lined with flattened cuboidal or squamous epithelium. Dermoids and mesenchymal inclusion cysts are included in this category. *False cysts* are more common, and usually result from trauma to the left upper abdomen. Histologically, they lack a true lining, although portions of the wall may consist of flattened cuboidal or squamous epithelium. The third type of cyst that may be encountered in the spleen is the *parasitic cyst,* usually caused by Echinococcus, which is often associated with calcification of the wall and eosinophilia in the peripheral blood.

Splenic cysts may give rise to a sense of fullness in the left upper quadrant and early satiety after ingesting food because of compression of the stomach. Angiography may help distinguish splenic cysts from splenic tumors.

Splenic Tumors. The most frequent tumors of the spleen are lymphocytic, lymphoblastic, or histiocytic lymphomas. Even though initial clinical examination may reveal no evidence of lymphoma elsewhere, the very nature of these disorders necessitates caution in designating splenic involvement by these generally systemic diseases as primary splenic tumors. Much less common are tumors of the vascular endothelium such as hemangiomas, lymphangiomas, and endothelial sarcomas. Rare primary splenic tumors include fibrosarcomas, leiomyosarcomas, or myomas involving the cap-

sule or trabecular framework; extremely rarely, one may encounter embryonic inclusions within the spleen. Again, angiography may be helpful in establishing the diagnosis.

Rupture of the Spleen. Trauma to the upper abdomen, such as an automobile accident, may cause the normal spleen to rupture. Less obvious reasons for splenic rupture may include spontaneous or postpalpation rupture of spleens enlarged because of infectious mononucleosis, sepsis (acute splenic tumor), abscess, or, rarely, leukemia. The hallmarks of splenic rupture include evidence of acute abdominal disease with sharp pain and muscle wall rigidity in the left upper quadrant, hemorrhage with shock, and pain which is commonly referred to the left shoulder and associated with splinting of the left diaphragm. This is a surgical emergency which should be dealt with immediately.

Aster, R. H.: Pooling of platelets in the spleen: Role in the pathogenesis of "hypersplenic thrombocytopenia." J. Clin. Invest., 45:645, 1966.

Battaxe, H. A., Watson, R. C., and Levin, D. C.: The angiographic appearance of splenic masses. Angiology, 23:316, 1972.

Boiger, L. E., Edhog, O., and Forsgren, L.: Splenectomy—indications and results. Acta Med. Scand., 192:213, 1972.

Christensen, B. E.: Pathophysiology of "hypersplenism syndrome." Scand. J. Haematol., 11:5, 1973.

Cormia, F. E., and Campos, L. T.: Infection after splenectomy. Ann. Intern. Med., 78:149, 1973.

Crosby, W. H.: Hypersplenism. Ann. Rev. Med., 13:127, 1962.

Crosby, W. H.: Hyposplenism: An inquiry into normal function of the spleen. Ann. Rev. Med., 14:349, 1963.

Dacie, J. V., Brain, M. C., Harrison, C. V., Lewis, S. M., and Worlledge, S. M.: Non-tropical idiopathic splenomegaly (primary hypersplenism): A review of the cases and their relationship to malignant lymphomas. Br. J. Haematol., 17:317, 1969.

Dameshek, W.: Hypersplenism. Bull. N.Y. Acad. Med., 31:113, 1955.

Das Gupta, T., Coombes, B., and Brashfield, R. D.: Primary malignant neoplasms of the spleen. Surg. Gynecol. Obstet., 120:947, 1965.

Eraklis, A. J., Kevy, S. V., Diamond, L. K., and Grass, R. E.: Hazard of overwhelming infection after splenomegaly in childhood. N. Engl. J. Med., 276:1225, 1967.

McIntyre, P. A., and Wagner, H. N., Jr.: Newer technics in hematology. *In* Progress in Hematology, Vol. 6. New York, Grune & Stratton, 1969.

Mitchell, J.: Lymphocyte circulation in the spleen. Marginal zone bridging channels and their possible role in cell traffic. Immunology, 24:93, 1973.

Nightingale, D., Prankerd, T. H. J., Richards, J. D. M., and Thompson, D.: Splenectomy in anaemia. Quart. J. Med., 41:261, 1972.

Sagoe, A. S.: Tropical splenomegaly syndrome. Long-term proguanil therapy correlated with spleen size, serum IgM, and lymphocyte transformation. Br. Med. J., 3:378, 1970.

Schwartz, S. I., Adams, J. T., and Bauman, A. W.: Splenectomy for hematologic disorders. *In* Current Problems in Surgery, May 1971.

Szur, L., Marsh, G. W., and Pettit, J. E.: Studies of splenic function by means of radioisotope-labeled red cells. Br. J. Haematol., 23:183, 1972.

Weed, R. I., and Weiss, L.: The relationship of red cell fragmentation occurring within the spleen to cell destruction. Trans. Assoc. Am. Physicians, 79:426, 1966.

Weiss, L.: The Spleen. *In* Histology. Third Edition. New York, McGraw-Hill Book Company, 1973, p. 445.

Section Fourteen. HEMORRHAGIC DISORDERS: DISORDERS OF PRIMARY HEMOSTASIS

Ralph L. Nachman

789. INTRODUCTION

The major hemorrhagic disorders are associated with malfunction of three physiologic systems either separately or in combination: (1) abnormalities of platelets, (2) abnormalities of blood vessels, and (3) abnormalities of plasma coagulation factors. Clinical disorders associated with qualitative or quantitative platelet defects and/or abnormalities of the blood vessel wall have been referred to as diseases of primary hemostasis or "purpuric syndromes." There are several important clinical and laboratory features which help differentiate this spectrum of diseases from those associated with disorders of coagulation factors (Table 1). Purpuric syndromes are characterized by capillary hemorrhages occurring chiefly in the skin and mucous membranes. Occasionally excessive bleeding may follow trauma; however, the usual lesions encountered are spontaneous petechiae and ecchymoses which result from a breakdown in the anatomic and physiologic integrity of small blood vessel walls. Gastrointestinal and genitourinary bleeding may occur spontaneously with either abnormalities of platelets or coagulation factors. Deep hematomas and hemarthroses are more frequently associated with a coagulation factor abnormality. It is important to note the relationship of excessive bleeding to antecedent trauma or surgery, such as circumcision, tonsillectomy, or tooth extraction. Recurrent bleeding for two to three days or more usually indicates an underlying coagulation disorder. In general, bleeding caused by platelet or blood vessel defects is immediate and responds to direct pressure. A strong familial history of a serious bleeding problem should clearly raise the possibility of a coagulation disorder; however, it is important to note that as many as one third of all hemophilic patients have a negative family history. Several simple bedside procedures are useful for the initial evaluation of a hemorrhagic disorder. The Rumpel-Leede vascular fragility test is usually positive in patients with a purpuric syndrome; however, the procedure is superfluous

in patients with spontaneous diffuse petechiae and ecchymoses The Duke bleeding time is also a valuable bedside test which can help differentiate patients with purpuric disorders from those with underlying coagulation abnormalities. The rebleeding phenomenon should not be confused with the prolonged primary bleeding time. Patients with hemophila may rebleed one to two hours after an essentially normal Duke or Ivy bleeding time. This results from the formation of a poorly formed friable clot owing to the deficiency of a coagulation factor.

An understanding of the physiology of primary hemostatic mechanisms is important for the interpretation of diagnostic laboratory tests and for the subsequent management of patients with purpuric disorders. The formation of a hemostatic platelet plug can be divided into several separate but interrelated stages. The initial event in the development of the primary plug occurs with great rapidity and involves the adhesion of circulating platelets to exposed subendothelial collagen fibers, microfibrils, or basement membrane at the site of vessel wall injury. The adhesion reaction is mediated by specific chemical and physical determinants on the collagen molecule and possibly by a platelet membrane enzyme system. ADP which is stored in platelet granules is released by a process analogous to endocrine gland secretion and leads to platelet aggregation (cohesion). A chain reaction of aggregating platelets releasing intracellular ADP which in turn recruits more platelets characterizes the growing plug. Platelet factor 3, a surface lipoprotein complex, and endothelial cell tissue factor become available at the site of the vessel injury probably owing to conformational changes of platelet and endothelial cell membranes. This soon results in the evolution of thrombin by activation of the intrinsic and extrinsic coagulation pathways. These biochemical events lead to consolidation and contraction of the platelet plug with eventual sealing of the injured vessel wall. The thrombin generated at the local site polymerizes fibrinogen, and the resulting fibrin reinforces the platelet mass at the periphery of the plug.

TABLE 1. Differentiation of Purpuric and Coagulation Disorders

Features	Purpuric Syndromes	Coagulation Disorders
Family history	Generally negative	Usually positive
Sex	More common in females	More common in males
Type of bleeding	Skin and mucosal surfaces	Visceral and intramuscular
	Petechiae and ecchymoses	Deep hematomas
	Spontaneous	Usually traumatic
Hemarthroses	Very rare	Frequent
Duration	Recent in onset	Usually lifelong
Bleeding time	Generally prolonged	Normal
Capillary fragility (tourniquet test)	Positive	Negative

QUANTITATIVE PLATELET ABNORMALITIES

790. THROMBOCYTOPENIA

Thrombocytopenia is the most common cause of hemorrhagic disease. Thus the peripheral blood of every patient who bleeds should be carefully examined. With experience, it is possible to approximate the platelet count by careful evaluation of a peripheral blood smear. Depending on the individual observer, the microscope, and the technique used in making the smear, there should be approximately three to ten platelets per oil immersion field. Smears prepared from "finger stick" blood samples show platelets which are less evenly distributed than smears from anticoagulated blood. Fewer than 50 platelets per 50 oil immersion fields usually suggests moderate to severe thrombocytopenia. With modern automated counting devices, the average normal platelet count varies from 200,000 to 400,000 per cubic millimeter.

The relationship of the platelet count and clinical bleeding is sometimes obscure. Some patients with severe thrombocytopenia may have little bleeding, but others with only a moderate decrease in platelet number present with a marked hemorrhagic diathesis. It is obvious that a number of contributing variables influence the integrity of the blood vessel wall. Sudden precipitous drops in platelet count, fever, and anemia appear to contribute significantly to petechial hemorrhage. Hormonal influences also can affect vascular integrity, as demonstrated by the beneficial effects of steroids in some patients in the absence of improvement in the platelet count. At very low levels, such as 10,000

platelets per cubic millimeter, major hemorrhagic manifestations such as central nervous system bleeding or massive gastrointestinal hemorrhage are more frequent. It is useful to categorize the many causes of thrombocytopenia in the framework of decreased production, decreased survival or excessive utilization, sequestration, and intravascular dilution (Table 2).

DECREASED PRODUCTION OF PLATELETS

Multiple anatomic as well as biochemical alterations may alter megakaryocyte number and function in the marrow. In such conditions, the erythroid and myeloid cellular elements may also be involved to varying degrees. Megakaryocyte depression from bone marrow infiltration may occur in leukemia, myeloma, carcinoma, lymphoma, granuloma, or myelofibrosis. Drugs, in particular the thiazide derivatives, ionizing radiation, and various toxins may cause major injury and megakaryocytic depletion. Familial aplastic anemia (Fanconi's anemia) with thrombocytopenia is a rare fatal childhood illness associated with multiple congenital and skeletal anomalies. A rare syndrome of infancy, congenital amegakaryocytic thrombocytopenia, is associated with bilateral absence of the radii. In congenital rubella, megakaryocytes are decreased in number with an associated decreased platelet production. In this disease the megakaryocyte may provide a preferred site for viral replication.

Impaired platelet production may also result from ineffective thrombopoiesis. Under these circumstances, adequate to increased numbers of megakaryocytes are present in the marrow; however, thrombocytopenia results from interference with the functional integrity of the marrow. This is seen in megaloblastic anemias, in paroxysmal nocturnal hemoglobinuria, and in various hereditary thrombocytopenias, including the Wiskott-Aldrich syndrome and the May-Hegglin anomaly.

DECREASED PLATELET SURVIVAL—INCREASED DESTRUCTION

Drug Purpura

Drugs must be considered a possible cause in every adult with thrombocytopenic purpura. Patients with drug purpura may develop hemorrhagic symptoms after weeks or even years of symptom-free use of an agent. Thrombocytopenia may develop within minutes to hours after administration of a drug to a sensitized patient. The bleeding at first is characterized by petechiae, purpura, occasionally hemorrhagic bullae of the oral mucosa, and not infrequently gastrointestinal and/or genitourinary hemorrhage. The petechiae do not itch, are not tender, and are not associated with wheals. In general the skin lesions are distributed over the lower extremities; they are not found on the soles or palms. In the majority of cases, the thrombocytopenic purpura will clear within a few days after removal of the offending drug. Purpura which persists for more than two to three weeks after drug exposure has been terminated should no longer be considered drug induced, and other conditions should be suspected. However, the duration of the purpura may be variable and

---

TABLE 2.   Thrombocytopenia

I. Decreased production
   A. Reduced marrow megakaryocytes
      Marrow infiltration
      Marrow hypoplasia—radiation, toxins, chemicals, drugs, idiopathic
      Fanconi's anemia
      Congenital amegakaryocytic thrombocytopenia
      Infection—congenital rubella
   B. Normal or increased marrow megakaryocytes
      Megaloblastic anemia
      Paroxysmal nocturnal hemoglobinuria
      Hereditary thrombocytopenia
         Wiskott-Aldrich syndrome
         May-Hegglin anomaly
II. Decreased platelet survival
   A. Increased destruction
      Drug-induced purpura
      Idiopathic thrombocytopenic purpura
      Post-transfusion purpura
      Neonatal purpura
      Secondary immunologic purpura
   B. Increased consumption
      Disseminated intravascular coagulation
      Hemangioma
      Thrombotic thrombocytopenic purpura
      Hemolytic-uremic syndrome
      Acute infections
III. Sequestration (splenomegalic states)
IV. Dilutional

depends to a large extent on the metabolic fate of the drug. Thus certain toxic agents such as gold remain in the body for long periods of time after the last injection. Many patients forget that they have been chronically ingesting various common remedies such as aspirin, sedatives, and/or various tranquilizers, which can cause thrombocytopenia.

Etiology and Pathogenesis. Many agents have been implicated as causes of thrombocytopenia (Table 3). These agents can produce thrombocytopenia by several different mechanisms. Thiazide derivatives, estrogens,

TABLE 3. Drugs Associated with Thrombocytopenic Purpura

I. Marrow suppression
   Thiazides, alcohol, estrogens
II. Direct cytotoxic effect
   Ristocetin
III. Immunologic mechanisms—peripheral destruction
   A. Etiologic relationship established
      Acetazolamide
      Allyl-isopropyl carbamide (Sedormid)
      Arsenical antiluetic drugs
      Carbamazepine
      Chlorothiazide
      Digitoxin
      Diphenylhydantoin sodium
      Hydrochlorothiazide
      Hydroxychloroquine
      Methyl dopa
      Novobiocin
      Para-aminosalicylic acid
      Quinidine
      Quinine
      Stibophen
      Sulfathiazole
   B. Etiologic relationship suspected but not confirmed
      Acetaminophen
      Aminopyrine
      Aspirin
      Butabarbitone
      Carbabutamide
      Chloramphenicol
      Chlorpheniramine maleate
      Chlorpromazine
      Chlorpropamide
      Codeine
      Desipramine
      Dextroamphetamine
      Digitalis
      Digoxin
      Disulfiram
      Erythromycin
      Ethyl-allyl-acetylurea
      Gold
      Iopanoic acid
      Isonicotinic acid hydrazide
      Meperidine
      Meprobamate
      Mercurial diuretics
      Penicillin
      Phenacetin
      Phenylbutazone
      Prednisone
      Prochlorperazine
      Promethazine
      Propylthiouracil
      Reserpine
      Streptomycin
      Sulfadiazine
      Sulfadimidine
      Sulfamethoxypyridazine
      Sulfamerizine
      Sulfisoxazole
      Tetracycline
      Thiouracil
      Tolbutamide

and alcohol may interfere with bone marrow megakaryocyte number and function. The antibiotic ristocetin may directly damage platelets in vivo. Among the drugs listed in Table 3, *particularly frequent offenders include quinidine, quinine, sulfonamides, and the thiazides.* One should have a high level of suspicion of drug sensitivity when thrombocytopenic purpura develops in a patient receiving any of these drugs. Widely used drugs such as aspirin, penicillin, and phenobarbital have also been reported as offenders. In effect, any drug taken by a patient is a possible cause of purpura.

The most common mechanism implicated in drug purpura is immunologic platelet destruction. In recent years, a convincing body of experimental and clinical evidence has been accumulated that clearly demonstrates the participation of the platelet in immunologic reactions. The external platelet surface is capable of nonspecifically adsorbing certain antibody drug complexes which then lead to platelet damage by an "innocent bystander" effect. According to this theory, the administered drug as hapten binds to a plasma protein or "carrier" to form an antigen. Antibodies stimulated by the immunogen bind to the drug, and these immune complexes secondarily interact with the platelet membrane, leading to cellular damage. Recent evidence also suggests that specific metabolic products of certain drugs rather than the primary agent may act as the offending immunogen.

Diagnosis. A careful history of drug ingestion is an absolute necessity in any patient with thrombocytopenia. In addition to the usual medications, specific questioning is necessary regarding intake of beverages which contain quinine. In general the purpuric lesions with thrombocytopenia develop within hours after exposure to the agent by a sensitized patient. There may be an increased percentage of circulating large young platelets in the peripheral blood which is indicative of increased platelet turnover. A number of laboratory tests have been utilized to demonstrate drug, platelet, and antibody interactions as evidence of drug purpura. Tests involving complement fixation and platelet factor 3 release have proved to be relatively sensitive. Inhibition of clot retraction in the presence of the suspected offending agent is the simplest to perform but only detects high titer antibody. These in vitro tests are based on the premise that the underlying mechanism of the drug purpura is platelet adsorption of immune complexes consisting of drug and antibody with subsequent secondary cell damage. Direct challenge of the patient by a test dose of suspected drug in vivo is potentially hazardous. No single test is capable of detecting all cases of drug purpura. The most sensitive tests are difficult to perform and require expert laboratory assistance.

Treatment. All drugs should be discontinued. Medications which are indisputably needed should be replaced with pharmacologically equivalent but chemically different preparations. Adrenal corticosteroids should be given for their beneficial effect on vascular integrity. Platelet transfusions should be used only for life-threatening hemorrhage.

Idiopathic Thrombocytopenic Purpura

Definition. *Acute.* Acute idiopathic thrombocytopenic purpura (ITP) is essentially a disease of young children, affecting both sexes equally. It is characterized by sudden onset of severe thrombocytopenic purpura in an otherwise healthy child, frequently occurring one to two weeks after a sore throat or ordinary cold. Acute ITP is seen most frequently between the ages of two and six years. The manifestations are extensive petechial hemorrhages and purpura with gingival, gastrointestinal, and genitourinary bleeding. There is frequently severe thrombocytopenia (platelet counts below 20,000 per cubic millimeter) with marked hyperplasia of bone marrow megakaryocytes. The spleen is usually not palpable. In over 80 per cent of the patients the disorder is self-limited, clearing spontaneously within two weeks. Patients should be treated with prednisone, 1 to 2 mg per kilogram of body weight, during the period of maximal thrombocytopenia. In some cases the thrombocytopenia may persist for two to six months. Approximately 10 to 15 per cent of affected children will develop chronic ITP, which eventually requires splenectomy.

Chronic. Chronic ITP is predominately a disease of young adults, affecting females three to four times as often as males. The disorder is characterized by insidious onset with a relatively long history of easy bruising and menorrhagia. Many patients give a history of mild to moderate bleeding after trauma or minor surgery such as dental extractions. The platelet count is usually in the range of 50,000 to 100,000 per cubic millimeter. Bone marrow examination reveals megakaryocytic hyperplasia with predominance of early young forms.

In a typical patient the physical findings are minimal except for petechiae and ecchymoses. There is no characteristic pattern of ditribution of the hemorrhagic lesions. The patient is afebrile, and in most cases the spleen is not palpable. The presence of an easily palpable spleen should direct attention away from the diagnosis of ITP. The disease may be present for a number of months to years and may be characterized by remissions and relapses. In most cases, the hemorrhagic complications are not life threatening; however, a rare individual may show central nervous system signs with intracerebral bleeding. In some patients the disorder appears to have cyclical characteristics, with striking exacerbations of systemic hemorrhagic symptoms with menstruation. These patients generally feel quite well except for complaints relating to the four or five days of hemorrhage per month.

Etiology and Pathogenesis. In approximately 85 per cent of cases, ITP is a disorder produced by a platelet autoantibody that develops in a patient with no evidence of underlying disease or significant exposure to drugs. For this reason, some authors now prefer to define this disease as *autoimmune thrombocytopenic purpura* (ATP).

Although platelet autoantibodies are difficult to demonstrate, a significant body of clinical and experimental evidence has suggested their presence. Thus pregnant women with ITP frequently give birth to thrombocytopenic infants, a situation strongly suggesting the transplacental transfer of antiplatelet antibody. Plasma from patients with ITP produces severe thrombocytopenia when infused into normal individuals. This plasma also produces thrombocytopenia in the donor individual when reinfused at a time of remission. The activity causing thrombocytopenia upon transfusion of ITP plasma has been identified as a 7S gamma globulin

which is absorbed by incubation with autologous and homologous platelets.

A number of in vitro test systems have been devised to demonstrate platelet antibodies in ITP. These include platelet agglutination, complement fixation, platelet factor 3 release, anti-gamma globulin consumption tests, and inhibition of labeled serotonin uptake. These tests are generally difficult to perform and are not yet part of routine laboratory studies. With sensitive in vitro systems it has been demonstrated that approximately 85 per cent of chronic ITP patients have antiplatelet antibodies. It is of interest that antibody production has been demonstrated in surgically removed spleens.

Diagnosis. The diagnosis of chronic ITP is in large part an exercise in clinical exclusion. This is because the in vitro tests used to demonstrate circulating antiplatelet antibodies are difficult to perform and are generally not available in most clinical centers. Thus the diagnosis is made by a consideration of the major clinical and laboratory hallmarks as outlined above, paucity of physical findings, absence of underlying systemic disorders, exclusion of other primary immunologic thrombocytopenic conditions, and, finally, response to therapy. In most patients, perhaps the most significant diagnostic differential involves the exclusion of primary drug purpura. It is useful initially to remove or replace all drugs for at least two to three weeks. Thrombocytopenia which persists beyond this period is only rarely associated with previous drug administration, with the possible exception of a gold preparation.

Therapy and Prognosis. Adrenal corticosteroids in a fairly high dose range, e.g., 60 mg of prednisone daily, are employed initially in an attempt to promote a significant rise in the platelet count and decrease bleeding. With steroid therapy, reduction in capillary fragility and decreased bleeding are often observed before an appreciable rise in the platelet count occurs. Most patients (approximately 70 per cent) with chronic ITP will respond to this therapy within two to three weeks. Unfortunately most of them will relapse within weeks to months after discontinuation of the steroids. Less than 15 per cent of adults with ITP will make a complete permanent recovery after an initial course of steroid therapy. In general, if significant clinical improvement does not occur within four to eight weeks or can be maintained only with toxic levels of steroids, splenectomy should be considered. For those patients who respond initially to steroids, the drug should be decreased gradually over several weeks so as to maintain the platelet count above 50,000 per cubic millimeter. In practical terms, most patients will require long-term doses of steroids which eventually lead to undesirable side effects. Thus unless the patient represents an unusual surgical risk, splenectomy should be performed.

Approximately 70 per cent of patients will achieve long-term and even permanent remissions after splenectomy. This is due to (1) removal of a major site of platelet destruction and (2) elimination of a major source of synthesis of platelet antibody. Most patients who enter remission after splenectomy show significant rises in the platelet count, often well above normal levels, within a few days. After surgery, up to 10 per cent of patients may require weeks or even months before a significant remission develops. Recent studies suggest that the effectiveness of splenectomy correlates with the response to prior corticosteroid therapy. A good or excellent response to splenectomy may be expected in a high percentage of patients who have shown a significant rise in the platelet count while on steroids.

Postsplenectomy failure with significant bleeding may respond to high-dose steroids even if the patient previously was refractory to the steroid effect. Immunosuppressive agents such as azathioprine and cyclophosphamide have proved useful in the treatment of these patients. These agents should also be considered for use in patients with symptomatic chronic ITP in whom splenectomy cannot be performed. As noted previously, a small group of women with ITP who do not respond to splenectomy may develop exacerbations of the hemorrhagic symptoms during the menses. Some of these patients show striking improvement in clinical manifestations after suppression of ovarian function with hormonal agents.

Platelet transfusions should be reserved for life-threatening hemorrhage in chronic ITP. Platelets should not be given prophylactically, because they will be rapidly destroyed by the circulating platelet antibodies.

Post-Transfusion Purpura

Post-transfusion purpura is a rare form of immunologic purpura which must be distinguished from ITP and drug purpura. The disease is characterized by sudden explosive onset of thrombocytopenic purpura about five to eight days after transfusion of whole blood. The disease develops because of the mismatching of an inherited platelet antigen with the subsequent development of a complement-fixing antiplatelet isoantibody. The antigen PL^{A1} is found in 98 per cent of the normal population and is absent from the platelets of the patient who develops the disorder. The process is self-limited; however, purpura may last up to six weeks. Conclusive diagnosis rests on the serologic demonstration of platelet antigen mismatching. Post-transfusion purpura should be suspected in any patient who develops sudden purpura in the absence of an overt underlying cause shortly after a blood transfusion. Owing to the danger of intracranial hemorrhage, the therapy consists of exchange transfusion and steroids in high dosage.

Neonatal Purpura

Neonatal thrombocytopenia may develop because of isoimmunization of the mother against fetal platelets with subsequent transplacental transfer of maternal antibody. The disease is the platelet analogue of erythroblastosis fetalis, with platelets rather than red cells serving as the antigenic stimulus. The infant shows generalized purpura at delivery, and platelet counts are usually below 30,000 per cubic millimeter. Intracranial hemorrhage has occurred in approximately 10 per cent of cases.

At least four well-defined platelet antigen systems have been elucidated and appear to be involved in the development of maternal-fetal incompatibility. These include the PL^{A1}, PL Gc Ly^{B1}, PL Gc Ly^{C1}, and PL^{E2} antigens. These antigens, which are distinct from erythrocyte antigens, are inherited as dominant characteristics. The B1 and C1 platelet antigens are shared by granulocytes and lymphocytes. Adrenal corticosteroids, transfusion with maternal platelets, and exchange transfusion have been tried in severe cases.

Secondary Immunologic Purpura

Idiopathic thrombocytopenic purpura may be associated with *autoimmune hemolytic anemia (Evans' syndrome)*. Patients with this disorder present with clinical and laboratory features of Coombs-positive hemolytic anemia and marked to moderate thrombocytopenia.

Autoimmune thrombocytopenia presenting in a manner identical to that of classic ITP occurs in approximately 10 per cent of patients with *systemic lupus erythematosus*. This entity may present as the only significant clinical feature of early lupus. For this reason, immunologic tests for lupus erythematosus should be performed on all patients who present with ITP.

A chronic ITP syndrome can be observed during the course of *chronic lymphocytic leukemia* and *malignant lymphoma*. It should be emphasized that the great majority of cases of thrombocytopenia associated with these diseases are secondary to marrow involvement. The pathogenesis in these rare cases appears to be the same as that described in the idiopathic (autoimmune) disorder. Certain postinfectious thrombocytopenic states, such as those occasionally seen with *rubella* or *infectious mononucleosis*, result from a temporary stimulation of circulating antibody to platelets. The antibody in some cases of infectious mononucleosis is a cold agglutinin with "i" specificity which coats platelets upon exposure to cold. The antibody-coated cells are sequestered in the spleen.

DECREASED PLATELET SURVIVAL—INCREASED CONSUMPTION

Disseminated Intravascular Coagulation

This group of disorders, which is discussed in Ch. 801, is generally associated with significant thrombocytopenia. The platelets are consumed throughout the vascular tree secondary to the generation of excessive amounts of thrombin in the circulation.

Cavernous Hemangioma (Kasabach-Merritt Syndrome)

Giant cavernous hemangioma of infancy is generally detected at birth. Thrombocytopenia, which may be severe, results from excessive consumption of circulating platelets on the damaged subendothelial surface of the neoplasm. Intravascular coagulation takes place within the tumor. Occasionally the tumors are located in visceral sites. In many of these the thrombocytopenia is the most prominent feature of the generalized coagulation disorder. Surgical excision of the tumor if possible and radiation have been used successfully in therapy.

Thrombotic Thrombocytopenic Purpura

Thrombotic thrombocytopenic purpura (TTP) is an acute disease which presents a clinical spectrum, including thrombocytopenic purpura, microangiopathic hemolytic anemia, transient fluctuating neurologic symptoms, kidney disease, and fever. Approximately 80 per cent of patients die within one month of onset of the illness. The most frequently observed symptoms are related to the fluctuating and, at times, bizarre central nervous manifestations and the severe hemorrhagic complications. The anemia is usually brisk, with hematocrits often below 20 per cent on initial examination. An important diagnostic feature is the striking microangiopathic peripheral blood picture; the blood smear shows an increased number of schistocytes, burr cells, and helmet-shaped red cell fragments. Careful evaluation of the coagulation parameters early in the illness does not support the premise that disseminated intravascular coagulation (DIC) has a primary role in this disorder. Later, as the illness becomes more severe and hepatic failure and sepsis occur, secondary DIC may be seen. Diagnostic confirmation of TTP requires histologic demonstration of a characteristic pathologic lesion: the deposition of hyaline thrombi within the lumina of arterioles and capillaries in the absence of vasculitis. These lesions are probably composed of aggregates of degenerating platelets and fibrin. The relationship of the platelet to the primary process in this disease remains unclear. Fibrin has been demonstrated in the thrombotic lesions of TTP by immunofluorescence techniques. Since fibrinogen constitutes approximately 10 per cent of the platelet proteins, focal platelet deposition on blood vessel walls would produce positive immunofluorescence reactions for fibrin. Radioisotope labeling studies have demonstrated decreased platelet survival but normal fibrinogen survival in patients with TTP.

The cause of TTP is unknown. The disorder should be considered a syndrome with multiple etiologic factors producing microcirculatory pathology resulting from the consumption of circulating platelets throughout the microvasculature at sites of vascular damage. In some cases, the primary lesion may reside in small blood vessels. Electron microscopic studies of capillaries have revealed subendothelial prethrombotic fibrin and accumulations of platelets. TTP has occurred in association with systemic lupus erythematosus and other collagen vascular disorders, supporting the possibility of an immune cause in some cases. Bartonella-like bacteria have been isolated from the blood of several patients with TTP. It is possible that other bacterial agents as well as viruses may act as intravascular platelet aggregating agents. Platelet aggregates which are formed in the circulation have been demonstrated to cause microvascular damage by deposition in small vessels and release of vasotoxic factors. Thus under some circumstances, the lesions of TTP could result from insults which primarily affect normal circulating platelets. Whether platelet aggregation is primary or secondary to vessel wall damage, platelet consumption is important in the disease process.

Acute TTP is a medical emergency. Therapy to date has been relatively ineffective, and the current approach is to some extent empirical. Steroids (60 to 100 mg of prednisone daily) and antiplatelet aggregating agents should be started as soon as the diagnosis is made. An effective antiplatelet aggregating combination includes combined dipyridamole and aspirin. If the clinical situation deteriorates, splenectomy should be performed. Anticoagulant therapy in general has not proved beneficial in this disorder.

Hemolytic-Uremic Syndrome

The hemolytic-uremic syndrome (*Gasser's syndrome*) is a disease of early childhood characterized by acute microangiopathic hemolytic anemia, thrombocytopenia, and renal failure. The explosive onset may follow a minor febrile illness or even prophylactic immunization. Neurologic symptoms are rarely seen, and the patients frequently have hemorrhagic diarrhea. The lesions are usually limited to the kidney and are characteristically focal thromboses of glomerular arterioles and capillaries with renal cortical necrosis. The pathogenesis of the hemolytic-uremic syndrome is unknown. Disseminated intravascular coagulation resulting from circulating immune complexes with deposition of circulating fibrin in the renal microvasculature has been considered as the most likely pathogenetic mechanism. Therapy has been primarily directed at management of the acute renal failure. Corticosteroids are probably not helpful. Heparin has appeared to be beneficial in some cases.

The hemolytic-uremic syndrome may also be seen in pregnant or postpartum women. The explosive onset of microangiopathic hemolytic anemia, thrombocytopenia, and acute renal failure may develop in the setting of premature separation of the placenta or toxemia of pregnancy. The pathologic lesions are identical to those seen in young children.

Acute Infections

Thrombocytopenia may occasionally develop during an acute viral or bacterial infection. Direct platelet damage caused by platelet-bacterium or platelet-virus interaction probably contributes significantly to thrombocytopenia. Extracellular toxins from both staphylococci and streptococci as well as endotoxins from gram-negative organisms lead to platelet damage and aggregation. In cases of severe sepsis, thrombocytopenia may in fact reflect consumption of circulating platelets in association with DIC. In contrast, the thrombocytopenia of some viral infections may be caused by suppression of megakaryocytic function, as is seen in congenital rubella.

SEQUESTRATION THROMBOCYTOPENIA

Thrombocytopenia may occur in any disorder associated with an enlarged spleen. The characteristic clinical picture is prominent splenomegaly with moderate thrombocytopenia (50,000 to 100,000 platelets per cubic millimeter). This entity has also been referred to as *hypersplenic thrombocytopenia*. Under normal circumstances, approximately one third of the total body platelet mass is in the spleen and the splenic platelet pool exchanges with the freely circulating platelets. In splenomegaly of any cause, the splenic platelet pool may be greatly expanded and up to 90 per cent of the platelets can be trapped at any one time. Thus a redistribution of platelets can occur, resulting in thrombocytopenia despite normal platelet production and normal platelet survival. In addition, young platelets tend to accumulate in the spleen to a greater extent than old platelets. The clinical picture will reflect the underlying etiology of the splenomegaly, e.g., cirrhosis with portal hypertension, myelofibrosis, or infiltrative disease such as Gaucher's disease or malignant lymphoma. The thrombocytopenia secondary to splenomegaly is rarely severe enough to produce hemorrhagic disease. Splenectomy, however, will generally restore a normal or even elevated platelet count.

DILUTIONAL THROMBOCYTOPENIA

Massive blood transfusions, extracorporeal circulation, and exchange transfusion may result in moderate thrombocytopenia because of blood volume replacement with platelet-poor banked blood. The severity of the thrombocytopenia is directly related to the number of transfusions.

791. THROMBOCYTOSIS

Thrombocytosis refers to clinical situations in which the platelet count is significantly elevated. Benign or secondary thrombocytosis usually occurs as a temporary event in the setting of another condition such as splenectomy, acute or chronic inflammatory disease, hemolytic anemia, acute hemorrhage, or iron deficiency, or as a response to exercise. Asymptomatic secondary thrombocytosis with platelet counts in the range of 700,000 to 1,000,000 per cubic millimeter has been reported in a number of patients with carcinoma, Hodgkin's disease, and other malignant lymphomas. The nature of the reactive thrombocytosis in these conditions is unknown, but it may represent a nonspecific megakaryocytic proliferative response to tissue necrosis. It is of interest that thrombocytosis has been noted after the use of drugs such as vincristine, which interferes with microtubules.

Essential thrombocythemia is characterized by spontaneous bleeding, at times alternating or coinciding with thrombotic episodes accompanied by a sustained elevation in the platelet count. The process may be considered one of the myeloproliferative diseases and can accompany or develop into chronic myelogenous leukemia, polycythemia vera, or myelofibrosis. The platelet count is usually in the range of 1,000,000 per cubic millimeter, and giant irregular forms and aggregates of platelets are seen on the peripheral smear. Platelet function studies such as the bleeding time, platelet factor 3 release, and platelet aggregation in response to epinephrine are frequently abnormal. The platelets are probably qualitatively defective; however, the precise mechanisms underlying the thrombotic and hemorrhagic symptoms are unknown. In some patients essential thrombocythemia has been unmasked after splenectomy for unrelated conditions. *Pseudohyperkalemia* is an interesting laboratory artifact seen in some of these patients. Serum potassium levels may be strikingly elevated in the absence of electrocardiographic evidence of hyperkalemia. In this circumstance the plasma potassium levels are normal, and the elevated serum levels are caused by release of potassium from platelets

during blood clotting. Clinically the hemorrhagic and thrombotic symptoms improve as the platelet count is lowered. Busulfan and other myelosuppressive agents have proved useful in the long-term management of these patients. Antiplatelet aggregating agents, such as aspirin and dipyridamole, may prove useful in preventing thrombotic complications.

792. QUALITATIVE PLATELET ABNORMALITIES

Several hemorrhagic disorders have been attributed to abnormalities in platelet function occurring in the presence of adequate numbers of circulating platelets. The abnormalities may result from (1) defects in the primary hemostatic process involving adhesion or cohesion, leading to ineffective platelet plug formation, and/or (2) defects in the procoagulant activity of platelets associated with abnormal platelet factor 3 availability. The bleeding time is probably the most useful in vivo test for rapid evaluation of platelet function. In addition, a number of in vitro test systems to monitor platelet aggregation and to measure the platelet adhesiveness to glass bead columns have helped to clarify these different defects. The presence of a qualitative platelet abnormality in a patient is established by the following criteria: (1) hemorrhagic history in the absence of a disorder of the coagulation factors, (2) normal platelet count, and (3) abnormal platelet function.

A large group of qualitative platelet disorders have not yet been satisfactorily characterized. Some exceedingly rare congenital disorders have been reported, including the *Bernard-Soulier syndrome,* a potentially fatal hemorrhagic condition with circulating giant lymphocytoid platelets. Both morphologic and functional platelet abnormalities have been observed in patients with certain inherited disorders of connective tissue, including *Ehlers-Danlos syndrome, osteogenesis imperfecta,* and *pseudoxanthoma elasticum.* Abnormal platelet function has been reported in the *Wiskott-Aldrich syndrome.* The more important diseases of abnormal platelet function are discussed below.

THROMBASTHENIA
(Glanzmann's Disease)

Thrombasthenia is a rare congenital hemorrhagic disease in which there is a profound aberration of the primary hemostatic process. The patients characteristically present with severe bleeding from mucous membranes, usually beginning in childhood. However, some suffer only a minor hemorrhagic problem. There is an autosomal recessive inheritance pattern. The bleeding time is markedly prolonged, and clot retraction is greatly reduced or absent. Platelets from these patients do not aggregate with ADP or thrombin. Although the precise nature of the platelet abnormality is unknown, defects in cellular size and shape as well as various enzyme abnormalities have been reported. Markedly diminished content of platelet fibrinogen in the presence of normal levels of plasma fibrinogen is a characteristic feature in most patients. The platelets also fail to provide surface platelet factor 3 activity after exposure to activating agents. If clinically significant bleeding occurs, they usually respond to therapy with platelet transfusions.

THROMBOPATHIA—DEFECTIVE ADP RELEASE

This is a relatively mild common platelet disorder. Patients present with easy bruising and mild to moderate postoperative bleeding, and the bleeding time may be moderately prolonged. Their platelets when studied in vitro respond normally to high ADP levels but show decreased aggregation with collagen and impaired aggregation with epinephrine. There are probably several types of abnormality within this group. For example, some patients appear to have decreased intracellular pools of ADP, whereas others have normal storage pools of ADP but are unable to release the nucleotide. The latter category resembles the defect seen after aspirin ingestion by normal subjects.

DRUG-INDUCED PLATELET ABNORMALITIES

Aspirin ingestion results in abnormal platelet function because of inhibition of the release of intrinsic platelet ADP. The bleeding time may be slightly prolonged, and platelet aggregation induced by collagen or epinephrine is abnormal. The mechanism by which aspirin inhibits ADP release is not known; however, acetylation of a platelet membrane protein may be an important component of the process. It is of interest that the effect of a single dose of aspirin may last for several days. In some individuals administration of small amounts of aspirin may prolong the bleeding time and lead to a significant hemorrhagic disorder, particularly if the patient is subjected to a surgical stress. This exaggerated aspirin response may reflect the unmasking of an underlying platelet functional abnormality. Patients with thrombocytopenia or blood coagulation disorders should avoid aspirin.

Other agents also can interfere with normal platelet function. Plasma expanders such as *dextran* and *hydroxyethyl starch* prolong the bleeding time, presumably by interrupting the normal process of adhesion. Numerous other agents currently used in clinical medicine adversely affect normal hemostasis. Included in this group are the anti-inflammatory agents *Butazolidin*, *sulfinpyrazone*, and *Indocin*, some *antihistamines*, various *local anesthetics*, *clofibrate*, and *dipyridamole*. Some of these pharmacologic agents or structural analogues may be useful as agents to counteract platelet aggregation in thrombotic disorders.

ACQUIRED PLATELET FUNCTIONAL ABNORMALITIES—SYSTEMIC DISEASE

Uremia. The bleeding time in uremic patients is frequently prolonged out of proportion to that caused by the moderate thrombocytopenia which is commonly present. The most consistent laboratory abnormalities include decreased platelet adhesiveness to glass bead columns and impaired release of the coagulant activity, platelet factor 3. Normal platelets in uremic plasma function abnormally, and the defect in uremia improves significantly after dialysis. It is therefore probable that the platelet functional aberration in uremia results from the accumulation of small molecular weight metabolic waste products.

Dysglobulinemia. Abnormal platelet function has been observed in patients with macroglobulinemia as well as in multiple myeloma. Macroglobulin probably coats the platelet surface and sterically interferes with the normal hemostatic reactions. Improvement has been noted in patients after plasmapheresis.

Defects in platelet aggregation with prolonged bleeding times have been seen in a number of systemic conditions such as *cirrhosis*, *systemic lupus erythematosus*, and *pernicious anemia*. The hemorrhagic symptoms in these conditions may be related to the associated qualitative platelet abnormalities.

793. VASCULAR PURPURA

A varied group of clinical syndromes are characterized by intrinsic abnormalities of the blood vessel wall which result in mucosal and skin hemorrhages in the absence of overt defects in platelet function and number or plasma clotting factor defects. These syndromes are listed in Table 4.

Among the most common examples is *purpura simplex*. This is seen in otherwise healthy females who present with frequent but relatively harmless purpuric lesions. The disorder is lifelong, and there is occasionally a positive family history. It is disturbing cosmetically, and there is no effective treatment. It is significant only that this benign condition should be distinguished from the more serious purpuric states.

Senile Purpura. This is a relatively harmless, common condition primarily affecting the elderly. Purpuric lesions are mainly localized over the back of the hands and the extensor surfaces of the forearms. Large superficial ecchymotic areas may develop after mild trauma. The lesions occur in thin parchment-like atrophic skin and are presumably related to the degeneration of sub-

TABLE 4. Causes of Vascular Purpura

Senile purpura
Dysproteinemia
   Macroglobulinemia
   Multiple myeloma
   Cryoglobulinemia
   Benign hyperglobulinemic purpura
Nonthrombocytopenic drug purpura
Henoch-Schönlein purpura
Hereditary connective tissue disorders
   Ehlers-Danlos syndrome
   Pseudoxanthoma elasticum
   Marfan's syndrome
   Osteogenesis imperfecta
Cushing's syndrome
Scurvy
Autoerythrocyte sensitivity

cutaneous elastic tissue. They are of little clinical significance.

Dysproteinemia. Vascular purpura may be seen in *macroglobulinemia, myeloma,* and *cryoglobulinemia.* As noted previously, the nonthrombocytopenic purpura may develop because of protein coating of the platelet surface as well as coating of endothelial vascular surfaces, leading to impairment in blood vessel integrity. Epistaxis is a common symptom in these patients. It is probable that platelet dysfunction as well as coagulation factor abnormalities contributes to the bleeding diatheses in patients with myeloma, particularly those of the IgA type. Hyperviscosity with sludging of red cells also contributes to capillary anoxia. In cryoglobulinemia, purpuric lesions appear after exposure to cold and are more frequent during the winter months.

Benign hyperglobulinemic purpura primarily affects middle-aged females who present with successive crops of petechiae on the legs occurring at variable intervals, leading to pigmentary changes in the skin. Occasionally local itching or urticaria precedes the petechial eruptions. In half the cases other conditions such as Sjögren's syndrome, disseminated lupus erythematosus, or rheumatoid arthritis are also present. The hypergammaglobulinemia is due to the presence of high titer IgG antiglobulins.

Nonthrombocytopenic Drug Purpura. Some of the agents listed in Table 3 (Ch. 790) may lead to purpura in the absence of thrombocytopenia. The chlorothiazides and chemically related compounds are probably the most common offenders. In these situations, it is probable that the vascular endothelium rather than the circulating platelet serves as a target tissue. Whether this is a true immunologic reaction remains to be determined. The bleeding disorder is usually mild, and the only necessary therapy is removal of the suspected offending agent.

Henoch-Schönlein Purpura. This allergic vasculitis occurs most frequently in children after a streptococcal infection or, occasionally, after ingestion of a sensitizing food or drug. The skin is invariably involved, usually with extensive elevated purpuric or ecchymotic lesions scattered over the extensor surfaces of the extremities. Initially, the skin lesion is urticarial in nature and gradually becomes hemorrhagic. The rash typically occurs in recurrent crops and may involve the face. Other systems frequently affected include the joints, especially knees and ankles, gastrointestinal tract, and kidneys. Intestinal complications include intramural hematomas and gross mucosal hemorrhage, both of which may be accompanied by severe colicky pain, hematemesis, and melena. Renal involvement with hematuria is seen in approximately 50 per cent of the patients. Chronic nephritis with uremia may also develop (see Ch. 611). In the younger patients, the disease is usually self-limited. Steroids have been used, particularly in the more severely ill patients with visceral involvement.

Hereditary Connective Tissue Disorders. Vascular purpura may be seen in certain inherited disorders of connective tissue, including the *Ehlers-Danlos syndrome, pseudoxanthoma elasticum, osteogenesis imperfecta,* and *Marfan's syndrome.* In some of these disorders abnormal platelet function has also been reported.

Cushing's Syndrome. Nonthrombocytopenic purpura predominantly distributed over the trunk and lower extremities is seen after prolonged administration of exogenous steroids as well as in patients with Cushing's syndrome. The nature of the vascular lesion is unknown; however, some observers believe that chronic exposure of the vasculature to steroids produces a catabolic effect which interferes with vascular integrity.

Scurvy. Chronic vitamin C deficiency is primarily a disease of extremes of age—the very young and the very old. Epistaxis, hematuria, and gastrointestinal bleeding are seen in infants. In adults, deep intramuscular hematomas are frequently encountered. In addition to the vessel wall defect, qualitative platelet defects may also contribute to the bleeding.

Autoerythrocyte Sensitivity. This unusual condition is seen only in women and is characterized by the spontaneous appearance of painful ecchymoses. The lesions occur over the anterior aspects of the upper and lower extremities and spread superficially. Many patients give a history of trauma preceding the onset of the ecchymoses. In general, the lesions appear over areas which are liable to superficial trauma. The etiology of the illness is not known; however, some evidence suggests that certain of these women are sensitive to their own red cells. Many of the patients have significant emotional difficulties, and the lesions at times may be self-inflicted.

794. HEREDITARY HEMORRHAGIC TELANGIECTASIA
(Osler-Weber-Rendu Disease)

Hereditary hemorrhagic telangiectasia is an inherited disorder associated with intermittent bleeding from vascular abnormalities scattered throughout the body, particularly on mucosal surfaces. Skin lesions appear as small, flattened telangiectases or dilated, raised small vascular nodules which blanch with pressure. The lesions are common on the face and in the mucous membranes of the tongue, lips, and nose. They are also found in the scalp, fingertips, conjunctival surfaces, vagina, and rectum. Visceral lesions are most common in the gastrointestinal tract, but the respiratory and genitourinary systems may also be involved. Approximately 20 per cent of the patients have pulmonary arteriovenous fistulas. Recurrent spontaneous epistaxis is the most common symptom. Severe gastrointestinal bleeding may also be a major clinical problem. The patients invariably have iron deficiency anemia which is sometimes severe. The pathologic lesions involving arterioles, venules, and capillaries are characterized by marked thinning of the vessel wall with ballooning and aneurysm formation. Management consists of symptomatic care of recurrent bleeding. Various plastic surgical procedures have been utilized to diminish the particularly troublesome recurrent episodes of epistaxis. Local pressure with packing is helpful. Systemic estrogen therapy has not proved particularly beneficial. All patients should be maintained on long-term iron administration.

Aster, R. H.: Thrombocytopenia due to enhanced platelet destruction. *In* Williams, W., Beutler, E., Erslev, H., and Rundles, R. (eds.): Hematology. New York, McGraw-Hill Book Company, 1972, Chap. 139, p. 1131.

Aster, R. H., and Keene, W. R.: Sites of platelet destruction in idiopathic thrombocytopenic purpura. Br. J. Haematol., 16:61, 1969.

Capra, D. J., Winchester, R. J., and Kunkel, H. G.: Hyperglobulinemic purpura. Studies on the unusual anti-γ globulins characteristic of the sera of these patients. Medicine, 50:125, 1971.

Horowitz, H. I., and Nachman, R. L.: Drug purpura. Semin. Hematol., 2:287, 1965.

Jaffé, E., Nachman, R., and Merskey, C.: Thrombotic thrombocytopenic purpura. Coagulation parameters in twelve patients. Blood, 42:499, 1973.

Karpatkin, S., and Siskind, G.: In vitro detection of platelet antibody in patients with idiopathic thrombocytopenic purpura and systemic lupus erythematosus. Blood, 33:795, 1969.

Marcus, A. J.: Platelet function. N. Engl. J. Med., 280:1213, 1278, 1330, 1969.

Nachman, R. L.: Disorders of primary hemostasis. *In* Mengel, C., Frei, T., and Nachman, R. L. (eds.): Hematology. Chicago, Year Book Medical Publishers, 1972, p. 600.

Shulman, N. R.: A mechanism of cell destruction in individuals sensitized to foreign antigens and its implications in autoimmunity. Ann. Intern. Med., 60:506, 1964.

Section Fifteen. HEMORRHAGIC DISORDERS: COAGULATION DEFECTS

Oscar D. Ratnoff

795. INTRODUCTION

A hemorrhagic disorder often appears when blood coagulation is impaired. Defective hemostasis may be caused by (1) inadequate production of one or more of the procoagulant substances of blood, (2) depletion of components required for clotting as a result of increased utilization, (3) the presence in blood of inhibitors of coagulation, or (4) activation of proteolytic mechanisms of plasma. Blood normally contains a relative abundance of each clotting factor, and hemorrhage is rarely the result of deficiency of one of these substances unless its concentration has been reduced to less than 50 per cent of the normal value. Abnormal bleeding may result from lack of each of the known clotting factors, with three exceptions. Hageman factor (factor XII) and Fletcher factor (plasma prekallikrein), proteins concerned with the initiation of blood clotting upon contact with foreign surfaces, are apparently not required for normal hemostasis. Depletion of calcium is not a cause of abnormal bleeding, because the cardiovascular and neuromuscular effects of profound hypocalcemia are incompatible with life. Deficiency of a single clotting factor is usually the result of an inherited disorder. Acquired coagulation defects are more likely to involve multiple components of the clotting system. In some clinical situations several mechanisms operate to impair hemostasis, and the extent to which each contributes may be difficult to analyze.

A knowledge of the physiology of blood clotting is essential in interpreting the results of laboratory tests useful in the diagnosis of hemostatic defects. Blood clots when fibrinogen (factor I) is converted to fibrin through the action of a proteolytic enzyme, thrombin (Fig. 1). Fibrinogen is a dimer, each half consisting of three subunits, $A\alpha$, $B\beta$ and γ chains. Thrombin splits off from each half of fibrinogen fibrinopeptides A and B, from the $A\alpha$ and $B\beta$ chains, respectively. What remains, fibrin monomer, then polymerizes to form insoluble strands of fibrin. The polymerization of fibrin is accelerated by calcium ions at physiologic concentrations, and probably by a heat-labile accelerator in normal plasma.

Under physiologic conditions, the molecules of fibrin are chemically bonded to each other by a second enzyme, fibrin-stabilizing factor (factor XIII), a transamidase which provides mechanical strength to the fibrin strands. Thrombin does not exist in detectable amounts in normal blood. When blood is shed, thrombin evolves through one or both of two convergent sequences of chemical reactions, the extrinsic and intrinsic pathways. Presumably, similar mechanisms operate to induce clotting in vivo. Thrombin formation via the extrinsic pathway is initiated by components of tissue known as tissue thromboplastin which interact with several plasma agents, factor VII, Stuart factor (factor X), proaccelerin (factor V), and calcium ions, to bring about the formation of a prothrombin-converting principle (Fig. 2). Blood also clots without the participation of tissue thromboplastin upon contact with certain negatively charged surfaces such as glass; in vivo, collagen and sebum may serve this function. This intrinsic pathway requires the successive participation of Hageman factor (factor XII), Fletcher factor, plasma thromboplastin antecedent (PTA, factor XI), Christmas factor (PTC, factor IX), antihemophilic factor (factor VIII), Stuart factor, and proaccelerin (Fig. 2). Some or all of these factors are "activated" during the clotting process. A prothrombin-converting principle, probably identical with that developed through the extrinsic pathway, evolves when calcium ions and phospholipids are available, the latter supplied by platelets and the plasma it-

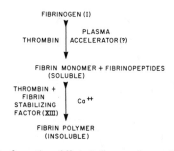

Figure 1. The formation of fibrin in human plasma. The site of action of the plasma accelerator, if this exists, is not known.

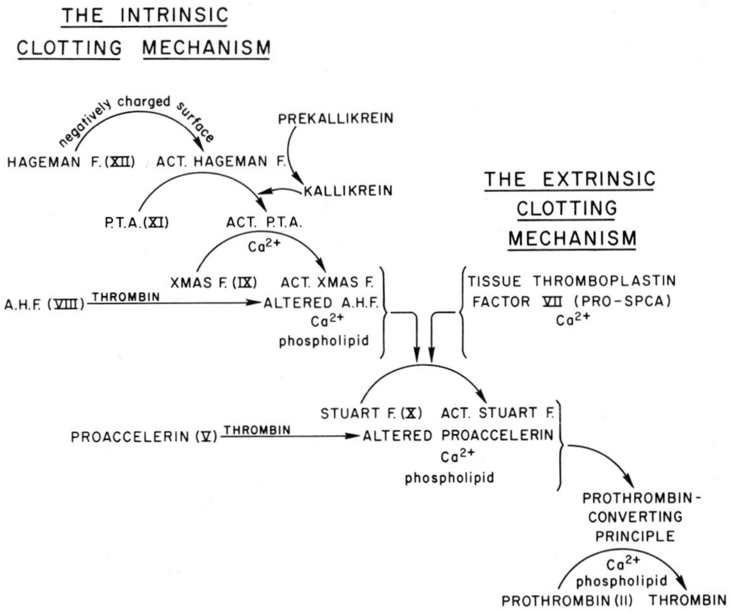

THE INTRINSIC CLOTTING MECHANISM

Figure 2. The intrinsic and extrinsic pathways for the formation of thrombin. Omitted from the diagram are inhibitors of the various steps. The phospholipid portion of tissue thromboplastin may function in the formation and action of the prothrombin-converting principle. The phospholipid for the intrinsic pathway is furnished by platelets and by the plasma itself. A proposed action of kallikrein on factor VII is not depicted.

self. Once the prothrombin-converting principle has formed, it liberates thrombin from its precursor, prothrombin (factor II), by an enzymatic process. In addition to its action on fibrinogen, thrombin promotes clotting in several ways, liberating phospholipid from platelets, activating fibrin-stabilizing factor from an inert precursor, and altering antihemophilic factor and proaccelerin so as to heighten their activity. Plasma contains potent inhibitors of the clotting process, of which those inhibiting thrombin, tissue thromboplastin, and the activated forms of Hageman factor, PTA, and Stuart factor are most clearly defined. It also contains the precursor of plasmin, a powerful proteolytic enzyme which can digest fibrinogen, fibrin, and other clotting factors as well as certain other substrates. The sole or principal site of synthesis of several clotting factors—namely, fibrinogen, prothrombin, factor VII, proaccelerin, Stuart factor, and Christmas factor—is the hepatic parenchymal cell. Vascular endothelium has been implicated in the synthesis of antihemophilic factor; the locus of synthesis of other factors is not certain.

The laboratory procedures used to differentiate disorders of blood clotting are based upon these physiologic considerations. Thus defects in the extrinsic pathway of coagulation are readily detected by measuring the one-stage prothrombin time, in which tissue thromboplastin and calcium ions are added to decalcified plasma, and the interval of time elapsing until clotting takes place is measured. Defects in the intrinsic pathway are reflected in the test tube by delayed clotting of whole blood, retarded "thromboplastin generation" (a misnomer for the evolution of the prothrombin-converting principle), deficient conversion of prothrombin to thrombin, i.e., prothrombin consumption, and a prolonged partial thromboplastin time, i.e., the clotting time of recalcified plasma in the presence of phospholipid to which an activator of Hageman factor, such as kaolin, is often added. The one-stage prothrombin time is normal in persons whose defect is restricted to the early part of the intrinsic pathway, before the participation of Stuart factor, but is prolonged if defects of the later parts of the

pathway are present. Defects in the conversion of fibrinogen to fibrin are measured by testing the effect of preformed thrombin on the clotting time of plasma, i.e., the thrombin time, whereas a deficiency of fibrin-stabilizing factor is detected by noting the solubility of fibrin in 5 molar urea or 1 per cent monochloroacetic acid, which cannot dissolve fibrin bonded by this factor.

The laboratory procedures available for investigation of defects of coagulation are often crude, nonspecific, and influenced by variations in technique. Accordingly, care is required in selection and performance of the tests and in interpretation of results. Assays are available for each of the known clotting factors. Final identification of a specific deficiency requires mixing of the patient's plasma with that of a patient with a known coagulation defect to determine whether correction occurs. Only fibrinogen can be measured in gravimetric terms, by its conversion to fibrin and by determination of the protein content of the clot.

Biggs, R. (ed.): Human Blood Coagulation, Hemostasis and Thrombosis. Oxford, Blackwell Scientific Publications, 1972.

Harker, L. A. (ed.): The Hemostasis Manual. 2nd ed. Philadelphia, F. A. Davis Company, 1974.

Poller, L. (ed.): Recent Advances in Blood Coagulation. London, J. & A. Churchill, Ltd., 1969.

Ratnoff, O. D. (ed.) Treatment of Hemorrhagic Disorders. New York, Harper & Row, 1968.

HERITABLE DISORDERS OF BLOOD COAGULATION

796. INTRODUCTION

The familial occurrence of a deficiency of each of the organic clotting factors is well established. The cause is either deficient synthesis or the synthesis of functionally defective factors. Transmission of the defect is genetically determined. In most instances, severe function deficiency of a single clotting factor is encountered in homozygotes in autosomal recessive traits and in male hemizygotes and female homozygotes in X-linked recessive disorders. In some cases, heterozygous carriers can be shown to have a reduced plasma level of the procoagulant, but, except in von Willebrand's disease, the deficiency is rarely sufficient to impair hemostasis. In one anomaly, dysfibrinogenemia, an autosomal dominant gene appears to be responsible for synthesis of a protein that may be normal in quantity but abnormal in structure and function. Rarely, familial deficiency of more than one clotting factor has been encountered. The genetic basis for multiple hemostatic defects is not understood.

797. CLASSIC HEMOPHILIA

Classic hemophilia, the best known of the familial disorders of blood coagulation, is the result of functional deficiency of antihemophilic factor (factor VIII). The plasma does not lack antihemophilic factor. Rather, it appears to contain a nonfunctional variant of this clotting factor. The abnormality is attributable to an X-linked recessive gene so that the disorder occurs almost exclusively in males. The sons of a male hemophiliac are unaffected and do not transmit the disease, although all his daughters are carriers. Heterozygous females do not bleed, but half their sons have hemophilia and half their daughters are carriers. Homozygous females, very rarely encountered, have the typical disease. The clinical manifestations vary from family to family, correlating with the intensity of the functional deficiency of antihemophilic factor, but within a family the degree of the bleeding tendency among affected members is about the same. A positive family history is obtained in only about two thirds of cases.

Clinical Manifestations. In severe hemophilia, in which virtually no functional antihemophilic factor is detectable in plasma, serious or lethal hemorrhage may occur in the neonatal period after circumcision, but bleeding from the umbilicus is unusual. In infancy, the bleeding tendency is frequently manifested by the appearance of cutaneous ecchymoses or hematomas in soft tissues, often after injuries so trivial as to be unnoted. Bleeding from the mouth, in particular from the frenum of the upper lip, is sometimes encountered in young children. After the early years of life, hemorrhages into the joints are characteristic. Increasing deformity, limitation of motion, and destruction of joints result from repeated hemarthroses, commonly the most disabling manifestation of the disease. The ankles, knees, and elbows are particularly likely to be involved, whereas the hands are usually spared. Bleeding is limited by the tension of the joint capsule, and ceases when the synovial space becomes distended. Hemorrhages into soft tissues are not similarly restricted, and may extend widely, dissecting through subcutaneous tissue, along fascial planes, or into muscles. Even enormous hematomas are usually reabsorbed, but sometimes they persist, leaving firm masses that calcify. Pseudotumors can produce symptoms by pressure on other structures, or

may erode bone and simulate neoplasms. Hemorrhages into the muscles sometimes cause contractures and deformities such as a claw hand. Bleeding into the lax tissues beneath the tongue, in the pharynx, or in the neck is particularly dangerous, because it may interfere with swallowing or may occlude the respiratory passage. Retroperitoneal hemorrhage can produce symptoms simulating those of appendicitis, or can give rise to other manifestations such as obstructive jaundice owing to occlusion of the common bile duct or fulminant hypertension from compression of the kidneys. Hemorrhage into the mesentery can cause abdominal pain, digestive symptoms, or even avascular necrosis of the bowel. Episodes of hematuria, often accompanied by ureteral colic, are common and tend to persist for weeks if untreated. Hemorrhage into the gastrointestinal tract may occur. Excessive bleeding is the rule after dental extraction or minor surgery, and tonsillectomy or major operative procedures may lead to fatal hemorrhage. Subdural hematomas and other hemorrhages into the central nervous system, although uncommon, are an important cause of disability or death, and may result from relatively trivial injury. Hematomas encroaching on nerve trunks may cause sensory loss or paralysis.

Only about half of hemophiliacs present this grim picture. Such individuals have little or no functional antihemophilic factor in their plasma. In others, in whom the concentration of this factor may be as high as 30 per cent of normal, the symptoms are proportionately milder, and bleeding may occur only after such challenges as injury, operative procedures, or dental extractions.

Diagnosis. Specific diagnosis can be established only by laboratory tests of blood coagulation, although the character of the bleeding and the family history provide important clues. Tests that detect abnormalities in the intrinsic pathway of coagulation usually give abnormal results, but the clotting time of whole blood may be normal in mildly affected patients. The prothrombin time, thrombin time, and bleeding time are normal. Proof of diagnosis requires the use of appropriate tests to demonstrate the functional deficiency of antihemophilic factor, preferably including an assay using the plasma of a known hemophiliac. A normal bleeding time helps to differentiate mild cases from von Willebrand's disease; careful analysis of the pattern of inheritance and tests of other relatives may be necessary. Further support for the diagnosis in doubtful cases can be obtained by demonstrating the presence of normal or elevated antigenic material related to antihemophilic factor in the plasma, typical of classic hemophilia, using antiserum raised in rabbits. All patients deficient in antihemophilic factor must be tested for the presence of circulating anticoagulants directed against this substance.

Treatment. Patients with hereditary hemorrhagic disease often have difficulty adjusting to the problems inherent in a disorder that poses unexpected threats to normal behavior and to life itself. As soon as the diagnosis is made, the patient or his parents should be instructed concerning the care, prognostic implications, and hereditary nature of his disorder. The parents should be encouraged to rear their afflicted children in as normal a way as is consistent with safety, for emotional crippling is as devastating as that resulting from hemorrhage. While the patient is too young to guard himself, the parents should arrange his environment so that it is as danger-free as possible, in order to lessen the need to restrain his behavior. As he grows older, the patient should be advised to indulge in such sports as swimming, running, tennis, and golf, and to avoid those involving body contact or predisposing to injury. The hemophiliac should prepare for a vocation which is not inherently dangerous; he and his parents should be reminded that hemophilia does not preclude a useful life in business or the professions. The object of therapy is to allow the patient to become a self-supporting adult, capable of caring for himself and living as full a life as possible.

The mainstay of therapy for episodes of bleeding is the transfusion of normal plasma or fractions of plasma rich in antihemophilic factor to correct temporarily the specific defect. The use of whole blood is restricted to the maintenance of blood volume after severe blood loss. Enough plasma or its fractions must be administered to raise the blood level of antihemophilic factor sufficiently to permit normal hemostasis. Once transfused, antihemophilic factor disappears rapidly from the circulation, only about half remaining after 10 to 12 hours, so that repeated transfusions must be given until bleeding has been controlled. Therapy with plasma or its fractions carries with it risks of transmitting hepatitis and of inducing the formation of circulating anticoagulants that specifically inhibit antihemophilic factor.

In the event of major injury or in preparation for surgical procedures, the plasma level of antihemophilic factor must be raised to at least 30 or 40 per cent that of a normal individual; lesser amounts may be adequate to control bleeding into joints or minor soft tissue hemorrhage. When only fresh or fresh-frozen plasma was available as a source of antihemophilic factor, adequate plasma levels of this substance were difficult to achieve without danger of circulatory overload except by exchange transfusion. Fortunately, during the last few years concentrates of antihemophilic factor that can be administered in a small volume have become generally available. One preparation in wide use is *cryoprecipitated antihemophilic factor,* separated during the cold thawing of fresh-frozen plasma. Plasma levels sufficient for adequate hemostasis can be achieved with the administration of the cryoprecipitate of 1 unit of plasma for each 4 kg of body weight, sustaining the plasma level of antihemophilic factor by administering half this amount every 12 hours. Larger doses may be needed if surgical procedures are undertaken. Another useful preparation is *lyophilized antihemophilic factor,* separated from plasma either by cryoprecipitation or by addition of glycine or other protein precipitants. Such material can be used under conditions in which frozen cryoprecipitated antihemophilic factor is not available. No rule of thumb can be provided as to how long therapy should be continued. In general, after surgery, dental extraction, or severe bleeding, concentrated antihemophilic factor is administered in the manner described for at least two days after all signs of bleeding have ceased, and the dose is then gradually decreased over the succeeding three or four days. Shorter courses of therapy are used when the danger of renewed bleeding is less threatening, as in most instances of hemarthrosis.

The availability of concentrates of antihemophilic factor has made it possible to abort hemorrhage more readily than was formerly possible without circulatory embarrassment. It has reduced the risk of surgical procedures and dental extractions in hemophiliacs. Indeed, in many patients, elective surgical procedures may be carried out, although surgery should be performed only in hospitals equipped to deal with this special problem.

This optimistic picture must be tempered by the fact that in as many as 20 per cent of severe hemophiliacs a circulating anticoagulant appears in plasma that specifically inactivates antihemophilic factor. The presence of this agent, which is an antibody directed against antihemophilic factor, vitiates the beneficial results of transfusion. Patients in whom this complication is present should under no conditions be subjected to surgery. Experimentally, immunosuppressive therapy has been attempted, but the results are usually disappointing.

If the bleeding site is accessible, *hemostasis* may be most effectively achieved by local measures. By appropriate use of local hemostatic agents such as bovine thrombin and the application of cold and gentle pressure, bleeding may often be controlled. These measures must be sustained, for recurrent bleeding is likely over a period of days. Dental extractions in particular require meticulous local measures. Extractions should be carried out only in the hospital and by dental surgeons with special training in the care of hemophiliacs. Except in patients with mild hemophilia, hemostasis should be enhanced by the transfusion of concentrates of antihemophilic factor. The administration of *epsilon-aminocaproic acid* (4 grams every four hours for ten days in adults) may reduce the need for transfusion therapy.

The transfusion of concentrated antihemophilic factor is also useful in aborting *bleeding into joints.* A single dose of cryoprecipitated antihemophilic factor, one bag for every 2 2/3 kg of body weight, combined with a short course of prednisone, 1 mg per kilogram daily for three days, with a maximum of 80 mg per day, followed by 0.5 mg per kilogram for two days, with a maximum of 40 mg per day, has been useful. Acutely swollen joints should be immobilized. Local chilling and application of elastic bandages may be beneficial, but the application of a constricting bandage is contraindicated. Aspiration of the joint is occasionally advantageous, and should be performed only after adequate transfusion therapy. Active motion without weight-bearing is essential after bleeding has stopped in order to prevent persistent limitation of motion. Careful use of physiotherapy, traction, and splints may be helpful in preventing and correcting deformities. Surgical correction of certain deformities has been successfully accomplished, but should be attempted only by experts and under the supervision of someone skilled in the transfusion therapy of hemophiliacs. Increased mobility of joints has sometimes been achieved by synovectomy.

Other forms of bleeding require special types of care. Particularly hazardous is bleeding into the soft tissues of the neck, in which tracheostomy, performed under the cover of transfusion therapy, may be needed. Hemophiliacs should not be given intramuscular injections, but venipunctures are not hazardous if performed with care. Immunization against tetanus is important, because bleeders are particularly prone to infection with this organism, but this is wisely delayed in severe hemophiliacs until the first course of replacement therapy. Immunization may be carried out without such preparation in mildly affected patients. Regular prophylactic care of the teeth should be provided. Bleeders should avoid the use of aspirin, because this agent may impair hemostasis. Acetaminophen, 0.65 gram every four hours in adults, and proportionately less in children, is a useful substitute.

Prognosis. The outlook for the hemophiliac has been greatly improved by modern methods of treatment. Those with moderately severe or mild hemophilia may seem so little affected that they live virtually normal lives, but even these patients may have exsanguinating hemorrhage after dental extraction, injury, or surgery. Those in whom the defect is more pronounced may require frequent admission to the hospital, and may be crippled by joint deformities. Some meet the challenge and are reasonably productive individuals, although others seem foredoomed to chronic invalidism. The life expectancy of hemophiliacs has lengthened with the availability of transfusion therapy, but death as the result of the complications of hemorrhage still occurs with disturbing frequency.

Detection of Carriers. Certain women in hemophilia families are necessarily carriers—the daughters of affected men, the mothers of more than one hemophiliac, and the mother of one hemophiliac who has other affected relatives. The carrier state in other women can be detected with a high degree of certainty by simultaneous measurement of functional antihemophilic factor and antigens related to this agent. In normal women, these two modalities vary from individual to individual, but in proportion. In contrast, in carriers, relative excess of antigenic material is nearly always present. Because of variation of functional antihemophilic factor titers both in normal women and in known carriers, this procedure alone successfully detects only a small proportion of carriers.

Biggs, R. (ed.): Human Blood Coagulation, Hemostasis and Thrombosis. Oxford, Blackwell Scientific Publications, 1972.

Biggs, R., and Macfarlane, R. G.: Treatment of Hemophilia and Other Coagulation Disorders. Oxford, Blackwell Scientific Publications, 1966.

Douglas, A. S. (ed.): Blood coagulation and fibrinolysis in clinical practice. Clinics in Haematology, Vol. 2, No. 1. London, W. B. Saunders, Ltd., 1973.

Hardisty, R. M., and Ingram, G. I. C.: Bleeding Disorders. Investigation and Management. Philadelphia, F. A. Davis Company, 1965.

Ratnoff, O. D. (ed.): Treatment of Hemorrhagic Disorders. New York, Harper & Row, 1968.

Rossi, E. D. (ed.): Symposium on Hemorrhagic Disorders. Medical Clinics of North America, Vol. 56, No. 1. Philadelphia, W. B. Saunders Company, 1972.

Spaet, T. H. (ed.): Progress in Hemostasis and Thrombosis. Vol. 1. New York, Grune & Stratton, 1972.

798. OTHER HERITABLE DISORDERS OF BLOOD COAGULATION

Von Willebrand's disease (vascular hemophilia) is a hemorrhagic disorder characterized by a long bleeding time and deficiency of antihemophilic factor (factor VIII). Both functional antihemophilic factor and antigens in plasma related to antihemophilic factor are reduced, and in proportion. The disease is transmitted by a dominant autosomal mutant gene, but has been detected more often in women than in men. The severity

of symptoms varies considerably among affected members of the same family, some of whom may be asymptomatic. Menorrhagia and postpartum bleeding are common. The patient may experience epistaxes and gingival bleeding in severe cases; cutaneous ecchymoses or hematomas may occur. Hemorrhage follows injury or surgical procedures. Hemarthroses are relatively uncommon, but visceral bleeding or severe and even lethal hemorrhage into the gastrointestinal tract has been observed. Occasionally, petechiae may be found.

A unique feature of von Willebrand's disease is the prolonged bleeding time, an abnormality not usually associated with other hemophilia-like diseases. The coagulation defect can be corrected in vitro by normal but not by hemophilic plasma. In contrast, transfusion of hemophilic as well as of normal plasma or serum is followed by a delayed but pronounced and protracted rise in the patient's plasma level of functional antihemophilic factor. A single unit of normal plasma may lead to the elevation of the antihemophilic activity of the patient's plasma to normal levels for many hours. Paradoxically, no corresponding rise in antigens related to antihemophilic factor occurs. These interesting observations are unexplained, although they suggest that the synthesis of antihemophilic factor takes place in at least two steps, the first of which is defective in von Willebrand's disease and the second in classic hemophilia. Whether the abnormality in bleeding time is due to a second plasma defect is disputed; the administration of plasma, but not of purified antihemophilic factor, is reported to shorten the bleeding time. Diagnosis is readily made when a markedly long bleeding time is encountered in a patient with functional deficiency of antihemophilic factor. Additionally, adhesion of platelets to glass beads is often impaired, although the specificity of this test is doubtful. Aggregation of platelets by the antimicrobial ristocetin, which occurs in normal or hemophilic platelet-rich plasma, is impeded in von Willebrand's disease. Sometimes, within a given family, affected individuals may be found in whom the bleeding time may be prolonged without significant deficiency of antihemophilic factor, or vice versa. Careful study of the patient's relatives may help to differentiate mild classic hemophilia from von Willebrand's disease. When the bleeding time is not significantly prolonged, recognition of the disease is facilitated by demonstration of a concomitant deficiency of antigens related to antihemophilic factor. Treatment of bleeding episodes consists of measures for local control of hemostasis and the administration of fresh blood, plasma, or cryoprecipitates of plasma, all of which contain the agent that induces synthesis of antihemophilic factor in von Willebrand's disease. Menorrhagia may be terminated by suppression of menstrual bleeding with hormonal preparations such as norethynodrel. During pregnancy, the titer of antihemophilic factor may rise to levels which would be normal in nonpregnant women, and parturition may occur without hemorrhage, although the bleeding time remains long.

Christmas disease is attributable to functional deficiency of Christmas factor (factor IX, plasma thromboplastin component), an abnormality transmitted by an X chromosome–linked gene. In most cases, patients seem unable to synthesize Christmas factor, whereas in a minority nonfunctional Christmas factor is demonstrable in plasma. The disorder typically occurs in males, and is less common than hemophilia, from which it is clinically indistinguishable. All the clinical manifestations of hemophilia are encountered in patients with Christmas disease. The disorder varies in severity from family to family, manifestations roughly paralleling the degree of the deficiency of Christmas factor measured in the laboratory. Heterozygous female carriers may have a partial deficiency of Christmas factor, and some have a mild bleeding tendency. A positive family history is obtained in only about two thirds of cases. Diagnosis is established by laboratory tests that demonstrate a defect in the early steps of the intrinsic pathway of thrombin formation, and by specific assay for Christmas factor, using a substrate plasma from a patient with known Christmas disease. Treatment is basically the same as for hemophilia, but cryoprecipitates of plasma lack Christmas factor. Christmas factor is relatively stable, so that the patient can be treated effectively with blood that has been stored under usual conditions in a blood bank. Large volumes of plasma are required to raise the level of Christmas factor sufficiently to provide normal hemostasis; thereafter smaller amounts will sustain the titer of this substance, because half the transfused Christmas factor is still present in the circulation after 20 or more hours. Concentrates of the vitamin K–dependent clotting factors, including Christmas factor, are now available, and can be used to provide large amounts of the missing factor without dangerous expansion of the circulating blood volume. These fractions, however, are often contaminated with hepatitis virus. In a few cases, the beneficial effects of transfusion are vitiated by the presence in the patient's plasma of a circulating anticoagulant, presumably an antibody directed against Christmas factor.

Plasma thromboplastin antecedent deficiency, a rare familial hemorrhagic disorder encountered in both sexes, is attributable to deficiency of PTA (factor XI). The disorder is inherited in an autosomal recessive manner; in most reported cases, the patients have been Jewish. Bleeding episodes often follow trauma or surgical procedures, but spontaneous bleeding occasionally occurs. Hemorrhage is usually less severe than in hemophilia, and hemarthrosis is rare. Sometimes the disorder is asymptomatic. Laboratory tests demonstrate a defect in the early steps of the intrinsic pathway of clotting, but the specific diagnosis is often difficult to establish even with appropriate tests, and requires careful confirmation, including matching the plasma with that of a patient known to have PTA deficiency. Transfusion of blood or plasma is used in the treatment of bleeding episodes. Since half of the infused PTA is still present in the circulation 60 hours after transfusion, correction of the defect is relatively simple.

Hageman trait is the hereditary deficiency of Hageman factor (factor XII). It occurs in both sexes, and is in most instances inherited as an autosomal recessive defect. Hageman trait is usually asymptomatic, although minor bleeding has occasionally been encountered. The diagnosis may be suspected when the clotting time is prolonged and a defect in the early steps of the intrinsic pathway is detected, but it can be established only by comparison with plasma of patients known to have this disorder. No treatment has been needed in reported cases, but in the event of hemorrhage normal plasma should be efficacious.

Fletcher trait is a rare, asymptomatic disorder of blood coagulation in which the intrinsic pathway of clotting is defective as demonstrated by prolongation of the partial thromboplastin time. The defect is due to a deficiency of Fletcher factor, apparently identical with a plasma prekallikrein, needed for the optimal action of Hageman factor upon PTA. No therapy is needed.

Parahemophilia, a familial bleeding disorder affecting both sexes, is caused by a functional deficiency of proaccelerin (factor V); in some cases, the plasma is said to contain normal amounts of a nonfunctional agent immunologically related to proaccelerin. The disease is inherited in an autosomal recessive manner. Spontaneous bleeding may occur at numerous sites, but the joints are rarely involved. Menorrhagia and postoperative bleeding may occur, but in some patients the disease is mild or latent. The clue to diagnosis is provided by a prolonged prothrombin time which is not shortened by plasma deficient in proaccelerin. A presumptive diagnosis can be made by demonstrating that the prothrombin time is shortened by addition of plasma from which the vitamin K–dependent clotting factors have been removed, but this test does not rule out a deficiency of fibrinogen. During surgical procedures or when abnormal bleeding is sufficiently severe to justify transfusion, fresh blood or plasma should be given in amounts adequate to maintain the plasma level of proaccelerin at about 25 per cent of normal; half the amount of proaccelerin infused disappears from the circulation in 12 to 36 hours.

Congenital deficiency of factor VII is transmitted in an autosomal recessive manner. Homozygous individuals of both sexes display a bleeding tendency of varying severity correlating with the severity of the deficiency. In some patients the plasma contains no material recognizable as nonfunctional factor VII, whereas in others a nonfunctional variant of the protein is present. Numerous hemorrhagic manifestations have been encountered, including umbilical bleeding in the neonatal period, epistaxis, ecchymoses, hemarthroses, menorrhagia, and hemorrhages into the gastrointestinal tract and central nervous system. The one-stage prothrombin time is prolonged, an abnormality that is not affected by plasma or serum from patients known to have factor VII deficiency. Factor VII is stable so that stored plasma is of therapeutic value. Large volumes of plasma, infused repeatedly, are required for effective hemostasis because of the rapid disappearance of factor VII from the circulation, half the amount infused being removed in only one or two hours; concentrates of the vitamin K–dependent clotting factors may also be used. Menorrhagia may be controlled by the administration of oral contraceptive agents.

Stuart factor deficiency, a rare congenital disorder of blood coagulation, is characterized by deficiency of Stuart factor (factor X), and is attributable to an autosomal mutant gene. Only homozygotes have a bleeding tendency, which is similar to that of congenital deficiency of factor VII. In some instances a functionally defective form of Stuart factor is demonstrable in plasma, whereas in others a true deficiency of this agent is apparently present. The prothrombin time is prolonged and is not shortened by plasma from patients with known Stuart factor deficiency. The clotting time of recalcified plasma is not shortened to a normal degree by the addition of Russell's viper venom, which requires Stuart factor for its procoagulant effect. Treatment is the same as that for factor VII deficiency, but transfusions have a much more prolonged action, half of the Stuart factor remaining in the blood after two or three days, so that transfusions need not be repeated as frequently.

Prothrombin deficiency, an extremely rare autosomal recessive trait, is clinically similar to factor VII and Stuart factor deficiencies. Two varieties have been discerned, a true deficiency of prothrombin and a condition in which nonfunctional prothrombin is detectable in plasma. The prothrombin time is prolonged and is not shortened by the addition of normal serum or of plasma from which the vitamin K–dependent clotting factors have been removed. The treatment of bleeding is the same as that for factor VII deficiency; about half of infused prothrombin disappears from the circulation in nine hours.

A rare anomaly has been described in which individuals have unusual *resistance to coumarin-like drugs.* As much as 20 times the usual dose is required to achieve a therapeutic effect. The disorder is inherited in an autosomal dominant manner. The mechanism underlying the defect is unknown, but in an analogous disease of rats, the microsomal membranes lack the normal capacity to bind warfarin.

Congenital deficiency of fibrinogen, a rare disorder occurring in both sexes, is apparently transmitted as an autosomal recessive trait. Clinical manifestations may begin at birth with hemorrhage from the umbilicus. In general, bleeding is hemophilia-like, except that permanent joint damage from hemarthroses is uncommon. Some patients have remarkably little bleeding, and even menstrual blood loss may not be excessive, but others have severe hemorrhages that can be fatal in early life. The blood does not clot even after the addition of thrombin, and little or no fibrinogen can be detected in plasma by physical, chemical, or immunologic methods. Bleeding episodes can be satisfactorily treated by intravenous administration of fibrinogen, either in the form of Cohn fraction I or of cryoprecipitates of plasma, in amounts sufficient to maintain a plasma fibrinogen level in excess of 100 mg per 100 ml. Several instances in which therapy has been impeded by the development of antibodies against fibrinogen have been reported. Strangely, death from obstruction of the pulmonary circulation by "thrombi" composed of platelets has been described.

Congenital dysfibrinogenemia is a recently described group of familial disorders in which fibrinogen is usually present in normal amounts, but is abnormal in structure and coagulability. The abnormality has occurred in both sexes and in consecutive generations, suggesting autosomal dominant inheritance. The anomaly appears to be different in different families. In some the release of fibrinopeptides is impeded; in others aggregation of fibrin monomers is defective; in one family chemical bonding by fibrin-stabilizing factor is impaired. The disorder is usually recognized because the prothrombin time is prolonged, reflecting the presence of the anomalous fibrinogen. The bleeding tendency is usually mild, although severe bleeding has been reported. In some patients wounds have dehisced, whereas in others a paradoxical thrombotic tendency has occurred. Clots are small and friable and form slowly upon the addition of thrombin to plasma, but fibrinogen concentration as measured immunologically is usually normal. In one family, in which recurrent thrombotic episodes were prevalent, the abnormal fibrinogen clot-

ted unusually rapidly upon the addition of thrombin.

Congenital deficiency of fibrin-stabilizing factor (factor XIII) is a rare disorder in which affected individuals have repeated episodes of serious bleeding after injury. Bleeding from the umbilicus is common. Hematomas, hemarthroses, hematuria, and habitual abortion have been described, and intracranial bleeding is a common cause of death. Sometimes wounds appear to heal slowly, occasionally breaking down repeatedly. The plasma of affected persons usually contains nonfunctional material antigenically similar to fibrin-stabilizing factor. The mode of inheritance of fibrin-stabilizing factor deficiency is not certain. In some families, the disorder is attributable to autosomal recessive mutant genes, whereas in others the syndrome seems limited to males. Diagnosis is established by demonstrating that clots of the patient's plasma are soluble in 5 molar urea or 1 per cent monochloroacetic acid, in contrast to normal clots which are insoluble. More sophisticated tests of the transamidation function of fibrin-stabilizing factor have been used. Transfusion of normal blood or plasma transiently corrects the hemorrhagic tendency and facilitates the healing of wounds.

Simultaneous congenital deficiency of several clotting factors has been repeatedly described. Only the *coexistent deficiencies of antihemophilic factor and proaccelerin* appear well established. The defect is probably inherited as an autosomal recessive trait. The bleeding tendency is usually mild, but should treatment of hemorrhage be needed, fresh-frozen plasma should be effective.

Biggs, R. (ed.): Human Blood Coagulation, Hemostasis and Thrombosis. Oxford, Blackwell Scientific Publications, 1972.

Biggs, R., and Macfarlane, R. G.: Treatment of Hemophilia and Other Coagulation Disorders. Oxford, Blackwell Scientific Publications, 1966.

Jackson, D. P., Beck, E. A., and Charache, P.: Congenital disorders of fibrinogen. Fed. Proc., 24:816, 1965.

Ratnoff, O. D. (ed.): Treatment of Hemorrhagic Disorders. New York, Harper & Row, 1968.

Rossi, E. D. (ed.): Symposium on Hemorrhagic Disorders. Medical Clinics of North America. Vol. 56, No. 1. Philadelphia, W. B. Saunders Company, 1972.

Spaet, T. H. (ed.): Progress in Hemostasis and Thrombosis. Vol 1. New York, Grune & Stratton, 1972.

ACQUIRED DISORDERS OF BLOOD COAGULATION

799.   VITAMIN K DEFICIENCY

Vitamin K is required for the synthesis of prothrombin, factor VII, Stuart factor, and Christmas factor. If a defiency of vitamin K is present, polypeptides are formed and, indeed, released into the plasma, but they lack clot-promoting properties. The role of vitamin K appears to be to transform these polypeptide chains to functional clotting factors.

If vitamin K is not available in adequate amounts, the plasma levels of these procoagulant substances fall and a hemorrhagic disorder ensues. The normal diet contains an abundance of vitamin K; deficiency rarely if ever can be attributed to inadequate diet alone. The bacteria of the intestinal tract synthesize relatively large amounts of the vitamin, which may contribute to the body's supply. Prolonged *oral administration of antibacterial agents* has been associated with depletion of vitamin K and a hemorrhagic disorder responsive to treatment with this vitamin. This syndrome is most likely to occur in patients undergoing parenteral feeding to whom no vitamin K is provided.

The infant at birth may be deficient in vitamin K and as a result may have *hemorrhagic disease of the newborn.* Melena is common, but bleeding may occur from numerous sites. In some cases transfusion is required, and hemorrhage may be fatal. The disorder is self-limited within a few days, because the minute amounts of vitamin K needed by the infant are provided in milk; cow's milk contains more vitamin K than human milk. The establishment of intestinal flora may contribute to the supply, and the administration of antimicrobial drugs to infants requiring correction of congenital gastrointestinal lesions may precipitate hemorrhagic disease of the newborn. The frequency of this disease can be lessened by administration of small amounts of vitamin K to the mother before delivery or to the infant at birth.

Naturally occurring compounds with vitamin K activity are fat soluble and are poorly absorbed from the intestine in the absence of bile salts. Bleeding that accompanies obstructive jaundice or biliary fistula is usually the result of impaired absorption of vitamin K and is promptly responsive to the parenteral injection of the vitamin. Vitamin K should always be given preoperatively in cases of biliary obstruction, for the first evidence of a hemorrhagic disorder often does not appear until the surgical procedure is performed. Deficiency of the vitamin of a degree sufficient to cause bleeding is encountered in *malabsorption syndromes* such as *sprue* or *celiac disease,* and is readily prevented by parenteral administration of vitamin K.

Derivatives of *coumarin* and *indandione* behave as antagonists of vitamin K. These substances, commonly employed in therapy of thromboembolic disease, impair synthesis of prothrombin and other vitamin K–dependent clotting factors. *Salicylates,* related in chemical structure to coumarin, may produce the same effect when given in large amounts; possibly *propylthiouracil* may have this action in rare instances. Hemorrhage associated with the administration of vitamin K antagonists is usually a complication of therapy. The possibility that hemorrhage complicating anticoagulant therapy is due to potentiation of vitamin K antagonists by other drugs—for example, phenylbutazone, allopurinol, chloral hydrate, salicylates, sulfonamides, glucagon, indomethacin, quinidine, clofibrate, or anabolic steroids—must be kept in mind. Some patients with an obscure hemorrhagic disorder have been discovered to have taken coumarin compounds surreptitiously or because these agents were dispensed in error. A characteristic of the coagulation defects produced by vitamin K antagonists is failure to respond rapidly to injection of large amounts of menadione, a synthetic derivative of naphthoquinone, which ordinarily has potent vitamin K activity; in contrast, vitamin K_1 (phytonadione) is promptly effective. Psychiatric treatment of patients suspected of ingesting coumarin compounds surreptitiously is imperative, because this bizarre behavior may be a manifestation of depression, and the patient may seek more effective means of committing suicide.

Bleeding associated with deficiency of prothrombin and related clotting factors is similar to that occurring with other coagulation defects. Cutaneous ecchymoses, epistaxes, hematuria, gastrointestinal bleeding, and postoperative hemorrhage are common, and intracranial hemorrhage may occur. The hemorrhagic disorder may be fatal.

Diagnosis of vitamin K deficiency is established by the demonstration of a significantly prolonged prothrombin time that is shortened within a few hours after administration of vitamin K.

Treatment consists of oral or parenteral administration of a preparation of the vitamin. For most deficiency states, including those associated with biliary obstruction and malabsorption syndromes, water-soluble derivatives of menadione (menadiol sodium diphosphate or menadione sodium bisulfite) are rapidly and completely effective in correcting the abnormalities of coagulation. An injection of 10 mg of the menadione preparation is adequate, but should be repeated at weekly intervals for patients with a persistent absorption defect. Menadione in moderate amounts can produce serious hemolytic anemia and kernicterus in the newborn, even if given to the mother before delivery. Vitamin K_1 (phytonadione) is preferable, and a single dose of 1 mg, given intramuscularly to the infant at the time of birth, is adequate to prevent hemorrhagic disease of the newborn. To overcome the effects of coumarin derivatives and related drugs, only vitamin K_1 is effective. It is given orally or intramuscularly in doses of 5 to 20 mg. Vitamin K_1 may be administered by slow intravenous injection, but this route should be avoided except in an urgent situation because of the possibility of untoward reactions. Immediate but transient correction of multiple deficiencies of the vitamin K–dependent clotting factors may be provided in life-threatening situations by transfusion of plasma or of concentrates of these factors.

Girdwood, R. H. (ed.): Blood Disorders Due to Drugs and Other Agents. Amsterdam, Excerpta Medica, 1973.

Rossi, E. D. (ed.): Symposium on Hemorrhagic Disorders. Medical Clinics of North America, Vol. 56, No. 1. Philadelphia, W. B. Saunders Company, 1972.

800. LIVER DISEASE

Diffuse hepatic disease often produces a hemorrhagic disorder. Ecchymoses and pretibial petechiae are common, and hemorrhage may occur from many sites; bleeding from surgical wounds is frequent. The bleeding tendency may have multiple causes, including vascular abnormalities, thrombocytopenia, and impairment of blood coagulation. Hypoprothrombinemia and deficiencies of the other vitamin K–dependent clotting factors are common; deficiencies of proaccelerin and PTA may contribute to the hemostatic defect. The catabolism of fibrinogen is often accelerated, and rarely, when parenchymal disease is severe, the concentration of plasma fibrinogen may be decreased. In some patients with advanced liver disease, depletion of plasma clotting factors and platelets may reflect diffuse intravascular coagulation. Another rarely encountered disturbance in chronic hepatic disease, particularly primary hepatoma, is the synthesis of a qualitatively abnormal form of fibrinogen which is converted to fibrin by thrombin at an abnormally slow rate. In cirrhosis of the liver, clots prepared from plasma or its euglobulin fraction dissolve abnormally rapidly, but evidence that this test tube phenomenon correlates with a bleeding tendency is insecure. Although the prothrombin time is usually prolonged in patients with hepatic disease who exhibit a bleeding tendency, the administration of vitamin K usually has little or no corrective effect. Transfusion of fresh blood or fresh-frozen plasma may provide transitory correction of the coagulative defect, but is usually not satisfactory in maintaining hemostasis. The use of currently available concentrates of the vitamin K–dependent clotting factors should be avoided, because fibrinolytic reactions have been described.

Ratnoff, O. D.: Disordered hemostasis in hepatic disease. *In* Schiff, L. (ed.): Diseases of the Liver, 3rd ed. Philadelphia, J. B. Lippincott Company, 1969, p. 147.

801. ACQUIRED HYPOFIBRINOGENEMIA AND SYNDROMES OF INTRAVASCULAR COAGULATION AND FIBRINOLYSIS

Deficiency of fibrinogen of a degree sufficient to cause abnormal bleeding is encountered in a number of different clinical syndromes. It occurs only rarely because of retarded production of fibrinogen and more often as a result of rapid utilization. A bleeding tendency encountered in some patients with *cyanotic congenital heart disease* is attributable in part to the very high hematocrit; the fibrinogen concentration of whole blood is so low that an adequate clot cannot form. Although fibrinogen is synthesized in the liver, *hepatic disease* is seldom the cause of profound deficiency.

Normal plasma contains, on the average, about 300 mg of fibrinogen per 100 ml, although individual variation is wide. During pregnancy, infection, inflammation, myocardial infarction, and other stresses, the concentration of fibrinogen in plasma may be much higher, an alteration principally responsible for the elevated erythrocyte sedimentation rate in these conditions. The biologic half-life of fibrinogen is about three days, but the nature of its normal catabolism is unknown. Neither consumption by intravascular coagulation, nor deposition at extravascular sites of inflammation, nor fibrinolysis by the proteolytic enzyme, plasmin, seems adequate to explain its continual destruction.

Plasmin is present in circulating plasma in the form of a protein precursor, plasminogen. In the test tube, this proenzyme can be converted to plasmin in many ways, including addition of streptokinase (a product of certain beta-hemolytic streptococci), urokinase (a proteolytic enzyme in normal urine), or a plasminogen activator found in many tissues, most impressively in the endothelium of venules and veins. Under certain conditions, the clotting process itself appears to initiate formation of plasmin, an effect mediated by activated Hageman factor via one or more intermediate agents. The long-recognized activation of plasminogen by incubation of plasma or its euglobulin fraction (that is, the

fraction insoluble at low ionic strength and low pH) with chloroform is apparently brought about through this Hageman factor–determined mechanism.

Plasmin can digest a wide variety of substrates, including fibrinogen, fibrin, antihemophilic factor, proaccelerin, gamma globulin, and corticotrophin (ACTH). It converts the first component of complement, C1, to its esterolytic form, $\overline{C1}$, and separates biologically active kinins, such as bradykinin, from their precursor in plasma, kininogen. Additionally, plasmin digests casein, gelatin, and certain synthetic esters of arginine and lysine, all of which have been used for in vitro assay of plasmin.

Plasma also contains several potent inhibitors of plasmin, notably $\alpha1$-antitrypsin, $\alpha2$-macroglobulin, and $\overline{C1}$ inactivator, a protein which also inhibits $\overline{C1}$, activated Hageman factor, activated PTA, and plasma kallikrein. Platelets, too, possess plasmin-inhibitory properties. Recent evidence also suggests that plasma may inhibit the activation of plasminogen.

Although purified fibrinogen and fibrin appear to be digested by plasmin at comparable rates, this is apparently not true in plasma. For example, fibrin formed in the presence of streptokinase dissolves rapidly, whereas the digestion of fibrinogen in an unclotted mixture of plasma and streptokinase proceeds more slowly. One likely explanation is that plasminogen, adsorbed to fibrin, can be converted to plasmin in situ and then induce fibrinolysis. Presumably, fibrinolysis takes place because the plasmin is physically separated from inhibitors of the activation of plasminogen and of plasmin itself. In unclotted plasma, these inhibitors protect fibrinogen from hydrolysis by plasmin. This phenomenon is of major importance in attempts at therapeutic dissolution of thrombi by the administration of plasminogen activators, with minimal digestion of circulating plasma proteins.

The digestion of fibrinogen by plasmin takes place by steps. The first cleavage of fibrinogen, whose molecular weight is about 340,000 D, splits this molecule into a fragment with a molecular weight of about 240,000 D (fragment X), which can still be clotted by thrombin, and several small fragments. Further digestion of fragment X leads ultimately to the formation of three incoagulable fragments, two with a molecular weight of about 83,000 D each (fragments D), and one with a molecular weight of about 50,000 D (fragment E). Similar fragments appear during the digestion of fibrin, but in this case fragment X is incoagulable. Fragments X and E are powerful anticoagulants, interfering primarily with polymerization of fibrin, apparently by forming complexes with monomeric units of fibrin, formed by the action of thrombin on fibrinogen. Clots formed in the presence of digestion products of fibrinogen and fibrin are structurally defective. The *degradation products of fibrinogen and fibrin (FDP)* also interfere with earlier stages of clotting, and perhaps with platelet aggregation, but the physiologic significance of these actions is unclear.

EXPERIMENTAL INTRAVASCULAR COAGULATION

When a massive amount of tissue thromboplastin or thrombin is injected intravenously into an animal, its blood clots, presumably because the extrinsic pathway of coagulation has been activated. Death ensues from circulatory obstruction. When, instead, the clot-promoting agent is injected slowly, the animal survives but its blood becomes incoagulable. The slower rate at which thrombin forms under these conditions results in slower, and perhaps incomplete, formation of fibrin, so that plasma may contain intermediates of fibrin formation, such as fibrin monomer, soluble fibrin polymers, or complexes of fibrin monomer and fibrinogen. These products are rapidly removed from the circulation by the reticuloendothelial system, whose cells then contain material recognizable immunologically as related to fibrinogen, whereas the circulating blood is depleted of this protein. Usually thrombi cannot be detected by microscopic examination, although occasionally the smallest blood vessels of the kidneys, adrenals, and other organs contain thrombi. Concomitant with the evolution of afibrinogenemia, the concentration of other clotting factors decreases, particularly prothrombin (presumably utilized in the formation of thrombin), proaccelerin, and antihemophilic factor (the latter two, perhaps, inactivated by thrombin). The platelet count falls, possibly because these cells are clumped by thrombin and removed from the circulation. Animals which have undergone experimental defibrination may undergo hemolysis, and their red blood cells may appear to have been fragmented, as if ruptured by intravascular strands of fibrin. Inconstantly, evidences of intravascular fibrinolysis may be detected, either by demonstration of products of digestion of fibrinogen or fibrin in the animal's serum, or by depletion of plasminogen, the precursor of the fibrinolytic enzyme, plasmin; direct evidence for the presence of fibrinolytic activity in the animal's plasma is more difficult to demonstrate. Nonetheless, fibrinolysis has been invoked as one cause for failure to find thrombi in animals injected with tissue thromboplastin; the plasma often acquires clot-inhibitory properties attributed to the presence either of degradation products of fibrin formed through the action of plasmin, or of complexes of these degradation products, fibrinogen, and dissolved fibrin monomers and polymers, in various combinations.

LABORATORY DIAGNOSIS OF INTRAVASCULAR COAGULATION

When intravascular coagulation has been extensive enough to induce hypofibrinogenemia or afibrinogenemia, rapid diagnosis may be made by observing the appearance of coagulating blood in a test tube. A simple qualitative test for hypofibrinogenemia is the addition of 1 ml of blood to 0.1 ml of bovine thrombin solution containing 1000 NIH units per milliliter. Unless virtually no fibrinogen is present, the blood clots quickly. The size of the clot can then be estimated by tapping the tube and observing the degree to which the clot retracts. The retracted clot may be so small that it is difficult to find among the extruded red blood cells and serum, leading to the misinterpretation that fibrinolysis has occurred. The existence of hypofibrinogenemia is confirmed by additional tests, including quantitative measurement of fibrinogen concentration.

In patients thought to have undergone intravascular coagulation, the thrombin time (that is, the time elapsing until a mixture of plasma and thrombin clots),

Disorders Accompanied by Intravascular Coagulation*

A. Hypofibrinogenemic or afibrinogenemic states:
1. Secondary to the introduction of extrinsic clot-promoting agents
   Amniotic fluid embolism
   Envenomation by snakebite
   Premature separation of the placenta
2. Secondary to intravascular elaboration of clot-promoting agents
   Acute hemolytic processes (e.g., mismatched blood transfusion)
   Extracorporeal circulation
   Massive arterial or venous thrombosis; pulmonary embolism
   Near drowning
3. Secondary to vascular injury, exposing clot-promoting tissues
   Purpura fulminans
   Sepsis with gram-positive or -negative organisms; septic abortion; Waterhouse-Friderichsen syndrome
   Infectious disease (e.g., generalized herpes simplex, dengue, cytomegalic inclusion disease, scrub typhus, Rocky Mountain spotted fever, miliary tuberculosis, subacute bacterial endocarditis, trypanosomiasis)
   Heat stroke
   Aortic aneurysm
   Traumatic shock; burns; head injury; surgical procedures
   Thrombotic thrombocytopenic purpura; hemolytic-uremic syndrome
4. Secondary to vascular stasis
   Giant hemangioma
   Hemangioendotheliosarcoma
   Cavernomatous transformation of veins
5. Pathogenesis uncertain (introduction of clot-promoting agents?)
   Malignancy (e.g., carcinoma of prostate, pancreas, etc., neuroblastoma, leukemia)
   Administration of L-asparaginase
   Acute pancreatitis
   Hydatidiform mole
B. Conditions in which intravascular coagulation has been implicated in the absence of hypofibrinogenemia:
1. Secondary to intravascular elaboration of clot-promoting agents
   Hemolytic processes (e.g., paroxysmal nocturnal hemoglobinuria)
   Rejection of organ transplants
2. Secondary to vascular injury
   Purpura fulminans
   Sepsis with gram-positive or -negative organisms
   Infectious diseases (e.g., exanthematous diseases, viral hemorrhagic fevers, influenza, rickettsial or mycotic disorders, falciparum malaria, bubonic plague, subacute bacterial endocarditis)
   Thrombotic thrombocytopenic purpura, hemolytic uremic syndrome, eclampsia
   Chronic glomerulonephritis, renal cortical necrosis, lupus erythematosus with renal disease, polyarteritis nodosum, nephrotic syndrome with proliferative glomerulonephritis
   Traumatic and anaphylactic shock, burns, surgical procedures
3. Secondary to vascular stasis
   Malignant hemangioendothelioma
4. Pathogenesis uncertain
   Malignancy (e.g., metastatic carcinoma of stomach, lung, breast, etc., especially mucin-producing tumors; Wilms' tumor)
   Idiopathic respiratory distress syndrome; hyaline membrane disease
   Cirrhosis of the liver
   Amyloidosis
   Fat embolism
   Poisoning with *Amanita phalloides*, mercuric oxide, alkyl phosphates, dichlorethane
   Cyanotic congenital heart disease
   Cardiogenic shock

*This tabulation is not all-inclusive; the classification is tentative, and the evidence supporting the existence of intravascular coagulation as an important component of the disease state varies in its cogency.

prothrombin time, and partial thromboplastin time may all be prolonged, both because necessary reactants have been depleted and because of the presence of clot-inhibitory agents. In some cases, intravascular coagulation may be suspected because the concentration of fibrinogen, although within the range found in normal individuals, is decreased below the level anticipated in the light of the patient's clinical condition. In parallel to the changes observed in laboratory animals, the platelet count may be reduced, and deficiencies of prothrombin, proaccelerin, and antihemophilic factor may be observed. Inconstantly, too, rapid dissolution of clots formed from plasma or its euglobulin fraction may suggest that *secondary fibrinolysis* has taken place. More frequently, the concentration of plasminogen may be diminished, as if this proenzyme had been converted to plasmin and then inactivated by its inhibitors in plasma, and the plasma may acquire inhibitory properties directed against the clotting process.

Direct evidence that intravascular coagulation has taken place has been provided in several ways. Thus free fibrinopeptide A, separated from fibrinogen through the action of thrombin, can be detected immunologically in the plasma of patients thought to be undergoing intravascular coagulation. Further, the incorporation of radioactive glycine methyl ester into a fraction of plasma rich in fibrinogen has been thought to reflect the presence of dissolved fibrin monomers or polymers; this ester is incorporated into fibrin, but not fibrinogen, through the action of fibrin-stabilizing factor. High molecular weight complexes, seemingly of fibrinogen and fibrin monomer, have been separated from plasma by physical means. And the half-disappearance time of intravenously injected radioactive fibrinogen is dramatically shortened in patients in whom intravascular coagulation is believed to be taking place. These four techniques are not yet firmly established, nor translated into practical methodology.

Indirect support for the existence of intravascular coagulation can be obtained by demonstrating that the patient's serum, normally devoid of fibrinogen, contains antigenic material related to this protein. Many techniques have been used to demonstrate these fibrinogen-related antigens (FRA), often called by the more restrictive term, fibrinogen degradation products (FDP), which implies that the materials identified are the product of the action of plasmin. Immunodiffusion, immunoelectrophoresis, tanned red blood cell hemagglutination inhibition, and agglutination of latex particles coated with heterologous antifibrin antiserum have all been used to detect fibrinogen-related antigens. Less reliably, gelation of plasma by addition of ethanol or protamine sulfate, or aggregation of certain strains of *Staphylococcus aureus* by the patient's serum may reflect the presence of dissolved polymers, particularly of fibrin monomer and fibrinogen but also, perhaps, of fibrin monomer and degradation products of the action of plasmin on fibrinogen or fibrin. Similarly, chilling plasma may induce precipitation of "cryofibrinogen," composed of complexes of fibrinogen and fibrin monomers. And in some patients evidences of intravascular damage to erythrocytes, similar to those seen in experimental animals undergoing defibrination, may be found.

The laboratory abnormalities described have been detected in the blood of patients undergoing disseminated intravascular coagulation. Similar changes, however, are observed in some patients with extensive localized thrombosis, for example, pulmonary embolism or aortic aneurysm.

HYPOFIBRINOGENEMIC SYNDROMES ASSOCIATED WITH LOCALIZED THROMBOSIS

Rarely, after massive arterial or venous thrombosis or pulmonary embolism, the blood is incoagulable, and marked thrombocytopenia is present. Presumably, the fibrinogen, platelets, and other clotting factors are depleted in the formation of thrombi. A similar coagulation defect may be encountered in *purpura fulminans,* a disease in which acute necrosis of superficial and peripheral parts of the body is associated with thrombosis at the sites of vasculitis in small blood vessels in the affected areas. This rare disorder, which is most prevalent in children and often follows shortly after an apparently banal infection, is usually self-limited, but its course may be aborted by administration of heparin, which inhibits further thrombin formation. Perhaps the rare instances of patchy *cutaneous necrosis during therapy with coumarin-like anticoagulants* have a similar pathogenesis, although hypofibrinogenemia has not been described in this situation. The lesions are most likely to appear at sites rich in fatty tissue, such as the breast and buttocks. The necrotic lesions are preceded by an evanescent, painful erythematous patch, and treatment with vitamin K_1 may abort the episode.

Unusually, hypofibrinogenemia has also been observed with *thrombotic thrombocytopenic purpura,* in which noninflammatory thrombosis of small blood vessels is associated with fever, acute hemolytic anemia, neurologic symptoms, thrombocytopenia, and acute renal failure (see Ch. 790); in this disorder, the administration of heparin is usually without benefit. Hypofibrinogenemia may occur in patients with *giant cavernous hemangioma, hemangioepithelioma,* or *cavernomatous transformation of veins,* particularly of the portal system; in these disorders, fibrin thrombi form in the relatively static blood within the vascular lesions. Other syndromes in which widespread thrombosis of relatively large vessels is commonplace, such as *paroxysmal nocturnal hemoglobinuria, sickle cell disease,* and *homocystinuria,* have not been associated with hypofibrinogenemia.

HYPOFIBRINOGENEMIC SYNDROMES ASSOCIATED WITH DIFFUSE INTRAVASCULAR CLOTTING

Hypofibrinogenemia or afibrinogenemia may be encountered in other disorders in which thrombosis may be difficult or impossible to demonstrate. In such cases, procoagulant substances are thought to be introduced into the bloodstream sufficiently slowly that massive thrombosis does not ensue. The fate of the fibrin that forms intravascularly is not clear. Perhaps, as is true in laboratory animals, fibrin is removed from the circulating blood by the reticuloendothelial system. Alternatively, soluble fibrin monomers or polymers, perhaps complexed with fibrinogen, are cleared from the bloodstream before insoluble fibrin strands can form, or fibrin is dissolved by plasmin, and the fibrin degradation products, some of which may be complexed with fibrinogen or fibrin monomer, are removed by the reticuloendothelial cells.

The clearest examples of defibrination by these mechanisms are *amniotic fluid embolism,* in which amniotic fluid and its contaminants enter the maternal bloodstream during parturition, *envenomation* by the bite of snakes whose venom contains procoagulant agents, and the administration of several hundred milliliters of *incompatible blood.* In this last circumstance, the products of lysis of the transfused cells may initiate intravascular coagulation and defibrinate the recipient's blood. Envenomation by the bite of the Malayan pit viper, *Agkistrodon rhodostoma,* has been extensively studied; the venom has a thrombin-like action upon fibrinogen, resulting in afibrinogenemia without any of the depletion of other clotting factors or platelets seen in other cases of intravascular clotting. These properties have led to its experimental use in the treatment of thromboembolic disorders.

Similar mechanisms have been evoked to explain hypofibrinogenemia in other disorders, although the evidence is more inferential. For example, hypofibrinogenemia has been encountered in patients with severe *sepsis,* particularly *septic abortion,* and *Waterhouse-Friderichsen syndrome.* In these syndromes, vascular damage may expose the circulating blood to subendothelial tissues which may induce thrombosis through activation of Hageman factor or localized aggregation of platelets. A wide variety of both gram-positive and gram-negative organisms have been implicated. The possibility that in some cases intravascular coagulation is part of the human counterpart of the generalized Shwartzman reaction has been advocated. Hypofibrinogenemia has been reported with peculiar frequency in individuals with *pneumococcal sepsis* who have asplenia, usually as the result of splenectomy, or splenic atrophy, such as occurs in sickle cell disease. Vascular damage may also be important in initiating disseminated intravascular coagulation in patients with *viral hemorrhagic fevers* or certain other infectious diseases.

Some cases of *premature separation of the placenta* may be complicated by hypofibrinogenemia; although the introduction of highly thromboplastic placental tissue into the maternal bloodstream has been invoked as an explanation, other mechanisms, such as the formation of a massive retroplacental clot, may be operative. The pathogenesis of hypofibrinogenemia in *prolonged retention of a dead fetus* or *neoplastic diseases* is less clear, although in such cases intravascular coagulation induced by procoagulants derived from the pathologic tissue has been surmised. *Metastatic carcinoma of the prostate* is the most frequent of the many neoplasms that may produce hypofibrinogenemia; this defect has also been encountered in patients with carcinoma of the breast, stomach, gallbladder, pancreas, lung, and colon, disseminated rhabdomyosarcoma, leukemia, most often of the acute promyelocytic type, and other tumors as well.

Hypofibrinogenemia, thrombocytopenia, and other coagulation defects have been encountered during various types of *extracorporeal circulation.* The apparatus may defibrinate the blood if insufficient heparin is employed. *Abnormal bleeding during cardiovascular surgical procedures* may have multiple causes, including the use of too much or too little heparin, as well as the operative procedure itself. Hypofibrinogenemia has also been observed during other surgical procedures, most frequently during pulmonary resection, although this is a rare complication. Hypofibrinogenemia may accompany *aneurysm of the aorta,* particularly *dissecting aneurysm,* presumably because the exposed subendothelial tissue is clot promoting. Widespread vascular damage may also explain the occurrence of hypofibrinogenemia in patients with *shock* of different origins and *heat stroke.*

Bleeding associated with the defibrinating syndromes is often severe, but the character of the bleeding, as well as the prognosis, is influenced by the nature of the underlying disease. Often, the first indication that defibrination is taking place is bleeding at the sites of arterial or venous puncture. In women with *premature separation of the placenta* or *amniotic fluid embolism,* major hemorrhage is usually from the uterus, although a generalized bleeding tendency may be evident. In patients with more chronic forms of hypofibrinogenemia, ecchymoses, hematoma formation, and bleeding from the gastrointestinal tract may be prominent. Patients with syndromes of diffuse intravascular coagulation may also have symptoms consequent upon the obstruction of the circulation by small thrombi; renal tubular and cortical necrosis caused by thrombosis in the smallest blood vessels are of the greatest moment.

Primary treatment of hypofibrinogenemia or afibrinogenemia caused by intravascular coagulation is that of the basic disease; if this can be eradicated or ameliorated, the coagulation defects are rapidly corrected. Thus the hypofibrinogenemia associated with *amniotic fluid embolism* is self-limited, whereas in patients with *premature separation of the placenta* or *retention of a dead fetus,* recovery follows shortly after the uterus is emptied. Severe bleeding associated with *carcinoma of the prostate* may subside, and the coagulation abnormalities may disappear within days of the institution of estrogen therapy. Transfusion of fresh blood is often required. Although administration of fibrinogen may be of temporary value and tide the patient over an acute episode of bleeding, if the basic pathologic process continues, the transfused fibrinogen is rapidly removed from the circulation and may participate in the formation of new disseminated thrombi. Moreover, the use of human fibrinogen preparations is all too often followed by serum hepatitis. In cases in which the primary disease cannot be treated, intravenous injection of heparin may impede intravascular defibrination by inhibiting the clotting process and raise the levels of depleted clotting factors. A typical course of therapy includes an initial dose of 50 to 100 units of heparin per kilogram of body weight, followed by 10 to 15 units per kilogram per hour, administered by intravenous infusion; more may be needed, and smaller doses may be appropriate if severe thrombocytopenia is present. This seemingly paradoxical approach to treatment is most effective when the disease is self-limited, as in the case of *extensive arterial or venous thrombosis* or *purpura fulminans,* or in cases of chronic defibrination, as in instances of *metastatic disease.* The risks of bleeding from operative wounds or the placental site limit the usefulness of heparin therapy in acute forms of hypofibrinogenemia.

DISSEMINATED INTRAVASCULAR COAGULATION WITHOUT HYPOFIBRINOGENEMIA

A widely held view is that many pathologic states may induce widespread intravascular coagulation, perhaps insufficient to cause significant hypofibrinogenemia, but adequate to bring about ischemic damage. Under such conditions, the thrombin time, prothrombin time, and partial thromboplastin time may be prolonged; serum may contain agents immunologically resembling fibrinogen; plasma may undergo coagulation upon addition of ethanol or protamine sulfate, and the platelet count may be depressed. In some patients, intravascular hemolysis may be detected, and the erythrocytes may have the morphologic characteristics of those of animals undergoing experimental defibrination, appearing fragmented and often triangular in shape. Such cells, often called *schistocytes,* are characteristic of *microangiopathic hemolytic anemia,* a state seen pre-eminently in *thrombotic thrombocytopenic purpura* and the *hemolytic-uremic syndrome.* In some cases, too, accelerated turnover of fibrinogen and platelets suggests that intravascular coagulation has occurred even though the blood levels of these substances may not be decreased because other compensating mechanisms are operative.

Application of these criteria has led to the assumption that myriad clinical disorders are accompanied by intravascular coagulation. Besides thrombotic thrombocytopenic purpura and the hemolytic-uremic syndrome, these diseases include fulminant *eclampsia* with hemolytic anemia and thrombocytopenia, *malignant hypertension, chronic glomerulonephritis, nephrotic syndrome* with proliferative glomerulonephritis, *renal cortical necrosis, cirrhosis of the liver, hyaline membrane disease, sepsis,* especially *meningococcemia* and *rickettsial* and *viral* disorders, *metastatic carcinoma, systemic lupus erythematosus, polyarteritis nodosum,* and *shock* of diverse origins. Intravascular coagulation has also been thought to be important in rejection of *organ grafts,* and may complicate *therapeutic abortion.* This by no means exhausts the disorders in which intravascular coagulation, disseminated or localized to specific organs, is thought to be an important feature (see accompanying table).

Evidences for the role of intravascular coagulation in the pathogenesis of these various disease states varies in degree of conviction. Particular criticism has been leveled at diagnostic reliance upon hemolysis or changes in red blood cell morphology, because these may occur in the absence of other changes associated with intravascular coagulation, and hemolysis may be the cause rather than the result of defibrination.

The beneficial effects of heparin in some cases of hypofibrinogenemia have led to its use in individuals in whom disseminated intravascular coagulation is suspected in the absence of hypofibrinogenemia. In some cases, a trial of heparin therapy, as outlined for patients with hypofibrinogenemic states, may be justified, and may be followed by clinical and laboratory improvement. In most instances, unfortunately, the results have been disappointing, and skepticism concerning the importance of disseminated intravascular coagulation in pathogenesis seems appropriate.

McKay, D. G.: Disseminated Intravascular Coagulation. An Intermediary Mechanism of Disease. New York, Hoeber Medical Division, Harper & Row, 1965.

Minna, J. D., Robboy, S. J., and Coleman, R. W. (eds.): Disseminated Intravascular Coagulation in Man. Springfield, Ill., Charles C Thomas, 1974.

Poller, I. (ed.): Recent Advances in Blood Coagulation. London, J. & A. Churchill, Ltd., 1969.

Rossi, E. D. (ed.): Symposium on Hemorrhagic Disorders. Medical Clinics of North America, Vol. 56, No. 1. Philadelphia, W. B. Saunders Company, 1972.

802. FIBRINOLYTIC STATES

An attractive hypothesis envisions that minor degrees of fibrinolytic activity operate under normal conditions to maintain the fluidity of blood by dissolving thrombi in the microcirculation. Evidence in support of this view is, however, equivocal. As measured in vitro, the fibrinolytic activity of blood or its euglobulin fraction is exaggerated in chronic hepatic disease, under such conditions of stress as traumatic shock, anxiety, electroconvulsive therapy or anoxia, and after the injection of certain vasoactive substances, for example, epinephrine or nicotinic acid. The enhanced fibrinolytic activity is thought to be due to the presence in plasma of circulating activators of plasminogen, perhaps derived from venous endothelium and, in the case of chronic hepatic disease, inadequately removed from the bloodstream by the liver. The clinical significance of these in vitro observations is uncertain, because the enhanced fibrinolytic activity is not ordinarily reflected in clinical symptomatology, and in vivo the array of inactivators of plasmin in plasma may limit the evolution of significant proteolytic activity. Moreover, demonstration of increased fibrinolytic activity in vitro usually requires the formation or presence of a fibrin clot, to which plasminogen and its activators may be adsorbed. Under these conditions, plasmin may form, physically separated from its inhibitors in plasma, allowing fibrinolysis to take place. In vivo, on the other hand, the array of inactivators of plasmin may limit the evolution of significant proteolytic activity.

Under the stress of intravascular coagulation, local fibrinolysis appears to be an important mechanism in dissolution of small thrombi. Here, as in vitro, plasmin may be capable of digesting clots without reaching effective levels in circulating plasma. Under these conditions, products of fibrinolysis may be found in circulating plasma, where they may inhibit the coagulation process and interfere with the polymerization of fibrin. Usually, direct evidence that fibrinolysis is taking place is meager, but fibrinolysis has been inferred from a fall in the concentration of plasminogen in plasma. The concentrations of antihemophilic factor and proaccelerin may also be decreased, and the patient's serum may contain antigenic material related to fibrinogen, possibly products of fibrinolysis but, as has been noted earlier, sometimes the result of incomplete clotting of fibrin. In some patients undergoing intravascular coagulation, fibrinolysis may be so extensive that clotted blood undergoes spontaneous dissolution within minutes or a few hours. This *secondary fibrinolytic state* is most often found in patients in whom defibrination is particularly severe, such as those with *amniotic fluid embolism, premature separation of the placenta, profound hemorrhagic shock,* or *neoplasms,* such as *metastatic carcinoma of the prostate* or *acute leukemia.* In some cases, despite the demonstration of potent fibrinolytic activity in vitro, the concentration of fibrinogen does not fall dramatically, recalling the observation noted earlier that fibrinolysis occurs more readily than fibrinogenolysis.

A few patients have been described who, under severe stress, have developed a fulminant hemorrhagic syndrome attributable to excessive fibrinolytic activity. Thus during laparotomy, blood may seem to ooze from every cut tissue; fibrinolysis may be so rapid that whole blood appears to be incoagulable, whereas the patient's plasma can be clotted by thrombin, only to redissolve within minutes. Although this rare syndrome has been ascribed to a *primary fibrinolytic state,* it is uncertain whether in fact the disorder does not reflect an episode of diffuse intravascular clotting in which fibrinolysis rather than thrombosis dominates the clinical picture. In contrast to the usual case of disseminated intravascular clotting, the platelet count may be normal; but other laboratory features, including prolongation of the thrombin time, prothrombin time, and partial thromboplastin time, depletion of clotting factors, and the demonstration of fibrinogen-related antigens in serum, do not distinguish the disorder from diffuse intravascular coagulation. If the diagnosis seems certain, the administration of large amounts of *epsilon-aminocaproic acid,* a drug which inhibits the activation of plasminogen, may be helpful. A typical regimen in an adult is 4 grams every four hours for two or three days. Unfortunately, this agent is strongly contraindicated in individuals undergoing intravascular coagulation, for it may stabilize thrombi which would otherwise dissolve. Thus great circumspection must be used in treating patients with suspected primary fibrinolysis with this agent.

A more certain primary fibrinolytic state may be induced during therapeutic attempts at dissolution of thrombi by administration of streptokinase or urokinase, activators of plasminogen. In such cases, more plasmin forms within the bloodstream than can be effectively neutralized by plasma inhibitors of this enzyme, and fibrinogen and other clotting factors may be depleted, without a concomitant fall in the platelet count. Hemorrhagic symptoms, apparently induced by excessive fibrinolytic activity, are a relatively common complication of experimental fibrinolytic therapy. If bleeding symptoms are alarming, therapy with epsilon-aminocaproic acid in the manner described for primary fibrinolytic states may be indicated, but caution must be exercised in its use, lest the thrombotic state for which therapy was initiated be worsened.

Local fibrinolysis after prostatectomy may lead to protracted and sometimes severe hematuria. The pathogenesis of bleeding under these conditions is uncertain; clots in the operative bed may be dissolved by plasmin, formed through the action either of urinary urokinase or of tissue activators in exposed prostatic tissue. Therapy with epsilon-aminocaproic acid is effective, and is not attended by the dangers inherent in the treatment of thrombotic states.

Douglas, A. S. (ed.): Blood coagulation and fibrinolysis in clinical practice. Clinics in Haematology, Vol. 2, No. 1. London, W. B. Saunders, Ltd., 1973.

Rossi, E. D. (ed.): Symposium on Hemorrhagic Disorders. Medical Clinics of North America, Vol. 56, No. 1. Philadelphia, W. B. Saunders Company, 1972.

803. ANTICOAGULANTS

The presence of an anticoagulant in the circulating blood causes a bleeding tendency that may be severe. This occurrence may follow parenteral administration of heparin, a substance that interferes with generation of the prothrombin converting principle as well as with the conversion of fibrinogen to fibrin. Heparin rapidly disappears from the circulation so that the hemorrhagic disorder subsides within an hour or two after intravenous injection is terminated. Rarely, inadvertent administration of heparin may be responsible for sudden, unexpected bleeding. A tentative diagnosis can be made by demonstrating that the patient's plasma clots abnormally slowly upon addition of thrombin (whose action is antagonized by heparin) but at a normal rate upon addition of Reptilase, i.e., the venom of *Bothrops atrox* (whose clotting action upon plasma fibrinogen is not blocked by heparin). A number of hemorrhagic disorders have been attributed to the production of heparin in vivo, but there are few if any cases in which this claim is supported by convincing evidence. Antiheparin agents, including protamine sulfate and toluidine blue, effectively counteract the action of heparin when given intravenously in precisely calculated amounts. Bishydroxycoumarin (Dicumarol) and related compounds are often referred to as anticoagulants, but they interfere with the synthesis of clotting factors and do not retard coagulation directly.

Endogenously produced anticoagulants are encountered under several circumstances and may produce a hemophilia-like disease. These circulating anticoagulants appear to be IgG antibodies, and they most often interfere with the early stages of coagulation. One frequently demonstrable in the plasma of patients with hemophilia specifically inactivates antihemophilic factor and is an antibody against this agent. An anticoagulant of similar nature and specificity sometimes occurs in the plasma of women after pregnancy, producing a hemophilia-like disorder. Hemorrhagic disease attributable to an apparently identical anticoagulant has appeared without obvious cause in persons who were previously healthy or who have a chronic disease. Comparable substances, specifically inactivating other clotting factors, have been encountered in patients with congenital deficiency of the clotting factor in question. A circulating anticoagulant occurring in the plasma of some patients with systemic lupus erythematosus is unusual, because it interferes with the conversion of prothrombin to thrombin; less commonly, patients with this disease have circulating anticoagulants against antihemophilic factor.

The presence of an anticoagulant is detected by demonstrating the retarding action of small proportions of the patient's plasma on the coagulation of normal blood or recalcified plasma. Circulating anticoagulants may disappear spontaneously, sometimes after a period of many months or years, but therapy is difficult. Because of the anticoagulant effect of the patient's plasma, transfusions do not correct the clotting defect. When bleeding is life threatening, exchange transfusion and the injection of massive amounts of the missing factor may be tried. The use of steroids or immunosuppressive agents has been disappointing. Patients with myeloma and with other diseases causing dysproteinemia may display impairment of blood coagulation attributable to the presence of the abnormal protein. The bleeding manifestations frequently associated with dysproteinemia are not, however, clearly related to retarded clotting.

Spaet, T. H. (ed.): Progress in Hemostasis and Thrombosis. Vol. 1. New York, Grune & Stratton, 1972.

Part XVII
DISEASES OF METABOLISM

804. INTRODUCTION

Nicholas P. Christy

The term "metabolism" used to be defined as the sum of the processes concerned in the building up and breaking down of living protoplasm, and as the chemical changes in living cells by which energy is provided for cellular work and for cellular repair. Such a definition depicts metabolism as a kind of cellular nutrition. Nowadays, the term is broadened to stand for "the sum of the processes by which a particular substance is handled . . . in the living body," i.e., the processes that are essential for survival, growth, maturation, and reproduction. Defined in this more general way, almost any disease is a "disease of metabolism" (from the Greek, μεταβολή, change; "metabolic" from μεταβολικός, changeable). After *trauma,* e.g., fracture of a hip, calcium may be lost from bone during prolonged immobilization, with accompanying hypercalcemia. An *infectious disease,* chronic pyelonephritis, may lead to renal insufficiency, uremia, and the familiar renal mismanagement of H^+, phosphate, and other ions; cholera is associated with tremendous gastrointestinal losses of sodium and water. *Hereditary diseases* of several systems are characterized by disordered "handling" of particular substances: in congenital adrenal hyperplasia, deficiency of one or another adrenal cortical enzyme results in reduced synthesis of cortisol, excessive secretion of androgens, and precocious virilism; the disordered synthesis of hemoglobin in sickle cell anemia, the classic "molecular disease," results in the specific amino acid difference in the beta chain that underlies the misshapen erythrocytes, the hemolysis, and the microinfarctions. A major clinical manifestation of a disease of *unknown etiology,* chronic pancreatitis, is steatorrhea with diarrhea, largely owing to deficiency of pancreatic exocrine secretion and the failure to hydrolyze triglycerides in the gut. Thus diseases of all systems and of diverse etiologies are metabolic diseases, in the sense that they show some change in the way the body deals with (metabolizes) a particular chemical substance.

Metabolism itself must be changeable; the internal environment is only relatively constant. In his famous and much quoted generalization, Claude Bernard said: "All the vital mechanisms, varied as they are, have only one object: that of preserving constant the conditions of life in the *milieu intérieur.*" But, as the American physiologist L. J. Henderson wrote in 1926, "This should not be thought of as absolute constancy, and it should be understood that variations in the properties of the internal environment may be both cyclical and adaptive, that is, functional. . . ." Normal metabolism thus operates to keep the cellular environment in a state appropriate to constantly changing conditions, e.g., growth, reproduction, and aging; changes in body temperature, hydration, and nutrition. It is a mistake to think of the constancy of the *milieu intérieur* as simply a ceaseless struggle of the cells to return to some fixed and immutable baseline. The baseline is continually changing. Abnormal metabolism (or disease), as defined by Bernard, can be viewed as a "perturbation or dislocation" of the mechanisms that make possible appropriate adjustments to change.

Part XVII contains an account of hereditary and acquired diseases characterized by derangement of the internal environment, diseases which have in common *disordered production or fate of a well-defined, specific chemical substance.** Consequences of these disorders are an excess or deficiency of that substance or a substance closely related to it. The excess or deficiency gives rise to a well-defined, specific clinical syndrome which involves either predominantly one or in some cases several organs or systems.

In Part XVII are placed most of the clinical conditions in which there is a demonstrated abnormality of a specific protein, either a "deficiency in a specific enzymatic activity . . . [or] a normal amount of a structurally abnormal protein" (see Ch. 7). Thus the various forms of glycogen deposition disease, galactosemia, pentosuria, Type I hyperlipoproteinemia, alcaptonuria, and xanthinuria are examples of the operation of the "one-gene, one-enzyme" hypothesis (Beadle and Tatum).

In addition, Part XVII includes examples of disorders of more than one gene (in association with envoronmental influences). The inheritance of gout may be polygenic. The endogenous hyperlipemias (Types IIb and IV hyperlipoproteinemia) represent several genotypes. There is heterogeneity of the mutations that lead to the enzyme deficiency present in the Lesch-Nyhan syndrome. The reader will observe that many of the diseases of metabolism are rare (not diabetes mellitus, with a prevalence in the United States of about 5 per cent, but, for example, primary hyperoxaluria, of which there are fewer than 200 reported cases) or of no clinical importance (fructosuria, pentosuria). If apologies are needed, one might offer these: (1) study of rare diseases has very often made possible a better understanding of normal metabolic processes (certain aminoacidurias); (2) discovery of some of these rare conditions early enough in life may lead to prevention of clinical disease simply by adjustment of the diet (galactosemia, phenylketonuria; (3) precise identification of a rare enzyme deficiency may lead to methods for replacement therapy with that enzyme (Fabry's disease); and (4) no disease is rare to the patient who has it.

Bernard, C.: An Introduction to the Study of Experimental Medicine (translated by H. L. Green). New York, Dover Publications, 1957, p. viii.

Bondy, P. K., and Rosenberg, L. E. (eds.): Duncan's Diseases of Metabolism. 7th ed. Philadelphia, W. B. Saunders Company, 1974.

Brady, R. O., Tallman, J. F., Johnson, W. G., Gal, A. E., Leahy, W. R., Quirk, J. M., and Dekaban, A. S.: Replacement therapy for inherited enzyme deficiency. Use of purified ceramidetrihexosidase in Fabry's disease. N. Engl. J. Med., 289:9, 1973.

Frimpter, G. W.: Aminoacidurias due to inherited disorders of metabolism. N. Engl. J. Med., 289:835, 895, 1973.

Garrod, A. E.: Inborn errors of metabolism (Croonian Lectures). Lancet, 2:1, 73, 142, 214, 1908.

---

*Part XXI includes conditions which are difficult to classify under standard categories and in which the biochemical defect is in most instances not completely understood (e.g., Marfan's syndrome, dysautonomia).

Seegmiller, J. E.: New prospects for understanding and control of genetic diseases. Arch. Intern. Med., 130:181, 1972.

Smith, L. H.: Pyrimidine metabolism in man. N. Engl. J. Med., 288:764, 1973.

Stanbury, J. B., Wyngaarden, J. B., and Fredrickson, D. S. (eds.): The Metabolic Basis of Inherited Disease. 3rd ed. New York, McGraw-Hill Book Company, 1972.

Tatum, E. L.: A case history in biological research. Science, 129:1711, 1959.

805. DISORDERS OF FLUID, ELECTROLYTE, AND ACID-BASE BALANCE

William B. Schwartz

Fluid and electrolyte disturbances usually occur as complications of an underlying illness, and the disorders to be considered in this chapter must therefore be viewed not as isolated entities but in the context of the specific clinical settings in which they appear.

As general background to the following discussion, it should be recalled that the water content of the body (approximately 50 to 60 per cent of body weight) is distributed between the intracellular and the extracellular compartments. Approximately two thirds of the water is within cells, and the remaining third is divided between the interstitial space and plasma, which together comprise the extracellular compartment. Water moves freely across cell boundaries, and for this reason changes in tonicity in one compartment induce a transfer of fluid that continues until a new steady state of osmotic equilibrium is established. By contrast, electrolytes are distributed in an asymmetric pattern, most of the ions in the extracellular fluid consisting of sodium, chloride, and bicarbonate and those in the intracellular fluid of potassium and organic anions. Except for the slight deviations attributable to the Donnan effect of the plasma proteins, the electrolyte compositions of plasma and interstitial fluid are virtually identical. Thus for clinical purposes plasma composition can be taken as representative of the entire extracellular compartment.

Ch. 601 and 602 summarize the renal regulation of electrolyte and acid-base equilibrium. In the present chapter relevant physiology will be presented entirely within the context of the clinical disorder under consideration.

DEPLETION OF VOLUME

The most common disturbance of fluid and electrolyte equilibrium is volume depletion. Loss of volume may occur from simple dehydration, but is seen more frequently in association with a combined loss of water and electrolytes.

Clinical Manifestations. The symptoms of volume depletion are few and nonspecific. The patient may complain of thirst, especially if the body fluids are hypertonic, but nausea, light-headedness, and weakness are perhaps the most frequent and troublesome manifesta-

tions. The major effects of volume depletion are on the circulation and on renal function. As plasma volume is diminished, blood pressure falls, heart rate rises, and a decrease in renal perfusion leads to oliguria and azotemia. When volume depletion is severe, profound shock becomes an immediate and serious threat to survival. The management of these clinical problems will be discussed after the individual causes of volume depletion have been considered.

Pathogenesis. The specific clinical circumstances in which volume depletion is encountered are listed in Table 1. These are discussed in the succeeding paragraphs.

Simple Dehydration (Loss of Water Without Electrolyte). The fluid requirement of the body is determined by the insensible losses through skin and lungs and by the amount of water that is required to excrete the daily solute load. Ordinarily the minimal intake that will serve to maintain water balance is 700 to 1000 ml per day. Thirst ordinarily serves to maintain water intake well above this basal level; but if weakness or disability sharply curtails fluid intake, dehydration will develop. The magnitude of the fluid deficit will be aggravated when insensible losses are increased by factors such as fever and hyperventilation or when urinary losses are abnormally large—for example, in uncontrolled diabetes insipidus.

Whenever water is lost in excess of electrolyte, hypertonicity and elevation of the serum sodium concentration accompany the depletion of volume. The clinical features and consequences of hypernatremia are discussed later in this chapter.

Combined Depletion of Water and Sodium. Severe volume deficits occur most commonly in patients who have suffered a combined loss of water and sodium, usually from the gastrointestinal tract, the kidneys, or the skin.

GASTROINTESTINAL LOSSES. Volume depletion may occur as the result of losses from any portion of the gastrointestinal tract. Gastrointestinal secretions normally amount to some 8 to 10 liters per day, and, if the body is deprived of a significant fraction of this total, severe volume depletion will result. Depletion is most commonly the consequence of vomiting, gastric drainage, or diarrhea. It also is seen with small-bowel drainage, ileostomy, colostomy, and pancreatic or biliary fistulas.

TABLE 1. Causes of Volume Depletion

Simple dehydration
  (Loss of water without electrolyte)

Combined depletion of water and sodium
  Gastrointestinal losses
    Vomiting
    Gastric or small bowel drainage
    Diarrhea
    Bowel fistulas (colostomy, ileostomy, etc.)
  Renal losses
    Chronic renal failure
    Diuretic phase of acute tubular necrosis
    Postobstructive nephropathy
    Adrenal insufficiency
    Osmotic diuresis
    Diuretics
  Skin losses
    Sweating
    Burns
  Paracentesis

Most gastrointestinal secretions are either isotonic or slightly hypotonic and, for this reason, enteric losses per se should not produce a striking change in serum sodium concentration. However, because serum sodium concentration is ultimately determined by over-all water balance (as influenced by fluid intake, skin losses, etc.), either hyponatremia or hypernatremia may be encountered.

RENAL LOSSES. Patients with *chronic renal failure* commonly have a reduced ability to conserve sodium, but the sodium-wasting tendency is seldom severe enough to become apparent if dietary intake of salt is normal. If salt intake is restricted, however, continued excretion of sodium and the associated loss of water may produce severe depletion of extracellular volume. Contraction of volume, in turn, causes a further reduction in glomerular filtration rate, and may even precipitate frank uremia. Sodium intake in the azotemic patient should not be curtailed, therefore, without careful sequential observations of body weight and sodium excretion.

An occasional patient wastes sodium even while ingesting a normal quantity of salt; most of these appear to have *medullary cystic disease* as their underlying renal lesion. In such cases of severe salt-wasting, the diet must be supplemented with sodium chloride if volume depletion is to be avoided. It is important to remember that in the patient with renal disease volume depletion should always be considered as a possible explanation for a sudden, otherwise unexplained increase in azotemia.

During the *diuretic phase of acute tubular necrosis* a defect in the ability of the damaged tubules to reabsorb sodium may lead to a considerable loss of sodium and water. Sodium wasting does not usually persist for more than several days, and is not likely to become clinically significant if the patient is taking a diet of normal salt content. At times it may be difficult to distinguish between an abnormal diuresis and the physiologic diuresis that will occur if an excessive quantity of fluid and electrolyte has been administered during the oliguric phase of the disease. If one is uncertain about the cause, treatment can ordinarily be delayed for a day or two until the issue is resolved either by the cessation of the diuresis or by the appearance of early signs of volume depletion. In this way an unnecessary and prolonged cycle of saline loading and saline loss can be avoided. A similar period of uncontrolled sodium and fluid loss by the kidney may be observed during *acute rejection episodes* after renal transplantation.

Postobstructive nephropathy occasionally produces severe sodium and volume depletion in patients in whom complete or nearly complete obstruction has been present for a prolonged period. The defect in sodium reabsorption results from tubular damage, and becomes manifest promptly after the relief of obstruction permits the filtered load of sodium to increase. Loss of salt may lead to an obligatory diuresis of as much as 5 or 10 liters per day and, thus, to an acute contraction of extracellular and plasma volume. Just as with the diuretic phase of acute tubular necrosis, the disorder is usually self-limiting, because the tubules generally recover their capacity to transport sodium within a few days.

Volume depletion consequent to excessive renal losses of fluid and electrolyte may also occur in the absence of structural renal disease. In patients with *adrenal insufficiency* (Addison's disease) a deficiency of salt-retaining steroids reduces the activity of renal transport mechanisms, and may allow large quantities of sodium and water to escape into the urine. Continued administration of *diuretics* to the patient who has been but is no longer edematous will also sometimes produce volume depletion.

Abnormal losses of sodium and water are also induced by the obligatory excretion of a large solute load. Such an osmotic diuresis is seen most frequently in association with the glycosuria of *diabetic ketoacidosis* (see Ch. 806) and of *nonketotic hyperosmolar coma*. This latter disorder typically occurs in middle-aged or elderly mild diabetics and is characterized by hyperglycemia, hyperosmolality, and profound dehydration. Blood sugar is often in the range of 1000 mg per 100 ml, but the disorder is readily distinguished from diabetic coma by the absence of ketoacidosis. Salt and water depletion caused by osmotic diuresis also sometimes occurs with administration of *tube feedings containing large quantities of protein*. Repeated infusions of *mannitol* may have the same effects.

SKIN LOSSES. Large losses of water and electrolyte from the skin may result either from excessive sweating or from burns. *Sweat* is a hypotonic solution normally containing no more than 50 mEq of sodium per liter, and for this reason sweating will produce a relatively larger deficit of water than of sodium. *Burns* can lead to two types of deficits: isotonic extracellular fluid may be lost by transudation; and water may be lost without electrolyte as the result of increased evaporation through damaged epithelium. An additional factor contributing to a severe depletion of circulating volume is the capillary damage that results in the interstitial accumulation of fluid, particularly during the first days after the burn has occurred. Such fluid loss, because it takes place internally, can readily be overlooked.

PARACENTESIS. An occasional patient with cirrhosis and ascites has been noted to develop circulatory collapse after *paracentesis*. Reduction of pressure within the peritoneal cavity may allow transudation of a large quantity of fluid with consequent contraction of plasma volume. Clinically significant contraction is not likely to occur in patients who have a substantial amount of peripheral edema, apparently because plasma volume can be readily replenished by transfer of fluid from the expanded interstitial space.

Diagnosis. The *history* is frequently of great value in an appraisal of the origin and magnitude of a volume deficit. The patient should be questioned closely about fluid intake and about losses of fluid that may have resulted from vomiting, diarrhea, sweating, polyuria, or other disturbances. In many cases, particularly when a reliable history is not available, *physical examination* is the single most valuable diagnostic tool. Reduction in turgor of the skin, particularly over the arms, legs, and face, is the most characteristic finding, and is usually accompanied by postural hypotension. The facies are usually pinched, and the tongue is dry. Lowered tension of the eyeballs, a rapid resting pulse, and hypotension in the recumbent position may be observed when dehydration is severe.

Laboratory findings are likely to be of less value. The serum sodium concentration reflects only the ratio of sodium to water and, whether low, normal, or high, gives no insight into the total volume of extracellular fluid present. Elevated hematocrit and hemoglobin concentrations suggest that plasma volume is contracted, but, unless the values before the acute illness are known, the interpretation of these data is likely to be difficult. The plasma creatinine concentration is sometimes helpful, because it may provide evidence of volume depletion and impairment of renal function even before the appearance of oliguria. The blood urea nitrogen level is a less useful index of renal dysfunction, because the urea concentration can be elevated by external factors, such as fever or an excess of adrenal corticoids.

Once the diagnosis of a sodium and water deficit has been made, measurements of sodium excretion may help to identify the source of the losses. If the depletion is of *extrarenal* origin, the contraction in volume will normally lead to relatively prompt and efficient conservation of sodium by the kidney. Increased secretion of aldosterone, a fall in glomerular filtration rate, and other as yet undefined factors augment sodium reabsorption and reduce sodium excretion to less than 5 or 10 mEq per day. If the excretion of sodium exceeds 30 to 40 mEq per day, it can generally be concluded that the losses are of *renal* origin and are the result of primary renal disease, Addison's disease, or osmotic diuresis. It should be noted, however, that if the contraction of volume is sufficiently severe to produce oliguria and a marked reduction in filtration rate, sodium excretion will sometimes fall to a low level even in disorders in which the underlying abnormality is defective renal conservation of sodium.

Treatment. The most serious threat to the patient with severe volume depletion is circulatory collapse, and the most immediate concern in treatment is restoration of an adequate blood volume and blood pressure. This goal can be accomplished most effectively by the rapid infusion of plasma (if the hematocrit is elevated) or blood. If neither plasma nor blood is available, isotonic saline solution should be given instead; saline is not an entirely satisfactory substitute, however, because a large fraction of administered salt and water is promptly lost from the circulation as it diffuses into the interstitial space.

After shock has been corrected, the remaining fluid and electrolyte abnormalities can be repaired in a more leisurely fashion. Close observation of skin turgor, body weight, blood pressure, and serum creatinine concentration will, together with available information concerning the volume and composition of the losses, provide the most reliable guide to replacement therapy. In some cases as much as 4 or 5 liters of fluid will be required to correct the volume deficit. If serum sodium is within normal limits (indicating a virtually equivalent deficit of sodium and water), repair should be carried out largely with isotonic saline solution, water without electrolyte being given only as needed to replace insensible and renal losses occurring during the period of treatment. Even if serum sodium concentration is moderately abnormal (as low as 130 mEq or as high as 150 mEq per liter), the same approach to therapy can be employed as in the patient with isotonic contraction of extracellular volume. If isotonic saline solution and modest quantities of water are administered, the kidney can be relied upon for final adjustment of both volume and tonicity. With gross deviations in sodium concentration, more specific measures will be necessary. Severe hyper-natremia will require the provision of considerably more water than salt and, conversely, severe hyponatremia (in the absence of edema) will call for correction, or partial correction, by administration of hypertonic sodium chloride solution. The management of hypernatremia and hyponatremia is discussed in detail later in this chapter.

The composition of the repair solutions must also allow for the presence of other electrolyte abnormalities. For example, if metabolic acidosis is present, the sodium deficit should be corrected in part with sodium bicarbonate rather than exclusively with sodium chloride.

Treatment of the patient with *nonketotic hyperosmolar coma* requires not only appropriate correction of the fluid and electrolyte deficits but also the administration of adequate amounts of insulin in order to deal with the hyperglycemia. Some observers have suggested that the amount of insulin required is less than that in the patient with diabetic ketoacidosis, but this question remains to be clarified.

Arieff, A. I., and Carroll, H. J.: Nonketotic hyperosmolar coma with hyperglycemia: Clinical features, pathophysiology, renal function, acid-base balance, plasma–cerebrospinal fluid equilibria and the effects of therapy in 37 cases. Medicine, 51:73, 1972.

Bricker, N. S., and Klahr, S.: Obstructive nephropathy. *In* Strauss, M. B., and Welt, L. G. (eds.): Diseases of the Kidney. 2nd ed. Boston, Little, Brown & Company, 1971, pp. 1018–1020.

Gault, M. H., Dixon, M. E., Doyle, M., and Cohen, W. M.: Hypernatremia, azotemia, and dehydration due to high-protein tube feeding. Ann. Intern. Med., 68:778, 1968.

HYPONATREMIA

Sodium is the ion present in highest concentration in the extracellular fluid, and sodium salts are thus the primary determinant of the osmolality (tonicity) of the extracellular compartment. Changes in sodium concentration thus have a major influence on the distribution of water between the intracellular and extracellular spaces.

Normally, serum sodium concentration is stabilized at approximately 140 mEq per liter by changes in water balance that occur in response to variations in plasma osmotic pressure. A slight increase in sodium concentration, and in osmotic pressure, leads to the release of antidiuretic hormone and to a retention of water that then restores normal tonicity. Conversely, a slight reduction in serum sodium concentration and osmotic pressure inhibits the release of hormone and permits any excess water to be excreted.

A variety of disturbances can lead to an abnormal and sustained reduction in serum sodium concentration. Retention of water without sodium, loss of sodium without a proportional loss of water, and redistribution of water between cells and extracellular fluid may each induce hyponatremia. As pointed out earlier, serum sodium concentration yields no direct information concerning the state of total sodium stores, but indicates only that there has been a disturbance in the ratio of sodium to water.

The specific causes of hyponatremia and the mechanisms that underlie their development are described in detail below. It is convenient, however, to consider first the clinical manifestations and the aspects of treatment that are common to all hypo-osmotic states.

Clinical Manifestations. The signs and symptoms of the hypo-osmotic state are those of *water intoxication,* and are apparently caused by movement of fluid from the extracellular space into the relatively more hypertonic cells. When serum sodium concentration falls to approximately 120 mEq per liter, the patient frequently becomes irritable and confused. More serious disturbances are seen if the sodium concentration falls to 110 mEq or below; the patient often becomes lethargic or comatose, and generalized convulsions develop. Death may result unless appropriate treatment is promptly instituted.

Treatment. Severe hyponatremia is best treated by the intravenous administration of hypertonic (5 per cent) sodium chloride. Elevation of serum sodium concentration to a level of 125 or 130 mEq per liter will ordinarily suffice to eliminate all evidence of central nervous system dysfunction. Full correction of hyponatremia need not and should not be carried out over a short time, because the sudden transfer of a large volume of fluid from the intracellular to the extracellular space is sometimes hazardous; an abrupt expansion of plasma volume may elevate central venous pressure and produce symptomatic pulmonary congestion, particularly in the patient with frank or latent heart disease.

Calculation of the amount of salt necessary to produce a given rise in sodium concentration must take into consideration the shift of water that will be induced by the increase in extracellular tonicity. As serum sodium concentration is elevated, water moves out of cells along the resulting osmotic gradient; the estimated sodium requirement must therefore be based on the need to restore tonicity throughout the total body water. The following is an illustrative example of this calculation, assuming an initial serum sodium concentration of 110 mEq per liter, a final concentration of 125 mEq per liter, and a body weight of 70 kg. Since approximately 50 per cent of the total body weight is water, the amount of sodium necessary to produce the desired change will be 35 liters × 15 mEq per liter, or approximately 500 mEq of sodium. The calculation can be summarized by the following equation:

$$[\text{Desired Na conc.} - \text{initial Na conc.}] \times 0.5 \text{ body weight} = \text{mEq of Na}$$

Pathogenesis. Table 2 lists the specific clinical circumstances in which a low sodium concentration is encountered. These are discussed in the succeeding paragraphs.

TABLE 2. Causes of Hyponatremia

1. Functional disorders leading to defective excretion of water
    Depletion of sodium and extracellular fluid volume
    Inappropriate secretion of antidiuretic hormone
    Addison's disease
2. Renal disease with defective excretion of water
    Acute renal failure with oliguria
    Chronic renal failure
3. Idiopathic hyponatremia
    Congestive heart failure
    Cirrhosis of the liver
4. Excessive water intake in the presence of normal renal function
    Psychogenic polydipsia
5. Hyponatremia without disturbance in water balance
    Accumulation of solute in the extracellular fluid
    Pseudohyponatremia

Functional Disorders Leading to Defective Excretion of Water. DEPLETION OF SODIUM AND EXTRACELLULAR VOLUME. Significant impairment of water excretion often results from severe depletion of sodium and volume, thus predisposing to the development of hyponatremia. If water is ingested or infused without electrolyte, the retention of a portion of this water leads to a fall in serum sodium concentration. This sequence of events accounts for the frequent occurrence of hyponatremia in conditions such as vomiting or diarrhea. It appears probable that a reduction in glomerular filtration rate, with a consequent reduced delivery of sodium and water to the distal nephron, accounts for the failure to excrete an appropriately dilute urine and for the persistence of hyponatremia.

In most patients with volume depletion, the water intake is not large enough to produce hyponatremia of great severity, serum sodium concentration decreasing by no more than 10 or 15 mEq per liter. In such cases the manifestations of volume depletion rather than hyponatremia usually dominate the clinical picture, and treatment should be aimed primarily at correction of extracellular volume rather than at elevating serum sodium concentration. As discussed earlier, if sodium concentration is only moderately reduced, correction of hyponatremia will occur as a by-product of expansion with isotonic saline solution; restoration of normal plasma volume will correct the renal defect in water excretion, and an augmented water output will then restore tonicity to normal.

INAPPROPRIATE SECRETION OF ANTIDIURETIC HORMONE. This term describes a condition in which hypotonicity of the plasma fails to suppress the release of antidiuretic hormone, with the result that renal excretion of water is impaired. The consequent expansion of extracellular volume not only causes dilution of body fluids but also induces a sodium diuresis and a negative sodium balance. The increase in sodium excretion in response to expansion of volume is apparently mediated by elevation of glomerular filtration rate and other as yet poorly defined factors (e.g., "third factor"). The combination of water retention and salt wasting produces a decrease in serum sodium concentration, serum levels occasionally falling to as low as 110 or even 100 mEq per liter.

The syndrome of inappropriate secretion of antidiuretic hormone (SIADH) has been noted most often in association with bronchogenic carcinoma of the oat cell type but has also been seen in patients with other malignant tumors (e.g., carcinoma of the pancreas). In such patients it appears that the production by the tumor of vasopressin or a vasopressin-like polypeptide is responsible for the abnormal fluid retention. The syndrome is also seen in a variety of other clinical settings, most notably in association with central nervous system disturbances (e.g., head injuries, brain tumors, encephalitis) and lung disease (e.g., cavitating tuberculosis, pneumonia). In each of these conditions, the retention of water apparently results from an aberrant stimulus to ADH release, that is, from a signal which bypasses the osmoreceptors of the hypothalamus. In addition, SIADH can occur in association with the administration of drugs, particularly chlorpropamide, vincristine, and cyclophosphamide. The syndrome occasionally occurs in the absence of a detectable underlying illness.

The following features are virtually diagnostic of SIADH: (1) hyponatremia with renal sodium wasting;

(2) normal tissue turgor and normal blood pressure; (3) normal blood urea nitrogen and creatinine concentrations; (4) normal adrenal function; and (5) specific gravity of the urine inappropriately high for a hypotonic subject, that is, in excess of 1.002 or 1.003. Edema is not a usual feature, because water retention does not ordinarily exceed 3 or 4 liters and because a large fraction of the retained fluid probably moves into cells.

It should be noted that although sodium loss is a classic feature of SIADH, the presence of a significant quantity of sodium in the urine is not a prerequisite for the diagnosis of the syndrome. As serum sodium concentration falls, a new balance is struck between the reduced filtered load of sodium and the reduced renal capacity for sodium reabsorption. Thus when a new steady state of serum sodium concentration has been achieved, the urine will become virtually sodium free if sodium intake is extremely low. The salt-wasting abnormality can, however, be readily unmasked by the administration of salt either by mouth or by vein.

When serum sodium concentration is so low that it produces signs of severe water intoxication (such as coma or convulsions), hypertonic sodium chloride solution should immediately be infused to raise plasma osmotic pressure. Since administered salt will rapidly be excreted if expansion of extracellular volume persists, one should also promptly undertake correction of the state of overhydration. Diuretic therapy with an agent such as furosemide is an effective means of producing such volume contraction and, when combined with hypertonic salt infusion, will produce a rapid and sustained elevation of serum sodium concentration.

If severe manifestations of water intoxication are not present, appropriate treatment consists simply of restricting fluid intake and allowing insensible and urinary losses of water to contract the volume of extracellular fluid. This program of management not only will restore the capacity for normal renal conservation of sodium but will also correct that component of hyponatremia which has developed as a consequence of dilution. Correction of that element of the hyponatremia caused by renal sodium loss does, of course, require provision of salt either by mouth or by vein. It should be emphasized that fluid restriction will not be effective unless it is stringent enough to produce a loss of several kilograms in weight. An intake of 400 to 500 ml per day over three to five days will usually accomplish this goal.

If the patient fails to conserve sodium subsequent to a large loss of weight, the diagnosis of SIADH must be called into serious question, and other disorders, in particular Addison's disease, must be considered. Addison's disease, it should be noted, can easily be overlooked unless one recognizes that sodium depletion in adrenal insufficiency need not be accompanied by volume depletion; in some patients the deficiency of cortisol causes an impairment of water excretion of such magnitude that, despite the loss of sodium, hydration remains normal. In such patients the clinical picture can closely mimic SIADH. For this reason, it is always advisable to carry out studies of adrenal function before concluding that the hyponatremia is due to inappropriate secretion of antidiuretic hormone.

In a disorder such as meningitis or pneumonitis, the water-excreting defect disappears as recovery from the underlying illness takes place. With permanent brain damage, or with carcinoma of the lung, the defect can persist indefinitely, and a moderate degree of water restriction may be necessary to prevent recurrence of severe hyponatremia and salt wasting.

Whether the transient water retention and hyponatremia frequently encountered in the postoperative state are the result of an inappropriate secretion of antidiuretic hormone remains to be determined.

Renal Disease with Defective Excretion of Water. During the oliguric phase of *acute renal failure* dilutional hyponatremia will regularly occur if fluid intake is not adequately restricted. The net loss of water from skin and lungs is normally about 400 to 500 ml per day, and if severe oliguria or anuria is present, administration of significantly more than this quantity (for example, 1000 to 1200 ml) will produce overhydration within a relatively short time.

Water intoxication is occasionally seen in *chronic renal failure,* and occurs primarily in patients who have been urged to ingest large quantities of fluid in an effort to increase urine volume and thus to promote urea excretion. Such attempts to force a diuresis not only may be hazardous, but also appear to have little beneficial effect on the clinical course, even when they produce a slight reduction in blood urea concentration.

Idiopathic Hyponatremia. Hyponatremia frequently appears without warning in the edematous patient entering the late stages of *congestive heart failure* or *cirrhosis of the liver.* In this setting it is an ominous prognostic sign that appears to be the reflection (rather than the cause) of the underlying clinical deterioration.

The factors responsible for this electrolyte disturbance have not been clearly defined. Salt depletion induced by diuretic therapy cannot be held accountable, because the edematous patient has a larger than normal quantity of sodium in his extracellular space and, in theory, could readily restore plasma sodium concentration to normal simply by excreting surplus water. Furthermore, the disorder has been observed in patients who have not received diuretics or in whom diuretics have failed to promote salt excretion. In some cases it can be demonstrated that retention of water is responsible for the hyponatremic state, but in others measurements of body weight give no evidence that fluid was retained during the period that sodium concentration fell. In the latter circumstance it has been proposed that a primary reduction in intracellular osmolality allows water to shift into the extracellular space and that the lowered osmotic pressure of the plasma is simply a passive reflection of the change in cellular tonicity. According to this thesis, failure to increase the excretion of water is explained by the absence of an osmotic gradient between plasma and the osmoreceptors of the hypothalamus.

In some patients with congestive heart failure or cirrhosis, the development of hyponatremia is apparently an indirect consequence of enhanced proximal reabsorption of sodium and water; the delivery of an abnormally small volume of glomerular filtrate from the proximal tubule to the distal nephron prevents the elaboration of a hypotonic urine and leads to pathologic water retention. Inappropriate secretion of antidiuretic hormone has also been invoked as a factor in the genesis of the hyponatremia, but clear support for this hypothesis has yet to be obtained.

As noted above, the appearance of hyponatremia in

the edematous patient is usually a grave prognostic sign. Even if the patient does not appear to be critically ill, prolonged survival is uncommon unless treatment directed toward improvement of the underlying cardiac or liver disease is successful. Elevation of the serum sodium concentration by either water restriction or the administration of hypertonic sodium chloride usually has no beneficial effect. Water restriction usually induces severe thirst before osmolality is restored to normal, and if the patient is then permitted to increase his fluid intake, he quickly re-establishes the hyponatremic state. The administration of hypertonic saline not only seems to be of little clinical value, but appears, in many instances, to hasten rather than retard the downward clinical course.

Hyponatremia of unknown cause is sometimes seen in seriously ill patients with a debilitating disease such as metastatic carcinoma or leukemia. Neither dehydration nor edema is present, and there is no evidence of extrarenal or urinary loss of sodium. The explanation for this disturbance is obscure.

Excessive Water Intake in the Presence of Normal Renal Function (Psychogenic Polydipsia). A syndrome virtually identical to that already described for inappropriate secretion of antidiuretic hormone may be produced by the ingestion of more water than the normal kidney can excrete; that is, more than 1000 or 1200 ml per hour. Intakes in excess of these amounts are unusual, but are occasionally seen in patients who have a severe psychiatric illness. In such cases the expansion of extracellular volume induced by the positive water balance leads to both hyponatremia and renal wasting of sodium. Characteristically, the urine is maximally dilute (specific gravity of 1.001), and it is this finding that unequivocally demonstrates that the syndrome is the result of excessive ingestion of water rather than of inappropriate secretion of antidiuretic hormone.

If signs of water intoxication are present, hypertonic saline solution should be given intravenously, but in most cases reduction of water intake and increased ingestion of salt will be the only treatment required.

Hyponatremia Without Disturbance in Water Balance. ACCUMULATION OF SOLUTE IN THE EXTRACELLULAR FLUID. Solutes such as glucose and mannitol, which do not distribute freely throughout body water, can accumulate in the extracellular space and create an osmotic gradient between cells and interstitial fluid. As a result, water shifts from the intracellular compartment, and the serum sodium concentration falls. Hyponatremia resulting from such a redistribution of fluid is a characteristic feature of the severe hyperglycemia seen in patients with uncontrolled diabetes mellitus; each 100 mg per 100 ml increment in blood sugar concentration above normal respresents the addition of slightly more than 5 milliosmoles of solute per kilogram to the extracellular compartment, and leads to a reduction in serum sodium concentration of approximately 1.5 mEq per liter. A blood sugar concentration of 1000 mg per 100 ml can thus be expected to lower sodium concentration from 140 to 126 mEq per liter. Failure to consider the role of hyperglycemia in the genesis of hyponatremia in the diabetic can lead to the administration of an excessive amount of sodium during the treatment of ketoacidosis.

The accumulation of mannitol in the extracellular fluid can also cause a shift of water sufficient to reduce serum sodium concentration. This problem is most likely to be encountered in the patient with acute renal failure in whom an unsuccessful attempt has been made to increase urine volume by repeated mannitol infusions.

Hyperosmolality will *not* produce hyponatremia if the solute distributes freely across cell membranes, and thus increases the osmolality of cells and interstitial fluid to a proportional degree. In uremia, for example, serum sodium concentration is unaffected by the hypertonicity induced by urea accumulation because urea penetrates cells readily, and its concentration is elevated throughout body water.

PSEUDOHYPONATREMIA. Pseudohyponatremia refers to a spurious reduction in sodium concentration resulting from a displacement of some fraction of plasma water by an abnormal accumulation of lipid or protein. Although plasma sodium concentration is usually measured as milliequivalents per liter of plasma, the physiologically significant measurement is the sodium concentration expressed as milliequivalents per kilogram of plasma water. Thus a sodium concentration of 140 mEq per liter, as measured on whole plasma, reflects an actual concentration of 150 mEq per kilogram of water in normal plasma containing 93 per cent water. Since the percentage of plasma that is water does not vary appreciably under most circumstances, reductions in plasma sodium concentration can generally be taken as reflecting a decrease in the sodium concentration per unit of plasma water and in the tonicity of extracellular fluid. On the other hand, if severe hyperlipemia (or hyperproteinemia) is present, the fraction of plasma that is water will be lower than normal, and a striking reduction in the sodium concentration per unit volume of plasma will be observed despite the absence of a significant change in the electrolyte concentration per kilogram of plasma water.

Hyperlipemia of sufficient magnitude to produce pseudohyponatremia occurs in a number of diseases, including diabetes mellitus, nephrotic syndrome, and biliary cirrhosis. In nearly all cases in which sodium concentration is reduced by lipidemia the plasma is frankly lactescent, and lactescence will thus often be the first finding that points to the correct diagnosis. *Hyperproteinemia* severe enough to cause pseudohyponatremia is a rare occurrence, and has been seen only in multiple myeloma. In this disease the plasma sodium concentration may be lowered to a value of 125 or 130 mEq per liter.

The contribution of an increased concentration of lipid or protein to a reduced plasma sodium concentration can be readily assessed by determination of plasma osmotic pressure (estimated from freezing-point depression). If osmotic pressure is normal despite the hyponatremia, it will be evident that the concentration of sodium in the aqueous phase of plasma is normal.

Aviram, A., Pfau, A., Czaczkes, J. W., and Ullmann, T. D.: Hyperosmolality with hyponatremia, caused by inappropriate administration of mannitol. Am. J. Med., 42:648, 1967.

Bartter, F., and Schwartz, W. B.: The syndrome of inappropriate secretion of antidiuretic hormone. Am. J. Med., 42:790, 1967.

Harrington, J. T., and Cohen, J. J.: Clinical disorders of urine concentration and dilution. Arch. Intern. Med., 131:810, 1973.

Langgard, H., and Smith, W. O.: Self-induced water intoxication without predisposing illness. N. Engl. J. Med., 266:378, 1962.

Leaf, A.: The clinical and physiologic significance of the serum sodium concentration. N. Engl. J. Med., 267:24, 1962.

Tarail, R., Buchwald, K. W., Holland, J. F., and Selawry, O. S.: Misleading reductions of serum sodium and chloride associated with hyperproteinemia in patients with multiple myeloma. Proc. Soc. Exp. Biol. Med., 110:145, 1962.

HYPERNATREMIA

Virtually all cases of hypernatremia result from a loss of water that produces a relative excess of sodium in the body fluids. Any hypotonic loss, such as that occurring with sweating or vomiting, will cause a modest degree of hypernatremia which will persist if adequate fluid replacement is not provided. Extreme elevations of plasma sodium concentrations (160 mEq per liter or above) are uncommon and are usually encountered in only one of three clinical settings: decreased or absent fluid intake, diabetes insipidus, or osmotic diuresis. Such extreme increases in tonicity of the extracellular fluid, when they occur, lead to marked cellular dehydration.

The most common cause of hypernatremia is a fluid intake that is inadequate to replace urinary losses and insensible losses of water from skin and lungs. This problem is most frequently encountered in the patient who is stuporous or who has some other disability that prevents him from drinking normally. In the comatose patient in whom *diabetes insipidus* develops after a head injury or a neurosurgical procedure, a large negative water balance is likely to appear with unusual speed. In most cases of diabetes insipidus, polyuria will quickly draw attention to the nature of the problem, but if solute intake is low, the diagnosis can readily be overlooked, because urine volume may not exceed 2 or 3 liters per day.

Osmotic loading can also produce severe hypernatremia. During osmotic diuresis water is lost in excess of sodium, and with sustained or repeated diuresis the serum sodium concentration sometimes rises to values greater than 175 mEq per liter. This sequence of events is often observed in comatose patients who are confronted with a massive urea load as the result of being given tube feedings containing large amounts of protein. In such patients maintenance of a normal urine volume by continued solute loading may sometimes obscure the fact that dehydration and hypertonicity are present. Under such circumstances, the progressive loss of weight, the physical signs of volume depletion, and the development of hypernatremia should draw attention to the correct diagnosis.

The specific signs and symptoms produced by a marked elevation of serum sodium concentration have not been clearly defined; most patients with hypernatremia are already seriously ill and the role of the hypertonicity, as distinguished from that of the underlying disease, is frequently difficult to evaluate. Clinical experience suggests, however, that when hypernatremia is encountered water should be administered (either orally or as 5 per cent glucose intravenously) in quantities sufficient to restore serum sodium concentration to normal. The quantity of water required must be calculated with an appreciation that hypertonicity is present not only in the extracellular fluid but throughout total body water. Thus a 70-kg man with a plasma sodium concentration of 170 mEq per liter will require a 20 per cent expansion of body water, that is, 8 liters of fluid, to restore serum sodium concentration to a normal value of 140 mEq per liter. Observations during the treatment of hypernatremia indicate that full correction should not be carried out rapidly, i.e., over a few hours, because a rapid reduction in tonicity may produce signs of water intoxication.

Gault, M. H., Dixon, E. E., Doyle, M., and Cohen, W. M.: Hypernatremia, azotemia, and dehydration due to high-protein tube feeding. Ann. Intern. Med., 68:778, 1968.

Leaf, A.: The clinical and physiologic significance of the serum sodium concentration. N. Engl. J. Med., 267:24, 1962.

Ross, E. J., and Christie, S. B. M.: Hypernatremia. Medicine, 48:441, 1969.

Weiner, M., and Epstein, F. H.: Signs and symptoms of electrolyte disorders. Yale J. Biol. Med., 43:76, 1970.

DISTURBANCES OF POTASSIUM EQUILIBRIUM

Potassium, the major intracellular cation, plays a significant part in control of osmotic pressure, and also serves as an essential activator in a number of enzymatic reactions. In addition, the potassium concentration of body fluids has an important influence on the excitability of both skeletal and cardiac muscle and on the structure and function of the kidneys. Disturbances in potassium equilibrium may therefore produce a wide range of clinical disorders.

The potassium concentration in extracellular fluid is normally 3.8 to 5 mEq per liter and in intracellular fluid approximately 150 mEq per liter. Since about 20 per cent of body weight is extracellular fluid, it can readily be calculated that only a small fraction of the 2500 to 3000 mEq of potassium within the body is contained in the extracellular space. On the other hand, changes in plasma potassium concentration often mirror changes in cellular potassium content, and plasma concentration thus usually provides a useful clinical guide to disturbances in potassium balance. Furthermore, relatively small absolute changes in extracellular concentration, by producing large differences in the ratio of intracellular to extracellular potassium, may have important effects on neuromuscular activity.

Despite the usual wide variations in dietary intake of potassium (40 to 120 mEq per day), plasma potassium concentration is normally stabilized within the narrow range of 4 to 5 mEq per liter by virtue of close renal regulation of potassium balance. As discussed earlier, renal potassium excretion is accomplished largely, if not exclusively, by a process of potassium secretion in the distal portion of the nephron; it has been demonstrated that essentially all filtered potassium is reabsorbed in the proximal tubule and that the potassium that appears in the urine is added to the filtrate by a distal process of sodium-cation exchange. Fecal excretion of potassium normally amounts to only a few milliequivalents per day and does not play a significant role in potassium homeostasis.

If a large potassium load is suddenly administered, renal mechanisms do not respond quickly enough to prevent a rise in serum potassium concentration to abnormal levels. Under such circumstances, sequestration of potassium within cells helps to prevent a dangerous degree of hyperkalemia. If renal function is normal, the elevation of serum potassium concentration usually persists only briefly.

The clinical aspects of disturbances in potassium metabolism will be considered under two headings, *potassium deficiency* and *potassium intoxication*.

Hypokalemia and Potassium Deficiency

Potassium deficiency may occur as the result of either *renal* or *extrarenal losses.* Typically, serum potassium concentration is reduced to a level of 2.5 to 3.5 mEq per liter, but with severe potassium depletion it may fall below 2 mEq per liter. In some circumstances, the reduction in potassium concentration is minimized or prevented by the concomitant presence of acidosis. Acidosis shifts the equilibrium between cells and extracellular fluid, tending to make serum potassium concentration high in relation to total body stores.

Hypokalemia can also occur without a loss of potassium from the body in the uncommon disorder known as *hypokalemic familial periodic paralysis.* This disorder is discussed in Ch. 480.

Pathogenesis and Diagnosis. Table 3 lists the common causes of potassium deficiency grouped according to whether the losses are of renal or extrarenal origin. As is evident from the table, a large variety of factors, including adrenal steroids, diuretics, and renal tubular disease, may promote abnormal renal excretion. Nearly all appear to increase sodium-potassium exchange in some fashion. *Adrenal steroids,* whether produced in excessive quantities by the body or given therapeutically, directly stimulate the sodium-cation exchange mechanism and thereby induce a urinary potassium loss. An excess of adrenal steroids resulting from overproduction is seen in *primary aldosteronism,* Cushing's syndrome, and various forms of *secondary aldosteronism* (see Ch. 850 to 852).

One uncommon cause of secondary aldosteronism and hypokalemia is *Bartter's syndrome.* This disease is characterized by juxtaglomerular hyperplasia, hypersecretion of renin, and metabolic alkalosis. Neither hypertension nor edema is present, and there is a subnormal pressor response to the administration of angiotensin. Renal salt wasting and accompanying hyponatremia are frequently striking features of the clinical picture.

Bartter's syndrome occurs most commonly in children and in some instances is familial in nature. The clinical manifestations of the disorder appear to result from an abnormal activation of the renin-angiotensin mechanism; nearly all the findings are accounted for by hyperplasia of the juxtaglomerular apparatus with a consequent excessive rate of renin production and of aldosterone secretion. The factors responsible for the juxtaglomerular hyperplasia have not been clearly defined, but several mechanisms have been proposed. It has been suggested, for example, that the stimulus to hyperplasia arises from a decreased responsiveness of

TABLE 3.   Causes of Potassium Deficiency

A. Renal
  1. Adrenal steroids
      Primary aldosteronism
      Secondary aldosteronism (including Bartter's syndrome
        and juxtaglomerular cell tumor)
      Cushing's syndrome
      Adrenal steroid therapy
  2. Diuretics
      Mercurials
      Ethacrynic acid
      Thiazides
      Furosemide
      Carbonic anhydrase inhibitors
  3. Renal tubular diseases
B. Extrarenal
  1. Vomiting
  2. Gastric drainage
  3. Diarrhea

blood vessels to angiotensin and a consequent chronic state of subclinical hypotension. Another postulate is that renal sodium wasting, with resulting chronic hypovolemia, produces the abnormal stimulus to the juxtaglomerular cells.

A disorder closely mimicking Bartter's syndrome has recently been observed in states of chronic volume depletion induced by vomiting, diarrhea, or diuretics. Juxtaglomerular hyperplasia, high rates of renin and aldosterone secretion, hypokalemic alkalosis, and a normal blood pressure are present, just as in the classic form of Bartter's syndrome. It thus appears that juxtaglomerular hyperplasia can be produced by a variety of stimuli and that a number of types of Bartter's syndrome will eventually be delineated.

Hypokalemia has also been observed as a cardinal feature of another disorder involving the juxtaglomerular apparatus, namely *juxtaglomerular cell tumor.* This tumor, as might be expected, produces excessive renin and thereby causes secondary aldosteronism and hypokalemic alkalosis. In striking contrast to Bartter's syndrome, however, blood pressure is markedly elevated rather than normal.

Studies of renal venous renin in the patient with a juxtaglomerular cell tumor will quickly identify one kidney as the source of the excessive renin production. Selective renal angiography will usually demonstrate the tumor, but in an occasional instance the lesion may be so small that it is overlooked; under such circumstances a decision regarding surgery must be made on the basis of the other clinical features. Blood pressure and electrolyte abnormalities usually return to normal shortly after the tumor is removed.

Renal potassium wasting and hypokalemia also occur as the result of *therapy with diuretics* such as thiazides, ethacrynic acid, and furosemide. These agents exert their effect on potassium balance by increasing the delivery of sodium to sodium-avid distal exchange sites and by thus accelerating the rate of sodium-potassium exchange. Diuretics which act through inhibition of carbonic anhydrase also cause potassium loss but exert their influence directly on the distal exchange mechanism; inhibition of carbonic anhydrase reduces the availability of hydrogen for exchange and thus enhances the exchange of sodium for potassium.

The derangements in function responsible for potassium wasting and hypokalemia in renal tubular diseases such as *renal tubular acidosis* are discussed in Ch. 619 to 624.

The only significant *extrarenal* route of potassium depletion is through the loss of gastrointestinal secretions. Gastric juice contains potassium in a concentration somewhat higher than plasma, and diarrheal fluid may have a potassium content as high as 50 to 60 mEq per liter. Thus prolonged vomiting, drainage of the upper gastrointestinal tract, or diarrhea typically produces a considerable deficit of potassium. If intake of potassium is poor, the severity of potassium deficiency will be further aggravated by renal losses; inefficient renal conservation allows considerable quantities of potassium to escape into the urine for as long as ten days or two weeks after potassium intake is lowered sharply. As much as 150 or 200 mEq can be lost before excretion is reduced to a level of less than 10 mEq per day.

In *hypokalemia of unknown origin* the quantity of potassium in the urine frequently provides the clue to the correct diagnosis. If a patient with persistent hypokalemia is excreting considerable quantities of potassium in the urine (30 mEq or more per day), the deficit is clearly of renal origin, and attention can therefore immediately be focused on those disorders listed under Section A of Table 3. Ordinarily the history and other clinical findings will clarify the etiology of such renal losses. There are several exceptions to this statement, however. A common problem, for example, is the evaluation of hypokalemia in the hypertensive patient who has received an agent such as a thiazide as part of his antihypertensive regimen. In such a patient it may be difficult to decide whether potassium deficiency is the result of diuretic therapy or is caused by primary aldosteronism. This question can usually be resolved by observation of the serum potassium level for at least several weeks after the drug has been discontinued.

In the patient with hypokalemia in whom potassium excretion is low (less than 15 mEq per day), the depletion is usually of extrarenal origin (Section B of Table 3). In nearly all such instances a history or other evidence pointing to gastrointestinal losses will easily be obtained, but sometimes the diagnostic problem is more difficult. Occasionally, a patient with *laxative-induced diarrhea* will deny both laxative ingestion and diarrhea, and it will then be necessary to obtain the relevant history from members of the family. Similarly, some patients with *psychogenic* or *self-induced vomiting* do not admit to their difficulties. Patients with *villous adenomas of the rectum* may also pose a diagnostic problem, because they usually have normally formed stools and, unless asked specifically, may neglect to mention the nearly continuous rectal leakage of mucus-like material which is characteristic of their illness. Accordingly, whenever unexplained chronic hypokalemia is associated with a low urinary potassium excretion, each of these uncommon disorders should be sought carefully.

Clinical Manifestations. The clinical effects of potassium deficiency may be manifested in one or more organ systems, including skeletal muscle, heart, kidneys, and the gastrointestinal tract. Perhaps the most serious disturbances are those affecting the neuromuscular system. At serum potassium concentrations in the range of 2 to 2.5 mEq per liter, muscular weakness is likely to occur, and with more severe hypokalemia the patient may develop areflexic paralysis. In this latter state respiratory insufficiency is an immediate threat to survival. The severity of the neuromuscular disturbance tends to be proportional to the speed with which the potassium level has declined. In an occasional instance, *myoglobinuria* has been noted in association with marked hypokalemia.

Finally, it should be noted that the patient who has developed potassium depletion as the result of diuretic therapy will sometimes demonstrate a low renal excretion of potassium even though the potassium loss was of renal origin. If diuretics are no longer being administered and if metabolic alkalosis is not present, the kidney will promptly begin to conserve potassium, and urinary excretion will remain low until the deficit is fully repaired.

Abnormalities in the electrocardiogram that commonly occur in hypokalemia are a sagging of the S-T segment, depression of the T wave, and elevation of the U wave (Fig. 1). With marked reductions in serum concentration, the T wave becomes progressively smaller,

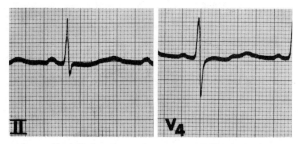

Figure 1. Typical electrocardiographic abnormalities induced by hypokalemia. (Serum potassium concentration 2.8 mEq per liter.) Note in lead II how the merger of the T and U waves might lead to the erroneous interpretation that the Q-T interval is prolonged.

whereas the U waves show increasing amplitude. In some cases the merging of a flat or positive T wave with a positive U wave may erroneously be interpreted as a prolonged Q-T interval. Ordinarily, there are no serious clinical consequences from the abnormalities in cardiac excitation, but in digitalized patients the sudden development of hypokalemia may precipitate serious arrhythmias.

Longstanding potassium depletion is apt to produce renal tubular damage—so-called *hypokalemic nephropathy*. This disorder is discussed in detail in Ch. 619. Potassium deficiency is believed to cause dysfunction of the smooth muscle of the gastrointestinal tract and in some patients has been held responsible for the development of *paralytic ileus*.

Potassium deficiency is also a regular concomitant of *metabolic alkalosis*. The role of potassium in the genesis and maintenance of alkalosis is considered later in this chapter.

Treatment. Under many circumstances potassium deficiency can be corrected by oral administration of potassium salts. The oral route should be used whenever feasible, because the relatively slow absorption from the gastrointestinal tract prevents a sudden large increase in serum potassium concentration of the sort that can occur during the injudicious administration of potassium intravenously. In this connection, it should be appreciated that correction of a typical deficit of 200 to 500 mEq requires the transfer through the extracellular compartment of a quantity of potassium that has the potential of raising serum concentration to well above lethal levels. For this reason, when potassium is administered intravenously, it should ordinarily be given at a rate not exceeding 15 to 20 mEq per hour and at a concentration no higher than 40 to 60 mEq per liter. It is also generally prudent to limit the supplement to 100 or 150 mEq per day and to use the serum potassium concentration as a guide to the need for further replacement. If acidosis is present, the serum potassium may be higher than is appropriate to the degree of potassium deficiency, and this discrepancy must be taken into account when treatment is planned. As acidosis is corrected, a more accurate appraisal of further potassium requirements will be possible. Unfortunately, there is no way of directly calculating the quantity of potassium that will be required for full replacement.

The *electrocardiogram* does not provide a reliable guide to the need for replacement therapy, but is extremely useful as a convenient and rapid means for determining whether an excessive quantity of potassium has been given. The electrocardiogram in hyperkalemia and potassium intoxication is discussed later.

The chloride salt of potassium is used almost exclusively for intravenous therapy, but it has fallen into some disfavor for purposes of oral administration because it often produces annoying upper gastrointestinal symptoms. Such symptoms can be avoided if potassium chloride is used in the enteric-coated form, but this mode of administration occasionally creates other problems. Dissolution of the enteric coating in the small intestine, and the resulting high local concentration of potassium on the mucosa, may produce ulceration, obstruction, or bleeding. For this reason, organic potassium salts, which are more palatable than potassium chloride and which can be given without an enteric coating (and without untoward local effects on the intestine), have come into widespread use. Potassium gluconate and potassium "triplex" (citrate, acetate, and bicarbonate) are among the agents frequently employed and are effective in patients who are not depleted of chloride. They are, however, relatively ineffective in repairing potassium deficiency when the patient is hypochloremic, alkalotic, and on a low-salt (low-chloride) intake. The explanation for this can be summarized as follows: In hypochloremic alkalosis a smaller than normal fraction of filtered sodium is reabsorbed with chloride and an increased fraction is reabsorbed by exchange with potassium and hydrogen. As long as hypochloremia and avidity for sodium persist, the accelerated rate of sodium-cation exchange forces a continued high rate of potassium excretion. For this reason, full repair of potassium deficiency cannot be achieved by administration of an organic potassium salt. Potassium must instead be provided as the chloride salt, or chloride must be made available in some other form, such as ammonium chloride or sodium chloride.

Hyperkalemia and Potassium Intoxication

Pathogenesis. Hyperkalemia is most often due to defective renal excretion of potassium. It may arise as the result of primary renal disease, deficiency of adrenal steroids, or the use of aldosterone antagonists (spironolactones) or other agents that inhibit sodium-potassium exchange by the tubule. Excessively rapid intravenous administration of potassium may also elevate plasma concentration to dangerous levels, as has been mentioned earlier in connection with the treatment of potassium deficiency. Potassium given by mouth rarely causes severe hyperkalemia unless renal function is severely impaired.

Hyperkalemia secondary to renal damage occurs frequently in *acute tubular necrosis* or in any other form of acute renal failure that is characterized by oliguria or anuria. In *chronic renal failure* potassium intoxication is usually encountered only in the terminal stages of the disease, but is sometimes seen earlier as a sequel to the inadvertent administration of potassium supplements. A deficiency of mineralocorticoid, caused either by *Addison's disease* or by *primary hypoaldosteronism,* a rare disorder, also impairs potassium secretion and may produce hyperkalemia.

The *spironolactones,* agents which are used in diuretic therapy for the purpose of antagonizing the sodium-retaining effects of aldosterone, do not usually cause significant elevation in serum potassium concentration. They do, however, impair the ability of the kidney to respond to a potassium load, and should not be given in conjunction with potassium supplements. The same caution concerning administration of potassium applies to patients receiving diuretic agents such as *triamterene* and *amiloride,* which also impair the exchange of sodium for potassium by the tubule.

Hyperkalemia also occurs in an uncommon and puzzling disorder known as *familial hyperkalemic periodic paralysis.* In individuals with this disorder, attacks can be induced by the ingestion of potassium. This disease is discussed in detail in Ch. 480.

Pseudohyperkalemia has been observed in a few patients with thrombocytosis secondary to a myeloproliferative disorder. The spurious elevation of serum concentration results from release of potassium from platelets during the coagulation process. Concentrations as high as 9 mEq per liter can be found in the serum at a time when plasma (platelet-free) has a normal potassium level. Similar spurious elevations in serum potassium concentration resulting from the release of potassium from white blood cells have also been reported in a few patients with chronic myelogenous leukemia. The possibility that one is dealing with pseudohyperkalemia should be considered whenever an elevated serum potassium concentration cannot otherwise be explained.

Clinical Manifestations. The clinical manifestations of potassium intoxication are related primarily to the heart and the neuromuscular system. *Electrocardiographic abnormalities* are the earliest and most frequent sign of disturbed membrane excitability, and are characterized by the development of tall, "tent-shaped" T waves, by decreased amplitude of the P waves, and later by atrial asystole (Fig. 2). Intraventricular block, with widening of the QRS complex, may lead to the development of a sine wave pattern and ultimately to ventricular standstill. Changes in the electrocardiogram usually appear when the serum potassium concentration reaches 7 to 8 mEq per liter, and cardiac standstill is likely to occur at a concentration of 9 to 10 mEq per liter. *Weakness* and *flaccid paralysis* appear only in association with severe hyperkalemia, but are not always present even at plasma levels sufficiently high to produce serious deterioration in the electrocardiogram. Indeed, death from cardiac arrest may occur even before muscular weakness is evident. For this reason the electrocardiogram is the single most important guide in appraising the threat posed by hyperkalemia and in determining how aggressive a therapeutic approach is necessary.

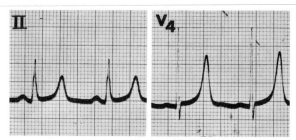

Figure 2. Typical electrocardiographic abnormalities induced by a moderate degree of hyperkalemia. (Serum potassium concentration 6.5 mEq per liter.) Note the typical "tent-shaped" T waves.

Treatment. The first goal in the treatment of severe potassium intoxication should be to promote the rapid transfer of potassium into cells in order to lower serum potassium concentration and prevent cardiac arrest. Two approaches to this goal are likely to prove effective. Infusion of glucose and insulin induces the cellular deposition of glycogen and at the same time brings about a shift of potassium to the intracellular space; 1 liter of a 10 per cent glucose solution with 30 to 40 units of insulin is generally employed for this purpose. In the acidotic patient further redistribution of potassium can be achieved by the administration of sodium bicarbonate (150 to 300 mEq). In many cases these measures will induce a striking reduction in plasma potassium concentration and prompt improvement in the electrocardiogram. In some instances the administration of calcium (as 2 grams of calcium lactate) is also useful, because calcium, though it has no effect on the plasma potassium concentration, opposes the cardiotoxic effects of potassium. It should be noted, incidentally, that calcium cannot be given in the same solution with sodium bicarbonate, because precipitation of the calcium ion will result.

Because the techniques described above do not remove potassium from the body and may be only temporarily effective, longer-term efforts should be directed toward promoting gastrointestinal losses of potassium. A cation-exchange resin in the sodium cycle, such as Kayexelate, will usually achieve this purpose if administered by mouth in a dose of 20 to 30 grams every six hours. Each gram of resin binds approximately 1 mEq of potassium, and within 24 hours a significant effect on plasma potassium concentration should be achieved. To enhance potassium loss and assure the rapid movement of the resin through the gastrointestinal tract, sorbitol, a nonabsorbable polyhydric alcohol, should be given in quantities sufficient to induce a soft or semiliquid bowel movement every few hours. The usual dose for this purpose is 20 ml of a 70 per cent solution three or four times a day. If the patient is unable to take medication by mouth, the resin can be administered by rectum as a retention enema of 100 grams in several hundred milliliters of water.

Hemodialysis is an efficient alternative means of removing excess potassium, but usually will not be required if the program outlined above can be implemented.

Cannon, P. J., Leeming, J. M., Sommers, S. C., Winters, R. W., and Laragh, J. H.: Juxtaglomerular cell hyperplasia and secondary hyperaldosteronism (Bartter's syndrome): a reevaluation of the pathophysiology. Medicine, 47:107, 1968.

Conn, J. W., et al.: Primary reninism. Arch. Intern. Med., 130:682, 1972.

Fleischer, N., Brown, H., Graham, D. Y., and Delena, S.: Chronic laxative-induced hyperaldosteronism and hypokalemia simulating Bartter's syndrome. Ann. Intern. Med., 70:791, 1969.

Ingram, R. H., and Seki, M.: Pseudohyperkalemia with thombocytosis. N. Engl. J. Med., 267:895, 1962.

Schwartz, W. B., and Relman, A. S.: Effects of electrolyte disorders on renal structure and function. N. Engl. J. Med., 276:383, 1967.

Welt, L. G., Hollander, W., and Blythe, W. B.: The consequences of potassium depletion. J. Chronic Dis., 11:213, 1960.

DISTURBANCES OF ACID-BASE EQUILIBRIUM

The pH of extracellular fluid normally ranges between 7.35 and 7.45, and is stabilized within these limits despite wide variations in the dietary load of acid or alkali. A large number of body functions are importantly influenced by the pH of body fluids, disturbances in acid-base regulation often having serious effects on metabolic activity, on the circulation, and on the central nervous system.

As background to a discussion of acid-base disturbances, it is instructive to consider briefly the way in which the body deals with the *normal daily acid load* and thus maintains a steady state of acid-base equilibrium. As food is oxidized, both carbon dioxide (carbonic acid) and nonvolatile acids such as sulfuric and phosphoric acids are added to the extracellular fluid. Immediate buffering within the interstitial fluid, plasma, and red blood cells minimizes the change in pH and permits large quantities of acid to be transferred to the lungs and kidneys for excretion. *Carbon dioxide* is excreted almost entirely by the lungs, and for this reason alveolar carbon dioxide tension is the prime determinant of Pco_2 in body fluids. With usual rates of carbon dioxide production, alveolar ventilation maintains the Pco_2 of blood at approximately 40 mm of mercury, that is, 1.2 millimoles of dissolved carbon dioxide per liter of plasma.

Nonvolatile acids are excreted solely by the kidney. The process by which this is accomplished is complex, because no significant fraction of the daily hydrogen ion load (some 50 to 100 mEq) can be excreted in an unbuffered form at the minimal urinary pH of 4.0 that the kidney can establish. Virtually all hydrogen must thus be removed as either *titratable acid* or *ammonium*. Acidification of the glomerular filtrate by a process of sodium-hydrogen exchange titrates buffers such as phosphate and also favors the diffusion of ammonia (NH_3) from the tubular cells to the lumen, where it reacts with hydrogen ions to form ammonium (NH_4^+). Bicarbonate generated in tubular cells as the result of acid excretion moves into peritubular blood and replenishes the bicarbonate stores that previously were depleted by the buffering of dietary acid. From all these considerations it is evident that derangements in either pulmonary or renal function, or the imposition of stresses that overwhelm normal regulatory mechanisms, can be expected to produce disturbances of acid-base equilibrium.

Because the carbonic acid–bicarbonate buffer pair is the major buffer system in the extracellular fluid, its parameters provide a meaningful and convenient expression of the acid-base status of the organism. The relation between pH and the bicarbonate and carbonic acid concentrations can be expressed in a general fashion according to the familiar Henderson-Hasselbalch equation,

$$pH = pK + \log \frac{HCO_3^-}{H_2CO_3} \tag{1}$$

where pK is the dissociation constant of carbonic acid. In the normal subject this expression will be

$$7.4 = 6.1 + \log \frac{24 \text{ mM/L}}{1.2 \text{ mM/L}} \tag{2}$$

Traditionally, disturbances in acid-balance equilibrium are considered in terms of a change in the ratio of bicarbonate to carbonic acid, but this approach, in the opinion of some, does not always provide the immediate and intuitive insight that can be derived from the following expression:

$$\begin{array}{c} 40 \text{ mm Hg} \\ \text{Pco}_2 \\ \searrow \searrow \\ H_2CO_3 \rightleftarrows H^+ + HCO_3^- \\ 1.2 \text{ mM/L} \quad pH \text{ } 7.4 \quad 24 \text{ mM/L} \end{array} \quad (3)$$

This equation allows ready visualization of the directional changes that can be anticipated in both metabolic and respiratory disturbances of acid-base equilibrium. It is apparent, for example, that a primary reduction in bicarbonate concentration (*metabolic acidosis*) will cause the reaction to shift to the right, thus increasing hydrogen ion concentration, whereas a primary elevation in bicarbonate concentration (*metabolic alkalosis*) will cause the reaction to shift to the left, thus decreasing hydrogen ion concentration. Respiratory disorders can be analyzed in the same fashion. A rise in Pco_2 increases the hydrogen ion concentration by shifting the reaction to the right (*respiratory acidosis*), and a fall has the reverse effect (*respiratory alkalosis*). In both metabolic and respiratory acid-base disturbances, the widest range of pH values compatible with life is approximately 6.8 to 7.8.

Metabolic Acidosis

Metabolic acidosis results whenever acid is added to the body, alkali is lost from the body, or impaired renal function prevents the excretion of the normal endogenous acid load. In each case the reduction in bicarbonate concentration is accompanied by a rise in hydrogen ion concentration, that is, a decrease in pH.

Physiologic Considerations. The normal organism confronted with a large acid load has a remarkable ability to maintain hydrogen ion concentration within tolerable limits until augmented excretion of acid (and concomitant regeneration of buffer stores) allows restoration of a normal plasma bicarbonate concentration. This resiliency is explained by the magnitude of the total body buffer capacity and the prompt respiratory adjustment of Pco_2.

Body buffers provide a large reservoir of hydrogen ion acceptors distributed through both the extracellular and intracellular compartments. In the extracellular space bicarbonate provides the bulk of the buffer capacity; hemoglobin and plasma proteins, though they make a significant contribution to the buffering ability of *blood,* are of little quantitative importance when viewed in terms of the entire extracellular compartment. Intracellular buffers, which consist largely of protein and organic anions, provide an additional buffer reserve that is responsible for sequestering half or more of an acid load and that thus serves the important function of protecting against lethal reductions in extracellular pH.

As the price for maintaining electroneutrality during cellular accumulation of hydrogen, both potassium and sodium are forced out of cells. If renal function is normal, the displaced potassium is ultimately lost in the urine. On the other hand, if renal function is impaired or if dehydration has reduced urine volume to oliguric levels, potassium will be retained and potentially dangerous elevations of serum potassium concentration may occur.

Respiratory compensation takes place promptly after the development of metabolic acidosis, an increase in both depth and rate of respiration lowering alveolar and arterial Pco_2. The magnitude of the fall in Pco_2 becomes larger as the reduction in bicarbonate concentration becomes greater, but respiratory defense is never sufficient to restore pH to normal.

Even with the most severe metabolic acidosis, Pco_2 does not fall below 10 mm of mercury because the physical effort required to produce a further increase in alveolar ventilation increases carbon dioxide production more rapidly than it does pulmonary gas exchange. Thus if bicarbonate concentration is very low and maximal reductions in Pco_2 have already been achieved, a slight further fall in bicarbonate concentration will produce a large decrement in pH.

The foregoing comments on respiratory defense have been based, of course, on the assumption that there will be a normal ventilatory response when metabolic acidosis occurs. Indeed, the clinical significance of a given reduction in plasma bicarbonate concentration is judged almost automatically (in the absence of pH measurements) on the basis of experience with the usual degree of respiratory compensation. In some circumstances, however, Pco_2 does not fall in the anticipated manner, and the increase in hydrogen ion concentration will therefore be far greater than is customary. This difficulty will be encountered if the respiratory center has been depressed by sedatives or other medications. It is also seen in the patient with pulmonary disease who, though able to maintain a normal Pco_2 under usual conditions, cannot increase alveolar ventilation to a significant degree under stress. In the patient with a plasma bicarbonate concentration of 10 mEq per liter, for example, normal respiratory compensation will usually reduce the Pco_2 to approximately 25 mm of mercury and keep the pH in the range of 7.20 to 7.25, whereas without a reduction in Pco_2 the pH would be 7.00. The measurement of pH or Pco_2 therefore is often important even in circumstances in which the diagnosis of metabolic acidosis is not in question.

Renal compensation is the final step in the defense against metabolic acidosis, but takes place slowly and does not contribute to the immediate protection of pH. Several days are required before excretion of ammonium and titratable acid rises sufficiently to regenerate bicarbonate and restore plasma concentration to normal. If renal function is impaired, or if underlying renal tubular disease is present, an even longer period may be required for correction to take place.

Pathogenesis (Table 4). *Large Acid Loads as a Cause of Acidosis.* Probably the most frequent cause of metabolic acidosis is the addition of a large acid load to the body fluids. *Diabetic ketoacidosis* is a familiar example of such a disturbance. In diabetic acidosis there is an imbalance between the production and utilization of

---

TABLE 4. Causes of Metabolic Acidosis

With Increase in Unmeasured Anions	Without Increase in Unmeasured Anions
Diabetic ketoacidosis	Diarrhea
Alcoholic ketoacidosis	Drainage of pancreatic juice
Salicylate poisoning	Ureterosigmoidostomy
Ethylene glycol poisoning	Carbonic anhydrase inhibitors
Methyl alcohol poisoning	Ammonium chloride
Paraldehyde (rarely)	Renal tubular acidosis
Lactic acidosis	
Renal failure	

beta-hydroxybutyric and acetoacetic acids, with the result that both accumulate in the extracellular fluid. Because these acids are almost completely dissociated at the pH of body fluids, nearly 1 millimole of bicarbonate is dissipated by the addition of each millimole of ketoacid.

Severe *ketoacidosis associated with alcoholism* has also been noted in nondiabetic patients. This disorder is seen in patients with chronic alcoholism who have been drinking heavily and who have eaten little or no food over several days. Typically such patients also have a history of protracted vomiting. Blood sugar is usually normal or mildly elevated. The acidosis, which is often severe, results from the accumulation of β-hydroxybutyric and acetoacetic acids (and sometimes lactic acid as well), but the severe ketosis can readily be overlooked because the ratio of β-hydroxybutyrate to acetoacetate in the plasma is unusually high; as a result, the nitroprusside test, which detects only acetoacetate, may be negative or only slightly positive. However, the characteristic history and the findings of a large "anion gap" should point strongly to the correct diagnosis.

Accumulation of lactic acid is now recognized as a relatively frequent cause of metabolic acidosis. *Lactic acidosis* is most often encountered in patients with circulatory failure caused by dehydration, hemorrhage, or endotoxic or cardiogenic shock. In these conditions the failure to supply sufficient oxygen to the tissues induces a shift from aerobic metabolism to anaerobic glycolysis and produces a lactic acidosis analogous to that occurring with severe exercise. Lactic acidosis may also occur in the absence of any obvious predisposing cause such as hypotension or hypoxemia. The onset is usually abrupt and without warning, and the acidosis is often of great severity. This syndrome of *spontaneous lactic acidosis* is seen in association with a variety of major illnesses, including diabetes mellitus, hepatic failure, subacute bacterial endocarditis, and leukemia. The etiology remains obscure. Lactic acid may also accumulate in significant quantities during *total fasting in the presence of obesity* and in *glycogen-storage disease*. Severe lactic acidosis has also been seen in association with *phenformin therapy* in diabetics and in association with the ingestion of huge doses of *isoniazid* (15 to 20 grams) taken by accident or in a suicide attempt.

Poisoning caused by the ingestion of *salicylates, methyl alcohol, ethylene glycol,* or (occasionally) *paraldehyde* leads to the accumulation of relatively strong and highly dissociated organic acids in the body fluids and to marked reductions in plasma bicarbonate concentration. The specific organic acids responsible for the acidosis in these disorders have not been adequately identified.

Metabolic acidosis can also result from the ingestion of mineral acid such as *ammonium chloride*. The release of hydrogen, as ammonium is converted by the liver to urea, makes the administration of ammonium chloride analogous to the administration of an equivalent quantity of hydrochloric acid. *Lysine hydrochloride* and *arginine hydrochloride* have the same effect on acid-base equilibrium, because they too deliver hydrochloric acid to the body fluids. Acidosis resulting from administration of acidifying salts is uncommon, however, because these agents are ordinarily administered only in conjunction with diuretic agents that tend to produce metabolic alkalosis.

Loss of Alkali as a Cause of Acidosis. Severe *diarrhea* frequently produces metabolic acidosis, because liquid stools usually contain bicarbonate in concentrations considerably higher than those in extracellular fluid. Loss of *pancreatic juice,* another highly alkaline solution, also leads to a reduction in plasma bicarbonate concentration. Acidosis of this latter origin is encountered almost exclusively in patients who have undergone prolonged drainage of a pancreatic fistula or of the upper portion of the small bowel.

Transplantation of the ureters into the sigmoid colon for the purpose of urinary diversion (*ureterosigmoidostomy*) leads to pooling of urine in the bowel, and sets into motion two physiologic events that tend to produce metabolic acidosis: movement of bicarbonate from plasma to urine in exchange for chloride directly depletes bicarbonate stores; and absorption of urinary ammonium from the bowel, with the consequent addition of hydrogen ions to the body fluids, further reduces plasma bicarbonate concentration. The more prolonged the period during which urine is in contact with the colonic mucosa, the larger will be these exchanges and the greater the compensatory increase in acid excretion that will be required. If kidney function is normal, this recycling can often be accomplished without serious disturbance in acid-base equilibrium. With impairment of kidney function, a common complication of ureterosigmoidostomy, severe acidosis is likely to occur. Acidosis can usually be avoided or minimized if the rectum is frequently emptied of urine, either voluntarily or by the use of a rectal tube.

Renal Dysfunction as a Cause of Acidosis. Inability of the diseased kidney to deal with the normal dietary load of nonvolatile acid will result in a positive acid balance and consequently in a reduction in plasma bicarbonate concentration. In *acute renal failure* the acid-base disturbance is usually transient and mild. In *chronic renal failure* metabolic acidosis is commonly present over an extended period and can be severe. In most patients with chronic renal failure the problem in acid excretion does not arise from any serious difficulty in acidifying the urine or in forming titratable acid, but is primarily the result of an inability to excrete normal quantities of ammonium. Defective renal reabsorption of bicarbonate is sometimes an additional contributory factor. Despite these abnormalities, plasma bicarbonate is usually stabilized at a level of 15 to 20 mEq per liter. This new steady state is achieved in part by the enhanced excretion of acid that accompanies the fall in plasma pH and in part by buffering of some portion of the acid load, probably by alkaline bone salts. The equilibrium is precarious, however, and any factor that increases either the intake or the production of acid (or induces a loss of alkali) is likely to precipitate a dangerous degree of metabolic acidosis.

In the foregoing discussion of renal acidosis, no mention has been made of the traditional view that retention of "acid anions" such as sulfate and phosphate is responsible for the reduction in plasma bicarbonate concentration. Such a view is inconsistent with modern concepts of physical chemistry that define an acid as any substance that donates hydrogen ions and a base as any substance that accepts hydrogen ions. In these terms substances such as sulfate and dibasic phosphate are actually weak bases rather than acids, and accumulation of these ions could not be expected to have a significant influence on either plasma bicarbonate concentration or pH. The tendency in many patients for bicarbonate to vary more or less reciprocally with the concentration of accumulated anions appears to be the fortuitous consequence of a parallel progression of glomerular and tubular damage, the reduction in filtration rate causing sulfate and phosphate retention, and the damage to tubules impairing acid excretion. It should also be realized that such a parallel change is not inevitable. In some patients, particularly those with chronic pyelonephritis, tubular capacity for acid excretion may be impaired at a time when glomerular filtration rate is only slightly reduced; under these circumstances the fall in plasma bicarbonate concentration is accompanied by an increase in chloride reabsorption that produces a state of so-called hyperchloremic acidosis.

Hyperchloremic acidosis is also seen in an uncommon form of renal dysfunction known as *renal tubular acidosis*. It is also observed in *Fanconi's syndrome*, a rare disease characterized by a multiplicity of tubular defects. These disorders are discussed in detail in Ch. 621 and 820, respectively.

Metabolic acidosis accompanied by hyperchloremia also follows the administration of *carbonic anhydrase inhibitors* such as acetazolamide. Carbonic anhydrase has an essential role in making hydrogen available for secretion by renal tubular cells, and inhibition of this enzyme impairs the cation-exchange process and reduces both sodium reabsorption and acid excretion. Carbonic anhydrase inhibitors, because of their ability to increase sodium excretion, were at one time widely used as diuretics. They proved, however, to be of relatively limited value because the modest diuresis which they produce is short lived; the prompt development of metabolic acidosis quickly impairs the effectiveness of these agents, and a rest period of several days must then be allowed to permit regeneration of bicarbonate and restoration of a normal plasma bicarbonate concentration.

Diagnosis. Hyperventilation is the only clinical finding characteristic of metabolic acidosis, and even this sign is sometimes difficult to detect. For example, patients with acidosis of long duration often appear to be breathing nearly normally at a time when measurements of Pco_2 demonstrate a striking increase in alveolar ventilation. Other clinical disturbances such as lethargy and coma are frequently seen in the patient with severe acidosis, but it is frequently difficult to decide whether these abnormalities are a manifestation of the acidosis per se or of the underlying disease, for example, diabetic acidosis or uremia.

In most cases, the history, in conjunction with the low plasma bicarbonate concentration and other routine chemical studies, will provide the basis for a tentative diagnosis of metabolic acidosis. However, since plasma bicarbonate concentration can also be reduced by primary hyperventilation (see below), a measurement of pH will be necessary in order to distinguish with certainty between respiratory alkalosis and metabolic acidosis. Subsequent measurements of pH will also serve the important function of providing a guide to effective clinical management.

Once the presence of metabolic acidosis has been documented, it is important to determine the exact cause. In many cases the cause is obvious, but in other

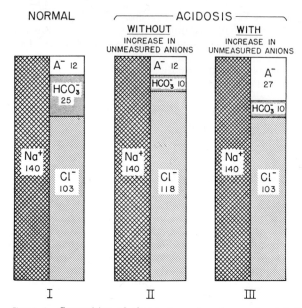

Figure 3. Composition of plasma in various forms of metabolic acidosis, with special reference to the concentration of unmeasured anions ("anion gap"). Column I shows that anions other than chloride and bicarbonate normally make up approximately 12 mEq per liter of the total anion content of plasma. Columns II and III indicate that acidosis can develop with or without an associated increase in concentration of unmeasured anions. The various causes of acidosis that will produce these patterns are listed in Table 4, and the way in which the "anion gap" can be used in differential diagnosis is discussed in the text.

instances it is obscure, and some rapid and systematic approach to differential diagnosis is invaluable. Particularly helpful is the calculation of the so-called "anion gap," or concentration of unmeasured anions, in plasma. This value, which is estimated by subtraction of the sum of chloride and bicarbonate concentrations from that of sodium, is normally about 10 to 12 mEq per liter (Fig. 3, column I), and represents negative charges contributed to plasma by ions other than chloride and bicarbonate (chiefly phosphate, sulfate, organic anions, and the anionic groups of plasma proteins).

In the patient with metabolic acidosis the reduction in bicarbonate concentration may or may not be accompanied by an increase in the "anion gap"; this distinction, which can be made on the basis of routine electrolyte measurements, immediately narrows the range of diagnostic possibilities (Table 4). If the concentration of unmeasured anions is increased (Fig. 3, column III), it can be concluded that hydrogen has been added to the body fluids with some anion other than chloride. This finding suggests a diagnosis of diabetic ketoacidosis, drug poisoning, renal failure, or lactic acidosis, and gives direction to further studies designed to identify the specific cause of the acid-base disturbance. Lactic acidosis is likely to pose the only special diagnostic problem, because in many hospitals lactate determinations are not yet routinely available. In nearly all cases, however, a tentative diagnosis of lactic acidosis can be made by exclusion of the other disorders characterized by an increased concentration of undetermined anions.

If, on the other hand, the "anion gap" is not increased (Fig. 3, column II), the reduction in bicarbonate concentration can clearly be attributed either to the accumulation of hydrogen with chloride or to a loss of bicarbonate. With the spectrum thus narrowed, it should again be relatively easy to identify the underlying disorder. A history of diarrhea, or of the ingestion of an acidifying agent such as ammonium chloride or acetazolamide, will often clarify the problem. The finding of a relatively alkaline urine and of nephrocalcinosis on roentgenographic examination of the abdomen will strongly suggest the diagnosis of renal tubular acidosis.

In some patients, of course, several causes of metabolic acidosis may be present simultaneously, and this possibility should not be overlooked. If, for example, the disappearance of ketonemia during the treatment of diabetic acidosis is not accompanied by restoration of a normal plasma bicarbonate concentration, the presence of a coexistent disorder such as lactic acidosis should be suspected.

Treatment. *General Principles.* Treatment should ordinarily be directed toward any reversible abnormality, such as ketosis or shock, which may be responsible for the acidosis. However, if the underlying disturbance is not amenable to treatment, or if acidosis is life threatening, alkali therapy will be necessary. Calculation of the amount of alkali to be administered must take into account not only the depletion of extracellular bicarbonate stores but also the magnitude of the intracellular acidosis. As mentioned earlier, a large fraction of an acid load is sequestered in cells, and restoration of normal acid-base equilibrium therefore involves repair of total body buffer stores. Estimates of alkali requirements should thus assume "distribution" of bicarbonate through a volume equivalent to 50 per cent of body weight. The calculation for full repair can be summarized by the following expression:

$$(25 \text{ mEq per liter} - \text{observed plasma HCO}_3 \text{ conc.})$$
$$\times 0.5 \text{ body weight (kg)} = \text{mEq of alkali}$$

The figure of 50 per cent for the distribution of bicarbonate is only approximate, but clinical experience has demonstrated that therapy based on this assumption usually induces a rise in plasma bicarbonate concentration close to the predicted level.

In most patients with severe acidosis immediate correction of the entire alkali deficit is unnecessary; if bicarbonate concentration is increased to 15 or 20 mEq per liter, plasma pH will be returned to a safe level, and renal adjustments (or continued treatment of the underlying metabolic abnormality) can be relied upon to complete the corrective process. More rapid correction may, in fact, be undesirable. If bicarbonate concentration is quickly restored to normal or nearly normal levels, blood pH may become frankly alkaline. This apparently paradoxical behavior is the consequence of persistent hyperventilation which often maintains a state of hypocapnia for as long as one or two days after bicarbonate stores have been replenished.

During the correction of metabolic acidosis, the movement of potassium into cells in exchange for hydrogen tends to lower serum potassium concentration. In the patient with hyperkalemia and potassium intoxication this serves a useful therapeutic purpose, as discussed earlier. If, however, serum potassium concentration is normal initially, the transfer of potassium from the extracellular fluid may produce hypokalemia and signs of potassium deficiency. This sequence of events has been noted with particular frequency during the correction of diabetic ketoacidosis, but it may also occur during the

repair of other acidotic states. For this reason careful clinical observation and occasional measurements of serum potassium concentration should be carried out in the course of treatment to determine the need for replacement of potassium deficits.

Special Problems in Management. Some of the disorders that cause metabolic acidosis present particular problems in management. This discussion considers such problems as they occur in lactic acidosis, diabetic ketoacidosis, and renal acidosis; salicylate poisoning and methyl alcohol poisoning are dealt with in detail in Ch. 26.

In metabolic acidosis resulting from the accumulation of either ketoacids or lactic acid there is the potential for prompt and full correction of the bicarbonate deficit without administration of exogenous alkali. In both diabetic and lactic acidosis, the anion that has accumulated in the body fluids, if fully oxidized, will regenerate an equivalent quantity of bicarbonate, and will restore plasma bicarbonate concentration to normal. A familiar physiologic example of this behavior is seen with the lactic acidosis of exercise; after exertion is discontinued, acidosis is rapidly corrected according to the following reaction:

$$\text{Na}^+ + \text{CH}_3\text{CH(OH)COO}^- + \text{HOH} + 3\text{O}_2$$
$$\rightarrow \underbrace{\text{Na}^+ + \text{OH}^-}_{} + \underbrace{3\text{CO}_2}_{} + 3\text{H}_2\text{O} \qquad (4)$$
$$\underbrace{}_{\text{Na}^-\text{HCO}_3^- + 2\text{CO}_2}$$

In *diabetic ketoacidosis* full and rapid oxidation of the organic anion occurs promptly after the administration of adequate quantities of insulin and glucose, and it is for this reason that most patients with ketoacidosis do not require alkali therapy. On the other hand, it is reasonable to administer small quantities of alkali if, at the time of admission, the patient is found to have acidosis of life-threatening severity. Such treatment will have an important influence on pH at a time before insulin can exert a significant effect, and will lead to only an inconsequential degree of alkalosis after ketosis has been fully corrected.

In the *ketoacidosis associated with alcoholism,* the only treatment necessary is administration of glucose and isotonic saline solution. Insulin is not required, but small amounts of bicarbonate should probably be given in the early phase of treatment if the metabolic acidosis is of life-threatening proportions.

The ease with which *lactic acidosis* can be corrected depends on the cause of the metabolic abnormality. If shock is responsible for the shift to anaerobic glycolysis, transfusions or other means of restoring blood volume and blood pressure will usually correct the acid-base disturbance. Lactic acidosis of unknown cause *(spontaneous lactic acidosis)* poses a completely different problem. Specific means for remedying the defect in lactate metabolism are not available, and one must therefore rely solely on alkali therapy. Treatment is often further complicated by the unpredictable response to administration of alkali; in some cases there is little or no rise in bicarbonate concentration despite administration of an amount of bicarbonate that, by usual estimates, would be more than sufficient to restore the plasma level to normal. The explanation for this "resistance" to therapy presumably lies in continued addition of lactic acid to the body fluids during the period of treatment.

In an occasional patient, the rate of addition of lactic acid to the body fluids may be so great that as much as 400 to 500 mEq of sodium bicarbonate must be administered over a period of a few hours in order to prevent the development of lethal acidosis.

On the other hand, bicarbonate concentration will sometimes rise spontaneously as a sudden increase in the oxidation of lactate regenerates large quantities of bicarbonate. In the patient who has previously been given alkali, frank metabolic alkalosis may be the result. For these reasons the acid-base status must be monitored closely during the course of therapy.

It should be emphasized that even when the acid-base disorder is well controlled, the majority of patients with spontaneous lactic acidosis do not survive. Any therapeutic approach directed toward the acid-base disturbance alone will obviously be far from satisfactory, because it deals with effect rather than cause. In this connection it should be noted that problems analogous to those seen in spontaneous lactic acidosis were encountered in the management of diabetic acidosis during the preinsulin era; resistance to alkali therapy was common, and death frequently occurred even after plasma bicarbonate concentration was restored to normal.

Chronic *renal acidosis* poses still a different problem. There is no accumulation of organic anion from which bicarbonate can be regenerated, and irreversible renal damage ordinarily precludes correction of the underlying tubular abnormality responsible for the acid-base disturbance. For this reason, reliance must be placed on alkali therapy alone. Fortunately, in most patients with renal insufficiency the degree of metabolic acidosis is not sufficiently great to demand treatment; reductions in bicarbonate concentration to 16 to 18 mEq per liter, which occur commonly, do not appear to cause symptoms or to aggravate the uremic syndrome. If, however, acidosis becomes severe, either sodium bicarbonate or sodium citrate should be given by mouth in doses of several grams per day; plasma bicarbonate concentration need not and, in fact, probably should not be raised to normal because of the risk of precipitating tetany if hypocalcemia is present. Sometimes the ingestion of alkali precipitates nausea or vomiting, and under these circumstances it may be necessary to discontinue treatment. Sodium bicarbonate is more likely than sodium citrate to produce gastrointestinal symptoms.

If the patient has a sodium-retaining state such as congestive heart failure, it is wise to defer administration of alkali as long as possible and, if treatment must be given, to restrict dietary sodium intake sharply.

The management of *renal tubular acidosis* and that of *Fanconi's syndrome* are discussed in Ch. 621 and 820, respectively.

Choice of an Alkalinizing Agent. Two agents, *sodium bicarbonate* and *sodium lactate,* have been widely employed in patients requiring the intravenous administration of alkali. Sodium lactate is usually an effective and satisfactory means of treatment, but has the disadvantage that it depends on the intervention of oxidative processes to make bicarbonate available (Equation 4). Thus if there is a defect in lactate metabolism, as in lactic acidosis, the prompt and quantitative conversion of lactate to bicarbonate cannot be relied upon. Bicarbonate, on the other hand, is ideally suited to the treatment of metabolic acidosis, because it directly replenishes depleted buffer stores. There thus appears no basis for the continued use of lactate in the treatment of acidotic states.

Bicarbonate can also be provided by the administration of *THAM* (tris-[hydroxymethyl]aminomethane), an organic buffer with a pK of 7.8, which reacts with carbonic acid according to the following equation:

$$THAM + H_2CO_3 \leftrightharpoons THAMH^+ + HCO_3^- \qquad (5)$$

It is not clear, however, that any advantage accrues from the administration of bicarbonate with, in effect, cationic THAM rather than sodium. THAM, or tris buffer, is toxic when given in large doses and furthermore may produce serious injury to tissue at the site of infusion because it must be administered as an intensely alkaline solution (pH 10). Parenthetically, it should be noted that the slight and transient reduction in carbon dioxide tension that follows an infusion of THAM is of no clinical significance in the patient with metabolic acidosis. The possible role of THAM in the treatment of *respiratory acidosis* will be discussed later in this chapter.

Metabolic Alkalosis

Metabolic alkalosis results from either an abnormal loss of acid or an excessive retention of alkali. In each case the rise in bicarbonate concentration induces a fall in hydrogen ion concentration, that is, an increase in pH.

Physiologic Considerations. As in metabolic acidosis, pH is defended to a significant extent by *tissue buffering*. In response to alkalinization of the extracellular fluid, hydrogen ions migrate from cells to extracellular space (in exchange for sodium and potassium), and thus mitigate the severity of the acid-base disturbance.

Respiratory compensation may serve as an additional mitigating factor. Diminished ventilation and a resulting rise in P_{CO_2} tends to restore a more normal ratio between the concentrations of carbonic acid and bicarbonate. Even with severe metabolic alkalosis, P_{CO_2} does not usually rise above 50 mm Hg, but values between 50 and 60 mm Hg are not rare, and in a very occasional patient P_{CO_2} may even reach a level of 65 mm Hg. In contrast to metabolic acidosis, however, the magnitude of the respiratory compensation is usually small, and becomes significant only when plasma bicarbonate concentration rises to 35 or 40 mEq per liter.

Renal excretion is the route for removal of excess alkali, and is thus ultimately responsible for the correction of metabolic alkalosis. Normally, the kidneys reabsorb approximately 25 mEq of bicarbonate per liter of glomerular filtrate, and when plasma concentration is elevated above this level by ingestion or infusion of alkali, the excess bicarbonate is rapidly and quantitatively excreted. Thus even a large alkali load induces only a transient alkalosis. The following theoretical example will serve to illustrate this point. If plasma bicarbonate is raised from 25 mEq per liter to 35 mEq per liter by alkali administration, approximately 10 mEq of bicarbonate will be excreted each time a liter of glomerular filtrate is formed. With a glomerular filtration rate of 180 liters per day, daily excretion would thus be 1800 mEq. Maintenance of the metabolic alkalosis would therefore require either the daily administration of 150 grams of sodium bicarbonate or the loss per day of 18 liters of gastric juice containing 0.1N HCl. Although such circumstances are rarely if ever encountered clinically, sustained elevations of plasma bicarbonate concentration do occur with considerable frequency. Indeed, plasma concentrations of 40 to 50 mEq per liter are seen even in patients who are neither receiving bicarbonate nor losing gastric juice. This finding clearly indicates that renal reabsorption of bicarbonate must be abnormally large, a conclusion borne out by the fact that the urine of the alkalotic patient typically has a pH in the acid range and contains virtually no bicarbonate. The problem confronting the physician therefore is the identification and correction of the cause of the defect in bicarbonate excretion.

Before the causes of metabolic alkalosis are considered, it seems desirable to review briefly the mechanism of bicarbonate reabsorption. Reabsorption of bicarbonate takes place by an indirect process involving the transport of sodium from the glomerular filtrate and the secretion of hydrogen into the lumen in its place. The addition of hydrogen to the filtrate converts bicarbonate to carbonic acid, but at the same time generates an equivalent quantity of bicarbonate in the renal tubular cells; the subsequent diffusion of this bicarbonate into the peritubular blood serves as the mode of bicarbonate "reabsorption." It is evident that any stimulus that increases the rate of sodium-hydrogen exchange will also increase bicarbonate reabsorption, and will sustain a metabolic alkalosis.

Pathogenesis (Table 5). A variety of clinical disturbances can produce metabolic alkalosis, but most of these can be grouped under the general headings of *losses from the upper gastrointestinal tract, diuretic therapy,* or *hyperadrenocorticism.* In each instance, as mentioned earlier, the urine is virtually free of bicarbonate, indicating that the rate of sodium-hydrogen exchange is increased. The nature of the mechanisms responsible for the enhanced bicarbonate reabsorption can perhaps best be understood by considering the renal adjustments that occur during vomiting or as the result of gastric drainage. As hydrochloric acid is lost from the stomach, bicarbonate is generated and plasma bicarbonate concentration rises, with the result that sodium formerly filtered with chloride is now filtered with bicarbonate. Because bicarbonate is not as readily reabsorbable as chloride, sodium reabsorption in the proximal tubule cannot proceed normally, and much of the newly generated bicarbonate is therefore delivered with sodium to distal exchange sites. Since the distal exchange sites, even when stimulated by a low sodium diet, cannot fully conserve this additional sodium, some sodium is initially lost into the urine with bicarbonate. A loss of potassium also occurs because a portion of the sodium which is conserved by the distal nephron is exchanged with potassium.

As sodium loss and contraction of the extracellular volume stimulate sodium reabsorption, and as the depletion of tubular potassium stores reduces the availability of this cation for exchange, sodium-hydrogen exchange is accelerated. As a result, all further sodium and bicarbonate that escapes proximal reabsorption is conserved and there is a sustained elevation of plasma bicarbonate concentration.

These same basic mechanisms account for the metabolic alkalosis seen with diuretic therapy in the edematous patient. Diuretic agents such as mercurials, furosemide, and ethacrynic acid block sodium chloride reabsorption and deliver sodium and chloride to sodium-avid exchange sites where some fraction of the sodium is exchanged with hydrogen and potassium. Hydrogen is therefore lost into the urine with chloride, and an equivalent quantity of bicarbonate is generated. As with gastric alkalosis, two conditions are required for maintenance of the high rate of sodium-hydrogen exchange and of the state of metabolic alkalosis. First, there must be a continued intense stimulus to sodium reabsorption; second, there must be a persistent deficiency of chloride which maintains the abnormally high ratio of bicarbonate to chloride in the glomerular filtrate.

The exact sequence of events leading to the rise in bicarbonate concentration in both *primary aldosteronism* and *Cushing's syndrome* remains to be determined, but the fundamental renal mechanisms at play are almost certainly the same as those responsible for the alkalosis seen with gastrointestinal losses or diuretic therapy. The syndrome of *posthypercapneic alkalosis* is discussed later in this chapter under Respiratory Acidosis.

Diagnosis. There are no signs or symptoms specific for metabolic alkalosis. The diagnosis is usually suspected because there is a history of vomiting, because therapy with diuretics or adrenal steroids has been given, or because the patient has undergone prolonged gastric drainage. Occasionally, an elevation of bicarbonate concentration is discovered accidentally in the course of routine measurements of serum electrolyte values. An unequivocal diagnosis of metabolic alkalosis can be made only after pH is shown to be increased, but, as a practical matter, an elevated bicarbonate concentration in a patient without significant pulmonary disease can be taken as virtually diagnostic.

The finding of unexplained metabolic alkalosis will sometimes lead to the diagnosis of *Cushing's syndrome* even when there are few, if any, clinical signs of the disease. This sequence of events is most likely to occur with adrenal hyperfunction associated with extra-adrenal neoplasms. The tumor most likely to produce this syndrome is bronchogenic carcinoma.

Treatment. The treatment of metabolic alkalosis (other than that caused by an excess of adrenal steroids) consists of correction of dehydration and of the various ionic deficits. It will be recalled from the discussion of the etiology of metabolic alkalosis that the combination of chloride deficiency and increased avidity for sodium is responsible for the abnormally high rate of bicarbonate reabsorption. Correction can therefore usually be accomplished promptly by administration of sodium chloride and water. Potassium chloride is also effective in the treatment of metabolic alkalosis and is particu-

---

TABLE 5.   Causes of Metabolic Alkalosis

Vomiting or gastric drainage
Diuretic therapy
   Mercurials
   Ethacrynic acid
   Thiazides
   Furosemide
Cushing's syndrome
Primary aldosteronism
Bartter's syndrome
Adrenal steroid therapy
Relief of chronic hypercapnia

larly useful in edematous states because sodium administration is usually contraindicated. Organic potassium salts, for example, "triplex" and gluconate, will not correct either alkalosis or potassium deficiency unless adequate amounts of chloride are available in the diet.

In cases of metabolic alkalosis of mild or moderate severity, the speed of correction of the acid-base disorder is not a critical factor. Slow correction over several days, achieved by the renal response to repair of the fluid and electrolyte deficit, usually represents optimal management. On occasion, however, an extreme degree of metabolic alkalosis may necessitate a more direct and intensive approach to therapy. In the Zollinger-Ellison syndrome, for example, continuous and massive losses of hydrochloric acid may elevate the plasma bicarbonate concentration to 60 mEq per liter or above. Under such circumstances, direct titration of the excess bicarbonate by the intravenous administration of hydrochloric acid, as ammonium chloride or arginine hydrochloride, may be imperative.

If ammonium chloride is used, it must be given slowly and under close observation, because if the rate of infusion exceeds the capacity of the liver to convert ammonium to urea, lethal ammonium intoxication may occur. This risk will be greatly increased if there is any element of underlying hepatic disease. Arginine hydrochloride has come into widespread favor as an alternative and safer means of providing hydrochloric acid intravenously.

In treating patients who are receiving diuretics that tend to produce metabolic alkalosis, it may at times be desirable to administer an acidifying salt by mouth. Ammonium chloride is the agent most commonly used for this purpose, and can be given without hazard if liver disease is not present. It is usually administered as an enteric-coated form, because it otherwise gives rise to unpleasant gastric symptoms. An amino acid salt such as lysine monohydrochloride is another useful vehicle for the oral provision of acid.

The management of alkalosis in the patient with hyperadrenocorticism *(Cushing's syndrome, primary aldosteronism)* poses a problem different from that encountered in more common clinical states. First, both the elevated plasma bicarbonate concentration and the hypokalemia persist despite a normal dietary intake of potassium, sodium, and chloride. Furthermore, even a large sodium chloride supplement does not correct the electrolyte abnormalities. Correction of both the alkalosis and potassium deficiency can, however, readily be accomplished over several days by administration of potassium chloride either by mouth or by vein. The explanation of this phenomenon remains obscure. Definitive treatment of the electrolyte disturbances associated with hyperadrenalism consists, of course, in the surgical removal of the offending adrenal tissue.

The alkalosis and potassium deficiency encountered in the syndrome of juxtaglomerular hyperplasia with secondary aldosteronism *(Bartter's syndrome)* has the characteristic of often being quite resistant to correction by potassium chloride. Daily supplements of several hundred milliequivalents of potassium may be necessary to hold the plasma bicarbonate concentration at normal or near-normal levels. In such instances spironolactone administration may be a useful adjunct to therapy.

Respiratory Acidosis

Respiratory acidosis results from any disturbance in ventilation that increases arterial Pco_2. An elevation of Pco_2 shifts the normal equilibrium of the bicarbonate–carbonic acid buffer system and increases the plasma hydrogen ion concentration (that is, it decreases pH). This effect on pH is mitigated, however, by a secondary *increase* in plasma bicarbonate concentration that is dependent on two mechanisms. During acute hypercapnia bicarbonate is generated by the titration of body buffers. With more prolonged elevation of Pco_2, additional bicarbonate is added to the extracellular fluid as the result of augmented renal acid excretion. A concomitant rise in the renal capacity for bicarbonate reabsorption permits conservation of the new bicarbonate and allows plasma concentration to be stabilized at an elevated level (Fig. 4). Experimental studies indicate that the complete process of renal adaptation requires several days or longer. It is apparent from these considerations that the extent of physiologic adjustment to a given degree of hypercapnia varies as a function of time and that intelligent appraisal of the acid-base changes in respiratory acidosis requires a knowledge of the duration of the ventilatory disturbance.

Pathogenesis. *Acute respiratory acidosis* occurs in a variety of clinical settings. Airway obstruction or hypoventilation resulting from central nervous system depression, neuromuscular disorders, or chest wall injuries are perhaps the most frequent causes. Acute hypercapnia may also occur as a result of decreased alveolar ventilation in disorders such as bacterial and viral pneumonias, aspiration pneumonitis, and pulmonary edema. Extreme respiratory acidosis is also often encountered in cardiopulmonary arrest.

Chronic respiratory acidosis is seen with progressive lung diseases such as emphysema or chronic bronchitis. The disturbance in gas exchange results from ventilation-perfusion mismatching and decreased effective alveolar ventilation. Pulmonary diseases characterized primarily by restrictive changes, such as pulmonary

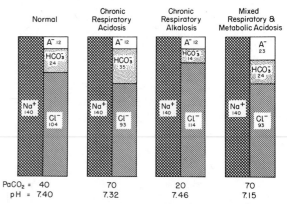

Figure 4. Composition of plasma in representative instances of chronic respiratory acid-base disorders. Note that in *chronic respiratory acidosis* plasma bicarbonate concentration is elevated, whereas in *chronic respiratory alkalosis* it is depressed; in each instance the change in bicarbonate concentration serves to minimize the effect on plasma pH of the abnormality in carbon dioxide tension. The column to the far right depicts a representative example of a *mixed respiratory and metabolic acidosis* in which the "anion gap" is elevated as the result of a disorder such as diabetic ketoacidosis or lactic acid acidosis.

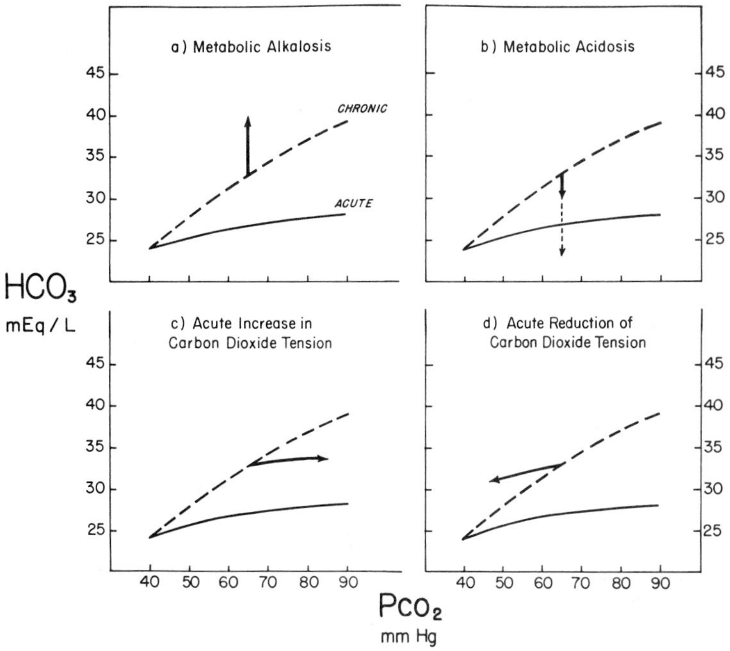

Figure 5. Schematic diagram of pathways followed by the acid-base disturbances that may complicate chronic respiratory acidosis. The *solid* lines represent the bicarbonate concentrations observed during acute hypercapnia in man, and the *dashed* lines the bicarbonate concentrations seen during chronic hypercapnia in the dog. The origin of each vector has been placed arbitrarily at a point depicting physiologically complete adaption to a Pco_2 of 65 mm of mercury. Each panel is discussed in detail in the text. (Reproduced by permission of the American Journal of Medicine.)

fibrosis, do not cause hypercapnia until late in the course of the illness.

Diagnosis. The tentative diagnosis of *acute respiratory acidosis* can often be made on clinical grounds alone if there is obvious impairment of ventilation. The definitive diagnosis depends, however, on demonstration that Pco_2 is elevated and that plasma pH is reduced. These measurements are of particular importance when clinical observation cannot be relied upon to reveal an impairment of gas exchange, as, for example, in the patient who is being artificially ventilated or who is suffering from intoxication with barbiturates or other central nervous system depressants.

Chronic respiratory acidosis should be suspected in any patient with the symptoms and physical findings of severe lung disease. Classically, the diagnosis rests on the finding of an elevated Pco_2 accompanied by a low pH. However, it is now recognized that in some patients with chronic pulmonary disease hypercapnia may occur in conjunction with a normal or even a high pH. Such values of pH have sometimes been interpreted as indicating full compensation or even "overcompensation" for the respiratory acidosis, but they are, in fact, almost always attributable to a complicating metabolic alkalosis (see below). This problem in interpretation illustrates the difficulty the physician faces in deciding whether a patient with chronic pulmonary insufficiency is suffering from respiratory acidosis alone or from a mixed disorder in which metabolic components are also present.

Hypercapnia and Mixed Acid-Base Disorders. Just as a variety of illnesses, e.g., vomiting, lactic acidosis, or diabetic ketoacidosis, may produce a metabolic acid-base disturbance in the normal subject, they can do the same in the patient with hypercapnia (Fig. 4). To recognize and quantitate the magnitude of a complicating metabolic disturbance in pulmonary insufficiency, *one must have prior knowledge of the pH and bicarbonate concentration appropriate to the given degree of uncomplicated hypercapnia.* Recent observations on changes in plasma composition during exposure of normal subjects

to various degrees of acute hypercapnia have provided a background for the appraisal of the acid-base status in *acute* respiratory acidosis. As shown in Figure 5, over a range of carbon dioxide tension up to 90 mm of mercury there is only a slight rise in plasma bicarbonate concentration. From this response curve and other available information, it appears that in uncomplicated acute hypercapnia of mild or moderate severity the bicarbonate concentration should lie between 25 and 30 mEq per liter. Concentrations above 30 mEq per liter indicate the presence of a complicating metabolic alkalosis, and those below 25 mEq per liter, the presence of a complicating metabolic acidosis.

Unfortunately, physiologic observations on the response to *chronic* hypercapnia are available only in the dog, but data on patients with chronic lung disease suggest that the pattern of response which has been defined experimentally is closely similar to that which occurs clinically. Figure 5 illustrates schematically how data on the adaptation to chronic hypercapnia can be utilized in the analysis of complex acid-base disorders. This figure contains four schematic diagrams depicting, by vectors, the ways in which the acid-base status in pre-existing chronic respiratory acidosis can be deranged. For purposes of discussion, the initial Pco_2 is assumed to be 65 mm of mercury.

Figure 5a contains the vector for a superimposed metabolic alkalosis. The bicarbonate concentration lies above the level appropriate for chronic adaptation to a Pco_2 of 65 mm of mercury, and indicates that there has been a pathologic loss of acid or retention of alkali. Such deviations of bicarbonate in the alkaline direction, occurring as a result of diuretics, steroid therapy, or vomiting, could have important clinical consequences, because an inappropriately high pH may diminish respiratory drive and aggravate the pre-existing degree of hypoxemia.

Figure 5b shows the pathway of a superimposed metabolic acidosis. A mild degree of metabolic acidosis, as indicated by the solid portion of the vector, will produce bicarbonate concentrations in the zone lying between the acute and chronic response curves. With a more severe metabolic disturbance, as shown by the dotted extension of the vector, the bicarbonate concentration will be depressed to a level below even the acute response curve.

Figure 5c demonstrates the sequence that will ensue when an acute increase in P_{CO_2} is superimposed on chronic hypercapnia. This disturbance occurs in association with such common complications as pneumonia, heart failure, and excessive sedation, all of which may further compromise alveolar ventilation. As an element of *acute* hypercapnia develops, body buffers can be expected to generate only a small additional amount of bicarbonate, and, as indicated by the vector, plasma bicarbonate concentration should follow a course roughly parallel to the acute titration curve. For a period of several days—that is, until there is renal compensation appropriate to the new level of hypercapnia—the bicarbonate concentration will remain at a point below the chronic response curve. It should be noted in Figure 5 that when either mild metabolic acidosis (Fig. 5b) or acute hypercapnia (Fig. 5c) is superimposed on chronic respiratory acidosis, the bicarbonate values will lie between the acute and chronic response curves. Obviously, the acid-base parameters per se cannot be used to differentiate these two complications, and additional clinical information will be required.

Figure 5d contains the vector resulting from a recent improvement in alveolar ventilation. A sudden fall in P_{CO_2} will titrate body buffers toward normal and induce a fall in bicarbonate concentration. This titration cannot be expected, however, immediately to erase the renal component of the initial increment in extracellular bicarbonate stores. Plasma bicarbonate concentration therefore will be high in relation to the P_{CO_2}, a condition that has been termed "*posthypercapneic alkalosis.*" If the diet contains sodium chloride or if the patient is given potassium chloride, the kidney will excrete the excess bicarbonate and the condition will disappear within several days. However, if chloride intake is low, metabolic alkalosis is likely to persist indefinitely. The physiologic mechanisms responsible for this behavior are the same as have already been discussed in connection with the metabolic alkalosis that results from vomiting or from diuretic therapy.

Treatment. The treatment of *acute respiratory acidosis* should be directed toward the underlying cause of the impaired ventilation. The measures required obviously will depend on the nature of the clinical problem. If, for example, alveolar gas exchange is impeded by bronchospasm, bronchodilators should be used. If inadequate ventilation is the result of a neuromuscular disturbance, artificial ventilation may be necessary.

The treatment of *chronic respiratory acidosis* should also be directed primarily toward improving alveolar ventilation, not toward the restoration of a normal pH. Bronchodilators, adrenal steroids, antimicrobials, postural drainage, and artificial ventilation all have a valuable place in therapy at one time or another in the course of the illness. The management of pulmonary insufficiency is dealt with in detail in Ch. 507, but a word of caution should be repeated here concerning the possible hazards of oxygen therapy in worsening chronic respiratory acidosis. In severe hypercapnia the sensitivity of the respiratory center to carbon dioxide may be diminished and, if this occurs, hypoxemia becomes the major stimulus to respiratory activity. If hypoxemia is then partially or totally corrected, ventilation often undergoes further serious impairment, hypercapnia becomes increasingly severe, and the patient can lapse into coma and die. Thus during oxygen therapy the patient must be watched closely to ensure that improvement in the degree of hypoxemia does not depress ventilation.

The use of an organic buffer such as THAM for the purpose of lowering P_{CO_2} (Equation 5) has little or nothing to recommend it; the rise in pH that follows the reaction of THAM with carbonic acid usually reduces minute ventilation and thus aggravates the pre-existing hypoxemia. This problem can be circumvented if the patient is given artificial ventilation, but even under such circumstances, THAM has little practical value; control of hypercapnia for more than one or two hours would require amounts of THAM far in excess of what can safely be administered.

Respiratory Alkalosis

Respiratory alkalosis results from any disturbance in ventilation that lowers arterial carbon dioxide tension. A reduction in P_{CO_2} shifts the normal equilibrium of the bicarbonate–carbonic acid buffer system and decreases the plasma hydrogen ion concentration (that is, it increases pH). This effect on pH is mitigated, however, by a secondary *decrease* in plasma bicarbonate concentration. During acute hypocapnia bicarbonate is removed from the extracellular fluid by a process of buffering in both blood and tissues, renal excretion of alkali playing only a minor role. During chronic hypocapnia there is a further reduction in bicarbonate concentration which is mediated largely if not entirely by the kidneys. If hyperventilation is sufficiently prolonged (as in persons living at high altitude), these adjustments are sufficient to restore plasma pH to normal or nearly normal levels (Fig. 4).

Pathogenesis. Probably the most common cause of respiratory alkalosis is the hyperventilation resulting from extreme anxiety. Other causes are central nervous system injury involving the respiratory center, artificial ventilation, fever, hepatic coma, and salicylate intoxication. Hypocapnia is also encountered in the early phase of pulmonary disease if a disturbance in the relation between ventilation and perfusion has produced hypoxemia and hyperventilation.

Finally, as discussed earlier, the persistence of respiratory compensation after the correction of metabolic acidosis may produce a picture indistinguishable chemically from a primary respiratory alkalosis.

Diagnosis. The presence of hyperventilation in a patient suffering from any one of the disorders considered under Pathogenesis should suggest the diagnosis of respiratory alkalosis. In many cases characteristic signs and symptoms provide evidence that one is dealing with primary hyperventilation rather than respiratory compensation for metabolic acidosis. Respiratory alkalosis produces a typical clinical syndrome in which the cardinal features are lightheadedness, numbness, tingling of the extremities, and circumoral paresthesia. In some patients, frank carpopedal spasm occurs.

The finding of an abnormally low plasma bicarbonate concentration and Pco_2 does not in itself distinguish between metabolic acidosis and respiratory alkalosis; the measurement of plasma pH is often vital to the differentiation. The problem of diagnosis sometimes is further complicated by the presence of a mixed acid-base disorder—that is, one with both respiratory and metabolic components. This combination occurs very often in salicylate poisoning.

Treatment. The treatment of respiratory alkalosis should be directed toward correction of the underlying disturbance responsible for the hyperventilation. In the patient with salicylism the goal is to promote removal of the offending drug. One can accomplish this purpose either by augmenting the renal excretion of salicylate (by means of urinary alkalinization and the administration of osmotic diuretics) or by hemodialysis. With injury to the central nervous system or with liver failure, the ability to correct respiratory alkalosis will be determined by the effectiveness of therapy directed toward the underlying pathologic process. The hyperventilation syndrome resulting from anxiety can often be effectively controlled if the patient rebreathes into a paper bag. If this fails, sedation will usually put an end to the acute episode. Recurrences can sometimes be prevented by reassurance and by explanation of the nature of the disorder to the patient, but if these techniques fail, psychotherapy may be indicated.

Arbus, G. S., Hebert, L. A., Levesque, P. R., Etsten, B. E., and Schwartz, W. B.: Characterization and clinical application of the "significance band" for acute respiratory alkalosis. N. Engl. J. Med., 280:117, 1969.

Brackett, N. C., Jr., Wingo, C. F., Muren, O., and Solano, J. T.: Acid-base response to chronic hypercapnia in man. N. Engl. J. Med., 280:124, 1969.

Levy, L. J., Duga, J., Girgis, M., and Gordon, E. E.: Ketoacidosis associated with alcoholism in nondiabetic subjects. Ann. Intern. Med., 78:213, 1973.

Oliva, P. B.: Lactic acidosis. Am. J. Med., 48:209, 1970.

Relman, A. S.: The acidosis of renal disease. Am. J. Med., 44:706, 1968.

Schwartz, W. B., van Ypersele de Strihou, C., and Kassirer, J. P.: Role of anions in metabolic alkalosis and potassium deficiency. N. Engl. J. Med., 279:630, 1968.

Seldin, D. W., and Rector, F. C.: The generation and maintenance of metabolic alkalosis. Kidney Int., 1:306, 1972.

DISORDERS OF CARBOHYDRATE METABOLISM

806. DIABETES MELLITUS

George F. Cahill, Jr.

General Considerations. *Diabetes mellitus* is a diagnostic term applied to a constellation of anatomic and biochemical abnormalities which share in common, as part of a syndrome, a disturbance in glucose homeostasis, which is secondary to a deficiency in the beta cells of the endocrine pancreas. This bulky and vague definition cannot be made more specific owing to the marked variability in the disorder. As was once said of syphilis, knowledge of diabetes and its sequelae touches on all areas of medicine.

The syndrome can be completely asymptomatic, or it can appear as an isolated disorder of any organ or system. Fulminant ketoacidosis, fatal unless immediately treated, may be the first sign. Often it is manifested by one of the long-term complications, such as foot ulcer, retinopathy, or proteinuria. Other pathologic states noted to be more frequent in diabetics as compared to the general population may be the clue. For example, the presenting event may be of a myocardial infarction in a young man, an unexpectedly large newborn or pruritus vulvae in the female, recurrent skin infections, or many other phenomena which at first glance appear unrelated. Diabetes mellitus is protean in its manifestations, and this variability is central to its diagnosis and treatment.

History. Descriptions of the disease were made 3000 years ago in Egypt. About 400 B.C., Charak and Susrut in India noted not only the sweetness of the urine but also the correlation between obesity and diabetes, the tendency of the disease to be passed from one generation to another through the "seed," and even two types of disease, one associated with emaciation, dehydration, polyuria, and lassitude, and the other characterized by "stout build, gluttony, obesity, and sleepiness." Near the beginning of the Christian era, the Romans Aretaeus and Celsus described the disease and gave it the name diabetes (= siphon) mellitus (melli = honey or sweet). Its correlation with gangrene was mentioned by the Arab, Avicenna, 1000 A.D. The sweetness of the urine was again described by Thomas Willis (1675). Dodson, 100 years later, demonstrated that the sweetness was due to sugar and suggested it was not formed de novo by the kidney, but rather that the kidney removed it from the body, a fact scientifically confirmed by the great French physiologist, Claude Bernard, in the mid-1800's.

In 1889 Von Mering and Minkowski first produced experimental diabetes by removing the dog's pancreas. Subsequently Opie (1901) noted changes in the islets of cells in the pancreas (the islets having been described by Langerhans in 1869) in humans dying with the disease. This led to attempts by many to prepare pancreatic extracts which would correct the deficiency. Active fractions were obtained by some, but not until 1921 did Banting and Best in Toronto achieve continuous success, and their discovery was rapidly applied to clinical therapy within six months of their first report. Until then, only a careful semistarvation diet with elimination of excess carbohydrate was even partially effective in prolonging life in the more insulin-deficient juvenile form of the disease, or in ameliorating the symptoms in many patients with the milder maturity-onset variety.

The Banting-Best era changed the outlook of the juvenile diabetic from certain death within two to three years to a nearly normal, albeit shortened, life expectancy. In 1936 the use of long-acting insulin was introduced, simplifying the management of the insulin-requiring diabetic. It became apparent at that time, however, that although insulin therapy prevented many of the acute metabolic problems such as ketoacidosis or those closely correlated with the hyperglycemia, e.g., pruritus vulvae or furunculosis, other sequelae such as retinitis, diabetic neuropathy, or renal glomerulosclerosis appeared in most patients with the juvenile form of the disease for two or more decades in spite of insulin therapy. These complications had been noted prior to the advent of insulin but were relatively unusual, because death from ketoacidosis or infection shortened the life of the patient before these could become manifest. Thus insulin, although a tremendous step forward, did not provide the total solution for the diabetic and his problem. Another development, although less significant than that of insulin, stemmed from the German observation during World War War II that certain sulfonamide derivatives lowered blood glucose, and subsequently Loubatières initiated trials in France which established their clinical efficacy. In 1955, oral sulfonylureas began to be generally used as hypoglycemic therapy in diabetics with the milder maturity-onset type of the disease.

Pathophysiology. Before discussing the etiology, epidemiology, pathology, and clinical aspects of diabetes, the metabolic effects of insulin in normal and abnormal states must be described. Simply, insulin is the animal's "fed" signal. After a large meal, the high circulating levels of insulin tell the body's tissues to take up and store fuel not required for immediate metabolic needs. An intermediate level of insulin resulting from a smaller intake signals the tissues to take up and store fuel less avidly. In contrast, a low level of insulin such as occurs during fasting tells the body that no fuel is entering, and the body's depots should therefore release

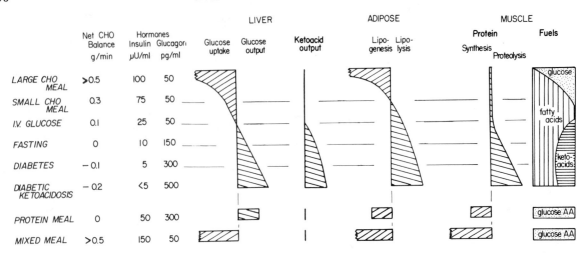

Figure 1. Insulin and glucagon levels and varying rates of organ metabolism as a function of net carbohydrate (CHO) balance in man. The progression from a large positive carbohydrate balance after a large CHO meal to a negative balance as in ketoacidosis forms a continuum of decreasing insulin levels and increasing glucagon levels. Relative metabolic fluxes after protein and mixed meals are also shown. Since the relative contributions of glucose or amino acids (AA) to muscle fuel are not known, these are not differentiated in the scheme.

their stored nutrients back into the blood. Insulin and its normal and abnormal metabolic effects form a continuum of metabolic events (Fig. 1), ranging from those seen when there is a total or near-total lack of insulin's metabolic effects (diabetic ketoacidosis) to those which occur when there are very high levels of insulin (after a large orally ingested mixed meal in a normal individual possessing adequate pancreatic beta cell reserve).

Body Fuels. As shown in Table 1 of Ch. 726, average man is about one fifth fat, which stores approximately a two- to three-month supply of calories. Carbohydrate reserves, in contrast, are minimal, about 70 grams (280 kcal) as liver glycogen and 200 grams (800 kcal) in muscle glycogen. Glucose in body fluids is even less, about 15 to 20 grams. Slightly more than 1 kcal per minute is required for basal metabolic needs in a normal resting adult; thus total available carbohydrate in the entire body provides less than one day's supply of fuel. Unlike carbohydrate and fat, there is no depot of protein purely for storage. All is being used for structure, for enzymes, or for other essential purposes. These points emphasize the role of fat as the primary energy storage depot in man and the minimal role of carbohydrate.

Tissue Fuel Utilization. In contrast to storage, in which fat predominates, fuel utilization by brain and, to a lesser degree, by certain other tissues requires a constant supply of glucose. Thus glucose concentration in normal man is confined to a zone between 50 and 150 mg per 100 ml, concentrations above the minimum required by brain and below that saturating the renal reabsorption capacity. Insulin plays the dominant role in maintaining glucose in this range. All other tissues are capable of using glucose and do so when ample amounts are present in the diet, but only if insulin levels are increased. Most of these, particularly fat and muscle, do not utilize glucose when insulin levels are low, and consume instead fat in the form of free fatty acids released from adipose tissue. The capacity of the endocrine pancreas to respond rapidly and adequately

to the nutritional state by its rate of insulin release is thus critical to fuel homeostasis.

FED STATE. After eating a mixed meal, gastrointestinal digestion hydrolyzes proteins to single amino acids and carbohydrates to simple sugars, and these enter the portal blood. The liver is easily permeable to all simple sugars and related molecules, and possesses specific enzymes for the phosphorylation and subsequent metabolism of these, particularly of galactose and fructose (see Ch. 808 and 811). Glucose is phosphorylated and incorporated into glycogen or metabolized by the liver both for its own energy needs and for fat synthesis. These processes require increased insulin levels. After a large carbohydrate-containing meal, much glucose also passes through to the periphery, and the increased insulin levels accelerate the transport of glucose across the muscle and adipose cell wall (Fig. 1).

In muscle, as in liver, glucose is rapidly phosphorylated and used for glycogen synthesis. It is also metabolized to lactate or pyruvate in the cell's cytosol and then, in the presence of adequate oxygen, to carbon dioxide by the cell's mitochondria to provide the bulk of the cell's ATP and, thereby, the muscle's energy needs. In adipose tissue, the augmented glucose uptake in the presence of high insulin levels is metabolized to pyruvate, but instead of the acetyl CoA from the pyruvate being oxidized to CO_2 for energy as in muscle, most is returned to the cytosol and long chain fatty acids are synthesized. In simple terms, the original potential energy available in glucose is converted into potential energy as fatty acid, and the fatty acids are then included, three at a time esterified to glycerol, as triglyceride, into the oil vacuole in the center of the fat cell. The net effect is transformation of a poor economy type of fuel expressed per unit weight as stored in tissues (carbohydrate) into a much more efficient form (fat).

The amino acids absorbed with the meal are removed by many tissues, particularly by muscle. It has been shown that insulin augments the transfer of certain amino acids across muscle cell membrane. Insulin also, when exposed to intact muscle, increases the protein-synthetic machinery inside the cell, and the net effect is to increase muscle protein. Thus, as was shown 50 years ago, insulin is anabolic, expanding the body's protein mass.

The third component of the diet, the ingested fat or triglyceride, is partly hydrolyzed in the gut lumen, absorbed by the mucosa where the triglyceride is resynthesized, and incorporated in association with several lipoproteins into a particle, or chylomicron, which is secreted into the lymphatics between the intestinal cells and then, via the thoracic duct, carried into the general circulation. A major part of these chylomicrons is removed in adipose tissue by an enzyme located at or near the fat-cell membrane, lipoprotein lipase, and this enzyme hydrolyzes the triglyceride to yield three free fatty acids, which, in turn, enter into the fat cell, and, like the fatty acid synthesized de novo from glucose, are esterified and incorporated as triglyceride into the central oil droplet. The acceptor for the intracellular re-esterification for fatty acids is glycerol phosphate derived from glucose metabolism. A high insulin level is necessary for the activity of lipoprotein lipase as well as to provide adequate glycerol phosphate for the intracellular esterification of the fatty acids.

In summary, in the "fed" state, a high insulin level is necessary for incorporation of glucose into liver and muscle glycogen, for muscle to consume glucose for energy needs, for both liver and adipose tissue to make fatty acid from glucose, for amino acids to be incorporated into muscle protein, for circulating chylomicrons to discharge their fatty acids into adipose tissue, and for these, in turn, to be re-esterified and incorporated into the triglyceride storage droplet in the middle of the cell.

INTRAVENOUS D AND W. Between the "fed" state, described above, and the fasted state is one in which small amounts of carbohydrate are ingested or administered. This is termed intravenous dextrose and water (IV D and W), because it is frequently employed during partial starvation in patients who cannot or should not be fed by mouth. Glucose, at 100 mg per minute, closely approximates the energy needs of the brain, about one fourth to one fifth the basal caloric need of the body, and thus its administration obviates the need for hepatic glycogenolysis or gluconeogenesis. The body achieves this by the beta cells slightly increasing insulin secretion as a response to the small increase in glucose concentration. This causes circulating insulin levels to rise sufficiently to decrease the release of amino acid from muscle and to prevent hepatic glycogenolysis and gluconeogenesis. It does not increase insulin concentration enough to open up muscle cell and adipose cell membranes to glucose utilization. Thus glucose is yet excluded from most tissues and spared for brain, and, most important, the breakdown of protein to provide precursor for glucose synthesis is no longer necessary. This is the basis for the well-known "nitrogen-sparing effect of carbohydrate." It must again be emphasized that this is achieved via levels of insulin slightly above those in simple fasting, and it is the beta cell which increases the insulin level, thanks to its exquisite sensitivity to the minimal but significant increase in blood glucose concentration.

FASTED STATE. As described above, man has minimal carbohydrate reserves, and these are rapidly depleted even during overnight fast. Between meals, glucose levels can be maintained by glycogenolysis, but during more prolonged periods of caloric deprivation, hepatic gluconeogenesis must be initiated to maintain adequate glucose concentrations. This is achieved by a reduction in beta cell release of insulin as glucose falls and thereby in reduced insulin levels, the low levels initiating (1) net muscle proteolysis, (2) the release of amino acids to the liver via the circulation, and (3) gluconeogenesis from these. Subsequently the glucose so produced is consumed by brain. Other tissues, such as renal medulla, red blood cells, peripheral nerve, and, to a limited degree, skeletal muscle, also utilize glucose, but mainly to pyruvate and lactate, and these are returned to the liver for resynthesis to glucose—the so-called Cori cycle. Some of the pyruvate is transaminated to alanine, which also participates in the cycle analogous to lactate and pyruvate. Thus brain is the major tissue metabolizing glucose completely to carbon dioxide and water and requiring gluconeogenesis from amino acids.

For a better understanding of fasting, and particularly of diabetes, more detail is necessary. As insulin level falls, muscle proteolysis outweighs synthesis, certain amino acids are metabolized in the muscle, and those which are glucogenic such as alanine are released. Liver, owing to low insulin and normal or high glucagon levels, is enzymatically poised in the direction of glucose synthesis, and the alanine and other glucogenic amino acids are made into glucose. This process requires both energy and hydrogen (reducing equivalent), and these are met by fat oxidation in the liver. The long-chain fatty acids, originally derived from adipose tissue, are partially oxidized to molecules of acetyl CoA, but few of these gain access for terminal combustion via the citric acid cycle to carbon dioxide for reasons not biochemically clarified. Instead they are condensed and exported from the liver, two at a time, as the *ketone bodies, acetoacetate* and *β-hydroxybutyrate*. Thus during fasting, coupled with gluconeogenesis is the production of ketoacids (ketone bodies).

Acetoacetate and β-hydroxybutyrate are readily utilized by muscle as fuel, and their rate of production by liver in simple fasting closely approximates their utilization, with little "spilling over" into the urine. However, after more than several days of fasting, peripheral tissues diminish their utilization of ketoacids, and their total level in blood rises to approximately 6 to 8 mM. In parallel with this increase is a gradual increase in cerebrospinal fluid ketoacids, sufficient in concentration to provide the major proportion of the brain's energy needs, displacing glucose utilization accordingly. This permits less gluconeogenesis and less mobilization of muscle protein as glucogenic precursor, and survival, thanks to this sparing of body nitrogen, is dramatically prolonged. All these are a result of a continuously low level of insulin, but it must be emphasized that insulin is still playing the central feedback role in the relationship between fuel utilization and mobilization.

Diabetes. With the metabolic states briefly described, it is apparent that abnormalities in insulin secretion must result in altered fuel homeostasis. If insulin secretion cannot be rapidly increased after ingestion of a meal, the rate of intestinal absorption (an insulin-independent process for carbohydrate, amino acid, and fat) will greatly surpass the peripheral uptake of all fuels, resulting in alimentary hyperglycemia, hyperaminoacidemia, and hyperlipemia. This is most easily tested by a simple glucose meal (glucose tolerance), whereby the blood level of glucose given orally or intravenously is followed over time. If insulin release is inadequate, the glucose level is high and remains higher for a longer time owing to failure of the body to receive an adequate "fed" signal. If the insulin deficiency is more marked and is insufficient to facilitate glucose ingress into muscle and adipose cells or glucose incorporation into liver glycogen, but yet enough to depress hepatic ketogenesis and gluconeogenesis, the glucose load will stay in the circulation. Glucose concentration then surpasses the renal threshold and spills into the urine, and dehydration, hypovolemia, and severe hyperglycemia ensue, possibly leading to hyperosmolar coma.

If the insulin deficiency is severe, irrespective of glucose concentration, peripheral amino acid release from muscle protein will provide the liver with more and more glucogenic substrate, and gluconeogenesis and ketogenesis will be rapidly increased. As in prolonged starvation, there is also a decreased peripheral ketoacid utilization, levels of β-hydroxybutyrate and acetoacetate rise quickly in the body, and life-threatening ketoacidosis occurs in addition to the marked hyperglycemia, dehydration, and volume deficiency.

Endocrine Pancreas. The entire carbohydrate, fat, protein, and lipid disorder, as seen in diabetic ketoacidosis, is precisely mimicked by acute pancreatectomy, by chemical destruction of the beta cells with agents such as alloxan or streptozotocin, or by administration of antibody to insulin. Subtotal destruction or removal of beta cells results in less severe degrees of diabetes. Likewise, postmortem examination of human pancreas has shown either total absence of beta cells in juvenile diabetics after several years of the disease or minimal reductions in number with variable nonspecific morphologic changes in the older, maturity-onset type of diabetic.

Little is known of the natural history of the beta cell. It appears early in the human embryo and continues to divide slowly through life. In states in which there is resistance to insulin's effects, beta cell hyperplasia may be noted. Why the diabetic cannot generate more beta cells to replace his deficiency is unknown, and this deficiency as well as a temporal delay in insulin release by the remaining cells may possibly be the primary underlying defect.

The beta cell responds both to the ambient concentration of *glucose* and to changes in glucose concentration by insulin release. This appears to be in two phases, one occurring almost immediately after the increase in glucose concentration and peaking in five to ten minutes, and a later phase occurring 15 to 30 minutes later and persisting as long as the glucose concentration remains elevated. Glucose taken by mouth elicits a greater insulin release than glucose infused parenterally; this is due to a hormonal effect in the gut during carbohydrate absorption which sensitizes the beta cells to release even more insulin in response to changes in glucose concentration. This gut hormone(s) has yet to be identified, but is probably similar to secretin; it also cross-reacts with some nonspecific antibodies to glucagon.

Amino acids also can provoke insulin release. Of particular interest are leucine and arginine, the former being an essential branched-chain amino acid which, in certain children, can induce excessive insulin release, causing symptomatic hypoglycemia (see Ch. 807). Arginine, as well as several other amino acids, also induces insulin release, and its administration has been used as one of a battery of research tests for assessing beta cell function. Eating a protein meal results in an apparently greater insulin release than one might expect from the constituent amino acids. This has been explained by the capacity of CCK-pancreozymin, the gut hormone released after protein ingestion to stimulate excessive pancreatic secretion, to affect also the endocrine pancreas by promoting insulin release from the beta cells (as well as glucagon from the alpha cells).

Other factors known to stimulate insulin release are the *sulfonylurea class of oral antidiabetic agents*, stimulation of parasympathetic nerves leading to the pancreas, and, to a lesser degree, elevated concentrations of fatty acids, ketoacids, and the potassium ion. The relative importance of innervation and these last-named factors appears to be less than that of glucose and amino acids in man. In other animals, such as the ruminants, ketoacids and related compounds are very active insulin secretagogues.

INSULIN.   Insulin is synthesized inside the beta cell as a single chain proinsulin of 86 amino acids which then folds back on itself; closure of sulfur bridges then follows (Fig. 2). As shown by Steiner in the mid-1960's, the "connecting peptide" is then split out, leaving two amino acid chains of 31 and 20 amino acids connected

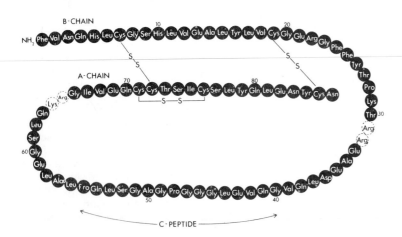

Figure 2. Probable sequence of human proinsulin, containing 86 amino acids in a single chain folded back on itself, with closure of 2 sulfhydryl bridges between the beginning and end as well as a bridge between amino acids 71 and 76. When the C-peptide (connecting peptide) is split out in the beta cell as the insulin is being collected into storage granules, the A and B chains are left connected by the sulfhydryl bridges. The eventual human A chain has 21 amino acids and the B chain 30 amino acids. The A-B chain insulin differs from pig insulin by a threonine (Thr) instead of an alanine at the end of the B chain. Many more differences exist in the connecting peptides between species; hence the higher antigenicity of the impure insulins. (Illustration courtesy of Dr. D. Steiner.)

by sulfur bridges. The insulin and connecting peptide are packaged together into granules; when the beta cell is stimulated to release insulin, the granules are brought to the surface of the cell, and insulin is discharged with the metabolically inert connecting peptide into the adjacent capillary. Normally a small amount of proinsulin is also released, but this hormone is either inactive or much less active than insulin itself. In abnormal states such as islet cell tumor or in diabetes, the proportion of proinsulin may be increased, a circumstance which has been helpful in diagnosis.

Insulin in blood is unbound. Approximately half is removed as it passes through liver, and most of the remainder is removed by the kidney, being small enough (5734 daltons) to be filtered and catabolized by the tubules on resorption. Thus insulin has a short half-life, approximately ten minutes. All data suggest that changes in its concentration are regulated by alterations in beta cell secretion, not by alterations in removal rates.

Insulin, like other peptide hormones, binds to specific receptors on cell membranes and elicits the release of one or more second messengers, which in turn alter enzyme levels and activities inside the cell. In muscle and adipose tissue, there is also a rapid acceleration of glucose transport across the cell wall after exposure to insulin, as well as augmented transport of certain amino acids and potassium into the cell and change in the membrane electrical potential. Which of these are primary insulin effects and which are secondary to one or more intracellular messengers remain to be established. In certain tissues, levels of cyclic AMP are reduced by insulin, but the numerous intracellular effects cannot be explained solely by the reduced level of cyclic AMP.

GLUCAGON. Glucagon is composed of a single strand of 29 amino acids and is secreted by the alpha cells in the islets. Its primary effect is to increase the activity of adenylcyclase in liver by reacting with sites on the liver cell membrane, and thereby to increase hepatic cyclic AMP. This in turn initiates activation of glycogen breakdown, by increasing the activity of the glycogen phosphorylase system and by decreasing the activity of the glycogen synthetase system (see Ch. 809). It also increases gluconeogenesis in the liver, again probably because of its effect on adenyl cyclase activity. The precise role of glucagon in man is as yet unclear, but it is probably important in the disposition of the amino acids in a pure protein meal. Its release is prompted by certain amino acids such as arginine and alanine and also by enteric hormones such as CCK-pancreozymin. Its level also increases in many states of stress, such as trauma, hypoglycemia, infection, exercise, and starvation. Unger has shown that at a given glucose concentration it is increased in diabetics as compared to nondiabetics, suggesting either a direct effect of insulin on the alpha cell or a primary alpha cell abnormality. Since destruction of the total pancreas or of beta cells specifically or removal of circulating insulin by administration of antibody in laboratory animals can produce the full-blown diabetic state, the role of glucagon, if any, may be minimal and secondary to that of insulin. In milder degrees of diabetes, its relatively increased level as compared to that of normals may play a role, but this has yet to be characterized.

Etiology. As known to the Hindis centuries ago, diabetes is familial. Environment also plays a large role, particularly overnutrition, as evidenced by the marked decrease in incidence of the disease in Europe during World War II. The geneticist's best tool, a comparison of identical versus fraternal twins, has been used several times, and a much higher concordance rate has been noted in identical twins, indicating an important genetic component. As mentioned before, the disease is a continuum ranging from a total or near total absence of insulin, resulting in death in two or three days in diabetic ketoacidosis, to a slightly elevated glucose level after a glucose load as compared to the disposition of a similar glucose load in a "normal" population. Terms used for either end of the spectrum include *"juvenile-onset"* or *"ketosis-prone"* for the markedly insulin-deficient, and *maturity-onset "mild"* or *"late-onset"* for the individual whose insulin release after a challenge is insufficient to effect normal glucose tolerance. Although most children exhibit the "juvenile-onset" form of diabetes, they can develop a very mild or "maturity-onset" type of the disease, and this latter predisposition, often associated with obesity, appears to be marked in certain families. Likewise, four fifths or more of all diabetics develop the "maturity-onset" type of the disease in later life and usually are overweight at diagnosis. Ketoacidosis is infrequent in this older-age-onset group, but does occur. Nonhereditary diabetes, such as that secondary to pancreatitis, should be considered when ketoacidosis develops early in diabetes in this older age group. Curiously, subjects in the eighth or ninth decade of life may also develop the juvenile type of diabetes, but this is infrequent.

Paradoxically, concordance for diabetes is much greater in identical twins developing the disease in middle or later life, approaching 90 to 100 per cent when tested by glucose tolerance. In the juvenile-onset type of diabetes, concordance, which occurs in approximately half of twin pairs, is within one or two years of the diagnosis in the first twin. If the second twin does not develop it within a few years, he frequently never will, suggesting juvenile-type diabetes to be less familial than the adult-onset type and possibly more influenced by environment—exactly the reverse of other inherited diseases, in which the more severe form appears to be more transmissible through heredity. Another strong possibility is that there are different forms of diabetes with a different genetic basis.

It has been suggested that juvenile diabetes may be due to viral destruction of beta cells, and British studies have shown juvenile diabetes to occur in clusters associated with certain common viral epidemics (e.g., group B, coxsackievirus). One still must note the greater prevalence of both types of diabetes in a given kindred as compared to the population as a whole, and this might be explained by a lesser capacity for beta cells to divide within the diabetic kindred. Although a single autosomal recessive was suggested at one time, a double dose being necessary for phenotypic expression, the inheritance is certainly polygenic. No difference in sex that cannot be attributed to the tendency of middle-aged females to be more obese in certain cultures has been consistently observed.

Siperstein has questioned whether a beta cell abnormality is the primary etiologic event, and his studies have shown offspring of two diabetic parents to possess significant thickening of the capillary basement membrane as shown by electron microscopic examination of tissues obtained by biopsy of the quadriceps muscle. Also it has been noted that fibroblasts of diabetic subjects grow less well in tissue culture, suggesting a more ubiquitous lesion in cell replication. Williamson has attributed Siperstein's observations simply to a progressive age-related thickening of the basement membrane. The subject remains controversial, but the high association with degenerative vascular disease suggests some underlying generalized tissue abnormality.

The high incidence of diabetes noted in many other hereditary diseases, such as Turner's and Werner's syndromes, and in various muscular disorders, such as amyotrophic lateral sclerosis, suggests the beta cell to be uniquely sensitive to inherent defects in metabolism, again possibly because of defective replication. Surprisingly, the body's most rapidly replicating cells, those in the gut mucosa and the hematopoietic cells, do not appear to be affected by such a replicative lesion in diabetic kindreds as would be true if this were fundamental in the diabetic pathogenesis. However, certain hematologic disorders such as Fanconi's anemia have a very high prevalence of diabetes both in affected subjects and in relatives. In certain multiple endocrine deficiencies an autoimmune process has been involved, but for other forms of diabetes, autoimmunity has not been adequately demonstrated.

Diagnosis.   The sine qua non for diagnosis is demonstration of the inability of a given subject to dispose appropriately of a glucose load, as evidence of a relative or absolute decrease in insulin release and circulating concentration. This legalistic description is, however, markedly qualified. Anxiety, prior carbohydrate deprivation, old age, acute illness, infection, delayed gastric emptying, certain pharmacologic agents,

hypokalemia, and many other factors can all result in abnormal glucose tolerance. A normal unstressed subject, having had adequate amounts of dietary carbohydrate (over 200 grams per day for several days), on ingesting 75 or 100 grams of glucose should have a venous whole blood glucose level below 110 mg per 100 ml before glucose ingestion, under 160 mg per 100 ml at one hour, and below 120 mg per 100 ml at two hours (Fig. 3). Capillary levels (mainly arterial) and levels in plasma (caused by the volume occupied by hemoglobin and red cell stroma) will be proportionally higher, and appropriate corrections should be made. The glucose is given as either pure glucose or commercially available flavored dextrins (i.e., Glucola), which are rapidly hydrolyzed to free glucose in the gut and then absorbed. The glucose may also be given intravenously, 0.5 gram per kilogram, and blood levels determined at several ten-minute intervals up to one hour after its rapid infusion. The per cent disappearance, calculated from half-life ($t\frac{1}{2}$) of blood glucose (e.g., the minutes elapsed when glucose levels decrease from 300 to 150 mg per 100 ml, as plotted semilogarithmically) is defined as:

$$K \left(\frac{\text{per cent disappearance}}{\text{minute}} \right) = \frac{0.69}{t\frac{1}{2} \text{ minutes}} \times 100$$

and should normally be greater than unity. This test has been utilized mainly as a research tool, because it bypasses the gut factor effect elicited by oral glucose. It has been found, however, to be clinically less discriminant than the oral glucose tolerance test.

Rarely, one is presented with a patient with classic diabetic retinopathy or nephropathy but a normal fasting glucose level, and even more rarely the same patient might have a normal glucose tolerance. Is this a diabetic? Probably yes, so the strict adherence to the legalistic glucose tolerance as being pathognomonic is not warranted. It is highly probable that this subject had had glucose intolerance at one time. This introduces a problem shared by most other diseases of the endocrine system, namely their fluctuating nature and capacity to remit and relapse without known cause.

Natural History and Definitions.   The disease may present as fulminant diabetic ketoacidosis at any age, but most frequently in childhood or adolescence. It is common for the disease then to remit, little or no insulin being required for several weeks to months, and then to recur as the remission ends. Glucose tolerance through the remission is usually abnormal, but occasionally it may even be normal. Also, the remission may last as long as one or two years, and very rarely the diabetes may not recur. Once the diabetes has recurred in the young individual, it may be relatively easy to manage with a simple morning injection of intermediate-duration insulin, but after several years the glucose levels become more difficult to manage, suggesting termination of all endogenous insulin release. Rubenstein and Steiner have shown connecting peptide (Fig. 2) to be present in plasma, suggesting that some endogenous insulin synthesis and secretion do persist through the early phases of the disease. The diabetes then becomes labile or "brittle" after endogenous insulin secretion ceases and requires more careful matching of diet and insulin, the latter usually necessary twice ("split-dose") instead of once a day.

In the maturity-onset type of diabetic, the insulin

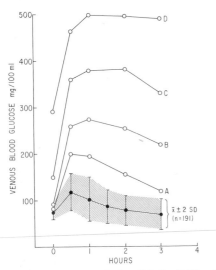

Figure 3.   Glucose tolerance tests in four diabetics (A–D) and range of values in 191 healthy controls. Shaded area shows range of two standard deviations in the normal population. Diabetics A and B have sufficient insulin for fasting glucose homeostasis, but an inability to increase insulin release appropriately. Diabetic C has fasting hyperglycemia and marked glucose intolerance. The late fall-off at the end of the curve may be due mainly to glucose loss in urine. Subject D, in whom the tolerance test was clinically unnecessary, is probably almost totally lacking in insulin, and, with this degree of fasting hyperglycemia, is a candidate for the development of ketoacidosis. In such a subject, glucose in the urine may even surpass the load given for the tolerance itself. (Unpublished data of R. Gleason and J. S. Soeldner.)

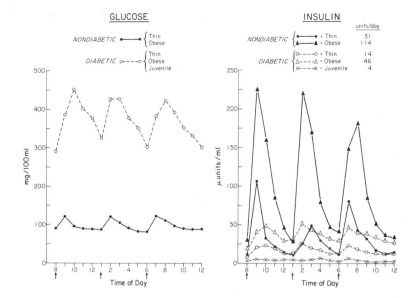

Figure 4. Glucose and insulin levels in five groups of subjects during 16 hours of the day. The glucose levels are lumped together into nondiabetics and diabetics. The diabetics were specifically selected to be those with a significant degree of fasting hyperglycemia. The obese diabetics show the marked hyperinsulinemia necessary to overcome their generalized resistance to insulin. The estimated peripheral insulin secretion rate in the obese diabetic is calculated as 114 units per day, almost four times that of the normal nonobese.

The obese diabetic has also a greater insulin secretion than does the normal, 46 units per day. The thin adult diabetic does less well than the normal, and the juvenile diabetic shows an almost total failure to increase the very meager insulin level after changes in fuel loads. (Data of S. Genuth.)

deficiency is less severe and may be evidenced only by glucose intolerance of varying degrees. Obesity, for as yet unexplained reasons, requires a higher insulin concentration and therefore a greater rate of insulin release for insulin to exert its metabolic effects (Fig. 4). Binding of insulin to various cells taken from experimentally obese animals has been shown to be decreased, as have the metabolic effects of insulin. Thus obesity unmasks diabetes (as do pregnancy and other endocrine disturbances associated with peripheral resistance to insulin). If the patient loses weight and normal glucose tolerance ensues, the patient is spoken of as a latent diabetic. This same term is applied to a mother with normal glucose tolerance post partum but a diabetic tolerance when pregnant. A "chemical diabetic" is one who is also asymptomatic at the time but has abnormal glucose tolerance or even an elevated fasting blood glucose value.

The maturity-onset type of diabetic, as just mentioned, may lose the glucose abnormality with weight loss, or, occasionally, may even lose it without weight loss by dietary therapy alone, meaning carbohydrate restriction. Conversely, the glucose intolerance may progress, with initial worsening of the glucose tolerance itself, followed by insufficient insulin to maintain normal fasting glucose concentrations, with exogenous insulin required to prevent ketoacidosis. Generally, however, the diabetes tends to remain at the severity at which the original diagnosis was made.

Incidence and Prevalence. Surveys in the United States have shown 1 to 2 per cent of the population to have documented diabetes and a similar number to have abnormal glucose tolerance without having been previously diagnosed. The "softness" of this statistic is grossly apparent in view of the "softness" of the criteria for diagnosis. In Michigan, 1 in 600 school children requires insulin; this is probably a good statistic for juvenile diabetes, but there are probably additional children with milder maturity-onset diabetes undiagnosed. In the total diabetic population, the juvenile type of diabetes comprises approximately 10 per cent, but again this is not a firm statistic, because many patients

who have insulin-requiring diabetes do not go into ketoacidosis without insulin but stabilize at a high glucose concentration, thanks to deficient yet significant endogenous insulin production. Thus the disease is a continuum between total insulin lack and the normal, and the characterization of the normal is made arbitrarily. With advanced age, a greater proportion of the population, as high as 40 to 60 per cent in the ninth decade, has abnormal glucose tolerance; so again the definition is arbitrary.

There are diverse cultural and racial differences in incidence and prevalence. Diabetes is rare in the Eskimo; in certain American Indians such as the Pima in Arizona, up to 50 per cent of the population develop diabetes. Similar high rates are observed in Asian Indians who have moved to South Africa and adopted a sedentary, high-caloric style of life. Ketoacidosis is less frequent to absent in these and in blacks in Africa or in the Oriental races, particularly homeland Japanese. The extent to which these differences are genetic on the one hand or environmental or nutritional on the other is under study.

Clinical Manifestations. The classic juvenile diabetic is a child with one or two weeks or longer of progressive polydipsia and polyuria, weight loss, lassitude, blurred vision, leg cramps, inattentiveness at school, irritability, and frequently a craving for sweet beverages. Such a child, if diabetes is undiagnosed, develops mild and then severe nausea, followed by vomiting, dehydration, stupor, coma, and finally death. The progression may be more rapid, particularly in infants or small children, or it may continue as the three "polys," polydipsia, polyuria, and polyphagia, for from weeks to months, with marked weight loss even to the point of emaciation. These latter subjects apparently still have some endogenous insulin production. Thus the initial presentation of the juvenile diabetic may be due to (1) ketoacidosis; (2) marked hyperglycemia, dehydration, and collapse without ketoacidosis, namely hyperosmolar coma; or (3) an intermediate between these two. Diabetic ketoacidosis always has some degree of hyperosmolarity.

If the insulin deficiency is less marked but fasting hyperglycemia and glucosuria are present, the patient may not be aware of the insidious onset of polydipsia and polyuria and may be brought to the physician's attention by superimposed infection. Females with glycosuria are particularly susceptible to bacterial and fungal infections of the vulva and vagina, with marked pruritus, excoriation, and bad odor. The hyperglycemia may predispose the subject to other soft tissue infection such as cellulitis, furunculosis, gingival abscess, otitis media, or paronychia. There is also a predisposition to other internal infective processes, such as appendicitis and cholecystitis, and particularly to pulmonary tuberculosis or systemic mycotic infections.

The patient with the milder, maturity-onset type of disease may be asymptomatic, and the diagnosis may be made by finding glycosuria or hyperglycemia or by glucose intolerance. The predisposition of diabetes to premature atherosclerosis frequently provokes medical attention, and the diabetes is then recognized. Myocardial infarction in a young man or, particularly, a woman in the reproductive age, premature peripheral vascular insufficiency, or occasionally diabetic neuropathy or nephropathy may be the first manifestation.

Eye. The ocular manifestations of diabetes are numerous. Hyperglycemia increases glucose concentration in the lens and optic humors, resulting in blurring of vision, weakness of accommodation, and myopia. Very rarely the lens itself may become opacified (the metabolic or *"snowflake" cataract*) presumably owing to sorbitol formation and accumulation; this may disappear after correction of the hyperglycemia. Another manifestation of acute or subacute diabetes is *lipemia retinalis,* the retinal arteries and veins appearing as if they contain cream of tomato soup rather than demonstrating their usual dark red color. Treatment of these conditions is directed to correction of the hyperglycemia (and hyperlipidemia) with appropriate therapy, namely insulin and diet, and other specific agents according to the type of hyperlipidemia.

More serious and much more prevalent are the *microvascular complications* of the chronic diabetic state. For example, about one sixth of all cases of acquired blindness are due to *diabetic retinopathy.* Approximately two thirds of diabetics with disease for 15 years and over 90 per cent of those with disease for three or four decades have evidence of retinopathy. It most often appears after ten years of known diabetes as an increased tortuosity and widening of the vessels, with scattered, barely visible dots caused by microaneurysms, usually about the macula or about the periphery of the temporal area. Later, small punctate hemorrhages may appear with "waxy" exudates which may either persist or disappear after months to years, leaving a small whitish scar, but with loss of visual elements in that area. Increased capillary permeability leads to extravasation of protein seen as fluffy "cottonwool" exudates, which also are variable, appearing and disappearing with time.

In the next phase, small new vessels may appear over the disc and along the nerves, and these may then grow into the vitreous. More ominous, they frequently rupture with large hemorrhages and, depending on whether the macular area is involved, with either loss of areas of vision or transient total blindness (Fig. 5). They usually undergo moderate to marked resorption with return of some vision until the next hemorrhage. However, these newly formed vessels, part of the syndrome of retinitis proliferans, usually portend an ominous prognosis unless treated. If there is hemorrhage anteriorly into the vitreous, resorption may be associated with contraction and tearing and detachment of the retina. However, the retinitis may arrest or even regress at any stage without known cause. More commonly, however, proliferating vessels usually lead to legal blindness in the affected eye within four to six years.

The microvascular disease is not limited to the retinal vessels but may also occur in the ciliary body and iris (*rubeosis iridis*), leading to occlusion of the outflow tract, resulting in open-angle neovascular glaucoma, or to hemorrhagic glaucoma after rupture of a vessel.

The pathogenesis of the retinal microangiopathy, as described by Kuwabara and Cogan, is a loss of the pericytes (mural cells) about the capillaries, followed by thickening and weakening of the wall forming the microaneurysm which, in turn, may rupture to cause the visible punctate hemorrhage. In addition shunt vessels surrounded by areas of capillary closure appear, and it is in these that microaneurysms frequently appear. Another theory postulates small capillary thromboses, vessel distention, rupture, and hemorrhage.

The Joslin Clinic staff and many other specialists have stressed the better visual prognosis in patients who control their diabetes with optimal insulin-carbohydrate homeostasis than in patients taking poorer care of their disease, especially for the first ten years of the disease. Rigid prospective studies on this point are not available, but the rapid acceleration of retinopathy noted in the diabetic decompensation with pregnancy or with infection supports the hypothesis. It is rare to see a patient with normal fundi who has had

---

Figure 5. *A*, Vitreous and preretinal hemorrhage from the disc area secondary to disc neovascularization.

B, Fibrous band resulting from going into a quiescent stage of retinopathy one year after slide *A* was taken. Patient maintained quiescent stage for eight years until he died a cardiac death.

C, Preretinal hemorrhages in region of macula which also has exudates and superficial hemorrhages. Note boat-shaped dependency type of hemorrhage.

D, Preretinal hemorrhage at site of frond of neovascularization. Note the new vessel fan underneath the boat-shaped preretinal hemorrhage. It is these new vessels which rupture spontaneously or with minimal stress.

E, Extensive fan of new vessels with fibrous network elevated forward into vitreous. Feeding vessels come from multiple arteries and veins at the retinal level, the entire process being analogous to an angioma.

F, Characteristic waxy exudates in macular zone accounting for decrease in vision, apparently due to incompetent capillaries and leaking from central areas of rings of waxy exudates where the red blotches are noted.

G, Fluorescein angiography in a diabetic, showing some very fine microaneurysms and some tiny areas of capillary closure but with good parafoveal network of vessels and 20/20 vision. These are early changes of diabetic retinopathy probably not seen on ophthalmoscopy. (Courtesy of Dr. L. Aiello.)

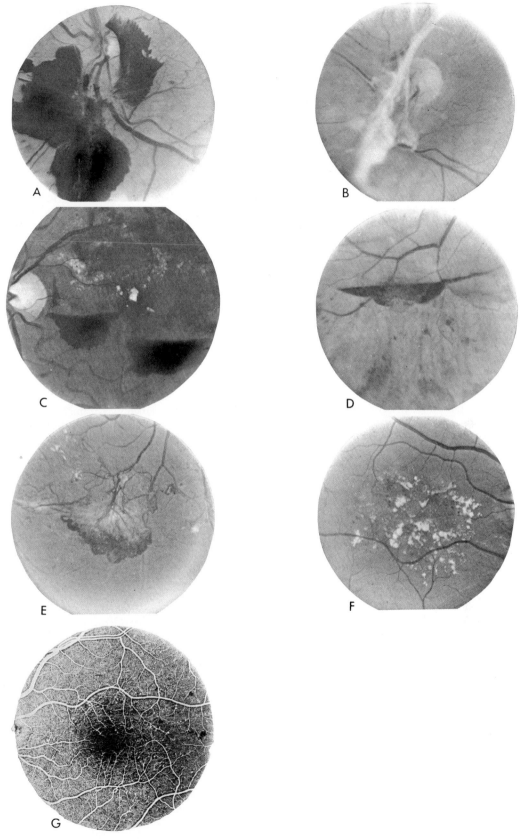

Figure 5. *See opposite page for legend.*

several episodes of ketoacidosis after 15 to 20 years of the disease; those with normal fundi after many years of the disease usually, but again not always, tend to be the "better controlled."

Treatment of the microangiopathy, if we adhere to the "control" hypothesis, calls for optimal treatment of the diabetes itself through adjustment of insulin and diet from the earliest recognition of the disease. Since many conscientious patients, even with the best effort, still develop retinopathy, numerous therapies, including various vitamins, dietary alterations, and hormones, have been used without effect.

An observation that a patient with diabetic retinopathy underwent remission after spontaneous pituitary necrosis prompted a wave of *pituitary ablative procedures* in the 1960's, including total surgical hypophysectomy, surgical section of the pituitary stalk, proton bombardment of the pituitary, transsphenoidal implantation of yttrium-90, freezing of the pituitary, and others, and a significant delay of the retinopathy or even improvement was observed in many. Many patients with hormonal evidence of total pituitary destruction nevertheless progressed, and a few others, in whom the pituitary was not destroyed, improved. The procedure has since been all but abandoned. It is still not clear why the procedure provided some benefit to the average patient; most authorities attribute its effect to reduction or removal of growth hormone.

Direct therapy of the fundus, using photocoagulation, has been a major advance. Patients with unilateral retinitis pigmentosa and diabetes were observed to have less diabetic retinopathy in the eye with the previous retinitis. This has prompted Aiello and Beetham and others to use the ruby laser to apply numerous scattered destructive lesions to the retina as the light is absorbed by the pigment layer, heating and coagulating the adjacent elements. These scattered lesions result in no field defect, and patients with early diabetic neovascularization have had progression of the disease halted or delayed, probably secondary to a diminished vascular need because of diminished tissue in the area treated. Similar results were previously obtained by Wetzig and others, using the polychromatic light of the xenon arc lamp. More recently a green source, the argon laser, has been used to specifically coagulate lesions in the vessels themselves, such as bleeding points, microaneurysms, or the newly forming vessels near or overlying the optic disc; optimal therapy involves treatment of both the specific lesions and the scattered destructive lesions described above.

The eye is occasionally the site of nerve lesions, most frequently the third, resulting in diplopia and strabismus. This disturbing lesion, probably caused by a small vascular infarction, may be preceded by severe pain; it usually reverses itself within several months. The pupil reaction, however, is maintained, because the infarct is usually with the nutrient vessels of the nerve, whereas the pupillary fibers on the outside of the nerve remain nourished by adjacent vessels. Finally, diabetics appear to be more susceptible to the common senile cataract, which appears at an earlier chronologic age and matures more rapidly than usual, and, as mentioned elsewhere, to infections of the eye. Corneal lesions are more pernicious than similar injuries in nondiabetics.

Kidney. The kidney is also a focal point for diabetes and its complications. The predisposition to infection makes pyelonephritis fairly frequent and serious, and the more severe renal infections may lead to papillary necrosis or perinephric abscess, grave conditions almost unique to the diabetic. For this reason urinary tract instrumentation such as catheterization should be avoided in a diabetic unless absolutely necessary, because subsequent infection is so often observed.

The main problem, however, is the *microangiopathy.* Proteinuria appears in two thirds of patients with diabetes for 20 years and portends progressive renal involvement, with uremia developing in the average patient in five years. Forty per cent of juvenile-type diabetics die from renal failure. Biopsies of kidneys in newly discovered diabetics by Lundbaek's group in Denmark have shown no demonstrable lesion, but after several years there is increased thickness of the capillary basement membrane and accumulation of material in the mesangial area as seen by the electron microscope, which then may become visible by standard light microscopy after 10 to 15 years. In some unfortunate patients, the nephropathy may be more rapid, occasionally leading to renal failure after only nine to ten years of diabetes. In a very fortunate few, and these appear to be those patients in whom the diabetes has been best controlled by insulin and diet, the signs or symptoms of nephropathy may not develop even after 50 years of the disease. With the progressive thickening and folding of the vascular basement membrane, composed of glycoprotein, as well as the mesangial accumulation of similar material, the lesion is seen as (1) a *nodular glomerulosclerosis* as described by Kimmelstiel and Wilson over 30 years ago, (2) a diffuse accumulation of glycoprotein in all areas of the glomerulus, or (3) a mixture of the two. Paradoxically, the thickened basement membrane is more permeable to macromolecules; hence the proteinuria. As the lesion progresses, entire glomeruli may become occluded, with loss of renal function, uremia, and death. Added to these microvascular lesions are the accelerated atherosclerosis and high frequency of hypertension and arteriolar nephrosclerosis in diabetics with nephropathy.

Beisswenger and Spiro have shown the accumulated material to be a specific complex glycoprotein and to contain an excess of hydroxylysine to which is attached a glucose-galactose disaccharide. Insulin-deficient laboratory animals show an increased activity in the enzymes involved in formation of this material, but the precise biochemical correlation between it and the diabetes awaits clarification. Transplantation of normal kidneys in experimentally diabetic animals has shown similar lesions to appear and to disappear with retransplantation back into nondiabetic animals.

As with retinopathy, treatment of diabetic nephropathy is directed to the treatment of the diabetes itself. Infection in the genitourinary system in particular, as well as any infection elsewhere with diabetic decompensation, tends to accelerate the nephropathy as well as the retinopathy. With renal failure, chronic dialysis and/or transplantation are the only direct forms of therapy; however, the generalized atherosclerosis makes vascular shunts difficult to create and maintain, and the diabetic's susceptibility to infection creates an even greater problem. Added to this, immunosuppression for transplantation poses such a risk that only subjects with advanced renal failure but otherwise in good condition should be considered as candidates. Basically, therefore, the treatment of diabetic nephropathy is no different from that of renal failure resulting from chronic glomerulonephritis, polycystic kidneys, or other causes; such treatment involves judicious use of diuretics and antihypertensives, a restricted protein diet, and careful adjustment of electrolyte intake.

Nervous System. Diabetes affects the nervous system in many ways as it does other organs and tissues. The marked predilection of the diabetic to atherosclerosis, particularly of medium-sized and small arteries, predisposes him to infarction. If the artery is to the spinal cord, *paraplegia* may result, a very infrequent but disastrous event. Rarely the occlusion may be to a nerve root, resulting in a radiculopathy confined to a dermatome. More frequently, a single peripheral nerve is involved, with sudden loss of sensory and motor function and pain. This may involve the ulnar or peroneal nerve or, more frequently, one of the oculomotor nerves, resulting in acute ophthalmoplegia of the facial nerve, producing Bell's palsy. Fortunately collateral circulation corrects most or all of the deficit and the mononeuropathy disappears in weeks or months.

By far the most frequent neurologic problem in diabetics is the *peripheral neuropathy* (see Ch. 465). This occurs in over 90 per cent of diabetics who have had the disease for one or more decades. The typical case presents after eight to twelve years of overt diabetes with a grossly symmetrical stocking-type of anesthesia, mainly of the lower extremities, producing decreased vibratory and fine-touch sensation and occasionally progressing after months to years to near-total or total anesthesia. Paradoxically, there may be marked hyperesthesia and pain, frequently nocturnal and occasionally excruciating in character. Fortunately for the patient, the progressive nature of the neuropathy provides relief of the pain after several months or occasionally a year or longer, resulting in hypesthesia to total anesthesia of the area, probably owing to total loss of sensory nerve function. Deep tendon reflexes in the lower extremity are almost always decreased to absent in these subjects. Many elderly subjects may exhibit similar changes; whether these are due to the diabetic syndrome associated with the mild glucose intolerance of the aged can be argued.

Histologic examination reveals segmental demyelinization. Experimental diabetes in animals is associated with an accumulation of sorbitol and fructose in peripheral nerves, probably in the Schwann cells, as well as delayed nerve conduction velocity. Whether this pathogenic sequence explains most instances of diabetic neuropathy is debatable, because the neuropathy occurs with almost equal frequency in diabetics without fasting hyperglycemia, particularly in older people; hence the biochemical basis remains conjectural. The similar findings in elderly subjects without diabetes suggest that the peripheral neuropathy is part of the accelerated senescence of the diabetic as manifested in the nervous system. Occasionally patients with marked hyperglycemia, peripheral pain, and delayed nerve conduction lose their symptoms and signs with reduction of glucose concentration, and this acute diabetic "neuropathy" is more probably related to the direct metabolic disorder of sorbitol and fructose accumulation.

The diabetic neuropathy may progress to total sensory anesthesia, and, as occurs to the hip and knee in syphilis with tabes, the safeguards of the normal foot to protect its structure by afferent signals is lost, and

chronic trauma to the joints leads to destruction, the so-called "*Charcot joint.*" Loss of position sense also leads to *ataxia*, the *pseudotabes of diabetes.* Likewise a callus may act as a foreign body, repeatedly injuring the anesthetized foot, leading to ulcer and infection, the "*neuropathic*" ulcer. Worse yet, the anesthesia of the foot prevents the patient from recognizing not only the aforementioned problem but also true foreign bodies such as thumb tacks. Daily inspection of the foot, careful and professional management of calluses and bunions, and properly fitted shoes are mandatory to prevent infection, ulcer, and subsequent amputation.

A peculiar syndrome, *diabetic amyotrophy,* usually occurring in middle-aged or older males, involves the anterior thigh muscles, frequently with pain; this may be due to some metabolic aberration at the nerve terminal. Like other mononeuropathy, it may persist without remission, but usually clears in 12 to 24 months.

The *autonomic nervous system* is also affected in the neurologic sequelae, involving both sympathetic and parasympathetic pathways. In the circulatory system this may be manifested as *orthostatic hypotension* caused by involvement of the afferent and efferent autonomic nerves. Decreased angiotensin production resulting from involvement of renal renin production may also contribute to the problem. *Decreased sweating* is also a common observation, although rarely *hyperhidrosis* may occur. *Impotence* in diabetic males is extremely frequent, again resulting from autonomic involvement; retrograde ejaculation is not uncommon. The gastrointestinal system is frequently affected, as evidenced by *delayed gastric emptying* (diabetic gastropathy), with nausea, anorexia, vomiting, and marked weight loss, not unlike that seen in a patient with mental depression or with gastrointestinal malignancy. The bowel itself, both small and large, may be involved, the former leading to a *malabsorption*-like syndrome and the latter to a distressing *diarrhea,* usually nocturnal, or, conversely, to *constipation* and occasionally *megacolon.* Also involved in the autonomic neuropathy is the *bladder,* leading to asymptomatic distention, occasionally with several liters of residual urine. This can be detected by enlargement of the lower abdomen and around-the-clock urination of small overflow volumes. Obviously, the predilection to urinary tract infection is marked in these subjects. Catheterization, unless essential, is contraindicated.

The treatment of all these disorders is depressingly nonspecific, namely better control of the diabetes. Paradoxically, many patients with peripheral neuropathy who are then placed into better carbohydrate-insulin homeostasis have a worsening of the neuropathy, possibly owing to transient improvement in the afferent nerves. In the specific problems, treatment is at best supportive. The patient with bladder involvement may need chronic catheterization or else genitourinary surgery to revise the outflow tract for better bladder decompression. Various cholinergic agents may be of help to the bladder dysfunction and also for the gastropathy. Occasionally antimicrobial drugs as well as anticholinergics may be palliative to the bowel disorder when diarrhea is severe.

The predisposition of the diabetic to *central nervous system vascular accident,* owing to the accelerated atherosclerosis, has already been mentioned. Of much interest, however, and not correlated with the vascular disease but purportedly associated with peripheral neuropathy is the frequent elevation of cerebrospinal fluid protein, occasionally to levels of 200 to 400 mg per 100 ml. In some patients the protein may be elevated without the neuropathy, and in others neuropathy may be present without the protein. Cellular elements, however, are low to absent, ruling out an infectious or other inflammatory process.

Skin. Dermatologic manifestations of diabetes result from the microvascular and macrovascular abnormalities, from the diabetic's predisposition to infection, and from the secondary lipid disorders in blood.

Necrobiosis lipoidica diabeticorum is a rare but dramatic skin condition, found more frequently in females than in males, which may even antedate the other clinical signs and symptoms of diabetes. Although usually in the pretibial area, it may appear elsewhere, particularly on the dorsum of the foot. The mature lesion is a clearly demarcated painless area of atrophic skin, usually deeply pigmented with small telangiectases about the border. Frequently it follows trauma to the area, but many times its appearance is unprovoked. The lesions, which start as red raised papules that coalesce and expand, may remain stationary or even regress without relation to other problems the patient may have. Many diabetics, particularly those of long standing, have a waxy hue of the skin, and small freckle-like brown spots are frequently seen over the lower extremities. Both these and the necrobiosis are probably due to a microangiopathy similar to that in the renal glomerulus and retinal capillary.

Macrovascular disease, or atherosclerosis, often involves the skin in the form of *gangrene* secondary to ischemia. Most commonly one or more toes are affected, but occasionally the entire foot or lower limb may be involved. Rarely the fingers or localized areas of skin anywhere on the body may be affected, probably secondary to occlusion of a small artery, the collaterals having been previously compromised by the same process.

Skin infections are extremely frequent, particularly if the patient is in poor control. The usual staphylococcal and streptococcal infections occur much more frequently than in nondiabetics and may lead to rapid and massive destruction unless antimicrobials are administered and the diabetes is brought under better control. Rectal abscesses, furunculosis, hidradenitis, cellulitis, and intertriginous infections caused by fungi such as dermatophytosis of the feet are all more frequent in the diabetic. Obviously, ischemic areas, especially the feet, are exquisitely susceptible to infection.

Xanthoma diabeticorum (eruptive xanthomatosis): A small percentage of uncontrolled diabetics have a marked elevation in circulating lipids. When triglycerides are chronically elevated, they accumulate not only in macrophages in liver and spleen but also as collections in the skin; these appear as clusters of raised papules, usually on a red base with a pale yellow center, and are referred to as eruptive xanthoma. Most often they are found over the buttocks and extremities, but they may appear anywhere. Diagnosis is made by finding the lipemia in the retinal vessels or by the turbidity or frank creaminess of the serum, and classification is made by electrophoresis into Type I (hyperchylomicronemia), IIb (mixed hypercholesterolemia and hyperchylomicronemia), IV (endogenous hypertriglyceridemia), or V (hyperchylomicronemia and endogenous hypertriglyceridemia) hyperlipidemias. If the diabetes is secondary to Type IV, standard diabetic treatment is indicated with restriction of dietary carbohydrates and, most important if the patient is overweight, a hypocaloric diet. Types IIb, IV, and V are also frequently associated with diabetes, and the hyperlipidemia and diabetes are treated according to the type and severity of each.

Atherosclerosis. Diabetes in all ages is associated with accelerated atherosclerosis. *Coronary insufficiency* in the premenopausal female is twenty times more common than that in the nondiabetic female. A *myocardial infarction* in a male under 40 is almost always associated with either diabetes or a familial lipid disorder. Fifty per cent of all diabetics die prematurely of myocardial infarction. In a diabetic with a myocardial infarction, five-year survival is limited to 30 per cent, whereas 60 per cent of a nondiabetic population would survive this period. *Peripheral arteries* are more severely affected, and gangrene of the feet caused by ischemia is 70-fold more frequent in diabetics. Many explanations have been offered for this accelerated atherosclerosis; one of these implicates defective lipoprotein metabolism. Approximately one fifth of all diabetics have an elevated circulating triglyceride level, mainly in the pre-beta region (endogenous hypertriglyceridemia), and these are diagnosed as Type IV hyperlipoproteinemics. Conversely, over 90 per cent of subjects with Type IV hyperlipoproteinemia have overt diabetes or glucose intolerance. Other lipid disorders, particularly Types IIb, III, and V, have an increased prevalence of diabetes (see Ch. 819). However, for the minimal or absent demonstrable circulating lipid abnormality present in most diabetics, their premature atherosclerosis is far out of proportion. Direct cholesterol synthesis in the vessels has been indicted, as has the basement membrane defect, leading to a microangiopathy of the vasa vasorum and then to atherosclerosis. As in the nondiabetic population, the pathogenic sequence is not clear.

Treatment poses a quandary, because most diabetic diets are restricted in carbohydrate, calling for a high fat intake which may contribute to the atherosclerosis. A compromise is usually suggested with a diet containing one half the calories as fat, but polyunsaturated in nature. For the specific dyslipidemias, clofibrate or nicotinic acid is used, as is cholestyramine. Interestingly, the waxy exudates in the retinal fundus have been significantly decreased with clofibrate therapy, but visual improvement has not been documented. Most important, the synergistic effect of smoking in augmenting vascular disorders with the diabetic predisposition makes *smoking abstinence* a most important part of therapy in any diabetic. Finally, although there is evidence that optimal diabetic control may mitigate the microvascular complications of diabetes, there is little evidence of any effect of control on the accelerated atherosclerosis, suggesting that this predisposition may be an inherent abnormality closely related to the inheritance of the diabetes itself but independent of the abnormality in insulin-glucose homeostasis.

Infection. At any stage of diabetes, infection is both a diagnostic indicator and a major threat. The reasons are manifold, including a decrease in macrophage mobility, a decrease in the potential of macrophages to phagocytose infectious particles, and the relative substrate richness of hyperglycemia itself for microorganisms. Added to these factors is decreased vascularity, particularly in the lower extremity, which makes infection an even greater threat. Noninvasive organisms, such as various fungi, find the diabetic a unique organism in which to flourish, similar to the patient with immunodeficiency caused by hereditary or acquired disorders. The diabetic is predisposed not only to soft tissue infection such as furunculosis, gingival abscess, or perinephric abscess, but also to meningitis, osteomyelitis, and many others. *Mucormycosis* occurs almost uniquely in the uncontrolled or ketoacidotic diabetic and is evidenced by a rapid invasive and destructive infection of the orbit or nasal sinuses eroding directly into major vessels, into the eye itself, and even into brain substance.

Lipoatrophic Diabetes. Patients with this relatively rare syndrome have a peculiar form of diabetes with minimal to absent ketoacidosis, marked resistance to insulin, hypermetabolism, and either congenital or acquired absence of grossly demonstrable adipose tissue. Other prominent features may include marked hyperlipidemia and hepatomegaly, leading to cirrhosis and occasionally to esophageal varices. There are frequently increased musculature, acanthosis nigricans, phlebomegaly, curly hair, thickened skin, and other peculiar anomalies such as cystic angiomatous lesions in bones, genital enlargement, and polycystic ovaries. How these diverse features (Lawrence's syndrome or the *Lawrence-Seip syndrome)* are genetically or metabolically interconnected is obscure. Treatment is symptomatic, and the marked insulin resistance usually makes insulin therapy ineffectual; however, most patients adapt to their marked polydipsia, polyuria, and glucosuria. Histologic examination may demonstrate a diminished number of scattered small adipose cells with minimal lipid. In the congenital variety the paucity of adipose tissue is evident at birth or soon thereafter, but the diabetes and other sequelae may not appear until several years later. In the later or acquired form, the adipose tissue may gradually atrophy through childhood, and again the diabetes occurs several years later. Both forms appear to be inherited as autosomal recessive traits. Hypotheses for this peculiar disorder include a lack of cellular receptors for insulin, a lack of intracellular effects of the insulin response itself, or possibly one or more factors produced in excess by the hypothalamus or pituitary which inhibit insulin's metabolic effects. (See Ch. 931.)

Secondary Diabetes. *Hemochromatosis.* Hemochromatosis is a hereditary disease resulting from iron deposition in various tissues such as liver, skin, and pituitary, and includes the endocrine pancreas (see Part XVI, Section Four). Treatment is directed to the hemochromatosis by iron depletion through phlebotomy and to the diabetes by standard insulin replacement and diet therapy, depending on the severity of the diabetes. Many patients require more insulin than might be expected from simple destruction of beta cells, and this relative insulin resistance may result from the accompanying liver disease.

Pancreatitis. The endocrine pancreas is also involved in the destruction and scarring that occur with acute and chronic pancreatitis. Thus diabetes occurring with episodic abdominal pain, periumbilical and boring through to the back, particularly in the alcoholic, and associated with elevations of circulating or urinary amylase, makes pancreatitis probable. Treatment of the diabetes is again as indicated by the severity of the disturbed carbohydrate homeostasis; with extensive destruction of the pancreas, total insulin replacement with split doses (two doses daily) of intermediate (with or without rapid-acting insulin) is indicated. The malabsorption resulting from exocrine deficiency may require oral pancreatic enzyme therapy. In patients with surgical removal of the pancreas because of tumor or, occasionally, pancreatic replacement by tumor or infection, therapy is similar to that for the patient pancreatectomized because of pancreatitis. Many patients in acute diabetic ketoacidosis may have transient elevations of amylase, possibly caused by mild pancreatitis associated with the acute metabolic decompensation, but residual pancreatic exocrine insufficiency is not observed.

Stress Diabetes. During severe stress, sufficient to increase circulating catecholamines and to activate sympathetic innervation of the endocrine pancreas, insulin release is suppressed and glucagon release provoked. The stress-induced hyperglycemia resulting from hepatic glycogenolysis serves to provide emergency fuel for anaerobic metabolism in muscle or in reparative tissue after trauma, without insulin promoting glycogen or fat synthesis from the glucose. Thus there is a true functional diabetes in severe trauma, septicemia, peritonitis, pneumonia, burns, stroke, and myocardial infarction, to name a few. Of course, if the patient had been a mild diabetic previously, the carbohydrate abnormality would be more marked or more easily unmasked. If parenteral glucose is administered, the hyperglycemia resulting from the absolute or relative lack of insulin may become extreme and the patient may progress into hyperglycemic hyperosmolar coma. These patients may have no evidence of diabetes before or after this episode. Should the hyperglycemia be greater than 400 mg per 100 ml, transient insulin therapy is advisable to prevent excess osmolarity. With lesser degrees of injury, or even with the physical incapacity associated with milder diseases, less severe depression of insulin release may occur, resulting in diabetic glucose tolerance; hence, for diabetes the diagnostic tolerance tests should not be performed until the patient is in good health with adequate nutrition and physical activity.

Acromegaly. Growth hormone administration provokes insulin resistance, and, likewise, excess endogenous growth hormone secretion requires a high concentration of insulin to maintain glucose homeostasis. In some series, 20 to 50 per cent of patients with acromegaly have been found to have either frank diabetes or glucose intolerance. In all patients there is a decreased sensitivity to administered insulin, as evidenced by a markedly decreased hypoglycemic effect of 0.1 unit of insulin per kilogram of body weight given intravenously. Before growth hormone immunoassays became available, diagnosis was made on clinical grounds and on the findings of enlargement of the sella turcica, elevated serum phosphate, and insulin resistance. Now any patient with suggestive acromegaloid features or evidence of postpubertal growth of extremities and jaw, thickening and coarsening of facial features and of skin, particularly fingers, increased sweating, and the many other signs or symptoms of excess growth hormone should be tested for diabetes and treated accordingly in addition to treatment for the acromegaly (see Ch. 832).

Cushing's Syndrome. Excess glucocorticoid, whether administered exogenously or secreted endogenously, may produce either glucose intolerance or frank clinical diabetes in one of five adults. Although there is a slight resistance to the metabolic effects of insulin, the glucose intolerance appears also to be related to increased gluconeogenesis and perhaps to a decrease in beta cell capacity to release insulin. Fajans and Conn have administered small doses of glucocorticoid followed by a glucose tolerance test the next morning as a test for latent diabetes, especially in subjects with strong family histories of diabetes.

Any diabetic, particularly one with early features suggestive of the rounded moon facies, buffalo hump, and truncal obesity, with abdominal striae, osteoporosis, hypertension, or psychosis, must be studied for adrenal hyperactivity. But the clinical challenge is in the less overt or earlier form of the syndrome, and this possibly should always be considered in any newly diagnosed diabetic (see Ch. 850). Again, the diabetes is treated according to its signs and symptoms, until the primary cause of the excess glucocorticoid is corrected. It is believed that most of these patients who require insulin have independent diabetes mellitus that has been aggravated by the excess glucocorticoid.

Other Endocrine and Metabolic Disorders. *Pheochromocytoma* is frequently associated with diabetes mellitus because of the suppression of insulin release from beta cells as well as the capacity for adrenal catechols to provoke hepatic glycogen breakdown and peripheral inhibition of glucose uptake. As in patients with major trauma and high levels of catecholamines, this type of diabetes probably may occur in an individual without inherent diabetes, never to return after removal of the tumor. *Thyrotoxicosis*, on the other hand, appears to be able to unmask latent diabetes mellitus, but its direct effect on carbohydrate metabolism is minimal and is possibly related to the relative starvation of the hypermetabolic patient. Also, accelerated gastric emptying and absorption may cause marked hyperglycemia early in an oral glucose tolerance test, similar to that seen in an individual with gastric resection. Other endocrinopathies that are diabetogenic include pregnancy (to be discussed) and the simulated pregnancy found in patients receiving exogenous estrogen. Many latent diabetics can be made overt if given *oral contraceptive agents*, and the estrogen moiety appears more diabetogenic than the progestin. The hypokalemia of *hyperaldosteronism* or during *diuretic therapy* diminishes insulin release from the pancreas and may contribute to diabetes or carbohydrate intolerance. Another factor leading to glucose intolerance is hyperlipidemia, but again many of these patients probably have independent diabetes, and the pathophysiologic relationship is obscure.

Finally, a large number of metabolic and endocrine disorders are associated with a higher incidence of diabetes than one might expect from the general population. These include the Prader-Willi syndrome, sexual ateliotic dwarfism, Schmidt's syndrome, Werner's syndrome, Refsum's syndrome, Friedreich's ataxia, optic atrophy and nerve deafness, Turner's syndrome, and many others. One wonders why the incidence of diabetes is so high in almost all chromosomal aberrations and inborn errors of metabolism. No clear answer is apparent.

Treatment. The specific treatment of diabetes depends upon the signs and symptoms of the individual patient presenting with the disease and can be subdivided accordingly. Since the spectrum has at one end fulminant ketoacidosis, which can result in death in coma within several days in the previously well-controlled subject omitting insulin (or in 24 to 48 hours in the child), and at the other end only a slightly abnormal glucose tolerance, the therapy is likewise varied. There is really no fixed regimen for any single patient, even one in ketoacidosis, so only general guidelines will be discussed.

In the terminal ketoacidotic patient in coma, the thready pulse, decreasing blood pressure, rapidly falling arterial pH, and rising Pco_2 (signifying inability to achieve compensation of the acidosis by hyperventilation) portend irreversible shock and death, and rapid heroic treatment is mandatory to reverse the fatal outcome. On the other hand, many patients will walk in with mild ketoacidosis, feeling poorly, without nausea or vomiting, but with a glucose level of 500 mg per 100 ml or higher and a total HCO_3 of 4 to 16 mEq per liter. A liter or two of saline plus 20 to 30 units of crystalline insulin intravenously or intramuscularly may be all that is necessary, as evidenced by correction of the metabolic disorder. This may be followed by the standard insulin dose eight to twelve hours later or, if these patients were not previously on insulin, by a small dose of intermediate-acting insulin (about 20 units) in order to initiate their standard replacement regimen.

The less severe type of diabetic, presenting with polydipsia and polyuria or with any of the sequelae, such as pruritus vulvae, may be handled by diet alone, particularly if over 30 to 40 years of age and overweight. By diet is meant a low calorie, carbohydrate-restricted regimen distributed between meals to avoid excessively large meals at any one time. Should this regimen not be effective in controlling hyperglycemia after one to two months' trial, insulin or one of the oral antidiabetic medications may be indicated in addition to the diet. If insulin is used, it is usually given as a single dose of one of the intermediate types, either NPH or lente, one half hour before breakfast, in order to supplement the endogenously produced insulin. The philosophy, of course, is the reciprocal of the normal physiology wherein the beta cells release insulin proportional to the composition and size of the ingested meal; in the diabetic, the meals are proportioned to match the rate of absorption of the injected intermediate-acting insulin (e.g., a smaller breakfast, a moderate-sized lunch, a mid-afternoon snack, a moderate-sized supper, and a small bedtime snack). Should a larger breakfast be desired, some crystalline insulin may be mixed with the intermediate insulin.

Since ketoacidosis is the most dramatic and life-threatening event, its treatment will be discussed first in greater detail.

Diabetic Ketoacidosis. As in most acute, life-threatening crises, the primary concern is lack of effective circulating volume. The marked hyperglycemia leads to marked glycosuria and an osmotic "washout" of water and electrolyte, mainly sodium and chloride. In addition, as a result of the elevated circulating levels of ketoacids, which are relatively poorly reabsorbed by the renal tubule from the glomerular filtrate, these relatively strong organic acids with pK's below 4 appear in the urine and are coupled with excretion of sodium, potassium, and ammonium, leading to further volume depletion. The ketoacidosis also leads to systemic acidosis, which, in itself, depresses cardiac contractility as well as the capacity of arterioles to respond to catecholamines, both the circulating epinephrine and the norepinephrine released locally from sympathetic nerve endings. Thus the thready pulse, hypotension, and poor organ perfusion reflect both hypovolemia and poor physiologic compensation to the decreased volume, the two processes enhancing each other's threat to survival.

Therapy first involves correct diagnosis; the history of polydipsia and polyuria in a patient with marked hyperglycemia and glycosuria together with the demonstration of excess ketoacid in plasma establishes the diagnosis. Usually the patient has omitted insulin because of intercurrent illness, with the mistaken thought that insulin is unnecessary if food is not eaten. Other explanations include the insulin resistance associated with infection or the first trimester of pregnancy, or even emotional stress. In the previously undiagnosed diabetic, the typical history may also include severe abdominal pain, frequently with a rigid, tender abdomen. The marked leukocytosis with immature granulocytes in the blood smear may make an acute surgical abdomen a reasonable diagnosis until the hyperglycemia, glycosuria, ketonemia, and ketonuria provide the correct cause.

In simplest terms, a large indwelling needle is inserted in a vein of the suspect patient, blood is drawn and checked for hyperglycemia by either an approximate bedside procedure (Testape or Reflectometer) or rapid automatic glucose determination, using glucose oxidose, and plasma or serum ketosis is assessed by a drop placed on one of several commercial preparations (e.g., Acetest, Ketotest, Ketostix). If hyperglycemia and marked ketosis are present, the diagnosis is immediately confirmed and therapy initiated.

The original needle inserted is obviously left in place after drawing the blood, and isotonic saline is run in at a rapid pace, because volume deficit is usually severe. If the patient is critically ill with marked hypotension and barely detectable peripheral pulse, plasma expanders such as plasma itself, albumin, or synthetic colloids can be given in order to improve the circulating hypovolemia. In this case, drawing of arterial gases and pH is mandatory; if the pH is below 7.1, sodium bicarbonate, 1 ampule (44 mEq), should be added to each liter of isotonic saline to help correct myocardial contractility as well as to improve vascular tone. With documentation of the hyperglycemia and the marked increase in ketone bodies, insulin should be given. The precise amount varies between clinics, but usually about five times the daily dose is given; for the average diabetic therefore approximately 200 units is given, half intravenously and half subcutaneously. Recently, some clinics have reported what they regard as improved results by giving 5 to 10 units per hour by continuous intravenous infusion or by giving 10 to 20 units hourly intramuscularly during the first hours of treatment. For the present the writer prefers to follow the philosophy that early vigorous reversal of the pathogenic sequence is indicated to spare life, and, once the progression of the metabolic lesion has been reversed, to proceed more slowly in making the final corrections in volume deficit and electrolytes. Of importance is the urinary loss of potassium during the development of ketoacidosis, owing partly to the osmotic diuresis and partly to loss of potassium from cells. With volume deficit, aldosterone is also called into play, and distal tubular exchange of potassium for sodium results in an even more marked deficit in body potassium. With the metabolic acidosis there is usually hyperkalemia, approximately 5 to 6.5 mEq per liter in spite of the total body deficit. An initial serum potassium of 4 to 5 mEq per liter or, more striking, of less than 4 mEq per liter signifies severe potassium deficiency. Therefore potassium, as the phosphate or chloride (preferably the phosphate), should be added to the infusion (40 mEq per liter), particularly after the insulin is injected, because that will accelerate potassium movement into cells, and life-threatening hypokalemia can ensue. Usually potassium administration can be withheld until glucose levels are shown to fall. If bicarbonate is administered because of severe acidosis and hypotension, the fall in potassium may be accentuated and replacement should be more vigorous.

Three or 4 liters of isotonic saline, with bicarbonate in the severely acidotic patient or with potassium in the patient predisposed to hypokalemia, may be given in the first two or three hours of therapy. If there is gastric atony with emesis of a black and frequently benzidine-positive fluid, gastric aspiration helps to return gastric compensation as well as lessening the risk of aspiration pneumonia. These patients may have a demonstrable succussion splash before decompression.

Except in very severe cases, when one may wish to monitor renal perfusion, urinary catheterization is contraindicated. The hyperosmolarity induced by the hyperglycemia exerts a protective effect on the kidney, and acute tubular necrosis after severe diabetic ketoacidosis is extremely rare. Electrocardiographic tracings help to monitor the physiologic effects of the potassium levels.

Of prime importance is close observation of the patient, together with the compilation of a detailed bedside flowsheet of all events: insulin administered, chemistries, pulse, blood pressure, and so forth. If blood glucose levels do not fall after the initial insulin injection, the infrequent but serious problem of insulin resistance may be present, requiring intravenous or subcutaneous injection of hundreds to thousands of units. This need to follow the glucose levels is one of the contraindications to giving exogenous glucose in the initial intravenous therapy until a significant insulin effect is observed, as evidenced by a definite fall in glucose concentration.

Although it appears more logical initially to administer hypotonic saline, since the patient has lost more water than electrolyte, isotonic saline provides a better defense for the maintenance of extracellular fluid volume. As glucose levels fall, thanks to insulin exerting its physiologic effects, the extracellular osmolarity falls and fluid tends to move into cells, decreasing, thereby, extracellular fluid volume; hence the preference for giving isotonic instead of hypotonic solutions initially. Also, the shift of water from the extracellular fluid into cells is shared by the central nervous system, leading tragically, but fortunately rarely, to cerebral edema and death. Hence, again, the principle in the treatment of diabetic ketoacidosis is to initiate treatment rapidly, in order to reverse the process and to correct circulatory fluid volume. Once the patient has begun to improve, the management can proceed more conservatively.

Should bicarbonate and potassium salts be added to

the infusate, 0.45 per cent sodium chloride can be used in the basic fluid in order to avoid overly hypertonic solutions.

As blood glucose levels fall, if potassium was not administered initially, it should be added subsequently, 1 ampule per liter (40 mEq) of solution, preferably as the phosphate salt. When the blood glucose level approaches the renal threshold of 180 to 200 mg per 100 ml, glucose as 5 per cent D/W or 5 per cent D/S can be infused in order to prevent hypoglycemia. The patient is returned to long-acting insulin therapy once the threat of hypoglycemia has passed.

Should the initial insulin therapy be ineffective as evidenced by a failure to reduce blood glucose levels in the first or second hour, a second injection must be given, and this is usually twice the first, unless the patient's condition has deteriorated markedly, in which case much larger doses should be given as well as alkali, volume expanders, and all other maneuvers used in the treatment of the patient in shock. If, however, the glucose level is decreased, for example, falling from 600 to 300 mg per 100 ml, a second insulin injection need not be given unless the progressive fall later ceases or glucose levels begin to increase, in which case a small second injection of insulin can be given, perhaps one quarter to one half the initial dose. Thus continuous monitoring and charting of blood glucose concentrations, first at hourly intervals and later at two-hour intervals, are essential. The availability of rapid bedside glucose techniques such as the glucose-oxidase analyzer has greatly simplified this task.

The precipitating event leading to ketoacidosis should always be kept in mind. Usually it is lack of understanding owing to poor education, the patient having omitted insulin when slightly ill from an upper respiratory infection or a gastrointestinal disturbance, believing that the decreased food intake obviated the need for daily insulin. Frequently, an unrecognized infection may provoke sufficient insulin resistance to tip the patient into ketoacidosis. Thus appendicitis, pyelonephritis, meningitis, and other disorders should be considered. The marked leukocytosis with immature forms associated with diabetic ketoacidosis makes exclusion of infection all the more difficult.

Alcohol is metabolized in liver to acetate which is then released for further metabolism by peripheral tissues. Thus alcohol compounds the rate of hepatic acetate production during fasting, particularly in the insulin-deficient diabetic, and severe ketoacidosis may occur with varying degrees of hyperglycemia. In the previously fasting nondiabetic, an alcoholic debauch may even provoke severe ketoacidosis with normal or low blood glucose levels. Thus a careful history is indicated, and in such a subject with severe ketoacidosis, glucose as well as electrolyte may be indicated in the initial therapy.

Hyperosmolar Coma. Coma, usually occurring in an elderly patient, with hyperglycemia caused by dehydration, prerenal azotemia, and marked but not total insulin deficiency, can mimic that of the subject in ketoacidosis. However, the Kussmaul respirations of severe acidosis and the smell of acetone are lacking owing to the low or absent ketonemia. On the other hand, if there are hyperventilation, a low pH, and low bicarbonate without demonstrable ketoacidosis, *lactic acidosis* is a probable diagnosis. The patient in hyperosmolar coma is treated like the patient in diabetic ketoacidosis with

an indwelling large needle in a peripheral vein through which isotonic saline is administered rapidly. The usual insulin resistance of ketoacidosis may be absent; if the hyperglycemia is in the range of 500 to 1000 mg per 100 ml or even higher, only 10 to 25 units of insulin need be first given intravenously. In these subjects, the requirement for isotonic as opposed to hypotonic fluid replacement is even more strongly indicated, because reduction of glucose levels markedly decreases extracellular osmoles and fluid entry into tissues will markedly compromise extracellular fluid volume as well as producing intracellular fluid overload, especially in the brain. Hence *hypotonic solutions should not be administered* until the patient's circulatory volume is stabilized, and then only slowly and judiciously. Also, as in ketoacidosis, the primary reason for the decompensation should be considered. Bronchopneumonia, myocardial infarction, and local or generalized infections are all included in the differential diagnosis. Again, with the decrease in glucose levels as treatment continues, potassium moves into cells and parenteral potassium replacement may be required. The needed amounts are usually far less than in ketoacidosis, but the same precaution, close observation with frequent monitoring such as precordial electrocardiographic tracings and serum electrolyte levels, is indicated.

Nonketotic or Nonhyperosmolar Patient. In the diabetic with marked fasting and postprandial hyperglycemia, the urgency of the aforementioned two syndromes is not present. In the young individual, particularly under age 20, with polyuria, thirst, and fasting hyperglycemia, insulin therapy is indicated, because deficiency of the hormone, although not as severe as in the patient with ketoacidosis, will eventually be complete or nearly complete. In an adolescent, 20 units of intermediate-duration insulin (lente or NPH) given each morning is a good start, followed by the adjustment of diet and insulin treatment based on urine and blood glucose levels. Since endogenous insulin secretion is moderately compromised, the diet is made to match the rate of insulin absorption within some structure as dictated by social convenience. Thus total calories might be distributed with two sevenths at breakfast, two sevenths at lunch, two sevenths at supper, and the other one seventh split between mid-afternoon and bedtime snacks. Many manuals and texts published by the American Diabetes Association and various hospitals and clinics describe this in further detail and should be

TABLE 1. Insulin in Clinical Usage*

	Peak Effect (Hours)	Duration of Effect (Hours)
Regular or crystalline	2–3	6–8
Semilente	3–6	10–14
NPH	6–10	16–24
Lente	6–10	16–24
Ultralente	10–16	36+
PZI (protamine zinc insulin)	10–16	36+

*Insulin preparations in the United States and their duration of action. They are available in 40, 80 and 100 units per milliliter, termed U40, U80 and U100 respectively. Standard and disposable syringes calibrated accordingly are available. The use of the two lower doses is being phased out in view of the simplicity of use of U100. Also available are U500 and U5000 for the rare patient with marked insulin resistance.

consulted for specifics. The patient is taught to test urine for glucose levels and to alter insulin and diet accordingly. If a larger breakfast is desired, or if the present insulin regimen does not cover the breakfast, regular or clear insulin can be added to the intermediate-duration insulin. Likewise, if there is glycosuria at bedtime, a short-acting insulin can be given before supper. Since the peak action of intermediate insulin is in the mid-afternoon, hypoglycemia at that time necessitates reduction of the dose (making sure the patient is not omitting the mid-afternoon snack). Conversely, late afternoon hyperglycemia necessitates increasing the morning dose of intermediate-duration insulin. Careful daily records should be kept by the patient of his urine sugar tests as well as hypoglycemic reactions, even if minimal.

If the patient does well through the day but has early morning hyperglycemia and glycosuria, a small injection of intermediate insulin may be necessary before supper or bedtime to carry through the night. This is usually not necessary in the juvenile diabetic in the first years of the disease, thanks to the small endogenous production of insulin. However, after about five years of disease all beta cell function has usually ceased, and the "split" dose of insulin, one in the morning and the other before supper, becomes the rule. In many juvenile-type patients, even the "split" dose with a most careful adherence to diet cannot adequately control the diabetes, and mild hyperglycemia is the compromise to prevent excessive hypoglycemic reactions. In these, occasional collection of a 24-hour urine with quantification of glucose may give an index of over-all control, with the hope that excretion is less than 5 to 10 per cent of dietary carbohydrate intake.

In the patient over 20 with marked fasting hyperglycemia, if not overweight but with minimal or mild ketosis, insulin therapy will also probably be necessary. If the patient is overweight, however, the insulin resistance of obesity calls for a trial of rigid dietary restriction and weight reduction, keeping close observation that he does not go into ketoacidosis. Rarely, a fat child without ketosis may fall in this group. Not infrequently, with weight loss, endogenous insulin becomes sufficient to maintain glucose homeostasis for at least several years, occasionally permanently. Too often, unfortunately, weight loss may be minimal because of failure to adhere to a calorically restricted diet; insulin or sulfonylurea therapy is then indicated. The insulin is usually given as a single injection of intermediate acting (NPH or lente) one half hour before breakfast and regulated according to urine and blood tests. Because urine glucose may represent hyperglycemia many hours previously, patients are usually advised to empty the bladder one half hour before the anticipated time of testing, to drink water, and then to void again—the "double-voided" urine specimen.

Oral Hypoglycemic Agents. Although weight reduction by caloric restriction is the ideal approach to the middle-aged overweight diabetic subject, it is almost universally unsuccessful. Thus in these patients, as well as in nonoverweight subjects with maturity-onset type diabetes, addition of the oral hypoglycemic agents is indicated should hyperglycemia persist, although, as discussed below, some controversy exists between experts in the field as to their value and contraindications.

TABLE 2.   Oral Agents

Sulfonylureas	Dosage	Duration of Effect (Hours)
Tolbutamide (Orinase)	0.5–3 grams/day	6–12
Acetohexamide (Dymelor)	0.25–1.5 grams/day	12–24
Chlorpropamide (Diabinese)	0.1–0.5 gram/day	24–48
Tolazamide (Tolinase)	0.1–0.75 gram/day	12–24
Glyburide (Micronase, Diabeta)	5–35 mg/day	12–24

Biguanides	Dosage	Duration of Effect (Hours)
Phenformin (Meltrol, DBI)	25–200 mg/day	4–6
Phenformin (Meltrol-50, DBI-TD)	50–200 mg/day	8–14

Table 2 lists the oral agents available in the United States. Those of the sulfonylurea type acutely increase insulin release from beta cells in man and in experimental preparations, and their chronic effect is allegedly through this same mechanism, but non-beta-cell effects have also been described, such as inhibition of hepatic glucose output. They differ from each other by their potencies, duration of action, and mechanism of elimination. Tolbutamide, the drug most commonly used, has a relatively shorter duration of action, and its lesser potency requires larger doses to be given as indicated in Table 2. Usually the patient is started on 1 to 2 grams per day, half in the morning and the other half in the evening. Tolbutamide is primarily metabolized to inert products by the liver and then excreted. Should its action not be reflected in lowered glucose levels, a larger dose (3 grams) can be given or else one of the other more potent and longer-acting agents. Acetohexamide is also metabolized by the liver, but its principal product retains hypoglycemic activity. Chlorpropamide, on the other hand, is excreted unchanged by the kidneys and is obviously contraindicated in renal insufficiency. Extremely infrequently these drugs cause skin rashes or other allergic manifestations; an even more rare but serious problem has been protracted hypoglycemia, particularly in elderly individuals, usually from the more potent, long-acting sulfonylureas. Other pharmacologic agents, such as anticoagulants and salicylates, compete with hepatic removal of the sulfonylurea (except chlorpropamide) and drug-drug interactions must always be considered when they are used. If the patient's abnormal glucose tolerance is successfully corrected toward normal or—more easily determined—a one- or two-hour postprandial glucose is less than 160 or 120 mg per 100 ml, respectively, the drug may be continued and later reduced in dosage or perhaps, after a year or so, terminated with the patient observed at quarterly or so intervals to see if glucose intolerance returns.

In a large multicenter study, the University Group Diabetes Project, sponsored by the National Institutes of Health and performed through the 1960's, it was demonstrated that middle-aged subjects on a fixed dose of one of the sulfonylureas, tolbutamide, although showing a small but significant lowering of blood glucose levels, had an increased incidence of sudden death, presumably resulting from myocardial infarction or arrhythmia. This study has limited the indiscriminate use of sulfonylureas, and has placed further emphasis on diet as the primary approach to the maturity-onset type of diabetic. Many experienced students of the disease question the significance of the study and continue to use the agents. Nevertheless, if one adheres to the hypothesis that hyperglycemia is deleterious, in that it leads to the microvascular complications, then the sulfonylureas may be indicated if their benefit outweighs the possible risk of increased myocardial instability. Certainly, in the elderly female with glycosuria, the correction of her discomfort associated with the glycosuria may far outweigh the theoretical increased risk of sudden death as found in the UGDP study. One is obviously hesitant to start older, debilitated individuals on insulin injections unless absolutely necessary, and in these the sulfonylureas may play an important role.

The biguanides, of which, at the time of this writing, only phenformin is available in the United States, apparently work independently of beta cell insulin release and thus can be used independently of or supplementary to the sulfonylureas. Their mode of action is not yet known, although many experimental metabolic effects have been demonstrated, such as delayed glucose absorption in the gut, augmented peripheral glucose uptake, and inhibition of gluconeogenesis. A predilection to lactic acidosis in patients receiving biguanides, has been described, and these agents are thereby contraindicated in elderly individuals with congestive failure or similar debilitated states. Their major use has been as an adjunct to the sulfonylureas when the latter have failed to reduce blood glucose levels sufficiently. A slight anorexigenic effect has also been attributed to the biguanides, with the suggestion that they might be all the more indicated in the obese diabetic. Thus persistent hyperglycemia and glycosuria in an individual on a full dose of one of the more potent sulfonylureas can be treated with one to two capsules of the longer-acting biguanide preparation, and a satisfactory hypoglycemic effect is frequently observed. This combined therapy is particularly useful in patients, such as those with visual problems, who are physically or emotionally unable to inject insulin. Unfortunately, a "metallic" taste in the mouth or even persistent nausea and, occasionally, vomiting may limit full usage of biguanide, and it is therefore logical to start with but a single capsule daily, increasing the dosage either until the desired metabolic effect is achieved or just before the gastrointestinal side effects are observed. In the same University Group Diabetes Project discussed above for tolbutamide, patients placed on phenformin given singly without sulfonylurea developed more hypertension and tachycardia than a placebo-treated control, and a significant increase in death from cardiovascular causes was recorded. These patients, however, were asymptomatic middle-aged diabetics, in whom dietary treatment should be the primary mode of therapy.

With both the sulfonylureas and biguanides, many patients may become refractory to their hypoglycemic effects after several years, and these "secondary failure" patients must be started on insulin therapy.

In the milder diabetic with normal fasting glucose and only intermittent or absent glucose in the urine, diet may be all that is necessary. This diet involves reduction or elimination of the easily and rapidly absorbed free sugars; hence no candy, preserves, cookies, or cakes may be eaten, and calories must be distributed throughout the day. Thus a typical diabetic diet of 2200 calories may be composed of 200 to 250 grams of carbo-

hydrate, 100 grams of protein, and the remainder as fat. Again, the standard diabetic texts and handbooks should be used for details such as caloric contents and types of foods as well as exchanges of similar types of foods to provide palatable variability in the diet.

Insulin Problems. The most frequent complication of insulin therapy is hypoglycemia, which can generally be prevented by readjustment of insulin type or dose and of diet. A well-controlled juvenile diabetic may experience occasional mild autonomic symptoms indicating a low glucose and respond by eating some carbohydrate, and this is not felt to be deleterious. In fact it may be helpful to demonstrate that ambient glucose levels are in the physiologic range. However, unconsciousness or convulsions are strongly contraindicated, and the insulin therapy is made less stringent in order to prevent these episodes. In many juvenile diabetics, hyperglycemia, as indicated by slightly positive urine tests, may be the compromise to prevent the physiologic and certainly the social consequences of hypoglycemia.

Allergy. Since insulin is a foreign protein, most patients experience slight reddening, discomfort, and occasionally itchiness at the site of injection after the first two or three weeks. These usually disappear in several weeks or months. In rare patients, the insulin may cause generalized hives and itching, requiring antihistamines, or, if more severe, desensitization to insulin according to schedules delineated in the standard diabetes texts. When allergy to insulin occurs, the patient is re-evaluated as to whether insulin per se is mandatory, because a more restricted diet with or without sulfonylureas or biguanides may suffice. In a juvenile, "ketotic type" diabetic, insulin is mandatory and desensitization must be performed. Also, as discussed under Insulin Resistance, the insulin preparation containing factors least foreign to man should be used.

Insulin Resistance. ANTIBODY-RELATED. Until 1972–73, commercially available insulin preparations contained small amounts of proinsulin and insulin with connecting peptide (C-peptide) still attached to the A or B chains, in addition to other contaminants such as insulin dimers. Thus all patients on daily insulin therapy for several weeks developed antibodies to insulin and these foreign proteins, since beef insulin and pig insulin differ from human insulin by 4 and 1 amino acids respectively. This antibody production, however, did not compromise the effectiveness of insulin except in about 1 in 1000 patients, in whom increasing amounts of insulin were necessary to saturate antibody binding sites in order to permit enough insulin to be physiologically active. By definition, patients receiving 200 units of insulin for two or more days were said to be insulin resistant. Many of these had been on and off insulin therapy on several occasions, an excellent antibody-inducing regimen. Treatment entailed use of the insulin closest in structure to man, pig insulin or pig insulin with the terminal beta-chain alanine removed, making it identical to human insulin minus the terminal beta-chain threonine. In some this decreased the daily insulin dosage, but in others with "resistance" little difference was observed.

In the early 1970's, insulin preparations without contaminants were prepared and found to be much less antigenic than those used formerly. This "single peak" insulin has induced less antibody formation, and the over-all incidence of insulin resistance on this preparation is much less, although its precise rate has yet to be determined. Thus patients with increasing insulin requirement should be started on "single peak" insulin (or "single component," an electrophoretically pure insulin) and, if available, with the amino acid sequence closest to that of man, namely pig.

Formerly, in those patients with insulin resistance, the insulin doses required for effective therapy frequently fluctuated. The patient might need several thousand units daily for several weeks; then because of unexplained alterations in insulin-antibody interrelationships, he might have frequent hypoglycemic reactions, with daily insulin needs being reduced to 100 or fewer units per day. This instability in management occasionally necessitated treatment with glucocorticoids to reduce antibody formation; indeed, even immunosuppressive therapy with antimetabolites was used in certain difficult cases in which management became extremely difficult.

ANTIBODY-UNRELATED. A non-antibody-related insulin resistance is seen in many metabolic states and these have been discussed under Secondary Diabetes. Rarely, a patient without prior immunization to insulin may require 100,000 units or more of insulin to correct the metabolic disorder. These patients are usually young females, and the precise metabolic defect is as yet unknown. It is for these rare patients that the physician must remember that preparations of U500 and U5000 are commercially available and may be life-saving.

OBESITY. In both laboratory animals and man, obesity is associated with a decreased metabolic response to exogenous and endogenous insulin. Decreased binding sites for insulin have been demonstrated on cell membranes from obese animals and man; Ogilvie, many years ago, found obese man to have true pancreatic hyperplasia at autopsy unless diabetes was present.

The hyperinsulinemia, both basal and postprandial, in obese man is shown in Figure 4. Since insulin degradation rates are equal in normal subjects and in the obese, the pancreas in the latter must secrete five to ten times more insulin to achieve fuel homeostasis. It is thus obvious that a deficient beta cell population is unmasked by obesity, and that, in any diabetic, obesity is a major problem. As discussed previously, the primary therapy in the obese diabetic is the hypocaloric weight-reducing diet. Many middle-aged obese diabetics may require 50 to 100 units of insulin daily, but with weight loss they may not require insulin, or possibly may not even need supplementary oral hypoglycemic agents. Only with weight loss in a given patient can the endogenous insulin secretory reserve be assessed.

SOMOGYI EFFECT. After a hypoglycemic reaction, counterregulatory processes such as increased sympathetic nerve activity and increased circulating catecholamines, glucagon, and cortisol and growth hormone (although the metabolic effects of these latter two are less than those of the first two) all induce peripheral insulin resistance as well as increasing hepatic glucose production from both glycolysis and gluconeogenesis. In addition, overzealous correction by oral intake of carbohydrate adds to the hyperglycemia. Thus as in starvation and diabetic ketoacidosis, the trend is toward hyperglycemia, and a larger than usual dose of insulin is necessary to correct the rebound. Occasionally another hypoglycemic reaction can follow and the sequence be repeated, resulting in marked metabolic swings of hyper- and hypoglycemia. This pattern has been emphasized by Somogyi, and his name is frequently applied to this diabetic instability. Therapy is to reduce the dose of the principal insulin injection and, unless already in use, to administer a second, smaller dose of intermediate-acting insulin before supper in order to "smooth out" the patient's metabolic state. In fact, a true "brittle" diabetic, one in whom glucose levels are highly unstable and unpredictable, is best treated by the "split" or double dose of insulin and occasionally might even do better on a third or, rarely, a fourth injection, judged according to premeal urine tests, the experience of the previous day or two, and anticipated meal size.

Lipoatrophy and Hypertrophy. Not infrequently, and most often in girls in their late teens, lipoatrophy is seen at sites of insulin injection. This disfiguring event, occurring in up to one third of all patients, is treated by rotating insulin injections to different sites; however, the new, purer insulin preparations have presumably decreased the incidence of this problem. In many cases, injection of the single peak or single component insulins has even reversed the lesion when injected into the same site.

The hypertrophy that occurs at the site of insulin injection of many diabetics, more often in males than in females, is a direct result of insulin's lipogenic action on fat cells. This can also be disfiguring and usually results from repetitive injections into the same site. Treatment is rotation of injection sites, using thighs, buttocks, abdominal wall, and triceps areas as loci, so that no one site is used more than once a week, even in a patient taking two injections daily.

Hypoglycemia. Any patient on insulin and occasional patients on oral hypoglycemic agents are subject to episodes of hypoglycemia. This is usually evident first as a disturbance in cerebration, such as inability to perform addition or subtraction, or mood changes, followed by parasympathetic signs and symptoms, salivation, hunger, and increased gastric motility. There may then be sympathetic hyperactivity, with sweating, tachycardia, piloerection, and anxiety. The pattern in a given patient may vary, and between patients it varies markedly. Bizarre behavior may arouse suspicion of alcohol or drug intoxication. As hypoglycemia becomes more severe, unconsciousness and convulsions occur which, if prolonged, may lead to severe organic deficit and possibly to an irreversible decorticate or decerebrate state or death. Patient education is most important. Deliberately causing a mild hypoglycemic reaction in a newly discovered and treated diabetic may be advisable so that he is aware of the symptoms and signs. Treatment is by administration of carbohydrate as candy or as a sweetened beverage; however, if the patient is stuporous, oral therapy of any sort must not be given because of danger of aspiration. Instead, glucagon, 1 mg given subcutaneously or intramuscularly by a trained family member or friend, or intravenously by a physician, causes sufficient glycogenolysis to elevate glucose transiently to awaken the patient, so further carbohydrate can be given by mouth. Thus glucagon should be in every diabetic kit. Of course, if the hypoglycemia occurs in a hospital or office setting, drawing a blood sample for glucose analysis can be done to document the diagnosis, and glucose (10 to 25 grams) can be given immediately intravenously, usually as a 50 per cent solution.

Symptoms and signs of hypoglycemia may occur literally within minutes and may rapidly progress to total unconsciousness. Thus any diabetic behaving in a bizarre fashion or, particularly, unconscious should be treated as if hypoglycemic until proved otherwise. Ketoacidosis, on the other hand, takes many hours to days to develop; in contrast to hypoglycemia, the patient appears and behaves chronically ill.

Patients on sulfonylureas, particularly the longer-acting agents, may also develop a severe and prolonged hypoglycemia requiring continuous intravenous glucose therapy for as long as two or three days. These are usually elderly patients with mild diabetes or with compromised renal function. As with insulin-induced hypoglycemia, the unconsciousness may be associated with a variable neurologic examination, including unilateral or bilateral Babinski reflexes and hyperactive or hypoactive deep tendon reflexes, and may mimic a cerebrovascular accident. A superimposed diabetic neuropathy may make the event all the more confusing, particularly because the deep tendon reflexes in the lower extremity may be decreased to absent.

If a patient taking insulin is found to need a progressive reduction in insulin dosage because of recurrent hypoglycemic episodes, particularly if the daily insulin requirement is less than 15 to 20 units, reasons other than simple fluctuations in insulin responsiveness should be considered. An islet cell tumor, partial hypopituitarism, adrenal insufficiency, hypothyroidism, and pregnancy are all possibilities, particularly pituitary disease, thanks to the diabetic's predilection for vascular infarction secondary to generalized atherosclerosis.

Pregnancy and Delivery. In the first trimester of pregnancy, a juvenile diabetic receiving insulin frequently needs a reduction in daily dosage owing to recurrent hypoglycemic episodes. In the second trimester, the diabetes tends to become more labile, and more insulin is needed. Ketoacidosis occurs more readily and, if severe, usually results in death of the fetus. Compounded with this lability, particularly in the third trimester, is the increased renal glomerular filtration rate, lowering the threshold and making urine tests less indicative of blood levels. Immediately after delivery there is a dramatic reduction in insulin need, literally within hours, but after one or two weeks the insulin requirement returns to the prepregnancy level.

The pregnant diabetic has a greater tendency to retain sodium and chloride, making her more susceptible to toxemia and to the development of hydramnios. The latter, caused by increased volume, may result in premature labor and delivery before maturation of the infant. Salt restriction and diuretics are indicated. Mothers with juvenile diabetes for less than ten years or with a milder maturity-onset type of diabetes have large babies, which may cause obstetrical difficulties. In a longstanding juvenile diabetic, particularly with microangiopathic complications or atherosclerosis as evidenced by calcified pelvic vessels, placental function may be decreased and the infant inadequately nourished and "small-for-dates." In both the hypermature or dysmature pregnancy there is a likelihood of sudden intrauterine death, and delivery prior to this catastrophic event is advised. However, the infant is also particularly subject to respiratory distress, and too early delivery is accordingly contraindicated. The thirty-seventh week is usually approximately optimal, but fetal movements, maternal hormone excretion (estrogen and estrogen metabolites, placental lactogen),

and amniotic fluid concentrations of pulmonary surfactants are all evaluated to select the best time for delivery.

The newborn possesses markedly hyperplastic pancreatic islets and is placed on intravenous dextrose and water to prevent prolonged and severe hypoglycemia. More important, the predisposition to the respiratory distress syndrome makes close supervision mandatory.

A successful obstetrical outcome results mainly from frequent observation of the pregnant patient and optimal insulin control of her diabetes, with weekly or twice-weekly visits and hospitalization for the last two to three weeks. Because diabetic complications such as retinopathy are frequently aggravated by pregnancy, delivery of one or certainly of two viable infants in a juvenile diabetic should raise consideration of measures to prevent further pregnancies.

General Principles in Diabetic Management. Since diabetes is a lifelong event, the patient must learn to become his own physician. This is accomplished through extensive education. If he is taking insulin, urine testing, with results recorded before each meal and at bedtime, is mandatory, and the insulin dose should be adjusted according to the previous one or two days' records. He is instructed to reduce insulin or take extra food before strenuous physical activity, or to increase insulin dosage in times of stress, whether it be physical or, occasionally, emotional, particularly as dictated by previous experience. Also if treated with insulin, he should be taught about insulin hypoglycemia and should always be in contact with someone who knows of his disease and the therapy of hypoglycemia. If he is traveling, identification bracelets or cards in the purse or wallet are mandatory. He should also be instructed in foot care, particularly if elderly and with peripheral vascular disease or neuropathy. For educating the young insulin-dependent diabetic, summer camps have been of great help; they have the additional advantage of exposing the child to others with the disease in order to minimize his inferiority as being "singled out." Finally, he should be especially warned of the threat of infection and of wounds, particularly of the lower extremities. The large number of juvenile and maturity-onset diabetics who have achieved major successes in all walks of life, including athletics, attests to the minimal impact of the disease in many. Unfortunately in many others, particularly with the juvenile-onset form of the disease occurring in childhood, inadequate or improper emotional support and guidance frequently result in gross maladjustment; these patients can become a burden to society as well as a major threat to their own well-being by neglect of their therapy.

Alberti, K. G. M. M., Hockaday, T. D. R., and Turner, R. C.: Small doses of intramuscular insulin in the treatment of diabetic coma. Lancet, 3:515, 1973.

Beisswenger, P. J., and Spiro, R. G.: Studies on the human glomerular basement membrane. Diabetes, 22:180, 1973.

Ellenberg, M., and Rifkin, H.: Diabetes Mellitus: Theory and Practice. New York, McGraw-Hill Book Company, 1970.

Fajans, S. S., and Sussman, K. E.: Diabetes Mellitus: Diagnosis and Treatment. Vol. III. New York, American Diabetes Association, 1971.

Gabbay, K. H.: The sorbitol pathway and the complications of diabetes. N. Engl. J. Med., 288:831, 1973.

Gamble, D. R., and Taylor, K. W.: Seasonal incidence of diabetes mellitus. Br. Med. J., 2:631, 1969.

Genuth, S. M.: Plasma insulin and glucose profiles in normal, obese, and diabetic persons. Ann. Intern. Med., 79:812, 1973.

Kilo, C., Vogler, N., and Williamson, J. R.: Muscle capillary basement membrane changes related to aging and to diabetes mellitus. Diabetes, 21:881, 1972.

Lundbaek, K.: Recent contributions to the study of diabetic angiopathy and neuropathy. Adv. Metab. Disord., 6:99, 1972.

Marble, A., White, P., Bradley, R. D., and Krall, L. P.: Joslin's Diabetes Mellitus. 11th ed. Philadelphia, Lea & Febiger, 1971.

Rimoin, D. L., and Schimke, R. W.: Genetic Disorders of the Endocrine Glands. St. Louis, C. V. Mosby Company, 1971.

Siperstein, M. D., Unger, R. H., and Madison, L. L.: Studies of muscle capillary basement membranes in normal subjects, diabetic and pre-diabetic patients. J. Clin. Invest., 47:1973, 1968.

Stanbury, J. B., Wyngaarden, J. B., and Fredrickson, D. S.: The Metabolic Basis of Inherited Disease. 3rd ed. New York, McGraw-Hill Book Company, 1972.

Steiner, D. G., and Freinkel, M. (eds.): Handbook of Physiology, Section 7, Endocrinology. Vol. I, Endocrine Pancreas. Washington, D.C., American Physiological Society, 1972.

Tattersall, R. B., and Pyke, D. A.: Diabetes in identical twins. Lancet, 2:1120, 1972.

Vracko, R.: Basal lamina layering in diabetes mellitus. Diabetes, 23:94, 1974.

807. HYPOGLYCEMIC DISORDERS

Norbert Freinkel

Homeostatic mechanisms are geared to preserve blood sugar within a narrow range. Fall of blood sugar to a concentration which elicits symptoms caused by glucose deprivation in the central nervous system constitutes hypoglycemia. It is a manifestation of homeostatic failure and can be caused by a variety of diseases. By arbitrary definition, hypoglycemia in adults has been equated with values for blood sugar below 40 mg per 100 ml (or plasma or serum glucose below 45 to 50 mg per 100 ml).

Because of intermittent eating, all human intermediary metabolism can be subdivided into two categories: the fed state and the fasted state. The fed state begins whenever we eat, and regulation at this time is designed to provide *synchronized* storage and anabolism from the ingested nutrients. When levels of circulating fuels have returned to pre-eating values, the fasting state is initiated. Regulatory processes are then geared to recall the various foodstuffs from stores in an integrated fashion that is parsimonious and yet appropriate to the prevailing needs for fuel in the central nervous system and periphery.

The pathophysiology of hypoglycemia and its attendant symptoms are substantially different in the fed state and in the fasting state. The distinctions justify classification of the hypoglycemic disorders on the basis of their relation to meals (see accompanying table).

HYPOGLYCEMIA IN THE FED STATE

Pathophysiology. Increased amounts of insulin can be demonstrated in the peripheral circulation within a few minutes after eating. Concentration of plasma insulin parallels the rise and fall of blood sugar. However, the decrement of insulin lags somewhat behind that of glucose so that normoglycemia is restored before circulating insulin returns to pre-eating levels.

Because of the anatomic location of the pancreas, insulin reaches the liver sooner and in greater amounts

Pathophysiologic Classification of Hypoglycemic Disorders

I. Hypoglycemia in the fed state ("overutilization" during the disposition of meals; reactive hypoglycemia)
  A. Relative excess of insulin
    1. Alimentary hyperinsulinism
    2. Reactive hypoglycemia of mild maturity-onset diabetes mellitus
    3. Leucine hypersensitivity of infancy and childhood
  B. Accumulation of metabolites which inhibit resumption of hepatic glucose output
    1. Fructose-1-phosphate aldolase deficiency (hereditary fructose intolerance)
    2. Galactose-1-phosphate uridyl transferase deficiency (galactosemia)
    3. Familial fructose and galactose intolerance
  C. Mechanism unknown
    1. Functional hypoglycemia

II. Hypoglycemia in the fasting state ("underproduction" during the metabolism of endogenous fuels; spontaneous hypoglycemia)
  A. Absolute production failure (intrinsic limitations in the hepatic capacity for glucose output)
    1. Diffuse hepatoparenchymal disease
    2. Defects in liver enzymes for
      a. Final common pathway
        (1) Glucose-6-phosphatase deficiency (glycogen storage disease, Type I)
      b. Glycogen turnover
        (1) Amylo-1,6-glucosidase deficiency (glycogen storage disease, Type III)
        (2) Defects in the phosphorylase enzyme system (glycogen storage diseases, Types VI and VIII)
        (3) Glycogen synthetase deficiency (aglycogenosis)
      c. Gluconeogenic formation of glucose-6-phosphate from smaller fragments
        (1) Pyruvate carboxylase deficiency
        (2) Fructose-1,6-diphosphatase deficiency
  B. Relative production failure (insufficient glucose output from in-

trinsically normal hepatocytes)
    1. Insulin excess
      a. Functioning pancreatic islet cell tumors
      b. Pancreatic islet cell hyperplasia
      c. Multiple endocrine adenomatosis (MEA I syndrome)
      d. Epithelioid tumors from foregut anlage
      e. Neonatal hypoglycemia in infants of diabetic mothers
      f. Neonatal hypoglycemia in erythroblastosis fetalis
    2. Deficiency of contrainsulin hormones
      a. Panhypopituitarism
      b. Primary hypoadrenocorticism
      c. Isolated deficiency of growth hormone
      d. Isolated deficiency of ACTH
      e. Hypothyroidism
    3. Limitations in the availability of gluconeogenic substrates
      a. Ketotic hypoglycemia of childhood
      b. Fasting hypoglycemia of late pregnancy
    4. Insulin-independent, supranormal removal of glucose
      a. Severe exercise
      b. Renal glycosuria
    5. Mechanism unknown
      a. Massive nonpancreatic tumors associated with hypoglycemia
      b. Neonatal hypoglycemia in low birth weight infants
      c. "Idiopathic hypoglycemia" of infancy and childhood

III. Hypoglycemia induced in the fasting state (pharmacological interruption of gluconeogenesis, fatty acid oxidation, or both)
  A. Induced insulin excess
    1. Administration of insulin
    2. Administration of oral hypoglycemic agents
  B. Direct inhibition, independent of insulin
    1. Alcohol hypoglycemia
    2. Ingestion of unripe ackee fruit ("Jamaican vomiting sickness"; hypoglycin intoxication)
  C. Mechanism unknown
    1. Salicylates

than any other structure. During an acute insulin secretory response to eating, net hepatic production of glucose is "turned off" almost immediately. It is "turned on" again when blood sugar returns to normal. However, even in normal subjects, there may be some lag resulting in a transitory hypoglycemic overshoot. The lag is exaggerated in those regulatory disturbances of the fed state which manifest themselves by symptomatic hypoglycemia during the disposition of meals. Such disorders reflect sluggish or thwarted resumption of hepatic glucose output with consequent prolongation of the period of net utilization of alimentary glucose (i.e., "overutilization").

Classification. In pediatric practice, hypoglycemia in reaction to eating may be caused by dietary components which produce excessive release of insulin (e.g., leucine sensitivity of infancy or childhood) or inhibitory metabolites which accumulate owing to inherited enzyme defects (e.g., galactose-1-phosphate in galactosemia; fructose-1-phosphate in hereditary fructose intolerance). However, in adults the hypoglycemias in the fed state are usually caused by one of the following three patterns of disturbed interactions between glucose and insulin during alimentation.

When prior *gastrectomy or surgical bypass of the pylorus* enables ingested glucose to have more rapid access to absorptive sites in the small bowel, the prompt rise in blood sugar may elicit secretion of insulin that is greater than normal, although appropriate to the hyperglycemia. Rapid utilization of glucose follows as blood sugar falls to pre-eating levels, and the "extra" insulin is not buffered by continuing absorption from a reservoir of carbohydrate within the gastrointestinal tract. This has been designated as "alimentary hyperinsulinism." An analogous situation can occur in normal persons when prolonged infusions of glucose sufficient to sustain hyperglycemia are abruptly terminated, or in patients undergoing hemodialysis when dialysates containing large amounts of glucose are withdrawn suddenly.

When *glucose absorption is normal and releases of insulin are sluggish,* attenuation of hepatic glucose output and net deposition of glycogen may be retarded, so that blood sugar rises more than normally. This can occur in mild, early maturity-onset diabetes mellitus and lead to another type of reactive hypoglycemia. The continuing stimulus to insulin secretion produces plasma levels of insulin that are high but perhaps subnormal in relation to the blood sugar. In such a setting of laggard islet cell response, relative hyperinsulinism may prevail once the utilization of glucose exceeds the rate of influx from the intestine.

More than two thirds of the hypoglycemias that occur in the fed state in adults remain unexplained and have been designated as *"functional hypoglycemia."* Herein, normal or exaggerated "hypoglycemic rebounds" with profound attendant symptoms may occur with seemingly normal rates of glucose absorption, disposition, and insulin release. Functional hypoglycemia is particularly frequent in thin, tense, hyperkinetic young women and tends to occur in subjects with vagotonia and compulsive, conscientious, and intense personality patterns. It may also be encountered in patients with peptic ulcer.

Signs and Symptoms. Signs and symptoms of the hypoglycemias in the fed state can be readily understood when viewed as "overutilization" during *non-steady-state conditions.* They are characterized by precipitous onset and by features of acute epinephrine release, e.g., tachycardia, tremulousness, sweating, weakness, anxiety, nervousness, and hunger. Although the hyperepinephrinemia is triggered by glucose deprivation in the central nervous system, the duration of hypoglycemia is usually too brief to elicit additional signs of central glucopenia other than faintness, inability to concentrate, and sometimes mental confusion or visual disturbance. Consciousness is almost always preserved. The hypoglycemia is evanescent and self-limited, because the extra insulin released in response to alimentation has a finite persistence and glycogen is deposited in the liver during the induction of the hypoglycemia. Thus as soon as sufficient counter-regulation is activated (the hyperepinephrinemia is one expression), glycogenolysis corrects the hypoglycemia.

However, such a benign course is not invariable. Hypoglycemic coma can occur in subjects with reactive hypoglycemia, especially when they are receiving therapy with autonomic blocking agents such as propranolol. Thus beta receptor blockade can impair the activated lipolysis and muscle glycogenolysis by which resistance to insulin may be induced and alternate fuels and gluconeogenic precursors mobilized during hypoglycemic rebound. Similarly, in subjects with compromised cardiovascular function, even evanescent hypoglycemia and hyperepinephrinemia may provoke angina, ectopic cardiac rhythms, pulmonary edema, and episodes of transient cerebral ischemia.

Diagnosis. Since *fasting* blood sugar is never abnormally low in the aforementioned disorders, diagnosis depends upon eliciting the hypoglycemia during reproduction of the fed state with oral tests of glucose tolerance. The time at which hypoglycemia becomes manifest depends on the factors that determine the hypoglycemic rebound. Thus in alimentary hyperinsulinism, hypoglycemia usually occurs one to three hours after glucose administration; in maturity-onset diabetes, the characteristic diabetic oral glucose tolerance curve is followed by transitory hypoglycemia during the fourth or fifth hour; and functional hypoglycemia is seen during the third or fourth hour. To maximize the diagnostic value of the test, blood samples are obtained at least every 30 minutes for five hours. The signs and symptoms ascribed to hypoglycemia should coincide with nadir values for blood sugar. Professional personnel should be in attendance throughout so that vital signs may be monitored regularly and blood sampled as soon as symptoms occur. The evanescent nadir may be missed by adherence to a fixed schedule of blood sampling even with intervals as short as 30 minutes. Increments in plasma cortisol should also be demonstrable 30 to 60 minutes after the symptomatic event and may be used as further evidence that the hypoglycemia threatens homeostasis. Rigid diagnostic criteria are imperative because neurasthenic symptoms unrelated to blood sugar, such as the hyperepinephrinemia of anxiety attacks, are easily confused with true reactive hypoglycemia. Particularly in functional hypoglycemia, oral glucose tolerance may be normal when tested in the hospital under conditions divorced from daily stresses, and abnormal only in a "real-life" outpatient setting. Hence a single negative glucose tolerance test need not exclude the diagnosis of hypoglycemia in the fed state; more frequent monitoring of blood sugars during symptomatic episodes may be required.

Treatment. General objectives are to dampen the elevations in blood sugar which elicit the subsequent excessive hypoglycemic rebounds. Multiple small feedings have constituted one approach. However, regular meal-eating with diets high in protein (120 to 140 grams), low in carbohydrate (75 to 100 grams), and sufficient in fat to maintain caloric adequacy have been more efficacious. Although long experience has corroborated that high protein, low carbohydrate diets diminish the frequency of all the hypoglycemias in the fed state, their mechanism of action remains unexplained.

Certain more specific therapies may be useful. Phenformin, a drug that slows absorption of glucose from the gastrointestinal tract, has been reported to help in alimentary hyperinsulinism. The postprandial hypoglycemia of early maturity-onset diabetes mellitus may be ameliorated by improving insulin-glucose interrelationships with weight reduction or oral hypoglycemic agents. However, the entity may also disappear spontaneously as the diabetes worsens and lesser absolute amounts of insulin are released in response to dietary stimulation. Reassurance and judicious use of mild sedatives or tranquilizers may be beneficial in functional hypoglycemia. In the light of existing knowledge, adrenocortical steroids have no place in the treatment of these hypoglycemic disorders.

SPONTANEOUS HYPOGLYCEMIA IN THE FASTING STATE

Pathophysiology. By the time of waking from overnight sleep, all energy requirements of the body are fulfilled from endogenous resources. Prevailing blood sugar then reflects a balance between the continuing utilization of endogenously derived glucose and the production of additional glucose via gluconeogenesis from smaller fragments to replace the glucose lost. The reliance of the brain on glucose for its oxidative demands determines the major metabolic objective of the fasted state, that is, to produce sufficient glucose for normoglycemia to be preserved. Since net production of glucose requires catabolism of structural protein, the second objective is to restrict utilization of glucose to a minimum. The following adaptations facilitate these objectives: (1) glucose utilization is restrained in most extracerebral tissues, and the more expendable fatty acids are substituted as oxidative fuels; (2) hepatic gluconeogenesis effects essentially complete recovery of lactic acid so that tissues which rely upon glycolysis for energy (e.g., red blood cells, renal medulla) can function without a *net* expenditure of glucose; and (3) hepatic ketogenesis generates lipid products which can cross the blood-brain barrier and replace glucose for *some* of the oxidative needs of the brain once *sufficient ketonemia becomes established.*

The net rate of glucose removal is the physiologic pacesetter for the equilibrium between glucose utilization and production by which normoglycemia is maintained in the fasted state. Hypoglycemia occurs when the liver is unable to "keep up" with rates of glucose removal.

As detailed elsewhere in this text, recent studies permit the relationships in adults to be formulated in quantitative terms. Splanchnic glucose output in normal man after overnight fast approximates 180 grams per day; 80 per cent of that is oxidized completely to carbon dioxide by nervous tissue, chiefly the brain, whereas the remainder undergoes only glycolysis with the formation of lactate which is recycled to glucose. Since postprandial hepatic glycogen averages only 70 to 75 grams, some de novo formation of glucose is mandatory even after overnight fast. The precursors for the net formation of new glucose have been estimated as originating approximately 50 per cent from amino acids (of which alanine accounts for more than half) and 10 per cent from glycerol derived during lipolysis.

Data are not available concerning the maximal capacity for gluconeogenesis in normal human liver. However, extrapolations from in vitro studies and infusions of gluconeogenic precursors suggest that the biosynthetic ceiling is several-fold greater than the aforementioned values. Thus normal regulation may be delimited largely by the factors which influence the extrahepatic generation of substrates for gluconeogenesis.

Classification. Spontaneous hypoglycemias in the fasting state represent "underproduction" of hepatic glucose and may be classified as "absolute" or "relative" (see table).

The "absolute" production failures are uncommon and arise when intrinsic anatomic or enzymic abnormalities in the liver compromise its capacity to elaborate enough glucose to offset normal rates of glucose utilization in the periphery. Limitations resulting from enzyme deletions are usually confined to pediatric practice. In adults, it used to be held that fasting hypoglycemia via "absolute" production failure occurs only with fulminant hepatic necrosis, very extensive destruction of parenchyma, or severe hepatic congestion secondary to heart failure. However, the recent finding of asymptomatic low blood sugars after overnight fast in patients with viral hepatitis suggests that less severe hepatic disease can cause hypoglycemia.

"Relative" production failures are far more common. They occur when normal hepatocytes cannot "keep up" with normal or supranormal rates of glucose utilization owing to functional restraints to hepatic glucose output, inadequate generation of endogenous substrates for gluconeogenesis, or both. In most instances, additive factors are operative. For example, direct inhibition of glucose release and ketogenesis in the liver may be combined with restrained lipolysis and protein catabolism and enhanced peripheral glucose utilization to effect the fasting hypoglycemia of insulin excess (see table).

Signs and Symptoms. The fasting hypoglycemias develop slowly, so that manifestations of acute epinephrine discharge are usually not observed. Instead, the clinical picture is dominated by signs and symptoms of more prolonged and severe glucose deprivation in the brain. These may range from confusion, disorientation, and memory lapses to psychotic behavior, paresthesias, transient paralysis, convulsions, and coma. Sclerotic cerebral vessels with selectively compromised blood supply may account for focal abnormalities such as hemiplegias and monoplegias. Vulnerability of different parts of the brain to glucopenia is in reverse order of phylogenetic development. Hence the cerebral cortex is affected first. However, no single constellation of nervous system involvement is diagnostic. Fasting hypoglycemia should be suspected whenever a neuropsychiatric or neurologic complex occurs repeatedly, especially *before breakfast* or after "skipped meals," and is ameliorated almost immediately by food. In these states, reactive hypoglycemia can also occur, presumably because the factors impairing glucose production during fasting may equally restrain resumption of hepatic glucose output during the postprandial hypoglycemic rebound.

Diagnosis. Diagnosis of fasting hypoglycemia presupposes that inadequate delivery of glucose to the brain can be duplicated by simply withholding all food. In normal subjects, normoglycemia and mental acuity are preserved even with prolonged fasting, although blood sugar stabilizes at somewhat lower plateaus from the second or third day onward. Sex differences become manifest after 24 hours; nadirs for plasma glucose averaging 66 mg per 100 ml in normal men compared with 48 mg per 100 ml in normal women have been observed during the second or third day of fasting. Hence criteria for "fasting hypoglycemia" based solely on arbitrary lower limits for normal blood sugar may require modification.

Certain findings may occur in all the fasting hypoglycemias without regard to etiology. For example, Whipple's triad of (1) symptomatic hypoglycemia, (2) low blood sugar, and (3) alleviation by glucose ingestion is not pathognomonic for any single entity. Similarly, exercise may precipitate symptomatic hypoglycemia in any of these disorders, because it promotes glucose utilization independent of insulin action and thereby overtaxes marginal glucose production. Procedures should be designed to differentiate between hypoglycemia resulting from insulin excess, lack of contrainsulin factors, or compromise of other factors which preserve the normal equilibrium between glucose production and utilization in the fasting state (see table).

For optimal interpretability, safety, and rigorous exclusion of pharmacologic lowerings of blood sugar by drugs or other *exogenous* agents, diagnostic evaluation should be conducted in the hospital.

FUNCTIONING ISLET CELL TUMORS

Functioning adenomas of the beta cells of the pancreatic islets are the most common cause of fasting hypoglycemia. They are usually single, although multiple adenomas have been reported in 4 to 10 per cent of the cases. Approximately 10 per cent are malignant and 0.5 to 1 per cent are ectopic, usually within the splenic hilum, pancreatic bed, or duodenal wall. A family history of diabetes mellitus is present in approximately 25 per cent of the cases. Peak incidence is encountered between ages 40 and 60; however, cases have been seen in all age groups, although with extreme rarity in infancy and early childhood. Single adenomas are distributed with equal frequency in the head, body, and tail of the pancreas. The incidence of benign adenomas shows no sex difference, whereas malignant functioning islet tumors may be more common in males. In certain instances, functioning islet cell tumors are associated with other endocrine adenomas, particularly in the pituitary, parathyroid, and adrenal (multiple endocrine adenomatosis, Type 1), so that search for multiple endocrinopathy should be instituted whenever disorders of any of these glands occur, especially on a familial basis. Peptic ulcer disease also deserves investigation, because it has been reported in 10 per cent of all islet cell tumor patients, and many believe that the Zollinger-Ellison

syndrome (see Ch. 640 to 644) and multiple endocrine adenomatosis may represent phenotypic variants of the same mutant gene.

Diagnosis. Specific diagnosis of functioning islet cell tumors requires demonstration of (1) inappropriately elevated insulin levels during hypoglycemia when food is withheld, and (2) excessive insulin release in response to certain islet secretagogues.

Levels of plasma total immunoreactive insulin above the upper limits of normal (25 μU per milliliter) in association with subnormal blood sugar occur in approximately two thirds of patients when blood samples are obtained after overnight fast on at least three separate days. Recognition that meaningful quantities of circulating insulin should no longer be demonstrable at plasma glucose levels of 30 mg per 100 ml has expanded the diagnostic potential of insulin measurements. In this context, "normal" insulin levels may be abnormal when associated with fasting hypoglycemia. Such inappropriate relationships between insulin and glucose may be unmasked by prolonging the period of dietary deprivation (and sampling blood repeatedly at six-hour intervals) whenever normoglycemia still prevails after overnight fast. The recent demonstration that proinsulin can account for a greater than normal proportion of fasting plasma total immunoreactive insulin (i.e., greater than 20 per cent) in some, but not all, patients with islet cell tumors may provide yet another diagnostically useful characterization. It should be emphasized that modest elevations of basal insulin per se can be encountered in a variety of states associated with insulin resistance, such as obesity or acromegaly. However, these are never associated with fasting hypoglycemia.

For provocative challenge with islet secretagogues, oral or intravenous glucose has proved unrewarding, and no characteristic patterns have emerged. On the other hand, the insulin secretory response to intravenous tolbutamide (1 gram dissolved in 20 ml of saline and given intravenously over two minutes) is supranormal (i.e., increments greater than 120 μU per milliliter above baseline) in approximately 80 per cent of patients with functioning islet cell tumors; leucine (0.2 gram per kilogram orally or intravenously) elicits greater than normal increases of plasma insulin (i.e., in excess of 30 μU per milliliter) in approximately 70 per cent; and the stimulated release of insulin that follows 1 mg of intravenous glucagon exceeds the peak normal response (i.e., greater than 130 μU per milliliter) in somewhat more than 50 per cent. Since maximal insulin responses occur early, within 3 to 30 minutes after administration of the secretagogue, diagnostic evaluation can be terminated before serious hypoglycemia supervenes. Although equally exuberant releases of insulin may follow tolbutamide or glucagon administration in obesity, acromegaly, pregnancy, and other states associated with heightened basal insulin secretion, the subsequent hypoglycemia is not commensurate with the hyperinsulinemia under such circumstances. Therefore both blood sugar and insulin values should be monitored during provocative tests for insulinoma.

Treatment. *Surgery* constitutes the treatment of choice. Preoperative attenuation of hypoglycemia may be achieved with 100 to 200 mg hydrocortisone per day and appropriate dietary supplementation. The nondiuretic benzothiadiazine, diazoxide, in doses of 200 to 800 mg per day has proved more effective, by inhibiting insulin secretion directly as well as by exerting peripheral actions. Because of its sodium-retaining properties, diazoxide should be combined with a natriuretic thiazide such as trichlormethiazide (2 to 4 mg per day). These medications should be discontinued two days preoperatively.

At surgery, the pancreas should be mobilized and explored carefully for single or multiple lesions that can be "shelled out." Preoperative localization by selective pancreatic arteriography has been successful in approximately 40 per cent of the limited number of instances in which it has been tried. Quite frequently, however, all efforts at visualization and palpation of the tumor fail. Under such circumstances, the tail and then the body of the pancreas should be excised sequentially, because this will remove a significant proportion of the insulinomas. Failure to find tumor on serial sectioning justifies subsequent excision of most of the head of the pancreas but avoiding duodenal and bile duct resection. Such surgical aggressiveness requires unequivocal preoperative diagnostic confidence—a circumstance that insulin immunoassays have made possible today. Monitoring of blood samples during surgery may also be helpful; a sharp rise in blood sugar within 30 minutes after excision of tumor affords presumptive evidence against residual functioning tumor in situ or additional tumors elsewhere.

Successful extirpation of tumor (or tumors) effects complete and prompt cure. However, nonresectable islet cell carcinomas may be functional and accompanied by hypoglycemia. Long-term symptomatic palliation with diazoxide and trichlormethiazide or hormones such as glucocorticoids, long-acting glucagon, or growth hormone has been tried. *Streptozotocin,* a broad-spectrum antimicrobial with relatively selective cytotoxicity for pancreatic beta cells, has proved more rewarding. In 52 patients with metastatic pancreatic islet cell carcinoma treated with streptozotocin, measurable response has been observed in 50 and 63 per cent of those with functional and nonfunctional tumors, respectively. Response included tumor regression, rectification of hyperinsulinism, and more than threefold improvement in survival. The renal and hepatic toxicities of streptozotocin, although appreciable, usually have been reversible.

EXTRAPANCREATIC NEOPLASMS ASSOCIATED WITH HYPOGLYCEMIA

Over 200 instances of massive extrapancreatic neoplasms (ranging from 1.5 to 20 pounds) associated with fasting hypoglycemia have been reported. Four major tumor groups have been involved. Approximately half have been mesothelial tumors (most commonly classified as fibromas, fibrosarcomas, spindle cell sarcomas, and leiomyosarcomas); 20 per cent have been malignant hepatomas; gastrointestinal carcinomas (particularly of the stomach, colon, and bile ducts) and adrenocortical carcinomas have each accounted for about another 10 per cent. The rest have been miscellaneous tumors. About 80 per cent of the tumors have been intra-abdominal.

Although the pathophysiology of this hypoglycemia is not fully understood, it has been associated in a number of cases with heightened glucose utilization by the tumor and restrained hepatic glucose output. Increased plasma immunoreactive insulin has not yet been demonstrated unequivocally with any of these neoplasms.

In this they differ from the smaller epithelioid tumors which are embryologically derived from the same foregut anlage as the islets. The latter on rare occasions have insulin secretory potential, and one bronchial carcinoid tumor has been described in which increased immunoreactive insulin was demonstrated in plasma as well as in primary and metastatic tumor tissue.

Massive extrapancreatic tumors associated with fasting hypoglycemia can be readily distinguished from insulinomas. Plasma immunoreactive insulin is low and usually appropriate to the prevailing hypoglycemia. Responses to tolbutamide and leucine are usually subnormal in terms of glucose as well as insulin, most likely because islet function has been dampened by the antecedent hypoglycemia.

Therapy should be directed toward total surgical excision, or as much tumoricidal ablation as possible. When such therapy is successful, the hypoglycemia has usually disappeared. Glucocorticoids, glucagon, growth hormone, and dietary manipulations have been helpful in managing the hypoglycemia during preparation for surgery and, occasionally, when tumor therapy has been unsuccessful. Diazoxide has been tried also; efficacy has been somewhat less than in other fasting hypoglycemias, perhaps because of the smaller role played by pancreatic insulin.

HYPOGLYCEMIA INDUCED IN THE FASTING STATE

Pathophysiology. The hypoglycemias which arise *spontaneously* in the fasting state must be differentiated from another group of disorders, the hypoglycemias *induced* in the fasting state. Here, an *exogenous* agent has been introduced which can block the endogenous realignments by which normoglycemia is preserved when food is withheld. The resulting hypoglycemia may persist for the duration of the biologic effectiveness of the exogenous agent and engender considerable diagnostic confusion in the unwary.

Classification and Manifestations. Two broad groups can be delineated: the hypoglycemias caused by *induced* insulin excess and those caused by drugs which directly impair homeostatic mechanisms, independent of insulin action (see table).

Induced insulin excess should always be suspected when hypoglycemic episodes have no well-defined, recurring pattern and when they involve individuals with ready access to hypoglycemic medications such as diabetics, relatives of diabetics, or medical and paramedical workers. The clinical picture in instances of *surreptitious or accidental administration of insulin* depends on the nature of the insulin involved. Short-acting preparations may elicit the hyperepinephrinemia and the clinical features characteristic of the hypoglycemias in the fed state. Contrariwise, long- or intermediate-acting preparations of insulin may effect a picture indistinguishable from the spontaneous hypoglycemias of the fasting state.

All the *sulfonylureas* have also been associated with life-threatening hypoglycemic comas, presumably owing to stimulation of excessive insulin release (see table). Vulnerability to this exaggeration of their action is greatest in the elderly, in newborns of diabetic mothers who have received sulfonylureas, and in subjects with reduced hepatic or renal capacities for metabolizing or excreting the drugs. Chlorpropamide has posed the greatest problem. As the longest-acting sulfonylurea, it has been implicated in 120 of the 220 known cases of coma caused by sulfonylurea drugs when used alone. The clinical hypoglycemic syndromes with all these agents have consisted of slowly evolving cerebral dysfunction progressing to coma.

Perhaps the most frequent cause of the hypoglycemias induced in the fasting state in adults is *ethanol* (see table). Although other factors may participate, the principal mechanism is by direct inhibition of gluconeogenesis resulting from the metabolism of alcohol in the cytoplasm of the liver. As each mole of ethanol is oxidized to acetaldehyde and then to acetate (or acetyl CoA) via alcohol and aldehyde dehydrogenase, respectively, two moles of NAD^+ are reduced. The ratio of $NADH/NAD^+$ thereby increases, a reductive environment supervenes, and NAD^+ is diverted from other reactions in the liver. Thus the citric acid cycle is restrained, and there is attenuation of the flux of precursors such as glycerol, lactate, and amino acids which enter the gluconeogenic sequence via NAD^+-dependent reactions. The duration of prior fasting required to lower blood sugar under such circumstances and the latency between imbibition and hypoglycemia depend upon (1) how much glycogen is present for sustaining hepatic glucose output while gluconeogenic renewal is blocked, and (2) how rapidly circulating glucose is being removed in the periphery. In normal adults, more than 24 hours of fasting are usually necessary; infants and children are far more vulnerable, and hypoglycemia may occur shortly after exposure to ethanol and after only minimal dietary deprivation.

The clinical signs differ little from other types of hypoglycemia occurring in the fasting state. However, the early mental changes are often mistaken for alcoholic inebriation so that help is not usually sought until patients become comatose. Even then, the transition from alcoholic stupor to hypoglycemic coma may be unsuspected. Hypothermia is common; trismus may be present; and convulsions are particularly prominent in infants and children. The relationship to prior ethanol ingestion need not be obvious. Alcohol oxidation is a linear function so that a relatively constant amount is oxidized per unit time. Therefore, depending upon initial intake, the generation of reducing equivalents within the liver may persist for many hours and at low blood alcohol levels. If there has been no intake of food, hypoglycemia can thus occur 6 to 20 hours after imbibition, and without any clinical signs of alcoholism.

The situation may be particularly complex and dangerous when several agents interact concurrently. For example, irreversible brain damage and even death have occurred from alcohol hypoglycemia in diabetic alcoholics who have received insulin during periods of spree drinking and dietary dereliction.

Salicylates warrant inclusion, because they account for most of the drug-induced hypoglycemias during the first two years of life. Because of the age group involved, salicylates have been associated with the greatest mortality of any hypoglycemic drug (33 per cent in 15 reported cases). The mechanism of hypoglycemic action remains unsettled (see table).

Diagnosis and Treatment. Recognition of hypoglycemia in these comatose patients is imperative. Failure to do so, and to treat accordingly, accounted for fatal ter-

minations in 25 per cent of the children and 11 per cent of the adults with alcohol hypoglycemia reported before 1962. As in all hypoglycemic comas, a high index of suspicion improves prognosis, and response to glucose is usually dramatic unless brain damage has been sustained. However, in the induced hypoglycemias, especially when caused by sulfonylureas, the effect of the drug may be prolonged, and continued administration of glucose, with frequent monitoring of blood sugar, may be necessary for several days. After the patient has been stabilized, it must be established whether the hypoglycemia in the fasting state was *spontaneous* or *induced*. This can only be done in a hospital, because rigorous supervision may be required to exclude *exogenous* agents (as in factitious hyperinsulinism). After the cause of induced hypoglycemia has been established, no definitive therapy may be required save for dietary instruction, psychiatric help when necessary, and other attempts to modify exposure to the offending agent. However, it must be appreciated that vulnerability to the hypoglycemic potential of drugs like alcohol is far greater in individuals in whom endogenous capacities for gluconeogenesis or lipolysis are already marginal. Therefore diagnostic work-up of the functions that influence blood sugar homeostasis in the fasting state is also indicated. Such evaluations have unmasked occult diseases (e.g., hypopituitarism, hypoadrenocorticism) in several instances.

Broder, L. E., and Carter, S. K.: Pancreatic islet cell carcinoma. Ann. Intern. Med., 79:101, 108, 1973.

Cahill, G. F., Jr.: Starvation in man. N. Engl. J. Med., 282:668, 1970.

Conn, J. W., and Pek, S.: Current concepts: On spontaneous hypoglycemia. Scope Monograph. Kalamazoo, Michigan, The Upjohn Company, 1970, pp. 1–33.

Felig, P., Brown, W. V., Levine, R. A., and Klatskin, G.: Glucose homeostasis in viral hepatitis. N. Engl. J. Med., 282:1436, 1970.

Freinkel, N., and Bleicher, S. J.: The physiologic basis for evaluation of "fasting hypoglycemias." Am. J. Surg., 105:730, 1963.

Freinkel, N., Cohen, A. K., Sandler, R., and Arky, R. A.: Alcohol hypoglycemia: A prototype of the hypoglycemias induced in the fasting state. *In* Proceedings of the VIth Congress of the International Diabetes Federation, Stockholm, July 30–August 4, 1967. Amsterdam, Exerpta Medica International Congress Series No. 172, 1969, pp. 873–886.

Freinkel, N., and Metzger, B. E.: Oral glucose tolerance curve and hypoglycemias in the fed state. N. Engl. J. Med., 280:820, 1969.

Merimee, T. J., and Fineberg, S. E.: Homeostasis during fasting. II. Hormone substrate differences between men and women. J. Clin. Endocrinol. Metab., 37:698, 1973.

Pagliara, A. S., Karl, I. E., Haymond, M., and Kipnis, D. M.: Hypoglycemia in infancy and childhood, Parts I and II. J. Pediatr., 82:365, 558, 1973.

Seltzer, H. S.: Drug-induced hypoglycemia. Diabetes, 21:955, 1972.

Sherman, B. M., Pek, S., Fajans, S. S., Floyd, J. C., Jr., and Conn, J. W.: Plasma proinsulin in patients with functioning pancreatic islet cell tumors. J. Clin. Endocrinol. Metab., 35:271, 1972.

Smith, H. M. (ed.): Diazoxide and the treatment of hypoglycemia. Ann. N.Y. Acad. Sci., 150:191, 1968.

Unger, R. H.: The riddle of tumor hypoglycemia. Am. J. Med., 40:325, 1966.

Yalow, R. S., and Berson, S. A.: Dynamics of insulin secretion in hypoglycemia. Diabetes, 14:341, 1965.

808. GALACTOSEMIA

Ernest Beutler

The galactosemias are disorders characterized by inability to metabolize galactose normally. When individuals with galactosemia ingest galactose, either in its free form or as the galactose-containing disaccharide, lactose, galactose and some of the products of its incomplete metabolism accumulate in the blood, tissues, and usually the urine. Two types of galactosemia may be distinguished: "classic" or *transferase deficiency galactosemia* caused by a lack of galactose-1-phosphate uridyl transferase activity, and *galactokinase deficiency galactosemia.*

CLASSIC GALACTOSEMIA

Etiology. "Classic galactosemia" is due to a marked deficiency of the enzyme galactose-1-phosphate uridyl transferase. This deficiency is inherited as an autosomal recessive disorder.

Incidence. The incidence of classic galactosemia is approximately 1 per 80,000 births in the white population. The incidence may be somewhat higher in the black population.

Pathogenesis. The galactose molecule is identical to the glucose molecule except for the relative position of the hydroxyl and hydrogen groups attached to the fourth carbon. However, the body is unable to utilize this sugar until it has been converted to glucose. Only one pathway for the metabolism of galactose has been clearly established. First, galactose is phosphorylated in the 1-position by ATP through the mediation of the enzyme galactokinase:

$$\text{Galactose} + \text{ATP} \xrightarrow{\text{galactokinase}} \text{galactose-1-P}$$

Next, the galactose-1-P formed exchanges with the glucose-1-P moiety attached to a uridine disphosphate carrier. This reaction is catalyzed by galactose-1-phosphate uridyl transferase (transferase):

$$\text{Galactose-1-P} + \text{UDPG} \xrightleftharpoons{\text{transferase}} \text{glucose-1-P} + \text{UDPGal}$$

Finally, the uridine diphosphogalactose (UDPGal) formed may be converted to uridine diphosphoglucose (UDPG) through the action of epimerase:

$$\text{UDPGal} \xrightleftharpoons{\text{epimerase}} \text{UDPG}$$

In classic galactosemia the absence of galactose-1-phosphate uridyl transferase activity results in accumulation of both galactose and galactose-1-P. Galactose may serve as a substrate for aldose reductase and for L-hexonate dehydrogenase. These enzymes oxidize NADPH, reducing galactose to its polyol derivative, dulcitol, to which cell membranes are relatively impermeable. In the lens of the eye, this creates an unbalanced osmotic force, resulting in excessive hydration. At the same time, it may deplete the lens of its supply of NADPH. The result of these changes is the irreversible precipitation of the lens protein with the formation of cataracts.

In addition, cirrhosis of the liver and mental retardation are characteristics of classic galactosemia. Since these changes do not occur in galactokinase deficiency (see below), it may be presumed that they are the result of galactose-1-phosphate accumulation.

Clinical Manifestations. Occasionally galactosemic infants may have cataracts at birth. More typically the symptoms of galactosemia begin within a few days or weeks of birth. The infant takes feedings poorly, vomits frequently, and may have diarrhea. Many galactosemic infants die in the first few weeks of life. The abdomen may enlarge owing to progressive hepatomegaly and ascites. Jaundice usually appears quite early, and the disorder has at times been mistaken for hemolytic disease of the newborn. Proteinuria and generalized aminoaciduria are constant findings. If they are not present at birth, cataracts may develop within a few weeks or, in some instances, not for many months. Mental retardation becomes evident as the infant matures. Administration of large galactose loads, as in the performance of galactose tolerance tests, may produce dangerous hypoglycemia.

Diagnosis. Classic galactosemia is diagnosed by demonstrating that galactose-1-P uridyl transferase activity is absent from the erythrocytes.

Treatment. The treatment of galactosemia consists of institution of a diet with a very low galactose content as soon as the diagnosis is established. Because milk contains a high concentration of lactose, a disaccharide of glucose and galactose, a milk substitute such as Nutramigen must be fed during infancy. Although the effectiveness of the low-galactose diet is established in infants, no data are available regarding the necessity for maintaining strict dietary control after the first few years of life. It is likely that the ingestion of small amounts of galactose is relatively harmless after the fifth or sixth year of life. However, until further evidence is available regarding the possible harmful effects of galactose when fed to older galactosemic children and adults, it is probably wise to continue a moderate degree of dietary restriction throughout life.

Prognosis. Untreated infants with classic galactosemia rarely survive more than a few months, and may succumb within a few days. A few cases first diagnosed in later childhood or early adult life are known. With the prompt institution of a low-galactose diet, the development of galactosemic children appears to be normal or nearly so. If treatment is delayed, however, some degree of permanent mental retardation and irreversible cataracts is often present. Signs of liver failure and growth retardation appear to respond promptly to therapy in most instances, however, and treated galactosemics generally survive into adult life.

Prevention. Galactosemia itself can only be prevented through genetic counseling. Heterozygotes for classic galactosemia have one half normal galactose-1-P uridyl transferase activity in their red cells. However, not all persons with this level of enzyme activity are carriers of galactosemia. Persons homozygous for another gene, that for the Duarte variant, also have one half of normal transferase activity, but may be differentiated from those heterozygous for galactosemia on the basis of the electrophoretic properties of the red cell enzyme.

Prevention of the clinical sequelae of galactosemia by early diagnosis and prompt institution of treatment is the most practical means of control. Microbiologic and enzymatic methods for the detection of galactose in the blood or in the urine have been developed and will detect most cases of classic galactosemia in the neonatal period. However, some false positive results are encountered, and false negative results will be found in infants who are so ill as to refuse their feedings. A fluorescent screening test which depends directly upon galactose-1-P uridyl transferase activity will reliably detect classic galactosemia even from cord blood. Prenatal diagnosis can be achieved by assaying cultured amniotic cells for galactose-1-P uridyl transferase.

Segal, S.: Disorders of galactose metabolism. *In* Stanbury, J. B., Wyngaarden, J. B., and Fredrickson, D. S. (eds.): The Metabolic Basis of Inherited Disease. 3rd ed. New York, McGraw-Hill Book Company, 1972, pp. 174–195.

Beutler, E., Matsumoto, F., Kuhl, W., Krill, A., Levy, N., Sparkes, R., and Degnan, M.: Galactokinase deficiency as a cause of cataracts. N. Engl. J. Med., 288:1203, 1973.

Kalckar, H. M., Kinoshita, J. H., and Donnell, G. N.: Galactosemia: Biochemistry, genetics, patho-physiology, and developmental aspects. Biol. Brain Dysfunct., 1:31, 1972.

GALACTOKINASE DEFICIENCY

Etiology. Galactokinase deficiency is a genetically determined disorder caused by an autosomally inherited enzyme deficiency.

Incidence. Only about 20 families with galactokinase deficiency have been described. However, the true incidence of the disorder is probably larger than this very small number of cases would suggest, because the disorder was first described only in 1965. Limited data suggest that the incidence may be of the order of 1 in 500,000 births, and that as many as 1 in 100 patients developing cataracts of unknown origin during the first year of life may have this defect.

Pathogenesis. Galactokinase catalyzes the first step of galactose metabolism (see above). In galactokinase deficiency, galactose accumulates in the body and produces cataracts through the same mechanism outlined under Classic Galactosemia.

It is uncertain whether only individuals with virtually total absence of galactokinase develop cataracts from galactokinase deficiency. Since galactose is the limiting enzyme in galactose metabolism, it is possible that repeated large galactose loads may result in lenticular damage even in individuals heterozygous for galactokinase deficiency who have one half normal galactokinase activity. An increased incidence of cataracts has been noted among heterozygotes in some families of galactokinase-deficient persons. However, most individuals heterozygous for galactokinase deficiency do not develop cataracts, and the link between partial galactokinase deficiency and cataracts cannot be considered to be firmly established.

Clinical Manifestations. The only clinical manifestation of galactokinase deficiency is the development of cataracts. After ingestion of galactose, elevated blood galactose levels and galactosuria may be found.

Diagnosis. The diagnosis of galactokinase deficiency should be considered in any person developing cataracts of unknown cause during childhood. The diagnosis is established by assaying the galactokinase activity of the red blood cells.

Treatment. The treatment of galactokinase deficiency consists of institution of a low-galactose diet (see above).

Prognosis. If a low-galactose diet is initiated at the time of birth or shortly thereafter, cataract formation is prevented. When cataracts are already present, some improvement may occur on institution of galactose restriction, particularly in the very young.

Prevention. The effects of galactokinase deficiency can be prevented by early detection and institution of a low-galactose diet. Detection of heterozygotes can be accomplished by measuring galactokinase activity in red cells. Genetic counseling can therefore be carried out with families in which a case of galactokinase deficiency has been found. Screening of the blood of neonates by methods which detect increased blood galactose level makes possible early detection so that treatment can be instituted promptly.

809. GLYCOGEN STORAGE DISEASE

J. B. Sidbury, Jr.

Definition. The glycogenoses are a group of heritable disorders of altered glycogen metabolism. Excluded are conditions associated with secondary glycogen accumulation such as Mauriac's syndrome and steroid therapy. A glycogen storage disease was the first inborn error of metabolism to be enzymatically defined. Cori's original classification into four types has been extended progressively to 13. Additions to the original classification have been made in the chronology of the enzymatic definition, except for Type 0 which is so designated because it is characterized by a deficiency of glycogen. Subtypes are designated to reflect different clinical presentation of the same enzymatic defect or when differences in the enzyme can be discerned without a distinguishing phenotypic pattern.

Etiology. The evidence available is compatible with autosomal recessive transmission except in Type IX which is sex linked. The symptoms associated with Types 0, I, III, IV, IX, XI, and XII can be ascribed to the inadequacy of liver glycogen availability, and the severity of symptoms is related to the degree of impediment in glycogen conversion to blood glucose. In Type IV the symptoms evolve from the resultant cirrhosis. The muscle glycogenoses, Types V, VII, VIII, and X, have symptoms resulting from the inadequacy of glycolysis in the muscle which is usually evident only with vigorous exercise.

Clinical Manifestations. The enzymatic deficiency of Type 0 results in inadequate rate of glycogen synthesis, and since the rate of degradation is normal, the inadequate glycogen stores are rapidly depleted and hypoglycemia results. Gluconeogenesis alone is inadequate in the infant to sustain the blood glucose. Symptoms are often not manifest until the frequency of feedings is decreased. The other *liver forms* of glycogenosis (see accompanying table) may have symptoms so similar as to be clinically indistinguishable, and the symptoms vary from difficult, symptomatic hypoglycemia and ketoacidosis to essentially asymptomatic hepatomegaly. Types I and III are more likely to be symptomatic, and the associated findings seen are susceptibility to infections, bleeding tendency, short stature, mild cushingoid features, excessive sweating, and eruptive xanthoma. Gout is unique to Type I, and it is not generally symptomatic until after puberty despite an elevation of uric acid throughout the course. The clinical management of the more symptomatic individuals is most difficult in the first five years of life. As a rule all symptoms and the hepatomegaly resolve with puberty or before in all the classic hepatic types except Type I. In patients with Type IV defect, death almost invariably supervenes as a result of the cirrhosis and portal hypertension before puberty. This is the only glycogen storage disease with splenomegaly.

The Enzymatically Defined Glycogenoses

Type	Defect	
0	UDPG-glycogen transferase	(L)
Ia	Glucose-6-phosphatase	(L)
Ib	Glucose-6-phosphatase, functionally	(L)
IIa,b	Lysosomal α-1,4-glucosidase	(M)
IIIa,	Amylo-1,6-glucosidase and/or	
b,c,d	oligo-1,4→1,4-glucantransferase*	(L)
IV	Amylo-1,4→1,6-transglucosylase*	(L)
V	Muscle phosphorylase	(M)
VI	Liver phosphorylase	(L)
VII	Phosphofructokinase	(M)
VIII	Phosphohexosisomerase	(M)
IX	Phosphorylase kinase	(L)
X	Phosphorylase kinase	(M)
XI	Phosphoglucomutase	(L)
XII	Cyclic 3′,5′-AMP dependent kinase	(L)

*Glycogen structure abnormal.
(L) Symptoms related to liver.
(M) Symptoms related to muscles.

The *muscle types* of glycogenosis, V, VII, VIII, and X, involve striated muscle. The symptoms may be first noted in early childhood (V, VII, and X) or not until the mature years (VIII). The day-to-day symptoms are unimpressive as are the physical findings, and these individuals are often labeled psychoneurotic for several years before the diagnosis is made. Vigorous exercise is associated with weakness, muscle cramps, and occasionally myoglobinuria. Symptoms tend to be slowly progressive. Seizures associated with myoglobinuria have been reported in individuals with the phosphorylase defect.

Type IIa designates classic *Pompe's disease* or generalized glycogenosis which is seen in infants who appear to be normal for the first two or three months of life and progress to flaccidity, absent reflexes, gross cardiomegaly, and death by one year of age. Patients with Type IIb, with apparently the same enzyme defect, do not have the heart involvement and present simulating relatively severe muscular dystrophy in the first few years of life or as a progressive myopathy in the teen years or later.

Diagnosis. The definitive diagnosis of glycogen storage disease is made by enzymatic assay of liver and/or muscle obtained by biopsy. The glycogen is characterized and the content determined. Enzymatic assays of leukocytes can be useful in Types III, IV, VI, and IX. Skin fibroblasts grown in culture have been shown to be useful in diagnosis and in the determination of heterozygosity in Types II and IV, and antenatal diagnosis is possible using these techniques. An antibody to glucose-6-phosphatase has been prepared which will detect the enzyme in the serum of normal individuals and gives no precipitin lines with the sera of patients with Type I glycogenosis. The response of blood glucose and lactate to the glucagon tolerance test is useful in that the blood glucose usually does not respond in Types I, III, and VI, and in Type I the lactate is high in the fasting state with a further increase in response to the glucagon. The red cell glycogen may be elevated markedly in Type III.

Types V, VII, VIII, and X are characterized by absence of rise in blood lactate consequent to anoxic exercise. This is performed by having the subject exercise the hand with the blood pressure cuff above the elbow inflated above systolic pressure and by obtaining blood from the antecubital vein at intervals for several min-

utes. The normal individual will have a two- to fourfold rise, whereas the muscle glycogen patients will have none. Type II glycogenosis patients show no abnormality of carbohydrate metabolism that can be approached through blood sampling. Electromyography can be helpful. In the muscle glycogenoses of impaired glycolysis, the signal becomes isoelectric after a period of vigorous exercise. The "dive bomber" effect is characteristically found in Type IIb glycogen storage. Type IIa muscle does not demonstrate a characteristic finding.

Treatment. Types I, II, III, and IV are the most likely to be management problems. Individuals with the Type I defect are at risk of severe ketoacidosis in association with infection in the early years. This complication, like the symptomatic hypoglycemia which is frequently seen, is best managed by frequent high carbohydrate feedings. Portacaval shunt has been found to relieve many of the biochemical aberrations, and preoperative intravenous hyperalimentation for two to three weeks reduces the operative risk. This approach should be considered only for the more severely ill patients. Patients with Type III glycogenosis and the occasional patient with the other forms of hepatic glycogenoses who are symptomatic will respond to a high protein diet with additional carbohydrates when symptomatic. Patients with Type IV glycogenosis are treated symptomatically as one would treat any other child with cirrhosis and portal hypertension. The infant with Type II glycogenosis is managed symptomatically. Digitalis is used for heart failure, but there is little evidence of its efficacy. Patients with glycogen myopathies associated with impaired glycolysis are symptomatic when engaged in vigorous exercise. They must be taught to modulate their activity and seek employment appropriate to their physical capacities. It is reported that fructose administration will help patients with Type VIII glycogen storage disease.

Cori, G. T.: Glycogen structure and enzyme deficiencies in glycogen storage disease. Harvey Lectures, 48:145, 1953.
Moses, S. W., and Gutman, A.: Inborn errors of glycogen metabolism. *In* Schulman, I. (ed.): Adv. Pediatr., 19:95, 1972.

810. PENTOSURIA
(Essential Pentosuria)

J. B. Sidbury, Jr.

Pentosuria is a clinically asymptomatic, rare, heritable abnormality of carbohydrate metabolism limited almost exclusively to Jews. It is transmitted as an autosomal recessive condition, with estimated incidence of 1:2000 to 1:5000 of the population at risk. Loading of the glucuronic acid cycle by oral administration of glucuronolactone will cause an increase in urinary 1-xylulose excretion in the homozygote and a lesser response in the heterozygote. Assay of the erythrocytes of affected individuals has demonstrated a deficiency of the specific NADP-linked xylitol dehydrogenase which converts 1-xylulose to xylitol and has further shown that the affinity of the mutant enzyme for NADP is significantly less than that from normal individuals. As a consequence of the enzyme reduction in the liver, affected individuals excrete 1 to 4 grams of 1-xylulose in the urine daily. The sugar can easily be distinguished from others by paper or thin-layer chromatography.

Glucose oxidase, which is the reagent in the dip-stick type of urine test, will not react with this sugar, whereas the reducing methods will. The practical importance of proper identification is in preventing the individual from being labeled a diabetic for treatment and insurance purposes.

Hiatt, H. H.: Pentosuria. *In* Stanbury, J. B., Wyngaarden, J. B., and Fredrickson, D. S. (eds.): The Metabolic Basis of Inherited Disease. 3rd ed. New York, McGraw-Hill Book Company, 1972, p. 119.
Wang, Y. M., and VanEys, J.: The enzymatic defect in essential pentosuria. N. Engl. J. Med., 282:892, 1970.

811. FRUCTOSURIA AND HEREDITARY FRUCTOSE INTOLERANCE

J. B. Sidbury, Jr.

Fructosuria (Essential Fructosuria). Fructosuria is an asymptomatic, rare, autosomal recessive condition resulting from a deficiency of fructokinase, which is the first reaction in the major pathway of fructose metabolism. The incidence of the condition is estimated to be 1:130,000. Fructokinase is normally found only in the liver, kidney, and intestinal mucosa. The diagnosis can be surmised by performing a fructose loading test determining the fructose rise in the blood by difference between total reducing substance and glucose and by identifying the fructose excreted in the urine by chromatography. Normally, under loading conditions the blood fructose will peak at one hour and not exceed 25 mg per 100 ml. No significant fructosuria occurs. Fructose will not react with glucose oxidase but will reduce copper sulfate, even at 80° C. The proper diagnosis is important to the patient in order to prevent his being labeled or treated as a diabetic.

Hereditary Fructose Intolerance. This is an autosomal recessive condition associated with a structural alteration of phosphofructoaldolase B. The adult will commonly note dyspepsia and anxiety with fructose ingestion but usually will have learned to avoid offending foods through personal observation. The untreated infant will have vomiting, failure to grow, hypotonia, jaundice, hepatosplenomegaly, ascites, bleeding disorder, hypoglycemia, hypophosphatemia, abnormal liver function tests, aminoacidemia, acidosis, uric acid elevation, proteinuria, mellituria (fructose and sometimes galactose and glucose also), and aminoaciduria. The clinical presentation and findings often make the differential diagnosis between this condition, tyrosinosis, and galactosemia very difficult indeed. Liver biopsy reveals portal and interlobar fibrosis without cellular infiltrate, steatosis, bile retention, and rosette formation. The reported pathology in the kidney is variable. The brain may show diminished neurons. The mechanism of the symptomatology is unclear when the defect is defined in terms of the inability to cleave fructose-1-phosphate to the corresponding trioses. That the symptoms might be similar to those of galactosemia is not surprising, because galactose-1-phosphate accumulates in the cells in galactosemia. In fructose intolerance fructose-1-phosphate accumulates in the liver and kidney, the two primary organs in which fructose is metabolized. Thus symptoms are secondary or tertiary phenomena. The hypoglycemia results from a marked decrease in glucose production by the liver very shortly

after fructose loading in these individuals. In spite of the recurrent hypoglycemia in infancy, the affected adults evaluated have had normal intelligence.

The defective enzyme, phosphofructoaldolase B or liver aldolase, has been shown to be decreased in total activity but more specifically to function in a manner analogous to aldolase A or muscle aldolase in that aldolase B normally demonstrates a 1:1 ratio of activity for fructose-1-phosphate and fructose-1,6-diphosphate, whereas aldolase A normally has a ratio of activity for these substrates of approximately 0.1 to 0.2. Kinetic studies of the mutant enzyme have shown a markedly reduced affinity for fructose-1-phosphate. Immunologically the mutant enzyme cross-reacts with the normal and quantitatively correlates with the activity for fructose diphosphate. The enzyme in the liver of parents showed no abnormality.

A presumptive *diagnosis* can be made in an individual whose symptoms are suggestive by an oral or intravenous loading test. Serious hypoglycemia can be induced; hence modified loading doses are recommended, e.g., 0.5 gram per kilogram of body weight orally or 0.25 gram per kilogram intravenously, or 3 grams per square meter of body surface area in children. Demonstrating resultant hypoglycemia, fructosemia, hypophosphatemia, and fructosuria constitutes presumptive evidence for the diagnosis. *Management*, once the diagnosis is made, is simply avoidance of fruits and foods with sucrose.

Froesch, E. R.: Essential Fructosuria and Hereditary Fructose Intolerance. *In* Stanbury, J. B., Wyngaarden, J. B., and Fredrickson, D. S. (eds.): The Metabolic Basis of Inherited Disease. 3rd ed. New York, McGraw-Hill Book Company, 1972, p. 131.
Nordmann, Y., and Schapira, F.: Intolérance au fructose. Biochimie, 54:741, 1972.
Odievre, M., Gantier, M., and Rieu, D.: Intolérance héréditaire au fructose du nourrisson. Arch. Franç. Péd., 26:433, 1969.

812. PRIMARY HYPEROXALURIA

Lloyd H. Smith, Jr.

Primary hyperoxaluria is a general term for two rare genetic disorders of glyoxylate metabolism productive of excessive synthesis and urinary excretion of oxalic acid. Both disorders are transmitted as autosomal recessive traits. The diseases are characterized by the onset in childhood of recurrent calcium oxalate nephrolithiasis or nephrocalcinosis, or both, usually leading to early death secondary to renal failure. At postmortem examination calcium oxalate may be found widely deposited in extrarenal sites, a condition known as oxalosis. More rarely, milder forms of the disease may be found in adults. Athough oxalate is an important constituent in approximately two thirds of all kidney stones, most adult patients with calcium oxalate nephrolithiasis excrete normal amounts of urinary oxalate.

Primary hyperoxaluria Type I (glycolic aciduria) represents a genetic defect in the soluble enzyme α-ketoglutarate: glyoxylate carboligase. The resulting accumulation of glyoxylate leads to its excessive oxidation to oxalate and its reduction to glycolate, both of which are excreted in increased amounts in the urine (more than 60 mg per 1.73 square meters per 24 hours each).

In *primary hyperoxaluria Type II* (L-glyceric aciduria) there is a defect in the enzyme D-glyceric dehydrogenase. Hydroxypyruvate accumulates and is reduced by lactic dehydrogenase (LDH) to L-glyceric acid, a compound which is undetectable in normal urine. The reduction of hydroxypyruvate to L-glycerate is probably coupled to the oxidation of glyoxylate to oxalate, both catalyzed by LDH. Each disease can be diagnosed by the characteristic pattern of metabolites in urine: Type I, oxalate and glycolate; Type II, oxalate and L-glycerate. Pyridoxine deficiency in laboratory animals and man also leads to hyperoxaluria and even oxalosis with a urinary pattern similar to that of the genetic disease Type I. With the onset of renal failure the clearance of oxalate is reduced (normally about 1.2 times the creatinine clearance) so that its urinary excretion may return to normal. The diagnosis may then be difficult to establish because of the unreliability of current methods for measuring serum oxalate.

No specific methods of treatment are now available. Efforts are directed toward reducing the amount of oxalate excreted and increasing its solubility. Large amounts of pyridoxine (200 to 400 mg per 24 hours) may decrease oxalate excretion in the Type I disease. Dilute urine should be maintained by forcing fluids, and a phosphate supplement seems to offer partial protection against stone formation. Attempts at renal homotransplantation have been disappointing because of rapid deposition of calcium oxalate in the transplanted kidney. A search for a more effective inhibitor of oxalate synthesis is being conducted.

An important cause of secondary hyperoxaluria has recently been found. Increased urinary excretion of oxalate and stone diathesis (in the absence of glycolic aciduria or L-glyceric aciduria) occurs in many patients who have small bowel disease and malabsorption. This form of acquired hyperoxaluria results from excessive absorption of dietary oxalate. It can be controlled by a low oxalate diet.

Boquist, L., Lindquist, B., Östberg, Y., and Steen, L.: Primary oxalosis. Am. J. Med., 54:673, 1973.

Chadwick, V. S., Modka, K., and Dowling, R. H.: Mechanism of hyperoxaluria in patients with ileal dysfunction. N. Engl. J. Med., 289:172, 1973.

Hockaday, T. D. R., Clayton, J. E., Frederick, E. W., and Smith, L. H., Jr.: Primary hyperoxaluria. Medicine, 43:315, 1964.

Williams, H. E., and Smith, L. H., Jr.: Disorders of oxalate metabolism. Am. J. Med., 45:715, 1968.

Williams, H. E., and Smith, L. H., Jr.: Primary hyperoxaluria. *In* Stanbury, J. B., Wyngaarden, J. B., and Fredrickson, D. S. (eds.): The Metabolic Basis of Inherited Disease. 3rd ed. New York, McGraw-Hill Book Company, 1972, p. 196.

DISORDERS OF LIPID METABOLISM

Richard J. Havel

813. INTRODUCTION

Changes in the concentration of lipids in blood plasma occur in a variety of disease states or as a result of inborn errors. In the former, they may provide a clue to diagnosis of the underlying condition. More important, deleterious consequences may occur in both, in-

cluding premature atherosclerotic vascular disease and recurrent pancreatitis. Taken together, the inborn hyperlipidemias are among the most common metabolic diseases. It is important to recognize them, because reasonably effective treatment is available which may prevent disability and delay death.

814. TRANSPORT OF LIPIDS IN THE BLOOD

Because of their insolubility in aqueous environment, essentially all lipids in blood plasma are in complexes (lipoproteins) containing amphiphilic substances which permit the dispersal of the lipids into small particles. The major lipids transported are fatty acids and cholesterol. Fatty acids exist as such in a complex with albumin and as esters of which the main transport form is triglyceride. The former are called free fatty acids (FFA) to indicate that their carboxyl groups are not in ester linkage. Cholesterol is also transported in the "free" state (alcohol group not in ester linkage) or esterified with fatty acids. The amphiphilic substances which coat the surface of microdroplets of the neutral lipids or form soluble complexes with them are mainly phospholipids and specific proteins.

Exogenous Fat (Triglyceride) Transport. Dietary fat, after hydrolysis to form partial glycerides and fatty acids, is absorbed from micelles containing conjugated bile acids. From these products, triglycerides are resynthesized in the mucosal cells of the small intestine, appear in particulate form in the Golgi region, and are secreted into the intestinal lacteals. In the lymph, they appear as chylomicrons and are delivered into the blood through the thoracic duct. Normally, chylomicrons are present only during active absorption of fat, because their life span in the blood is only a few minutes. Triglycerides in chylomicrons are removed primarily in tissues other than the liver which contain on the endothelial surface of their capillaries an enzyme, lipoprotein lipase, which hydrolyzes the triglycerides to FFA and glycerol. These products readily diffuse across the capillary and other cell membranes where they are stored or oxidized.

Endogenous Fat Transport. Triglycerides, derived from fat transported in the blood or synthesized from nonlipid precursors, are stored mainly in adipose tissue. Normally, these triglycerides are hydrolyzed to FFA and glycerol at a variable rate controlled by the action of hormones and the adrenergic innervation of the tissue on a "hormone-sensitive" lipase. Catecholamines and growth hormone increase lipase activity, whereas insulin reduces it. The FFA, as albumin complexes, are rapidly transported to various tissues to be oxidized or stored temporarily as lipid esters. They are also the major precursors of endogenous plasma triglycerides, secreted continuously by the liver in particles similar to, but smaller than, chylomicrons (very low density, pre-beta lipoproteins, VLDL; Fig. 1). In the postprandial state, these triglycerides may be derived from dietary fatty acids or from fatty acids synthesized de novo in the liver; in the fasting state, they are derived mainly from plasma FFA. This pathway appears to provide a mechanism for exporting excess fatty acids to sites of storage or oxidation. The metabolism of VLDL-

PROPERTIES OF PLASMA LIPOPROTEINS

CLASS	HDL	LDL	VLDL			CHYLOMICRONS		
· DIAMETER (Å)	100	200	300	500	800	800	2000	5000
· DENSITY	1.06–1.21	1.006–1.063	0.95 – 1.006			0.94		
· ELECTROPHORETIC MOBILITY	α_1	β	PRE-β			ORIGIN		
PER CENT · COMPOSITION								
· PROTEIN	50	20	15	7	4	4	2	1
· PHOSPHOLIPIDS	25	25	25	18	13	13	8	3
· CHOLESTEROL (FREE + ESTERS)	20	50	45	22	13	13	8	3
· TRIGLYCERIDES	5	5	15	53	70	70	82	93

Figure 1. Properties of plasma lipoproteins. (From Havel, R. J.: Adv. Intern. Med., 15:117, 1969.)

triglycerides resembles that of chylomicrons, but their disposal is less efficient, and they remain in the blood for a considerably longer period.

Transport of Cholesterol. Cholesterol (both free and esterified) is also transported in chylomicrons. The esterified cholesterol remaining in chylomicrons, "remnants," which are formed when triglycerides are taken up in various extrahepatic tissues, is removed in the liver. The free cholesterol may also be removed in the liver; alternatively, it may be transferred to high density lipoproteins (HDL), where it receives a fatty acid residue from lecithin in a transesterification catalyzed by the enzyme lecithin–cholesterol acyl transferase. Eventually, these esters are also taken up in the liver. The transferase may also promote the transport of cholesterol transferred to HDL from various tissues.

Role of Apolipoproteins. Three major groups of apoproteins (termed A, B, and C apoproteins) have essential roles in lipid transport. The C apoproteins are transferred from HDL to newly secreted triglyceride-rich lipoproteins. One of them facilitates the hydrolysis of triglycerides by lipoprotein lipase. One of the A apoproteins has a similar role in the action of lecithin-cholesterol acyl transferase in HDL. The B apoprotein is essential for the formation of VLDL and chylomicrons. In the process of metabolism of triglycerides and cholesterol in chylomicrons and VLDL, this apoprotein appears in low density, beta lipoproteins (LDL). Normally, LDL contain most of the cholesterol and cholesteryl esters present in blood plasma; the latter presumably are transferred to LDL from HDL after they are

synthesized through the action of lecithin-cholesterol acyl transferase.

Fredrickson, D. S., Levy, R. I., and Lees, R. S.: Medical progress. Fat transport in lipoproteins—an integrated approach to mechanisms and disorders. N. Engl. J. Med., 276:34, 1967.

Glomset, J. A., and Norum, L. R.: The metabolic role of lecithin–cholesterol acyltransferase: Perspectives from pathology. *In* Advances in Lipid Research, Vol. 11. New York, Academic Press, 1973, p. 1.

Havel, R. J.: Mechanisms of hyperlipoproteinemia. *In* Holmes, W. F., Paoletti, R., and Kritchevsky, D. (eds.): Pharmacological Control of Lipid Metabolism. New York, Plenum Press, 1972, p. 57.

815.   CLASSIFICATION AND ANALYSIS OF PLASMA LIPOPROTEINS

Plasma lipoproteins can be separated by electrophoresis or in the ultracentrifuge into the four main classes shown in Figure 1. In most disorders involving plasma lipoproteins, these classes do not differ substantially from normal in gross chemical and physical properties so that they are classified as hyper- or hypolipoproteinemias. In some states, lipoproteins differing from those normally comprising the bulk of a given class may accumulate; these are classified as dyslipoproteinemias.

For most clinical purposes, relatively simple methods will characterize these states. Two approaches are now

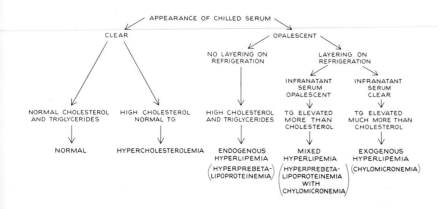

Figure 2. Evaluation of hyperlipoproteinemias with simple techniques. (From Havel, R. J.: Adv. Intern. Med., 15:117, 1969.)

generally used. In both, the concentration of cholesterol and triglycerides is measured in fasting serum or plasma. From the actual and relative values of these constituents, certain inferences can be made concerning the lipoprotein class or classes involved. For better subclassification of the hyperlipemias (increased concentration of triglycerides), it is necessary to establish whether their source is *exogenous* (chylomicrons), *endogenous* (VLDL), or *mixed* (chylomicrons plus VLDL). This can usually be achieved by evaluating lactescence of serum chilled overnight in a refrigerator, because chylomicrons tend to form a creamy layer spontaneously, whereas VLDL do not (Fig. 2). Additional studies that can be used include electrophoresis on a supporting medium, such as paper, agarose gel or cellulose acetate, or measurement of light scattering before and after passing diluted serum through a microporous filter. The last-named method has the advantage of simultaneously providing a quantitative estimate of triglyceride concentration. In some instances, particularly in certain dyslipoproteinemias, classification may be uncertain so that additional methods are needed. However, combined information gained from examination of the patient and from the simple laboratory tests will permit classification in almost all cases.

Beaumont, J. L., Carlson, L. A., Cooper, G. R., Fejfar, Z., Fredrickson, D. S., and Strasser, T.: Classification of hyperlipidaemias and hyperlipoproteinaemias. Bull. WHO, 43:891, 1970.
Havel, R. J.: Hyperlipidemia: The significance and management. Modern Medicine, January 24, 1972.

816. NORMAL REGULATION OF PLASMA LIPOPROTEIN CONCENTRATION

Apart from chylomicrons, all lipoprotein classes are present in blood plasma at all times. Among these, the concentration of VLDL, the carrier of endogenous triglycerides, is most variable and is a function rate of hepatic triglyceride synthesis. This rate, in turn, depends upon rate of uptake of FFA from the blood or synthesis of fatty acids from glucose, and also upon the extent to which the fatty acids are oxidized or converted to triglycerides. Ingestion of glucose initially causes a rapid fall in level of VLDL, presumably related to the accompanying decrease in mobilization of fat from adipose tissue. After one to three days on a high carbohydrate, low fat diet, VLDL level tends to rise. The extent to which this reflects increased hepatic triglyceride synthesis or impaired removal of triglycerides in extrahepatic tissues is uncertain. Ingestion of foodstuffs in excess of need is accompanied by rapid increase in level of VLDL. In addition, in stable obesity, VLDL levels are increased. This has been equated with associated insulin resistance and hyperinsulinism, but the precise mechanism is not clear (see Ch. 723). Increased triglyceride and VLDL levels accompany several other states in which insulin resistance and hyperinsulinism are present.

Plasma levels of LDL and HDL tend to fall as VLDL levels rise, presumably because some components of these lipoprotein species also are constituent parts of VLDL. The concentration of HDL is regulated by sex hormones and hence is sex dependent; increases are

produced by estrogens and a fall by androgens. The level of LDL is also moderately sensitive to caloric intake, but is influenced more by specific dietary factors. In particular, fats containing saturated fatty acids and cholesterol increase the level of this cholesterol-rich lipoprotein. Substantial differences in lipoprotein levels occur in various population groups throughout the world. The major cause of these differences, which occur predominantly in cholesterol-rich LDL, appears to be dietary (see also Ch. 723).

Conner, W. E., Stone, D. B., and Hodges, R. E.: The interrelated effects of dietary cholesterol and fat upon human serum lipid levels. J. Clin. Invest., 43:1691, 1964.
Havel, R. J.: Caloric homeostasis and disorders of fuel transport. N. Engl. J. Med., 287:1186, 1972.

817. INBORN ERRORS OF LIPOPROTEIN METABOLISM

HYPERLIPOPROTEINEMIAS

Whereas characterization of the lipoprotein class or classes responsible for hyperlipoproteinemia in a patient is generally straightforward, establishment of a definitive diagnosis in inherited forms of hyperlipoproteinemia frequently is difficult and may not be possible. There are two major reasons for this. First, lipoprotein concentrations vary with time in an affected individual as well as among affected family members. Second, a given abnormality may represent more than one disorder and pattern of inheritance. Thus both monogenic and polygenic disorders may lead to the same phenotype. The most widely used system of classification, introduced by Fredrickson, defines six patterns or phenotypes: I, elevated chylomicrons; IIa, elevated LDL; IIb, elevated LDL and VLDL; III, elevated beta-migrating VLDL with increased content of cholesterol; IV, elevated VLDL; and V, elevated VLDL and chylomicrons. In the three most common types, IIa, IIb, and IV, classification by this system frequently fails to identify a specific disorder. Thus an obese individual, initially classified as Type IV, may, with sufficient loss of weight, be classified as Type IIa. Further, individuals classified as Type IV may belong to kindreds in which IIa, IIb, and IV all occur commonly; in other kindreds all affected individuals belong to Type IV. Fortunately, treatment of such individuals may be determined simply from quantitative estimation of serum cholesterol and triglycerides, as described earlier, after exclusion of the acquired disorders described below.

Familial Hyperbetalipoproteinemia
(Hypercholesterolemia, Type IIa Hyperlipoproteinemia)

Familial hyperbetalipoproteinemia, inherited as a mendelian dominant trait, is characterized by increased concentration of LDL of normal composition. Xanthomas in the tendons, particularly the Achilles, plantar, patellar, and digital extensors of the hands, as well as tuberous xanthomas, xanthelasmas, and early onset of corneal arcus, are frequently encountered. In adults, serum cholesterol concentration usually exceeds 350 mg per 100 ml. Its prevalence is not established, but it may occur in up to 1 per cent of the American population.

Etiology and Pathogenesis. The specific molecular or enzymatic defect responsible for the increased concentration of LDL is unknown, but recent studies suggest the presence of a cellular defect in the regulation of 3-hydroxy-3-methylglutaryl reductase, the enzyme controlling the rate-limiting step in cholesterol biosynthesis.

Clinical Manifestations. The hyperlipoproteinemia is present from birth or shortly thereafter, and is generally detected as hypercholesterolemia with little or no increase in triglycerides; the xanthomas usually do not appear until after puberty. The patient may not be aware of the presence of large xanthomas in the Achilles or plantar tendons, and the latter may be missed by the physician unless the tendon is put under tension by having the patient extend his toes. Small xanthomas of the extensor tendons of the hands are best detected by observing the tendon while the patient flexes and extends the finger, and small xanthomas in the Achilles tendon are detected by palpation of irregular contour, usually in the central region. Xanthelasmas (raised, yellow plaques about the eyelids near the inner canthus) and corneal arcus are not diagnostic, because they may also be seen in individuals with no discernible abnormality of plasma lipoproteins. The incidence of premature coronary heart disease is several times that of control populations in countries with a "western" culture, and the incidence of peripheral atherosclerotic occlusive disease is also increased. In the homozygous states, the disease is much more severe, with large xanthomas occurring in childhood, together with "malignant" atherosclerotic disease, including calcific aortic stenosis. A possible variant of the disease is seen in the Near East in which early occurrence of large xanthomas is common.

Diagnosis. Hypercholesterolemia without hypertriglyceridemia in the absence of known cause, such as hypothyroidism, is not sufficient basis for making a diagnosis unless the cholesterol level exceeds 400 mg per 100 ml. Presence of characteristic xanthomas is diagnostic, and demonstration of familial occurrence (at least one parent should have hyperbetalipoproteinemia) provides strong presumptive evidence. Some individuals or families may have moderate hypertriglyceridemia (Type IIb). This must be distinguished from familial dysbetalipoproteinemia, described below. Most normotriglyceridemic individuals whose cholesterol level is 275 to 325 mg per 100 ml (also classified as Type II hyperlipoproteinemia) have a different disorder, which may be polygenic (see Ch. 819).

Treatment. No simple method has been devised to reduce lipoprotein levels to normal. Some reduction can be achieved by a diet restricted in saturated fats and cholesterol, with sufficient polyunsaturated fats to provide a total fat intake of 30 to 35 per cent of calories. Nonabsorbable bile acid–binding substances, such as cholestyramine (15 to 30 grams daily in divided doses with meals), are more effective. Large doses of nicotinic acid (5 to 12 grams daily in divided doses) may also be effective. These drugs may in some cases reduce lipoprotein levels to normal. Surgical bypass of the terminal 150 cm of the ileum, which also prevents absorption of bile acids, generally gives good results. Frequent, loose stools are generally produced by this operation. In post-

menopausal women, estrogens may provide some improvement. Thyroxine and its analogues, especially d-thyroxine (4 to 8 mg daily) and the ethyl ester of p-chlorophenoxyisobutyrate, occasionally give good results. Xanthomatous lesions regress slowly; tendinous lesions seldom disappear. It is reasonable to begin treatment in childhood, although it has not been established that reducing the lipoprotein level will prevent or delay onset of ischemic vascular disease.

Familial Dysbetalipoproteinemia
(Broad-Beta Disease, Type III Hyperlipoproteinemia)

Definition. Familial dysbetalipoproteinemia is characterized by accumulation of abnormal beta lipoproteins, which resemble normal pre-beta migrating VLDL in size and flotation characteristics, but differ from them in composition. Planar xanthomas, particularly in the palmar and digital creases, are peculiar to this form of primary hyperlipoproteinemia, but tuberous, tuberoeruptive, and tendinous lesions also occur. It is much rarer than familial hyperbetalipoproteinemia; in the older literature, it was frequently called *xanthoma tuberosum*. The mode of inheritance is uncertain.

Etiology and Pathogenesis. The abnormal lipoprotein contains predominantly the B apoprotein together with a basic protein, unusually rich in arginine, in particles with more cholesteryl ester and less triglyceride than normal VLDL. Its electrophoretic mobility is also abnormal, encompassing the beta and extending toward the pre-beta region ("broad beta"). This lipoprotein is thought to represent remnant-VLDL which accumulate because of abnormality in the mechanism responsible for uptake of cholesteryl esters in the liver.

Clinical Manifestations. The disorder is seldom discovered before early adult life and is usually manifested by appearance of xanthomas when the patient gains weight. The patient may be unaware of the characteristic planar xanthomas which are yellow to orange and tend to fill the palmar and digital creases; they may also appear over the dorsal surfaces of the hands. The tuberous xanthomas tend to be smaller and more numerous than in hyperbetalipoproteinemia and are often confluent and surrounded by an erythematous halo ("tuberoeruptive"). They occur most commonly over the knees and elbows and on the buttocks. Tendinous lesions are usually in the extensors of the hands. Premature coronary and peripheral atherosclerotic vascular disease are quite common. Overt diabetes mellitus is seldom seen, but slight degrees of glucose intolerance usually can be detected, as in the other forms of endogenous hypertriglyceridemia described below.

Diagnosis. Combined hypercholesterolemia and hypertriglyceridemia are always present. The levels of these two lipids are often similar, and they change rapidly with alterations in diet. Most patients have the characteristic planar xanthomas which, in the absence of obstructive biliary tract disease, are pathognomonic. The serum is usually lactescent. Lipoprotein electrophoresis shows a "broad-beta" pattern with normal or reduced content of alpha lipoproteins. Slight chylomicronemia is often present when hyperlipoproteinemia is severe. Spurious "broad-beta" bands may be seen in other states, particularly in some of the secondary hyperlipemias. Definitive laboratory diagnosis requires additional tests, such as ultracentrifugation of serum at its own density to demonstrate "floating-beta" lipoproteins.

Treatment. The mainstay of treatment is diet. In obese subjects, caloric restriction is almost always very effective. The diet should be restricted in simple sugars and in cholesterol but not in fat, which should provide 40 to 50 per cent of calories. Concentration of cholesterol and triglycerides will usually fall almost to normal. For patients who will not adhere to a dietary program and for the few who respond inadequately, the ethyl ester of p-chlorophenoxyisobutyric acid, 500 mg four times daily, will almost always produce a good response. Xanthomas invariably regress or disappear with effective reduction in lipid levels. There is some evidence that atheromatous lesions also regress (see Ch. 819). This disorder is greatly aggravated by hypothyroidism, in which a similar lipoprotein may accumulate. For this reason, thyroid function should always be carefully evaluated.

Primary Hyperlipemias

Exogenous Hyperlipemia
(Bürger-Grütz Syndrome, Type I Hyperlipoproteinemia)

Definition. This rare disease, inherited as a recessive trait, is characterized by accumulation of chylomicrons proportional to intake of dietary fat and manifested by recurrent acute pancreatitis, usually beginning in childhood.

Etiology and Pathogenesis. This disorder is caused by deficient activity of lipoprotein lipase with resultant defective removal of triglycerides from the blood. Hydrolytic activity with the characteristic properties of this enzyme on lipoprotein-bound triglycerides is almost absent in blood plasma obtained a few minutes after intravenous injection of heparin, although another lipase, thought to be derived from the liver, is present. In one family, no lipoprotein lipase activity could be demonstrated in adipose tissue.

Clinical Manifestations. Chylomicronemia develops as soon as fat is ingested, and the disorder has been diagnosed during the first week of life. Pancreatitis is very common, and many patients diagnosed in adult life have a history of bouts of abdominal pain in childhood. Abdominal pain, not definable as pancreatitis, has been reported frequently, but causes other than pancreatitis have not been established. Other complications, described rarely, include melena and pretibial ulcers. Like the pancreatitis, they may result from ischemia related to agglomeration of chylomicrons in capillaries. Hepatosplenomegaly, presumably the result of phagocytosis of chylomicrons by reticuloendothelial cells, is common, and hypersplenism has been described. Foam cells may be found in the bone marrow. The endogenous hyperlipemia occurring normally during pregnancy is greatly magnified and may lead to repeated attacks of pancreatitis. In infants and children especially, eruptive xanthomas—small yellow papules in the skin, surrounded by an erythematous halo—may occur when lipemia is severe. Lipemia retinalis—whitish reflection from retinal arterioles and venules—can usually be detected when triglyceride levels in plasma exceed 3000 mg per 100 ml and becomes florid with levels above 5000 mg

per 100 ml. Other xanthomas do not occur, and premature atherosclerotic vascular disease has not been described. Carbohydrate metabolism is normal.

Diagnosis. Markedly lactescent blood plasma in a young patient with severe midabdominal pain and no history of alcoholism is presumptive evidence for this disorder or one of the other primary hyperlipemias. In exogenous hyperlipemia, the chylomicrons rise to form a creamy layer when the serum is allowed to stand overnight in the refrigerator and the infranatant serum is usually limpid. Triglyceride concentration is increased far more than that of cholesterol, and the chylomicron band predominates on electrophoresis. Triglyceride levels fall dramatically when intake of dietary fat is severely restricted for two to three days. Lipolytic activity, measured in blood plasma obtained ten minutes after intravenous injection of 0.2 mg of heparin per kilogram of body weight, is reduced, and activity sensitive to inhibition by 0.5 M NaCl (a characteristic of lipoprotein lipase) is virtually undetectable.

Treatment. The only established measure is restriction of dietary fat ("saturated" and "polyunsaturated" fats are equivalent) sufficient to reduce fasting triglyceride levels to 500 mg per 100 ml or less. This usually requires an intake of no more than 30 grams per day by adults. On this regimen, xanthomas disappear and pancreatitis is uniformly prevented. Pretibial ulcers have also healed, and hypersplenism has subsided on this regimen. Once pancreatitis occurs, recurrence is very common when large amounts of fat are ingested and may happen within hours. During pregnancy, complete elimination of fat from the diet may be necessary to control hyperlipemia and minimize the possibility of pancreatitis.

Endogenous Hyperlipemia
(Types IIb and IV Hyperlipoproteinemia)

Definition. The term endogenous hyperlipemia encompasses a group of disorders, frequently shown to be familial, which are common in middle life. These disorders are characterized by accumulation of VLDL of normal composition and electrophoretic mobility and by insulin resistance. In some kindreds, the trait appears to be an autosomal dominant. The concentration of VLDL depends upon several environmental factors, and the true prevalence is unknown.

Etiology and Pathogenesis. Secretion of hepatogenous triglycerides in VLDL varies with quantity and quality of food intake, including ethanol, and with neural and hormonal responses to stress. These responses are generally magnified in endogenous hyperlipemia, in which there is evidence for impaired catabolism of VLDL-triglycerides as well as increased hepatic secretion, but the nature of these abnormalities is not known. Evidence that severity of the hypertriglyceridemia is related to hyperinsulinism and insulin resistance, together with the fact that gain in weight, which increases insulin resistance, almost uniformly increases the hyperlipemia, indicates a close relationship with disordered carbohydrate metabolism. The concentration of LDL may be low, normal, or elevated. In the latter case, the disorder is usually called combined hyperlipidemia (Type IIb). As indicated earlier, in some kindreds hyperlipoproteinemic individuals may have elevated LDL, elevated VLDL, or both, whereas in others all those affected have only elevated VLDL. The endogenous hyperlipemias evidently represent several genotypes which condition the responses of VLDL and LDL to common environmental influences.

Clinical Manifestations. Most commonly, the disorder is detected when patients with ischemic vascular disease are screened for metabolic abnormalities. Although endogenous hyperlipemia is commonly found in individuals who develop such disease prematurely, the incidence of vascular complications has not been established. The great majority of patients are at least moderately obese when hyperlipemia is found, but only a few have fasting hyperglycemia. With severe hyperlipemia, eruptive xanthomas and pancreatitis may occur, as in exogenous hyperlipemia.

Diagnosis. The disorder should be suspected in obese subjects with premature vascular disease. It is diagnosed presumptively when fasting serum is lactescent with no layering on standing. When serum cholesterol is normal or is less than half the concentration of triglycerides, VLDL alone are generally increased. When serum cholesterol is elevated and equal to or greater than the triglyceride level, both LDL and VLDL are increased. Numerous other causes of endogenous hyperlipemia must be excluded (see Ch. 818).

Treatment. Effective measures are available to reduce the level of VLDL, but it has not been shown that atherosclerotic lesions regress or that the progress of ischemic vascular disease is slowed. For obese patients, caloric restriction alone usually produces rapid reduction of serum triglycerides, often almost to normal. The diet should also be restricted in simple sugars as described for familial dysbetalipoproteinemia. If cholesterol remains elevated, dietary measures used to reduce LDL should also be employed. Ethyl ester of p-chlorophenoxyisobutyrate may be used for individuals with inadequate dietary response, as in familial dysbetalipoproteinemia. When added after the patient has responded partially to a dietary program, it usually reduces triglycerides further, but cholesterol levels often remain unchanged, indicating an increase in level of LDL at the expense of VLDL. Since there is no evidence that such a change is beneficial, treatment with the drug should be discontinued in such patients. Drugs used to reduce the level of LDL in familal hyperbetalipoproteinemia, such as cholestyramine, nicotinic acid, and d-thyroxine, may then be employed.

Mixed Hyperlipemia
(Type V Hyperlipoproteinemia)

Definition. This is a rare disorder of adolescence and adult life, in which VLDL and chylomicrons of normal composition accumulate in the blood on ordinary diets. It is usually accompanied by overt, insulin-independent diabetes mellitus and often by eruptive xanthomas and recurrent acute pancreatitis.

Etiology and Pathogenesis. The metabolic abnormalities in this disorder partake of both endogenous and exogenous hyperlipemia. In familial cases, insulin resistance is usually accompanied by fasting hyperglycemia, and postheparin lipolytic activity in plasma is often somewhat reduced. Possibly, multiple genetic defects are present which combine insulin resistance with defective activity of lipoprotein lipase. Some patients with endogenous hyperlipemia may accumulate chylomicrons when their lipemia is severe, particularly with ingestion of substantial quantities of ethanol; in these cases, the chylomicronemia may represent an "overload" phenomenon. In others, the distinction between endogenous and mixed hyperlipemia is blurred.

Clinical Manifestations. The disorder usually presents in adolescence or early adult life with recurrent attacks of obscure abdominal pain, sometimes definable as acute pancreatitis. At onset of pain, lipemia is usually severe. Eruptive xanthomas are often present and frequently are confluent. As in exogenous hyperlipemia, hepatosplenomegaly and lipemia retinalis are often found. Overt hyperglycemia is only occasionally severe enough to produce symptoms of diabetes, and evidences of microangiopathy are usually absent. Hyperuricemia is also common. Obesity is frequent but by no means universal. In some patients, evidences of premature atherosclerotic vascular disease may be found, but incidence is not known to be increased.

Diagnosis. Markedly lactescent serum, which separates into a creamy layer with persistent lactescence in the infranatant serum, provides presumptive evidence for mixed hyperlipemia. This can be confirmed by nephelometry or electrophoresis. Alcoholic hyperlipemia must be considered, particularly in patients presenting with abdominal pain, and diabetic hyperlipemia must be ruled out when hyperglycemia is severe and accompanied by ketoacidosis. Differentiation from exogenous hyperlipemia usually presents no problem and depends on the accompanying severe endogenous hyperlipemia, hyperglycemia, and normal or slightly reduced lipolytic activity in postheparin plasma.

Treatment. For obese patients, restriction of caloric intake and ethanol usually reduces levels of both chylomicrons and VLDL effectively. For patients of normal body weight, avoidance of intermittent excesses of sugars, fat, or ethanol generally provides some improvement. The hyperglycemia usually responds to the caloric restriction or to addition of sulfonylurea drugs. Neither the sulfonylureas nor insulin, however, have a specific effect on the hyperlipemia. The ethyl ester of p-chlorophenoxyisobutyrate, given as described for familial dyslipoproteinemia, may be effective in some patients not responding to diet. Nicotinic acid, in doses of 1 to 2 grams three times daily, is frequently useful. As in exogenous hyperlipemia, recurrent pancreatitis is prevented by effective reduction of lipoprotein levels, and eruptive xanthomas disappear.

Fredrickson, D. S., and Levy, R. I.: Familial hyperlipoproteinemia. *In* Stanbury, J. B., Wyngaarden, J. B., and Fredrickson, D. S. (eds.): The Metabolic Basis of Inherited Disease. 3rd ed. New York, McGraw-Hill Book Company, 1972, p. 531.

Goldstein, J. L., and Brown, M. S.: Familial hypercholesterolemia: Identification of a defect in the regulation of 3-hydroxy-3-methylglutaryl coenzyme A reductase activity associated with overproduction of cholesterol. Proc. Natl. Acad. Sci. USA, 70:2804, 1973.

Havel, R. J., and Kane, J. P.: Drugs and lipid metabolism. *In* Elliott, H. W. (ed.): Annual Review of Pharmacology. Vol. 13. Palo Alto, Calif., Annual Review, Inc., 1973, p. 287.

Havel, R. J., and Kane, J. P.: Primary dysbetalipoproteinemia: Predominance of a specific apoprotein species in triglyceride-rich lipoproteins. Proc. Natl. Acad. Sci. USA, 70:2015, 1973.

Levy, R. I., et al.: Dietary and drug treatment of primary hyperlipoproteinemia. Ann. Intern. Med., 77:267, 1972.

Slack, J., and Nevin, N. D.: Hyperlipidaemic xanthomatosis: I. Increased risk of death from ischaemic heart disease in first degree relatives of 53 patients with essential hyperlipidaemia and xanthomatosis. II. Mode of inheritance in 55 families with essential hyperlipidaemia and xanthomatosis. J. Med. Genet., 5:4, 8, 1968.

Strisower, E. H., Adamson, G., and Strisower, B.: Treatment of hyperlipidemias. Am. J. Med., 45:488, 1968.

Thompson, G. R., and Gotto, A. M.: Ileal bypass in the treatment of hyperlipoproteinemia. Lancet, 2:35, 1973.

HYPOLIPOPROTEINEMIAS

These conditions are exceedingly rare, but they have considerable importance for the light that they shed on normal functions of plasma lipoproteins.

Abetalipoproteinemia
(Bassen-Kornzweig Syndrome)

This disease, inherited as an autosomal recessive, is characterized by complete absence of LDL, VLDL, and chylomicrons. The absence of the B protein appears to be accompanied by virtually complete loss of ability to transport triglycerides in the blood. It is manifested by severe malabsorption, beginning in early childhood, followed by progressive ataxia, nystagmus, distal sensory loss, weakness, and visual impairment with scotomas. These are related, respectively, to inability to deliver triglycerides into the intestinal lymph; demyelination of spinocerebellar tracts, posterior columns, and, occasionally, peripheral nerves; and pigmentary retinal degeneration ("atypical retinitis pigmentosa"). Other findings include peculiar thorny or spiny red cells (acanthocytes) and fatty liver (resulting from failure to export triglycerides in very low density lipoproteins). This disorder is also discussed in Ch. 438 and in Part XIV, Section Three.

Diagnosis is established by finding very low cholesterol concentration (about 50 mg per 100 ml) and almost no triglycerides in blood plasma in an individual with one or more of the characteristic symptoms. The disorder should be considered in any patient with hereditary ataxia. On paper electrophoresis only alpha lipoproteins are present, and blood smears or wet preparations show the characteristic acanthocytes. Treatment is limited to restriction of ordinary fat and supplementation with fat-soluble vitamins. Medium-chain triglycerides are well tolerated. Such measures have not been shown to alter the progressive and disabling course of the disease.

Hypobetalipoproteinemia

A few families have been described with low concentrations of beta lipoproteins. Some patients have had acanthocytes and late onset of neuromuscular difficulties.

Tangier Disease
(Alpha-Lipoprotein Deficiency)

This disorder, in the homozygous state, leads in childhood to diffuse deposition of cholesterol esters in reticuloendothelial tissues, with enlargement of liver, spleen, and lymph nodes, and especially to grossly enlarged tonsils with a characteristic orange color. Foam cells may be found in the bone marrow. In adults, flocculent corneal infiltrates may occur. Usually, the disorder does not affect growth, nutrition, or general health. Electrophoretic or ultracentrifugal examination shows almost no alpha lipoproteins or HDL, and one of the A proteins is reduced to about 1 per cent of the normal level. Heterozygotes have low concentrations of HDL but no other detectable abnormalities. In homozygotes, levels of LDL tend to be reduced, although

those of triglycerides and VLDL are high. No treatment is available. There is limited evidence that premature vascular disease may develop.

Lecithin–Cholesterol Acyltransferase Deficiency

This disorder has been found only in a few individuals in Scandinavia. Affected subjects have proteinuria, anemia, and corneal deposits of lipids. HDL are almost absent, levels of VLDL and chylomicrons are variably increased, and abnormal lipoproteins bearing some resemblance to those found in cholestasis are present (see Biliary Obstruction in Ch. 818). Cholesteryl esters comprise less than 10 per cent of total cholesterol in plasma (normal value about 72 per cent) and are found almost entirely in the triglyceride-rich lipoproteins. Their fatty acids are much more saturated than those produced normally by the plasma enzyme lecithin–cholesterol acyltransferase, and this enzyme cannot be detected. Other findings include foam cells in the bone marrow and renal glomeruli and increased concentration of cholesterol and lecithin in the red blood cells. The relationship between the enzyme deficiency and the various clinical and chemical abnormalities is uncertain.

Fredrickson, D. S., Gotto, A. M., and Levy, R. I.: Familial lipoprotein deficiency. *In* Stanbury, J. B., Wyngaarden, J. B., and Fredrickson, D. S. (eds.): Metabolic Basis of Inherited Disease. 3rd ed. New York, McGraw-Hill Book Company, 1972, p. 493.
Gjone, E., and Norum, K. R.: Familial serum cholesterol ester deficiency. Acta Med. Scand., 183:107, 1968.

818. ACQUIRED DISORDERS OF LIPOPROTEIN METABOLISM

HYPERLIPOPROTEINEMIAS

These conditions are important as clues to diagnosis or because they may be associated with premature atherosclerotic vascular disease.

Hyperbetalipoproteinemia

Hypothyroidism. Hyperbetalipoproteinemia is a characteristic finding in myxedema; hypothyroidism must be considered in all patients with this abnormality. All forms of hyperbetalipoproteinemia are accompanied by hypercarotenemia, but this is particularly striking in myxedema because of the additional defect in conversion of carotene to vitamin A. Occasionally, increased levels of VLDL are also present.

Dietary. Moderate degrees of hypercholesterolemia may occur in subjects ingesting large amounts of cholesterol, usually in eggs and dairy products.

Nephrotic Syndrome. Hyperbetalipoproteinemia is frequently observed in nephrotic states when serum albumin concentration falls below 3 grams per 100 ml. As the level of albumin falls below 1.5 grams per 100 ml, concentration of VLDL rises to produce the characteristic nephrotic hyperlipemia. Treatment is that of the underlying disorder.

Resolving lipemias. As levels of chylomicrons or VLDL are reduced in various hyperlipemic states, the concentration of LDL usually rises, presumably reflecting the removal of triglyceride with liberation of constituent B protein and associated lipids. Such hyperbetalipoproteinemia may persist for days to weeks and can lead to confusion if the sequence is not appreciated.

Hyperadrenocorticism. Hyperbetalipoproteinemia of moderate degree is commonly seen in Cushing's syndrome and subsides with appropriate treatment.

Endogenous and Mixed Hyperlipemias

Diabetic Hyperlipemia. Mixed hyperlipemia is characteristic of prolonged insulin deficiency with ketosis. It is generally accompanied by fatty liver and by weight loss and other evidences of a catabolic state. It is not ordinarily seen with acute diabetic ketoacidosis. Defective removal of triglycerides and reduced lipolytic activity in postheparin plasma can be demonstrated. Eruptive xanthomas and lipemia retinalis are commonly seen. With administration of adequate insulin, triglyceride levels fall rapidly and cholesterol levels more slowly. Diabetic hyperlipemia must be differentiated from primary endogenous hyperlipemia and especially mixed hyperlipemia with its frequent associated hyperglycemia. These states are not accompanied by ketosis or wasting and do not respond to insulin.

Alcoholic Hyperlipemia. This lipemia, usually mixed, is seen in chronic alcoholics with fatty liver and good hepatic function. Diversion of fatty acids entering the liver to triglyceride synthesis accompanies oxidation of ethanol to acetate and appears to be the most important abnormality, but decreased activity of lipoprotein lipase has also been implicated. Some of these patients have underlying primary hyperlipemias, and ingestion of ethanol is an important factor aggravating primary endogenous and mixed hyperlipemias. The association of jaundice and hemolytic anemia with hyperlipemia has been described in patients with alcoholism (Zieve's syndrome), but it has not been shown that the features of this triad are causally interrelated. Pancreatitis and hyperlipemia may also coexist. It is unlikely that pancreatitis causes the hyperlipemia, because the association is confined almost entirely to alcoholics in whom these complications can occur separately. This situation must be clearly distinguished from occurrence of pancreatitis as a complication of one of the primary (usually exogenous or mixed) hyperlipemias.

Hyperlipemia in Glycogen Storage Disease Type I. Endogenous or mixed hyperlipemia is consistently found in children and adults. It is related both to increased hepatic secretion of triglycerides in VLDL and decreased activity of lipoprotein lipase. Measures decreasing delivery of absorbed carbohydrate to the liver may be helpful.

Hyperlipemia in Lipodystrophy. Hyperlipemia is consistently observed in generalized as well as in partial forms of lipodystrophy. The mechanism is not understood, especially in partial lipodystrophy; but, as in primary endogenous hyperlipemia, insulin resistance and hyperinsulinism are associated phenomena.

Stress Hyperlipemia. In a variety of situations, increased secretion of catecholamines, together with growth hormone and ACTH, can lead to hyperlipemia by increasing mobilization of fatty acids from adipose tissue to liver with resultant increased secretion of triglycerides in VLDL. Such hyperlipemia, appearing soon after myocardial infarction, can lead to confusion with primary endogenous hyperlipemia.

Administration of Contraceptive Steroids. Mild endogenous hyperlipemia is commonly produced by the estrogenic component of estrogen-progestogen mixtures and is associated with insulin resistance, hyperinsulinism, and decreased lipolytic activity in postheparin plasma.

Other Causes. Endogenous hyperlipemia has been described in uremia, after renal homotransplantation, and in hypopituitarism, Niemann-Pick disease, Gaucher's disease, Werner's syndrome, and hepatoma. The prevalence of hyperlipemia is increased in gout.

Dyslipoproteinemias

Biliary Obstruction. A low-density lipoprotein which has not been detected in health appears in the plasma of patients with extrahepatic or intrahepatic biliary obstruction. It is a spherical vesicle about 400 Å in diameter, the wall of which is a lipid bilayer composed of a 1:1 molar mixture of cholesterol and phospholipids, together with a small amount of C apoproteins. This "cholestasis lipoprotein" or "LP-X" can be detected in virtually all patients with biliary obstruction, but very high levels are most characteristic of the early stages of primary biliary cirrhosis and are frequently accompanied by eruptive and planar xanthomas and xanthelasmas. Bile acid-binding agents, such as cholestyramine, may reduce the concentration of the lipoprotein. Spontaneous subsidence of the hyperlipoproteinemia and disappearance of xanthomas usually signify failing hepatic parenchymal cell function in primary biliary cirrhosis.

Paraproteinemias. The abnormal globulins in patients with multiple myeloma and macroglobulinemia may be associated with lipid. In some cases, lipoprotein-globulin complexes have been demonstrated with accompanying hyperlipemia and various xanthomas.

HYPOLIPOPROTEINEMIAS

The secondary states are characterized chiefly by hypobetalipoproteinemia and are the result of malnutrition, malabsorption, or parenchymal liver disease. Presumably they reflect decreased transport of exogenous and endogenous triglycerides, so that formation of LDL is decreased. Reduced concentrations of LDL also occur in healthy individuals when intake of calories and saturated fats is habitually low.

Bagdade, J. D., Porte, D., and Bierman, E. L.: Diabetic lipemia. A form of acquired fat-induced lipemia. N. Engl. J. Med., 276:427, 1967.

Beck, P.: Contraceptive steroids: Modifications of carbohydrate and lipid metabolism. Metabolism, 22:841, 1973.

Earley, L. E., Havel, R. J., Hopper, J., Jr., and Grausz, H.: Nephrotic syndrome. Calif. Med., 115:23, 1971.

Glueck, C. J., Kaplan, A. P., Levy, R. I., Greten, H., Gralnick, H., and Fredrickson, D. S.: A new mechanism of exogenous hyperglyceridemia. Ann. Intern. Med., 71:1051, 1969.

Hamilton, R. L., Havel, R. J., Kane, J. P., Blaurock, A., and Sata, T.: Cholestasis: Lamellar structure of the abnormal human serum lipoprotein. Science, 172:475, 1971.

Havel, R. J., Balasse, E. O., Kane, J. P., and Segel, N.: Splanchnic metabolism in von Gierke's disease (glycogenosis type I). Trans. Assoc. Am. Physicians, 82:305, 1969.

Piscatelli, R. L., Vieweg, W. V. R., and Havel, R. J.: Partial lipodystrophy: Metabolic studies in three patients. Ann. Intern. Med., 73:963, 1970.

819. HYPERLIPOPROTEINEMIA IN ATHEROSCLEROTIC VASCULAR DISEASE

Although atherosclerosis develops under the influence of a variety of factors, the role of plasma lipoproteins may be decisive in the muscular arteries supplying the heart and lower extremities. Plasma levels of LDL, VLDL, or both, tend to be elevated in patients with occlusive atherosclerotic disease in these vessels, particularly before the sixth decade. The level of cholesterol, which closely reflects that of LDL in large population groups, is a powerful predictor of the incidence of, and mortality from, coronary artery disease in middle-aged men. Retrospective studies indicate that the level of triglycerides, which closely reflects the level of VLDL, is also associated with premature ischemic vascular disease, but prospective studies suggest that solitary elevation of triglycerides is a less powerful predictor than elevation of serum cholesterol alone.

The level of serum cholesterol is subject to strong familial influence even in the absence of a major gene effect, such as that operating in familial hyperbetalipoproteinemia. The influence could be environmental, but genetic data suggest that multifactorial inheritance is mainly operative. However, the level of serum cholesterol (and that of LDL) is also influenced by content of cholesterol and saturated fats in the diet. In industrialized countries, where intake of these nutrients is large, cholesterol levels are substantially higher than in underdeveloped countries where habitual intake of animal fat is low. The much lower incidence of coronary artery disease in underdeveloped countries is consistent with the putative role of LDL-cholesterol in the early development of the atherosclerotic plaque.

In the absence of the major gene effects described in Ch. 817, the level of serum triglycerides is less subject to familial influence. The substantial effects of caloric intake and ethanol on serum triglyceride concentration accord with this fact and suggest that sporadic cases of mild to moderate hypertriglyceridemia largely reflect alterations in lipid transport produced by nutritional or other environmental influences.

Recent studies of survivors of myocardial infarction indicate that hyperlipoproteinemia occurs in about half of those under the age of 50. More than half of the hyperlipoproteinemic survivors, in turn, appear to carry major gene defects. Familial hyperbetalipoproteinemia accounts for only about one fifth of these; the remainder have endogenous hyperlipemia, usually with associated elevation of LDL cholesterol (combined hyperlipidemia). Families in whom most affected individuals have combined hyperlipidemia are more common than families characterized by elevation of VLDL alone; however, many affected individuals in families with combined hyperlipidemia have solitary elevation of VLDL, and some may have only elevated LDL. These variations presumably reflect the influence of obesity, diet, and other factors on lipid transport as described in Ch. 816. In addition, polygenic hypercholesterolemia and sporadic cases of hypertriglyceridemia are also common among survivors of myocardial infarction, so that a genetic diagnosis is seldom possible without extensive studies of the patient's family. The major exception to this situation is the patient with severe hyperbetalipoproteinemia (cholesterol exceeding 350 mg per 100 ml);

such individuals frequently have tendinous xanthomas. In them, the diagnosis of familial hyperbetalipoproteinemia can generally be made with confidence and with the knowledge that dietary measures alone will be of limited benefit. In all other situations, diets designed to reduce the level of VLDL or LDL may be recommended as described earlier, with drug therapy reserved for those individuals who do not respond adequately.

The important question of whether reduction of lipoprotein levels will prevent progression or cause regression of atherosclerotic lesions has not been answered convincingly. Regression of experimentally induced atherosclerosis occurs in animals under some circumstances, and recent studies suggest that reduction of dietary cholesterol and saturated fats may delay death from ischemic vascular disease in survivors of myocardial infarction and in elderly men. In patients with primary dysbetalipoproteinemia, more direct evidence of regression of occlusive lesions in muscular arteries of the leg has recently been obtained in subjects treated with diet and clofibrate. Thus specific dietary or pharmacologic treatment of hyperlipoproteinemia is probably indicated in established coronary artery disease and peripheral atherosclerotic vascular disease as well as for prophylaxis.

Since the risk of developing coronary artery disease is a graded function of the concentration of LDL-cholesterol, the presence of normal levels of cholesterol and triglycerides in survivors of myocardial infarction cannot be taken to exclude a major influence of plasma lipoproteins in the pathogenesis of their disease. Statistical normality of LDL-cholesterol level in industrialized countries should therefore not be confused with the level consistent with maintenance of health. Rather, levels in the range of 90 to 130 mg per 100 ml serum (equivalent to total cholesterol level of 140 to 180 mg per 100 ml) may be normal in this context. The relative immunity of premenopausal women to complications of atherosclerosis may result from their lower levels of LDL. This is not reflected in the level of total serum cholesterol, because the level of HDL-cholesterol is higher in premenopausal women than in men. These differences presumably result from actions of sex hormones and disappear after the menopause.

Immediately after myocardial infarction, the concentration of VLDL tends to rise as a result of increased fat mobilization produced by secretion of "stress" hormones and increased sympathetic nervous activity. At the same time, the level of LDL-cholesterol may fall as a result of reduced caloric and fat intake. Therefore evaluation of the nature and magnitude of associated hyperlipoproteinemia should be postponed for two to three months after the acute episode.

Carlson, L. A.: Serum lipids in men with myocardial infarction. Acta Med. Scand., 167:399, 1960.

Goldstein, J. L., Hazzard, W. R., Schrott, H. G., Bierman, E. L., and Motulsky, A. G.: Hyperlipidemia in coronary heart disease: I. Lipid levels in 500 survivors of myocardial infarction. II. Genetic analysis of lipid levels in 176 families and delineation of a new inherited disorder, combined hyperlipidemia. III. Evaluation of lipoprotein phenotypes of 156 genetically defined survivors of myocardial infarction. J. Clin. Invest., 52:1533, 1544, 1569, 1973.

Kannel, W. B., Garcia, M. J., McNamara, P. M., and Pearson, G.: Serum lipid precursors of coronary heart disease. Human Pathol., 2:129, 1971.

Turpeinen, O.: Control of atherosclerosis: Progress in primary diet trials. In Jones, R. J. (ed.): Atherosclerosis. Proceedings, Second International Symposium. New York, Springer-Verlag, 1970, p. 572.

Zelis, R., Mason, D. T., Braunwald, E., and Levy, R. I.: Effects of hyperlipoproteinemias and their treatment of the peripheral circulation. J. Clin. Invest., 49:1007, 1970.

820. INBORN ERRORS
OF AMINO ACID
METABOLISM

Charles R. Scriver

HYPERAMINOACIDURIA

General Comments. A certain amount of L-aminoaciduria, representing less than 2 to 3 per cent of the total urinary nitrogen, is a normal phenomenon. A small fraction, usually less than 5 per cent, of the filtered load of the amino acids in plasma is not absorbed completely by the proximal portion of the renal tubule and is excreted in the urine. In the healthy person, the efficiency of renal tubular transport for the individual amino acids is related to their chemical and steric structure, the amount in the glomerular filtrate, and the sex, age, and physiologic state of the subject. Data for normal range and mean values of endogenous renal clearance rates, plasma levels, and urinary excretion rates of approximately 20 L-amino acids are now available for infants, children, and adults, both male and female, in fasting and nonfasting states. Advances in the knowledge of aminoaciduria have come primarily from the development of chromatographic methods, which allow rapid qualitative screening and reliable quantitative estimation of the complex amino acid composition of physiologic fluids.

Renal tubular absorption of amino acids is mediated by reactive sites which are believed to be membrane proteins, and whose catalytic relationships to the individual amino acids observe Michaelis-Menten kinetics. This means that the transport mechanism is saturable (equivalent to the T_m) and is susceptible to competitive and noncompetitive inhibition. The specificity of the site (protein) is genetically controlled.

Flux of the site–amino acid complex transfers the amino acid across the membrane (a directional process) by a mechanism which either is coupled to metabolic reactions which produce energy (nondirectional reactions) or elicits coupled fluxes in the same or opposite direction of other solutes.

Abnormal aminoaciduria will result when there is an acquired or hereditary disturbance of cellular metabolism or transport of amino acids. The known hyperaminoacidurias (Table 1) can be classified according to four basic mechanisms:

1. *Saturation:* Substrate is at elevated concentration and approaches or exceeds the capacity of the system ("overflow" aminoaciduria).

2. *Competition:* One substrate itself at elevated concentration competes with other members for access to the system ("combined" aminoaciduria).

3. *Modification of reactive site(s):* Substrate(s) not transported efficiently because access to the system is modified ("renal" aminoaciduria).

4. *Inhibition of substrate transfer:* Impaired energy-dependent processes, coupled to the transfer of substrates across membrane ("renal" aminoaciduria).

In some diseases, e.g., in Group III of Table 1, gene mutation affects amino acid transport in both the renal tubule and the intestine. Furthermore, it appears that the individual mechanisms required for transport of each amino acid can be grouped into at least five major gene-controlled and nonoverlapping systems, each having a particular *preference for a group of amino acids* normally found in plasma and usually elucidated in a particular aminoacidopathy. Another series of reactive sites *recognizes individual amino acids,* one site for each of the protein amino acids. Yet *another series permits transepithelial absorption of oligopeptides* in the intestine, with hydrolysis following uptake of the peptides. The *group-specific sites* used by free amino acids, and particularly evident through the inborn errors of amino acid metabolism, are classified as follows:

1. *The β-amino system:* β-alanine, β-aminoisobutyric acid, and taurine (viz., hyper-β-alaninemia).

2. *The α-amino systems:*

   a. "Basic" system: lysine, arginine, ornithine (and cystine, although not as a "basic" amino acid, viz., cystinuria).

   b. "Acidic" system: aspartic, glutamic.

   c. Neutral-I system: prolone, hydroxyproline, and glycine (viz., hyperprolinemia and renal iminoglycinuria).

   d. Neutral-II system: the remaining neutral α-amino acids (viz., Hartnup disease).

It is usually possible to classify the aminoaciduria by analyzing the amino acid content of plasma and urine collected conjointly (Table 1). Chromatographic techniques will reveal the details of hyperaminoaciduria more accurately than any other method. The recognition of a specific aminoaciduria can provide an accurate clinical diagnosis for which there may be appropriate therapy.

Scriver, C. R., and Rosenberg, L. E.: Amino Acid Metabolism and Its Disorders. Philadelphia, W. B. Saunders Company, 1973.

THE HYPERPHENYLALANINEMIAS

Mass screening of newborn infants in recent years has shown that all that is hyperphenylalaninemia is not necessarily phenylketonuria. Hence this section has been broadened to include mention of several hyperphenylalaninemic phenotypes evident in the human race. As position papers of their time, the conference reports edited by Anderson and Swaiman (1968) and by Bickel et al. (1971) should be read to supplement this brief discussion.

Metabolism of Phenylalanine. L-Phenylalanine is an essential amino acid for man. In infancy half or more of its dietary intake is used for protein synthesis, and the remainder is oxidized to tyrosine by hydroxylation in the liver. As body size increases, the phenylalanine intake increases from 1/2 gram per day at birth to as much as 4 grams daily in the older child and adult; at the same time that the rate of growth slows, a larger fraction of phenylalanine is catabolized to tyrosine, and the amount required for anabolism decreases proportionately. Any impairment of oxidation, without change in the other parameters, will cause the phenylalanine free pool to enlarge and its plasma concentration to rise above the normal maximum (1.2 mg per 100 ml). When this happens, other minor pathways of phenylalanine catabolism are called upon, and increased amounts of normal minor metabolites will appear in body fluids.

The key step in L-phenylalanine catabolism, namely, hydroxylation to tyrosine, has received much attention. This complex reaction involves several genes which control various components. Not surprisingly, several types of hyperphenylalaninemias are known; further variants will undoubtedly be discovered in the future.

Classic Phenylketonuria

Definition. The disease was first described by Følling in 1934. In its fully expressed form, there is persistent hyperphenylalaninemia in excess of 1 mMolar (16.5 mg per 100 ml), mental retardation (in most cases), and excessive urinary excretion of phenylpyruvic acid and other phenylalanine derivatives. The condition is autosomal recessive, being the result of complete absence of phenylalanine hydroxylase activity. If mass screening of newborn infants for this trait and genetic counseling are to be effective, the patient with classic untreated phenylketonuria should become an oddity, often mentioned but rarely seen in modern medical practice.

Prevalence. The homozygote occurs once in about 12,000 live births in Caucasians, with significant variation in frequency among ethnic groups. The disease is rare in the black and in the Ashkenazic Jew; in the latter cases, the mutation may not be allelic with the gene causing Caucasian phenylketonuria.

Clinical Manifestations. The most important and consistent feature is mental retardation. This becomes evident at six months of age, and in later childhood 98 per cent of untreated patients have an I.Q. below 70. Phenylketonuric patients are clinically normal at birth, distinguishable only by hyperphenylalaninemia, which is established in the first postnatal week. Other manifestations, such as seizures (often with the hypsarrhythmic EEG pattern), psychotic behavior, eczema, dermatographia, "mousy" odor (owing to excretion of phenylacetic acid), and pigment dilution, are found in untreated patients. None of these are seen in patients who benefit from early diagnosis and proper treatment.

The Metabolic Error. Homozygotes are almost completely lacking in phenylalanine hydroxylase activity; heterozygotes have partial activity, sufficient to maintain normal phenylalanine metabolism under ordinary circumstances.

Phenylalanine accumulates when the catabolic pathway is blocked, and is found in excessive amounts in blood, urine, and cerebrospinal fluid. Minor pathways are then overutilized, and, characteristically, phenylpyruvic acid is formed and excreted in urine. Additional compounds such as the lactic and acetic derivatives and the glutamine conjugate are also formed and excreted. Orthohydroxylation can occur and the corresponding ortho series of metabolites may be present.

Excessive amounts of phenylalanine and its derivatives can inhibit other enzymes. As a result disturbances of tyrosine and tryptophan metabolism occur. Diminished formation of catecholamines, melanin, and serotonin is observed in untreated phenylketonuria.

The cause of mental retardation in phenylketonuria is still unknown. It is probably due to many chemical abnormalities which occur as a consequence of the disturbed chemical environment during the critical early postnatal stage of brain development.

Diagnosis. Recognition of the trait should result from early postnatal detection of hyperphenylalaninemia. Subsequent studies to assess the degree of hyperphenylalaninemia, the dietary phenylalanine tolerance, and the persistence of the trait will help to distinguish it from other genetic variants affecting phenylalanine metabolism. Testing of the urine and ferric chloride (a few drops of 5 per cent solution in 0.1N HC1 added to 1 to 2 ml urine) is not recommended for diagnosis in the newborn, because this test requires the excretion of phenylpyruvic acid, whose formation is dependent on transamination of phenylalanine; the latter function may not mature for at least three weeks after birth, even in full-term babies. All current newborn screening programs employ a specific microbiologic assay, fluorometric assay, or partition chromatography to detect excess phenylalanine in a few microliters of capillary blood collected from the heel of the infant.

Treatment. Replacement or induction of phenylalanine hydroxylase is not feasible. Partial liver transplantation from a normal homozygote or heterozygote would give the patient a stable source of enzyme, and perhaps this mode of treatment will be possible in the future. At present dietary restriction of phenylalanine is the only practical therapy. By means of semisynthetic diets containing a low-phenylalanine hydrolysate, it is possible to restrict L-phenylalanine intake to about 250 to 500 mg daily while providing the recommended amounts of other essential amino acids and of calories and other nutritional factors. Close supervision of this treatment is important, and is best performed at centers experienced with such regimens.

Reduction of hyperphenylalaninemia to about 4 to 12 mg per 100 ml (relaxed regimen), when begun within 60 days of birth, will allow normal physical and mental development. Delayed or inadequate treatment impairs normal mental development. There is no agreement whether dietary treatment should be continued after the fifth year of life when human brain growth is complete. Female homozygous phenylketonurics should be treated during pregnancy to prevent harm to the fetus from intrauterine hyperphenylalaninemia.

Hyperphenylalaninemic Variants

The following phenotypes behave as independent autosomal recessive traits. Their recognition is important in order to avoid confusion with classic phenylketonuria and subsequent inappropriate treatment and counseling.

Atypical Phenylketonuria (Mild Variant). This variant is characterized by its high dietary tolerance for phenylalanine, which allows the patient to ingest between 700 and 2000 mg of the amino acid in the diet. Phenylalanine hydroxylase deficiency in the liver is probably incomplete; impaired intestinal absorption or excessive renal or fecal loss of phenylalanine does not account for the different phenotype.

Transient Phenylketonuria. Several sibships are known in which disappearance of the phenylketonuric phenotype and restoration of normal or nearly normal dietary phenylalanine tolerance occur spontaneously during infancy or childhood. The precise enzymatic basis for the phenotype has not been established.

Benign Persistent Hyperphenylalaninemia. This trait was first observed in families of Mediterranean origin but now also in other ethnic groups, including Jews. The concentration of phenylalanine in plasma of homozygotes consuming normal diets is usually less than 1 mMolar (16.5 mg per 100 ml). Mental and physical development is normal without treatment in these subjects.

TABLE 1. Hereditary and Acquired Aminoacidopathies:* Classified According to Mechanism and Preferred Fluid for Detection

Group IA: Primary defect in catabolism
Low renal clearance of amino acid
Hyperaminoaciduria by saturation of transport system
Detection preferable in plasma

Condition or Disease	Amino Acids Affected	Abnormal Enzyme	Comment
I.A.1 *Common perinatal (adaptive) traits*			
Neonatal hyperphenyl-alaninemia*	Phenylalanine	Phenylalanine hydroxylating system (?)	Benign; may respond to folic acid; often occurs with tyrosinemia
Neonatal tyrosinemia†	Tyrosine	p-Hydroxy-phenyl pyruvic acid hydroxylase (EC 1.14.2.2)	Benign; responds to ascorbic acid and reduced protein intake
Hypermethioninemia†	Methionine	ATP: 1-methionine S-adenosyl transferase (?) (EC 2.5.1.6)	Benign; usually found with high protein intake
Hyperhistidinemia†	Histidine	L-Histidine ammonia lyase (?) (EC 4.3.1.3)	Benign; related to high protein intake
I.A.2 *Inherited aminoacidopathies*			
1. The hyperphenylalaninemias			
(i) "Classic" phenylketonuria	Phenylalanine	L-Phenylalanine tetrahydropteridine; oxygen oxidoreductase (4-hydroxylating) (EC 1.14.3.1) (residual activity <1%)	(i) Plasma phenylalanine >16 mg/100 ml; causes mental retardation; when treated, L-phenylalanine tolerance in diet is 250–500 mg phe/day
(ii) "Atypical" phenylketonuria†	Phenylalanine	L-Phenylalanine tetrahydropteridine: oxygen oxido-reductase (4-hydroxylating) (EC 1.14.3.1) (residual activity >1%)	(ii) Plasma phenylalanine >16 mg/100 ml; similar to (i), but dietary tolerance for L-phenylalanine is >500 mg/day
(iii) "Transient" phenylketonuria†	Phenylalanine	L-Phenylalanine tetrahydropteridine: oxygen oxido-reductase (4-hydroxylating) (EC 1.14.13.1)	(iii) Plasma phenylalanine >16 mg/100 ml; change in status to (iv), or normal, several months or years after birth
(iv) "Benign" hyperphenylalaninemia†	Phenylalanine	L-Phenylalanine tetrahydropteridine: oxygen oxido-reductase (4-hydroxylating) (EC 1.14.3.1)	(iv) Plasma phenylalanine <16 mg/100 ml; on normal diet; benign trait
2. The hypertyrosinemias			
(i) Tyrosinosis (Medes)	Tyrosine	L-tyrosine: α-ketoglutarate amino transferase (?) (EC 2.6.1.20)	One case known; myasthenia gravis, probably incidental finding
(ii) Hypertyrosinemia†	Tyrosine	Soluble (cytosol) tyrosine aminotransferase	One case; associated developmental retardation
(iii) Hereditary tyrosinemia†	Tyrosine (and methionine)	p-HPPA hydroxylase (EC 1.14.2.2) Primary or secondary defect?	Hepatic cirrhosis, and renal tubular failure, eventually fatal; responds to tyrosine restriction
3. The hyperhistidinemias			
(i) "Classic" form†	Histidine (alanine in some cases)	L-Histidine ammonia lyase (EC 4.3.1.3.) (liver and skin)	Usually associated with mental retardation and speech defect
(ii) Variant form	Histidine	L-Histidine ammonia lyase (EC 4.3.1.3) (liver only)	As above
4. The branched-chain hyperaminoacidemias			
(i) "Classic maple syrup urine disease"†	Leucine isoleucine, valine, allo-isoleucine	Branched-chain α-keto acid; lipoate oxidoreductase (acceptor acylating) (EC 1.2.4.-) (<2 per cent of normal)	Postnatal collapse, mental retardation in survivors; early diet therapy effective
(ii) Intermittent form	Same	Same (2–15 per cent of normal)	Intermittent symptoms; development may be otherwise normal
(iii) Mild form	Same	Same	Unremittent; milder than (i)
(iv) Thiamin-responsive	Same	Same	Mild form; B_1-responsive (10–20 mg/day)
(v) Hypervalinemia	Valine	Valine amino-transferase (EC 2.6.1.-)	Retarded development and vomiting; responds to diet
(vi) Hyperleucinemia	Leucine/isoleucine	Leucine-isoleucine transferase (EC 2.6.1.-)	Retarded development
(vii) Others§			

TABLE 1.   Hereditary and Acquired Aminoacidopathies:* Classified According to Mechanism and Preferred Fluid for Detection (*Continued*)

Group IA: Primary defect in catabolism
Low renal clearance of amino acid
Hyperaminoaciduria by saturation of transport system
Detection preferable in plasma

Condition or Disease	Amino Acids Affected	Abnormal Enzyme	Comment
5. Sulfuraminoacidemias (i) Homocystinuria‡	Methionine and homocystine	L-Serine hydrolase (deaminating); ("cystathionine synthetase") (EC 4.2.1.13)	Usually associated with thromboembolic disease, mental retardation, ectopia-lentis, and Marfan phenotype; some cases respond to Vitamin B_6
(ii) Cystathioninuria‡	Cystathionine	L-Homoserine hydrolyase (deaminating) (EC 4.2.1.15)	Probably benign trait; vitamin B_6 corrects biochemical trait in most patients
6. The hyperglycinemias (i) Ketotic form†	Glycine and other glucogenic acids	Propionyl-CoA; carbon dioxide ligase (ADP) (EC 6.4.1.3)	Ketosis, neutropenia, mental retardation; often fatal
(ii) Nonketotic form†	Glycine	"Glycine decarboxylase" (?)	Different trait; poor prognosis
7. Sarcosinemia‡	Sarcosine (ethanolamine)	Sarcosine: oxygen oxidoreductase (demethylating) (EC 1.5.3.1)	Benign trait (probably)
8. The hyperprolinemias (i) Type I†	Proline	L-Proline: NAD(P) 5-oxido-reductase, ("proline oxidase") (EC 1.5.1.2) (partial defect)	Benign trait, which is sometimes associated with hereditary nephritis
(ii) Type II	Proline	"Δ^1-pyrroline-5-carboxylate dehydrogenase"? or more complete deficiency of oxidase?	Benign trait, sometimes associated with CNS disease; ΔPC excreted in urine; proline concentration greater than Type I
9. Hydroxyprolinemia	Hydroxyproline	"Hydroxyproline oxidase"	Two cases, associated with CNS disease; others normal
10. The hyperlysinemias (i) Type I	Lysine (and glutamine)	Lysine: α-ketoglutarate: triphospho-pyridine nucleotide (TPNH), oxidoreductase (ϵ-N-[L-glutaryl 1-2]-L-lysine forming)	Associated with mental retardation and hypotonia
(ii) Type II	Lysine, arginine (NH_3)	(Partial defect of above [10, i]) or different enzyme?	Hyperammonemia symptoms, related to protein intake
(iii) Saccharopinuria‡	Lysine, saccharopine, citrulline	"Saccharopinase"(?)	First case associated with mental retardation and short stature
11. Pipecolicacidemia‡	Pipecolic acid	"Pipecolate oxidase" (?)	Hepatomegaly and mental retardation
12. The hyperammonemias (i) Type I	Glycine, glutamine	ATP: carbamate phosphotransferase (EC 2.7.2.2)	
(ii) Type II†	Glutamine (and orotic acid)	Carbamoylphosphate: L-ornithine carbamoyl-transferase (EC 2.1.3.3.)	Type II is X-linked; it and the autosomal recessive diseases show ammonia intoxication, protein intolerance, hepatomegaly, vomiting, etc.; ASAuria also has trichlorrhexis nodosa
(iii) Hyperornithinemia	Ornithine	Unknown	
(iv) Citrullinemia†	Citrulline	L-Citrulline: L-aspartase ligase (AMP) (EC 6.3.4.5)	
(v) Argininosuc-cinicaciduria‡	ASA	L-Argininosuccinate argininelyase (EC 4.3.2.1)	
(vi) Argininemia	Arginine	"Arginase": L-Arginineamidino hydrolase (EC 3.5.3.1)	
(See also 10, Type II)			
13. Glutamicacidemia	Glutamate	Unknown	X-linked mental retardation; possibly the same as Menkes' (kinky hair) syndrome
14. The hyperalaninemias	Alanine	(i) Pyruvate dehydrogenase (EC 4.1.1.1) decarboxylase (EC 1.2.4.1) deficiency	Lactic acidosis, intermittent ataxia, mental retardation

(Table continued on following pages)

TABLE 1.   Hereditary and Acquired Aminoacidopathies:* Classified According to Mechanism
and Preferred Fluid for Detection (Continued)

Group IA: Primary defect in catabolism
Low renal clearance of amino acid
Hyperaminoaciduria by saturation of transport system
Detection preferable in plasma

Condition or Disease	Amino Acids Affected	Abnormal Enzyme	Comment
		(ii) Pyruvate carboxylase deficiency (EC 6.4.1.1)	Intermittent lactic acidosis, intermittent hypoglycemia
15. Aspartylglucosaminuria	Glucoasparagines	2-acetamido-1-(β^1-L-aspartamido)-1,2-dideoxyglucoseamido hydrolase	Lysosomal disease? mental retardation
16. "Glutathionemia"	Glutathione or related peptide	γ-Glutamyl-transpeptidase deficiency	Mental retardation associated with finding

1.A.3 *Nutritional and other diseases which may affect amino acids in plasma*

Protein-calorie malnutrition	Tryptophan/leucine / isoleucine/valine $\downarrow$; tyrosine/glycine/ proline $\uparrow$		Severity of change related to severity of malnutrition
Prolonged fasting	Alanine $\downarrow$; threonine; glycine $\uparrow$		Early fasting does not show same pattern
Obesity	Leucine/isoleucine/ valine/phenylalanine/ tyrosine $\uparrow$; Glycine $\downarrow$		Reflects insulin insensitivity
Hepatitis	Methionine/tryosine $\uparrow$		Reflects severity of liver disease

Group IB: Primary defect in catabolism
High renal clearance of amino acid
Hyperaminoaciduria by saturation
Detection preferable in urine

Condition or Disease	Amino Acids Affected	Abnormal Enzyme	Comment
1. (a) Hypophosphatasia	Phosphoethanolamine	? Deficiency of o-phosphoryl-ethanolamine phospho-lyase (EC 4.2.99.-)	"Rickets" unresponsive to vitamin D; craniosynostosis; hypercalcemia
(b) Pseudohypophosphatasia	Phosphoethanolamine	"Alkaline phosphatase" activity present but altered (Km mutant)	(Same as 1a)
2. β-Aminoisobutyricaciduria	βAIB	?	Benign polymorphic trait
3. Hyper-β-alaninemia	β-Alanine	β-Alanine transaminase?	Seizures; somnolence; mental retardation
4. Carnosinemia	Carnosine	Carnosinase	Seizures and mental retardation
5. Pyroglutamicaciduria	5-oxo-L-proline (pyrrolidone-2-carboxylic acid)	Overproduction secondary to defective glutathione synthesis?	5-O-P in urine; origin in kidney ?

See also homocystinuria (I.A.2.5.i), cystathioninuria (I.A.2.5.ii), and argininosuccinicaciduria (I.A.2.12.v)

Group II: Primary defect in catabolism; secondary defect in transport
Hyperaminoaciduria of combined origin (saturation and competition)
Detection possible in plasma and urine

Disease	Amino Acids Affected in Plasma	Amino Acids Present in Urine	Comment
1. Hyperprolinemia Types I and II	Proline	Proline plus hydroxyproline and glycine	See I.A.2.8; competition occurs on iminoglycine transport system (see III, 2)
2. Hyper-β-alaninemia	β-Alanine	β-Alanine plus βAIB and taurine	See I.B.3; competition occurs on β-amino transport system
3. Hyperlysinemia	Lysine	Lysine plus ornithine and arginine	See I.A.2.10; competition occurs on "dibasic" transport system (see III, 1)

TABLE 1. Hereditary and Acquired Aminoacidopathies:* Classified According to Mechanism and Preferred Fluid for Detection (*Continued*)

Group III: Primary defect in membrane transport site
High renal clearance of amino acid
Detection possible only in urine

Disease or Trait	Amino Acids Affected	Abnormal Transport System	Comment
III.A *Common perinatal (adaptive) traits*			
1. Neonatal iminoglycinuria	Proline, hydroxyproline, and glycine	Low capacity system for proline; same for glycine	Iminoaciduria persists about 3 months; glycinuria persists 5–6 months
III. B. *Hereditary traits*			
1. Cystinuria†	Dibasics and cystine	High capacity, diaminomonocarboxylic (involving cysteine during efflux only)	
a. Type I	In homozygote, not in heterozygote	Kidney plus gut	Cystine stone formation in urinary tract is major hazard
b. Type II	In homozygote and heterozygote	Kidney plus gut	
c. Type III	In homozygote and heterozygote	Kidney (plus gut, partial or normal)	
2. Hypercystinuria	Cystine only	Substrate-specific system for cystine	
3. Renal iminoglycinuria†	Proline, hydroxyproline, and glycine	High capacity system for imino acids and glycine	
a. Type I		Kidney and gut	
b. Type II		Kidney alone	Benign trait
4. Hartnup disease†	Neutral mono-amino acids and monocarboxylic acids (except imino acids and glycine)	High capacity system shared by neutral amino acids	Pellagra-like symptoms under condition of marginal protein nutrition
a. Type I		Kidney and gut	
b. Type II		Kidney only	
5. Blue diaper syndrome	Tryptophan	Low capacity system for specific amino acid (in the intestine)	Hypercalcemia
6. Methionine malabsorption	Methionine		Mental retardation

Group IV: Generalized inhibition of transport processes
High renal clearance of substrates
Detection best in urine

Primary Abnormality	Aminoaciduria and Other Findings	Comment
1. Acquired		
e.g., Degraded tetracyclines, salicylates, heavy metals, vitamin D deficiency, scurvy, etc.	Generalized aminoaciduria, plus combinations of glucosuria, hyperphosphaturia, etc. (Fanconi's syndrome)	Early removal of toxin or correction of deficiency usually followed by recovery of normal transport function
2. Hereditary		
Galactosemia	Generalized + galactosuria	Can be induced by galactose feeding and treated by removal of galactose
Oculocerebro-renal syndrome	Generalized + phosphaturia and renal tubular acidosis	X-linked glaucoma, hypotonia, and mental retardation; defect in ammonia synthesis?
Other Fanconi syndromes, related to:	Generalized + loss of glucose, phosphate, K, bicarbonate, water, etc.	Symptoms related to functional defect (Po₄ and K loss, etc.) plus primary disease
a. Cystinosis		a. Cystine storage; recessive gene
b. Idiopathic (infants)		b. No cystine storage; sporadic cases
c. Idiopathic (adults)		c. Recessive inheritance; no cystinosis
d. Luder-Sheldon variety		d. Onset in late childhood
e. Secondary to Wilson's disease		e. Onset in late childhood
f. Secondary to tyrosinemia (Baber's syndrome)		f. Onset usually in late infancy
g. Others, including fructosemia (aldolase deficiency)		g. Differentiate from f

*Table refers only to those conditions associated with perturbation of the normal content of ninhydrin-reactive metabolites in plasma or urine.
†These conditions have been detected by screening methods applied in the newborn period of life.
‡Urine screening is probably preferable in these conditions.
§A number of disorders of branched-chain amino acid catabolism cause accumulation of substances which are ninhydrin-negative. These compounds can usually be detected by gas-liquid chromatographic methods.
EC=Enzyme classification number.

Recognition of the trait is important, for it must not be confused with phenylketonuria.

Anderson, J. A., and Swaiman, K. F. (eds.): Proceedings of a Conference on Phenylketonuria and Allied Disorders. U.S. Department of Health, Education, and Welfare, Social and Rehabilitation Service, Children's Bureau. U.S. Government Printing Office, 1967–0–282–371.

Bickel, H., Hudson, F. P., and Woolf, L. I. (eds.): Phenylketonuria and Some Other Inborn Errors of Amino Acid Metabolism. Biochemistry, Genetics, Diagnosis, Therapy. Stuttgart, Georg Thieme Verlag, 1971.

Justice, P., O'Flynn, M. E., and Hsia, D. Y.: Phenylalanine-hydroxylase activity in hyperphenylalaninaemia. Lancet, 1:928, 1967.

BRANCHED-CHAIN AMINOACIDURIA

Maple Syrup Urine Disease. The colloquial term describes a characteristic odor of patients with *branched-chain ketoaciduria, and aminoacidopathy*. The disease is autosomal recessive, and its apparent rarity may reflect, in part, missed diagnoses in patients dying in infancy. Severe hypotonia, apnea, feeding difficulty, and hypoglycemia appear in the first week of life, progressing to seizures, decorticate rigidity, severe mental retardation, and death. At least three variants with episodic illness or mild mental retardation presenting in later infancy have been reported.

The primary enzymatic defect is a block in decarboxylation of branched-chain α-keto acids; consequently leucine, isoleucine, alloisoleucine, and valine and their equivalent α-keto acids and α-hydroxyacids accumulate after birth; symptoms are primarily related to abnormal leucine metabolism. The aminoacidopathy can be detected in blood and urine within the first week of life; the enzyme defect can be assayed in leukocytes and in cultured skin fibroblasts.

The disease responds to dietary control of leucine, isoleucine, and valine intake, the best results following the earliest possible treatment. One variant is responsive to thiamin at ten times the normal daily intake.

Hypervalinemia. Symptoms of vomiting, blindness, and retardation of physical and mental development in a single Japanese infant were reported, which improved abruptly with a valine-restricted diet. Valine transaminase is the defective enzyme; hence only valine accumulates in body fluids.

HYPERHISTIDINEMIA

Many cases of this rare and apparently autosomal recessively inherited disease are now known. Inactivity of the enzyme histidase, which nonoxidatively deaminates histidine to uraconic acid, can be detected in skin biopsy material. Accumulation of histidine (and sometimes of alanine) above normal levels and depressed serotonin levels are found in blood; increased excretion of imidazolepyruvic acid and a positive ferric chloride test are found in urine. The risk of mild mental retardation and/or short auditory memory span, reflected as delayed speech development, is apparently about 1 in 2. Low-histidine therapy is feasible and, in view of the risk of delayed mental development, is probably indicated.

THE HYPERPROLINEMIAS AND HYDROXYPROLINEMIA
(Iminoacidopathies)

Hyperprolinemias. *Type I* (L-proline oxidase deficiency) is a recessively inherited condition. Proline is the only amino acid elevated in plasma, but a "combined" aminoaciduria involving proline, hydroxyproline, and glycine is found. In *Type II* hyperprolinemia the block is apparently at the second step in proline degradation (Δ-pyrroline-5-carboxylate dehydrogenase); the pyrroline derivative is also excreted in urine. Type I hyperprolinemia is sometimes associated with familial hematuric nephropathy, but pedigree studies show that prolinemia and nephropathy are not the consequences of a single gene effect; seizures also occur in both types of hyperprolinemia.

Hydroxyprolinemia. Mental retardation was the principal finding in the first patient described. The enzymes for free hydroxy-L-proline catabolism are distinct from those for L-proline, and the deficient enzyme is a hydroxyproline-specific "oxidase." Subsequent patients have been free of clinical symptoms.

DISEASES OF THE UREA CYCLE

A number of enzymes are involved in the incorporation of ammonia and its delivery as urea. Differences in their relative activity (Table 2) and their location in the cell may account for some of the differences in clinical severity of the inborn errors of the urea cycle. In addition to the catalytic steps, two transport steps across the mitochrondrial membranes are involved, one of which delivers citrulline to the cytoplasm from the mitochondria, the other returning ornithine to the mitochondrion. *Carbamyl phosphate synthetase deficiency* is an intramitochondrial disease with severe hyperammonemia and a rapidly fatal course after birth; inheritance is probably autosomal recessive. *Ornithine transcarbamylase deficiency* is an X-linked disease, with males severely, even fatally, affected and females exhibiting a variable range of clinical symptoms as expected in an X-linked trait. *Citrullinemia* and *argininosuccinicaciduria* are each autosomal recessive, their names identifying the substrate which accumulates in the presence of their respective enzyme deficiencies. *Argininemia* is an autosomal recessive disorder of the last step of the cycle. *Ornithinemia* is yet another apparently autosomal recessive disease of the cycle in which the defective catalytic reaction (perhaps the transport step) has not yet been identified.

Each disease of the urea cycle is accompanied by a set of similar findings which include hyperammonemia, metabolic alkalosis, failure to thrive, convulsions, hepatomegaly, and mental retardation. A fatal outcome is common.

The severity of symptoms and biochemical imbalance varies with the site of the defect and with its completeness. It is interesting that most patients maintain normal or nearly normal urea synthesis, presumably

TABLE 2. Enzymes in Urea Cycle and Relative Activities*

Carbamyl phosphate synthetase	4.5
Ornithine transcarbamylase	163.0
Argininosuccinic acid synthetase	1.0
Argininosuccinic acid lyase	3.3
Arginase	149.0

*From Scriver, C. R., and Rosenberg, L. E.: Amino Acid Metabolism and its Disorders. Philadelphia, W. B. Saunders Company, 1973.

reflecting a partial block only in the urea cycle compensated for by marked substrate accumulation. Symptomatic treatment with low protein diet and prevention of ammonia intoxication is sometimes feasible. Careful genetic counseling, coupled with the option for prenatal diagnosis in some of the diseases, is recommended.

DISORDERS OF METHIONINE DEGRADATION

Homocystinuria. The full spectrum of clinical features of this autosomal recessive disease is diagnostic: ectopia lentis, downward and forward, mental retardation, lax ligaments, lengthened extremities, malar flush, and fine sparse hair; death from thromboembolic phenomena is frequent. Late-surviving patients have ocular, skeletal, and vascular changes likened to those of Marfan's syndrome (see Ch. 933). Cystathionine synthetase is deficient; its substrate, homocysteine, and the precursor, methionine, accumulate; the product, cystathionine, is deficient in brain. Homocysteine is oxidized and excreted in urine as homocystine, where it can be detected by the cyanide-nitroprusside test. Early dietary therapy with methionine restriction (and cystine supplementation) has apparent benefit. Some patients respond to large doses of pyridoxine (vitamin B_6).

Cystathioninuria. This condition is transmitted in autosomal recessive fashion. It appears to be a benign and not uncommon condition often found in patients with other diseases that attract attention first. Acquired cystathioninuria also occurs secondary to hepatic failure and neuroblastoma. In the hereditary form, the presumed heterozygote exhibits modest elevation, and the homozygote has marked elevation of cystathionine levels in body fluids related to a deficiency of cystathionine-cleaving enzyme activity. Biochemical improvement with pyridoxine therapy demonstrates that the cleaving enzyme is present in the patient's tissues, but is inactive until an excess of pyridoxal-5-phosphate is available, indicating a specific defect in co-factor binding by the apoenzyme.

β-AMINOISOBUTYRICACIDURIA

β-Aminoisobutyric acid (β AIB) is a derivative of thymine and valine metabolism. High urinary excretion (more than 100 μM per gram total N) occurs in some humans who are probably homozygous for a gene controlling β AIB metabolism. In these subjects, plasma levels of β AIB are elevated; the renal clearance rate of the natural isomer, D-(-), β AIB, exceeds that for inulin, indicating net renal "secretion" of β AIB; probenecid can suppress excretion. Hyperexcretors are common in the Mongolian race but infrequent (approximately 5 per cent) in Caucasians; the adaptive significance for the mutation is unknown. Increased β AIB excretion can also be acquired under catabolic stress.

RENAL HYPERAMINOACIDURIAS

Certain hyperaminoacidurias reflect impairment of specific transport systems; the transport lesion is frequently demonstrable in the gut as well as in the kidney. The renal clearance rates of affected amino acids are high, and their plasma levels are low or normal, rather than elevated.

Cystinuria. Three homozygous cystinuric phenotypes are now recognized; in all, there is elevated urinary excretion of cystine, lysine, ornithine, and arginine. In Type I, gut transport of the four amino acids is also abnormal; the heterozygote has normal aminoaciduria (complete recessive). Type II has defective gut transport of the basic amino acids but not of cystine; the heterozygote has elevated urinary lysine and cystine (incomplete recessive). Type III has normal gut transport; the heterozygote phenotype is "incomplete." The exact mechanism of the hyperaminoaciduria is unclear; net tubular "secretion" of the affected amino acids in patients may indicate exaggerated back-flux from cell into urine.

Genetic classification of patients now extends to include "genetic compounds," that is, individuals who resemble homozygotes in their findings but who have inherited two *different* mutant alleles (e.g., I-III, I-II, or II-III).

Urinary cystine calculi are the predominant clinical problem, related to the poor aqueous solubility of cystine in acid urine. Prevention of calculi formation and attendant complications can be attained with copious free water excretion throughout day and night and the use of sodium bicarbonate (10 to 30 grams per day). Rapid solubilization of cystine by formation of a mixed disulfide with D(-) penicillamine (0.5 to 1.0 gram every six hours) may be useful in some patients. Cystinuric patients also have modest growth retardation, perhaps related to fecal and urinary loss of lysine. In a few children severe growth failure and generalized intestinal malabsorption occur with cystinuria as a particular syndrome.

Hartnup Disease. Episodic clinical features include pellagra-like symptoms with photosensitive dermatitis, cerebellar ataxia, and psychosis. Biochemical findings include reduced blood levels of tryptophan metabolites, e.g., nicotinic acid and serotonin, and a fluctuant increase in urinary excretion of indolic acids and derivatives. A constant transport defect for certain neutral α-amino acids is demonstrable in kidney and intestine. The abnormal "indoluria" is dependent on intestinal flora degrading unabsorbed L-tryptophan, with absorption and renal excretion of the products. Defective intracellular transport of tryptophan may account for the deficiency of its endogenous metabolites. Good protein nutrition, normal general intestinal health, and nicotinamide supplements (40 to 200 mg per day) can maintain good general health of the patient.

Proline-Hydroxyproline-Glycinuria (Iminoglycinuria). This finding is normal in early infancy. Failure of the group-specific transport system to develop has been observed as a frequent, benign autosomal recessive trait. Presence or absence of an associated intestinal transport defect indicates at least two mutant genotypes.

FANCONI'S SYNDROME

The term "Fanconi's syndrome" describes a disturbance of proximal renal tubular function of multiple causation and comprising generalized hyperaminoaciduria, renal glucosuria, and hyperphosphaturia, as well as renal loss of potassium, bicarbonate and water, and other substances conserved by the proximal tubule. Fanconi's syndrome should be considered as the final result of any one of many possible primary insults to proximal tubular function (see Group IV aminoacidurias, Table 1). The patient's symptoms reflect the disturbance of tubular function, in addition to the primary cause of the syndrome. Osteomalacia is a particularly prominent clinical finding primarily reflecting phosphate wasting. Acidosis accompanies the bicarbonate loss, whereas muscular weakness may be a prominent manifestation of hypokalemia.

Fanconi's syndrome may be inherited or acquired. The various hereditary forms are predominantly recessive, different alleles being responsible for the different diseases causing the syndrome. For example, cystinosis is a recessive, inherited disease, with cystine accumulation occurring in tissues and accompanied by the syndrome that first appears about six months after birth. The idiopathic Fanconi syndrome in adults is a recessively inherited disorder of early middle age. Acquired causes are numerous; deteriorated tetracycline (epianhydrotetracycline) is an interesting example of a toxic cause of the syndrome.

The syndrome appears to follow inhibition of cellular mechanisms sustaining transport function in the proximal tubule. As a result, the tubular capacity for transport is impaired. In severe cases, morphologic changes also occur, with reduction in cell organelles and cell mass of the proximal portion of the proximal convoluted tubule (swan-neck lesion). There is considerable experimental evidence that solutes enter urine in excess not only because of impaired absorption but also by backflux from renal cells after entry into kidney tissue from peritubular capillaries.

The disturbance of proximal tubular function results in the alterations in urine and plasma composition referred to above. The final levels of expression of the syndrome are more peripheral, and are related to both the disturbances in renal physiology and the primary causes of the syndrome. Pitressin-resistant diabetes insipidus is sometimes diagnosed in children before the syndrome is recognized. There may also be evidence for the primary cause of the syndrome, e.g., cystine crystals in the cornea, Kayser-Fleischer rings of Wilson's disease, a history of exposure to antimicrobial drugs or toxins, or other affected family members.

Treatment.   Attempt to eliminate the primary cause, e.g., removal of exogenous toxic agents or deficiency states. Other primary conditions may be ameliorated, e.g., removal of milk in galactosemia or removal of copper in Wilson's disease.

Offset the disturbance in tubular physiology. Osteomalacia is readily treated, and prevented, with oral phosphate supplements (1.0 to 2.0 grams phosphorus per day, equivalent to 20 grams of "neutral" phosphate salt); supplemental vitamin D_2 may also be required in doses adjusted to the patient's need. Shohl's solution, 30 ml three times daily for adults, usually controls the acidemia. Hypokalemia may be corrected with potassium salts (as phosphate or citrate). Adequate fluid intake is indicated to prevent dehydration.

Efron, M. L.: Aminoaciduria. N. Engl. J. Med., 272:1058, 1107, 1965.
Nyhan, W. L. (ed.): Amino Acid Metabolism and Genetic Variation. New York, McGraw-Hill Book Company, 1967.
Scriver, C. R., and Rosenberg, L. E.: Amino Acid Metabolism and Its Disorders. Philadelphia, W. B. Saunders Company, 1973.

THE HYPERGLYCINURIAS

Six forms of isolated hyperglycinuria are known:

1. Hyperglycinemia with "overflow" hyperglycinuria.

a. Type I (ketotic): Vomiting, acetonuria, neutropenia, thrombocytopenia, and leucine intolerance occur in the neonatal period; retardation of growth and mental development follow if the infant survives. The findings to a lesser or greater degree are found in propionicacidemia (propionyl CoA carboxylase deficiency), methylmalonicacidemia (methylmalonyl CoA mutase deficiency), and a disorder of isoleucine catabolism (β-ketothiolase deficiency). Restriction of dietary protein intake may be helpful.

b. Type II (nonketotic): There is severe developmental and mental retardation. Conversion of glycine to carbon dioxide, methylenetetrahydrofolate, and ammonia is apparently impaired.

2. Renal glycinurias.

a. Impaired renal conservation of glycine occurs as the heterozygous phenotype in one form of familial iminoglycinuria.

b. Resistant rickets and renal hyperglycinuria occur in association with (i) hyperphosphaturia, (ii) hyperphosphaturia and glucosuria (both renal).

c. Dominantly inherited, asymptomatic renal glycinuria with renal glucosuria has been reported from Switzerland.

ALCAPTONURIA AND OCHRONOSIS

Definition.   Alcaptonuria (homogentisicaciduria) is a disorder of tyrosine metabolism which results from deficiency of the enzyme homogentisic acid oxidase. Alcaptonuria is the predecessor of ochronosis, the condition which results from chronic deposition of an oxidized brown-black pigment of homogentisic acid in connective tissue, causing spondylosis and arthropathy. Alcaptonuria is one of the inborn errors of metabolism originally described by Garrod, and the first disease for which autosomal recessive inheritance was proposed.

Pathogenesis.   Homogentisic acid (2,5-dihydroxyphenylacetic acid) is normally oxidized in liver and kidney to maleylacetoacetic acid. In the absence of this reaction, homogentisic acid accumulates in tissues, and is secreted into urine by alcaptonuric subjects. There is no significant homogentisicacidemia, because the compound is rapidly secreted by kidney, its renal clearance greatly exceeding the glomerular filtration rate. The damage to connective tissue characteristic of ochronosis results from prolonged exposure to homogentisic acid. Its oxidized pigment, benzoquinoneacetic acid, is believed to polymerize to form a melanin-like pigment, which binds irreversibly with collagen. It has been suggested that such binding cross-links collagen, thus altering its physicochemical properties, which in turn leads to the degenerative changes observed in ochronosis. Although alcaptonuria may be detected in the newborn period, changes in connective tissue do not appear until adulthood, perhaps because the enhanced remodeling of connective tissue during childhood and adolescence removes the chemically modified collagen.

Diagnosis.   Homogentisicaciduria is present from birth onward, and its intensity is proportional to the dietary intake and catabolism of phenylalanine and tyrosine. With modern sanitation patients may not know for many years that their urine can darken on standing. Thus the diagnosis usually rests on clinical suspicion, a family history, and chemical tests.

Urine. Freshly voided urine is normal in appearance; darkening occurs slowly from the exposed surface downward on standing in air, and rapidly when made alkaline. Homogentisic acid reduces Benedict's reagent to a brown-orange color, and produces a purple-black reaction with ferric chloride reagent. Large amounts of ascorbic acid may give false positive reactions with these chemical tests, and it will prevent spontaneous darkening. Coloration of urine caused by bile, porphyrins, myoglobin, and hemoglobin should be distinguished. Homogentisic acid can be confirmed by chromatography and a specific enzymatic method.

Ochronosis

Deposition of brown-black pigment in connective tissue is the legacy of prolonged exposure to homogentisic acid. It can occur in dermis and sweat glands, conjunctiva and cornea, sclera, pinna, tympanic membrane, and ossicles of the middle ear, laryngeal and tracheal cartilages, heart valves, genitourinary tract, tendons, large diarthrodial joints, and spine. Pigment granules occur as both intracellular and extracellular deposits. Characteristically the pinnae are stiff and opaque to transillumination; the corneas are black; conduction hearing loss may accompany involvement of tympanum and ossicles. Renal stones and prostatic calculi occur but usually do not cause renal disease, although prostatitis may be caused by alcaptonuria. Heart disease is not more frequent in alcaptonuria despite pigmentation of the endocardium and intima of the aorta.

Ochronotic Arthropathy. The most serious complication of ochronosis is arthropathy. Unlike rheumatoid disease, it spares the small joints of hands and feet. Onset of arthropathy is earlier and more severe in males, and the knee is the most frequently and severely affected peripheral joint. Spondylosis, which is very often present, appears slowly with pain and stiffness, usually in the low back. Ultimately involvement of the lumbar and thoracic spine results in loss of motion and disappearance of the normal lumbar lordosis. Herniation or calcification of the intervertebral discs is also characteristic. As a consequence of ochronotic arthropathy, the typical patient assumes a wide-based stance with forward stoop, rigid spine, and flexed hips and knees.

Roentgenographic examination reveals narrowing of the intervertebral spaces, disc calcification, and gradual fusion of vertebral bodies. However, the annular ossification ("bamboo spine") of ankylosing spondylitis is not seen. In the peripheral joints there may be evidence of synovial effusion and osteochondral bodies in the knee joint; the osteophytes and periarticular cystic changes of osteoarthritis are not prominent. With time, degenerative changes occur, with narrowing of the joint space, eburnation, sclerosis, and calcification of adjacent tendons.

Prognosis. Life expectancy is normal. Alcaptonuria and ochronotic pigmentation are symptomless manifestations of homogentisic acid accumulation. Patients with the disease usually marry noncarriers, and will transmit the trait, with a 1 in 2 probability, to their offspring.

Treatment. There is no specific treatment for alcaptonuria. Limitation of phenylalanine and tyrosine intake would be of theoretical value to prevent homogentisic acid accumulation, but such lifelong dietary treatment is not feasible. The reducing agent, vitamin C, impedes oxidation and polymerization of homogentisic acid and large amounts in the diet might delay ochronotic changes. Occupations which stress the spine and large joints should be avoided. Families expressing this autosomal recessive trait should be given appropriate genetic counseling.

Garrod, A. E.: The incidence of alkaptonuria. A study in chemical individuality. Lancet, 2:1616, 1902.

LaDu, B. N.: Alcaptonuria. *In* Stanbury, J. B., Wyngaarden, J. B., and Fredrickson, D. S. (eds.): The Metabolic Basis of Inherited Disease. 3rd ed. New York, McGraw-Hill Book Company, 1973, pp. 308–325.

LaDu, B. N., Zannoni, V. G., Laster, L., and Seegmiller, J. E.: The nature of the defect in tyrosine metabolism in alcaptonuria. J. Biol. Chem., 230:251, 1958.

O'Brien, W. M., LaDu, B. N., and Bunim, J. J.: Biochemical, pathologic and clinical aspects of alcaptonuria, ochronosis and ochronotic arthropathy. Am. J. Med., 34:813, 1963.

Stoner, R., and Blivaiss, B. B.: Reaction of quinone of homogentisic acid with biological amines. Arthritis Rheum., 10:53, 1967.

DISORDERS OF PURINE METABOLISM

Lloyd H. Smith, Jr.

821. GOUT

Definition. Gout represents a group of *genetic* diseases of purine metabolism or excretion ordinarily identifiable by *hyperuricemia.* When clinically manifest, gout presents as an acute inflammatory *arthritis,* the accumulation of sodium urate deposits as *tophi, uric acid nephrolithiasis,* or *renal failure.* These manifestations can occur in any combination. This definition, which must remain arbitrary until the pathogenesis of each gouty syndrome has been more firmly established, has several points of emphasis which will be discussed more fully later in this chapter. First, it emphasizes the genetic or familial origin of gout. This attribute has long been recognized. Galen attributed gout to "debauchery, intemperance, and an hereditary trait," and Sydenham emphasized its early occurrence in patients "when they have received the ill seeds of this disease from their parents by inheritance." Second, gout is defined here in terms of its chemical derangement, essentially hyperuricemia. This is analogous to the diagnosis of diabetes mellitus as essential hyperglucosemia. The clinical manifestations are complications of hyperuricemia (or hyperuricaciduria) which may or may not occur in the individual patient. It has been estimated that these complications in some combination occur in only 10 to 20 per cent of individuals with hyperuricemia, the incidence increasing in rough proportion to the level of serum uric acid. Finally, the definition emphasizes the heterogeneity of gout. Several different diseases lead to the common feature of persistent hyperuricemia (see Pathogenesis and Table 1).

In a sense all of us have inappropriate hyperuricemia

because of two errors in evolution. Uricase catalyzes the conversion of relatively insoluble urate to soluble allantoin, which would be a much more appropriate end product for the mammalian kidney. The evolutionary retention of this enzyme would have obviated both gout and uric acid nephrolithiasis. A second error compounds the first. The mechanism by which the human kidney excretes uric acid is complex, including glomerular filtration, tubular reabsorption, and tubular secretion. The net result is renal retention of more than 90 per cent of that filtered. At equilibrium, the same amount of uric acid is presumably excreted but at the cost of relative hyperuricemia. Renal tubular reabsorption of filtered uric acid is not present in other primates, which therefore have serum uric acid levels of less than 0.05 mg per 100 ml. The suggestion has been made that renal retention might help to modulate bursts of uric acid excretion owing to purine ingestion, and also might shunt more urate into the gut for bacterial destruction. Whether this is true or not, it seems clear that gout represents an exaggeration of a genetic legacy of hyperuricemia common to all.

History. Gout has figured largely in history, perhaps rivaled only by pandemics of infectious diseases and mental illness. Its classic manifestations were noted in classical times, and the occurrence of osseous tophi and uric acid stones has allowed archeologic diagnoses to be made with confidence. Hippocrates, who recognized and described podagra, devoted three of his aphorisms to the disease, saying in effect: 28, Eunuchs do not take the gout, nor become bald; 29, Women do not take the gout until their menses be stopped; 30, Young men do not take the gout until they indulge in coition. Galen described tophaceous gout and commented upon the familial occurrence of the disease. The term gout, derived from the Latin word *gutta*, came into usage during the Middle Ages to reflect a theory of pathogenesis that this form of arthritis resulted from the "dropping" of a poisonous "*noxa*" into the joint. It is interesting to see the recent confirmation of this theory and the identification of sodium urate microcrystals as the *noxa*. In the seventeenth century, Thomas Sydenham (1683), sometimes called the Shakespeare of gout, wrote clinical descriptions of the disease which have yet to be improved on. He wrote with an authority based on intense personal experience with gouty arthritis and stones. Uric acid was first discovered as a component of stones by Scheele in 1776 (designated lithic acid), followed two decades later by its identification in tophi by Wallaston (1797). In the middle of the nineteenth century the elder (A. B.) Garrod developed a crude but ingenious method for estimating uric acid in serum (crystallization on a linen fiber), and found it to be elevated in patients with gout, demonstrating for the first time the chemical hallmark of the disease. His postulate that acute gouty arthritis was due to deposits of sodium urate was convincingly supported by the work of Freudweiler (1899), who demonstrated the inflammatory potential of sodium urate microcrystals and leukocytic phagocytosis of such crystals in acute gout. This contribution was lost in the sediment of subsequent investigations, the phenomenon of *microcrystalline synovitis* being independently rediscovered within the past few years. In 1931, the younger (A. E.) Garrod proposed that gout should be classified as one of the inborn errors of metabolism. Over the past two decades studies in many laboratories, notably those of Buchanan, Greenberg, Seegmiller, and Wyngaarden, have elucidated the pathways of purine biosynthesis and degradation and the controlling mechanisms for modulating the appropriate rate of control of purine metabolism. It is against this background that current studies of pathogenesis, to be reviewed below, are being conducted.

The history of gout has been intermingled with sociologic and cultural variables as well as the march of medical and biochemical progress. From earliest observations the disease has been associated with dissipation and venery. Even gouty Sydenham wrote, "the gout generally attacks those aged persons who have spent most of their lives in ease, voluptuousness, high living, and too free use of wine and other spirituous liquors." It gradually became a disease in caricature in the eighteenth and nineteenth centuries, used by novelist, satirist, and political cartoonist alike as symbolic of medical retribution for excessive indulgence of natural appetites. Ambrose Bierce defined gout as "a physician's name for the rheumatism of a rich patient." The disease gradually won grudging respect ("disease of kings and king of diseases") because of its remarkable association with men of genius and exceptional achievement. An incomplete list of those alleged to have suffered from the gout includes Alexander the Great, Louis XIV, Isaac Newton, William Harvey, Martin Luther, John Calvin, Leonardo da Vinci, Samuel Johnson, and Benjamin Franklin. It is an amusing sequel that several recent studies have confirmed positive statistical corre-

lations of serum uric acid levels and intelligence or social status. In this context it is unkind to recall, with Hippocrates, that gout is rare in the premenopausal female.

Genetics of Gout. Family aggregation of clinical gout has been observed since the first clinical descriptions of the disease in antiquity. Gout has appeared in an irregular pattern both in successive generations and in sibships. A positive family history for clinical gout is found in about 10 to 20 per cent of patients with the primary disorder. Attempts have been made to use hyperuricemia as a more precise marker for the presence of the gouty trait. Within the restrictions imposed by the statistical uncertainties of the boundary between normal and abnormal serum urate levels (Fig. 1), hyperuricemia has been found in 15 to 25 per cent of close relatives of patients with clinical gout. It is sometimes stated that primary gout is transmitted as an autosomal dominant with incomplete penetrance. The pattern of inheritance of hyperuricemia has varied so widely that it may be polygenic in origin. Many variables affect the phenotypic expression of the gouty trait: age, sex, diet, and renal function. It is noteworthy that in the form of gout in which a specific enzyme defect of purine metabolism has been most clearly established, the syndrome of hypoxanthine–guanine phosphoribosyltransferase deficiency, the genetic transmission has been established as that of a sex-linked recessive trait. Glycogen storage disease Type I, which is associated with a specific form of secondary renal gout, is transmitted as an autosomal recessive trait. It seems probable that the mode of inheritance of other forms of gout will not be clearly established until genetic markers more specific than hyperuricemia are available. This must await clarification of the pathogenesis of the various gouty syndromes in more specific phenotypic terms.

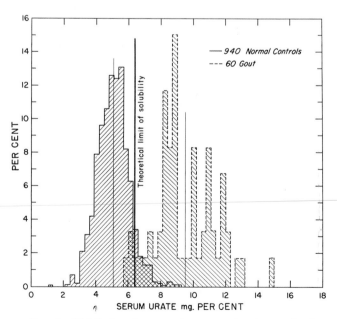

Figure 1. Distribution of serum urate concentrations in normal and gouty male subjects and calculated limit of solubility of sodium urate in serum. (From Seegmiller, J. E.: Diseases of purine and pyrimidine metabolism. *In* Bondy, P. K., and Rosenberg, L. E. [eds.]: Duncan's Diseases of Metabolism. 7th ed. Philadelphia, W. B. Saunders Company, 1974.)

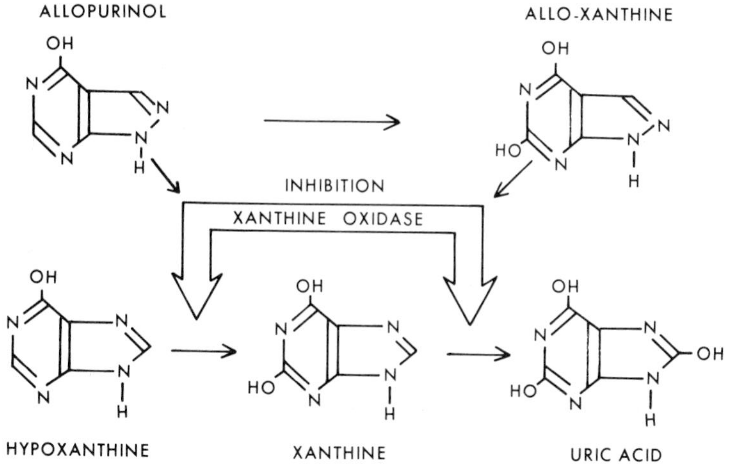

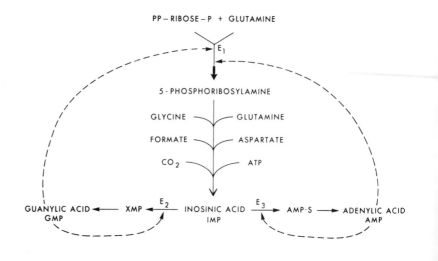

Figure 2. Pathway of uric acid synthesis catalyzed by xanthine oxidase and the site of action of allopurinol.

Pathogenesis. It has been established for over 100 years (A. B. Garrod) that the hallmark of gout is hyperuricemia. All of the clinical manifestations of gout, with the single exception of uric acid nephrolithiasis, derive from the cystallization of sodium urate from extracellular fluids where it has accumulated in a supersaturated concentration. No one has shown that sodium urate in solution is toxic. There are several questions which relate to the pathogenesis of gout: What leads to the accumulation of urate in extracellular fluid? What are the variables in its precipitation? How do sodium urate crystals lead to inflammatory arthritis?

The Cause of Hyperuricemia. The accumulation of any metabolite in excess must result from one (or a combination) of four variables: increased absorption, decreased metabolism, decreased excretion, or increased biosynthesis. There is no evidence that gouty patients habitually ingest excessive purines or have an increased avidity for purine absorption. Elimination of purine ingestion usually results in a reduction of serum urate of about 0.6 mg per 100 ml in normal subjects and about 1.0 mg per 100 ml in gouty patients. Under experimental conditions, ingestion of a diet very high in nucleic acids may lead to hyperuricemia in normal subjects comparable to gouty levels. In summary, absorption of preformed purines from dietary sources may modify extracellular urate levels, but does not represent a primary cause of gout.

Uric acid is the end product of purine metabolism, most of it being excreted as free urinary urate. Recent studies have indicated at least two mechanisms by which it is partially destroyed in man. Leukocytes contain verdoperoxidases capable of degrading uric acid to allantoin and carbon dioxide. Of much greater importance quantitatively, uric acid is secreted into the gut where uricolysis is carried out by bacterial enzymes. Approximately one quarter of that synthesized daily is degraded through these mechanisms. Studies in gout have not supported decreased uricolysis as a mechanism for hyperuricemia. In fact, with high urate concentrations, especially after the onset of renal insufficiency, excretion into the gut, and uricolysis there, may be enhanced as an important second line of defense. Particular attention has therefore been directed toward increased synthesis or decreased excretion as primary mechanisms for hyperuricemia in gout.

Uric acid is synthesized from xanthine and from hypoxanthine (via xanthine), these successive oxidations being catalyzed by xanthine oxidase (Fig. 2). The free purine bases bear complex metabolic relationships to various pools of purine nucleotides. In part the free bases are reutilized to form functioning nucleotides; in part they are converted to uric acid for excretion. Be-

Figure 3. De novo pathway of purine nucleotide biosynthesis and the feedback control mechanisms (— — — →). E_1, Glutamine 5-phosphoribosylpyrophosphate amidotransferase; E_2, inosine 5′-phosphate dehydrogenase; E_3, adenylsuccinic acid (AMP-S) synthetase; XMP, xanthosine 5′-phosphate.

cause of this reutilization, sometimes called "salvage synthesis," uric acid synthesis, as reflected in urinary excretion and intestinal destruction, represents only a part of the purine nucleotide turnover rate. At equilibrium, however, that part should approximate the the de novo synthetic rate of purine nucleotides. Small amounts of hypoxanthine, xanthine, and other trace purines are normally excreted in the urine as well. Several methods have been widely applied in an attempt to determine whether there is excessive purine synthesis in gout: measurement of urate excreted on a low purine diet, use of isotopic urate to determine its pool size and turnover rate, and study of the time course of incorporation of a purine precursor, usually glycine, into urate (Fig. 3). Each of these methods is subject to limitations which cannot be detailed here. The following information has emerged from such studies. In normal man the daily rate of production of uric acid on a low purine diet averages about 750 mg. The miscible pool of uric acid is about 1.0 to 1.3 grams, so that two thirds to three fourths of the body pool turns over daily. Urinary excretion of urate varies widely even during dietary regulation, averaging in men 426 ± 81 mg per 24 hours. The difference between the estimated production rate of urate and that excreted in the urine represents uricolysis, mostly by bacterial action in the gut.

By use of these methods, evidence for excessive synthesis of uric acid has been obtained in about two thirds of patients with primary gout. Overproduction is readily understood in patients with diseases resulting in increased tissue breakdown, e.g., myeloid metaplasia, polycythemia vera, and leukemia. The hypoxanthine-guanine phosphoribosyltransferase deficiency syndrome will be discussed later in this chapter as the biochemical basis for excessive purine synthesis in one form of gout. The first step unique to purine nucleotide biosynthesis and the major site of metabolic regulation is that of the synthesis of phosphoribosylamine, catalyzed by the enzyme glutamine 5-phosphoribosyl-pyrophosphate (PRPP) amidotransferase:

$$\text{Glutamine} + \text{PRPP} + \text{H}_2\text{O} \xrightarrow{\text{Mg}^{++}} \text{glutamic acid} + \\ \text{5-phosphoribosylamine} + \text{pyrophosphate}$$

There are several possibilities for loss of normal rate control at this regulatory site; these include excessive concentrations of the substrate glutamine, PRRP, or both, a genetic alteration in the enzyme rendering it less sensitive to normal feedback control by purine nucleotides, or a partial deficiency of one of the nucleotides (adenylic, guanylic, and inosinic acids) which, in concert, exert allosteric modulation of the enzyme (Fig. 3). Recent work from two laboratories has demonstrated increased activity of PRPP synthetase in a few patients with gout, presumably driving purine synthesis by excessive availability of PRPP. Glutamate but not glutamine is raised in the plasma of a number of gouty patients. It can be anticipated that future studies will document further heterogeneity in the mechanisms by which purine synthesis is enhanced in various types of overproduction gout.

In about one third of patients with gout there is no evidence for overproduction of uric acid by any of the methods now available. Evidence suggests that these patients have an inherited disorder (or group of disorders) of the renal tubule resulting in decreased urate clearance as the cause of hyperuricemia. Renal clearance of urate is a complex function of filtration, tubular reabsorption, and tubular secretion. There is partial binding of urate to plasma proteins, but this does not seem to represent a significant fraction under physiologic conditions at 37° C. Using the assumption that urate is completely filterable at the glomerulus, there is net tubular reabsorption of 90 to 95 per cent. Urate which is excreted is in part and perhaps in toto that secreted by the tubule. Patients with "renal gout" exhibit reduced clearances of urate, the differences being most evident when compared to normal controls with dietary induction of comparable plasma levels of uric acid. The differences have not always been striking, and in some cases may be difficult to interpret because of early impairment of renal function by gout. In renal gout reduced net clearance of urate probably results from a defect in its tubular secretion, although enhanced tubular reabsorption of urate has not been excluded. In theory, an increase in the bound fraction of urate would also reduce clearance by reducing that filtered. An impaired tubular secretion of urate might be an intrinsic defect of the transport mechanism, which has not yet been clarified biochemically. It might also result from a genetic or acquired metabolic disorder in some other pathway which leads to the accumulation of a metabolite which secondarily interferes with tubular urate secretion. An example of this latter mechanism is the hyperuricemia associated with the lactic acidosis of Type I glycogen storage disease (see Ch. 809). Idiopathic renal gout might similarly result from the accumulation of other uric acid transport inhibitors not yet identified. When over-all reduction of renal function occurs, as happens not infrequently in gout, hyperuricemia is further exacerbated, and an increased percentage of urate is excreted into the gut for uricolysis.

In summary, the important causes of persistent hyperuricemia are those of excessive synthesis and decreased renal clearance. This allows for a rational classification of gout as shown in Table 1. Such a classification reflects only a progress report. Although hypoxanthine–guanine phosphoribosyltransferase deficiency and PRPP synthetase excess represent the only types of metabolic gout for which specific enzymatic defects have been established, new defects in the rate control mechanisms will almost certainly be established shortly, possibly as abnormalities of phosphoribosyl-

TABLE 1.   Classification of Hyperuricemia
and Gout

I. Metabolic gout—excessive synthesis
  A. Genetic
    1. Hypoxanthine–guanine phosphoribosyltransferase deficiency
     —Lesch-Nyhan syndrome or incomplete forms
    2. Excessive activity of 5-phosphoribosylpyrophosphate
     synthetase
    3. Other defects of rate control
  B. Acquired—excessive tissue turnover
II. Renal gout—reduced clearance
  A. Genetic— ↓ renal tubular secretion?
    1. Idiopathic
    2. Lactic acidosis—glycogen storage disease Type I
  B. Acquired
    1. Inhibition of urate transport—drugs, metabolites (lactic acid,
     β-hydroxybutyric acid)
    2. Renal failure

pyrophosphate amidotransferase. Similarly, the genetic types of renal gout will probably prove to be more heterogeneous in future studies. A variety of drugs (notably the chlorothiazide diuretics) and metabolites (lactate, β-hydroxybutyrate) diminish urate clearance in the normal kidney, and may precipitate clinical gout.

Precipitation of Urate. Uric acid is not toxic to man in its soluble state. Although hyperuricemia has been associated epidemiologically with a number of conditions, e.g., coronary artery heart disease and hypertension, there is no evidence that it has any pathogenic relationship to those disorders. Uric acid seems to produce disease "physically" rather than "chemically" when precipitated as sodium urate at pH 7.40, or as uric acid in acidic urine. Its precipitation as amorphous sodium urate, which may occur in virtually any tissue in the body except for the central nervous system, results in tophi with tissue disruption and destruction but with minimal inflammatory response. Its precipitation as microcrystals of critical size in certain tissues, especially in synovial tissues and spaces, leads to an acute inflammatory reaction to be described below. Its precipitation in the renal distal collecting tubules as uric acid may rarely lead to acute renal failure. The precipitation of uric acid in a protein matrix in the renal pelvis, or more rarely in the ureter or bladder, leads to uric acid nephrolithiasis.

Sodium urate is soluble in human plasma to a concentration of only about 7 mg of urate per 100 ml. Values above this denote supersaturated solutions, although sodium urate may remain in supersaturated solution with considerable stability. Why do some patients with serum uric acid levels of 9 mg per 100 ml have severe tophaceous gout or acute gouty arthritis or both, whereas others may maintain similar levels for years or even for life with no evidence of precipitation, i.e., of clinical gout? The reasons for these differences in threshold of precipitation are not known. One recently described variable is that of protein binding of urate in plasma to a specific α_1-α_2 globulin (Alvsaker) and to albumin. The report that some patients with tophaceous gout have reduced protein-binding of urate is provocative but has not been confirmed. Furthermore, the importance of protein-binding of urate remains to be established.

The solubility of urate in urine decreases with increasing acidity because of the shift to free uric acid. The titration curve is such that the undissociated uric acid increases to 85 per cent at pH 5.0. At this pH only 6 to 8 mg of urate is soluble per 100 ml of urine so that supersaturation is required to excrete an average uric acid load in a normal urine volume. The solubility increases 20-fold at pH 7.0 over that at pH 5.0. Three factors are therefore important in the urinary precipitation of uric acid: urine volume, the amount of urate excreted per 24 hours, and urine pH. It is possible that the availability of stone matrix and the level of stabilizing substances in urine may also play important roles.

Cause of Acute Gouty Arthritis. The four clinical manifestations of gout are those of tophaceous deposits, acute gouty arthritis, uric acid nephrolithiasis, and gouty kidney with various degrees of impairment of renal function. Of these clinical manifestations or complications associated with hyperuricemia, acute inflammatory arthritis is that which has been most obscure in its pathogenesis. Garrod the elder, in the second of his

ten propositions on "the true nature or essence of gout" (1859), wrote: "Investigations recently made in the morbid anatomy of gout prove incontestably that true gouty inflammation is always accompanied with a deposition of urate of soda in the inflamed part." This proposition was strongly supported by the experimental work of Freudweiler (1899), who was able to produce inflammation with sodium urate crystals and observe their subsequent presence in leukocytes. For many years, however, this work was ignored because of evidence which seemed to indicate that retention of uric acid, the seemingly obvious basis of tophi, was unrelated to the sudden acute attacks of inflammatory arthritis. Several pieces of evidence supported that view. The onset of acute attacks bore no relation to changes in serum urate levels. Joints severely involved with tophaceous deposits were often free from acute attacks. Despite its almost specific therapeutic effectiveness, colchicine had no demonstrable effect on urate metabolism. During reductions of serum urate levels with uricosuric drugs, attacks of acute gouty arthritis were fairly often exacerbated. Because of these and other observations, major attention was directed toward alternative explanations, such as abnormalities in the metabolism of trace purines.

Within the past few years gouty arthritis has been clearly shown to be an inflammatory reaction to microcrystals of sodium urate, mediated by a series of chemical changes accompanying phagocytosis of the crystals by leukocytes. The presence of sodium urate microcrystals in synovial fluid from gouty joints during acute inflammation, both free and in leukocytes, is so con-

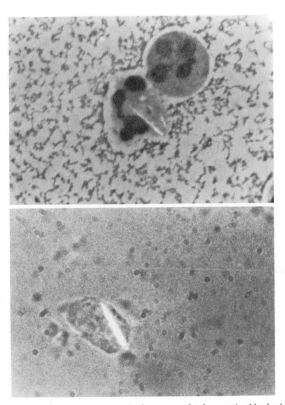

Figure 4. Sodium urate monohydrate crystals phagocytized by leukocytes in synovial fluid from acute gouty arthritis examined by polarized light. (Reproduced with permission of Dr. Daniel J. McCarty, Jr.)

stant as to be of diagnostic value (Fig. 4). This was the key observation that led to the experiments supporting the early Garrod-Freudweiler concept. The injection of sodium urate microcrystals into joints of normal controls or gouty patients produces typical gout responsive to colchicine. Aspiration of these joints demonstrates phagocytosis of some of the injected crystals. In fact, no experimental gouty arthritis can be produced in laboratory animals in the absence of leukocytes. The inflammatory reaction of microcrystalline synovitis is a nonspecific one, being produced by injection of other crystals of appropriate size and shape, such as sodium orotate or calcium pyrophosphate.

The exact mechanism by which sodium urate crystals initiate inflammation has not been established. The crystals can activate Hageman factor, and in this way initiate the chain of events resulting in bradykinin synthesis. Bradykinin levels are raised in synovial fluid from gouty joints, but injection of carboxypeptidase B, which destroys bradykinin, does not prevent experimental gout. The requirement for leukocyte-crystal interaction was noted above. Uric acid has been found to be leukotactic. Phagocytosis of the crystals leads to increased metabolic activity of the leukocyte, release of lysosomal enzymes, and increased lactic acid production. Interesting studies on the molecular basis of crystal-induced inflammation have been carried out recently (Weissmann, McCarty). Phagocytosis of sodium urate crystals leads to rapid destruction of the phagolysosome membrane, releasing its hydrolytic enzymes into the cell cytoplasm. This results in cell lysis. The original crystal, the hydrolytic enzymes, and the cytoplasmic enzymes from the destroyed leukocyte are released into the surrounding tissue. This crystal-membrane interaction, which can be simulated with artificial lipid membranes ("liposomes") as well, is thought to result from hydrogen bonding between the rigid crystal and elements in the lipid membrane surface, leading to breaks in its continuity. The attack of the leukocyte on the sodium urate crystal is therefore both suicidal and counterproductive, setting in motion an inappropriate inflammatory response which is injurious to the host.

Although the biochemical events of inflammation are poorly understood, the establishment of the general mechanism of microcrystalline synovitis has allowed a rational explanation of acute gouty arthritis. Still unexplained are the mechanisms by which the acute attack is initiated, i.e., what leads to the presumed burst of microcrystallization at a given time. How are the known precipitating events of acute gouty arthritis, which may be roughly grouped together as stresses, translated into microcrystallization?

The model of leukocyte-crystal interaction may offer an explanation for the action of colchicine. As stated, in the therapeutic range colchicine has no effect on net purine metabolism as reflected in levels of extracellular uric acid or in its excretion. On the other hand, colchicine diminishes leukocyte migration and modifies many of the metabolic concomitants of phagocytosis in the leukocyte. The use of such an in vitro model may allow the rational development of other therapeutic agents in the future.

Clinical Manifestations. As previously stated, the clinical manifestations of gout can be arbitrarily divided into four categories: acute gouty arthritis, tophaceous gout, uric acid nephrolithiasis, and gouty kidney. Although the basic metabolic abnormalities of genetic gout must be presumed to have been present since conception, clinical gout is extraordinarily rare before the rise in extracellular uric acid levels which accompany puberty in the male. Exceptions to this are seen in the juvenile gout of the Lesch-Nyhan syndrome and in glycogen storage disease Type I. Clinical gout usually makes its appearance in middle life in men, although the majority of patients with hyperuricemia never exhibit these complications. As observed by Hippocrates, clinical gout in women rarely occurs before the menopause, at which time there is a further rise in uric acid levels. In most series, gout in women accounts for only 5 to 10 per cent of cases.

The epidemiology of gout and hyperuricemia has received increasing attention beyond the genetic studies of families. The positive statistical correlation of uric acid levels with education, intelligence, and social status was pointed out above. Exceptionally high frequencies of hyperuricemia have been found in Filipinos (in the United States but not in the Philippines), in Maoris, and in the natives of the Marianas Islands. The over-all incidence of clinical gout in the United States has been estimated as 3 patients per 1000 population. As a generality it has been stated that gout makes up about 5 per cent of arthritis.

Acute Gouty Arthritis. Acute gouty arthritis is the most frequent first clinical manifestation of the disease. It has been eloquently described by many who have endured it, but by none more effectively than Sydenham, who wrote, "it [the affected part] is not able to bear the weight of the cloths upon it, nor hard walking in the chamber." He further alluded to the pain as being "like the gnawing of a dog." Acute gouty arthritis often follows a precipitating event: surgery, injury, alcohol ingestion, dietary excess, emotional stress, or even the minor stress of excessive walking. In view of the current concept of the pathogenesis as that of microcrystalline synovitis, such stress must somehow be translated into localized sodium urate crystallization, or must alter the tissue reaction to such crystals. Since sodium urate usually exists in a supersaturated solution in the gouty patient, the initiating event need introduce only a single crystal focus for seeding a cascade of precipitation. Some of the precipitating events, such as starvation and alcohol ingestion, increase urate levels by inhibition of renal urate excretion through the accompanying ketosis and lactic acidosis, respectively. The particular association of gout with spirituous liquors, legendary in medieval history ("in the young wine goes to the head; in the aged it goes to the feet"), therefore finds some scientific basis at the level of the renal tubule. A particularly puzzling and important kind of exacerbation of acute gouty arthritis is that which frequently occurs during early stages of treatment designed to lower extracellular urate levels. This may complicate the use of uricosuric agents or of allopurinol, to the great distress of both patient and physician. It has been difficult to explain the exacerbation of gout in the face of a falling urate concentration. It is possible that mobilization of amorphous tophaceous deposits may allow for local precipitation of the microcrystals conducive to inflammation. The frequent occurrence of this complication may occasionally obviate or delay effective treatment.

Gout usually presents as a sudden, exquisitely painful arthritis. After a few premonitory twinges the onset of inflammation may occur within minutes with severe arthritis within a few hours. Typically a patient may retire for the night in good health, yet be awakened a few hours later with excruciating pain in the affected joint. He may develop podagra (gouty arthritis of the first metatarsophalangeal joint) with such rapidity that he is unable to remove his shoe in time. More rarely the warning signals of impending arthritis develop into a crescendo pattern ending in the acute attack.

Gouty arthritis exhibits a marked predilection for the larger joints, particularly in the feet and ankles. Hippocrates described podagra, which still represents the most frequent site of involvement (Fig. 5). This may reflect the trauma of weight-bearing which in the normal foot produces the greatest force per unit area (pressure) there. Other frequent sites of early attacks are the ankle, the instep, or occasionally the knee. Less frequently the elbow, wrist, or metacarpophalangeal joints are the sites of gouty arthritis. The hips, shoulders, and spine are very rarely the sites of microcrystalline synovitis, and almost never the sites of initial involvement. Gouty arthritis is usually monoarticular, especially in the earliest attacks. Some patients may have marked tophaceous gout with bone and articular destruction and few if any attacks of acute gout. Involvement of a joint by tophi does not seem to predispose that area to acute attacks, and some clinicians have even suggested that tophaceous areas enjoy relative immunity from acute inflammation.

Acute gouty arthritis is characterized by severe inflammation, not only in the joint itself but typically in the periarticular tissues and skin. The presence of heat, marked swelling, exquisite tenderness, and rubor extending well beyond the immediate vicinity of the joint capsule has often led to the erroneous diagnosis of septic arthritis or cellulitis. Occasionally lymphangitis may be evident. The skin over the area of inflammation is usually tense and shiny, and after subsidence of the attack undergoes superficial desquamation as is seen in erysipelas. Systemic signs of inflammation may include fever, leukocytosis, and elevation of the sedimentation

rate which may further suggest an infectious etiology. The severity of the associated pain has been referred to above, and commands respect and attention rather than the traditional jocularity. When untreated, an attack of acute gouty arthritis usually subsides gradually over a period of one to two weeks. Generally there are no residual signs or symptoms; more rarely, stiffness persists, or a second flareup supervenes before there is complete recovery.

As stated, only about one of six patients with hyperuricemia will eventually have one or more of the complications of clinical gout. Moreover, the clinical course of gout after an initial attack of acute arthritis is highly variable. Some patients have only a single attack of monoarticular arthritis and then remain free of symptoms despite the persistence of hyperuricemia. More often, after a symptom-free interval, but usually within the first year, there is recurrence of an attack. In Gutman's series, 62 per cent have had recurrences within the first year, 16 per cent in one to two years, 11 per cent in two to five years, 4 per cent in ten years, and 7 per cent, no recurrence as yet during prolonged follow-up. In the usual pattern, subsequent attacks come with increasing frequency over the years unless prophylactic measures are taken, with gradual reduction in the duration of the symptom-free intervals (sometimes called intercritical gout). In about one third of patients, the number of attacks occurring each year has remained constant, and, rarely, there has been a spontaneous decline in frequency with increasing age of the patient. When attacks become more frequent they also tend to become more severe, both in the extent and duration of the inflammation and in the number of joints affected. The patient may reach a state at which he is rarely free of gouty inflammation, and at which even with subsidence of an acute attack there is enough residual swelling, stiffness, and pain in the involved joints to give permanent disability not responsive to the measures usually effective in acute attacks.

Tophaceous Gout. Sodium urate may accumulate in virtually any tissue in the body with the exception of the central nervous system, where the concentration is reduced by the blood-brain barrier. Tophi occur most

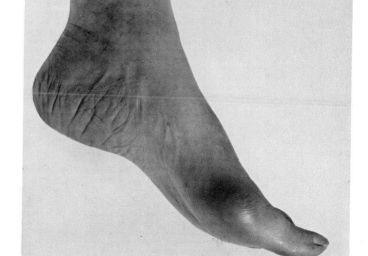

Figure 5. Acute gouty arthritis of great toe.

often in and around joints in cartilage, bone, bursae, and subcutaneous tissue. As foreign bodies, these deposits elicit a low-grade chronic inflammatory process with disruption of tissues and fibrosis. Destruction of tissue is particularly evident in cartilage and bone, leading to radiolucent "punched-out" lesions of bone and gross deformities of joints (Figs. 6 and 7). Deposits of sodium urate may be massive, particularly in the hands and feet and around the olecranon bursa. Subcutaneous deposits may be easily visible as yellowish-white excrescences, which on occasion may erode through the skin and discharge a pale paste composed largely of crystalline needles of sodium urate. In advanced cases, deposits of several hundred grams may lead to grotesquely deformed extremities. Rarely, involvement of the heart has been observed with tophi causing conduction disturbances. A frequent site of tophaceous deposits is the external ear, especially in the helix and antihelix. The local factors that control the sites of crystallization are not known. Massive tophi may be found in the hands, feet, and elbows with none of the typical auricular deposits. Conversely, the external ear may be the only site of visible tophi over many years of gouty diathesis. As stated above, recent work suggesting that patients most susceptible to tophi may have reduced protein binding of urate has not been confirmed.

About one half of all patients with clinical gout have visible tophi at some stage of their disease. Other patients may have more diffuse deposition of sodium urate without local nodules or infiltrates demonstrable by physical or radiologic examination. The destruction and gross distortion of articular structures (cartilage, bone, capsule, synovial membranes) by tophi leads to a form of chronic gouty arthritis which compounds the stiffness, pain, and fibrosis that may follow repeated attacks of acute gouty arthritis. Although symptomatic and objective improvement may occur with proper therapy, this late stage of destructive gout cannot be completely reversed. One of the objectives of modern management is to prevent the excessive accumulation of urate that results in tophaceous destruction and connective tissue reaction.

Uric Acid Nephrolithiasis. Kidney stones are very common. It has been estimated that 1 in every 1000 inhabitants of the United States is hospitalized annually because of a kidney stone. This figure does not include those whose stones remain in situ or are passed without hospitalization. In large series it has been found that 5 to 10 per cent of all kidney stones in adults are composed mainly of uric acid deposits within a protein matrix. Uric acid may serve as the nidus for a stone of mixed composition, in particular in association with calcium oxalate. Pure uric acid stones are radiolucent, being demonstrable only by the use of contrast media. Other radiolucent stones, so-called matrix stones which are predominantly proteinaceous and xanthine stones, are extremely rare.

Most patients with uric acid stones do not have clinical gout. On the other hand, patients with gout are much more likely to have stones. The frequency of stones in primary or genetic gout has been estimated at 15 to 20 per cent, and in secondary overproduction gout (e.g., myeloid metaplasia, polycythemia vera) at 35 to 40 per cent. Stone formation may occur at any stage in the disease, as the first manifestation of gout or as a late complication in the course of crippling arthritis. Stones may be infrequent or, rarely, they may be the main problem, with almost constant uric acid gravel and superimposed episodes of acute renal colic from passage of larger stones.

As noted earlier, the absolute amount of uric acid excreted per 24 hours is only one of the factors conducive to stone formation. A concentrated acidic urine increases the likelihood of stones at any level of uricaciduria. Some investigators have reported that patients with gout, and certain other patients with uric acid stone diathesis, habitually excrete more acid urine. It is postulated that this reflects a shift toward increased titratable acidity rather than ammonia excretion because of a relative defect in renal ammonia production. These data have been both confirmed and denied, perhaps an indication in part of the difficulty in choosing proper controls.

Gouty Renal Disease. A selective defect in urate

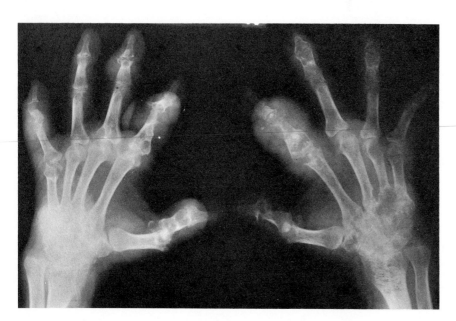

Figure 6. Chronic gouty arthritis with tophaceous destruction of bone and joints.

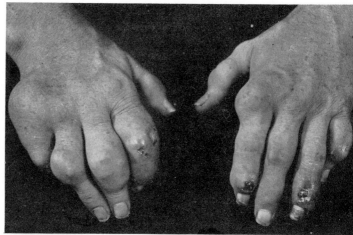

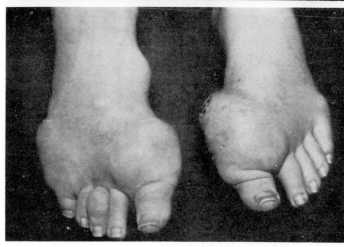

Figure 7. Advanced tophaceous gout, with ulcerations.

excretion may be the basic defect in possibly one third of all patients with gout. Extracellular urate rises non-specifically in all patients with renal insufficiency, uric acid representing one component of nonprotein nitrogen. The onset of renal failure in gout tends to exacerbate the disease, especially the frequency and severity of tophaceous deposits. More generally, renal tubular reabsorption of urate in man, as opposed to other primates, leads to inappropriate urate retention without which there would be no gout. The kidney therefore plays a significant role in the pathogenesis and progression of gout.

Conversely, gout may impair renal function and lead to death in uremia. The so-called gouty kidney represents a variable mixture of factors. Sodium urate may crystallize in the renal interstitial tissue, especially in the pyramids, with tissue destruction and distortion and a low-grade inflammatory reaction leading to fibrosis. In addition to this primary lesion, uric acid stones lead to obstruction with hydronephrosis and increased susceptibility to chronic pyelonephritis, a complication quite often found in late-stage gouty kidney. Finally, gout, or at least hyperuricemia, carries a statistical association with accelerated vascular disease and hypertension, so that nephrosclerosis may contribute in some measure to impairment of renal function. There are no characteristic clinical or laboratory find-

ings to distinguish gouty kidney from chronic glomerulonephritis except for the association of the former with clinical gout. The question whether gout (i.e., hyperuricemia) ever leads to renal failure in the absence of the other three manifestations of the disease, i.e., arthritis, tophi, and stones, is pertinent to the prophylactic treatment of patients discovered to have essential hyperuricemia (considered here to be gout without complications). Gouty kidney in the absence of these manifestations of clinical gout is extraordinarily rare, and even then the entity may be open to question because of variable interpretations of renal pathology. One unusual family has been described in which this syndrome occurred.

A particular form of uric acid nephropathy may be found in the absence of clinical gout. With sudden exceptionally high levels of uric acid excretion, seen almost exclusively after chemotherapeutic or radiation therapy of certain malignant myeloproliferative disorders, crystals may occlude the distal collecting tubules, leading to acute renal failure. These intraluminal crystals are uric acid rather than sodium urate, precipitate in the distal tubule in which maximal concentration and acidification occur, and lead to intranephronic hydronephrosis. This complication is easy to prevent with fluids, alkalinization of the urine, and allopurinol inhibition of urate synthesis. Oliguria, once

TABLE 2.   Diseases Associated with Gout

1. Myeloproliferative disorders
2. Psoriasis
3. Sarcoidosis
4. Glycogen storage disease Type I (glucose-6-phosphatase deficiency)
5. Diabetes mellitus
6. Hyperparathyroidism
7. Chronic renal disease—glomerulonephritis, pyelonephritis, hereditary nephropathy
8. Lead poisoning

established, usually follows a course similar to that seen with acute renal failure secondary to shock or to an incompatible blood transfusion.

Diseases Associated with Gout (Table 2). Several diseases have been described in association with gout. In some cases, the relationship seems to be clear pathogenically, as outlined in the classification of gout in Table 1. Some associations have not yet been so explained. Many diseases which lead to continued tissue synthesis and breakdown may produce hyperuricemia and clinical gout because of the resulting increased turnover of nucleic acids and functional nucleotides. This form of secondary or acquired metabolic gout is that seen with polycythemia vera, myeloid metaplasia, chronic leukemia, mast cell disease, extensive psoriasis, and sarcoidosis. The triad of sarcoidosis-psoriasis-gout has been described in a small number of patients, although this may represent the fortuitous coincidence of two quite common diseases, both of which may be productive of secondary gout. Severe gout may be a major complication in surviving patients with glycogen storage disease Type I because of the constant lactic acidosis which inhibits renal tubular urate secretion. Studies with isotopic glycine also suggest excessive synthesis of urate in this disease. It has been suggested that this may result from excessive synthesis of PRPP, one of the substrates for the rate-limiting initial step in purine synthesis catalyzed by glutamine 5-phosphoribosylpyrophosphate amidotransferase. The hyperuricemia of starvation has a similar mechanism in that β-hydroxybutyrate, as one of the ketone bodies, also inhibits renal urate excretion. The association of gout and diabetes mellitus is not a strong one. Three to 5 per cent of patients with gout have diabetes, but this figure is not far from that of the incidence of diabetes in the general population when adjusted for age. Some diabetic patients considered to have atypical gout in the past in fact have pseudogout, as described in Ch. 97. Over the last decade several clinics have documented a high incidence of hyperuricemia and clinical gout in patients with primary hyperparathyroidism even in the absence of renal failure. This relationship is obscure, because the hyperuricemia has not always responded to successful surgical treatment of the hyperfunctioning parathyroid glands. Hyperuricemia may also be found in hypothyroidism. Renal insufficiency is a common cause of hyperuricemia. It is surprising how rarely this results in clinical gout in view of the high concentrations of uric acid which may be found. It may be that hyperuricemia in uremia does not have sufficient duration, i.e., time at risk, to result in a high incidence of sodium urate precipitation. Uremia may also interfere in some way with the crystallization potential of sodium urate, as it does for bone salts in osteoid, or diminish the inflammatory response to such crystals when they occur. Garrod commented upon the association of lead poisoning and gout in his treatise of 1876, and this has been repeatedly confirmed in subsequent reports. Saturnine gout, as it has been called, occurs late in the course of chronic plumbism. The mechanism has not been established but it has been supposed that enhanced breakdown of tissue, including the erythropoietic series, is the origin of excessive urate synthesis in lead poisoning. Hyperuricemia has also been described in Down's syndrome and in nephrogenic diabetes insipidus.

Pseudogout. The syndrome of pseudogout, also called *chondrocalcinosis articularis,* is considered as a separate entity in Ch. 97.

Hypoxanthine–Guanine Phosphoribosyltransferase (HG-PRT) Deficiency. The X-linked genetic disease HG-PRT deficiency is a form of gout associated with overproduction of urate in which a specific enzymatic defect has been clearly established. It is important beyond its relative infrequency, because (1) the enzymatic defect can be demonstrated as a cause of excessive purine synthesis; (2) the mechanism of genetic transmission is known, in contrast to other forms of gout except for glycogen storage disease Type I; and (3) in its complete form it produces a distinct clinical picture with neurologic abnormalities: the Lesch-Nyhan syndrome.

In 1964, Lesch and Nyhan described a distinctive syndrome characterized by mental retardation, choreoathetosis, spasticity, weakness, and compulsive self-mutilation. Patients with this syndrome generally appear normal at birth but show evidence of neurologic deficits and retarded mental development within the first few months of life. Bizarre self-mutilation of extremities, lips, and other oral structures may require constant restraint of the patient, despite the evident pain which accompanies this uncontrollable self-destructive process. These patients often develop uric acid stones and gouty nephropathy which may lead to death in uremia. In contrast, gouty arthritis rarely occurs despite very high levels of extracellular urate. The severity of the neurologic damage usually leads to institutionalization, and most patients with the Lesch-Nyhan syndrome die in childhood, although a few survive to early adult life. Some of the patients have had a megaloblastic anemia resistant to the usual hematinic agents. The enzyme HG-PRT is coded on the X chromosome and the disease is transmitted as an X-linked recessive with no clinical phenotypic expression in hemizygous females. As predicted in the Lyon hypothesis, mothers of children with the Lesch-Nyhan syndrome can be shown by tissue culture of their fibroblasts to exhibit mosaicism, with one cell population deficient in HG-PRT and one in which there is normal enzymatic activity.

The Lesch-Nyhan syndrome as defined above represents one end of the clinical spectrum associated with HG-PRT deficiency. There are some patients who have some incomplete deficiency of HG-PRT with severe clinical gout, marked by excessive synthesis of urate, but without the characteristic mental and neurologic derangements. A minority of these patients have exhibited some neurologic abnormalities: mild spastic quadriplegia, cerebellar ataxia, dysarthria, and seizures. This group of patients, like those with the Lesch-Nyhan syndrome, have been particularly susceptible to uric acid stones as a consequence of the excessive uricaciduria. As might be anticipated, genetic transmission of partial HG-PRT deficiency resembles that of the Lesch-Nyhan syndrome, with relative constancy of phenotypic expression within a given family.

In the catabolism of purine nucleotides, free bases are released as adenine, guanine, and hypoxanthine. In part these undergo deamination and further oxidation to uric acid via hypoxanthine and xanthine, these oxidations being catalyzed by xanthine oxidase. In part, the free bases are reutilized, being coupled with PRPP to form purine nucleotides, a process sometimes described as "salvage synthesis" to distinguish it from de novo synthesis from simple precursors (Fig. 8). To the extent that salvage synthesis preserves the purine bases, the requirement for de novo synthesis is reduced, and at equilibrium urate synthesis and excretion are correspondingly reduced. One enzyme, HG-PRT, catalyzes the salvage synthesis of inosine-5′-phosphate and guanosine-5′-phosphate from hypoxanthine and guanine, respectively. A separate enzyme, A-PRT, catalyzes the synthesis of adenosine-5′-phosphate from adenine (and PRPP). The Lesch-Nyhan syndrome is secondary to a selective, almost complete deficiency of HG-PRT, the activity of adenine PRT being normal, or, more often, significantly increased. By immunologic techniques HG-PRT protein has been found to be present in normal amounts in the Lesch-Nyhan syndrome, indicating that the decrease in enzyme activity is secondary to a structural mutation. The defect, most conveniently shown in hemolysates of erythrocytes, has also been found in fibroblasts and brain. The enzyme activity is normally found in highest concentration in the basal ganglia, a major site of neurologic deficit in the Lesch-Nyhan syndrome. In HG-PRT deficiency, tissue levels of PRPP are increased. Uric acid synthesis is massively increased, with urinary excretion in the range of 50 mg per kilogram per 24 hours (normal being about 6). Patients with partial deficiency of HG-PRT also have severe overproduction gout, with levels of uric acid excretion intermediate in amount between the normal range and those found in the Lesch-Nyhan syndrome (about 20 to 25 mg per kilogram per 24 hours). This excessive purine synthesis probably results from inadequate allosteric inhibition of phosphoribosylamidotransferase, the rate-limiting first step in the biosynthetic sequence, because of reduced tissue levels of guanosine-5′-phosphate and inosine-5′-phosphate. The mechanism of neurologic injury has not been established. It may represent localized purine starvation owing to the inability of de novo synthesis to keep pace with the demands generated by failure of salvage synthesis. It is also possible that the resulting high levels of oxypurines (hypoxanthine and xanthine) in the central nervous system are injurious.

The diagnosis of the Lesch-Nyhan syndrome offers no difficulties when the typical neurologic and mental deficits are combined in a male with marked hyperuricemia, and in particular with grossly abnormal uricaciduria. Partial HG-PRT deficiency may be suspected in a male patient with severe gout, possibly with minor neurologic abnormalities, who excretes uric acid in an amount greater than 0.75 times that of creatinine. The final diagnosis can best be made by enzymatic assay of a hemolysate preparation, preferably sent to one of the laboratories engaged in research on purine metabolism. Therapy is ineffective in preventing or reversing neurologic damage, but may reduce the complications directly related to urate accumulation and excretion, as described below.

Diagnosis. The diagnosis of acute gouty arthritis rarely offers difficulties when there is sudden onset of typical inflammatory involvement of a susceptible joint in a patient with hyperuricemia. Rarely, the serum uric acid concentration may be within the upper range of normal at the time of measurement (Fig. 1), or the arthritis may be atypical in its location or persistence. Rapid response of the pain and inflammation after administration of colchicine is so characteristic as to be of diagnostic usefulness. Some response of rheumatoid arthritis or sarcoid arthritis has been described with colchicine, but the effects are not so dramatic as those in gout. Demonstration of the typical needle-shaped birefringent crystals of sodium urate in leukocytes of synovial fluid is diagnostic of gout. With proper technique, intraleukocytic sodium urate crystals are found in over 95 per cent of aspirates from joints affected by acute gout (Fig. 4). Although use of a polarizing microscope is preferable, sodium urate crystals can also be demonstrated in centrifuged, heparinized joint fluid by examining the sediment with an ordinary microscope. Positive identification of the crystals may be achieved by incubation of the synovial fluid preparation with uricase. The particular characteristics of pseudogout or *chondrocalcinosis articularis* are described in Ch. 97. Occasionally, gout may simulate infectious arthritis or be confused with monarticular rheumatoid arthritis. Examination of the joint fluid, measurement of serum uric acid, and response to colchicine should suffice to establish the diagnosis.

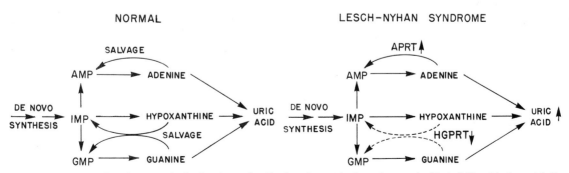

Figure 8. Pathways for salvage synthesis of purine nucleotides from free purine bases in normal subjects (left) and in the metabolic abnormality of hypoxanthine-guanine phosphoribosyltransferase (HG-PRT) deficiency (right). APRT, Adenine phosphoribosyltransferase.

A classification of types of gout according to path-ogenesis has been outlined in Table 1. It is clearly important to determine whether gout is secondary to a myeloproliferative disorder, renal failure, or drug or metabolite interference with renal tubular secretion or urate. In the study of the average patient with idiopathic gout, in the absence of the aforementioned disorders, it is not necessary to establish whether the disease is metabolic (overproduction) gout or renal (underexcretion) gout in order to institute proper treatment. In the absence of clear-cut hyperuricaciduria on a low purine diet, this further classification is still a laborious procedure requiring isotopic studies.

Treatment. Genetic gout cannot be cured, but its phenotypic expression can usually be modified and progression of its clinical complications controlled or reversed. The therapeutic program differs according to the complications present. Generally, in the majority of patients, the treatment of gout is now quite adequate with the introduction of potent uricosuric drugs and allopurinol, and more skilled use of colchicine as a prophylactic agent. The purpose of every therapeutic program is to prevent the complications of gout or, failing complete prophylaxis, to treat each complication specifically when it occurs.

Acute Gouty Arthritis. Although acute gouty arthritis is self-limited in duration, the severity of the pain and the persistence of the untreated inflammatory process over one to two weeks call for early intervention. The earlier the onset of treatment, the more likely a rapid response. The affected joint should be placed at rest. Usually the degree of pain will demand this, and on occasion specific medication, i.e., a narcotic, for pain may be required. Four types of drugs have been utilized with repeated success in the treatment of acute gout: colchicine; phenylbutazone, indomethacin, and glucocorticoids (or ACTH).

Colchicine is still widely used and is a relatively specific agent for the treatment of acute gout. A number of regimens can be used. It is recommended that an initial dose of 1.0 mg be given orally, followed by 0.5 mg every hour until the relief of pain or the onset of diarrhea. These responses often occur more or less spontaneously. No more than 6.0 mg of colchicine should be given for an acute attack; no more than that should be given over a 72-hour period. Colchicine may also be given intravenously (2.0 mg given in 20 ml of saline over a ten-minute period) instead of orally, with less gastrointestinal reaction, and repeated if necessary after an interval of four to six hours. Not more than 5.0 mg should be administered intravenously within a 24-hour period. Diarrhea is the most frequent complication of colchicine therapy and often requires treatment, e.g., paregoric, for rapid relief. Colchicine is excreted by the kidney and should be used cautiously in uremia. Large amounts of colchicine may cause transient leukopenia. The probable mechanism of action of colchicine has been discussed earlier. Because of the frequent occurrence of gastrointestinal symptoms during its use, colchicine has been replaced by the anti-inflammatory agent phenylbutazone as the first drug of choice in the treatment of acute gouty arthritis in many if not most clinics.

Phenylbutazone (Butazolidin) or *oxyphenbutazone* (Tandearil) is given in a dose of 200 mg four times a day for two days, with rapid tapering to discontinuation over the following two days. With such brief therapeutic periods, toxicity is minimized. *Indomethacin* (Indocin) may be given in amounts of 50 mg three times daily with early resolution of an acute attack, but it may produce more side effects. Glucocorticoid (or ACTH) therapy is not recommended for routine use in acute gouty arthritis because of variability in response and the high incidence of rebound arthritis after its discontinuation. ACTH has proved to be useful in postoperative gout when parenteral therapy is mandatory. Here it may be given as 40 units by slow intravenous drip on the first day, combined with 40 units of ACTH gel intramuscularly on each of the first three days.

When effective treatment has been given, improvement in symptoms usually begins within 6 to 12 hours, with virtually complete remission within 24 to 48 hours. In about 5 to 10 per cent of patients, no rapid relief is obtained, especially if treatment is begun late in the course, and the resolution of the inflammatory arthritis is more gradual. The use of uricosuric agents is not indicated in the management of acute gout.

One of the purposes of therapy is to prevent acute attacks of arthritis. By experience, patients may become aware of stressful experiences or dietary or alcoholic excesses which precipitate attacks, and in this way be able to avoid them. The proper use of uricosuric agents or allopurinol will lower urate levels below the saturation concentration over time, and in this way help to prevent the crystallization which precedes attacks. The short-term effect of such treatment, however, usually leads to exacerbation of gouty arthritis during periods of mobilization of urate deposits. Gutman has established the usefulness of daily colchicine (0.5 mg once or twice a day) as a simple measure to prevent acute attacks in patients subject to recurrent arthritis. Colchicine prophylaxis is not recommended for patients with a single attack (which may never recur) but should be instituted for all patients with frequent attacks of arthritis. Finally, the importance of aborting acute attacks by the use of colchicine or phenylbutazone during the earliest premonitory symptoms should be stressed. This will be the responsibility of the patient himself.

Tophaceous Gout. There are two ways to remove or reduce the size of tophi: surgical removal or redissolving sodium urate crystals. In extracellular fluid, sodium urate crystals can be dissolved only by lowering urate below the saturation level (approximately 7 mg per 100 ml, assuming normal protein binding). The rate of redissolving sodium urate bears a direct relationship to the degree of unsaturation achieved, although it may be modified by blood supply, fibrosis, and the area of crystal surface exposed. Two methods are in general use to lower urate levels: the use of uricosuric drugs to increase renal clearance, and the use of allopurinol to inhibit urate synthesis. Dietary restriction may help to reduce urate synthesis from preformed purines, but with the advent of the aforementioned methods of treatment it has become less important. In theory, an ideal approach to treatment would be to increase urate excretion into the gut (normally one fourth to one third of that synthesized) for bacterial uricolysis. No agent has yet been found which selectively increases gut excretion of urate.

Two uricosuric agents are most often employed, *probenecid* (Benemid) or *sulfinpyrazone* (Anturan). Either of these drugs should be started in small amounts with forced fluids and mild alkalinization of the urine (if no contraindications exist), in order to prevent uric acid stone formation. If the patient has been subject to acute arthritis, prophylactic colchicine should be administered simultaneously to anticipate the exacerbation of gouty arthritis during the early phases of uricosuric therapy. Probenecid should be started at a dose of 0.25 gram twice daily, gradually increasing over a two-week period to a maintenance dose of 0.5 gram two or three times daily. A few patients, particularly those with reduction in renal function, may require 2.5 to 3.0 grams daily in order to reduce serum urate to satisfactory levels, preferably lower than 6.0 mg per 100 ml. Sulfinpyrazone may be used as an alternate in beginning doses of 50 mg twice daily, gradually increasing to a maintenance dose of 100 mg three to four times daily. Exceptionally, sulfinpyrazone may be required in doses of 200 mg four times daily for effective uricosuria. In general, both drugs are well tolerated. The most frequently reported reactions are those of gastrointestinal intolerance and drug-induced dermatitis. Very rarely, marrow suppression and hepatic necrosis have been reported. Although uricosuric in large doses, salicylates should not be used in the treatment of gout. At usual therapeutic levels they may primarily inhibit renal tubular secretion of urate and therefore be uricoretentive.

The availability of *allopurinol* (Zyloprim) has introduced a new approach to the treatment of gout. This analogue of hypoxanthine and its oxidation product allo-xanthine competitively inhibit xanthine oxidase, and in this way reduce the oxidation of hypoxanthine to xanthine and of xanthine to uric acid (Fig. 2). The human kidney clears hypoxanthine and xanthine much more efficiently than uric acid, so that their extracellular fluid concentrations do not rise commensurately with the fall in urate. The total amount of purine bases excreted is generally somewhat reduced, owing probably to increased reutilization of the oxypurines for salvage synthesis of nucleotides. Furthermore, the more equitable distribution of purines excreted among the three metabolites reduces the tendency toward urinary saturation by either xanthine or uric acid (hypoxanthine being highly soluble). Allopurinol is usually given in divided doses of 300 to 600 mg per day. As in the case of uricosuric drugs, its use may initially increase the number of acute attacks of gouty arthritis unless colchicine prophylaxis is used. The pharmacologic production of xanthinuria, an analogue of the genetic disorder, has rarely resulted in difficulties from xanthine stone formation, notably in two patients with the Lesch-Nyhan syndrome and in a few patients being treated with antineoplastic agents. The nucleotide of allopurinol is formed in vivo, and inhibits the enzyme orotidylic decarboxylase with secondary orotic aciduria and orotidinuria. This partial inhibition of pyrimidine synthesis has not been shown to be adverse, and no incorporation of allopurinol nucleotide into nucleic acid as a possible mutagenic agent has been found. Toxic effects of allopurinol are rare (3 to 5 per cent of patients), and consist of dermatitis, fever, headache, diarrhea, transitory leukopenia, and elevation of serum transaminase enzymes of hepatic origin. Intramuscular crystals of xanthine and oxipurinol have been described in patients receiving allopurinol. The significance of this observation in terms of ultimate toxicity is not clear.

The availability of two general methods of treatment allows choice in the management of tophaceous gout or marked hyperuricemia productive of acute gout. It is recommended that uricosuric agents be given an initial trial in treatment, allopurinol being withheld for more specific indications. Probenecid has been widely used for over 20 years, whereas the use of allopurinol, although the known toxic effects are few and rarely severe, represents the introduction of a foreign purine base and nucleotide with which there has been extensive experience for only eight or nine years. This expression of some therapeutic restraint in the use of allopurinol is a conservative position, for there is a definite trend toward using this agent in the initial treatment of hyperuricemia. Allopurinol is definitely indicated for certain patients: when uricosuric treatment proves ineffective in lowering the extracellular urate level sufficiently (to less than 6 mg per 100 ml); when there are toxic reactions to uricosuric drugs; when tophaceous gout is particularly severe (which often accompanies some degree of renal functional impairment and poor response to uricosuric agents); or when there have been recurrent uric acid stones. In general, the allopurinol regimen is more effective in rapidly lowering urate levels without the added hazard of passing extra uric acid through the kidney and urinary tract. Although a uricosuric drug may be used in conjunction with allopurinol, this is not usually wise, because probenecid may increase urinary excretion of allopurinol and alloxanthine, making it less effective, and may also decrease the excretion of the oxypurines. Combined treatment has been used successfully for patients with severe tophaceous gout with good renal function when neither drug alone has sufficed to lower urate levels adequately.

With prolonged treatment, remarkable reversal of tophaceous gout may be obtained. Treatment should then be continued for life to prevent recurrence of hyperuricemia and its complications.

Gouty Kidney. There is no specific way to treat gouty kidney when renal failure has occurred. There is rarely any evidence of improvement in renal function when urate values are reduced enough to mobilize tophaceous deposits. Treatment is limited to control of pyelonephritis if it exists, prevention of further stone formation, lowering extracellular urate levels by the methods previously described in order to prevent further injury, treatment of hypertension to modify the progress of nephrosclerosis, and the general metabolic measures used to treat any patient with diminished renal function. With early diagnosis and treatment, renal failure is becoming a much rarer complication of gout. With uremia, the dose of allopurinol used should be lower.

A particular form of gouty kidney, acute tubular blockade by uric acid with oliguria or anuria, can be prevented in patients being treated with cytotoxic agents by the use of fluids, alkalinization of the urine, and, in particular, full doses of allopurinol *before* the treatment of the myeloproliferative disorder. If anuria occurs, the usual measures for the treatment of acute renal failure should be instituted in anticipation of tubular regeneration over a 10- to 14-day period.

Uric Acid Stones. As previously described, the tendency to form uric acid stones is a function of the concentration of free uric acid, as opposed to sodium urate, in urine. Preventive measures attempt to reduce uric acid concentration by increasing urine volume (forcing of fluids, particularly at night), increasing urine pH (administration of sodium citrate or bicarbonate to maintain urine pH greater than 6), or reducing urate excretion (allopurinol). In most patients, fluids and mild alkalinization suffice to prevent uric acid stones. When uricaciduria is marked, when excess sodium is contraindicated, or when these measures are not successful, the use of allopurinol offers a specific method for the prevention of uric acid stones. As stated, the theoretical possibility of substituting xanthine stones for uric acid stones exists, but this complication has so far occurred only in the Lesch-Nyhan syndrome.

Essential Hyperuricemia. In this chapter, essential hyperuricemia is considered to be gout without complications. The incidental discovery of elevated serum urate values in the absence of any of the clinical manifestations of gout has increased with the broader use of screening laboratory determinations. One of the most vexing problems facing the physician is whether asymptomatic hyperuricemia should be treated. There are few firm data on which to base a decision. Although hyperuricemia is associated epidemiologically with hyperlipidemia, hypertension, obesity, glucose intolerance, and accelerated vascular disease, there is no evidence that it is primary in any of these derangements, or that lowering uric acid levels affects their course. Similarly, gout may lead to renal failure, but documentation of gouty kidney in the absence of other clinical manifestations is exceedingly rare. Finally, only a minority of patients develop complications of gout despite a lifetime of hyperuricemia in the postpubertal period, although the incidence of complications is roughly proportional to the degree of sodium urate supersaturation in extracellular fluid. Because of these uncertainties, it does not seem justified to start therapy for life in essential hyperuricemia. On the other hand, when serum uric acid values are consistently above 9.0 mg per 100 ml, the degree of supersaturation is such that the incidence of complications is perhaps 90 per cent. It would seem reasonable to treat such patients with uricosuric agents, or allopurinol, in order to maintain safer uric acid levels.

Garrod, A. B.: A Treatise on Gout and Rheumatic Gout. 3rd ed. London, Longmans, Green & Co., Ltd., 1876.

Gutman, A. B., and Yü T.-F.: Uric acid nephrolithiasis. Am. J. Med., 45:756, 1968.

McCarty, D. J., Jr.: Mechanisms of the crystal deposition diseases—gout and pseudogout. Ann. Intern. Med., 78:767, 1973.

Rieselbach, R. E., and Steele, T. H.: Influence of the kidney upon urate homeostasis in health and disease. Am. J. Med., 56:665, 1974.

Seegmiller, J. E. (ed.): Symposium on clinical and biochemical features of X-linked uricaciduria. Arch. Intern. Med., 130:181, 1972.

Seegmiller, J. E.: Diseases of purine and pyrimidine metabolism. In Bondy, P. K., and Rosenberg, L. E. (eds.): Duncan's Diseases of Metabolism. 7th ed. Philadelphia, W. B. Saunders Company, 1974, p. 655.

Smyth, C. J., and Percy, J. S.: Comparison of indomethacin and phenylbutazone in acute gout. Ann. Rheum. Dis., 32:351, 1973.

Steele, T. H.: Control of uric acid excretion. N. Engl. J. Med., 284:1193, 1971.

Watts, R. W. E., Scott, J. T., Chalmers, R. A., Bitensky, L., and Chayen, J.: Microscopic studies on skeletal muscle in gout patients treated with allopurinol. Quart J. Med., 40:1, 1971.

Weissman, G.: Crystals, lysosomes, and gout. Adv. Intern. Med., 19:239, 1974.

Weissman, G., and Rita, G.: Molecular basis of gouty inflammation: Interaction of monosodium urate crystals with lysosomes and liposomes. Nature (New Biol.), 240:167, 1972.

Wyngaarden, J. B.: The metabolic defects of primary hyperuricemia and gout. Am. J. Med., 56:651, 1974.

Wyngaarden, J. B., and Kelley, W. N.: Gout. In Stanbury, J. B., Wyngaar-
den, J. B., and Fredrickson, D. S. (eds.): The Metabolic Basis of Inherited Disease. 3rd ed. New York, McGraw-Hill Book Company, 1972, p. 889.

Yü, T.-F.: Milestones in the treatment of gout. Am. J. Med., 56:676, 1974.

822. XANTHINURIA

Xanthinuria is a rare genetic disorder secondary to deficiency of xanthine oxidase. Approximately a dozen cases have been described, and some of these have not been fully investigated. It is probably transmitted as an autosomal recessive trait, although this has not been firmly established and there is no method now available for detection of heterozygotes. Deficient activity of xanthine oxidase has been demonstrated in liver and gut mucosa in xanthinuria. The normal function of this enzyme is to catalyze the oxidation of hypoxanthine to xanthine and of xanthine to uric acid.

Most patients with xanthinuria have been asymptomatic, being discovered in the investigation of hypouricemia (serum urate less than 1 mg per 100 ml). Three patients had xanthine kidney stones, which resemble uric acid stones in their radiolucency. Two of the patients had muscle cramps, made worse by exercise, and were found on muscle biopsy to have intracellular crystals of xanthine and hypoxanthine. Although one patient with xanthinuria had hemochromatosis, no other patients have shown abnormal avidity for iron absorption.

The diagnosis is established by the demonstration of hypouricemia and hypouricaciduria with increased excretion of hypoxanthine and xanthine. In xanthinuria these oxypurines are usually excreted in amounts somewhat less than the normal value for uric acid. Hypoxanthine is partially reutilized to form inosine-5'-phosphate, a reaction catalyzed by hypoxanthine guanine phosphoribosyltransferase, the enzyme which is deficient in the Lesch-Nyhan syndrome. Xanthinuria is simulated pharmacologically by the use of allopurinol which is a competitive inhibitor of, as well as a substrate for, xanthine oxidase. (See Ch. 821.) Hypouricemia may also occur in proximal renal tubular disease (Fanconi's syndrome, Wilson's disease) and during treatment with uricosuric agents. Uricosuric agents include aspirin, x-ray contrast agents, and glyceryl guaiacolate. Hypouricemia has been described repeatedly in association with neoplastic diseases. It has also been described in several healthy individuals who had an isolated defect in renal tubular reabsorption of urate (clearance of urate 1.3 times creatinine clearance), similar to that found in the Dalmatian coach hound and in primates other than man. Probably a few patients have had xanthine stones or mixed stones containing xanthine as one component in the absence of the genetic disease. The solubility of hypoxanthine prevents its precipitation in the urinary tract.

Treatment is usually not required. A program for the prevention of xanthine stones would be similar to that for uric acid stones, i.e., forcing fluids, alkalinization of the urine (although the enhancement of solubility of xanthine by alkalinization is not as great as that of urate), and possibly a low purine diet if the above does not suffice. Despite the very low levels of xanthine oxidase, studies on a single patient suggest that allopurinol might increase the amount of oxypurine excreted as the more soluble hypoxanthine.

Engelman, K., Watts, R. W. E., Klinenberg, J. R., Sjoerdsma, A., and Seegmiller, J. E.: Clinical, physiological and biochemical studies of a patient with xanthinuria and pheochromocytoma. Am. J. Med., 37:839, 1964.

Seegmiller, J. E.: Xanthine stone formation. Am. J. Med., 45:780, 1968.

Seegmiller, J. E.: Hereditary xanthinuria. *In* Bondy, P. K., and Rosenberg, L. E.(eds.): Duncan's Disease of Metabolism. 7th ed. Philadelphia, W. B. Saunders Company, 1974, p. 739.

Wyngaarden, J. B.: Xanthinuria. *In* Stanbury, J. B., Wyngaarden, J. B., and Fredrickson, D. S. (eds.): The Metabolic Basis of Inherited Disease. 3rd ed. New York, McGraw-Hill Book Company, 1972, p. 992.

823.   DISORDERS OF PYRIMIDINE METABOLISM

Lloyd H. Smith, Jr.

Pyrimidine nucleotides share equally with purine nucleotides the chemical chore of transmitting genetic information for reproduction or for phenotypic expression within the cell. They also function in the intermediary metabolism of lipids and carbohydrates. Only a few disorders of pyrimidine metabolism have been recognized.

Hereditary orotic aciduria is a rare genetic disorder of pyrimidine metabolism characterized by megaloblastic anemia resistant to the usual hematinic agents, leukopenia, failure of normal growth and development, and the continued excessive urinary excretion of orotic acid. Orotic acid is highly insoluble and often forms a heavy sediment of urinary crystals which may on occasion result in ureteral or urethral obstruction. The disorder, which is transmitted as an autosomal recessive trait, is usually characterized by reduced activities of two consecutive enzymes in pyrimidine biosynthesis, orotate phosphoribosyltransferase (OPRT) and orotidine 5'-phosphate decarboxylase (ODC). A single patient has been described with isolated deficiency of ODC. There is a prompt and sustained hematologic and general clinical response to oral uridine (2 to 4 grams per day), which must be continued indefinitely as replacement therapy. The disease has attracted special attention because it represents a block in the de novo pathway of pyrimidine synthesis, is an example of a double enzyme defect, and produces a requirement for replacement of a normal metabolic intermediate, uridine.

Orotic aciduria, without the characteristic hematologic abnormalities, also occurs in *ornithine transcarbamylase deficiency*. It is presumed that this results from the overflow of carbamyl phosphate from urea synthesis (partially blocked in this disease) to pyrimidine synthesis.

Excessive urinary excretion of orotic acid and orotidine occurs during treatment with *allopurinol* or *6-azauridine*. Metabolic products of both compounds inhibit orotidine 5'-decarboxylase activity.

Beta-aminoisobutyric aciduria is a benign hereditary disorder of thymine catabolism which occurs in 5 to 10 per cent of Caucasians and in a much higher percentage of Asians. The defect presumably lies in the transamination of beta-aminoisobutyric acid to methylmalonic acid semialdehyde. The aminoaciduria which results, representing the only known disorder of pyrimidine catabolism, has no known biologic disadvantage.

Smith, L. H., Jr.: Pyrimidine metabolism in man. N. Engl. J. Med., 288:764, 1973.

Smith, L. H., Jr., Huguley, C. M., Jr., and Bain, J. A.: Hereditary orotic aciduria. *In* Stanbury, J. B., Wyngaarden, J. B., and Fredrickson, D. S. (eds.): The Metabolic Basis of Inherited Disease. 3rd ed. New York, McGraw-Hill Book Company, 1972, p. 196.

Weissman, S. M.: Human pyrimidine metabolism. J.A.M.A., 195:27, 1966.

Part XVIII
DISEASES OF THE ENDOCRINE SYSTEM

824. INTRODUCTION

Nicholas P. Christy

FUNCTIONS OF THE ENDOCRINE SYSTEM

Like the nervous system, the endocrine system provides mechanisms by which the mammalian organism adapts itself to a constantly changing environment. Parts of the endocrine system may indeed be regarded as extensions of the nervous system: the adrenal medulla, which secretes epinephrine in response to environmental change, is of ectodermal origin, arising from the neural crest; many environmental stimuli cause cells in the hypothalamus to secrete neurohumoral peptides which are carried in the hypothalamic-hypophysial portal venous system to cells in the anterior pituitary, which then secrete growth hormone, adrenocorticotrophin, or gonadotrophins (see Ch. 826). These two glands, the adrenal medulla and the anterior pituitary, are particularly clear examples of endocrine organs whose secretions mediate between the external and internal environments. Less dramatic but no less important examples are the neurohypophysial response to changes in hydration and the fluctuations of adrenocortical secretion of aldosterone with changes in dietary Na+. These and the other endocrine glands, by steady or by waxing and waning secretion of hormones, wield an important *regulatory* influence on cellular metabolism (see Ch. 806).

Again like the nervous system, the endocrine system has both *vegetative* and *adaptive* functions. The essential roles of pituitary growth hormone and thyroxine on normal growth and the effects of the sex steroids, testosterone and estradiol, on the gradual and orderly maturation of the secondary sex characters are examples of *vegetative* activity. Rapid *adaptive* functions are numerous: insulin secretion in response to hyperglycemia; epinephrine secretion during profound hypoglycemia; antidiuretic hormone secretion in the presence of increased osmolarity of the plasma; and the instantaneous hypersecretion of pituitary adrenocorticotrophic hormone (ACTH) in response to many noxious stimuli, of growth hormone to severe muscular exercise, and of aldosterone to hemorrhage-induced hypovolemia. It is apparent that both the vegetative and adaptive, that is, the slowly acting and rapidly acting functions are in effect homeostatic (see Ch. 804). However, it is probably a mistake to think of the endocrine system as a system in a rigid sense. It is true that the endocrine organs are all by definition ductless glands which secrete hormones that have many actions at sites remote from those glands. It is also true that several hormones may conspire to affect single, well-defined functions or substances. For instance, it can be shown that all the following hormones have the capacity to influence the concentration of blood glucose: pituitary growth hormone, ACTH, thyroxine, cortisol, epinephrine, insulin, and glucagon. Pituitary growth hormone, ACTH, cortisol, aldosterone, and antidiuretic hormone all influence serum Na+ concentration. But in any of these groupings, it is difficult to know in a given set of circumstances which hormone is quantitatively the most important and to calculate accurately how the several hormones, with their complementary, supplementary, synergistic, or opposing actions, operate together to regulate the serum concentration of glucose or Na+. Further, it is hard to see, for example, how epinephrine secretion by the adrenal medulla relates to the secretion of parathyroid hormone, how growth hormone secretion bears on thyroxine secretion, and how aldosterone and gonadotrophins inter-relate. There are at least as many examples of independent as of interdependent functions among the endocrine glands. Therefore it seems most reasonable not to regard the endocrine glands as such a tightly integrated system as the anatomically distinct nervous system, but rather as a loose group of secretory organs, arising from different embryologic sources, having made their appearance at different stages in evolution, and possessing a broad range of functions, some separate and distinct and some interdigitated. These regulatory functions are exerted by circulating chemical substances upon biochemical processes of all cells and tissues.

The *disorders of the endocrine glands* become clinically apparent through excessive, deficient, or untimely secretion of a hormone, owing either to primary disease of the endocrine gland or to an abnormal secretion by that gland in response to disease of some other organ (see Categories of Endocrine Disease, below). All endocrine diseases have this property in common: the secretion of the hormone is not regulated or is improperly regulated by the control mechanisms that operate under normal conditions; that is, the production of the hormone is *autonomous, anarchic,* or *inappropriate,* a state of affairs that leads to disordered homeostasis.

BIOCHEMISTRY AND MODE OF ACTION OF HORMONES

The *chemical nature* of human hormones is now well known. The substances are amines (epinephrine), amino acids (thyroxine), peptides (vasopressin or antidiuretic hormone), proteins (pituitary growth hormone, parathyroid hormone), and steroids (aldosterone). Many hormones have been chemically synthesized, e.g., epinephrine, thyroxine, most of the steroids, and even some of the peptides and proteins, as vasopressin, oxytocin, thyrotrophin-releasing hormone (TRH), and ACTH. For some of the hormones of high molecular weight, e.g., growth hormone, amino acid sequences have been worked out; knowledge of the structures of thyrotrophin and the gonadotrophins is still not complete. Methods have now been developed for accurate measurement of nearly all the important human hormones. These chemical techniques, although difficult and time consuming, are enormously superior to the indirect or biologic assay methods investigators and clinicians used to rely on. The chemical methods, including the revolutionary radioimmunoassay techniques introduced by Berson and Yalow, have now made it possible to quantify the plasma or urinary concentrations of virtually all the known hormones. These advances have put endocrine diagnosis on a firm footing, and have enabled workers in the field not only to measure blood levels but also to determine secretory rates or production rates of several classes of hormones. Thus it is now possible to measure accurately the daily secretion rate of steroid hormones, e.g., aldosterone and cortisol, and even to estimate the daily turnover rate of such protein hormones as growth hormone and ACTH.

Despite intensive study by many workers, the mode of action of hormones is still not completely understood. There is a good deal of information about the *structural determinants of hormonal activity,* e.g., the number, sequence, and identity of the amino acids that determine the immunologic reactivity and the biologic potency of the ACTH molecule (see Ch. 828). Small changes in the molecular structure of hormones profoundly affect their biologic activity and metabolism, both qualitatively and quantitatively; for example, among the steroid hormones, cortisone, with a ketone group at the carbon-11 position of the steroid nucleus, is quite inactive in vitro, whereas cortisol, the principal adrenocortical glucocorticoid of man, which differs structurally from cortisone only by having a hydroxyl (-OH) instead of a ketone group (-O) at carbon-11, is highly active; among the thyroid hormones, L-thyroxine has a half-time in plasma twice that of its stereoisomer, D-thyroxine, and ten times its calorigenic potency. What is not yet definitely known is the exact chemical form of any hormone that is active at the cellular level; it remains to be shown how the known alterations of any hormone molecule brought about by peripheral metabolism are necessary steps in hormone action.

The significance of the *physical state* of a given hormone in the *plasma* is also not clear. The conventional view is that only the portion of a hormone that is *not* bound to a plasma protein is "active" in the sense that only the unbound, "free" form is available to cells. There is some evidence to support this view. Under various conditions—e.g., rare hereditary abnormalities in the serum concentration of certain α-globulins, pregnancy, estrogen therapy, nephrotic syndrome, severe hepatic disease, and several acute illnesses—there are definite changes in the plasma levels of thyroxine-binding globulin or of corticosteroid-binding globulin. Yet, although these changes give rise to easily measurable changes in *total* serum concentration of thyroxine or cortisol, there is no clinical evidence of an altered thyroid or adrenal state, presumably because the "free" thyroxine and "free" cortisol levels are not significantly abnormal.

The biochemical mode of action of hormones at the cellular level is discussed in detail in Ch. 825.

UBIQUITY OF HORMONAL EFFECTS

Since all hormones circulate in the blood, their actions are to be found everywhere. The effects of disordered endocrine function impinge upon most organs and systems. Some examples are the characteristic changes in the skin, central nervous system, muscles, gastrointestinal tract, heart, and blood vessels (increased susceptibility to atherosclerosis) in severe *hypothyroidism;* the changes in the psyche, the eyes, the regulation of blood glucose (hypoglycemia), the blood pressure, water metabolism, and the structure and function of the sexual apparatus in fully developed *pituitary insufficiency;* and the changes in the psyche, central nervous system (lethargy, coma), muscles, gastrointestinal tract (constipation, ileus), kidneys (stones), and skeleton that are characteristic of *hyperparathyroidism.*

Many acute and chronic diseases impinge on the endocrine glands. Examples are such changes as increased adrenocortical and adrenal medullary secretion of cortisol and epinephrine during *acute myocardial infarction,* increased aldosterone secretion in the accelerated phase of *hypertension,* decreased pituitary gonadotrophin secretion with hypogonadism accompanying the inanition and emotional disorder of *anorexia nervosa* (see Ch. 724), and the secondary hyperparathyroidism of *renal insufficiency* (see Ch. 890).

Looking at endocrine disease from another point of view, many common symptoms and signs may be parts of endocrine syndromes. *Hypertension* is common in acromegaly and *Cushing's syndrome;* not all patients with these diseases can be diagnosed on inspection. Fixed hypertension is also present in *pheochromocytoma, aldosteronism, renal artery stenosis,* and in some patients with *congenital adrenal hyperplasia.* In the differential diagnosis of *coma,* one must consider the hypercalcemia of *hyperparathyroidism,* the hypoglycemia associated with *islet cell tumors* or *panhypopituitarism,* and the severe water intoxication sometimes associated with the syndrome of *inappropriate secretion of antidiuretic hormone.* Serious *psychologic disturbance,* including psychosis, may be an important feature of *pituitary insufficiency, hypothyroidism, hyperthyroidism, hyperparathyroidism,* any of the *hypoglycemias, Addison's disease,* and *Cushing's syndrome.*

The aim here is to sensitize the reader to the systemic but less obvious signs of endocrine disease; he does not need to be reminded that the patient with clear signs of thyrotoxicosis may have disease of an endocrine gland.

CATEGORIES OF ENDOCRINE DISEASE

In the light of the discoveries made during the past two decades, it is no longer enough to think of endocrine disease simply as too much or too little hormone. For clinical purposes, the following may be a helpful classification:

Primary Hyperfunction of Endocrine Glands. Most diseases in this group are due to *benign tumors* of endocrine glands, such as the pituitary adenoma of acromegaly, the "toxic adenoma" which produces hyperthyroidism, the parathyroid adenoma of hyperparathyroidism, the insulin-secreting islet cell adenoma of the pancreas, benign pheochromocytoma, and the adrenal cortical adenoma of Cushing's syndrome. *Malignant hormone-secreting tumors* of the anterior pituitary and thyroid are extremely rare, but cancers of the parathyroids, islet cells, adrenal medulla, and adrenal cortex are occasional causes of severe and intractable endocrine disease. No more is known about the etiology of these endocrine cancers than about that of any other cancer.

There are hyperfunctional states *not associated with endocrine tumors*. An example is Graves' disease or toxic diffuse goiter, which was formerly believed to be due to pituitary oversecretion of TSH. It is not; plasma TSH concentrations are low (see Ch. 837).

Secondary Hyperfunction of Endocrine Glands. This term defines overactivity of a "target" gland owing to *hyperfunction of the anterior pituitary.* Cushing's syndrome not associated with adrenal tumor is caused by excessive and unremitting ACTH secretion; there are very rare instances of hyperthyroidism associated with TSH overproduction by pituitary tumors.

Primary Hypofunction of Endocrine Glands. Primary glandular failure is the usual cause of endocrine deficiency syndromes. The etiology is often obscure. Fibrosis or even absence of the anterior pituitary has been discovered at autopsy *without anatomic evidence of any cause.* Destruction of a gland by formation of *autoantibodies* to that gland has been postulated as a cause of the hypothyroidism of Hashimoto's thyroiditis, and also as a cause of hypoparathyroidism and of "idiopathic" Addison's disease. Autoantibodies to thyroid, parathyroid, and adrenals have indeed been demonstrated in many patients with these disorders, but it is not clear whether the antibodies are the primary cause of the glandular destruction or are secondary consequences, arising from damage to the glands by unknown agents. There has been recent interest in the possibility that delayed or cellular hypersensitivity related to abnormal "lymphoid recognition" may play a part, especially in cases of polyglandular insufficiency. *Tumors* may destroy a gland. Breast cancer and lymphomas may metastasize or spread to invade the neurohypophysis or supraoptic nuclei, giving rise to diabetes insipidus; chromophobe adenoma is the most common cause of anterior pituitary insufficiency. Several cancers, especially lung cancer, very often metastasize to the adrenals, but rarely cause enough destruction to produce adrenocortical insufficiency. *Infections* are not very common causes of glandular failure: tuberculosis and syphilitic gummas used to be occasional causes of pituitary destruction, but are now museum pieces; tuberculosis, histoplasmosis, and blastomycosis may destroy the adrenals with ensuing Addison's disease. *Chromosomal disorders,* such as Klinefelter's syndrome and gonadal dysgenesis (Turner's syndrome), are not rare as causes of primary gonadal deficiency in phenotypic males and females (see Ch. 859 and 867).

Secondary and Tertiary Failure of Endocrine Glands. This term means failure of the gonads, thyroid, or adrenals owing to *pituitary insufficiency.* Although it is true that the growth hormone–secreting and gonadotrophic functions of the pituitary are usually the first to drop out during the course of destructive pituitary disease, and, as a corollary, if only one function is affected, it is likely to be either growth (hypopituitary dwarfism) or gonadal function, the other functions, i.e., thyrotrophic or adrenocorticotrophic, may fail singly or in any combination (see Ch. 831). The key to diagnosis is to study the patient carefully for the presence of pituitary disease in every instance of growth failure, hypogonadism, hypothyroidism, or hypoadrenocorticism. There may be good clinical evidence to implicate or rule out pituitary involvement, but, if not, assessment of thyroid or adrenal response to TSH or ACTH or direct measurement by radioimmunoassay of the trophic hormones in plasma or urine will clarify the diagnosis. When the anterior pituitary insufficiency is the result of hypothalamic disease, the target gland failure is defined as "tertiary," e.g., "tertiary hypothyroidism" (see Ch. 826).

"Functional" Disorders of the Endocrine Glands. The response of endocrine glands to certain disease states may be clinically important or clinically trivial. Important endocrine responses are the secondary hyperparathyroidism of renal failure, leading to renal osteodystrophy; and the secondary aldosteronism of portal cirrhosis and of the nephrotic syndrome with ascites and edema—aldosterone is an important contributing factor in edema formation. Responses which are either trivial or not yet of proved clinical significance are altered metabolism of thyroxine in liver disease and in patients acutely ill from a variety of causes; the altered metabolism of cortisol in portal cirrhosis; the altered metabolic disposition of androgens in thyroid disease and acute intermittent porphyria; and many others.

Failure of an End-Organ to Respond to a Hormone. There are several examples of this in human medicine. One is *nephrogenic diabetes insipidus,* a heritable defect in which the kidney fails to respond to vasopressin in the face of adequate secretion of vasopressin by the supraoptic nuclei. Another is *pseudohypoparathyroidism,* a hereditary disease characterized by renal and osseous resistance to measurable effects of parathyroid hormone (PTH), which is secreted in normal or greater than normal amounts by normal or hyperplastic parathyroids. In both these diseases, the respective hormones, vasopressin and PTH, fail to activate the adenylate cyclase system of the appropriate renal tubular cells; there is no rise in cyclic AMP and no metabolic effect of the hormone. Still another type of failure of end-organ response, the so-called *pseudohypoparathyroidism type II,* is characterized by adequate cyclic AMP response to PTH but absence of phosphaturia or rise in serum calcium concentration. The inference is that there is a failure to receive the intracellular cyclic AMP "message." A third example is the syndrome of *testicular feminization,* a developmental defect in which "target tissues" are unresponsive to endogenous or administered androgen. In this entity the mechanism of end-organ failure has not been worked out.

Production by an Endocrine Gland of an Abnormal or Unusual Hormone. Such lesions are characteristic of the inborn errors of metabolism. In *congenital adrenocortical hyperplasia,* deficiencies of C-21 and C-11 hydroxylases cause metabolic blocks in the synthesis of cortisol, with the additional result that several cortisol precursors, e.g., pregnanetriol and 17α-hydroxyprogesterone, normally present in very small amounts, are secreted in amounts much greater than normal, as are C_{19} androgens. In *goitrous cretinism* enzymic blocks in the synthesis of thyroxine give rise to thyroidal secretion into the bloodstream of large quantities of mono- and diiodotyrosines. In "T_3 *thyrotoxicosis*" hyperthyroidism is present and serum PBI and thyroxine concentrations are normal; for unknown reasons the goiter or thyroid nodule apparently synthesizes excessive quantities of the normally less abundant hormone, triiodothyronine

(T_3). A form of hypoparathyroidism *("pseudoidiopathic hypoparathyroidism")* has been described in which the glands secrete a biologically ineffective PTH, possibly because of a defect in conversion of proparathyroid hormone to an active form.

Production of a Hormone by a Nonendocrine Organ. Cancers of many organs (lung, thymus, pancreas) may produce substances that cannot be chemically or immunologically distinguished from normal endocrine products, usually proteins, such as ACTH, MSH, gonadotrophins, erythropoietin, and others. The clinical features and hypotheses concerning the mechanisms by which these "hormones" are secreted are discussed in Ch. 870.

Prostaglandins. The status of *prostaglandins* is not yet clear. These 20-carbon, unsaturated, cyclic fatty acids were originally found in seminal fluid, but are now known to be present in most tissues and biologic fluids. At least 16 prostaglandins have been isolated and described. Their effects are widespread and varied. In addition to many actions on the central nervous, cardiovascular, and gastrointestinal systems and the kidney, the prostaglandins have many effects upon the endocrine organs. Prostaglandins have been shown to affect the hypothalamus–anterior pituitary "axis," to augment pituitary growth hormone release in vitro, to mediate the effect of luteinizing hormone on the ovary, to exert a lytic effect on the corpus luteum, to alter thyroidal response to TSH, and to affect adrenal cortical steroidogenesis. Prostaglandins have been shown to mimic the "hormonal" effects of cyclic AMP and, under certain conditions, to attenuate cyclic AMP effects. The *physiologic* importance of the prostaglandins in regulating endocrine function remains to be worked out. Although their actions often appear to be "hormonal," there is still no agreement as to whether they should be considered hormones.

Iatrogenic Endocrine Disease. By far the most common of these is iatrogenic Cushing's syndrome caused by administration of ACTH or cortisol and its derivatives in pharmacologic doses for many allergic, inflammatory, and neoplastic diseases. In the United States, there are hundreds of thousands of patients receiving long-term steroid therapy. An unknown number of these are getting very large doses (more than 50 mg per day of cortisol, or equivalent), and an unknown proportion of them have overt hyperadrenocorticism. The features of this entity are the physical signs of spontaneously occurring Cushing's syndrome, but with a lesser incidence in the iatrogenic form of diabetes, hypertension, and psychosis, and a higher incidence of peptic ulcer and certain rarer untoward effects, e.g., pseudotumor cerebri, glaucoma, pancreatitis, and "aseptic necrosis" of the hip joint. In addition, an unpredictable and probably small number have enough suppression of pituitary-adrenal function to be important in times of intercurrent acute illness or surgical emergency. The writer has developed elsewhere the idea that these patients are addicted to corticosteroids (see References; also Ch. 849). The point is that one should be as ungenerous as possible in the dosage of corticosteroids.

Prescription of sex hormones and thyroid hormone to patients without gonadal or thyroidal deficiency rarely produces iatrogenic disease, but there have been instances of surreptitious thyroxine ingestion leading to thyrotoxicosis. Overenthusiastic use of estrogen may induce endometrial hyperplasia and breakthrough bleeding; some patients are apparently hypersensitive to methyl testosterone, which may cause cholestatic jaundice. The abnormalities in glucose tolerance, serum triglycerides, and liver function tests and the increased incidence of thromboembolic disease associated with administration of oral contraceptives have become familiar.

The protein hormones are sometimes troublesome. There are more than 80 reported instances of anaphylaxis owing to ACTH. For further details about the toxicity of hormonal products, the reader is referred to textbooks of pharmacology. The keys to successful hormone therapy are accurate diagnosis and great restraint in dosage.

HORMONES AS MEDICINES

Hormones are legitimately given to patients in three sets of circumstances: (1) for replacement of lost functions, (2) as tests of endocrine function, and (3) to achieve a pharmacologic purpose.

Replacement Therapy. This is probably the most gratifying use of hormones to both patient and physician, and is the easiest to defend. So long as an endocrine deficiency is clearly and definitely demonstrated, in most instances a realistic goal owing to the availability of good chemical tests for most hormonal diseases, the physician can achieve brilliant clinical results with small doses of hormones. Cortisol for adrenal insufficiency, thyroid hormone USP or thyroxine for hypothyroidism, and human growth hormone for hypopituitary dwarfism are all given in amounts very close to the estimated daily production rates of the respective hormones. It is common practice to give too much cortisone to patients with primary or secondary adrenal insufficiency, i.e., enough to induce signs of mild Cushing's syndrome; daily doses of not more than 10 to 25 mg per day are usually quite sufficient. With thyroid hormone replacement, restraint is also necessary, especially in older people with coronary artery disease, in whom the maintenance dose should be attained gradually. The writer believes that triiodothyronine is never indicated for treatment of longstanding myxedema; too many older patients with atherosclerosis have had bouts of severe coronary insufficiency or even myocardial infarction when this rapidly acting hormone is given. Triiodothyronine may have a place in the treatment of myxedema coma (see Ch. 839).

Replacement dosages of sex hormones have been arrived at by "clinical experience." In the writer's experience, treatment to develop deficient secondary sex characters is best given just before or at the expected time of puberty. If replacement therapy with estrogen or testosterone is delayed until late in the second or well into the third decade, the induced sexual development is suboptimal. This puts a premium on early diagnosis as the basis for early treatment.

Few protein hormones are used routinely in treatment. Although it would be theoretically most correct, say in hypopituitarism, to replace absent trophic hormones by giving gonadotrophins, TSH or ACTH, this is not practical, owing to antibody formation, short supply, and the need for parenteral administration. Gonadotrophins are given only in short courses to induce ovulation in women (see Ch. 867); to stimulate ovarian or testicular function over a long period of time is cumbersome, so sex hormones, which can be administered orally, are used instead. Treatment of secondary hypothyroidism and hypoadrenalism is much more easily done with thyroid hormone and cortisone; allergic reactions to ACTH have been alluded to above. Parathyroid hormone from human sources is not available; vitamin D and calcium salts are simpler to give. The only protein hormone other than insulin that is generally used as replacement therapy is human growth hormone, because there is still no satisfactory substitute for it.

Testing. TSH and ACTH are useful for assessing thyroidal and adrenal response in differentiating between primary and secondary deficiencies of these glands, and the triiodothyronine suppression test of thyroidal ^{131}I uptake is a useful adjunct in diagnosis of some patients with hyperthyroidism. These testing procedures entail the direct chemical or physical measurement of a hormone or of a glandular function. Such methods have largely superseded indirect methods of estimating endocrine activity (e.g., the BMR and the eosinophil count). Some of the older techniques, being provocative tests, were potentially dangerous, e.g., the water-loading and salt withdrawal tests for Addison's disease. These should now be abandoned.

By testing, the writer does not mean the administration of a hormone as a *therapeutic trial,* that is, to determine by the patient's response whether he has or does not have an endocrine deficiency. This approach may be tolerable in an emergency, as for a patient in acute shock when there seems to be some possibility of adrenocortical insufficiency and there is no time for careful chemical study. Under any other conditions, failure to establish a diagnosis is an inexcusable basis for giving hormonal therapy.

Hormones Given to Achieve a Pharmacologic End. Hormones customarily are given to patients in high doses to achieve some pharmacologic, not physiologic, goal in three sets of circumstances: treatment of diseases in which large doses of hormones are *often beneficial;* treatment of diseases for which large doses of hormones are *possibly* or *sometimes beneficial;* and treatment of diseases for which large doses of hormones are *never beneficial* or of very doubtful value.

Beneficial Uses. The obvious examples are of course ACTH and cortisol and its congeners. Although ACTH is usually associated with fewer serious untoward effects and with less danger of a "withdrawal syndrome" when treatment is stopped, the corticosteroids are preferred because of the convenience of the oral route of administration, more flexibility in spacing of doses, shorter action, the larger doses attainable, and the absence of serious allergic reactions. The ideal use of high-dosage corticosteroids is in acute, self-limited diseases such as serum sickness owing to penicillin allergy or bouts of status asthmaticus. In serious inflammatory diseases such as pemphigus, ulcerative colitis, acute rheumatic fever, and lupus erythematosus, in hematologic disorders such as acute lymphoblastic leukemia of childhood, and in bronchial asthma of allergic origin, among other conditions, there is good evidence that corticosteroids often alter the course of the disease in a favorable direction. As in giving any other medicinal agent, the physician has to balance the probability of benefit from corticosteroid therapy against the disability or danger incurred by giving the patient corticosteroids, with the attendant risk of iatrogenic Cushing's syndrome. To make this semiquantitative judgment,

the doctor has to have the fullest possible knowledge of the *natural history* of what he proposes to treat, that is, the natural course of the disease untreated (Feinstein).

Possibly or Sometimes Beneficial Uses. The efficacy of corticosteroids in such disorders as scleroderma and endotoxin shock remains arguable. The same statement applies to the use of testosterone or estrogen, or both, in the treatment of postmenopausal osteoporosis (q.v.); the use of vasopressin or mineralocorticoids in the management of idiopathic postural hypotension; administration of small doses of corticosteroids to women with "acquired adrenal virilism," an entity which may or may not exist; and many others. In this group of diseases, further work is needed toward an understanding of pathogenesis; only this will provide a rational basis for giving or withholding treatment.

Uses That Are Never Beneficial. These uses are derived by the trial and error method, with emphasis on the latter. Examples are numerous; outstanding ones are the widespread administration of thyroid hormone for obesity, for fatigability, and for infertility and menstrual disturbances, the use of estrogens to treat frigidity in the female, and the use of testosterone for impotence in the male. The major objection to such therapies is that they are ineffective. Further, they are often expensive and raise false hopes. The physician must resist the temptation to keep trying one hormonal remedy after another in the hope that something will work. "The empiricist," said Claude Bernard, "is never at a loss." It is the patient who loses.

HORMONES AND MAGIC

By now, it is apparent to the reader that endocrinology is inseparable from the rest of internal medicine. Until the 1920's, endocrinology was entirely an empirical branch, not quite respectable, not quite accepted as professional, lurking on the outskirts of medicine. The endocrinologist dealt with patients who were too fat, too thin, too short, too tall, too tired, too hairy, or not hairy enough. With the discovery of insulin in 1922, with the elucidation of the structures of thyroxine and the steroid hormones in the next decade, and with good studies of hormone metabolism in the period from 1950 to the present, there began to be a firm scientific basis for the practice of endocrinology. But three factors have contributed to the persistence of empiricism. One was the isolation and synthesis of cortisone and cortisol and their derivatives; it is easier to list the diseases for which these compounds have not been given than those for which they have been at least tried. Second is the dramatic and gratifying clinical response that follows administration of a hormone in a deficiency state, or the surgical removal of a hyperfunctioning gland. The physician is sometimes irresistibly tempted to achieve such magical results even when the diagnosis of endocrine deficiency or excess is not firmly established. The third factor, a corollary of the second, is that endocrine diagnostic procedures are time consuming, technically difficult, and sometimes not available locally, and that the data produced are not always easy to interpret. The physician grows impatient. Enough has been said previously about the need for accurate diagnosis as an essential basis for endocrine replacement therapy. Accuracy is equally essential for establishing a diagnosis of glandular hyperfunction; since most of the treatments for such conditions are ablative, the physician should be on solid ground before consigning the patient to such major surgical procedures as thyroidectomy, parathyroidectomy, partial pancreatectomy, or adrenalectomy. Fortified by accurate diagnosis, the endocrinologist no longer has any excuse to treat blindly or to practice magic.

Bloodworth, J. M. B. (ed.): Endocrine Pathology. Baltimore, Williams & Wilkins Company, 1968.
Christy, N. P. (ed.): The Human Adrenal Cortex. New York, Harper & Row, 1971.
Cope, C. L.: Adrenal Steroids and Disease. 2nd ed. Philadelphia, J. B. Lippincott Company, 1972.
Deane, H. W., and Rubin, B. L. (eds.): The Adrenocortical Hormones. Part 3. Handbook of Experimental Pharmacology, Vol. XIV/3. Berlin, Springer-Verlag, 1968.
Drezner, M., Neelon, F. A., and Lebovitz, H. E.: Pseudohypoparathyroidism, Type II: A possible defect in the reception of the cyclic AMP signal. N. Engl. J. Med., 289:1056, 1973.
Edmonds, M., Lamki, L., Killinger, D. W., and Volpé, R.: Autoimmune thyroiditis, adrenalitis and oophoritis. Am. J. Med., 54:782, 1973.
Ezrin, C., Godden, J. O., Volpé, R., and Wilson, R. (eds.): Systematic Endocrinology. Hagerstown, Md., Harper & Row, 1973.
Gardner, L. I. (ed.): Endocrine and Genetic Diseases of Childhood. Philadelphia, W. B. Saunders Company, 1969.
Labhart, A. (ed.): Klinik der inneren Sekretion. 2nd ed. Berlin, Springer-Verlag, 1971.
Nusynowitz, M. L., and Klein, M. H.: Pseudoidiopathic hypoparathyroidism. Hypoparathyroidism with ineffective parathyroid hormone. Am. J. Med., 55:677, 1973.
Rimoin, D. L., and Schimke, R. N.: Genetic Disorders of the Endocrine Glands. St. Louis, C. V. Mosby Company, 1971.
Schwartz, T. B., Ryan, W. G., and Becker, F. O. (eds.): The Year Book of Endocrinology. Chicago, Year Book Medical Publishers, 1973.
Sterling, K., Refetoff, S., and Selenkow, H. A.: T_3 thyrotoxicosis. Thyrotoxicosis due to elevated serum triiodothyronine levels. J.A.M.A., 213:571, 1970.
Sutherland, E. W.: Studies on the mechanism of hormone action. Science, 177:401, 1972.
Werner, S. C., and Ingbar, S. H. (eds.): The Thyroid. 3rd ed. New York, Harper & Row, 1971.
Wilkins, L.: The Diagnosis and Treatment of Endocrine Disorders in Childhood and Adolescence. 3rd ed. Springfield, Ill., Charles C Thomas, 1965.
Williams, R. H. (ed.): Textbook of Endocrinology. 5th ed. Philadelphia, W. B. Saunders Company, 1974.
Wilson, D. E. (ed.): Symposium on prostaglandins. Arch. Intern. Med., 133:29, 1974.
Wurtman, R. J. (ed.): Symposium: Biogenic amines and endocrine functions. Fed. Proc., 32:1769, 1973.

825. MODE OF ACTION OF HORMONES

John N. Loeb

The physiologic effects of the endocrine secretions have long been recognized as among the most dramatic in clinical medicine. The conspicuous consequences of castration in the male have been known since ancient times, and by the mid-nineteenth century the results of ablation of various other endocrine tissues had begun to be appreciated. By the end of the first quarter of the present century most of the currently recognized syndromes of endocrine hypersecretion had been described as well, and at the present time it is recognized that an enormous diversity of metabolic processes, exerting profound effects on growth and differentiation, are under endocrine control.

In recent years there has been a concerted effort to understand the biochemical mechanisms by which these processes are regulated, and in particular to account, in molecular terms, for the diverse and dramatic effects of the endocrine secretions on structure and function. The development of sensitive biochemical techniques has permitted a shift in focus from simple observations of hormonal effects to efforts at defining mechanisms by which such effects are mediated. It is becoming increasingly clear that, despite the variety of their physiological effects, the fundamental modes of action of many hormones are similar. This chapter outlines some of the patterns which are beginning to emerge and discusses some of their implications.

PROPERTIES COMMON TO ALL HORMONES

As non-neuronal carriers of information between different organs, hormones must interact specifically and reversibly with target cells, and this interaction must have the capacity to result in widespread cellular effects. The fact that hormones are normally present in extraordinarily low concentrations (e.g., 10^{-11} to 10^{-8} molar) moreover requires that target tissues be sensitive to even minute changes in hormone concentration. It follows that hormone–target cell interactions must have at least two characteristics: *specificity,* and the capacity for *amplification* of an initial hormone signal in terms of subsequent biochemical events. These two characteristics will be discussed in some detail below for different classes of hormones.

STEROID HORMONES

A general model for the mode of action of a steroid hormone is shown in Table 1. After secretion, the hormone, either alone or complexed to a specific plasma-binding protein, circulates to its target cell. The free hormone then diffuses into the cytoplasm, where it becomes attached to another specific binding protein called a "receptor" protein. This attachment results in a steroid-receptor complex which has a high affinity for a specific region of the nuclear chromatin (DNA–histone protein complex). The steroid-receptor complex then enters the nucleus, becomes attached to this region of the chromatin, and, through mechanisms still unknown, interacts with the chromatin to bring about an increased rate of transcription (synthesis) of specific messenger RNA (mRNA). The resulting mRNA molecules leave the nucleus and enter the cytoplasm where they are "translated" into molecules of corresponding specific protein (see Part IV). These latter proteins, at least some of which are enzymes, then influence specific intracellular biochemical pathways and account for the ultimate "biologic effects" of the hormone. In recent years a number of steroid hormones have been studied, and in all instances their mechanism of action, insofar as it has been elucidated, appears to conform to this model.

CATECHOLAMINE, POLYPEPTIDE, AND PROTEIN HORMONES

In contrast to the steroid hormones, which must reach the cell *nucleus* before influencing cellular events, many other hormones exert their biochemical effects by

TABLE 1.   Outline of Modes of Action of Some Different Classes of Hormones

Hormone Class	Location of Receptor	Primary Result of Interaction with Receptor		Consequences
Steroids ? Thyroid hormones	Target cell cytoplasm	Steroid-receptor complexes in cytoplasm migrate to nucleus, bind to specific region(s) of chromatin, and result in increased rate of synthesis ("transcription") of specific mRNA molecules	mRNA molecules migrate to cytoplasm, where they are "translated" into molecules of protein (e.g., specific enzymes) →	Changes in enzyme concentrations, which can then influence the rates of specific biochemical events within the cell
Catecholamines Polypeptides Most proteins	Target cell outer membrane	1. Modification of adenyl cyclase activity: a. Stimulation of cAMP synthesis (e.g., catecholamines, majority of polypeptide and protein hormones—see Table 2)	Increased intracellular concentration of cAMP →	Changes in enzyme activities, changes in cell permeability, etc. (effects of cAMP dependent upon nature of particular target cell—see Table 2)
		b. ? Inhibition of cAMP synthesis (e.g., to account for known effects of insulin on liver and fat cell cAMP levels)	Decreased intracellular concentration of cAMP →	Increased rate of liver glycogen synthesis; decreased rate of gluconeogenesis, glycogenolysis, and lipolysis
		2. ? Direct effect on membrane transport processes (e.g., effects of insulin on glucose uptake by adipose tissue and skeletal muscle)	Increased rate of glucose entry →	Increased rate of glucose utilization and glycogen synthesis

interacting directly with the external cell surface. These latter hormones include many polypeptide and protein hormones as well as the catecholamines, and in these instances the hormone receptors, instead of being located in the cytoplasm of the target cell, appear to be located in the external cell membrane ("plasma membrane") itself. As shown in Table 1, the result of the interaction of one of these hormones with its receptor in the cell membrane depends upon the nature of the hormone. As first shown by the brilliant work of Sutherland, a large number of membrane-active hormones exert their effects by interacting specifically with the enveloping cell membrane to activate *adenyl cyclase,* an enzyme present in the membranes of a great variety of cells. Activation of adenyl cyclase causes an increased rate of synthesis of 3′,5′-cyclic adenosine monophosphate ("cAMP") from ATP. This mechanism leads to an increase in the intracellular concentration of cAMP and accounts for the action of the catecholamines and of most polypeptide and protein hormones for which mechanisms are currently known. An increase in cAMP concentration in a target organ can have diverse and important biochemical consequences which depend upon the cell type and which account for the physiologic effects of the hormone on its target tissue. The diversity of these effects is illustrated in Table 2. In contrast to the steroid hormones, the effects of which require new RNA and protein synthesis (see above), the catecholamine and most of the polypeptide hormones act directly to influence the activity of pre-existing enzyme systems. Many of their physiologic effects can thus be observed almost instantaneously (e.g., those of epinephrine), in contrast to those of the steroid hormones which often require many minutes or longer to become clinically apparent (e.g., the effects of hydrocortisone).

Insulin, in contrast to the hormones discussed in the preceding paragraph, is known to produce a *decrease* in the cyclic AMP content of several tissues. Although it is possible that a fall in intracellular cAMP accounts for many of the effects of insulin on the liver and adipose tissue, it is by no means clear that it explains *all* the biologic effects of the hormone. Other important effects of insulin, such as the stimulation of glucose uptake by

skeletal muscle, appear thus far to take place in the absence of any demonstrable change in adenyl cyclase activity or total intracellular cAMP concentration and may instead reflect direct and independent effects of the hormone on membrane transport processes. Two other examples of protein hormones whose mechanism of action remains unclear are growth hormone and calcitonin.

TABLE 2.   Some Hormonal Responses Dependent Upon an Activation of Adenyl Cyclase

Hormone	Target Tissue	Response
Catecholamines	Liver	Activation of phosphorylase Inactivation of glycogen synthetase
	Skeletal muscle	Activation of phosphorylase Inactivation of glycogen synthetase
	Heart	Activation of phosphorylase Positive inotropic response
	Adipose tissue	Lipolysis
	Salivary gland	Amylase secretion
	Kidney	Renin production
	Pineal gland	Melatonin synthesis
Glucagon	Liver	Activation of phosphorylase
	Pancreatic beta cell	Insulin release
	Adipose tissue	Lipolysis
ACTH*	Adrenal cortex	Steroidogenesis
	Adipose tissue	Lipolysis
LH (ICSH)*	Corpus luteum	Steroidogenesis
	Testis	Steroidogenesis
Angiotensin	Zona glomerulosa	Steroidogenesis
Vasopressin	Renal collecting tubule	Increase in permeability to water
TRH*	Anterior pituitary	TSH release
TSH*	Thyroid	Thyroid hormone release
Gastrin	Gastric parietal cell	Production of HCl
Parathormone	Renal tubule	Excretion of phosphate
	Bone	Calcium mobilization

*ACTH, adrenocorticotrophic hormone; LH (ICSH), luteinizing hormone (interstitial cell–stimulating hormone); TRH, thyrotrophin-releasing hormone; TSH, thyroid-stimulating hormone (thyrotrophin). (Modified after Sutherland, E. W., et al.: Circulation, 37:279, 1968.)

SPECIFICITY OF HORMONAL EFFECTS; "AMPLIFICATION" OF HORMONAL SIGNALS

Two characteristics of hormonal effects have already been mentioned: their *specificity* and the fact that hormones exert their biochemical effects at extremely low molecular concentrations. Both characteristics will be considered briefly as they apply to the two different models for hormone action presented above. In the first model, that for *steroid hormone* action, specificity resides in the affinity of the steroid hormone for its appropriate receptor protein in the cytoplasm of the target tissue. Thus tissues which are estrogen sensitive contain an estrogen-binding receptor protein in their cytoplasm, whereas those which are unresponsive to estrogen do not. "Amplification" of the initial steroid signal can occur at several subsequent steps: interaction of the steroid-receptor complex with the nuclear chromatin can bring about the transcription of more than one molecule of mRNA from a given DNA gene; each of these can then be translated into many enzyme molecules, each of which in turn can catalyze the transformation of many molecules of intracellular substrate into product.

The model presented for *those hormones which operate through cAMP* provides a similar opportunity for both specificity of hormone effect and amplification of the hormonal signal. The mechanisms, however, are different. In the case of the polypeptide and catecholamine hormones, specificity is determined not only by the presence or absence of specific hormone receptors in a cell membrane, but also by the response of that cell to an increased level of cAMP once adenyl cyclase has been activated (see, e.g., Table 2 and References). Mechanisms by which the adenyl cyclase system can amplify an initial hormonal signal are described under the following heading.

CYCLIC AMP

Biologic Effects. The effects of changes in the intracellular concentration of cAMP depend upon the nature of the cell in which these changes occur. Thus in various cells an increase in intracellular cAMP may affect enzyme activities (for example, that of phosphorylase in liver or muscle), may affect permeability of the external cell membrane (as in the renal collecting tubule), may influence gene transcription, or, in certain tissues, may actually stimulate the production or release of certain hormones (see Table 2). The generation of cAMP in response to a hormonal signal at the surface of the cell permits the conversion of an external hormonal signal into a new kind of *(intracellular)* signal, referred to by Sutherland as a "second messenger," and can greatly amplify the original hormonal signal; by stimulating adenyl cyclase activity, a single hormone molecule can potentially cause the synthesis of many molecules of cAMP, which in turn can produce a whole cascade of events within the cell. Both the complexity of these events and their extraordinary rapidity, despite this complexity, are illustrated by the familiar example of hepatic glycogenolysis in response to epinephrine. The steps involved are illustrated in Figure 1; the many steps which intervene between the binding of epinephrine to receptor sites in liver cell membranes and the clinical "result" (an elevation of the blood sugar) are evident.

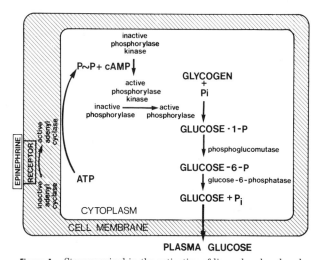

Figure 1. Steps required in the activation of liver phosphorylase by epinephrine resulting in glycogenolysis and hyperglycemia. The activation of phosphorylase is only one of the consequences of an increased level of cAMP in the liver, and the precise mechanism by which cAMP produces a shift in the balance between inactive and active phosphorylase in favor of the active form is still somewhat conjectural for this tissue. ($P \sim P$, pyrophosphate; P_1, inorganic phosphate; enzymes are indicated in small type.)

Regulation of Intracellular Cyclic AMP Concentration. The intracellular concentration of cAMP is controlled both by regulation of its rate of synthesis and by regulation of its rate of degradation. Degradation of cAMP occurs via a phosphodiesterase which rapidly hydrolyzes cAMP (3′,5′-cyclic AMP) to the noncyclic monoester 5′-AMP. It has been found that many substances not conventionally considered hormones are capable of affecting intracellular cAMP levels and hence of mimicking the effects of certain hormones (Fig. 2). Epinephrine and theophylline, for example, have very different primary biochemical actions, yet through entirely different mechanisms they both cause an in-

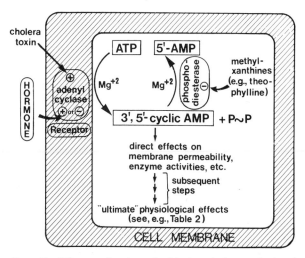

Figure 2. Influence of various physiologic and pharmacologic substances on the formation and degradation of cyclic AMP. → ⊕ implies stimulation; → ⊖ implies inhibition. Prostaglandins may also affect adenyl cyclase activity, but whether they result in an increase or a decrease in the level of cyclic AMP depends upon target cell type. (Modified after Sutherland, E. W., et al.: Circulation, 37:279, 1968.)

creased concentration of cAMP in many cells. In view of this "final common path" it is not surprising that many of the familiar physiologic effects of theophylline and epinephrine (e.g., tachycardia, positive inotropic effect, dilatation of the coronary arteries, bronchodilatation, nervousness, sweating, glycogenolysis, lipolysis) are so similar.

OTHER HORMONES

The modes of action of certain other hormones remain obscure. Perhaps the most conspicuous example is that of the thyroid hormones, thyroxine and triiodothyronine, which, despite the relative simplicity of their chemical structures, exert their biologic effects by mechanisms still unclear. Although early effects of thyroid hormones include both stimulation of nuclear RNA synthesis and stimulation of mitochondrial protein synthesis and oxygen consumption, and although some of the latter effects can be mimicked by the addition of thyroid hormones to isolated mitochondria in vitro, recent reports of specific nuclear hormone-binding sites suggest the nucleus as a primary site of action. There is evidence that the calorigenic effect of these hormones may be mediated by an increased utilization of ATP in the process of intracellular sodium extrusion, but this phenomenon, in contrast to effects on nuclei and mitochondria, is a relatively late consequence of thyroid hormone administration. (See References for further discussion of some current hypotheses about thyroid hormone action.)

HORMONE STRUCTURE AND SPECIFICITY

The relation between hormone structure and specificity is imperfectly understood, but studies of the relation between molecular structure and function in simpler systems suggest concepts that may apply to hormones and their target-cell receptors. In most of the systems studied so far it appears that the number of indispensable functional groups per molecule is small. For steroid hormones, for example, it is probable that the steroid nucleus itself functions little more than as a rigid spacer to hold essential functional groups in fixed relation to each other. Thus the stilbestrol molecule, a potent but nonsteroidal synthetic estrogen, bears only superficial resemblance to estradiol except in the relative (and fixed) positions of its phenolic hydroxy groups.

In the more complex polypeptide hormones it is possible that one portion of the molecule is responsible for specific binding to a membrane receptor, while another portion interacts with adenyl cyclase to stimulate the synthesis of cAMP. Thyroid-stimulating hormone (TSH) and luteinizing hormone (LH), for example, both exert their biologic effects by stimulating adenyl cyclase in their respective target tissues. Both hormone molecules consist of subunits made up of two different proteins, and one of these two subunits is identical in both hormones. It is tempting to speculate that the subunit which is shared in common contains the site that interacts with adenyl cyclase, whereas the other subunit, which is different in the two hormones, contains the determinants for their tissue specificity.

It now seems likely that those hormone molecules which act by influencing cAMP synthesis and which have tissue specificity contain not only functional groups capable of interacting with adenyl cyclase, but also functional groups which confer an affinity for specific receptors in their target cell membranes. An ingenious and attractive, though still unproved, hypothesis has recently been advanced by Beers and Reich. They have suggested that certain essential tyrosinyl, histadyl, and tryptophanyl residues in the polypeptide hormones may represent the evolutionary descendents of three "primeval" adenyl cyclase–stimulating amines, epinephrine, histamine, and serotonin, and that these amino acids may play an analogous role in the stimulation of adenyl cyclase in target tissues. The rest of the polypeptide molecule is regarded as an elaborate appendage which has been acquired in the course of evolution to confer necessary tissue specificity and to maintain the amino acid at the adenyl cyclase–active site in an appropriate three-dimensional orientation. Epinephrine, for example, is a simple amine and stimulates adenyl cyclase in a great variety of target cells (see, e.g., Table 2); in contrast, the specificity of a substance like parathormone may, by this hypothesis, be attributed to the acquisition of a portion of the molecule which is capable of binding to a more restricted range of target tissues, and which may in fact be at some distance from the site which interacts with adenyl cyclase.

"PHYSIOLOGIC" VS. "PHARMACOLOGIC" EFFECTS

The diversity of the human hormones and their striking tissue specificity are apparent. With the ready availability of many of these hormones in pure form, and with the present ability of the biochemist to detect even subtle effects, an ever-increasing number of hormonal "effects" are being described. One must be cautious in interpreting some of these observations, particularly those made at hormone concentrations which greatly exceed those present in the normal organism. At high concentrations of hormone it is possible that certain exquisite end-organ specificities are simply overcome; under such conditions occasional "anomalous effects" on "surprising" target organs may have little *physiologic* significance.

Buchanan, J., and Tapley, D. F.: Thyroid hormones: Subcellular effects. *In* Werner, S. C., and Ingbar, S. H. (eds.): The Thyroid: A Fundamental and Clinical Text. New York, Harper & Row, 1971, p. 90.
Cahill, G. F., Jr.: Glucagon (editorial). N. Engl. J. Med., 288:157, 1973.
Ismail-Beigi, F., and Edelman, I. S.: The mechanism of the calorigenic action of thyroid hormone: Stimulation of Na⁺ + K⁺-activated adenosine triphosphatase activity. J. Gen. Physiol., 57:710, 1971.
Jesen, E. V., and DeSombre, E. R.: Estrogen-receptor interaction. Science, 182:126, 1973.
Lefkowitz, R. J.: Isolated hormone receptors: Physiologic and clinical implications. N. Engl. J. Med., 288:1061, 1973.
Levine, R.: Action of insulin: An attempt at a summary. Diabetes, 21 (suppl.): 454, 1972.
Loeb, J. N.: Models for hormone action. *In* Christy, N. P. (ed.): The Human Adrenal Cortex. New York, Harper & Row, 1971, p. 191.
Maddaiah, V. T.: A model for hormone specific activation of adenyl cyclase. J. Theor. Biol., 25:495, 1969.
O'Malley, B. W.: Mechanisms of action of steroid hormones. N. Engl. J. Med., 284:370, 1971.
Oppenheimer, J. H., Koerner, D., Schwartz, H. L., and Surks, M. I.: Specific nuclear triiodothyronine binding sites in rat liver and kidney. J. Clin. Endocrinol. Metab., 35:330, 1972.
Pitot, H. C., and Yatvin, M. B.: Interrelationships of mammalian hormones and enzyme levels in vivo. Physiol. Rev., 53:228, 1973.
Robison, G. A., Butcher, R. W., and Sutherland, E. W.: Cyclic AMP. New York, Academic Press, 1971.

Roth, J.: Peptide hormone binding to receptors: A review of direct studies in vitro. Metabolism, 22:1059, 1973.

Samuels, H. H., and Tsai, J. S.: Thyroid hormone action in cell culture: Demonstration of nuclear receptors in intact cells and isolated nuclei. Proc. Natl. Acad. Sci. (USA), 70:3488, 1973.

Sutherland, E. W.: Studies on the mechanism of hormone action. Science, 177:401, 1972.

Sutherland, E. W., Robison, G. A., and Butcher, R. W.: Some aspects of the biological role of adenosine 3′,5′-monophosphate (cyclic AMP). Circulation, 37:279, 1968.

Thompson, E. B., and Lippman, M. E.: Mechanism of action of glucocorticoids. Metabolism, 23:159, 1974.

Tomkins, G. M., Gelehrter, T. D., Granner, D., Martin, D. W., Samuels, H. H., and Thompson, E. B.: Control of specific gene expression in higher organisms. Science, 166:1474, 1969.

826. THE CONTROL OF ANTERIOR PITUITARY SECRETION

Seymour Reichlin

Although the anterior pituitary gland lacks a direct nerve supply, the secretion of each of its hormones is under the control of the central nervous system. Through specialized secretory neurons localized in the ventral hypothalamus, the function of the pituitary and, in turn, of its target glands becomes responsive to changes in the external and internal environment. In addition, the neurohumoral connections of the anterior pituitary are important in the "feedback" regulation of a number of hormones such as cortisol, the gonadal steroids, thyroxine, and prolactin, and serve as part of the integrated mechanism by which behavioral and metabolic adaptation to the external environment is accomplished.

During the last few years, as the importance of neural factors in the control of pituitary secretion has become increasingly apparent, a division of study of endocrinology has developed which is termed *neuroendocrinology*. This area deals mainly with the interaction of neural and hormonal factors in endocrine and metabolic control systems.

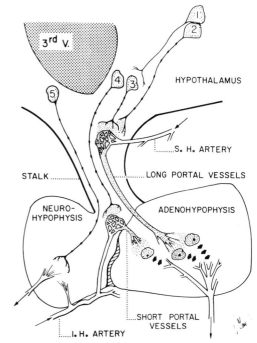

Figure 1. The functional elements of control of the hypothalamic-pituitary unit. Two general types of neurons are involved in anterior pituitary regulation. One type, the peptidergic neuron, forms the releasing hormones (shown here as No. 3, ending in the median eminence, and No. 4, ending in the pituitary stalk), both in relation to the capillary plexus of the hypophysial-portal vessels. These neurons (corresponding to the designation "tuberohypophysial" neurons) are neurosecretory. That is, they combine the function of excitable electrical tissue and secretory function and serve as "neuroendocrine transducers" (Wurtman, 1971) to convert neural information to hormonal information. Their function is analogous to the function of the classic supraopticohypophysial neuron (No. 5), the structure responsible for secretion of vasopressin. The second type of neuron is the link between the rest of the brain and the peptidergic neuron. These are largely monaminergic and are believed to end on the cell body of the peptidergic neuron in a conventional manner (No. 1), or to end on the axon terminus of the peptidergic neuron (No. 2) in a manner termed by Schneider and McCann "axo-axonic." Abbreviations: S.H., superior hypophysial; I.H., inferior hypophysial; 3rd V., third ventricle. (From Gay, V.: Fertility and Sterility, 23:50, 1972.)

HYPOTHALAMIC NEUROSECRETION: HYPOPHYSIOTROPHIC NEURONS

The pituitary gland and hypothalamus are closely related anatomically, as may be seen in Figure 1. This relationship has both embryologic and functional significance. The neural lobe develops as a downgrowth of axons from the diencephalon, whose cells of origin are located in the paraventricular and supraoptic nuclei of the hypothalamus. These nerve fibers pass as unmyelinated axons through the neural stalk and terminate in the neural lobe. Like neurons elsewhere, supraopticohypophysial and paraventriculohypophysial neurons are electrically excitable, conduct action potentials, and are responsive to neurotransmitters. Unlike most other neurons, these cells are neurosecretory, that is, they synthesize hormonal substances which are released into blood vessels for action at a remote site rather than locally at synapses, as is characteristic of most neurons. Hormones of the neurohypophysis are synthesized

mainly in cell bodies located in the hypothalamus and pass in granule form (associated with a protein carrier substance) to the nerve endings in the neural lobe, where they are stored. Neurosecretory neurons thus manifest the properties of both nerve and gland. These cells, of which the neurohypophysial neurons are the classic example, have been termed by Wurtman "*neuroendocrine transducers.*" Cells of this type are the major effector links between the nervous system and the endocrine gland. Although the neural lobe lies close to the anterior lobe of the pituitary and neurohypophysial secretory products are identifiable in blood reaching the pituitary, the secretions of the neurohypophysis (oxytocin, vasopressin, neurophysin) have no established regulatory action in the anterior lobe but are released into the systemic circulation to affect remote tissues such as the kidney, breast, and uterus.

The phylogenetically more primitive neuroendocrine "transducer" for anterior pituitary control is located within the median eminence of the hypothalamus.

Nerve endings here contain "hypophysiotrophic" hormones; these substances, also called *"releasing factors,"* reach the anterior pituitary through a specialized system of capillaries and veins, the hypophysial-portal circulation. The cells of origin of the median eminence neurons are clustered around the medial-basal hypothalamus in the so-called hypophysiotrophic area. They resemble neurohypophysial neurons in being electrically active, pharmacologically excitable, and responsive to a wide variety of nerve impulses arising from other sites in the brain and to feedback hormonal stimuli. Neuron endings of the stalk–median eminence region (tuberohypophysial neurons) and the associated blood vessels have been likened to the posterior lobe and can be looked upon as a "median eminence gland"; taken together, these structures constitute the "final common pathway" for neural control of the anterior pituitary gland.

This outline of anterior pituitary regulation is the *portal vessel chemotransmitter hypothesis.* According to this view, lesions of the hypothalamus (and of the portal vessel complex of the stalk) reduce most anterior pituitary functions by causing a deficiency of releasing factors. Direct electrical stimulation of the tuberohypophysial neurons, or reflex activation of these neurons, caused, for example, by emotional stress, activates the anterior pituitary by the release of hypophysiotrophic hormones.

Initially based on indirect physiologic experiments, this hypothesis has been established by demonstration of hypothalamic substances which selectively affect each of the known pituitary hormones. These are CRF (corticotrophin-releasing factor), TRF (TRH) (thyrotrophin-releasing factor), GHRF (growth hormone–releasing factor), LRF (LRH) (luteinizing hormone–releasing factor), FSHRF (follicle-stimulating hormone-releasing factor), and PRF (prolactin-releasing factor). Because the existence of these substances seems so well established, it has been proposed that they be called releasing hormones. Inhibitory hypophysiotrophic hormones have also been identified. These are PIF (prolactin inhibitory factor) and GHRIF (growth hormone release inhibitory factor [somatostatin]). MSH secretion by intermediate lobe cells (which do not form a definite anatomic subdivision in the human subject) appears to be regulated by both excitatory (MSHRF) and inhibitory factors (MSHIF).

The chemical nature of TRF, now termed thyrotrophic-releasing hormone (TRH), was identified in 1969 as a tripeptide amide, pyroglutamyl histidyl prolineamide (Fig. 2). The chemical nature of LRF (LRH) was identified in 1971 as a decapeptide (Fig. 2), the amino terminal of which (like TRH) is pyroglutamic acid and the carboxyl terminal an amide. A substance with powerful growth hormone release inhibitory activity, chemically identified in 1973 as a linear peptide composed of 14 amino acids (Fig. 2), was named by its discoverers *somatostatin.* The chemical nature of the MSH-regulating peptides is still somewhat uncertain, but fractions of oxytocin (the terminal tripeptide, and the five-membered ring tocinoic acid) have been reported to have powerful effects on MSH secretion in various test situations. Although the primary activity of the aforementioned chemically identified releasing hormones is related to the original bioassay properties used in purification and identification, it is now apparent that there are certain

pyroGlu-His-Pro Amide

TRH, Thyrotrophin-releasing hormone

pyroGlu-His-Trp-Ser-Tyr-Gly-Leu-Arg-Pro-Gly Amide

LRH, Luteinizing hormone–releasing hormone, gonadotrophin-releasing hormone, GnRH

H-Ala-Gly-Cys-Lys-Asn-Phe-Phe-Trp-Lys-Thr-Phe-Thr-Ser-Cys-OH

GHRF-IF, Somatostatin

Figure 2. Structural formulas of the established hypophysiotrophic hormones.

crossover effects of these hormones. Thus TRH is a potent releaser of prolactin in man and certain other species and releases GH in some acromegalics. LRH releases FSH as well as LH and may therefore be the only gonadotrophin-releasing hormone (GnRH) for regulation of both of these gonadotrophins. Somatostatin inhibits TSH secretion as well as somatotrophic hormone secretion and, when given in "pharmacologic" doses, inhibits pancreatic secretion of glucagon and insulin. The chemical nature of CRF and GHRF has not been identified.

In the human subject, TRH and LRH have been widely used for physiologic and diagnostic studies of pituitary function.

One of the important consequences of these discoveries is that means have now been provided for selective manipulation of the secretion of TSH, LH-FSH, prolactin, and GH.

BIOGENIC AMINE CONTROL OF HYPOPHYSIOTROPHIC FUNCTIONS

The hypophysiotrophic neurons are in turn innervated by specialized monaminergic neurotransmitter neurons (Fig. 1), the principal ones of which secrete dopamine, norepinephrine, and serotonin. It appears probable, though not completely established, that norepinephrine stimulates the secretion of LRH, TRH, and GHRF, and that dopamine stimulates the secretion of PIF. There is evidence that serotonin may inhibit the secretion of PIF and of TRF. A noradrenergic link in the regulation of CRF appears to be inhibitory. Since the central nervous biogenic amine network is also involved in the regulation of affective states (such as depression), many drugs commonly used as psychopharmacologic agents, e.g., reserpine and phenothiazines, may alter anterior pituitary function. Clinical examples of such effects are irregular menstrual cycles or anovulation in women (owing to blockade of the cyclic discharge of LRH), galactorrhea (owing to inhibition of PIF release), and inhibition of reflex somatotrophin release (owing to inhibition of GHRF). Certain of the drug effects have been used to test hormonal secretion. For example, chlorpromazine and other phenothiazines stimulate prolactin release and have been used as a means of testing prolactin secretory reserve. Chlorpromazine has been used to treat acromegaly, because it lowers GH levels in some cases, presumably through changes in secretion of GHRF. L-Dopa, a drug used in the treatment of Parkinson's disease, which increases central nervous system concentration of dopamine, brings about the release of GH and the inhibition of prolactin secretion. In acromegalics L-dopa may paradoxically inhibit growth hormone secretion.

Hormonal feedback effects are also involved in the control of the hypophysiotrophic neurons. The relative importance of hypothalamic and pituitary feedback appears to differ to some degree from one system to another. The pituitary-thyroid axis is the best worked out of these control systems. Thyroid hormone regulates TSH secretion through a direct inhibitory effect on the anterior pituitary. These inhibitory effects are opposed by the stimulatory effect of hypothalamic drive brought about by TRH secretion. TRH secretion, a neurogenic function, is responsive to a variety of neural signals, including those involved in temperature regulation. It has been proposed that the secretion of TRH may also be stimulated by thyroid hormone as a *positive* feedback effect, although the opposite effect of thyroid hormone has also been reported to occur.

Gonadotrophic hormone secretion is regulated by a complex interaction of ovarian or testicular hormone feedback on both the pituitary and hypothalamus. Evidence has been adduced in man which shows that LRH secretion may be stimulated by the positive feedback effects of estrogen on the hypothalamus. Estrogenic hormones inhibit pituitary responsiveness to LRH, but can also transiently *sensitize* the pituitary to releasing hormone, depending upon the effects of time and dose. In addition to this hormonal interaction, gonadotrophin secretion is subject to "open-loop" effects such as emotional stress (which in the human can inhibit ovulation), and in animals such as the rabbit copulation can trigger reflex ovulation.

Growth hormone secretion is almost exclusively controlled by the central nervous system. Estrogenic hormones appear to sensitize the pituitary to the growth hormone–releasing factor, and metabolic (as well as stress-related) events are mediated at the level of the hypothalamus. An important aspect of GH regulation is so-called short-loop feedback control. Plasma GH itself is capable of inhibiting the secretion of GHRF.

Prolactin secretion, like GH secretion, is largely regulated by the nervous system; there is a short-loop feedback control, and estrogen also appears to sensitize the pituitary to the effects of PRF.

Cortisol feedback inhibition of the pituitary-adrenal axis appears to act primarily on the median eminence of the hypothalamus, but there is an important negative feedback effect on the pituitary, and cortisol may also act on suprahypothalamic neural structures. Some workers believe that all feedback control is directed at the pituitary and that results of experiments in which intrahypothalamic injection of cortisol was effective in inhibiting ACTH were due to transport of the cortisol via the median eminence to the pituitary.

An important recent insight is that pituitary secretion of growth hormone, prolactin, and ACTH is regulated by intrinsic brain rhythms related to the sleep-wake cycle or to changes in lighting, rather than by specific homeostatic requirements. Nocturnal GH secretion (largely related to early deep sleep) accounts for more than half of total daily GH secretion, values at night approaching the levels found in acromegaly. Nocturnal prolactin secretion begins about the same time that GH secretion does but appears to last longer. The

secretion of ACTH with a peak in the early morning hours is linked to the day-night lighting cycle. Nocturnal rhythms for TSH and (under certain circumstances) gonadotrophins have also been shown. Disturbances in sleep-related hormonal secretion may be the earliest indication of incipient or mild hypothalamic-pituitary disturbance. Proper evaluation of total endocrine function under physiologic or pathologic states must take into account these diurnal rhythms.

NEUROENDOCRINE DISEASES OF THE PITUITARY GLAND

It is apparent that any consideration of the neuroendocrine diseases of the pituitary overlaps the descriptions of diseases of the pituitary itself (see Ch. 830 to 832). The following paragraphs emphasize, primarily, neuroendocrine disorders of the anterior pituitary.

In the context of the foregoing description of the hypothalamic-pituitary unit, disorders of pituitary se-

TABLE 1.   Endocrine Syndromes of Hypothalamic Origin

Hypophysiotrophic hormone deficiency:
  Surgical pituitary stalk section
  Basilar meningitis and granuloma, sarcoidosis, tuberculosis,
    sphenoid osteomyelitis, eosinophilic granuloma
  Craniopharyngioma
  Hypothalamic tumor
    Infundibuloma
    Teratoma (ectopic pinealoma)
    Neuroglial tumors, particularly astrocytoma
  Maternal deprivation syndrome
  Isolated GHRF deficiency
  Hypothalamic hypothyroidism
  Panhypophysiotrophic failure

Disorders of regulation of LRH and FRH:
  Female
    Precocious puberty
    Delayed puberty
    Neurogenic amenorrhea
      Pseudocyesis
      Anorexia nervosa
      "Functional amenorrhea"
      "Functional oligomenorrhea"
      Drug-induced amenorrhea
  Male
    Precocious puberty
    Fröhlich's syndrome
    Olfactory-genital dysplasia (Kallmann's syndrome)

Disorders of regulation of prolactin-inhibiting hormone (nonpuerperal galactorrhea):
  Tumor
  Sarcoid
  Drug-induced
  Reflex
    Herpes zoster of chest wall
    Post-thoracotomy
    Nipple manipulation
    Spinal cord tumor
  "Psychogenic"
  Chiari-Frommel syndrome
  Hypothyroidism
  CO_2 narcosis

Disorders of regulation of CRF:
  Paroxysmal ACTH discharge (Wolff's syndrome)
  Loss of circadian variation
  Cushing's disease?

Hypersecretion of GHRF:
  Acromegaly?

cretion can be viewed as occurring at many "levels" of function. Defects may arise resulting from destruction of the pituitary itself (as by a tumor), or from genetically determined deficiency of a particular type of pituitary cell. At a higher level, disorders may arise through disruption of the stalk–median eminence neurons or of their essential vascular channels to the anterior pituitary gland. Such destruction of the "final common path" of anterior pituitary regulation occurs after surgical stalk section, in tumors of the stalk region, e.g., craniopharyngioma, infundibuloma, or teratomas, and in such inflammations as sarcoidosis. In precocious puberty, the tonically active inhibitory system which determines the time at which the hypophysiotrophic neurons will become active may be destroyed or inactivated too soon. Disease may also arise from abnormal stimulation of the hypophysiotrophic neurons. In Table 1 the major endocrine diseases of hypothalamic origin are listed.

Hypophysiotrophic Hormone Deficiency

Introduction of TRH and LRH into clinical medicine has made it possible to identify several syndromes of hypophysiotrophic neuron failure. Isolated TSH deficiency secondary to isolated TRH deficiency has been identified as a rare cause of thyroid failure. This disorder has been termed *"hypothalamic hypothyroidism"* or *"tertiary"* hypothyroidism. Isolated LRH deficiency accounts for the endocrine deficiency in many patients with isolated gonadotrophic deficiency, as in Kallmann's syndrome (hypogonadotrophic hypogonadism with hyposmia). Isolated GHRF deficiency appears to underlie the growth hormone secretory failure in the bulk of patients with idiopathic dwarfism. There also appears to be a disorder of "panhypophysiotrophic failure" in which all pituitary functions are lost. Most children with idiopathic panhypopituitarism fall into this category.

Hypophysiotrophic deficiency can be induced by destruction of the hypophysiotrophic area of the hypothalamus, of the stalk, or of the vascular supply to the anterior pituitary. The association of hypophysiotrophic deficiency with abnormal EEG's, and a history of birth trauma in some cases, or its occurrence as a congenital loss of hypophysiotrophic secretion, suggests an analogy with other forms of birth injury.

Under most circumstances, acquired hypophysiotrophic deficiency (as in surgical stalk section) results in a moderate to severe degree of pituitary failure, but the extent of endocrine deficit is not as extreme as that seen after hypophysectomy. This residuum of function (which is readily duplicated in laboratory animals) has been thought in the past to represent the "autonomous" capacity of the pituitary to function independent of the hypothalamus. With the identification of syndromes of hypophysiotrophic failure, as in "hypothalamic hypothyroidism" and panhypophysiotrophic failure, has come the recognition that pituitary deficiency as severe as that observed after hypophysectomy can at times follow loss of hypothalamic function. It is probable that most of the so-called pituitary autonomy after stalk section is the result of residual hypothalamic hypophysiotrophic function.

The main endocrine manifestations of hypothalamic failure are variable loss of TSH secretion, abolition of gonadotrophin secretion, loss of normal GH secretory responses to hypoglycemia and other stimuli, and loss of normal sleep pattern. Circadian and tonic baseline corticotrophin secretion is abolished, as is feedback control by circulating cortisol levels, but the response to certain kinds of stress, such as pyrogens, may be retained, suggesting that there are extrahypothalamic sites of formation of CRF. In sharp contrast to the hypophysectomized patient, individuals with hypothalamic disease usually have high circulating levels of prolactin owing to loss of PIF influence. Galactorrhea develops in about one fourth of women after section of the pituitary stalk, although all have elevated prolactin levels in plasma. The most sensitive signs of hypothalamic damage appear to be loss of diurnal GH rhythms, loss of GH secretory responses to stress, and the capacity to have an ovulatory surge of LH secretion.

Disorders of Regulation of GHRF

In addition to idiopathic hypophysiotrophic failure and specific damage to the hypothalamus or stalk, growth hormone deficiency may arise on a psychogenic basis in the so-called maternal deprivation syndrome (MDS). Such patients, generally children from grossly disturbed homes, may fail to grow despite adequate food intake. When they are brought into the hospital and given a degree of tender, loving care, growth rate returns to normal. GH secretion is impaired or absent in such children, and they do not respond to the usual stimuli such as hypoglycemia or arginine infusion. Since this disturbance is reversible after psychologic management, it has been concluded that a functional inhibition of the hypophysiotrophic GH-regulating neurons has taken place in these children. Deprivation in infants can cause severe marasmus.

In adults a somewhat analogous situation is seen in severe "monopolar" depression. Failure to release GH in response to hypoglycemia or to L-dopa administration suggests that in such patients there is an abnormality in central hypophysiotrophic function. In the light of modern ideas about the role of biogenic amines in determination of affective states, it is believed that the GH unresponsiveness in depression may be a reflection of abnormalities in central noradrenergic pathways in the hypothalamus.

In addition to GH unresponsiveness, some children with MDS may have unresponsive pituitary-adrenal function with loss of the circadian rhythm and of the response to the metyrapone test of ACTH reserve.

Excessive GHRF secretion has been proposed to be the cause of some cases of acromegaly.

Disorders of Regulation of GnRH

The concept of "levels" of neurogenic disruption of pituitary control is best illustrated in abnormalities of secretion of the gonadotrophins. Deficiency of both LH and FSH occurs after destruction of the hypophysiotrophic neurons. But disturbances also occur if the hypophysiotrophic neurons are themselves abnormally stimulated. The characteristic pattern of male gonadotrophin regulation is one of tonic low-level secretion of LH and FSH which leads to growth, development, and maturation of the spermatozoa, a process taking place over a 70-day period. The characteristic pattern of human female regulation is that of the recurring menstrual cycle, dependent upon a recurring surge of LH secretion which is in turn dependent upon cyclic secretion of estrogens by the ovary. In certain forms of hypothalamic disease, the characteristic normally recurring cyclic pattern of LH secretion may be lost. Because this often occurs transiently in a setting of severe psychologic stress, as after incarceration in concentration camps, in bombing attacks, or after minor stress such as going away to school, and develops in the absence of evident structural disease of the pituitary or hypothalamus, it is probable that loss of LH cycling may be an acquired psychologic disorder. The terms "functional amenorrhea," "functional oligomenorrhea," and "hypothalamic amenorrhea" have been applied to such cases. These probably represent a neural inhibition of normal estrogen-induced LRH secretion. A similar correlation appears likely in pseudocyesis, most often a manifestation of hysteria, and in anorexia nervosa. In about half the cases of anorexia nervosa, amenorrhea begins coincident with the disturbance in eating, and for this reason must be regarded as a concomitant rather than a consequence of inanition. Resumption of menstrual cycling does not occur until the patient has returned to a "critical weight," thus supporting the role of nutritional factors in this disease.

Besides these more obvious psychogenic changes in menstrual function, many women with "secondary" amenorrhea are encountered who have no apparent psychologic distress, but in whom the pattern of menstrual irregularity, amenorrhea, and oligomenorrhea is similar to that seen in the neurogenic syndromes. In one series, fully one fourth of the women in this category who were placed into a research study after one year or more of anovulation developed normal cycles within a month of their entry into the research project.

Next to pregnancy, "functional" amenorrhea is the most common cause of a secondary failure to menstruate. A clear-cut differential diagnosis between functional amenorrhea and disease of the anterior pituitary or hypothalamus can now be made. The patient with pituitary or hypothalamic disease most often has more than one trophic hormone deficiency, may have evidence of local pituitary damage, e.g., enlarged sella by x-ray, visual field defects, and behavioral or other neurologic abnormalities of the hypothalamus. Sixty to 80 per cent of patients with "functional" amenorrhea release luteinizing hormone after treatment with the drug clomiphene. Synthetic LRH stimulates LH and FSH release in patients whose disease is due to hypothalamic and not pituitary disorder. In patients with longstanding LRH deficiency, the pituitary may become relatively resistant to LRH. Repeated injections are required to restore normal responsivity. This finding indicates that LRH stimulates either the synthesis of LH or the secretory machinery for LH, or both, a conclusion supported by laboratory studies.

Drug-induced anovulation should be borne in mind as a cause of amenorrhea. Reserpine and the phenothiazines are particularly common causes. Patients who fail to resume normal menses after discontinuance of contraceptive pills ("post-pill amenorrhea") usually have underlying functional abnormalities of the pituitary-gonad axis evident before taking the pill. Such patients release LH in response to LRH. Excessive prolactin secretion (as in certain chromophobe adenomas) has recently been recognized as a cause of amenorrhea. Prolactin is thought to inhibit hypothalamic secretion of LRH. The tumor may not be detectable by usual neuroradiologic diagnostic methods, and cures have been achieved by removal of very small adenomas by microsurgical techniques.

Gonadotrophin regulatory difficulties may arise from loss of hypophysiotrophic function, from failure of the intrinsic cycling mechanism, and, at a higher functional level, from precocious or delayed development of sexual maturation. The timing of the onset of puberty is a neural function, and involves a patterned development of brain analogous to the patterns of development of other brain functions such as crawling, sitting, or walking and the development of abstract ability. Both delayed and accelerated puberty can be observed. When sexual function is normal in other respects, the term *precocious puberty* is applied, in contradistinction to the condition arising from primary secretory abnormalities of the gonads, properly termed *pseudoprecocious puberty*. All true precocious puberty is neurogenic in origin. In males, more than half the cases are due to brain lesions which directly or indirectly impinge upon the hypothalamus. In girls, fewer than 10 per cent have demonstrable lesions, although a high proportion have EEG abnormalities and may be regarded as suffering from mild degrees of brain damage.

In the male, primary isolated gonadotrophin failure is a well recognized cause of delayed puberty. In one type, there is an association with failure to develop rhinencephalic brain structures, manifested clinically by hyposmia. Such cases have been termed olfactory-genital dysplasia (Kallmann's syndrome), and appear to be due to failure to develop hypophysiotrophic function, because the patients usually respond to injections of LRH, albeit sluggishly. Cases of isolated gonadotrophic failure resulting from intrinsic pituitary disease have also been identified.

Disorders of Regulation of PIF

Many conditions cause lactation unrelated to pregnancy (nonpuerperal galactorrhea). Certain chromophobe pituitary tumors may secrete prolactin (Forbes-Albright syndrome) and induce lactation. Hypothalamic disturbance or "psychogenic" factors are important causes of galactorrhea. Causes listed in Table 1 have in common a presumed deficiency of prolactin inhibitory hormone, whether caused by irritation of the neural pathways involved in normal suckling reflexes (herpes zoster, nipple stimulation, post-thoracotomy) or by drugs, encephalopathy, hypothyroidism, or direct damage to the hypothalamus or stalk. Still uncertain is the relative frequency of small chromophobe adenomas as a cause of prolactin hypersecretion. Improved criteria for making the diagnosis of chromophobe adenoma are being developed. Values for prolactin over 150 ng per millimeter are very suspicious for tumor.

USE OF THE HYPOTHALAMIC HORMONES IN DIAGNOSIS OF ANTERIOR PITUITARY DISEASE

Synthetic TRH and LRH have been widely used for diagnostic purposes. The intravenous injection of TRH (15 to 800 μg; usual dose, 400 μg) is followed within five minutes by a rise in TSH which peaks between 15 and 45 minutes (Fig. 3). Changes in TSH secretion lead to a detectable increase in T_3 and a slight and less consist-

RESPONSE TO I.V. TRH 800 μg IN HUMANS

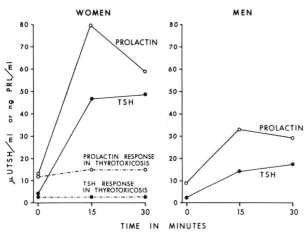

Figure 3. Effect of TRH on plasma TSH and prolactin in the human. (Data replotted from Bowers, C. Y., Friesen, H. G., Hwang, P., Guyda, H. J., and Folkers, K.: Biochem. Biophys. Res. Comm., 45:1033, 1970.) This figure illustrates the response of plasma TSH to injection of TRH in normal men and women and in patients with thyrotoxicosis. Note that the response is greater in women than in men, and is abolished by the thyrotoxic state. The latter effect is due to thyroxine- and triiodo-thyronine-induced inhibition of response at the pituitary level. TRH also acts as a prolactin-releasing hormone, and, like the TSH response, it is blocked by the administration of thyroxine, or the spontaneous occurrence of thyroid hormone excess.

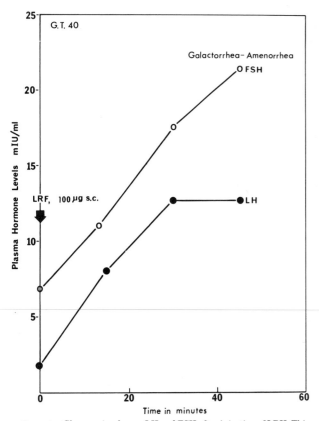

Figure 4. Changes in plasma LH and FSH after injection of LRH. This patient with a chromophobe adenoma of the pituitary had been amenorrheic for 15 years. Plasma prolactin levels (not shown) were 365 ng per ml. The prompt and striking response to LRH indicates that the amenorrhea was secondary to hypophysiotrophic failure, in this case owing to prolactin-induced inhibition of LRH secretion.

TABLE 2.* Changes in Plasma LH and FSH After Intravenous Injection of a Standard Test Dose of 100 μg of LRH

	LH (μIU/ml)	FSH (μIU/ml)
Males	83.9 ± 42.7	9.3 ± 4.4
Females		
Adult premenopausal	61.8 ± 26.2	5.2 ± 2.2
Menopausal	154.4 ± 46.9	49.1 ± 19.3

*From Hashimoto, T., Miyai, K., Izumi, K., and Kumahara, Y.: J. Clin. Endocrinol. Metab., 37:910, 1973.

ent increase in T_4. Mean responses in normal men are slightly less than in normal women, presumably owing to the estrogen sensitization of the anterior pituitary. In one series of normal subjects, mean maximal increment ±S.D. after 400 μg was 16.0 μU per ml ±2.5; in another, mean response to 500 μg was 25 μU ±10 of TSH. In normal people, prolactin levels also rise (Fig. 3), and in many acromegalics (unlike the normal) GH levels may also rise. Pituitary failure causes a loss of the response to TRH or a reduction in response, and in patients with TRH hypophysiotrophic failure the response may be slightly delayed in onset, but may rise higher, presumably owing to the associated hypothyroidism. This test thus permits the differentiation between pituitary and hypothalamic forms of secondary hypothyroidism. Because of the fact that thyroid hormone inhibits the pituitary, the response to TRH is also abolished in patients being treated with thyroid hormone, or in individuals with hyperthyroidism which may be so mild as to be barely detectable (Fig. 3). This response, in fact, is a very sensitive test for mild degrees of hyperthyroidism. Recovery of TSH responsiveness may be very much delayed (as long as six weeks) after a course of thyroxine treatment.

The administration of 20 to 500 μg of LRH (usual dose 100 μg subcutaneously or intravenously) is followed by a prompt rise in LH and a somewhat less marked and much more delayed rise in FSH (Fig. 4). Many patients will show only the LH response to the lower doses. There may be a shift in these responses according to prior hormonal state. In one well-studied series of patients, normal values ± S.D., as shown in Table 2, were obtained for peak increment in plasma gonadotrophins after intravenous injection of 100 μg of LRH.

Responses are abolished in patients with pituitary failure, and they may be excessive if the patient is in a state of increased gonadotrophic secretion, e.g., in menopausal or certain hypogonadal states. Individuals with hypothalamic failure may have reduced LH secretory responses to LRH, but these values return toward normal after repeated injections of the releasing hormones. The administration of estrogen in usual therapeutic doses usually causes a transient increase in the sensitivity of the pituitary to LRH in women, and a decrease in men.

Side effects after TRH include mild nausea and a sense of urinary urgency. "Allergic" symptoms have occasionally been observed, but no serious reactions have been reported, and even these mild symptoms are prevented if the material is injected over a two-minute period instead of as a single rapid "bolus." No side effects have been observed after LRH injection.

TREATMENT

Treatment of granulomatous disease of the hypothalamic region consists of treating the specific disease, e.g., adrenal corticosteroids for sarcoidosis; these have been effective in some cases. Surgery for tumors of this region may entail a high risk. Decision about the best therapeutic method depends upon the nature of the tumor (cyst, craniopharyngioma, infundibuloma) as best one can interpret it clinically and radiographically, the precise location of the tumor, and the presence or absence of encroachment on important nearby structures, e.g., the optic chiasm. (For the treatment of pituitary tumors that rise up out of the pituitary fossa and impinge upon the hypothalamus, see Ch. 830).

Bardin, C. W., Ross, G. T., Rifkind, A. B., Cargille, C. M., and Lipsett, M. B.: Studies of the pituitary–Leydig cell axis in young men with hypogonadotropic hypogonadism and hyposmia: Comparison with normal men, prepubertal boys, and hypopituitary patients. J. Clin. Invest., 48:2046, 1969.

Bowers, C. Y., Schally, A. V., Hawley, W. D., Gual, C., and Parlow, A.: Effect of thyrotropin-releasing factor in man. J. Clin. Endocrinol. Metab., 28:978, 1968.

Frohman, L. A.: Clinical neuropharmacology of hypothalamic releasing factors. N. Engl. J. Med., 286:1391, 1972.

Gual, C.: Clinical effects and uses of hypothalamic releasing and inhibiting factors. In Ganong, W. F., and Martini, L. (eds.): Frontiers in Neuroendocrinology. New York, Oxford University Press, 1973, pp. 89–131.

Guillemin, R.: Hypothalamic hormones: Releasing and inhibiting factors. Hosp. Prac., 8:111, 1973.

Kastin, A. J., Schally, A. V., Gual, C., Midgley, A. R., Jr., Bowers, C. Y., and Diaz-Infante, A., Jr.: Stimulation of LH release in men and women by LH-releasing hormone purified from porcine hypothalami. J. Clin. Endocrinol. Metab., 29:1046, 1969.

Martin, J. B.: Neural regulation of growth hormone secretion. N. Engl. J. Med., 288:1384, 1973.

Martini, L., and Ganong, W. F. (eds.): Neuroendocrinology. New York, Academic Press, Vol. 1, 1966; Vol. 2, 1967.

Martini, L., and Ganong, W. F. (eds.): Frontiers in Neuroendocrinology. New York, Oxford University Press, Vol. 1, 1969; Vol. 2, 1971; Vol. 3, 1973.

McCann, S. M., and Porter, J. C.: Hypothalamic pituitary-stimulating and -inhibiting hormones. Physiol. Rev., 49:240, 1969.

Reichlin, S.: Hypothalamic-hypophysial function. In Scow, R. (ed.): Proceedings of the Fourth International Congress of Endocrinology. Amsterdam, Excerpta Medica, 1973.

Sawyer, C. H., and Gorski, R.: Steroid Hormones and Brain Function. The UCLA Forum in Medical Sciences, Nuber 15. University of California Press, 1971.

Siler, T. N., VandenBerg, G., and Yen, S. S. C.: Inhibition of growth hormone release in humans by somatostatin. J. Clin. Endocrinol. Metab., 37:632, 1973.

THE ANTERIOR PITUITARY
(Adenohypophysis)

Nicholas P. Christy

827. INTRODUCTION

Diseases of the anterior pituitary manifest themselves in two ways: mechanically, when space-occupying pituitary tumors impinge upon adjacent structures; and functionally, when there is deficient or excessive secretion of some or all of the several hormones secreted by the gland.

History. The pituitary gland was first described by Vesalius in 1543. The earliest known artistic representation of pituitary disease is found in a sculptured figure on the Rheims Cathedral (thirteenth century): one of the gargoyles has distinctly acromegalic features. Good clinical and pathologic descriptions of acromegaly were provided by Verga (1864) and Fritzsche and Klebs (1884). Pierre Marie (1886) named the disease "acromegaly" because of the hypertrophy of the extremities. The pituitary tumor was recognized by Minkowski (1887) and by Broca (1888). In 1900, Benda ascribed the disorder to eosinophilic adenoma of the hypophysis.

Hypofunction of the pituitary was suspected by Lorain (1871), who associated dwarfism with pituitary destruction in man. Simmonds (1914) described the necropsy findings in an emaciated woman who proved to have extreme atrophy of the anterior pituitary and ovarian fibrosis and splanchnomicria. He correctly attributed the clinical picture to pituitary destruction, which he later showed could also result from tuberculosis or tumor (1916). Many later authors described clinical features now interpreted as those of pituitary insufficiency in patients with tumors of the infundibulum and chromophobe adenomas of the anterior lobe (Honlinger, Cushing and others, 1923–1938). The association of pituitary destruction with the puerperium was definitely established by H. L. Sheehan (1937–1949). He demonstrated acute pituitary necrosis in women dying shortly after difficult labor. He also traced the syndrome of chronic hypopituitarism and pituitary atrophy to episodes of postpartum hemorrhage, and showed that cachexia is not an essential feature of the syndrome.

Experimental elucidation of the functions of the pituitary began with Aschner's demonstration (1909) that hypophysectomy caused arrest of growth in young animals. Splanchnomicria was found in hypophysectomized animals (Livon and Peyron, 1912), and P. E. Smith observed failure of growth after hypophysectomy in the frog and the rat (1916–1926). In 1921, Evans and Long made the important observation that administration of pituitary extracts restored normal growth in the hypophysectomized animal and that large amounts of such growth-promoting extracts produced gigantism in the rat. Smith (1927–1930) described the repair by hypophysial extracts of the gonadal, thyroidal, and adrenocortical atrophy that follows hypophysectomy. He also showed the distinctive effects of destruction of the pituitary (hypopituitarism) as opposed to the hypothalamus (obesity).

The last four decades have witnessed rapid progress in knowledge of the physiologic and biochemical effects of ablation of the pituitary in animals and man. The work of many investigators has led to methods for the extraction of progressively purer pituitary hormones for physiologic study and clinical use, to knowledge of the chemical structure of several, to the total synthesis of at least two (ACTH, MSH) and to the measurement of all in plasma by radioimmunoassay (Berson and Yalow). Current experimental and clinical interest centers around the central nervous system control of anterior pituitary function (Harris and others), especially the role of the hypothalamic "releasing hormones" (see Ch. 826).

Anatomy. The adult pituitary gland weighs 0.4 to 0.9 gram, averaging about 0.6 gram. It enlarges during pregnancy, and after repeated pregnancies may attain a weight of 1.0 to 1.5 grams; the weight tends to decrease in old age. The gland rests in the bony sella turcica and is bounded superiorly by the tough diaphragma sellae, a lamina of the dura mater. The pituitary stalk perforates the diaphragma and connects the pituitary to the hypothalamus; it contains the neurosecretory fibers, which pass from the supraoptic and paraventricular nuclei to the posterior pituitary (neurohypophysis) and the complex arterial and hypothalamic-hypophysial portal venous system, which serves as the functional connection between the nuclei of the hypothalamus and the anterior pituitary. For clinical purposes, the *gross anatomy* of the pituitary is the anatomy of the sella turcica; roentgenographic changes in that structure provide evidence of pituitary enlargement in the form of increase in the linear measurements of the sella and erosion, demineralization, or displacement of its bony borders. The normal sella can be oval, round, or flat. In normal adults, the anteroposterior diameter (sagittal plane) should not exceed 17 mm, the vertical diameter should not be greater than 14 mm, and the normal width (frontal projection) is about 19 mm. Measured roentgenographically, the calculated area of the normal adult pituitary fossa (sagittal plane) does not exceed 130 sq mm; the volume is about 1100 cu mm. Even when sellar measurements are normal, pituitary tumor is suspected if there is suprasellar calcification (Fig. 1), elevation or

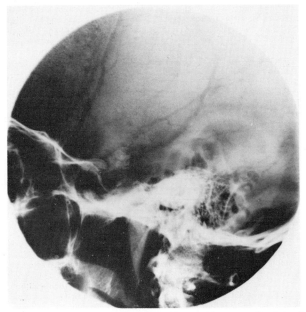

Figure 1. Craniopharyngioma in a 69-year-old woman. The lateral (sagittal) film of the skull shows suprasellar calcification and a normal-sized sella with depression of the sellar floor and some flattening of the dorsum sellae.

destruction of the anterior or posterior clinoids, demineralization or depression of the floor of the sella (Fig. 1), or "ballooning" of the fossa.

The pituitary fossa is enlarged in many but not all instances of intrasellar tumor; intrasellar calcification may be present. The fossa is also large in some suprasellar tumors with intrasellar extension, e.g., craniopharyngioma, metastases to the sella (as from carcinoma of the breast or prostate), longstanding increase of intracranial pressure from any cause, the so-called "empty sella syndrome," and hypothyroidism (see Ch. 830). The fossa is often small in patients with postpartum pituitary necrosis (Sheehan's syndrome), hypopituitary dwarfism without pituitary tumor, and myotonic muscular dystrophy. Rarely observed in presumably normal people, the significance of the small sella is not clear. Roentgenographic changes in the base of the skull may involve the sella in several disorders, e.g., osteoporosis, Paget's disease, Hand-Schüller-Christian disease, and Hurler's syndrome.

When pituitary tumors extend upward through the diaphragma sellae they encroach upon the optic chiasm to produce the familial bitemporal hemianopia. When such tumors impinge on the pituitary stalk or the diencephalon there may be symptoms of hypothalamic involvement (diabetes insipidus, galactorrhea). Such upward extensions can often be seen roentgenographically with the use of pneumoencephalography or carotid artery angiography.

The *microscopic anatomy* of the anterior pituitary is complex. The classic concept of secretory acidophilic (eosinophilic) and basophilic cells and functionless chromophobes has to be modified in the light of recent data. There appear to be five or six distinct kinds of cells; it is probable that each pituitary hormone is secreted by one of the distinct cell types. Somatotrophic cells are acidophils which secrete growth hormone. The pituitary

tumors associated with acromegaly (excessive secretion of growth hormone) are usually composed of acidophils; sometimes the tumors consist of acidophils mixed with chromophobes, chromophobes alone, or cells which have features of both types of cell ("amphophils"). Another kind of acidophil has been identified in the primate and human pituitary. This larger acidophil (known as "lactotrophic" or "mammotrophic") can be distinguished from the growth hormone–secreting acidophil by special stains. Increased numbers of these cells, now accepted as *prolactin*-secreting, are found in the pituitaries of pregnant and lactating women and patients with galactorrhea. A recognizable type of basophil secretes gonadotrophins; there is some evidence that two distinct subtypes of basophils are associated with FSH and LH secretion. Gonadotrophin-secreting basophils are few or absent in childhood, but increase in number at puberty; there are subtle changes during the menstrual cycle; marked changes are observed after castration and menopause. The thyrotrophin-secreting cell is another identifiable type of basophil. The number of these cells increases, and the morphology changes with thyroprivic states. The corticotrophin- (ACTH-) secreting basophil, known as the (R) basophil, probably also secretes MSH in man; the human pituitary lacks a definite intermediate lobe, the source of MSH secretion in lower animals. The pituitary tumors described by Cushing in hyperadrenocorticism are basophilic. In the absence of pituitary tumor, the most notable feature of pituitary cytology in patients with Cushing's syndrome is in the basophils; the cytoplasm becomes hyalinized ("Crooke's change"), a change also found in patients whose hyperadrenocorticism is due to very large doses of administered adrenocortical steroids. In the rather aggressive pituitary tumors that occur after bilateral adrenalectomy in 10 to 15 per cent of patients with Cushing's syndrome associated with bilateral adrenal cortical hyperfunction (owing to oversecretion of ACTH by the pituitary), the cell type is a distinctive kind of chromophobe which often has the capacity to secrete MSH as well as ACTH (see Ch. 850).

Adams, J. H., Daniel, P. M., and Prichard, M. M. L.: Observations on the portal circulation of the pituitary gland. Neuroendocrinology, 1:193, 1965/66.

Bergland, R. M., Ray, B. S., and Torack, R. M.: Anatomical variations in the pituitary gland and adjacent structures in 225 human autopsy cases. J. Neurosurg., 28:93, 1968.

Daughaday, W. H.: The adenohypophysis. In Williams, R. H. (ed.): Textbook of Endocrinology. 5th ed. Philadelphia, W. B. Saunders Company, 1974, p. 31.

Harris, G. W., and Donovan, B. T. (eds.): The Pituitary Gland, 3 vols. Berkeley, University of California Press, 1966.

Meador, C. K., and Worrell, J. L.: The sella turcica in postpartum pituitary necrosis (Sheehan's syndrome). Ann. Intern. Med., 65:259, 1966.

New, P. F. J.: The sella turcica as a mirror of disease. Radiol. Clin. North Am., 4:75, 1966.

Ney, R. L.: The Anterior Pituitary Gland. In Bondy, P. K., and Rosenberg, L. E. (eds.): Duncan's Diseases of Metabolism. 7th ed. Philadelphia, W. B. Saunders Company, 1974, p. 961.

Russfield, A. B.: Adenohypophysis. In Bloodworth, J. M. B. (ed.): Endocrine Pathology. Baltimore, Williams & Wilkins Company, 1968, p. 75.

828.   THE HORMONES OF THE ANTERIOR PITUITARY

Seven *protein* or *peptide hormones* have been isolated from human pituitary tissue: growth hormone, prolactin, follicle-stimulating hormone, luteinizing hormone, thyrotrophin, adrenocorticotrophin and melanocyte-stimulating hormone. Each is regulated by the *releasing hormones of the hypothalamus* which stimulate the secretion of pituitary peptides; it is not yet certain that the releasing factors act to increase the synthesis of pituitary hormones. *Hypothalamic inhibitory factors* also exert an important regulatory influence. The tonic control of prolactin secretion is exerted by prolactin-inhibiting factor (PIF), and there are inhibitory peptides for growth hormone ("somatostatin") and MSH.

Pituitary hormones act directly (prolactin) or through "second messengers." The growth-promoting activity of growth hormone is probably via an intermediary protein, "somatomedin" (see below); the gonadotrophins, TSH and ACTH, stimulate hormone synthesis in their corresponding target glands via cyclic AMP.

Largely controlled by the central nervous system (see Ch. 824 and 826), the anterior pituitary hormones profoundly affect growth, maturation, and metabolism. The paragraphs immediately following deal with the chemistry, physiology, and regulation of these hormones under normal conditions; pathologic states are discussed in Ch. 829.

Brazeau, P., Vale, W., Burgus, R., Ling, N., Butcher, M., Rivier, J., and Guillemin, R.: Hypothalamic peptide that inhibits the secretion of immunoreactive growth hormone. Science, 179:77, 1973.

Frohman, L. A.: Clinical neuropharmacology of hypothalamic releasing factors. N. Engl. J. Med., 286:1391, 1972.

GROWTH HORMONE
(Somatotrophin)

Pituitary growth hormone is the substance that, secreted or given in excessive amounts, induces gigantism and acromegaly in animals and man; its absence results in failure to grow. The hormone exerts a major influence on somatic growth in man from an early stage of infancy. It also has widespread metabolic effects in both young and adult subjects.

Chemically, human growth hormone (HGH) is a single-chain peptide containing 190 amino acids whose sequence is now known; the molecular weight is 21,500.

Within the substance of the gland and in the plasma, HGH is heterogeneous, existing in at least two forms. "Orthodox" HGH (the 21,500 peptide) has in common with prolactin and placental lactogen several segments of identical amino acid sequence; all three hormones may be phylogenetically descended from a single primordial peptide. The daily production rate is about 500 μg per day.

The physiologic effects of HGH are many. The salient action is anabolic. In the hypophysectomized, dwarfed animal, GH administration induces symmetrical growth of the skeleton (chondrogenesis and osteogenesis), the musculature, and viscera. Several effects of HGH on cartilage appear to operate through the obligatory intermediate, *"sulfation factor"* or *"somatomedin,"* a protein of molecular weight 8000 whose site of origin is the liver. Somatomedin is thought to play a vital role in HGH-induced skeletal growth. Optimal growth response also requires the presence of thyroid hormone and insulin. HGH causes both cellular hypertrophy and hyperplasia; there is an increased rate of cellular mitosis, as well as an increase in tissue and organ weight. The hormone induces accelerated transport of specific amino acids into cells, stimulates synthesis of messenger and ribosomal RNA, and influences the activity of several enzymes.

HGH augments protein anabolism in hypophysectomized or hypopituitary human subjects. Nitrogen retention occurs within 24 to 48 hours; BUN concentration falls even earlier, within 12 to 24 hours. Nitrogen storage is great (3 to 4 grams per day) for the first several days of treatment, then falls to an amount compatible with growth requirements, about 0.3 gram of nitrogen retained per day in children 9 to 13 years of age. Linear growth can be induced in hypopituitary dwarfs (see Pituitary Insufficiency in Childhood, in Ch. 831).

HGH brings about changes in electrolyte and water metabolism. Tissue protein and water are increased. Phosphorus and potassium are stored, the latter in amounts larger than can be accounted for by the estimated quantity of new tissue formed. Moderate sodium retention occurs. Hypercalciuria is the rule, but most studies of calcium metabolism indicate an over-all positive calcium balance.

The increase in tissue mass induced by administration of HGH is not accompanied by fat deposition. The hormone is in fact adipokinetic. Although many other pituitary hormones have fat-mobilizing properties, e.g., prolactin, thyrotrophin, corticotrophin, MSH, and several other peptides, HGH appears to be the major adipokinetic principle of the human anterior pituitary. Administration of this hormone to hypophysectomized man rapidly stimulates the release of fat from adipose tissue, with a rise in plasma free fatty acids. This HGH effect on fat metabolism may operate in the anabolic response by ensuring a supply of calories, yet sparing protein breakdown through gluconeogenesis. In acromegalic patients, fat deposition is notably absent; obesity is extremely rare.

HGH also affects carbohydrate metabolism. The hormone is well known to be diabetogenic; many acromegalics have diabetes. The diabetic state is characterized by fasting hyperglycemia, impaired glucose tolerance, insulin resistance, lipemia, and ketosis. HGH given to normal subjects produces only minor changes; in diabetics the diabetes is often substantially exacerbated. Nondiabetic and diabetic subjects are much more sensitive to this effect of growth hormone after hypophysectomy.

The closely interrelated effects of HGH on fat and carbohydrate metabolism may be of great importance in concert with insulin, not only in promoting growth but also in maintaining homeostasis during feast or famine.

Most important observations have followed the recent development of accurate methods for the measurement of HGH in serum by radioimmunoassay (see Ch. 829). The findings have provided new insights into the role of the hormone in the growth of children. Basal serum concentrations and secretion rates are slightly higher in young children and adolescents than in older children or adults. It is now clear that HGH is required for the normal growth rate of infants but not of the fetus; growth hormone–deficient mothers bear children of normal birth weight.

The serum concentration of HGH in *adults* is extremely labile, responding to a variety of stimuli, and being spontaneously secreted in periodic bursts, probably under the influence of the CNS. Serum values rise at the onset of deep sleep. Rapid rises in the serum levels of HGH are induced by hypoglycemia, fasting, and exercise; in some obese subjects these responses are blunted. HGH response to hypoglycemia is inhibited by corticosteroids. Hypoglycemia-induced rises in HGH level are quickly suppressed when glucose is given. Ambulation raises the serum levels of HGH in women, not in men; estrogen administration reproduces this increase. Increases in ambulatory (not basal) serum levels of growth hormone occur during the luteal phase of the menstrual cycle. Growth hormone also participates in the response to *stress*, e.g., surgery, but the pattern of response differs from that of ACTH; this suggests that the neural pathways influencing the two hormones are different. Infusion of amino acids, ACTH, glucagon, and large amounts of catecholamines and oral administration of L-dopa also stimulate HGH secretion. The production rate of HGH is subnormal in hypothyroidism, raised in hyperthyroidism.

Apart from the obvious value of measuring serum levels of HGH for the diagnosis of hypopituitarism and acromegaly, the aforementioned findings have clearly shown that HGH is not secreted at a uniform rate in adults. The lability of response to many metabolic events indicates that the hormone is not functionless in adults, as formerly thought, but participates in the day-to-day regulation of organic metabolism.

The use of the hormone in treatment of HGH deficiency is discussed in Ch. 831 under Pituitary Insufficiency in Childhood.

Berson, S. A., and Yalow, R. S.: Radioimmunoassay of peptide hormones in plasma. N. Engl. J. Med., 277:640, 1967.
Catt, K. J.: Growth hormone. Lancet, 1:933, 1970.
Daughaday, W. H.: Sulfation factor regulation of skeletal growth: A stable mechanism dependent on intermittent growth hormone secretion. Am. J. Med., 50:277, 1972.
Glick, S. M., Roth, J., Yalow, R. S., and Berson, S. A.: The regulation of growth hormone secretion. Rec. Prog. Hormone Res., 21:241, 1965.
Li, C. H.: Hormones of the adenohypophysis. Proc. Am. Philosoph. Soc., 116:365, 1972.
Martin, J. B.: Neural regulation of growth hormone secretion. N. Engl. J. Med., 288:1384, 1973.
Yalow, R. S., Varsano-Aharon, N., and Berson, S. A.: HGH and ACTH secretory responses to stress. Horm. Metab. Res., 1:3, 1969.

PROLACTIN
(Lactogenic Hormone)

Because of many chemical and biologic similarities to HGH, prolactin was not recognized as a separate hormone in man until recently. Human prolactin is now definitely established as a distinct hormone, distinguishable from HGH. The evidence is this: the human pituitary during pregnancy and lactation and in galactorrhea contains many acidophils that are unlike HGH-secreting acidophils; patients with galactorrhea do not have high plasma HGH concentrations; plasma HGH is not raised in lactating women; normal postpartum lactation occurs in mothers with isolated HGH deficiency; pituitary tumors from women with galactorrhea have been shown to contain large amounts of prolactin activity not neutralizable with anti-HGH antiserum; bioassay experiments have indicated high prolactin activity in the presence of low immunoassayable HGH in normal and pathologic lactation; and prolactin has been found to be immunologically distinct from HGH.

In women, prolactin governs growth, development, and milk formation in the breast. These effects require the presence of estrogens, progestogens, adrenocortical steroids, insulin, and perhaps HGH. The physiologic role of prolactin in men is not yet clear.

The hormone is a single polypeptide chain (molecular weight about 23,000) containing 198 amino acids; its chemical similarity to HGH and human placental lactogen (HPL) has been described above.

Prolactin has more than 20 physiologic actions in animals and man, most of them related to reproduction. Apart from its effect on the primate breast, prolactin controls cutaneous "milk" secretion in certain teleost fish, the renal osmoregulatory adaptation of salmon migrating to fresh water, hormone secretion by the corpus luteum in some rodents, and broodpatch formation in birds. In man, prolactin has growth-promoting (and nitrogen-retaining) effects similar to but much weaker than those of HGH; the hormone may also induce renal sodium, potassium, and water retention. The role of prolactin in human breast cancer is now under intense study.

Prolactin is secreted throughout the day in *periodic bursts* unrelated to those of HGH. Plasma levels are lowest during the waking hours, rising 60 to 90 minutes after the onset of sleep and reaching highest concentrations at 5 to 7 A.M. Plasma levels do not vary from day to day throughout the normal *menstrual cycle,* but rise progressively during *pregnancy;* there are sharp rises during *breast feeding.*

Many *physiologic stimuli* elicit increased secretion of prolactin. These include suckling in postpartum women, stimulation of the nonlactating breast (women show a greater response than men), strenuous physical exercise, sexual intercourse in women (most striking when orgasm occurs), profound hypoglycemia, and surgical stress; plasma prolactin values fall with prolonged fasting. Several *pharmacologic agents* alter plasma prolactin levels. Rises follow the administration of TRH, estrogens (but not progesterone), arginine, phenothiazines and other tranquilizing drugs (which sometimes cause galactorrhea), and reserpine. L-Dopa, nicotine, and ergot alkaloids induce falls in plasma prolactin concentration. Chlorpromazine and L-dopa appear to exert their effects by respectively inhibiting and stimulating the hypothalamic secretion of PIF.

Frantz, A. G.: The regulation of prolactin secretion in humans. *In* Ganong, W. F., and Martini, L. (eds.): Frontiers in Neuroendocrinology. New York, Oxford University Press, 1973, p. 337.
Friesen, H. G.: Prolactin: Its physiologic role and therapeutic potential. Hosp. Pract., 7:123, 1972.
Friesen, H. G., Guyda, H., Hwang, P., Tyson, J. E., and Barbeau, A.: Functional evaluation of prolactin secretion: A guide to therapy. J. Clin. Invest., 51:706, 1972.
Hwang, P., Guyda, H., and Friesen, H. G.: A radioimmunoassay for human prolactin. Proc. Nat. Acad. Sci. U.S.A., 68:902, 1971.
Kleinberg, D. L., and Frantz, A. G.: Human prolactin: Measurement by in vitro bioassay. J. Clin. Invest., 50:1557, 1971.
Schwartz, T. B.: Prolactin. *In* Schwartz, T. B. (ed.): The Year Book of Endocrinology. Chicago, Year Book Medical Publishers, 1973, p. 7.
Tyson, J. E., Friesen, H. G., and Anderson, M. S.: Human lactational and ovarian response to endogenous prolactin release. Science, 177:897, 1972.

FOLLICLE-STIMULATING HORMONE
(FSH)

Follicle-stimulating hormone is the pituitary hormone essential for the normal cyclic growth of the ovarian follicle and for restoration of follicular growth in the hypophysectomized female; it stimulates spermatogenesis in the male without significant influence on the androgen-secreting interstitial cells of the testis. For optimal effect upon both ovary and testis, FSH seems to require the presence of luteinizing hormone (LH).

The molecular weight of human FSH is not finally established; estimates vary between 24,000 and 35,000. It is a glycoprotein, containing 7 per cent carbohydrate. Sialic acid is an integral part of the molecule; biologic activity is lost on exposure to neuraminidase. The purest preparations contain slight LH activity. FSH comprises two subunits: an α subunit which resembles the α subunits of LH and human chorionic gonadotrophin (HCG), and a unique β subunit in which the specific biologic activity of FSH probably resides.

Administration of purified human FSH to amenorrheic women elicits increased secretion of estrogens and

may stimulate the ovary to polycystic enlargement; given together with HGC, FSH sometimes provokes spermatogenesis. Discussion of the use of human gonadotrophins in the treatment of infertility in men and women is found in Ch. 859 and 867.

Gonadotrophin concentrations are low in the pituitaries and in the plasma and urine of infants and young children. The hormones rise to reach detectable levels well before puberty. In adult women, the values are about the same as those for men during the preovulatory (follicular) and postovulatory (luteal) phases of the menstrual cycle. In adult men, FSH and LH are secreted in arrhythmic, pulsatile bursts (like ACTH [q.v.]), during sleep, but without relation to the phasic peaks of HGH and prolactin secretion.

Secretion of Gonadotrophins During the Normal Menstrual Cycle. Hypothalamic control of FSH and LH secretion by one or more hypothalamic releasing factors is discussed in Ch. 825, and the role of positive and negative feedback control of gonadotrophin release by estrogens and progesterone is dealt with in Ch. 866. This chapter sets out the pattern of hormone secretion during the normal menstrual cycle. Figure 2 shows the cyclic secretion of FSH, LH, estradiol, and progesterone. During the early *follicular phase,* plasma FSH rises from its nadir during menstruation, and then, while estrogen secretion is rising, falls toward mid-cycle. In this phase, plasma LH progressively rises toward mid-cycle. Just after the peak level of estrogen, now thought to stimulate gonadotrophin (LH) release, both FSH and LH reach their maximal secretion rate (day 0 in Fig. 2); the average daily production rates of FSH and LH are 15 and 30 μg per day, respectively, increasing 10- to 15-fold at *mid-cycle,* when *ovulation* occurs. Values for plasma FSH and LH then decline through the *luteal phase* (FSH being lowest when progesterone levels are high), LH rising slightly as estrogen and progesterone values fall just before menses.

Unopposed by the negative feedback action of gonadal hormones, plasma and urinary FSH values are high, as in ovariectomized and postmenopausal women. In females, the negative feedback is in part due to estrogen inhibition of hypothalamic gonadotrophin-releasing hormone; in the male, the inhibiting testicular hormone may be elaborated by the seminiferous tubule, testosterone being a weak suppressor of FSH secretion.

SECRETION OF PITUITARY AND OVARIAN HORMONES
IN THE NORMAL MENSTRUAL CYCLE

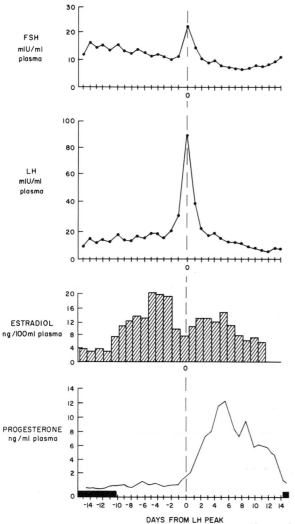

Figure 2. Notice the fall of plasma estradiol values on the day before the midcycle peak of FSH and LH. Plasma estradiol and progesterone concentrations both rise during the luteal phase after the midcycle "surge" of gonadotrophin. The luteal rise in progesterone is reflected by a rise in basal body temperature (BBT) and increased urinary excretion of pregnanediol. The black bar denotes menses. (Adapted from Yen, S. C. C., Vela, P., Rankin, J., and Littell, A. S.: J.A.M.A., 211:1513, 1970; and Catt, K. J.: Lancet, 1:1097, 1970.)

Albert, A.: Bioassay and radioimmunoassay of human gonadotrophins. J. Clin. Endocrinol. Metab., 28:1683, 1968.

Baghdassarian, A., Guyda, H., Johnson, A., Migeon, C. J., and Blizzard, R. M.: Urinary excretion of radioimmunoassayable luteinizing hormone (LH) in normal male children and adults, according to age and stage of sexual development. J. Clin. Endocrinol. Metab., 31:428, 1970.

Catt, K. J.: Reproductive endocrinology. Lancet, 1:1097, 1970.

Rifkind, A. B., Kulin, H. E., and Ross, G. T.: Follicle stimulating hormone (FSH) and luteinizing hormone in the urine of prepubertal children. J. Clin. Invest., 46:1925, 1967.

Ross, G. T., Cargille, C. M., Lipsett, M. B., Rayford, P. L., Marshall, J. R., Strott, C. A., and Rodbard, D.: Pituitary and gonadal hormones in women during spontaneous and induced ovulatory cycles. Recent Prog. Horm. Res., 26:1, 1970.

Rubin, R. T., Kales, A., Adler, R., Fagan, T., and Odell, W.: Gonadotropin secretion during normal sleep in normal adult men. Science, 175:196, 1972.

Schally, A. V., Nair, R. M. G., Redding, T. W., and Arimura, A.: Isolation of the luteinizing and follicle-stimulating hormone-releasing hormone from porcine hypothalami. J. Biol. Chem., 246:7230, 1971.

Vande Wiele, R. L., Bogumil, J., Dyrenfurth, I., Ferin, M., Jewelewicz, R., Warren, M., Rizkallah, T., and Mikhail, G.: Mechanisms regulating the menstrual cycle in women. Recent Prog. Horm. Res., 26:63, 1970.

LUTEINIZING HORMONE OR INTERSTITIAL CELL–STIMULATING HORMONE
(LH or ICSH)

Luteinizing hormone is essential for ovulation, for the formation of the corpus luteum, and for stimulation of steroid hormone secretion by that structure. Acting alone, it does not produce follicular growth; to be effective, LH requires the prior action of FSH on the follicle. Human LH is assumed to be the luteotrophic hormone; there is evidence that the corpus luteum has an intrinsic life span that is not much influenced by pituitary hormones. LH also stimulates the growth and secretory activity of the testicular interstitial cells. This interstitial cell–stimulating activity is sufficient to correct the testicular endocrine defect of hypophysectomy, producing androgen secretion and maintenance of the secondary sex organs. The steroidogenic action of LH on the corpus luteum and the Leydig cells is mediated by cyclic AMP. Spermatogenesis in man requires the synergism of FSH.

Like FSH, LH is a glycoprotein. Human LH (ICSH) has a molecular weight estimated at about 28,000. It is composed of two subunits, designated α and β; the α subunit is chemically similar to that of FSH and TSH, so that the hormonal specificity of LH probably resides in the β subunit. The hormone has been little used therapeutically; the more readily available human chorionic gonadotrophin (HCG), which also contains an α subunit similar to that of human LH, has predominantly LH properties and is used instead.

The circadian and cyclic secretion of LH is described above (see FSH). Partly through their action on the elaboration of hypothalamic FSH/LH-releasing hormone, testosterone, estrogen, and progestogens inhibit the secretion of LH. In men testosterone lowers plasma LH levels; in women estrogen-progestin combinations (as in antiovulatory drugs) suppress the mid-cycle "surge" of LH and reduce LH secretion in the postmenopausal state. Conversely, LH values are high in castrate men and postmenopausal women. It appears that the concentration of circulating estrogen in the follicular phase of the menstrual cycle *stimulates* LH release.

Lipsett, M. B., Cargille, C. M., and Ross, G. T.: Reproductive endocrinology: Methodologic advances and clinical studies. Ann. Intern. Med., 72:933, 1970.
Marsh, J. M., Butcher, R. W., Savard, K., and Sutherland, E. W.: The stimulating effect of luteinizing hormone on adenosine-3′,5′-monophosphate accumulation in corpus luteum slices. J. Biol. Chem., 241:5436, 1966.
Rathnam, P., and Saxena, B. B.: Subunits of luteinizing hormone from human pituitary glands. J. Biol. Chem., 246:7087, 1971.
Schalch, D. S., Parlow, A. F., Boon, R. C., and Reichlin, S.: Measurement of human luteinizing hormone in plasma by radioimmunoassay. J. Clin. Invest., 47:665, 1968.

THYROTROPHIN
(Thyrotrophic or Thyroid-Stimulating Hormone, TSH)

Throtrophin repairs the atrophy of the thyroid gland that follows hypophysectomy. The hormone also restores the ability of the thyroid to synthesize and secrete thyroxine and triiodothyronine. If given in large doses to normal or hypophysectomized animals or man, thyrotrophin evokes the morphologic and secretory changes of hyperthyroidism. TSH elicits a rapid release of thyroxine and triiodothyronine from the gland; the content of colloid is reduced, and the quantity of organic iodine is decreased.

Thyrotrophin is a glycoprotein, containing hexose and glucosamine. The molecular weight is about 28,000; there are two subunits, the α subunit being essentially identical to the α subunit of LH and similar to those of FSH and HCG, and the β subunit comprising the hormone-specific properties. The linear amino acid sequences of the two subunits are known. There is evidence that the TSH molecule is heterogeneous. The hormone stimulates many metabolic processes in the thyroid, e.g., the uptake and oxidation of glucose, the production of TPNH, and many others. The rapid discharge of thyroxine from the thyroid follicles is in part due to the action of TSH upon a proteolytic enzyme that accelerates the release of the hormone from the intrafollicular protein thyroglobulin. Within 24 hours after the administration of TSH, hypertrophy and hyperplasia of the thyroid epithelium occur. The weight of the thyroid increases. TSH augments the capacity of the thyroid to take up iodide, to convert iodide to organic iodine, and to synthesize thyroxine. These effects can be reproduced by cyclic AMP; this and other evidence indicates that the nucleotide is an important mediator of TSH action on the thyroid.

Hypothalamic TRH appears to be the most important regulator of TSH secretion; the daily production rate of TSH is about 100 μU. Circadian rhythm of plasma TSH levels in man is slight, and, in contrast to other anterior pituitary hormones, TSH secretion remains remarkably constant in the face of many kinds of stimuli. Except for a transitory increase in early neonatal life, there is no age-related change in plasma TSH values; they are the same in both sexes and do not change in response to exercise, the stress of surgery, or the administration of vasopressin, glucagon, arginine, or, surprisingly, antithyroid drugs. Corticosteroids suppress TSH secretion, and prolonged exposure to cold slightly increases it. Thyroxine and triiodothyronine also exert important effects on the hypothalamic and pituitary control of TSH secretion; values are high in primary hypothyroidism and low in naturally occurring and iatrogenic hyperthyroidism (see Ch. 837).

Bovine thyrotrophin and synthetic TRH are available for medical use; diagnostic tests of thyroid function are discussed in Ch. 829.

Anderson, M. S., Bowers, C. Y., Kastin, A. J., Schalch, D. S., Schally, A. V., Snyder, P. J., Utiger, R. D., Wilber, J. F., and Wise, A. J.: Synthetic thyrotropin-releasing hormone. N. Engl. J. Med., 285:1279, 1971.
Hershman, J. M., and Pittman, J. A.: Control of thyrotropin secretion in man. N. Engl. J. Med., 285:997, 1971.
Pierce, J. G., Liao, T., Howard, S. M., Shome, B., and Cornell, J. S.: Studies on the structure of thyrotropin: Its relationship to luteinizing hormone. Recent Prog. Horm. Res., 27:165, 1971.
Shenkman, L., Mitsuma, T., and Hollander, C. S.: Modulation of pituitary responsiveness to thyrotropin-releasing hormones by triiodothyronine. J. Clin. Invest., 52:205, 1973.
Utiger, R. D.: Radioimmunoassay of human plasma thyrotropin. J. Clin. Invest., 44:1277, 1965.

ADRENOCORTICOTROPHIN
(ACTH, Corticotrophin)

Adrenocorticotrophin repairs the adrenocortical atrophy and failure to synthesize steroid hormones that follow hypophysectomy. In most species, ACTH administration causes hypertrophy and hyperplasia of the adrenal. The main effect appears to be upon the fascicular and reticular zones. The hormone stimulates the synthesis and release of cortisol, corticosterone, and androgens; it also elicits a moderate increase in the secretory rate of aldosterone, but this increase is not sustained. Large amounts of exogenous corticotrophin cause enlargement and hyperemia of the adrenal, and hemorrhagic infarction has occurred rarely.

The chemical nature of adrenocorticotrophin is known. It is a single polypeptide made up of 39 amino acids. Smaller fragments of the ACTH peptide, e.g., that containing amino acids 1 to 20, have full biologic potency. The complete hormone has been synthesized; its molecular weight is 4567, its potency 100 to 140 units per milligram. ACTH exists in two forms in the pituitary; "big ACTH" may serve as a precursor, whereas "little" ACTH (molecular weight 4500) is the circulating, biologically active hormone. One international unit, equal to 1 USP unit, is the biologic activity of 1 mg of international standard. The daily production rate of ACTH in man is small, about 10 μg per day.

The action of the hormone upon the adrenal cortex is complex. It stimulates increased mitotic activity. The increase in steroidogenesis is the result of an increase in the rate of steroid biosynthesis, not simply of accelerated release of steroid into the bloodstream. The precise point in the biosynthetic pathway at which corticotrophin acts is debatable; the increased steroid production may be mediated by ACTH stimulation of a particular messenger RNA. An important mechanism by which ACTH induces increased steroid synthesis is its capacity to stimulate the synthesis of active adrenocortical phosphorylase by raising the concentration of cyclic AMP in the gland. The increased phosphorylase activity makes available more glucose-6-phosphate from the hexose monophosphate shunt, thus providing larger quantities of NADH (TPNH), a compound essential for the synthesis and hydroxylation of steroids.

Corticotrophin has extra-adrenal actions. It stimulates the release of free fatty acids from adipose tissue; the importance of this effect is unknown. In large doses it causes darkening of the skin.

In man, the short-term administration of adrenocorticotrophin causes a rapid increase in the secretion of cortisol, reflected by an abrupt rise in plasma cortisol concentration. This effect has proved useful in the diagnostic assessment of adrenocortical response, as has the biologic and immunologic assay of ACTH in human serum. Radioimmunoassay measurements of plasma ACTH concentration have confirmed earlier ideas about the extraordinary lability of this hormone in response to physiologic and pathologic stimuli. Plasma ACTH undergoes a free-running circadian cycle under CNS (hypothalamic CRF) influence. The hormone is secreted in episodic bursts, with highest levels tending to be in the early morning; a nadir is reached by late evening. Plasma cortisol levels roughly reflect this circadian rhythm. Hospitalized patients not acutely ill often have ACTH concentrations higher than normal, and severely ill patients occasionally show extremely elevated levels. Plasma ACTH rises in addisonian and adrenalectomized patients and in response to metyrapone, and falls when suppressive doses of adrenocortical steroids, e.g., dexamethasone, are given (see Ch. 845). Stressful stimuli, such as surgery under general anesthesia, electro-

shock, and hypoglycemia, and the administration of histamine and vasopressin are usually followed by raised plasma ACTH concentrations.

The long-term effects of adrenocorticotrophin in human subjects are the same as those produced by cortisone, cortisol, and their synthetic analogues. In contrast to the adrenocortical steroids, corticotrophin evokes sensitivity reactions, but antihormone formation does not occur. Corticotrophin brings about a greater degree of sodium and water retention, more androgenicity, and a more constant elevation in serum cholesterol than do steroids. Large doses elicit the stigmata of Cushing's syndrome (e.g., osteoporosis, hyperglycemia, psychosis). The unpleasant symptoms associated with abrupt withdrawal of steroid therapy are said to occur rarely after a course of ACTH therapy.

Adrenocorticotrophin regulates the growth, structural integrity, and steroid secretion of the adrenal cortex. This constantly changing regulatory influence is exerted by central nervous system control of the anterior pituitary and by a reciprocal relation between the amounts of circulating cortisol and ACTH. In man, noxious stimuli such as acute illness or severe and prolonged emotional disturbance provoke an increased or abnormally regulated output of adrenocortical steroids, mediated via an increased rate of endogenous corticotrophin release.

ACTH is available for diagnostic purposes in lyophilized and repository (with gelatin or zinc) forms. Two synthetic ACTH preparations are also available in unmodified and repository forms: α^{1-24} ACTH (Synacthen, Cortrosyn), and α^{1-18} ACTH (see Ch. 829 and 846). ACTH has also been used *therapeutically,* but most clinicians think that the diseases which respond to hyperadrenal therapy are more simply managed with corticosteroids than with ACTH.

Berson, S. A., and Yalow, R. S.: Radioimmunoassay of ACTH in plasma. J. Clin. Invest., 47:2725, 1968.
Grahame-Smith, D. G., Butcher, R. W., Ney, R. L., and Sutherland, E. W.: Adenosine-3′,5′-monophosphate as the intracellular mediator of the action of adrenocorticotrophic hormone in the adrenal cortex. J. Biol. Chem., 242:5535, 1967.
Weitzman, E. D., Fukushima, D., Nogiere, C. Roffwarg, H., Gallagher, T. F., and Hellman, L.: Twenty-four hour pattern of the episodic secretion of cortisol in normal subjects. J. Clin. Endocrinol. Metab., 33:14, 1971.

MELANOCYTE-STIMULATING HORMONE
(MSH)

MSH produces darkening (addisonian pigmentation) in human skin. Two MSH peptides have been identified in pituitary tissue. The smaller and more potent molecule, α-MSH, is made up of 13 amino acids and has a molecular weight of 1823; it is found in the pituitaries of pigs, cows, and monkeys, and may be present in the neurohypophysis of man. The characteristic human peptide, β-MSH, contains 22 amino acids and has a molecular weight of 2734. α-MSH has a common 13-amino acid sequence with ACTH; β-MSH a 7-amino acid sequence. These partial identities of structure may account for common physiologic properties among the three molecules: ACTH has a slight pigmentary effect on skin; both MSH molecules and ACTH are adipokinetic; both MSH's have weak adrenal-stimulating activity. Studies of plasma β-MSH concentration in man have shown that the hormone undergoes a circadian rhythm in normal subjects and that its secretion is regulated by the same factors that control ACTH. Metyrapone raises and adrenocortical steroids depress plasma β-MSH levels.

The functional significance of human β-MSH is unknown. Plasma values are the same in pigmented and nonpigmented races, and are normal in albinism and in several diseases characterized by increased dermal pigmentation.

Abe, K., Nicholson, W. E., Liddle, G. W., Orth, D. N., and Island, D. P.: Normal and abnormal regulation of β-MSH in man. J. Clin. Invest., 48:1580, 1969.

Lerner, A. B., and McGuire, J. S.: Effect of alpha- and beta-melanocyte stimulating hormones on skin colour of man. Nature (London), 189:176, 1971.

829. ASSESSMENT OF ANTERIOR PITUITARY FUNCTION

Clinical Detection of Pituitary Disease. Clinical suspicion of hypopituitarism must be entertained in patients with short stature, delayed puberty, primary and secondary amenorrhea, sterility, and hypothyroidism. Typical ocular findings or the incidental discovery of an enlarged pituitary fossa (as in a skull film taken for head injury) also require diagnostic study of pituitary function (see below).

Functional Detection of Pituitary Disease. This is based on measurement of hormones in plasma or urine. In addition to detection of abnormally high or low levels of pituitary hormones, such measurements permit an evaluation of abnormal *regulation* of pituitary hormone secretion (see Ch. 824). *Direct* measurement of pituitary hormones is made when possible, as for growth hormone and gonadotrophins; *indirect* evaluation of TSH and ACTH is usually done by measuring the hormones of glands that are under their trophic control, because the methods are more generally available, e.g., thyroidal response to TSH, adrenocortical response to ACTH (see below).

GROWTH HORMONE

Radioimmunoassay of plasma growth hormones is becoming a routine procedure, and can be done at many medical centers and commercial laboratories. This is the most direct method for detecting hypopituitary states and acromegaly. In *hypopituitary dwarfism,* radioimmunoassay for growth hormone has superseded the crude indirect indices that clinicians have had to rely on, e.g., measurements of body proportions, chromosomal analysis, roentgenographic estimate of bone age, and laborious exclusion of all other causes of short stature. In pituitary dwarfism, basal plasma HGH values of less than 1.0 ng per milliliter may be found; these low values are not diagnostic, because the normal range is 0 to 5 ng per milliliter. One must demonstrate failure of growth hormone to respond to a stimulus, e.g., hypoglycemia. When suspicion is strong, the starting dose of insulin should be 0.05 unit per kilogram, given intravenously; if the hypoglycemia is inadequate, the dose can be increased to 0.1 or even 0.15 unit per kilogram, given under careful supervision to avoid prolonged hypoglycemia. Adequate stimulus requires a lowering

of blood glucose to one half the basal value or to 40 mg per 100 ml for at least ten minutes; if this condition is satisfied, patients without growth hormone deficiency show a rise in HGH value of at least 7 ng per milliliter above the basal level 60 minutes after injection. *Failure of growth hormone response to hypoglycemia is the most common laboratory abnormality in adult hypopituitarism, and is characteristic only of the dwarfism associated with growth hormone deficiency.* Certain amino acids also have the property of inducing growth hormone release; intravenous administration of neutralized arginine hydrochloride, 0.5 gram per kilogram, is preferred by some workers, because one avoids possibly dangerous hypoglycemia. The rise in growth hormone value is again 7 ng per milliliter above the resting levels.

In *acromegaly* also, HGH radioimmunoassay has begun to replace the highly unsatisfactory indirect methods clinicians have struggled with for years: histologic changes in the cartilage of the costochondral junction, measurement of serum phosphorus, PBI, urinary calcium, hydroxyproline excretion, and so forth. Basal plasma HGH may be in the range of 50 to more than 100 ng per milliliter. Many patients with untreated acromegaly fail to show a sharp drop in plasma HGH concentration, as do normal people, after administration of glucose (given as for a standard glucose tolerance test, blood samples being taken for glucose and growth hormone determinations at 30-minute intervals for at least three hours). It will require protracted follow-up studies of acromegalic patients before and after treatment and careful correlation with clinical findings, e.g., acral growth, to assess the usefulness of this nonresponse to hyperglycemia as an index of "acromegalic activity." In some acromegalics, plasma HGH paradoxically *rises* in response to glucose.

Glucagon and L-*dopa* have been recently introduced as provocative tests of HGH adequacy. Both have the virtue of simplicity. One mg of glucagon is given subcutaneously or intramuscularly; in normal subjects plasma HGH rises to 8 ng per milliliter or more within two to three hours. L-Dopa, 0.5 gram, is given orally; normal subjects raise HGH levels more than 5 ng per milliliter with a peak rise at 90 minutes. Response is said to be subnormal or absent in pituitary disease. These two maneuvers are promising but require further trial.

Eddy, R. L., Gilliland, P. F., Ibarra, J. D., Jr., McMurry, J. F., Jr., and Thompson, J. Q.: Human growth hormone release: Comparison of provocative test procedures. Am. J. Med., 56:179, 1974.

Fraser, R.: Human pituitary disease. Br. Med. J., 2:449, 1970.

Mitchell, M. L., Byrne, M. J., Sanchez, Y., and Sawin, C. T.: Detection of growth hormone deficiency: The glucagon stimulation test. N. Engl. J. Med., 282:539, 1970.

Nelson, J. C., Kollar, D. J., and Lewis, J. E.: Growth hormone secretion in pituitary disease. Arch. Intern. Med., 133:459, 1974.

Rabkin, M. T., and Frantz, A. G.: Hypopituitarism: A study of growth hormone and other endocrine functions. Ann. Intern. Med., 64:1197, 1966.

PROLACTIN

The development of sensitive bioassay and radioimmunoassay measurements for plasma prolactin has introduced a new and useful method for evaluating pituitary disease and *galactorrheic states.* Normal values are the same for adult men and women, usually less than 15 ng per milliliter, with an extreme upper limit of 25 ng per milliliter. Plasma prolactin is usually elevated in patients who have had *pituitary stalk section,* owing to interference with the action of hypothalamic PIF (see Ch. 826). A finding of major importance is detection of high plasma prolactin levels in patients with various kinds of *pituitary tumors,* often in the absence of galactorrhea and when all other pituitary hormones are low and there is clinical panhypopituitarism. The mechanism is either mechanical interference with PIF action or actual oversecretion of prolactin by the pituitary tumor. Plasma prolactin measurement may turn out to be valuable as an early hormonal sign of "nonfunctional" chromophobe adenoma. Raised prolactin levels are usually but not always found in patients with *galactorrhea:* e.g., in the *Chiari-Frommel syndrome* (postpartum amenorrhea and low gonadotrophin levels), *Del Castillo's syndrome* (amenorrhea and low gonadotrophin levels but not in relation to parturition), the *Forbes-Albright syndrome* (the same but associated with chromophobe adenoma), and the *"oversuppression" syndrome* (the same after cessation of antiovulatory medication), occasionally in *acromegaly,* and rarely in *primary hypothyroidism* (especially when the pituitary is enlarged) and injury to the chest wall. Prolactin levels are often high in renal failure but are usually normal in gynecomastia.

Provocative tests have been devised to distinguish between hypothalamic and pituitary disorders of prolactin secretion: stimulation with TRH and chlorpromazine and suppression with L-dopa. Panhypopituitary patients have low plasma prolactin levels which fail to respond to all three tests; patients with hypothalamic involvement respond abnormally to one or more of the three agents. Details of protocols and interpretation are given by Tolis et al.

Besser, G. M.: Galactorrhea. Br. Med. J., 1:280, 1972.

Forsyth, I. A., Besser, G. M., Edwards, C. R. W., Francis, L., and Myres, R. P.: Plasma prolactin activity in inappropriate lactation. Brit. Med. J., 2:225, 1971.

Frantz, A. G., Kleinberg, D. L., and Noel, G. L.: Studies on prolactin in man. Recent Prog. Horm. Res., 28:527, 1972.

L'Hermite, P., Copinschi, G., Golstein, J., Vanhaelst, L., Leclercq, R., Bruno, O. D., and Robyn, C.: Prolactin release after injection of thyrotropin-releasing hormone in man. Lancet, 1:763, 1972.

Tolis, G., Goldstein, M., and Friesen, H. G.: Functional evaluation of prolactin secretion in patients with hypothalamic-pituitary disorders. J. Clin. Invest., 52:783, 1972.

GONADOTROPHINS
(FSH and LH)

Biologic assay of urinary gonadotrophin is useful in distinguishing primary from secondary gonadal failure after the expected age of puberty. In the former, urinary gonadotrophin titers are elevated; in the latter (resulting from pituitary deficiency), levels are not detectable. Results of urinary gonadotrophin (human pituitary gonadotrophin) assays, done by the mouse uterine weight or rat ovarian weight method, are expressed in mouse uterine units (muu) or rat units (RU). In the mouse assay, a reported value of "positive at 20 muu" means that one twentieth of the extract of a 24-hour urine just produced a definite response in the injected mice. If one twentieth of a 24-hour urinary extract produces a definite response in the rat assay, results are reported as "20 RU per 24 hours." The rat assay is the more sensitive; normal people occasionally have undetectable values in the mouse assay. There is no official reference

TABLE 1. Plasma Gonadotrophin Values as Measured by Radioimmunoassay in Normal People (with the "2nd IRP–Human Menopausal Gonadotrophin" as Standard)

	FSH, mIU/ml	LH, mIU/ml
Children	3–19	5–15
Adult males	3–42	3–32
Adult females		
Follicular phase	10–18	7–27
Mid-cycle	20–30	70–100
Luteal phase	6–18	7–22
Postmenopausal	35–215	0–90

standard for this bioassay. Representative mean values for the rat assay are as follows: adult men, 10; women in the follicular and luteal phases, 7; women at mid-cycle, 15; postmenopausal women, 75 – all values being expressed in RU per 24 hours. Corresponding figures for the mouse assay are 35, 20, 55, and 200 – all expressed in muu per 24 hours. In pituitary insufficiency, urinary gonadotrophins are usually undetectable; this abnormality is one of the earliest laboratory signs to appear in the course of the disease.

The highly sensitive radioimmunoassays for plasma FSH and LH are becoming available for routine clinical use, and they may very well supplant the bioassay methods in time. As expected, values are low or undetectable in pituitary insufficiency and high in primary gonadal failure. The normal ranges for various stages of the reproductive cycle are set out in Table 1.

Use of FSH and LH radioimmunoassay measurements has permitted sharper diagnostic accuracy in *delayed puberty* and the identification of patients with *hypogonadotrophic hypogonadism,* e.g., isolated FSH deficiency and gonadotrophin deficiency associated with *anosmia* or *hyposmia (Kallmann's syndrome),* in some of whom the defect may be in the synthesis or release of gonadotrophin-releasing factor (FSH-LH/RF). *Provocative tests* which entail administration of FSH-LH/RF or clomiphene have been used in attempts to distinguish hypothalamic from pituitary hypogonadotrophism. Clomiphene may be therapeutically effective in some patients with gonadotrophin deficiency. (For detailed protocols, see references.)

Hamiliton, C. R., Henkin, R. I., Weir, G., and Kliman, B.: Olfactory status and response to clomiphene in male gonadotrophin deficiency. Ann. Intern. Med., 78:47, 1973.

Marshall, J. C., Harsoulis, P., Anderson, D. C., McNeilly, A. S., Besser, G. M., and Hall, R.: Isolated pituitary gonadotrophin deficiency: Gonadotropin secretion after synthetic luteinizing hormone and follicle stimulating hormone–releasing hormone in man. Br. Med. J., 2:643, 1972.

Newton, J., Ramsay, I., and Marsden, P.: Clomiphene as a test of pituitary function. Lancet, 2:190, 1971.

Rabin, D., Spitz, I., Bercovici, B., Bell, J., Laufer, A., Benveniste, R., and Polishuk, W.: Isolated deficiency of follicle-stimulating hormone: Clinical and laboratory features. N. Engl. J. Med., 287:1313, 1972.

Saxena, B. B., Beling, C. G., and Gandy, H. M. (eds.): Gonadotropins. New York, John Wiley & Sons, 1972.

THYROTROPHIN
(TSH)

Radioimmunoassay for serum thyrotrophin is becoming available for general clinical use; normal values are

0.5 to 11.5 μU per milliliter. The values in primary myxedema, as expected, are high, falling to normal when thyroid hormone is given, and are undetectable in Graves' disease (see Ch. 837). A *provocative test*, in which 200 to 500 μg of TRH is given intravenously and plasma TSH rise is measured 30 to 60 minutes later, has permitted differentiation between "hypothalamic" and pituitary hypothyroidism. TSH rise may be normal in the former and absent in the latter. In intrinsic pituitary disease, the basal TSH level is low; if this measurement cannot be obtained, an acceptable method for distinguishing primary myxedema from secondary thyroid deficiency is the thyrotrophin stimulation test. The most reliable technique seems to be measurement of 24-hour ^{131}I uptake by the thyroid before and after intramuscular administration of bovine TSH, 10 USP units per day intramuscularly for three days. In primary myxedema, there is no response; normal subjects respond briskly; patients with myxedema secondary to pituitary failure respond, but subnormally. Exceptions are some patients with Sheehan's disease of long duration, who may be unresponsive.

Burke, G.: The thyrotrophin stimulation test. Ann. Intern. Med., 69:1127, 1968.

Costom, B. H., Grumbach, M. M., and Kaplan, S. L.: Effect of thyrotropin-releasing factor on serum thyroid-stimulating hormone. J. Clin. Invest., 50:2219, 1971.

Foley, T. P., Jr., Owings, J., Hayford, J. T., and Blizzard, R. M.: Serum thyrotropin responses to synthetic thyrotropin-releasing hormone in normal children and hypopituitary patients. J. Clin. Invest., 51:431, 1972.

Nelson, J. C., Johnson, D. E., and Odell, W. D.: Serum TSH levels and the thyroidal response to TSH stimulation in patients with thyroid disease. Ann. Intern. Med., 76:47, 1972.

Pittman, J. A., Haigler, E. D., Hershman, J. M., and Pittman, C. S.: Hypothalamic hypothyroidism. N. Engl. J. Med., 285:844, 1971.

Shenkman, L., Mitsuma, T., Suphavai, A., and Hollander, C. S.: Triiodothyronine and thyroid-stimulating hormone response to thyrotropin-releasing hormone. Lancet, 1:111, 1972.

ADRENOCORTICOTROPHIN
(ACTH)

Measurement of the ACTH secretion of the pituitary is usually done *indirectly* by testing adrenocortical response. A safe and specific method is intravenous administration of 25 units of lyophilized ACTH in 500 ml of 0.9 per cent saline over a four-hour period. Five per cent glucose in water should not be used as a diluent, because it may aggravate pre-existing hyponatremia. In primary adrenocortical failure (Addison's disease) there is no response of plasma corticosteroids; in pituitary deficiency with secondary adrenal failure, response is present but subnormal. Equally useful is intravenous infusion of ACTH over several days with measurement of urinary steroid excretion; some workers think this is a more certain method for differentiating primary and secondary adrenal insufficiency. It is prudent to give 0.5 to 1.0 mg of dexamethasone orally to obviate untoward reactions to ACTH. Use of the synthetic corticotrophins avoids these reactions, but results are not yet standardized. The nonspecific methods, insulin tolerance test and water loading, can be dangerous and are not recommended.

Four other methods have been used to assess pituitary ACTH release; like the ACTH-response test described above, the index is rise or failure to rise of plasma or urinary corticosteroid values. Three of the methods entail stimulation of ACTH release by giving a more or less noxious stimulus: insulin-induced hypoglycemia, vasopressin, and bacterial pyrogen. Although it is true that patients with hypopituitarism show absent or subnormal rises in plasma cortisol concentration after all three of these, there is no agreement about which is the most discriminating or the most sensitive. The insulin, vasopressin, and pyrogen tests have not found favor as clinical methods in this country. The fourth method, the metyrapone test, a measure of pituitary ACTH reserve, is described in Ch. 845 and 848. To make certain that the adrenal has the capacity to respond to ACTH, a standard ACTH response test should be done before metyrapone is given. In a few patients with severe hypopituitarism, metyrapone blockade of adrenocortical biosynthesis coupled with poor or absent ACTH reserve has resulted in clinically significant adrenal insufficiency. In patients with possibly advanced hypopituitarism, "coverage" with 0.5 to 1.0 mg of dexamethasone is therefore a reasonable safeguard during a metyrapone test.

Biologic assay and radioimmunoassay of plasma ACTH, although not yet available for clinical purposes, are *direct* techniques which have yielded valuable information about the fluctuations of this hormone. Normal values are a mean of about 0.3 mU per 100 ml by bioassay and a mean of 22 pg per milliliter by radioimmunoassay (normal range, 12 to 80 pg per milliliter). Values are occasionally ten times higher than those in severely ill patients; as expected, levels are low or not detected in hypopituitarism. The changes in plasma ACTH concentration that occur in the various forms of Cushing's syndrome are discussed in Ch. 850.

Christy, N. P., Wallace, E. Z., and Jailer, J. W.: The effect of intravenously administered ACTH on plasma 17,21-dihydroxy-20-ketosteroids in normal individuals and in patients with disorders of the adrenal cortex. J. Clin. Invest., 34:899, 1955.

Staub, J. J., Jenkins, J. S., Ratcliffe, J. G., and Landon, J.: Comparison of corticotrophin and corticosteroid response to lysine vasopressin, insulin, and pyrogen in man. Br. Med. J., 1:267, 1973.

Wood, J. B., Frankland, A. W., James, V. H. T., and Landon, J.: A rapid test of adrenocortical function. Lancet, 1:243, 1965.

MELANOCYTE-STIMULATING HORMONE
(MSH)

A radioimmunoassay for plasma β-MSH has been developed but is not used for clinical purposes. Normal levels are 20 to 110 pg per milliliter. The values are raised in untreated Addison's disease and congenital adrenal hyperplasia, and fall during corticosteroid administration. Plasma β-MSH is slightly elevated, as is plasma ACTH, in the "pituitary" form of Cushing's syndrome (see Ch. 850), and is very much elevated in patients who develop pituitary tumors and dermal hyperpigmentation after bilateral adrenalectomy for this disease. Elevations of plasma β-MSH tend to parallel those of plasma ACTH, and large amounts of each peptide have been found in extracts of hormone-secreting tumors (see Ch. 870). A new finding of great interest is the detection of raised plasma β-MSH levels in patients with parkinsonism; this raises the possibility that β-MSH functions as a neuroregulatory hormone.

Abe, K., Nicholson, W. E., Liddle, G. W., Island, D. P., and Orth, D. N.: Radioimmunoassay of β-MSH in human plasma and tissues. J. Clin. Invest., 46:1609, 1967.

Shuster, S., Thody, A. J., Goolamali, S. K., Burton, J. L., Plummer, N., and Bates, D.: Melanocyte-stimulating hormone and parkinsonism. Lancet, 1:463, 1973.

830. DIAGNOSIS AND TREATMENT OF PITUITARY TUMORS

Epidemiologic studies indicate that there are 2500 newly diagnosed pituitary tumors per year in the United States. Tumors of the pituitary may be *asymptomatic.* In an autopsy study of 1000 "normal" pituitaries, adenomas were found in nearly 25 per cent, over half being chromophobic, more than a quarter basophilic, and the rest (7.5 per cent) acidophilic. Although some pathologists believe, on the basis of special stains, that most pituitary tumors are chromophilic and contain stainable, possibly hormone-secreting granules, the majority of tumors are chromophobic by conventional light microscopy, whatever implication this may have for their secretory capacities. Thus in a recent collection of nearly 1000 cases of known pituitary adenoma, 98 per cent were chromophobic, the remaining 2 per cent being acidophilic. Malignant chromophobe adenomas are rare. Extrasellar and suprasellar cysts and tumors, especially gliomas of the optic chiasm and craniopharyngiomas, are less common tumors that may involve the pituitary, either by direct extension into the pituitary fossa or by impingement upon the adjacent hypothalamus or pituitary stalk.

Patients with pituitary tumor are more likely to seek medical aid because of visual or neurologic symptoms than for complaints of endocrine dysfunction. In a recent series, about three quarters of the patients had headaches (not by themselves sufficiently typical to be diagnostic); two thirds had impairment of visual fields, and the same proportion had impairment of visual activity; about 40 per cent complained of decreased libido, and one third had diplopia, decrease in potency, dizziness (postural hypotension), change in distribution of sexual hair, or intolerance to cold. By far the most common visual field defect is *bitemporal hemianopia,* occurring in 70 to 80 per cent of patients; it is noteworthy that about 15 per cent of patients with this defect are unaware of it. Paralysis of cranial nerves III, IV, and VI usually denotes a large tumor extending outside the sella turcica. Among *endocrine symptoms,* about 90 per cent of patients give a history of some degree of gonadal insufficiency on careful questioning, about 80 per cent have symptoms of thyroid failure, and perhaps half give evidence of adrenocortical deficiency. Even when pituitary tumors rise up out of the sella turcica and exert pressure on the diencephalon, they rarely cause *hypothalamic symptoms;* diabetes insipidus and disorders of sleep or temperature regulation are rare and do not occur unless the diencephalon is grossly damaged. About one eighth of patients may have symptoms caused by *"pituitary apoplexy"* (abrupt hemorrhage into the tumor).

Physical findings in pituitary tumor are also more

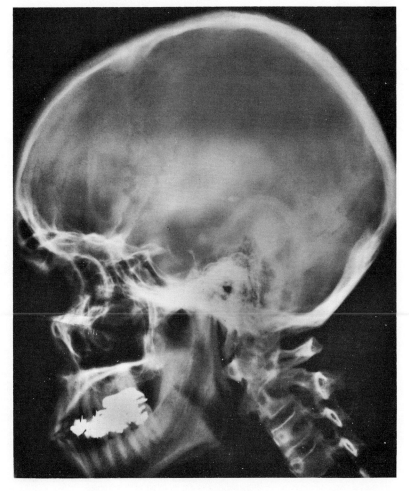

Figure 3. Chromophobe adenoma in a 36-year-old man. Roentgenogram of the skull shows moderate enlargement of the sella (24 mm in the anterior-posterior diameter, 16 mm in depth on the original film). The sellar floor shows a double contour, indicating uneven downward growth of the tumor, which depresses one side of the sella more than the other. The dorsum sellae is thin; the posterior clinoids are intact. The texture and appearance of the skull and facial bones are normal (cf. acromegaly, Fig. 4).

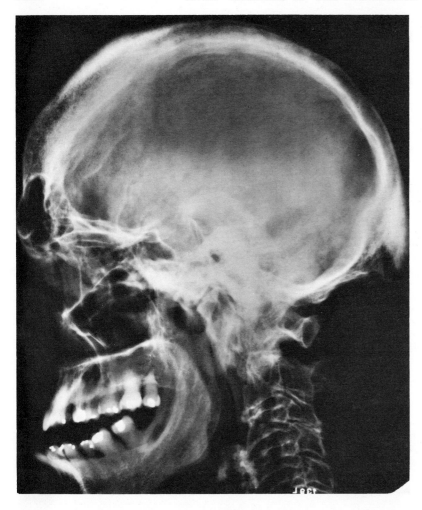

Figure 4. Skull roentgenogram typical of acromegaly; 66-year-old woman with acromegaly of 43 years' duration. Radiotherapy to sella within five years of onset. Intermittent increases in the acral parts. No symptoms of endocrine deficiency (serum protein-bound iodine normal, normal blood glucose two hours after a meal). The film shows thickening and hyperostosis of the cranial vault and occipital protuberance, and overdevelopment of the frontal sinuses. As is not uncommonly true in acromegaly, the sella is only slightly enlarged (18 mm. in the sagittal plane). The dorsum sellae is pneumatized. Prognathism is indicated by the overlapping lower teeth.

Figure 5. X-ray of the hands in acromegaly. There is tufting of the distal phalanges, but the most characteristic finding is increase in soft tissue mass.

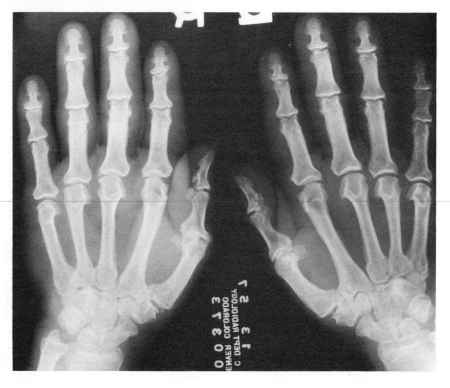

commonly related to the eyes than to the endocrine system. In addition to bitemporal hemianopia, up to 85 per cent of patients can be shown to have reduced visual acuity, more than half have optic atrophy, and one third have cranial nerve palsies. About two fifths of patients are found to have loss of body hair, and a third or fewer have changes in the skin or genital atrophy.

Roentgenographic detection (see Anatomy in Ch. 827) should be based on frontal as well as sagittal views of the skull and sella. In addition to changes in the length and depth of the pituitary fossa, the examiner looks for erosion or destruction of the anterior and posterior clinoids and of the tuberculum sellae, suprasellar calcification (chromophobe adenoma, craniopharyngioma), and "double floor" of the sella, seen when a tumor extends downward unevenly (Fig. 3). Laminagraphy may show intrasellar calcification or extension of a tumor into the sphenoid sinus. Carotid artery angiography and particularly pneumoencephalography may show quite accurately the degree of upward extension of an intrasellar tumor; these procedures, at least the latter, should always be done before craniotomy for pituitary tumor, and are also necessary guides in the design of a radiotherapeutic program. In *acromegaly,* plain films of the skull show not only enlargement of the sella turcica in 80 to 90 per cent of patients, but also thickening of the calvarium, enlargement of the paranasal sinuses, and widening of the mandibular angle with prognathism (Fig. 4). Films of the hands disclose gross increase in the mass of soft tissue, a more characteristic finding than tufting of the distal phalanges (Fig. 5). Spinal films may reveal anterior lipping of vertebral bodies; lateral films of the os calcis often show thickening of the heel pad.

Chromophobe Adenoma. *Natural History.* These tumors may occur in adolescence but are most common between the ages of 30 and 60, with equal distribution between men and women. They are the largest of pituitary tumors, having a tendency to extend upward for a considerable distance. The clinical picture is variable. The tumors may be asymptomatic; the symptoms may be predominantly ocular or neurologic; or *endocrine symptoms* and signs may predominate, the most common being secondary gonadal failure (amenorrhea, decreased frequency of shaving, impotence), with evidence of secondary thyroidal and adrenocortical failure being less common and occurring later in the course. *Galactorrhea* may be the only endocrine symptom (Forbes-Albright syndrome) or may coexist with elements of hypopituitarism. Recent studies have called attention to the possibility that longstanding *primary hypogonadism* or *hypothyroidism* may give rise to pituitary enlargement, owing to chromophobe adenoma in most cases (Bower; Lawrence et al.). In contrast, there are rare instances of *oversecretion* of a *pituitary* hormone, e.g., TSH, by a chromophobe adenoma.

Treatment. It is now clear that chromophobe adenoma must be treated; it is not safe to manage "expectantly" a patient suspected to have this lesion. A recent study has shown that of 16 such patients left untreated, 14 eventually required treatment, and during the observation period (6 months to 15 years) growth of the adenoma produced further and irreversible damage in 8. The best treatment appears to be *surgery,* followed by *conventional radiotherapy* (4000 to 5000 rads over five to six weeks); this method yields a control rate of about 75 per cent. Surgery (mortality rate 5 to 7 per cent) is

mandatory if there is evidence of recent or rapid growth of the adenoma or if there is a major threat to vision. Since surgery alone is followed by an appreciable recurrence rate, radiotherapy should be added. In selected cases, radiotherapy alone may suffice. Preliminary results suggest that treatment with *heavy particles* (protons, α-particles) may be as effective as conventional radiotherapy for this tumor; the method is available only at those few centers that have cyclotrons.

Treatment of *galactorrhea* is either *surgical* or *pharmacologic.* If the tumor is large and threatens vision, surgery must be done. Hardy has had considerable success with *transsphenoidal* removal of laterally located prolactin-secreting microadenomas without producing hypopituitarism (Kohler and Ross). With or without pituitary tumor, treatment of galactorrhea with L-*dopa* and *ergot alkaloids* has shown promise, eliciting falls in plasma prolactin levels and, after several weeks, suppressing the inappropriate lactation.

Acidophilic Adenoma with Acromegaly. *Natural History and Pathogenesis.* There is some evidence that acidophilic tumors may arise through an abnormality in HGHRF secretion by the hypothalamus. The course and prognosis of this lesion are more unfavorable than used to be thought. Life expectancy is reduced; in one series half the patients were dead before age 50 and nearly 90 per cent by age 60; among 194 patients followed for up to 30 years in London, the death rate was almost twice that in a matched group of patients without acromegaly (see Ch. 832). Treatment is therefore mandatory, even in "mild" cases without ocular or neurologic symptoms.

Treatment. Several modes of therapy are available; each is more or less effective and more or less hazardous. As Gorden and Roth have put it (Kohler and Ross): "At the present time patients are treated largely on the basis of regional expertise or preference. No single mode of therapy has emerged as ideal or clearly preferable. All therapeutic modalities to date leave some patients with distinctly elevated growth hormone concentrations." *Conventional pituitary radiation* (4000 to 5000 rads over five weeks) probably controls tumor growth in over 70 per cent of patients; if one is willing to wait, plasma HGH values will fall somewhat by one to two years after radiation and will be reduced by nearly 80 per cent after 3 to 6 years, with some values in the normal range; untoward effects are not common. Treatment with *heavy particles* (4500 to 6500 rads over 11 days) sometimes produces dramatic results; there are more untoward effects than with conventional external radiation. The method works best when there is no major extrasellar extension of the tumor. Plasma HGH falls to levels below 10 ng per milliliter within two years after radiation in about three fourths of patients; at these levels metabolic improvement is almost always seen.

More in Europe than in the United States, *transsphenoidal implantation of radioactive isotopes* (^{90}Y, ^{198}Au) into the pituitary has found favor. There are many reports of beneficial effect, with resolution of soft tissue and osseous abnormalities and reduction of plasma HGH levels, but there is an appreciable rate of complications (meningitis, CSF rhinorrhea), and a still higher rate may be expected during the developmental phase at a given institution.

Many *surgical approaches* have been tried. *Transfrontal hypophysectomy* is effective and has a mortality rate of well under 5 per cent in experienced hands; the difficulty is in achieving total removal of the tumor, for short of that plasma HGH values remain elevated. *Transsphenoidal* removal, especially of small adenomas, may be highly successful in skilled hands; in a recent series of 40 patients, 25 had clinical "cure" with return of plasma HGH to normal levels, and 10 showed improvement with substantial falls of plasma HGH; there was one late postoperative death. Both *stereotaxic* and *transsphenoidal cryohypophysectomy* have also been used in small numbers of patients.

A number of *pharmacologic agents* have been tried: *estrogens, chlorpromazine, progestins,* and *somatostatin* (HGH-inhibiting hormone). These drugs may prove to be suitable in selected "mild" cases; further trials over long periods will be required for full evaluation of efficacy.

Basophilic Adenoma with Cushing's Syndrome. *Natural History.* These tumors are *small,* being rarely visible radiographically. If the sella is enlarged, it is most likely owing to a chromophobe adenoma; those occurring after bilateral total adrenalectomy for Cushing's syndrome have chromophilic granulations, are aggressive, and may secrete ACTH and β-MSH with dermal pigmentation (Nelson's syndrome).

Treatment. Conventional external pituitary radiation (up to 4000 rads) in Cushing's syndrome may yield results better than the 30 to 40 per cent of incomplete or temporary remissions that could be achieved in the past (Orth and Liddle). In *Nelson's syndrome,* tumors may be aggressive or malignant, and require more radiation; with *heavy particles,* doses of 12,000 to 16,000 rads have been given with control of most tumors. In the faster-growing adenomas, particularly those with large extrasellar extension, *surgery* is required.

Transsphenoidal surgery for removal of these tumors, especially when small (microadenomas), has corrected the ACTH and β-MSH oversecretion and controlled the tumor without producing hypopituitarism. When there is a large suprasellar component, the *transfrontal* approach is preferable.

Craniopharyngioma (Rathke's Pouch Tumor, Adamantinoma). Although they may first appear in adult life, most of these tumors become manifest in childhood. Signs of increased intracranial pressure, changes in visual fields and acuity, and slowing or cessation of growth in late childhood are typical; because of the suprasellar location of the major portion of the tumor mass, *hypothalamic symptoms,* especially *diabetes insipidus,* occur occasionally. About 80 per cent of craniopharyngiomas display suprasellar calcification on x-ray (Fig. 1); the sella may be normal, eroded, or enlarged. Since these tumors are cystic (lined with squamous or columnar epithelium not resembling pituitary cells), they are not very radiosensitive; *transfrontal surgery* is usually indicated.

Multiple Endocrine Adenomatosis. *Clinical Characteristics.* Acidophilic or chromophobic adenomas of the pituitary are occasionally accompanied by functioning islet cell tumors of the pancreas and adenomas of the parathyroids and adrenal cortex. Intractable peptic ulcer (hypergastrinemia, Zollinger-Ellison syndrome; q.v.) is often associated. The disorder is familial in many instances. Presenting symptoms may be those of pituitary tumor (ocular, neurologic, acromegaly), hypoglycemia, hyperparathyroidism (e.g., renal colic), or gastrointestinal hemorrhage. Acromegaly with hypertension has been associated with surgically proved, primary *aldosterone-secreting adrenal adenoma.* It is probably more correct to regard multiple endocrine adenomatosis as a complex of separate genetic abnormalities than as a series of consequences of a single primary disease. This syndrome (known as multiple endocrine adenomatosis Type I or MEA I) should not be confused with MEA Type II: medullary carcinoma of the thyroid, pheochromocytoma, and parathyroid hyperplasia (also known as Sipple's syndrome) which is transmitted as an autosomal dominant trait with a high degree of penetrance (see Ch. 837 and 843).

Treatment. This syndrome may present the physician with a nice problem in deciding which tumor to treat first. Generally, the pituitary tumors are not so

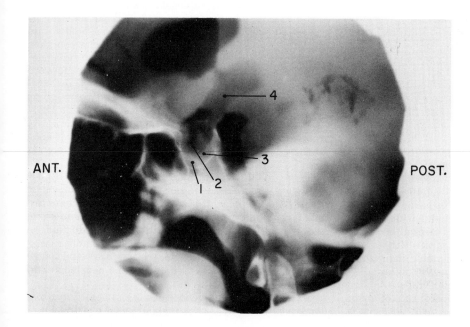

ANT.   POST.

Figure 6. "Empty sella" in a 56-year-old woman. Pneumoencephalogram, lateral (sagittal) view of the sella which shows depression of the sellar floor (1). The striking abnormality is downward extension of air (2) into the sella; the pituitary is flattened downward and posteriorly (3). Normally, no air should enter the sella. If an intrasellar tumor were present, one would expect it to elevate the air column above the sella and encroach upward upon the third ventricle (4).

threatening as the others; unless there is a major or rapidly progressive impairment of vision, treatment of the pituitary adenoma or of acromegaly can wait. Obviously, the gastrointestinal problem, the hypoglycemia, or the hypercalcemia will have to be attacked first, depending upon which is the most acute or the most incapacitating.

The "Empty Sella" Syndrome. *Pathogenesis and Clinical Characteristics.* In an unknown proportion of cases, enlargement of the pituitary fossa as seen on lateral x-rays of the skull is not due to pituitary tumor. In a recent study, nearly a third of enlarged sellae were found on pneumoencephalography to contain not too much but too little pituitary tissue (Fig. 6). One autopsy series has revealed a 5.5 per cent incidence of this lesion in nearly 800 presumably normal people, the space above the pituitary remnant being replaced by a subarachnoid sac filled with cerebrospinal fluid. "Empty sella" may occur as a consequence of Sheehan's syndrome or of necrosis of a pituitary adenoma, either spontaneous or after x-irradiation. The sella may be radiologically enlarged or normal. The pathogenesis is debated. Possible mechanisms include a defective diaphragma sellae through which an outpouching of subarachnoid membrane may descend, and medial kinking of the internal carotids compressing the "waist" of the dorsum sellae, with consequent expansion ("ballooning") of the pituitary. The *clinical picture* may show *no endocrine abnormality* or *frank hypopituitarism.* Usually symptoms of pituitary deficiency are not prominent, but one or more defects in anterior pituitary hormone secretion can be shown by test. There seems to be a curious predisposition to "empty sella" in obese middle-aged women who have had many children.

Diagnosis and Treatment. This lesion emphasizes the need for *pneumonencephalography* in all cases of enlarged sella (Fig. 6) in which radiotherapy is contemplated; such treatment, directed to an unsuspected empty sella, is likely to produce a permanent CSF fistula. If an empty sella is found, the only therapy required is replacement of lost hormonal functions if any are shown to exist.

Ballard, H. S., Frame, B., and Hartsock, R. J.: Familial mulitple endocrine adenoma–peptic ulcer complex. Medicine, 43:481, 1964.

Besser, G. M., Parke, L., Edwards, C. R. W., Forsyth, I. A., and McNeilly, A. S.: Galactorrhea: Successful treatment with reduction of plasma prolactin levels by brom-ergocryptine. Br. Med. J., 2:669, 1972.

Bower, B. F.: Pituitary enlargement secondary to untreated primary hypogonadism. Ann. Intern. Med., 69:107, 1968.

Brisman, R., Hughes, J. E. O., and Holub, D. A.: Endocrine function in nineteen patients with empty sella syndrome. J. Clin. Endocrinol. Metab., 34:570, 1972.

Craven, D. E., Goodman, D., and Carter, J. H.: Familial multiple endocrine adenomatosis: Multiple endocrine neoplasia, type I. Arch. Intern. Med., 129:567, 1972.

Fürst, E.: On chromophobe pituitary adenoma. Acta Med. Scand. (Suppl. 452), 1966.

Hall, R., Schally, A. V., Evered, D., Kastin, A. J., Mortimer, C. H., Tunbridge, W. M. G., Besser, G. M., Coy, D. H., Goldie, D. J., McNeilly, A. S., Phenekos, C., and Weightman, D.: Action of growth-hormone-release inhibitory hormone in healthy men and in acromegaly. Lancet, 2:581, 1973.

Hamilton, C. R., Jr., Adams, L. C., and Maloof, F.: Hyperthyroidism due to thyrotropin-producing pituitary chromophobe adenoma. N. Engl. J. Med., 283:1077, 1970.

Keiser, H. R., Beaven, M. A., Doppman, J., Wells, S., Jr., and Buja, L. M.: Sipple's syndrome: Medullary thyroid carcinoma, pheochromocytoma, and parathyroid disease. Ann. Intern. Med., 78:561, 1973.

Kohler, P. O., and Ross, G. T. (eds.): Diagnosis and Treatment of Pituitary Tumors. New York, American Elsevier Publishing Company, 1973.

Kolodny, H. D., Sherman, L., Singh, A., Kim, S., and Benjamin, F.:

Acromegaly treated with chlorpromazine: A case study. N. Engl. J. Med., 284:819, 1971.

Lawrence, A. M., and Kirsteins, L.: Progestins in the medical management of active acromegaly. J. Clin. Endocrinol. Metab., 30:646, 1970.

Lawrence, A. M., Wilber, J. F., and Hagen, T. C.: The pituitary and primary hypothyroidism: Enlargement and unusual growth hormone secretory responses. Arch. Intern. Med., 132:327, 1973.

Lawrence, A. M., Pinsky, S. M., and Goldfine, I. D.: Conventional radiation therapy in acromegaly: A review and reassessment. Arch. Intern. Med., 128:369, 1971.

Lawrence, J. H., Tobias, C. A., Linfoot, J. A., Born, J. L., Lyman, J. T., Chang, C. Y., Manougian, E., and Wei, W. C.: Successful treatment of acromegaly: Metabolic and clinical studies in 145 patients. J. Clin. Endocrinol. Metab., 31:180, 1970.

LeMay, M.: The radiologic diagnosis of pituitary disease. Radiol. Clin. North Am., 5:303, 1967.

Neelon, F. A., Goree, J. A., and Lebovitz, H. E.: The primary empty sella: Clinical and radiographic characteristics and endocrine function. Medicine, 52:73, 1973.

Orth, D. N., and Liddle, G. W.: Results of treatment in 108 patients with Cushing's syndrome. N. Engl. J. Med., 285:243, 1971.

Roth, J., Gorden, P., and Brace, K.: Efficacy of conventional pituitary irradiation in acromegaly. N. Engl. J. Med., 282:1385, 1970.

Snyder, N., III, Scurry, M. T., and Deiss, W. P.: Five families with multiple endocrine adenomatosis. Ann. Intern. Med., 76:53, 1972.

831. HYPOPITUITARISM

PITUITARY INSUFFICIENCY IN THE ADULT

Definitions. Hypopituitarism is the clinical condition resulting from destruction of the anterior pituitary; it is accompanied by secondary atrophy of the gonads, thyroid, and adrenal cortex. The term *panhypopituitarism* has been used to designate total absence of all the known pituitary secretions. *Simmonds' disease* is used synonymously. The term *Sheehan's disease* describes hypopituitarism resulting from postpartum necrosis of the gland. The designation *pituitary insufficiency* is inclusive.

Etiology, Pathology, and Pathogenesis. The most common cause of pituitary insufficiency in adult life is *pituitary tumor,* particularly chromophobe adenoma; the most common cause of *very severe* adult hypopituitarism is probably postpartum necrosis of the gland. The pathogenesis is debated. The common denominator is obstetric accident. According to Sheehan, peripheral vascular collapse is followed by spasm of local vessels, then thrombosis, and then infarction. McKay holds that the primary event is not arteriolar spasm but thrombosis of pituitary vessels as part of generalized intravascular coagulation. Neither view accounts for the peculiar susceptibility of the pituitary to damage in the postpartum period. The well-demarcated infarctions are small or nearly total. Sheehan and Summers have shown that pituitary insufficiency does not occur unless the lesion is very large. The late lesion is fibrosis with residual small nests of normal chromophils.

Lesions other than tumors (see Ch. 830) are fibrosis of unknown cause, granulomas, which may be nonspecific, syphilitic, or tuberculous, and aneurysms of the *internal carotid artery.* Ischemic necrosis has occasionally followed acute infection (usually associated with diabetes mellitus), meningitis, basal skull fracture, and septic cavernous sinus thrombosis. In some patients the primary defect may be in the hypothalamus (e.g., sarcoidosis, metastatic cancer, idiopathic).

General pathologic findings in pituitary insufficiency include widespread *splanchnomicria* with particularly striking atrophy of the gonads, thyroid, and adrenal cortex.

Clinical Manifestations and Natural History. The speed of onset of pituitary insufficiency depends upon the nature and size of the lesion. When *postpartum necrosis* of the pituitary is extensive and severe, acute symptoms such as *diabetes insipidus* and *hypoglycemia* occur during the puerperium and may be only transitory; the patient may suddenly die within weeks, probably as a consequence of acute adrenocortical insufficiency. More commonly, the onset after obstetric accident is slow, occurring over months to years. The first symptom is usually failure to lactate; pubic and axillary hair fails to grow; menses do not return owing to gonadal failure, or the periods are scanty and transitory; amenorrhea follows. Libido is lost. Symptoms of *thyroid and adrenocortical failure* occur later as a rule than do those of ovarian deficiency, but *there is no set pattern.* General

deterioration ensues. Patients become weak, easily fatigued, indifferent to their surroundings, slothful, and negligent of household duties. *Personality changes* range from mild idiosyncrasies to frank psychosis. Intolerance of cold, as in primary hypothyroidism, may be extreme. *Hypopituitary coma* with hypotension and hypothermia, probably in most instances resulting from *hypoglycemia,* may have its onset gradually with no apparent cause, or rapidly in response to minor illness. At times collapse is preceded by clinical manifestations of *adrenal crisis* with nausea, vomiting, high fever, and hypotension. Although *anorexia* is a prominent feature in some patients, cachexia is uncommon and is a terminal event in the neglected patient. Pre-existing diabetes is on rare occasions ameliorated abruptly, with sudden lowering of the insulin requirement, after pituitary destruction ("Houssay phenomenon").

The *physical examination* discloses a fair state of nutrition as a rule (Fig. 7). The skin is thin, smooth, cool and pale, with fine wrinkling about the eyes (geroderma). The dry, scaly skin and puffy face of primary myxedema are unusual but occur on occasion. Pubic and axillary hair is absent or sparse. The pulse is slow and thin, the blood pressure low. Symptomatic hypotension on orthostasis is common. The breasts may appear well preserved, but genital atrophy is the rule.

General *laboratory examination* shows a moderate normochromic anemia that is less striking than the pallid appearance suggests. Roentgenogram of the skull is normal (there is no expanding intrasellar lesion). Blood glucose concentration is often low. The serum sodium concentration may be 120 mEq per liter or lower without symptoms of adrenal insufficiency. Hyponatremia is probably related to hemodilution owing to inadequate excretion of water, which in turn is due to deficient cortisol secretion. Episodic hyponatremia in patients with pituitary insufficiency is correlated with measurable water retention (increased total body water), not with sodium depletion. The level of serum potassium is normal. As in the hypophysectomized animal or man, the aldosterone function of the adrenal cortex is fairly well preserved; the hypopituitary patient responds to salt withdrawal by a slow but adequate increase in aldosterone secretion and consequent retention of sodium. In very severe hypopituitarism with complete adrenal destruction, this capacity may be lost. The urinary 17-ketosteroids and corticosteroids are decreased. The basal metabolic rate is low, and serum protein-bound iodine is depressed; but thyroidal uptake of ^{131}I is often inexplicably normal even when the patient is clinically hypothyroid.

The typical clinical picture becomes obvious as late as 15 to 20 years after the obstetric accident. Acute adrenocortical failure with or without superimposed infection is the chief cause of death in untreated patients.

Expanding intrasellar tumors—e.g., chromophobe adenoma—may have a similar insidious onset. The clinical picture and natural history are discussed in Ch. 830. In patients with intrasellar tumor, both the chief complaint and the ultimate cause of death are more commonly mechanical results of the adenoma than of pituitary failure.

Diagnosis. A history of postpartum hemorrhage, symptoms and signs of an intracranial tumor with chiasmal pressure, or evidence of multiple glandular deficiencies should raise the question of hypopituitarism. Diagnosis is difficult early in the course of the

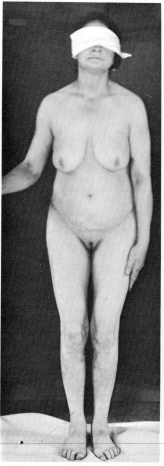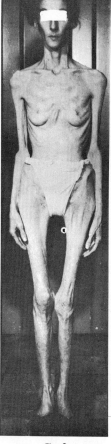

Fig. 7   Fig. 8

Figure 7. A patient with documented hypopituitarism 21 years after postpartum necrosis of the pituitary. Pubic and axillary hair is gone. Notice the absence of cachexia. Compare with Figure 8. (Reproduced by permission from Sheehan, H. L., and Summers, V. K.: Quart J. Med., 42:319, 1949.)

Figure 8. The patient is a 30-year-old unmarried woman with anorexia nervosa who had lost 55 pounds (compare with the good nutritional state of the patient with hypopituitarism, Fig. 7). Pubic hair was present and menses continued but were scanty and irregular. (Reproduced by permission from Bliss, E. L., and Branch, C. H. H.: Anorexia Nervosa. New York, Paul B. Hoeber, Inc., 1960.)

disease, before symptoms and signs of deficiency of more than one target gland are definite. Hypopituitarism should be suspected in patients with onset of gonadal failure in adult life. Amenorrhea occurring in a fertile woman before the expected age of menopause requires inquiry about obstetric hemorrhage in the past. Loss of axillary and pubic hair and atrophy of the external genitalia make hypopituitarism likely in a relatively young woman with amenorrhea. In men, loss of previously normal libido and potency and loss of body hair with or without genital atrophy are suggestive; roentgenogram of the skull shows sagittal stretching or ballooning of the sella if a pituitary tumor is present. Reduced visual acuity, optic atrophy, and bitemporal hemianopia provide evidence of suprasellar expansion of an intrasellar mass (see Ch. 830). Failure of sexual development late in the second decade raises the question of hypopituitarism in either sex.

In the *differential diagnosis,* primary gonadal failure and primary hypothyroidism must be considered. *Primary gonadal failure,* in the *male* especially, may resemble pituitary insufficiency. The degree of eunuchoidism (disproportionately long arms and legs owing to late closure of the epiphyses of the long bones) depends on the age of onset of hypoleydigism, being extreme if early, absent if late. Many males with gonadal failure have the fine, pale, wrinkled skin of hypopituitarism, but thyroid and adrenal function is normal. *Anorexia nervosa* is not difficult to differentiate, because only gonadotrophic deficiency is present and the degree of emaciation is extreme (Fig. 8; see Ch. 724).

Levels of urinary gonadotrophin are elevated in testicular deficiency, undetectable in pituitary failure. Klinefelter's syndrome (seminiferous tubule dysgenesis) is easily distinguished. In the female the same principles apply: The level of urinary gonadotrophin is undetectable in hypopituitarism, high in natural menopause. *Primary myxedema* is generally characterized by more noticeable dryness and puffiness of the skin, and the serum cholesterol tends to be higher. In hypothyroidism resulting from pituitary failure, other glandular deficiencies are often present and should be sought. Measurement of thyroidal response to thyrotrophin may be helpful (see Ch. 829). *Primary adrenocortical failure* (Addison's disease) is not hard to differentiate. The skin is darkly tanned (MSH) rather than pale, gonadal function is often normal, and thyroidal function is unimpaired, unless Hashimoto's thyroiditis is associated (Schmidt's syndrome). Diagnosis of this entity is discussed in Ch. 846. Primary adrenal failure is ruled out, and subtle adrenal insufficiency caused by pituitary failure is diagnosed by measuring the response of plasma or urinary corticosteroids to intravenous corticotrophin. This constitutes more specific evidence of adrenal deficiency than do low urinary steroid values, which are reduced in a great variety of chronic, debilitating diseases.

Treatment. *Long-term medical management* of the patient with hypopituitarism consists of careful replacement of lost functions. (Management of intrasellar mass lesions is discussed in Ch. 830.) Trophic hormones are not used because of expense and the bother of daily injections. By far the most important defect is that of the *adrenal cortex;* acute adrenal crisis may come on abruptly and without warning, and may lead to death. Under ordinary conditions, cortisone or hydrocortisone (10 to 25 mg per day in two divided doses, by mouth) provides a sense of well-being and adequate protection against hypotension, hypoglycemia, and water and electrolyte imbalance. Small doses are preferred, because patients with hypopituitarism have a peculiar susceptibility to the effects of larger doses of corticosteroids (peptic ulcer, facial rounding, psychosis) possibly because of coexisting secondary hypothyroidism in which metabolism of corticosteroids is much delayed. Added salt and a mineralocorticoid are only occasionally required. In the female, diethylstilbestrol, 0.5 to 1.0 mg per day for 20 days of each month, provides good maintenance of developed secondary sex characters and, in time, leads to an artificial menstrual cycle. Induction of ovulation in women with hypopituitarism is discussed in Ch. 867. In the male, a fair degree of libido and potency can be conferred by androgens (methyltestosterone, 20 to 30 mg per day orally; testosterone propionate, 25 to 100 mg two to three times per week by intramuscular injection; or a long-acting ester once per month intramuscularly). Thyroid replacement should be started with small doses (8 to 15 mg per day of USP thyroid orally), which are gradually increased over a period of several weeks; for optimal effect a dose as large as 0.180 gram may be needed. Roughly equivalent doses of L-thyroxine are 0.1 to 0.2 mg per day. It is probably wise to begin corticosteroid therapy first, because adrenal crisis has allegedly been precipitated by vigorous treatment with thyroid hormone.

Treatment of an acute illness or management during a surgical procedure, e.g., craniotomy for intrasellar tumor, is essentially that of adrenal crisis. Thyroid hormone is not necessary. *Corticotrophin should never be relied upon,* because the degree of endogenous adrenal response is unpredictable. Correct treatment is hydrocortisone (100 to 300 mg per day of a water-soluble ester in isotonic saline intravenously). It is better to err on the side of *moderately* excessive doses, because untoward reactions are not likely to occur during the few days of vigorous treatment generally required; the dose should be reduced as quickly as possible to the maintenance level. If in an emergency there is doubt concerning the presence of secondary hypoadrenalism, one should assume that it exists rather than attempt a time-consuming laboratory evaluation of adrenal status. If *diabetes insipidus* occurs postoperatively, treatment is as set out in Ch. 834.

Keller, P. J.: Induction of ovulation by synthetic luteinizing-hormone releasing factor in infertile women. Lancet, 2:570, 1972.

Martin, L. G., Martul, P., Connor, T. B., and Wiswell, J. G.: Hypothalamic origin of idiopathic hypopituitarism. Metabolism, 21:143, 1972.

McKay, D. G.: Pituitary. Disseminated Intravascular Coagulation. New York, Hoeber Medical Division, Harper & Row, 1965, pp. 405, 460.

Sheehan, H. L., and Davis, J. C.: Pituitary necrosis. Br. Med. Bull., 24:59, 1968.

Sheehan, H. L., and Summers, V. K.: The syndrome of hypopituitarism. Quart. J. Med., 42:319, 1949.

Sherman, B. M., Gorden, P., and diChiro, G.: Postmeningitic selective hypopituitarism with suprasellar calcification. Arch. Intern. Med., 128:600, 1971.

Stocks, A. E., and Powell, L. W.: Pituitary function in idiopathic haemochromomatosis and cirrhosis of the liver. Lancet, 2:298, 1972.

Warren, M. P., and Vande Wiele, R. L.: Clinical and metabolic features of anorexia nervosa. Am. J. Obstet. Gynecol., 117:435, 1973.

DEFICIENCY OF SINGLE ANTERIOR PITUITARY HORMONES

It is hard to determine in an individual case whether there is isolated deficiency of a pituitary hormone or whether one is observing an early stage of what will ultimately be panhypopituitarism. Whereas some *pituitary dwarfs* are panhypopituitary, others have *isolated HGH deficiency,* either of pituitary or hypothalamic origin. Patients who have Hand-Schüller-Christian disease with short stature have also been shown to have isolated HGH deficiency. It is not yet known whether women who have failure of postpartum lactation are deficient in *prolactin* secretion. Idiopathic isolated gonadotrophin failure exists in several forms, with or without anosmia, in men and women (see Ch. 867). *Isolated deficiencies of TSH and ACTH* have been reported; in one instance of the latter, pituitary basophils were virtually absent. Isolated corticotrophin deficiency has been found as part of the hypothalamic disorder of acute intermittent porphyria.

The most common form of isolated ACTH deficiency occurs in patients receiving *long-term corticosteroid therapy,* which is discussed in Ch. 849. Prolonged treatment with thyroid hormone and antiovulatory drugs usually induces *self-limited* TSH and gonadotrophin deficiency; rarely, the latter persists ("oversuppression syndrome"; see Ch. 867).

Treatment. Thyrotrophin and adrenocorticotrophin deficiencies are usually treated with thyroid hormone (or thyroxine) and corticosteroids, respectively. Administration of purified human FSH and HCG is effective in the induction of ovulation in hypopituitary women and, sometimes, spermatogenesis in men (see Ch. 857 and 867).

Braunstein, G. D., and Kohler, P. O.: Pituitary function in Hand-Schüller-Christian disease: Evidence for deficient growth-hormone release in patients with short stature. N. Engl. J. Med., 286:1225, 1972.

Christy, N. P.: Iatrogenic Cushing's syndrome. *In* Christy, N. P. (ed.): The Human Adrenal Cortex, New York, Harper & Row, 1971, p. 395.

Males, J. L., Townsend, J. L., and Schneider, R. A.: Hypogonadotropic hypogonadism with anosmia – Kallmann's syndrome. Arch. Intern. Med., 131:501, 1973.

Miyai, K., Azukizawa, M., and Kumahara, Y.: Familial isolated thyrotropin deficiency with cretinism. N. Engl. J. Med., 285:1043, 1971.

Spitz, I. M., Diamant, Y., Rosne, E., Bell, J., David, M. B., Polishuk, W., and Rabinowitz, D.: Isolated gonadotropin deficiency: A heterogenous syndrome. N. Engl. J. Med., 290:10, 1974.

Tagatz, G., Fialkow, P. J., Smith, D., and Spadoni, L.: Hypogonadotropic hypogonadism associated with anosmia in the female. N. Engl. J. Med., 283:1326, 1970.

Waxman, A. D., Berk, P. D., Schalch, D., and Tschudy, D. P.: Isolated adrenocorticotropic hormone deficiency in acute intermittent porphyria. Ann. Intern. Med., 70:317, 1969.

HYPOPHYSECTOMY-INDUCED HYPOPITUITARISM

Since 1952, pituitary ablation has been used as a palliative treatment for metastatic cancer and for diabetic retinopathy.

The metabolic consequences of hypophysectomy in man are familiar. They are repaired by hormonal replacement therapy. If diabetes insipidus is present, it is treated with vasopressin as set forth in Ch. 834. Loss of gonadotrophic function, observed as disappearance of detectable urinary gonadotrophin, occurs within a week after hypophysectomy. Gonadal steroids are not given, especially to patients with cancer, because hypogonadism may be an important part of the palliative therapy. Loss of thyrotrophic function is apparent from fall of serum PBI values to myxedematous levels at one week and of thyroidal uptake of ^{131}I at two weeks after pituitary ablation. If hypophysectomy is incomplete, these indices decline, only to return to normal within a month after surgery. Loss of adrenocorticotrophic function is notable only if hypophysectomy has been virtually total. Some investigators believe that the metyrapone test and measurement of plasma prolactin concentration are the most sensitive indices of completeness of hypophysectomy.

Conventional medical treatment consists of thyroid USP in daily doses of 0.120 gram and cortisone acetate, 25 mg or less, both given by mouth.

Methods for pituitary ablation are numerous: transfrontal and transsphenoidal hypophysectomy, cryosurgery, stereotaxic radiofrequency surgery, pituitary stalk section, implantation of radioactive gold or yttrium (^{198}Au, ^{90}Y), and external delivery of heavy particles (proton beam) from the cyclotron. It is not yet possible to decide which of these techniques is the safest or the most effective. It is also not clear why pituitary ablation is effective at all; there is evidence that adequate palliation may not be closely or uniquely related to the degree of reduction in growth hormone or prolactin secretion.

The present position can be summarized in this way. Carefully selected patients with advanced, widespread metastases from cancer of the breast have objective remissions in bony, cutaneous, and pulmonary metastases in about 50 per cent of cases treated with surgical hypophysectomy. In metastatic prostatic cancer, remissions occur in fewer than half the patients. The methods which bring about less complete ablation of the pituitary tend to be associated with lower remission rates (see Ch. 877).

In patients with diabetic retinopathy, surgical hypophysectomy is rarely done now (see Ch. 806). It is ineffective in proliferative retinopathy, and in several series the remission rate of hemorrhages and exudates is about the same in hypophysectomized as in untreated groups of patients.

Juret, P.: Endocrine Surgery in Human Cancers. 2nd ed. Springfield, Ill., Charles C Thomas, 1966.

Krieger, D. T., Sirota, D. K., and Lieberman, T.: Cryohypophysectomy for diabetic retinopathy: Ophthalmological and endocrine correlation. Ann. Intern. Med., 72:309, 1970.

Ray, B. S.: Hypophysectomy as palliative treatment. J.A.M.A., 200:974, 1967.

PITUITARY INSUFFICIENCY IN CHILDHOOD

Lesions involving the pituitary in childhood cause *dwarfism;* like that of gonadotrophin, secretion of HGH appears to be more sensitive to impairment than the thyrotrophic or adrenocorticotrophic functions of the pituitary. Pituitary insufficiency is an uncommon cause of short stature, accounting for fewer than 10 per cent of instances. About two thirds of pituitary dwarfs have no evidence of pituitary tumor; usually there is no evidence of an anatomic lesion. The lesion may in some cases be hypothalamic. Idiopathic hypophysial *fibrosis* has been occasionally observed. Of the tumors, *craniopharyngioma* (adamantinoma) is the most common. This neoplasm arises from fragments of oral epithelium remaining from the embryologic invagination (see Ch. 830). Other causes are *suprasellar cysts* and *Hand-Schüller-Christian disease.* Reversible isolated HGH deficiency has been documented in children with the maternal deprivation syndrome.

Diagnosis of pituitary dwarfism is often difficult early in life. The infant's size may be normal at birth. Growth does not stop entirely, but is obviously retarded in early infancy. Evidence of thyroid and adrenocortical insufficiency, e.g., hypoglycemic attacks, is strongly suggestive, but may be subtle or absent. If, however, the patient reaches the early years of the second decade with continued retardation of growth and complete failure of sexual development, suspicion of pituitary dwarfism is raised. The physical examination discloses relatively normal proportions. The facies is childish, but the skin may become wrinkled early, imparting an incongruous aspect of aging. Laboratory study shows absence of urinary gonadotrophin, reduced concentration of serum protein-bound iodine, and subnormal response of plasma corticosteroids to intravenous adrenocorticotrophin. Idiopathic hypopituitary dwarfism may occur either as an isolated, recessively inherited deficiency of growth hormone, or sporadically. When sporadic, the deficiency may involve growth hormone alone or several pituitary hormones.

The *differential diagnosis* of pituitary dwarfism includes constitutional retardation of growth and delay in the onset of puberty (see Ch. 857); in the latter condition, the family history is often positive, evidence of thyroidal and adrenocortical insufficiency is lacking, and in time normal growth and maturation take place. *Systemic and other endocrine diseases* may cause dwarfism; among these are chondrodystrophy, rickets, Hurler's syndrome, intestinal malabsorption, chronic renal disease, hypoxia associated with congenital cardiac malformations, hypothyroidism, and sexual precocity with premature fusion of the epiphyses. These conditions are distinguished by the inappropriately short extremities, osseous deformities, overt malnutrition and evidence of fat intolerance, gross proteinuria and nitrogen retention, cyanosis and heart murmur, mental deficiency and other stigmata of cretinism, or precocious development of the genitalia. D. W. Smith has presented a list of 52 conditions associated with short stature, some of which are recognized at a glance by seasoned pediatricians; Smith also lists the very numerous systemic diseases in which growth retardation is observed.

One of the most difficult disorders to distinguish from pituitary dwarfism before puberty is *primordial dwarfism*. The patients, also known as sexual ateliotic (incomplete) dwarfs, become miniature adults, often capable of producing normal offspring. McKusick and his co-workers have shown that in some of these patients the failure to grow in association with normal gonadal and secondary sexual development and normal thyroid and adrenal function is due to a deficiency of end-organ response to growth hormone. With radioimmunoassay measurements of serum growth hormone, it is possible to define four subgroups of ateliotic dwarfs, some of whom fail to raise sulfation factor (somatomedin) activity when HGH is administered. It is interesting that the African pygmy also has subresponsiveness to administered growth hormone, whereas endogenous growth hormone release is apparently normal (Table 2). The differentiation of pituitary dwarfism in the female and *gonadal dysgenesis (Turner's syndrome)* may be difficult before puberty; patients with this disorder are phenotypic females who often have associated congenital anomalies (webbed neck, coarctation of the aorta) and short stat-

TABLE 2. Classification of Pituitary Dwarfism*

I. *HGH undetectable:*
   A. Idiopathic hypopituitarism (primary disorder of pituitary or secondary to deficiency of hypothalamic HGHRF)
      1. Panhypopituitarism
      2. Isolated HGH deficiency (may be familial)
   B. Organic hypopituitarism
      1. Tumors
      2. Trauma
      3. Infection
      4. Hand-Schüller-Christian disease
   C. HGH unreactive immunologically, partially active biologically (Merimee's Type II ateliotic dwarf)
      1. Absent HGH response to provocative tests
      2. Evidence that endogenous HGH has some activity
      3. Resistance to exogenous HGH (including no rise in somatomedin)
      4. Autosomal dominant inheritance in some cases

II. *HGH detectable but ineffective:*
   A. Laron dwarf
      1. Normal plasma HGH response to provocative tests
      2. Plasma HGH normal or high
      3. Deficient generation of somatomedin when HGH is given
   B. African pygmy
      1. Normal plasma HGH response to provocative tests
      2. Plasma HGH normal
      3. Somatomedin low and showing no rise when HGH is given

*Compiled from many sources by Dr. C. A. L. Abrams of the Pediatric Service, The Roosevelt Hospital, and the Department of Pediatrics, The College of Physicians and Surgeons, Columbia University. See references to the text (Merimee, Najjar).

ure; the distinguishing features are less immature facies, less delay in epiphysial closure, slight but definite growth of pubic hair at puberty, a frequently negative (male) chromatin pattern on buccal smear, and, after the age of 9 to 13, an elevated rather than absent titer of urinary gonadotrophin (see Ch. 867). Recognition of *progeria* is easy; this rare idiopathic condition is characterized by retardation of growth, baldness, loss of subcutaneous fat, premature fusion of epiphyses, and atherosclerosis or arterial calcification, all occurring within the first few years of life. The life span is short; there is no evidence of endocrine disease.

As indicated in Ch. 829, the best way to detect growth hormone deficiency is to test the response of serum growth hormone values to insulin-induced hypoglycemia. If a metabolic ward is available, demonstration of a sharp increase in nitrogen retention in response to administered growth hormone is diagnostic of classic idiopathic HGH deficiency (see also Table 2). Analysis of the growth curve determines whether or not to subject the patient to elaborate testing procedures.

As to *treatment*, a moderate degree of linear growth can be achieved in pituitary dwarfs through the administration of thyroid hormone in combination with gonadal steroids. Impressive skeletal growth can be induced with the administration of purified human growth hormone. The optimal dose is about 20 to 45 mg per month (see Tanner et al.). This therapy is limited by the short supply of the hormone; if it is used, gonadal steroids should not be given until maximal linear growth is attained so that epiphysial closure will not occur; thyroid hormone augments the somatotrophic effects. Crawford and his colleagues have set out detailed criteria for diagnosis and treatment of pituitary dwarfism and have described the response to growth hormone. The hormone causes only minimal if any increase in linear growth rate in children whose short stature is not due to deficiency of HGH. Since growth hormone should therefore be reserved for patients with growth hormone deficiency, a high premium is placed upon accurate diagnosis.

Goodman, H. C., Grumbach, M. M., and Kaplan, S. L.: Growth and growth hormone: II. A comparison of isolated growth hormone deficiency and multiple pituitary hormone deficiencies in 35 patients with idiopathic hypopituitary dwarfism. N. Engl. J. Med., 278:57, 1968.

Grumbach, M. M., and Kaplan, S. L.: The pathogenesis of growth hormone deficiency. Proceedings of the XIII International Congress of Pediatrics, 15:10, 1971.

Lacey, K. A., and Parkin, J. M.: Causes of short stature: A community study of children in Newcastle upon Tyne. Lancet, 1:42, 1974.

Laron, Z., Pertzelan, A., Karp, M., Kowaldo-Silbergeld, A., and Daughaday, W. H.: Administration of growth hormone to patients with familial dwarfism with high plasma immunoreactive growth hormone: Measurement of sulfation factor, metabolic and linear growth responses. J. Clin. Endocrinol. Metab., 33:332, 1971.

Merimee, T. J., et al.: An unusual variety of endocrine dwarfism: Subresponsiveness to growth hormone in a sexually mature dwarf. Lancet, 2:191, 1968.

Merimee, T. J., Hall, J. D., Rimoin, D. L., and McKusick, V. A.: A metabolic and hormonal basis for classifying ateliotic dwarfs. Lancet, 1:963, 1969.

Merimee, T. J., Rimoin, D. L., and Cavalli-Sforza, L. L.: Metabolic studies in the African pygmy. J. Clin. Invest., 51:395, 1972.

Najjar, S. S., Khachadurian, A. K., Ilbawi, M. N., and Blizzard, R. M.: Dwarfism with elevated levels of plasma growth hormone. N. Engl. J. Med., 284:809, 1971.

Root, A. W., Rosenfield, R. L., Bongiovanni, A. M., and Eberlein, W. R.: The plasma growth hormone response to insulin-induced hypoglycemia in children with retardation of growth. Pediatrics, 39:844, 1967.

Silver, H. K., and Finkelstein, M.: Deprivation dwarfism. J. Pediatr. 70:317, 1967.

Smith, D. W.: Compendium on shortness of stature. J. Pediatr., 70:463, 1967.

Tanner, J. M., Whitehouse, R. H., Hughes, P. C. R., and Vince, F. P.: Effect of human growth hormone treatment of 1 to 7 years on growth of 100 children with growth hormone deficiency, low birthweight, inherited smallness, Turner's syndrome, and other complaints. Arch. Dis. Child., 46:745, 1971.

832. HYPERPITUITARISM

ACROMEGALY

Definition. Acromegaly is a chronic disease of middle life characterized by overgrowth of bone, connective tissue, and viscera in response to prolonged and excessive secretion of adenohypophysial growth hormone. The term "acromegaly" denotes the typical enlargement of acral or distal parts of the body—the hands, feet, face, and head.

Etiology. The increased secretion of growth hormone results from overactivity of the acidophil cells of the pituitary. The evidence for excessive growth hormone is that (1) similar pathologic changes are produced in animals by administration of the hormone, and (2) increased concentrations of growth hormone have been detected in plasma of patients with acromegaly. Hyperactivity of the anterior pituitary is deduced from (1) the almost invariable necropsy finding of pituitary enlargement, (2) histologic observation of overgrowth of the acidophilic cells, and (3) the clinical improvement that frequently follows destruction of the gland.

Incidence and Prevalence. Acromegaly is a rare disorder with about 300 new cases per year being discovered in the United States. The sexes are affected equally often. Acromegaly starts most commonly in the third and fourth decades; a few patients trace the start

of acromegaly to adolescence. Some 30 acromegalic children have been reported.

Pathology and Pathogenesis. Acidophilic or mixed acidophilic and chromophobe adenoma is found in 75 per cent or more of autopsied patients with acromegaly. Rarely, acidophil cell hyperplasia is observed, malignancy almost never. The growth of the tumor may obliterate normal cells. The assumption is that if hypopituitarism occurs, it is a result of atrophy of normal pituitary tissue owing to the pressure of the tumor. Over 90 per cent of adenomas cause sufficient enlargement of the sella turcica to be visible in roentgenograms of the skull. Sellar enlargement may be minimal or gross. Upward extension rarely produces clinical evidence of hypothalamic involvement, e.g., diabetes insipidus, but invasion of the optic tracts of chiasm is of clinical significance (visual field changes, optic atrophy) in about 60 per cent of patients.

The excessive secretion of growth hormone affects virtually all organs and tissues. The response of cartilage and bone is obvious and distinctive. The histologic appearance of chondrogenesis and osteogenesis is somewhat disorderly. The cartilaginous and bony response occurs at points of special sensitivity, e.g., mandible, zygoma, ribs, and clavicles. The uneven growth is thought to be due to the effect of pressure or of muscular traction. Increased *chondrogenesis* is most obvious in hypertrophy of the costal cartilages, which contributes to the increased circumference of the thorax. *Acromegalic arthritis,* affecting chiefly the large joints and the spine, resembles osteoarthritis and results from proliferation of deep layers of joint cartilage with thinning of articular cartilages. Hypertrophy of nasal and aural cartilage accounts for part of the enlargement of nose and ears. *Osteogenesis* from the thickened periosteum is accelerated; absorption of bone is also rapid; late in the disease *osteoporosis* may be striking. There is overgrowth of the supraorbital ridge. The anterior temporal ridge advances with forward growth of the lateral portions of the orbit, expansion of the frontal sinuses, and forward displacement of the zygoma. Overgrowth of the maxilla lengthens the face, and the teeth are separated by heaping up of alveolar bone. The ramus of the mandible grows longer; the angle between ramus and body opens out to produce mandibular prognathism. The ribs and clavicles widen and reach a length 2 to 3 inches greater than normal. The *long bones* thicken and become massive. The humerus and femur may be lengthened, and the latter may be deformed by bowing. The vertebral bodies are increased in the anteroposterior diameter; the greatest changes occur in the thoracic spine with deposit of new bone upon diaphyses, particularly anteriorly; this change makes forward flexion of the spine difficult.

The visible *enlargement of distal parts* is chiefly due to proliferation of soft tissue, not bone. Subcutaneous connective tissue is grossly increased, giving the characteristic thick and fleshy appearance of the *hands* and *feet,* enlargement of the *lips,* and *accentuation of skin folds.* The skin itself is greatly thickened; there are increased sweating and seborrhea; hirsutism occurs in a few female patients. The *tongue* may be so large as to protrude from the mouth.

Widespread splanchnomegaly is the rule. The heart, lungs, liver, spleen, and intestines are variously enlarged two- to fivefold. The kidneys are enlarged by the growth of individual nephrons; studies of renal function indicate increased glomerular filtration rate and proximal tubular activity. The endocrine glands participate in the splanchnomegaly. A possible role of accompanying oversecretion of trophic hormones is not proved. The gonads, although often functioning subnormally and showing histologic evidence of failure, may be large. The *adrenal cortex* is hyptertrophied, and nodules are often found. The *thyroid* may be eight to nine times the normal size; goiters are diffuse or nodular. True hyperthyroidism is uncommon. The *parathyroids* are usually enlarged, and adenomas occur. Although there is generalized enlargement of tissues and organs and a considerable gain in weight, obesity is almost unknown, possibly because of the adipokinetic effect of growth hormone. The muscles enlarge somewhat but without conspicuous hypertrophy; edema and deposition of mucopolysaccharide in muscle have been reported; atrophy is a late finding.

Clinical Manifestations and Natural History. The onset of acromegaly is usually so insidious and so subtle that it escapes detection by the patient and his intimate associates. The gradualness and subtlety of onset are such that a third of the patients seek medical help for unrelated diseases, being unaware of their acromegaly. In Davidoff's series of 100 patients, the mean age of onset was estimated as 27 years, but the mean age at which the patients presented themselves was over 40; this average lapse of 13 or 14 years implies chronicity and a generally slow course. Careful analysis of the history reveals that early symptoms are related to peripheral effects of growth hormone or, much less commonly, to the mechanical pressure of the intrasellar tumor. Even before the obvious changes in appearance are noticed patients may complain of excessive sweating, paresthesias of the hands and feet, and pain and stiffness of the slowly expanding fingers and toes. Arthralgias are common. Accounts of hypersexuality and greatly increased muscular strength early in the course of the disease are rare. Complaints of hypogonadism (amenorrhea, loss of libido) are common. Headache may be extremely severe; the mechanism is not clear, because, in many instances, there is little clinically detectable enlargement of the pituitary tumor. Impairment of visual acuity or symptomatic encroachment upon visual fields occurs in over 60 per cent of patients at one time or another.

The *clinical picture* of advanced acromegaly is easily recognized on physical examination, but the changes are occasionally subtle. The typical acromegalic is large and burly; in late stages the forward carriage of the head, prognathism, kyphosis, bowing of the legs, and rolling gait are distinctive. The features are blunt and coarse, the nose and ears large; the brow is prominent and the jaw prognathous; the facial wrinkles are exaggerated; the lips are full. The skin is thick and hairy, the voice husky and cavernous. The hands and feet are enlarged; shaking hands with an acromegalic patient gives the startling impression of losing one's hand in a mass of dough. The superficial veins of the extremities are thick and prominent. The thoracic cage is widened and deepened and thoracic kyphosis is present. Galactorrhea is an occasional finding in both men and women.

Most routine *laboratory data* are within normal limits. The basal metabolic rate is elevated in more than half the patients, but other evidence of hyperthyroidism (increased thyroidal uptake of ^{131}I or level of serum PBI) is usually lacking even when the thyroid is palpably enlarged. Appraisal of adrenocortical function reveals normal plasma cortisol values, normal response to ACTH, occasionally increased excretion of urinary 17-ketosteroids or corticosteroids, and sometimes raised cortisol secretory rate and a degree of adrenal refractoriness to suppression by dexamethasone. Urinary gonadotrophin titer is normal or reduced; semen analysis generally shows oligospermia. Despite the reported increased insulin activity of acromegalic plasma, glycosuria or glucose intolerance is found in about a third of acromegalic subjects and frank diabetes in about one fifth. The diabetes is usually mild and somewhat resistant to insulin, but management of the diabetes presents no unusually difficult problems, and ketoacidosis is rare. Hypercalciuria is a common finding, and hypercalcemia occurs in a few patients; in some this abnormality is apparently due to hypersecretion of growth hormone, because it disappears with successful treatment of the acromegaly. However, in others the hypercalcemia persists and can be shown to be due to associated hyperparathyroidism as part of the syndrome of *multiple endocrine adenomatosis.*

As the disease progresses, muscular weakness (predominantly of proximal muscle groups) supervenes; kyphosis increases, partly because of osteoporosis. Visual impairment may become aggravated to the point of blindness. Partial or total pituitary insufficiency may ensue. The course is extremely variable; it is hard to know with accuracy the natural history, because the onset is usually so insidious and because most patients have received some sort of treatment. Life expectancy is reduced (see Ch. 830). The course may be fulminant, resulting in death within three years (usually because of tumor growth in younger patients), or benign and intermittent, lasting 50 years or longer. Death comes from the tumor (expansion, hemorrhage into its substance, "pituitary apoplexy"), cardiac failure (owing to "acromegalic heart disease"), or the effects of hypertension (found in 20 to 50 per cent of patients) or degenerative vascular disease. The causes of death in years past were diabetes and hypopituitarism; these are now rarely lethal because of the availability of adequate treatment.

Diagnosis. The typical acromegalic is recognized at a glance. *The great need is a means of early diagnosis.* If acromegaly is suspected, a history of increasing size of gloves and shoes and of increasingly poor fit of dentures provides useful clues. Tightness of old rings is suggestive; comparison of the patient's features with old photographs is helpful. Roentgenogram of the skull and tests of the visual fields usually give confirmatory evidence.

The differential diagnosis rarely presents difficulties. The large tongue, hoarse voice, and periorbital edema may suggest myxedema, but the other physical and laboratory abnormalities of hypothyroidism are absent. Patients with pachydermoperiostosis, some of whom look quite acromegalic, do not have involvement of the pituitary, and plasma HGH values are normal. Some patients receiving anticonvulsants for long periods may develop "acromegaloid" coarsening of the features. The articular pains of acromegaly are usually distinguishable from those associated with other forms of arthritis by the typical acromegalic aspect.

There is no generally satisfactory method for the *indi-*

rect assessment of the *secretory activity* of the adenoma. History of recent acral enlargement is the best evidence of active secretion, and some clinicians believe that excessive sweating and seborrhea are good guides. Laboratory data are disappointing. Elevation of serum phosphorus follows administration of human growth hormone, but is an unreliable index of "activity" of the disease in acromegaly. The same may be said of the glucose tolerance test and basal metabolic rate. Some investigators consider the insulin tolerance test useful. Biopsy of costal cartilage may show active endochondral bone formation. Urinary excretion of hydroxyproline is increased. None of these laboratory indices has been conclusively proved to correlate closely with the clinical course of the disease. If plasma growth hormone measurements cannot be made, one must rely on a synthesis of historical, physical, and laboratory findings. Without documentary evidence of recent acral growth, judgment of secretory activity is highly subjective.

The use of *radioimmunoassay of plasma growth hormone* is the method of choice for *direct* assessment of the secretory activity of the acidophilic tumor. It is known that most untreated acromegalics have high concentrations. After hypophysectomy these fall, often to normal, but sometimes they remain elevated, presumably when hypophysectomy is not complete. After pituitary radiation, levels often do not fall. Not enough data are yet available to allow a complete appraisal of growth hormone response to physiologic stimuli (hypoglycemia, glucose administration) as a measure of "activity" in acromegaly. What is needed is careful correlation (over a period of years) of plasma growth hormone levels with objective studies of acral growth. Such studies will reveal the value of plasma growth hormone measurements as indices of secretory activity. At the moment, it appears that sharp falls in basal plasma growth hormone value, or recovery of growth hormone responsiveness to administered glucose, are closely related to clinically arrested disease.

Treatment. Treatment is discussed in detail in Ch. 830. No single method has been shown to be ideal (Fig. 9).

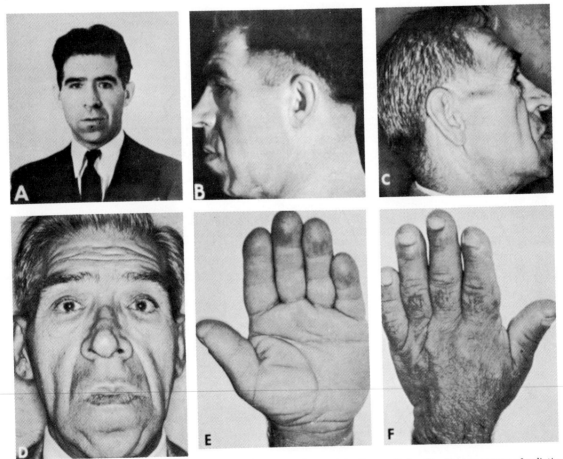

Figure 9. Evolution of acromegaly. *A,* Age 38, within a year after onset of the disease. *B,* Age 55, after two courses of radiation therapy to sella; disease has progressed with moderate coarsening of features: thickening of lips, enlargement of nose and ears. *C, D,* Age 64, 26 years after onset, after a third series of x-ray treatments to sella (total dose of radiation to the pituitary, 10,000 rads); nose and ears have enlarged further, supraorbital ridge and zygoma have become more prominent, and jaw is more prognathous; frontal view shows deepening of skin wrinkles (temporal atrophy is a result of x-irradiation). *E, F,* Age 64, volar and dorsal aspects of hand, showing broadened fingers and characteristically "meaty" appearance owing to gross increase in soft tissue, not bone (compare Fig. 5). The patient died 12 years later at age 76 of cardiac and respiratory failure. By that time diabetes mellitus and hypopituitarism (thyroid and adrenocortical deficiency) had developed and were treated, but the last plasma HGH measurement, six years before death, was still elevated, 27 ng per ml.

Clinicopathological Conference: A case of acromegalic heart disease. Br. Med. J., 1:718, 1973.

Davidoff, L. M.: Studies in acromegaly: III. The anamnesis and symptomatology in one hundred cases. Endocrinology, 10:461, 1926.

Falconer, M. A., and Davidson, S.: Coarse features in epilepsy as a consequence of anticonvulsant therapy: Report of cases in two pairs of identical twins. Lancet, 2:1112, 1973.

Goldfine, D., and Lawrence, A. M.: Hypopituitarism in acromegaly. Arch. Intern. Med., 130:720, 1973.

Gordon, D. A., Hill, F. M., and Ezrin, C.: Acromegaly: A review of 100 cases. Can. Med. Assoc. J., 87:1106, 1962.

Mastaglia, F. L., Barwick, D. D., and Hall, R.: Myopathy in acromegaly. Lancet, 2:907, 1970.

Strauch, G., Vallotton, M. B., Touitou, Y., and Bricaire, H.: The renin-angiotensin-aldosterone system in normotensive and hypertensive patients with acromegaly. N. Engl. J. Med., 287:795, 1972.

GIGANTISM

Gigantism is arbitrarily defined as height exceeding 78 to 80 inches or, in children, exceeding a height three standard deviations above the mean for age. This rare disorder has been conventionally regarded as the childhood counterpart of acromegaly, i.e., as oversecretion of growth hormone by a pituitary adenoma in a growing organism *before closure of the epiphyses.* However, acromegaly occurs in young children. It is reasonable to doubt a pituitary cause when (1) there is no evidence of acromegaly, (2) the sella is not enlarged, or (3) there is a strong familial history of unusually tall stature suggesting constitutional gigantism. A form of "cerebral gigantism" is described in children; associated features are macrocrania, large extremities, large hands and feet, evidence of cerebral dysfunction, and normal values and normal response of plasma growth hormone. An additional cause of tall stature is hypogonadism or late puberty, resulting in prolongation of the period of linear growth because of delayed epiphysial closure. In such patients, the bodily proportions are eunuchoidal, with a lower segment greater than the upper segment and arm span greater than height.

In those giants who are acromegalic (about 50 per cent), management is that of acromegaly. Treatment of the pituitary adenoma must be vigorous. The radioimmunoassay for growth hormone provides more accurate assignment of cause in gigantism and a more objective criterion as a guide to management

Baumann, G., Cain, J. P., and Dingman, J. F.: Gigantism with hypopituitarism: A re-evaluation. Am. J. Med., 53:805, 1972.

Haigler, E. D., Jr., Hershman, J. M., and Meador, C. K.: Pituitary gigantism: A case report and review. Arch. Intern. Med., 132:589, 1973.

Hook, E. B., and Reynolds, J. W.: Cerebral gigantism. Endocrinological and clinical observations of six patients, including a congenital giant, concordant monozygotic twins, and a child who achieved adult gigantic size. J. Pediatr., 70:900, 1967.

Ludwig, G. D., Chaykin, L. B., and Escueta, A. V.: Cerebral gigantism with intermittent fractional hypopituitarism and normal sella turcica. Ann. Intern. Med., 67:123, 1967.

POSTERIOR PITUITARY

Alexander Leaf

833. ANTIDIURETIC HORMONE

Normal Physiology. Antidiuretic hormone is produced in nuclei of the anterior hypothalamus. The major source of this hormone is the supraoptic nuclei, but contributions from the paraventricular and filiform nuclei are thought to be added. The hormone produced in these neural centers is transported by a process of neural secretion down the supraopticohypophysial tract to the neurohypophysis or posterior pituitary where the hormone is stored until released into the blood according to the state of hydration of the subject.

The antidiuretic hormone in man was identified by du Vigneaud as the octapeptide arginine vasopressin. The hormone is released normally in response to osmotic stimuli; a rise in concentration of solute, largely the salts of sodium, in the plasma or extracellular fluid, serves as the stimulus for release of vasopressin from the neurohypophysis. The hormone circulates to the kidney where its major action is on the epithelium lining the collecting ducts. In the presence of vasopressin this epithelium becomes more permeable to water so that water is transported from the tubular lumen to the more concentrated peritubular fluids. This serves to reduce urine volume and increase its concentration, thereby conserving body water. Dilution of plasma or extracellular fluids, as occurs after water ingestion, inhibits release of antidiuretic hormone. The dilute luminal fluid entering the distal convoluted tubule is excreted with little modification in concentration, with the result that a copious flow of dilute urine characterizes the absence of antidiuretic hormone. This rids the body of any excess of water.

The thirst center is functionally and anatomically closely related to the antidiuretic mechanism. Andersson has shown that osmotic or electrical stimulation of the anterior portion of the supraoptic nuclei creates a sensation of thirst; dilution of plasma inhibits thirst. The integrated activity of thirst and antidiuretic mechanism serves to regulate the concentration of body fluids as follows:

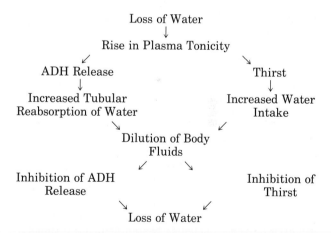

This double negative feedback system works with remarkable effectiveness to preserve the concentration of sodium in the serum between some 136 and 143 mEq per liter. Since intracellular fluids are in osmotic equilibrium with the extracellular fluids, this mechanism regulates the tonicity of the body fluid compartments.

In addition to the usual osmotic stimuli regulating release of vasopressin, other factors may affect this process. Pain and emotional states have been associated with antidiuresis, as have a number of pharmacologic agents which act to release the hormone. These include cinchoninic acid, acetylcholine, nicotine, morphine, barbiturates, ferritin, and bradykinin. Alcohol may inhibit release of antidiuretic hormone, but the effect is weak and is often obscured. Physiologically, reduction in the effective plasma volume appears to be a stimulus for secretion of antidiuretic hormone; at least this has been documented after acute large blood loss.

It is now appreciated that in a considerable number of clinical conditions there is an apparent inappropriate secretion of substances possessing antidiuretic activity. The adjective "inappropriate" is used to indicate that neither osmotic nor circulatory (volume) stimuli are responsible for the excessive persistent antidiuretic activity. Furthermore, the antidiuretic substances may not arise in all instances from the neurohypophysis but may be secretory products of the tumors or inflammatory tissue which give rise to the syndrome of inappropriate antidiuretic hormone secretion (see Ch. 805).

Andersson, B.: Polydipsia, antidiuresis and milk ejection caused by hypothalamic stimulation. *In* Heller, H. (ed.): The Neurohypophysis. London, Butterworth Scientific Publications, 1957.

Bartter, F. C., and Schwartz, W. B.: The syndrome of inappropriate secretion of antidiuretic hormone. Am. J. Med., 42:790, 1967.

du Vigneaud, V.: Hormones of the posterior pituitary gland: oxytocin and vasopressin. *In* The Harvey Lectures 1954–1955. New York, Academic Press, 1956.

Leaf, A.: The clinical and physiologic significance of the serum sodium concentration. N. Engl. J. Med., 267:24, 77, 1962.

Leaf, A., Bartter, F. C., Santos, R. F., and Wrong, O.: Evidence in man that urinary electrolyte loss induced by pitressin is a function of water retention. J. Clin. Invest., 32:868, 1953.

Schwartz, W. B., Bennett, W., Curelop, S., and Bartter, F. C.: A syndrome of renal sodium loss and hyponatremia, probably resulting from inappropriate secretion of antidiuretic hormone. Am. J. Med., 23:529, 1957.

Verney, E. B.: The absorption and excretion of water: The antidiuretic hormone. Lancet, 2:739, 781, 1946.

834. DIABETES INSIPIDUS

Etiology. Diabetes insipidus is an uncommon disturbance resulting from any condition which damages the neurohypophysial system. Idiopathic cases constitute the major group, comprising approximately 45 per cent. The idiopathic condition may become manifest at any age and affect either sex. It is unusual in infancy, but may commence in early childhood. Familial diabetes insipidus is very uncommon, but may occur in infancy or childhood and affect either sex. The condition has been noted in seven generations of one family. Familial diabetes insipidus is to be distinguished from nephrogenic diabetes insipidus, which is a renal tubular defect, inherited largely by males, in whom the affected tubules are unresponsive to antidiuretic hormone.

Head trauma (accidental or neurosurgical) and neoplasms (primary or metastatic) are the major causes of acquired diabetes insipidus. Of the metastatic tumors, breast cancer seems to have a special predilection for the hypothalamic area. Other rarer etiologic factors include sarcoidosis, birth injuries, eosinophilic granuloma, and a variety of local infections. Even with lesions directly in the hypothalamus, diabetes insipidus is rare, because a small fraction of normal tissue suffices to protect against manifest dysfunction. Since the posterior and anterior pituitary have separate blood supplies, infarction of the latter need not be associated with failure of the former; a space-occupying lesion is suspect when insufficiency of both occurs.

Clinical Manifestations. The polyuria and polydipsia can be so dramatic that adult patients may remember an exact date or even hour when symptoms started. The fluid exchanges may reach the distressing proportions of 5 to 10 liters or more per 24 hours. The specific gravity of the urine is usually 1.001 to 1.005; corresponding concentrations will be about 100 to 200 mOsm per liter. With restriction of fluid intake the specific gravity may reach 1.010, or even slightly higher with severe water lack, and urine concentration may increase to 300 mOsm per liter. Urine slightly hypertonic to serum has been produced experimentally in the complete absence of antidiuretic hormone by greatly reducing the glomerular filtration rate. The elaboration of a hypertonic urine by a patient with diabetes insipidus during severe dehydration or with acute reduction of the glomerular filtration rate from any cause need not therefore indicate the presence of residual neurohypophysial function.

Other than the annoyance of polyuria and polydypsia, there may be no evidence of ill health or of other physiologic disturbance associated with the condition, unless the patient suffers from the underlying local or systemic disease which has destroyed the neurohypophysial system. The assumption that patients with diabetes insipidus suffer from severe dehydration is not supported by measurements of serum sodium or total solute concentrations. A slight elevation of sodium and total solute concentrations of serum has been demonstrated statistically, but the overlap in individual cases is such as to make these determinations of little assistance diagnostically: 297 ± 12 mOsm per liter (S.D.) for diabetes insipidus and 285 ± 4 mOsm per liter (S.D.) for normal persons. As long as the patient's thirst center remains intact, the total solute concentration of the body fluids will be preserved close to normal values, but at the expense of polydipsia and the large fluid exchange characteristic of the condition. After a period of water restriction, these differences may be accentuated and have greater diagnostic value.

With unconsciousness resulting from trauma or anesthesia, the inability of the patient to demand water may be fatal. This situation may occur at the onset of diabetes insipidus secondary to head injury or intracranial surgery, and is one of the causes of hypernatremia after trauma to the head. A careful record of urine volumes and urine and serum concentrations in patients with acute head trauma and coma will prevent the occurrence of severe dehydration.

Differential Diagnosis. A patient with persistent polyuria and urine of low concentration may have one or more of three basic disturbances: (1) inability of the kidney to elaborate a concentrated urine despite adequate vasopressin, (2) deficient vasopressin, or (3) persistent excessive water intake. Any condition which disturbs the renal concentrating mechanism, rendering it unresponsive to vasopressin, may produce polyuria. Hypercalcemia, potassium depletion, or renal failure (both chronic and acute) may impair maximal concentrating ability, but none of these conditions cause the urine to be persistently hypotonic, and in only a few patients does the resulting polyuria suggest diabetes insipidus. These conditions are readily excluded in establishing the diagnosis of diabetes insipidus. The rare nephrogenic diabetes insipidus results from a failure of the renal tubule to respond to vasopressin. Patients with uncontrolled diabetes mellitus may exhibit extreme polyuria and polydipsia, but the specific gravity of the urine is high, although its osmolality may not be over 300 mOsm per liter; the large contribution which glucose makes to the specific gravity accounts for this seeming discrepancy.

Although it is evident that polyuria in diabetes insipidus is primary to polydipsia, compulsive water drinking may give rise to a condition which closely mimics diabetes insipidus. Chronic ingestion of large volumes of water impairs the renal concentrating mechanism, making it sometimes quite difficult to distinguish this psychogenic disturbance from true diabetes insipidus.

Several special procedures have been devised to assist in establishing the diagnosis of diabetes insipidus in patients with polyuria and polydipsia. They all test ability to respond to osmotic stimuli by elaboration of a concentrated urine, whether failure to do so is the consequence of a lack of endogenous vasopressin or of an inability of the renal tubules to respond to the hormone.

Water restriction with observation of urine volume and concentration constitutes the simplest test. Weight should be followed to avoid the hazards of incurring loss of more than 3 to 5 per cent of body weight. Small children and infants are especially liable to serious circulatory disturbances if dehydration is allowed beyond this limit. A normal subject may be expected to reduce urine flow to less than 0.5 ml per minute and increase urine concentration to greater than 800 mOsm per liter (corresponding to a specific gravity of 1.020 or above). In patients with diabetes insipidus, urine volumes well above this limit persist, and urine concentration remains below 200 mOsm per liter (specific gravities of 1.001 to 1.005) until advanced states of dehydration are present. Unfortunately, the differences are often not so clear, and patients with neurohypophysial insufficiency may concentrate their urine to 300 to 400 mOsm per liter (specific gravities of 1.008 to 1.014) with marked dehydration.

Another means of increasing plasma osmolarity to test the release of antidiuretic hormone is by the infusion of hypertonic solutions. After an initial hydrated state is established, 2.5 per cent sodium chloride is infused intravenously at a rate of 0.25 ml per minute per kilogram of body weight for 45 minutes. Urine flow is measured at 15-minute intervals. If neurohypophysial and renal functions are normal, urine flow will drop promptly to 25 per cent or less of control.

If either the water deprivation test or the infusion of hypertonic saline fails to reduce urine flow or to increase urine concentration, as expected, the ability of the patients' kidneys to respond to exogenous vasopressin must be demonstrated, in order to separate nephrogenic causes from hormone deficiency. For this purpose 5mU per minute of aqueous vasopressin (vasopressin injection, USP) may be administered intravenously for at least one hour by a slow drip, or 5 units of the long-acting vasopressin tannate in oil may be administered intramuscularly. An injection of the latter material in the evening, with urine samples collected on arising the following morning and hourly for three successive hours thereafter, should induce maximal concentration.

These simple measures will readily distinguish diabetes insipidus from nephrogenic causes of diminished response to vasopressin. To distinguish true diabetes insipidus from compulsive water drinking may be more difficult, because continued polydipsia lowers the maximal urinary concentrations achievable after dehydration, infusions of hypertonic saline, or exogenous vasopressin. Barlow and de Wardener have pointed out that a normal subject with intact neurohypophysis will achieve a higher urinary concentration after water deprivation than after administration of vasopressin without water restriction. The patient with diabetes insipidus has just the opposite response, i.e., higher urine concentration after vasopressin than after water restriction. Patients with psychogenic polydipsia respond in this regard normally; whatever the absolute value of urine concentration they achieve, concentrations during dehydration will exceed those attained after injections of vasopressin. In addition to the laboratory studies it should be remembered that compulsive water drinking to a degree which is confused with diabetes insipidus constitutes a severe psychogenic disorder. Clinical evaluation is usually rewarding in revealing other neurotic symptoms supporting the suspicion of a serious personality or behavioral disturbance.

Treatment. If symptoms are mild, no therapy may be warranted, although a thorough search for underlying causative factors should be conducted. When symptoms interfere with sleep or interrupt work, treatment is indicated. Replacement therapy intramuscularly with long-acting vasopressin in oil (1.0 ml ampule contains 5 units per milliliter; 0.5 to 1.0 ml injected every 24 to 72 hours, as necessary to control polyuria) is generally reserved for the more severe cases, whereas an aqueous nasal spray, self-administered as necessary every two to six hours, may suffice to alleviate symptoms. The oral hypoglycemic agent chlorpropamide has been found to enhance the antidiuretic activity of residual endogenous antidiuretic hormone; 100 to 500 mg once daily will usually relieve polyuria and polydipsia in patients with incomplete neurohypophysial failure. Thiazide diuretics—250 mg of chlorothiazide two or three times daily—presumably by sustaining a condition of persistent mild salt depletion, will blunt a water diuresis, and in patients with diabetes insipidus may reduce urine flow by some 50 per cent. In patients with nephrogenic diabetes insipidus this form of antidiuretic agent is also effective.

Barlow, E. D., and de Wardener, H. E.: Compulsive water drinking. Quart. J. Med., 28:235, 1959.

Coggins, C. H., and Leaf, A.: Diabetes insipidus. Am. J. Med., 42:807, 1967.

Dashe, A. M., Cramm, R. E., Crist, C. A., Habener, J. F., and Solomon, D. H.: A water deprivation test for the differential diagnosis of polyuria. J.A.M.A., 185:71, 1963.

Leaf, A.: Diabetes insipidus. In Astwood, E. B. (ed.): Clinical Endocrinology, I. New York, Grune & Stratton, 1960.

Williams, R. H., and Henry, C.: Nephrogenic diabetes insipidus: Transmitted by females and appearing during infancy in males. Ann. Intern. Med., 27:84, 1947.

835.   THE PINEAL

Seymour Reichlin

The pineal gland was discovered more than 20 centuries ago, and its function has long been a matter of scientific and philosophic speculation. Arising embryologically from ependyma lining the roof of the third ventricle, the pineal consists of parenchymal cells supported by a meshwork of neuroglia. In the adult, the gland weighs between 100 and 180 mg and is a cone-shaped organ lying in the groove formed by the superior colliculi. Although connected to the epithalamus by a peduncle, the pineal does not receive a direct nerve supply from this source. Instead, it is innervated by postganglionic nerve fibers which arise in the cervical sympathetic ganglia and travel along the great vein of Galen. A number of humorally active substances have been isolated from the pineal. In addition to norepinephrine, serotonin, histamine, and melatonin are found. Melatonin is formed by a series of enzymatic steps from tryptophan (Fig. 1). One of the intermediates is serotonin, which in turn is converted to N-acetylserotonin by the enzyme N-acetyl transferase; the conversion of N-acetylserotonin to melatonin is accomplished by the enzyme hydroxy-o-methyl transferase (HIOMT). Measurement of the activities of these enzymes has been used to study the factors controlling melatonin synthesis and, by inference, melatonin secretion. Both enzyme activities are influenced by alterations in the light-dark cycle (in rats and other laboratory forms), a change mediated by a special retinal-hypothalamic neural pathway (the inferior accessory optic tract) which does not involve the visual cortex. It was initially believed that the HIOMT enzyme was the rate-limiting step for melatonin synthesis. More recent work indicates that the acetyltransferase system is more important, but both enzymes may be involved in final control of pineal secretion. Enzymic activity of the pineal gland and its secretory function are regulated by noradrenergic nerve endings on pinealocytes (Fig. 2). Beta norepinephrine receptors activate adenyl cyclase with the formation of cyclic AMP through the classic second messenger mechanism. The activated ATP-protein kinase is believed to promote the formation of the melatonin-synthesizing enzymes. Norepinephrine also stimulates pineal uptake of the precursor tryptophan (Fig. 2). Although melatonin is a potent hormone in lower animals (it causes contraction of granules dispersed in melanocytes) and inhibits gonadotrophic and possibly thyrotrophic function through actions at the hypothalamic level, it has no known action in man. Lacking a method for measurement of melatonin in peripheral blood, there is no clear evidence for changes in pineal secretion of melatonin in the human

subject under any of the conditions in which the activity of the pineal is altered in the laboratory animal. Recent development of a radioimmunoassay for melatonin may change this situation. Recently, three of the hypothalamic releasing factors have also been demonstrated. These are TRH, LRH, and somatostatin. The functional significance of these findings is unknown.

The pineal gland has no known function in man but becomes of clinical significance because of the occurrence of calcification and of tumor formation. Calcific nodules termed *acervuli* form in a matrix of ground substance secreted by pinealocytes. This process begins in early childhood and becomes increasingly evident by roentgenography beginning in the second decade of life. Calcification has no known effect on pineal function, as inferred from the fact that the characteristic enzymes of the pineal (HIOMT, monoamine transferase, and histamine N-methyl transferase) maintain normal concentrations throughout life.

Pineal tumors are rare, and their classification and nature are still disputed by pathologists, some of whom believe that the pineal cell in situ or situated in ectopic regions of the brain (chiefly the infundibular area) can give rise to neoplasms. The most common pineal cell tumor is the parenchymal tumor, classified as a pineoblastoma or pineocytoma according to the degree of differentiation. Convincing evidence that at least certain of these tumors are truly of pineal origin comes from the finding by Wurtman and collaborators that tissue from a parenchymal and from an ectopic pinealoma contained the marker enzyme HIOMT. Pineal cell tumors may also resemble seminomas of the testis (seminomatous pinealomas); the relationship of these tumors to teratomas is not well understood. The pineal also gives rise to teratomas of dermoid type and to tumors of the supporting structures such as gliomas, astrocytomas, and endothelial tumors.

Pinealomas occur mainly in young males. The symptoms and signs of the tumor reflect both local effects on the brain and, in a minority of cases, more remote changes in sexual maturation. Enlargement of a mass in the pineal region compresses the aqueduct of Sylvius and distorts the quadrigeminal plate. Internal hydrocephalus gives rise to characteristic manifestations of

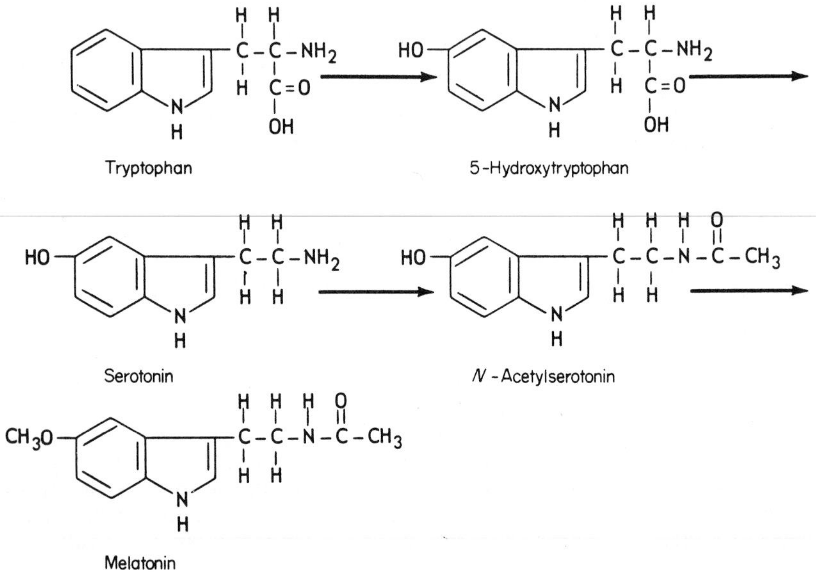

Figure 1. Biosynthesis of melatonin from tryptophan in the pineal gland. Step 1 is catalyzed by tryptophan hydroxylase; Step 2 by L-aromatic amino acid decarboxylase; Step 3 by N-acetylating enzyme; and Step 4 by HIOMT. (From Wurtman, R. J., Axelrod, J., and Kelly, D.: The Pineal. New York, Academic Press, 1968, p. 60.)

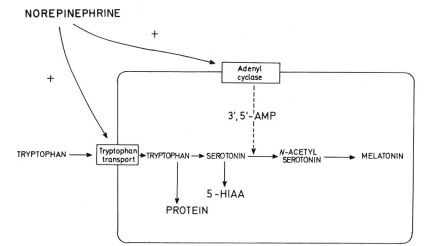

Figure 2. The effect of norepinephrine on tryptophan metabolism in the pineal. 5-HIAA = 5-hydroxyindole acetic acid. (From Shein, H. M.: *In* Wolstenholme, G., and Knight, J. (eds.): The Pineal Gland. London, Churchill Livingstone, 1971.)

increased intracranial pressure such as headache, vomiting, papilledema, and disturbance of sensorium. Pressure on the superior colliculi causes conjugate paralysis of upward gaze (Parinaud's syndrome). Disturbances of gait, resulting from either hydrocephalus or possibly cerebellar damage, are also observed.

Pineal tumors arising in male children may, in about one third of cases, cause precocious puberty; over-all, however, pineal tumors are exceedingly rare and are therefore a relatively rare cause of sexual precocity. The mechanism of effect of the tumor on gonadotrophic function is controversial. It has been suggested that the pineal secretes a hormone which tonically inhibits onset of sexual maturation; destruction of the pineal permits the earlier development of puberty. In support of this hypothesis is the finding in laboratory animals that melatonin injections delay puberty, that tumors destroying the pineal are three times as likely to cause precocious puberty as are parenchymal tumors, and that some cases of precocious puberty occur in the absence of local brain damage.

On the other hand, there is impressive evidence that pineal tumors, like certain other types of hypothalamic tumors, cause precocious puberty by direct physical damage to the gonadotrophin-regulating areas of the brain. For example, Bing and co-workers found that whenever precocious puberty was caused by a pineal tumor, neuroanatomic evidence indicated extension beyond the pineal region with internal hydrocephalus or invasion of the third ventricle or hypothalamus. Clinical evidence of hypothalamic involvement, e.g., diabetes insipidus, polyphagia, somnolence, obesity, or behavioral disturbance, was observed in 71 per cent of cases. These clinicopathologic correlations strongly support the view that neoplasms of the pineal gland produce sexual precocity indirectly through involvement of the hypothalamus. In a few cases, precocity or infantilism (also reported to occur) may prove to be due to altered pineal hormone secretion, but convincing evidence of this occurrence has not yet been adduced.

A special type of pinealoma is sufficiently distinctive to be noted here. "Ectopic" pinealomas arising from pineal rests in midline areas most commonly occur in the region of the infundibulum and produce diabetes insipidus, compression of the optic chiasm, and hypopitui-

tarism. Precocious puberty may also occur in such patients.

Treatment of pineal tumors is generally unsatisfactory. Because of their critical location in the epithalamic region above the midbrain, or in the infundibulum, surgical removal is hazardous and usually impossible. Most of them are radiosensitive, and respond at least partially to deep x-ray therapy. A few apparent radiotherapeutic cures have been reported, but the long-range prognosis is poor.

Wolstenholme, G. E. W., and Knight, J. (eds.): The Pineal Gland. Ciba Foundation Symposium. Edinburgh and London, Churchill Livingstone, 1971.

Wurtman, R. J., Axelrod, J., and Kelly, D. E.: The Pineal. New York, Academic Press, 1968.

THE THYROID

Leslie J. DeGroot

836. INTRODUCTION

Thyroid hormone serves as a metabolic thermostat, regulating the level of biochemical activity of most tissues. In general, malfunction of the thyroid gland leads to two sets of symptoms: those related to the local effects of a mass in the neck, and the generalized effects of an excess or deficiency of hormone. Illnesses involving this gland are relatively common medical disorders and, excluding diabetes, account for nearly four fifths of endocrine disease.

DEVELOPMENT AND ANATOMY

The embryonic thyroid gland develops from segments of the fourth pharyngeal pouches, joined by a midline anlage from the base of the tongue. During the first three months of growth, the thyroid gland is unable to synthesize and release thyroid hormone. Accordingly, if hormone is needed in this period, the fetus must depend upon the maternal supply of thyroid hormone. By the end of the first trimester, the gland has assumed its adult shape and position, concentrates iodide, synthesizes thyroglobulin, and functions under the control of the fetal pituitary. During the remainder of intrauterine life, the gland produces the hormone required for the developing fetus. If necessary because of malfunction of the fetal gland, the fetus derives some hormone from the maternal circulation, but it is not established whether an adequate supply reaches the fetus when maternal hormone levels are in the normal range for pregnancy. During the first 18 or 20 years after birth, the gland doubles in size three to four times to attain a weight of 15 to 20 grams. In the absence of disease or changes in iodine supply, the size and function of the gland remain relatively constant throughout life until advanced age, when hormone production gradually diminishes.

The normal thyroid gland is butterfly shaped, firm, smooth, and red-brown. It consists of two elongated lobes on either side of the trachea connected by a thin isthmus of tissue at or below the level of the cricoid cartilage. (Often, a remnant of the lingual anlage, the pyramidal lobe, extends superiorly from one side of the isthmus. Under normal circumstances, this is too small to be detected by external palpation.) The fine structure consists of numerous follicles, each approximately 300 μ in diameter and made up of clusters of cells surrounding a colloid-filled luminal space. The colloid is a mixture of proteins, of which thyroglobulin comprises about 80 per cent.

The thyroid cells are 15 μ high; the borders facing the lumen have microvilli, thought to be involved in secretory and resorptive activities. In hyperplastic glands the cells are taller, and colloid space is reduced. Certain cells do not contact the luminal surface and have slightly different staining properties; these perifollicular or "C-cells" secrete the hormone calcitonin and are involved in regulation of calcium metabolism. The parathyroid glands occur as two pairs, one posterior to the upper poles of the thyroid and the other below or embedded in the substance of the lower poles. The recurrent laryngeal nerves pass immediately beneath the lower poles of the thyroid, or are sometimes embedded in the substance of the thyroid gland. Occasionally bits of normal-appearing thyroid tissue are present adjacent to the gland.

PHYSIOLOGY OF THE THYROID

It is best to view the thyroid gland as part of a system designed to provide a constant supply of hormone to somatic cells. Thyroid hormone is transported from blood to the peripheral tissues, where it produces its characteristic metabolic stimulation, and is in turn degraded. The thyroid gland replenishes this supply by secreting about 75 μg of tetraiodothyronine (thyroxine, T_4) and 25 μg of triiodothyronine (T_3) daily. If the hormone supply to tissue is depleted, the change is sensed by the pituitary (and possibly the hypothalamus), which increases the secretion of thyroid-stimulating hormone (TSH). TSH increases secretion of hormone by the thyroid gland in a feedback control system until the circulating level of hormone returns to the original level and suppresses TSH to its control level.

Iodide Metabolism (Fig. 1). Iodine bears a unique relation to thyroid physiology, because the element is a major and characteristic constituent of the hormones.

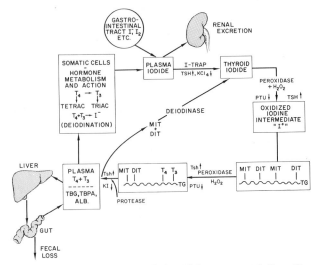

Figure 1. The iodide cycle and thyroid hormone metabolism. The pathway includes iodide absorption, thyroid trapping, oxidation by peroxidase, iodination of tyrosine and intramolecular coupling, proteolysis, plasma hormone transport, and finally hormone action and metabolism with recirculation of iodide.

The average daily American diet contains 150 to 600 μg of iodide, depending in part on the consumption of certain varieties of bread, which may contain much iodate, and milk, which may contain considerable iodide. Another major source is iodized salt. Most forms of ingested iodine are reduced to iodide in the gastrointestinal tract before absorption. Absorption is usually complete in one hour. Iodide is cleared from plasma by the salivary glands and gastric parietal cells into their secretions, but normally this iodide is recycled to plasma. Iodide is cleared unidirectionally by the kidney from plasma at a rate of about 30 ml per minute. The normal thyroid clears plasma iodide at a rate of 4 to 12 ml per minute. The TSH feedback control system regulates the clearance rate to provide the gland with enough iodide for hormone production, and this control point is probably the prime determinant of thyroid hormone production. If iodide intake is low and thyroid uptake of iodide is diminished, thyroxine production is reduced and the level of hormone in plasma falls. TSH secretion is then increased and augments iodide clearance by the thyroid gland. Under the influence of TSH or in thyroid hyperactivity of thyrotoxicosis, clearance may be elevated 5 to 20 times the normal range. With augmented levels of iodide ion in the body, e.g., during therapy with Lugol's solution, thyroid clearance falls to a fraction of a milliliter per minute. The thyroid cells actively transport iodide and maintain a concentration gradient of 20 to 1 over the level in plasma. The iodide concentration process is blocked competitively by perchlorate or thiocyanate ions. These drugs can thus interfere with formation of thyroid hormone. They are also used to establish the presence of elevated amounts of free iodide in the gland (see below).

Hormonogenesis. As rapidly as iodide is transported into the normal thyroid cell it is oxidized by a peroxidase and bound to tyrosine residues present in thyroglobulin. This iodination process takes place near the apical cell border, either in secretory vesicles before liberation of thyroglobulin to colloid or inside the colloid space. The iodine acceptor protein, thyroglobulin, is a huge glycoprotein of 670,000 molecular weight. Each thyroglobulin molecule contains about 120 tyrosine residues and, after iodination, 26 atoms of iodine. The iodination of the tyrosyl residues in thyroglobulin leads to the production of monoiodotyrosine (MIT) and diiodotyrosine (DIT) in the peptide chain. Then two iodotyrosyl groups couple to form an iodothyronine (T_3 or T_4), still within the peptide chain of thyroglobulin. In the iodine-replete gland, each thyroglobulin molecule contains about one iodothyronine molecule (T_3 or T_4). The ratio of T_4 to T_3 molecules is about 4 to 1.

Hormone Secretion. As thyroglobulin is iodinated and coupling of iodotyrosines occurs, some molecules are hydrolyzed to release hormone and others are stored in the colloid for days or weeks. Resorption from colloid occurs by pinocytosis; microvilli or pseudopods on the surface of the thyroid cell surround a small fragment of colloid, and a droplet is thus formed within the cell. The colloid droplet then fuses with a lysosome, producing a phagosome within which thyroid protease hydrolyzes thyroglobulin to its component amino acids. MIT and DIT are released and deiodinated by a dehalogenase present in the microsomal fraction of the cell; the liberated iodide is reincorporated into new MIT and DIT in thyroglobulin. The thyroxine and triiodothyronine released from thyroglobulin are secreted into blood, along with some unhydrolyzed thyroglobulin, small amounts of iodotyrosines, and small amounts of iodide. The thyroid also iodinates other proteins, including a protein very similar to serum albumin, and secretes this iodinated protein into the circulation. Other particulate and soluble iodoproteins are formed in the gland, but their metabolic role is unknown. Some T_4 may be monodeiodinated to form T_3 within the thyroid cell.

Hormone Transport. The T_4 and T_3 secreted by the gland are transported in plasma largely bound by non-covalent bonds to plasma proteins. Of these, the main and most specific hormone-binding protein is thyroxine-binding inter-alpha-globulin, or TBG. Approximately 70 per cent of T_4 in the blood is carried by this protein. Perhaps 15 per cent of thyroxine is bound to thyroxine-binding prealbumin (TBPA), and the remainder is bound to albumin. Triiodothyronine is less tightly bound to TBG, and insignificant amounts bind to TBPA. T_4 binds firmly to the proteins; only 0.04 per cent of the hormone exists free in solution at any one time. The plasma protein–hormone interaction is reversible. The binding proteins control distribution of hormone between serum and cells, serve as a reservoir constantly replenishing free hormone, and also prevent the iodinated thyronines from being excreted in urine. Free hormone gains access to cells and appears to be the metabolically important fraction. The level of TBG is raised by estrogen treatment and lowered by testosterone. TBG is rarely absent or present in excess on a congenital basis, and its formation is depressed in serious malnutrition or liver disease. In these conditions there may be wide variations in the total thyroid hormone content of plasma, but since the absolute level of free hormone remains constant, the patients remain metabolically normal (Fig. 2).

Free hormone penetrates cells and controls the feedback mechanism in the hypothalamus and pituitary. Approximately one third of the extrathyroidal hormone is loosely bound in the liver. The hormone slowly penetrates most other tissues, reaching an equilibrium within tissue (e.g., muscle) in two or three days.

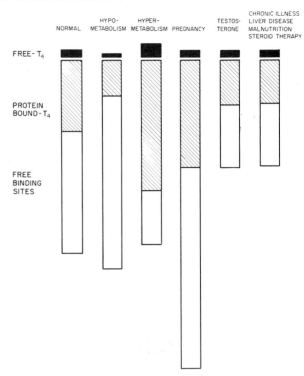

Figure 2. Variations in plasma hormone level. Plasma T_4 (and T_3) is largely bound to protein, whose capacity for holding the hormone is partially saturated. The small fraction of free hormone regulates metabolism. Variations in total hormone primarily reflect the protein bound fraction, and must be combined with analysis of the fraction that is free in order to assess properly that hormone which is active on body tissues.

T_4 leaves the blood with a disappearance half-time of about six days, and T_3 with a half-life of approximately one day. The usual ratio of T_4 to T_3 secreted by the thyroid is 4 to 1. Because of the difference in T_4 and T_3 binding to plasma proteins and metabolism, the ratio of T_4 to T_3 in plasma is about 40 to 1. About 30 per cent of T_4 is converted to T_3 by monodeiodination in peripheral tissues. A significant fraction of this T_3 returns to plasma. T_4 may be considered to be a plasma hormone, or pro-hormone, and T_3 the main tissue hormone. T_3 is less firmly bound to plasma proteins, and enters the cells much more rapidly. T_3 is somewhat selectively taken up and bound by receptor molecules in the cell nuclei. Because of extensive conversion of T_4 to T_3, and the threefold greater metabolic potency of T_3 in comparison to T_4, a large proportion of the metabolic stimulation caused by the hormones may be due to T_3.

Metabolic Action. The exact metabolic action of the hormone is unclear. In animals made hypothyroid by ablation of the gland, administration of thyroid hormone is followed by stimulation of liver nucleic acid synthesis in about 12 hours, increased protein synthesis in 24 hours, and increased mitochondrial oxidative phosphorylation, reaching a peak within two to seven days. Coincident with this increased synthetic and oxidative activity in the cell, the activity of many enzymes, including alpha-ketoglutarate dehydrogenase and isocitrate dehydrogenase, is stimulated.

Usually several hours elapse before any action of the

hormone is observed after administration to animals or man. After a single dose, peak action is seen within two to five days, and gradually decays over a period of two to three weeks. T_3 has a slightly more rapid onset of action than T_4, and its action is more rapidly dissipated. It is of interest that some tissues (brain, spleen, and testes) do not appear to respond to thyroxine.

Treatment of animals with large doses of thyroid hormone or addition of thyroid hormone in vitro induces uncoupling of mitochondrial oxidative phosphorylation. For years one theory of the primary action of thyroid hormone action has centered around this phenomenon. There are two objections to this theory. (1) The change from the sluggish metabolic activity of the hypothyroid state to the normal or mildly hyperactive state induced by administration of physiologic doses of thyroid hormone to animals is accompanied by an increased rate of oxidative phosphorylation *without* loss of efficiency. (2) Studies of mitochondria taken by biopsy from patients with severe hyperthyroidism have shown increased metabolic activity but normally coupled oxidative phosphorylation.

Many other actions of thyroid hormone have been observed, including stimulation of protein synthesis in isolated mitochondria and microsomes, inhibition of pyridine nucleotide-linked dehydrogenases, and swelling of mitochondria.

Recent studies indicate that T_3 and, to a lesser extent, T_4 are accumulated rapidly in the nuclei of responsive tissues and are found tightly but noncovalently linked to a protein associated with chromatin. Although no specific effects of this T_3-protein complex are known, it is postulated that the complex may modulate nuclear RNA synthesis, leading to subsequent increases in protein synthesis and enzyme actions.

Thyroid hormone seems to differ in its mechanism of action from the peptide hormones which act on the adenyl cyclase system at the cell membrane, or the steroid hormones which cause an almost immediate stimulation of nuclear RNA synthesis.

Thyroid Hormone Metabolism. A major portion of T_4 is metabolized by monodeiodination in peripheral tissues to form T_3. In fact T_4 is considered by some as only a pro-hormone, but evidence indicates that T_4 can independently affect tissue metabolism. In any event, T_4 to T_3 conversion must be considered a very important aspect of normal hormone metabolism. In a few instances (in the fetus, in severe illness), low serum and tissue T_3 levels occur in the absence of clinical hypothyroidism. The significance of these findings is not clear.

T_4 and T_3 are metabolized to form butanol-insoluble iodoprotein, some of which may be covalently bound hormone. This material is formed in the microsomal fraction of cells, and some in plasma. Most likely it is a degradative product of thyroid hormone. The alanine side chain of the molecule is metabolized to the acetic acid and pyruvic acid derivatives, analogues which are significantly less active than the parent compound. The hormone is also metabolized extensively by deiodination without rupture of the ether linkage. In some tissues the ether linkage is broken with formation of a hydroquinone and protein-bound DIT. As a final result of metabolism, the hormone is deiodinated and the iodide is returned to plasma to follow the same fate as newly absorbed dietary iodine.

Approximately 10 to 20 per cent of hormone is lost in the feces after secretion by the liver as glucuronide and in other conjugates. A small amount of hormone derived from free T_4 and T_3 in plasma is cleared by the kidneys to urine.

Feedback Control. Each day the thyroid releases approximately 60 to 100 μg of hormonal iodide, of which three fourths is thyroxine and one fourth triiodothyronine. If production falls because of inefficiency in the gland or diminished iodide supply, the level of free hormone in blood decreases, and this alteration is detected by the pituicytes which synthesize increased TSH. The signal recognized by the pituicyte requires RNA and protein synthesis. It is presumed that T_3 and T_4 exert the same sort of metabolic activity on the tissues involved in feedback control as they do in other cells and that this metabolic process constitutes the feedback signal.

In turn, the feedback control of T_4 on the pituitary is modulated by the hypothalamus. Neural centers in the hypothalamus synthesize and secrete the tripeptide pyro-glutamyl-histidyl-proline amide known as thyrotrophin-releasing hormone (TRH). This hormone travels down the hypophysial-portal vessels and stimulates TSH release. There is a delicate balance between the TRH stimulation and T_3-T_4 feedback inhibition of the pituicyte; excess of either can overcome the effect of the other.

TRH is needed for normal tonic control of TSH secretion, as evidenced by the hypothyroidism occurring when the hypothalamus is damaged and TRH is no longer formed. However, the physiologic control of TRH is unclear. Secretion may be altered in response to neural stimuli or cold, but there is no evidence that an excess or deficiency of thyroid hormone alters secretion of TRH. TRH is also a potent stimulant of pituitary prolactin release, but its exact role in the physiologic control of prolactin synthesis and secretion is unknown.

TSH Action on the Thyroid. TSH released by the pituitary binds to a receptor on the thyroid cell membrane and initiates a sequence of reactions, including stimulation of adenyl cyclase and formation of increased intracellular cyclic adenosine monophosphate (cAMP). It is believed that this cAMP "second messenger" somehow mediates all the metabolic stimulatory actions of TSH, including increased uptake and binding of iodide, increased thyroglobulin synthesis, increased colloid resorption, proteolysis, and hormone release.

Other Controls of Thyroid Function. As described above, pituitary TSH is the main regulator of thyroid function. The adrenal gland exerts some control; excess cortisol depresses pituitary production of TSH, possibly by blunting the pituitary sensitivity to TRH. Cortisol also directly depresses the level of TBG in plasma, and augments urinary excretion of iodide. Pregnancy, associated with its increased estrogen production, augments the level of circulating TBG, and increases the concentration of circulating T_4 and T_3. However, the turnover rate of the hormone in blood is proportionately decelerated, so that net hormone utilization remains unchanged. Androgens have a converse effect. Severe illness and stress appear to accelerate thyroid hormone disappearance from plasma. Thyroid hormone utilization is also accelerated in animals by exposure to cold and in man by conditioning to strenuous exercise.

In a very real sense, the average daily intake of iodide controls thyroid function. The feedback control system is designed to maintain a constant level of serum T_4 and T_3. To achieve this the gland must accumulate a constant amount of iodide each day. Thus variations in iodide intake are countered by reciprocal changes in thyroid activity (uptake and binding of iodide, for example) which achieve homeostasis.

THYROID FUNCTION TESTS

In examining a patient with thyroid disease, one seeks to determine the level of tissue metabolic activity and the nature of the thyroid disease. The most direct measure of metabolic activity is the basal metabolic rate (BMR), but the wide range of normal values and the changes in the BMR caused by nonthyroidal factors make the determination of limited diagnostic value. There is no other good approach to assaying the peripheral action of thyroid hormone, although numerous measurements can be made. The serum cholesterol is elevated in hypothyroidism and depressed in hyperthyroidism. The relaxation half-time of the deep tendon reflexes is sometimes shortened below 240 msec in hyperthyroidism, and characteristically prolonged beyond 360 msec in hypothyroidism. Plasma tyrosine levels are elevated in hyperthyroidism, urinary hydroxyproline excretion is depressed in hypothyroidism, and CPK, SGOT, and LDH are elevated in hypothyroidism. None of these tests are useful for definitive diagnosis, because they are nonspecific and similar alterations can be caused by other disease processes.

Protein-Bound Iodine. Lacking a good measure of hormone action in the tissues, most physicians turn to a measure of thyroid hormone in blood. The standard determination for years was the serum protein-bound iodine (PBI) or butanol-extractable iodine (BEI). In the past decade, direct measurements of serum T_4 and T_3 by competitive displacement (T_4D and T_3D) or radioimmunoassay (T_3-RIA and T_4-RIA) have been developed and have replaced PBI and BEI because of their unique specificity. When combined with a measure of saturation of TBG by hormone, such as thyroxine dialyzable fraction (per cent DT_4) or resin uptake (T_3RU), a measure of serum-free thyroxine (FT_4) or triiodothyronine (FT_3) is obtained. The latter values are the most precise measures of thyroid hormone supply to tissues that are currently available.

The PBI measures all iodine in serum precipitable by protein-denaturing agents. Ordinarily this consists mainly of thyroid hormone, but if large quantities of iodide are present, or if any of the roentgenographic contrast medium used for gallbladder examinations, intravenous pyelograms, or arteriograms is present in plasma, the level is falsely elevated. Iodoproteins, formed by the thyroid in augmented amounts in some conditions, e.g., thyroiditis, are also precipitated. Nevertheless, the test is useful as a screening examination and is still widely available. The normal range is 4 to 8 μg of iodine per 100 ml. It is wise to determine total plasma iodine as well; if the level is no more than 2 or 3 μg per 100 ml above the PBI, it can be assumed that contamination with excess quantities of free iodide is not present. The butanol-extractable iodine (BEI) procedure is technically more sophisticated and is more specific for thyroid hormone because it excludes iodoproteins. If the PBI exceeds the BEI by more than 20 per cent, abnormal amounts of iodoprotein are present. Neither of these tests is widely used for diagnosis at present.

Serum Thyroxine and Triiodothyronine. A competitive protein-binding assay for thyroxine, similar in principle to the radioimmunoassay of peptide hormones, is widely available. The technique is in practice like the resin uptake test. T_4 is extracted from a serum sample. The T_4 of the plasma sample is then mixed with isotope-labeled T_4 in a standard TBG-containing solution, and its capacity to displace some of the radioactive-labeled hormone from the TBG to a resin is quantitated, by comparison to a standard curve made with known amounts of T_4. The test is technically demanding, but is extremely useful because it is specific for tetraiodothyronine and triiodothyronine. In practice it measures mainly T_4, because so little T_3 is present in plasma. Serum T_4 by displacement analysis (T_4D) is usually 4 to 10 μg per 100 ml, expressed as quantity of thyroxine, not iodide. Serum T_3 can also be measured specifically by this technique if the T_3 is first extracted from serum and separated chromatographically from T_4.

Specific antibodies to T_4 and T_3 have been generated, allowing radioimmunoassay of T_4 (T_4-RIA) and T_3 (T_3-RIA). These techniques are gradually becoming available in most medical centers and commercial laboratories. T_4 (RIA) results are similar to T_4(D). The levels of T_3 reported from various laboratories have varied widely, but most results suggest that normal T_3 (RIA) is about 140 (100 to 200) ng per 100 ml. Usually T_4 and T_3 vary concordantly. Under some circumstances (limited availability of iodine, diminished peroxidase, thyroid hyperplasia), excess T_3 may be produced relative to T_4. Thus measurement of T_3 (RIA) may ultimately replace T_4 (D) or T_4 (RIA) as the standard measure of serum hormone.

Variation in total T_4 or T_3 in serum may occur because of excess or diminution of hormone supply, or because of increase or decrease in serum TBG. Changes in hormone supply represent chemical thyrotoxicosis or hypothyroidism. Increased TBG resulting from pregnancy, estrogen administration, or heredity, or decreased TBG or TBPA resulting from liver disease, severe malnutrition, severe illness, steroids, or testosterone is accompanied by concordant alterations in T_4 and T_3 but reciprocal alterations in per cent free T_4 and T_3, resulting in normal quantities of FT_4 and FT_3. To differentiate between these two possible causes of high or low serum thyroid hormones, one must make an independent assessment of the level of TBG, or measure per cent DT_4 (Fig. 2).

T_3 Resin Uptake (T_3RU). Serum is incubated with a trace amount of labeled T_3 and a resin. Uptake of the tracer by the resin varies directly with total serum T_4 and T_3 and per cent FT_4 if TBG levels are normal, and inversely with serum TBG if it is altered. Resin uptake is *inversely* proportional to, and can be used as an estimate of, unoccupied TBG and varies *directly* with free hormone fraction.

Per Cent FT_4. Serum plus a labeled T_4 tracer is dialyzed to equilibrium against a buffer. The dialyzable fraction, normally ± 0.04 per cent of the total T_4, represents the free hormone fraction.

Free Thyroid Hormone. Multiplication of the total serum $T_4 \times$ per cent FT_4 yields FT_4, the actual concentration of free—non-protein-bound—T_4. The usual range is 1.5 to 3.5 ng per 100 ml. The same measure can be derived for T_3 (FT_3) if T_3 concentration and per cent FT_3 are available.

In most laboratories advantage is taken of the relationship of the resin uptake to per cent FT_4 in order to calculate an "index," as first suggested by Clark and Horn. Total $T_4 \times \dfrac{\text{Patient's } T_3 \text{ RU}}{\text{Standard } T_3 \text{ RU}}$ equals the free thyroxine index (FTI), which is a very good approximation of free T_4 and correlates exactly with FT_4.

FT_4 or FTI constitutes the best available contemporary measure of hormone supply to tissues, is independent of variations in plasma thyroid hormone binding proteins, and is not affected by excess iodide or iodide-containing compounds.

Two problems must be remembered when performing function tests. Excess iodine in any form may elevate the PBI and BEI and depress the radioactive iodide uptake test. Roentgenographic contrast dyes may for a short time depress the radioactive uptake test, and for periods of weeks or months falsely elevate the PBI and BEI. Alterations in binding proteins caused by heredity, hormones, illness, liver disease, or malnutrition can cause increases or decreases in the PBI, BEI, serum thyroxine, and T_3 values without altering the level of free thyroid hormone.

Radioactive Iodine Uptake. Another commonly used measure of thyroid activity is the thyroidal radioactive iodide uptake (RAIU). The patient is given a trace dose of radioactive iodide, and the fraction accumulated in the gland is determined at 2, 6, or 24 hours, the last of these being the most widely used end-point. The normal uptake is inversely dependent upon available iodide supply. In areas where the iodide intake is 150 to 200 μg per day, it ranges from 20 to 50 per cent. In most of the United States, an increase in iodide in the diet up to 400 to 600 μg per day has reduced the normal range to 10 to 25 per cent. This procedure measures the activity of the thyroid trapping and binding process, which can be augmented owing to excess TSH stimulation or because of inherent thyroid hyperactivity. The RAIU is characteristically elevated in areas of iodide deficiency.

Perchlorate Discharge Test. The presence of trapped but unbound iodide in the thyroid gland can be ascertained by administering 1 gram of $KClO_4$ orally two hours after a ^{131}I tracer. Discharge of more than 10 per cent is characteristic of thyroid organification defects of congenital (e.g., Pendred's syndrome) or acquired (e.g., Hashimoto's thyroiditis) types (Fig. 3).

Serum TSH Assay. Measurement of serum TSH by RIA is now a standard and useful determination. Normal TSH varies from undetectable to 8 μU per milliliter. TSH is characteristically suppressed by exogenous or endogenous excess of thyroid hormone. Elevations of 20 to 400 μU per milliliter occur in primary thyroid failure of any cause. Mild elevations (10 to 20 μU) are of less certain significance and may represent mild hypothyroidism or euthyroidism (compensated hypothyroidism) achieved by the elevated TSH. Undetectable or normal TSH levels are found in pituitary hypothyroidism, hypothalamic damage, and in almost all patients with thyrotoxicosis.

Tests for Specific Conditions. The nature of the disease process affecting the thyroid can be evaluated by a number of other procedures.

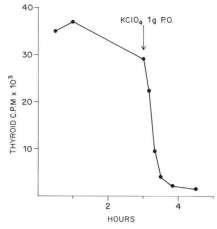

Figure 3. $KClO_4$ discharge test. In the usual test thyroid RAIU is measured sequentially over two to three hours after a tracer dose of ^{131}I. One gram of $KClO_4$ is given orally, and thyroid uptake determinations are continued. In this patient with organification defect resulting from complete lack of peroxidase, $KClO_4$ caused nearly complete release of accumulated iodide, indicating that the tracer existed in the gland as iodide and had not been bound in the normal manner to thyroglobulin.

T_3 Suppression Test. A high thyroid ^{131}I uptake caused by endogenous TSH can be reduced in most circumstances to or below the normal range by administration of 100 μg of triiodothyronine daily for one week. Serum T_4 will also be lowered, and its determination is useful when administration of radioiodine is contraindicated (e.g., pregnancy). Thyroid activity is not suppressible in most patients with active Graves' disease (see Ch. 837). This response is seen whether the basal RAIU is elevated or normal and is accepted as the most characteristic abnormality in this illness. However, nonsuppressibility also occurs in the closely related syndrome of Hashimoto's thyroiditis and if autonomous functioning thyroid nodules are present.

TSH Stimulation Test. The presence of functioning thyroid tissue can be evaluated by administration of 5 units of TSH subcutaneously daily for three days, with a radioactive iodide uptake test (and sometimes a scan) before and after. TSH should raise the radioactive

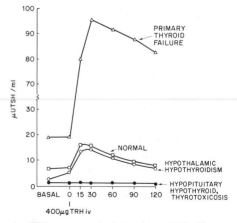

Figure 4. TSH responses to intravenous TRH. The normal rapid elevation of plasma TSH after TRH is obliterated in thyrotoxicosis, by thyroid hormone administration, or in pituitary destruction. An excessive response occurs in primary thyroid failure.

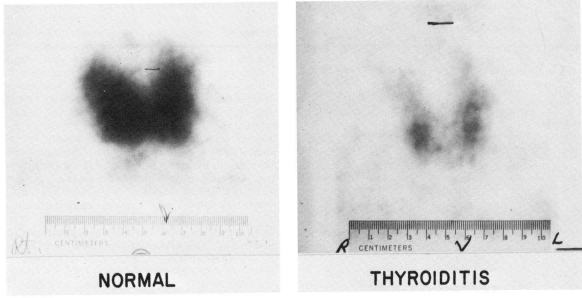

NORMAL   THYROIDITIS

Figure 5. Fluorescent thyroid scan. Fluorescence induced by [241]Americium indicates distribution and concentration of stable [127]I in the normal gland. By contrast, the gland affected by Hashimoto's thyroiditis is nearly devoid of iodine.

iodide uptake to a normal level or at least double it in a patient whose basal function is low because of deficient TSH. The test is also useful for demonstrating normal tissue which has been suppressed by a functioning "hot" nodule.

TRH Test (Fig. 4). The ability of the pituitary to secrete TSH can be elevated by administration of 400 μg of TRH intravenously and measuring serum TSH during the subsequent 90 minutes. Hypothalamic hypothyroidism is associated with normal basal TSH, responding normally to the administration of exogenous TRH. Primary thyroid failure is associated with a high basal level of TSH hyper-responsive to TRH. Hypothyroidism resulting from pituitary failure causes low serum TSH and absent TRH response. Administration of replacement doses of T_4 or T_3 or excess endogenous or exogenous T_4 or T_3 obliterates the response to TRH.

Antibodies and LATS. Autoimmunity against thyroid antigens can be demonstrated by measuring antithyroglobulin antibodies by the tanned red cell agglutination procedure, or antithyroid microsomal antibodies by the immunofluorescent, complement fixation, or tanned red cell agglutination methods. Positive tests are found in Hashimoto's thyroiditis, primary thyroid failure, and Graves' disease.

Long-acting thyroid stimulator (LATS), measured by a bioassay described in Ch. 837, is characteristic of Graves' disease.

Thyroid Scans. A scintiscan performed after administration of [199]Te or radioactive iodide provides anatomic localization of functioning thyroid tissue. Adenomas may appear inactive ("cold") or hyperactive ("hot"). Graves' disease and Hashimoto's thyroiditis show diffuse uptake, whereas multinodular goiter gives a mottled picture. Uptake outside the thyroid identifies aberrant thyroid tissue, metastatic thyroid cancer, and struma ovarii.

Recently, fluorescent scanning with a [241]Am source has been developed. This technique identifies concentration and distribution of the stable [127]I present in the gland (Fig. 5). It is a useful technique when radioisotopes should be avoided (children, pregnant women, lactation). In addition, it provides another independent index of thyroid function. The Hashimoto's gland is characteristically and diagnostically found to be devoid of stored iodine. Also, the thyroid can be shown to have a normal appearance and iodine content in pituitary hypothyroidism and when uptake of a tracer is suppressed by administration of exogenous hormone or iodide.

Needle Biopsy. Needle biopsy of the thyroid is a useful procedure in properly selected cases and can provide a histologic diagnosis when all other techniques fail.

Initial Selection of Function Tests. In most thyroid diseases careful history and physical examination lead to the diagnosis, and laboratory procedures serve to confirm the clinical impression. In the initial evaluation of most patients, it is useful to measure the serum thyroxine, the free thyroxine index, and occasionally the radioactive iodine uptake. A scan can be done at the same time if there is a question of nonuniformity of gland function raised by history or examination of the neck. The TSH level should be checked if hypothyroidism is suggested. The test for antithyroglobulin antibodies is also useful in the initial evaluation of many patients. To follow the progress of therapy, the most useful procedures are serial determinations of serum thyroxine. Frequent measurement of the patient's weight also constitutes an excellent measure of whole body metabolism.

Further tests are dictated by the progress of the evaluation. Many specialized assays are available if needed to define unusual congenital or acquired diseases.

Davis, P. J.: Factors affecting the determination of the serum protein bound iodine. Am. J. Med., 40:918, 1956.
DeGroot, L. J.: Kinetic analysis of iodine metabolism. J. Clin. Endocrinol. Metab., 26:149, 1966.
Dowling, J. T., Appleton, W. G., and Nicoloff, J. T.: Thyroxine turnover during human pregnancy. J. Clin. Endocrinol. Metab., 27:1749, 1967.

Dumont, J. E.: The action of thyrotropin on thyroid metabolism. Vitam. Horm., 29:287, 1971.

Hershman, J. M., and Pittman, J. A.: Utility of the radioimmunoassay of serum thyrotrophin in man. Ann. Intern. Med., 74:481, 1971.

Hoffer, P. B., Gottschalk, A., and Refetoff, S.: Thyroid scanning techniques: The old and the new. Curr. Prob. Radiol., 2:5, 1972.

Kaplan, S. L., Grumbach, M. M., Friesen, H. G., and Costom, B. H.: Thryotropin-releasing factor (TRF) effect on secretion of human pituitary prolactin and thyrotropin in children and in idiopathic hypopituitary dwarfism. J. Clin. Endocrinol. Metab., 35:825, 1972.

Lieblick, J., and Utiger, R. D.: Triiodothyronine radioimmunoassay. J. Clin. Invest., 51:157, 1972.

Oppenheimer, J. H.: Role of plasma proteins in the binding, distribution and metabolism of the thyroid hormones. N. Engl. J. Med., 278:1153, 1968.

Ormston, B. J., Garry, R., Coyer, R. J., Besser, G. M., and Hall, R.: Thyrotrophin releasing hormone as a thyroid function test. Lancet, 2:10, 1971.

Rapoport, B., and DeGroot, L. J.: Current concepts of thyroid physiology. Semin. Nucl. Med., 1:265, 1971.

Robin, N. I., Hagen, S. R., Collaco, F., Refetoff, S., and Selenkow, H. A.: Serum tests for measurement of thyroid function. Hormones, 2:266, 1971.

Roitt, I. M., and Doniach, D.: Thyroid autoimmunity. Br. Med. Bull., 16:152, 1960.

Sterling, K., and Brenner, M. A.: Free thyroxine in human serum. Simplified measurement with the aid of magnesium precipitation. J. Clin. Invest., 45:153, 1966.

Taunton, O. D., McDaniel, H. G., and Pittman, J. A.: Standardization of TSH testing. J. Clin. Endocrinol. Metab., 25:266, 1965.

Vale, W., Burgus, R., and Guillemin, R.: On the mechanism of action of TRF: Effects of cycloheximide and actinomycin on the release of TSH stimulated in vitro by TRF and its inhibition by thyroxine. Neuroendocrinology, 3:34, 1968.

Wolff, J.: Transport of iodide and other anions in the thyroid gland. Physiol. Rev., 44:45, 1964.

837. GRAVES' DISEASE AND HYPERTHYROIDISM

Hyperthyroidism refers to a state of heightened thyroid gland activity associated with the production of excess quantities of thyroid hormone. The clinical state is also referred to as *thyrotoxicosis*. Most commonly hyperthyroidism is part of a syndrome which may include goiter, exophthalmos, and pretibial myxedema, known as *Graves' disease* or *Basedow's disease*. Thyrotoxicosis can also be caused by excessive production of hormone by a *single "toxic" nodule,* by a *toxic multinodular goiter,* by occasional *functioning thyroid carcinomas,* or by *medication*. Rarely, it is caused by a TSH-secreting pituitary adenoma, is associated with acromegaly, occurs because of production of TSH-like material in trophoblastic tumors or embryonal cell carcinomas, or is due to hyperfunctioning teratoma (struma ovarii).

Incidence. Hyperthyroidism is not a reportable condition, so exact data on incidence are unavailable. Incidence is probably in excess of 3 per 10,000 adults per year. It is largely a disease of adult women, with a sex ratio of approximately 5 to 1. Peak incidence is between 30 and 50 years of age.

Etiology and Pathogenesis. The manifestations of Graves' disease fall into two categories: (1) the primary disease involving the thyroid (plus eyes and skin), and (2) the circulatory, neurologic, and metabolic abnormalities, described below, which are secondarily caused by excess thyroid hormone produced by the thyroid gland impinging on tissues.

There are two recurring themes in discussions of the etiology of Graves' disease: (1) It may be the result of

emotional trauma, or (2) it may be an "autoimmune" disease. The previous impression that the thyroid in Graves' disease was responding to excess TSH is erroneous, because TSH in plasma of patients with this disorder is characteristically reduced or absent, apparently suppressed by increased circulating thyroid hormone.

For decades it has been suggested that Graves' disease is induced by emotional stress, because of the frequency with which physicians obtain a history of emotional trauma occurring before the onset of hyperthyroidism. Characteristically the event is a marital problem or death of a loved one. Although such testimonials are frequent, the meager factual data available are inconclusive. Psychiatric evaluations indicate that there is nothing special about the individual who becomes a victim of Graves' disease, and that the incidence of emotional stress in these patients is comparable to that in a control population. Perhaps, in the individuals who report a stressful circumstance, Graves' disease was already present and made the emotional reaction more dramatic. Also, the patient suffering from Graves' disease has anxiety and tremulousness as a result of the illness; these symptoms may be misinterpreted as causal.

Autoimmunity directed against thyroid antigens is currently thought to be the most probable cause. Antibodies directed against endogenous thyroid antigens were detected in patients with Hashimoto's thyroiditis in 1956, and several thyroid antibody-antigen systems have since been found in patients with thyroiditis, idiopathic myxedema, and Graves' disease (see Ch. 838). Sixty to 80 per cent of patients with Graves' disease have antibodies directed against thyroglobulin or against thyroid microsomes. In addition, Adams and Purves described in 1956 a factor (long-acting thyroid stimulator, LATS), present in the serum of about half the patients with Graves' disease, which stimulated the release of hormone from the prelabeled thyroid of a test animal. LATS is now known to be a polyclonal gamma globulin, probably an autoantibody directed against a component of the thyroid cell membrane. LATS can be neutralized by reacting with antibodies prepared against 7S human IgG. LATS adsorbs to thyroid microsomes, but the reaction is not entirely specific and does not require complement. In addition to causing release of hormone, LATS stimulates increased synthesis of nucleic acids and proteins, increases incorporation of phosphate into phospholipids, stimulates glucose metabolism, and causes thyroid growth. A contemporary interpretation is that LATS is an autoantibody which mimics the action of TSH and stimulates the synthesis and release of thyroid hormone. In patients whose thyroids are capable of responding to such a trophic stimulus, LATS may be the mediator of hyperthyroxinemia. LATS crosses the placenta and is the cause of transient hyperthyroidism in some neonates born to mothers who have high circulating levels of the antibody.

LATS is, however, found in at most 80 per cent of patients with Graves' disease, and its presence or level does not correlate uniformly with thyroid hyperactivity. Recent data suggest that there may be other "thyrotrophic" antibody systems present which can be detected in different assays. One of these is the "human thyroid stimulator" (HTS) of Onaya et al.; another possible factor is the "LATS protector" of Adams.

In addition to circulating antibodies (humoral immune response), there is much evidence for cell-mediated immunity (CMI) in Graves' disease, as well as in Hashimoto's thyroiditis and primary myxedema. The CMI is probably involved in a cell-destructive response. Our theory is that Graves' disease is due to autoimmunity, and that its manifestations represent a balance between the stimulatory or blocking effect of circulating antibodies such as LATS and HTS and the cell-destructive effects of CMI.

Exophthalmos has also been related to autoimmunity. In serum of patients with exophthalmos, a factor causing experimental exophthalmos in animals is found. Various reports also indicate an abnormality in binding of gamma globulin from exophthalmic patients to orbital antigens, and two studies indicate that patients with exophthalmos have CMI against these antigens.

Why the body should develop a humoral antibody and CMI response active against its own tissues remains unknown. There is no evidence for an abnormal antigen in these conditions, or for an abnormal sequestration or release of antigen. Because of the association of thyroid autoimmunity with immunity against several other organs of the body, it seems possible that Graves' disease is basically a manifestation of deranged immune homeostasis.

Much evidence indicates that *a strong hereditary factor is involved in Graves' disease, Hashimoto's thyroiditis, and myxedema,* and that the three diseases are intimately related. Patients with Graves' disease and thyroiditis usually have a family history positive for the same condition. Thyroid autoantibodies, including LATS, are found in relatives of patients with these diseases. The incidence of any one of the other two diseases is increased in relatives of patients who have one of the three. Some patients appear to have a combination of thyroiditis and Graves' disease that has been called "Hashitoxicosis."

Another intriguing bit of circumstantial evidence related to etiology is the occasionally reported occurrence of Graves' disease after consumption of desiccated thyroid for weight reduction. It is as if the ingestion of thyroid hormone somehow conditioned the body to a high level of the substance and "demanded" continued thyroid hyperfunction after the exogenous hormone was withdrawn.

Iodine administration occasionally induces hyperthyroidism. This Jod-Basedow phenomenon typically occurs in areas of endemic goiter when iodinization of salt is introduced, but can occur after administration of iodine to patients in nonendemic areas. Apparently the thyroid was functioning autonomously at a hyperactive level before the introduction of iodine, but was unable to manifest hyperthyroidism owing to the limitation of hormone synthesis imposed by the low iodide intake.

Little is known about other causes of hyperthyroidism. The etiology of the toxic nodular goiter, the toxic solitary nodule, or the hyperfunctioning thyroid carcinoma is related to the problem of tumor formation. Hyperthyroidism found in association with acromegaly may be due to increased TSH production, although this has not been established. Hyperthyroidism associated with trophoblastic tumors is due to the production of a trophic substance by the tumor. Placental thyrotrophin is a normal placental product; a slightly different protein is formed in excess in patients with hydatidiform mole and in choriocarcinoma. It is immunologically related to bovine thyrotrophin, but does not cross-react with antibodies to human thyrotrophin.

Pathology. The main pathologic abnormality in Graves' disease is evident in the size of the thyroid cells. The cells are tall, and the size of the average follicle is reduced. Small amounts of colloid are present in the lumen. The picture is analogous to a gland under intense TSH stimulation. In addition there is characteristically an infiltration of mononuclear cells, mainly small lymphocytes and some plasma cells, and lymphoid germinal centers may be apparent. Sometimes the process shades into a picture characteristic of Hashimoto's thyroiditis. There is generalized lymph node hyperplasia, the thymus is enlarged, and the proportion of active thymic tissue is increased. Active germinal centers are also found in the thymus, and the histology is similar to that of myasthenia gravis or lupus erythematosus. The muscles are usually microscopically normal, but occasionally the cells are atrophic, multiple nuclei are present, striations are indistinct, and a lymphocyte infiltrate is apparent. Hepatic changes include cellular edema, focal necrosis, and lymphocyte infiltrates. The epidermis and dermis are thinned. Bones may show osteoporosis or osteomalacia. Pathology of the eye and "localized myxedema" are described below.

Clinical Manifestations. In many patients the changes are so obvious as to be inescapable; in others the subtlety of the disease defies anything except a laboratory diagnosis. The patient may notice weakness, increased fatigue, insomnia, weight loss, or tremulousness. The skin becomes fine and moist, and there is excess perspiration. The hair thins, and the nails become thin and brittle. Increased tolerance to cold or decreased tolerance to moderate heat is noted. Friends observe that the eyes are prominent, and the patient appears to be staring. Double vision, blurred vision, burning, tearing, and decreased visual acuity may occur. Often the patient finds a mass in the neck, although this produces few local symptoms. A hyperactive heart, palpitations, dyspnea on exertion, and ankle edema may be evident, usually in the absence of congestive failure. Weight loss occurs despite increase in appetite. There may occasionally be abdominal pain reminiscent of an ulcer and frequent loose bowel movements. Subdeltoid bursitis may occur. Menstrual periods become scanty, the cycle is shortened, some periods may be missed, and fertility is reduced. Usually libido is not altered. Thirst and polyuria are sometimes noted. Weakness of the muscles is prominent; it may be the primary symptom in older persons who have had chronic low-grade thyroid hyperfunction for months or years. Such patients report that they cannot climb stairs or get up easily from a chair. Pruritus is frequently noticed, and occasionally hives occur.

On examination the patient appears anxious, tremulous, and restless, and is typically quick to cooperate. The hair is fine and thin, and females may show some temporal recession of the hairline. The skin feels moist, hot, thin, or even silky, and pigmentation may be increased. Vitiligo, especially of the hands and feet, is present in about 7 per cent of cases. The nails are thin, and the hyponychium is often seen to have receded, forming an irregular concave erosion under the distal portion of the nail. This change (onycholysis or Plummer's nails) is most typically found bilaterally on the fourth digit. The elbows are sometimes red, as are the palms.

The eyes may appear prominent, and the sclera is visible above the iris on upward or downward gaze (lid lag). The lids may be grossly puffy. Proptosis (forward displacement of the globes in the orbits) may be evident, and if severe the lids may not close adequately. Edema of the scleral conjunctiva may form loose pockets filled with clear liquid (chemosis). Extraocular muscle function may be diminished, often first with a loss of upward gaze, and later with a fixed strabismus caused by contracture of a damaged muscle. In severe cases total loss of ocular motility and convergence are present. With proptosis the edge of the lacrimal gland may be felt bulging below the supraorbital ridge. The beefy red insertion of the lateral rectus can sometimes be seen. Depending on the severity of the process, there may be papilledema or hemorrhages and exudates in the retina. Visual acuity may be severely reduced.

The thyroid typically is enlarged, usually three to four times the normal size, although rarely the gland may be of normal dimensions. Usually the gland is symmetrically involved and may be lobulated. It characteristically feels rather firm and beefy, and often the pyramidal lobe is palpable. Lymph nodes are often present in the supraclavicular fossae and may be tender. A systolic bruit may be heard over the thyroid or palpated ("thrill") in very vascular glands.

The precordium is hyperactive, and the heart sounds are intensified. A systolic murmur is usually audible, and sometimes a scratching systolic sound (Lerman's sound) is heard in the second or third left intercostal space. Murmurs present before the onset of thyroid disease are louder. Occasionally murmurs suggestive of mitral insufficiency or stenosis are audible; they disappear after hyperthyroidism is controlled. Tachycardia is usually present, and there is an increased propensity to atrial fibrillation. Axillary lymph nodes are frequently palpable; on examination of the abdomen, the spleen or liver or both may be minimally enlarged. Muscle strength and bulk may be reduced. Reflexes are exaggerated in speed and strength.

Rarely, typical attacks of hypokalemic periodic paralysis occur during severe hyperthyroidism, especially in young men of Oriental extraction.

Occasionally patients develop severe hyperthyroidism but present few classic manifestations. In this picture, termed *masked hyperthyroidism,* to which older people are most prone, the tremor, anxiety, and hyperkinesis may be lacking. Instead, the patient is apathetic, sometimes mentally confused, or obtunded. There may be extreme weakness and muscle atrophy. The skin may not be thinned, and the sweating and eye signs may also be lacking. Usually, however, tachycardia, goiter, and low-grade fever are present. A coincidental atrial fibrillation and weight loss should suggest this diagnosis.

Diagnosis. The flagrant case with all the characteristic manifestations is usually recognized by laymen who refer the patient to the physician for therapy. Other patients do not present with more than a few of the signs and symptoms of Graves' disease, and in these patients laboratory studies become critical. Diagnosis begins with the history and physical examination. Serial weights should be recorded, because progressive loss of weight is a strong clue to the diagnosis. To prove the diagnosis, the serum thyroxine (or better, the free

thyroxine index) and RAIU are probably the most useful tests. The BMR, cholesterol, T_3RU, and reflex time may occasionally be helpful. The antithyroglobulin or antimicrosomal antibody tests are useful, because a positive test indicates that the patient has some variety of thyroid autoimmune disease. Often patients develop a normochromic and normocytic anemia with 9 to 11 grams of hemoglobin per 100 ml. Alkaline phosphatase may be elevated because of increased rate of bone turnover, and serum calcium, urinary calcium, and hydroxyproline excretion may be increased. Bilirubin is occasionally elevated. Roentgenograms of the skull and views of the orbits should be obtained if there is a question of an intracerebral or orbital space-occupying lesion, especially if unilateral exophthalmos occurs before the onset of hyperthyroidism. All the tests must be carefully evaluated in the light of the patient's known iodide intake, exposure to radiographic contrast media, and medications. If there is doubt about the diagnosis, a T_3 suppression test may be useful. *Nonsuppressibility of the thyroid is considered the most characteristic feature of Graves' disease.*

T_3 Toxicosis. In some patients who have clinical symptoms suggestive of hyperthyroidism, but in whom the radioactive iodide uptake and serum thyroxine are normal, measurement of elevated plasma triiodothyronine may confirm the condition known as "T_3 toxicosis." This condition can be the presenting feature of Graves' disease, but is more frequently found in patients with an autonomous nodule or residual tissue after radioiodide (RAI) or surgical therapy, or in areas of iodine deficiency. Some reports indicate that as many as one tenth of patients have T_3 toxicosis without elevated T_4 levels. This has not been the author's experience. Although it is imperative to remember that T_3 toxicosis can explain the unusual case, the great majority of patients present with both high T_4 and high T_3, and cause no difficulty in diagnosis by the more commonly available serum T_4 measurement.

It is especially important to consider this diagnosis in elderly patients who have atrial fibrillation or congestive heart failure. Other diagnostic hints are unexplained diarrhea, severe muscle weakness, bursitis, and vitiligo of the hands and feet.

Severe pulmonary disease, anxiety, carcinoma, malabsorption, cirrhosis, and myasthenia can have features similar to thyrotoxicosis, and must be considered in the differential diagnosis.

In this age of dependence upon chemistry, it is not rare to be faced with a patient who has negligible signs and symptoms but in whom an elevated T_4 or T_3 has been detected by chance. In such patients it is wise to establish as carefully as possible the presence or absence of disease by RAIU, T_3 suppression test, and FT_4 or FT_3 levels, and then to observe events for a period of time. The process may subside, show evidence of damage to cardiac, hepatic, or osseous tissues, indicating need for treatment, show no change, or progress gradually into overt thyrotoxicosis.

In fact, major reliance is placed on the laboratory tests. A significant elevation of FT_4 or FT_3 can alone be the determining feature of Graves' disease and demand therapy.

The RAIU, formerly a very useful test, is now of less value because elevated intake of iodide has depressed the normal and thyrotoxic values and confused the area of overlap between them. It is not necessarily required for diagnosis, but is useful when planning RAI therapy and with a scan when defining autonomous thyroid function caused by an adenoma or multinodular goiter.

Differentiation from Other Mitochondrial Diseases. The symptoms and signs of thyrotoxicosis are due to hypermetabolism, and theoretically could be mimicked by any cause of uncontrolled mitochondrial function. In fact few conditions have been reported in which mitochondrial oxidative phosphorylation is disturbed, and only one syndrome has caused confusion in diagnosis. A unique illness suggestive of thyrotoxicosis was reported by Luft. Weakness, excessive perspiration, marked hypermetabolism, and weight loss led to thyroidectomy, but induction of overt hypothyroidism failed to control the illness. Muscle mitochondria from this patient were unusually abundant and large, and had excessive crista formation. Respiration was not controlled as in normal tissues, and uncoupled oxidative phosphorylation was demonstrated. The cause of this illness is unknown.

Other cases that less clearly represent mitochondrial disease have been described, but none resemble thyrotoxicosis. Distorted mitochondria in hepatocytes and a defect in electron transport between dehydrogenases and the cytochromes have been observed in the fatal congenital "cerebro-hepato-renal syndrome." Abnormal increased, diminished, and absent muscle mitochondria have been detected in various idiopathic myopathies, in steroid-induced myopathy, and in cardiac muscle in experimental left ventricular failure. Experimental iron deficiency can lower tissue cytochrome content, and copper deficiency may be associated with diminished cytochrome oxidase. The clinical correlates of these observations are unknown. Considering the importance of mitochondria in cell homeostasis, they so far appear to be remarkably immune from disease-related pathology.

Therapy. The choice of therapy for hyperthyroidism resulting from Graves' disease has been debated for decades, and final resolution is not yet in sight. During the period from 1950 to 1970, sentiment gradually swung to the use of RAI in most adults because of its simplicity and absence of surgical complications or hospitalization. When hypothyroidism was observed to occur in 40 to 70 per cent of patients in the 5- to 10-year period after treatment with "conventional" doses of RAI, many clinics adopted a "low dose" [131]I treatment program. This clearly reduced the incidence of early hypothyroidism, but is associated with a need for multiple doses and continued treatment of many patients with various other agents over one to five years. Dissatisfaction with ^{131}I has swung the pendulum, to some extent, back toward surgery. In fact this treatment is now the author's first choice for most young adults through age 40. Although the three common treatments for hyperthyroidism are excellent, each has its built-in disadvantages and none of the therapies can be considered ideal.

Radioactive Iodide. For adults older than 25, administration of radioactive iodide appears to be a satisfactory form of treatment. So far there is no evidence that this therapy causes an increased incidence of leukemia or significant somatic damage. Hypothyroidism, attributable to an "overeffective" treatment, is a disadvantage and will be discussed below. The radiation dose delivered to the gonads during treatment is similar to that given during an intravenous pyelogram or barium enema and is probably inconsequential. Patients have now been treated with this agent for nearly three

decades, and there is still no evidence of ^{131}I-induced tumor formation. Evidence on this point must continually be accumulated, but for the moment it does not appear that radiation of the adult thyroid with ^{131}I leads to subsequent thyroid malignancy.

A major difficulty with radioactive iodine treatment has been the onset of hypothyroidism, either immediately or long after the treatment. The incidence of hypothyroidism may approach 40 to 70 per cent after ten years. Most patients are now treated with a dose of radioactive iodide approximately half that used five or ten years ago, in an effort to diminish the incidence of hypothyroidism.

Therapy is planned to deliver a retained dose of 40 to 100 μC per estimated gram of weight at 24 hours, the dose per gram increasing with thyroid size from 20 to 100 grams. With this dose, many patients do not achieve immediate euthyroidism, and require ancillary therapy such as administration of potassium iodide solution or an antithyroid drug if hyperthyroidism is not controlled within two or three months. These agents should be continued for 6 to 12 months, because the full effect of radiation is not obtained until then. At the end of 6 or 12 months, the potassium iodide or the antithyroid drug or both are discontinued, and if hyperthyroidism recurs, a second treatment of radioactive iodide is given. Thirty to 50 per cent of the patients need a second treatment, and occasionally a third dose is required (Fig. 6). In selected individuals, in whom it is imperative that hyperthyroidism be rapidly controlled, a two- to threefold larger dose is administered, and re-treatment is given at three months if required. If prompt control is necessary, antithyroid drug and then KI can be instituted within one day of administration of the therapeutic ^{131}I dose, with loss of about one fifth of the radiation effect. Control of the disease with this combined treatment is usually achieved in one to four weeks.

All women in the reproductive age who are to receive

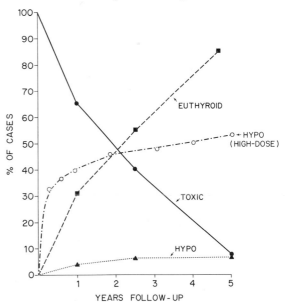

Figure 6. Graphic representation of current therapeutic results achieved with "low-dose" [131]I therapy of thyrotoxicosis. Although hypothyroidism is infrequent in the first five years, many patients remain toxic for a prolonged period after initial therapy. The high and progressively increasing incidence of hypothyroidism after "high-dose" therapy is also indicated.

radioactive iodide must be questioned for possible pregnancy or lactation, which are contraindications to this treatment. It is best to give the radioactive iodide shortly after a menstrual period. Women should be advised to avoid pregnancy for a period of at least one year, because the possible need for re-treatment will not be eliminated before this time has elapsed.

There was a recent wave of interest in the use of ^{125}I for therapy, on the basis that it would be less likely to produce hypothyroidism. The few reported trials do not establish any improved efficacy of ^{125}I over [131]I.

Antithyroid Drugs. Children and young adults are best treated initially by a long-term course of antithyroid drug. Patients with small goiters, recent onset of disease, and mild symptoms respond most frequently to this therapy and are thus the preferred candidates. Usually propylthiouracil, 100 mg every eight hours, or methimazole, 10 mg every eight hours, is given orally. If this is not effective within two to four weeks, the dose may be doubled. Rarely, 1 gram of propylthiouracil or 100 mg of methimazole will be needed daily. It is imperative that the patient be instructed to take the medication at the scheduled times. Antithyroid drugs have a short duration of action, and one of the main causes of treatment failure is that patients do not adhere to a rigorous time schedule. As a response is obtained, the dose is progressively lowered to 50 or 100 mg of propylthiouracil every 12 hours, or a comparable dose of methimazole. Many patients can be maintained on a single daily dose of medication. Some physicians prefer to maintain a higher dose of the antithyroid drug and to add replacement doses of thyroid hormone in order to avoid hypothyroidism. Overtreatment with antithyroid drugs will of course block formation of thyroid hormone, lower the T_4, and cause a TSH response. This is usually evident in rapid enlargement of the thyroid.

Symptoms of thyrotoxicosis usually abate within two to six weeks, and the patient should be metabolically normal after this period of time. The thyroid gland, in the absence of induced hypothyroidism, either remains at the original size or gets smaller. The latter is a favorable prognostic sign. Another favorable prognostic sign is return of thyroid suppressibility after administration of T_3 (T_3 suppression test), which has been documented to occur in some patients as early as eight weeks after the start of antithyroid drug treatment. The medication is continued for one to two years and then is gradually discontinued. Half the treated patients will enter a prolonged remission. Others will relapse within 1 to 12 months, and are either re-treated with the same drug or given an alternative form of therapy. The incidence of remission is higher after the first year of therapy, and decreases among patients who have failed to remit with each subsequent year of treatment.

During antithyroid drug administration, patients must be carefully monitored for occurrence of side effects such as pruritus, rash, and epigastric pain, and for the more serious but less frequent occurrence of neutropenia or even agranulocytosis. A mild skin rash may disappear spontaneously. Pruritus can be treated by the addition of an antihistaminic drug. A severe rash calls for discontinuation of the antithyroid drug. It is often useful to institute therapy with an alternative antithyroid medication, because cross-reactions do not always occur. The leukocyte count should be checked at each visit during administration of antithyroid drugs. Occa-

sionally, a count as low as 3500 cells per cubic millimeter may be observed spontaneously in patients with thyrotoxicosis. If, however, the blood count falls from a normal range down to a level of 3500 or lower during therapy, the antithyroid drug should be discontinued. Occasionally agranulocytosis develops, requiring intensive care in a hospital, but is usually reversible.

Surgery. Subtotal thyroidectomy performed by a skilled surgeon is also very effective. It is the preferred therapy in children who fail to respond to antithyroid drugs or have had adverse reaction to the drug, in young adults who do not wish to pursue a prolonged course of treatment, in patients who are apprehensive about the possible adverse effects of radioactive iodide, in patients who have huge thyroids, and in patients whose glands are believed to harbor a carcinoma. As the initial mode of treatment for adults of 20 to 40 years, it usually offers the most prompt return to normal function. Although no hard data can be offered, it also seems preferable to RAI therapy in patients with marked exophthalmos. The procedure is accompanied by a mortality rate of less than 1 in 1000, an incidence of permanent hypothyroidism in from 5 to 40 per cent, recurrence of thyrotoxicosis in 5 per cent or more (depending on the extent of the initial resection), occasional instances of damage to the recurrent laryngeal nerves and parathyroids, need for hospitalization, and considerable expense. Patients should be rendered euthyroid with an antithyroid drug in preparation for surgery, and should be given potassium iodide (saturated solution of potassium iodide, 2 drops twice daily) or Lugol's solution (ten drops twice daily) for a period of one to two weeks before the operation. Iodide decreases vascularity of the gland and makes the surgical procedure less difficult. Induction of euthyroidism before surgery is imperative, because cardiac arrhythmias during surgery are frequent in patients with thyrotoxicosis.

Iodine. Iodine was introduced for control of hyperthyroidism 50 years ago but is rarely used today as the sole treatment. When given in doses of greater than 6 mg per day, iodide blocks further formation of iodotyrosines (Wolff-Chaikoff effect), and diminishes release of thyroid hormone by inhibiting proteolysis of thyroglobulin. Most patients are benefited initially by iodide, although some respond only partially, and some have an exacerbation of their illness despite continuation of iodine. Iodine treatment may induce hypothyroidism, especially in patients who have previously been treated with surgery or radioactive iodide. Addition of iodine to the regimen of patients who are already receiving antithyroid drugs has been known to induce a severe exacerbation of hyperthyroidism. At present the three more certain and well defined modes of treatment described above seem preferable to the use of potassium iodide, but it is probable that further study of this treatment will be forthcoming in future years, especially in treatment of mild hyperthyroidism.

Potassium perchlorate is rarely used at present for control of hyperthyroidism because of its reported association with fatal aplastic anemia.

Cortisone and immunosuppressive treatments have been tried experimentally, but no data indicate that they are appropriate for routine use.

Ancillary Treatments. Most patients benefit from a period of rest, a good diet, and added vitamins and calcium. The response to a few days in a hospital bed is often remarkable even before specific therapy is instituted. Phenobarbital, diazepam, and reserpine are useful for sedation.

Much recent interest has been given to propranolol as a specific therapy because of its ability to counteract the alleged beta-adrenergic mediated features of thyrotoxicosis. Although the mechanism may be uncertain, in doses of 10 to 40 mg by mouth four times daily, propranolol will reduce tachycardia and provide a beneficial calming effect in some patients. The author believes it is a useful drug, but does not find it to be more than an adjunct to usual therapy.

Therapy in Pregnancy. The choice of therapy in pregnancy is between antithyroid drug and surgery during the middle trimester. At present most patients are probably treated by administration of antithyroid drugs, although there is no certain superiority of one method. It is advisable to use the smallest dose necessary to bring the FTI into the high normal range, that is, between 9 and 13, if this coincides with a remission of symptoms. This precaution is taken because induction of fetal hypothyroidism by the antithyroid drug could result in mental damage. Therapy is followed by measurement of the FTI, or FT_4. These tests avoid the problem of interpreting the effect of pregnancy on T_4 and T_3 (high TBG). An alternative (although not preferred) program is to continue the antithyroid drug and to institute coincident therapy with thyroid hormone. Since this method exposes the fetus to a higher level of antithyroid drug than is needed in the absence of added hormone, and since there is no evidence that the added hormone has any protective effect, it is not recommended.

Therapy in Children. Thyrotoxicosis in children is usually less severe than in adults. Restlessness, inability to concentrate, weight gain or loss, emotional lability, and poor performance at school may be the presenting signs. Exophthalmos is rarely severe, and pretibial myxedema does not occur.

After surgery, there is a pronounced tendency for the disease to recur, unless an extensive subtotal resection is done; this increases the likelihood of postoperative hypothyroidism. RAI is avoided in individuals under the age of 25, if possible, because of the belief that children are most susceptible to induction of tumors. Thus individuals under age 25 are typically given a one- to two-year trial of antithyroid drugs before considering an alternative approach. Sometimes the drugs are continued for four to seven years if a remission does not occur after one year, in an attempt to delay a more drastic form of therapy until the child is older. Subtotal resection is an appropriate alternative therapy if a one- to two-year trial of drug treatment fails to induce remission or if the child is unable for some reason to maintain a drug regimen satisfactorily over the required months or years. RAI has been used only rarely, when some problem such as a severe reaction to both propylthiouracil and methimazole occurred, preventing adequate preparation for surgery and making the radiation hazard the least of the several evils.

Prognosis. Untreated hyperthyroidism can result in death from inanition, congestive heart failure, and other causes. All three major forms of therapy should result in prompt control of hyperthyroidism, and most patients subsequently lead a normal life. It is interesting to observe that none of the treatments are directed toward the cause of the illness. There is a tendency for a patient who responds to antithyroid drugs (less so to surgery) to have recurrence of the illness years later. This rarely if ever occurs in patients who have been adequately treated with radioactive iodide. *Delayed onset of hypothyroidism must always be watched for,* and therefore patients who have been treated with surgery, RAI, or antithyroid drugs should be followed indefinitely at yearly intervals. The prognosis for the ophthalmologic and dermatologic complications of Graves' disease is not so sanguine. Often these complications persist for years or even decades and may be incapacitating. As set out below, their course seems to be little influenced by the course of hyperthyroidism.

COMPLICATIONS OF GRAVES' DISEASE

Ophthalmopathy. Mild lid retraction and stare are probably effects of hyperthyroxinemia and in themselves are inconsequential. The remaining abnormalities of Graves' ophthalmopathy (described previously) appear to be due to infiltration of the retro-orbital tissues, extraocular muscles, and lacrimal gland by lymphocytes, plasma cells, and polymorphonuclear leukocytes, as well as an increase in tissue water, mucopolysaccharides, and mucoproteins. The extraocular muscles are often swollen to five or ten times their normal diameter, and the muscle fibers may be largely destroyed, leading in time to contractures. The lacrimal gland may likewise be severely swollen and damaged, although keratitis sicca does not appear. The initial presentation is as a cosmetic defect owing to proptosis and lid edema, often with tearing, burning, or retrobulbar pain. As the condition increases, the patient's difficulties include diplopia, susceptibility to infection, and the more severe complications such as loss of visual acuity, corneal ulceration, and panophthalmitis. Occasionally the process presents essentially as retrobulbar neuritis with loss of vision and few other signs. Infiltrative ophthalmopathy may occur at any time in relationship to the hyperthyroidism of Graves' disease. Most typically it develops with the onset of hyperthyroidism and subsides coincident with therapy. Changes of infiltrative ophthalmopathy are present in 10 to 20 per cent of patients with Graves' disease, and severe progressive ("malignant") exophthalmos occurs in 2 to 3 per cent.

The cause of this complication is unknown. Plasma of patients with progressive exophthalmos has been found to contain a factor which stimulates exophthalmos in certain test animals; the material is known as exophthalmos-producing substance (EPS). Some data suggest that EPS may be a fragment of TSH. Although LATS is present more frequently in patients with exophthalmos and typically in higher titers than in the average patient with Graves' disease, there is no evidence that LATS itself causes exophthalmos. No localization of gamma globulin in orbital tissue has been recognized, and retro-orbital tissue does not bind and neutralize LATS. Gamma globulin from exophthalmic patients is reported to bind to retrobulbar antigens in what may be a pseudoimmunologic reaction. These patients also have CMI against orbital antigens. Thus the belief exists that exophthalmos is an autoimmune phenomenon, but the cause and nature of the antigen are unknown. Although there is usually little diagnostic confusion, some degree of exophthalmos may occur in Cushing's syndrome, Turner's syndrome, and cirrhosis. Orbital tumor, sphenoid ridge meningioma, and thrombosis of the cavernous sinus must also be considered in reaching a diagnosis, especially when the exophthalmos is unilateral, and differentiation from other causes of optic neuritis must be considered.

Treatment. Patients with any degree of exophthalmos should be reassured that the process is almost invariably self-limiting. The eyes usually return to an essentially normal condition, although some degree of proptosis may persist. Useful local measures include shielding the eyes from excessive light and dust, avoidance of smoke and other irritants, and instillation of 10 per cent methylcellulose. Patients may find it useful to sleep with the head of the bed elevated, and to cover the eyes at night with cold saline compresses. If proptosis is severe, the lids may be taped together with cellophane tape which holds a piece of wet gauze and Saran Wrap over the eyelids. Diuresis (chlorothiazide, 500 mg every day) may be useful. Diplopia can be alleviated in part by covering one eye with a patch or obscuring one lens of the patient's glasses. Any sign of infection should be treated by appropriate antimicrobial ointments or, if necessary, by parenteral administration of antimicrobial drugs. If proptosis is severe, muscle function is progressively lost; if vision deteriorates, glucocorticoids may be helpful. Most patients who have active exophthalmos respond, whereas those who have stable changes do not. A common starting dose is 20 to 40 mg of prednisone daily in divided doses, although occasionally, and especially in patients with retrobulbar neuritis, doses up to 120 mg daily may be required. This medication induces Cushing's syndrome. It should be given for a few weeks, after which an attempt should be made to reduce the dose gradually. Sometimes improvement can be maintained with 10 to 20 mg of prednisone daily or every other day The response is variable, ranging from none at all to a complete remission of muscle paresis, papilledema, improvement in visual acuity, and recession of exophthalmos.

In patients resistant to steroids but requiring therapy, a Kronlein lateral decompression may be useful. In some clinics, other operative procedures such as the Naffziger supraorbital decompression or decompression into the antrum and ethmoids may be performed. The results are unpredictable, but often improvement is gained, and a few patients respond dramatically. In more chronic cases, operations on the muscles may restore binocular vision, and recession of the levator palpebrae superioris can help alleviate a disturbing stare. Muscle surgery, however, should not be done during the stage of progression but should be reserved for a time when fibrosis has occurred and diplopia is stable.

Lateral tarsorrhaphy is useful in patients whose eyes become damaged because the lids do not close during sleep. It provides some protection against corneal abrasions and infection and, sometimes, cosmetic benefits but has little effect on the basic process.

When these procedures have been exhausted, one sometimes resorts to methods whose basis is speculative. Some patients have been treated with azathioprine. Total surgical ablation of the thyroid followed by radioactive iodide has been proposed as being univer-

sally effective, but reports from several clinics indicate that it has no predictable effect on exophthalmos. Hypophysectomy, hypophysial stalk section, x-ray treatment of the pituitary, and x-ray treatment to the posterior aspects of the orbits have all been espoused, but none is of consistent value. The latter procedure, used extensively in earlier years, has been resuscitated recently by several thyroidologists who report sufficiently frequent successes to make it a possible first-line therapy, useful before steroids.

The *course and prognosis* of this illness are difficult to predict. In general, patients whose thyroid disease is successfully controlled will in time do well, although they may go through a period of severe discomfort. Typically, in 6 to 18 months, the activity of the process appears to abate, and there is subsequent slow but progressive evolution toward normality. Rarely sight is severely impaired or even lost, despite the administration of steroids and use of local x-ray and decompressive surgery. In general it is best to treat coincident hyperthyroidism by the most logical means irrespective of the ophthalmologic complication, and to maintain the patient in a *euthyroid* state after the initial control of the thyrotoxicosis. It is possible that RAI therapy, perhaps by inducing release of antigens and an augmented immune response, may exacerbate exophthalmos. With considerable reservation about the scientific basis for the recommendation, surgery or antithyroid drug therapy is preferred over RAI by the author for patients who have evidence of possibly dangerous exophthalmos.

Pretibial Myxedema (Fig. 7). In the simplest form, pretibial or localized myxedema presents as a firm bulging over the lateral aspect of the lower leg, just above the lateral malleolus. Often the skin is shiny and has an orange-peel appearance. The deposits may extend from an area of a few centimeters to involve multiple areas or even the entire anterior leg and foot. Occasionally, similar deposits can be found on the abdomen, hands, or face. Histologically there is an infiltration of mucopolysaccharide and mucoprotein material in the dermis, an increase in fluid, fraying of connective tissue fibers, and increase in collagen. The pattern is very similar to that observed in thyroid hormone deficiency, although there is no evidence that local thyroid hormone deficiency is present. There is a characteristic increase in hyaluronic acid in the lesions and also in uninvolved skin. The process almost invariably occurs in patients who have exophthalmos. It typically is first noted during the onset of hyperthyroidism, but may occur without associated hyperthyroidism and even in some patients whose thyroid appears to have been destroyed by thyroiditis and who are euthyroid or hypothyroid. Usually the process is not incapacitating, and except for its cosmetic disadvantage it requires no therapy. Topical application of triamcinolone ointment under Saran Wrap may be temporarily useful. It is striking that patients with this lesion characteristically have high and sometimes remarkable levels of serum LATS. If LATS disappears, so does the pretibial myxedema. Nevertheless, no etiologic relationship with LATS or other autoimmunity has been shown.

Thyroid Storm. Sudden severe exacerbation of hyperthyroidism may occur as a feature of the basic disease process or because of coincident infection, trauma, or surgery. Without treatment, and even with

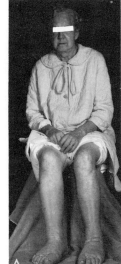
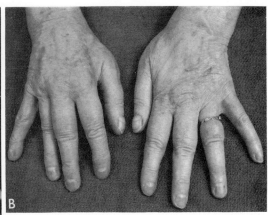

Figure 7. *A,* An example of severe "localized myxedema" involving the entire legs, feet, and hands, and coincident exophthalmos. *B,* Deposits of localized myxedema on the dorsum of the second, third and fourth digits, which are unusual manifestations of this condition.

therapy, the illness carries a *high mortality.* The patients develop severe hyperkinesis, tachycardia, hyperpyrexia, vomiting, and shock, and may drift into coma. Dehydration may be prominent.

If the diagnosis seems reasonable, treatment of the hyperthyroidism should begin at once, pending laboratory confirmation. Oral or parenteral blocking doses of an antithyroid drug should be given, followed in one hour with potassium iodide. The latter agent should cause a rapid remission in the symptoms of hyperthyroidism, and it is active in the presence of a methimazole block. The prior introduction of an antithyroid drug block ensures that the gland will not be flooded with iodide and guards against a subsequent flare of the illness. If the patient is not obtunded, sedatives such as phenobarbital (60 mg intramuscularly every four to six hours) or reserpine (1 to 3 mg every eight hours) should be given. Propranolol, 10 to 40 mg every six hours orally, or 2 to 10 mg every four hours intravenously, has recently been introduced for therapy of this condition and probably is useful, although experience is limited. This drug should be given with caution in the presence of congestive heart failure. Dehydration should be treated by appropriate fluid supplementation. Cultures should be taken to exclude infection, and antimicrobial therapy given as indicated. Adrenocortical steroids (50 to 100 mg of hydrocortisone intramuscularly every six hours) are given empirically. Occasionally plasma, blood, or norepinephrine is required to support the circulation. Hyperthermia can be treated by cooling. Digitalization may be needed to control congestive heart failure.

Treatment in the Presence of Heart Disease. Usually this complication occurs in older patients who would typically receive RAI. The FTI usually decreases progressively after RAI therapy, and no exacerbation of the heart disease (angina, congestive heart failure, myocardial infarction, arrhythmia) is seen. But if there is concern about therapy because of the gravity of the heart disease, several not very certain approaches can be suggested. RAI, followed in 24 hours by methimazole and then Lugol's solution, is probably safe and effective. Multiple low doses of RAI can be used, but therapeutic response is delayed.

Buhler, U. K., and DeGroot, L. J.: Effect of stable iodine on thyroid iodine release. J. Clin. Endocrinol. Metab., 29:1546, 1969.

Das, G., and Krieger, M.: Treatment of thyrotoxic storm with intravenous administration of propranolol. Ann. Intern. Med., 70:985, 1969.

Goldfischer, S., Moore, C. L., Johnson, A. B., Spiro, A. J., Valsamis, M. P., Wisniewski, H. K., Ritch, R. H., Norton, W. T., Rapin, I., and Gartner, L. M.: Peroxisomal and mitochondrial defects in the cerebro-hepato-renal syndrome. Science, 182:62, 1973.

Graves' Disease—1972. Second F. Raymond Keating, Jr., Memorial Symposium, April 14 and 15, 1972. Mayo Clinic Proceedings, November and December, 1972, pp. 803–995.

Lamki, L., Row, V. V., and Volpe, R.: Cell-mediated immunity in Graves' disease and in Hashimoto's thyroiditis as shown by the demonstration of migration inhibition factor (MIF). J. Clin. Endocrinol. Metab., 36:358, 1973.

Luft, R., Ikkos, D., Palmieri, G., Ernster, L., and Afzelius, B.: A case of severe hypermetabolism of non-thyroidal origin with a defect in the maintenance of mitochondrial respiratory control: A correlated clinical, biochemical, and morphological study. J. Clin. Invest., 41:1776, 1962.

McKenzie, J. M.: Humoral factors in the pathogenesis of Graves' disease. Physiol. Rev., 48:252, 1968.

Munro, R. E., Lamki, L., Row, V. V., and Volpe, R.: Cell-mediated immunity in the exophthalmos of Graves' disease as demonstrated by the migration inhibition factor (MIF) assay. J. Clin. Endocrinol. Metab., 37:286, 1973.

Nofal, M. M., Beierwaltes, W. H., and Patno, M. E.: Treatment of hyperthyroidism with sodium iodide I[131]. J.A.M.A., 197:605, 1966.

Rapoport, B., Caplan, R., and DeGroot, L. J.: Low dose sodium iodide I[131] therapy in Graves' disease. J.A.M.A., 224:1610, 1973.

Sterling, K., Refetoff, S., and Selenkow, H. A.: T₃ toxicosis—thyrotoxicosis due to elevated serum triiodothyronine levels. J.A.M.A., 213:571, 1970.

Wilson, W. R., Theilen, E. O., Hege, J. H., and Valenca, M. R.: Effects of beta-adrenergic receptor blockade in normal subjects before, during, and after triiodothyronine-induced hyperthyroidism. J. Clin. Invest., 45:1159, 1966.

838. THYROIDITIS

Three types of thyroiditis are recognized: chronic, acute, and subacute. Chronic thyroiditis is not an infection nor, in the usual sense, an inflammation, and therefore the name may be inappropriate. Two varieties are defined by pathologists: lymphocytic thyroiditis and Riedel's struma. In lymphocytic thyroiditis (Hashimoto's thyroiditis, struma lymphomatosa), the thyroid is replaced to a varying degree by lymphocytes forming germinal centers and fibrous tissue, leading to goiter, parenchymal destruction, and thyroid hormone insufficiency. Riedel's thyroiditis (ligneous thyroiditis) is a possibly related, slowly progressive fibrosis of the thyroid, of great rarity. These two processes will be considered separately, with the main emphasis on Hashimoto's thyroiditis.

HASHIMOTO'S THYROIDITIS

Etiology and Pathogenesis. Hashimoto's thyroiditis is thought to be an autoimmune disease. In 1956, Doniach and Roitt, and Witebsky, coincidentally discovered antibodies to thyroid antigens in patients with this illness. The thyroid antigen-antibody systems that are now known include (1) antibodies reacting with thyroglobulin, usually detected by the tanned red cell agglutination test; (2) antibodies reacting with a component of thyroid cytoplasm, detected by the immunofluorescent technique, by a complement-fixing reaction with thyroid microsomes, or by a variation of the tanned red cell technique; and (3) antibodies reacting with a colloidal antigen which is distinct from thyroglobulin. When antibodies against thyroglobulin and thyroid cell cytoplasm are both measured, about 95 per cent of patients with Hashimoto's thyroiditis have a positive titer in one or both tests, and frequently the titers are very high.

Thyroiditis with a similar histologic pattern can be induced by immunization of animals with thyroid tissue. The experimentally induced disease cannot be transferred from animal to animal by serum, but can be transferred in inbred guinea pigs by transfer of lymphocytes. This observation, as well as the poor correlation of circulating antibody titers with the course of the disease, suggested that *cell-mediated immunity* (CMI) was important in the destruction of thyroid cells. This has been abundantly confirmed in the past few years by studies demonstrating CMI by in vitro techniques such as leukocyte migration inhibition assay and lymphotoxin assay. Patients with thyroiditis, primary thyroid failure, and Graves' disease are found to have lymphocytes presensitized to thyroid antigens. The antigens are associated with particulate fragments of the cell. CMI is most obvious in patients with primary myxedema, and is less intense in patients with thyroiditis or Graves' disease.

Why individuals should produce antibodies against thyroid antigens remains a mystery. It might be supposed that an abnormal antigen exists in the cells, but none has been found. It has been suggested that thyroglobulin or other thyroid antigens are normally hidden from the organism during fetal life when immune tolerance is established, and that subsequent escape of the thyroglobulin from the thyroid follicle could induce immunity in the adult. This seems unlikely, because thyroglobulin normally circulates in the blood. Possibly viral infection or other injury could alter thyroid tissue and produce neoantigens. There is a strong hereditary pattern for the illness, and the propensity to produce antibodies is transmitted as a dominant trait. Further, thyroiditis is associated with a number of other possibly autoimmune diseases, including pernicious anemia, idiopathic adrenal insufficiency, rheumatoid arthritis, Sjögren's syndrome, ulcerative colitis, lupoid hepatitis, disseminated lupus erythematosus, and hemolytic anemia. The relationship to pernicious anemia is especially prominent. Fifty per cent of patients with pernicious anemia have antibodies against thyroid tissue antigens, and the converse is also true. There is also an associated increased incidence of antibodies against parathyroid tissue, and possibly of antibodies against the pancreas and ovary. These observations suggest that some ill-understood hereditarily defined abnormality in immune homeostasis occurs in these patients, predisposing them to develop reactivity to self-antigens.

In the author's view, Graves' disease, Hashimoto's thyroiditis, and myxedema are variants of a common process. Among the relatives of patients with one of these three diseases, it is typical to find examples of the other two. The histology of Graves' disease shades into that of Hashimoto's thyroiditis, and the histology of idiopathic thyroid failure is interpreted by some as the end-stage of lymphocytic and fibrotic replacement of the thyroid. Antibody titers against thyroid cell antigens are high in each condition. It is as if an abnormality in immune homeostasis were at the root of each illness, possibly triggered by some environmental factor. Perhaps with the development of antithyroglobulin and anticytoplasmic antibodies, plus a cell-mediated response, Hashimoto's thyroiditis occurs. If the destructive cell-mediated response is severe, the process may go on to thyroid failure. If, in addition to or in the absence of the other antibodies, LATS or other thyroid-stimulating antibodies are formed, and if the thyroid is capable of responding, thyroid hyperplasia and hypersecretion occur with the picture of Graves' disease. Although this formulation is by no means universally accepted, it embodies the thinking of many workers in the field.

Pathology (Fig. 8). On gross inspection the thyroid appears pale yellow-tan and has a lumpy surface. The normal thyroid structure is replaced with dense infiltration by lymphocytes, and lymphoid germinal centers are evident. The remaining thyroid tissue often shows hyperplasia, with small empty follicles. The cells frequently are enlarged and eosinophilic. In many specimens, fibrosis is prominent. The thymus is characteristically enlarged, and germinal centers are seen. There may be lymph nodes showing reactive hyperplasia in the area surrounding the thyroid.

Clinical Manifestations. This illness occurs with an incidence roughly similar to that of Graves' disease. There is good evidence that it has tripled in frequency in the past three decades. Hashimoto's thyroiditis may present with thyroid enlargement or symptoms of hypothyroidism. The disease is 20 times as frequent in women as in men. It can occur even in young children, but is most common between ages 30 and 50. In children the process is occasionally seen to subside spontaneously. In other instances, extensive destruction of the gland can lead to thyroid failure and growth retardation (Fig. 8). Most characteristic is the thyroid enlargement, which varies from two to five times normal, averaging 30 to 50 grams. The gland may be soft, normal, or firm, and there is no thrill or bruit. The surface may feel lobulated, but distinct nodules are usually not found. Their presence suggests that a mass of lymph nodes is present or that a thyroid adenoma or malignancy is present. Typically the pyramidal lobe is palpable. Sometimes patients complain of choking or difficulty in swallowing or of a sensation of local pressure, but usually the goiter is asymptomatic. Rarely, the illness proceeds more rapidly, and there are pain and tenderness in the thyroid gland. The trachea is charac-

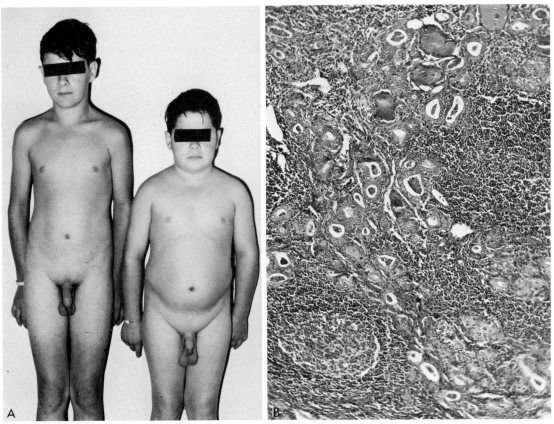

Figure 8. *A,* Identical twins, age 12, both of whom developed Hashimoto's thyroiditis. One boy ceased growing at age 8 and was hypothyroid. *B,* Biopsy specimen from one twin, showing small hyperplastic residual follicles, fibrosis, and lymphocytic infiltration. (Photographs provided by Dr. Frank Milgram.)

teristically in the midline. The remainder of the physical examination is unremarkable unless there are signs of hypothyroidism.

The presence of an asymptomatic diffuse thyroid enlargement (with a palpable pyramidal lobe) in a middle-aged woman who appears to be euthyroid is indicative of Hashimoto's thyroiditis. The serum thyroxine may be normal or depressed, depending on the stage of development of the process. The PBI may be low, normal, or elevated owing to butanol-insoluble iodinated albumin in plasma. This can be detected by simultaneous determination of the PBI and BEI, or the PBI and serum T_4. The RAIU test may be elevated, normal, or low, but usually is normal unless the patient has developed hypothyroidism. Other tests of thyroid function reflect the ability of the thyroid to produce hormone. Characteristically, the scintiscan shows an enlarged thyroid with a smooth outline and diffuse distribution of the isotope. Fluorescent scans show a diminution or virtual absence of thyroid-stable iodine. The diagnosis can be made if the tanned red cell (TRC) agglutination titer is positive at a greater than 1:2560 dilution or if there is a very strongly positive test for anticytoplasmic antibodies. However, only 60 per cent of the patients have a positive TRC, and only 95 per cent are positive if both tests are performed. If it seems imperative that the diagnosis be established and the antibody response is not in the diagnostic range, needle biopsy is both safe and effective. A diagnostic piece of tissue will be obtained in perhaps 80 per cent of the biopsies. Failure of

radioactive iodide uptake to rise after administration of TSH is also suggestive, indicating the syndrome of low thyroid reserve. Further, some patients will show a positive perchlorate discharge test. Occasionally there are striking elevations of the serum gamma globulin.

Therapy. In patients with thyroid deficiency, therapy with thyroid hormone is indicated. It is also useful to give replacement therapy to euthyroid individuals who have developed a goiter causing a cosmetic defect or local symptoms, or to prevent further thyroid enlargement. In young patients, treatment results in disappearance of the goiter, but in older persons whose thyroid enlargement has been present for a prolonged period, it may have little effect. When the thyroid is minimally enlarged, it is debatable whether therapy is indicated. Serial biopsies have shown that the histologic picture may not change over a decade. Further, there is no evidence that the process tends to spread to other organs.

Usually therapy is with thyroid hormone, although there are reports of other approaches. In children steroid therapy causes diminution of goiter and suppresses antibody titers, but the entire process recurs when therapy is withdrawn. This approach does not appear to have merit.

Prognosis. There is a tendency for the involved thyroid to enlarge slowly and for hypothyroidism to develop. Spontaneous thyroid atrophy may occur, and it is hypothesized that this sequence may be the cause of "idiopathic" myxedema.

RIEDEL'S THYROIDITIS

In Riedel's thyroiditis, a very uncommon condition, the gland is replaced by a mass of dense, infiltrative fibrotic tissue which extends into the capsule of the thyroid, the trachea, and the surrounding strap muscles. Patients seek attention because of local symptoms such as choking or difficult swallowing, because a small goiter is observed, or because of hypothyroidism. The disease is more frequent in women than in men and characteristically occurs after age 40. Some circumstantial evidence suggests that it is a variant of Hashimoto's thyroiditis. Patients have been observed who first had typical lymphocytic thyroiditis but later had the histology of Riedel's struma. On examination, the thyroid is found to be of normal size, reduced in bulk, or moderately enlarged, and is unusually firm and densely adherent to the trachea. Thyroid function tests reveal normal function or hypothyroidism. There is no specific diagnostic test, and antibody titers to thyroid antigen are not elevated in this condition as in Hashimoto's thyroiditis.

Diagnosis is usually made at operation, when the surgeon finds fibrotic thyroid tissue bound to the trachea. Often the process suggests a sclerosing carcinoma, and the diagnosis is made on frozen sections. The only known therapy is surgery if pressure symptoms are sufficient to warrant this approach. The gland may be resected or the isthmus may be exposed and divided, allowing the two halves of the gland to fall laterally, thus avoiding tracheal constriction. Since resection may cause loss of the parathyroids or recurrent laryngeal nerve, simple division of the isthmus and mobilization of the lateral lobes is the preferred approach. Thyroid hormone therapy may be required.

An association has been suggested between this process and sclerosing cholangitis, mediastinal fibrosis, and periureteral fibrosis (see Ch. 107). Since some of these processes may respond to steroid administration, it is possible that this would be a useful therapy in Riedel's thyroiditis; information on this therapeutic approach is not available.

ACUTE THYROIDITIS

Acute and subacute thyroiditis are etiologically unrelated. Both are transient inflammatory reactions involving the thyroid, and they are clinically distinct from chronic thyroiditis. "Acute thyroiditis" (acute infectious thyroiditis, suppurative thyroiditis) means an uncommon condition in which the thyroid gland is invaded by pathogenic bacteria. This occurs as part of a cellulitis in the neck or because of infection of a cyst in a multinodular goiter. Usually the patient presents with fever, pain in the neck, and a mass involving the thyroid area. The area is erythematous and tender to palpation. Often only one portion of the thyroid is involved, and contiguous infection is evident. The leukocyte count is elevated. The serum thyroxine is normal. On scintiscan there may be some depression of radioiodine uptake in a portion of the thyroid, but RAIU is usually normal.

Cultures should be taken and appropriate antimicrobials administered. With suitable therapy, the process subsides rapidly. Occasionally resection of a portion of the thyroid is indicated.

SUBACUTE THYROIDITIS

Subacute thyroiditis (granulomatous thyroiditis, acute thyroiditis, De Quervain's thyroiditis) is an inflammatory condition of the thyroid causing painful enlargement, lasting over a period of weeks or months, with a prominent tendency to relapse. Its incidence is not known, but it appears to be about one tenth as common as Graves' disease.

Etiology. Subacute thyroiditis frequently occurs two to three weeks after viral upper respiratory infection. This association suggests that the thyroiditis represents an immunologic response to the viral infection. Other data imply that direct viral invasion of the thyroid may be the cause. Thyroiditis has occurred in outbreaks of mumps, and the mumps virus has been cultured from the thyroid. Numerous other attempts at viral culture have been negative. Volpe finds that most patients have antiviral antibody titers which are high at the time of diagnosis, and tend to fall progressively over subsequent weeks. Antibodies are frequently found against common pathogens such as echovirus, coxsackievirus, and adenovirus, and often one finds significant changes in titers against two or even three viral antigens. The reported occurrence with mumps virus or in mumps epidemics may represent one possible etiology, but is not the most common. The causation remains obscure.

Pathology. The thyroid may be enlarged with dense infiltration by polymorphonuclear cells, lymphocytes, and plasma cells. Fibrosis is prominent. Many pyknotic thyroid follicular cells are apparent. The follicular structure is often destroyed, and in its place are found small granulomas with giant cells. There is poor correlation between the histologic abnormalities, which may be extreme, and the clinical picture.

Clinical Manifestations. Subacute thyroiditis may be painful and disabling, but it does not last long. The patient usually notices gradual onset of severe pain and tenderness involving one or both sides of the lower neck, sometimes localized to the thyroid. The process may begin in one lobe and travel over several days to the other. There may be fullness and the sensation of pressure. Pain typically radiates up the lateral aspects of the neck and into the jaw and ear. Swallowing may be uncomfortable, causing the patient to choke over saliva. There are often mild fever, sore throat, malaise, and fatigue. Sometimes the process is entirely asymptomatic.

On examination the thyroid is enlarged and often extremely tender. The process may be restricted to one portion of a lobe or may involve the entire gland. Lymph nodes are usually not enlarged. Sometimes the patient develops symptoms and signs of mild hyperthyroidism, but usually the clinical status is that of euthyroidism or rarely hypothyroidism. The disease tends to remit spontaneously or because of therapy, only to recur after a period of two to three weeks, and this cycle may recur several times. Over the course of one to twelve months the process finally subsides.

Diagnosis. The typical history of pain and the tender enlargement of the thyroid are highly suggestive of subacute thyroiditis. The leukocyte count may be elevated to 15,000 to 20,000, or may be normal. The sedimentation rate is characteristically high, and may reach 100 mm per hour (Westergren). Anemia is said to accompany the illness, although the cause is unknown.

On scan, RAIU is suppressed in the involved portion of the gland, which may be one lobe or the entire thyroid, and the RAIU is often zero. Fluorescent scanning shows the involved thyroid tissue to have lost all iodine stores. The PBI, T_4, and FTI may be elevated because of iodoprotein or excess thyroid hormone released during the acute phase of the illness, making the patient thyrotoxic. During recovery, the TSH and RAIU may be transiently elevated while T_4 is depressed, and then over a period of two to three months all tests return to normal. Antibody titers against thyroid antigens may be transiently demonstrable, but they rarely if ever reach the levels found in Hashimoto's thyroiditis, and the responses are not sustained.

This process can usually be differentiated from acute thyroiditis because of the localization to the thyroid, absence of signs of infection, characteristically high sedimentation rate, and depressed radioactive iodide uptake. Occasionally, aspiration biopsy may be necessary to prove the diagnosis. Rarely, Hashimoto's thyroiditis presents with a rather acute and painful onset, and it may be difficult to make the distinction short of biopsy. Sometimes the diagnosis of Graves' disease is suggested by a painless goiter and thyrotoxicosis, but in these cases the patient fails to have the appropriate history or physical evidence of long-term thyrotoxicosis. Exogenous iodine can depress RAIU in Graves' disease to near zero, offering another source of confusion. Serial observations over a few weeks will identify the proper diagnosis.

Therapy. In mild cases the inflammatory process subsides spontaneously, and all that is needed is mild analgesia. Aspirin, up to 6 grams daily, is useful in suppressing the pain. It is probably advantageous to give desiccated thyroid if the disease has gone on for more than a few days, because TSH stimulation may exacerbate the process. If the illness does not subside with these simple measures, corticosteroids are useful; 20 to 40 mg of prednisone is given daily for a period of one to four weeks, with progressive diminution of the dose as symptoms are controlled. Often withdrawal of steroids is followed by exacerbation of the process, and such a cycle may recur several times before the illness eventually subsides. Rarely, a chronic, tender enlargement of the thyroid persists despite therapy and requires surgical resection.

Prognosis. In the author's experience, all patients with subacute thyroiditis, with the exception of one who required surgery, have eventually returned to normal thyroid function and become asymptomatic. It is reported that up to 10 per cent of the patients develop permanent hypothyroidism.

Bastenie, P. A.: Contribution à l'étiologie du myxoedème spontane de l'adulte. Bull. Acad. R. Med. Belg., 9:179, 1944.
Calder, E. A., McLeman, D., Barnes, E. W., and Irvine, W. J.: The effect of thyroid antigens on the in vitro migration of leukocytes from patients with Hashimoto's thyroiditis. Clin. Exp. Immunol., 12:429, 1972.
DeGroot, L. J., Hall, R., McDermott, W. V., and Davis, A. M.: Hashimoto's thyroiditis, a genetically conditioned disease. N. Engl. J. Med., 267:267, 1962.
Greene, J. N.: Subacute thyroiditis. Am. J. Med., 51:97, 1971.
Ling, S. M., Kaplan, S. A., Weitzman, J. V., Reed, G. B., Costin, G., and Larding, B. H.: Euthyroid goiter in children: Correlation of needle biopsy with other clinical and laboratory findings in chronic lymphocytic thyroiditis and simple goiter. Pediatrics, 44:695, 1969.
McConahey, W. M., Keating, F. R., Jr., Beahrs, O. H., and Woolner, L. B.: On the increasing occurrence of Hashimoto's thyroiditis. J. Clin. Endocrinol. Metab., 22:542, 1962.
McMaster, P. R. B., and Lerner, E. M.: The transfer of allergic thyroiditis in histocompatible guinea pigs by lymph node cells. J. Immunol., 99:208, 1967.
Rapoport, B., Block, M. B., Hoffer, P. B., and DeGroot, L. J.: Depletion of thyroid iodine during subacute thyroiditis. J. Clin. Endocrinol. Metab., 36:610, 1973.
Roitt, I. M., and Doniach, D.: Thyroid autoimmunity. Br. Med. Bull., 16:152, 1960.

839. HYPOTHYROIDISM AND MYXEDEMA

Hypothyroidism (Gull's disease) refers to the morbid state characterized by progressive slowing of all bodily activities owing to deficiency in thyroid hormone. The severest form is known as myxedema because of the characteristic infiltration of the skin by nonpitting, mucinous edema.

Etiology. Probably most cases of *"idiopathic"* hypothyroidism and myxedema develop as the end-stage of Hashimoto's thyroiditis. The histologic pattern confirms this suggestion; antithyroglobulin and anticytoplasmic antibody are frequently present in high titers, and progress from Hashimoto's thyroiditis to hypothyroidism can be observed. More commonly, thyroid failure occurs because of administration of RAI to control the thyrotoxicosis in Graves' disease or after subtotal thyroidectomy for Graves' disease, multinodular goiter, or Hashimoto's thyroiditis. Hypothyroidism sometimes occurs as part of the presentation of Graves' syndrome, with coincident exophthalmos and pretibial myxedema. Less frequently, hypothyroidism occurs as the only feature of hypopituitarism because of isolated failure of the pituitary to produce TSH or because of damage in the hypothalamus inhibiting TRH secretion. Hypothyroidism is reported to occur in 10 per cent of patients who have had subacute thyroiditis (see Ch. 838). Some patients with multinodular goiter are hypothyroid. Hypothyroidism is also found in patients with congenital metabolic defects of thyroid hormone synthesis, is sometimes caused by severe iodine deficiency in areas of endemic goiter, and can be induced by medications such as the antithyroid drugs, resorcinol, or para-aminosalicylic acid. In some individuals, administration of iodine (more than 6 mg per day) induces inhibition of thyroid hormone synthesis and release, with the development of goiter and hypothyroidism.

Pathogenesis and Pathology. Whatever the cause of thyroid hormone deprivation, the effects are similar. Over a period of months and years, there is progressive infiltration of the skin by mucoprotein and mucopolysaccharides, giving a puffy appearance. Similar deposits of mucopolysaccharide are reported to occur under the sarcolemma of striated muscle. Muscle fibers become frayed, and the cells may become necrotic. Effusion can occur in any serosal space. Thickening of joint capsules and joint effusion also occur. There is a generalized decreased rate of nucleic acid and protein synthesis, and almost all enzyme systems are reported to be underactive.

In idiopathic myxedema the thyroid is replaced by scar tissue containing a few scattered thyroid cells and many lymphocytes. In secondary hypothyroidism resulting from pituitary failure, the thyroid is small, with flattened, cuboidal epithelium and acini filled with colloid. In other conditions the pathology is that of the primary process. In goiter resulting from metabolic defects in hormone formation or the action of thyroid blocking drugs or iodide, the characteristic picture is extreme hyperplasia, which may look much like papillary adenocarcinoma.

Clinical Manifestations. Quite typically the patient has no complaints. He or, more commonly, she may be brought to the doctor because someone else recognized unusual sluggishness, weight gain, or sleepiness. Sometimes the presenting symptom is edema or menorrhagia. We have seen several women whose menorrhagia, caused by myxedema, was treated first by hysterectomy and only later by thyroid hormone. The symptoms and signs are in proportion to the severity and duration of the illness. In advanced cases the diagnosis is obvious. The patient notices fatigue and somnolence, often falling asleep at inopportune times. There is marked increase in sensitivity to cold. Hearing may be diminished. The eyes are puffy or watery. The hair is brittle, sparse, and coarse; curl tends to be lost. The eyebrows are sparse, and the outer third may be missing. The skin is thickened and dry, and sweating rarely occurs. There is generalized thickening and puffiness of the face and extremities; pitting is not characteristic, but may occur in the presence of fluid retention or congestive heart failure. True obesity is not characteristic. The patients have a jocular air about them, their answers to questions often being delayed and seemingly humorous but inappropriate. As a group they tend to be uncomplaining and hardly recognize the marked change that may have occurred in their appearance and behavior. The tongue is thick, and papillae may be atrophic, especially if there is coincident pernicious anemia, which occurs in 12 per cent of patients with idiopathic thyroid failure. The thyroid may be absent or palpable, depending on the etiology. The heart is quiet, the pulse is slow, and diastolic blood pressure may be elevated. Although pericardial effusion is frequently present, physical signs of tamponade are rarely if ever found. Pleural effusion may occur, and the abdomen may be distended by ascites. These fluids may have a high specific gravity. The patient complains of severe constipation, and ileus and megacolon have been reported. Irregular menstrual pattern and severe menorrhagia frequently occur in younger women. Deep tendon reflex relaxation time is markedly prolonged. Other neurologic signs include diminished hearing, paresthesias, vertigo, and ataxia with lateral column signs. Often the skin shows perifollicular keratoses. The nails may be thickened. Joint stiffness, thickening of the joint capsules, joint effusion, arthritis, and bursitis are occasionally seen.

Overt *psychosis* may develop as a manifestation of prolonged and severe myxedema. Hallucinations, disorientation, paranoia, and attempted suicide have been reported. With substitution therapy, the psychosis usually clears, although some patients never regain sanity. Occasionally patients develop overt psychosis as therapy is introduced. The name "myxedema madness" has been applied to these conditions.

The degree of abnormality is by no means always as great as that described. In mild hypothyroidism it may be impossible to make a clinical distinction from the normal state.

Diagnosis. In the classic case the diagnosis can be confirmed at the bedside by evaluation of the slow relaxation time of the Achilles tendon reflexes. Other tendon jerks are less reliable. The PBI and serum T_4 are characteristically low, as is the RAIU, except in individuals who have a block in thyroid hormone formation as a cause of their thyroprivia. Both the T_4 and the RAIU tend to be less severely depressed in patients with hypothyroidism of pituitary origin, and in these subjects the values tend to overlap the normal range. The RAIU is not a very useful test now, because normal values (down to 10 per cent) overlap the values found in hypothyroid patients. The BMR is depressed, the serum cholesterol and carotene are elevated, and there may be marked elevation of the enzymes GOT, LDH, and CPK. Uric acid is sometimes elevated. The EKG shows slow rate and low voltage. Most patients have anemia. This may be due to menorrhagia causing iron deficiency or to coincident pernicious anemia, or may be normocytic or macrocytic and be related solely to hypothyroidism. Pernicious anemia, nephritis, uremia, and mongolism are occasional causes for confusion in differential diagnosis.

After the conclusion is reached that the patient is hypothyroid, it is imperative that the cause be evaluated. It there is atrophy of thyroid tissue, the presence of thyroiditis may be ascertained by tests for antithyroglobulin and anticytoplasmic antibodies. Goiter and a positive $KClO_4$ discharge test may be found in hypothyroidism caused by congenital metabolic defects, including Pendred's syndrome and Hashimoto's thyroiditis. Pituitary dysfunction should be considered unless there is strong evidence incriminating primary thyroid failure. In primary thyroid failure, the sella turcica is usually normal, but it may be enlarged in cretins and in some adults with longstanding myxedema. Plasma cortisol is normal, although ketosteroid and hydroxycorticoid excretion is depressed, and the adrenal response to metyrapone may be delayed and low. Follicle-stimulating hormone is characteristically elevated in postmenopausal women with primary thyroid failure, but is occasionally low, returning to an elevated level after therapy with thyroid hormone has been started. Growth hormone should be present in primary thyroid failure, but the response to insulin hypoglycemia is often depressed. TSH is characteristically very high in primary thyroid failure, often 20 to 1000 μU per milliliter. Absent or normal TSH and a failure to respond to exogenous TRH indicate pituitary damage. Hypothyroidism and a normal TSH which responds to exogenous TRH identify "hypothalamic hypothyroidism." This condition may be the cause of most instances of secondary hypothyroidism in children, and can be acquired by trauma or neoplastic lesions.

Therapy. Treatment with desiccated thyroid is a remarkably satisfactory therapeutic maneuver. Usually it is advantageous to initiate treatment with a low dose of hormone, such as 15 or 30 mg of USP desiccated thyroid daily or the equivalent dose of one of the synthetic mixtures of T_4 and T_3 (liotrix). Subsequent increments of 15 or 30 mg are made at intervals of 7 to 14 days, until a full replacement dosage is reached in two to three months. Marked improvement should be seen with 30 mg. The usual replacement dosage is 90 to 120 mg of desiccated thyroid daily given in one dose, although a range of 60 to 200 mg per day is found, with some dependence upon patient's size. Equivalent doses of L-thyroxine (100 μg = 60 mg USP desiccated thyroid) or L-triiodothyronine (37.5 μg = 60 mg USP desiccated thyroid), may be used for replacement therapy. If desiccated thyroid or liotrix is used to achieve replacement therapy, the FTI should be in the normal range when the patient is optimally replaced. Using thyroxine alone, the T_4 or FTI will be in the upper range of normal or slightly elevated. When T_3 is given, the T_4 or FTI will be near zero even when replacement is quite adequate.

In patients who have congestive heart failure, previous myocardial infarction, or angina pectoris, it is best to initiate therapy very gradually. Often such conditions are exacerbated by therapy, although some patients cease to have angina pectoris on replacement of the hormone. Triiodothyronine is theoretically useful because of the more rapid disappearance of its effect should toxicity be encountered, but in most patients, replacement with desiccated thyroid or liotrix is preferred, because with these medications the T_4 is within the normal range during adequate therapy and is a useful guide.

The best guide to treatment is the patient's and the physician's progressive re-evaluation of the clinical status. There should be a return to a normal and steady weight, a disappearance of all symptoms, and a feeling of well-being. Severe myalgias and arthralgias may occur during therapy, but disappear gradually if therapy is continued. It is sometimes useful to increase the dose until symptoms of thyroid hormone excess appear and then return to a slightly lower dose, in order to be certain that sufficient medication is administered. Once the dosage is established, the patient may take exogenous hormone for years or decades without change. Patients must be cautioned to continue taking the medication indefinitely, for some will feel that treatment is no longer needed once well-being has been restored. It is especially important that women be urged to continue the medication without interruption and at the same dosage level throughout pregnancy. Dosage need not be changed in preparation for or during surgery.

Prognosis. The prognosis for treatment of hypothyroidism in the ambulatory patient is excellent; usually there is a complete return to normal health.

SPECIAL PROBLEMS IN HYPOTHYROIDISM

Myxedema Coma. As myxedema worsens, the affected individual becomes more and more lethargic, and episodes of apparent sleep may become frequent, culminating in severe obtundation or even coma from which the patient cannot be aroused. In other instances coma develops abruptly during an intercurrent illness such as pyelonephritis, pneumonia, or cellulitis. Patients with severe myxedema may develop sepsis with minimal symptoms, no fever, and little leukocytosis.

Typically, if a history is available, it is that the patient had previous surgery or radioactive iodine therapy for hyperthyroidism, did well for a number of years afterward, but then over five or ten years gradually lapsed into hypothyroidism, finally developing coma. Often such people have received replacement therapy with thyroid hormone, but have for some reason discontinued it.

The mechanism of myxedema coma is unknown.

Blood flow to the brain is diminished, but oxygen consumption is allegedly not diminished. Altered cortical activity is apparent in sluggish mentation and slowing of the alpha rhythm of the EEG. The pathologic correlates of these changes are not well known. Progressive hypothermia, hypoglycemia, and carbon dioxide retention may be specific causes of coma in some patients.

The clinical manifestations are fundamentally those of severe myxedema, as described before. Localizing neurologic signs are characteristically absent. The reflexes are symmetrical and depressed, and the relaxation time is delayed. Babinski reflex may be evident. Often the patients are severely obtunded rather than comatose, and they are typically disoriented. It may be possible to arouse the patient from his stupor, only to have him immediately slip back into a depressed state. The temperature should be carefully recorded, and may be as low as 29.5 to 30.5° C.

The diagnosis is usually suggested by physical examination which reveals signs of advanced hypothyroidism and cutaneous myxedema. The scar of a thyroidectomy, a history of previous thyroid surgery or radioactive iodide treatment, and a history of thyroid therapy are important diagnostic clues. The thyroid is impalpable or replaced by fibrous tissue. Careful search should be made for precipitating causes such as infection of the lungs or urinary tract, as well as other causes of coma, e.g., cerebrovascular accidents, renal and hepatic failure, and drug ingestion. The last-named cause is important, because hypothyroid patients are excessively sensitive to the usual doses of barbiturates and opiates. Diagnosis rests on finding abnormally low blood levels of thyroid hormone, but usually these tests are not immediately available. Clinical judgment is called for in the interim; this can sometimes be supplemented by measurement of the deep tendon reflex relaxation time. Severe hyponatremia and hypoglycemia may occur as a manifestation of primary or secondary thyroid failure. The usual measures needed for differential diagnosis of primary and secondary thyroid failure, including FTI, antibody tests, TSH levels, measurement of plasma cortisol, skull films, and measurement of plasma LH and FSH, should be carried out. Carbon dioxide retention should be excluded, if necessary, by arterial gas determination, because hypoventilation may induce coma in some patients. If the diagnosis seems probable but cannot be established at the time the patient is admitted, it is best to institute treatment without a diagnosis because of the urgency of the condition.

The appropriate treatment remains a matter of debate. Failure has consistently been reported in patients treated with very slow supplementation of thyroid hormone, and an impressive series of successes has been reported in patients given a massive intravenous dose of T_4 or T_3 in an attempt to return the circulating thyroid hormone to normal levels without delay. Approximately 300 μg of thyroxine is administered intravenously and 100 to 200 μg is given daily thereafter with monitoring of the plasma thyroid hormone blood levels. Hypothermia is best treated by covering the patient with warm blankets and allowing endogenous body heat to bring up the temperature gradually. Rapid warming by means of electrical blankets or hot baths has resulted in shock and death. Appropriate antimicrobial therapy should be given if there is evidence of infection. If there is carbon dioxide retention, the patient should be placed on a respirator to provide an adequate ventilatory exchange. If there is any suggestion of pituitary failure, shock, or hyponatremia suggestive of adrenal steroid insufficiency, the patient should be given 100 to 200 mg of hydrocortisone intravenously. Occasionally blood pressure must be supported by transfusions or by use of norepinephrine. Fluid and electrolyte therapy should be given with caution; since cutaneous and respiratory losses are extremely small, 600 to 1000 ml of fluid per day, of which one third to one half is a balanced electrolyte solution, is sufficient. Overhydration is the major problem in therapy and often leads to congestive failure, cerebral edema, and death. Hyponatremia should be treated preferably by fluid restriction rather than by administration of hypertonic saline, because with thyroid hormone therapy excess stored salt in myxedema tissue is mobilized and may precipitate congestive failure.

If the patient survives the critical first few days and is able to take medication orally, replacement therapy can be switched to any standard preparation of thyroid hormone. The blood thyroxine level should be checked to assay adequacy of replacement.

Despite some advances in understanding of the precipitating causes of this illness, therapy remains unsatisfactory, and mortality rates of 50 to 90 per cent are reported.

Myxedema Heart. Cardiomegaly and congestive failure often accompany myxedema. The EKG shows low voltage, flattened T waves, and occasionally first degree AV block. Is there a specific variety of heart disease associated with thyroid hormone deficiency? Obviously patients who develop myxedema may be in the older age groups expected to have a high incidence of hypertension and coronary artery disease. The coexistence of mild hypertension, which may be alleviated by therapy with thyroid hormone, has previously been noted. Another and probably more common cause of presumptive cardiomegaly is the frequent pericardial effusion found in this illness. The pericardial effusion is usually functionally insignificant, but rare instances of cardiac tamponade have been reported.

Atherosclerosis was for many years thought not to be accelerated by hypothyroidism, but present evidence indicates that there is an association between these two conditions.

In addition, it appears that severe myxedema can be associated with a specific cardiac lesion, evident pathologically as an edema of the myocardium, deposition of mucopolysaccharides and mucoproteins between the cells, fraying of cardiac myofibrils, and death and necrosis of cells. Probably this represents a very advanced stage of myxedema, and these changes are not found in most patients dying of myxedema coma.

Although the effusion, decreased cardiac output, and EKG changes are manifestations of hypothyroidism per se, most instances of heart failure associated with myxedema are probably due to coexistent organic heart disease. Occasionally the problem may not be overt before institution of therapy because of the lesser cardiac output required in the hypothyroid patient. With therapy increased demands are put upon the heart, and congestive failure, angina, and even myocardial infarction may occur.

Begg, T. B., and Hall, R.: Iodide goiter and hypothyroidism. Quart. J. Med., 32:351, 1963.

Bland, J. H., and Frymoyer, J. W.: Rheumatic syndromes of myxedema. N. Engl. J. Med., 282:1171, 1970.
Holvey, D. N., Goodner, C. J., Nicoloff, J. T., and Dowling, J. T.: Treatment of myxedema coma with intravenous thyroxine. Arch. Intern. Med., 113:89, 1964.
Sanders, V.: Neurologic manifestations of myxedema. N. Engl. J. Med., 266:547, 1962.

840. MULTINODULAR GOITER

Multinodular goiter refers to an enlargement of the thyroid associated with more than one identifiable nodule. In fact the condition more specifically refers to a replacement of the normal homogeneous cytostructure of the thyroid by a collection of nodules of variegated histologic pattern, ranging from colloid-filled cysts and colloid adenomas to follicular and fetal adenomas. There may be some residue of histologically normal thyroid between the lumps, but more typically the structure between the more discrete adenomatous nodules consists of follicles with distended colloid-filled lumina. Often there is considerable associated fibrosis, sometimes there is calcification in the fibrous tissue or in the nodules, and hemorrhage into the nodules may be evident. Sometimes there is lymphocytic infiltration.

Etiology. The causation of this condition is not known with certainty, but there is evidence that mild deficiency in thyroid hormone production with consequent long-term stimulation of the gland (by TSH?) is one etiology. In areas of iodide deficiency, children under age 10 typically have diffuse enlargement of the thyroid, which on histologic examination shows a pattern of follicles distended with colloid and low cuboidal epithelium. Between ages 10 and 20, there is a gradual transformation of the process into the multinodular structure. Alternate periods of iodide deficiency with thyroid hyperplasia, and iodide sufficiency with involution, may lead first to colloid goiter and later to the typical multinodular goiter. Experimental proof of this theory in man is lacking. Presumably the hypertrophy of the thyroid in the iodide-deficient areas is due to TSH stimulation, but why this should lead to a colloid goiter rather than to hyperplasia is uncertain. For some reason the iodide-deficient gland forms excessive poorly iodinated thyroglobulin which is resistant to hydrolysis by intrathyroidal proteases, and thus accumulates.

Another possible cause is an inherited partial defect in hormone synthesis. Some patients with typical multinodular goiter secrete a large proportion of the iodide from the thyroid in a butanol-insoluble form, apparently an iodinated protein. These patients are usually euthyroid. Multinodular goiter tends to occur with high incidence in some kindreds. It has been generalized from this evidence that mild forms of metabolic defects in hormone synthesis, or perhaps the heterozygous carrier state for such a defect, may lead to the development of sporadic multinodular goiter.

Prevalence. The prevalence of multinodular goiter is related to geography, age, and heredity, among other factors. In iodide-deficient areas, multinodular goiter may occur in most individuals. In the United States a conservative estimate of the prevalence of palpable multinodular goiter among adults is 2 per cent, but this is probably low. Identical pathologic changes in the thyroid which do not produce gross enlargement of the gland are present in a much higher proportion of individuals at autopsy.

Clinical Presentation. Most commonly the condition exists throughout life and is not detected. In some patients enlargement and nodularity of the thyroid are found on routine physical examination. Since the incidence is 10 to 20 times as great in women as in men, and since it develops and progressively increases in size during life, it is often found in females of 50 to 70. Usually the condition is asymptomatic, but with progressive growth there may be a visible enlargement in the neck; tracheal compression, producing a sensation of choking or coughing; and occasionally pressure on the recurrent laryngeal nerve or edema, causing hoarseness. Sometimes there is hemorrhage into a cyst, producing sudden enlargement and tenderness in one area of the goiter. The problems of thyrotoxicosis and malignancy are discussed below.

Diagnosis. The diagnosis of multinodular goiter is usually made on the basis of physical examination. In its most typical form, the goiter feels like a bunch of grapes. The nodules vary in size from 0.5 to several centimeters in diameter and are of variable consistency. The patients are usually euthyroid on clinical examination, and this is confirmed by measuring the serum T_4 or FTI and the RAIU. Single nodules and Hashimoto's thyroiditis are the most common sources of confusion with multinodular goiter. Extensive development of one portion of the gland may lead to the impression of a single nodule; up to half of all thyroid enlargements thought to be single nodules turn out at operation to be multinodular goiters. The gland of Hashimoto's thyroiditis may have a lobulated texture, making it impossible to distinguish from multinodular goiter. Thyroid scintiscan may be useful if it shows a mottled distribution of radioisotope in the gland. Fluorescent thyroid scans show the same mottled distribution of stable iodine, in contrast to the uniform and diminished stable iodine in the gland of thyroiditis. Roentgenographic examination of the neck may give evidence of broad septate calcification or ringlike calcification in nodules. Often the trachea is deviated because of pressure by the goiter; this is rare in Hashimoto's thyroiditis. If diagnosis is imperative and cannot be made on the basis of the examinations already mentioned, needle biopsy is useful.

Therapy. Small nodular goiters in euthyroid subjects require no therapy. However, the natural history is progressive enlargement, and therefore it is appropriate to place patients on permanent therapy with desiccated thyroid in the hope that this will suppress TSH and prevent further enlargement of the gland. This should be done with careful observation, because some of the glands become autonomous, and the additional metabolic effect of exogenous hormone occasionally causes thyrotoxicosis. If the gland is grossly enlarged and causes a cosmetic defect or tracheal compression, resection may be indicated. Subsequently such patients should be placed on replacement therapy, because there is a pronounced tendency for regrowth. Sudden swelling and pain in the gland owing to hemorrhage into a cyst usually subside spontaneously over several weeks, and can be treated with analgesics. Nodular goiters that have progressively enlarged and have become displaced below the clavicles (substernal goiter) may cause tra-

cheal compression and should be resected. Such lesions can usually be removed through a cervical incision. Long-term pressure on the trachea occasionally produces tracheomalacia. The cartilaginous rings of the trachea are destroyed with a loss of normal rigidity. In such patients it is imperative that the function of the trachea be examined during inspiration and expiration at operation. Occasionally it is necessary that a tracheostomy be performed. The tracheostomy tube is left in place for 10 to 14 days to induce a fibrous reaction in the trachea and give it some rigidity.

Prognosis. The prognosis in untreated multinodular goiter is for slow enlargement of the gland. Administration of thyroid hormone may prevent progressive growth. It is also typical for longstanding multinodular goiter to develop autonomy and produce clinical hyperthyroidism.

COMPLICATIONS OF MULTINODULAR GOITER

Toxic Nodular Goiter. Many years ago Plummer observed that after nodular goiters had been present for an average of 17 years, thyrotoxicosis tended to develop. This may be due to the coincident occurrence of Graves' disease in the normal tissue between the nodules, but more often it is due to the uncontrolled hyperfunction of one or more nodules in the multinodular gland. In areas of endemic goiter this is the most common cause of hyperthyroidism, especially when iodine supplementation is first introduced into a previously deficient area. It is presumed that nodules developing because of TSH stimulation eventually become autonomous. Also, some autonomously functioning nodules in which hormone production has been limited by restricted iodine supplies are, in the presence of iodide supplementation, able to augment greatly the production of thyroid hormone. Patients with toxic nodular goiter are typically elderly, and symptoms are often minimal. Although the pathophysiology does not differ from that of other forms of thyrotoxicosis, congestive heart failure, atrial fibrillation, and muscle weakness tend to be prominent. The diagnosis should be suspected in any individual with a multinodular goiter and symptoms suggestive of hyperthyroidism, especially if heart failure or atrial fibrillation is present. The RAIU and serum T_4 may be in the high normal range or elevated. The diagnosis is further substantiated by a thyroid scan which localizes radioactivity to one or more of the nodules of the gland. In some of these patients it has been shown that there is a preferential secretion of T_3, leading to an increased ratio of T_3 to T_4 in blood. If the thyrotoxicosis is caused primarily by the excess T_3, the serum T_4 level may be normal. This diagnosis can be partially corroborated by observing failure of suppressibility of the gland, but must be confirmed by direct measurement of T_3.

Toxic multinodular goiter may be treated either by thyroidectomy after appropriate preparation with antithyroid drugs and potassium iodide or by administration of larger doses of radioiodine than are used in the treatment of Graves' disease, typically 10 to 15 mCi. Hypothyroidism is rarely produced because the isotope is distributed unevenly throughout the gland, and some portions are spared from radiation. The gland usually shrinks, but does not disappear. If the patient has significant heart disease, it is best to pretreat with antithyroid drugs before giving RAI, or to use multiple small doses of isotope (5 mCi every two to three months) until euthyroidism is achieved. Release of stored hormone after vigorous RAI therapy can otherwise precipitate congestive failure or infarction.

Administration of small doses of iodine (1 to 4 mg per day) occasionally induces thyrotoxicosis in previously euthyroid individuals with multinodular goiter. The thyrotoxicosis may be transient or may require treatment.

The Cancer Problem. Although the vast proportion of patients with multinodular goiter are never referred for evaluation or for surgery, the occurrence of sudden growth of one area of a multinodular gland, the palpation of an unusually firm area, or the development of hoarseness may raise the question of malignancy. Patients who come to surgery are obviously highly selected because they have developed symptoms that brought them to a physician and that were considered significant enough for referral to a surgeon. Among those who are operated upon, the incidence of verified carcinoma, usually papillary adenocarcinoma, varies from 2 to 20 per cent. Because of this frequency, some physicians view the presence of multinodular goiter as sufficient indication for thyroidectomy. The gross illogic of this reasoning can be seen by some simple calculations. If 2 per cent of the population have multinodular goiter and 10 per cent of these have thyroid malignancy, at least 400,000 papillary cancers would be present in the United States. In fact it is known that the prevalence of multinodular goiter is much greater than the figure used. In contrast, only 5000 thyroid cancers are detected annually, and the majority of these are found in patients whose thyroids are normal except for the malignancy. Because of this, it seems more logical to accept multinodular goiter as a measure of assurance that malignancy is not present. Multinodular goiter should not be resected because of a general fear of malignancy, but thyroidectomy is logical in the presence of signs that in themselves are suggestive of malignant change. In contrast, glands harboring a single nodule carry a real increase in risk of thyroid carcinoma.

Mortensen, J. C., Woolner, L. D., and Bennett, W. A.: Gross and microscopic findings in clinically normal thyroid glands. J. Clin. Endocrinol. Metab., 15:1270, 1955.

Sokal, J. E.: The incidence of thyroid cancer and the problem of malignancy in nodular goiter. *In* Astwood, E. B. (ed.): Clinical Endocrinology. New York, Grune & Stratton, 1960, Vol. 1, pp. 168–178.

Vagenakis, A. G., Wang, C. A., Burger, A., Maloof, F., Braverman, L. E., and Ingbar, S. H.: Iodide-induced thryotoxicosis in Boston. N. Engl. J. Med., 287:523, 1973.

Vander, J. B., Gaston, E. A., and Dawber, T. R.: The significance of nontoxic thyroid nodules. Ann. Intern. Med., 69:537, 1968.

Veith, F. J., Brooks, J. R., Grigsby, W. P., and Selenkow, H. A.: The nodular thyroid gland and cancer. A practical approach to the problem. N. Engl. J. Med., 270:431, 1964.

841. ENDEMIC GOITER

In the United States the average iodide intake is 200 to 600 μg or more per day, and detectable thyroid enlargement occurs in 2 to 4 per cent of adults. In contrast, in areas where iodide deficiency is present, as evidenced by urinary iodine excretion below 50 μg per day, the incidence of palpable enlargement of the thyroid increases in inverse relation to the average urinary iodide excretion. Endemic goiter exists in many mountainous areas of the world, including the Andes, central New Guinea, and Switzerland, as well as in many lowland areas such as the Baltic Plains and Zaïre. In almost all well-studied endemics, the cause is deficient iodide in the soil and water, leading to deficient iodide intake. Presumably, iodide privation leads to diminished production of thyroid hormone, which is sensed by the pituitary, resulting in augmented secretion of TSH, and thus to increased thyroidal clearance of plasma iodide. With this there is also growth (both hyperplasia and hypertrophy) of the thyroid. The thyroid strives to gain the necessary 60 to 100 μg of iodide needed daily for hormonogenesis, and does so by accumulating almost all the iodide ion entering the vascular compartment, either from the diet or from degradation of hormone within the body. The uptake of a radioactive tracer is 90 to 98 per cent in some endemic areas. Initially the gland is diffusely enlarged, and the histologic picture in adolescence is a "colloid goiter" with large follicles and flat cuboidal epithelium. In time the picture changes into the multinodular goiter described previously; the histology is identical with that of sporadic multinodular goiter found in other regions. Usually diffuse goiter predominates in youth, and multinodular goiter in older persons. The incidence is higher in women than in men unless the endemic is unusually severe. In some areas, practically all adults have thyroid enlargement.

Pathogenesis. The biochemical abnormalities that lead to the formation of multinodular goiters in response to iodide deficiency are not known. Alternate periods of iodide deficiency and repletion may lead to hyperplasia and involution and produce the picture of endemic goiter. TSH is elevated in some severe endemics, but in Argentina adults have been found to have endemic goiter in the presence of normal levels of plasma TSH. Possibly these people had elevated TSH levels earlier in their lives, or perhaps owing to iodide deficiency the gland is more sensitive to TSH. The thyroglobulin of endemic goiters is iodine poor and characteristically has an excess of MIT over DIT, and the content of T_4 and T_3 tends to be low. Possibly these alterations of iodide content or distribution in the amino acids of thyroglobulin lead to abnormalities in degradation of thyroglobulin and produce the picture of a colloid-filled goiter.

Goitrogens. In a few instances factors other than iodide deficiency operate to cause endemic goiter. Thus a factor present in water appears to be associated with an endemic in Colombia. Thiocyanates are derived from some plants, e.g., cassava eaten in Central Africa. Potent goitrogens related in action to the thioureas are found in some plant species and are transmitted through cow's milk to humans in Tasmania and Finland. As fascinating as these examples are, they account for only a minute fraction of endemic goiter, a condition that involves many millions of people throughout the world.

Clinical Manifestations. Patients with goiter in endemic zones present with thyroid enlargements that may be diffuse or nodular and that vary in size from barely detectable to as large as the head (Fig. 9). In some places monstrous enlargement of the thyroid is accepted as normal. Usually such individuals, when adult, are euthyroid, and thus appear to have adapted to iodide deficiency by growth of the goiter. All the problems related to thyroid enlargement, such as dysphagia, respiratory difficulty, tracheal deviation and compression, and cosmetic problems may of course be associated with the thyroid enlargement. Occasionally, in severe endemics, some people are hypothyroid clinically and by laboratory examination. In contrast to the condition known as endemic cretinism, described below, patients with endemic goiter do not have neurologic signs or gross mental retardation. Aside from what might be considered by foreigners a cosmetic blemish, endemic goiter itself is inconsequential to most adults with this condition. However, there is evidence, discussed below, that the neural complications of iodide privation may be important.

Diagnosis. The diagnosis of endemic goiter is best made by study of a population group. The characteristic feature is reduced excretion of iodide in the urine. Iodide excretion is often 30 to 50 μg per day, although values as low as 5 μg per day have been recorded. RAIU values are elevated to the 70 to 95 per cent range.

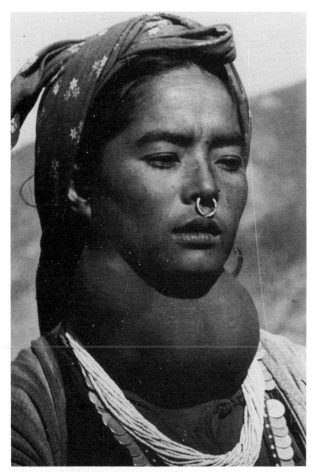

Figure 9. A young woman from the Nepalese village of Wapsa which has severe iodine deficiency and a high incidence of endemic goiter. (Photograph kindly provided by Professor Kaye Ibbertson of the University of Auckland, Private Bag, New Zealand.)

Thyroid hormone in blood, as measured by the PBI or T_4, is normal, or rarely is depressed, and the patients are hypothyroid. The T_4 may be low in the presence of euthyroidism; these patients maintain normal metabolism by producing relatively more T_3. The findings of diminished urinary iodide, augmented thyroid uptake, and high incidence of goiter are sufficient to incriminate iodide as the cause of the endemic. If iodide intake is sufficient, i.e., above 100 μg per day in the presence of endemic goiter, some other cause must be sought, such as a goitrogenic agent in foodstuffs.

Treatment. The best treatment for endemic goiter is iodine prophylaxis applied to the entire population group. The most convenient approach is salt iodinization, adding about 50 μg of iodide per gram of salt as iodate or as potassium iodide. Another approach is to inject population groups with iodinated poppyseed oil. This provides a depot of 1 to 2 grams of potential iodide, and is sufficient to supply iodide for one to four years. Treatment with desiccated thyroid should prevent further enlargement of the goiters and suppress diffuse goiters in children. It usually has little effect on the multinodular goiters of adults. Local symptoms caused by massive enlargement of the thyroid may require thyroidectomy.

Thyrotoxicosis is rarely seen in areas of severe endemic goiter, apparently because the limitation of iodide supply prevents its development. Occasionally it does occur, and may be difficult to recognize because RAIU values are elevated even in "normal" subjects. The PBI or serum T_4 may be elevated, or may be normal if the patient secretes an excess of T_3. After administration of iodine in salt or by injection, some patients develop thyrotoxicosis. Sometimes this process (Jod-Basedow) is self-limiting, but therapy with antithyroid drugs, radioactive iodide, or surgery may be required.

There is no convincing evidence that carcinoma occurs with increased frequency in areas of endemic goiter, but there is a strong suggestion that a higher proportion of the tumors that do occur are poorly differentiated or sarcomatous.

ENDEMIC CRETINISM

This term refers to defective individuals having a typical constellation of signs and symptoms found with increased frequency in areas of severe endemic goiter. If recognized shortly after birth and if the children are hypothyroid, there is a typical appearance with increased hair, low forehead, puffy features, umbilical hernia, enlarged tongue, and sluggish behavior. Other abnormalities may be detected: deaf-mutism, mental retardation, and evidence of spastic paraplegia. These may occur with or without overt hypothyroidism, or as individual entities. If there is continued hypothyroidism, retarded growth and retarded bone age and epiphysial stippling occur. The individual may be goitrous, or no thyroid tissue may be present. In childhood, most endemic cretins achieve a euthyroid metabolic state, but stunted growth, deaf-mutism, mental subnormality, and diplegia give evidence of the syndrome. Endemic cretinism is probably caused by severe iodide deficiency leading to hypothyroidism in both mother and child during fetal development. Athyrotic individuals born to normal mothers in nonendemic zones rarely if ever develop the full-blown syndrome, apparently because significant quantities of thyroid hormone are transported from the mother to the fetus across the placenta. When investigated during childhood or adult life, endemic cretins may be hypothyroid or euthyroid. Treatment of euthyroid adult cretins with thyroid hormone has had no beneficial effect on mental function, deafness, or neurologic damage. The only known therapy is iodine prophylaxis, as described above for endemic goiter. Studies by Fierro in Ecuador suggest that in severe endemics associated with cretinism, mental subnormality may afflict a much larger portion of the population. Thus the effects of endemic iodide deficiency, goiter, and cretinism appear to be even more devastating than was previously known, making iodine prophylaxis of crucial importance in these areas.

Butterfield, I. H., Black, M. L., Hoffmann, M. J., Mason, E. K., and Hetzel, B. S.: Correction of iodine deficiency in New Guinea natives by iodized oil injection. Lancet, 2:767, 1965.

Dumont, J. E., Ermans, A. M., and Bastenie, P. A.: Thyroidal function in a goiter endemic. IV. Hypothyroidism and endemic cretinism. J. Clin. Endocrinol. Metab., 23:325, 1963.

Ermans, A. M., Bastenie, P. A., Galperin, H., Beckers, C., Van Den Schrieck, H. G., and DeVisscher, M.: Endemic goiter in the Uele region. II. Synthesis and secretion of thyroid hormones. J. Clin. Endocrinol. Metab., 21:996, 1961.

Fierro-Benitez, R., Penafiel, W., DeGroot, L. J., and Ramirez, I.: Endemic goiter and endemic cretinism in the Andean region. N. Engl. J. Med., 280:296, 1969.

Stanbury, J. B. (ed.): Endemic Goiter. Scientific Publication No. 193. Washington, D.C., Pan American Health Organization, 1969, p. 447.

Stanbury, J. B., and Kroc, R. L. (eds.): Human Development and the Thyroid Gland. Relation to Endemic Cretinism. New York, Plenum Press, 1972.

842. METABOLIC DEFECTS IN THYROID HORMONE FORMATION, TRANSPORT, AND ACTION

CONGENITAL METABOLIC DEFECTS IN THYROID HORMONE FORMATION
(Sporadic Goitrous Hypothyroidism or Goitrous Cretinism)

The biosynthesis of thyroid hormone proceeds via transport of iodide into the thyroid, binding of iodide to tyrosine in thyroglobulin, coupling of iodotyrosines, subsequent proteolysis of thyroglobulin with release of iodotyrosines and thyronines, intrathyroidal deiodination of iodotyrosines and reutilization of their iodide, and release of thyroid hormone to the blood. Specific enzymatic defects causing diminished efficiency in the formation of thyroid hormone have been identified as several of these steps. The various genotypes usually produce a common phenotype, characterized by the presence of a hyperplastic thyroid plus hypothyroidism or euthyroidism.

Defect in Iodide Trapping. A few patients have been recognized with hyperplastic thyroid glands and congenital hypothyroidism associated with inability to transport iodide into the thyroid and thyroidal uptake of tracer isotope near zero. Thyroid tissue from such patients, studied in vitro, is unable to establish an iodide concentration gradient. The patients also fail to transport iodide into saliva and gastric juice; this observation forms the basis of a simple test for the defect. The concentration of iodide in saliva is compared with that in plasma two hours after administration of a radioactive iodide tracer. In affected individuals the ratio is 1, whereas in normal individuals and in presumed heterozygotes it is from 10 to 100. Thyroid tissue of these patients contains the other enzymes needed for hormone synthesis. It should be remembered that the usual cause for failure of iodide uptake during a tracer test is that the gland is saturated by exogenous iodine, rather than a faulty iodide-concentrating mechanism.

Iodide Organification Defect. The most common defect in hormone synthesis is at the iododide-binding step. The patients are able to transport and concentrate iodide in the thyroid, but the iodide is not bound to tyrosine in thyroglobulin. Iodide in the thyroid remains in equilibrium with that in plasma, and as iodide in plasma is cleared to the urine, the free thyroidal iodide gradually returns to plasma. Such patients have an elevated thyroid uptake shortly after administration of a tracer and a low uptake at 24 hours. The iodide content of the gland is greatly reduced. Reduced amounts of iodinated compounds are formed or released to plasma. T_4 is low.

A defect in binding can be identified by administration of potassium perchlorate two hours after administration of a radioactive iodide tracer. The potassium perchlorate will effectively block the iodide transport mechanism. If there is a large pool of free intrathyroidal iodide, potassium perchlorate will cause a release of this material to plasma, with a dramatic drop in the thyroid iodide content. A release of 10 per cent or more of the iodide present at two hours is considered a positive test.

A variant of this condition is found in association with congenital nerve deafness (Pendred's syndrome). This condition is transmitted as a mendelian dominant, but is expressed to varying degrees. Deafness ranges from complete through nearly normal hearing, and hypothyroidism may be severe or thyroid function may be normal.

The biochemical basis of the organification defect syndromes has been identified in patients studied in the author's laboratory. Some patients have diminished or absent peroxidase. Others have an abnormal peroxidase apo-protein which fails to bind the hematin prosthetic group firmly; thus the enzyme is not fully active. In other patients, an abnormality of thyroglobulin synthesis results in a diminished quantity of iodide acceptor. Other proteins are iodinated, but apparently inefficiently, resulting in a buildup of free intrathyroidal iodide and failure to produce iodothyronines.

"Coupling" Defect. Some individuals with congenital goiter have large, hyperactive thyroids and low thyroid hormone in plasma. Large amounts of MIT and DIT are found in their thyroglobulin. An abnormality of the coupling process is implied by these observations, but it is by no means certain what this abnormality is. It could, for example, be an abnormality in energy supply, an abnormality in the structure of the thyroglobulin, or perhaps lack of peroxidase enzyme related to the coupling process. It is currently believed that there is no "coupling enzyme," rather that peroxidase mediates this process as well as initial iodination of thyroglobu-

lin. Although patients with congenital thyroid disease, hypothyroidism, low plasma T_4, and plentiful iodotyrosines in the thyroid must have a defect of the coupling process, a more exact definition will require new information about the normal synthetic process.

Iodotyrosine Dehalogenase Defect. Thyroglobulin is degraded in the thyroid by a combination of protease and peptidases, and each amino acid of the thyroglobulin peptide chain is thus separated. Normally the iodotyrosines are deiodinated by a dehalogenase present in the microsomes. The liberated iodide is reutilized for the iodination of tyrosine to form more MIT and DIT. Each day about four times as much iodide goes through this cycle as enters the thyroid from the blood. Some patients have a specific defect of the dehalogenase. In the most carefully studied cases, the enyzme defect also exists in other tissues. Because of the defect in the thyroid, iodotyrosine is liberated from the gland into the blood. Because of lack of the enzyme in other tissues, iodotyrosines are not deiodinated, but are excreted in the urine. This iodide loss causes marked hypothyroidism and thyroid enlargement. The disease can be diagnosed by the identification of labeled iodotyrosines in plasma or urine after administration of a radioactive iodide tracer. Also, infused iodotyrosine is not deiodinated, but is excreted unchanged in the urine. Parents of affected individuals, who are presumed to be heterozygous, often show a minor abnormality in their ability to deiodinate iodotyrosine.

Butanol-Insoluble Iodide Defect. Many patients with congenital or familial thyroid enlargement and hypothyroidism have in their plasma iodine insoluble in acidified butanol, and thus not T_4 or T_3. This material is formed in the thyroid, and is of heterogeneous nature. Some glands secrete large amounts of iodinated albumin, prealbumin, or both. Others seem to secrete iodinated proteins that do not react with antihuman albumin serum, and do react in part with antithyroglobulin antibodies. Possibly these are abnormal subunits or fragments of thyroglobulin. The iodoproteins usually contain mainly MIT and DIT and no T_4 or T_3.

This inefficient utilization of glandular iodine restricts the formation of T_4 and causes thyroid hyperplasia. The basic abnormality is poorly understood. There may be inadequate production of normal thyroglobulin. Other proteins may then gain access to the gland and be iodinated. Another possibility is an abnormality in the proteolytic enzymes of the thyroid so that iodinated subunits of thyroglobulin are released to plasma. Attempts to identify defective protease activity have been inconclusive.

Epidemiology. The metabolic defects in hormone synthesis occur sporadically or in family groupings. Affected siblings may be identifiable, and occasionally parents are found to have a minor metabolic abnormality. Typically there is inbreeding in the family. The metabolic defects usually represent the expression of a homozygous recessive genetic abnormality. The exception to this is in Pendred's syndrome, which is inherited as a mendelian dominant.

Pathology. Typically there is marked hyperplasia of the thyroid. The gland is beefy, the cells are columnar, there is little or no colloid, and hypervascularity is marked. The extreme hyperplasia may take on the appearance of a papillary carcinoma. In other instances the longstanding thyrotrophin stimulation to the gland results in change into a carcinoma, metastases, and death. Disease, other than in the thyroid, depends upon the degree of hypothyroidism. In Pendred's syndrome there is in addition nerve deafness, but information on the nature of the lesion is lacking.

Clinical Presentation. Patients present a common phenotype. Usually the illness is not suspected at birth but becomes apparent within the first few months or, more frequently, during childhood. If the illness is severe, the child will develop evidence of hypothyroidism. There is symmetrical enlargement of the thyroid from two to ten times normal size. The gland is usually very vascular, and typically a bruit and thrill are present. The signs and symptoms of hypothyroidism are those described previously. The presence of metastases, including pulmonary infiltrates, indicates malignant change in the goiter.

Diagnosis. The diagnosis is suggested by observation of a hyperplastic thyroid in an individual who is apparently euthyroid or hypothyroid. The iodide-trapping defect can be demonstrated by the inability of the gland to accumulate iodide during a tracer uptake study. A corroborative finding is lack of concentration of iodide in the saliva. An iodide organification defect can be shown by a positive perchlorate discharge test and hypothyroxinemia. The iodotyrosine dehalogenase defect can be identified by chromatography revealing iodotyrosine in plasma and urine after administration of a tracer. The butanol-insoluble iodoprotein defect is detected by an abnormal difference between the PBI and BEI or between the PBI and serum T_4 iodine. Normally the difference is no more than 20 per cent. In patients with the syndrome, the BEI or T_4 iodine may be only 30 to 40 per cent of the PBI. Identification of the labeled protein can be made by electrophoresis of plasma or thyroid proteins obtained at biopsy after administration of a radioiodide tracer.

Therapy. Since the patients have a goitrogenic response to TSH caused by deficiency of thyroid hormone, the obvious therapy is to replace thyroid hormone. This corrects existing hypothyroidism and in children usually results in complete regression of the goiter. In older people in whom multinodular goiter has developed, there may be little change in size. In patients with the iodide trapping or dehalogenase defects, administration of a few drops of Lugol's solution daily will compensate for the defect. Development of thyrotoxicosis during iodide therapy for dehalogenase defect has been reported.

Prognosis. It is imperative that individuals with these syndromes be treated with suppressive doses of thyroid hormone or potassium iodide, as indicated, for the duration of their lives. Inadequate therapy will allow continued TSH stimulation of the gland, and malignant degeneration may occur. In general the patients and parents can be reassured that if the defect has been detected early so that there is no neurologic abnormality, treatment will result in normal health and longevity. Further, it is highly unlikely that progeny will be affected if there is no inbreeding.

DEFECTS IN HORMONE TRANSPORT

Occasionally patients have a great elevation or depression of blood thyroid hormone in the absence of corresponding clinical symptoms, owing to the presence of abnormal quantities of thyroxine-binding globulin (TBG). In well-studied kinships, the abnormalities have been shown to be transmitted as X-linked traits. Thus the affected or "carrier" females are typically heterozygous, and affected males are homozygous. In families with hypo-TBG-nemia, the males have extremely low or undetectable levels of TBG, with PBI or T_4 values in the range of 1 to 2 μg per 100 ml. Affected females usually have about half-normal TBG and PBI or serum T_4 values. The abnormality is the altered production of a normal protein, because no protein immunologically related to TBG is found in the serum of TBG-deficient subjects and turnover of labeled normal TBG injected into these subjects is similar to turnover in unaffected individuals. The decrease in total bound hormone in the plasma of such patients is counterbalanced by an increased fraction of free hormone. The absolute free hormone concentration is therefore normal, and the patients are eumetabolic. Aside from the confusion caused in the interpretation of laboratory tests, there is no known physiologic abnormality associated with this defect.

A few individuals have been reported with elevations of TBG to approximately two times normal and gross elevation of serum T_4. Again this appears to be genetically X-linked, with affected males exhibiting TBG elevation about twice that of affected (carrier) females. The patients are euthyroid, and no change in the availability of thyroid hormone to tissues can be shown.

The possibility of genetically induced decreased or (rarely) increased TBG should always be kept in mind when a thyroid hormone test reveals a level that appears to be discordant with the observed clinical state and no hormonal or disease-related cause exists. Measurement of absolute free T_4 content, or of the FTI, will indicate that the amount of functioning thyroid hormone in the plasma is normal. Another way to show the nature of the condition is by measurement of the T_4 carrying capacity of TBG. Evaluation of other members of the family will help verify the diagnosis.

HEREDITARY RESISTANCE TO THE ACTION OF THYROID HORMONE

Three of eight children in one reported sibship have apparent resistance to the action of thyroid hormone. The children have a characteristic facial appearance, retarded growth, delayed bone age, stippled epiphyses, deaf-mutism, and elevated thyroid hormone concentration in blood. The hormone in blood is T_3 and T_4, and there is no abnormality of binding proteins. Their thyroids produce about five times the normal amount of hormone daily, and this quantity is likewise degraded in the peripheral tissues. They appear to be euthyroid. A large body of laboratory data supports the conclusion that these children are resistant to the action of thyroid hormone. In compensation, an increased quantity of hormone is made available to the peripheral tissues. Even with this, some organs (e.g., the ears and bones) receive an insufficient supply of hormone. It is hypothesized that the hypothalamus shares in the decreased sensitivity. Studies designed to identify the basic enzymatic defect have not been revealing, and no therapy

has been devised. Conceivably, treatment of the mothers of such individuals with large doses of thyroid hormone during early pregnancy would be advantageous to the neurologic development of the fetus.

DeGroot, L. J., and Stanbury, J. B.: The syndrome of congenital goiter with butanol insoluble serum iodine. Am. J. Med., 27:586, 1959.

Lissitzky, S., Bismuth, J., Codaccioni, J. L., and Cartouzou, G.: Congenital goiter with iodoalbumin replacing thyroglobulin and defect of deiodination of iodotyrosines. Serum origin of the thyroid iodoalbumin. J. Clin. Endocrinol. Metab., 28:1797, 1968.

Niepomniszcze, H., Castells, S., DeGroot, L. J., Refetoff, S., Kim, O. S., Rapoport, B., and Hati, R.: Peroxidase defect in congenital goiter with complete organification block. J. Clin. Endocrinol. Metab., 36:347, 1973.

Niepomniszcze, H., DeGroot, L. J., and Hagen, G. A.: Abnormal thyroid peroxidase causing iodide organification defect. J. Clin. Endocrinol. Metab., 34:607, 1972.

Refetoff, S., DeGroot, L. J., Benard, B., and DeWind, L. T.: Studies of a sibship with apparent hereditary resistance to the intracellular action of thyroid hormone. Metabolism, 21:723, 1972.

Refetoff, S., Robin, N. I., and Alper, C. A.: Study of four new kindreds with inherited thyroxine binding globulin abnormalities. Possible mutations of a single gene locus. J. Clin. Invest., 51:848, 1972.

Stanbury, J. B., and Chapman, E. M.: Congenital hypothyroidism with goiter. Absence of an iodide-concentrating mechanism. Lancet, 1:1162, 1960.

Stanbury, J. B., Kassenaar, A. A. H., Meijer, J. W. A., and Terpstra, J.: The occurrence of mono- and di-iodotyrosine in the blood of a patient with congenital goiter. J. Clin. Endocrinol. Metab., 15:1216, 1955.

843. THYROID NEOPLASMS

Thyroid neoplasms are adenomas and malignant tumors. Pathologically, adenomas are classified into fetal, follicular, Hürthle cell, and papillary forms. Carcinomas are usually grouped into papillary, follicular, mixed, Hürthle cell, medullary, and anaplastic varieties. Lymphoma and lymphosarcoma are also found in the thyroid.

Etiology. As in all other neoplasms, the exact etiology is unknown. In the case of thyroid cells, it is certain that both radiation and TSH stimulation may be in some way involved. After the original observation by Duffy and Fitzgerald, a relation between x-ray to the pharyngeal or thymic area in early childhood and subsequent development of thyroid carcinoma (usually papillary) was well documented. In children who develop thyroid carcinoma under the age of 20, this association is characteristically present. Although the tumors are presumed to occur because of x-ray damage to the thyroid, it is possible that the pathogenesis involves damage to the immunologic surveillance system of the thymus, or that the response is fundamentally due to x-ray damage to the thyroid with subsequent TSH hypersecretion. Another known relationship is between chronic TSH stimulation and the formation of invasive thyroid carcinoma, best identified in patients with congenital metabolic defects. A third relationship is to a variety of the multiple endocrine adenomatosis syndrome (Type 2), involving pheochromocytoma and medullary thyroid carcinoma, which is transmitted as a dominant genetic trait. Multiple cutaneous neuromas are also seen in association with this syndrome, and occasionally parathyroid adenomas. Many thyroid tumors are known to be TSH dependent, in that administration of suppressive doses of thyroid hormone leads to decrease in or regression of the malignancy. The exact relation of x-ray or TSH to induction of autonomous growth is unclear, although it is presumed to involve a mutational change with deletion of genes that restrict growth of the thyroid cells.

Little is known about the development of thyroid adenomas, although it may be presumed that the same sort of change that causes thyroid carcinoma is involved in the pathogenesis of adenomas. Thyroid adenomas, or at least nodularity, are present with increased frequency in patients who have received x-ray therapy to the thymus, and adenomas are produced in laboratory animals subjected to long-term TSH stimulation. Multiple follicular adenomas are occasionally found in family groups. Although adenomas may develop into thyroid carcinomas, this is not a common process.

A high incidence of thyroid carcinoma has been found in patients coming to surgery with multinodular goiter. The reasons for this have been discussed in Ch. 840. It has been stated for years that the incidence of thyroid cancer in Graves' disease is diminished, but this is not certain. In a recently reported large series, 0.5 per cent of patients undergoing thyroidectomy for Graves' disease were found to have papillary thyroid carcinoma.

THYROID ADENOMAS

Pathology. Adenomas are new growths of thyroid tissue having a homogeneous histologic pattern, surrounded by a capsule composed of fibrous tissue or compressed normal cells. They may present as single structures in otherwise normal glands or, less frequently, as two or three discrete adenomas, or they may be a feature of the multinodular goiter. The most common variety is the follicular adenoma, composed of large colloid-filled follicles with flattened cuboidal epithelium. A common variety of this growth has large colloid-filled follicles and an ill-defined capsule, leading to its designation as a "colloid nodule." Whether or not these are true adenomas is debated. Occasionally there may be degeneration, and the adenoma is then cystic and filled with a gelatinous material. Evidence of old or recent hemorrhage into a degenerating adenoma is common. Some adenomas have the histologic appearance of normal thyroid tissue. Adenomas with smaller follicles and more cellularity are termed fetal or embryonal and are occasionally transitional forms between adenomatous and carcinomatous growths. In the Hürthle cell adenoma the cells are eosinophilic and have the appearance of liver cells. All of these are variants of the follicular adenoma. Papillary "adenomas" have characteristic fronds of cells projecting into a sparsely filled lumen; these may in fact be carcinomas.

Clinical Presentation. *The clinical problem most often presented by the thyroid adenoma is management of a solitary thyroid nodule.* This may be asymptomatic, or, less commonly, may be brought to attention because of hoarseness, pain, or difficulty in swallowing. Single nodules may be present in 2 per cent of the adult population. They are much less frequent in men than in women. It is certain that most remain without significant danger for long periods of time.

The problem is in differentiation of such lesions from thyroid cancer. In the vast majority of persons, the clinical finding is limited to a nodule in an otherwise normal gland. On clinical and laboratory examination,

most patients are euthyroid, although some are clinically toxic. RAIU and scanning studies may show that the nodule is "cold" (most commonly), that it is equal in uptake of radioactive iodide to that of the normal tissue, or that it concentrates radioactive iodide selectively. Some of the "hot" nodules produce excessive hormone and suppress the normal gland, or produce clinical thyrotoxicosis. Nodules may be "cold" because they are biochemically unable to transport radioactive iodide into the thyroid or are unable to bind it, but most frequently they are "cold" because they are cystic. If the nodule is "cold," is unusually firm, is fixed to the trachea or surrounding structures, is irregular in contour, or is known to have recently grown, or if cervical nodes are felt, the likelihood of malignancy is increased. However, it is certain that clinical examination and isotope scanning cannot segregate carcinomas from benign adenomas. Carcinoma may occur in nodules that are clinically "hot" on scanning; from 3 to 10 per cent of carcinomas are warm or hot by this technique. Solitary nodules in the thyroids of children and men are particularly dangerous. It cannot be taken for granted that a nodule known to have been present for a few years is benign. Further, it is probably not advantageous to treat such lesions for a long time with desiccated thyroid in an attempt to suppress their growth, because this rarely causes disappearance of the nodule. Short-term therapy before surgery may be of value since it makes the lesion more discrete and facilitates a localized resection. Positive diagnosis of cancer can be made in the infrequent medullary carcinomas by detection of elevated thyrocalcitonin levels, if this assay is available.

Since clinical differentiation between benign and malignant lesions is very difficult, and since most physicians are reluctant to perform a needle biopsy for diagnosis of possible neoplasm, *a logical approach is to resect most single nodules unless there is a clear contraindication to surgery.* The operative procedure is usually subtotal lobectomy if the lesion appears to be benign and if there are no observable lymph nodes. Frozen sections are made; if the diagnosis of adenoma is confirmed, no further procedure is done. If the lesion is malignant, a more extensive procedure is carried out, as discussed below. Patients who have a subtotal resection for a benign adenoma should be placed on permanent thyroid hormone replacement therapy. *Up to half the "single nodules" subjected to surgery are found to be multinodular goiters, and from 10 to 20 per cent are diagnosed by the surgical pathologist as thyroid carcinoma.*

A significant fraction of thyroid nodules, perhaps one third, are largely cystic. This differentiation can sometimes be made by palpation, and by echograms. Some surgeons are currently treating lesions thought to be cystic by aspiration, and early results indicate that this may effectively reduce the nodule. Other physicians are performing diagnostic needle biopsy to select lesions for surgery. Both these approaches carry the possible objections of spreading tumor or of false negative diagnosis. However, the techniques now being employed on a trial basis may prove beneficial; if so, they will greatly alter the indications for surgery noted above.

THYROID CARCINOMAS

Papillary Carcinoma. Nearly 80 per cent of thyroid carcinomas are papillary tumors, and there is debate over whether a benign papillary adenoma actually exists. The tumors have fronds of cellular tissue projecting into slitlike lumina containing scant or no colloid. Other portions of the lesion may show differentiation into a relatively normal follicular structure. The lesions are frequently very small and often are found as incidentally observed microscopic tumors in glands removed for some other lesion. Papillary tumors tend to metastasize early to lymph nodes in the neck, often when the primary tumor cannot be detected by physician examination or by scanning. The tumor remains confined to cervical lymph nodes for a long time, but may invade locally into strap muscles and the larynx, and metastasize to lungs. The histologic patterns of the primary and metastatic disease may be quite different, with follicular elements in either area. Growth tends to be partially dependent on TSH. The disease is less aggressive in individuals under age 40. Ten-year survival with various forms of therapy is 80 to 90 per cent.

Up to two thirds of the thyroid tumors in the differentiated papillary group cannot be categorized as either purely papillary or follicular, but are mixed. These tumors behave more or less like pure papillary lesions. It is impossible to tell which element has metastasized, and there may be major discrepancies in architecture and function between the primary and the metastatic deposits.

Follicular Carcinoma. Follicular thyroid carcinoma varies in appearance from relatively normal-looking thyroid tissue, to microfollicular structures, large follicles, or areas of solid, rather anaplastic-appearing tumor. Often some areas have Hürthle cell changes. These tumors metastasize early via the bloodstream to lung and bones. The tumors are TSH responsive and tend to pick up and metabolize iodide and to form thyroid hormone. Occasionally the unchecked biosynthetic activity of the tumor results in clinical thyrotoxicosis. The ten-year survival in patients with this illness is approximately 50 per cent.

Hürthle cell carcinoma tends to invade and metastasize locally in the neck. It has a morbidity approximately like that of follicular carcinoma.

Medullary Carcinoma. Medullary cell carcinoma is derived from the "C" cells, or calcitonin-secreting parafollicular cells of the thyroid. These tumors form sheets of cells with large nuclei. There is usually extensive deposition of amyloid and considerable fibrosis; lymphocyte infiltration may also be prominent. The tumors tend to metastasize locally to the neck and finally to the lungs and soft tissues. Their course is like that of follicular carcinoma, despite their undifferentiated "solid tumor" appearance. The tumors are associated with pheochromocytoma and a variety of other endocrine syndromes. It is clear that they produce calcitonin and rarely cause hypocalcemia. In response to this they may induce parathyroid adenomas. The tumors may also secrete "hormonal" polypeptides and, through this mechanism, may cause Cushing's syndrome and may produce excess serotonin. A history of familial cancer, pheochromocytoma, or hypocalcemia should suggest this diagnosis, and assay for calcitonin should be done.

Anaplastic Carcinomas. Anaplastic thyroid cancer ranges from small cell tumors through carcinosarcomas, giant cell tumors, and epidermoid tumors. These tend to invade locally and behave much as malignant

neoplasms in any other portion of the body. Survival is usually less than 10 to 20 per cent after one year.

Lymphoma and lymphosarcoma may also involve the thyroid. It is doubtful that this is related to the occurrence of Hashimoto's thyroiditis. The mortality rate depends upon the histologic nature of the lesion.

Treatment of Thyroid Cancer. The selection of patients for operation has been discussed above. Patients with a neck mass thought to be due to thyroid cancer, or those with a thyroid mass plus cervical nodes, should have *thyroidectomy* unless some contraindication to surgery is present. At surgery diagnosis is made on the basis of examination of the primary lesion by the physician, resection of lymph nodes, and examination of frozen sections. If the lesion is differentiated (papillary or follicular cancer) and is confined to the thyroid, a total lobectomy is done on the involved side, resection of the lymph nodes in the tracheoesophageal groove is carried out, and a subtotal resection is performed on the opposite side. If there is evidence of multicentricity, a more radical resection is performed. If the lesion involves the thyroid and has metastasized to the neck, a total thyroidectomy is done, with preservation of the parathyroids by careful dissection or transplantation, and a homolateral limited neck dissection is performed. Occasionally patients will present with metastatic disease. If there is proved thyroid cancer with a solitary metastasis, it may be profitable to extract both the thyroid and the metastasis, because some patients will survive for a long time. In preparation for surgery and after surgery, patients with thyroid cancer should be on hyperphysiologic doses of thyroid hormone in order to suppress endogenous TSH. Many tumors are TSH dependent, and this therapy will prevent growth or actually cause tumor involution over years or decades.

If there is definite evidence of lymph node involvement or metastases, the patients are given one or more doses of 50 mCi ^{131}I to ablate residual thyroid tissue. If uptake in the metastasis can be demonstrated by scanning techniques after stimulation by endogenous or exogenous TSH, then patients are given courses of approximately 150 mCi of radioactive iodide-131 at intervals of three months (Fig. 10). Except when receiving ^{131}I therapy, all should receive thyroid hormone in doses sufficient to induce mild clinical hyperthyroidism. Some spectacular cures of metastatic thyroid cancer are obtained by ^{131}I, but all too frequently tumor uptake is low or declines with treatment, and there is a gradual overgrowth of tumor which does not concentrate isotope.

Medullary thyroid cancer is treated by surgery followed by x-ray therapy to the neck, because this tumor rarely concentrates radioactive iodide.

Anaplastic thyroid cancer is treated by local dissection to the extent possible. A radioactive iodide scan should be performed, but it is most unlikely that these tumors will concentrate radioactive iodide. Roentgen therapy is useful. After surgery, patients are placed on suppressive doses of thyroid hormone. Patients with lymphoma or lymphosarcoma are usually treated by surgery combined with postsurgical radiotherapy. The long-term survival is excellent in the lymphomas, and is perhaps 50 per cent at ten years in lymphosarcoma.

Recent reports indicate that the antitumor agents bleomycin and adriamycin may be useful in treating

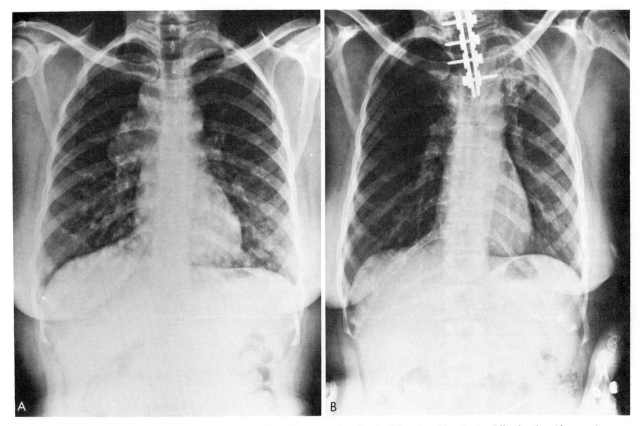

Figure 10. *A*, Chest roentgenogram demonstrating pulmonary and mediastinal deposits of functioning follicular thyroid cancer in a 43-year-old woman. *B*, Two years and 450 mC ¹³¹I later, the original nodules are invisible. However, nonfunctioning osseous metastasis has destroyed the body of D2 requiring a steel brace to alleviate spinal cord compression.

thyroid cancer unresponsive to surgery, ¹³¹I, or x-ray therapy.

Black, B., Yadeau, R., and Woolner, L.: Surgical treatment of thyroidal carcinomas. Arch. Surg., 88:610, 1964.

Buckwalter, J.: Surgical treatment of thyroid carcinoma. Arch. Surg., 98:597, 1969.

DeGroot, L. J., and Paloyan, E.: Thyroid carcinoma and radiation. J.A.M.A., 225:487, 1973.

Duffy, B. J., Jr., and Fitzgerald, P. J.: Cancer of the thyroid in children: A report of twenty-eight cases. J. Clin. Endocrinol. Metab., 10:1296, 1950.

Leeper, R. D.: The effect of ¹³¹I therapy on survival of patients with metastatic papillary or follicular thyroid carcinoma. J. Clin. Endocrinol. Metab., 36:1143, 1973.

Melvin, K. E. W., Miller, H. H., and Tashjian, A. H.: Early diagnosis of medullary carcinoma of the thyroid gland by means of calcitonin assay. N. Engl. J. Med., 285:1115, 1971.

ADRENAL CORTEX

Grant W. Liddle

844. THE ADRENAL STEROIDS AND THEIR FUNCTIONS

The function of the adrenal cortex is to secrete hormonal steroids, and the major disorders of the adrenal cortex arise from deficiencies or excesses of one or another of the adrenal steroids.

Table 1 lists the major adrenal steroids, their most abundant metabolites, their functions, and the clinical consequences of steroid deficiencies or excesses.

It has been known since the publication of Thomas Addison's classic monograph in 1855 that the adrenal cortex is essential for life. The two essential hormones are cortisol and aldosterone. The former provides resistance to a variety of stresses and maintains the activity of a number of enzyme systems; the latter enables the organism to withstand salt deprivation. In the quantities normally secreted, all the other adrenal steroids may be regarded as relatively weak or inactive precursors, metabolites, or by-products of cortisol and aldosterone. Cortisol and aldosterone are, indirectly, self-regulating, because each one is capable of initiating a series of physiologic events that result in the suppression of their respective stimulators.

Although cortisol and aldosterone are essential for life, when secreted in excessive quantities they can be life threatening. Beyond the scope of this chapter is the fact that supraphysiologic doses of cortisol and certain of its synthetic analogues can be used to modify the courses of a wide variety of nonendocrinologic disorders, particularly inflammatory and allergic processes.

Cortisol is the most important product of the human adrenal cortex in the sense that it is the one steroid that corrects most of the pathophysiologic effects of adrenalectomy when given in doses comparable to the amounts normally secreted. Cortisol is synonymous with hydrocortisone (the official pharmaceutical term) and, chemically, is $11\beta,17\alpha,21$-trihydroxy-pregn-4-ene-3,20-dione. It is closely related to *cortisone*, the glucocorticoid first produced synthetically on a large enough scale for widespread use as a therapeutic agent. Chemically, cortisone differs from cortisol in only one small detail: it has an 11-keto group instead of an 11β-hydroxyl group. This small chemical difference is extremely important biologically, however, for cortisone itself is lacking in biologic activity. It becomes effective in the body only because it can be converted to cortisol.

Cortisol is secreted by the zona fasciculata in response to adrenocorticotrophic hormone (ACTH). A specific biosynthetic step that is catalyzed by ACTH is the conversion of cholesterol to pregnenolone (3β-hydroxy-pregn-5-ene-20-one). Pregnenolone is then transformed by a series of adrenal enzymes to progesterone → 17α-hydroxyprogesterone → 11-deoxycortisol → cortisol. An inborn error in one of these enzymes or pharmacologic inhibition of one of them diminishes the efficiency of cortisol production and results in hypersecretion of the precursor occurring immediately before the inhibited step.

Upon entering the circulation, cortisol is reversibly bound to an α_2-globulin, transcortin. The major process of metabolic inactivation is carried out in the liver and involves reduction of ring A: Cortisol → dihydrocortisol → tetrahydrocortisol → tetrahydrocortisol glucuronide. The glucuronide is rapidly excreted by the kidneys. Some of the cortisol is oxidized to cortisone and then reduced and excreted as tetrahydrocortisone glucuronide. Tetrahydrocortisol and tetrahydrocortisone are the two most abundant end-products of cortisol metabolism; together, they account for almost 50 per cent of the total disposition of cortisol.

A widely used method for measuring cortisol in biologic fluids is the Porter-Silber reaction, utilizing the chromogenicity of the product resulting from the combination of phenylhydrazine with steroids having 17,21-dihydroxy-20-keto side chains (17-hydroxycorticosteroids, 17-OHCS). Normally, cortisol is the only major 17-OHCS in plasma, and tetrahydrocortisol and tetrahydrocortisone are the only major 17-OHCS in urine.

Another simple method for estimating plasma cortisol is based on the fact that it fluoresces; the fluorogenic steroid method is not applicable to the measurement of tetrahydrosteroids. Urinary tetrahydrocortisol and tetrahydrocortisone can be oxidized to 17-ketosteroids by bismuthate and are, therefore, 17-keto*genic* steroids

TABLE 1.   Properties of the Major Adrenal Steroids

Steroid	Regulated by	Major Metabolites*	Methods of Measurement	Major Actions	Clinical Consequences of Deficiency	Clinical Consequences of Excess
Cortisol	ACTH	Tetrahydro-cortisol Tetrahydro-cortisone	17-OHCS (Porter-Silber) Fluorogenic 17-KGS	Suppression of ACTH and MSH Protein catabolism Impairs glucose utilization Stabilizes lysosomes Suppresses inflammation Na retention K excretion	Hyperpigmentation (high ACTH, MSH) Fasting hypoglycemia Anorexia and vomiting Weight loss Apathy Impaired water excretion	Impaired glucose tolerance Thinning of skin Ecchymoses Poor wound healing Osteoporosis Weakness Hypertension Impaired growth Central obesity
Aldosterone	Angiotensin K,Na ACTH Volume	Tetrahydro-aldosterone Aldosterone-18-glucuronide	Isotopic	Na retention K excretion	Hypotension Hyponatremia Hyperkalemia	Hypertension Hypokalemia
Deoxycorticosterone (DOC)	ACTH	Tetrahydro-DOC	Isotopic	Na retention K excretion		Hypertension Hypokalemia
Dehydroisoandrosterone	ACTH	Androsterone Etiocholanolone	17-KS	Weakly androgenic and anabolic	Lack of axillary hair in women	Virilization of women and children
Unidentified androgens	ACTH			Androgenic	Lack of axillary hair in women	Virilization of women and children
Unidentified estrogens	ACTH			Estrogenic		Feminization in men and children
Substance S	ACTH	Tetrahydro-S	17-OHCS 17-KGS			
17α-OH-progesterone	ACTH	Pregnanetriol	17-KGS			
Corticosterone	ACTH	Tetrahydro-corticosterone	Isotopic			

*Methods such as 17-OHCS, 17-KS, and 17-KGS are not specific; isotopic and chromatographic methods are used in specific identification of individual steroids.

(17-KGS). This method is somewhat less specific than the Porter-Silber reaction; nevertheless, it is widely used for estimating cortisol metabolites.

Cortisol is ubiquitous as a physiologic regulator; hardly a tissue in the body is unaffected by this hormone. Cortisol influences the level of activity of certain enzymes. It restrains the secretion of ACTH and melanocyte-stimulating hormone (MSH) by the pituitary. It accelerates the catabolism of protein and the hepatic metabolism of amino acids. It increases the appetite and promotes the deposition of fat in the facial, cervical, and truncal portions of the body. It retards the uptake of glucose by muscle cells and promotes hepatic gluconeogenesis from amino acids, pyruvate, lactate, and bicarbonate. It stabilizes lysosomes and suppresses a variety of inflammatory processes. It stimulates a number of electrolyte transport systems. As will become apparent in the discussions of Addison's disease and Cushing's syndrome, most of the manifestations of these clinical disorders can be understood in terms of inadequacies or exaggerations of the physiologic actions of cortisol.

Aldosterone is secreted by the zona glomerulosa in response to angiotensin, potassium, and ACTH. Like cortisol, it is metabolized by the liver to an inactive tetrahydro derivative; but, in addition, about 10 per cent is conjugated by the liver and kidneys to aldosterone-18-glucuronide. This is an acid hydrolyzable conjugate which recovers its identity as biologically active aldosterone when exposed to acid, a fact which has been exploited in the measurement of urinary aldosterone. Aldosterone is extremely potent, and the concentrations encountered in clinical situations are so low that they can be measured precisely only with highly sophisticated isotopic methods.

The physiologic effects of aldosterone stem from its property of stimulating transport of electrolytes by epithelial cells of the sweat glands, gastrointestinal tract, and, of greatest importance, the nephron. In response to aldosterone all these tissues tend to conserve sodium and lose potassium. Aldosterone deficiency leads to sodium depletion, loss of extracellular fluid, hypovolemia, and hypotension. An excess of aldosterone leads to sodium retention, expansion of extracellular volume, and hypertension.

11-Deoxycorticosterone (DOC) is normally secreted at about the same rate as aldosterone (of the order of 0.1 mg per day), but since it has only about one thirtieth the mineralocorticoid potency of aldosterone it is usually of little physiologic importance. DOC normally occurs in the biosynthetic pathway as a precursor of corticosterone and aldosterone, but in certain varieties of congenital adrenal hyperplasia it may be secreted in quantities sufficient to cause hypertension. It is metabolized to tetrahydro-DOC, but the quantities of either DOC or its metabolite that appear in biologic fluids are so small that isotopic techniques are usually required to measure them.

Dehydroisoandrosterone, a weakly androgenic 17-ketosteroid, is the most abundant steroid secreted in response to ACTH. A small portion is excreted as such; some is excreted in the form of androsterone and etiocholanolone; a minute portion is converted to testosterone. Dehydroisoandrosterone is the major precursor of the urinary 17-ketosteroids. Except in states in which it is secreted in grossly excessive quantities, such as

virilizing congenital adrenal hyperplasia, it is of little physiologic importance.

11-Deoxycortisol (Reichstein's substance S) is the immediate precursor of cortisol and is, therefore, produced in response to ACTH. Normally, it is retained by the adrenal long enough to undergo 11β-hydroxylation, resulting in formation of cortisol. Inefficiency of 11β-hydroxylase can occur as an inborn error of metabolism (hypertensive congenital adrenal hyperplasia), in carcinomatous adrenals, and as a consequence of treatment with an 11β-hydroxylase inhibitor (metyrapone). It has little biologic activity. Like cortisol it has a 17,21-dihydroxy-20-ketone side chain and is, therefore, measurable either as a 17-OHCS or as a 17-KGS.

17α-Hydroxyprogesterone is the cortisol precursor preceding the formation of 11-deoxycortisol and is under the regulatory control of ACTH. It has little biologic activity, and probably has no important role in the clinical manifestations of virilizing congenital adrenal hyperplasia. It is normally secreted in trivial quantities, but in the most common variety of congenital adrenal hyperplasia (21-hydroxylase deficiency) it is secreted in large amounts. This steroid is metabolized to a tetrahydro derivative, pregnanetriol, which is excreted in the urine and is of diagnostic value: a large excess of urinary pregnanetriol is practically pathognomonic of virilizing congenital adrenal hyperplasia owing to 21-hydroxylase deficiency. Although pregnanetriol is not a 17-OHCS by the Porter-Silber reaction, it is a 17-KGS and thus contributes to the nonspecificity of the latter as an index of cortisol production.

845. REGULATION OF ADRENAL STEROID SECRETION

The adrenal cortex may be regarded as two related but distinct organs. The inner portion of the cortex (zona fasciculata and zona reticularis) is under the control of ACTH and secretes all the adrenal steroids except aldosterone. The outer portion of the cortex (zona glomerulosa) secretes aldosterone in response to angiotensin, potassium, and ACTH.

ACTH activates adrenal adenyl cyclase, stimulating the formation of adenosine-3′,5′-monophosphate (cyclic AMP). Cyclic AMP is thought to activate an enzyme system that catalyzes the conversion of cholesterol to 20α-hydroxy-cholesterol, which in turn is converted to pregnenolone. The latter serves as a precursor for all hormonal steroids. The pattern of steroids secreted depends upon the enzymatic makeup of the adrenal cortex. Under normal circumstances the most abundant secretory products of the human adrenal cortex are cortisol and dehydroisoandrosterone, but a deficiency of one of the enzymes involved in the conversion of pregnenolone to its normal derivatives results in increased secretion of the biosynthetic intermediates occurring before the impaired step. Such distortions of adrenal secretory patterns are observed in congenital adrenal hyperplasia, in certain adrenal neoplasms, and during treatment with pharmacologic inhibitors of adrenal enzymes.

Since the secretory activity of the adrenal cortex is directly controlled by ACTH, many questions concerning the regulation of adrenal steroid secretion can be transformed into questions of what controls the secretion of ACTH. In brief, there are three major determinants of ACTH secretion in man. The *first* of these is the level of cortisol. Of all the products of the human adrenal cortex, only cortisol has significant ACTH-regulating potency. The higher the cortisol level, the greater is its restraining influence on ACTH secretion; the lower the cortisol level, the less the restraint on ACTH secretion. A *second* factor governing the secretion of ACTH is the sleep schedule. In people in the habit of sleeping at night, plasma ACTH (and cortisol secretion) begins to rise at about 2 A.M. It crests at about the time of awakening; then during the day it falls irregularly to low values during the evening. Thus there is a "diurnal rhythm" in the secretion of ACTH. The *third* factor governing the secretion of ACTH has been referred to as stress. Such experiences as pyrogenic reactions, acute hypoglycemia, electroconvulsive treatments, and major surgical operations bring about increases in ACTH secretion. Whether various stresses influence ACTH secretion through a common mechanism or separate mechanisms is unknown.

For practical purposes, in people with normal adrenal responsiveness, the plasma cortisol concentration can be used as an indirect index of ACTH secretion. Within the physiologic range of ACTH concentrations the adrenal response is directly proportional to the amount of ACTH reaching it. The cortisol secretory response to ACTH begins within minutes and continues as long as the plasma ACTH concentration is maintained. Once ACTH secretion has ceased, the plasma ACTH concentration falls with a half-time of about ten minutes; and once cortisol secretion has ceased, the plasma cortisol concentration falls with a half-time of one to two hours.

The secretion of aldosterone is only partially under the control of ACTH. Large amounts of ACTH induce increases in aldosterone transiently; but if ACTH is administered for more than two or three days, aldosterone secretion diminishes to pretreatment levels. Aldosterone is also influenced by potassium; depletion of bodily potassium diminishes aldosterone secretion. Impressive increases in aldosterone secretion can be brought about simply by depletion of bodily sodium, thus inducing hypovolemia. Hypovolemia of any cause induces renal production of renin, which catalyzes the generation of angiotensin; and angiotensin stimulates adrenocortical secretion of aldosterone. It is currently thought that the renin-angiotensin system is the principal regulator of aldosterone secretion in most of the conditions grouped under the heading Secondary Aldosteronism (see Ch. 852).

846. ADDISON'S DISEASE
(Primary Adrenal Cortical Insufficiency)

Incidence and Etiology. Addison's disease has been estimated to occur with an incidence of 1 case per 100,000 population. It is usually caused by granulomatous destruction or idiopathic atrophy of the adrenal cortex. Clinical adrenal insufficiency usually does not occur

unless at least 90 per cent of the adrenal cortex has been destroyed. The most common granulomatous disease destroying the adrenal cortex is tuberculosis, but, in certain regions, disseminated fungal infections are almost equally common. Idiopathic atrophy of the adrenal cortex is thought by some to be a consequence of an autoimmune process. All other causes of Addison's disease are decidedly rare. They include amyloidosis, adrenal apoplexy, and destruction of the adrenal cortex by metastatic tumor.

Pathogenesis. From the foregoing comments, it should be apparent that Addison's disease commonly arises in association with other significant disease processes. Thus the patient with Addison's disease resulting from granulomatous destruction of his adrenal glands should be considered to have had hematogenous spread of a tuberculous or fungal infection, and should be carefully surveyed for evidence of an active infection of other organs, particularly the genitourinary and respiratory systems. Patients with "autoimmune" atrophy of their adrenals have an increased probability of having other diseases such as diabetes mellitus, hypothyroidism, and hypoparathyroidism. Patients with Addison's disease preceded by the nephrotic syndrome should be suspected of having amyloidosis.

The pathology of the granulomatous adrenal was described in masterful detail in a monograph written in 1931 by Rowntree and Snell. Of interest to physiologists in later years was the fact that the few remaining adrenal cells were often "arranged in adenoma-like nodules . . . suggesting . . . compensatory hypertrophy." All the pathophysiologic consequences of Addison's disease can now be understood in terms of deficiencies of cortisol, aldosterone, and adrenal androgen.

Cortisol deficiency results in increased pituitary secretion of ACTH and melanocyte-stimulating hormone (MSH), and these pituitary hormones are responsible for the mucocutaneous accumulation of melanin in classic Addison's disease. Cortisol deficiency also results in loss of appetite, loss of vigor, inability to maintain adequate blood glucose levels during prolonged fasting, inability to excrete a load of free water with normal rapidity, and inability to withstand severe or even rather minor stresses without going into shock.

Aldosterone deficiency renders the distal convoluted tubule of the nephron unable to carry out cation exchange at a normal rate. Consequently, there is failure to conserve sodium and excrete potassium normally. As a result of sodium wastage, there is depletion of extracellular fluid volume, blood volume decreases, blood pressure falls, cardiac output falls, and heart size diminishes. This process may culminate in peripheral vascular collapse, and is a prominent feature of addisonian crisis. Hyponatremia results from failure to conserve sodium and, as noted before, impaired ability to excrete a water load. Impaired ability to excrete potassium causes serum potassium concentrations to rise. If serum potassium concentrations exceed about 7 mEq per liter, disturbances of cardiac electrophysiology occur, manifested by sharp peaking of the T waves of the electrocardiogram and cardiac standstill in diastole.

Adrenal androgen deficiency is of no consequence in the male, because testicular androgen production suffices to induce adequate virilization. In women, however, the adrenal is responsible for a major portion of the total production of androgen, and loss of adrenal function results in a decreased growth of axillary and pubic hair.

The clinical manifestations of Addison's disease are usually insidious, and often exist in mild form for several weeks or months before correct diagnosis leads to proper treatment. Throughout this time, however, the patient with severely compromised adrenal function is in jeopardy of fatal addisonian crisis, either through progression of the chronic abnormalities or through superimposition of some acute stress such as fasting (vomiting), injury (surgical operation), or infection.

The mechanisms of death are peripheral vascular collapse (shock) and hyperkalemic cardiac standstill; perhaps hypoglycemia plays a role in some cases.

Clinical Manifestations. One can hardly do better than to quote or paraphrase the clinical descriptions in the monographs by Addison and by Rowntree and Snell, written before synthetic steroids became available to alter the natural course of Addison's disease. Addison wrote:

> The patient, in most of the cases I have seen, has been observed gradually to fall off in general health; he becomes languid and weak, indisposed to either bodily or mental exertion; the appetite is impaired or entirely lost; ...the pulse small and feeble...excessively soft and compressible; the body wastes...slight pain or uneasiness is from time to time referred to the region of the stomach, and there is occasionally actual vomiting...it is by no means uncommon for the patient to manifest indications of disturbed cerebral circulation.... We discover a most remarkable, and, so far as I know, characteristic discoloration taking place in the skin,—sufficiently marked indeed as generally to have attracted the attention of the patient himself, or of the patient's friends.... It may be said to present a dingy or smoky appearance, or various tints or shades of deep amber or chestnut-brown.... The body wastes...the pulse becomes smaller and weaker, and ...the patient at length gradually sinks and expires.

In their experience with 108 cases of Addison's disease, Rowntree and Snell noted that asthenia, weight loss, gastrointestinal symptoms (anorexia, nausea, vomiting, and abdominal pain), and hypotension were almost always part of the syndrome. Hyperpigmentation was present in most cases and was described in such terms as "a suntan which does not wear off . . . tinged somewhat with blue or gray . . . dirty in appearance." The exposed portions of the body (hands, face, neck, and arms), points of pressure and friction, nipples, freckles, recently formed scars, genitalia, and creases of the palms often showed exaggerated pigmentation. Brown, blue, or gray spots on the lips and buccal mucous membranes were common.

Nowadays, earlier diagnosis and specific therapy make it possible to correct the compensatory hypersecretion of ACTH and MSH before development of prominent mucocutaneous hyperpigmentation, so that this manifestation may disappear in the patient who has been treated for a long time. Hyperpigmentation is not present in all untreated patients, so one should not take the position that the absence of characteristic hyperpigmentation rules out the diagnosis of Addison's disease.

The mental state of the untreated addisonian patient was frequently characterized as "asthenia, languor, exhaustion, or disinclination to physical or mental effort." Less frequently, irritability, confusion, and delusions were noted. Almost invariably the patients lacked the vigor to carry on productive lives.

Fever was not found in "uncomplicated" cases of Addison's disease. When it did occur it was attributable to coexisting infection.

It is of historical interest that the laboratory abnormalities of Addison's disease as listed by Rowntree and Snell were limited to such items as gastric achlorhydria, elevated serum urea, and delayed excretion of phenolsulfonphthalein and water. It was only later that hyponatremia and hyperkalemia were recognized as being commonplace abnormalities in the chemical profile of Addison's disease.

It is important to remember that Addison's disease often occurs in association with other diseases. Since the clinical manifestations of Addison's disease are shared by many other debilitating disorders, it is easy to overlook the possible presence of Addison's disease while attributing all the manifestations to some coexisting condition. Fortunately, it is now possible to establish with certainty whether a patient has Addison's disease with a specific test for adrenocortical reserve, and this should be carefully performed without hesitation whenever the possibility of Addison's disease seems realistic, for example, in any patient with a syndrome of hypotension, weakness, anorexia, and weight loss.

Diagnosis and Differential Diagnosis. To establish the diagnosis of Addison's disease one should measure the steroid secretory response to a standard dose of ACTH. A standard test, which has a number of modifications, all valid in experienced hands, is to give 50 units of ACTH as a constant intravenous infusion for eight hours and measure the resulting rise in plasma cortisol. Individuals with normal adrenal glands should respond with increases in plasma cortisol to at least 30 μg per 100 ml. Addisonian patients show little or no increase in plasma cortisol, which is usually less than 15 μg per 100 ml both before and during the infusion of ACTH. Intermediate (subnormal) responses are observed in patients with adrenocortical insufficiency secondary to hypopituitarism or prolonged corticosteroid therapy; these conditions can be distinguished from Addison's disease by demonstrating that repetitive treatment with ACTH, over several successive days, induces a stepwise increase in adrenal steroids until normal values are attained. Among the acceptable modifications of this standard test are procedures employing intramuscular injection of a good quality of depot ACTH and measurement of urinary 17-OHCS, 17-KGS, or 17-ketosteroids. The crucial point is that the patient with Addison's disease has little or no adrenocortical capacity to respond to ACTH (Fig. 1).

Treatment. The most important principles to observe in the management of Addison's disease are (1) that only two adrenal hormones, cortisol and aldosterone, are vitally important; (2) that the physiologic requirements for these two hormones fluctuate; (3) that cortisol substitution therapy should never be totally withdrawn unless it can first be demonstrated that the diagnosis of Addison's disease was erroneous, and (4) that sodium chloride must be administered in liberal quantities in order to correct extracellular fluid depletion.

Treatment of Addisonian Crisis. The patient in addisonian crisis is in immediate danger of losing his life because of glucocorticoid deficiency, extracellular fluid depletion, and hyperkalemia. Without delay, he should be treated with an intravenous infusion of physiologic sodium chloride; the infusion should be given rapidly, on the assumption that the patient probably has a deficit of at least 20 per cent of his extracellular volume (at least 3 liters in the adult). A water-soluble glucocor-

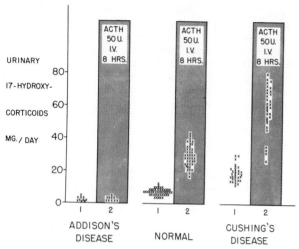

Figure 1. Urinary 17-OHCS:(1) during a control day and (2) during a day on which 50 units of ACTH was administered intravenously over a period of eight hours. In contrast to normal subjects and patients with Cushing's disease, patients with Addison's disease have low steroid values on both days.

ticoid such as hydrocortisone phosphate, 100 mg, should be added to the infusion. Within a few hours, if the electrolyte imbalance is corrected, the endocrinologic crisis may be considered to be over, and therapy should be adapted to meet the patient's current needs; if there is no stressful complication, the dose of glucocorticoid may be reduced to the physiologic range of approximately 20 mg of hydrocortisone daily; but if the patient is stressed, larger doses will be required. An attempt should be made to determine whether the crisis might have been precipitated by some stress such as an infection, and if so, this should be treated specifically.

If the diagnosis of Addison's disease has not previously been established and the patient's illness is suggestive of addisonian crisis, one should without delay initiate therapy and, at the same time, carry out a definitive diagnostic test for Addison's disease. Physiologic sodium chloride solution should be administered as outlined above. Instead of adding hydrocortisone phosphate to the saline infusion, one should add the potent water-soluble glucocorticoid dexamethasone phosphate, 4 mg. This will be equivalent to 100 mg of hydrocortisone in biologic potency, but will not obscure the adrenal response to an infusion of ACTH. To the intravenous infusion one may add ACTH in a dose sufficient to assure that the patient receives at least 5 units each hour for eight hours. Plasma cortisol should be measured prior to the addition of ACTH and again toward the end of the ACTH infusion. An adequate rise in plasma cortisol in response to ACTH excludes the diagnosis of Addison's disease; a negligible adrenal response confirms the diagnosis.

Chronic Treatment of Intercritical Addison's Disease. Therapeutic strategy in Addison's disease aims at simulating normal rates of secretion of cortisol and mineralocorticoid. Normal adults secrete about 20 mg of cortisol per day, and adults with Addison's disease usually require approximately 20 mg of cortisol (hydrocortisone) daily in the form of medication; it may be administered orally or parenterally in single or divided doses. Various synthetic glucocorticoids may be substi-

tuted for hydrocortisone, providing that proper adjustment is made for their differences in biologic potency.

Normal adults receiving unrestricted diets usually consume 100 to 300 mEq of sodium daily, and while on such diets they secrete approximately 0.1 mg of aldosterone daily. Aldosterone is not available for therapeutic use, but a synthetic mineralocorticoid, fludrocortisone (9α-fluorohydrocortisone), is available, and a tablet containing 0.1 mg taken once daily usually suffices as an aldosterone substitute. Another useful preparation is *desoxycorticosterone pivalate,* a slowly absorbed suspension given intramuscularly in doses of about 50 mg (2 ml) per month. A patient who has a history of hypertension prior to the onset of Addison's disease may not require mineralocorticoid replacement therapy as long as he receives glucocorticoids and ordinary amounts of dietary sodium. No addisonian patient will do well, however, without an ample intake of sodium chloride.

Children with Addison's disease require smaller doses of steroids than adults. The daily cortisol dose should be about 12 mg per square meter of body surface. If the child's linear growth does not proceed normally, it should be assumed that the dose of cortisol might be excessive, and the dose should be adjusted downward. The dose of mineralocorticoid should be adjusted as necessary to maintain normal blood pressure.

Treatment During Stresses. The maximal response of the normal pituitary-adrenal system to extreme stress results in the secretion of 200 to 500 mg of cortisol per day. This is the dosage range of hydrocortisone phosphate to be administered parenterally to patients undergoing bilateral adrenalectomy or to addisonian patients undergoing extensive surgical procedures. Hydrocortisone phosphate administered parenterally in doses of 100 mg every four to six hours should suffice as glucocorticoid replacement therapy in any severely stressed addisonian patient. As the stress subsides, the dose of hydrocortisone should be diminished accordingly. For example, after a major surgical operation, the daily dose of hydrocortisone can usually be decreased by decrements of 50 per cent each day until the usual dosage employed in chronic substitution therapy is reached.

For one reason or another, severely stressed patients usually do not consume adequate diets. It is important that addisonian patients be given at least 1 liter of physiologic sodium chloride solution daily until they resume their normal diets; a particularly hazardous period in convalescence is that during which orders are ordinarily given for the patient to take a "soft diet" or "surgical liquids." During this period the patient often does not even take all that is offered and may become depleted of extracellular fluid.

Mild stresses such as minor surgical operations and injuries require only minor increases in corticosteroid therapy. Usually a two- to fourfold increase in glucocorticoid treatment on the day of the stress will suffice. Oral medications may be used if they can be retained. Again, it is important that the addisonian patient who is fasting or vomiting be given parenteral sodium chloride solution.

Treatment in the Presence of Infection. In the presence of infection, it is particularly important that glucocorticoid dosage should simulate the cortisol secretion rate of the similarly infected but endocrinologically normal person. Overtreatment might impair the patient's mechanisms for defending against invading microorganisms, whereas undertreatment might predispose the infection-stressed patient to addisonian crisis. As a rule, an endocrinologically normal person secretes no more than 20 to 100 mg of cortisol per day in response to infection. This then is the hydrocortisone dosage range that is appropriate for the addisonian with an intercurrent infectious illness. A practical rule is to be guided by the patient's body temperature. If it is in excess of 39° C, the dose of hydrocortisone should be increased to whatever amount is needed to reduce the temperature to less than this level. If the temperature is normal, the hydrocortisone dosage should be lowered until maintenance doses are reached. If the temperature is between 38 and 39° C, it may be assumed that the dose of hydrocortisone is appropriate (presumably between 20 and 100 mg per day). It is of utmost importance that infections be specifically diagnosed and specifically treated as quickly as possible.

Mineralocorticoid vs. Sodium Chloride Therapy. Mineralocorticoids are used in treating intercritical adrenal insufficiency in order to assist the well-fed patient in maintaining adequate sodium stores without taking supplemental sodium chloride. Ordinary doses of mineralocorticoids do not adequately protect the addisonian patient from sodium and extracellular fluid depletion during periods of fasting or vomiting. Once sodium depletion has occurred, it must be corrected by the administration of sodium chloride; if adequate attention is given to this matter, upward adjustment of mineralocorticoid dosage (simulating the normal aldosterone secretory response to sodium depletion) will be unnecessary. Patients who sustain losses of sodium chloride but who are still capable of retaining oral medication, e.g., patients who sweat excessively, may be given supplemental sodium chloride tablets in doses of 2 grams two to four times daily.

Identification Bracelet and Injectable Hydrocortisone. The patient with Addison's disease should wear an identification bracelet stating his name, nearest kin's name and telephone number, and physician's name and telephone number. It should also state: "I have adrenal insufficiency. In any emergency involving injury, vomiting, or loss of consciousness, the hydrocortisone in my possession should be injected under my skin, and my physician should be notified." The patient should carry a small, clearly labeled kit containing 100 mg of hydrocortisone phosphate solution in a sterile syringe ready for injection. Even if never used, the bracelet and kit are of educational value to the addisonian patient who must understand that his survival depends upon the timely use of steroids.

Prognosis. With the advent of synthetic corticosteroids the prognosis of Addison's disease became radically altered from one of almost certain fatal termination within months (rarely years) to one of normal activity and life expectancy. The well-treated addisonian patient should have essentially normal steroid and electrolyte values under all circumstances; therefore he should not be incapacitated or have his life expectancy shortened by the fact that he has Addison's disease. All of the author's addisonian patients are productively employed unless they suffer from some additional disorder which is in some way incapacitating. Addisonians must, however, face the perils of emergencies in which they are incapable of caring for themselves and in which they might depend upon the assistance of others to assure that the essential steroids and electrolytes are administered. Their prognosis might also be limited by other diseases sometimes associated with Addison's disease, such as tuberculosis, histoplasmosis, diabetes mellitus, or amyloidosis. Most of the addisonian patients who have been discovered since synthetic cortisone became generally available are still living, and there are no accurate data to indicate whether Addison's disease per se, when adequately treated, alters life expectancy.

ADRENAL INSUFFICIENCY SECONDARY TO BILATERAL ADRENALECTOMY

Adrenal insufficiency secondary to bilateral adrenalectomy is one variant of Addison's disease which should never present any diagnostic difficulty inasmuch as it is iatrogenic. Treatment is the same as that outlined under Addison's Disease.

847. ADRENAL APOPLEXY

Hemorrhagic infarction of the adrenal glands can occur in the course of meningococcal septicemia (Waterhouse-Friderichsen syndrome) or as a complication of anticoagulant therapy. The occurrence of hypotension in either of these clinical settings should alert the physician to the possibility of adrenal apoplexy, and treatment similar to that outlined under the heading Treatment During Stresses (Ch. 846) should be undertaken on an emergency basis. Specific treatment for the underlying disorder (meningococcemia or coagulation defects) should also be carried out without delay. If the patient survives, he may at some later date undergo a standard test for adrenocortical reserve in order to determine whether steroid replacement therapy can be withdrawn safely.

Although the adrenal glands are hemorrhagic in the Waterhouse-Friderichsen syndrome, hypotension, shock, and death in this condition are usually not attributable to adrenal insufficiency. Cortisol should be given in large doses, because it is impossible to rule out adrenal insufficiency within the time that is available to initiate decisive therapy; the patient who might have true adrenal insufficiency in association with adrenal apoplexy should not be denied the benefits of adequate cortisol therapy.

848. ADRENAL INSUFFICIENCY SECONDARY TO HYPOPITUITARISM

Definition and Incidence. Since normal adrenal function is dependent upon the stimulatory action of ACTH secreted by the pituitary, it follows that any disorder in which the pituitary is damaged in such a way as to reduce ACTH secretion to subnormal values leads to secondary adrenocortical hypofunction. This situation is encountered in approximately 1 of 1000 patients admitted to hospitals. (See Ch. 831.)

Pathogenesis. Whether associated with tumor, infarction, infection, histiocytosis, surgical resection, or intensive irradiation, loss of pituitary function is attributable to loss of pituitary tissue or to interruption of the connections between the hypothalamus and the pituitary. The degree of hypopituitarism is variable from patient to patient, ranging from such profound deficiencies as to be incompatible with survival to such mild deficiencies that special tests of pituitary reserve are required to demonstrate an abnormality.

Absence of ACTH results in decreased secretion of cortisol and adrenal androgen, but aldosterone secretion remains relatively intact. Cortisol deficiency results in loss of appetite, loss of vigor, inability to maintain adequate blood glucose levels during prolonged fasting, inability to excrete free water with normal rapidity, and inability to withstand severe stresses without going into shock. Hyponatremia is commonly encountered in patients with hypopituitarism who have been given liberal amounts of fluid, and it is directly attributable to the difficulty these individuals have in excreting free water. If they are given glucocorticoid so that they can excrete water adequately, they can be shown to have the capacity to adapt to simple sodium chloride deprivation by increasing their aldosterone secretion sufficiently to enable them to excrete urine that is virtually sodium free.

Absence of adrenal androgen is itself of little consequence; but when adrenal insufficiency is secondary to hypopituitarism, it is usually accompanied by a deficiency of gonadotrophins with secondary hypogonadism and a consequent decrease in testicular secretion of testosterone. Therefore, in contrast to Addison's disease, in which only the adult female shows evidence of androgen deficiency, in hypopituitarism patients of either sex are likely to exhibit manifestations of androgen deficiency.

Clinical Manifestations. There are several similarities and a few important differences between hypopituitarism and Addison's disease with regard to their clinical manifestations. Like the addisonian, the patient with hypopituitarism "falls off in general health; he becomes languid and weak, indisposed to either bodily or mental exertion; the appetite is impaired...and there is occasionally actual vomiting." Fasting may lead to hypoglycemia, and hypoglycemic symptoms (including loss of consciousness) are probably more common in untreated hypopituitarism than in Addison's disease. A liberal intake of water may lead to severe hyponatremia and manifestations of water intoxication such as confusion, incoordination, stupor, and convulsions. Severe stress may precipitate peripheral vascular collapse.

In contrast to the addisonian, the patient with hypopituitarism does not show mucocutaneous hyperpigmentation (this abnormality, in Addison's disease, is a consequence of *excessive* secretion of the pituitary hormones ACTH and MSH). Unlike the addisonian, the patient with hypopituitarism can tolerate simple sodium deprivation without developing shock or hyponatremia. In addition to the manifestations of adrenal insufficiency, the patient with hypopituitarism usually exhibits manifestations of hypogonadism and hypothyroid-

ism, and may show other evidence of pituitary or intracranial disease, e.g., erosion of the sella turcica and temporal visual field defects.

Diagnosis and Differential Diagnosis. The diagnosis of secondary adrenal insufficiency is established by the demonstration that cortisol levels in blood and cortisol metabolite levels in urine are subnormal and that they can be induced to rise to normal or above normal by repetitive treatment with ACTH over a period of one to three days. Urinary 17-ketosteroids are also subnormal, but rise in response to ACTH.

Primary adrenal insufficiency (Addison's disease) is easily differentiated from secondary adrenal insufficiency by the failure of steroids to rise substantially regardless of the dosage or duration of treatment with ACTH.

It is advisable to measure both plasma and urinary steroids in order to avoid pitfalls in differentiating secondary adrenal insufficiency from certain disorders of cortisol metabolism in which a normal relationship between plasma and urinary corticosteroids is lacking. Thus in primary hypothyroidism, hepatic insufficiency, and severe renal insufficiency, and during treatment with drugs that alter the extra-adrenal metabolism of cortisol (diphenylhydantoin, aminoglutethimide, amphotericin, o,p'-DDD, triparanol), the urinary 17-OHCS do not adequately reflect cortisol secretion rates and are falsely low in relation to plasma cortisol levels. In these situations, plasma cortisol concentrations accurately reflect cortisol secretion under basal conditions and in response to ACTH, whereas urinary 17-OHCS might falsely suggest the presence of secondary adrenal insufficiency. In contrast, there is a familial disorder in which plasma transcortin concentrations are subnormal, even though cortisol secretion rates, plasma free cortisol concentrations, and urinary 17-OHCS are all normal. In this situation, plasma cortisol concentrations alone might erroneously suggest the presence of secondary adrenal insufficiency.

Various clinical clues are also helpful in arriving at a correct diagnosis of secondary adrenal insufficiency, e.g., hypothyroidism with normal responsiveness to thyrotrophin, hypogonadism with subnormal gonadotrophin levels in plasma or urine, or growth failure with consistently negligible levels of growth hormone in serum (even after provocative maneuvers such as arginine infusion or insulin-induced hypoglycemia). Other evidence of pituitary disease, such as erosion of the sella turcica or a history of postpartum hemorrhage, should also alert the physician to the possibility that the patient might have hypopituitarism, subnormal ACTH production, and secondary adrenocortical deficiency.

A mild degree of ACTH deficiency can exist with normal or slightly subnormal plasma and urinary corticosteroids and normal or slightly subnormal responses to ACTH. Such mild degrees of ACTH deficiency are referred to as limited pituitary reserve, and are characterized by failure of the pituitary to secrete normal quantities of ACTH (and therefore a failure of the adrenal glands to secrete normal quantities of corticosteroids) in response to stress or to standard test doses of metyrapone.

Treatment. Secondary adrenocortical insufficiency requires cortisol replacement therapy in the same doses and under the same conditions as outlined for Addison's disease (see Ch. 846). Mineralocorticoid therapy is unnecessary. An identification card and hydrocortisone phosphate for emergency use should be employed as in Addison's disease.

If the patient suffers from hypogonadism, hypothyroidism, or diabetes insipidus, these conditions should be treated with androgens or estrogens, thyroid, or pitressin, as outlined in Ch. 859, 839, and 834, respectively.

Prognosis. As in the case of Addison's disease, the prognosis in secondary adrenal insufficiency is excellent if intelligent use is made of hormones for replacement therapy and if the primary basis for the hypopituitarism is not otherwise incapacitating or life threatening (see Ch. 831).

849. ADRENAL INSUFFICIENCY SECONDARY TO PITUITARY-ADRENAL SUPPRESSION BY CORTICOSTEROIDS

Prolonged administration of glucocorticoids or prolonged secretion of cortisol by an adrenal tumor in quantities sufficient to cause Cushing's syndrome consistently causes suppression of ACTH secretion and consequent adrenocortical atrophy. Withdrawal of steroid therapy or removal of the adrenal tumor results in adrenal insufficiency. Diagnosis should not be difficult in view of the physician's or surgeon's role in bringing about the condition. If the hypercortisolism has been severe and has existed continuously for at least one year, the course of pituitary-adrenal recovery may be slow, requiring several months for completion. Early in the course the basal corticosteroid levels, the adrenal response to ACTH, and the pituitary-adrenal response to metyrapone are all subnormal, simulating adrenal insufficiency secondary to hypopituitarism. Treatment consists of giving a physiologic dose of hydrocortisone, 20 mg once daily, to prevent symptoms of adrenal insufficiency. Over a period of months this dose can gradually be reduced to 5 mg daily and finally withdrawn altogether as pituitary-adrenal function gradually returns to normal. Until pituitary-adrenal recovery is complete, one should treat the patient as if he had hypopituitarism during periods of stress or infection (see Ch. 831).

850. CUSHING'S SYNDROME

Definition. Cushing's syndrome is the clinical and metabolic disorder resulting from a chronic excess of glucocorticoids. *Cushing's syndrome medicamentosus* is a common iatrogenic disorder caused by any of several synthetic glucocorticoids. Spontaneous Cushing's syndrome, on the other hand, is caused solely by cortisol, the only glucocorticoid produced in significant quantities by the human adrenal cortex.

Etiology. Normally, cortisol is not secreted except in response to ACTH, and ACTH is not secreted in the presence of supraphysiologic levels of cortisol. Therefore the very occurrence of Cushing's syndrome implies a disorder in the regulation of cortisol or ACTH secretion: either the adrenal gland has acquired the capability of secreting cortisol in the absence of ACTH, or ACTH secretion is not normally suppressible by cortisol. There are three well-established causes of Cushing's syndrome. *First,* adrenocortical tumors can secrete cortisol autonomously, that is to say, in the virtual absence of ACTH. The tumors may be carcinomas, solitary adenomas, or (rarely) multiple adenomas. *Second,* certain nonpituitary neoplasms secrete ACTH, which stimulates the adrenal cortices to secrete supraphysiologic quantities of cortisol. This clinical entity is sometimes referred to as the ectopic ACTH syndrome (see Ch. 870). *Third,* pituitary function can become disordered so that ACTH is secreted in excessive quantities, thus stimulating excessive secretion of cortisol by the adrenals. This condition is referred to by the specific term Cushing's disease. The pituitary can be normal in appearance, contain a small basophil adenoma, or contain a large chromophobe adenoma; regardless of the morphologic appearance of the pituitary, virtually all patients with excessive pituitary ACTH show similar patterns of ACTH secretion. There is loss of normal diurnal rhythmicity, relative but not absolute resistance to suppression by glucocorticoids, and increased secretion of ACTH in response to a reduction of cortisol levels to normal.

Incidence. Cushing's syndrome resulting from adrenal tumor occurs in approximately 1 of every 10,000 hospital admissions. Cushing's disease occurs in approximately 1 of every 4000 admissions. The incidence of the ectopic ACTH syndrome is difficult to estimate, because it is frequently overlooked. There is evidence that ectopic ACTH might be produced by as many as 8 per cent of visceral carcinomas. Careful screening of patients with nonpituitary tumors might reveal the production of ectopic ACTH to be the most common cause of hypercortisolism.

Pathogenesis. The major features of Cushing's syndrome are understandable in terms of the known actions of cortisol. When present in excessive quantities, this hormone accelerates the catabolism of protein and stimulates the hepatic uptake and deamination of amino acids. It also inhibits the transport of amino acids into extrahepatic tissues. As a consequence of these actions, prolonged high concentrations of cortisol cause clinical manifestations of protein wasting. Children show retardation of linear growth. Wasting of the integument and increasing capillary fragility result in ecchymoses. Cutaneous striae form in areas where the skin is stretched by an accumulation of adipose tissue. In extreme cases, wasting of muscle results in pronounced weakness. Wasting of bone matrix results in osteoporosis.

Abnormally high levels of cortisol alter the body's responses to injury and infection. Cortisol stabilizes lysosomal membranes, thus diminishing the tendency of injured tissues to perpetuate their own damage. It suppresses the sticking of leukocytes to endothelial surfaces, and diminishes the accumulation of leukocytes at sites of tissue injury. It inhibits the diapedesis of white blood cells and impairs their migration through tissues. In high concentrations over long periods of time, cortisol impairs antibody production and inhibits the proliferation of lymphocytes. Thus almost every aspect of the normal cellular response to injury or infection is suppressed by high concentrations of cortisol, leaving the patient with impaired capacity to limit the spread of invading organisms.

Cortisol promotes potassium excretion and sodium retention by stimulating cation exchange by the distal convoluted tubules. A severe excess of cortisol can result in depletion of bodily potassium to such a degree that hypokalemia, electrocardiographic abnormalities, muscular weakness, and impairment of renal concentrating capacity develop. Retention of sodium and elevated blood pressure occur. Steroid hypertension, like other varieties of hypertension, leads to left ventricular hypertrophy and predisposes the patient to congestive heart failure and strokes. Even without frank congestive heart failure, some patients experience expansion of their extracellular fluid volumes to the point of edema.

In addition to stimulating the formation of new glucose from amino acids, lactate, pyruvate, and bicarbonate, cortisol impairs the action of insulin in transporting glucose across cell membranes. Consequently, abnormally high amounts of cortisol tend to raise the level of blood glucose; this is most readily apparent in the prolongation of hyperglycemia after a glucose load; a minority of patients with hypercortisolism have abnormally high fasting blood glucose levels (see Ch. 806).

Adrenal carcinomas that secrete cortisol usually secrete significant quantities of adrenal androgen as well. In men this is of no clinical consequence, but in women and children it gives rise to virilism. Benign adenomas that cause Cushing's syndrome are somewhat less likely to produce excessive quantities of androgen. Mild virilism, usually amounting to nothing more than acne, thinning of scalp hair, and some degree of facial hirsutism, is common in women with Cushing's disease or the ectopic ACTH syndrome. In these disorders the increased levels of ACTH result in increased production of adrenal androgens as well as cortisol.

Although Cushing's syndrome is due entirely to an excess of corticosteroids, one must realize that the clinical illness of the patient may be affected by other factors as well. This is readily apparent in the ectopic ACTH syndrome when the clinical picture is usually dominated by other effects of the ACTH-secreting tumor. These patients often have a degree of weakness out of proportion to the severity of their hypercortisolism, and they often lose weight, in contrast to patients with classic features of Cushing's syndrome.

Clinical Manifestations. The clinical manifestations of Cushing's syndrome are familiar to every physician who has seen a patient treated with large doses of a cortisol-like steroid for several weeks or longer. In addition to the picture of cortisol excess, there will, in some patients, be features of virilism and mineralocorticoid excess as well. The frequencies of various clinical manifestations in Cushing's syndrome are listed in Table 2.

General Appearance and Physiognomy. The typical patient with Cushing's syndrome has central obesity, with rounding of the face, thickening of the fat pads in the supraclavicular fossae, and thickening of the thoracicoabdominal panniculus (Fig. 2). In longstanding cases, the abdominal obesity can progress to grotesque proportions while the extremities remain remarkably slender. People with pre-existing obesity from other causes can, of course, develop Cushing's syndrome; under such circumstances it is difficult to decide on clinical grounds

TABLE 2.   Frequency of Clinical Manifestations in Cushing's Syndrome

	Per Cent
Impaired glucose tolerance	94
Central obesity	88
Hypertension	82
Oligomenorrhea	72
Osteoporosis	58
Purpura and striae	42
Muscle atrophy	36
Hirsutism	30
Edema	20
Hypokalemia (unprovoked)	18
Kidney stones	12
Psychotic mentation	6

alone whether the patient has Cushing's syndrome and, if so, to what extent his obesity is attributable to the steroid excess. Patients with malignant tumors often show little or no obesity, even though their steroid levels are high and other features of Cushing's syndrome are fully expressed.

Cutaneous Manifestations. The face and neck often have a ruddy hyperemic appearance. Trivial trauma often results in ecchymosis. In advanced cases, the skin

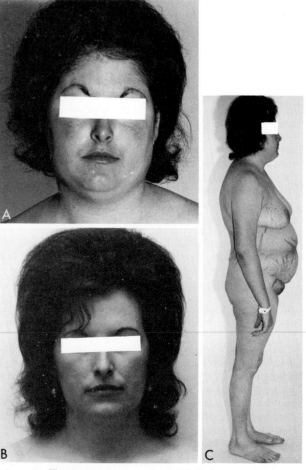

Figure 2. The appearance of a patient with Cushing's syndrome (*A*) before and (*B*) one year after removal of an adrenal adenoma. (*C*) Profile, before treatment.

over the forearms and legs becomes thin, having the appearance of parchment. Slight injury to the skin can result in purpuric extravasation of blood; the sites of venipunctures sometimes show extensive subcutaneous hemorrhage. Removal of adhesive tape sometimes denudes the delicate skin of the patient with the advanced protein-wasting of Cushing's syndrome. Wounds heal slowly and often become the sites of indolent infections. In areas where the weakened skin is stretched by the underlying accumulation of fat (particularly the abdomen, shoulders, and hips), wide purplish striae may form.

The reaction to infection is attenuated in Cushing's syndrome. Superficial fungal infections, e.g., tinea versicolor, occur in about 20 per cent of cases. In more severe cases, bacterial infections are not well confined in the form of discrete abscesses of short duration, but are more likely to be chronic and to give rise to cellulitis and bacteremia. This is a dangerous situation which may escape notice, because the patient with Cushing's syndrome often has less discomfort and experiences less of a febrile reaction than would ordinarily be expected with a given degree of infection.

Largely as a function of an associated excess of androgens, acne and hirsutism commonly occur in patients with Cushing's syndrome. The hirsutism is usually slight, downy, and distributed over the cheeks and shoulders, but coarse hairs may appear in the beard area and on the chest and abdomen. In men, of course, this aspect of hyperadrenocorticism is unnoticed.

Reproductive Functions. Most women with Cushing's syndrome have oligomenorrhea. Although it is difficult to evaluate with certainty, many of them may have diminished fertility; however, this is by no means uniform. Men with Cushing's syndrome are sometimes said to be troubled with impotence; this is certainly not always so, and might not be related to the hyperadrenocorticism when it does occur. Infertility is probably not a feature of Cushing's syndrome in men.

Musculoskeletal Manifestations. Children with Cushing's syndrome experience arrest of linear growth. If obesity in a child is associated with growth arrest, the possibility of Cushing's syndrome should receive strong consideration; continued normal linear growth is strong evidence that the child's obesity is not due to Cushing's syndrome. Insidious atrophy of the skeleton results in mild hypercalciuria and, in time, in frank osteoporosis. Severe osteoporosis of the vertebral bodies may result in bulging of intervertebral discs, giving the appearance of codfish vertebrae in lateral roentgenographic views. Compression fractures with anterior wedging of the vertebral bodies result in kyphosis and loss of height. Pathologic fractures of ribs and hips occasionally occur.

In severe Cushing's syndrome, muscular atrophy may progress to such an extent that the patient is too weak to rise from a squatting position without assistance. Muscular weakness is usually not noticeable in milder cases.

Cardiovascular and Renal Manifestations. Most patients with Cushing's syndrome have hypertension, the course and complications of which are similar to those of essential hypertension. Edema can occur as a manifestation of congestive heart failure, but in 10 to 20 per cent of cases, mild edema occurs in the absence of congestive failure.

Hypokalemia with hypochloremic alkalosis occurs spontaneously in about 10 to 20 per cent of the cases (usually those with the most severe excesses of steroid secretion), and may occur in others as a complication of diuretic therapy.

Renal lithiasis can occur in chronic cases of Cushing's syndrome.

Hematologic Features. Some patients with Cushing's syndrome have erythrocytosis, granulocytosis, lymphopenia, and eosinopenia.

Carbohydrate Tolerance. Impaired carbohydrate tolerance occurs in more than 90 per cent of cases of Cushing's syndrome. In the majority it is manifested merely by a failure of the blood glucose to return to normal fasting levels during the first three hours after a glucose load. In about 20 per cent it is manifested as clinical diabetes mellitus.

Psychologic Abnormalities. Alterations of mood are common in Cushing's syndrome. Many patients feel irritable and weep with little provocation. A few experience psychotic mentation with delusional content. A few patients are depressed, and some attempt suicide. Manic and hypomanic behavior may also occur.

Diagnosis and Differential Diagnosis. It is important for the physician to know when to suspect Cushing's syndrome and then how to prove or disprove the diagnosis, keeping in mind the need for economy and precision. Taken singly, the various clinical manifestations of Cushing's syndrome are not very specific. Thus only a minute percentage of all hypertensive patients have Cushing's syndrome; only a minute percentage of diabetic patients have Cushing's syndrome; only a minute percentage of patients with renal lithiasis have Cushing's syndrome, and so forth. The coexistence of multiple clinical manifestations greatly increases the probability that a given patient might have hypercortisolism. If one encounters a patient with a single manifestation of Cushing's syndrome, he should always ask himself if hypercortisolism could be present; but if no other symptoms or signs of the syndrome can be found in the course of a complete medical evaluation, it will usually be unrewarding to pursue this line of investigation. Here we are discussing only probabilities, and should recognize that rare examples of hypercortisolism have been unequivocally diagnosed in the virtual absence of clinical manifestations.

Under certain conditions, one can make a clinical diagnosis quite confidently. For example, a patient with protein wasting (osteoporosis, easily denuded skin) and centripetal obesity probably has hypercortisolism. A child who simultaneously develops central obesity and experiences arrest of linear growth probably has Cushing's syndrome. Osteoporosis occurs commonly in patients beyond the age of 50 and is of limited value in diagnosis in this group; but osteoporosis in children and young adults should make one alert to the possibility of Cushing's syndrome. Although impaired glucose tolerance, taken by itself, is not especially suggestive of Cushing's syndrome, *normal* glucose tolerance is rare in Cushing's syndrome (about 10 per cent) and is therefore useful in discounting the probability of hypercortisolism. Patients with tumors of any organ and unprovoked hypokalemia should be suspected of having hypercortisolism, regardless of lack of obesity or signs of protein wasting.

Whenever the suspicion of Cushing's syndrome cannot be dismissed confidently, one should proceed with assays of plasma cortisol or urinary 17-hydroxycortico-steroids under basal conditions and during treatment with standard small doses of dexamethasone. At this point, a reliable laboratory with well-established ranges of normal values is indispensable. Equally important is close supervision of the patient so that specimens are collected properly, so that stresses or medications which might lead to high steroid values are avoided, and so that the physician knows that the dexamethasone is taken as prescribed.

Normal subjects have plasma cortisol concentrations of 8 to 25 μg per 100 ml in the morning and less than 8 μg per 100 ml in the evening. Patients with untreated Cushing's syndrome almost always have plasma cortisol concentrations in excess of 15 μg per 100 ml at all times. Normal subjects have urinary 17-OHCS of 3 to 7 mg per gram of urinary creatinine. Patients with untreated Cushing's syndrome almost always have urinary 17-OHCS in excess of 10 mg per gram of creatinine.

In response to small doses of dexamethasone (0.5 mg every six hours for two days), normal subjects show decreases in plasma cortisol to less than 5 μg per 100 ml and excrete less than 2 mg of 17-OHCS per gram of creatinine. Under similar conditions, patients with Cushing's syndrome almost always maintain plasma cortisol concentrations above 8 μg per 100 ml and excrete more than 3 mg of 17-OHCS per gram of creatinine.

Having established the fact that a patient has hypercortisolism, the physician must then determine whether it is caused by autonomous adrenal function, ectopic secretion of ACTH, or inappropriate secretion of pituitary ACTH. There are many useful guides in making this differential diagnosis, but the most reliable approach is to perform a large-dose dexamethasone suppression test and then, if pituitary-adrenal suppressibility cannot be demonstrated, to perform an assay for plasma ACTH if this measurement is available. The purpose of the large dose of dexamethasone is to determine whether adrenal function is under pituitary control. In almost all cases of Cushing's syndrome caused by inappropriate secretion of ACTH by the pituitary, it is possible to suppress adrenal function distinctly and reproducibly (though not necessarily profoundly) by administering dexamethasone in doses of 2 mg every six hours for two days. If a distinct, reproducible decrease in adrenal function does not occur, one should assume that adrenal function is autonomous or that it is under the control of ectopic ACTH. The distinction between these two disorders can be made by assaying plasma ACTH. In patients with autononous adrenal function, plasma ACTH concentrations should be subnormal; but in patients with the ectopic ACTH syndrome plasma ACTH is high-normal or distinctly elevated (Fig. 3). The reason for emphasizing the importance of reproducibility in the large-dose dexamethasone suppression test is to avoid diagnostic errors that might result if spontaneous decreases in tumor activity should occur or if inadequate urine collections happen to be made at the same time as the administration of dexamethasone. Such coincidences should not be reproducible, but suppression of pituitary ACTH secretion should be. Frequently it is unnecessary to carry out the large-dose dexamethasone test, because all the information one requires can be derived from an analysis of the results

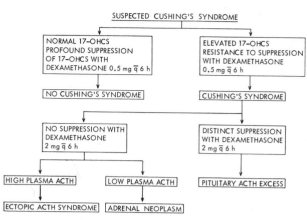

Figure 3. Diagnostic flow sheet for Cushing's syndrome.

of the small-dose test. Many patients with an excess of pituitary ACTH show partial suppression of their steroid output in response to 0.5 mg of dexamethasone every six hours. Definite, reproducible suppression of adrenal function with any dose of dexamethasone implies that adrenal function is under the control of the pituitary.

Blind reliance upon a single set of laboratory values is not to be recommended; for example, high levels of estrogen, such as those encountered in pregnancy or during treatment with oral contraceptives, lead to elevations of plasma cortisol by raising the concentration of cortisol-binding globulin, but there is no increase in cortisol secretion rate or in urinary 17-OHCS. Hyperthyroidism can lead to accelerated removal of cortisol from the circulation and a compensatory increase in cortisol secretion rate, accompanied by an increase in urinary 17-OHCS, but plasma 17-OHCS values are not elevated. Awareness of the total clinical condition and use of more than one dimension in evaluating adrenal function should protect one from making diagnostic errors.

Although the approach described above is the most economical and reliable method of establishing a definitive diagnosis of Cushing's syndrome, the following points may often offer additional help (Fig. 4):

1. Patients with Cushing's disease almost invariably respond to metyrapone with increased secretion of ACTH and total 17-OHCS (the increase in 17-OHCS is attributable to a large increase in 11-deoxycortisol). Patients with Cushing's syndrome caused by adrenal tumor do not respond to metyrapone with increased 17-OHCS production. Patients with the ectopic ACTH syndrome vary in their responses; some show increases in 17-OHCS and others do not.

2. In patients with hypercortisolism, a grossly disproportionate elevation of urinary 17-ketosteroids is highly suggestive of adrenal carcinoma. The same may be said if more than 30 per cent of the urinary 17-OHCS are made up of 11-deoxy-cortisol and its tetrahydrometabolite.

3. Virtually all patients with Cushing's disease respond to exogenous ACTH with large increases in cortisol secretion; this is also true of patients with the ectopic ACTH syndrome unless their basal levels of cortisol are very high. Patients with Cushing's syndrome resulting from adrenal carcinoma almost never

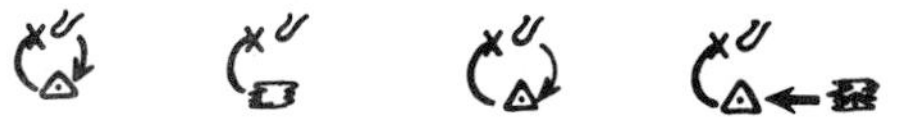

	NORMAL	ADRENAL TUMOR	"CUSHING'S DISEASE"	ECTOPIC ACTH SYNDROME
PLASMA CORTISOL	10-25 μg% RHYTHMIC	HIGH, NO RHYTHM	HIGH, NO RHYTHM	HIGH, NO RHYTHM
PLASMA ACTH	0.1 - 0.4 mU%	LOW	HIGH	HIGH
17-OHCS RESPONSE TO ACTH	3-5 FOLD RISE	+, 0	+	+, 0
RESPONSE TO METYRAPONE	2-4 FOLD RISE	0	+	+, 0
RESPONSE TO DEXAMETHASONE	0-3 mg/d	NO FALL	PARTIAL FALL	NO FALL
PLASMA ACTH AFTER ADRENALEC-TOMY, ON NORMAL CORTISOL	NORMAL	LOW	HIGH	HIGH

Figure 4. Typical cortisol, ACTH, and urinary 17-OHCS values in normal subjects and in the hypercortisolism associated with (a) adrenal tumor, (b) Cushing's disease (pituitary ACTH excess), and (c) the ectopic ACTH syndrome. (From Liddle, G. W.: Am. J. Med., 53:638, 1972. By permission.)

respond to brief infusions of ACTH. Patients with cortisol-secreting adenomas vary in their responses; about half of them respond and half do not.

4. Adrenal carcinomas are usually so inefficient in producing steroids that they do not cause Cushing's syndrome until they have become large enough to be readily demonstrated by intravenous urography or arteriography; some are so large that they can be palpated through the anterior abdominal wall by the time the patient exhibits Cushing's syndrome.

Treatment. The prime therapeutic objectives in Cushing's syndrome are to reduce cortisol levels to normal and to eradicate any associated tumors. Secondary objectives are to avoid producing hormonal deficiencies and to avoid making the patient chronically dependent upon medication. All these objectives can be achieved in some patients in each of the three categories of Cushing's syndrome. In many cases, however, compromises must be made. Sound therapeutic strategy begins with precision in diagnosis.

In Cushing's disease, ideal therapeutic results can be achieved in about 25 per cent of cases by irradiation of the pituitary with about 4500 R. Although this mode of therapy was abandoned in many medical centers when the availability of cortisone substitution therapy made it feasible to perform bilateral adrenalectomy, it remains the only form of therapy that offers the patient a chance of achieving all the therapeutic objectives listed above. The author has 24 patients who have been in remission from 1 to 17 years after pituitary irradiation. None of the patients appear to have developed deficiencies of any pituitary hormones as a consequence of therapy. There are only three drawbacks to this therapeutic approach. First, one must be certain that his diagnosis is correct; pituitary irradiation is clearly inappropriate for patients with adrenal tumors or for patients with the ectopic ACTH syndrome. Second, many patients do not respond, and ultimately require other therapy. Third, the results of pituitary irradiation are not apparent for one to four months; and the patient with fulminant hypertension, rapidly progressive osteoporosis, or psychosis not well controlled by psychoactive drugs should be treated more aggressively.

A technical advance in pituitary irradiation has been achieved recently through careful use of a cyclotron to deliver intensive irradiation to a sharply localized region. Through this means, it is possible to deliver 10,000 R to the pituitary gland with little risk of injury to neighboring structures. Information thus far available indicates that this form of therapy might cure at least two thirds of the patients with Cushing's disease; however, there is at least a small risk of producing hypopituitarism, a problem that did not arise in connection with conventional irradiation with less than 5000 R.

Only three other modes of therapy have been consistently effective in Cushing's disease. With each of them, normalization of cortisol is usually achieved, but the patient incurs life-threatening hormonal deficiencies which require lifelong substitution therapy. Bilateral adrenalectomy is most widely practiced. Substitution therapy with a glucocorticoid (and usually a mineralocorticoid) must begin at the time of adrenalectomy and continue for the duration of the patient's life. The principles of substitution therapy are outlined in Ch. 846. Subtotal adrenalectomy is not to be recommended because of the likelihood of recurrence of hyperadrenocorticism and the frequent impossibility of finding and removing all the regenerative remnant from a scarred mass of perinephric fat at a second operation.

Hypophysectomy and subtotal ablation of the pituitary by means of transsphenoidal microdissection, cryosurgery, or the implantation of radioactive gold or yttrium have been mastered in several medical centers. These forms of therapy carry the risk of producing hypopituitarism and are therefore not be be recommended for the young patient to whom reproductive capacity and normal growth are, obviously, important matters.

Selective destruction of the zona fasciculata and zona reticularis without the induction of aldosterone deficiency can be achieved with prolonged administration of the adrenocorticolytic drug mitotane (o,p'-DDD). This mode of therapy is attended by at least minor gastrointestinal side effects and entails the risk of producing virtually complete loss of glucocorticoid secretory capacity unless the physician is able to follow the patient closely enough to adjust the dose of o,p'-DDD so that plasma cortisol concentrations remain within the optimal range. The advantage of this form of treatment, apart from the avoidance of operative risks, is the preservation of the aldosterone secretory mechanism so that the patient is not so vulnerable to sodium depletion as is the totally adrenalectomized patient.

In the ectopic ACTH syndrome, ideal therapeutic results can be achieved only if the ACTH-secreting tumor can be completely removed. Thus far this has been possible in only a score of cases. In those cases in which the ACTH-secreting tumor cannot be removed, it is still possible to curtail the hypercortisolism by treatment with metyrapone. This drug inhibits the final step in cortisol synthesis and leads to secretion of the biologically weak precursor, 11-deoxycortisol. One can start with small doses of 250 mg every eight hours and increase them if necessary to achieve the desired reduction of cortisol production (under these circumstances the simplest way to estimate cortisol levels is to measure plasma fluorogenic steroids). Doses in excess of 500 mg every six hours are rarely required. Bilateral adrenalectomy or o,p'-DDD therapy might be employed in selected patients in whom the hypercortisolism offers a more immediate threat to life than does the ACTH-secreting tumor. It should be borne in mind that o,p'-

DDD so alters the extra-adrenal metabolism of cortisol that the measurement of urinary 17-OHCS is unreliable in evaluating cortisol secretion; the patient's progress should be followed by measurements of plasma cortisol.

The only completely satisfactory treatment of Cushing's syndrome resulting from adrenal tumor is the surgical removal of the tumor. Most tumors are benign and unilateral, and removal of the tumor-bearing gland is curative. It is essential that the patient be supported with glucocorticoids during and for several days after the operation, because chronic suppression of ACTH production will have resulted in atrophy of the non-tumorous adrenal. A regimen similar to that employed during bilateral adrenalectomy is appropriate. Post-operatively, glucocorticoid therapy should be progressively reduced so that within a week or so the patient receives only 20 to 30 mg of cortisol per day. This supportive therapy should be withdrawn gradually over the ensuing year. It is possible during this period to give the entire daily steroid supplement as a single dose in the morning, thus permitting the pituitary-adrenal system to escape from the suppressive influence of cortisol for a portion of each day. On this schedule the daily dose of cortisol can gradually be reduced from 30 mg to 5 mg and then discontinued altogether. Throughout this first year the physician and patient should be alert to the possible need for increased cortisol dosage in the event of an acute stress. The principles of therapy in this situation are the same as those described for patients with adrenal insufficiency. After steroids have been withdrawn for a time, the patient's recovery of normal pituitary-adrenal function can be verified by a metyrapone test. A normal response should indicate that the patient no longer needs to be concerned about pituitary-adrenal insufficiency.

Approximately 5 to 10 per cent of patients with Cushing's syndrome resulting from benign adrenal adenomas have bilateral tumors. These patients require bilateral adrenalectomy followed by lifelong treatment, as for Addison's disease.

Although adrenal surgery is curative in some patients with adrenal carcinoma, a majority have either apparent or occult metastases by the time they seek medical attention. In about two thirds of these patients, the adrenocorticolytic drug o,p'-DDD will induce a temporary remission of hyperadrenocorticism, and about one half of these experience regression of tumor mass for several months to a few years. The dose ranges from 3 to 10 grams per day, depending upon the severity of gastrointestinal side effects. If measures to control growth of the tumor are unsuccessful, it is still possible to control hypercortisolism with metyrapone given in divided doses totaling 1 to 2 grams daily. In patients with adrenal tumors, overtreatment with adrenal inhibitors can result in adrenal insufficiency; this can be avoided by erring on the side of undertreatment or by giving 0.5 mg of dexamethasone daily as a supportive measure.

Significance of Virilism in Association with Cushing's Syndrome. Clinical and chemical evidences of androgen hypersecretion are not uncommon in Cushing's syndrome. Although not a highly reliable rule, it is usually true that when a patient with Cushing's syndrome exhibits marked evidence of androgen excess, the cause is likely to be adrenocortical carcinoma. In other varieties of Cushing's syndrome, virilism is usually mild or inapparent.

The most important question to be settled early in the evaluation of any patient with virilism is whether or not this is associated with hypercortisolism, for virilism associated with hypercortisolism should be managed according to the principles outlined above for Cushing's syndrome, but virilism without hypercortisolism represents an entirely different group of disorders requiring drastically different treatment (see Ch. 853, 854, 858, and 867).

851. PRIMARY ALDOSTERONISM

Definition, Etiology, and Incidence. Narrowly defined, "primary aldosteronism" is the constellation of chemical and clinical abnormalities resulting from the "autonomous" hypersecretion of aldosterone. The words "primary" and "autonomous" are employed to set this condition apart from "secondary aldosteronism," which refers to hypersecretion of aldosterone in response to a known stimulus such as angiotensin. Usually primary aldosteronism is due to an aldosterone-secreting adenoma (Conn's syndrome), but occasionally it is associated with adrenal hyperplasia or with morphologically normal adrenals (idiopathic hyperaldosteronism).

The incidence of primary aldosteronism is a subject of controversy. Conn has suggested that it might be present in 7 per cent of patients who otherwise appear to have essential hypertension. Others believe it to be less common, perhaps occurring in 1 per cent of the hypertensive population. It has been reported in about twice as many females as males.

Pathogenesis. Virtually all the features of primary aldosteronism are attributable to the fact that aldosterone promotes the conservation of sodium and the excretion of potassium.

Excessive conservation of sodium leads to expansion of extracellular volume, elevation of the blood pressure, and suppression of renin production. In the absence of circulatory insufficiency, modest expansion of extracellular volume leads to physiologic adjustments which enable the excretory system to come into equilibrium with the sodium intake; progressive expansion of extracellular volume is thus avoided, and overt edema is absent or only slight. (These adjustments are sometimes referred to as the "escape phenomenon.")

Excessive excretion of potassium can result in potassium depletion, hypokalemic alkalosis, muscular weakness, areflexia, tetany, paresthesias, electrocardiographic abnormalities (S-T depression, flattening of T waves, and appearance of U waves), idioventricular arrhythmias, and kaliopenic nephropathy, with impaired renal concentrating capacity that cannot be corrected by vasopressin. Despite the hypokalemia, urinary potassium excretion usually exceeds 30 mEq per day. Since potassium secretion in the distal convoluted tubule is, in part, a function of the quantity of sodium reaching that portion of the nephron, a high sodium intake tends to exaggerate the potassium-wasting process, and a low sodium intake tends to mask it.

The action of aldosterone in promoting the conservation of sodium and the rejection of potassium is observable not only in the kidney but in all epithelialized organ systems which carry on cation exchange. Thus in hyperaldosteronism one can often demonstrate depression of the sodium:potassium ratio in sweat, saliva, and gastrointestinal secretions.

Apart from the relatively rare patients who develop alarming ventricular arrhythmias or incapacitating muscular weakness as a result of potassium depletion, the great dangers of primary aldosteronism are the common complications of hypertensive cardiovascular disease: cardiac hypertrophy, congestive heart failure, strokes, and progressive impairment of renal function. Although uncommon, malignant hypertension can occur as a complication of primary aldosteronism and can be associated with either elevated or suppressed plasma renin activity.

Clinical Manifestations. All patients who have been proved to have primary aldosteronism have had hypertension. This is somewhat tautologic because physicians do not usually consider the diagnosis in the absence of hypertension. Nevertheless, the clinical importance of primary aldosteronism is in the main related to hypertension and its sequelae. There are no characteristics of the hypertension of primary aldosteronism that are helpful in distinguishing it from "essential" hypertension.

The coexistence of hypertension and *unprovoked* hypokalemia is highly suggestive of primary aldosteronism. Indeed, in some studies as many as 50 per cent of patients with this combination of abnormalities have ultimately been shown to have primary aldosteronism. In a large percentage of patients the hypokalemia is asymptomatic. In an uncertain but probably small percentage it is not demonstrable at all. The clinical manifestations of potassium depletion have been summarized under Pathogenesis. Another possible consequence of potassium depletion in primary aldosteronism is impairment of carbohydrate tolerance.

Diagnosis and Differential Diagnosis. In practice, the diagnosis of primary aldosteronism usually begins with the recognition that the patient has hypertension. Serum potassium should be determined on several occasions while the patient is on a liberal sodium intake and is not receiving kaliuretic drugs (diuretics) or experiencing diarrhea or vomiting. The finding of unprovoked hypokalemia in association with hypertension calls for measurements of aldosterone and renin. If the aldosterone secretion rate is elevated, it may be assumed that the patient has either primary or secondary aldosteronism. If plasma renin activity is suppressed, one may assume that the patient has primary rather than secondary aldosteronism. Anecdotal evidence indicates that some patients have coexistent primary and secondary aldosteronism, but it is impossible to diagnose primary aldosteronism with certainty until the secondary aldosteronism has been corrected and it can be demonstrated that the hypersecretion of aldosterone persists in spite of subnormal plasma renin activity.

Hypokalemia is not an essential feature of primary aldosteronism, but the diagnosis is not easy to establish in its absence, when total reliance must be placed on the aldosterone and renin determinations. There is no substitute for a sophisticated and reliable laboratory if one is to practice competently in this area of medicine.

Conditions that can lead to concomitant hypertension and hypokalemia include malignant hypertension, Cushing's syndrome (especially the ectopic ACTH syndrome), congenital adrenal hyperplasia caused by 17-hydroxylase deficiency or 11-hydroxylase deficiency (see below), ingestion of large quantities of licorice, and a familial renal disorder simulating primary aldosteronism but with negligible aldosterone secretion (Liddle, Bledsoe, and Coppage). Except for the last condition, all these disorders should be recognizable in the course of a routine evaluation, which includes a determination of 17-OHCS.

Once the diagnosis of primary aldosteronism has been established by demonstrating that, under carefully standardized conditions, the patient has an abnormally high aldosterone secretion rate and abnormally low plasma renin activity, one would like to know whether the hypersecretion of aldosterone is unilateral or bilateral. If the source of aldosterone is a unilateral adenoma, the condition can usually be cured by unilateral adrenalectomy with the expectation that the contralateral adrenal gland will then function normally. If the source of aldosterone is bilateral (with or without adenomas), the disorder usually cannot be surgically corrected short of bilateral adrenalectomy, and this is too high a price to pay in view of the fact that medical therapy with the mineralocorticoid antagonist spironolactone will generally correct both the hypokalemia and the hypertension of primary aldosteronism.

Unfortunately, the art of distinguishing between unilateral and bilateral hypersecretion of aldosterone is not highly developed. Kahn and Melby have found it possible to determine which of the two adrenal glands contains an aldosterone-secreting adenoma by catheterizing the adrenal veins (via a femoral vein) and measuring aldosterone concentrations in the adrenal effluents before and after brief injection of angiotensin. This procedure is not generally useful owing to the extraordinary expertise that is required in placing the adrenal venous catheters properly. Adrenal venography has been used to demonstrate the location of aldosterone-secreting tumors, but this procedure carries the danger of rupturing the adrenal vein. Scanning of adrenals with radioactive iodocholesterol has been used to demonstrate the location of a small number of adenomas, but this procedure is not highly reliable and is still limited to a few centers where active investigative programs are in progress. Robertson has developed a computer program for distinguishing between unilateral adenoma and bilateral hypersecretion, combining a large variety of clinical and laboratory data, but the applicability of the program to patients in other medical centers does not yield distinctions having the reliability that Robertson found in his original study in Scotland, presumably because other medical centers employ somewhat different standard conditions for collecting and reporting their data. In summary, most medical centers still find it necessary to explore both adrenals surgically in order to determine whether primary aldosteronism is attributable to unilateral or bilateral hypersecretion of aldosterone.

Treatment. Unless the patient is a poor surgical risk, the treatment of choice in primary aldosteronism is surgical excision of an adenomatous adrenal gland. During the weeks prior to operation the patient's hypertension and potassium depletion should be corrected by treatment with the aldosterone antagonist spironolactone in doses of 200 to 400 mg daily. Both glands are exposed, inspected, and palpated before a decision is made as to what should be resected. If one gland is found to contain an adenoma, it should be removed, and the contralateral gland should be left intact. If no adenoma can be found, one gland may be removed and sectioned carefully in search of a small tumor; if one is found, nothing further is required. If a tumor is not found in the first gland to be removed, half of the second gland may be resected in search of an adenoma. Even if an adenoma is not encountered, the operation should be terminated at this point rather than risk permanent adrenal insufficiency.

Patients who are poor surgical risks, those who are unwilling to undergo adrenal exploration, and those whose hyperaldosteronism persists after subtotal adrenalectomy should be treated chronically with spironolactone in doses of 100 to 400 mg daily.

Prognosis. Without treatment, patients with primary aldosteronism will sooner or later have the disabling and fatal complications common to hypertensive cardiovascular disease in general; they have been known to die of strokes, congestive heart failure, and renal insufficiency. Within several days to several months after the successful removal of an aldosterone-secreting tumor, 70 per cent of the patients become normotensive, 25 per cent exhibit significant lowering of blood pressure but not to normal levels, and only 5 per cent are unimproved. Correction of the electrolyte disturbance is uniformly observed after correction of the aldosterone excess. Adequate treatment with spironolactone is almost equally effective in correcting the hypertension and potassium depletion of primary aldosteronism, but not infrequently it leads to gynecomastia, impotence, or menstrual irregularity.

852. SECONDARY ALDOSTERONISM

The normal response of the adrenal cortex to increased stimulation by the renin-angiotensin system is to secrete increasing quantities of aldosterone. The aldosterone, in turn, promotes sodium conservation and potassium excretion. The retention of sodium results in expansion of extracellular volume and tends to restrain further production of renin. In many circumstances the renin–angiotensin–aldosterone–sodium-volume sequence can be viewed teleologically as a compensatory mechanism designed to support the blood flow to the kidney by expanding extracellular volume. Thus severe dehydration, sodium depletion, hemorrhage, hypoalbuminemic states, renal arterial constriction, and sequestration of blood on the venous side of the circulation are all conditions in which blood flow to the kidney is diminished, calling forth increased production of renin and aldosterone. Secondary aldosteronism, then, is not a disease but, rather, is a response of the normal adrenal to physiologic demands arising in the course of a variety of disease processes, notably the nephrotic syndrome and hepatic cirrhosis.

853. CONGENITAL ADRENAL HYPERPLASIA

General Considerations, Definition, Etiology. Steroidal hormones are derived from cholesterol through a long series of enzymatically controlled steps. Each enzyme system carries the biosynthetic process one step along the pathway from ultimate precursor through an orderly series of intermediates to the final, biologically potent derivative. Many of these enzyme systems are common to both the zona fasciculata and zona glomerulosa, and some are important in the biosynthesis of gonadal androgens and estrogens as well as corticosteroids.

An inborn error in an adrenal enzyme system which impairs the efficiency of any step in the biosynthesis of cortisol or aldosterone can lead to congenital adrenal hyperplasia. Impairment of cortisol synthesis leads to a compensatory increase in ACTH secretion by the pituitary, and impairment of aldosterone synthesis leads to a compensatory increase in the production of renin and angiotensin. These trophic hormones stimulate the production of cortisol and aldosterone precursors and induce hyperplasia of the adrenal cortex. If the block in cortisol or aldosterone biosynthesis is not complete, and if the compensatory increase in ACTH or renin secretion is adequate, the resultant production of cortisol and aldosterone may be within the normal range. However, the chemical hallmark of an intra-adrenal enzyme deficiency would still be evident: a distortion of steroid secretory pattern with conspicuous overproduction of the intermediates that occur in the biosynthetic pathway immediately prior to the blocked step. The clinical manifestations of congenital adrenal hyperplasia are determined in part by the biologic properties of the biosynthetic intermediates which are excessively secreted and in part by the degree of deficiency of cortisol, aldosterone, or gonadal steroids.

Beyond the fact that the enzymatic defects that lead to congenital adrenal hyperplasia are genetically determined, little is known about their etiology. The pattern of familial occurrence is usually consistent with the view that congenital adrenal hyperplasia is inherited as a recessive trait. Within any one family, the same enzyme appears to be defective in all affected members.

Varieties of Congenital Adrenal Hyperplasia. Thus far, six varieties of congenital adrenal hyperplasia have been described, each resulting from impaired function of a different enzyme (Fig. 5).

Deficiency of 20α-Hydroxylase. The first step in the conversion of cholesterol into hormonal steroids is 20α-hydroxylation. Impairment of this process results in clinical adrenal insufficiency and, in the male fetus, incomplete differentiation of the external genitalia. The adrenal glands are hyperplastic and contain high concentrations of cholesterol. This is an extremely rare disorder.

Deficiency of 3β-Hydroxysteroid Dehydrogenase. This too is a rare disorder; it is characterized by genital ambiguity in infants of either sex. The explanation for this is that these patients have impaired capacity to transform Δ^5 steroids into Δ^4 steroids. Cortisol, aldosterone, and the potent androgens are all Δ^4 compounds; therefore these hormones are subnormal in this disorder, and affected patients have clinical adrenal insufficiency. Males have inadequate genital differentiation owing to lack of testicular androgen during fetal life. In response to increased levels of ACTH, both males and females secrete superabundant amounts of the Δ^5 steroids, pregnenolone and dehydroisoandrosterone. Although the latter is not a very strong androgen, it is secreted in large enough quantities to cause partial masculinization of the external genitalia of the female fetus. Both males and females therefore have adrenal

GLAND	ENZYME	ENZYME DEFICIENCY RESULTS IN:	
		UNDERPRODUCTION OF:	OVERPRODUCTION OF:
Adrenal and Gonad	20 - Hydroxylase	Cortisol, Aldosterone, 17-KS, Testosterone, Estrogen	Cholesterol
Adrenal and Gonad	3-OH-Dehydrogenase	Cortisol, Aldosterone, Testosterone, Estrogen	Pregnenolones, 17-KS
Adrenal and Gonad	17- Hydroxylase	Cortisol, 17-KS, Testosterone, Estrogen	DOC and Corticosterone
Adrenal	21 - Hydroxylase	Cortisol, Aldosterone	17-OH-Progesterone, 17-KS
Adrenal	11 - Hydroxylase	Cortisol, Aldosterone	DOC, Substance S, 17-KS
Adrenal	18 - Hydroxylase	Aldosterone	Corticosterone

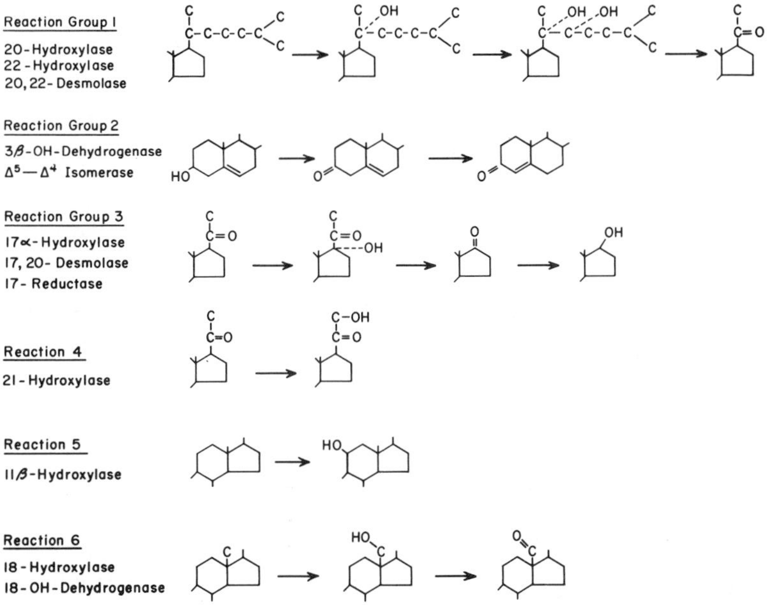

Figure 5. Summary of the enzymatically regulated reactions through which cholesterol is converted to hormonal steroids. A deficiency of each enzyme results in underproduction of certain important adrenal or gonadal hormones and overproduction of their precursors and by-products.

insufficiency, ambiguous genitalia, and elevated urinary 17-ketosteroids (derived from dehydroisoandrosterone).

Deficiency of 17 α-Hydroxylase. Congenital adrenal hyperplasia resulting from a deficiency of 17α-hydroxylase has only recently been described; it is undoubtedly a very rare disorder but is nevertheless important because it represents a curable cause of hypertension. Cortisol synthesis is impaired at the step where progesterone is converted to 17α-hydroxyprogesterone. Androgen and estrogen synthesis, whether by the adrenal, ovary, or testis, also depend upon hydroxylation at the 17α-position prior to cleavage of the 17-20 carbon-carbon bond. Thus impairment of 17α-hydroxylation leads to a deficiency of estrogen and androgen. The patient with 17-hydroxylase deficiency has subnormal cortisol production, a compensatory increase in ACTH, and a consequent increase in the secretion of 17-deoxycorticosteroids, the most prominent of which are DOC and corticosterone. The excessive mineralocorticoid results in hypertension and suppression of renin production; aldosterone production is subnormal. Estrogen and androgen deficiencies result in sexual infantilism and compensatory increases in gonadotrophin secretion.

Deficiency of 21-Hydroxylase. The most common variety of congenital adrenal hyperplasia is attributable to a deficiency of 21-hydroxylase activity. This condition affects approximately one person in 10,000 of our general population. Cortisol synthesis is impaired at the step at which 17-hydroxyprogesterone should be converted to 11-deoxycortisol, and aldosterone synthesis is impaired at the step where progesterone is normally converted to 11-deoxycorticosterone. If the defect is

severe, the patient during the first weeks of life may show signs of adrenocortical insufficiency such as salt-wasting, dehydration, hypotension, shock, prerenal azotemia, hyponatremia, hyperkalemia, vomiting, hypoglycemia, and poor tolerance to stress. Plasma ACTH and renin levels are high. Plasma concentrations of melanocyte-stimulating hormone (β-MSH) are also raised, and occasionally the patient may exhibit mucocutaneous hyperpigmentation. Hypersecretion of 17-hydroxyprogesterone is of no clinical consequence, but it results in the excretion of a diagnostically specific urinary metabolite, *pregnanetriol.*

Adrenal androgens do not require 21-hydroxylation for their synthesis, and as part of the adrenal response to high levels of ACTH they are produced in excessive quantities. Chemically, this is reflected in excessive levels of urinary 17-ketosteroids. The clinical consequence is virilization. The precise clinical manifestations of virilism depend upon the sex of the patient, the age at which the androgen excess occurs, and the severity of the androgen excess. In the male fetus, testicular production of androgen is sufficient to bring about completely masculine differentiation of the genitalia, and even a large excess of adrenal androgen has no obvious effect on genital differentiation or growth. The female fetus, though lacking gonadal androgen, is nevertheless very sensitive to androgens. In females with virilizing congenital adrenal hyperplasia, an excess of adrenal androgen results in partial masculinization of those portions of the genitourinary system that are the last to undergo differentiation. The abnormalities include the development of a urogenital sinus, fusion of labioscrotal folds, and hypertrophy of the clitoris. In extreme cases the external genitalia may be so ambiguous that on superficial examination the patient appears to be a male with hypospadias and bilateral cryptorchidism. In general, female infants with the most profound deficiencies of cortisol and aldosterone (the so-called salt-wasters) are likely to have conspicuous genital abnormalities, and the diagnosis should be suspected at birth, well in advance of any clinical difficulty from adrenal insufficiency. Salt-wasting males, on the other hand, lacking abnormalities of genital differentiation, are unlikely to attract special attention until they are in trouble with vomiting, dehydration, and other consequences of adrenal insufficiency. A positive family history, however, sometimes assists the pediatrician in considering the diagnosis before clinical complications arise.

Unless he or she succumbs or is treated, the patient with 21-hydroxylase deficiency grows rapidly and becomes quite muscular; at some time between two and ten years of age, pubic and axillary hair appear; this is followed by facial hirsutism and deepening of the voice. Investigation at this time reveals that the bone age is advanced beyond the height age, which, in turn, is advanced beyond the chronologic age. Early epiphysial closure foredooms the patient to short stature during adult life.

Clinically, the male patient may appear normal except for precocious puberty. The untreated female patient, however, does not undergo true pubertal changes but simply shows slowly progressive virilization; she lacks the feminization, mammary development, uterine development, and menstrual cycles that are a part of true puberty in the female.

The definitive diagnosis of 21-hydroxylase deficiency is based upon the demonstration of excessive quantities of pregnanetriol in the urine together with *easy* suppressibility of pregnanetriol and 17-ketosteroids by administration of glucocorticoids. This maneuver aids in distinguishing patients with congenital adrenal hyperplasia from those with Cushing's syndrome and those with adrenal tumors.

Deficiency of 11β-Hydroxylase. The second most common variety of congenital adrenal hyperplasia is attributable to a deficiency of 11β-hydroxylase. Fewer than 100 cases have been recognized thus far. The final step in cortisol synthesis is impaired so that cortisol secretion is subnormal, ACTH secretion is excessive, and the biologically inactive precursor of cortisol, *11-deoxycortisol,* is secreted in large quantities. Normally, corticosterone is secreted by the zona fasciculata in quantities of the order of 2 mg daily, but in patients with 11β-hydroxylase deficiency the final step in corticosterone synthesis is impaired, and large quantities of *11-deoxycorticosterone (DOC)* are secreted. DOC is a mineralocorticoid having about one thirtieth the potency of aldosterone. When secreted in quantities of several milligrams daily, DOC induces hypertension. Renin and aldosterone levels are low.

Adrenal androgens do not require 11β-hydroxylation for synthesis, and they are produced in excessive quantities as part of the adrenal response to high levels of ACTH. The consequent virilization is similar in its pathogenesis to that observed in patients with 21-hydroxylase deficiency.

The clinical manifestations of 11β-hydroxylase deficiency are simply those of hypertension and virilism. Plasma and urinary 17-OHCS are elevated because 11-deoxycortisol and its tetrahydro derivative behave like cortisol and its tetrahydro derivatives in chemical tests based on the presence of the 17,21-dihydroxy-20-keto configuration. Despite the elevation of 17-OHCS, this condition should not be confused with Cushing's syndrome, because plasma fluorogenic steroids should be normal or low in 11β-hydroxylase deficiency, the elevated steroids should be *readily* suppressible by the administration of glucocorticoids, and the clinical features of central obesity, protein wasting, and impaired carbohydrate tolerance are absent. The history of lifelong abnormalities together with *easy* suppressibility of the high steroid levels should distinguish 11β-hydroxylase deficiency from an adrenal tumor.

Deficiency of 18-Hydroxysteroid Dehydrogenase. This rare disorder results in a selective impairment of the final step in aldosterone biosynthesis. As a consequence the patient suffers excessive sodium loss, dehydration, and hypotension; there is a compensatory increase in formation of the aldosterone precursor 18-hydroxycorticosterone.

Treatment of Congenital Adrenal Hyperplasia. The major abnormalities in congenital adrenal hyperplasia stem from deficiencies of cortisol or aldosterone or both. Compensatory increases in secretion of ACTH or renin or both then stimulate overproduction of the precursors or by-products of these important steroids. The rationale of therapy is to provide physiologic quantities of glucocorticoid and mineralocorticoid, thus correcting the deficiency state, suppressing the trophic hormones, and curtailing the secretion of steroid precursors and by-products.

The technique of treatment is similar to that employed in adrenal insufficiency. For the first several days it is advisable to employ slightly greater than physiologic doses of glucocorticoid in order to hasten the involution of the hyperplastic, very responsive adrenal cortex. Thereafter only physiologic doses are required, and overtreatment must be assiduously avoided so that growth will not be inhibited.

In those varieties of congenital adrenal hyperplasia that are characterized by the excessive excretion of 17-ketosteroids, glucocorticoid dosage should be adjusted from time to time so as to bring daily 17-ketosteroid excretion to approximately 1 mg for each year of chronologic age, up to 12 years. More profound suppression of 17-ketosteroids is not necessary to prevent progression of virilism, but would be indicative of excessive glucocorticoid dosage. During intercurrent stressful illnesses, corticosteroid doses should be adjusted upward in the same manner and for the same reason as in treating adrenal insufficiency.

Several steroid preparations are available, and with proper consideration of relative potencies, effective routes of administration, and duration of effect, one can substitute one glucocorticoid for another and one mineralocorticoid for another at will. Many patients do well on approximately 12 mg of hydrocortisone and 0.06 mg of 9α-fluorohydrocortisone per square meter of body surface per day. In any case, the dosage must be adjusted to suit individual requirements; the objectives of therapy are to avoid adrenal insufficiency, to normalize 17-ketosteroid excretion, and to maintain normal blood pressure.

Certain therapeutic considerations are peculiar to the specific varieties of congenital adrenal hyperplasia. Mineralocorticoid therapy is required only for patients with salt-wasting varieties of congenital adrenal hyperplasia and not for those with the hypertensive varieties. Glucocorticoid therapy is not required in treating 18-hydroxysteroid dehydrogenase deficiency. Estrogen and androgen therapy may be needed to induce secondary sex characteristics in patients with 17α-hydroxylase deficiency, those with 20α-hydroxylase deficiency, or those with 3β-hydroxysteroid dehydrogenase deficiency.

Plastic surgery to correct gross abnormalities of the external genitalia should be carried out before the age of two years, by which time the child's psychosexual identity should be unambiguously established.

Prognosis. Without treatment, patients with various salt-wasting forms of congenital adrenal hyperplasia are unlikely to survive infancy. Patients with the hypertensive varieties also have decreased life expectancy. Many experience psychosexual problems arising from pseudohermaphroditism in the females and precocious puberty in the males.

If recognized early and treated properly, patients with any variety of congenital adrenal hyperplasia should theoretically be able to live normal lives. This is true for the patients with 21-hydroxylase and 11β-hydroxylase deficiency, except that they have usually not attained normal height. It appears that reproductive functions will be normal if proper treatment is started before adulthood. It is of interest that a child whose bone age has advanced beyond about 13 years before suppressive treatment with glucocorticoids is instituted will exhibit adult pituitary-gonadal relationships (females will undergo breast development and establish their menstrual cycles) when glucocorticoid treatment is finally begun; this is true even if the chronologic age is only seven or eight years.

The other varieties of congenital adrenal hyperplasia have less favorable prognoses. In 17α-hydroxylase deficiency, reproduction will probably not be possible even though the hypertension can be controlled and all other clinical manifestations of steroid deficiency corrected. The survival of patients with deficiencies of 20α-hydroxylase or 3β-hydroxysteroid dehydrogenase has been unaccountably poor up to the present time.

854. VIRILIZING TUMORS

Adrenal tumors that produce a clinically significant excess of androgen along with cortisol have been discussed in Ch. 850. Somewhat less common are adrenal tumors that secrete androgen without significant quantities of cortisol. Most of these tumors are malignant, and the majority are large and have metastasized by the time they are clinically apparent. The clinical hallmark of such tumors is virilization; this manifestation, of course, is limited to children and women; adult males usually recognize no increased virilization as a result of even large excesses of the relatively weak adrenal androgens. The common chemical hallmark of a purely virilizing tumor is the excessive excretion of 17-ketosteroids. This is a remarkably uniform characteristic of adrenal carcinomas. Several adrenal carcinomas have, probably erroneously, been reported as being nonfunctioning simply because they did not give rise to clinical virilization. Evidence was inadequate to support this conclusion, however, whenever 17-ketosteroid excretion was not measured.

It is not sufficient just to measure urinary 17-keto-

steroids; under basal conditions one should also carry out dexamethasone suppression tests and demonstrate that urinary 17-ketosteroids can reproducibly be reduced to less than 6 mg per day within three days before concluding that an adrenocortical carcinoma is nonfunctioning.

Suprarenal "masses" that are discovered accidentally during roentgenographic examinations almost never prove to be adrenal cortical tumors if basal 17-OHCS and 17-ketosteroids are normal and normally suppressible, and they almost never prove to be adrenal medullary tumors if catecholamines are consistently normal.

Virilizing adrenal tumor must be differentiated from congenital adrenal hyperplasia, Cushing's syndrome with virilism, ovarian tumor, idiopathic hirsutism, and precocious puberty. This can be accomplished by a history of late onset of first clinical manifestations, absence of Cushing's syndrome, presence of a palpable abdominal mass, abnormal resistance to suppression of 17-ketosteroids with dexamethasone, absence of ovarian mass, and presence of an adrenal mass on urography or arteriography.

Treatment is with surgical resection and with o,p'-DDD. A sizable minority responds favorably to each mode of therapy, at least temporarily.

855. FEMINIZING ADRENAL TUMORS

Feminization as a clinical manifestation of adrenal tumor is exceedingly rare. The most common sign is gynecomastia, and this is one of the least common causes of gynecomastia. The diagnosis is made by the observation of other signs of adrenal overactivity, e.g., hypertension, demonstration of excessive estrogen in the urine, and demonstration of a suprarenal mass by intravenous urography or arteriography. If positively diagnosed, the tumor may be treated by surgical resection, and, if this fails, with o,p'-DDD. Experience is too limited to support a generalization as to prognosis.

Addison, T.: On the constitutional and local effects of diseases of the suprarenal capsules. London Med. Gaz., 43:517, 1849, 1855.
Bartter, F. C., Albright, F., Forbes, A. P., Leaf, A., Dempsey, E., and Carroll, E.: The effects of adrenocorticotropic hormone and cortisone in adrenogenital syndrome associated with congenital adrenal hyperplasia: An attempt to explain and correct its disordered hormonal pattern. J. Clin. Invest., 30:237, 1951.
Baulieu, E. E., and Robel, P. (eds.): Aldosterone: Prague Symposium. Oxford, Blackwell Scientific Publications, 1964.
Blizzard, R. M., and Kyle, M.: Studies of the adrenal antigens and antibodies in Addison's disease. J. Clin. Invest., 42:1653, 1963.
Bongiovanni, A. M., Eberlein, W. R., Goldman, A. S., and New, M.: Disorders of adrenal steroid biogenesis. Recent Prog. Horm. Res., 23:375, 1967.
Christy, N. P. (ed.): The Human Adrenal Cortex. New York, Harper & Row, 1971.
Conn, J. W., Knopf, R. F., and Nesbit, R. M.: Clinical characteristics of primary aldosteronism from an analysis of 145 cases. Am. J. Surg., 107:159, 1964.
Cope, C. L.: Adrenal Steroids in Disease. 2nd ed. Philadelphia, J. B. Lippincott Company, 1972.
Cushing, H.: The basophil adenomas of the pituitary body and their clinical manifestations (pituitary basophilism). Bull. Johns Hopkins Hosp., 50:137, 1932.
Eisenstein, A. B. (ed.): The Adrenal Cortex. London, J. & A. Churchill, Ltd., 1967.
Gabrilove, J. L., Sharma, D. C., Wotiz, H. H., and Dorfman, R. I.: Feminizing adrenocortical tumors in the male: A review of 52 cases including a case report. Medicine, 44:37, 1965.

Glaz, E., and Vecsei, P.: Aldosterone: International Series of Monographs in Pure and Applied Biology. New York, Pergamon Press, 1971.

Graber, A. L., Ney, R. L., Nicholson, W. E., Island, D. P., and Liddle, G. W.: Natural history of pituitary-adrenal recovery following long-term suppression with corticosteroids. J. Clin. Endocrinol. Metab., 25:11, 1965.

Liddle, G. W.: Tests of pituitary-adrenal suppressibility in the diagnosis of Cushing's syndrome. J. Clin. Endocrinol. Metab., 20:1539, 1960.

Liddle, G. W., Bledsoe, T., and Coppage, W. S., Jr.: A familial renal disorder simulating primary aldosteronism but with negligible aldosterone secretion. Trans. Assoc. Am. Physicians, 76:199, 1963.

Liddle, G. W., Island, D., and Meador, C. K.: Normal and abnormal regulation of corticotropin secretion in man. Recent Prog. Horm. Res., 18:125, 1962.

Orth, D. N., and Liddle, G. W.: Results of treatment in 108 patients with Cushing's syndrome. N. Engl. J. Med., 285:243, 1971.

Rowntree, L. G., and Snell, A. M.: A Clinical Study of Addison's Disease. Mayo Clinic Monographs. Philadelphia, W. B. Saunders Company, 1931.

Temple, T. E., and Liddle, G. W.: Inhibitors of adrenal steroid biosynthesis. Ann. Rev. Pharmacol., 10:199, 1970.

Thorn, G. E. (ed.): Symposium on the adrenal cortex. Am. J. Med., 53:No. 5, 1972.

THE TESTIS*

Mortimer B. Lipsett

856. INTRODUCTION

FETAL DEVELOPMENT

The primordial gonad arises in the urogenital ridge from intermediate mesoderm during the fifth week of gestation. Early in its development, the bipotential primitive gonad (Fig. 1) is composed of two unipotential mesodermal primordia, each with a distinct physiologic as well as morphologic capacity: (1) a cortical component, consisting of the germinal epithelium; and (2) a medullary component, made up of the primary sex cords derived from the germinal epithelium, and mesonephric and blastemal elements. A third constituent, the primordial germ cell, which appears to be bipotential, arises in an extragonadal site and migrates to the gonads. The cortical component can differentiate only as an ovary, and the medullary component only as a testis (Fig. 1); normally, the dominant element follows the genetic sex of the zygote, and the recessive element retrogresses.

When the gonad destined to become a testis begins to differentiate in a male direction during the seventh to eighth week of embryonic life, the cortical component involutes. Within the medulla, seminiferous tubules form from the primary sex cords and anastomose with the rete testis and testicular ducts, and Leydig cells develop. Leydig cells proliferate predominantly during the first half of gestation, but then gradually involute, persisting until shortly after birth. With morphologic differentiation, the Leydig cells acquire the capacity to synthesize testosterone, and this steroid hormone has been found in the fetal testis.

---

*In the four previous editions this chapter was written by Dr. Melvin M. Grumbach, who has kindly given me permission to include portions of this material. M.B.L.

ACCESSORY SEX STRUCTURES

Fetal castration experiments in placental mammals have clarified the regulation of development of the accessory sex structures. Jost and others demonstrated that castration of male fetuses at an early critical period prevented the differentiation of male structures and led to entirely female development of ducts, urogenital sinus, and external genitalia. These studies, in the light of recent observations of anomalies of sex in man, support the notion that a fetal testicular morphogenetic substance causes regression of the müllerian (female) duct system and that testosterone, which does not have this property, brings about masculinization of the urogenital sinus and external genitalia.

Intrinsic or extrinsic factors that adversely affect any stage of the mechanisms of sex determination and sex differentiation can lead to sexual anomalies. Most disorders of sexual differentiation can be understood by reference to the separate action of each of these fetal testicular substances. These disorders will be discussed in Ch. 859 and 860.

CHEMISTRY AND PHYSIOLOGY OF THE TESTICULAR HORMONES

The testicular hormone *testosterone*, secreted from the Leydig cell, has the primary role in the development and maintenance of the male accessory sex organs, prostate, and seminal vesicles, in the elaboration of semen, and in the development of masculine secondary sexual characteristics. These properties define a class of substances, the androgens; the important androgen secreted by the testis is testosterone. Recent evidence suggests that the 5α reduced derivative of testosterone, 5α-dihydrotestosterone, may be the active form of the hormone at the nuclear receptor within the male accessory sex structures, and is responsible for inducing growth of these organs.

The adrenal cortex secretes little testosterone. The weak androgenic potency of adrenocortical steroids such as androstenedione and dehydroepiandrosterone can be attributed to their conversion to testosterone in small yield.

The contention that testosterone is the principal testicular androgen has been confirmed by the measurement of this steroid in human spermatic vein blood. Healthy young men secrete about 7 mg of testosterone per day. From animal experiments in which the seminiferous tubules were destroyed without affecting the Leydig cells, it has been concluded that testosterone originates in the Leydig cells, although the seminiferous tubule has a weak capacity for testosterone synthesis. Clinical signs of androgen deficiency are absent in certain testicular disorders in man associated with defective seminiferous tubules but with intact Leydig cells.

Pathways for the biosynthesis of testosterone by the Leydig cell resemble those in other steroid-synthesizing glands. Precursors such as acetate and cholesterol are converted enzymatically to testosterone via 17-hydroxypregnenolone and 17-hydroxyprogesterone. The testis can also aromatize testosterone to estradiol. In adult man 15 to 20 μg of estradiol is secreted daily; an additional 25 to 30 μg is produced peripherally by aroma-

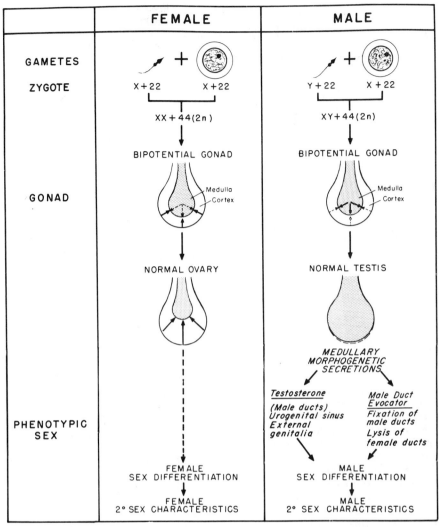

Figure 1. Diagrammatic scheme of human sex determination and differentiation. (Modified from Grumbach, M. M.: *In* Astwood, E. B. (ed.): Clinical Endocrinology I. New York, Grune & Stratton, Inc., 1960.)

tization of blood testosterone in other tissues. Estrone, however, is predominantly a product of adrenal cortical secretions.

The liver is the main site of catabolism of testosterone and of the conjugation of its known metabolites with glucuronic or sulfuric acid; other tissues play a less important role in its metabolism. The major identifiable urinary metabolites are the 17-ketosteroids androsterone and etiocholanolone, which are excreted principally as glucuronides and account for 20 to 40 per cent of the testosterone secreted. A small amount of testosterone (0.2 to 2 per cent) is excreted as testosterone glucuronide.

The two functions of the testis, the synthesis of testosterone and sperm production, are under the control of the hypothalamic-pituitary unit. Luteinizing hormone (LH) acts on the Leydig cell to induce testosterone synthesis, although FSH may synergize to a limited extent. FSH is necessary to initiate spermatogenesis, but it is uncertain whether it has any other role in the process.

The seminiferous tubule is a target tissue for androgen, and there are many data showing that the high concentration of testosterone in the fluid bathing the tubule is functionally important. In hypophysectomized man or monkey it has been shown that spermatogenesis continues if intratesticular testosterone concentration is maintained by human chorionic gonadotrophin (HCG) administration or testosterone implants, respectively. The identification of a tubular androgen-binding protein regulated by FSH may be the link that connects FSH, androgen, and spermatogenesis.

Testosterone exerts a negative feedback on LH secretion, although it is not clear whether the steroid combining at the hypothalamic receptor sites is testosterone or one of its metabolites, dihydrotestosterone or estradiol. The hypothalamus has the capacity to metabolize testosterone to dihydrotestosterone and estradiol. Plasma FSH is also suppressed by testosterone, but an additional factor, derived probably from the Sertoli cell, also modulates FSH secretion. Thus plasma FSH and LH are high in the absence of Leydig cell secretions, but FSH alone is increased when there is severe seminiferous tubule disease. These relationships are shown diagrammatically in Figure 2.

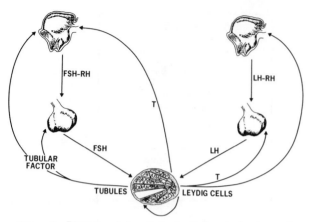

Figure 2. Diagram of hypothalamic-pituitary-testis interactions. (From Lipsett, M. B., and Sherins, R. J.: The testis. *In* Bondy, P. K., and Rosenberg, L. E. [eds.]: Duncan's Diseases of Metabolism. 7th ed. Philadelphia, W. B. Saunders Company, 1974.)

EVALUATION OF TESTICULAR FUNCTION

Clinical Assessment. A clinical estimate of the adequacy of androgen production may be obtained by ascertaining the degree of development of the penis and scrotum, size of the prostate, general maturity and status of male secondary sex characteristics, habitus and skeletal proportions, muscular development, and sexual potency. This assessment has limitations in the mature adult, however, because regression of secondary sexual characteristics is slow even after complete loss of Leydig cell function. Furthermore, distribution of facial and body hair can be highly variable owing to differences in responsiveness of these skin appendages to hormonal stimulation. In this regard, the American Indian, the black African, and some Orientals have sparse or absent facial and body hair despite normal testicular function and plasma testosterone concentration.

Urinary 17-Ketosteroids. About 80 per cent of the urinary 17-ketosteroids (17-KS) is derived from adrenocortical steroids that have little intrinsic androgenic activity. Less than 3 mg daily is derived from Leydig cell secretions. Androsterone and etiocholanolone, the principal urinary metabolites of testosterone, are also metabolites of adrenocortical 11-deoxysteroids. Thus, since urinary 17-KS are an index chiefly of adrenal cortical function, they cannot be used to assess testicular function. Testosterone, which has a hydroxyl group at carbon atom 17, is not a 17-ketosteroid.

The normal range of 17-KS excretion in men is 8 to 25 mg per day (mean, 15 mg). Before puberty only small amounts are detectable in urine. In adult men and women after the third decade, urinary 17-KS decrease gradually owing to lessening adrenal secretion of dehydroepiandrosterone. The excretion of 17-KS may be reduced in eunuchoidism, although the values obtained in such patients are often within the normal range. In panhypopituitarism the function of both the testis and the adrenal cortex is impaired, and the excretion of urinary 17-KS is greatly decreased. Low values are also frequently found in chronic debilitating disease and renal insufficiency. Measurement of urinary 17-KS has little clinical value in disease of the testis or adrenal cortex except as a screening test for congenital adrenal hyperplasia and adrenal tumors (see Ch. 853 to 855).

Urinary Estrogens. It was suggested by Maddock and Nelson that the increase in urinary estrogen after the administration of chorionic gonadotrophin (a placental gonadotrophin with LH-like activity) could be a useful index of Leydig cell function. It has been shown recently that the Leydig cell is the source of almost all of the plasma estradiol in men. Nevertheless, neither measurement of plasma estradiol concentration or that of urinary estrogen excretion is a practical index of Leydig cell function.

Plasma and Urinary Testosterone. The measurement of plasma and urinary testosterone, the latter as the glucuronide conjugate, provides reliable indices of Leydig cell function. The production rate of testosterone can be estimated, but the method is too cumbersome for routine use. Young adult males excrete 40 to 100 μg per day of testosterone glucuronide; women excrete less than 6 μg, and boys before puberty less than 0.5 μg. The concentration of testosterone in plasma of young adult men ranges from 0.3 to 1.2 μg per 100 ml (mean 0.65 μg per 100 ml), and the concentration in women varies from 0.034 to 0.06 μg per 100 ml (mean, 0.054 μg per 100 ml). More than 95 per cent of testosterone in plasma is bound to a specific β-globulin, and thus only 1 to 2 per cent is available for diffusion into cells. The administration of HCG to adult men induces a rise in plasma and urinary testosterone; this procedure has been used to assess the responsiveness of the Leydig cell and to distinguish between primary and secondary testicular disease.

Plasma and Urinary Gonadotrophins. Only a small proportion of the FSH and LH secreted daily appears in the urine in a biologically active form. The normal range of gonadotrophin excretion by the mouse uterine weight method is 10 to 100 mouse uterine units per day, and by the rat ovarian weight method 5 to 20 rats units per day. The common bioassays of urinary gonadotrophins measure the combined excretion of LH and FSH and cannot therefore give meaningful information about variations in individual hormones. Further, the imprecision of the measurements is such that only successive determinations will permit a statement about low or normal levels. Gonadotrophins are detectable by bioassay in 15 per cent of samples obtained randomly from prepubertal children and are diminished or absent in hypogonadism secondary to pituitary or hypothalamic disturbances and frequently in chronic debilitating disease, malnutrition, and starvation. The excretion of gonadotrophin is increased in many but not all primary testicular disorders. In general, elevated levels appear to be related to the degree of damage to the seminiferous tubules, reflecting increased urinary FSH.

The advent of radioimmunoassay procedures has led to the development of sensitive, accurate, practical methods for measurement of these glycoproteins in serum and urine. Determination of plasma or urinary FSH and LH is a useful diagnostic procedure replacing urinary gonadotrophin bioassay. The values obtained by immunoassay are expressed in terms of International Units of the Second International Reference Preparation (2nd IRP) of human menopausal gonadotrophin or in ng of a human pituitary FSH and LH standard. The mean plasma FSH concentration in adult men is 11.7 mIU per milliliter (range 4 to 27 mIU per milliliter) and the mean plasma LH concentration is 9.1 mIU per milliliter (range 4 to 18.9 mIU per milliliter) in terms of the 2nd IRP-HMP (see Ch. 828 and 829).

Plasma FSH levels remain fairly constant throughout the day; nonsystematic pulsatile fluctuations of LH are commonly noted. It has been estimated that 200 to 300 IU of each hormone is secreted daily; of this only 5 to 20 IU is excreted in the urine.

Assessment of Hypothalamic-Pituitary Gonadotrophin Release. Clomiphene citrate, an analogue of the nonsteroidal estrogen chlorotrianisene, is an estrogen antagonist and competes with both androgen and estrogen at hypothalamic receptor sites. When administered to normal men by mouth, 100 to 200 mg per day for five to seven days, it evokes a mean increase in the concentration of plasma FSH of 130 per cent and of plasma LH of 160 per cent. It also induces a rise in urinary FSH and LH and of plasma testosterone. Little or no increase in FSH or LH secretion is elicited in men with pituitary disease.

The recent identification and synthesis of a hypothalamic decapeptide with predominantly LH-releasing activity has enabled the physician to establish pituitary responsiveness directly (see Ch. 829). It may prove valuable in distinguishing between normal and decreased pituitary synthesis of gonadotrophins.

Testicular Biopsy. This procedure can be of great value in the diagnosis and prognosis of testicular disorders. It provides information concerning primarily the gametogenic function of the testis—the status of the seminiferous tubules and the stages of spermatogenesis. Biopsy examination of the testis is of use in diagnosis of tubular disease, in assessing processes of sperm maturation, and in distinguishing azoospermia resulting from obstruction to the passage of sperm from azoospermia of other causes.

Examination of Semen. Specimens of semen for analysis are usually obtained two to three days after the last ejaculation. The volume of the specimen, the total number of sperm, and the motility and morphology of the sperm are determined. The minimal number of sperm necessary for normal fertility is unknown, but a total sperm count of 60 million may be considered normal. Less than this in general means decreased fertility. Because of the wide variations in sperm count among several specimens from the same patient, evaluation of therapy requires long control periods. Assessment of motility and morphology may require examination of many specimens to establish an accurate baseline.

Sex Chromatin Pattern. The number of X chromosomes in the sex chromosome complex can be assessed indirectly by cytologic methods because of sexual dimorphism in the nuclear structure of somatic cells. Preparations suitable for examination can be obtained from smears of buccal mucosa, skin biopsy specimens, or blood (see Ch. 13). This test is widely used in the investigation of abnormalities of sex differentiation, particularly of males with defective testes and azoospermia or severe oligospermia. When a chromatin-positive (female-type) nuclear sex chromatin pattern is detected in a phenotypic male with bilateral testes, it suggests that an associated congenital primary testicular disorder may be present (see Ch. 859).

Instances have been described in which some of the nuclei from phenotypic males or females contained two or more sex chromatin bodies. The maximal number of sex chromatin bodies in somatic nuclei is equivalent to one less than the number of X chromosomes in the sex chromosome complex. For example, XO and XY individuals have chromatin-negative (male-type) somatic nuclei (no chromatin bodies), whereas a high proportion of diploid nuclei in individuals with XX or XXY sex chromosome constitution contain a maximum of one sex chromatin body. Similarly, in XXX females and XXXY males a maximum of two bodies is found in somatic nuclei.

It has been found that quinacrine hydrochloride, an acridine derivative, when utilized as a stain, produces intense fluorescence of the Y chromosome in interphase nuclei, in metaphase preparations, and in sperm. This discovery makes it possible to detect XYY, XXYY, and other double Y syndromes by the simple buccal smear technique.

857. PUBERTAL DEVELOPMENT IN THE MALE

There are wide variations in the age of onset, duration, and sequence of events that characterize the biologic pattern of male puberty. In normal boys signs of puberty may appear at any age between 10 and 17 years; the average age of onset is 12 to 13 years. Once initiated, the major changes are usually completed or well advanced in three to four years; in a small percentage of normal persons, maturity is not attained until the age of 21, and rarely thereafter.

A substantial body of evidence suggests that the stimulus for release of pituitary gonadotrophin at puberty originates in the hypothalamus and is mediated by a neurohormonal secretion, LH-releasing hormone (LHRH). It seems likely that a certain level of physiologic maturation, presumably including the central nervous system, is necessary before this complex and incompletely understood mechanism is activated. This level of development can be best correlated with the degree of osseous and epiphyseal development (bone age) rather than with the chronologic age. Of interest is the observation that small amounts of FSH and LH are secreted by prepubertal children. There is good evidence in animals as well as some data in man showing that the hypothalamic-pituitary-testicular negative feedback mechanism is operative and set at a low level before pubescence.

The sequence of events that marks the pubertal period starts with an acceleration in the growth of the testes and scrotum. The initial increase in testicular size is largely attributable to changes in the seminiferous tubules, which occupy about 90 per cent of the volume of the testis. After initial acceleration of testicular growth, there is an increase in the size of the penis, the appearance of pubic hair, which has at first a transverse growth, and gradual enlargement of the prostate and other accessory organs and glands. It should be noted that the increase in testis size precedes the first appearance of pubic hair by approximately two years and peak height velocity by three years, and is an important clinical feature in ascertaining onset of early puberty. With pubescence, pulsatile and increased release of LH is observed, first at night and then throughout the 24 hours.

Concomitantly, usually between the ages of 13 and 15, an acceleration of growth takes place. This adolescent growth spurt is completed in about three years and, in boys, accounts for an average increment in height of about 8 inches (4 to 12 inches) and a gain in weight of about 40 pounds.

It is necessary that the physician be cognizant of the wide range of normality of the pubertal process in time of onset, intensity, and duration, and also of normal variations in the degree of development of the secondary sex characteristics. In normal men, the pitch of the voice, the size of the external genitalia, the amount of body hair, and the body habitus vary from individual to individual, and are largely attributable to genetic factors and not to differences in the secretion of testosterone.

Delayed Adolescence. Commonly, failure to undergo sexual maturation by the average age is ascribable to the normal variation in pubertal development. Delayed adolescence, although inherently a benign condition, is often a severe psychologic handicap to the patient and a cause of parental anxiety. Many of these boys are short, and a delay of several years in osseous development is not uncommon. Frequently there is a history of late onset of puberty in other members of the family. Retardation of puberty may also be due to inadequate dietary intake or to chronic illness, because these may be associated with diminished secretion of pituitary gonadotrophin.

Pubertal failure or arrest in pubertal development secondary to pituitary-hypothalamic dysfunction or gonadal disease must be excluded in cases of delayed puberty. To exclude pituitary tumor, roentgenographic examination of the skull and careful examination of the fundi and visual fields are required, as well as search for other signs of neurologic involvement in boys who are significantly delayed in their sexual development, particularly when this is accompanied by stunting of growth. It is advisable to assess other pituitary functions (see Ch. 829), especially if the delayed maturation is accompanied by short stature or a decreased rate of growth. In addition, a buccal smear for sex chromatin and determination of urinary or plasma gonadotrophins may clarify the clinical situation. The response to clomiphene will not differentiate between delayed puberty and hypogonadotrophic hypogonadism, because both groups are clomiphene unresponsive. LHRH usually causes LH release in both groups so that the response to this agent also is not diagnostic.

Treatment. Treatment should be directed toward correction of the basic disturbance, e.g., measures to improve nutrition or surgical removal or irradiation of a pituitary neoplasm. Substitution therapy with male sex hormone should be started at about 13 or 14 years of age so that the onset of the patient's maturation coincides with that of his contemporaries. The use of this regimen does not preclude subsequent induction of spermatogenesis with FSH in those individuals with hypogonadotrophic hypogonadism.

Less well defined is the treatment of boys in whom no apparent etiologic factor is found. Many will mature spontaneously before 17 years of age and merely represent an extreme of the normal range. Indiscriminate use of hormonal treatment in this group is unwise, and a conservative approach is indicated. Nonetheless, at times, sociopsychologic considerations may make it expedient to treat such boys. A therapeutic trial with human chorionic gonadotropin, 500 to 1000 IU three times weekly injected intramuscularly, or with a testosterone preparation for three to six months will cause virilization, and often maturation will progress after treatment is discontinued.

858. SEXUAL PRECOCITY

Isosexual precocity in boys is defined as the occurrence of signs of masculinization before the age of ten years. Skeletal maturation is accelerated and the epiphyses fuse at a premature age, leading to short stature in adult life. On the other hand, mental and dental development are not precocious. Sexual precocity occurs about three times more frequently in girls than in boys. There are four main causes of isosexual precocity in boys: *cerebral, adrenocortical, testicular,* and *extra-endocrine tumors secreting HCG.*

The cerebral causes of sexual precocity may be functional or organic. They are associated with premature activation of the hypothalamic-pituitary mechanism and the release of pituitary gonadotrophic hormones. This form, designated true precocious puberty or complete isosexual precocity, is manifested by maturation of the Leydig cells and spermatogenesis.

True precocious puberty may be caused by organic lesions of the brain either directly or indirectly involving the posterior hypothalamus, such as hypothalamic and pineal tumors, hamartoma of the tuber cinereum, craniopharyngioma, hydrocephalus, postencephalitic lesions, congenital defects, tuberous sclerosis, and neurofibromatosis. The *McCune-Albright syndrome* of sexual precocity, polyostotic fibrous dysplasia, and pigmented areas of skin is rare in boys. The mechanism whereby such lesions activate the hypothalamic-pituitary secretion of gonadotrophins is unknown. Cerebral lesions, particularly tumors, accompanied by precocious puberty may affect other hypothalamic functions, causing diabetes insipidus, bulimia, obesity, somnolence, emotional lability, or disturbances in temperature regulation. Diabetes insipidus in association with precocious puberty is a syndrome that tends to occur in the presence of an aberrant pinealoma. Involvement of the optic nerves or visual pathways causes visual disturbances. In some instances signs of puberty precede the onset of detectable neurologic involvement, and a prolonged period of observation with repeated careful neurologic examinations, roentgenograms of the skull, and determinations of the visual fields is necessary before it is possible to exclude cerebral neoplasm. When no organic cause is found, the condition is described as *idiopathic precocious puberty;* in some instances, it is transmitted as a sex-limited autosomal dominant trait. In the idiopathic cases, seizure disorders and abnormal electroencephalographic patterns are appreciably more frequent than in normal children.

In all varieties of true precocious puberty, the excretion of urinary 17-ketosteroids rises slowly to normal adolescent values; initially, levels are between 2.5 and 4.0 mg per day. Plasma and urinary testosterone values are increased, because Leydig cell secretion is stimulated. In contrast to precocious pseudopuberty, pituitary gonadotrophin is excreted in the urine; frequently, however, this is not detectable early except by the more sensitive radioimmunoassay procedures for FSH and LH. The pulsatile secretion of LH that normally occurs with pubescence has been noted in precocious puberty. Medroxyprogesterone acetate, a synthetic long-acting progestin, administered intramuscularly, is occasionally of value in the management of patients with idiopathic precocious puberty by virtue of its capacity to inhibit pituitary LH secretion. Rarely, extrapituitary neoplasms, such as hepatoma, that secrete a HCG-like gonadotrophin cause isosexual precocity.

In other forms of isosexual precocity not related to intracranial causes, the testes remain immature, in contrast to the enlarged phallus, and true puberty does not occur. Accordingly, this type has been called *incomplete sexual precocity* or *precocious pseudopuberty*.

The most common cause of incomplete sexual precocity in boys is adrenocortical hyperfunction resulting from congenital virilizing adrenal hyperplasia or a virilizing adrenocortical tumor. With few exceptions the testes remain prepubertal in size despite enlargement of the penis and scrotum and development of other secondary sexual characteristics. An ectopic nodule of hyperplastic adrenal tissue is occasionally palpable in the testis, sometimes bilaterally, and may be confused with Leydig cell tumor, especially in rare instances in which striking enlargement of the testis is found. The excretion of 17-KS is increased in relation to chronologic age, and urinary pregnanetriol is high (see Ch. 853).

Interstitial cell tumor of the testis is a rare cause of isosexual precocity. In almost all reported cases the tumor has been unilateral, and the contralateral testis is immature. Gynecomastia is occasionally present. The excretion of 17-KS varies from 3 to 64 mg per day. Plasma testosterone concentration has generally been in the normal male range, although an occasional high value has been reported. Spermatogenesis has been observed in the tubules surrounding the tumor only, thereby confirming the importance of high intratesticular androgen concentrations for spermatogenesis.

Iatrogenic sexual precocity has been produced by the administration of male sex hormone, but is seen most frequently in boys who have been treated with large doses of HCG for cryptorchidism.

859. HYPOGONADISM

Hypogonadism may refer to a decrease in either the endocrine or the gametogenic function of the testis or to both. Hypogonadism is most commonly classified as primary or secondary, depending on the site of the defect. Primary hypogonadism is due to testicular disease, whereas secondary hypogonadism is a result of hypothalamic-pituitary disease. The excretion or blood level of gonadotrophins is normal or high in primary hypogonadism, and is decreased in secondary hypogonadism. Of common occurrence are primary lesions of the testis involving only spermatogenesis, resulting in infertility. On the other hand, when testosterone secretion is deficient, spermatogenesis is impaired.

Androgen Deficiency. The clinical signs of androgen deficiency depend upon the age of onset and upon severity and duration of the deficiency. Total loss of testicular androgenic function, usually secondary to surgical castration or congenital defects of the testes, before or during early puberty results in eunuchoidism in adulthood. Eunuchoidism causes disproportionate growth of the long bones owing to delay in epiphysial closure. The span exceeds the height by several inches, and the distance between the symphysis pubis and the sole (lower segment) measures more than 55 per cent of the height. Tall stature is common, but not invariable. (The characteristic skeletal proportions of the eunuch are not pathognomonic and may be found in otherwise normal men.) The shoulders tend to be narrow and, although the habitus may be lean or obese, excessive fat deposition often occurs about the pectoral region, hips, thighs, and lower abdomen. Muscular development is poor. Except for the appearance of sparse pubic hair, secondary sex characteristics fail to appear, and the voice remains juvenile. Gynecomastia occurs in association with Klinefelter's syndrome and with male pseudohermaphroditism. Acne and baldness do not occur. Sex drive and potentia are absent or greatly reduced. The hematocrit and hemoglobin levels are characteristic of those for women and increase with administration of androgen.

The effects on somatic and sexual development of partial loss of testicular androgenic function are less striking and vary greatly in degree. Characteristic of the milder forms of eunuchoidism are the scant growth of facial hair and a female distribution of pubic hair. In men who have attained sexual maturity, castration does not result in complete regression of secondary sexual characteristics, and the signs of androgen deficiency are less conspicuous. The most common signs are reduction in prostatic size, diminished rate of growth of the beard and body hair, the appearance of fine wrinkles around the eyes, and a pasty, sallow complexion. Semen volume is reduced. Potentia and libido, although usually diminished, occasionally persist. There may be vasomotor phenomena, including hot flushes.

The most useful substances for the treatment of androgen deficiency are the preparations of testosterone that are available in forms suitable for intramuscular, oral, and buccal or sublingual administration. The mode of administration depends, for the most part, on the preference of the patient and the cost.

Esterification of testosterone with organic acids potentiates its activity when injected as an oily solution. Testosterone propionate in doses of 25 to 50 mg by intramuscular injection two or three times weekly is usually adequate for replacement therapy. However, longer-acting esters are available that can be administered less frequently. One dose of 200 to 400 mg of testosterone cyclopentylpropionate or testosterone enanthate is highly effective when injected at two- to four-week intervals.

Methyltestosterone is an effective preparation for oral and buccal or sublingual use. It is usually administered in doses of 50 mg (30 to 75 mg) orally or about 25 mg per day by sublingual absorption. It is not metabolized to 17-KS as is testosterone. No potent protein anabolic steroid lacking androgenic properties in man is available at present, although intensive efforts have been made to obtain one.

Undesirable effects of androgens include edema caused by retention of extracellular electrolyte (an uncommon effect except with use of large doses or in elderly persons with diminished cardiac reserve), polycythemia, acne, gynecomastia, depression of spermatogenesis in some fertile men when administered in large doses, and premature closure of the epiphyses. Rarely, methyltestosterone causes intrahepatic cholestatic jaundice. Androgen therapy may be contraindicated in patients with carcinoma of the prostate.

PRIMARY HYPOGONADISM
(Primary Failure of the Testis)

The problem of classification of primary hypogonadism has not been entirely resolved, because the etiology of many of the disorders in this group is uncertain. Primary hypogonadism may result from genetic and developmental defects, such as seminiferous tubule dysgenesis and Laurence-Moon-Biedl syndrome, or from other causes: trauma, destruction of spermatogonia after orchitis, exposure to ionizing radiation, chemotherapy, and surgical castration. Disorders in this group may or may not be accompanied by androgen deficiency, although in some eunuchoidism is a constant or frequent feature. Disorders of spermatogenesis characterized only by oligospermia and infertility are likewise examples of primary hypogonadism. The excretion of gonadotrophin is normal or increased, depending, apparently, upon the integrity of some component of the seminiferous tubules. Increase of plasma FSH signifies severe tubular damage.

Klinefelter's Syndrome; Seminiferous Tubule Dysgenesis

This syndrome was described in 1942 by Klinefelter, Reifenstein, and Albright and is characterized classically by small, firm testes, azoospermia, gynecomastia, and elevated urinary gonadotrophins. The features become apparent during early puberty, and also include eunuchoidism. Histologically there are atrophy and hyalinization of the seminiferous tubules; Leydig cells tend to occur in large clumps and are apparently increased in number, but total Leydig cell volume is probably normal. The tubules are lined by Sertoli cells; rarely, germ cells are present in isolated tubules. The cause of the syndrome is a developmental defect of the gonad associated with and probably resulting from a sex chromosome abnormality. More recently Klinefelter's syndrome and its variants have been defined by the single constant finding of an increase in the number of X chromosomes in at least one cell line.

The discovery in 1956 that most persons with the classic features of Klinefelter's syndrome are chromatin positive, followed by the detection of sex chromosome abnormalities, served to identify an especially well-defined disorder caused by a nonfamilial, genetically determined gonadal defect. In accordance with this observation and the histopathologic characteristics of the testicular lesion, the term "seminiferous tubule dysgenesis" has been suggested. This disorder, which occurs sporadically, is an important cause of male infertility and a common type of sexual anomaly. The results of several large surveys of newborns in nurseries indicate that the frequency of chromatin-positive seminiferous tubule dysgenesis is of the order of 1 in 500 newborn males.

The most frequent clinical feature of Klinefelter's

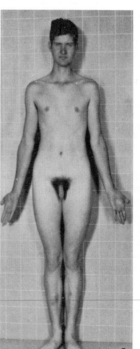
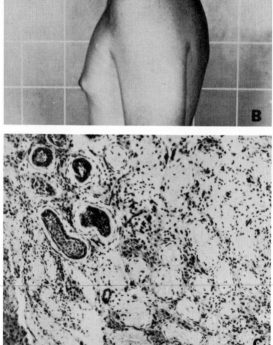
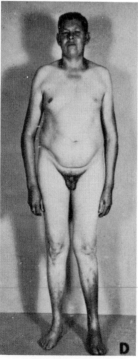

Figure 3. *A* and *B,* Typical 19-year-old phenotypic male with chromatin-positive seminiferous tubule dysgenesis (Klinefelter's syndrome). This patient had a positive sex chromatin pattern and an XXY karyotype. His 17-ketosteroid excretion was 11.2 mg per 24 hours, and his urinary gonadotrophin excretion was more than 100 mu. These patients vary widely in their habitus and degree of virilization. This patient is well virilized, but had long extremities with eunuchoidal proportions and exhibited gynecomastia. The testes measured 1.8 × 0.9 cm and were small and firm. Testicular biopsy, *C,* revealed a severe degree of hyalinization of his seminiferous tubules and Leydig cell hyperplasia. *D,* Forty-eight-year-old man with chromatin-positive Klinefelter's syndrome who came to medical attention only because his severe leg varicosities were thought to reveal a "female trait." (From Van Wyk, J. J., and Grumbach, M. M.: Disorders of sex differentiation. *In* Williams, R. H. (ed.): Textbook of Endocrinology. 4th ed. Philadelphia, W. B. Saunders Company, 1968.)

syndrome is the small size of the testes, the long diameter usually being less than 2 cm. The testes are firmer than normal owing to hyalinization of the tubules. Gynecomastia is present in fewer than 50 per cent of cases, and eunuchoidism is variable. Patients with this disorder are often tall, and the skeletal proportions frequently are eunuchoid as a consequence of the disproportionately long lower extremities, even though epiphysial fusion is not delayed and skeletal maturation usually follows the normal male pattern (Fig. 3). Cryptorchidism and hypospadias are infrequent. Mental retardation and psychopathic behavior are not uncommon, and there is often evidence of poor social adaptation. This disorder has been reported in association with mongolism and with leukemia. It has been suggested that chronic pulmonary disease and varicose veins are more prevalent in affected adults. The frequency of impaired glucose tolerance and of mild diabetes is inreased.

The excretion of urinary gonadotrophin is almost invariably increased, and plasma FSH is always increased as a result of the extensive tubular disease. Plasma LH may be either high or normal, depending perhaps on whether Leydig cell function is normal. In general, urinary 17-KS are within the normal range. The plasma concentration of testosterone is often low, and may increase only slowly with the daily administration of human chorionic gonadotrophin for four to five days.

The abnormality of the sex chromosomes in chromatin-positive Klinefelter's syndrome, characterized by an XXY sex chromosome constitution and a chromosome number of 47, was first demonstrated in 1959 by Jacobs and Strong and by Ford and his associates. Subsequently, less common types of sex chromosome abnormalties have been reported in this disorder. These include phenotypic males with the genotypes 48,-XXYY; 48,XXXY; or 49,XXXXY, which have been found so far only in mentally retarded persons. Unusually tall stature has been found in the XXYY group, along with a tendency to more aggressive and delinquent behavior. The 48,XXXY sex chromosome complex is associated with two sex chromatin bodies in a proportion of diploid somatic nuclei, and the 49,-XXXXY constitution with three sex chromatin bodies. In addition to mental retardation, the XXXXY men have had severe congenital malformations, including very small, usually undescended testes, hypoplastic external genitalia, minor skeletal deformities, including radioulnar synostosis, and other congenital anomalies. It seems that with increasing numbers of X chromosomes, the severity of the abnormalities increases.

Instances of sex chromosome mosaicism have also been described in which at least two populations of cells with different cell chromosome complexes were found in the same individual, e.g., XY/XXY (one cell line with an XY sex chromosome complex and another with an XXY sex chromosome complex), XY/XXXY, XX/XXY, and XXXY/XXXXY. Sex chromosome mosaics arise from a mitotic error in an early division after fertilization in a zygote that originally had either a normal or an abnormal sex chromosome constitution. The detection of a chromatin-positive sex chromatin pattern on buccal smear should not by itself be used as incontrovertible evidence of sterility. Active spermatogenesis was found in the testes of an XY/XXXY mosaic, and additional examples of potential fertility may be found in chromatin-positive males with other forms of sex chromosome mosaicism, especially XY/XXY. In several carefully studied men with Klinefelter's syndrome, only an XX sex chromosome constitution was found. The maternal origin of the two X chromosomes suggests that a Y chromosome was present early in ontogeny and was lost or more likely translocated to an X chromosome or autosome, or that these men were mosaics and the Y-bearing cell line has escaped detection.

The typical XXY sex chromosome constitution of seminiferous tubule dysgenesis may arise from an abnormality of meiosis during gametogenesis or from a mitotic error in the fertilized zygote (see Ch. 13 to 16). The positive association of this disorder with advanced maternal age and the results of surveys of color blindness (a sex-linked recessive trait) and of the Xg blood group suggest a maternal origin with nodisjunction occurring during oogenesis. Using X-linked markers, a paternal origin of one X has been established in several informative pedigrees, nondisjunction during spermatogenesis giving rise to an XY-bearing sperm and fertilization yielding an XXY zygote. More complex sex chromosome anomalies may arise from meiotic or mitotic errors, or from a combination of both.

The gonadal defect is a consequence of the abnormal sex chromosome constitution. The single Y chromosome is a sufficiently powerful male determiner to suppress the cortical component (ovarian anlage) of the primordial gonad despite the presence of two (or even four) X chromosomes. The fetal testes that develop may have either an adequate number or a deficiency of germ cells, but bring about normal male differentiation of the genital tract. At puberty, if the function of the Leydig cells is adequate, male secondary sexual characteristics develop, but the seminiferous tubules lack or are severely deficient in germ cells. Tubular hyalinization usually does not begin until the later prepubertal period. It seems likely that the characteristic appearance of the testes in adolescent and adult cases depends on the direct or indirect action of pituitary gonadotrophins from the onet of puberty on an inherently defective testis, which, before this time, shows only subtle signs of an abnormal histologic structure.

Treatment. If there is evidence of androgen deficiency, testosterone replacement is indicated. Mastectomy may be necessary in some patients, primarily for cosmetic reasons. It should be noted that testosterone treatment may produce transient increase in gynecomastia and nipple tenderness.

Chromatin-Negative Klinefelter's Syndrome

This term is a misnomer and was bestowed before the fundamental distinction was made on the basis of karyotype. The small testes and azoospermia suggest the Klinefelter phenotype. The testicular lesion resembles that of Klinefelter's syndrome, but it should be remembered that the testis can react to injury in only a limited number of ways. The patients have none of the associated anomalies seen in Klinefelter's syndrome, but hypogonadism is sometimes present. It is probable that so-called chromatin-negative Klinefelter's syndrome is the end-stage of several different disease processes, the final result being hyalinization of the tubules with loss of spermatogonia. Some of these patients may be unrecognized mosaics with one cell line bearing an XXY karyotype and would thus be classified as

Klinefelter's syndrome. Plasma testosterone levels have varied from normal to low.

XYY Syndrome

Although the XYY syndrome is discussed under the topic of primary hypogonadism, in fact primary hypogonadism is unusual in XYY subjects. The XYY syndrome is characterized by a chromosome complement of 47 with an extra Y chromosome and a sex chromatin–negative buccal smear that contains nuclei with two small fluorescent Y chromatin masses, and is estimated to occur in 1 per 500 to 1 per 1000 male births. Newborn males and young boys with this syndrome have a normal phenotype. A number of associated characteristics have been reported in the adolescent and adult XYY male. These include tall stature (often over 6 feet), severe acne, and skeletal abnormalities, e.g., radioulnar synostosis. In studies of criminals with a history of aggessive crimes, an increased frequency of the XYY genotype has been noted. On the other hand, some adult XYY males are physically and mentally normal.

Although the extra Y apparently confers the potential for increased stature, Leydig cell function and plasma and urinary testosterone concentrations have been normal.

Germinal Aplasia
(Sertoli-Cell-Only Syndrome)

This condition is characterized by seminiferous tubules lined with Sertoli cells, little or no tubular fibrosis, and absent germinal cells. The patients are first seen by the physician because of sterility. Leydig cell function is normal. Azoospermia is an invariable finding. The testes are normal or moderately reduced in size. Urinary gonadotrophins are usually increased owing to increased FSH excretion, and plasma FSH is increased four- to fivefold, whereas LH levels are within normal limits. The sex chromosome constitution is XY. Germinal aplasia probably is a developmental defect; but the lesion has also been described after exposure of the testes to ionizing radiation and after extensive chemotherapy with cytotoxic agents. There is no treatment for the spontaneous form, but the lesion after damage to the spermatogenic epithelium may be reversible.

Myotonic Muscular Dystrophy

Testicular atrophy, occurring in middle age, is found in about 80 per cent of affected men with myotonic dystrophy. This syndrome is characterized by myotonia, muscle wasting, frontal baldness, and lenticular opacities. In the series of Drucker et al., signs of androgen deficiency occurred in 18 per cent of the patients and gynecomastia in 12 per cent. The excretion of urinary gonadotrophins was usually normal. The histology of the testis shows tubular fibrosis, hyalinization, and disordered spermatogenesis. There are other metabolic abnormalities which, in association with the testicular findings, have been described as accelerated aging.

Anorchia

Absence of both testes in phenotypic males has been described but is exceedingly rare. Careful surgical exploration is required to establish the diagnosis. Unilateral anorchia is more common, and may result from testicular atrophy after herniorrhaphy, from attempted orchiopexy, or from a developmental disturbance, in which case there may be associated anomalies of the genitourinary tract. Arrest at an early stage of pubescence has been described in association with anorchia. In a few cases, catheterization of the spermatic vein revealed a testosterone gradient, suggesting that a nidus of Leydig cells in the expected position of the testis remained functional.

Infertility

In many testicular lesions, the defect involves only spermatogenic function and results in infertility. Endocrine manifestations are absent. Either the semen lacks sperm or the number or quality of sperm is impaired. Testicular biopsy has a major role in differentiating the various disturbances in spermatogenic activity and in determining prognosis. Azoospermia is usually associated with severe tubular fibrosis, germinal aplasia, or spermatogenic arrest, and oligospermia with germinal cell desquamation, hypospermatogenesis, incomplete spermatogenic arrest, and less severe forms of tubular fibrosis. In general, only azoospermia or severe oligospermia is associated with increased plasma FSH concentrations. In most cases the cause is unknown. Azoospermia may also result from obstruction in the afferent ducts secondary to gonorrhea, tuberculosis, or a nonspecific infection. Absence or atresia of the vas deferens and a rudimentary epididymis are common bilateral lesions in boys with cystic fibrosis, but may occur spontaneously. Hypospermatogenesis is of unknown cause and is not accompanied by other measurable abnormalities.

Sterility is a common sequel of bilateral cryptorchidism and may occur in association with unilateral cryptorchidism. Sterility may follow orchitis caused by mumps, gonorrhea, brucellosis, leprosy, or occasionally other systemic infection; it may result from radiation of the testes or treatment with chemotherapeutic agents; it may be of developmental origin, as in seminiferous tubule dysgenesis. Even relatively minor illnesses may cause profound depression in sperm count. Starvation and chronic debilitating diseases associated with inanition adversely affect spermatic function. Estrogen and androgen administration also inhibit spermatogenesis by suppression of gonadotrophins with concomitant decrease in intratesticular testosterone concentration.

Treatment of Infertility in the Male.   Although important advances have been made in the evaluation of spermatogenic function, treatment of infertility caused by primary testicular disease is unsatisfactory. The results of therapy of hormonally normal men with testicular defects of spermatogenesis by the use of large doses of androgenic steroids, gonadotrophins, pregnenolone, thyroid hormone, clomiphene, and vitamin preparations have been unsuccessful. Claims of success in the treatment of oligospermia with human gonadotrophins usually stem from a lack of appreciation of the variability of the sperm count. In published reports the dose of FSH has been about 75 IU three times a week. Since subjects with oligospermia have normal plasma FSH concentrations, their daily FSH production rates are 200 to 300 IU. Thus the "treatment" does not increase FSH "production rate" to a significant extent.

The intermittent use of large doses of testosterone to take advantage of the "rebound effect" on spermatogenesis has not been established as efficacious.

SECONDARY HYPOGONADISM

Secondary hypogonadism is due to decreased secretion of gonadotrophins, and may result from neoplastic, inflammatory, traumatic, vascular, and degenerative lesions involving the pituitary or hypothalamus. These lesions include such entities as pituitary adenoma, craniopharyngioma, astrocytoma, infarction, carotid aneurysm, granulomas such as tuberculosis, histiocytosis X, and hemochromatosis. In many instances, the nature of the underlying lesion is not known. A functional and reversible depression of gonadotrophin secretion occurs in malnutrition, in chronic disease states associated with inanition and nutritional deficiencies, and in some patients with myxedema. High concentrations of androgen and estrogen, as in the adrenogenital syndrome, may cause secondary hypogonadism by suppression of gonadotrophin secretion. Excessive estrogen, either from ingestion or endogenous, as from a feminizing adrenal tumor, depresses the secretion of pituitary gonadotrophin. The testicular atrophy and gynecomastia that occur in some patients with severe liver disease have been ascribed by some to increased levels of estrogen. Decreased gonadotrophin secretion may also result from the nutritional and metabolic disturbances accompanying hepatic cirrhosis.

Decreased secretion of pituitary gonadotrophins occurs either as an isolated defect, *hypogonadotrophic hypogonadism,* or, more commonly, in association with a deficiency of growth hormone and other anterior pituitary hormones. On the other hand, hypoadrenocorticism or hypothyroidism secondary to pituitary failure is rarely found without concurrent involvement of gonadotrophic function and secondary hypogonadism. Although only LH secretion may be impaired, usually secondary hypogonadism is characterized clinically by both inadequate androgenic function and, with rare exceptions (see below), absent or deficient spermatogenesis.

The clinical manifestations vary with age of onset, degree of the deficiency, and whether there is coexistent deficiency of other anterior pituitary hormones. Hypopituitarism occurring during childhood, commonly designated "pituitary dwarfism," results in proportionate dwarfism and complete sexual infantilism. The characteristic features of prepubertal or pubertal gonadotrophic failure are eunuchoid habitus, small testes, lack of development of secondary sexual characteristics, an increased frequency of anosmia or hyposmia, low or absent gonadotrophins, low 17-ketosteroid excretion, low plasma testosterone concentration, and failure of response to clomiphene. Kindreds have been described in which the pattern of inheritance was consistent with either an X-linked or sex-linked dominant trait or as an autosomal recessive trait. The absence of gynecomastia, regarded by some as a salient feature, is of no clinical value in differentiating primary from secondary hypogonadism. It is important to detect organic disease of the pituitary region. Such evaluation should include study of the visual fields, roentgenography of the sella turcica, and, when indicated, such procedures as tomography of the sella, pneumoencephalography, and carotid and venous angiography.

A familial form of isolated hypogonadotrophic hypogonadism limited to males occurs in association with anosmia or hyposmia *(Kallmann's syndrome)* and is transmitted as either an X-linked or a sex-linked dominant trait. Aplasia of the olfactory lobes has been found in autopsied cases. Leydig cell responsiveness to HCG in some of these patients may be decreased. Both familial and sporadic forms of isolated FSH and LH deficiency are known, and these may be associated with a variety of somatic anomalies and neurologic defects. Although the response to LHRH has been variable, the data suggest that hypothalamic synthesis or release of LHRH is impaired in some of these patients.

The testis in patients with hypogonadotrophic hypogonadism remains infantile, the tubular diameter being the same as that of the fetal testis. When the pituitary function is decreased in adult life, tubular collapse, fibrosis, and hyalinization occur at variable times after the onset of gonadotrophic failure.

Isolated LH Deficiency. Pasqualini and Bur described a group of eunuchoidal men with relatively normal-sized testes and some spermatogenic function. Later, McCullagh applied the term "fertile eunuch" to patients with this syndrome. The patients are not fertile, however, because spermatogenesis is decreased, and libido and potentia are absent. Leydig cells are absent or hypoplastic, and androgen deficiency is always present. The excretion of urinary gonadotrophin is usually normal. However, the concentration of plasma LH and the excretion of urinary LH are low or undetectable, whereas the secretion of FSH is normal. Chorionic gonadotrophin stimulates Leydig cell function and ameliorates the androgen deficiency. These patients have an isolated deficiency of LH, which may arise from an abnormality in the hypothalamus (and the synthesis or release of LHRH) or in the pituitary gland. A kindred with two affected brothers has been reported. Rarely, a pituitary tumor or idiopathic delayed adolescence may manifest itself as isolated LH deficiency.

The pathogenesis of the testicular atrophy that follows injury to the spinal cord is uncertain. Both primary and secondary hypogonadism have been described in the Laurence-Moon-Biedl syndrome.

Treatment. A physiologic approach to the treatment of secondary hypogonadism characterized by decreased spermatogenesis requires the use of gonadotrophins. Unfortunately, FSH preparations derived from animal sources are not consistently effective and, when injected repeatedly, stimulate antibody formation that reduces the effect of the hormones. Although human pituitary FSH is not available commercially, gonadotrophin prepared from menopausal urine has been used successfully in combination with chorionic gonadotrophin to induce spermatogenesis in patients with hypogonadotrophic hypogonadism. Here, 75 IU of FSH three times a week has induced normal spermatogenesis. Testosterone cannot be used in place of HCG, because intratesticular testosterone concentrations do not reach the levels attained when the Leydig cells are stimulated. HCG stimulates the Leydig cells to secrete androgen, but must be administered at frequent intervals (three to four times a week). It does not have a direct effect on the seminiferous tubules, although in a few instances of partial gonadotrophic failure spermatogenic as well as Leydig cell function improved after its use. HCG has been effective in maintaining spermatogenesis after hypophysectomy for diabetic retinopathy. When only androgen substitution therapy is needed, one of the long-acting testosterone preparations is preferred.

860. MALE PSEUDOHERMAPHRODITISM

Male pseudohermaphroditism may be considered a form of fetal hypogonadism, because those fetal structures normally responsive to androgen develop incompletely or not at all. Depending on the degree of androgen deficiency, the adult phenotype may range from almost normal female to male with minimal abnormalities. Male pseudohermaphroditism is most often familial and is transmitted either as a sex-linked autosomal dominant or as a sex-limited recessive trait manifest in the male.

SYNDROME OF TESTICULAR FEMINIZATION

This form of familial male pseudohermaphroditism deserves detailed consideration because the pathophysiology illuminates areas of hormone action and fetal regulation. The patients have primary amenorrhea, absent or sparse axillary and pubic hair, female external genitalia, a short blind vaginal pouch, absence of uterus and usually of the male genital ducts, and undescended or labial testes. The phenotypic women are usually tall, have good breast development, and show cornification of the vaginal mucosa. The karyotype is 46 XY.

The cause of the syndrome is a congenital resistance to androgens. Exogenous androgens have been shown to be ineffective in causing axillary or pubic hair growth, virilization, or nitrogen retention. From studies of rat and mouse models of this syndrome, it is probable that the androgen resistance is due to absence of the cytosol androgen-binding protein receptor present in androgen-responsive tissues. This receptor is also present normally in the male gonaducts. In its absence, the male fetus receives no effective androgenic stimulus, resulting in failure of fusion of the genital folds and swellings to form penis and scrotum, respectively, and a lack of posterior migration of the labioscrotal folds. The fetal testicular inducer of müllerian duct regression is not an androgen and continues to be secreted by the fetal testis in this syndrome. Thus, since the upper third of the vagina is a müllerian duct derivative, it regresses and the vagina remains short. Wolffian duct derivatives such as the vas deferens, however, are induced by androgen and therefore are usually absent in this syndrome.

The hormonal relationships in the adult are likewise of interest. Plasma testosterone concentrations are within the normal range for men. Plasma LH is increased, presumably because of end-organ resistance of hypothalamic receptors. Plasma FSH is normal, however, suggesting that feedback is normal owing to a combination of normal estradiol concentration and "tubular factor."

The testes in these patients have tubules containing only Sertoli cells and showing considerable peritubular fibrosis. Spermatogenesis is rare. The Leydig cells appear hyperplastic.

Treatment consists of orchiectomy, because the risk of cancer in these gonads is several times that of gonads in the normal individual. The patients should receive replacement doses of an estrogen such as 0.5 mg of diethylstilbestrol or 0.05 mg of ethinyl estradiol daily to prevent the vasomotor instability characteristic of castration and to maintain normal female secondary sexual characteristics.

OTHER FORMS OF MALE PSEUDOHERMAPHRODITISM

When androgen secretion or effect is decreased during fetal development, the male infant shows varying degrees of ambiguity of the external genitalia. The most extreme example of this would be testicular feminization. The family reported by Lubs et al. has a lesser degree of abnormality because the children were raised as girls but the genitalia were ambiguous. In *Reifenstein's syndrome* and the patients reported by Gilbert-Dreyfus, the phenotype was male. The former syndrome is characterized by severe hypospadias, incomplete fusion of the labioscrotal folds, and gynecomastia. In the latter syndrome, the abnormalities were similar but less marked. Virilization at pubescence in these patients was slow or incomplete, and spermatogenesis was quantitatively decreased. The pathologic physiology of these syndromes has been clarified by Wilson, who showed that decreased 5α-reductase activity with resultant decreased dihydrotestosterone formation would selectively alter the external genitalia.

There have been a few reports of patients with hypospadias and gynecomastia. These may be examples of the least severe form of the syndrome.

861. CRYPTORCHIDISM

The terms "cryptorchidism" and "undescended testes" are used synonymously to designate testes that have never descended into the scrotum. Unilateral cryptorchidism is approximately four times as common as bilaterally undescended testes. A cryptorchid testis may be situated in the abdomen, within the inguinal canal, or in an ectopic position outside the scrotum and the normal pathway of descent. The majority of undescended testes are inguinal. To avoid needless treatment, it is essential to distinguish this condition from retractile testes, which lie in the lower or upper scrotum and are withdrawn into the inguinal region and occasionally into the abdomen by slight stimulus.

The testes usually descend into the scrotum about the eighth fetal month; but occasionally descent is delayed until shortly after birth. Incomplete descent is common in premature male infants. Scorer found undescended testes at birth in 3.4 per cent of 1500 full-term male infants; during the first month of life 50 per cent of the undescended testes reached the scrotum. In a prospective study of the incidence of congenital anomalies by McIntosh and associates, only 0.5 per cent of 2793 liveborn male infants had undescended testes at 12 months of age. The incidence of unilateral and bilateral cryptorchidism in large series of adult males has been variously estimated at 0.2 to 0.4 per cent. Spontaneous descent occurs frequently during the first year of life and is less common after this age.

The etiology is not understood. Not infrequently a normal testis resides in the superficial inguinal pouch, its descent arrested by Scarpa's fascia. However, the cryptorchid testis is often dysgenetic. In rare instances, unilateral or bilateral cryptorchidism is the only overt anatomic abnormality of the external genitalia in individuals with fetal testicular dysfunction.

Diagnosis. The most difficult aspect of diagnosis is distinguishing the true undescended testis from the more common retractile testis of childhood; repeated examinations may be necessary, especially in obese boys. It is important to ascertain by careful inquiry whether the testes have at any time been observed in the scrotum. In cryptorchidism the ipsilateral side of the scrotum is empty and poorly developed. The patient should be carefully examined while standing, squatting, and in a recumbent position, in a warm room and with warm hands. Bimanual examination and palpation while the patient performs a Valsalva maneuver or while the examiner applies pressure to the lower abdomen are also useful procedures. In boys with retractile testes, elicitation of the cremasteric reflex often results in a localized puckering of the scrotal skin. If the testis is palpated in the normal pathway of descent, gentle manipulation should be used in an attempt to displace it into the scrotum. Such mobile testes do not require therapy and will remain in the scrotum with the advent of puberty. Failure to palpate a testis on multiple occasions suggests that the testis is intra-abdominal, atrophic, or absent.

Treatment. The treatment of undescended testes is a vexing and controversial subject; experienced observers differ in their approach to the problem. Major considerations are (1) the potential fertility of the undescended testis, (2) the likelihood of spontaneous descent, and (3) the propensity of the undescended testis to undergo malignant change.

It is well established that during or after puberty the undescended testis shows degenerative changes that eventually proceed to atrophy. With good reason these changes have been ascribed to the deleterious effect of the higher temperature of an extrascrotal environment on the testes, especially on the germinal epithelium. The tubules gradually undergo progressive fibrosis and loss of germinal elements, although androgenic function may persist for many years. These degenerative changes may also be manifestations of a dysgenetic testis. This distinction is important, because the risk of cancer in the dysgenetic gonad is considerably greater than in the normal gonad.

Men with bilateral undescended testes are sterile. However, general agreement is lacking as to the age at which the fertility potential of the cryptorchid testis is impaired. A lag in development of the seminiferous tubules and, in some instances, a mild degree of fibrosis in testes retained after the age of six to ten years have been observed. The significance of these changes is uncertain, but after puberty irreversible degenerative changes frequently occur.

The incidence of cancer in undescended testes is considerably greater than in scrotal testes, and more so in abdominal than in inguinal testes. Although precise statistics are not available, the over-all risk appears to be small, with the exception of the dysgenetic, frequently undescended gonads of intersexes, which are especially prone to malignant degeneration.

The most important problem in the treatment of patients with cryptorchidism is the age at which it is advisable to attempt correction. Treatment consists of orchiopexy or of the administration of HCG followed by orchiopexy when necessary. It is generally agreed that therapy must be started before pubescence if irreparable testicular damage is to be prevented, but opinions differ about the optimal age for treatment. In the more common unilateral cryptorchid, the scrotal testis, if normal, is adequate for fertility. Treatment is recommended for cosmetic reasons, to facilitate examination for neoplasm, and as additional insurance against infertility in the event that the scrotal testis is defective or impaired at a later age.

In bilateral cryptorchidism preservation of fertility is the major consideration. Here the risk of damage to the testis by orchiopexy, which even in experienced hands is not negligible, must be weighed against the possibility of infertility if surgical treatment is delayed too long. When bilateral orchiopexy is followed by atrophy of the testes, the patient will be eunuchoid as well as sterile. Since many undescended testes descend before puberty, it is justifiable to delay treatment until nine years of age unless the testis is ectopic or associated with a hernia.

In some cases hormonal therapy is effective and orchiopexy is unnecessary. It is the opinion of most that testes that descend with such therapy would have descended spontaneously at puberty under the stimulus of endogenous gonadotrophin. To minimize a theoretical risk of damage to the tubule, short intensive courses of 4000 units of HCG administered intramuscularly daily for three days or 4000 units three times a week for three weeks may be used. Hormonal treatment is contraindicated when the testis lies outside the normal pathway of descent.

If the undescended testis is atrophic and biopsy examination at the time of surgery shows irreversible changes, it is generally advisable to perform orchiectomy, provided that the contralateral testis is in the scrotum. This also applies to a testis that, despite all attempts at mobilization, cannot be brought into the scrotum.

862. IMPOTENCE

Impotence is a complicated problem that may be either relative or complete and may involve any phase of the sexual act. Although it is a symptom of androgen deficiency and of genitourinary or neurologic disease, in most instances it is psychic in origin. Multiple sclerosis, tabes dorsalis, and diabetic neuropathy are commonly associated with impotence. Impotence without apparent impairment of libido has been described in patients with temporal lobe lesions. Ganglionic blocking agents, used in the therapy of hypertension, are also a notable cause of impotence. When impotence is the principal complaint of a patient, it is usually the result of an emotional disturbance, and androgen therapy is valueless and at times may add to the psychic trauma. Several recent studies show clearly that, in men as well as in women, stress can decrease gonadotrophic secretion and thereby affect androgen secretion and spermatogenesis (see Ch. 867).

863. "MALE CLIMACTERIC"

The spontaneous occurrence of a male climacteric is still controversial. Although in women during the fifth or sixth decade ovarian failure with a compensatory rise in gonadotrophin excretion is an anticipated and physiologic accompaniment of the aging process, spontaneous testicular deficiency of sufficient degree to produce symptoms is an exceedingly rare occurrence. Many of the symptoms ascribed to this syndrome are common in psychoneurotic syndromes in middle-aged and elderly men. The diagnosis should be documented by finding an increased excretion of gonadotrophin and a low concentration of plasma testosterone, and should be confirmed by obtaining a therapeutic response to androgen therapy, but not to placebos. Plasma testosterone concentrations show little change until after 70 years of age. However, increasing concentrations of testosterone-binding globulin (TeBG) are associated with the gradually decreasing concentration of plasma-free testosterone that has been noted after the age of 50. A progressive increase in plasma LH levels after age 50 has been described.

864. ORCHITIS

Acute orchitis, a common complication of mumps, is a rare occurrence in the course of other specific infectious diseases (see Ch. 125).

Chronic orchitis is associated with painless, hard, sometimes nodular enlargement of the testis. *Syphilis,* the most common cause, may produce an interstitial orchitis in which the testis is characteristically smooth and wooden in consistency ("billiard ball" testis); involvement is frequently bilateral. Other causes include *tuberculosis, leprosy, brucellosis, glanders,* and certain parasitic infections such as *filariasis* and *bilharziasis.* In these diseases, Leydig cell function almost always remains intact, but severe tubular destruction may result.

865. TUMORS OF THE TESTIS

Tumors of the testis are uncommon, comprising about 0.7 per cent of all forms of cancer in the male, occur in about 0.002 per cent of men, and frequently are malignant. The greatest incidence occurs in the third and fourth decades. Testicular tumors may arise from any of the cellular components of the testis or their embryonal precursors.

Considerable uncertainty applies to classification, especially of those neoplasms whose origin has been ascribed to the totipotent germ cell. Melicow has suggested the classification shown in the accompanying table.

GERMINAL TUMORS

Most common are germinal tumors, and, of these, seminoma exceeds in frequency all other testicular tumors. *Seminoma,* although usually fairly uniform in

Tumors of Testis: Classification

I. Primary tumors
  A. Germinal
    1. Seminoma
    2. Embryonal tumors
      a. Embryoma
      b. Choriocarcinoma
      c. Embryonal carcinoma
      d. Teratocarcinoma
      e. Adult teratoma
    3. Combinations of seminoma and embryonal tumor and of the various types of embryonal tumors
    4. Gonadal tumors in intersexes (gonadoblastomas)
  B. Nongerminal tumors
    1. Interstitial cell tumor
    2. Sertoli cell tumor
    3. Tumors of testicular stroma: fibroma, lipoma, etc.
II. Secondary tumors
  A. Lymphoma, plasmacytoma, leukemia, etc.
  B. Metastatic carcinoma

cellular architecture, may contain embryonal elements such as chorionic syncytium in the primary growth or in metastatic lesions. In contrast to the embryonal tumors, which tend to invade the spermatic cord and to metastasize early, especially to lung, seminomas in general are relatively slow growing and commonly invade the iliac and periaortic lymph nodes before generalized dissemination is demonstrable. In addition, seminomas are frequently highly radiosensitive, whereas embryonal tumors are usually resistant to radiotherapy. The significantly increased incidence of germinal tumors, particularly seminoma, in undescended testes and in the dysgenetic gonads of intersexes has been discussed above.

Many patients with germinal tumors excrete increased amounts of chorionic gonadotrophin. This may almost always be attributed to the presence of trophoblastic elements in the tumor. Response to therapy or evidence of recurrence may be monitored by measurement of plasma HCG levels.

INTERSTITIAL CELL TUMORS

Tumors of this type are rare, occur at any age, and are usually but not invariably benign. The tumors are small and often difficult to palpate. In boys interstitial cell tumors cause sexual precocity but not true puberty, because spermatogenesis is absent in the contralateral testis. The only recognizable endocrine manifestation in the adult is gynecomastia, which has been observed in about 10 per cent of cases. Malignant interstitial cell tumors that retain their steroid-synthesizing capacities have been reported.

Bardin, C. W., Ross, G. T., and Lipsett, M. B.: Site of action of clomiphene citrate in men: A study of the pituitary–Leydig cell axis. J. Clin. Endocrinol. Metab., 27:1558, 1967.

Bardin, C. W., Ross, G. T., Rifkind, A. B., Cargille, C. M., and Lipsett, M. B.: Studies of the pituitary–Leydig cell axis in young men with hypogonadotropic hypogonadism and hyposmia: Comparison with normal men, prepubertal boys, and hypopituitary patients. J. Clin. Invest., 48:2046, 1969.

Bergada, C., Cleveland, W. W., Jones, W. H., and Wilkins, L.: Variants of embryonic testicular dysgenesis. Bilateral anorchia and the syndrome of rudimentary testes. Acta Endocrinol., 40:521, 1962.

Bowen, P., Lee, S. N. C., Migeon, C. J., Kaplan, N. M., Whalley, P. J., McKusick, V. A., and Reifenstein, E. C., Jr.: Hereditary male pseudohermaphroditism with hypogonadism, hypospadias, and gynecomastia. Ann. Intern. Med., 62:252, 1965.

Brasel, J. A., Wright, J. C., Wilkins, L., and Blizzard, R. M.: An evaluation of seventy-five patients with hypopituitarism beginning in childhood. Am. J. Med., 38:484, 1965.

Clermont, Y.: Kinetics of spermatogenesis in mammals: Seminiferous epithelium cycle and spermatogonial renewal. Physiol. Rev., 52:198, 1972.

Court Brown, W. M.: Males with an XYY sex chromosome complement. J. Med. Genet., 5:341, 1968.

Davidson, J. M.: Neuroendocrine mechanisms in the control of spermatogenesis. J. Reprod. Fertil., 2:103, 1967.

Dorfman, R. I., and Shipley, R. A.: Androgens: Biochemistry, Physiology, and Clinical Significance. New York, John Wiley & Sons, 1956.

Drucker, W. D., Blanc, W. A., Rowland, L. P., Grumbach, M. M., and Christy, N. P.: The testis in myotonic muscular dystrophy: A clinical and pathologic study with a comparison with the Klinefelter syndrome. J. Clin. Endocrinol. Metab., 23:59, 1963.

Faiman, C., Hoffman, D. L., Ryan, R. J., and Albert, A.: The "fertile eunuch" syndrome: Demonstration of isolated luteinizing hormone deficiency by radioimmunoassay technique. Mayo Clin. Proc., 43:661, 1968.

Faiman, C., and Ryan, R. J.: Radioimmunoassay for human follicle stimulating hormone. J. Clin. Endocrinol. Metab., 27:444, 1967.

Federman, D. D.: Abnormal Sexual Development. Philadelphia, W. B. Saunders Company, 1967.

Foss, G. L., and Lewis, F. J. W.: A study of four cases with Klinefelter's syndrome, showing motile spermatozoa in their ejaculates. J. Reprod. Fertil., 25:401, 1971.

French, F. S., Baggett, B., Van Wyk, J. J., Talbert, J. M., Hubbard, W. R., Johnston, F. R., and Weaver, R. P.: Testicular feminization: Clinical, morphological and biochemical studies. J. Clin. Endocrinol. Metab., 25:661, 1965.

Howard, R. P., Sniffen, R. C., Simmons, F. A., and Albright, F.: Testicular deficiency: A clinical and pathologic study. J. Clin. Endocrinol. Metab., 10:121, 1950.

Jost, A.: Problems of fetal endocrinology. Recent Prog. Horm. Res., 8:379, 1953.

Kelch, R. P., Jenner, M. R., Weinstein, R., Kaplan, S. L., and Grumbach, M. M.: Estradiol and testosterone secretion by human, simian, and canine testes, in males with hypogonadism and in male pseudohermaphrodites with the feminizing testes syndrome. J. Clin. Invest., 51:824, 1972.

Kessler, S., and Moss, R. H.: The XYY karyotype and criminality: A review. J. Psychiatr. Res., 7:153, 1970.

Lipsett, M. B., and Sherins, R. J.: The Testis. In Bondy, P. K., and Rosenberg, L. E. (eds.): Duncan's Diseases of Metabolism. 7th ed. Philadelphia, W. B. Saunders Company, 1974.

Mancini, R. E., Seiguer, A. C., and Perez Lloret, A.: Effect of gonadotropins on the recovery of spermatogenesis in hypophysectomized patients. J. Clin. Endocrinol. Metab., 29:467, 1969.

Marshall, W. A., and Tanner, J. M.: Variations in the pattern of pubertal changes in boys. Arch. Dis. Child., 45:13, 1970.

Martin, F. I. R.: The stimulation and prolonged maintenance of spermatogenesis by human pituitary gonadotrophins in a patient with hypogonadotrophic hypogonadism. J. Endocrinol., 38:431, 1967.

Melicow, M. M.: Classification of tumors of the testis. J. Urol., 73:547, 1955.

Moore, K. L. (ed.): The Sex Chromatin. Philadelphia, W. B. Saunders Company, 1966.

Nowakowski, H., and Lenz, W.: Genetic aspects in male hypogonadism. Recent Prog. Horm. Res., 17:53, 1961.

Odell, W. D., Ross, G. T., and Rayford, P. L.: Radioimmunoassay for luteinizing hormone in human plasma or serum: Physiological studies. J. Clin. Invest., 46:248, 1967.

Paulsen, C. A.: The testes. In Williams, R. H. (ed.): Textbook of Endocrinology. 4th ed. Philadelphia, W. B. Saunders Company, 1968.

Paulsen, C. A., Gordon, D. L., Carpenter, R. W., Gandy, H. M., and Drucker, W. D.: Klinefelter's syndrome and its variants: A hormonal and chromosomal study. Recent Prog. Horm. Res., 24:321, 1968.

Pearson, P. L., Borrow, M., and Vosa, A. G.: Technique for identifying Y chromosomes in human interphase nuclei. Nature, 226:78, 1970.

Rifkind, A. B., Kulin, H. E., and Ross, G. T.: Follicle-stimulating hormone (FSH) and luteinizing hormone (LH) in the urine of prepubertal children. J. Clin. Invest., 46:1925, 1967.

Rosemberg, E., and Paulsen, C. A. (eds.): The Human Testis. New York, Plenum Press, 1970.

Santen, R. J., and Paulsen, C. A.: Hypogonadotropic eunuchoidism. I. Clinical study of mode of inheritance. J. Clin. Endocrinol. Metab., 36:47, 1973.

Scorer, C. G.: The descent of the testis. Arch. Dis. Child., 39:204, 1964.

Steinberger, E.: Hormonal control of mammalian spermatogenesis. Physiol. Rev., 51:1, 1971.

Swanson, D. W., and Stipes, A. H.: Psychiatric aspects of Klinefelter's syndrome. Am. J. Psychiatry, 126:814, 1969.

Van Thiel, D. H., Sherins, R. J., and DeVita, V. T., Jr.: Evidence for a specific seminiferous tubular factor affecting follicle-stimulating hormone secretion in man. J. Clin. Invest., 51:1009, 1972.

Van Wyk, J. J., and Grumbach, M. M.: Disorders of sex differentiation. In Williams, R. H. (ed.): Textbook of Endocrinology. 4th ed. Philadelphia, W. B. Saunders Company, 1968.

Walsh, P. C., Madden, J. D., Harrod, M. J., Goldstein, J. L., MacDonald, P. C., and Wilson, J. D.: Familial incomplete male pseudohermaphroditism, Type 2. N. Engl. J. Med., 291:944, 1974.

Wilson, J. D., and Gloya, R. E.: The intra-nuclear metabolism of testosterone in the accessory organs of reproduction. Recent Prog. Horm. Res., 26:309, 1970.

THE OVARIES

Nathan Kase

866. OVARIAN STRUCTURE AND FUNCTION

The human ovary has a dual physiologic responsibility: (1) development and release of ova and (2) elaboration of estrogen and progesterone. From menarche to menopause both these activities are bound to the cycle of follicle development, ovulation, corpus luteum formation, and regression. In reality each ovary is a heterogeneous, cyclically changing tissue containing subunits with differing properties. During their brief interval of dominance each subunit defines the function of the total organ. The sequential appearance of each unit and their respective gametogenic and endocrine performances are directed by pituitary secretion of varying quantities of gonadotrophins: follicle-stimulating hormone (FSH) and luteinizing hormone (LH). Release of these factors is controlled by a specific neurosecretory substance or substances originating in hypothalamic nuclei that are sensitive to "feedback" levels of circulating ovarian hormones.

The ovary contains specialized cells in the cortical and medullary areas that may contribute to abnormal ovarian function in certain pathologic conditions, but its major elements are the follicle and corpus luteum. The follicle consists of the ovum and two layers of tissue surrounding it: an inner band of granulosa cells without blood vessels, and an outer vascularized mantle of theca cells. At any given time in the preovulatory phase a number of follicles display varying degrees of developmental maturity: cystic changes, hormonal activity, and atresia. The factors responsible for the selection of one to attain full maturity and ovulation while others atrophy are unknown. Morphologic clues indicating development of a follicle are the degree of thecal proliferation and vascularity and the ratio of granulosa layer thickening to cystic distention of the antrum. The formation of a true corpus luteum is a direct consequence of final maturation and ovulation of the follicle. The ruptured follicle is transformed by proliferation, vascularization, and luteinization of the granulosa into the yellow body that characterizes the last two weeks of an ovulatory cycle. Contrary to evidence obtained in other mammals, the human corpus luteum appears to possess an inherent life span of two weeks, during which it is sustained by modest postovulatory pituitary secretion of LH. After this period, the corpus luteum recedes unless renewed major trophic stimulation appears in the form of human chorionic gonadotrophin originating in a flourishing mass of syncytiotrophoblasts associated with an implanted conceptus.

OVARIAN HORMONE FUNCTION—THE ENDOMETRIAL CYCLE

It is helpful to consider the function of ovarian hormones relative to their ability to provide an appropriate milieu for fertilization, implantation, and nutrition of the early embryo. Before menstruation has ceased, preparation for a more successful ovum is resumed. FSH and small quantities of LH renew follicle growth and augment estrogen secretion. Under the influence of estradiol and estrone, endothelial and mucosal repair takes place. In the ensuing fortnight continued estrogen stimulation produces growth of glands and spiral arterioles. These vessels remain unbranched to the periphery where a terminal capillary network is formed. Accompanying this proliferation, endometrial expansion is accomplished by accumulation of ground substance and modest edema of the stroma. This estrogen-induced phenomenon unfolds the collapsed stromal reticulum. In this way follicle estrogen produces an endometrium with sufficient height, vascularity, and concentrations of glycogen and protein to satisfy the early requirements of the anticipated embryo. Furthermore, estrogen-dependent changes in cervical mucus aid sperm migration.

The midcycle preovulatory peak of estrogen probably signals the release of pituitary LH. The brief surge of this gonadotrophin induces acute follicle distention. By unknown mechanisms necrosis of the thinned follicle wall occurs, leading to capsular rupture and permitting extrusion of the ovum. The corpus luteum is formed, and secretion of progesterone rapidly increases. This hormone and sustained levels of estrogen combine to inhibit further LH secretion.

In the absence of a conceptus, at day 12 post ovulation, the corpus luteum recedes and hormone levels wane. With stromal cell shrinkage and loss of ground

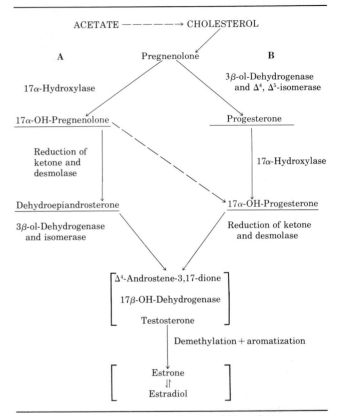

Figure 2. Pathways of ovarian steroid biosynthesis.

substance, the endometrium thins. The vessels buckle, and diminished peripheral blood flow is reduced further by tonic vasoconstriction of spiral arterioles. Localized peripheral ischemia and fragmentation occur, with progressive hemorrhage and disruption of superficial zones of the endometrium. With the loss of the peripheral binding epithelium, menstruation begins.

The ranges of peptide and steroid hormone concentrations and their interrelationships during an ovulatory cycle are shown in Figure 1.

OVARIAN STEROID BIOSYNTHESIS

It is clear that appropriate target organ processes are dependent on periodic variations in the quantity and type of hormone emanating from the ovary. How does the ovary accomplish the initial production of microgram quantities of estrogen and then milligram secretion of progesterone? The in vitro analyses of Ryan, using isolated follicles and corpora lutea and radioactive steroid precursors, contributed significantly to the understanding of these processes. This work confirmed the accumulated evidence bearing on the dominance of two biosynthetic pathways leading to estrogen production in the ovary. These routes (A and B) are depicted in Figure 2. Route A provides for conversion of pregnenolone to estrogen via a pathway in which the 3β-ol,Δ^5 characteristic is maintained to the C_{19} stage. On the other hand, route B projects immediate conversion of pregnenolone to progesterone (change from Δ^5-3β-ol to Δ^4-3 ketone in ring A) prior to loss of sidechain and estrogen generation. Ryan's data suggest that, whereas the corpus luteum utilizes the pathway via proges-

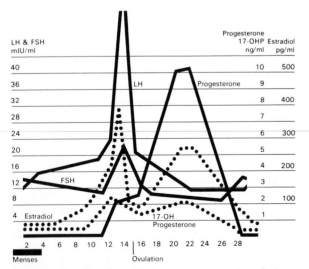

Figure 1. Steroid and peptide hormone concentrations during an ovulatory menstrual cycle. (From Speroff, L., Glass, R. H., and Kase, N. G.: Clinical Gynecologic Endocrinology and Infertility. Baltimore, Williams and Wilkins Company, 1973.)

terone (*B*), the follicle employs route *A*, bypassing formation of this biologically active intermediate. Individual cell studies have shown that granulosa and theca cells have similar biosynthetic capabilities and that only quantitative differences exist between these tissues. Apparently both granulosa and theca cells are necessary for adequate steroid production in biologic studies.

There are broader endocrine implications in the biosynthetic mechanisms depicted in the figure. With certain notable exceptions, such as the 11-hydroxylation property of the adrenal cortex, it is apparent that all steroid-producing organs make steroids in roughly the same manner. The biosynthetic pathways require the presence of biologically active steroids other than those typically secreted by a gland, but these are normally not apparent clinically. However, disordered activity of these pathways in certain ovarian disease leads to abnormal levels of secretion of these active intermediates with clinically demonstrable hormone effects.

Hisaw, F. L.: Development of the graafian follicle and ovulation. Physiol. Rev., 27:95, 1947.

Rock, J., Garcia, C.-R., and Menkin, M.: A theory of menstruation. Ann. N. Y. Acad. Sci., 75:831, 1959.

Ross, G. T., et al.: Pituitary and gonadal hormones in women during spontaneous and induced ovulatory cycles. Rec. Prog. Horm. Res., 26:1, 1970.

Ryan, K., and Smith, O. V.: Biogenesis of steroid hormones in the human ovary. Rec. Prog. Horm. Res., 21:367, 1965.

Schally, A. V., et al.: Gonadotropin-releasing hormone: One polypeptide regulates secretion of luteinizing and follicle stimulating hormones. Science, 173:1036, 1971.

Schally, A. V., et al.: The hypothalamus and reproduction (current developments). Am. J. Obstet. Gynecol., 114:423, 1972.

Vande Wiele, R. L., et al.: Mechanisms regulating the menstrual cycle in women. Rec. Prog. Horm. Res., 26:63, 1970.

867. OVARIAN DISORDERS PERTINENT TO GENERAL MEDICINE

EVALUATION OF OVARIAN FUNCTION

The simple existence of ovarian function may be inferred from the development and maintenance of the breasts and the internal and external genitalia. However, a range of ovarian secretion essential to the full activity of these organs is more critically expressed by the periodic phenomenon of ovulatory menstruation. With the corpus luteum's inherent life span of two weeks, an implicit termination point for each cycle is provided in the menstruation resulting from estrogen and progesterone withdrawal and the recycling surge of FSH.

It is helpful to group disorders of ovarian function within the following descriptive categories:

Sexual precocity: the onset of menses before the age of ten years or development of breasts or pubic (not vulvar) hair growth before the age of eight years. Although these elements may appear as isolated manifestations, this general term usually applies to premature appearance of all three aspects of sexual maturation.

Primary amenorrhea: the delay of menarche beyond the age of 18. Statistically 5 per cent of girls initiate menses after 16 and 1 per cent after age 18. In the presence of breast development, pubic hair growth, and a normal adolescent growth spurt, diagnostic evaluation of delayed menarche may be postponed until 18.

Secondary amenorrhea: the cessation of uterine bleeding at any age in women who have previously menstruated. The elapsed interval of amenorrhea necessary for the diagnosis cannot be rigidly defined, and is often dictated by other clinical factors. However, if the patient has not bled within a length of time equivalent to three or four of her normal cycles, then investigation is warranted.

Oligomenorrhea: a recurrent prolongation of intermenstrual intervals leading to a decreased frequency of menses (three to six per year). This irregularity is commonly seen in postmenarchal and premenopausal women. In the absence of other signs and symptoms, intensive work-up is not required at these times. Evaluation is in order in other age groups because anovulatory infertility is frequently associated with this menstrual anomaly.

Hypomenorrhea: a diminution in the quantity of menstrual flow based on tampon or napkin requirement. It is of little diagnostic significance if found as a solitary problem. Investigation beyond a physical examination, which includes a pelvic examination and cytologic smear, is unnecessary.

Hypermenorrhea: a definite relative increase in duration or quantity (or both) of menstrual flow that occurs at normal cycle intervals. A subgrouping called *polymenorrhea* designates menstrual flow close to normal in quantity and duration but which recurs too frequently (less than 21 days apart). Each group requires immediate gynecologic assessment. Because each is frequently associated with anovulation, endocrine evaluation may also be in order.

AIDS TO DIAGNOSIS

The clinical categories just described represent a spectrum of abnormal ovarian function which appears clinically as changes in sexual development, menstrual regularity, and ovulation. Such malfunction may be caused by primary ovarian disease, abnormal stimulation of the ovary by other glands, disease of target organs, or systemic disease. Steps to appropriate diagnosis begin with a complete history and physical examination, including careful examination of the pelvic organs and external genitalia. When properly selected, certain procedures and laboratory tests can be of great diagnostic assistance.

Pituitary Gonadotrophin Function. Pituitary gonadotrophins may be measured by bioassay or by radioimmunoassay. The bioassay requires a 24-hour urine collection from which gonadotrophins are extracted by a process including acidification, kaolin absorption and elution, followed by acetone precipitation. The extract is diluted and injected into immature female mice, and the increase in the weight of the mouse uterus is measured. The assay depends on the FSH and LH in the extract to stimulate the immature mouse ovaries to produce estrogen. The greatest dilution of the urine extract which causes a 100 per cent increase in uterine weight is the titer of gonadotrophins, and the result is expressed in mouse uterine weight units (muu) per 24 hours. Less than 6 muu per 24 hours indicates normal prepubertal levels or adult hypogonadotrophism. A castrate or postmenopausal level is greater than 200 muu per 24 hours.

This assay is notoriously unreliable and has been al-

TABLE 1. Values for Gonadotrophins in Serum

Clinical State	Serum FSH	Serum LH
Normal adult female	5–30 mIU/ml, with ovulatory midcycle peak two times baseline	5–20 mIU/ml, with ovulatory midcycle peak three times baseline
Hypogonadotrophism (prepubertal, hypothalamic and pituitary dysfunction)	Less than 5 mIU/ml	Less than 5 mIU/ml
Hypergonadotrophism (postmenopause, castrate, ovarian failure)	Greater than 40 mIU/ml	Greater than 25 mIU/ml

most entirely replaced by specific radioimmunoassays for FSH and LH in serum. It must be remembered (Fig. 1) that wide swings in gonadotrophin levels are typical of ovulatory cycles. Table 1 depicts the ranges of gonadotrophins in various clinical circumstances.

Ovarian Function. Tests that are based on biologic effects of ovarian hormones are simply performed, providing immediate and valuable data at little cost to the patient. Therefore more costly laboratory evaluations of hormone excretion or blood concentrations are rarely required for clinical purposes.

Gonadal Hormone Effects. CORNIFICATION OF VAGINAL EPITHELIUM. The percentage of fully cornified cells is related to ovarian estrogen production. Because cytologic criteria and staining methods vary from center to center, no normal values can be given. However, because other factors affect this evaluation (progesterone, cortisone, and androgen diminish, although digitalis increases cornification), the stage of the cycle as well as current therapy must be considered in evaluation of test results.

Endometrial biopsy tests endometrial responsiveness as well as the existence of appropriate ovarian hormone secretion during the cycle. Evaluation must take into consideration the stage of the cycle when the biopsy specimen is taken.

In addition to the quantity and clarity of *cervical mucus,* the development of an arborization pattern in a dried specimen *(the "fern" test)* indicates the presence of estrogen. Correlation with cycle dates is essential, for secretion of progesterone inhibits this phenomenon.

The *basal body temperature* will demonstrate the occurrence of ovulation if serial readings are taken throughout a cycle. Based on the mild thermogenic properties of progesterone, a sustained postovulatory rise of temperature (0.3° C or more) of two weeks' duration indicates corpus luteum function. Retrospectively, the timing of ovulation in the cycle can be estimated from the date when the effect of progesterone first appeared.

PROGESTERONE WITHDRAWAL BLEEDING. If menses can be induced after administration of progesterone or a nonestrogenic derivative, this event indicates prior ovarian estrogen secretion and its proliferative or "priming" effect on the endometrium.

Gonadal Hormone Plasma Concentrations. The normal levels for total plasma estrogens or estradiol and plasma progesterone vary with the time in the menstrual cycle when the blood sample is drawn. (For the pattern of these variations, see Fig. 3.) The normal ranges of plasma gonadal steroids as measured by radioimmunoassay are depicted in Table 2.

Gonadal Hormone Excretion. TOTAL URINARY ESTROGENS PER 24 HOURS. The measurement of estrogen in a 24-hour urine sample is useful in guiding replacement FSH-LH therapy for the induction of ovulation. The range of estrogen excretion during various clinical states is shown in Table 3.

URINARY PREGNANEDIOL EXCRETION. Pregnanediol is the main urinary metabolite of progesterone but accounts for only 7 to 20 per cent of total progesterone production. Measurement of this metabolite in urine has been used to document ovulation and the presence and well-being of early pregnancy. The range of excretion of pregnanediol is seen in Table 4.

URINARY PREGNANETRIOL EXCRETION. Although not exclusively a metabolite of gonadal hormone production, the concentration of this metabolite of 17α-OH-progesterone in a 24-hour urine specimen is useful in the diagnosis of adrenocortical hyperplasia. In normal circumstances urinary pregnanetriol excretions in children and adults are within the ranges shown in Table 5.

Other Tests. Other tests of importance include those that estimate *adrenal cortex and thyroid activity.* Specific details concerning interpretation of results and the diagnostic manipulations involved are given in other sections of this text. Dysfunction of either organ may have pronounced effects on ovarian and target organ physiology.

HUMAN CHORIONIC GONADOTROPHIN. Secretion of human chorionic gonadotrophin (HCG) by the syncytiotrophoblast cells of the placenta is directed predominantly into the maternal circulation. The assay of HCG in maternal urine has been the basis of many pregnancy tests since the original Aschheim-Zondek test.

These bioassays depend upon the response of ovaries or testes in immature animals to the gonadotrophic properties of HCG when present in urine. The endpoints were increased gonadal weight, hyperemia, or response in sex organs to increased gonadal steroidogenesis induced by HCG. The expulsion of ova or sperm in amphibia was also a widely used clinical assay. These biologic tests have been entirely replaced

TABLE 2. Values for Plasma Estrogens and Progesterone

Cycle Phase	Total Estrogen or Estradiol	Progesterone
Follicle phase	25– 75 pg/ml	Less than 1 ng/ml
Midcycle peak	200–600 pg/ml	
Luteal phase	100–300 pg/ml	5– 20 ng/ml
Pregnancy, first trimester	1– 5 ng/ml	20– 30 ng/ml
Pregnancy, second trimester	5– 15 ng/ml	50–100 ng/ml
Pregnancy, third trimester	10– 40 ng/ml	100–400 ng/ml

TABLE 3. Values for Urinary Estrogen

Clinical Circumstance	Total Urinary Estrogen/24 Hours
Prepubertal	0– 5 μg/24 hr
Follicle phase	10– 25 μg/24 hr
Midcycle peak	35–100 μg/24 hr
Luteal phase	25– 75 μg/24 hr
Postmenopausal	5– 15 μg/24 hr

by the clinical application of immunoassays for HCG in urine – the urinary chorionic gonadotrophin (UCG) test.

Three types of immunologic assays are used: hemagglutination-inhibition, complement-fixation, and radioimmunoassay. In the hemagglutination-inhibition reaction, the presence of HCG in maternal urine inhibits an agglutination reaction between HCG-coated red cells and the antisera. In some commercial methods latex particles are used in place of red cells. A rapid although less sensitive slide test using latex particles is available, but the two-hour red cell test is more reliable. A first morning voided urine specimen is preferred.

HCG and LH are similar in structure, and considerable immunologic cross-reaction exists. The sensitivity of most commercial HCG assays is limited to 1000 IU per liter of urine to avoid false positive cross-reactions with LH. Because of the limitations in sensitivity, a positive test does not appear until ten days to two weeks after the missed menstrual period. From that point the levels of HCG rise to an average peak of 100,000 IU per liter at 10 weeks' gestation, and then declines over the next four weeks to 20,000 IU per liter, at which point excretion levels are sustained for the remainder of the pregnancy.

Patients with *hydatidiform moles* generally display urinary HCG levels around 300,000 IU per liter. *Choriocarcinoma* may be associated with levels in the millions of IU. Although absolute levels are helpful, they are not absolutely diagnostic of disease. Multiple gestations may also show high levels of UCG excretion.

A semiquantitative estimation of HCG in a 24-hour urine may be useful in evaluating threatened abortion or ectopic gestation. A low or declining level of UCG indicates a poor prognosis for an intrauterine pregnancy, whereas a low level of HCG (below 5000 IU per liter of urine) is commonly seen when the pregnancy test is positive in ectopic pregnancy.

Three weeks after a spontaneous or therapeutic abortion, the urinary pregnancy test should reverse to negative. Before that time positive tests may still be encountered.

Clinical assays. *In* Speroff, L., Glass, R. H., and Kase, N. G.: Clinical Gynecologic Endocrinology and Infertility. Baltimore, Williams & Wilkins Company, 1973, pp. 226–250.

TABLE 4. Values for Urinary Pregnanediol

	Urinary Pregnanediol/24 Hours
Follicle phase	Less than 1 mg
Luteal phase	2–5 mg
Pregnancy, 20 weeks	40 mg
Pregnancy, 30 weeks	80 mg
Pregnancy, 40 weeks	100 mg

TABLE 5. Values for Urinary Pregnanetriol

	Urinary Pregnanetriol/24 Hours
Children	Less than 0.5 mg
Adults	0.2 to 2–4 mg (upper limits vary with laboratory)

PUBERTY

The initiation of menstrual function in humans occurs with greatest frequency at age 12 or 13, but there is a considerable "normal" variation in the time of its onset. When menstruation begins before the age of 10 or after 16, a decision must be made whether the precocious or delayed menarche is a physiologic variant or whether it is due to some abnormality. Furthermore, since menarche is but one of several important changes associated with puberty and a variation in its timing is by no means the only feature of disease, it is useful to review the characteristic sequence of female puberty.

The *first sign of puberty* is generally the appearance of the *breast bud.* Pubic hair quickly follows breast development, but appearance of axillary hair is normally delayed as much as two years. At about the time of breast development the adolescent growth in linear height begins, and over the next year of peak growth a girl will grow 6 to 11 cm. In the typical pubescence, within two years of initiating this growth spurt, the first menstruation, i.e., the menarche, occurs.

Because the growth of pubic and axillary hair is almost certainly due to an increased production of adrenal androgens at puberty, this event is often referred to as *adrenarche* as well as pubarche. Premature thelarche (premature breast development) as an isolated biologic event is less common. The etiology of these events is not understood at present; gonadotrophin and estrogen levels are not elevated.

Although pubescence has been described in terms of the two-year sequence – increased linear growth rate, breast development, pubarche, and menarche – varying patterns occur frequently and are not necessarily indicative of dysfunction or disease.

Certain aspects of the neuroendocrine mechanism involved in normal puberty have been uncovered. It has been shown that the anterior pituitary of infants contains adequate quantities of gonadotrophins and that an intact pituitary is essential for the prepubertal development and maintenance of the gonads. Removal of the ovaries in this age group is associated with increased gonadotrophin excretion, the formation of castration cells in the pituitary, and enlargement of the gland. These changes can be prevented by estrogen therapy in very low doses. Therefore the small quantity of estrogen secreted prepubertally is sufficient to inhibit all but a small clinically undetectable quantity of gonadotrophin release. Further indirect evidence that this central inhibition is the critical mechanism in the *normal* delay of sexual maturation can be seen in the fully responsive competence of the premenarchal ovary to exogenous gonadotrophin therapy. Certain areas in the hypothalamus are believed to be responsible for this temporary extreme sensitivity to inhibiting levels of circulating steroids. It has been suggested that neoplastic and vascular disorders that alter hypothalamic function probably reverse this low threshold inhibition and lead to precocious puberty.

SEXUAL PRECOCITY

Precocity may be due to organic or constitutional (idiopathic) causes. Ninety per cent of patients with this symptom will fall in the latter category despite thorough evaluation. However, it is essential that these cases be distinguished from those with lesions of the brain or the rare diseases of ovary and adrenal that produce premature development.

Constitutional Sexual Precocity. This is due to the premature release of the adult sequence and levels of gonadotrophin, which are sufficient to initiate prematurely the normal physiologic and endocrine processes of breast development, appearance of pubic and axillary hair, and menstruation. Although it is assumed that hypothalamic inhibitory influences have been diminished, the precise inciting factor is unknown. Diminished secretion of inhibitory quantities of melatonin by the pineal gland is suggested as one possible etiologic factor. Generally the normal, orderly, albeit more rapid appearance of breast development, pubic hair growth, and then menarche is found in the five- to eight-year age group. However, menarche may be the first symptom noted and may occur as early as three months of age. The usual sequential maturation pattern may be altered or only partially displayed. Although not all patients will ovulate, biologic manifestations of ovulation rule out precocity based on gonadotrophin-independent estrogen production by ovarian or adrenal disease. Estrogen production from any source is likely to induce accelerated linear growth and advancement of bone age, which is seen best in roentgenograms of carpal bones, knee, and elbow. Although these children are temporarily taller than their normal counterparts, premature closure of epiphyses produces a final height that is less than normal. Thus the diagnostic criteria for a constitutional etiology of precocity include the sequence of secondary sex characteristics, advanced bone age, adult levels of estrogen and gonadotrophin, normal urinary adrenal metabolites, and normal neurologic examination and skull films. Optimal therapy (reversible suppression of gonadotrophins without peripheral target organ stimulation) may be achievable with long-acting nonestrogenic depomedroxyprogesterone acetate. This potent progestational agent, when administered in large doses (400 mg) intramuscularly monthly for three months and then once every three months, provides long-term inhibition of gonadotrophin secretion. Pubic hair does not disappear, but further menstruation, breast development, and growth may be inhibited. The response to progestins is not uniformly positive; it is not possible to determine which child will respond favorably in advance of therapy.

These children present a serious emotional and social problem not only because they are distinctly different from their contemporaries, but also because they are insufficiently mature emotionally to cope with the sexual interest they provoke in others. That they are capable of reproduction has been demonstrated many times, but most dramatically in the case of a Peruvian girl, Lena Medina, who was delivered of a normal child by cesarean section at five and a half years of age.

Precocity Due to Organic Causes. *Cerebral Lesions.* A variety of brain disorders produce sexual precocity secondary to premature gonadotrophin release, presumably by the abolition of the inhibitory effects of the hypothalamus. Although the anatomic location of these inhibitory centers is uncertain, three general groups of tumors may cause precocity: lesions in the tuber cinereum, lesions in the posterior hypothalamic mammillary body area, and lesions destroying the pineal. In addition, disorders indirectly affecting hypothalamic function (internal hydrocephalus, encephalitis, meningitis, and cranial trauma) may be associated with precocity. Differential diagnosis of this type of precocity from the constitutional variety cannot be achieved by endocrine survey. Only after intensive neurologic, roentgenographic, and pediatric evaluation and follow-up reappraisal will proper diagnosis be made.

Organic Precocious Pseudopuberty Due to Adrenal and Ovarian Hyperfunction. The term pseudopuberty defines the basic difference between precocity resulting from premature gonadotrophic activity (constitutional, central types) and those lesions in which adrenal and ovarian estrogen stimulates target organs. In the latter, gonadotrophin is absent, and therefore ovulation does not occur.

Although certain elements of premature maturation (pubic hair, bone age advancement) appear in adrenal disorders, the masculinization and rarity of vaginal bleeding (delayed menarche is usual) make the diagnosis relatively simple. Isosexual pseudopuberty is more commonly associated with estrogen-producing ovarian tumors. Although the diagnosis of tumor is always considered, it is rarely confirmed. Only 5 per cent of *granulosa tumors* occur before true puberty. The presence of a palpable adnexal mass and the absence of urinary gonadotrophin, ovulation, and regular cyclic bleeding support the diagnosis. In addition, the exceedingly rare *choriocarcinoma, teratoma, or dysgerminoma* of the ovary may be associated with pseudopuberty. However, these will sometimes pose a diagnostic complication. The production of chorionic gonadotrophin by these tumors will give falsely elevated adult levels of "FSH" in mouse uterine weight tests and elevated serum LH values in routine radioimmunoassay, in addition to positive pregnancy tests. The finding of an ovarian mass calls for laparotomy.

Albright's syndrome, consisting of cystic bone lesions, patchy skin pigmentation, and sexual precocity, is grouped with pseudopuberty in that gonadotrophin excretion and ovulation are absent. Normal puberty and ovulation follow and fertility is not decreased.

Greulich, W. W., and Pyle, S. L.: Radiographic Atlas of Skeletal Development of The Hand and Wrist. Stanford, Calif., Stanford University Press, 1950.

Pedowitz, P., Felmus, L. B., and Mackles, A.: Precocious pseudopuberty due to ovarian tumors. Obstet. Gynecol. Survey, 10:633, 1955.

Van Der Werff Ten Bosch, J. J.: Isosexual precocity. In Gardner, L. I. (ed.): Endocrine and Genetic Diseases of Childhood. Philadelphia, W. B. Saunders Company, 1969.

DISORDERS OF MENSTRUAL FUNCTION

Delayed Menarche and Primary Amenorrhea

Menarche may be delayed beyond the age of 16 years on a constitutional basis and often as a familial trait. In these instances there is no demonstrable organic lesion, and with time normal periods appear. However, some cases of delayed menarche are not benign, and these bring up the vexing problem of which patients in this age group require intensive work-up. In general, delayed menarche accompanied by any of the following signs requires full evaluation to prevent worsening of the underlying condition, which is only initially presenting as delayed menstruation: absence of other secondary sexual characteristics, symptoms and signs of outflow tract incompetence, systemic disorders (neurogenic, obesity, cachexia, thyroid and adrenocortical disease), psychiatric disorders, or signs of abnormal chromosomal constitution.

Lacking these associated conditions, delayed menarche may be managed by sympathetic reassurance of the likelihood of eventual establishment of normal menses.

If menarche is delayed beyond the age of 18, *primary amenorrhea* is said to exist. The diagnostic investigation of this entity is best oriented to assessment of the various anatomic sites involved in the generation and transport of menstrual fluid. These include the vaginal tract, uterus, ovaries, pituitary, and hypothalamus.

Mechanical Obstruction. Mechanical obstruction at the hymen or in the vaginal or cervical canal will prevent drainage of uterine secretions. Such stenosis is usually congenital but may be secondary to infection. Outward signs of menses are absent, but periodic vaginal or lower abdominal pain and the presence of a mass on rectal or vaginal examination are observed. Depending on the site and duration of obstruction, hematocolpos, hematometra and/or hematosalpinx are present.

Absence or Unresponsiveness of the Endometrium. This presents as primary amenorrhea. Agenesis of the uterus is rare, as are the "acquired" lesions such as tuberculosis, uterine schistosomiasis, and postsepsis obliteration of the endometrium and uterine cavity, which render this organ incapable of reacting to normal cyclic levels of estrogen.

Primary Hypogonadism. Amenorrhea is the basic symptom of primary hypogonadism. The most common cause of primary ovarian failure is *Turner's syndrome (gonadal dysgenesis).*

The chromosomal anomaly in gonadal dysgenesis is the presence of only one X chromosome in all cell lines (X chromosome monosomy). The individual is referred to as 45,X or frequently as XO. Despite absence of gonadal development, these patients are phenotypic, albeit immature, females. The clinical facets of the syndrome are well known; these include short stature (48 to 58 inches), sexual infantilism, streak gonads, increased carrying angle, shield chest, pterygium colli, a tendency to form keloids, intestinal telangiectasias, prominent epicanthal folds, micrognathia, dental malocclusion, anomalies of the ocular muscles, and multiple skin nevi. Mental retardation is seen in many patients. In addition to renal anomalies, coarctation of the aorta and short fourth metacarpals are seen. The streak gonad is composed of fibrous tissue containing no follicles or ova and devoid of medullary components.

Although the diagnosis is usually not made until puberty when amenorrhea with castration levels of urinary gonadotrophin, lack of sexual development, and short stature become evident retrospectively, the history will show that the patient weighed less at birth than expected by gestational age and that she tended to be below average weight and body length throughout childhood. At birth, some of the stigmata of the Bonnevie-Ullrich syndrome, i.e., lymphedema of the dorsum of the hands and feet, cutis laxa, and low hairline on the neck, may indicate the presence of this condition.

The incidence of 45,X is 0.04 per cent of newborn females.

A large variety of mosaic patterns is seen with gonadal dysgenesis. From analysis of various combinations, it appears that short stature is related to loss of the short arm of one X chromosome. Thus X, XXp, and XXqi are all short individuals. Xqi designates an isochromosome for the long arms, and Xp deletion of the short arm. The loss of the long arm of one of the X chromosomes is associated with amenorrhea and streak gonads, but these patients are not short and do not have other malformations. Thus loss of material from the short arms of the X chromosomes leads to short stature and other stigmata of Turner's syndrome. Streak gonads result if either the long or the short arm is missing. This would suggest that normal ovarian development requires two loci, one on the long arm and one on the short arm; loss of either results in gonadal failure.

Menstrual function and reproduction in a patient with Turner's phenotype must be due to a mosaic complement such as a 46,XX line in addition to 45,X. Multiple X females (47,XXX) have normal development and reproductive function, although mental retardation may be more frequent. Secondary amenorrhea or eunuchoidism, or both, may be seen, depending on the initial amount and rapidity of loss of follicular apparatus.

In gonadal dysgenesis, the gonadal structures are streak gonads. In *mixed gonadal dysgenesis,* testicular tissue may be present. Mosaicism is the likely underlying abnormality, even if it is not detected in the cell line studied. Ambiguous genitalia are produced if testicular tissue is present. In this instance, gonadectomy is necessary both to avoid further heterosexual development if sex assignment is female and to avoid neoplastic change in the testicular tissue even if sex assignment is male.

In Noonan's syndrome affected males and females have apparently normal chromosome complements and normal gonadal function. The phenotypic appearance of the female is that of a patient with Turner's syndrome: short stature, webbed neck, shield chest, and cardiac malformations. The cardiac lesion in the male phenotype is different from that in the female. Pulmonic stenosis is most frequent in Noonan's syndrome, as opposed to aortic coarctation in Turner's syndrome. Apparently, this syndrome results from a mutant gene or genes. These patients have been referred to as male Turner's syndrome or Turner's syndrome with normal chromosomes.

A disorder of ovarian function evidenced morphologically by polycystic changes, although more commonly associated with secondary amenorrhea (see below), may also produce primary amenorrhea.

Adrenal and Thyroid Disease and Diabetes Mellitus. These may be accompanied by primary amenorrhea or, more commonly, secondary amenorrhea, despite the presence of normal ovaries.

Inadequate Gonadotrophins. Although ovaries and external genitalia may be otherwise normal, menses will not appear if gonadotrophin stimulation of these organs is insufficient or absent. Causes of this hypogonadotrophic hypogonadism are best considered according to their anatomic distribution. Intrasellar lesions such as pituitary cysts, tumors, and infarction may interfere not only with gonadotrophin secretion but also with the entire range of pituitary responsibilities. On the other hand, depending on a tumor's initial size and growth tendencies, amenorrhea may be the first sign of a disorder that by further encroachment gradually progresses to panhypopituitarism. Except for growth hormone, gonadotrophin secretion appears to be the most sensitive to adverse changes in intrasellar pressures and blood flow.

Suprasellar disorders also produce primary or secondary amenorrhea by diminishing gonadotrophin release. Aneurysm of the internal carotid artery, tumor, and internal hydrocephalus with expansion of the third ventricle are among the lesions reported. Hypogonadism, diminished adrenal and thyroid function, and short stature are seen in these conditions.

Amenorrhea due to isolated hypogonadotrophism without eventual impairment of other trophic hormones is common. The frequent association of this physiologic aberration (which reverses spontaneously in a high proportion of cases) with severe systemic illness, obesity, and emotional trauma should be noted.

A rare female condition presenting itself as hypogonadotrophic hypogonadism, primary amenorrhea, and anosmia is *Kallmann's syndrome.* In addition to amenorrhea, these patients display infantile sex development, low serum LH values, and a normal female karyotype. Although the patient may be unaware of her inability to perceive odors (perfumes, coffee grounds), inability to perceive certain food tastes may be the first clue that leads to further testing.

"Testicular Feminization Syndrome." This syndrome consists of chromatin-negativity, primary amenorrhea, mature feminine appearance, and abdominal, inguinal, or labial testes. The name is unfortunate, for many studies have shown that the basic defect is not in testicular steroid production or metabolic clearance, but is an interference in the mechanism of action of androgen at the target tissue level. Inability to form the biologically active dihydrotestosterone at the target was a suggested explanation for androgen insensitivity in these subjects, but this theory has not been confirmed. Impaired function or insufficient concentration of androgen protein receptors in target cells is the current preferred explanation for defective androgen activity. As a result of the metabolic abnormality (whatever it may be), axillary and pubic hair are scant, the clitoris is small, and although only rudimentary oviducts are present and the uterus is absent, there is no wolffian duct stimulation. Exogenous androgen does not masculinize these patients. Differentiation of the complete syndrome from an incomplete type displaying clitoral enlargement, inactive gonads, and variably androgen-sensitive target tissue can be accomplished. Patients with a deficit in testicular 17-dehydrogenase activity have impaired testosterone production and appear clinically as the incomplete syndrome. Therapy in either form of the syndrome is castration and sufficient exogenous estrogen to maintain serviceable external genitalia in support of the female sex role with which these patients permanently identify.

Because the diagnostic evaluation and therapy of the lesions involved in primary and secondary amenorrhea are similar, these matters will be discussed in later paragraphs.

Albright, F.: Polyostotic fibrous dysplasia. J. Clin. Endocrinol. Metab., 7:307, 1947.

Asherman, J. G.: Traumatic intrauterine adhesions and their effects on fertility. Int. J. Fertil., 11:49, 1957.

Bardin, C. W., Bullock, L. P., Shearins, R. J., Mowszowicz, I., and Black-
burn, W. R.: Androgen metabolism and mechanism of action of male pseudohermaphroditism: A study of testicular feminization. Rec. Prog. Horm. Res., Vol. 29, 1973.

Frank, R. T.: Formation of artificial vagina without operation. Am. J. Obstet. Gynecol., 35:1053, 1938.

Goebelsmann, U., Horton, R., Mestman, J. H., Arce, J. J., Nagata, Y., Nakamura, R. M., Thorneycroft, I. H., and Mishell, D. R., Jr.: Male pseudohermaphroditism due to testicular 17β-hydroxysteroid dehydrogenase deficiency. J. Clin. Endocrinol. Metab., 36:867, 1973.

Jones, H. W., Jr., and Scott, W. W.: Hermaphroditism, Genital Anomalies and Related Endocrine Disorders. Baltimore, Williams & Wilkins Company, 1971.

List, C. F., Dowman, C. E., Bagchi, B. K., and Bebin, J.: Posterior hypothalamic hamartomas and gangliogliomas causing precocious puberty. Neurology, 8:164, 1958.

Neu, R. L., and Gardner, L. I.: Clinical aspects of abnormalities of the X and Y chromosomes. Clin. Obstet. Gynecol., 15:141, 1972.

Summit, R. L.: Turner's syndrome and Noonan's syndrome. J. Pediatr., 74:155, 1969.

Van Der Werff Ten Bosch, J. J.: Isosexual precocity. *In* Gardner, L. I. (ed.): Endocrine and Genetic Diseases of Childhood. Philadelphia, W. B. Saunders Company, 1969.

Secondary Amenorrhea

A change in the frequency of menstruation is a sensitive indicator of ovarian dysfunction. Therefore the most serious form of menstrual aberration is the appearance of secondary amenorrhea. Its onset may be marked by the abrupt cessation of previously normal cycles, or it may follow menses of diminishing frequency (oligomenorrhea). It is well to remember that certain physiologic states predispose to amenorrhea. Absence of periodic menstruation in any adult female should suggest the possibility of pregnancy. Furthermore, amenorrhea of varying length will frequently be associated with the puerperium and the immediate postmenarchal and premenopausal periods. Finally, the menopause is an irreversible state of ovarian inactivity and amenorrhea.

Not all instances of secondary amenorrhea have a hormonal basis. As noted in the discussion of primary amenorrheas, acquired anatomic disorders must be considered in the differential diagnosis of absent menstruation. Stenotic lesions obstructing the egress of uterine discharge may result from scarring induced by infection, chemical burns, and operative trauma. Similarly, endocervical carcinoma may diminish the caliber of the cervical canal. As always, pelvic examination is essential to proper evaluation of absent menses. Destruction of the endometrium also produces amenorrhea despite the presence of normal cyclical ovarian hormone secretion. This condition may result from tuberculous endometritis or may be secondary to overzealous curettage performed to reverse unremitting hemorrhage occurring at abortion, post partum, or at withdrawal from prolonged anovulatory cycles. In the latter instances of iatrogenic endometrial failure, investigation of the uterine cavity by means of hysterography may reveal cavitary distortions and obliteration due to uterine synechia *(Asherman's syndrome).* Operative disruption of uterine defects and intensive estrogen therapy may reverse this situation. Finally, temporary endometrial inactivity may be inadvertently induced with the use of newer progestational agents, particularly of the long-acting intramuscular type (depomedroxyprogesterone acetate). Protracted release of hormone leads to persistent amenorrhea and typical progestin-induced endometrial morphologic changes. Although most cases spontaneously reverse within a few months, periods may not recur for years.

These local matters aside, the major diagnostic issue

in secondary amenorrhea is evaluation of the integrity of the pituitary-ovarian servomechanism. Unfortunately, pituitary-ovarian relationships do not adhere to an "all or none" principle. If one assumes adequate gonadotrophin stimulation, it appears that not all cycles are ovulatory or of equal length. Some cycles are climaxed by ovulation only after a prolonged preovulatory phase. Other cycles may be anovulatory, although cycle length shows no variation. The basic question in the pathogenesis of this relative hypogonadism is whether anovulation is due to inadequate or improper gonadotrophic stimulation or to an inherent unresponsiveness of certain follicles. As the follicle grows, intraovarian factors potentiate or diminish the response of the follicle to the stimulatory effect of FSH. Estradiol, by a local effect, enhances the follicle growth and differentiation response to FSH. Inhibition of this reactivity is observed with androgens.

Although clinical experiments with exogenous gonadotrophin therapy indicate some ovarian control over follicle maturation, most cases showing anovulatory amenorrhea and "normal" gonadotrophins are probably ascribable to improper synchrony and amount of gonadotrophin stimulation. Abnormal quantity or sequence of gonadotrophin secretion may result from local disturbances of the hypothalamic-hypophysial control mechanisms induced by emotional stress, precipitous weight changes, and systemic disease. On the other hand, these control centers may be misdirected by feedback levels of hormones of unusual type and quantity resulting from thyroid disease, adrenocortical disease, functioning ovarian tumors, and probably ovarian dysfunctions such as the Stein-Leventhal syndrome. Undoubtedly these conditions also affect ovarian reactivity to gonadotrophins, leading to disturbed or arrested follicle maturation seen in systemic disease as well as local pelvic disorders, including chronic pelvic infection, endometriosis, and uterine fibromyomas. Finally, absence of gonadotrophin secretion results from a variety of insidiously destructive intrasellar and suprasellar disorders. As in primary amenorrheas, these lesions may produce isolated gonadotrophic insufficiency, which at first results in decreased ovulation frequency but progresses through anovulation, amenorrhea, and hypoestrogenism to panhypopituitarism.

Pituitary and Suprasellar Lesions. Altered menses may be the earliest sign of an otherwise asymptomatic pituitary tumor. At first, small lesions interfere with cyclic variations in gonadotrophin release, but serum levels of gonadotrophins are unaffected. However, with increasing size and encroachment on production sites, diminished or absent gonadotrophin supervenes. Eventually further enlargement leads to more obvious neurologic, ophthalmic, and roentgenologic signs. At this point other trophic hormone deficiencies occur, leading to the complex endocrine metabolic derangements of panhypopituitarism. Aneurysm of the internal carotid artery, tumor of the third ventricle, glioma of the optic chiasm, obstruction of the aqueduct of Sylvius, and meningioma of the floor of the anterior fossa may simulate pituitary tumor and produce amenorrhea. Similarly, functioning tumors of the pituitary are often associated with specific clinical patterns of acromegaly, inappropriate galactorrhea, or Cushing's disease, as well as amenorrhea. Extensive non-neoplastic pituitary damage may result from necrosis associated with postpartum hemorrhage or obstetric shock. In studies spanning three decades concerning this entity, Sheehan has shown that almost total destruction of the anterior pituitary substance must exist before panhypopituitarism occurs. It is therefore understandable that a prolonged course of progressive deterioration is seen in a variety of lesions of the central nervous system. Gonadotrophic function is the first deficiency to appear clinically, although impaired growth hormone reaction to arginine or insulin-induced hypoglycemia is an earlier but usually occult event. Less often, only gonadotrophin inadequacy exists. Although this may be associated with persistent lactation (see below), other patients have perfectly normal trophic responses save for gonadotrophin inadequacy (psychogenic stress, obesity, and variants of anorexia nervosa). A relatively uncommon finding is the patient with an enlarged sella not caused by tumor expansion but filled with cerebrospinal fluid. In this anatomic variant called the *"empty sella syndrome,"* the pituitary is flattened and compressed by fluid pressure. Endocrine problems are mild, but owing to the special vulnerability of gonadotrophins, anovulation and amenorrhea are likely clinical manifestations.

Ovarian Lesions. Two major causes of ovarian amenorrhea are (1) inability of the ovary to react to appropriate gonadotrophic stimulation and (2) ovarian production of abnormal quantities of steroids, disrupting central nervous system control of cyclic gonadotrophin.

Irreversible ovarian failure is characterized by diminished ovarian steroid hormones and high total urinary gonadotrophins. *Premature menopause* exists when cessation of menses occurs before the age of 40 and is associated with the findings of hypergonadotrophic hypogonadism. The pathogenesis of this impairment of ovarian function is unknown. Somewhat better understood is the ovarian failure associated with the various forms of gonadal dysgenesis. In these instances reactive ovarian substrate is either absent or rapidly depleted, resulting in hypogonadism. It is important to remember that not all these patients have primary amenorrhea, and some (as many as 20 per cent) are chromatin positive.

The *polycystic ovary syndrome (Stein-Leventhal syndrome)* is perhaps the best example of arrested ovarian follicle maturation associated with noncyclic "dampening" of the pituitary-ovarian servomechanism. To be sure, infrequent anovulatory cycles may occur in normally menstruating, fertile women. As has been noted, some women exhibit varying degrees of reversible hypogonadism characterized by limited fertility and irregular cycles. The Stein-Leventhal syndrome therefore is the severest form of a spectrum of ovarian follicular disorders associated with anovulation.

As originally described in 1935, this syndrome consists of menstrual abnormality, either oligomenorrhea or amenorrhea, anovulatory infertility, and the development of hirsutism, which occurs in about half the patients. Though insidiously progressive facial hirsutism and acne may exist, and a male pubic escutcheon may be found, other signs of masculinization are absent. Obesity is no longer considered an important feature of the condition. The ovaries are bilaterally enlarged by the presence of multiple follicular cysts (never more than 1 cm in diameter), which lie just beneath a thickened, smooth, and pale ovarian capsule. Each rotund, expanded ovary is equal in size to or is larger than the uterine fundus, which is often smaller than normal. Microscopically, the ovaries reveal hyperplastic fibrosis of the cortical stroma and unusual thickening and luteinization of the theca cells surrounding the ubiquitous follicle cysts. Evidence of ovulation (corpora lutea) is rarely found. This finding is reflected in the endometrium, which is proliferative or hyperplastic. Patients with concomitant endometrial carcinoma have been reported.

Although the structural changes of the ovary were once thought to be pathognomonic of the syndrome, similar ovarian changes have been found in association with other disorders, such as adrenocortical hyperplasia, to which anovulatory amenorrhea is secondary. Indeed, *any condition leading to chronic anovulation in which some gonadotrophin function is retained is associated with polycystic changes in the ovary.*

Ovulatory cyclicity depends on the repetitive success of a series of exquisitely integrated biologic events linking ovarian and CNS-pituitary function. Three basic mandatory recycling events can be depicted: (1) The negative feedback relationship of estradiol with FSH results in the initial rise of gonadotrophin during menses that propels maturation of the follicle. (2) The positive feedback relationship of estradiol with LH is the ovulatory trigger. The fully mature follicle, by its timely and sizable production of estrogen, signals its readiness to ovulate in this fashion. (3) The resulting corpus luteum at the conclusion of its inherent life span of two weeks in the absence of a pregnancy will signal resumption of the next cycle by the acute withdrawal of its estrogen and progesterone production.

Anovulation, the loss of cyclicity, results if the CNS-pituitary system for gonadotrophin secretion is impaired by failure to perceive or act upon appropriate steroidal signals; if steroid feedback is inappropriate by timing availability, the individual follicle units do not respond appropriately. In these ways, any one of a large number of etiologic possibilities may be responsible for anovulation. By far the most common cause is "hypothalamic" dysfunction induced by disease, drugs, environment, or emotional stress. Inappropriate feedback may result from adrenocortical disease, ovarian tumors, or disorders of metabolic clearance of signal steroids, as may exist in liver disease and obesity. Finally, gonadal unresponsiveness is seen in acute, severe pelvic infection and in endometriosis, as well as in conditions associated with excess of androgen.

Anovulation represents a spectrum of malfunction in the CNS-pituitary-ovarian axis. In contrast to the characteristic fluctuations in the normal cycle, a "steady state" of tonic gonadotrophin and estrogen is seen (Fig. 3). Polycystic ovaries are consistently found in these circumstances.

From Figure 3 it will be seen that in the patient with chronic anovulation the average daily production of estrogen is increased, and the circulating levels of estrogen are relatively constant. This results in slightly depressed levels of FSH and slightly elevated levels of LH. The condition is self-sustaining. As a follicle cyst undergoes atresia, the small, brief FSH increment leads to its replacement by an inadequately stimulated and therefore developmentally arrested follicle cyst. But the atresia does not mean termination of steroidogenic activity of the theca remnants of the follicle. The stromal compartment of the human ovary is derived chiefly from atretic follicles and has been shown to be capable of secreting significant amounts of androstenedione and testosterone when stimulated by LH.

By these mechanisms the classic picture of the polycystic ovary is attained—numerous follicles, none ovulatory, and dense stromal tissue. The loss of recycling signals has resulted in a hormonal steady state featuring tonic estrogenicity, increased androgen production, and anovulation.

Because the morphology of the ovary is predictable and is the end result of many disorders, least likely of which is primary to the ovary, the various endoscopic and radiologic efforts to "prove" the polycystic state are unnecessary. All efforts of the physician should be turned to diagnosis and therapy of a syndrome likely to cause infertility, hirsutism, and dysfunctional uterine

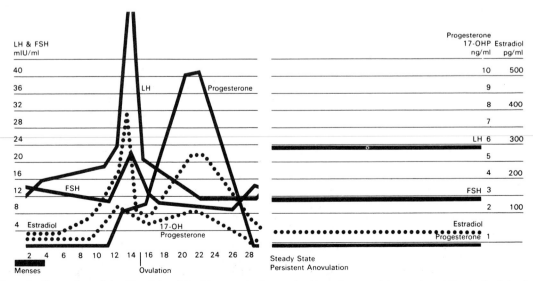

Figure 3. Comparison of steroid and gonadotrophin concentrations and patterns in an ovulatory cycle and the steady state of persistent anovulation. (From Speroff, L., Glass, R. H., and Kase, N. G.: Clinical Gynecologic Endocrinology and Infertility. Baltimore, Williams and Wilkins Company, 1973.)

bleeding. At the moment, the diagnosis of the Stein-Leventhal syndrome (see below) is made by exclusion of adrenocortical and pituitary abnormality.

Adrenal Disease. For more detailed description of these entities the reader is referred to Ch. 844 to 855.

Thyroid Disease. The practice of administering small doses of thyroid hormone preparations to basically euthyroid women with menstrual irregularities unfortunately is still prevalent. Delay of adequate work-up thus incurred compounds the basic physiologic irrationality of this approach. In fact, only patients with advanced thyroid disease display menstrual irregularities. In hyperthyroidism, as toxicity deepens the menses become less frequent, amenorrhea indicating a severe disorder. On the other hand, though oligomenorrhea is sometimes seen in hypothyroidism, menometrorrhagia is the rule, particularly in myxedema. In hypothyroidism secondary to hypopituitarism, of course, amenorrhea is a constant finding.

Systemic Disease. Throughout the discussion of the amenorrheas, it has been emphasized that details of the etiologic mechanisms involved are lacking. This issue is most acute in the consideration of the evolution of ovarian dysfunction secondary to chronic illnesses such as hepatic and renal disease, diabetes, or anemia. In addition to glands of internal secretion, the adequacy of organ systems involved in hormone conjugation, binding, and transport, extraction and excretion, inactivation by metabolism, interconversions of form, and interchange between anatomic pools of differing accessibility critically influence the total effective tissue concentrations of biologically active material.

Asherman, J. G.: Amenorrhea traumatica. J. Obstet. Gynaecol. Br. Emp., 55:23, 1948.

Bardin, C. W., and Lipsett, M. B.: Testosterone and androstenedione blood production rates in normal women and women with idiopathic hirsutism and polycystic ovaries. J. Clin. Invest., 46:891, 1967.

Kirschner, M. A., Bardin, C. W., Hembree, W. C., and Ross, G. T.: Effect of estrogen administration on androgen production and plasma luteinizing hormone in hirsute women. J. Clin. Endocrinol. Metab., 30:727, 1970.

MacDonald, P. C., Grodin, J. M., and Siiteri, P. K.: The utilization of plasma androstenedione for estrone production in women. Proc. Int. Congr. Endocrinol., 184:770, 1969.

Rice, B. V., and Savard, K.: Steroid hormone formation in the human ovary. IV. Ovarian stromal compartment: Formation of radioactive steroids from acetate and action of gonadotropins. J. Clin. Endocrinol. Metab., 25:593, 1966.

Schindler, A. E., Ebert, A., and Friedrich, E.: Conversion of androstenedione to estrone by human fat tissue. J. Clin. Endocrinol. Metab., 35:627, 1972.

Sheehan, H. L., and Stanfield, J. P.: The pathogenesis of postpartum necrosis of the anterior lobe of the pituitary gland. Acta Endocrinol., 37:479, 1961.

Stein, I. F., and Leventhal, M. L.: Amenorrhea associated with bilateral polycystic ovaries. Am. J. Obstet. Gynecol., 29:181, 1935.

Yen, S. S. C., Vela, P., and Rankin, J.: Inappropriate secretion of follicle-stimulating hormone and luteinizing hormone in polycystic ovarian disease. J. Clin. Endocrinol. Metab., 30:435, 1970.

Evaluation of Amenorrhea

Although understanding of the multiple interdependent factors that regulate menstrual function is admittedly incomplete, current concepts of neuroendocrine target organ relationships permit a relatively simple and precise localization of defective components. This program involves sequential testing of the major elements that produce a menstrual cycle: the endometrium, the ovary, and the hypothalamic pituitary unit

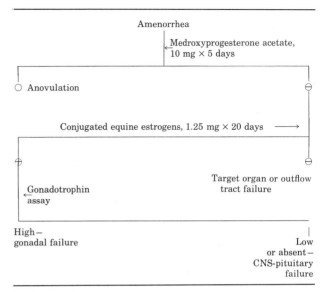

Figure 4. Suggested "flow sheet" made for clinical evaluation of amenorrheas.

(Fig. 4). Estimates of modifying systems such as the thyroid and the adrenal cortex are also essential.

The determination of ovarian function can be achieved by a summation of information gathered from basal body temperature curves, appropriately timed cervical changes in mucus, vaginal cornification indexes, endometrial biopsy, and progesterone withdrawal bleeding. Fifty to 100 mg of progesterone intramuscularly for two days or medroxyprogesterone acetate, 5 to 10 mg orally for three days, will induce vaginal bleeding in a previously amenorrheic patient if the endometrium has been primed by ovarian estrogen. In this case the integrity of the entire system short of ovulation is confirmed. However, if flow after progesterone withdrawal does not occur and the possibility of endometrial failure is eliminated by the appearance of vaginal bleeding after 21 days of 1.25 mg conjugated equine estrogens daily orally, then the lack of estrogen production is due to either ovarian or pituitary failure. If serum gonadotrophins are low or absent, pituitary failure is suggested, and neurologic, roentgenologic, ophthalmologic, and laboratory estimates of its competence are indicated. The anticipated availability of a decapeptide with gonadotrophin-releasing attributes, LRF, will be useful in the differentiation of hypothalamic versus pituitary disease as the cause of hypogonadotrophism. A positive reaction to LRF would indicate hypothalamic dysfunction and not intrinsic pituitary disease. Similar use of TRF stimulation of TSH has been found helpful in thyroid disorders (see Ch. 836 to 843). If gonadotrophins are high, reflecting diminished feedback inhibition, ovarian failure is diagnosed. If confirmation of the diagnosis is desired, challenge of the ovary with exogenous human gonadotrophin can be employed.

Using this technique, amenorrheas can be classified according to the specific area of pituitary-ovarian derangement uncovered: (1) hypergonadotrophic hypogonadal amenorrhea (ovarian failure), (2) hypogonadotrophic hypogonadal amenorrhea (pituitary failure), or (3) normogonadotrophic normoestrogenic amenorrhea (anovulation). With definition of these categories, appropriate therapy and management can be evolved.

Treatment of Amenorrhea

The therapy of inadequate ovarian hormone function depends not only on the degree of hormonal failure, but also on the therapeutic objectives. Certainly menstruation is not a necessity, for its absence does not represent a threat to the life expectancy of the patient. Therefore except in the treatment of infertility, and possibly in rare psychologic situations, a patient need not be treated solely for the purpose of recreating menstrual cycles. On the other hand, certain patients who show other evidence of estrogen deficiency, such as loss of secondary sex characteristics, deserve substitutive therapy. At no time should artificial cycles be instituted without preliminary investigation to uncover serious underlying lesions.

Hypergonadotrophic Hypogonadism. The patient with gonadal dysgenesis should be given cyclic exogenous estrogen therapy indefinitely for development and maintenance of adequate secondary sexual characteristics. The transformation induced by cyclic estrogen therapy in these otherwise anatomically, biologically, and cosmetically handicapped patients is particularly gratifying. Among the oral regimens available, 1.25 mg of conjugated equine estrogens daily for 21 days is satisfactory; during the last five days of treatment, the addition of 5 mg daily of medroxyprogesterone acetate orally provides endometrial stability and controlled withdrawal flow.

The woman with premature ovarian failure (before the age of 40 years) presents a somewhat different therapeutic problem. In this situation replacement medication is required to sustain systems already developed and dependent upon ovarian hormone secretion. Patients of this type are concerned not only about secondary amenorrhea and the termination of their reproductive capabilities but also about the usual severe vasomotor symptoms that attend this type of ovarian failure. These *hot flashes* are not seen in primary hypogonadism, although gonadotrophins are elevated in both conditions. Probably as a consequence of these disabilities and the fear of further restrictions, there are various subjective symptoms such as depression, anxiety, and loss of libido. No satisfactory treatment of this condition exists at present except substitution therapy with estrogen. Control of vasomotor instability, preservation of a serviceable vagina, and maintenance of other feminine aspects, including menses, are possible with cyclic conjugated equine estrogens (Premarin, 125 mg every day), or ethinyl estradiol (Estinyl, 0.05 mg every day). Again, the terminal addition of a progestin after 21 days of estrogen is advantageous. It should be noted that these doses of estrogen stimulate menstrual function and are higher than necessary for nonmenstrual metabolic requirements. This point comes into active consideration when determining what, if any, therapy should be given for ovarian failure occurring after the age of 40.

Menopause. The menopause is a physiologic and not a pathologic phenomenon. Menstruation ceases for a variety of reasons at other times of life, but after 40 the ovary becomes atrophic and ceases to respond to gonadotrophic stimulation. No amount of gonadotrophic stimulation can produce activity in the menopausal ovary. It becomes small, pale, and more wrinkled. The few remaining follicles undergo atresia so that none are found within a few years after cessation of menses.

Diminution of all ovarian elements proceeds, resulting in a firm structure one third the size of the active organ.

Vasomotor instability and genital atrophy are the only clinical symptoms definitely associated with ovarian aging that occurs when otherwise the woman may be active, healthy, and vital physically, emotionally, and mentally. However, because of improved general health, women can expect to live for 20 to 25 years beyond the menopause, and interest has increased in the possible amelioration of certain disease states associated with the menopause by administration of exogenous estrogen therapy. Whether actual causal relationships exist between certain disorders and diminished estrogen secretion has not been established. Nevertheless, beneficial effects on extragenital organs and prevention of atherosclerosis and osteoporosis have been claimed.

A statistical rise in coronary atherosclerosis in postmenopausal women has been ascribed to estrogen deficiency. Castration performed before natural menopause also has been associated with increased coronary and peripheral vascular disease. The ability of estrogen to reverse abnormal serum lipids in laboratory animals as well as in human subjects is a possible mechanism by which treated castrates may have a lower incidence of abnormal electrocardiograms and hypertension than untreated women.

However, *excessive therapy* has been observed to pose increased risks. Studies of the preventive effects of estrogens for heart attacks have yielded variable results. Administration of 10 mg of conjugated estrogens per day appeared to be associated with beneficial survival statistics but revealed a disturbing incidence of early vascular accidents. In the Coronary Drug Project, 5 mg conjugated estrogen therapy was associated with an excess of nonfatal myocardial infarctions over controls. In the Stroke Study, estrogens were associated with increased recurrent cerebral accidents and myocardial infarctions rather than protection against these two insults.

Postmenopausal osteoporosis is also believed to be related to estrogen deficiency. Estrogen induces positive calcium balance and reduces bone resorption, but bone formation also drops within three to nine months after initiation of therapy. Although there is no net increase in bone mass in the osteoporotic woman, estrogen would seem to stabilize bone turnover at a new and slower rate. However, there is no *prospective* evidence that estrogen can prevent osteoporosis. Appropriate diet and exercise are certainly also involved in bone matrix biology. Conclusive proof is lacking that diminished estrogen is a factor in this and other age-related disorders such as arthritis, muscular weakness, migraine headache, and stomatitis. On the other hand, atrophic changes in the distal urinary tract, particularly in the urethra, which result in urinary frequency, burning, and occasionally stress incontinence, are reversible by the administration of local or systemic estrogen. Finally, estrogen controls the often embarrassing and sometimes disabling irritations of atrophic vaginitis and vulvitis.

In the postmenopausal situation, in which menstrual function is not required, only small doses of cyclic estrogen are necessary for appropriate therapy. Conjugated estrogen, 0.625 mg daily for three weeks of every four, is sufficient. Despite the ease of administration and its obvious physiologic and clinical value, estrogen therapy has often been limited in duration or actively avoided. The reason for this restraint is the concern that protracted estrogen treatment will induce neoplastic changes in estrogen-sensitive aging tissues. The contribution of endogenous estrogen to the pathogenesis of uterine and breast carcinoma is still speculative, but suspicion has been aroused, particularly as to the effects of unopposed estrogen in the stimulation of endometrial disease. Clearly, indiscriminate use of this hormone in high doses without periodic evaluation is condemned. On the other hand, if therapy is given within the restrictions stated, there is more evidence in favor of than against its use.

In this regard the importance of frequent medical evaluations in this age group should not be understated. In addition to the opportunities such interviews present for continual psychologic support of the apprehensive patient, the full physical examination performed on these occasions may uncover basic organic disease, the symptoms of which have been incorrectly minimized by the woman as further evidence of "a change of life."

Hypogonadotrophic Hypogonadism. Before embarking on a therapeutic program in this form of amenorrhea, the physician must have assured himself of the absence of various intracranial diseases that inhibit or destroy gonadotrophin secretion.

In the absence of neoplastic, vascular, or congenital anomaly to account for disruption in pituitary function, there is usually a history of some stressful circumstance as the precipitating event. Improved dietary habits or psychotherapy may result in return of ovulatory cycles. In fact, the frequency of spontaneous remission is so high that simple observation is often satisfactory. However, when amenorrhea is prolonged and is associated with incipient atrophy of dependent organs and infertility, or is accompanied by lactation, more active therapeutic measures must be undertaken.

Inappropriate Lactation—Galactorrheic Syndromes. Galactorrhea refers to the inappropriate mammary secretion of milky fluid that is not immediately related to pregnancy or the needs of a neonate. The quantity of secretion is not an important criterion. Galactorrhea may involve both breasts, or one or the other breast consecutively or alternately. Amenorrhea does not necessarily accompany galactorrhea, even in the most serious disorders.

A variety of eponymic designations have been applied to variants of the lactation syndromes. These are based on the association of galactorrhea with intrasellar tumor (Forbes, Henneman, Griswold, and Albright, 1954), antecedent pregnancy with inappropriate persistence of galactorrhea (independently reported by Chiari and Frommel in 1852), and the absence of previous pregnancy (Argonz and del Castillo, 1953). In all these types, the association of galactorrhea with eventual amenorrhea was observed. On the basis of currently available information, categorization of individual cases according to these eponymic guidelines neither is helpful nor permits discrimination of patients who will eventually develop serious intrasellar lesions.

The differential diagnosis of galactorrhea syndromes is a difficult and complex clinical challenge. The difficulty arises from the multiple factors involved in the control of prolactin release. In most pathophysiologic systems, the final common pathway leading to galac-

torrhea is an inappropriate augmentation of prolactin release.

Prolactin is a polypeptide secreted from the anterior pituitary and has a half-life of 15 to 30 minutes. Prolactin is apparently under a chronic, tonic inhibition owing to hypothalamic secretion into the pituitary portal system of prolactin-inhibiting factor (PIF). The following considerations are important in differentiation of causes of excess prolactin:

1. *Excessive estrogen* (as may be administered in birth control pills) can lead to milk secretion via hypothalamic suppression, causing inhibition of PIF and consequent release of pituitary prolactin. Progesterone, on the other hand, seems to have a restraining effect, perhaps by a stimulatory effect on the hypothalamus leading to production of PIF.

2. Prolonged intensive *suckling* can also release prolactin, via hypothalamic reduction of PIF control of prolactin. Similarly, thoracotomy scars, cervical spinal lesions, and herpes zoster can induce prolactin release by activating the afferent sensory neural arc.

3. A variety of *drugs* can also inhibit hypothalamic PIF. There are nearly 100 phenothiazine derivatives with indirect mammotropic activity. In addition, many phenothiazine-like compounds, reserpine derivatives, amphetamines, and a variety of other drugs can initiate galactorrhea via hypothalamic suppression (thioxanthenes, diazepines, butyrophenones, α-methyldopa).

4. *Emotional stresses* (presumably capable of increasing hypothalamic PIF and diminishing prolactin secretion) can also inhibit hypothalamic PIF and induce the secretion of prolactin and galactorrhea. Severe anxiety and trauma often occur in temporal relation to the onset of galactorrhea. The posthysterectomy or menopausal onset of this symptom is a rare but known entity.

5. *Hypothalamic lesions,* stalk lesions, or compression—events that physically reduce production or delivery of PIF to the pituitary—can release excess prolactin, leading to galactorrhea (see Ch. 826).

6. *Hypothyroidism* (juvenile or adult) can be associated with galactorrhea. The mechanism of this relationship requires the introduction of a positive hypothalamic material (prolactin-releasing factor, PRF) that can release, not inhibit, pituitary secretion of prolactin. PRF exists in various fowl (e.g., pigeon, chicken, duck, turkey, and the tricolored blackbird). Although the identity of this material has not been elucidated or its function substantiated in normal human physiology, in pathologic situations such as hypothyroidism, thyrotrophin-releasing hormone (TRH) may be active as a PRF. Synthetic TRH is a potent stimulant of prolactin secretion in man. With diminished circulating levels of thyroid hormone, hypothalamic TRH is produced in excess and as such may act as a PRF to release prolactin from the pituitary. Adult hypothyroidism associated with galactorrhea is well known. In juvenile hypothyroidism, prepubertal breast development and galactorrhea may be seen. Reversal with thyroid hormone therapy is strong circumstantial evidence in support of this thesis.

7. Also acknowledged as a rare cause of galactorrhea is *Cushing's disease.* It is not known whether the direct effect of excessive free cortisol enhances otherwise nonstimulating levels of prolactin secretion to cause galactorrhea, or whether hypothalamic-pituitary dysfunction

involves not only increased corticotrophin-releasing hormone but also excess PRF or reduced PIF.

8. Increased prolactin release may be the consequence of prolactin elaboration and secretion from *pituitary tumors* which function independently of the otherwise appropriate restraints exerted by PIF from a normally functioning hypothalamus. This dangerous tumor with endocrine, neurologic, and ophthalmologic liabilities makes the differential diagnosis of persistent galactorrhea a major clinical challenge. Beyond prolactin production, the tumor may also suppress pituitary parenchyma by expansion and compression, interfering with other trophic hormones (see Ch. 830).

9. *Ectopic production of prolactin* has been reported in one patient without galactorrhea and with a bronchogenic carcinoma, and in one patient with galactorrhea and a hypernephroma. An occult carcinoma, although a remote possibility, should be considered.

Symptoms of galactorrhea may antedate the recognition of intrasellar tumors by many years. It is recognized that a mean duration of 10 to 12 years of galactorrhea and amenorrhea may precede the radiologic demonstration of a pituitary adenoma. As a result, follow-up must be prolonged and zealous. Furthermore, the criterion of antecedent pregnancy does not necessarily suggest that a different pathophysiologic process is involved in the galactorrhea. Cases of pituitary adenoma which did not alter competent gonadotrophin secretion are known, and conception has occurred in some of these patients.

Galactorrheic women with pituitary tumors shown by x-ray can demonstrate withdrawal from progesterone and even have menses and ovulate, as stated above. Obviously, the presence of galactorrhea is not incompatible with gonadotrophin release. However, in the majority of patients a single lesion is sufficiently extensive or critically placed to impair both mechanisms and, on rare occasions, other trophic hormones (TSH, ACTH).

Therefore regardless of the clinical circumstances, in galactorrhea of six months' to one year's duration, a pituitary tumor must be considered. The longer the follow-up, with the progressive exclusion of other benign causes, the higher the incidence of tumor diagnosis in persistent galactorrhea.

ENDOCRINE MANIPULATIONS TO RULE OUT PITUITARY TUMOR. In a large retrospective study of pituitary failure owing to tumors, a sequence of trophic hormone loss was found. Growth hormone, gonadotrophins, TSH, and ACTH are lost over time in roughly that order. Loss of ACTH and TSH is a very late occurrence in the course of the disease. From these data, it can be reasoned that loss of growth hormone in the face of galactorrhea may give early diagnosis of suspected tumor before x-rays of the sella are abnormal. However, normal adults do not show symptoms from loss of growth hormone. Furthermore, normal values for growth hormone are low, and stimulation of growth hormone secretion is required for measurement. Inability to stimulate growth hormone response may indicate the presence of a pituitary tumor. Growth hormone rises during hypoglycemia induced by insulin or during an infusion of arginine. A rise above 10 ng per milliliter (the units may vary from laboratory to laboratory) in response to arginine is strong but not conclusive evidence against tumor-related galactorrhea.

L-DOPA RESPONSE. L-Dopa (0.5 gram four times a day) may be administered to galactorrheic patients with high prolactin blood levels. L-Dopa enters the hypothalamus and is decarboxylated to form dopamine, which then activates PIF release. If prolactin levels fall after L-dopa, tumor-dependent production of prolactin may be ruled out and hypothalamic dysfunction is the probable cause of the galactorrhea.

LRH RESPONSE. LRH has now been synthesized and administered to human subjects to induce surges of LH. Pregnancies have been induced in previously infertile women by appropriate LRH therapy. If LRH administration causes a rise in peripheral LH, a pituitary tumor is unlikely as a cause of galactorrhea and amenorrhea.

Differential diagnosis proceeds by excluding the several causes of galactorrhea. Current clinical practice depends on repeated yearly x-rays of the sella turcica, and ophthalmologic surveillance of visual fields. Endocrine survey of TSH, ACTH, and calcium metabolism should be performed as clinically warranted. L-Dopa, LRH, and growth hormone provocative tests should be performed when and if available. In severe hypogonadism, hormone replacement is appropriate. Fertility can be achieved with clomiphene or human menopausal gonadotrophins, and recently pregnancy has been reported with the use of ergot alkaloids.

If pregnancy ensues, careful follow-up is required to avoid intragestational expansion of the tumor or acute hemorrhage with abrupt hypopituitarism, compression of optic tract or chiasma, or hypothalamic disruption.

The earlier a tumor is diagnosed, the better the treatment result. Early diagnosis and extirpation preclude unnecessary progressive endocrine, neurologic, and ophthalmologic complications. Better tumor therapy is possible if tumors are small and completely intrasellar. In this favorable circumstance, a transnasal frontal approach (transsphenoidal) is possible with direct visualization of the sellar contents. Aspiration of the tumor, good hemostasis, and preservation of residual pituitary tissue can be achieved in experienced hands. Smaller postoperative doses of radiation therapy are an added benefit. Finally, early diagnosis and specific therapy avoid the hazards of induction of ovulation and pregnancy in the presence of an occult tumor.

Gonadotrophin Therapy. HUMAN PITUITARY FOLLICLE-STIMULATING HORMONE (HPFSH) AND HUMAN CHORIONIC GONADOTROPHIN (HCG) THERAPY. In 1958 Gemzell reported the use of a human pituitary preparation that stimulated follicular growth and estrogen production in amenorrheic women. The material was extracted from pituitary tissue collected at autopsy and partially purified by ammonium sulfate fractionation. When assayed against relatively specific standards, it revealed combined FSH and LH potencies, but with the former dominating the biologic activity. Ovulation occurs during HCG administration. Dose size and duration are adjusted according to the ovarian response noted. In limited trials it has been found that more than 90 per cent of patients ovulated once or several times, and more than 50 per cent became pregnant. The limited availability of material (requiring approximately 10 pituitaries to produce an ovulation with this system) has been its major disadvantage.

HUMAN MENOPAUSAL URINARY GONADOTROPHIN (HMG-FSH, PERGONAL). Although menopausal urine has been recognized as a potential source of gonadotrophins (FSH activity by animal studies) since 1930, toxic reactions precluded utilization in human investigations. Acceptable material is now available clinically as Pergonal, which contains 75 units of FSH and 75 units of LH potency per ampule. Toxic and allergic reactions have been eliminated. At least 90 per cent of appropriately selected patients ovulate, and 50 to 70 per cent achieve pregnancy. The usual dose required is 8 to 12 days of 2 ampules of human menopausal gonadotrophin (HMG) per day, followed by 10,000 units of HCG. However, variable ovarian reactivity has been encountered. In addition to monitoring HMG-induced ovarian stimulation by biologic expressions of estrogen (cervical mucus changes), urinary estrogen excretion has proved to be useful. An excretion range between 100 μg and 200 μg total estrogen is the goal of HMG therapy, at which time the ovulatory dose of exogenous HCG can be applied. In this range, an optimal ratio between induced pregnancy rate and incidence of serious side effects (hyperstimulation and multiple pregnancy) is expected.

The results of species-specific FSH (as HMG) therapy (two to five courses) are 90 per cent ovulation, 50 to 70 per cent pregnancies, 20 per cent abortion, 20 per cent multiple gestation (15 per cent twins, 5 per cent three or more), and 1 per cent serious side effects (hyperstimulation).

SIDE EFFECTS OF GONADOTROPHIN THERAPY. Certain side effects have been noted that may limit general application of these agents. The reactions encountered are attributable to the effects of ovarian enlargement and production of unusual quantities of ovarian hormones. These consist of abdominal pain, bloating, pressure, nausea, and general malaise. Acute distention can even cause ovarian rupture and hemorrhage. Because many of the reactions are self-limiting, nonsurgical supportive therapy is advised, laparotomy and conservative surgery short of castration being reserved for the deteriorating circumstance. In this regard hypovolemic shock resulting from a syndrome of severe ascites and hydrothorax has been recognized. Additional expressions of ovarian hyperstimulation are the frequency of abortion and multiple pregnancy and the consequent diminution in fetal salvage noted in all series. Finally, it has become clear that gonadotrophin therapy is effective only during the treatment interval. Regardless of frequency of ovulation or the occurrence of pregnancy, patients revert to pretreatment hypogonadal status upon cessation of therapy or conclusion of pregnancy. For this reason gonadotrophin induction of ovulation is currently withheld until other modes of treatment have failed.

Normogonadotrophic Normoestrogenic Anovulation. In this type of amenorrhea, the chain of events leading to normal ovulation and menstruation is upset by the absence of the midcycle surge of LH. Lacking progesterone secretion, continued unopposed estrogen stimulation leads to hyperplasia of the endometrium. For this reason amenorrhea may be punctuated by prolonged, sometimes severe uterine hemorrhages (*metropathia hemorrhagica*) that require special attention. In addition, infertility further complicates this syndrome. Clearly the correction of both these circumstances is found in the return of recurrent ovulation.

Correction of Menstrual Pattern. There may be no specific requirement for reproductive function, but the inconvenience and uncertainty of the menstrual pattern

prompt the patient to seek hormonal regulation of her cycle. In the absence of serious underlying disease, this may be accomplished by inducing progesterone withdrawal flow with an oral progestin such as 10 mg of medroxyprogesterone acetate for five days after an interval of endogenous estrogen stimulation. Two to five days after progestin withdrawal, menses will appear. Retreatment with progestin should be delayed for sufficient time (six weeks) to determine whether spontaneous ovulation will return. Only in cases of too frequent menstruation (polymenorrhea) is the disadvantage of complete cycle coverage by combined estrogen and progestin (as in the birth control medications) acceptable. Medication should be withdrawn periodically, because spontaneous correction may have occurred during therapy.

When severe dysfunctional bleeding occurs, an effort must be made to obtain an endometrial biopsy, but curettage is not essential. Regardless of the duration or severity of flow, anovulatory bleeding of this type is treated by converting the proliferative endometrium to a secretory endometrium from which limited withdrawal flow will occur. Three to four times the contraceptive doses of oral 19-nor steroids will rapidly diminish dysfunctional bleeding with complete cessation within 12 hours. Therapy is then continued, and is gradually tapered to allow an interval for blood replacement as well as general, gynecologic, and hematologic evaluation. The possibility of underlying disorders of coagulation must always be considered. After withdrawal flow, contraceptive doses of 19-nor steroids must be resumed for two to three cycles. The initial use of high doses of estrogen intravenously (Premarin, 25 mg) before progestin conversion is limited to those cases in which bleeding has been prolonged or severe and immediate cessation is required. On the other hand, if agents such as 19-nor steroids do *not* control abnormal flow, then pathologic bleeding is diagnosed and curettage is mandatory.

Reversal of Anovulation. Obviously, correction of proved adrenocortical and thyroid disease will reverse associated anovulation. The drug Clomid (a synthetic nonsteroidal analogue of chlorotrianisene) has proved useful in the treatment of diagnostically nonspecific anovulation. It has almost entirely replaced the low-dose corticosteroid regimens and has virtually eliminated the need for operative wedge resection of the ovaries to achieve resumption of ovulation. Using 50 to 100 mg daily for five days of each cycle, induction of ovulation is achieved in patients with intermediate follicle maturation arrest but with sufficient function to secrete some estrogen. The drug's mode of action is not understood, although it appears to enhance both endogenous gonadotrophin secretion and ovarian synthesis of estrogen. In properly selected patients, 80 per cent can be expected to ovulate and approximately 50 per cent become pregnant. The percentage of pregnancies per number of induced ovulatory cycles is 15 per cent. The multiple pregnancy rate in accumulated national statistics is approximately 8 per cent, almost entirely twins. The abortion rate is 20 per cent. The incidence of congenital anomalies is not increased as a result of Clomid-induced ovulation. There is no evidence that the effect of Clomid is long lasting; it is considered to be limited to the cycle in which the drug is used. The side effects are similar to those of the gonadotrophins and are related to increased ovarian size, hormone production, and multiple pregnancies. In the event that Clomid (after gradually increased doses over four to six months) is unsuccessful, then bilateral wedge resection of the ovaries or HMG plus HCG therapy is advised. Because all the therapies cited present some risk to the patient and none guarantee lasting results, other aspects of the fertility potential of the involved couple must be fully evaluated before ovulation induction is undertaken.

Argonz, J., and del Castillo, E. B.: A syndrome characterized by estrogenic insufficiency, galactorrhea, and decreased urinary gonadotropin. J. Clin. Endocrinol. Metab., 13:79, 1953.

Chard, T.: The Chiari-Frommel syndrome: An experiment of nature. J. Obstet. Gynaec. Br. Commonw., 71:624, 1964.

Coronary Drug Project Research Group: The coronary drug project: Initial findings leading to modifications of its research protocol. J.A.M.A., 214:1303, 1970.

Engel, T., Jewelewicz, R., Dyrenfurth, I., Speroff, L., and Vande Wiele, R. L.: Ovarian hyperstimulation syndrome: Report of a case with notes on pathogenesis and treatment. Am. J. Obstet. Gynecol., 112:1052, 1972.

Forbes, A. P., Henneman, P. H., Griswold, G. C., and Albright, F.: Syndrome characterized by galactorrhea, amenorrhea, and low FSH. J. Clin. Endocrinol. Metab., 14:265, 1954.

Furman, R. H.: Coronary heart disease and the menopause. In Menopause and Aging. NIH, 1973, pp. 39–52.

Furman, R. H.: Menopausal effects on calcium homeostasis and skeletal metabolism. In Menopause and Aging. NIH, 1973, pp. 59–66.

Hack, M., Brish, M., Serr, D. M., Insler, V., Salomy, M., and Lunenfeld, B.: Outcome of pregnancy after induced ovulation: Follow-up of pregnancies and children born after gonadotropin therapy. J.A.M.A., 211:791, 1970.

Kase, N., Mroueh, A., and Buxton, C. L.: Pergonal therapy of anovulatory infertility. Am. J. Obstet. Gynecol., 100:2, 1968.

Kase, N., Mroueh, A., and Olson, L. E.: Clomid therapy for anovulatory infertility. Am. J. Obstet. Gynecol., 98:1037, 1967.

Lawrence, A. M., and Hagen, T. C.: Ergonovine therapy of nonpuerperal galactorrhea. N. Engl. J. Med., 287:150, 1972.

Malarkey, W. B., Jacobs, L. S., and Daughaday, W. H.: Levodopa suppression of prolactin in nonpuerperal galactorrhea. N. Engl. J. Med., 285:1160, 1971.

Rabkin, M. T., and Frantz, A. G.: Hypopituitarism: A study of growth hormone and other endocrine functions. Ann. Intern. Med., 64:1197, 1966.

Taymor, M. L., Yussman, M. A., and Gminski, D.: Estrogen monitoring in ovulatory induction. Fertil. Steril., 21:759, 1970.

Turkington, R. W.: Inhibition of prolactin secretion and successful therapy of the Forbes-Albright syndrome with L-dopa. J. Clin. Endocrinol. Metab., 34:306, 1972.

Veterans Administration Cooperative Study: An evaluation of estrogenic substances in the treatment of cerebral vascular disease. Circulation, 33(5) SII:2–3, May 1966.

INVESTIGATION OF INFERTILITY

Approximately 10 per cent of married couples in the United States are unable to conceive. The cause of infertility varies with geographic and socioeconomic factors, but some general statements can be made regarding the frequency of certain etiologic factors. Of 100 couples in whom a definite disorder is identified, approximately 40 will show a male factor deficiency, 20 a female hormonal defect, 30 a female tubal disorder, and 10 a cervical defect. Ten to 20 per cent of couples with infertility remain undiagnosed as to the cause of their problem. Because investigation of infertility in the female is time consuming and expensive, evaluation of the male factor is carried out first.

Male Factor. The most important procedure is the analysis of the semen. Although some estimate of sperm can be made from postcoital cervical examinations, before any final conclusion of deficiency is made, three separate masturbatory specimens should be examined for volume, sperm count, motility, morphology, and viability. A normal ejaculate is considered to have a volume not less than 1 ml and not more than 6 ml, 60 per cent active forms after two hours, 60 per cent normal morphology, and at least 20 million sperm per milliliter. If counts are below 20 million, full urologic and medical investigation is warranted. Regardless of count, the male partner should be questioned and instructed when necessary in the development of appropriate sexual and social habits.

Female Factor. Once it is established that ovulation regularly occurs (by means of basal body temperature curves, appropriately timed examination of cervical mucus, endometrial biopsy, and pregnanediol excretion), investigation of the female attempts to certify functional and anatomic competence of the reproductive tract to permit union of sperm and ovum in the ampulla of the oviduct.

The postcoital test is performed at the expected date of ovulation, not less than 2 and not more than 16 hours after intercourse. A specimen of endocervical mucus is inspected for clarity, ferning, elasticity, and the number and activity of spermatozoa. In this way the adequacy of coital position, intromission, and ejaculate content, as well as the cervical environment, can be evaluated. Sperm survive in mucus that is abundant, clear, and elastic. The presence of this type of mucus is indicative of adequate local cervical and ovarian function. Repeatedly poor postcoital examinations, despite documented ovulation, make examination of the male factor and coital habits imperative. Furthermore, anatomic abnormalities of the cervix or hostile mucus resulting from erosions, infections, and other local disorders of the cervix should be investigated and specifically treated.

Tubal competence is evaluated by tubal insufflation with carbon dioxide (the Rubin test), by roentgenographic demonstration of patency by hysterosalpingography, or by direct visualization by laparoscopy or culdoscopy. Each serves distinct functions and should be included in the definitive infertility work-up.

The *Rubin test* is best performed before ovulation. It involves transcervical introduction of carbon dioxide under a carefully monitored flow rate and pressures and insufflation of gas through the uterus and the ostia of the tubes into the peritoneal cavity. A positive test (indicating tubal patency) involves demonstration of gas under the diaphragm by the appearance of referred shoulder pain. The insufflation occurs at a gas pressure usually less than 120 mm of mercury. If tubal blockade exists, escape of gas is prevented and the pressure readings rise continuously to above 200 mm of mercury. At this point the test should be discontinued. It must be remembered that a single negative test is not diagnostic, because functional occlusion (tubospasm) is frequently encountered. Multiple studies are essential and may be undertaken with paracervical block local anesthesia. On the other hand, a positive Rubin test does not rule out the presence of distortions of the tube or tubal-ovarian junction secondary to pelvic adhesions. For this reason if infertility persists in the face of positive tubal insufflation, then ancillary tests of tubal competence are required.

Hysterosalpingography is ordinarily performed by instillation of 3 to 6 ml of radiopaque oil into the uterine cavity and oviducts under fluoroscopic observation. In this way defects in the uterine cavity that may interfere with implantation and alteration in tubal architecture can be visualized and permanently recorded. The presence of peritubal adhesions may be diagnosed by the dye diffusion pattern about the tubal ostia at the time of examination and 24 hours later.

Laparoscopy (which has virtually replaced culdoscopy) accompanied by tubal insufflation with methylene blue is probably the most effective means of diagnosing peritubal and pelvic adhesions producing infertility. Combined with salpingography, these procedures offer detailed information as to the feasibility and type of corrective adnexal surgery to be undertaken.

Uterine factors were once considered important elements in infertility. However, current views no longer give significance to the multiple anatomic variations in uterine displacement from the usual anterior position. However, abnormalities of the uterine cavity, such as congenital anomalies and submucous myomas, deserve surgical repair if associated with otherwise unexplained infertility.

FERTILITY CONTROL
(Population Control)

Discussion of the need for population control is beyond the scope of this text. Obviously, once the public health issues of the demographic gap and its consequences are put aside, the basic issue remains the acceptability of the form of fertility control offered to the individual couples. If 100 women of proved fertility are exposed to pregnancy for one year, approximately 80 pregnancies will result. Clearly, then, *any* method of contraception is more effective than none. It must be remembered that significant discrepancies always exist between the theoretical and practical effectiveness of any contraceptive method, as is illustrated by experience with the "rhythm" method. The fertile phase (requiring sexual continence) is estimated as extending from the eighteenth day before the onset of the earliest likely menstruation up to and including the eleventh day before the onset of the latest likely menstruation. The method assumes that ovulation occurs about 14 days before menstruation, that spermatozoa can fertilize for 48 hours after intercourse, and that the ovum can be fertilized for about 24 hours after it emerges from the ovary. The method depends on motivation to accumulate menstrual records for one year before use and to remain continent during the fertile period. Studies of the effectiveness of this method reveal pregnancy rates of about 15 conceptions per 100 years of exposure. Although this is about double the conception rates with mechanical devices (condom, diaphragm), it represents an important reduction compared with the projected rate of 80 which would have been expected. All physicians must be prepared to teach this method as long as a substantial proportion of the population is limited by religious belief to this method alone.

When considering the other available contraceptive modalities, it is apparent that with advancing scientific knowledge and public awareness the traditional, folklore-based methods (douche, withdrawal, household spermicides) have given way to proved methods of prevention. Vaginal jellies, foams, diaphragms, and condoms are all safe and fairly reliable. Their relative acceptability varies geographically and according to social class. Their application and use are described in Calderone's manual.

Two modern methods of contraception have altered worldwide concepts of conception control. These are the oral ovulation-inhibiting steroid "pill" and the intrauterine device (IUD).

Oral Hormonal Control of Ovulation. Clinical trials with contraceptive steroids began with combined agents in 1958 and sequential pills in 1962. At least 20 million women are current users of these medications in the world at large. Evaluation of coincidental medical problems and side effects continues to be a pressing issue. As synthetic steroids, these agents induce a pharmacologic state posing a long-term challenge to the physiologic reserve of the recipient. Thus far, the contraceptive action has not been separated from wide-ranging biochemical and metabolic liabilities.

The progestational agents in steroid contraceptives are derived from two basic groups: 19-nortestosterones and 17-acetoxy progesterones. The estrogen components are either ethinyl estradiol or its 3-methyl ether, mestranol. The substituents attached to the basic steroid structures confer the property of activity by the oral route and increased potency, presumably because of longer half-lives, reflected by metabolic clearance.

It is the progestational agent which provides the main contraceptive action in the combination pills, principally by the negative feedback action on the hypothalamus; this action inhibits secretion of the gonadotrophin-releasing factor. In addition, the progestational agent produces an endometrium which is hostile to implantation of the ovum, a decidualized bed with atrophied glands. Furthermore, cervical mucus becomes thick and impervious to the migration of spermatozoa into the uterus.

The estrogen in combination pills serves two purposes. First, the negative feedback of the progestin is enhanced by the presence of estrogen. Second, estrogen provides the structural support for endometrial stability and avoidance of irregular shedding and breakthrough bleeding. Estrogen also suppresses early FSH stimulation of the ovary with diminished follicle development but with no reduction in over-all rate of follicular atresia (thereby negating the possibility of pregnancies late in life).

The sequential medications take advantage of this negative feedback attribute of estrogen in the early phase of the cycle as the exclusive basis of contraceptive efficacy. A terminal five days of progestin after the estrogen is used to yield more predictable and orderly menstrual desquamation. Although less effective than combined agents in early trials, restriction of the pill-free interval to seven days, regardless of bleeding patterns, has brought sequential efficacy up to the combined level (0.1 per cent failure rate). A continuing liability inherent in sequential medications is their dependence on higher doses of estrogen with a consequent higher rate of disturbed metabolism.

Despite almost 100 per cent contraception, concerns over short- and long-term effects of these medications have restricted acceptability and usage. These effects are related to general metabolic and target organ effects of the steroids involved.

1. *Oncogenic potential.* A major concern is whether prolonged steroidal usage will increase the incidence of uterine (corpus and cervix) and breast cancer. Although duration of application has not yet been sufficient to permit absolute statements, the anticipated effect on uterine cancer is reduction in the case of endometrial

disease because of the protective chemotherapeutic effect of progestin, and earlier diagnosis and presumed higher cure rates in disease of the cervix because of the improved screening inherent in the periodic examinations carried out in women receiving antiovulatory medication.

No definite relationship exists between estrogen therapy and the etiology of human breast cancer. However, anxiety lingers owing to the effect of estrogen on breast carcinoma incidence in rats and mice and a similar effect of progestins (of the C-21 progesterone family) in beagle dogs. There has been no increase in mortality in the Connecticut registry since the introduction of estrogen or contraceptive steroid therapy. Current practice does not exclude steroid contraception in women with chronic mastitis or fibrocystic disease. Although these steroids are contraindicated in women with treated breast cancer, there is no evidence that normal women with a family history of breast cancer should be excluded from therapy.

2. *Thromboembolic disease.* The striking rise in the incidence of thromboembolic phenomena since 1958 has affected both sexes. However, it seems indubitable that steroidal birth control medication has increased the risk to users beyond that of controls. A series of retrospective studies in England revealed a six- to sevenfold greater risk to users, with older women (35 to 44 years) incurring double the risk of 20- to 34-year-old users. The British findings also indicated that the mortality from pulmonary embolism and cerebral thrombosis was seven times higher among pill recipients. An American study concluded that the risk of thromboembolism was 4.4 times higher in pill users, with no differential risk with age. No increase in cerebrovascular accidents was found in this study.

Despite differences between studies, the general view is that the estrogenic component (more than 75 μg) of birth control pills increases the risk of venous thrombosis, pulmonary embolism, and cerebral thrombosis, but not coronary thrombosis. There is no indication that study individuals who were affected were especially susceptible; hence the level of risk is believed to be higher in all users. Older women and patients anticipating or recovering from elective surgery should avoid these medications.

It should be emphasized that the onset or exacerbation of severe headaches, usually of the migraine type, is an indication to discontinue the pill. Women experiencing cerebrovascular accidents seem to have experienced prodromal warning by the onset of severe headaches as long as three months before the ischemic episode.

3. *Carbohydrate metabolism.* Glucose tolerance is impaired in 15 to 40 per cent of women receiving birth control pills, and in these women plasma levels of insulin as well as blood sugar are elevated. Generally, the effect of the pill is to increase peripheral resistance to insulin action. Most women can meet this change by increasing insulin secretion without detectable change in glucose tolerance. Those with limited insulin response have abnormal glucose tolerance. The derangement in carbohydrate metabolism may also be affected by estrogenic influences on lipid metabolism, hepatic enzymes, and elevation of plasma-free cortisol levels.

The clinical significance of the elevated blood sugar remains uncertain. It may be a functional change, not deleterious per se and completely reversible. On the other hand, there may be a persisting diabetogenic effect. One preliminary report revealed that four of five class A diabetics (abnormal glucose tolerance while pregnant) remained diabetic after discontinuation of oral contraception. Obese women, or women with strong diabetic family histories, can be given steroidal contraception, but alternatives should be seriously explored.

Clinically, it is particularly necessary to offer women with frank diabetes birth control. This may be given under supervision, because the effect on insulin requirement is neither consistent nor predictable.

4. *Lipid metabolism.* Progestins have no apparent effect on lipids, whereas estrogens increase plasma triglycerides and phospholipids. Because these changes can be seen in subjects on fat-free diets, estrogen either increases hepatic lipogenesis or impairs removal into adipose tissue by inhibiting heparin action on lipase activity. The clinical significance of these changes is not known. In women with strong family histories of coronary disease, periodic measurement of triglyceride levels while on contraceptive pills seems a wise precaution.

5. *Hypertension and the renin-angiotensin system.* The first report of hypertension in a woman receiving birth control pills appeared in 1962 (Brownrigg) and was later well documented by Laragh in 1967. The mechanism of the hypertension is thought to involve the renin-angiotensin system. Plasma angiotensinogen is eight times normal in women receiving birth control pills, but hypertension is usually avoided by a compensatory reduction in plasma renin concentration. The susceptible patient, however, cannot achieve this decrease, and hypertension develops. Usually, blood pressures return to normal three to six months after stopping treatment. It would appear that women with pre-existing hypertension or marginal cardiac reserve should seek alternative modes of contraception.

6. *Liver.* Estrogen influences the synthesis of hepatic DNA and RNA, hepatic cell enzymes, serum enzymes formed in the liver, and plasma proteins. Estrogenic hormones also affect hepatic lipid and lipoprotein formation, the intermediary metabolism of carbohydrates, and intracellular enzyme activity. The active transport of biliary components is impaired by a large number of estrogens and some progestins. Cholestatic jaundice and pruritus are occasional complications of the pill and are similar to the recurrent jaundice of pregnancy. BSP retention is abnormal in 20 per cent of users, and serum alkaline phosphatase is elevated in 2 per cent; but SGOT elevation, if persistent, is not caused by the pill. Pre-existing acute and chronic cholestatic hepatic diseases are contraindications to the use of steroidal contraception. Cirrhosis and previous hepatitis do not seem to be aggravated.

7. *Adrenal cortex.* For some time it has been known that estrogen increases cortisol-binding globulin, transcortin. It has been thought that the increase in plasma cortisol while taking birth control medication was due to increased binding by the globulin without increase in the concentration of free cortisol. Recently, free cortisol has also been shown to be elevated in people taking these steroids. The prolonged effects of this elevation are unknown. The pituitary-adrenal reaction to stress is unimpaired, although the adrenal reaction to metapyrone may be subnormal (owing to estrogen-influenced conjugation of metapyrone).

8. *Other metabolic effects.* Gastrointestinal effects, breast discomfort, and weight gain remain common disturbing effects of birth control pills. Fortunately, these are most intense in the early months of use and usually disappear thereafter. Weight gain on medication is very common but responds to caloric restriction. For some patients, weight gain is a particularly discouraging symptom because of the additional burden of periodic fluid retention.

Chloasma, an increase in facial pigment, was at one time found in as many as 5 per cent of users but is less commonly seen with the current reduction of the steroid content of pills. Once chloasma does appear, it fades slowly and incompletely. Skin-blanching medications may be useful in cosmetically burdened women.

Oral contraception may inhibit the absorption of folate polyglutamates, and prolonged use may lead to megaloblastic anemia in patients with folic acid–deficient diets. Pyridoxine deficiencies may also be seen.

Hematologic effects reported include increased fibrinogen, increased sedimentation rates, increased serum total iron-binding capacity, and a decrease in prothrombin time.

In some women, mental depression or reduction in libido, or both, may require search for an alternative contraceptive method.

Contraindications. The absolute contraindications for oral contraception are previous thromboembolic disease, cholestatic liver disease, estrogen-dependent tumors, sickle cell anemia, and other disorders associated with predisposition to thrombosis (valvular heart disease, arrhythmias, leukemia, polycythemia). Treatment with special observation is indicated in multiple sclerosis, otosclerosis, uterine fibroids, hypertension and other cardiac diseases, diabetes, porphyria, lupus erythematosus, and migraine or unusual headaches. Treatment should be withheld in young women with incomplete epiphysial closure and women who are breast feeding.

Intrauterine Devices for Contraception. With increased use and experience, pregnancy rates in users of various intrauterine spiral or loop devices vary from 2 to 5 per 100 woman years, and therefore tend to be similar to rates observed for other mechanical contraceptives. Obviously the advantage of this mode of contraception is that it minimizes the factor of patient error and is therefore suited to large-scale application in the lower socioeconomic groups. A complicating factor is the often unnoticed expulsion of the device, with consequent loss of contraceptive protection. Pregnancy has occurred with the device in place. The disturbing incidence of intermenstrual spotting, menorrhagia, reproductive tract infection, and perforation of the uterus detracts from the acceptability of these devices. Furthermore, contraindications to their application include distorting fibromyomas and adnexal disease.

The mechanism of action is not understood. In rats the devices affect ovum transport, in rabbits implantation and postimplantation stages are affected, and in monkeys tubal ova are lost. Objective studies of associated alterations in human physiology have not appeared. Their usefulness to date has been in large-scale programs requiring minimal patient cooperation.

Beck, P.: Effects of gonadal hormones and contraceptive steroids on glucose and insulin metabolism. *In* Salhanick, H. A., Kipnis, D. M., and Vande Wiele, R. L. (eds.): Metabolic Effects of Gonadal Hormones and Contraceptive Steroids. New York, Plenum Press, 1969, p. 97.

Brownrigg, G. M.: Toxemia in hormone-induced pseudopregnancy. Can. Med. Assoc. J., 87:408, 1962.

Crane, M. G., Harris, J. J., and Winsor, W., III: Hypertension, oral contraceptive agents, and conjugated estrogens. Ann. Intern. Med., 74:13, 1971.

Feinleib, M., and Garrison, R. J.: Interpretation of the vital statistics of breast cancer. Cancer, 24:1109, 1969.

Hertz, R.: Experimental and clinical aspects of the carcinogenic potential of steroid contraceptives. Int. J. Fertil., 13:273, 1968.

Inman, W. H. W., and Vessey, M. P.: Investigation of deaths from pulmonary, coronary and cerebral thrombosis and embolism in women of child-bearing age. Br. Med. J., 2:193, 1968.

Laragh, J. H., Sealey, J. E., Ledingham, J. G. G., and Newton, M. A.: Oral contraceptives, renin, aldosterone, and high blood pressure. J.A.M.A., 201:918, 1967.

Masi, A. T., and Dugdale, M.: Cerebrovascular diseases associated with the use of oral contraceptives. Ann. Intern. Med., 72:111, 1970.

Mears, E.: Pregnancy following antifertility agents. Int. J. Fertil., 13:340, 1968.

Rock, J., Pincus, G., and Garcia, C. R.: Effects of certain 19-nor steroids on the normal human menstrual cycle. Science, 124:891, 1956.

Royal College of General Practitioners: Oral contraception and thromboembolic disease. J. R. Coll. Gen. Pract., 13:265, 1967.

Salhanick, H. A., Kipnis, D. M., and Vande Wiele, R. L. (eds.): Metabolic Effects of Gonadal Hormones and Contraceptive Steroids. New York, Plenum Press, 1969.

Sartwell, P. E., Masi, A. T., Arthes, F. G., Greene, G. R., and Smith, H. E.: Thromboembolism and oral contraception: An epidemiological case-control study. Am. J. Epidemiol., 90:365, 1969.

Szabo, A. J., Cole, H. S., and Grimaldi, R. D.: Glucose tolerance in gestational diabetic women during and after treatment with a combination-type oral contraceptive. N. Engl. J. Med., 282:646, 1970.

Vessey, M. P., and Doll, R.: Investigation of relation between use of oral contraceptives and thromboembolic disease. Br. Med. J., 2:199, 1968.

Vessey, M. P., and Doll, R.: Investigation of relation between use of oral contraceptives and thromboembolic disease. A further report. Br. Med. J., 2:651, 1969.

COUNSELING IN GYNECOLOGY

The emphasis in the preceding discussions has been directed to analysis of changes in the primary ovarian function of ovulation. In these concluding paragraphs some mention of the physician's role in sexual counseling must be made.

Whereas deep-seated sexual problems are usually discussed in psychiatry teaching programs in the medical curriculum, ordinarily no instruction is given the medical student in the normal aspects of sexual life or in its commonly occurring abnormalities. The physician therefore enters practice without benefit of the usual guidelines of diagnosis and management that he has developed for most of the other disorders he will be called upon to see. However, because of his professional status he is often asked for advice in sexual matters and, owing to the uncertainty of applying his own intuitive perception to these matters, the physician usually avoids comment. Unfortunately, this attitude compounds the official silence with which these subjects are treated by schools, religious groups and families.

As a result of the important observations and clinical activities of Masters and Johnson, recorded in two widely read volumes, a factual description of the biophysical progression of male and female sexual response associated with orgasm as well as an approach to diagnosis and therapy of sexual dysfunction is available. Using rapid (two-week) therapeutic methods involving instructional and interpretive interactions between the dysfunctional couple and a male and female co-therapy team, an over-all treatment success rate of 80 per cent has been achieved in the four main categories of human sexual inadequacy: premature ejaculation, male impotence, female orgasmic deficiency, and vaginismus.

In general, the direction of therapy, regardless of the type of presenting distress, is based upon the premise that subjective appreciation of sexual responsivity derives from positive pleasure in sensory experience. For the sexually dysfunctional individual the sensory deprivation originates in one of several possibilities: fear and apprehension of sexual situations, denial of personal sexual identity, rejection of partner or the circumstance of sexual encounter, and lack of sexual awareness through either emotional or physical fatigue or preoccupation. It is not known what special susceptibility causes only a fraction of individuals exposed to these traumas to undergo protracted sexual dysfunction.

The therapist's role is to provide an accurate "mirror" of professional objectivity and knowledge to the troubled couple. In doing this, myths and misconceptions are dismissed, and fear of poor performance, lack of goal orientation, and the notion of the patient as a "spectator" in sexual activity are eliminated. Furthermore, since there appears never to be a purely unilaterally dysfunctional partner, the couple must be trained to communicate needs and exchange sexual vulnerabilities. Thus a nonverbal and verbal signal system is established to maximize pleasure, excitation, mutual satisfaction, and avoidance of stereotyped performance. In this process of reorientation, education, and physical direction, exploration without performance pressures, development of "sensate focus," and carefully graded escalation of sexual involvement comprise the therapeutic sequence.

Orgasmic Dysfunction — Male. *Premature ejaculation* exists if the male cannot control the onset of his ejaculation for a sufficient length of time during intravaginal containment to satisfy his partner in at least 50 per cent of coital opportunities. Obviously, this problem also affects female function. It limits her ability to express sexual reactions and to achieve satisfactory relief of mounting sexual tensions, inevitably leading to frustration at "just being used." On the other hand, the rapid conclusion of sexual contact is a welcome relief from involvement in unpleasant and unrewarding service. The derivations of this self-centered male expression of need appear to be initial teenage exposures to prostitutes, exclusive reliance on "heavy petting" and coital simulation, and dependence on withdrawal as a contraceptive technique. Under all these circumstances there was no need either to learn ejaculatory control or to undertake responsibility for the partner's reactions and responses. Apparently, masturbation practices do not play an etiologic role.

Therapy by "squeeze technique" and gradual resumption of coital contact have led to almost complete therapeutic success (98 per cent).

Male impotence is classified as *primary* when a male has never been able to achieve and/or maintain an erection qualitatively sufficient to accomplish coital connection. His erection may be achieved but then dissipated without ejaculation. This male may masturbate successfully. Masters and Johnson assign certain events in adolescence as factors influencing the formation of primary impotence. These include untoward maternal influences, the psychosocial restrictions of religious orthodoxy, homosexual functioning, and

personal devaluations from experiences with prostitutes. These events lead in a very few men to a longstanding and deep concern about subsequent sexual performance. Therapy has been successful along the general lines outlined above with the augmenting use of replacement partners or partner surrogates.

Secondary impotence is said to exist if at least one successful coital intromission has occurred; as many as several hundred may have been experienced before the onset of secondary impotence. Inability to obtain or maintain a satisfactory erection for coitus normally occurs as an accompaniment to fatigue or distraction. However, if 25 per cent of opportunities are not achieved, then secondary impotence exists. Among the etiologic factors involved are premature ejaculation, alcoholism, excessive dominance of either parent, homosexuality, and religious orthodoxy. Only rarely are physiologic causes (diabetes, neurologic disease, drug intake, genitourinary problems) found as responsible for impotence. All too often the effect of inadequate counseling is a precipitating or prolonging factor.

The treatment of impotence is directed at combating the male's personal insecurity and his feelings that "nothing can be done," that the problem is unique to the patient, that the partner is viewed as a liability leading to disability, and that the problem must be kept secret even from the therapist. In therapy, the patient must be convinced that he can never "will" an erection. As fears of sexual performance are reduced, the patient's concept of being a spectator of his own dysfunction is diminished. The female partner must also be supported and instructed. Thorough discussion, discovery of sensate focus (the opportunity to think and feel sexually without orientation to performance), sharing mutual genital manipulation and masturbation pleasures with verbal and nonverbal communication, and a "tease" technique in graded resumption of coital opportunities lead to repair of sexual dysfunction in 60 to 70 per cent of cases.

Orgasmic Dysfunction — Female. The physician may incorrectly assume that the "modern" girl is well versed in genital anatomy and physiology and the technique of the sexual act. Practical experience indicates that in many instances the young woman approaching marriage knows too little and has the disturbing notion, perhaps by conditioning from her mother's experience, that marital sex for the female is overrated, exploitative, and sinful. In such instances, without adequate counseling for both partners, repeated dissatisfaction may confirm these attitudes and set the pattern for a lifetime of maladjusted performance of a "wifely duty." Although it may appear too simple a solution for a problem of such magnitude, the physician can help the couple to avoid this situation by tactful and sympathetic review of basic facts during premarital examinations or any other occasion requiring medical consultation.

The fear of genital injury or expectation of pain and hemorrhage owing to rupture of the hymen during sexual intercourse poses a threat to achievement of vaginal-oriented orgasm. Such preconceived attitudes can be dispelled by the assurance of the physician that the pelvic examination just performed reveals anatomically adequate external and internal genitalia. Some pain is usually experienced on entry into the vagina, but lubrication, a considerate partner, and repeated experience favor prompt resolution of this difficulty.

Because mutual precoital sexual excitement is imperative, varying patterns of stimulation as well as coital techniques must be encouraged and instruction given. Every effort must be made to motivate both partners to seek this result by experimentation and frank discussion. In this situation affectation of false modesty or "man of the world" all-knowing attitudes should be discouraged. In 223 dysfunctional couples, 107 had bilateral impairment in which an anorgasmic female was paired with a male who was a premature ejaculator.

It must be made clear that, no matter how satisfactory the circumstances, few women experience orgasm regularly. Often this misunderstanding, if uncorrected, provokes undue concern and tension that may produce further diminution in satisfaction, a change in coital frequency, substitution of clitoral orgasm, or pretending satisfaction when none occurs. Once these patterns are set, reconditioning for vaginal orgasm is possible but only after a long and difficult period of adjustment. Some of the factors leading to the initial lack of coital orgasm are fear of pregnancy, the possibility of discovery by parents or children, economic and social pressures, poor health, and fatigue. All these profoundly influence both partners' interest in and response to intercourse. Possibly the most common factor in the development of aversion to sexual intimacy in the somewhat older married woman is that over the years these intimacies have tended to follow a monotonous, routine sameness of time, place, and practice. Reluctance to discuss the matter with her husband or with her physician abets the situation. The alert physician can usually suspect this problem from the patient's response during history taking and the nature of her physical complaints. Again sympathetic but informative discussions will bring a more open and intelligent outlook on the part of the patient, and whereas no quick cure exists, reorientation of sexual practice and renewed motivation can occur, with an increasing degree of satisfaction derived. Coaching the couple in the recognition of the female indicators of sexual arousal and the sequence leading to achievement of orgasm is particularly helpful. Delay of coitus until extragenital and genital responses in the female (generalized skin flush, retraction of the clitoris, ballooning of the vagina, color changes in the labia) will increase the frequency of coital orgasm, release female sexual tension, and make the anxious, uncertain couple more confident and eager for sexual contact. The therapeutic use of testosterone and alcohol in the sexually frigid woman is not recommended. The effects are temporary and only serve to postpone the necessary personal examination that must be carried out. *Cantharis vesicatoria* (Spanish fly) is a severe irritant to the clitoris and has no place in therapeutics.

Sometimes problems appear to be so complicated and deep seated that psychiatric help is worthwhile. Fortunately these are rare. However, if sexual frigidity appears to have the malicious motivation of deprivation, if sexual intercourse and practice are revolting prospects, or if the woman displays pronounced aggressive or homosexual tendencies, psychiatric evaluation is in order.

Vaginismus is a constriction of the outer third of the vagina by spastic involuntary contractions of the muscles of the pelvic floor. This occurs in reaction to imagined, anticipated, or real attempts at vaginal penetration. As a result, penile penetration is exceedingly difficult or impossible and coitus is rare or the marriage is unconsummated. It is not infrequently found in association with a male partner who suffers from primary impotence or other male dysfunction. In addition, religious orthodoxy, early psychosexual trauma (e.g., rape), recurrent vaginitis or dyspareunia caused by endometriosis, pelvic inflammatory disease, postoperative adhesions, or homosexual preferences are seen as contributory factors. Therapy of the primary pathologic problem and vaginal dilators lead to nearly 100 per cent therapeutic success.

Masters, W. H., and Johnson, V. E.: Human Sexual Response. Boston, Little, Brown & Company, 1966.
Masters, W. H., and Johnson, V. E.: Human Sexual Inadequacy. Boston, Little, Brown & Company, 1970.

868. THE ADRENAL MEDULLA AND SYMPATHETIC NERVOUS SYSTEM

Karl Engelman

The sympathetic nervous system is made up of cellular elements distinguished by their embryologic derivation from neural crest cells and by their distinct chemistry and pharmacology relating to the synthesis and release of the postsynaptic neurotransmitter catecholamine compounds. The cells are found widely distributed throughout the body with major foci located in the central nervous system as well as in ganglia associated with the thoracolumbar segments of the spinal cord. Peripheral sites of localization include the innervation of the heart, blood vessels, smooth muscle of the gastrointestinal tract, sweat and salivary glands, adipose tissue, and adrenal medulla.

Alterations of sympathetic nervous system activity may lead to a wide variety of clinical manifestations. Within the central nervous system, abnormalities result in changes of mood and emotional status as well as movement and tremor disorders. Peripheral manifestations include deficits in vasomotor control with resultant hypo- or hypertension, and altered motility and secretory activity of other visceral organs. In addition, tumors may develop from sympathetic neural tissue, producing clinical syndromes dependent upon the biochemical and pharmacologic activity of the hormones synthesized and released from these cells.

HORMONES OF THE ADRENAL MEDULLA AND SYMPATHETIC NERVOUS SYSTEM

The hormones of the sympathetic nervous system are dopamine, norepinephrine, and epinephrine; the last-named is primarily synthesized and released by the adrenal medulla. These compounds are classified chemically as *catecholamines,* because they are amine derivatives of the catechol (dihydroxybenzine) nucleus. In common usage the term is usually applied only to norepinephrine and epinephrine, because they have the most clearly identified peripheral effects, whereas to date the primary physiologic role of dopamine has been localized to the central nervous system. The accepted pathway for synthesis of these hormones was first postulated by Blaschko in 1939, and the intermediate steps with the related enzymes are shown in Figure 1. The rate-limiting step in the pathway is hydroxylation of the amino acid precursor tyrosine to form dihydroxyphenylalanine (dopa), a reaction under feedback control by end-product (norepinephrine) inhibition.

Synthesis of the catecholamines is a unique capability of sympathetic nervous tissue; except for the enzyme aromatic-L-amino acid decarboxylase, the biosynthetic enzymes are found only within sympathetic nervous cells. This anatomic distribution is further specialized in that the enzyme required for the conversion of norepinephrine to epinephrine is found solely within the adrenal medulla. Tyrosine hydroxylase and dopamine beta-hydroxylase (DβH) are found almost universally in sympathetic neural cells where synthesis normally terminates with norepinephrine. On the other hand, the adrenal medulla contains very large quantities of both norepinephrine and epinephrine, the latter comprising 70 to 80 per cent of the total. These catecholamines are normally stored within sympathetic nerve terminals in intracellular granules which migrate to the cell membrane at the time of neural activity and discharge the amines.

When catecholamines are released from sympathetic tissues other than the adrenal medulla, the primary route of physiologic inactivation of their activity is effected by an active transport mechanism which returns

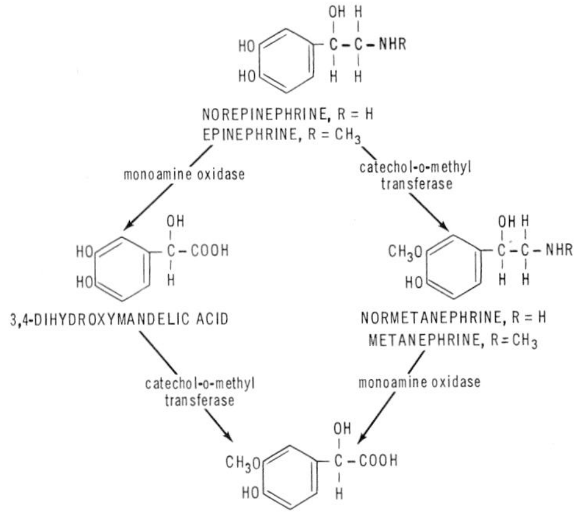

Figure 2. Major routes of catecholamine metabolism.

the unaltered catecholamine into the nerve ending. Either the residual hormone is metabolized locally, or a small portion may diffuse away to appear in the circulation where it may be further metabolized (liver) or excreted unchanged by the kidney. In contrast, catecholamines released from either the adrenal medulla or hormone-producing tumors appear directly in the circulation and manifest their peripheral effects as a result of their concentration in plasma instead of their local tissue concentrations. The primary routes of catecholamine metabolism are accounted for by enzymatic processes shown in Figure 2. For circulating catecholamines, the major route is via O-methylation by the enzyme catechol-O-methyltransferase, followed by oxidative deamination via aldehyde dehydrogenase and monoamine oxidase. In contrast, catecholamines metabolized either within the sympathetic nerve cells or in sympathetic tumors are in large part initially converted by oxidative deamination, followed by O-methylation. In either case, the initial metabolic product is pharmacologically inactive, and the major end product of metabolism is VMA.

The catecholamines and their metabolites are primarily excreted in the urine, and VMA makes up 75 to 80 per cent of the total. The methoxyamines (metanephrines) comprise 10 to 15 per cent, and free catecholamines in the urine usually represent less than 1 per cent of the quantity released. Quantitatively, norepinephrine and its metabolites make up 80 per cent of the total, with epinephrine and its metabolites comprising the balance. Under usual circumstances and with normal activity, humans excrete from 10 to 70 μg of norepinephrine and from 5 to 30 μg of epinephrine per 24 hours. After adrenalectomy the excretion of epinephrine decreases to minimal values, whereas norepinephrine excretion is little changed. Normal excretion of the methoxyamines (normetanephrine plus metanephrine) ranges from 0.3 to 1.3 mg per 24 hours and that of VMA from 2.0 to 6.8 mg per 24 hours.

Pharmacology. Important quantitive differences between epinephrine and norepinephrine, relating to the proportionately greater beta-adrenergic potency of epinephrine, are observed when small doses (5 to 10 μg per minute) are administered intravenously to humans. Although a potent direct vasoconstrictor in some vascular beds, epinephrine produces over-all vasodilatation and

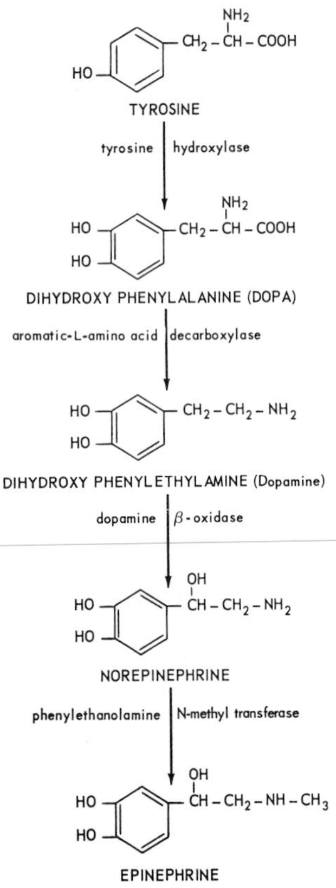

Figure 1. Biosynthetic pathway of the catecholamines.

a decrease in peripheral resistance as well as striking increases in cardiac output and heart rate. Systolic blood pressure is increased, but diastolic pressure remains unchanged or falls, and there is little change in the mean arterial pressure. In contrast, norepinephrine causes an increase of both systolic and diastolic pressure owing to generalized vasoconstriction. Although norepinephrine also has potent beta-sympathomimetic activity, the predominating rise in pressure leads to reflex slowing of the heart, resulting in little change or decrease in cardiac output. When very large doses of norepinephrine or epinephrine are infused into humans or are released from catechol-producing tumors, these differences in physiologic activities of the hormones are usually muted.

Both norepinephrine and epinephrine produce profound metabolic effects, including increased lipolysis and oxygen consumption, elevation of body temperature, and hyperglycemia caused by increased glycogenolysis, as well as inhibition of insulin release from the pancreas. Many of the varying alpha- and beta-sympathetic effects of these hormones have recently been shown to be mediated through changes in the adenyl cyclase system. Current theory holds that beta-sympathomimetic effects are primarily induced by stimulation of adenyl cyclase and increased cyclic-AMP generation, whereas alpha-adrenergic effects inhibit adenyl cyclase activity.

Under normal conditions secretion of epinephrine and norepinephrine by the adrenal medulla is probably not of great physiologic significance. Although hormone production from this sympathetic tissue achieves greater importance during conditions of considerable stress, as in insulin hypoglycemia, the role of the adrenal medulla in normal physiology appears to be mainly supportive in nature. Deficiency states are not generally noted in patients who have had total adrenalectomy with adequate adrenocortical replacement. On the other hand, neuropathic or pharmacologic interruption of the nonadrenal sympathetic tissues appears to produce profound effects most notable in vasomotor control and propulsive activity of the hollow viscera. Among the more commonly encountered clinical conditions in which there is disorder in the sympathetic nervous system are idiopathic orthostatic hypotension and the Riley-Day syndrome (familial dysautonomia), conditions in which both sympathetic and parasympathetic functions are abnormal (see Ch. 471). In addition, results of recent investigations tend to implicate an increase in sympathetic nervous system activity as a causative factor in a significant number of patients with what has previously been called essential hypertension.

PHEOCHROMOCYTOMA

Pheochromocytoma is a catecholamine-producing tumor arising from cells of the sympathetic nervous system and producing a readily recognizable distinctive clinical syndrome which can in most instances be attributed to excessive production of the sympathetic hormones by the tumor. The first clinical description of the syndrome is credited to Labbé and his associates in 1922, and successful surgery for this condition was first performed in 1927 by Dr. Charles H. Mayo.

The most distinctive feature is hypertension. Although pheochromocytoma is responsible for far less than 1 per cent of all patients with hypertension, its importance and notoriety derive from the fact that the clinical features of the disease are dramatic. Although potentially lethal if undiagnosed and untreated, it is curable in about 90 per cent of cases.

Pheochromocytomas may arise from any sympathetic nerve tissue within the body, with the exception of catecholamine-producing cells within the central nervous system. In general, patients with pheochromocytoma tend to be young; most diagnoses are made in patients between 5 and 25 years of age. In young women the diagnosis is frequently made during pregnancy, in part because the blood pressure is taken more frequently then and in some measure because the enlarging uterus may produce pressure on the tumor, inducing more frequent attacks. The tendency to develop pheochromocytoma may be inherited in association with certain other hereditary neuroectodermal disorders. It is known that patients with von Recklinghausen's disease and associated disorders have a high incidence of pheochromocytoma within the family. Furthermore, pheochromocytomas can be inherited in association with medullary carcinoma of the thyroid and a tendency to parathyroid hyperfunction resulting from hyperplasia or multiple parathyroid adenomas *(Sipple's syndrome)*. In some instances these patients also manifest multiple mucocutaneous neuromas as well as generalized ganglioneuromatosis of visceral organs (Fig. 3). These conditions are inherited as autosomal dominant traits, and the pheochromocytomas are almost always multiple, including bilateral adrenal tumors.

Pathology. More than 95 per cent of pheochromocytomas arise within the abdominal and pelvic cavities. The majority are found in one or both adrenal glands,

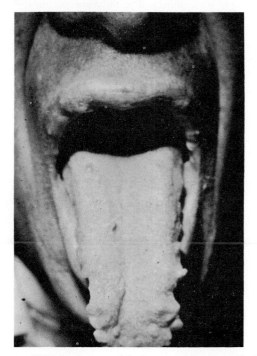

Figure 3. Multiple neuromas of the tongue and lips in a patient with bilateral multiple adrenal pheochromocytomas, medullary carcinoma of the thyroid, exstrophy of the bladder, and multiple visceral ganglioneuromas.

but other sites of origin include embryologic rests of neural crest tissue found usually in association with major arteries. Areas of predilection for extra-adrenal tumors include the paravertebral sympathetic ganglia, and in particular those at the bifurcation of the aorta which make up the organ of Zuckerkandl. Very rarely, tumors arise from sympathetic ganglia within the wall of the urinary bladder, producing distinctive symptoms which should strongly suggest this diagnosis. The majority of those arising in the chest are in paravertebral sympathetic ganglia. Very rarely they have been found to arise from the aortic body area. Other chemodectomas, especially of the carotid body, may produce increased amounts of catecholamines and the clinical syndrome of pheochromocytoma, but the majority of these do not appear to produce hormone syndromes. Extremely rare catecholamine-producing tumors may arise from sympathetic tissue in association with the vagus nerve. Collectively, these tumors, known as glomus jugulare tumors, are formed along the base of the skull in the area of the jugular foramen and within the mastoid and temporal bones and the middle ear. Most glomus jugulare tumors are nonfunctional, but very rarely they may produce the entire pheochromocytoma syndrome.

Most patients have single benign pheochromocytomas, but multiple primary tumors may be found in up to 20 per cent of patients. These appear to predominate in patients with familial inheritance of the tumor, and they usually are adrenal medullary tumors (Fig. 4). An occasional patient may present with both an adrenal medullary and ectopic tumor. Malignant tumors are found in fewer than 10 per cent of patients. The definition of malignancy cannot be made on the histologic appearance of the tumor. Frequently, benign tumors present with bizarre nuclear and cellular patterns which under normal circumstances would be considered evidence of malignancy. The only acceptable definition of malignancy rests on the finding of tumor tissue in areas where pheochromocytomas would not normally arise, e.g., in the liver, bone, lymph nodes, lung, and marrow.

Benign tumors vary in size from less than a gram to almost a kilogram in weight; most are in the range of 15 to 100 grams. The smallest tumors are usually found in association with other large tumors, especially in the hereditary cases (Fig. 4). Solitary tumors less than 10 grams in size rarely produce symptoms. They are highly vascular and usually well encapsulated. On cut surface the color may vary from gray to red. In the larger tumors there may be central areas of necrosis and fibrosis. The cells are polygonal or spheroidal with granular cytoplasm and are often arranged in masses separated by connective tissue. Multinucleate and bizarre-looking cells are frequently observed even in what are considered to be benign tumors. When unfixed sections are exposed to chromium salts, the tissue may take on a brown color owing to a chemical reaction with the catecholamine containing intracellular granules, thus giving rise to the term "chromaffin cells." The catecholamine content is generally greater than that of the adrenal medulla, usually in the range of 1 to 10 mg per gram of tumor. All tumors contain increased quantities of norepinephrine, but fewer than 50 per cent appear to synthesize epinephrine as well. The majority of those containing epinephrine appear to arise from the adrenal medulla. This is in contrast to the catecholamine content of densely sympathetically innervated tissues such as heart and brain, which contain 5 to 10 μg of norepinephrine per gram of tissue.

Clinical Manifestations. The most common finding is *hypertension* which is classically described as being paroxysmal in character, occurring in association with palpitations, tachycardia, a feeling of malaise and apprehension, and excessive sweating. Many patients are persistently hypertensive, having superimposed paroxysmal rises in blood pressure, and an approximately equal number have fluctuating blood pressures, normal at times and hypertensive at others (Fig. 5). Most patients with pheochromocytoma will be hypertensive on at least 50 per cent of readings. Patients who have attacks only at intervals of several days to several weeks are extremely rare, and probably comprise less than 1 per cent of the total group. Symptoms usually occur spontaneously and vary considerably in frequency, se-

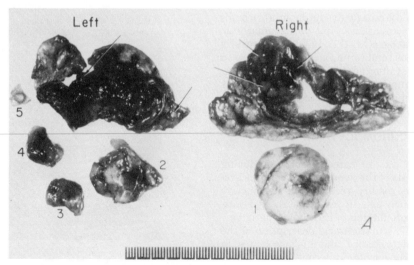

Figure 4. Bilateral adrenal medullary pheochromocytomas from a patient with Sipple's syndrome. The five largest tumors have been extirpated from the specimens, and an additional five tumors, each measuring approximately 2 mm in diameter, are depicted by the arrows on the specimens.

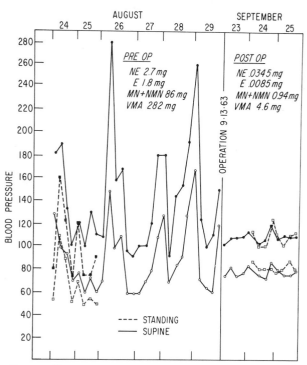

Figure 5. Pattern of blood pressure in a patient with pheochromocytoma. Note variability of blood pressure and presence of orthostatic hypotension prior to therapy and surgery.

tracerebral hemorrhage, cardiac failure, or hyperpyrexia, all of which may result in death.

In rare instances only special manifestations will suggest this diagnosis in a patient who might otherwise be thought to have essential hypertension. Of prime importance in such cases are the presence of *excessive sweating* or *hypermetabolism with weight loss* unexplained by overactive thyroid function and the presence of *orthostatic hypotension* in a hypertensive patient not receiving antihypertensive drugs (Fig. 4). This manifestation is found in approximately 70 per cent of patients with pheochromocytoma and reflects a paradoxical impairment of normal autonomic reflex responses to standing despite the excessive catecholamine production by the tumor. The former attribution of the orthostatic hypotension to hypovolemia appears not to be substantiated. *Polycythemia* has been noted in several such individuals, explained by the finding of high plasma and tumor concentrations of erythropoietin. Other important features of the syndrome include *impaired glucose tolerance* which may be misdiagnosed as diabetes mellitus, *paradoxical pressor responses* to autonomic blocking agents such as guanethidine, and *enhanced pressor responses* to sympathomimetic agents such as the amphetamines and commonly used nasal and bronchial decongestants. Severe *constipation* is found in some individuals—presumably because of the marked inhibitory effect of the catecholamines on bowel motility and enhanced sphincter tone. For unknown reasons the incidence of *cholelithiasis* is markedly increased in patients with pheochromocytoma, and it is not unusual to make this diagnosis even in young adult males who would not otherwise be expected to have it.

Additional clinical features relate to the *inherited disorders which may be found in association with pheochromocytoma.* Most prominent among these are the neurocutaneous syndromes associated with *von Recklinghausen's disease* and *Sipple's syndrome.* In the latter, diarrhea and remarkable flushing resulting from prostaglandin and serotonin production by the tumor may simulate certain aspects of the carcinoid syndrome, and biochemical evidence for hyperparathyroidism exists when secondary parathyroid hyperplasia or tumor induction occurs.

Untreated, the disease may progress in a manner similar to other forms of hypertension, although it is relatively unusual for patients to present with advanced atherosclerotic changes or renal impairment. The primary mode of death in the untreated patient is a cardiovascular or intracerebral catastrophe associated with a severe rise in blood pressure. In some instances chronic congestive heart failure caused by a metabolic cardiomyopathy (*"catecholamine cardiomyopathy"*) may be the most serious clinical manifestation, even in patients who may be normotensive or only mildly hypertensive.

Diagnosis. Recognition of the variety of clinical features associated with pheochromocytoma should provide the most important asset in suspecting this diagnosis in a patient. Often included in the differential diagnosis are essential hypertension, hyperthyroidism, diabetes mellitus, and a variety of psychoneurotic conditions. Once the diagnosis is suspected, it can usually readily be confirmed.

Pharmacologic Tests. Historically, pharmacologic tests were the primary means of confirming or exclud-

verity, and duration in different patients. They often occur while the patient is at rest, or may be precipitated by emotional upset, postural changes or bending, physical exertion, and eating. Attacks coincidental with micturition suggest that the patient has a primary bladder tumor. Before an attack patients may experience apprehension, frequently associated with abdominal or low back pain discomfort which evolves with palpitations, pounding headache, and even angina pectoris. Occasional patients will describe a peculiar, poorly defined sensation of tightness beginning in the lower abdomen and rising through the thorax into the neck and through the head at the onset of attacks. Because of the peculiar nature of many of the symptoms and the frequency with which these patients are manifestly anxious or tremulous, it is not uncommon for them to be labeled as having psychiatric disorders. Observers will frequently note tremulousness and pallor or flushing of the face and extremities as well as dilatation of the pupils and marked diaphoresis. Blood pressures recorded during severe attacks may exceed 300 mm Hg, and after the attack the patient may complain of prostration, lassitude, or fatigue. In some instances a "shocklike" state has been recorded in which peripheral blood pressure has not been obtainable. Although shock and myocardial infarction may occur as a result of a severe attack, frequently the inability to obtain a peripheral blood pressure is due to severe peripheral vasoconstriction. Under these circumstances central blood pressures are usually very high, and very strong central pulses are usually palpable in the axillary or carotid arteries. In rare instances when intense vasoconstriction persists for long periods of time, necrosis and ulceration of tissue may occur. The most serious complications of severe attacks are myocardial infarction, in-

ing the diagnosis of pheochromocytoma in patients suspected of having this condition. More recently, with the general availability of good biochemical assays for catecholamines and metabolites, the use of pharmacologic tests has been relegated to a secondary or even lesser role in the evaluation of this condition.

Although they are no longer recommended as primary diagnostic maneuvers, it is still worthwhile to recognize the nature, attributes, and limitations of pharmacologic tests. *Provocative tests* produce a significant rise in blood pressure after the administration of stimulating drugs; *blocking tests* were thought to be diagnostic by virtue of a selective decrease in blood pressure after administration of certain alpha-adrenergic blocking agents.

Among the stimulatory tests which have been used, the test with which there is greatest experience involves the intravenous injection of 25 to 50 μg of histamine base (available as histamine phosphate solution, 275 μg per milliliter, equivalent to 100 μg per milliliter of histamine base) and the monitoring of blood pressure. Administration of this dose of histamine usually causes flushing, pounding headache, tachycardia, and, frequently, a rise in blood pressure. It is generally accepted that a blood pressure rise of greater than 40 mm Hg, and of more than 20 mm Hg greater than the rise produced by a cold pressor test, indicates a positive response. False positive and false negative responses have each been observed with an incidence of 20 to 30 per cent. Dangers of the test include the precipitation of a severe hypertensive crisis with resulting sequelae or the induction of asthmatic attacks in sensitive individuals. Because of the danger of inducing a severe paroxysm of hypertension, the alpha-adrenergic blocking drug phentolamine (see below) should always be available for prompt intravenous administration. Most patients find this test a most unpleasant experience because of the severe headache usually associated with it. It should not be undertaken in patients whose blood pressure is 170/100 mm Hg or higher. The mechanism by which histamine injection induces enhanced pressor responses in pheochromocytoma is not well understood. Direct release of catecholamine from the tumor by histamine and enhanced discharge of greatly increased sympathetic nerve stores of catecholamines after the acute hypotension produced initially by the histamine-induced vasodilatation have been offered as hypotheses for these events.

Two other provocative tests are still undergoing evaluation. One involves the injection of the indirectly acting sympathomimetic agent, *tyramine,* which has been shown to produce enhanced pressor responses in patients with pheochromocytoma. Advantages of the tyramine test include its safety and lack of unpleasant side effects, because no headache is produced and smaller transient pressor responses are required for a positive diagnosis (20 mm rise in systolic pressure in response to 1000 μg tyramine base); a disadvantage in common with other pharmacologic tests is the fact that there are 10 to 15 per cent false negative responses; false positive responses are extremely rare. The intravenous use of *glucagon* (1 mg) has also been proposed as a diagnostic test with the claim that enhanced pressor responses are produced in patients with pheochromocytoma. The mechanism by which glucagon induces a blood pressure rise in these patients is not understood, and this test

has also been found to have a significant number of false positive and false negative responses.

The only suppressive or vasodepressor test which still has any common usage is the *Regitine (phentolamine) test.* When this alpha-blocking drug is injected into a hypertensive patient with pheochromocytoma, a significant and sustained fall in blood pressure usually occurs. When a dose of 5 mg is given intravenously, phentolamine usually causes a fall of systolic pressure by greater than 35 mm Hg. Although false negative responses rarely occur with this test except in patients who are normotensive, false positive responses may occur, especially in patients who have received sedatives or other antihypertensive drugs, or in those who are uremic. In very sensitive patients, and especially in those whose tumors produce excessive amounts of epinephrine, the fall in blood pressure may be very severe, and shock may be produced as a result of inhibition of the alpha-mediated vasoconstrictor effects, leaving unopposed the beta-mediated vasodilatation; for this reason a preliminary test dose of 1 or 2 mg is suggested. A number of instances have been observed and reported in which this severe reduction of blood pressure has resulted in ischemic infarction of the tumor, with subsequent central hemorrhage, necrosis, and rupture, resulting in serious hazard to the patient.

Chemical Tests. Because of the hazards associated with pharmacologic tests and the significant number of false positive and false negative responses, their use is now discouraged, and the preferred method of confirming the diagnosis of pheochromocytoma is by demonstration of excessive urinary excretion of the catecholamines and their metabolites. Reliable methods are generally available for the measurement of norepinephrine and epinephrine (either singly by specific tests or as a combined total expressed as norepinephrine equivalents), the metanephrines (combined normetanephrine plus metanephrine), and VMA. In almost all patients with pheochromocytoma, analysis of any 24-hour urine collection will reveal increased excretion of all these substances (Fig. 6). The upper limit of normal excretion of these compounds is usually exceeded by an increase of twofold or more for all compounds. In both instances in which the values were at the upper limits of normal or within the normal range, the urines were analyzed more than eight years after their collection, and it appeared likely that chemical destruction of the compounds in the intervening period might have accounted for the relatively low values.

Despite the fact that almost all patients with pheochromocytoma always have increased urinary excretion of catecholamines and metabolites, there are very rare patients who truly have intermittent attacks on very infrequent occasions. These patients constitute less than 1 per cent of the total group, and they will invariably have normal 24-hour urinary excretion values between attacks. In such cases it is possible to make the diagnosis only by collecting carefully timed urine collections over short periods in association with a documented attack. In this way it is usually possible to demonstrate a marked increase in urinary catecholamine excretion for the one- to two-hour period after an attack and then return to normal baseline values. It has been noted in these instances that, although the total excretion rate of free catecholamines may not rise to abnormal levels, if the catecholamine content in these speci-

URINARY EXCRETION OF CATECHOLAMINES AND METABOLITES IN PHEOCHROMOCYTOMA

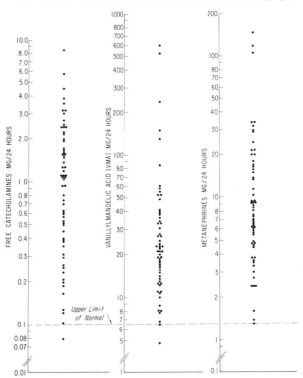

Figure 6. Distribution of excretion values for catecholamines and metabolites determined on single 24-hour urine collections in 64 patients with pheochromocytoma. The vertical axis depicts values on a logarithmic scale.

mens is specially fractionated into norepinephrine and epinephrine, it is usually possible to show a significant rise in either one or the other compound when the data are expressed as an hourly excretion rate.

Determination of plasma concentrations of catecholamines is extremely difficult (see Tumor Localization, below). Although levels are usually very high in patients with pheochromocytoma, there is significant overlap with values that may be obtained with excitement and emotional disturbance and those seen in patients with essential hypertension and depression. Thus this test is not diagnostic and should not be generally performed.

Because certain drugs interfere with one or another of the chemical determinations producing either real or apparent increases or decreases in values, it is important that the therapy of the patient be kept in mind

when specific tests are ordered for screening for this condition. Drugs in common use and the changes which they produce are noted in the accompanying table. Despite the use of any of these drugs, it is possible to adequately screen a patient for the disease without restricting drug therapy. This is especially important in patients with hypertension who might be receiving methyldopa or monoamine oxidase (MAO) inhibitors, and in whom discontinuation of therapy would result in hazardous rises in blood pressure. For many years, it has been advocated that severe dietary restriction be practiced for several days prior to the collection of a urine sample for VMA determination. This requirement was necessary because the rather crude screening tests relied upon color reactions with phenolic acids, and these food constituents resulted in false positive test results. However, for more than a decade there have been available better spectrophotometric or electrophoretic assays which are specific for VMA and which do not require dietary restriction. Laboratories which accept values in the range of 10 to 14 mg per 24 hours as being normal are using crude screening tests, and specimens should not be sent to them for this assay, because the normal VMA excretion should not exceed 6.5 to 7.0 mg per 24 hours.

Tumor Localization. Although the surgeon is understandably concerned about direct localization of the tumor prior to operation, experience with many cases has taught us that precise preoperative localization is of little significance, and some of the maneuvers involved in acquiring the information may be quite dangerous to the patient as well as being costly and often misleading. The essential question concerns the body section in which the tumor is to be found. Since almost all pheochromocytomas are found within the abdominal and pelvic cavities, the major preoperative diagnostic attempts to localize the tumor should be directed at *excluding* the presence of an intrathoracic pheochromocytoma or one arising from the neck or in the skull. Such conditions are readily determined by palpating the area of the carotid bifurcations for the presence of a large, hard mass. Functioning intracranial glomus jugulare tumors should be suspected by the presence of deficits in cranial nerves VII to XII or by the appearance of tumor tissue in the outer or middle ear which can readily be seen by otoscopic examination. In almost all instances in which chest x-rays were obtained in patients having intrathoracic pheochromocytomas, the tumor was readily seen as a posterior mediastinal paravertebral mass. To exclude the presence of such tumors, all patients with pheochromocytoma should have chest fluoroscopy as well as routine and oblique x-rays of the

Urinary Values and Interfering Drugs

Metabolite	Normal Excretion Rate (mg/24 hr)	Usual Range in Pheochromocytoma (mg/24 hr)	Drug	Drug Effect on Excretion Rate
1. Free catecholamines	< 0.1	0.2–4.0	Methyldopa	False increase
			L-Dopa	False increase
2. Metanephrines (normetanephrine plus metanephrine)	< 1.3	2.5–40	MAO inhibitors	Increase
3. Vanillylmandelic acid (VMA)	< 6.8	10–250	MAO inhibitors	Decrease
			Clofibrate (Atromid–S)	False decrease
			Nalidixic acid (NegGram)	False increase

chest. Intra-abdominal pheochromocytomas present no problem of localization at the time of operation (see Treatment, below), and large tumors can usually be demonstrated by the relatively noninvasive technique of intravenous pyelography with laminagrams of the renal and retroperitoneal areas. If the tumor is not seen, evidence of its presence by distortion of the renal contour or shift in the position or axis of the kidney or ureter gives strong indication of its position. Retroperitoneal instillation of air or CO_2 as a means of outlining a tumor has now been largely discarded as dangerous, often misleading, and rarely revealing small tumors which would not otherwise be found at exploration. Arteriography may readily define large tumors, but small or ectopic tumors may be missed, and the hazard and cost of the procedure do not seem to justify its routine use.

In exceptional cases, routine preoperative evaluation and thorough surgical exploration will fail to identify tumor tissue, and in such circumstances it may be necessary to perform venous catheterization of the superior and inferior vena cava as well as their major tributaries to collect blood samples for catecholamine determination. These assays are extremely difficult and can be performed accurately in only a few research laboratories, so such problem patients are best handled by experts. Demonstration of a step-up in plasma catecholamine concentrations at any particular level indicates the probable area in which the venous drainage of the tumor enters the major veins. It is noteworthy that falsely elevated values may be produced inadvertently by the person performing the catheterization if radiopaque dye is instilled into the adrenal veins under sufficient pressure to cause local tissue damage. This will result in sufficient catecholamine release from normal adrenals to simulate tumor secretion. Values obtained from the hepatic vein may be most helpful in evaluating the patient for possible hepatic metastases. Under normal circumstances, hepatic venous effluent should have a very low catecholamine concentration because of metabolism of these compounds in the liver. When values obtained from this source are as high as or higher than those obtained from other systemic veins, this is indication of hepatic metastases which are releasing catecholamines beyond the portal circulation.

Although cholecystography is not specifically a localizing procedure for the pheochromocytoma, all patients about to undergo surgery for this condition should have a preoperative oral cholecystogram to determine the possible presence of gallstones which might be removed after tumor resection.

Treatment. The objective of therapy of pheochromocytoma is prevention of the physiologic and metabolic effects of the catecholamines secreted by the tumor. The preferred mode of therapy is complete surgical excision of the single or multiple tumors, and this can be achieved successfully in approximately 90 per cent of the patients. In the remainder, who either have metastatic disease or are not operative candidates for reasons of serious medical complications, pharmacologic therapy can prove very effective in reversing the symptoms of the disease and markedly prolonging life. Regardless of the ultimate form of therapy, pharmacologic therapy will have to be instituted in almost every patient. Adequate control of the effects of catecholamines is necessary before surgery, because the greatest danger to the patient exists during induction of anesthesia and in-

traoperative manipulations, when life-threatening or lethal rises in blood pressure and arrhythmias may occur as a result of tumor stimulation. Two categories of adrenergic blocking drugs are useful in such cases: those which competitively block the peripheral effects of circulating catecholamines, and several still experimental drugs which have proved useful in competitively inhibiting the synthesis of the catecholamines by the tumor. The competitive peripheral sympathetic blocking drugs may be further divided into two groups: the alpha- and beta-sympathetic blockers. The *alphablockers* (dibenzylene and phentolamine) compete primarily with the peripheral vasoconstrictor effects of the catecholamines, thus reducing blood pressure, and they also are effective in blocking the alpha-mediated inhibition of insulin release. Dibenzylene (phenoxybenzamine) is a very long-acting drug which may be administered orally once or twice daily. The usual dose range necessary for the control of most patients is from 20 to 100 mg per day. Occasional patients may require larger doses. The onset of action is rapid, and maximal effect from a single dose is usually achieved in one to two hours. Phentolamine, although also available in an oral dose form, is primarily used intravenously because of its short duration of action. Aside from its use in the diagnostic vasodepressor test, phentolamine is primarily useful as acute adjunctive therapy to control severe hypertensive crises during surgery. Again, it should be noted that patients whose tumors produce significant amounts of epinephrine may produce exaggerated hypotensive responses to alpha-blockers.

The only *beta-sympathetic blocker* available for use in the United States at this time is propranolol. Its primary salutary effect is as a specific antagonist of the catecholamine-induced arrhythmias and tachycardia, although it is not usually suggested for use for the latter condition unless the pulse rate is above the range of 110 to 120 beats per minute. Propranolol may be administered either orally or intravenously. Patients with pheochromocytoma are extremely sensitive to its effects, because its use in this condition for disturbances of cardiac rate and rhythm is specifically related to the causative agent (excess of catecholamine stimulation), unlike other instances in which the drug may be used. Oral doses of 5 to 10 mg every six hours are frequently sufficient to reduce heart rate and abolish arrhythmias. During surgery, doses in the range of 0.5 to 2.0 mg may be used intravenously to control arrhythmias when they present a danger or produce adverse hemodynamic effects. Because of the negative inotropic effects of this drug, it must be used with caution, especially in patients who have catecholamine cardiomyopathy and who may be thrown into severe congestive failure by very small doses. Paradoxical rises in blood pressure are usually produced when beta-blockers, such as propranolol, are administered to patients whose tumors produce epinephrine. Under these circumstances, the drug blocks the beta-mediated vasodilatation which occurs primarily in muscle vasculature, thus producing a net increase in peripheral resistance by converting epinephrine pharmacologically into norepinephrine ("epinephrine reversal"). Both types of adrenergic blockers are effective in reducing the sweating and hypermetabolism associated with this condition.

In contrast to the selective effects produced by the adrenergic blocking drugs, experimental competitive inhibitors of the rate-limiting step in catecholamine synthesis, the conversion of tyrosine to dopa (catalyzed by the enzyme tyrosine hydroxylase), produce a panoramic effect, because all catecholamine actions are reduced in proportion to the inhibition of hormone synthesis. To date, the most effective of these experimental drugs has proved to be the tyrosine analogue alpha-methyl-para-tyrosine. In doses of 2.0 to 4.0 grams per day, this drug has resulted in inhibition of catecholamine synthesis by as much as 85 to 90 per cent and essentially complete reversal of all the deleterious effects of the tumor. Limitations in its use have been the production of sedation and diarrhea in some patients and the very low solubility of the drug in urine so that patients receiving larger doses have developed evidence of crystalluria. Despite these shortcomings and its lack of general availability, this drug appears to be the pharmacologic treatment of choice for pheochromocytoma.

After control of the physiologic abnormality produced by the pheochromocytoma, the patient may be explored. Successful surgery depends on a concerted and prearranged team effort, comprising the surgeon, anesthetist, and internist-pharmacologist. The procedure is greatly facilitated by constant electronic monitoring of blood pressure and the electrocardiogram so that appropriate use of blocking drugs may be made to counter any sudden changes in pressure or rhythm. Drugs to control catecholamine effects in the preoperative management of the patient should not be discontinued prior to the day of surgery, and the fear that they may produce untoward effects during surgery appears to be unsubstantiated. Preanesthetic medications should be limited to sedation the evening before surgery, but the use of atropine or other anticholinergic drugs as a routine may present problems because of the tachycardia produced by these compounds. Satisfactory anesthesia has been achieved with combinations of nitrous oxide and ether, as well as with the use of the newer halogenated hydrocarbon gases. Halothane has proved especially useful because it blocks the alpha-adrenergic vasoconstriction. In common with other halogenated hydrocarbons, it does seem to enhance the development of cardiac arrhythmias in the presence of excessive catecholamine secretion. Cyclopropane is contraindicated for anesthesia in these patients because of its marked arrhythmic effects. Propranolol should be available for rapid intravenous administration in case serious disturbances of cardiac rhythm occur. Doses in the range of 0.5 to 2.0 mg usually suppress dangerous rhythm disturbances for sufficient periods of time to permit the tumor to be removed and the surgery to be completed. Lidocaine is also useful in this regard, but its duration of effectiveness is very short compared to that of propranolol. If hypertensive crises occur during surgery despite preoperative preparation, small doses of phentolamine (1 to 5 mg) should be given rapidly intravenously for rapid blood pressure control.

When the tumor is thought to be within the abdominal cavity, exploration should be done whenever possible through an anterior transabdominal approach, rather than by a retroperitoneal flank incision which might be a more usual procedure for an adrenal tumor. The more difficult anterior approach is advocated because of the likelihood of multiple tumors being found at the time of surgery, some of which might not be suspected after preoperative testing. This approach permits direct visualization and palpation of both adrenal glands as well as all the other common sites from which

these tumors may arise between the floor of the pelvis and the diaphragm. Even when tumors have not been located by diagnostic procedures before surgery, it is usually not difficult for the surgeon to locate small ectopic masses. Direct digital stimulation of tumor tissue, even when inapparent to the surgeon and transmitted through other organs, usually results in significant changes in cardiac rate and rhythm or blood pressure. When these occur, careful selective palpation with monitoring of vital signs will readily lead the surgeon to the tumor. Multiple and bilateral adrenal pheochromocytomas occur almost universally in patients with Sipple's syndrome, and in most instances total bilateral adrenalectomy must be performed or residual tumor tissue will be left behind (Fig. 4). However, multiple ectopic tumors must be suspected in *all* patients, and despite the removal of a large tumor, patients must be thoroughly explored to exclude other foci. Great care must be taken in the dissection of these tumor masses, because they bleed profusely when incised. In a number of instances, it appears that metastases have spread as a result of incision or rupture of a tumor and implantation of otherwise benign cells throughout the field of surgery.

After removal of all tumors, blood pressure almost invariably falls to hypotensive levels. The mechanism of this hypotension is thought to relate to persistent impairment of autonomic reflexes and not to hypovolemia. Nonetheless, all blood loss should be replaced quantitatively during the course of surgery. In anticipation of final severance of the tumor blood supply, rapid expansion of intravascular volume by the administration of plasma or plasma substitute (5 per cent albumin in normal saline) has been found most effective in sustaining a normal blood pressure at this time. This maneuver has proved much more effective than pressor drug infusions which are frequently difficult to discontinue for hours to days after surgery and have sometimes led to the demise of the patient in what was called "intractable shock." When volume expansion has been used in a large series of patients, use of pressor drugs has not been necessary, and the clinical course after removal of the tumor has been more stable.

During the first postoperative day, most patients will become hypertensive, especially in the period in which they are experiencing pain as they emerge from the effect of anesthesia. The usual cause of this hypertension is a combination of the cardiovascular responses to stress and iatrogenic hypervolemia induced in the course of treatment of the hypotensive reaction. This rise in blood pressure is usually unresponsive to intravenous administration of phentolamine; although it usually diminishes rapidly over the period of the ensuing day, it may be treated with parenteral administration of a rapidly acting diuretic such as furosemide or ethacrynic acid. Other causes of postoperative hypertension include inadvertent damage to a kidney or ligation of a renal artery or one of its branches during the course of surgery, or the presence of residual pheochromocytoma tissue, persisting either as additional undiscovered benign primary tumors or as metastases. Even in the immediately postoperative patient, a radioactive renal scan may be performed relatively readily, and it should indicate any major difficulty with a kidney which might be responsible for the hypertension. When residual pheochromocytoma is suspected, postoperative urine collections should be obtained for catecholamine or metabolite assays in an attempt to determine whether the previously elevated values have returned to normal. Since most patients normally excrete increased quantities of these compounds for four to five days after surgery, the collection should be delayed until the end of the first postoperative week so that the results of the tests are interpretable. Before discharge from the hospital, all patients who have undergone surgery for pheochromocytoma should have repeat analyses to determine the adequacy of surgery. Follow-up determinations, initially at six-month and then at yearly intervals, seem adequate to exclude development of new tumors or metastases unless clinical symptoms indicate an earlier re-evaluation. When the patient has associated evidence of von Recklinghausen's disease or Sipple's syndrome, it is mandatory to extend the investigation to members of the family, especially those who are hypertensive, in an attempt to discover other cases. Even in apparently sporadic cases, hypertensive members of the family should have screening tests performed on their urine in an attempt to exclude this potentially curable form of hypertension.

In patients who cannot undergo surgery or who are not cured by surgery, prolonged therapy with either the adrenergic blocking agents or alpha-methyl-tyrosine has proved successful in controlling the signs and symptoms of the disease. This is especially important because most patients with malignant pheochromocytoma die as a result of cardiovascular catastrophes rather than because of the directly aggressive nature of the cancer. Indeed, most patients with this condition have exceedingly slow-growing tumors, and patients with documented metastases have been treated successfully for more than ten years, often without evident progression. These tumors have uniformly proved unresponsive to treatment with either high-voltage radiation or other chemotherapeutic agents.

OTHER TUMORS ARISING FROM SYMPATHETIC TISSUES

Depending upon the state of differentiation of primitive neural crest cells, sympathetic tissues may contain either immature pluripotential cells or cells which have differentiated into mature ganglion cells or adrenal medullary pheochromocytes. Tumors may arise from cell types which run the whole gamut of this differentiation. The most common are classified as ganglioneuromas or neuroblastomas, the latter originating from more primitive cell types. It is not unusual to encounter multiple cell types within any particular tumor, and the pathologic classification usually is based upon the predominant cell morphology. Although certain clinical features have been associated with the presence of these tumors (evidence of vasomotor instability, flushing, fever, and diarrhea), they generally have been considered to be nonfunctional tumors in contrast to the pheochromocytomas. However, during the past decade it has been demonstrated that these tumors not only produce catecholamines, their precursors, and metabolites, but are also capable of producing other hormones which may contribute to clinical syndromes. There appears to be some correlation between the degree of differentiation of the primary cell types of the tumor and the pattern of catechol excretion. Those which are primarily composed of immature cells tend to excrete relatively larger quantities of dopa, dopamine, and their primary metabolites, whereas the most mature tumors tend to excrete relatively greater quantities of norepinephrine and its metabolites. Regardless of the nature of the tumor, VMA and metanephrine values are almost universally increased and serve as excellent screening and diagnostic tests in confirming the diagnosis preoperatively (Fig. 7).

Ganglioneuromas are usually well encapsulated and rarely malignant. They may arise from any of the sympathetic ganglia, and they are frequently found in childhood as prominent posterior mediastinal paravertebral masses. Less commonly, they arise in the adrenal medulla or para-aortic sympathetic ganglia in the abdomen, and they also may be found in association with sympathetic ganglia in the bowel wall. This latter occurrence is especially notable among those patients with the familial inheritance of Sipple's syndrome in association with multiple cutaneous neuromas and multiple visceral ganglioneuromas. The tumor is composed of mature ganglion cells which are surrounded by connective tissue containing nerve fibers.

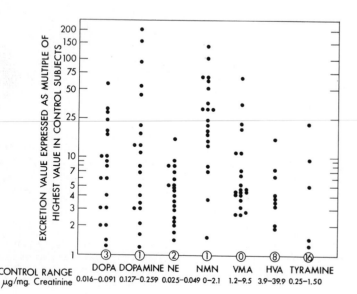

Figure 7. Excretion values for catecholamines and their precursors and metabolites in 21 patients with neuroblastoma, sympathoblastoma, and ganglioneuroma are expressed on a logarithmic scale as multiples of the highest value obtained in normal control subjects. The circled values corresponding to a multiple of 1 indicate the number of instances in which the values were normal.

Neuroblastomas are highly malignant tumors occurring during infancy and early childhood; except for Wilms' tumor, they are the most common retroperitoneal tumors in children. They arise most commonly in the adrenal medulla, but they may also develop in other sympathetic ganglia within the thorax or abdomen. They metastasize early with widespread involvement of lymph nodes, liver, bone, lung, and marrow. When the tumor is diagnosed prior to obvious metastases, the prognosis is often good, but with metastases prognosis is poor despite the extensive use of radical surgery, deep x-ray therapy, and chemotherapeutic agents. As with patients with ganglioneuroma, these patients may demonstrate marked diarrhea in addition to other systemic effects. The demonstration in these patients of very high concentrations of prostaglandins within both tumor tissue and plasma lends considerable support to the hypothesis that the gastrointestinal manifestations and flushing may be related to tumor production of these fatty acid hormones. Recent experimental evidence relating to the elaboration of increased quantities of a hormone stimulating nerve growth (nerve growth factor, NGF) has raised questions about the role of this trophic hormone in eliciting this disease. Similarly, studies on the production of tumor immunity have suggested the possibility that immune mechanisms may be developed as more effective modes of therapy.

Catalona, W. J., Engelman, K., Ketcham, A. S., and Hammond, W. G.: Familial medullary thyroid carcinoma, pheochromocytoma, and parathyroid adenoma (Sipple's syndrome), study of a kindred. Cancer, 28:1245, 1971.

Conference on the Biology of Neuroblastoma. J. Pediatr. Surg., 3: Part 2, 1968.

Cooperman, L. H., Engelman, K., and Mann, P. E. G.: Anesthetic management of pheochromocytoma employing halothane and beta-adrenergic blockade. A report of 14 cases. Anesthesiology, 28:575, 1967.

Engelman, K.: Assay of plasma catecholamines; an approach to evaluating altered sympathetic activity in essential hypertension. *In* Laragh, J. H. (ed.): Hypertension Manual. New York, Yorke Medical Books, 1973, p. 605.

Engelman, K., Horwitz, D., Ambrose, I. M., and Sjoerdsma, A.: Further evaluation of the tyramine test for pheochromocytoma. N. Engl. J. Med., 278:705, 1968.

Engelman, K., Horwitz, D., Jéquier, E., and Sjoerdsma, A.: Biochemical and pharmacologic effects of alpha-methyl-tyrosine in man. J. Clin. Invest., 47:577, 1968.

Gifford, R. W., Kvale, W. F., Maher, F. T., Roth, G. M., and Priestley, J. T.: Clinical features, diagnosis, and treatment of pheochromocytoma: A review of 76 cases. Mayo Clin. Proc., 39:281, 1964.

Regulation of catecholamine metabolism in the sympathetic nervous system (New York Heart Association Symposium). Pharmacol. Rev., 24:161, 1972.

Sandler, M., Karim, S. M., and Williams, E. D.: Prostaglandins in amine-peptide–secreting tumours. Lancet, 2:1053, 1968.

Schimke, R. N., Hartman, W. H., Brout, T. E., and Rimoin, D. L.: Syndrome of bilateral pheochromocytoma, medullary thyroid carcinoma, and multiple neuromas. N. Engl. J. Med., 279:1, 1968.

Sjoerdsma, A., Engelman, K., Waldmann, T. A., Cooperman, L. H., and Hammond, W. G.: Pheochromocytoma: Current concepts of diagnosis and treatment. Ann. Intern. Med., 65:1302, 1966.

Studnitz, W. von, Kaser, H., and Sjoerdsma, A.: Spectrum of catecholamine biochemistry in patients with neuroblastoma. N. Engl. J. Med., 269:232, 1963.

869. THE CARCINOID SYNDROME

Karl Engelman

Definition. Carcinoid tumors and the often bizarre and distinctive clinical features manifested by patients with this rare disease have been clinical and scientific enigmas for almost three quarters of a century. Tumors of the gastrointestinal tract composed of cell types now associated with carcinoid tumors had been known since the early 1800's, and were generally thought to be benign tumors of little clinical importance. In 1907, Oberndorfer postulated that these tumors were a morphologic entity, and although he thought them to be malignant tumors on the basis of their cellular appearance, he thought they behaved in a very indolent and benign manner. For this reason he coined the name "karzinoid" (carcinoma-like) to emphasize their malignant appearance but benign nature. At various times they were thought to be derivatives of autonomic nerve tissue, as well as several types of intestinal mucosal cells. Masson advanced the hypothesis in 1928 that carcinoid tumors arose from argentaffin cells (Schmidt's cells, Kulschitzky's cells) which are normal constituents of the intestinal mucosa near the base of the crypts of Lieberkühn. The term argentaffin derives from the fact that many of these cells reduce and fix certain silver salts in pathologic preparations. It was not until the early to mid-1950's that studies by Thorson, Waldenström, and others suggested that the constellation of signs and symptoms in patients harboring this tumor might be related to production of hormones. Initially, both serotonin and histamine were found in large quantities in most carcinoid tissues, and the clinical features of the patients were ascribed to production of these hormones. With time and study of an increasing number of patients, it has been necessary to revise earlier concepts on the basis of demonstrated tumor production of additional vasoactive substances such as the kinin peptides and prostaglandins. Furthermore, it is now possible to define several subsets of the originally described clinical syndrome, based on specific variants of clinical features, anatomic site of origin of the primary tumor, and the related biochemical differences in the tumors as manifested by their secretion products.

Pathology. In general, the carcinoid *syndrome* occurs only in relation to malignant tumors which have metastasized, usually with extensive hepatic implants. The most common primary tumor is a small lesion of the terminal third of the ileum, although other sites include other areas of the small and large bowel, the pulmonary bronchial tree, gastric mucosa, pancreas, common bile ducts, and ovaries. Carcinoid tumors of the appendix are rarely malignant and almost never cause the carcinoid syndrome; carcinoids of the rectum are frequently multicentric in origin, usually nonfunctional, and rarely malignant.

Diarrhea and intestinal obstruction are the most common gastrointestinal symptoms associated with carcinoid disease, but it is extremely rare that these symptoms are produced either mechanically or metabolically by the primary tumor itself. The primary tumor is often a very small, innocuous-looking lesion which can rarely be found by radiographic procedures. When the disease is diagnosed on the basis of the production of the typical syndrome, it is unusual for the primary tumor to constitute more than 1 per cent of the tumor mass in the body. Mechanical impairment of gastrointestinal tract continuity and function is usually attributable either to local sclerosing metastases in the bowel wall which kink and obstruct the bowel or to extensive mesenteric lymph node metastases which eventually sclerose and coalesce to shorten the mesentery and impair the blood supply of the bowel. At its end-stages, the bowel often has the appearance of a parachute in which the shrouds have been pulled tightly toward the center so that the loops of small bowel are kinked, narrowed, and usually relatively fixed in position at a central retroperitoneal point. Contributing to this process is an unusual proliferation of fibrous tissue which is one of the yet unexplained unusual manifestations of the carcinoid syndrome. Other areas in which dense fibrosis may occur—entirely without evidence of local tumor growth—include peritoneal and pleural surfaces and the endocardium of the heart chambers and heart valves. When there is extensive involvement of the peritoneal surfaces, retroperitoneal and pelvic fibrosis may result in obstruction of urinary drainage and simulate retroperitoneal fibrosis (see Ch. 107). One of the original reports of this disease described a pelvic examination in a woman with longstanding carcinoid syndrome. By both rectal and pelvic manipulation the entire pelvic floor was described as absolutely fixed by rock-hard tissue, with the examiner commenting: "it was as though one placed one's hand into a plaster of Paris cast of the pelvic organs." At autopsy the hard mass was found to be dense fibrous tissue and not tumor.

Other fibrotic lesions with considerable clinical significance involve the endocardial aspects of the heart and associated great vessels. Minimal to massive fibrotic proliferation occurs mainly on the right side of the heart and involves the valvular surfaces as well as the endocardium of the heart chambers. Lesser degrees of involvement on the left side of the heart occur under circumstances of longstanding carcinoid syndrome, but they occur earlier in patients who have primary bronchial lesions and when there is an atrial septal defect with a right-to-left intracardiac shunt. Pathologically, the distribution of the fibrosis is distinctive and readily differentiated from that which occurs with the more common endomyocardial fibroelastosis and generalized myocardial fibrosis. The unique features of this fibrotic lesion are that it does not disrupt the internal elastic lamina of the myocardial and heart valves and that the fibrosis appears in apposition to the endocardial surface. There is a peculiar predilection for fibrosis on the underside of the heart valves, upstream from the blood flow (i.e., on the ventricular surface of the tricuspid valve and the pulmonary arterial surface of the pulmonic valve). Initially, the predominant functional lesion produced by this fibrotic process is valvular stenosis followed by valvular insufficiency.

The peculiar and extensive fibrosis frequently observed in the carcinoid syndrome both within the cardiovascular system and on peritoneal surfaces remains unexplained. Several lines of evidence indicate that serotonin may be implicated in this feature of the syndrome. When introduced into fibroblast tissue culture, serotonin results in marked stimulation of cellular growth and fiber production. Furthermore, the serotonin antagonist methysergide, used in treatment of migraine headache, occasionally causes extensive retroperitoneal fibrosis with ureteral obstruction. More recently, Graham has reported that chronic methysergide therapy may also produce endocardial and valvular lesions indistinguishable from that of the carcinoid disease, lending further support to the hypothesis that these lesions may be related in some way to serotonin metabolism.

Clinical Manifestations.   The carcinoid syndrome, be-cause of its variable clinical features, is frequently undiagnosed for many years after the initial onset of symptoms. The clinical features may be considered in relation to the organ systems involved.

Vasomotor.   One of the cardinal features of the carcinoid syndrome is *flushing,* chiefly occurring over the face and neck and in sun-exposed areas. The onset of flushing may be sudden and may range from a bright red to a violaceous hue. Facial and periorbital edema, tachycardia, hypotension, and pulmonary and gastrointestinal symptoms frequently accompany a flush. Black patients, in whom the change in color may be less apparent, frequently report a feeling of warmth or intense heat, and vascular dilatation is usually very apparent in the bulbar conjunctivae. Certain distinctive features of the flush, including anatomic distribution, temporal relationships, and color, vary with the anatomic site of the primary tumor (see Variant Syndromes, below). Precipitating stimuli include ingestion of food and especially alcohol, pain, physical activity, and emotional upset. In common with the finding that emotional stimuli resulting in sympathetic nervous system activation induce flushing, studies have shown that small doses of intravenous catecholamines, especially those with alpha-sympathetic activity, are potent flush-provoking agents. Although this phenomenon has been proposed as a diagnostic test for the carcinoid syndrome, the associated hypotension or shock produced by the massive flushing reaction may be life threatening to the patient, and the use of this pharmacologic test is not to be encouraged. When patients have experienced flushing for several years, they usually develop fixed cutaneous changes in the areas in which flushing occurs. These changes include the development of multiple fine telangiectasias and a fixed purple hue, usually over the malar areas, the nose, the upper lip, and the chin. The findings are somewhat like the malar telangiectasia which develops in patients with longstanding mitral stenosis.

Gastrointestinal.   Recurrent attacks of mild to explosive diarrhea, abdominal pain, bloating, and severe tenesmus are common. Frequently, the loose bowel movements and symptoms of hypermotility, especially when mild, are misdiagnosed for years as functional bowel disease. Nausea and vomiting may also develop, especially in association with evidence of small bowel obstruction. Right upper quadrant tenderness is common, and when hepatic metastases grow to massive size an additional feature may be the episodic development of severe right upper quadrant pain, fever, right shoulder pain, leukocytosis, and all the features of an acute abdomen. Although the diagnosis of a perforated abdominal viscus must be entertained and evaluated, most commonly these features represent hemorrhage and necrosis within tumor which seems to have outgrown its blood supply with resultant peritonitis. Treated conservatively with small bowel suction and other supportive measures, the patient may be sustained during a period of a week to ten days, during which the entire syndrome evolves and disappears. Surgery for this condition is rarely necessary. *Peptic ulcer disease* also appears to occur more commonly in patients with carcinoid syndrome than in the general population.

Cardiopulmonary.   Blood pressure in patients with carcinoid syndrome is usually normal or low, especially during flushing attacks when severe *hypotension* and even life-threatening shock may occur. *Hypertension* has rarely been found in association with the carcinoid syndrome, despite the widely held clinical impression that this is a feature of the disease. Although experience with functioning bronchial carcinoids is limited, this variant of the carcinoid syndrome may be an exception, because a significant number of these patients have been found to be mildly to moderately hypertensive. Cardiac involvement (see Pathology, above) is a progressive complication which occurs late in the disease. In general, as a result of the predominantly right-sided lesions, evidence of right-sided congestive heart failure becomes a serious problem and a common cause of death. Edema as a result of these cardiac diseases may be enhanced by hypoproteinemia which commonly results from severe diarrhea, protein loss, and replacement of liver by tumor. Auscultatory evidence of pulmonic stenosis and tricuspid stenosis and insufficiency can usually be demonstrated in patients with long-standing carcinoid disease. Murmurs indicating left-sided heart involvement are less common, except in patients with bronchial carcinoid or atrial septal defect. Pulmonary symptoms caused by primary heart failure are rare except in those with predominantly left-sided lesions, but bronchospasm and wheezing in association with flushing attacks are seen in 20 to 30 per cent of the patients. In some instances this may be indistinguishable from bronchial asthma, and the use of glyceryl guaiacolate–containing expectorants may further complicate diagnosis by yielding false positive tests for urinary serotonin metabolites (see Diagnosis, below).

Nutritional. Chronic weight loss, often unremitting and leading to cachexia, may be attributed not only to the catabolic effects of the tumor, but also to the severe diarrhea frequently resulting in malabsorption syndromes. Satisfactory control of the diarrhea is usually beneficial with regard to both the sense of well-being and the development of positive nitrogen balance. Patients with far-advanced carcinoid disease with extensive metastases sometimes develop the signs and symptoms of pellagra, including dementia and typical skin lesions in sun-exposed areas. The development of niacin deficiency has a dual etiology. First, patients with poor nutrition have a decreased intake of niacin and its amino acid precursor, tryptophan. Second, the carcinoid tumor which effectively forms 5-hydroxyindole compounds from tryptophan diverts dietary tryptophan from the kynurenine–nicotinic acid pathway to production of serotonin and its metabolites (see Chemistry, below).

Malignant carcinoid tumors have also been associated with a variety of ectopic hormone production syndromes. The bronchogenic tumors have been more commonly associated with peptide hormone synthesis than have the ileal or other tumors. In addition to the production of prostaglandins and 5-hydroxyindole compounds, excessive ectopic production of parathyroid hormone, gonadotrophins, ACTH, insulin, and probably growth hormone have all been documented.

Chemistry. The biochemical hallmark of malignant carcinoid tumors is excessive production of *5-hydroxyindole compounds*. The biosynthetic pathway for these is illustrated in Figure 8. The essential amino acid tryptophan is hydroxylated to 5-hydroxytryptophan (5-HTP) by the enzyme tryptophan hydroxylase, the rate-limiting step in serotonin synthesis. Within the tumor (except

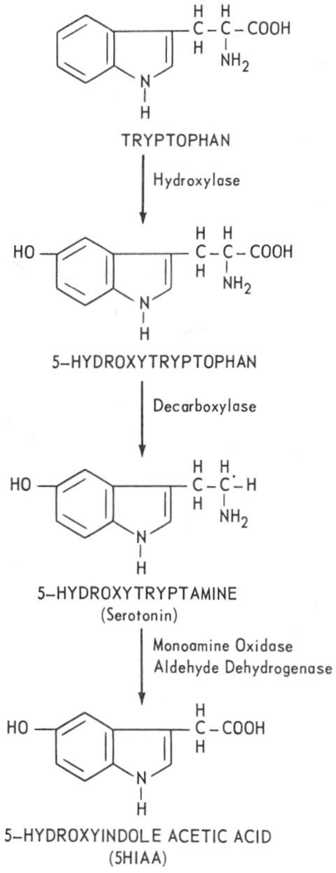

Figure 8. Synthesis and metabolism of serotonin.

in gastric carcinoid—see below) the 5-HTP is further metabolized to serotonin (5-HT), its pharmacologically active metabolite. Small quantities of serotonin are normally produced in the body, major depots being the gastrointestinal mucosa, the brain, and the platelets. In the last-named, the serotonin is thought to be synthesized elsewhere and merely stored in the platelet granules in high concentrations as a result of an active transport process which traps the amine. Normally, less than 1 per cent of total dietary tryptophan (1000 to 1500 mg per day) is converted to 5-hydroxyindole compounds, but when very large masses of malignant carcinoid tissue are found in the body, as much as 600 to 1000 mg of 5-HIAA may be excreted in the urine daily. This may represent almost all the dietary tryptophan available to the patient, especially in those who have severe gastrointestinal symptoms, anorexia, diarrhea, and poor food intake; this accounts for the development of niacin deficiency and pellagra (see above). When the clinical condition results in the inability to eat, the urinary 5-HIAA values fall to low values only to rise after dietary tryptophan ingestion increases, thus demonstrating the limiting relationships of dietary tryptophan on niacin and serotonin synthesis. Excessive quantities of histamine may also be synthesized by carcinoid tumors, especially those of gastric origin.

Physiology. The pharmacologic effect of serotonin as a smooth muscle agonist has long been considered responsible for the hyperperistalsis, diarrhea, and bronchial constriction of the carcinoid syndrome. Although initially the serotonin was also thought to be related to the severe flushing, this hypothesis does not fit with the known effects of serotonin as a peripheral vasoconstrictor and the observations that infusions of serotonin do not reproduce these features of the syndrome. Elegant experiments and observations by Peart and co-workers demonstrated that the flushing phenomenon is indirectly mediated by sympathetic stimulation. Subsequent work by Oates and others showed that sympathetic stimulation resulted in the appearance in the blood of the kinin peptide bradykinin after catecholamine stimulation of the tumor. The catecholamines were shown to activate a tumor enzyme—kallikrein—which in its active form was capable of cleaving the decapeptide lysyl-bradykinin from a circulating α_2-globulin precursor, kininogen. After release of the decapeptide and its appearance in the hepatic vein effluent, it is converted to the potent vasoactive nonapeptide bradykinin in the plasma. Although infusions of bradykinin could reproduce the carcinoid flush, it was not possible to demonstrate increased kinin levels in some patients with more severe flushing. Subsequently, it was shown that carcinoid tumors also produced very large quantities of vasoactive fatty acid hormones, prostaglandins, which could also explain some of the flushing.

Diagnosis. As with pheochromocytoma, the diagnosis in a patient with carcinoid syndrome should be suspected on the basis of appearance of distinctive clinical features. Confirmation of the diagnosis can be achieved preoperatively by demonstration of increased 5-hydroxyindole production. Since approximately 99 per cent of serotonin infused intravenously is converted to 5-HIAA, this metabolite rather than the hormone should be measured in the urine of patients suspected of this disease. Both qualitative and quantitative tests are available for the assay of 5-HIAA in urine.

The *qualitative screening test,* as originally described by Sjoerdsma, is a simple procedure requiring only 0.2 ml of urine from any random voiding. Indole compounds in the urine are converted to colored derivatives by the addition of nitrosonaphthol reagent. After extraction with an organic solvent, the color in the aqueous layer is compared with that of a blank sample to which water was added instead of the urine sample. A positive test is indicated by the presence of a faint to deep purple color in the aqueous layer, depending upon the quantity of indole compounds present in the urine sample. Assuming a normal daily urine volume of 1000 to 1500 ml, this qualitative screening test will not be positive unless the patient is excreting 30 to 50 mg of 5-HIAA per 24 hours (Fig. 9). Thus since the upper limit of normal for 5-HIAA excretion is 9 mg per 24 hours, some patients with this disease may have a false negative screening test when their urinary 5-HIAA excretion is less than 50 mg per day total.

Although some laboratories have attempted to use the screening test in a quantitative way by determining the optical density of the aqueous supernatant in a spectrophotometer, the limitations of the assay do not permit such modification. Under these circumstances the test will commonly yield false positive results. The reason for these aberrant findings is that the nitrosonaphthol reagent will react with any indole compounds in the urine (not just 5-hydroxyindoles), and a greater apparent amount of 5-HIAA will be thus determined. However, there is a relatively simple specific *quantitative test* for 5-HIAA which employs certain modifications of the screening test and which will yield accurate absolute results. The complete 24-hour urine collection, rather than a random urine sample, is required for this deter-

mination, because the calculation of 5-HIAA excretion will now be based upon its total content in the sample as opposed to relative concentrations in a single voided sample. Certain dietary precautions must be taken. Food which contains large quantities of serotonin (bananas, pineapples, walnuts, red plums, avocados) must be restricted from the diet or 5-HIAA excretion will be increased spuriously. In addition, drugs such as mephenesin and especially cough preparations containing glyceryl guaiacolate (see Cardiopulmonary, above) yield metabolites which result in color formation, producing false positive tests by both the qualitative and quantitative assays. Phenothiazines, frequently used for the prevention or treatment of flushing, interfere with the test reaction, reducing the color yield, and could produce false negative tests. Patients with malignant carcinoid usually excrete 5-HIAA in the range of 50 to 500 mg daily. Rare patients will excrete values closer to the upper limit of normal, and these must be distinguished from certain patients with nontropical sprue who have been known to have moderately elevated (10 to 15 mg per 24 hours) 5-HIAA excretions.

Except in a peculiar variant of the carcinoid syndrome in which 5-HTP is the primary product of tumor secretion (see Gastric Tumor, below) urinary serotonin is rarely increased significantly, because the serotonin is so readily converted to 5-HIAA. Thus in the vast majority of patients with carcinoid, determinations of serotonin in urine are of little value. Serotonin in the blood is carried almost exclusively in platelets, and in most patients with carcinoid syndrome total blood or platelet serotonin is high, but these determinations are not diagnostic and should not be part of the general workup. Bidirectional paper chromatography of urinary indole compounds may be a useful adjunct to determining the specific biochemistry of carcinoid tumors. This procedure is readily done in most research biochemistry laboratories. In patients with gastric or other 5-HTP–producing tumors, increased quantities of serotonin and 5-HTP may be demonstrated as well as large increases of 5-HIAA.

Histologic confirmation of the diagnosis may be obtained by biopsy of the primary tumor or metastases. However, the constellation of the typical clinical features, increased 5-HIAA excretion in the urine, and demonstration of metastases—especially to the liver by indirect means such as physical examination, abnormal liver enzyme levels, abnormal liver scan, and evidence of other distant metastases—is usually sufficient to confirm the diagnosis without invasive procedures such as exploration or liver biopsy. This may be especially important because of the limitation of treatment of the patient and the probability of intra-abdominal complications requiring future surgery (see Prognosis and Therapy, below).

Variant Syndromes. *Ileal Tumor ("Classic Carcinoid Syndrome").* The majority of patients with carcinoid syndrome have a primary tumor on the terminal portion of the ileum metastatic to the liver, producing typical symptoms of flushing, diarrhea, valvular heart disease, and, in a significant minority of patients, asthmatic attacks. Flushing is usually episodic with a red to cyanotic coloration (Fig. 10). Duration of flushing varies from 1 to 30 minutes, and in patients with more advanced disease it may be relatively constant. Right-sided heart lesions and right-sided heart failure predominate. 5-Hydroxyindoles in the urine appear almost

Fig. 9

Fig. 10

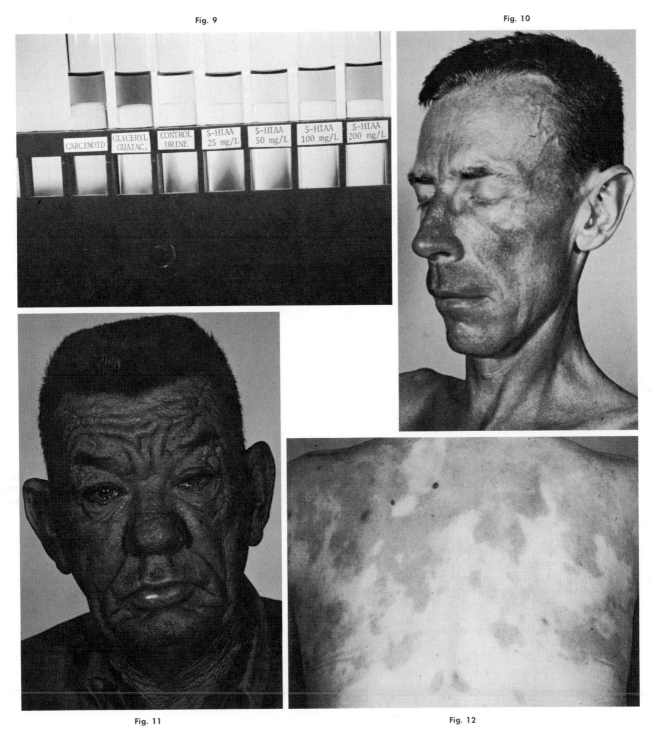

Fig. 11

Fig. 12

Figure 9. Qualitative screening test for carcinoid (tubes, left to right): carcinoid patient excreting approximately 200 mg 5-HIAA per day; color reaction in normal subject taking 15 ml cough preparation containing glyceryl guaiacolate on the previous day; normal urine; and the same urine to which had been added 5-HIAA to give the final concentration noted on each tube. The color of a positive test is first detected visually at a 5-HIAA concentration of approximately 50 mg per liter.

Figure 10. Classic or ileal carcinoid flush.

Figure 11. Bronchial carcinoid flush.

Figure 12. Gastric carcinoid flush.

exclusively as 5-HIAA. Metastases to regional mesenteric lymph nodes with massive involvement of the liver always occur prior to the onset of typical clinical symptoms; metastasis to bone or other peripheral tissues is rare. Abdominal pain, especially in association with intestinal obstruction, is common, and irremediable intra-abdominal mechanical lesions or resistant right-sided heart failure are usually the causes of death.

Bronchial Tumor. Carcinoid tumors of the bronchial tree are generally nonfunctioning and are removed after incidental finding of a solitary pulmonary lesion. Rarely, when systemic signs and symptoms are produced by this tumor, there are a number of unique clinical features which distinguish it from the usual ileal tumor syndrome. The most important is the nature of the flushing episodes. With functioning bronchial carcinoids, the flushes are a livid red, and they are of devastating severity, frequently lasting for hours to days. Hypotension is common during severe flushes, often resulting in oliguria or anuria, and patients may have to be treated acutely with intravenous volume-expanding fluids and large doses of glucocorticoids in an attempt to abort the attack and to sustain the circulation. Marked chemosis, tearing, nasal discharge, and excessive salivation are fairly constant concomitants. During the intense flushes patients frequently develop swelling of the entire face, and, unlike other carcinoid flushes, this flush may involve most of the body. Left-sided cardiac lesions may develop, along with or before right-sided lesions. As with the ileal variant, systemic symptoms rarely occur without distant metastases, especially in the liver. In common with other carcinoids derived from embryologic foregut areas (stomach, bile duct, and pancreas), metastases to bone are common, and they are frequently osteoblastic in nature. Biochemically, these tumors may produce both serotonin and 5-HTP, so the pattern of urinary 5-hydroxyindole excretion products may more closely resemble that of the gastric carcinoid variant (see below). In addition, other endocrine syndromes may be produced by these tumors, most notably Cushing's syndrome resulting from ACTH production by the tumor. In contrast to other forms of the carcinoid syndrome, between flushing attacks these patients have a tendency to be hypertensive. Headaches are also prominent in contrast to other carcinoid variants, and marked enlargement of lacrimal, parotid, and submaxillary and submandibular salivary glands may develop with time. Patients who survive the disease for several years tend to develop thickening and creasing of the skin about the face and forehead. Rhinophyma is prominent, and the fixed, thickened, hard skin folds of the upper face and forehead lend the semblance of "leonine facies" (Fig. 11). It is notable that Graham has recently observed that patients with longstanding migraine headaches, a disease postulated to be related to an abnormality of serotonin metabolism, develop the same peculiar facial features.

Gastric Tumor. The syndrome associated with primary tumors of gastric origin is distinctive from other carcinoid syndromes in both clinical and biochemical features. The flush is characterized by raised, wheal-like lesions of a reddish-brown coloration with variegated borders (Fig. 12). These lesions may occur on any part of the body and frequently are migratory, sometimes involving the palms and soles where they may become intensely pruritic. Metabolic products of these tumors also differ from the other varieties. Oates

and Sjoerdsma, acting on the previous suggestions by Sandler and Waldenström, were able to demonstrate in a patient with gastric carcinoid that although the major 5-hydroxyindole excretion product was 5-HIAA, this constituted only about 60 per cent of the total 5-hydroxyindoles in the urine as opposed to more than 99 per cent in the usual carcinoid patient. Studies by bidirectional paper chromatography of small samples of the urine revealed excretion of large quantities of serotonin and 5-HTP. Quantitatively, the serotonin comprised 25 per cent of the total and the 5-HTP, 17 per cent. These workers suggested that the tumor was incapable of decarboxylating 5-HTP to serotonin (see Fig. 8) and that 5-HTP was the secretion product of the tumor. The explanation for the subsequent metabolism of the 5-HTP to serotonin, and eventually to 5-HIAA, was that the 5-HTP was further decarboxylated in peripheral tissues by this fairly ubiquitous enzyme. The serotonin formed in tissues other than the kidney would be quantitatively metabolized to 5-HIAA, and the serotonin synthesized in the kidney itself would be the primary source of the great increase in urinary serotonin. Subsequent studies in which 5-HTP was infused into noncarcinoid patients resulted in the same excretion pattern of 5-hydroxyindoles found in the gastric carcinoid syndrome. This lent substantial indirect evidence in support of the original hypothesis, and our subsequent demonstration of the absence of the enzyme aromatic-L-amino acid decarboxylase in a gastric carcinoid tumor fully confirmed it. In addition, Oates and Sjoerdsma demonstrated much increased urinary excretion of histamine in two patients with the carcinoids, whereas this finding was uncommon in other patients with the carcinoid syndrome. The unique pruritic, wheal-like flushing which occurs with the gastric carcinoid may therefore be related to histamine production.

"Noncarcinoid" Tumor. Typical features of the carcinoid syndrome may occur with what are considered to be noncarcinoid tumors. Most common among these is *medullary carcinoma of the thyroid* (see Pheochromocytoma, above, and Ch. 843) which, in addition to producing calcitonin, has also been shown to produce increased quantities of prostaglandins and serotonin. Carcinoid-like flushing and multiple watery bowel movements may be common features in patients with these tumors, especially when the primary thyroid tumors are very large or when there are multiple metastases. Urinary 5-HIAA values as high as 300 to 600 mg per 24 hours have been recorded, although usually the values are little, if at all, increased. As yet, there have been no reports of extensive fibrotic lesions in the endocardium and other tissues in association with the medullary thyroid carcinoma. *Tumors of ovarian origin* have also been implicated in this syndrome. Usually these arise from ovarian teratomas and differ from other carcinoid variants in that all the typical symptoms of ileal carcinoid as well as fibrotic thickening of endocardium and mesothelial cavity linings may occur, but notably without metastases in the liver or other organs. It is argued that this is probably related to the fact that the venous drainage of the tumors is not via the portal system; thereby tumor products are introduced directly into the general circulation. This could explain the otherwise universal finding that abdominal carcinoids do not produce systemic symptoms until extensive hepatic metastases have developed.

Tumors of the common bile duct or pancreatic islets may produce biochemical and clinical features of the carcinoid syndrome. In common with other carcinoid tumors of embryologic foregut origin (bronchial and gastric), these tend to produce both 5-HTP and serotonin. In addition, it is predominantly foregut tumors which are associated with ectopic production of other polypeptide hormones. Because of the similarity of the biochemical and clinical features of many of the tumors producing the carcinoid syndrome, there has been growing acceptance of the hypothesis that all these tumors arise from cells of similar embryologic anlage with pluripotential endocrine function, and the nature of the hormone production may depend on the state of derepression of the cellular genetic material in any given tumor.

Prognosis and Therapy. Patients with malignant carcinoid syndrome frequently have symptoms for at least several years before the diagnosis is made, and it is not unusual for them to survive for 10 to 15 years after the initial diagnosis. The course is frequently characterized by spontaneous remissions and exacerbations, although the over-all status progresses slowly and inexorably. With proper nutritional and pharmacologic therapy, and with the exercise of surgical restraint, these patients can usually be carried for long periods of time before they succumb to cardiac or hepatic failure or to complications of mechanical obstruction in the gastrointestinal tract. Above all, it must be understood by the physician, the patient, and his family that this must be considered a chronic disease, and the diagnosis of malignancy, even with widespread hepatic metastases, does not carry with it the dire immediate implications of other bowel tumors with similar distribution. Because the patients frequently suffer periods of severe pain, often requiring hospitalization for days to weeks, the physician must enlist the aid, cooperation, and understanding of the patient in his care. In view of the expected protracted course and its inevitable outcome, the psychologic aspects of patient care are extremely important and may prove most taxing for the physician.

Except in rare instances in which a primary bronchial or ovarian tumor may cause symptoms of the carcinoid syndrome in the absence of metastases, patients cannot be cured by surgery. Indeed, in the usual ileal case the eventual clinical course of the patient may be seriously prejudiced by an attempt to remove large segments of small bowel and its attached mesentery in an attempt to remove as much tumor as possible from the abdominal cavity. Not uncommonly in such instances, patients who have had tolerable or controllable diarrhea prior to surgery develop problems of malnutrition and fluid and electrolyte loss postoperatively owing to marked increase in the number and magnitude of watery bowel movements. This change in the course of the disease may be attributable to decreased bowel area for absorption of nutrients, fluid, and electrolytes. Resection of the distal ileum also compromises the enterohepatic circulation of bile salts which in themselves may constitute a potent cathartic if increased quantities are permitted to enter the large bowel by virtue of the loss of the terminal small bowel where they usually are reabsorbed. If a patient is explored for diagnostic reasons or to attempt to remedy an area of small bowel obstruction, the surgeon should carry out the minimal resection necessary to restore continuity. It may be necessary on several occasions to resort to surgery to relieve areas of obstruction. Frequently, the most effective measures to be employed are to create one or several enteroenterostomies to bypass areas of obstruction while retaining as much absorptive surface of small bowel as is possible. Hypotension, especially during surgery, is a serious problem in patients with carcinoid disease and requires special consideration of the pharmacology of vasopressor substances. Most sympathomimetic pressor drugs produce *paradoxical hypotension* in patients with carcinoid syndrome because of their ability to induce flushing and severe peripheral vasodilatation via the activation of tumor kallikrein and bradykinin synthesis. Only two vasopressor compounds—methoxamine (Vasoxyl) and angiotensin II (Hypertensin)—may be used safely. Prophylactic treatment with corticosteroids may prevent flushes by endogenous sympathetic mechanisms, and thus hypotensive episodes may be minimized during the operation.

The results of chemotherapy and irradiation have generally been unrewarding in patients with the carcinoid syndrome regardless of the site of origin. In common with many other slow-growing tumors, this condition seems to be unresponsive to these forms of treatment. Isolated reports of temporary responses to *cyclophosphamide* (Cytoxan), *methotrexate, phenylalanine mustard,* or oral administration or hepatic artery perfusion with *5-fluorouracil* or *cytosine arabinoside* (Cytosar) have also been rarely useful. More recent enthusiasm for the use of *streptozotocin* has also appeared to be ill substantiated when examined critically. Since few of these cases respond favorably to single or multiple doses of chemotherapeutic agents, the most common effect of such therapy is to further exacerbate the disease and produce the complications frequently associated with the use of these drugs in other conditions. In many instances the death of patients has been hastened by use of cytotoxic drugs.

Nonetheless, significant control of some of the clinical complications of the carcinoid syndrome may be achieved by other pharmacologic agents which do not directly affect tumor growth. Basic to all therapy is the maintenance of adequate nutrition with vitamin supplementation, especially of niacin (see Chemistry, above) and other vitamins. Although low roughage diets are commonly suggested for patients with chronic diarrheal states, modification of food intake does not uniformly provide relief for patients with the carcinoid syndrome. Frequently, the patient's own experience is best relied upon, and it is suggested that he be permitted to select foods which seem not to exacerbate his symptoms.

Flushing attacks may be controlled or diminished by the use of *antiadrenergic drugs* and those which have antikinin properties. Phenothiazine compounds which have alpha-adrenergic blocking activity, such as prochlorperazine (Compazine), 5 to 10 mg, or chlorpromazine (Thorazine), 25 to 50 mg, orally every six hours, may be helpful in reducing the incidence of flushing, and the alpha-adrenergic blocker dibenzyline in a dose of 10 to 50 mg daily may prove very effective. Beta-sympathetic blocking drugs have no effect on the flushing. Naturally, reducing the intake of alcohol and other known stimulants to flushing may reduce the need for prophylactic and therapeutic use of other drugs. Only in the most extreme cases should glucocorticoids be used for the treatment of flushing. Their use (10 to 40 mg of prednisone per day) should be reserved for unusually severe and protracted periods of flushing which may occur at times in the ileal carcinoid syndrome, usually in association with necrosis of liver metastases, or for those patients with bronchial carcinoids whose continuous flushing may be life threatening. In the latter instance it is frequently necessary to use suppressive doses of steroids chronically, thus subjecting the patient to the added morbidity associated with hyperadrenocorticism.

Diarrhea and tenesmus are best treated with the use of conventional antidiarrheal drugs, sometimes in association with specific serotonin antagonists. Belladonna alkaloids, camphorated tincture of opium (paregoric), or kaolin- and pectin-containing compounds may prove useful early in the disease for those who have mild diarrhea, but in most patients more potent agents are required. The most generally useful drugs in the treatment of severe diarrhea are the more concentrated opium alkaloids such as diphenoxylate (Lomotil), 1 or 2 tablets every three or four hours, or tincture of opium, 6 to 20 drops every three to four hours. When patients have many daily bowel movements, it is usually desirable to administer these on a regular schedule rather than on a demand basis. If diarrhea does not respond to these more conservative measures, the specific serotonin antagonists cyproheptadine (Periactin), 4 to 12 mg every six hours, or methysergide (Sansert), 2 to 4 mg three to four times daily, may be tried. Use of the latter, even though often successful, is to be discouraged because of the severe complications relating to both fluid retention and the development of fibrotic lesions of the retroperitoneal area, heart valves, and other tissues which are known to be a complication of its use and which would be presumed to be accelerated in a patient with the carcinoid syndrome. In patients with the gastric carcinoid syndrome, the use of methyldopa (Aldomet), 250 to 500 mg every six to eight hours, has been found uniquely useful in reducing the diarrhea. The effect of the drug in this circumstance is by its activity as an aromatic-L-amino acid decarboxylase inhibitor which reduces the peripheral conversion of the tumor product 5-HTP to serotonin. An undesirable side effect of the methyldopa in these patients would be the associated reduction of blood pressure in what is usually already a hypotensive state. Although there have been no reports to date of the use of alpha-methyldopa hydrazine (Carbidopa) for this purpose, this would seem to be a more desirable and effective drug to achieve these effects. Currently, this compound is being used as an adjunct to L-dopa therapy in Parkinson's disease (see Ch. 365). Since the drug does not produce hypotension, it should be more effective in treatment and produce fewer complications. For patients whose diarrhea is exacerbated by resection of small bowel with resultant bile salt–enhanced diarrhea, oral cholestyramine (Sequestran), 4 to 8 grams every six hours, may prove useful by its ability to bind and inactivate the bile salts.

It has been thought that the diarrhea in the carcinoid syndrome is due to excessive serotonin production. The most direct evidence has been demonstration that specific inhibition of serotonin synthesis has resulted in reduction of diarrhea with little effect on flushing or other manifestations. Although the effect of decarboxylase inhibition with methyldopa may prove successful in the gastric variant syndrome, this mode of therapy has not generally proved effective in the majority of tumors which produce serotonin. Discovery of a specific inhibitor of the enzyme tryptophan hydroxylase, the

rate-limiting step in serotonin synthesis, has provided the opportunity to test this hypothesis. Parachlorophenylalanine, when administered in doses of up to 3 grams daily, has proved uniquely successful in reducing 5-hydroxyindole production by as much as 90 per cent while concomitantly producing reduction or complete remission of diarrhea. Other manifestations of the syndrome do not seem to have been affected by this therapy. Unfortunately, a majority of patients using it for more than six weeks develop allergic reactions, and then its use must be discontinued. Nonetheless, it offers the hope that a compound with similar mechanism of action may be discovered which will prove effective in symptomatic treatment.

Adamson, A. R., Peart, W. S., Grahame-Smith, D. G., and Starr, M.: Pharmacological blockage of carcinoid flushing provoked by catecholamines and alcohol. Lancet, 2:293, 1969.

Engelman, K., Lovenberg, W., and Sjoerdsma, A.: Inhibition of serotonin synthesis by parachlorophenylalanine in patients with the carcinoid syndrome. N. Engl. J. Med., 277:1103, 1967.

Graham, J. R.: Cardiac and pulmonary fibrosis during methysergide therapy for headache. Am. J. Med. Sci., 254:23, 1967.

Melmon, K. L., Sjoerdsma, A., and Mason, D. T.: Distinctive clinical and therapeutic aspects of syndromes associated with bronchial carcinoid tumors. Am. J. Med., 39:568, 1965.

Oates, J. A., and Sjoerdsma, A.: A unique syndrome associated with secretion of 5-hydroxytryptophan by metastatic gastric carcinoid. Am. J. Med., 32:333, 1962.

Peart, W. S., Robertson, J. I. S., and Andrews, T. M.: Facial flushing produced in patients with carcinoid syndrome by intravenous adrenaline and noradrenaline. Lancet, 2:715, 1959.

Roberts, W. C., and Sjoerdsma, A.: The cardiac disease associated with carcinoid syndrome (carcinoid heart disease). Am. J. Med., 36:5, 1964.

Sandler, M.: The role of 5-hydroxyindoles in the carcinoid syndrome. *In* Garattini, S., and Shore, P. A. (eds.): Advances in Pharmacology. Vol. 6, Part B (Biological role of indolealkylamine derivatives: Pharmacology, behavior, and clinical aspects). New York, Academic Press, 1968, p. 127.

Sandler, M., Karim, S. M. M., and Williams, E. D.: Prostaglandins in amine-peptide–secreting tumors. Lancet, 2:1053, 1968.

Torvick, A.: Carcinoid syndrome in a primary tumour of the ovary. Acta Pathol., 48:81, 1960.

870. ENDOCRINE SYNDROMES ASSOCIATED WITH CANCER

Nicholas P. Christy

Neoplasms are often associated with systemic symptoms and signs not explained by local spread or distant metastases. Extreme cachexia in the presence of a small nonmetastatic tumor and glucose intolerance, more often subtle than obvious, are familiar. Many other examples, involving various systems, can be cited (Table 1). These have been observed in all classes of neoplasms: carcinomas, sarcomas, lymphomas, and leukemias. It is not yet possible to ascribe all these effects to humoral agents elaborated by the tumors, although many substances have been postulated, including bradykinin, kallikrein, and others.

There are now plausible humoral explanations for well-defined endocrine syndromes associated with cancer (Table 2). The weight of evidence is that the tumors themselves, although not arising from glandular tissue, secrete and release substances with the

TABLE 1.   Remote Systemic Manifestations of Nonmetastatic Cancer*

Syndrome	Site of Tumor	Humoral Agent Shown to Be Secreted by Tumor
Dermatologic		
Acanthosis nigricans	Breast, colon, lung, stomach	
Dermatitis herpetiformis	Breast, lymphomas, ovary, stomach, uterus	
Dermatomyositis (over age 40)	Breast, lung, ovary, stomach	
Herpes zoster	Several	
Hyperpigmentation	Lung, thymus, others	MSH
Hypertrichosis	Several	
Ichthyosis	Several	
Scleroderma (over age 40)	Breast, lung, ovary, stomach	
Gastrointestinal		
Hepatomegaly without metastases	Hypernephroma	
Zollinger-Ellison syndrome	Pancreas (non-β islet cells)	Gastrin
Hematologic		
Anemia (without blood loss or infection)	Many	
Eosinophilia	Breast, colon, lymphomas, pancreas, stomach	
Erythrocytosis	Adrenal medulla, cerebellum, kidney, liver, uterus	Erythropoietin
Fibrinogen deficiency	Lung, prostate	
Hemolytic anemia	Many cancers, leukemia, lymphoma	
Intravascular coagulopathy	Many	
Leukoerythroblastic and leukemoid reactions	Breast, prostate	
Red cell aplasia	Thymus	
Thrombocytosis	Colon, Hodgkin's disease	
Metabolic		
Disturbances in protein metabolism		
Amyloidosis	Several	
Cryofibrinogenemia (bleeding, thrombosis)	Prostate, others	
Hypoalbuminemia, raised α- and γ_2-globulins	Many	
Macroglobulinemia, cryoglobulinemia, cold agglutinins	Mesothelioma, others	
Galactorrhea	Hypernephroma, lung	+†
Gynecomastia, sexual precocity	Lung, liver	+†
Hyperadrenocorticism	Lung, pancreas, thymus, others	+†
Hypercalcemia	Lung, kidney, ovary, others	+†
Hyperglycemia	Many	
Hypoglycemia	Mesoderm, liver	
Inappropriate water retention	Lung, pancreas	+†
Neurologic		
Cortical cerebellar degeneration	Breast, cervix, colon, lung, breast	
Encephalopathy	Lung, breast	
Myasthenia-like syndrome	Lung, breast	
Myelopathy	Lung, breast	
Myopathies	Lung, breast	
Peripheral neuropathy	Lung, breast	
Subacute spinocerebellar degeneration	Lung, breast	
Renal		
Membranous glomerulonephritis	Several	
Skeletal		
Digital clubbing	Lung	
Pachydermoperiostosis, acromegaloid features	Lung	
Pulmonary hypertrophic osteoarthropathy	Lung, mesothelioma of pleura	
Vascular		
Arterial thrombosis	Hypernephroma	
Carcinoid syndrome	Carcinoid of bronchus	5-Hydroxytryptophan, histamine
	Carcinoid of appendix, cecum, small intestine	5-Hydroxytryptamine (serotonin)
Marantic endocarditis	Lung, pancreas, stomach	
Venous thrombosis, thrombophlebitis	Breast, cervix, lung, ovary, pancreas	

*Data adapted from Greenberg, E., et al., Am. J. Med., 36:106, 1964; and Ross, E. J., Br. Med. J., 1:735, 1972.
†See Table 2.

biologic properties of natural hormones. There are also instances of tumors that originate in endocrine tissue but secrete the "wrong" hormone: e.g., rare cancers of the thyroid and adrenal medulla secreting ACTH, testicular tumors secreting gonadotrophin. The syndromes are not always obvious. The hyperthyroidism that accompanies choriocarcinoma (Table 2) is more chemical than clinical, and many patients with oat cell carcinoma of the lung have laboratory evidence of hyperadrenocorticism, viz., elevated urinary and plasma 17-hydroxycorticosteroid values, exaggerated response of the latter to administrated ACTH, and abnormal diurnal variation of plasma corticoids, but do not have clinically detectable Cushing's syndrome. *The point is that there probably are associated with cancer a great many biochemical abnormalities which may turn out to*

TABLE 2. Endocrine Syndromes Associated with Cancer*

Syndrome	Hormone-Like Activity	Sites of Primary Tumor
Cushing's syndrome	ACTH	Lung (oat cell), pancreas (islet cell), thymus, thyroid, others
Dermal hyperpigmentation	α- and β-MSH	Lung (oat cell), pancreas, thymus
Galactorrhea	Prolactin	Hypernephroma
Hypercalcemia	PTH†	Lung (squamous cell), kidney, ovary, uterus, others
Hyperthyroidism	"TSH" (HCG‡)	Choriocarcinoma, embryoma of testis, hydatidiform mole, lung
Hypoglycemia	Insulin-like (not insulin)	Mesenchyme, liver, adrenal cortex, others
Inappropriate antidiuresis	ADH (vasopressin)	Lung (oat cell), cerebellum, duodenum, lymphoma
Precocious puberty, feminization	FSH, LH	Liver, lung
Precocious puberty, gynecomastia	HCG‡	Adrenal cortex, liver, pineal, testis

*Adapted from Lipsett, M. B., et al., Ann. Intern. Med., 61:733, 1964; Bower, B. F., and Gordan, G. S., Ann. Rev. Med., 16:83, 1965; Omenn, G. S., Ann. Intern. Med., 72:136, 1970; and Ross, E. J., Br. Med. J., 1:735, 1972.
†PTH = Parathyroid hormone.
‡HCG (also written hCG) = human chorionic gonadotrophin.

be useful as signals of clinically important problems. For example, lung carcinoma has been shown to secrete the placental proteins human chorionic somatomammotrophin and placental alkaline phosphatase.

The evidence that tumors secrete and release hormones is not perfect, but it is good. What is required for proof is roughly analogous to Koch's postulates as applied to the etiologic significance of a microbe. There must be (1) coexistence of tumor and an endocrine syndrome; (2) a demonstration in blood or urine of the causative hormone; (3) demonstration of large quantities of that hormone in the tumor and evidence that the hormone does not come from its "usual" glandular site; (4) ideally, demonstration in vitro of the tumor's capacity to make large amounts of the hormone; and (5) disappearance of, or definite improvement in, the endocrine syndrome upon removal of the tumor.

(1) Coexistence of neoplasms and endocrine syndromes is generally accepted; there are now many reported cases, and the syndromes are of at least 11 distinct and recognizable types (Table 2). (2) Greatly elevated concentrations of hormone activity have been shown by biologic or radioimmunoassay in blood of patients with tumors, e.g., of ACTH in association with Cushing's syndrome, gonadotrophins with precocious puberty, and erythropoietin with erythrocytosis (Table 2). One of the major imperfections in the data is that none of the hormones associated with tumors has been absolutely proved chemically to be identical with the natural product. The ACTH produced by tumors includes an ACTH similar, if not identical, to pituitary ACTH, but also N-terminal and C-terminal fragments. Tumor MSH differs in molecular weight from pituitary MSH. PTH (parathyroid hormone) of tumor origin contains a ratio of the various forms of immunoreactive PTH different from that found in hyperparathyroidism. However, the biologic behavior of some of the hormones is so nearly that of the native substance that for clinical purposes there seems no reason to doubt that many of the hormone-like materials elaborated by the tumors are nearly the same as those made by glands. (3) Very high concentrations of these hormones or hormone-like activities have been measured directly in tumors associated with endocrine syndromes, not in most other tumors: ACTH, MSH, gonadotrophins, chorionic gonadotrophin, prolactin, ADH, parathyroid hormone, glucagon, gastrin, and erythropoietin. In one case of presumed gonadotrophin-secreting bronchogenic carcinoma, secretion was proved by showing a higher concentration of FSH in the venous effluent from the tumor than in its arterial supply. With respect to ACTH, high concentrations have been found in plasma and tumor, low concentrations in the pituitary; the inference is that the tumor secretes massive amounts of ACTH, adrenocortical hyperplasia follows, and the induced hypercortisolism suppresses synthesis of ACTH by the pituitary. Similarly, several patients have had tumors containing gonadotrophin, gonadotrophinuria, and reduced pituitary gonadotrophin. (4) In one malignant thymoma associated with Cushing's syndrome, cells propagated in tissue culture continued to produce ACTH for weeks. (5) There are now many instances of cure or definite remission of endocrine syndromes after successful removal of the associated tumor. For example, Liddle et al. have reported nine surgical cures of Cushing's syndrome by removal of the "ACTH"-producing tumor. Dermal hyperpigmentation has disappeared after tumor removal in several cases of MSH-producing cancer. Radiation to a presumably ADH-secreting lung tumor has brought about temporary remission of inappropriate water retention in at least one case, and there are now several reported remissions of hypercalcemia after removal of a "parathyroid hormone"–secreting tumor. The primary role of the tumor in the secretion of the hormone is further strengthened by return of the hypercalcemia in some of these patients when the tumor recurred.

Incidence. Endocrine and metabolic disturbances associated with cancer and not attributable to metastases are not rare. In a large, unselected series of patients with proved bronchogenic carcinoma, the combined incidence of hypercalcemia, gynecomastia, inappropriate ADH secretion, and Cushing's syndrome was 8.5 per cent.

Pathogenesis. The evidence for tumor secretion and release of hormones, mostly polypeptides, is convincing. The mechanisms by which neoplastic tissue manages to synthesize complex molecules with hormonal activity are still conjectural. The prevailing view is that the neoplastic cells in a characteristic process of dedifferentiation lose certain genetic depressor mechanisms so that normally inhibited genetic information is expressed. This hypothesis now appears more tenable than the theory of the "sponge," i.e., the taking up of materials (hormones) from the circulation by the tumor. It is also conceivable that the cancer cell produces a large array of polypeptides, some of which, by chance, have an amino acid sequence capable of bringing about a recognizable biologic activity which can be measured. The matter is discussed by Ross.

Terminology. These endocrine manifestations have

been termed "ectopic," as in the "ectopic ACTH syndrome" (Liddle). The term is appropriate only when the site of the tumor presumably secreting the hormone is clearly not in the organ that ordinarily secretes that hormone, as in an oat cell carcinoma of the lung secreting ACTH, an ovarian tumor secreting parathyroid hormone–like peptide, or a pancreatic tumor secreting serotonin. The term is not appropriate in hyperthyroidism associated with "TSH"-secreting choriocarcinomas, because placental chorionic gonadotrophin has thyrotrophic properties which account for the thyroid-stimulating effects of these tumors; in erythrocytosis associated with renal carcinoma or renal cyst, because the normal kidney synthesizes an erythropoietin; or in carcinoid tumors associated with argentaffin tumors of the small intestine, because this tissue is a normal site of serotonin production.

Clinical Manifestations and Treatment (Table 2). There are practical reasons for recognizing the associations of endocrine syndromes with neoplastic disease. (1) Frequently, the endocrinopathy antedates the appearance of the tumor, and thus may serve as a diagnostic clue to neoplastic disease. (2) The endocrine disorders may be life threatening, as hypoglycemia or hypercalcemia, or severely disabling, as Cushing's syndrome, and yet amenable to palliative treatment. (3) Successful removal of tumor may cure the endocrine syndrome as well as the cancer. (4) Differences in clinical and biochemical behavior of these tumor-associated endocrinopathies from those associated with the classic glandular hyperfunctional states often make a differential diagnosis possible. The general characteristics of the tumor-associated endocrine syndromes are that the hormone is secreted in *anarchic* fashion, that is, secretion is not regulated by the normal control mechanisms; and, as indicated above, the locus of secretion is *displaced* to a site not ordinarily involved in hormonal synthesis.

The discussion that follows emphasizes comparison of the endocrine syndromes associated with cancer with the classic patterns of hormone overproduction in order to facilitate differential diagnosis.

Cushing's Syndrome. Clinically evident hypercortisolism has been observed in association with oat cell carcinomas of the lung, thymomas, noninsulin-producing islet cell tumors of the pancreas, pheochromocytomas, and tumors of the thyroid, ovary, prostate, parotid, liver, and neural tissue. A few hundred instances of this association have been reported, and subtle chemical evidence of hypercortisolism has been found in many more, especially with carcinoma of the lung (see above). Large quantities of ACTH have been thoroughly characterized in plasma and in some tumors. In isolated instances of lung and pancreatic cancer, peptides with the properties of corticotrophin-releasing factor (CRF) have been detected along with ACTH. That the capacity to synthesize ACTH may be a more general property of tumors can be inferred from the finding of Liddle et al. that about 8 per cent of unselected visceral carcinomas not associated with clinically apparent Cushing's syndrome contained considerable amounts of the hormone.

The most important point to be made about the clinical features of Cushing's syndrome associated with nonendocrine tumors is that they are often *subtle*. Patients may show the classic features, but most do not. The absence of obesity and striae is probably a function of the weight loss accompanying the cancer. Patients with all forms of Cushing's syndrome have an equal incidence of glucose intolerance and hypertension, about 90 per cent. But in the syndrome associated with tumor, the onset is faster and the sex incidence favors men, whereas the "pituitary" form of Cushing's disease and adrenal adenoma are far more common in women. Patients with the tumor-related form rarely have osteoporosis, probably because the clinical course of the tumor is short. Generalized dermal hyperpigmentation is common in the tumor form, because of the huge quantities of ACTH secreted by the cancer, or of MSH, which may also be produced in large amounts. Severe hypokalemia and weakness, as well as edema, are also more common in this form of the disease, and are best explained by the enormous quantities of cortisol secreted by the hyperplastic adrenals. Hypokalemia is not due to aldosteronism; the secretion of aldosterone is normal or low. In the other forms of Cushing's syndrome, the patients die of infection or the effects of hypertension; in the tumor form, the usual cause of death is the cancer. At necropsy, the adrenals are enormously hypertrophied, and the pituitary contains subnormal amounts of ACTH.

The laboratory evidence of hypercortisolism is definite and extreme. Plasma cortisol values (ca. 80 μg per 100 ml) and urinary 17-hydroxycorticosteroid and 17-ketogenic steroids may be ten times normal, all much higher than in the "pituitary" or adrenal adenoma forms of Cushing's syndrome. Provocative tests show autonomous cortisol secretion owing to autonomous ACTH secretion by the tumor; urinary steroids do not rise when metyrapone is given, and do not fall in response to dexamethasone. Differentiation from primary adrenocortical carcinoma, also characterized by very high steroid values, can be made by failure to find a suprarenal mass radiographically, and by measuring plasma ACTH concentration; it is very low in adrenal cancer, very high in the presence of ACTH-secreting tumor (see Ch. 850).

To recapitulate: an ACTH-secreting tumor, most likely to be in lung, thymus, or pancreas, should be suspected in any patient with subtle or borderline clinical signs of Cushing's syndrome who has lost, not gained, weight, who has weakness and severe hypokalemia, and whose plasma or urinary corticosteroid values are extremely high.

Management, ideally, is total removal of the tumor, which has been followed by remission of the Cushing's syndrome in several cases. Therefore a vigorous effort should be made to excise tumors completely; some are relatively benign, e.g., bronchial adenomas. If this is not possible, palliative x-radiation or chemotherapy of the cancer is carried out, and chemical palliation of the hyperadrenocorticism can be tried with o,p'-DDD, metyrapone, aminoglutethimide, or combinations of these drugs (see Ch. 850). If the effects of hypercortisolism, e.g., hypokalemia, are incapacitating, bilateral total adrenalectomy may be done, and has in some cases provided good relief.

Dermal Hyperpigmentation. Generalized hyperpigmentation of the skin, resembling that of Addison's disease, may occur with oat cell carcinoma of the lung, thymoma, neurogenic tumors, or tumors of the ovary, pancreas, and prostate. Raised concentrations of α-MSH and β-MSH have been measured in plasma by radioimmunoassay; most of the pigmentary effect is due to the β-MSH, which has also been found in the associated cancers. Some tumors in this group have been shown to secrete both excessive MSH and ACTH, with resulting addisonian dermal pigmentation and Cushing's syndrome. Several patients have shown disappearance or diminution of dermal pigment when tumors were successfully removed.

Gynecomastia, Precocious Puberty. About 5 per cent of male patients with lung cancer have gynecomastia, but in only a few have elevated gonadotrophin values been detected in blood or urine. Tumor types are "large cell" carcinomas, epidermoid, anaplastic, and oat cell carcinomas, and adenocarcinoma. In some of the patients with gynecomastia, raised levels of urinary estrogens have also been found, possibly a result of adrenal or testicular stimulation by gonadotrophin secreted from the tumor; in some cases, striking hypertrophic pulmonary osteoarthropathy has also been present. Its relation to gonadotrophin or estrogen excess is not yet clear.

Evidence that the tumor is indeed the site of gonadotrophin secretion is convincing (see above). When analyzed by radioimmunoassay, the gonadotrophin has been usually LH, on one occasion FSH. There is one report of a patient with galactorrhea whose hypernephroma was shown to secrete prolactin.

Spider angiomas and pulmonary osteoarthropathy may or may not accompany gynecomastia. In such cases, careful search for a pulmonary tumor by roentgenography should be done, and measurements made for urinary estrogens and for urinary gonadotrophins (by bioassay) or plasma LH (by radioimmunoassay). Failure to suppress high urinary or plasma gonadotrophin levels by administration of large amounts of estrogen for several days may turn out to be a useful diagnostic test.

Treatment is unsatisfactory. The tumors are very malignant and have not been surgically curable. Radiation and chemotherapy are ineffective. It remains to be seen whether methotrexate will reduce gonadotrophin production, as it does in trophoblastic tumors (see below).

Another group of tumors has been associated with secretion of HCG. In addition to benign or malignant tumors of the placenta, these are choriocarcinomas of the pineal or testis, hepatoblastoma of the liver, and adrenocortical carcinoma. A recent survey has disclosed high levels of plasma HCG, usually without clinical signs, in 12 per cent of a series of patients with cancer. With testicular tumors (by far the most common) excluded, the incidence becomes about 7 per cent, with cancers of the gastrointestinal tract or breast, multiple myeloma, and malignant melanoma the next most frequent. *The interesting point here is the possible value of measurements of HCG as markers in attempts at early detection of cancer* (see above).

The clinical manifestations, when present, are gynecomastia in the adult male and isosexual precocity in children. In boys, the testes have been enlarged in some, and all show testicular interstitial cell hyperplasia histologically. The gonadotrophin has the characteristics of HCG, and has been found in high concentration in the urine, serum, and tumors. In a very few cases, gonadotrophin levels have been temporarily lowered by methotrexate which had variable effects on the tumor itself. So far, these tumors have all been fatal.

Hyperthyroidism. In addition to the rare association of hyperthyroidism with tumors of the gastrointestinal tract, hematopoietic system, lung, and other organs, several patients have been identified in whom thyrotoxicosis coexisted with metastatic disease of trophoblastic origin (choriocarcinoma or hydatidiform mole) and, in a few cases, with metastatic embryonal cell carcinoma of the testis. Together with the expected finding of high titer of urinary HCG, these patients have thyrotrophic activity in plasma and tumor tissue. The best current evidence indicates that this thyroid-stimulating activity is an intrinsic property of HCG or of a glycoprotein molecule chemically and immunologically similar to HCG. The *clinical manifestations* of hyperthyroidism are usually minimal; many patients have no symptoms, and the rest have only mild symptoms of thyrotoxicosis. All have tachycardia, but other physical signs of the endocrinopathy, e.g., goiter, are generally absent, although laboratory evidence—raised serum PBI and high thyroidal uptake of ^{131}I—is definite. These indices can be controlled with antithyroid drugs or iodides, but most striking is the favorable response of both clinical and laboratory signs of hyperthyroidism to treatment with methotrexate, which is also capable of causing regression of these tumors. The presence of mild thyrotoxicosis, seen in fewer than 10 per cent of women with trophoblastic neoplasms, does not affect prognosis of the tumor.

Inappropriate Antidiuresis. Excessive sodium excretion in patients with lung cancer was first reported in 1938, but not until 1957 did Bartter and Schwartz and their co-workers attribute this abnormality to water retention resulting from abnormally regulated secretion of ADH. Studies done in the last decade have disclosed ADH-like activity in several tumors taken from patients with the syndrome of inappropriate ADH secretion; the tumors have been mostly oat cell carcinomas of the lung, with a few others, e.g., pancreatic and duodenal carcinoma. The ADH-like activity has not been completely characterized, but resembles in physical, chemical, and biologic properties human pituitary ADH, i.e., arginine vasopressin. In some (so far, a minority of) patients, plasma values for arginine vasopressin have been found to be high.

The clinical manifestations of hyponatremia may be minimal or absent, probably because the abnormality has developed slowly. Often, hyponatremia is a chance finding during routine study of a patient with lung cancer. To prove the entity, one has to show a urine hypertonic with respect to plasma, normal GFR, and normal adrenocortical function, i.e., absence of adrenocortical insufficiency. The extracellular space, if measured, is found to be expanded. The pathogenesis of this pattern of abnormalities is discussed in Ch. 805. Treatment with hypertonic salt is useful only as an emergency measure, e.g., for coma or convulsions owing to profound hyponatremia; the only effective medical therapy for long-term use is restriction of water intake to less than 1 liter a day. In a few patients, the water and electrolyte abnormality has undergone temporary remission with successful palliative treatment of the tumor by x-radiation or chemotherapy.

Hypercalcemia. The hypercalcemia of malignant disease may be due to four mechanisms: (1) osteolytic lesions of bone associated with widespread metastases, as from carcinoma of the thyroid, prostate, or lung, or lymphoma; (2) osteolysis in the absence of bony metastases, associated with some carcinomas of the breast which presumably elaborate sterols related to vitamin D; (3) osteolysis in the absence of bony metastases, in association with tumors which appear to secrete a parathyroid hormone (PTH)–like substance; and (4) osteolysis without bony metastases in the presence of tumors which secrete some humoral substance other than parathyroid hormone or proparathyroid hormone, i.e., a substance or substances not detectable by radioimmunoassays for the various forms of these hormones (see Powell et al.). Tumors have been squamous cell carcinomas of the lung and other organs, and carcinomas of the kidney, ovary, uterus, pancreas, and colon. Evidence for primary secretion of parathyroid hormone by the neoplasm has come from demonstration of immunoreactive PTH in plasma of patients with nonparathyroid tumors and hypercalcemia, from the detection of PTH-like substance in the tumors, disappearance or diminution of hypercalcemia upon tumor removal, and reappearance of the electrolyte abnormality with recurrence of the cancer.

The clinical features of hypercalcemia are presented in detail in Ch. 872. The important clinical point is that the hypercalcemia associated with PTH-secreting tumor of nonendocrine tissue is more likely to manifest itself as lethargy, weakness, anorexia, nausea, and vomiting, and less likely to appear as renal stones or bone disease. Patients with the "ectopic PTH syndrome" are more apt to lose weight and to be anemic.

Separation of these patients from those with hyperparathyroidism by laboratory tests may be difficult. Both may have extreme hypercalcemia, low or normal serum phosphorus, elevated plasma values for PTH, and unresponsiveness of hypercalcemia to corticosteroids; but careful examination, laboratory study, and roentgenographic search, e.g., by chest films and intravenous pyelography, will disclose most of the nonparathyroid tumors. Riggs et al. and Arnaud have discussed the diagnostic difficulties in the use of PTH radioimmunoassays for detection of this immunoheterogeneous substance.

The *treatment* of hypercalcemia is discussed in Ch. 872.

It has been recently postulated that *hypophosphatemic osteomalacia* in the presence of benign hemangiomas may be due to a humoral substance (not PTH) that increases renal clearance of phosphate.

Hypoglycemia. The association of severe fasting hypoglycemia with certain neoplasms, especially very large retroperitoneal or intrathoracic tumors, is well established. Most of the tumors are fibromas or sarcomas, sometimes of huge size—up to 10 kg; others are hepatoma, adrenocortical carcinoma, adenocarcinoma of stomach and colon, undifferentiated bronchial carcinoma, and bronchial carcinoid. As for the mechanism of hypoglycemia, there is some evidence against excessive glucose utilization by the tumor and against stimulation by the tumor of insulin secretion by the pancreas, removal of which does not affect the hypoglycemia. The prevailing view is that the tumor secretes a hypoglycemia-producing substance, which, with only a few exceptions, is not demonstrable as high levels of immunoreactive insulin in plasma or tumor, but only as "insulin-like" activity. The secretory role of the tumor is affirmed by surgical "cure" of the hypoglycemia in about 20 patients whose tumors have been successfully removed.

The hypoglycemia is indistinguishable clinically and by most of the provocative tests from that associated with islet cell adenoma or carcinoma of the pancreas. However, almost all patients with nonpancreatic tumors lack high plasma insulin values, and the presence of a large tumor is usually apparent.

Treatment is best done by excising the tumor; even incomplete removal may relieve the hypoglycemia temporarily. Failing this, palliative measures must include continuous feeding of carbohydrate and administration of corticosteroids, diazoxide, and possibly glucagon (see Ch. 807).

Carcinoid Syndrome. This, the only definite example of an "endocrine" syndrome owing to production of a humoral agent that is not a polypeptide, is discussed in Ch. 869.

Erythrocytosis; Zollinger-Ellison Syndrome. These syndromes, caused by tumor secretion of gastrin and erythropoietin, respectively, are discussed in detail in Ch. 730 and Ch. 640 to 644.

Multiple Hormones Produced by a Single Tumor. Several tumors have been reported which apparently secrete two or even three distinct hormones. The pulmonary and thymic tumors secreting both ACTH and MSH have already been mentioned. A few patients with hepatoma have had both hypoglycemia and polycythemia, and islet cell tumors of the pancreas have been described with coexisting hypoglycemia and carcinoid syndrome, and with Cushing's syndrome and carcinoid syndrome. Three hormones, ACTH, MSH, and gastrin, were found in a single pancreatic tumor, and in one patient with an islet cell carcinoma of the pancreas there was chemical or good clinical evidence for secretion by the tumor of six hormones: gastrin and glucagon ("appropriate" hormones for the pancreas), ACTH, MSH, ADH, and parathyroid hormone.

Amatruda, T. T., Jr.: Nonendocrine secreting tumors. *In* Bondy, P. K., and Rosenberg, L. E. (eds.): Duncan's Diseases of Metabolism. 7th ed. Philadelphia, W. B. Saunders Company, 1974, p. 1629.

Arnaud, C.: Parathyroid hormone: Coming of age in clinical medicine. Am. J. Med., 55:577, 1973.

Baumann, G., Lopez-Amor, E., and Dingman, J. F.: Plasma arginine vasopressin in the syndrome of inappropriate antidiuretic hormone secretion. Am. J. Med., 52:19, 1972.

Braunstein, G. D., Vaitukaitis, J. L., Carbone, P. P., and Ross, G. T.: Ectopic production of human chorionic gonadotrophin by neoplasms. Ann. Intern. Med., 78:39, 1973.

Gordan, G. S., and Roof, B. S.: "Humors from tumors": Diagnostic potential of peptides. Ann. Intern. Med., 76:501, 1972.

Liddle, G. W., Nicholson, W. E., Island, D. P., Orth, D. N., Abe, K., and Lowder, S. C.: Clinical and laboratory studies of ectopic humoral syndromes. Rec. Prog. Horm. Res., 25:283, 1969.

Orth, D. N., Nicholson, W. E., Mitchell, W. M., Island, D. P., and Liddle, G. W.: Biologic and immunologic characterization and physical separation of ACTH and ACTH fragments in the ectopic ACTH syndrome. J. Clin. Invest., 52:1756, 1973.

Plimpton, C. H., and Gellhorn, A.: Hypercalcemia in malignant disease without evidence of bone destruction. Am. J. Med., 21:750, 1956.

Powell, D., Singer, F. R., Murray, T. M., Minkin, C., and Potts, J. T.: Nonparathyroid humoral hypercalcemia in patients with neoplastic diseases. N. Engl. J. Med., 289:176, 1973.

Riggs, B. L., Arnaud, C. D., Reynolds, J. C., and Smith, L. H.: Immunologic differentiation of primary hyperparathyroidism from hyperparathyroidism due to nonparathyroid cancer. J. Clin. Invest., 50:2079, 1971.

Ross, E. J.: Endocrine and metabolic manifestations of cancer. Br. Med. J., 1:735, 1972.

Unger, R. H.: The riddle of tumor hypoglycemia. Am. J. Med., 40:325, 1966.

PARATHYROID

G. D. Aurbach

871.   PARATHYROID HORMONE AND CALCITONIN

Parathyroid hormone, the principal humoral regulator of calcium metabolism in man, has been characterized definitively as a polypeptide 84 amino acids in length. The complete structure of the bovine and porcine hormones and part of the sequence of human parathyroid hormone are known and active analogues of the hormones have been synthesized. It is now recognized that biosynthesis of the hormone proceeds through a prohormone molecule 90 amino acids in length (Fig. 1). Immediately after synthesis the prohormone is converted within the gland to the 84 amino acid polypeptide for storage and subsequent secretion. Radioimmunoassays show that calcium is the primary factor controlling secretion of the hormone. A fall in blood calcium concentration provokes secretion of the hormone, which in turn causes an increased rate of transfer of calcium from bone and glomerular filtrate to the extracellular fluids. The hormone also causes increased urinary excretion of phosphate by direct action on the kidney (possibly by inhibition of the reabsorption of phosphate). These physiologic effects on both calcium and phosphate are accounted for by a single hormonal molecule. The mechanism of action of parathyroid hormone is mediated by cyclic 3',5'-adenosine monophosphate (3',5'-AMP) produced through direct specific hormonal activation of the enzyme adenylate cyclase in bone and kidney. The consequent increase in concentration of 3',5'-AMP in the renal cortex and bone activates other intracellular processes which account for the physiologic actions of the hormone. The increase in concentration of 3',5'-AMP induced by parathyroid hormone in the renal parenchyma is manifested also by increased urinary excretion of 3',5'-AMP.

Calcitonin is another polypeptide hormone involved in regulation of calcium and bone metabolism. The structures of the calcitonins are known, syntheses have been completed, and radioimmunoassays have been developed, but the physiologic significance of calcitonin for normal man is still uncertain.

Calcitonin is secreted from the parafollicular cells found in the mammalian thyroid but related embryologically to the ultimobranchial body of lower vertebrate species. The rate of secretion of calcitonin is a direct function of the concentration of calcium in plasma, whereas parathyroid hormone is secreted at a rate inversely proportional to calcium concentration. The hypocalcemic action of calcitonin is effected through an inhibition of resorption of mineral from bone, and the physiologic actions of this hormone seem to be mediated through the adenylate–cyclic AMP system.

Diseases of the parathyroid gland include hyperparathyroidism and hypoparathyroidism. Pseudohypoparathyroidism encompasses the general clinical and laboratory features of hypoparathyroidism but is an abnormality not of parathyroid gland function but of the receptor tissue for parathyroid hormone. Medullary carcinoma of the thyroid is a complex pathophysiologic state in which the tumor secretes excessive amounts of

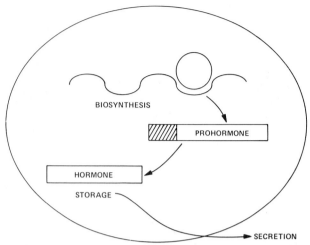

Figure 1. Schematic representation of biosynthesis of hormone within cell of parathyroid gland. The prohormone (90 amino acids in length) is synthesized and then released from the ribosome. After release the N-terminal 6 amino acids (represented by the shaded area) are cleaved enzymatically from the molecule, yielding the parathyroid hormone molecule (84 amino acids in length) which is stored in the gland and released therefrom upon physiologic stimulus. After elaboration of the intact hormone (84 amino acids) into the circulation and interaction with peripheral target tissues (kidney and bone), the hormone is metabolized further to biologically inactive but radioimmunologically detectable fragments.

calcitonin with high concentrations of calcitonin in plasma. Primary hyperparathyroidism, pheochromocytoma, Cushing's syndrome, and multiple neuromas are found associated in some cases of the syndrome.

Aurbach, G. D.: Isolation of parathyroid hormone after extraction with phenol. J. Biol. Chem., 243:3179, 1959.

Aurbach, G. D., and Chase, L. R.: Cyclic 3',5'-adenylic acid in bone and the mechanism of action of parathyroid hormone. Fed. Proc., 29:1179, 1970.

Aurbach, G. D., Keutmann, H. T., Niall, H. D., Tregear, G. W., O'Riordan, J. L. H., Marcus, R., Marx, S. J., and Potts, J. T., Jr.: Structure, synthesis and mechanism of action of parathyroid hormone. Recent Prog. Horm. Res., 28:353, 1972.

Brewer, H. B., Jr., and Ronan, R.: Bovine parathyroid hormone: Amino acid sequence. Proc. Natl. Acad. Sci. U.S.A., 67:1862, 1970.

Chase, L. R., and Aurbach, G. D.: Renal adenyl cyclase: Anatomically separate sites for parathyroid hormone and vasopressin. Science, 159:545, 1968.

Copp, D. H., Cockcroft, D. W., and Kueh, Y.: Calcitonin from ultimobranchial glands of dogfish and chickens. Science, 158:924, 1967.

Deftos, L. J., Lee, M. R., and Potts, J. T., Jr.: A radioimmunoassay for calcitonin. Proc. Natl. Acad. Sci. U.S.A., 60:293, 1968.

Hirsch, P. F., Gauthier, G. F., and Munson, P. L.: Thyroid hypocalcemic principle and recurrent laryngeal nerve injury as factors affecting the response to parathyroidectomy in rats. Endocrinology, 73:244, 1963.

Hirsch, P. F., and Munson, P. L.: Thyrocalcitonin. Physiol. Rev., 49:548, 1969.

Niall, H., Keutmann, H., Sauer, R., Hogan, M., Dawson, B., Aurbach, G. D., and Potts, J. T., Jr.: The amino acid sequence of bovine parathyroid hormone. I. Hoppe-Seyler's Z. Physiol. Chem., 351:1586, 1970.

Potts, J. T., Jr., Niall, H. D., Keutmann, H. T., Brewer, H. B., Jr., and Deftos, L. J.: The amino acid sequence of porcine thyrocalcitonin. Proc. Natl. Acad. Sci. U.S.A., 59:1321, 1968.

Sherwood, L. M., Mayer, G. P., Ramberg, C. F., Jr., Kronfeld, D. S., Aurbach, G. D., and Potts, J. T., Jr.: Regulation of parathyroid hormone secretion: Proportional control by calcium, lack of effect of phosphate. Endocrinology, 83:1043, 1968.

872.   HYPERPARATHYROIDISM

Definition.   Primary hyperparathyroidism is the clinical condition caused by excessive and incompletely regulated secretion of hormone from the parathyroid glands. The manifestations, which may include hypercalcemia, tissue calcification, and osteitis fibrosa cystica, represent the result of excessive parathyroid hormone action on bone and kidney.

Etiology. Hypersecretion of parathyroid hormone as a manifestation of primary parathyroid disease may be caused by adenomas, single or multiple, primary chief cell or clear cell hyperplasia, or carcinoma of the glands. In over 80 per cent of the cases primary hyperparathyroidism is attributable to a single parathyroid adenoma, and in less than 2 per cent carcinoma of the parathyroid gland is the cause. Other cases are about equally divided between clear cell hyperplasia, chief cell hyperplasia, and multiple adenomas. An analogous syndrome can result from ectopic production of parathyroid hormone by nonparathyroid tissue. *Secondary hyperparathyroidism* develops as a compensatory mechanism in any abnormal state tending to produce true hypocalcemia; this state may occur in hypovitaminosis D, vitamin D–dependent rickets, malabsorption of calcium, chronic renal disease, hyperphosphatemia, or renal tubular acidosis. There are no known factors to which development of primary hyperparathyroidism can be attributed. There is a suggestion that prolonged, progressive secondary hyperparathyroidism may evolve into autonomous primary hyperparathyroidism in some cases of chronic renal disease, but there is no evidence that parathyrotrophic substances exist in either normal or abnormal physiology. Several families with autosomal dominant hyperparathyroidism have been reported; thus a genetic factor is involved in some cases.

Incidence. Recent surveys validate earlier projections that better diagnostic methods and wider clinical awareness promote discovery of new cases. Automated laboratory facilities now make possible routine analysis of serum calcium for all patients in the clinic and hospital populations. In one center routine analyses were performed on a large series of patients, and it was found that the incidence of hyperparathyroidism was as high as one case per thousand.

Pathology. Usually parathyroid adenomas vary in size from 1 to 5 grams, but occasionally very large tumors, 50 grams or more, may develop. In general, large tumors are more likely to be associated with clinically evident bone disease, marked hypercalcemia, very high concentrations of parathyroid hormone in plasma, and short interval between development of symptoms and establishment of diagnosis. Histologic examination usually shows chief cells and some water-clear cells; sometimes the latter are predominant. Rarely adenomas are composed of oxyphil cells. Hyperplasia may be of the chief cell or water-clear cell type. Occasionally adenomas of other endocrine glands are found in hyperparathyroidism (multiple endocrine adenomatosis; see Clinical Manifestations, below). The effect of the disease is manifested in the bones as osteitis fibrosa cystica generalisata (see Ch. 890). When the kidneys are affected, nephrolithiasis or nephrocalcinosis is apparent; pyelonephritis often complicates the course of the kidney disease.

Muscle biopsy frequently shows neuropathic (not myopathic) atrophy of type II muscle fibers. This denervation-type structural change (probably secondary to a metabolic lesion in the nerve itself) parallels the severity of muscle weakness in hyperparathyroidism.

Pancreatitis, acute or chronic, is recognized as a possible complication of hyperparathyroidism. About half of the patients with advanced hyperparathyroidism examined at autopsy show calcification in the pancreas. It is possible that chronic hypercalcemia contributes to the development of pancreatitis, but the actual mechanism of this association has not been established.

Pathologic Physiology and Chemistry. Hypersecretion of parathyroid hormone from adenomatous or hyperplastic glands is expressed in acceleration of the normal physiologic actions of the hormone on bone and kidney. The effect on bone leads to an increase in rate of resorption of calcium from bone, and in more severe cases to pathologic development in bone of osteitis fibrosa cystica. The effect on the kidney causes an increase in rate of resorption of calcium from the glomerular filtrate as well as increased renal clearance of phosphate from plasma with consequent hypophosphatemia. The renal concentrating ability may decrease, resulting in polyuria and polydipsia. Hypercalcemia results from the actions of the hormone on bone and kidneys. The urinary excretion of 3′,5′-AMP is greater than normal.

Most new cases of hyperparathyroidism discovered in the clinic show little or no detectable bone disease. This finding may be attributable to more widespread and precise determinations of serum calcium with consequent discovery of earlier and milder forms of the disease and greater general recognition of the problem. Some early or mild cases become clinically apparent chiefly by nephrolithiasis and hypophosphatemia, with little or no hypercalcemia or skeletal abnormality.

Although hypercalcemia is principally a manifestation of the effects of the hormone on bone and kidney, calcium absorption from the gastrointestinal tract is increased as well. Recent studies indicate that this effect on the gut may be influenced through effects of parathyroid hormone on the renal metabolism of vitamin D. Parathyroid hormone stimulates the renal mechanism that converts 25-hydroxy–vitamin D to 1,25-dihydroxy–vitamin D. This latter metabolite, formed in the kidney, acts on the intestine, causing increased absorption of calcium.

The classic laboratory manifestations of primary hyperparathyroidism are low serum phosphate and high serum calcium. Frequently 24-hour excretion of calcium is high because of significant hypercalcemia, even though the renal clearance of calcium is relatively reduced. Hypercalciuria, with calcium excretion in excess of intake, is particularly apparent when diets low in calcium are given. Generally a diet low in calcium is given for three days, and then total urinary calcium is determined for 24-hour periods. Normal subjects should not excrete in excess of 175 mg per 24 hours when taking a diet containing 150 mg of calcium. The alkaline phosphatase in plasma may be high in hyperparathyroidism when there is significant bone disease; this is probably a manifestation of increased bone formation, a compensatory mechanism for the high rate of bone resorption induced by excessive parathyroid hormone secretion. Other manifestations of increased bone resorption are increased urinary excretion of hydroxyproline and pyrophosphate. Kinetic studies utilizing radioactive calcium frequently show evidence of increased bone metabolism.

Clinical Manifestations. The disease tends to segregate into three categories in terms of clinical presentation. In the mildest form there may be no symptoms or signs, and discovery is made only through routine determination of serum calcium. The second category develops insidiously, sometimes over a period of years, and presents predominantly as renal colic. In the third group the course of the disease is more rapid, with development of marked hypercalcemia, weight loss, vomiting, debility, and bone pain, sometimes with pathologic fracture. Debility, weight loss, anemia, and elevated sedimentation rate may be so prominent in the severe form of the disease as to suggest malignancy. The most frequent symptoms of the disease in general are weakness, fatigability, and renal colic. Epigastric pain, neurologic abnormalities, and constipation are also common. Hypercalcemia may cause polydipsia, polyuria, anorexia, nausea, and vomiting. Neurologic abnormalities include impaired mentation, loss of memory for recent events, depression, emotional lability, hyperactive deep tendon reflexes, sensory loss for pain and vibration, and proximal muscle weakness, particularly in the lower extremities. There may also be abnormal movements (resembling fasciculations) of the tongue, glossal atrophy, ataxic gait, hoarseness, dysphagia, anosmia, and abnormal flexor reflex. Careful clinical examination may elicit neurologic abnormalities even in patients who are otherwise asymptomatic.

Still other symptoms cannot be clearly related to distinct pathophysiologic mechanisms. There may be burning in the throat or abdomen, vague malaise, back or coccygeal pain, or dry skin. Occasionally headache or pruritus is the sole presenting complaint. It is of inter-

est in this regard that the pruritus of uremia may be dramatically relieved after removal of parathyroid glands showing secondary hyperplasia. Anemia, elevated erythrocyte sedimentation rate, and hypertension also are each observed in 25 per cent or more of the cases.

Hypercalcemia may depress sensitivity to electrical stimuli of ganglia and peripheral nerves (Erb's sign). Shortening of the Q-T interval (between the onset of the Q wave and the beginning of the T wave) in the electrocardiogram is found in some patients with hypercalcemia. Prolonged hypercalcemia may lead to calcification in the eye displayed as "*band keratopathy*," opaque material appearing in vertical lines parallel to and within the limbus, or as conjunctival crystals without the limbus or under the eyelids. Detection of these may require examination by slit lamp.

Bone disease in hyperparathyroidism, osteitis fibrosa cystica, may be recognized by roentgenographic examination (Fig. 2); it sometimes causes bone pain or pathologic fracture. Roentgenographically, bone disease may appear as generalized osteopenia, loss of the lamina dura about the teeth, erosion of the distal ends of the clavicles, bone cysts (Fig. 2B), "brown tumors" of bone, epulis of the jaw, or subcortical bone resorption, most readily observed in the phalanges (Fig. 2A) or distal clavicles. Chondrocalcinosis (Fig. 2B) may also be found by roentgenography.

Hypercalciuria may lead to *nephrolithiasis* and passage of calcium oxalate or calcium phosphate stones with or without renal colic. In other instances

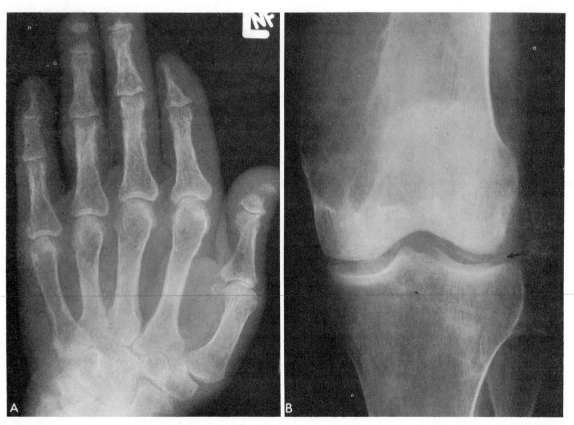

Figure 2.   Roentgenographic signs in hyperparathyroidism. *A*, Bone resorption. There is severe bone resorption with general loss of mineral, thinning of the cortices, marked subperiosteal resorption along the cortical surfaces of the proximal and distal phalanges, and gross resorption of the distal phalangeal tufts. *B*, Cysts (osteitis fibrosa cystica) in femur and tibia in subject with severe hyperparathyroidism. Also note intra-articular chrondrocalcinosis (thin line of calcification in knee joint indicated by arrow).

nephrocalcinosis may develop, sometimes causing progressive renal failure. Infection may complicate either type of renal disorder.

Peptic ulcers are common in hyperparathyroidism, and may reflect a potentiating effect of hypercalcemia on acid secretion. An association between acute or chronic *pancreatitis* and hyperparathyroidism is recognized more and more frequently. One should be aware that hyperparathyroidism may exist in any case of pancreatitis, and may be masked by the acute lowering of serum calcium in pancreatitis.

In addition to pancreatitis and peptic ulcer, several other diseases may be associated with primary hyperparathyroidism. Hypertension occurs in up to 50 per cent of cases. It cannot be clearly related to any particular factor (e.g., associated renal disease) and does not often regress after surgical cure. There is an increased incidence of ill-defined arthralgia as well as of gout and pseudogout. The latter is associated with intra-articular deposition of calcium pyrophosphate crystals. Discovery of pseudogout should suggest possible coexistence of primary hyperparathyroidism. Primary hyperparathyroidism may exist as part of the multiple endocrine adenomatosis syndrome. In such cases pituitary and pancreatic tumors may produce associated endocrinopathies. These include acromegaly or hypopituitarism caused by pituitary tumors, peptic ulceration caused by excessive gastrin secretion (Zollinger-Ellison syndrome), or hypoglycemia resulting from secretion of insulin by pancreatic tumors. Hyperparathyroidism may also occur in another type of endocrine adenomatosis consisting of pheochromocytomas, parathyroid adenomas, and medullary carcinoma of the thyroid (see Ch. 876). Each of the two types of multiple endocrine adenomatosis syndromes may be familial. Sporadic cases of hyperparathyroidism have also been observed in association with hyperthyroidism, sarcoidosis, Albright's fibrous dysplasia of bone, Paget's disease, Cushing's syndrome, and malignancy.

Metabolic acidosis occurs in about one fourth of patients, with hyperchloridemia and low serum bicarbonate. The acidosis can be attributed to impaired tubular reabsorption of bicarbonate and parallels the increase in phosphate clearance. It may become worse in the immediate postparathyroidectomy period when hypophosphatemia is accentuated. A similar defect in proximal tubular reabsorption of bicarbonate may occur in a number of metabolic disorders characterized by secondary hyperparathyroidism or cellular depletion of phosphate, or both. The abnormality can be documented by carrying out a test for T_m of bicarbonate reabsorption. Eventually metabolism returns to normal after surgical removal of hyperplastic or adenomatous parathyroid glands. Hypercalcemia in cancer is less likely to be associated with acidosis; indeed, metabolic alkalosis may be expressed in this disorder. Hypokalemia and hypomagnesemia also are occasionally observed in hyperparathyroidism. The hypokalemia is attributed to decreased distal tubular reabsorption of potassium and may be made worse by treating subjects with high doses of phosphate by mouth. Phosphate depletion may also account for decreased magnesium reabsorption.

Differential Diagnosis. Hypercalcemia, demineralizing disease of bone, and nephrolithiasis are clinical problems that commonly suggest the diagnosis of hyperparathyroidism. *Hypercalcemia* may be expressed in diverse metabolic, endocrine, or malignant diseases,

including hyperparathyroidism, several types of cancer, sarcoidosis, milk-alkali syndrome, vitamin D intoxication, hyperthyroidism, acute adrenal insufficiency, and a rare disease, hypophosphatasia. Thiazides can produce a slight increase in serum calcium, and the widespread use of these drugs may increase significantly the number of mildly hypercalcemic subjects requiring diagnosis. In Paget's disease or osteoporosis, hypercalcemia may develop upon prolonged bed rest. Hypercalcemia may occur in malignancy as a consequence of one or more etiologic factors: osteolytic metastases causing hypercalcemia through local resorptive influence of the lesions in bone; production by the tumor of substances (e.g., prostaglandins) capable of inducing bone resorption and hypercalcemia ("pseudohyperparathyroidism"); production of an abnormal blood protein (which may explain hypercalcemia in some cases of multiple myeloma) which is capable of binding calcium, the increase in serum calcium being attributable simply to a higher concentration of bound calcium in the plasma compartment; or "ectopic" hyperparathyroidism, in which a nonparathyroid tumor produces parathyroid hormone itself. The last-named may be particularly difficult to diagnose, because the laboratory findings do not differ from those of hyperparathyroidism caused by parathyroid adenoma or hyperplasia; blood calcium is high, blood phosphate is low, and the alkaline phosphatase may be elevated. (Development of metabolic acidosis, however, seems to occur less frequently in ectopic than in primary hyperparathyroidism.) The "pseudohyperparathyroid" syndrome (production of a unique bone-resorbing humoral substance unrelated to parathyroid hormone) is also associated with hypophosphatemia, but there is no detectable parathyroid hormone by immunoassay either in the tumor or in plasma. The question of malignancy with hypercalcemia requires extensive studies to ascertain the true nature of the disease. Severe cases of true primary hyperparathyroidism may present particular diagnostic problems, because the disease itself can cause anemia, weight loss, debility, and increased erythrocyte sedimentation rate suggestive of malignant disease.

Paget's disease of bone, osteoporosis, osteomalacia, multiple myeloma, and malignancies metastatic to bone show varying degrees of skeletal demineralization. The roentgenographic appearance in each of these disorders, though, is more or less characteristic. In osteoporosis, the serum calcium, phosphate, and alkaline phosphatase are normal. Extensive Paget's disease is attended by an increase in serum alkaline phosphatase, but phosphate and calcium in blood are normal except during periods of immobilization, when hypercalcemia may develop. Examination of bone marrow is helpful in excluding multiple myeloma, and is occasionally of value in diagnosing lymphoma or metastatic malignancy. Analysis of plasma and urine for myeloma proteins should be routine in suspected cases. Osteomalacia may be caused by hypovitaminosis D, resistance to vitamin D, intestinal malabsorption syndromes, or renal tubular acidosis. In these conditions, serum calcium is normal or low, sometimes with tetany; blood phosphate is low; and the alkaline phosphatase is elevated. The differential diagnoses of hyperparathyroid bone disease (osteitis fibrosa cystica), osteomalacia, fibrous dysplasia of bone, Paget's disease, and osteoporosis are discussed also in Part XIX.

Secondary hyperparathyroidism in chronic renal dis-

ease may produce the histologic picture of osteitis fibrosa cystica. In general, serum phosphate is high and there is a tendency to hypocalcemia. Occasionally, however, primary hyperparathyroidism may become superimposed upon chronic renal failure. This complication becomes evident by an increase in serum calcium to the high normal or hypercalcemic range. In this event hyperplastic or adenomatous parathyroid glands should be removed surgically.

Development of nephrolithiasis with calcium phosphate or calcium oxalate stones, particularly when associated with hypercalciuria, requires clinical testing to rule out primary hyperparathyroidism. "Idiopathic hypercalciuria" with recurrent nephrolithiasis may be associated with hypophosphatemia, making the distinction more difficult. This category may still include some patients with bona fide hyperparathyroidism. Repeated tests of serum calcium are essential in reaching the correct conclusion. In some cases in which the diagnosis has been doubtful, hyperparathyroidism is obvious at the follow-up examination 6 to 12 months later.

Diagnostic Investigations. Hypercalcemia is almost always present in primary hyperparathyroidism. Indeed, hypercalcemia per se, detected in a general clinic population, can be attributed on chance alone to primary hyperparathyroidism in almost half the cases. Although malignancy is an equally common cause of hypercalcemia in the general population, hypercalcemia associated with hypophosphatemia and a long relatively benign clinical history makes the diagnosis of primary hyperparathyroidism more likely. In any one patient, though, particularly with an early or mild case, serial analyses may show fluctuations of serum calcium into the normal range. In rare instances hypomagnesemia or vitamin D deficiency may mask hyperparathyroidism. Correction of the magnesium or vitamin D deficiency in these cases allows the hypercalcemia to be expressed. In general, though, the finding of high serum calcium is the laboratory test most likely to lead to the diagnosis. Several further investigations based on assessing the secretion or actions of parathyroid hormone help establish the diagnosis.

Several tests have been based on the known physiologic action of parathyroid hormone in causing increased phosphate clearance (and decreased tubular reabsorption of phosphate, TRP). Although these procedures are constantly modified in attempts to obtain greater diagnostic accuracy, none offer sufficient specificity to be of regular clinical value.

Prednisone Suppression Test. Hypercalcemia in sarcoidosis or vitamin D intoxication is particularly amenable to correction with corticosteroid therapy; subjects with the milk-alkali syndrome may respond also. These observations form the basis of a test that is helpful in differentiating among several types of hypercalcemia. Usually either prednisone, 60 mg daily, or hydrocortisone, 120 mg daily, is given in divided doses for ten days. The hypercalcemia of hyperparathyroidism, ectopic or primary, almost invariably is resistant to the effects of this treatment. The response in other types of hypercalcemia is more variable. The milk-alkali syndrome and hypervitaminosis D both respond to withdrawal of the offending agents, and the hypercalcemia of sarcoidosis may respond to therapy with chloroquine. In general, the clinical, laboratory, and roentgenographic features cited under diagnosis of the particular disease should lead one to the proper diagnosis in the other disorders listed. Hypercalcemia in hyperthyroidism is best treated by correcting the hyperthyroid state. Hypercalcemia that persists in the euthyroid state suggests the coexistence of hyperparathyroidism.

Urinary Excretion of Cyclic AMP. Parathyroid hormone exerts its effects on target tissues by activating adenylate cyclase and causing thereby an increase in tissue concentration of cyclic 3′,5′-AMP. Part of the cyclic 3′,5′-AMP accumulating within renal cells in response to parathyroid hormone is excreted in the urine; this nephrogenous contribution to the urinary excretion of cyclic 3′,5′-AMP in man is approximately 40 to 50 per cent of the total excreted. In primary hyperparathyroidism the mean urinary excretion of 3′,5′-AMP is elevated, and conversely in hypoparathyroidism the rate of excretion is low. After surgical correction of hyperparathyroidism, the rate of excretion falls to normal; this is a reliable index of successful surgery. The ratio of cyclic AMP to creatinine in the urine in normal subjects is 1.3 to 4.2 (average 2.7) μmoles per gram of creatinine. In hyperparathyroid patients cyclic AMP excretion averages 5.2 (standard deviation 2.2) μmoles per gram of creatinine. Thus although there is a highly significant increase in excretion of the cyclic nucleotide in hyperparathyroidism, there is nevertheless considerable overlap with results for normal subjects. On the other hand, a high ratio of cyclic AMP to creatinine in the urine in association with clinical hypercalcemia is highly suggestive of hyperparathyroidism, primary or ectopic. Certain nonparathyroid cancers producing hypercalcemia are associated with low rates of cyclic AMP excretion, reflecting suppressed PTH secretion, and thus can be distinguished from hyperparathyroidism.

Radioimmunoassay for Parathyroid Hormone. Radioimmunoassays for parathyroid hormone have been developed in several laboratories, but radioimmunoassay alone, particularly in random peripheral plasma samples, does not afford an absolute diagnostic index for primary hyperparathyroidism. After the hormone is secreted from the gland, it undergoes degradation to fragments in the periphery. One of the principal fragments remaining is immunologically reactive but biologically inert. This fragment (derived from the carboxyl two thirds of the molecule) disappears relatively slowly from the circulation and accumulates to an even greater extent in chronic renal disease. Moreover, some antisera are relatively more reactive than others with the carboxyl terminus of the molecule. Thus results for radioimmunoassays in peripheral plasma samples vary from one laboratory to another simply on the basis of differences in antisera employed in the assay as well as differences in renal function in any particular patient. Nevertheless, in hyperparathyroidism, use of the assay usually shows abnormally high concentrations (particularly relative to calcium content of plasma) of hormone in the plasma. Hypercalcemia from causes unrelated to parathyroid hormone is associated with undetectable hormone in plasma. Moreover, the immunoassay is particularly applicable to studies on samples obtained by selective venous catheterization. Blood drawn directly from the thyroid veins contains hormone immediately as it is secreted and before it has undergone degradation in the periphery. This procedure allows preoperative localization of abnormal parathyroid tissue and helps establish the exact diagnosis before surgery. The diagnosis of primary hyperparathyroidism is definitive on laboratory grounds alone in any case in which each of the following criteria are fulfilled: (1) hypercalcemia, (2) normal or high concentration of parathyroid hormone in peripheral plasma, and (3) detection of a high concentration of parathyroid hormone in the venous system draining the thyroid bed.

High concentrations of hormone in peripheral plasma have been found also in cases of hyperparathyroidism resulting from ectopic production of hormone by nonparathyroid tumors as well as in secondary hyperparathyroidism and pseudohypoparathyroidism. The difficulty of precise analysis for parathyroid hormone in peripheral plasma will undoubtedly be lessened by developing assays more specific for the active form. Ultimately it is likely that the radioimmunoassay (or possibly a radioreceptor assay) will become the principal diagnostic test for hyperparathyroidism. In particular, measurement of the secretory responses to induced hypo- or hypercalcemia should provide definitive tests for the differential diagnosis of primary and secondary hyperparathyroidism.

Preoperative Localization of Abnormal Parathyroid Tissue. Several methods have been proposed for identification of parathyroid adenomas before surgery. Occasionally large glands have been identified simply on esophagography; other procedures that have been used include scanning with 75selenium-labeled methionine, intraoperative vital staining with toluidine blue, thermography, and arteriography (Fig. 3). None of these methods have been highly successful. The advent of the radioimmunoassay for parathyroid hormone, coupled with selective venous catheterization, has provided a means for more specific localization. Highly accurate localization of adenomas is possible when each of the

thyroid veins can be selectively catheterized. Radioimmunoassays on samples obtained through the catheter show high gradients of parathyroid hormone concentration in the particular veins draining the lesion. Parathyroid hyperplasia, on the other hand, is frequently associated with a significant hormone gradient in each of the superior and inferior thyroid veins. In cases requiring repeated surgery for hyperparathyroidism, selective venous catheterization should be considered strongly before undertaking a further operation. In such instances, arteriography should be carried out as well in an attempt to delineate the thyroid venous anatomy as well as to uncover lesions representing potential parathyroid tissue.

Prognosis. Untreated, hyperparathyroidism with significant hypercalcemia may cause progressive renal impairment and ultimately death. Occasionally severe hypercalcemia develops rapidly ("hyperparathyroid crisis") and causes an immediate threat to life. On the other hand, the disease may exist in mild form without symptoms, and it is probable that some patients in apparently excellent health harbor hyperfunctioning parathyroid adenomas for decades and die of unrelated causes.

Uncomplicated primary hyperparathyroidism is correctable definitively by surgery. Occasionally a second adenoma becomes apparent after initial resection was apparently successful. When primary hyperplasia of the parathyroid glands is the cause and insufficient tissue has been resected, recurrence of the disease will show itself by return of preoperative symptoms and signs.

Treatment. *Hypercalcemia* (from whatever cause) that is neither severe nor progressive requires treatment directed only toward correction of the underlying

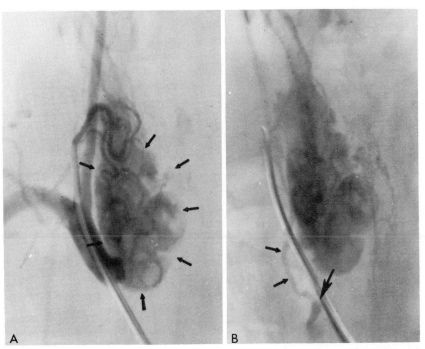

Figure 3. Arteriographic localization of large parathyroid adenoma. *A,* Arrows outline large parathyroid adenoma filled by radiographic dye injected into right inferior thyroid artery. This phase of the arteriographic study shows also a rich arterial vascular plexus within the gland. *B,* Late phase of arteriographic study, showing vein (delineated by arrows) draining the adenoma. Subsequent selective venous sampling showed a very high gradient for parathyroid hormone concentration at the point marked by the large arrow.

disease state. On the other hand, progressive and severe hypercalcemia *("hypercalcemic crisis")* leads to marked weakness, mental deterioration, coma, progressive uremia, and death within a short period. Several methods have been proposed for control of progressive hypercalcemia which may be so severe as to require emergency attention. Intravenous infusions of EDTA, sodium sulfate, or phosphate salts have been recommended, but each of these may produce hazardous side effects. Phosphate by mouth is effective in doses equal to those given intravenously, and there is probably less danger in this approach. Dehydration is often an important contributory factor in the development of progressive hypercalcemia and uremia. It is therefore important to restore extracellular fluids parenterally. Intravenous saline and furosemide are highly effective in reducing hypercalcemia. Sodium competes with calcium for reabsorption in the distal renal tubule, and furosemide potentiates this effect. Together furosemide and saline cause a marked increase in renal clearance of calcium and reduction of hypercalcemia.

One should also begin treatment with phosphate by mouth. For the first few days the equivalent of 2 grams of elemental phosphorus should be given in divided doses four times daily. Capsules can be prepared containing 190 mg of potassium dihydrogen phosphate plus 800 mg of disodium hydrogen phosphate. This provides 0.22 gram of elemental phosphorus per capsule. After three to five days when control of hypercalcemia has begun to be effective, the dosage of phosphorus should be reduced to 1 to 1.5 grams daily. Calcium, phosphate, and blood urea nitrogen should be monitored regularly to assure that the desired effect is obtained. It is best not to allow the blood phosphorus concentration to exceed 6 mg per 100 ml. Some patients with primary hyperparathyroidism have been maintained with nearly normal blood calcium for periods up to six months, pending clarification of other complications before parathyroidectomy. However, this form of treatment should be regarded as temporary; at the earliest possible moment, definitive therapy for the underlying disease should be instituted. Phosphate therapy may cause hypokalemia in these patients, requiring administration of potassium supplements. Calcitonin has not proved to be generally efficacious in controlling hypercalcemia.

Surgery is the only definitive treatment yet devised for primary hyperparathyroidism. In very mild cases it may be deferred, but only if frequent and regular observation of the patient is possible. It is the author's view that treatment should be deferred only so long as the patient is completely asymptomatic, can return for frequent evaluation, shows no clinical symptom or sign of the disease, and maintains a serum calcium concentration under 11.5 mg per 100 ml. Otherwise parathyroidectomy should be performed by a surgeon qualified by extensive experience. It is essential that the highest possible rate of success be obtained at the *initial* surgical procedure. As would be expected, multiple explorations for parathyroid adenomas carry increased risk and expense, as well as greater difficulty for the surgeon, particularly when scarring from earlier surgery is significant. One side of the neck should be searched meticulously first. If an obvious adenoma plus a normal gland is found on that side, the adenoma should be removed and the wound closed. This leaves the contralateral side undisturbed and suitable for ac-

curate exploration at a future time in the unlikely event this becomes necessary.

If the lesion is not found initially, the surgeon should extend the procedure to the contralateral side and should try to identify all four parathyroid glands, biopsying each for rapid histologic confirmation. Positive identification is important if subsequent surgical exploration becomes necessary and also provides for the possible existence of diffuse hyperplasia which is an indication for removal of seven eighths of all parathyroid tissue found. In rare instances there are more than four hyperplastic or adenomatous glands.

If neither hyperplastic nor adenomatous glands are found in the neck, a mediastinal exploration should be considered at a later date. Mediastinal tumors account for approximately 20 per cent of parathyroid adenomas; 95 per cent of them lie superiorly embedded in or attached to the mediastinal fat pad. As such, they are readily removable along with the fat pad through the routine neck incision. Thus only 1 per cent of all parathyroid adenomas should require a sternal splitting procedure. This conclusion is borne out by the observation that virtually all missed adenomas, discovered at subsequent surgical explorations, prove to be in the neck. Arteriography and selective venous catheterization (see Preoperative Localization, above) should be carried out before a second surgical procedure. The results of surgery can be assessed readily with serial analyses of serum calcium, and by following urinary excretion of cyclic $3',5'$-AMP, which decreases to normal after successful parathyroidectomy.

Postoperatively, tetany may be expected in patients who show significant bone disease. This may require treatment at intervals with 10 per cent calcium gluconate (10 to 30 ml in 500 to 1500 ml of saline) intravenously and administration of vitamin D, 50,000 units or more daily by mouth, until severe hypocalcemia shows signs of control. Adequate dietary intake of calcium (at least 1 gram daily) should be assured; if necessary, calcium lactate capsules should be given by mouth. Therapy should be withdrawn as rapidly as clinical progress allows. Almost invariably, remaining parathyroid tissue recovers normal function; definite signs of recovery are usual within seven to ten days. It is best to allow some degree of hypocalcemia during the recovery period as long as symptoms are controlled, because hypercalcemia would tend to inhibit recovery of remaining parathyroid tissue. Excessive therapy with calcium by vein or vitamin D by mouth is neither necessary nor desirable.

Other complications in the postoperative period include temporary worsening of renal function or metabolic acidosis (see above), hypomagnesemia, pancreatitis, and gout or pseudogout. The physician should be particularly alert to the potential for the last two of these in subjects with intra-articular calcification or history of prior attacks.

Albright, F., Aub, J. C., and Bauer, W.: Hyperparathyroidism. J.A.M.A., 102:1276, 1934.

Albright, F., and Reifenstein, E. C., Jr.: The Parathyroid Glands and Metabolic Bone Disease. Baltimore, Williams & Wilkins Company, 1948.

Aurbach, G. D., and Potts, J. T., Jr.: The parathyroids. *In* Levine, R., and Luft, R. (eds.): Advances in Metabolic Disorders. New York, Academic Press, 1964, p. 45.

Aurbach, G. D., Mallette, L. E., Patten, B. M., Heath, D. A., Doppman, J. L., and Bilezikian, J. P.: Hyperparathyroidism: Recent studies. Ann. Intern. Med., 79:566, 1973.

Berson, S. A., and Yalow, R. S.: Parathyroid hormone in plasma in adenomatous hyperparathyroidism, uremia, and bronchogenic carcinoma. Science, 154:907, 1966.

Berson, S. A., Yalow, R. S., Aurbach, G. D., and Potts, J. T., Jr.: Immunoassay of bovine and human parathyroid hormone. Proc. Natl. Acad. Sci. U.S.A., 49:613, 1963.

Bilezikian, J. P., Doppman, J. L., Shimkin, P. M., Powell, D., Wells, S. A., Heath, D. A., Ketcham, A. S., Monchik, J., Mallette, L. E., Potts, J. T., Jr., and Aurbach, G. D.: Preoperative localization of abnormal parathyroid tissue: Cumulative experience with venous sampling and arteriography. Am. J. Med., 55:505, 1973.

Boonstra, C. E., and Jackson, C. E.: Hyperparathyroidism detected by routine serum calcium analysis. Ann. Intern. Med., 63:468, 1965.

Dohan, P. H., Yamashita, K., Larsen, P. R., Davis, B., Deftos, L., and Field, J. B.: Evaluation of urinary cyclic 3',5'-adenosine monophosphate excretion in the differential diagnosis of hypercalcemia. J. Clin. Endocr., 35:775, 1972.

Goldsmith, R. S.: Differential diagnosis of hypercalcemia. N. Engl. J. Med., 274:674, 1966.

Goldsmith, R. S., and Ingbar, S. H.: Inorganic phosphate treatment of hypercalcemia of diverse etiologies. N. Engl. J. Med., 274:1, 1966.

Lafferty, F. W.: Pseudohyperparathyroidism. Medicine, 45:247, 1966.

Mallette, L. E., Bilezikian, J. P., Heath, D. A., and Aurbach, G. D.: Primary hyperparathyroidism: Clinical and biochemical features. Medicine, 53:127, 1974.

Marx, S. J., Powell, D., Shimkin, P. M., Wells, S. A., Ketcham, A. S., McGuigan, J. E., Bilezikian, J. P., and Aurbach, G. D.: Familial hyperparathyroidism: Mild hypercalcemia in at least nine members of a kindred. Ann. Intern. Med., 78:371, 1973.

Moldawer, M. P., Nardi, G. L., and Raker, J. W.: Concomitance of multiple adenomas of the parathyroids and pancreatic islets with tumor of the pituitary: A syndrome with familial incidence. Am. J. Med. Sci., 228:190, 1954.

Muldowney, F. P., Carroll, D. V., Donohoe, J. F., and Freaney, R.: Correction of renal bicarbonate wastage by parathyroidectomy. Quart. J. Med., 40:487, 1971.

Neelon, F. A., Birch, B. M., Drezner, M., and Lebovitz, H. E.: Urinary cyclic adenosine monophosphate as an aid in the diagnosis of hyperparathyroidism. Lancet, 1:631, 1973.

Patten, B. M., Bilezikian, J. P., Mallette, L. E., Prince, A., Engel, W. T., and Aurbach, G. D.: Neuromuscular disease of hyperparathyroidism. Ann. Intern. Med., 80:182, 1974.

Powell, D., Singer, F. R., Murray, T. M., Minkin, C., and Potts, J. T., Jr.: Nonparathyroid humoral hypercalcemia in patients with neoplastic diseases. N. Engl. J. Med., 289:176, 1973.

Segre, G. V., Habener, J. F., Powell, D., Tregear, G. W., and Potts, J. T., Jr.: Parathyroid hormone in human plasma. J. Clin. Invest., 51:3163, 1972.

Sherwood, L. M., O'Riordan, J. L. H., Aurbach, G. D., and Potts, J. T., Jr.: Production of parathyroid hormone by nonparathyroid tumors. J. Clin. Endocr., 27:140, 1967.

Wermer, P.: Endocrine adenomatosis and peptic ulcer in a large kindred. Inherited multiple tumors and mosaic pleiotropism in man. Am. J. Med., 35:205, 1963.

873. HYPOPARATHYROIDISM

Definition. Hypoparathyroidism is the syndrome characterized by deficient secretion of parathyroid hormone, with consequent hypocalcemia.

Etiology. In most instances hypoparathyroidism is the consequence of mechanical injury to or removal of parathyroid glands during surgery for primary thyroid disorders or occasionally parathyroid disorders. Idiopathic hypoparathyroidism is rare; approximately 100 cases are known. It is usually recognized in childhood or adolescence and, in distinction to pseudohypoparathyroidism, it may be associated with pernicious anemia, ovarian failure, moniliasis, or Addison's disease; it occurs with equal incidence in males and females, and rarely is familial.

Pathology. In postsurgical and most cases of idiopathic hypoparathyroidism there is complete absence of the parathyroid glands. There may be calcification in the basal ganglia and cataracts. The bones may be abnormally dense, and the calvarium may be thickened.

Idiopathic hypoparathyroidism may represent an autoimmune disease.

Pathologic Physiology and Chemistry. The physiologic consequences of insufficient secretion of parathyroid hormone are low blood calcium, high blood phosphate, and a low rate of phosphate clearance into the urine. Attendant upon hypocalcemia is a very low concentration of calcium in the urine. As a general rule, the clearance of calcium into the urine approaches zero as its concentration in blood falls below 7 mg per 100 ml.

Hypocalcemia in hypoparathyroidism is a manifestation of the reduced rate of bone resorption in the absence of sufficient parathyroid hormone. The diminished concentration of calcium in extracellular fluid leads to increased neuromuscular excitability and tetany. Hyperphosphatemia in this disorder is primarily attributable to lack of the hormone effect on phosphate clearance by the kidney. The rate of urinary excretion of 3',5'-AMP is reduced, but in distinction to pseudohypoparathyroidism there is a normal response to exogenous parathyroid hormone.

Clinical Manifestations. The principal symptoms of hypoparathyroidism are due to a low concentration of calcium in the extracellular fluid. Hypocalcemic tetany is manifested by numbness and tingling in the fingers and toes and around the lips, and sometimes by laryngeal stridor with "crowing" inspiration, dyspnea, and cyanosis. In severe tetany, cramps of individual muscle groups occur in the hands and feet as carpopedal spasms. The differential diagnosis of tetany is discussed below. There may also be convulsions or abdominal pain, nausea, and vomiting. Epileptiform attacks are a striking symptom of hypoparathyroidism. Usually the seizures are of a grand mal type, but they are not always preceded by aura, loss of consciousness, involuntary trauma, or incontinence. The electroencephalogram may show abnormalities typical of idiopathic epilepsy. The seizures and usually the abnormal electroencephalographic pattern associated with tetany respond to treatment with calcium, whereas the latter is without effect in idiopathic epilepsy. Sometimes seizures of the petit mal type are expressed. Other cases may display choreiform movements, and in general there is increased sensitivity in hypoparathyroidism to the dystonic reactions of phenothiazine drugs.

Mental abnormalities may occur in hypoparathyroidism. Irritability, emotional lability, moroseness, impairment of memory, mental confusion, lethargy, depression, and mental deficiency have been described.

Papilledema, sometimes associated with increased intracranial pressure, may also accompany the hypocalcemia of hypoparathyroidism. These manifestations as well as the electroencephalograms return to normal when hypocalcemia is corrected. Cataracts are a characteristic consequence of chronic hypoparathyroidism. Other forms of ectopic calcification may be exhibited in the basal ganglia or subcutaneous tissues. The calvarium may be thickened.

Patients with idiopathic hypoparathyroidism may display abnormalities of the ectodermal structures, including the teeth, skin, nails, and hair. A characteristic feature of hypoparathyroidism early in life is blunting of the roots of the teeth and dysplasia of the enamel. The nails may be malformed and brittle and show transverse grooves. In addition, there is a significant incidence of moniliasis in idiopathic hypoparathyroidism, and when this involves the nails they become pitted and flaky in appearance. The transverse grooves, but not moniliasis, disappear when the serum calcium is corrected toward normal. The hair is thin, there may be patchy alopecia, and the skin is sometimes coarse and dry.

Diagnosis. Complaints of numbness and tingling in the extremities and around the mouth should suggest tetany. "Latent" tetany may be detected by eliciting Chvostek's sign by tapping over the facial nerve. A positive response consists of twitching of the muscles about the mouth and sometimes the nose and eyelids. Trousseau's sign is sought by producing ischemia with a cuff inflated above systolic pressure for three minutes. Characteristically, carpal spasm becomes evident during the course of the test. In latent tetany one may find increased sensitivity to galvanic current in producing muscle contraction (Erb's sign). The electrocardiogram may show a prolonged Q-T interval as a consequence of hypocalcemia.

Patients with atypical epilepsy, other manifestations of increased neuromuscular irritability, or bizarre mental symptoms should be investigated for possible hypoparathyroidism. Obviously a history of prior thyroid surgery should alert one to this possibility. Tetany associated with Addison's disease, pernicious anemia, or moniliasis should immediately suggest a diagnosis of idiopathic hypoparathyroidism. Each of these diseases may be caused by or associated with autoimmunity. Autoantibodies to parathyroid as well as ovarian, thyroid, or gastric tissue have been detected in some of these cases.

Prognosis. Hypoparathyroidism that follows thyroid or parathyroid surgery may often be transient. One should try withdrawing therapy several months postoperatively in such cases before it is concluded that permanent hypoparathyroidism exists. The prognosis is excellent with full life expectancy in established cases adequately treated. Untreated, the subject with hypoparathyroidism may suffer the discomfort and morbidity of muscular spasms, convulsions, cataracts, and mental impairment. It is not certain that cataracts can be prevented in hypoparathyroidism by correction of hypocalcemia early in the course of the disease. Epileptiform seizures are generally alleviated as hypocalcemia is corrected.

Treatment. Acute hypocalcemic tetany requires treatment with intravenous calcium, for example, calcium gluconate, 10 per cent solution (10 to 30 ml in 500 to 1500 of saline) given as necessary to control the symptoms. At the same time vitamin D, 50,000 to 100,000 units daily by mouth, should be given. Adequate intake of at least 1 to 2 grams of calcium by mouth should be assured, and sometimes further supplementation with 15 grams of calcium lactate (equivalent to 2 grams of calcium) in divided doses is necessary. The amount of vitamin D and calcium should be gradually reduced as serum calcium approaches normal. Crystalline dihydrotachysterol may be used instead of vitamin D and is advantageous in cases of toxicity because it is cleared more rapidly from the body. The commercial preparation *A.T.-10* shows variable potency and is not recommended for therapy. In the absence of parathyroid hormone, vitamin D may cause an inordinately high rate of excretion of urinary calcium with the danger of nephrolithiasis. If regulation is difficult by reduction of calcium and vitamin D intake, the hypercalciuria may be controlled by giving phosphate

by mouth. Sulkowitch's test is not of value in the management of these patients; quantitative analyses for 24-hour excretion of calcium are required.

874. PSEUDO-HYPOPARATHYROIDISM AND PSEUDOPSEUDO-HYPOPARATHYROIDISM

Definition. *Pseudohypoparathyroidism* is a clinical state of hypoparathyroidism characterized by normal secretion of hormone from the parathyroid glands, but with a genetic defect in the receptor tissues so that there is little or no response to the action of the hormone. The defect is transmitted as a sex-linked dominant trait, and is associated with characteristic abnormalities of physiognomy and growth. The genetically related disorder *pseudopseudohypoparathyroidism* (see below) represents an incomplete form of the syndrome, shows the constitutional features without the chemical findings of hypoparathyroidism, and may occur in the same families with pseudohypoparathyroidism.

Etiology and Genetics. Recent clinical investigations in this disorder as well as current studies on the mechanism of action of parathyroid hormone have shed light on the pathophysiology in this syndrome. The original hypothesis of Albright and his associates that the receptor tissues, bone, and kidney are unresponsive to parathyroid hormone still best accounts for the endocrinopathology of this disorder. Other hypotheses such as secretion of a biologically inactive form of parathyroid hormone, circulating antibodies to the hormone, or secretion of excessive amounts of calcitonin have been tested without substantiation. The direct action of parathyroid hormone on the kidney is reflected in the urinary excretion of cyclic 3',5'-AMP. Normal subjects show a marked increase in excretion of the nucleotide after injection of parathyroid hormone. Pseudohypoparathyroidism is characterized by a defective response to exogenous parathyroid hormone in terms of urinary excretion of 3',5'-AMP. The most reasonable interpretation of this finding, and the probable explanation for the disorder, is the genetic transmission of defective or deficient receptor–adenylate cyclase complex in the renal cortex and perhaps bone of those subjects.* These subjects, when hypocalcemic, secrete parathyroid hormone at increased rates reflected in high concentrations of the hormone in peripheral plasma. The secretory rate responds normally, though, to blood calcium.

The genetics of the disorder is currently best explained by a sex-linked dominant mode of inheritance. The sex incidence ratio is female to male 2:1; no instances of male-to-male transmission of the complete syndrome have been documented with biochemical test-

---

*It is possible that the defect does not involve the receptor itself or the enzyme adenylate cyclase. In one instance, the only case in which adenylate cyclase from renal tissue was tested directly, there appeared to be a normal in vitro response to parathyroid hormone. Other biochemical abnormalities, such as defective nucleotide or phospholipid regulatory site on the enzyme or a defect distal to generation of cyclic nucleotide, have not been excluded. However, these patients respond normally to exogenous dibutyryl cyclic 3',5'-AMP, and thus it seems that the metabolic defect must be at a site prior to formation of cyclic 3',5'-AMP.

ing. Possibly the short stature characteristic of the syndrome is also attributable to an abnormal X chromosome. Genetic studies of sex-linked disorders indicate that in order to achieve normal height two functional sex chromosomes are required; that is, both the X chromosomes in females or both X and Y in males must be normal in the segments controlling growth. Pseudopseudohypoparathyroidism, in females at least, may reflect genetic mosaicism with a relatively greater degree of inactivation of the abnormal X chromosome.

Incidence. Pseudohypoparathyroidism and its incomplete variant pseudopseudohypoparathyroidism are rare. The average case is recognized earlier in life than is idiopathic hypoparathyroidism. Approximately 100 cases of pseudohypoparathyroidism and still fewer cases of the variant have been reported.

Pathology. The parathyroid glands are normal or hyperplastic. Shortening of the carpal and metatarsal bones and metastatic calcification, including calcification of the basal ganglia, occur. Also, there may be thickening of the calvarium, defective enamel of the teeth, dental aplasia, coxa vara, coxa valga, and bowing of the long bones. Cataracts are common.

Pathologic Physiology and Chemistry. The clinical chemical findings, hypocalcemia, hyperphosphatemia, and a low urinary calcium, are qualitatively similar but sometimes milder than those found in idiopathic or postoperative hypoparathyroidism. However, in pseudohypoparathyroidism, biologically active hormone under normal secretory control is elaborated from the parathyroid glands, but the receptor tissues do not respond. Exogenously administered parathyroid hormone causes little or no effect. Other endocrinopathies may coexist. Hypothyroidism (particularly that caused by selective pituitary TSH deficiency), diabetes mellitus, hypomenorrhea, or gonadal dysgenesis may be found associated with pseudohypoparathyroidism. Conversely, moniliasis, Addison's disease, and pernicious anemia, which may be associated with idiopathic hypoparathyroidism, have not been found in cases of pseudohypoparathyroidism.

Clinical Manifestations. The symptoms and signs of pseudohypoparathyroidism encompass those of hypoparathyroidism plus certain unique abnormalities of physiognomy and growth. Mental retardation, short, stocky, obese stature, and round facies are characteristic. The hands and feet are usually disproportionately short, resulting in about 75 per cent of cases from shortening of one or more metacarpal and metatarsal bones. This is readily recognized when the fist is clenched, thereby causing a dimple over the head of the affected bone. Less frequently, shortening of the phalanges or uniform brachydactyly may occur. The calvarium is thickened in over one third of the patients. There may be delayed dentition, defective enamel, or complete dental aplasia. Less common defects include abnormally dense or lucent bones, exostoses, coxa vara, coxa valga, bowing of the ulna, radius, tibia, and fibula, and loss of "tubulation" of the long bones. Calcification occurs in the basal ganglia and in the dentate nucleus, and there may be actual ossification as well as calcification in the skin, subcutaneous tissue, and deep connective tissues. Cataracts are also common. Most cases of true pseudohypoparathyroidism show the abnormalities of physiognomy and growth originally described by Albright and his associates.

Diagnosis. The diagnosis is established by the characteristic constitutional changes, by the clinical and laboratory abnormalities of hypoparathyroidism, and by testing the response to purified parathyroid hormone or parathyroid extract given intravenously. The earlier test for pseudohypoparathyroidism based on measurement of urinary phosphate excretion did not allow clear-cut separation of pseudohypoparathyroidism from normal subjects who vary widely in response; determination of 3',5'-AMP in the urine affords virtually complete differentiation between the two groups. Normal subjects, but not those with pseudohypoparathyroidism, show a marked rise (to give 3',5'-AMP-to-creatinine ratios greater than 15 μmoles per gram) in the rate of excretion of urinary 3',5'-AMP within 15 to 45 minutes after injection of 200 U.S.P. units of parathyroid hormone intravenously. There is no overlap of results between normal subjects and those with the disease. Baseline excretion of cyclic AMP is lower than normal in patients with idiopathic, postsurgical, and pseudohypoparathyroidism, but higher than normal in pseudopseudohypoparathyroidism. The last-named group comprises patients with the physiognomy of pseudohypoparathyroidism but a normal response to parathyroid hormone. Parathyroid hormone in peripheral plasma is high (as long as hypocalcemia is not corrected) in pseudohypoparathyroidism, in contrast to other forms of hypoparathyroidism in which it is undetectable. Some patients previously categorized as having pseudohypoparathyroidism associated with intestinal malabsorption syndromes, osteitis fibrosa cystica, or both, should be re-examined with the newer diagnostic procedures. It is the author's view that opinions should be deferred pending further tests before accepting a patient with atypical family history or clinical findings as a true example of pseudohypoparathyroidism.

Treatment. In general the treatment of pseudohypoparathyroidism is the same as that of hypoparathyroidism. Usually hypocalcemia is easier to control in pseudohypoparathyroidism, although occasional patients seem relatively resistant to vitamin D and require unusually high doses to achieve normal blood calcium.

875. TETANY

Tetany may develop in hypocalcemia, alkalosis, potassium deficiency, and occasionally hypomagnesemia. The symptoms and signs of tetany are discussed in Ch. 873. In addition to the information obtained by clinical examination, the laboratory findings are particularly important in diagnosing the cause of tetany. In hypoparathyroidism the serum phosphate is high, whereas in the hypocalcemic states of rickets or osteomalacia serum phosphate may be below normal. Urinary calcium is low in all these states. Tetany caused by alkalosis is associated with normal serum phosphate and calcium and normal urinary excretion of calcium, but the blood pH is high. Alkalotic tetany may occur in hyperventilation, usually a manifestation of psychoneurosis, and can be corrected by inducing the patient to reduce the respiratory rate or breathe into a paper bag.

Metabolic alkalosis, caused by persistent vomiting, hypokalemic alkalosis, or excessive treatment with alkali, may also produce tetany. In excessive treatment with alkali, the serum calcium and phosphate are normal as long as there is no renal impairment, but the serum pH is high. Tetany is produced by overcorrection

Differential Diagnosis of Tetany

Cause	Serum			Urine	
	Ca	P_i	pH	Ca	pH
Hypocalcemia					
Hypovitaminosis D		↓	N		—
Resistance to	N or ↓	↓	N		—
vitamin D		↓	N		—
Intestinal					
malabsorption					
Hypoparathyroidism		↓	↑	N	—
Hypomagnesemia	N or ↓	N or ↑	N	N or ↓	—
Alkalosis					
Respiratory	N	N	↑	N	
Metabolic	N	N	↑	N	

Ca = Calcium. P_i = Phosphate. N = Normal. (−) = Indeterminate.
↑ = High. ↓ = Low.

of acidosis in chronic renal disease. In such a condition, there is a tendency to hypocalcemia as well as hyperphosphatemia. In respiratory alkalosis plasma bicarbonate is low or normal, whereas in metabolic alkalosis plasma bicarbonate is high. The history should suggest the appropriate diagnosis in cases of excessive intake of alkali or excessive loss of gastric acid. The diagnosis is supported by finding a high concentration of bicarbonate in the serum and an alkaline urine. Treatment is directed at checking the cause. Hypokalemic alkalosis may appear in primary aldosteronism or treatment with corticosteroid analogues, and calls for correction of hormone excess and repletion of body potassium. Neonatal hypocalcemia may occur after asphyxia in premature infants, or in the progeny of diabetic or hyperparathyroid mothers. This last is a transient phenomenon secondary to hypercalcemia attendant upon primary hyperparathyroidism in the mother. Hypomagnesemia is a rare cause of tetany refractory to treatment with calcium; magnesium deficiency in those instances should be corrected.

Albright, F., Burnett, C. H., Smith, P. H., and Parson, W.: Pseudohypoparathyroidism—an example of the "Seabright-Bantam syndrome." Endocrinology, 30:922, 1942.

Aurbach, G. D., and Potts, J. T., Jr.: The parathyroids. In Levine, R., and Luft, R. (eds.): Advances in Metabolic Disorders. New York, Academic Press, 1964, p. 45.

Bell, N. H., Avery, S., Sinha, T., Clark, C. M., Jr., Allen, D. O., and Johnston, C., Jr.: Effects of dibutyryl cyclic adenosine 3',5'-monophosphate and parathyroid extract on calcium and phosphorus metabolism in hypoparathyroidism and pseudohypoparathyroidism. J. Clin. Invest., 51:816, 1972.

Blizzard, R. M., Chee, D., and Davis, W.: The incidence of parathyroid and other antibodies in the sera of patients with idiopathic hypoparathyroidism. Clin. Exp. Immunol., 1:119, 1966.

Bronsky, D., Kushner, D. S., Dubin, A., and Snapper, I.: Idiopathic hypoparathyroidism and pseudohypoparathyroidism: Case reports and review of the literature. Medicine, 37:317, 1958.

Chase, L. R., Melson, G. L., and Aurbach, G. D.: Pseudohypoparathyroidism: Defective excretion of 3',5'-AMP in response to parathyroid hormone. J. Clin. Invest., 48:1832, 1969.

Harrison, H. E., Lifshitz, F., and Blizzard, R. M.: Comparison between crystalline dihydrotachysterol and calciferol in patients requiring pharmacologic vitamin D therapy. N. Engl. J. Med., 276:894, 1967.

Tashjian, A. H., Jr., Frantz, A. G., and Lee, J. B.: Pseudohypoparathyroidism: Assays of parathyroid hormone and thyrocalcitonin. Proc. Natl. Acad. Sci. U.S.A., 56:1138, 1966.

876. CALCITONIN AND MEDULLARY CARCINOMA OF THE THYROID

Medullary carcinoma of the thyroid (see also Ch. 843) arises from the parafollicular cells of the thyroid which derive embryologically from the final or ultimobranchial cleft. These particular cells of the ultimobranchial cleft may, like chromaffin tissue, take origin initially in the neural crest. In submammalian vertebrates the ultimobranchial cells remain separate as the ultimobranchial gland, whereas in mammals the anlage merges with the embryological thyroid, In either instance, the cells derived from the ultimobranchial cells constitute the gland that synthesizes and secretes calcitonin. Medullary carcinoma may be sporadic or familial and is part of a syndrome (the so-called "multiple endocrine adenomatosis, type 2") encompassing hyperplasia or adenoma of the parathyroid glands, sometimes expressed as primary hyperparathyroidism, pheochromocytoma, multiple neuromas, and Cushing's syndrome. Abnormally high concentrations of calcitonin are found in medullary thyroid tumors as well as in plasma taken from these patients.

Incidence. Medullary carcinoma of the thyroid accounts for 5 to 10 per cent of the cases of thyroid cancer. In the familial form it follows the autosomal dominant form of inheritance.

Pathology. Histologically this tumor differs from other cancers of the thyroid in that the cells resemble parafollicular cells, there is often amyloid infiltration, and there are no papillary folds, follicles, or polymorphonuclear infiltrates in the tissue. (Sometimes artifacts of fixation look like papillary folds in sections.) The tumor usually does not appear to be encapsulated, and may show areas of calcification. The tissue does not take up radioactive iodine. As noted above, pheochromocytoma or parathyroid hyperplasia or adenoma may be associated with medullary carcinoma of the thyroid.

Pathologic Physiology. Although many of these tumors elaborate calcitonin at a high rate, hypocalcemia is unusual, perhaps because parathyroid hormone is secreted as a compensatory mechanism (secondary hyperparathyroidism). Moreover, as stated above, there may be frequent occurrence of primary hyperparathyroidism in the syndrome. It is possible that the development of primary hyperparathyroidism represents induced autonomy in the glands as a consequence of prolonged chronic secondary hyperparathyroidism. On the other hand, calcitonin, at least under experimental conditions, can directly stimulate secretion of parathyroid hormone; hyperparathyroidism might thus arise as a consequence of prolonged effects of calcitonin acting as a secretagogue. The concentration of histaminase in serum frequently is increased in metastatic medullary carcinoma.

Measurements by radioimmunoassay or bioassay show that hypercalcemia induces secretion of calcitonin from normal parafollicular cells as well as from medullary carcinoma tissue. In addition, glucagon or gastrin, injected intravenously in pharmacologic doses, causes secretion of calcitonin in some species as well as in patients with medullary carcinoma. These responses to calcium, glucagon, or gastrin are valuable in conjunction with radioimmunoassay as diagnostic tests for the syndrome. Completely asymptomatic cases in the familial syndrome have been detected by this means. Indeed, thyroid C-cell "hyperplasia" has been discovered in some family members showing abnormal secretory responses to calcium.

Clinical Manifestations, Prognosis, and Treatment. Medullary carcinoma may become evident simply as a mass in the thyroid or by the clinical expression of the associated endocrinopathies, pheochromocytoma, primary hyperparathyroidism, or Cushing's syndrome. The tumor, local or metastatic, may be hard or tender, and sometimes is calcified to a degree detectable by x-ray. Severe diarrhea may occur, possibly related to elaboration by the tumor of prostaglandins, serotonin, or calcitonin, any of which can stimulate intestinal secretion. Other conditions occasionally associated with the syndrome include buccal or orbital neuromas, peculiar facies, megacolon, or Marfan's syndrome–like habitus. Medullated nerves in the cornea are detected in some cases on slit lamp examination. The tumor often spreads locally, and metastases may grow to huge size. There is not yet sufficient experience to project the natural clinical course in this disorder. The tumor is refractory to treatment with radioactive iodine or antithyroid drugs, and usually to external radiation as well. At this time surgery represents the best approach, and should consist of wide excision, avoiding local seeding with tumor fragments. Isolated metastases may also be amenable to surgery. Persistent high concentrations of calcitonin in plasma reflect residual unresected tumor or metastases.

Aurbach, G. D., Potts, J. T., Jr., Chase, L. R., and Melson, G. L.: Polypeptide hormones and calcium metabolism. Ann. Intern. Med., 70:1243, 1969.

Cunliffe, W. J., Black, M. M., Hall, R., Johnston, I. D. A., Hudgson, P., Shuster, S., Gudmundsson, T. V., Joplin, G. F., Williams, E. D., Woodhouse, N. J. Y., Galante, L., and MacIntyre, I.: A calcitonin-secreting thyroid carcinoma. Lancet, 2:63, 1968.

Foster, G. V.: Calcitonin (thyrocalcitonin). N. Engl. J. Med., 279:349, 1968.

Hazard, J. B., Hawk, W. A., and Crile, G., Jr.: Medullary (solid) carcinoma of the thyroid—a clinicopathologic entity. J. Clin. Endocr., 19:152, 1959.

Hennessy, J. F., Gray, T. K., Cooper, C. W., and Ontjes, D. A.: Stimulation of thyrocalcitonin secretion by pentagastrin and calcium in two patients with medullary carcinoma of the thyroid. J. Clin. Endocrinol. Metab., 36:200, 1973.

Keiser, H. R., Beaven, M. A., Doppman, J., Wells, S., Jr., and Buja, M.: Sipple's syndrome: Medullary thyroid carcinoma, pheochromocytoma and parathyroid disease: Studies in a large family. Ann. Intern. Med., 78:561, 1973.

Melvin, K. E. W., Tashjian, A. H., Jr., and Miller, H. H.: Studies in familial (medullary) thyroid carcinoma. Recent Prog. Horm. Res., 28:399, 1972.

Steiner, A. L., Goodman, A. D., and Powers, S. R.: Study of a kindred with pheochromocytoma, medullary thyroid carcinoma, hyperparathyroidism and Cushing's disease: Multiple endocrine neoplasia, type 2. Medicine, 47:371, 1968.

Tashjian, A. H., Jr., and Melvin, K. E. W.: Medullary carcinoma of the thyroid gland: Studies of thyrocalcitonin in plasma and tumor extracts. N. Engl. J. Med., 279:279, 1968.

Tubiana, M., Milhaud, G., Coutris, G., Lacour, J., Parmentier, C., and Bok, B.: Medullary carcinoma and thyrocalcitonin. Br. Med. J., 4:87, 1968.

Wolfe, H. J., Melvin, K. E. W., Cervi-Skinner, S. J., Saadi, A. A., Juliar, J. F., Jackson, C. E., and Tashjian, A. H., Jr.: C-cell hyperplasia preceding medullary thyroid carcinoma. N. Engl. J. Med., 289:437, 1973.

877. MEDICAL TREATMENT OF HORMONE-DEPENDENT CANCERS

Philip K. Bondy

INTRODUCTION

It is always best to cure a malignant tumor by local excision, destruction with radiation, or both. However, if the tumor has already metastasized, local treatment alone is of course inadequate, and attempts to slow down the growth rate or eradicate the tumor require systemic therapy. The factors controlling tumor growth are not clear, but in some instances the endocrine environment may be important. In general, endocrine manipulations are most useful in tumors of hormone-sensitive organs, e.g., breast and prostate.

The application of endocrine treatment should not be considered as separate from the use of other modalities but should be part of an integrated approach, including surgery, radiotherapy, and chemotherapy as well. Thus the best results are obtained when treatment is planned from the beginning by an experienced team of people who are familiar with current knowledge and are constantly evaluating those results. There is no place for the lone entrepreneur in modern cancer treatment.

CANCER OF THE BREAST

This is a very common disease (incidence about 70 per 100,000 women per year; prevalence about 100 per 100,000 women per year). Incidence is higher in certain families and in childless women, and is reduced by early pregnancy. It is bilateral in 4 to 10 per cent of women when first seen, suggesting a multicentric origin. In spite of this, early diagnosis is desirable and regular examination should be carried out, especially in childless women over 30 years old, when family history is positive, or when a previous breast cancer has occurred. Diagnosis should be confirmed histologically. The prognosis is somewhat better in well-differentiated tumors, or when there are extreme lymphocyte infiltration and lymph node histiocytosis.

Treatment. The first step in designing treatment is to determine accurately the *distribution* of the tumor. Local disease is usually treated by surgery, supplemented by radiation if local lymph nodes are involved. If the primary tumor is too large for safe surgical treatment, radiation (sometimes followed by local surgery) is proper initial treatment. This local approach cannot be defended (except for palliation of painful or ulcerated masses) if there is evidence of distant dissemination. All patients should therefore have a skeletal roentgenographic survey, chest x-ray, and bone scan before surgery is planned. Further, it appears that the urinary excretion of more than 40 mg of hydroxyproline per gram of creatinine may indicate the presence of skeletal metastases. Elevation of the serum concentration of carcinoembryonic antigen suggests the presence of metastases, but a normal level does not exclude them.

Decisions about the type of surgery to perform and whether or not to irradiate the breast and nodes prophylactically are beyond the scope of this chapter (see textbooks of surgery). The design of medical treatment of inoperable or disseminated cancer rests on at least the following four factors:

Status of Ovarian Function. Castration is associated with tumor regression in about one third of premenopausal patients, whereas postmenopausal patients most commonly respond to the administration of estrogen. Cessation of menstrual flow is not by itself a safe guide, however. Many women continue to secrete estrogens for some time after their menses stop, and amenorrhea in younger women is not necessarily associated with depressed ovarian function. Thus if the estrogen levels of urine or plasma remain high, such women should be considered "premenopausal" even though they no longer have menstrual flow. Demonstration of a high plasma level of follicle-stimulating hormone (FSH) in perimenopausal or amenorrheic women may prove to be the best method for establishing the presence of true menopause.

Sensitivity of the Tumor to Hormones. Clinically, this must be determined chiefly by assessing the effects of castration or administration of hormones, although there is good evidence that tumors which lack in their cytoplasm the protein which binds estrogen are unlikely to respond to hormonal manipulation. Clinical response is definite only when tumor masses shrink in volume by 50 per cent or more. Symptomatic improvement without objective change is a treacherous criterion. Changes in urinary hydroxyproline or plasma carcinoembryonic antigen can usually be trusted as indicators; more specific indices are needed.

Disease-Free Interval after Excision. The outlook is better if this is more than two years.

Distribution of the Metastases. Involvement of soft tissues, for example, tends to respond to estrogens in postmenopausal women, whereas bone involvement is more responsive to androgens and chemotherapy. Local skin metastases in postmenopausal women respond to norethisterone more often than to any other endocrine treatment.

A general plan of treatment like that shown in the accompanying figure provides a consistent approach to treatment. Although experts may differ in details, the pattern outlined is widely accepted. Several points deserve comment.

1. *Prophylactic castration* is not recommended. It provides some extension of the disease-free interval but no prolongation of life. On the other hand, castration before recurrence interferes with evaluation of the response to ovarian ablation. Since this response determines the probability of subsequent response to endocrine treatment, a good deal of assurance is lost in the design of subsequent treatment schedules if early oophorectomy is carried out.

2. The *method of oophorectomy* is unimportant; surgery provides a quicker response than x-ray castration, at the expense of an additional operation. If the patient is desperately ill, surgery is probably preferable. Otherwise, some clinicians prefer irradiation.

3. *Chemotherapy* is seen in this scheme as a last resort. Usually, *successful* endocrine treatment provides longer remissions than chemotherapy; but the possibility of combining chemotherapy with endocrine treatment has not yet been adequately explored. It has been the writer's practice to combine quadruple chemotherapy (see below) with the appropriate endocrine manipulation from the very beginning in patients with a bad prognosis, i.e., those with a short disease-free interval or with extensive involvement of the viscera.

4. Success of *hypophysectomy* depends on the completeness of excision. In some instances, prolactin secretion has persisted even when growth hormone secretion has been abolished. In such patients, therapeutic failure may occur. This would indicate incompleteness of the operation. After hypophysectomy, the plasma prolactin level should be monitored for a year or more before it is decided that complete excision has taken place. The effect of removing prolactin cannot be evaluated unless it is known that the hormone is totally absent.

5. The postoperative treatment of patients lacking adrenals or pituitaries is discussed in Ch. 836 and 841.

There is much interest now in the possibility of controlling growth of breast cancers by suppressing *pituitary prolactin* secretion pharmacologically. At present, the only drug approved for use in the United States which has this effect is L-dopa, but its effects are too transient to make it practical. Preliminary reports

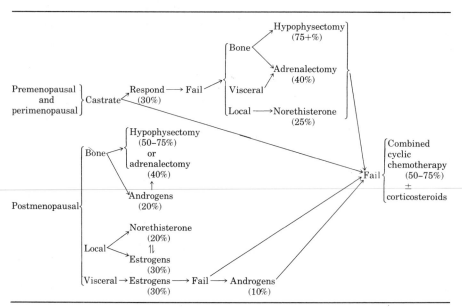

A generally accepted flow sheet for treating advanced cancer of the breast. The percentage figures represent the expected response of the group of patients receiving the treatment indicated above it. Thus hypophysectomy would be expected to produce about 75 per cent improvement in the premenopausal group which had responded to castration previously. In some clinics chemotherapy is given very early, along with or preceding endocrine treatment (see text). No mention is included of techniques which have not yet been adequately evaluated, e.g., anti-estrogens and pharmacologic suppression of prolactin secretion.

suggest that, in rare instances, it may reduce the growth rate of mammary tumors if given in maximal tolerated doses four or more times daily. Other drugs under preliminary investigation include the ergocornine and ergocryptine groups and some of their derivatives. As this is written, their use is not yet approved by the Food and Drug Administration. They are much more effective in animals than is L-dopa, and they may prove useful in the future.

Most textbooks state that cancer of the breast is unresponsive to *chemotherapy*, but this is incorrect. At least half the patients have a useful response to properly designed chemotherapy, although duration of the response may not be more than a few months. On the other hand, there is probably no hope of producing a cure of disseminated cancer with endocrine manipulations, whereas the possibility exists that cure might be achieved if the right pattern of chemotherapy could be found. Thus experiments to design effective treatment schedules are of great importance.

This approach to treatment may be used under several circumstances. A clinical trial is now in progress in the United States to determine whether *prophylactic administration* of phenylalanine mustard (Melphalan) to patients with extensive lymph node involvement will reduce the incidence or defer the development of metastases. Early reports suggest that metastases appear less frequently after this treatment than in controls.

Most oncologists agree that chemotherapy should be given to patients who have never responded to endocrine treatment, or who have escaped from an earlier response. Since one fourth to one third of tumors respond to alkylating agents, methotrexate, vinca alkaloids, or 5-fluorouracil, a combination of all four is often used. The writer's group has given cyclophosphamide, 500 mg, 5-fluorouracil, 500 mg, methotrexate, 50 mg, and vincristine, 2 mg, by a series of single injections one after another in the order listed, over a few minutes, repeating treatment every three weeks, provided that the blood count is satisfactory. This is a safe program, but it is probably less effective when compared with Edelstyn's schedule which spreads equivalent treatment over five days. Prolonging the duration of each treatment for five days increases the danger of bone marrow depression, however. New schedules including adriamycin are now being studied.

A few oncologists believe that treatment with chemotherapeutic agents should begin as soon as a diagnosis of dissemination has been made. Some (like Edelstyn) believe that chemotherapy should precede and supersede endocrine treatment. Others, including the author, feel that the two should be integrated. Further experience is needed.

Prognosis. In those women who respond, the mean duration of improvement after castration is about a year, and the maximum is several years. Response is more likely after a long disease-free interval and in patients with bone metastases. Patients younger than 35 may respond less often.

Estrogen treatment is about twice as likely to be effective as androgen in the postmenopausal woman. Androgens present few complications aside from masculinization; this is minimized by using one of the synthetic steroids, e.g., nandrolone.

A curious but useful effect is sometimes seen when endocrine treatment is discontinued after the patient has escaped from its effects. Withdrawal of treatment sometimes results in a second regression; but when the tumor resumes its growth a third regression can rarely be produced by resuming the original hormonal treatment.

Complications of Hormonal Treatment. Any endocrine treatment may cause a sudden, life-threatening rise of serum calcium, especially in patients with many lytic deposits in bone. This is combated by stopping treatment and by generous hydration; oral prednisolone, 10 mg four times daily, or cortisol, 100 mg intravenously every six hours. Mithramycin, 25 μg per kilogram intravenously at 48-hour intervals for not more than three doses, will safely reduce the serum calcium if these measures fail. The risk of hypercalcemia may be minimized by starting estrogen treatment at low doses (0.1 mg of diethylstilbestrol) for one to two weeks. Even a single course of quadruple chemotherapy usually restores the serum calcium value to normal, even though estrogen treatment is continued. If treatment is successful, rapid healing of osteolytic areas may cause hypocalcemia; this requires treatment with intravenous calcium salts and oral vitamin D until the rate of recalcification slackens off.

Large doses of diethylstilbestrol often cause nausea and vomiting. Conjugated mixed estrogens (Premarin) cause fewer gastrointestinal disturbances if they are given first in oral doses of 2.5 to 5 mg daily. Patients usually tolerate diethylstilbestrol after a week or so in doses of 0.5 mg thrice daily. There is rarely an advantage to larger doses.

Continuous administration of estrogens may cause breakthrough uterine bleeding, but this is unusual. If it occurs, cyclic courses are advisable. Edema may occur during estrogen treatment, and can be managed by diuretics. Increased pigmentation often occurs and is harmless. Thrombophlebitis may be a serious hazard, but whether the danger outweighs the advantage of treatment is not yet known.

In addition to these methods of treatment, radiation should always be available, to toleration, for relief of bone pain or of brain metastases. Proper support of the psyche, nutrition, and bone marrow should be provided.

Cancer of the Breast in Males. Malignant breast tumors are very rare in men; but when they occur they are usually much more aggressively malignant than in women. The same principles apply for treating the disease in men as in women, except that castration is generally considered to be an essential part of treatment regardless of age.

CANCER OF THE PROSTATE

This is a very common tumor, affecting between 14 and 46 per cent of all adult males in various autopsy series, but in most instances the tumor is localized and not of clinical significance. About 36 per 100,000 population have clinically significant tumor. In the United States there are about 17,000 deaths and 25,000 new cases per year. About 50 per cent of the clinically important cases can be diagnosed on rectal examination; the remainder are recognized from histologic examination of tissue removed at prostatectomy for benign prostatic hypertrophy. Once the diagnosis is suspected, histologic confirmation is essential, either by prostatectomy or by needle biopsy of suspicious nodules. After the diagnosis is established, the stage of the tumor's growth should be established.

Four stages are generally recognized:

1. Entirely intraprostatic, and too small to be suspected by physical examination or clinical laboratory methods.

2. Apparent on physical examination, but entirely confined to the prostate.

3. Confined to the pelvis. Here the tumor may have spread to other tissues in the pelvis but has not yet metastasized to distant points or bone.

In stages 1, 2, and 3, acid and alkaline phosphatase levels are not elevated in the serum, and skeletal x-ray, lymphogram and isotope scanning of bone are negative. In these stages, there is hope of cure by surgery, radiation therapy, or both combined.

4. Distant metastases. Serum acid phosphatase is elevated in about two thirds of these patients. In those with skeletal metastases diagnosed by skeletal x-rays or bone scan, the alkaline phosphatase may also be elevated. These patients can no longer be cured by local treatment.

Treatment. The principles applicable to treating cancer of the breast are also appropriate for prostatic carcinoma. So long as the tumor is localized, every reasonable effort should be exerted to cure the tumor by surgery, radiation, or both. Chemotherapy or hormonal manipulations should be considered only when local methods are no longer applicable. By the same reasoning, local treatment should not be pushed beyond palliative levels if evidence of distant spread is already available. Careful staging is therefore essential before a decision about appropriate treatment can be made.

Since growth of prostatic cells is dependent on the presence of androgens, it was reasonable for Huggins and his colleagues to try the effects of *castration* on the growth of prostatic tumors (1941). About 80 per cent of cases respond to androgen deprivation by reduced bone pain and size of the tumor masses. In some cases, skeletal metastases may begin to show radiographic evidence of healing. In almost all, the elevated acid phosphatase drops somewhat, but this is an unreliable index of overall response of the tumor, because tumor cells produce less acid phosphatase, even though they may not die, when androgenic stimulation is removed.

Since castration has unpalatable emotional connotations even for aged men, administration of *estrogens* has sometimes been substituted for orchidectomy, with comparable symptomatic results. The dose schedule is much the same as for tumors of the breast. Some patients respond to estrogens after response to castration has disappeared. In spite of this, there is no evidence that castration, estrogens, or both together actually prolong life. They must be considered purely palliative measures. It is therefore especially noteworthy that the United States Veterans Administration Co-operative Urological Research Group found that administration of estrogens increased the death rate from cardiovascular causes by about 75 per cent, more than canceling a modest (25 per cent) reduction in mortality from the cancer. Since neither estrogens nor castration prolongs life, neither should be used except to relieve pain or urinary tract obstruction; even in these situations, the beneficial effects of radiation to local disease of bone or pelvis should be exploited before hormonal manipulation is tried. If a decision is made to turn to hormone therapy, castration is preferred, because it is not as-

sociated with the increased cardiovascular complications seen in estrogen-treated patients. If castration loses its useful effect, and the symptoms cannot be controlled by conventional methods or radiotherapy, low doses of estrogens (1 or 2 mg of diethylstilbestrol daily) may be tried. This dose is probably less risky than full 5 mg doses. *Adrenalectomy* and *hypophysectomy* offer no advantages after castration has failed.

The place of *cytotoxic chemotherapy* is less well established in prostatic cancer than in cancer of the breast; but it is the writer's impression that several agents, including cyclophosphamide and methotrexate, sometimes give relief of bone pain, suggesting a response. Objective evidence of reduced tumor size or increased longevity is not at hand. Further studies of chemotherapeutic combinations are needed in this disease.

CANCER OF THE THYROID

Well-differentiated thyroid carcinomas are often under pituitary control, and their growth can be blocked and the metastatic masses may disappear if secretion of thyroid-stimulating hormone (TSH) is suppressed. This is accomplished by giving replacement doses of thyroxine or equivalent hormone combinations of thyroxine and triiodothyronine. Suppression may continue for very long periods with control of the cancer. The matter is discussed in more detail in Ch. 843.

OTHER ENDOCRINE CANCERS

There is no evidence that suppressing pituitary ACTH secretion controls the growth or activity of carcinomas of the adrenal cortex, whether functional or not. Endocrine manipulations are ineffective in treating tumors of other endocrine organs. The influence of pituitary growth factors and insulin on tumors of nonendocrine tissues has not yet been established. The cytotoxic effects of *adrenocortical steroids* are used in treating lymphomas, Hodgkin's disease, and other tumors and to ameliorate secondary effects of tumors such as dermatomyositis, neuropathy, and hemolytic disease. They may also relieve pressure by reducing the inflammatory zone surrounding tumor masses, e.g., in cerebral metastases.

Byar, D. P.: Treatment of prostatic cancer: Studies by the Veterans Administration Co-operative Urological Research Group. Bull. N.Y. Acad. Med., 48:751, 1972.

Canellos, G. P., Devita, V. T., Gold, G. L., Chabner, B. A., Schein, P. S., and Young, R. C.: Cyclical combination chemotherapy for advanced breast cancer. Br. Med. J., 1:218, 1974.

Edelstyn, G. J. A., and Macrae, K. D.: Cyclical combination chemotherapy in advanced breast cancer. Br. J. Cancer, Vol. 28, 1973.

Huggins, C., and Hodges, C. V.: Studies on prostatic cancer: Effect of castration, of estrogen, and of androgen injection on serum phosphatase in metastatic carcinoma of the prostate. Cancer Res., 1:293, 1941.

Jensen, E. V., Block, G. E., Smithe, S., Kyser, K., and DeSombre, E.: Estrogen receptors and breast cancer response to adrenalectomy. Natl. Cancer Inst. Monogr., 34:55, 1971.

Stoll, B. A.: Endocrine Therapy in Malignant Disease. Philadelphia, W. B. Saunders Company, 1972.

Veterans Administration Co-operative Urological Research Group: Treatment and survival of patients with cancer of the prostate. Surg. Gynecol. Obstet., 124:1011, 1967.

878. BONE PHYSIOLOGY AND CALCIUM HOMEOSTASIS

Robert P. Heaney

Duality of Skeletal Function. The skeleton functions as both a structural and a calcium homeostatic organ. Diseases that affect bone both alter the supporting function of the skeleton and have far-reaching effects on calcium homeostasis; conversely, derangements of calcium homeostasis are inevitably reflected in bone as a supporting tissue. Although it would be difficult to conceive of terrestrial existence without the mechanical support provided by a rigid endoskeleton, the fact is that the tissue, bone, evolved in exclusively aquatic vertebrates, in which there probably was no selective advantage conferred by a rigid endoskeleton. The principal evolutionary significance of bone lies in the fact that it has afforded higher vertebrates the ability to regulate the concentration of calcium and phosphate ions in body fluids. This primitive ability remains a fundamental property of the modern human skeleton, and reminds us of this by occasionally exerting its primacy over the much more obvious structural role of the tissue.

Whereas parathyroid hormone, discussed at length in Ch. 871, exerts the primary endocrine control over calcium homeostasis, it is bone that provides the principal end-organ by which this homeostasis is effected. This action depends upon two fundamental properties of bone tissue: (1) the physical-chemical equilibrium between the solid phase bone mineral and calcium ions in the body fluids, and (2) the continuous structural remodeling of bone with its associated deposition and removal of large quantities of calcium and phosphorus.

Bone Structure and Composition. Bone consists of a highly organized system of cells embedded in a matrix composed of a fibrous protein, collagen, encrusted with tiny calcium phosphate crystals. Cells occupy 2 to 3 per cent of the total volume, but are evenly distributed through the bone and interconnected by a series of canaliculi, so that no volume of interstitial bony material is more than a fraction of a micron from a cell or its processes, and no bone cell is more than 100 microns from a capillary. In fully mineralized bone the protein matrix accounts for half the volume and one third the weight of the intercellular material, and the crystals comprise most of the remainder. Mucopolysaccharides make up about 5 per cent of the organic matrix, and although quantitatively a minor component of bone, they probably contribute significantly to matrix maturation and mineralization. The collagen fibers in adult human bone are not randomly arranged, but are oriented to resist the mechanical forces which the organ must withstand. Furthermore, the intimate association of fibrous protein and ultramicroscopic crystals constitutes what, in materials engineering, has been termed a "two-phase" material. The breaking strength and elasticity of bones depend not only on their mass and shape, but as well on the intrinsic mechanical properties of this two-phase system and on changes that occur in those properties as the material ages. Although still poorly understood, it is probable that some of the symptoms and signs of the diseases to be described in the following pages represent qualitative abnormalities in the bone material itself.

The mineral component of bony material is a calcium-phosphate generally considered to possess the crystal structure of hydroxyapatite. There is an additional carbonate component which may comprise as much as 8 per cent of bone ash and which is currently believed to be present both as $CaCO_3$ and as limited carbonate substitution in or on the apatite crystal. The calcium carbonate phase is acid labile, even in vivo, and is depleted during systemic acidosis. When initially deposited, bone mineral appears crystallographically amorphous and gradually matures to the characteristic apatitic pattern.

Bone Formation. Bone is deposited on free surfaces by osteoblasts that synthesize collagen and secrete it onto the bone-forming surface. Soon after secretion the soluble collagen molecules aggregate into spatially oriented insoluble fibrils. The factors that control their orientation are not well understood, but bioelectrical fields of the magnitude known to be produced in bone by applied mechanical stress have been shown to influence the orientation of collagen fibrils in vitro. Osteoblasts deposit a layer of matrix about $1\ \mu$ in thickness per day. There is about a ten-day lag before mineralization occurs, so that a normal osteoid seam averages $10\ \mu$ in thickness. Under control of the parent osteoblast the matrix undergoes a complex series of biochemical changes, which ultimately lead to crystal nucleation and growth. This process includes changes in the mucopolysaccharide component of the matrix and appearance of lipid-staining material at the calcification front. These and other changes are reflected in distinct layers and sequences recognizable only by special stains. Alkaline phosphatase has long been associated with active bone formation and can be detected both within osteoblasts and extracellularly in the superficial layers of newly deposited matrix, but not more deeply at the calcification front itself. Despite many attractive hypotheses, no clearly definable role of this enzyme has been found, and its association with active bone formation remains largely circumstantial.

Once maturation is complete, the collagen fibril becomes capable of initiating the deposition of mineral, in a specific crystalline pattern, from the ions present in the bathing fluid. These crystals are formed both within and upon the fibril and are oriented along its length. Crystal growth displaces the water that originally occupied 50 per cent of the volume of unmineralized matrix. Approximately three fourths of the ultimate mineral content may be deposited within a few hours. The remaining mineral enters more slowly, largely because the decrease in free water severely limits diffusion, and thus completion of mineralization may require weeks or even months.

Once nucleation occurs, mineral is extracted from the surrounding fluid with great efficiency. This appears to be explained by the fact that the solubility product of hydroxyapatite is considerably lower than the $Ca \times P$ ion product in extracellular fluid, and thus crystal growth occurs as rapidly as blood flow can transport mineral to the site. On the other hand, spontaneous precipitation of calcium phosphates from the body fluids does not normally occur in other tissues because, though supersaturated with respect to the ultimate mineral phase of bone, these fluids are undersaturated with respect to the mineral crystalline forms that calcium phosphate is known to assume when precipitated at physiologic pH. The extraordinary beauty of this arrangement lies in the fact that mineralization thus occurs only at sites specifically rendered mineralizable by formation of an *improbable* nucleating configuration, and in the fact that one and the same body fluid carries a great surplus of mineral when in the presence of such a nucleating center, but is indefinitely stable – indeed undersaturated – elsewhere.

An important consequence of this mineralization scheme is the demand for mineral created by nucleated, but as yet incompletely mineralized bone. This demand amounts to a kind of "mineralization debt," analogous to the lactic acid debt of anaerobic muscle work, and will inevitably lower the concentration of calcium in body fluids unless specifically offset by homeostatic adjustment. Indeed, this continuing demand, which cannot apparently be modulated after it is initiated, is quantitatively the largest single stress to which the calcium homeostatic system must respond. Normally new bone mineralization utilizes 300 to 500 mg of calcium daily, an amount greater than the total calcium content of the entire blood volume. This demand may increase by as much as two orders of magnitude in diseases in which active bone formation occurs, such as severe osteitis fibrosa, and is partially responsible for the "bone hunger" and associated hypocalcemia that are sometimes seen after removal of a parathyroid adenoma.

Bone Resorption. Resorption occurs by virtually simultaneous dissolution of both mineral and matrix, and is produced both by large multinucleated cells known as osteoclasts and by osteocytes (which enlarge their lacunae in response to parathyroid stimulation). Osteoclasts are short lived and do their work quickly. The space eventually to be filled by a new haversian system can be tunneled out of cortical bone in less than 10 per cent of the time required by osteoblasts to fill it in with new bone. This means that large quantities of mineral can be released from the skeleton in short periods of time. The mechanisms by which bone solids are solubilized are largely unknown. Collagenase and a variety of lysosomal proteases are involved in matrix hydrolysis, and large quantities of H^+ are consumed in solubilization of the mineral (approximately one proton for each calcium ion). The H^+ production derives from both organic acids and carbonic anhydrase, and is both dependent upon and stimulated by O_2 levels in the bathing fluids. Carbonic anhydrase has been specifically localized to osteoclasts, and its inhibitors can directly reduce bone resorption.

Control of Bone Remodeling. Teleologically, bone remodeling serves both homeostatic and structural needs. By processing large quantities of mineral each day it establishes an input-output system capable of being adapted to calcium deficiency or excess by comparatively minor adjustments of the balance between formation and resorption. Structurally it allows the bone to reshape itself to meet new forces and, even more fundamental, it continually renews its aging interstitial material and thus maintains optimal mechanical properties.

The control of bone formation and resorption, i.e., structural bone turnover, is exerted at two levels: in intrinsic bone cellular activity and in the superimposed systemic influences such as those produced by hormones, nutrition, and systemic disease. The former is the more important; unfortunately, it is still poorly understood.

Systemic Control. Growth hormone and thyroid hormone stimulate osteoblast activity and osteoblastic recruitment from osteoprogenitor cells, whereas adrenal corticoids, malnutrition, fever, and a variety of systemic diseases decrease both new matrix production and the osteoblast-mediated ripening of the osteoid seam. Androgens and estrogens, previously thought to stimulate osteoblastic activity, have been shown to exert their effect, instead, by suppressing bone resorption, and if they have any effect on osteoblasts at all, probably suppress them to a minor extent. None of these effects can be considered homeostatic, either from the point of view of the skeleton as a structural unit or from the point of view of the extracellular fluid calcium ion level, simply because there exist no known feedback loops from the skeletal effects to the control of hormone secretion.

Homeostatic control of bone turnover is exerted by parathyroid hormone and calcitonin, which are concerned not with skeletal homeostasis, but with the maintenance of calcium ion concentration in the extracellular fluid. Parathyroid hormone secretion is inversely related to extracellular fluid calcium ion levels, and hormone action is exerted on at least three independent end-organs: bone, intestinal mucosa, and renal tubule. The intestinal absorptive effect is mediated through control of vitamin D metabolism (see below). All three effects function to raise the concentration of calcium ion in extracellular fluid. In bone the most obvious effect of the hormone is a stimulation of bone resorption, with consequent release of calcium and phosphorus. In cases of severe parathyroid dysfunction there is commonly also an increase of new bone formation that parallels the more immediate change in resorption. In the intestinal mucosa parathyroid hormone is indirectly responsible for control of calcium absorption. The efficiency of calcium absorption, which, in the adult, is about 30 per cent, may rise to over 90 per cent in hyperparathyroidism and fall to nearly zero in hypoparathyroidism. In the kidney parathyroid hormone effects are twofold: a decrease in tubular phosphate reabsorption (discussed elsewhere in this text) and an increase in tubular calcium reabsorption. The renal effects occur within minutes and the bone effects within hours, whereas the intestinal response requires days to become apparent. Although all three responses have the same general effect, the renal response seems best suited for emergency adjustment, the bone response represents the largest reserve capacity of the three, and the intestinal response seems designed more to restore total body calcium balance than to adjust the level of calcium ion in extracellular fluid.

A variety of factors modulate parathyroid hormone effects on bone resorption. Mechanical stresses, gonadal steroids, high concentrations of calcium or phosphate, calcitonin, fluoride, and the diphosphonate compounds all depress resorptive response to a given level of parathyroid hormone. Some act at the level of mesenchymal activation (such as the gonadal steroids), some at the existing resorptive cellular machinery (such as calcitonin), and some at the mineral level itself (such as fluoride), but the ultimate effect of each is a shift in the dose response curve of parathyroid-mediated bone resorption in the direction of resistance. On the other hand, disuse, heparin, increased oxygen tension, and local inflammation all enhance resorptive response to parathyroid hormone. The significance of these interactions lies not in calcium homeostasis (for plasma calcium regulation takes place despite these alterations of PTH responsiveness, simply by compensatory adjustment of parathyroid hormone secretion rate), but in the bone mass itself. Enhanced responsiveness leads to negative calcium balance, reduced responsiveness to positive balance.

Calcitonin suppresses bone resorption, by inhibiting both osteocytes and osteoclasts. Its immediate effect is reduction in release of calcium and phosphorus from bone; hence in the fasting state it produces a fall in both plasma calcium and phosphate. Although secreted in small quantities at normal plasma calcium levels, it is normally released in response to hypercalcemia and probably finds its chief role in normal physiology in moderating absorptive hypercalcemia. This is most important in infancy, when absorbed milk calcium might otherwise inundate the infant's small extracellular fluid volume and thus produce serious hypercalcemia. The effect of calcitonin on skeletal mass in man is unknown, but it is to be expected that long-term overproduction or exogenous administration would lead to increased skeletal mass. (Calcitonin has, in fact, been indirectly implicated in the hyperostosis of bulls fed a milking ration.)

Intrinsic Control. Apparently the two most important elements of local control are mechanical forces and local blood flow, the latter with its associated regulation of nutrient supply, pH, and O_2 tension. Increased blood flow is associated with osteoclastic resorption, and vascular stasis with increased osteoblastic activity. The effects of mechanical forces are profound. A bone or bony region subjected to heavy use will increase its mass and revise both its internal structure and external shape so as to resist applied forces; conversely, disuse leads rapidly to decrease in mass and loss of specific architectural features. Normally, muscle mass and skeletal mass maintain a ratio of approximately 10:1.

Both the nature of the signal that mechanical forces transmit to bone cells and the nature of the cellular response are largely unknown. However, bone exhibits many of the features of a semiconductor and has been shown to generate and maintain small electrical fields when deformed by externally applied forces. These fields are of the same magnitude as those shown to be capable of orienting collagen fibril aggregation and those controlling limb bud regeneration in amphibia. Thus it is possible that both cellular activity and extracellular organization of matrix fibrils may be determined by local electrical fields. The distribution of stresses within bone and associated induced electrical fields and altered blood flow are so complex and so heterogeneous that turnover may be intense at one site and only a few millimeters distant may be virtually at a standstill.

Envelope-Specific Remodeling. The foregoing statements, although applicable in a general way, must be further modified to incorporate a most important component of intrinsic control, namely envelope-specific remodeling. Because the bony material is exterior to the cells, all bone remodeling must take place from bone surfaces. These surfaces comprise three virtual envelopes, periosteal, haversian (intracortical), and trabecular-endosteal, and the behavior of bone cells on each of these envelopes exhibits distinct differences, despite common systemic

influences. Aging, hormones, drugs, and diseases are all characterized by discrete envelope-specific remodeling patterns. These patterns are useful both for classification and recognition of bone diseases and for adequate understanding of bone pathophysiology.

In normal adult bone something less than 5 per cent of the free surface of all three envelopes is involved in remodeling at any time. When a microscopic site on one of these envelopes becomes a remodeling locus, events always proceed in an orderly sequence, which consists first of mesenchymal activation, followed next by osteoclastic erosion into the bone surface, and finally by osteoblastic repair. The entire sequence normally requires from 3 to 12 months to go from start to completion at any given site. At any remodeling site, wherever located, resorption always precedes and appears to be a necessary preliminary to formation. The three bony envelopes differ primarily in the balance between resorption and formation which occurs in this remodeling sequence and in how the process responds to systemic and hormonal stimuli.

Except for modeling of external contours associated with growth, the periosteal surface normally exhibits a preponderance of formation over resorption, and hence constitutes an expanding envelope throughout life. There is a brief period in adolescence, most marked in females, when the endosteum is also predominantly a forming surface, at which time the bony cortex is thickened by apposition from both sides; but through most of life the endosteal-trabecular envelope is predominantly a resorbing surface. On the haversian envelope, however, resorption and formation are normally balanced so that replaced bone is approximately equivalent to removed bone.

Although treated in greater depth in the following chapters some examples of envelope-specific patterns may help to illustrate this concept. Postmenopausal and corticosteroid osteoporosis are both exclusively disorders of the endosteal envelope; whereas hyperparathyroidism, either primary or the parathyroid effect seen in osteomalacia and renal osteodystrophy, produces activation of all three envelopes, with resorption predominating. Growth hormone also activates all three envelopes, but causes formation to dominate. In fact growth hormone is the only known, naturally occurring agent able to convert the adult endosteum to a predominantly forming surface.

Vitamin D. Both the plant and animal D vitamins (ergo- and cholecalciferol, respectively) are first hydroxylated at the 25-position by a specific liver enzyme system, and then, in the kidney, further hydroxylated at the 1- or the 24-position. The 1,25-dihydroxy compound (1,25-HCC) is the active form of the vitamin, mediating the control of intestinal calcium absorption and acting to facilitate parathyroid hormone effects on bone resorption. There appears to be continuous renal hydroxylation of 25-OH cholecalciferol; the synthetic balance between the 1,25- and the 24,25-derivatives is controlled by the level of parathyroid hormone. High parathyroid hormone levels favor the 1,25-derivative, which in turn increases intestinal calcium absorption and enhances the parathyroid hormone effect on bone resorption. No significant biologic activity has yet been associated with the 24,25-derivative. It is possible that the parathyroid effect on hydroxylation may be indirect, i.e., mediated through the plasma phosphate levels, inasmuch as lowered plasma phosphate has the same effect on directing hydroxylation to the 1,25-derivative as does an elevated parathyroid hormone level.

Calcium absorption from the intestine is associated with a transport protein with a high affinity for calcium (calcium-binding protein), and 1,25-HCC is necessary for production of this material in most species studied to date. Nevertheless, much uncertainty remains both as to the actual cellular mechanism of vitamin D action and as to the tissues most affected by vitamin D deficiency. Plainly vitamin D is necessary for intestinal calcium absorption, and most particularly for the absorptive responses to low calcium intake or high parathyroid hormone levels. There is no general agreement, however, whether vitamin D is necessary for osteoid maturation or epiphyseal cartilage growth and maturation, each of which is retarded in vitamin D deficiency states. Attempts to explain each of these effects as a result of calcium absorptive defects are unconvincing, and it seems safest to assume a direct dependence of each of these cell types on vitamin D until such is clearly shown to be unnecessary. Curiously, the renal tubular effects of parathyroid hormone on calcium and phosphate transport seem to be independent of vitamin D.

Age Changes in Bone. In general, after the fourth decade, bone mass declines at an average rate of 5 to 10 per cent per decade. Although certain individuals may be exempted from this decline, it appears to be universally true of all populations and racial groups studied, regardless of nutritional or environmental factors. The decline appears to coincide with, or at least be accelerated at the time of, menopause in women, and the rate of loss is greater in women than in men, but it nevertheless occurs in both sexes.

Bourne, G. H. (ed.): The Biochemistry and Physiology of Bone. 2nd ed. New York, Academic Press, 1971.

Frost, H. M.: Bone Remodeling and Its Relationship to Metabolic Bone Disease. Springfield, Ill., Charles C Thomas, 1973.

Harris, W. H., and Heaney, R. P.: Skeletal Renewal and Metabolic Bone Disease. Boston, Little, Brown & Company, 1970.

McLean, F. C., and Urist, M. R.: Bone. 3rd ed. Chicago, University of Chicago Press, 1968.

Vaughn, J.: The Physiology of Bone. New York, Oxford University Press, 1970.

THE OSTEOPOROSES

Robert P. Heaney

879. INTRODUCTION

Definition. The term osteoporosis, literally "bone porosity," designates a deficiency of bone tissue per unit volume of bone as an organ. The deficiency relates only to the structural function of bone, not to its calcium homeostatic role. The bone that remains is considered to be normal by both chemical and ordinary histologic criteria. The fibrous and fatty marrow that fills the voids once occupied by bone is also normal, and there is no obvious morphologic evidence of osteoblastic or osteoclastic dysfunction. These requirements exclude many specific entities also associated with quantitative reduction in a qualitatively normal bone mass, such as hyperparathyroidism, multiple myeloma, and carcinoma metastatic to bone. Thus these features *describe* osteoporosis, rather than *define* it, because osteoporosis is not so much the presence of an abnormal bone condition as it is the absence of a normal quantity of bone.

Morphologic and Roentgenographic Characteristics. The decrease in bone mass expresses itself as loss of normal cortical thickness, and as thinning, fragmentation, and loss of trabeculae. The external dimensions of the involved bone do not change (except as a consequence of fracture). The cortical thinning is usually readily visible on roentgenograms of long bones. Decreased roentgenographic density is an unreliable sign, and thus early changes in primarily cancellous bone, such as the pelvis and spine, are hard to evaluate. As the disease advances, one can discern increased contrast between the end plates and bodies of vertebrae, relative accentuation of vertical trabeculae, biconcave compression of the end plates (producing the characteristic "codfish" vertebrae), herniation of the nucleus pulposus into the bodies of the vertebrae (Schmorl's nodes), and, finally, vertebral compression fractures. The involved bodies are usually wedged anteriorly, especially in the thoracic region, but sometimes uniform collapse or even posterior body wedging is seen, depending on the region of the spine involved. The neural arch invariably remains intact.

Except for the purely local osteoporoses such as those associated with inflammation or disuse, most osteoporoses are generalized diseases involving the entire skeleton, and, if carefully sought, roentgenographic evidence of decreased bone mass can be found in all bones examined, including the skull, the long bones, and the hands and feet. Decreased cortical thickness of the femur and of the metacarpal, metatarsal, and phalangeal bones is a common accompaniment of vertebral osteoporosis and usually, though not always, parallels the latter in severity. The combined thickness of the two cortices usually amounts to more than 45 per cent of total shaft diameter in these bones; values less than this are indicative of decreased bone mass. Disproportionately more severe bone loss in the largely cancellous bone of the central skeleton usually signifies a rapidly developing osteoporosis, whereas more uniform bone loss means slow development. When the degree of bone loss becomes extreme, macroscopic regions of cancellous bone may present a cystlike appearance roentgenographically.

Microscopically the bone shows no abnormalities by usual criteria. Increased marrow mast cell counts have been noted in all types of osteoporosis evaluated to date. This is of interest because of the known potentiation of endogenous parathyroid hormone by heparin and because bone loss of osteoporosis occurs primarily at the endosteal envelope, which is also the sole bony interface with the bone marrow. However, it is not known whether the mast cells precede the onset of the osteoporotic process or are a response to it.

General Pathophysiologic Considerations. Many useful analogies can be drawn between osteoporosis and anemia. Like anemia, osteoporosis is not a specific disease entity but is instead a quantitative deficiency of a normal body constituent. It is the end result of many quite different pathophysiologic processes. The one element common to all these mechanisms is that, in the transition between normal bone and osteoporotic bone, the resorptive component of bone turnover must exceed new bone formation. But, again like anemia, this destructive imbalance can proceed at high, low, or normal rates of bone turnover. The osteoporosis of Cushing's syndrome develops at low rates of new bone formation; postmenopausal and senile osteoporoses usually develop at normal or near normal absolute rates of bone turnover; and disuse osteoporosis, peri-inflammatory osteoporosis, and the osteoporoses of acromegaly and hyperthyroidism develop at high rates of bone turnover. Indeed, the rate of bone turnover is largely an irrelevant consideration; the only important matter is why resorption is higher than formation. This problem is more difficult than it appears, because it implies a knowledge of the mechanisms by which formation and resorption are matched and bone mass is preserved in normal persons. This information is not yet available.

One thing, however, seems certain: the elements of calcium ion homeostasis are involved in the pathogenesis of osteoporosis, at least as unwitting participants if not as originators of the process. Significant bone loss cannot develop at low remodeling rates; hence tonic parathyroid secretion, which is quantitatively the major determinant of normal bone remodeling, becomes involved either actively or passively in development of any osteoporosis. The components of calcium homeostasis constitute a kind of final common pathway for skeletal remodeling, and most, if not all, modalities altering the remodeling balance between formation and resorption exert their effects either directly via parathyroid hormone or by altering bony end-organ responsiveness to parathyroid hormone.

Certain animal species, notably rats, kittens, puppies, and lions, all develop osteoporosis when placed on low calcium diets. The animals show clear evidence of increased parathyroid hormone secretion, and the osteoporosis can be prevented by prior parathyroidectomy. The excess bone resorption and consequent osteoporosis are homeostatically mediated and represent not so much a homeostatic derangement as a quite appropriate consequence of normal calcium ion regulation. Bone is resorbed to meet mineral needs that the animal cannot obtain from its food. Comparable calcium-deficiency osteoporosis undoubtedly exists in man, but there is no evidence that it is common, and efforts to implicate calcium deficiency as a *primary* cause of most types of human osteoporosis have not been successful.

Nevertheless, the clear implication to be drawn from continued parathyroid secretion during development of most human osteoporosis is that this secretion is necessary to sustain normal calcium ion levels. Some fraction of the calcium resorbed from bone is lost from the body, not because it is present in excess, but for some other reason, and the extra resorption, mediated by parathyroid hormone, comes about precisely to compensate for this loss. It is in this fashion that the calcium homeostatic system becomes implicated in osteoporosis even when there is no evidence of absolute dietary calcium deficiency. The reasons for this calcium wastage are uncertain, but there is a growing body of evidence that changes in the intrinsic responsiveness of the three parathyroid hormone end-organs, and most specifically bone itself, to endogenous parathyroid hormone may account for inefficient calcium conservation. It is worth stressing that the sought-for effect need not be great; net calcium loss of as little as 50 mg per day will reduce the skeletal mass by 15 to 20 per cent per decade.

880. POSTMENOPAUSAL AND SENILE OSTEOPOROSIS

Definition and Etiology. Postmenopausal and senile osteoporosis differs in no way from the foregoing general description. By definition it is found only in postmenopausal women and in elderly persons of both sexes. These patients exhibit a remarkably homogeneous clinical picture and differ in several important respects from patients with specific osteoporoses in which known causal factors can be found. The cause of postmenopausal and senile osteoporosis is unknown. Nor is it known whether clinical osteoporosis is distinct from the universal age-related bone loss which occurs in both men and women, or whether it is simply a consequence of starting with a skeleton at the low end of the bone mass spectrum. The rate of bone loss in women after the menopause is much greater than in men of the same age, and the suppressive effect of gonadal hormones – particularly estrogen – on activation of bone remodeling foci would appear to explain this sexual dimorphism. Nevertheless there is at best only a very weak correlation between age at menopause and onset of osteoporotic symptoms. Thus the normal decrease in estrogen secretion after menopause probably plays no more than a secondary or permissive role in the etiology of osteoporosis. The common finding of osteoporosis in young women with gonadal agenesis (45,X syndromes) is believed to represent an additional manifestation of the genetic defect rather than of endocrine deficiency.

Incidence. Postmenopausal and senile osteoporosis is the most common of all metabolic bone diseases. Satisfactory population studies have not yet been made, but available work suggests that approximately one fourth of all white females in the United States develop clinically significant osteoporosis. (By this is meant that they show the structural consequences of diminished bone mass: compression fractures, "codfish" vertebrae, Schmorl's nodes, dorsal kyphosis, and decreased stature). Furthermore, at least three fourths of all elderly people with fractures of the upper femur have pre-existing osteoporosis, presumably as the predisposing cause of fracture. In the two decades from age 50 to age 70 osteoporosis is predominantly a disease of women. By age 80 the disease is also common among males, although it usually causes less disability than in women. Among women living in the United States, the disorder is most common in those of northern European extraction; it is less common in those of southern European ancestry and still less common in Negroes. Because of both racial and sexual protection, the disease is rare among Negro males of any age. Japanese, both in Japan and in the United States, have a high incidence of osteoporosis. These racial differences appear to be related primarily to differences in normal adult bone mass, rather than to protection against age-related bone loss. Thus the adult Negro male has the largest initial bone mass and has therefore the largest structural reserve against the development of osteoporosis.

Pathogenesis. Many physiologic differences have been found between osteoporotics and comparable normal persons, but their relation to the pathogenesis of osteoporosis is uncertain. Studies of the population at risk have not been made, nor have individual women been studied long enough to determine whether these abnormalities precede the development of the disease. In comparison with normal persons, osteoporotics have been observed to consume 20 to 30 per cent less calcium in their diet, to absorb a smaller fraction of the ingested calcium, to have 40 per cent higher calcium requirements simply to achieve a balance between intake and output, to fail to reduce their urinary calcium normally when placed on low calcium diets, to possess lower circulating vitamin D levels, and to have subnormal growth hormone release in response to hypoglycemic challenge. Urinary estrogen excretion and vaginal epithelial cornification are both somewhat lower in osteoporotics than in age-matched controls, and, in addition, alterations in the excretion pattern of steroid metabolites have been described which suggest lower androgen production.

Although "normal" adults are able to adapt to calcium intakes below 500 mg per day, some otherwise apparently healthy persons fail to achieve calcium balance on low intakes. There is no doubt that calcium deficiency can cause osteoporosis and that some of the patients in this group represent the end result of prolonged deficiency. Nevertheless, the disease occurs also in patients with higher than average intakes, and it seems safest to conclude that, in the group as a whole, inefficient calcium conservation serves at most as a contributory cause rather than as the primary factor in the development of osteoporosis.

Within the bone itself, quantitative studies of remodeling have shown wide variations in osteoblastic new bone formation rates, from well above to well below age-specific normal values. For the most part cell-level bone formation is subnormal, but because more than normal remodeling sites are usually present, it turns out, at the organ-level, that bone-remodeling rates are very nearly normal (although the variance of this measure is significantly larger than normal). It is not certain what role, if any, these changes play in the development of clinical osteoporosis.

Clinical Manifestations. The principal manifestations of osteoporosis are vertebral compression with resultant kyphosis and loss of vertical height, back pain, and susceptibility to fractures (particularly fractures of the upper femur and distal radius). The vertebral compression is often asymptomatic, and probably no more than one third of all patients with the disease actively seek medical aid. The vertebral collapse and kyphosis exaggerate the downward angulation of the ribs and produce prominent horizontal skin folds over the lower chest and abdomen. These folds, particularly in thin people, are a clear indicator of vertebral collapse. The lower ribs may actually ride into the pelvic brim. Occasionally when this occurs the patient experiences severe flank pain, which is relieved by hyperextension of the spine or by surgical excision of the lower costal cartilages. Presumably the pain arises from the costal perichondrium.

Osteoporosis is an important predisposing factor in fractures, particularly those associated with minimal trauma. Hip fracture is a major cause of death and disability in the elderly, and it is probable that most such fractures are due to osteoporosis. Other bones are also more fragile, and fractures are often seen in the pubic and ischial rami, in the rib cage, and in the humerus. The fractures heal normally in all cases except those in which the original bone was so attenuated that the fracture completely destroyed the residual bony scaffolding. This sometimes happens in intertrochanteric and femoral neck fractures.

The back pain is of two types: an acute, sometimes severe pain, well localized to the midline over a restricted region of the spine, that disappears over a period of weeks, and a much more chronic, diffuse, aching pain. The former is related to new compression fractures or to extension of old collapse, and usually disappears as the associated soft tissue and periosteal damage heals. Occasionally the pain precedes roentgenographic evidence of fracture by several days or weeks. Patients commonly relate the attacks of pain to physical exertion, such as bending forward or lifting heavy objects, but weight bearing is not always found, and some patients incur fractures simply by turning over in bed. On physical examination, point tenderness can be found on percussion or pressure over the involved vertebrae. There are commonly associated paravertebral muscle spasm and tenderness. The more chronic pain is found only in a minority of patients, may not be related to the osteoporosis at all, or may be due to associated muscle spasm or to degenerative arthritis aggravated by malaligned weight-bearing forces. It is usually aggravated by prolonged standing or sitting and is relieved by lying down.

Diagnosis. The roentgenographic changes in postmenopausal and senile osteoporosis have been described. The plasma calcium, phosphorus, and alkaline phosphatase are normal, and the urine calcium is usually normal. Bone biopsy reveals only thinning of the cortex and attenuation and fragmentation of trabeculae, both of which are hard to evaluate in a single biopsy sample. The biopsy is of value, however, not because it is characteristic of osteoporosis, but because it excludes certain other disorders. The principal differential considerations include the specific osteoporoses such as that due to Cushing's syndrome, diffuse skeletal involvement with multiple myeloma, hyperparathyroidism, osteogenesis imperfecta (which in mild forms may first manifest itself in adult life), and metastatic malignancy. Despite a common misconception to the contrary, osteomalacia is not a cause of diffuse skeletal atrophy, and it does not present a clinical or roentgenographic picture similar to osteoporosis.

The clinical picture of Cushing's syndrome or of hyperthyroidism is usually sufficiently obvious so that little confusion with postmenopausal or senile osteoporosis should occur. Rarely, however, patients with these endocrinopathies may present with predominantly skeletal manifestations. Myeloma is excluded by examination of the bone marrow (which can be performed on the same specimen removed for bone biopsy), by electrophoretic separation of the plasma proteins, and by search for Bence Jones protein in the urine. Normal plasma calcium, phosphorus, and alkaline phosphatase serve to exclude hyperparathyroidism and those malignant conditions that mimic parathyroid hyperfunction. Metastatic malignancy presents a differential problem principally when it is a cause of vertebral compression fracture. In such patients, skeletal roentgenographic surveys may demonstrate more characteristic metastatic lesions in other bones. Further, the finding of apparently osteoporotic compression fractures in younger patients, particularly males, or of involvement of the neural arch should suggest a neoplastic cause for the lesion.

An important feature of osteoporotic pain is that it is associated with fracture. Back pain at a site remote from vertebral compression, or in a spine simply osteoporotic but without compression fractures, is usually not due to osteoporosis. In addition to the painful bony disorders just described, the clinician should also exclude certain nonskeletal causes of back pain such as pancreatitis, posterior penetration of a duodenal ulcer, and posterior abdominal malignancies.

Treatment. Treatment in osteoporosis is directed at arresting and stabilizing the condition and at symptomatic relief, support, and rehabilitation of the patient.

Because the pain of acute episodes subsides spontaneously as the compression fracture heals, all treatments may *appear* to work. Nevertheless, no treatment has been conclusively shown to increase bone mass in a representative group of patients. Some help in retarding further bone loss or in increasing the functional capacity of the patient may be afforded by mineral supplements, gonadal hormones, and physical therapy. A number of other agents, including fluoride, phosphates, calcitonin, and the diphosphonate compounds, are still under investigation.

Because virtually all patients conserve calcium poorly, a high calcium intake is sometimes recommended as the cornerstone of any therapeutic regimen. The risk of hypercalciuria with such treatment is negligible. Calcium intake should be at least 1500 mg per day; if derived from the diet, this requires the ingestion of at least one quart of milk per day, which is more than most osteoporotic patients will accept. It is usually necessary to employ supplemental medicinal calcium, which is available in a variety of forms, including the gluconate, lactate, phosphate, carbonate, and glycerophosphate salts. All are absorbed equally well except for the carbonate, which is poorly absorbed in the presence of achlorhydria. There is suggestive, but still inconclusive, evidence that retention is better if supplemental phosphate is also provided; thus the phosphate salts may be preferable to the others. In some patients, particularly those with low urine calcium excretion, vitamin D in doses from 1000 to 10,000 IU per day appears to aid calcium retention.

Estrogens and androgens, alone or in combination, have been shown to improve calcium balance and possibly also to decrease the incidence of fracture. Dosage regimens vary greatly; adequate therapy is probably provided by ordinary replacement doses, i.e., 0.05 to 0.1 mg of ethinyl estradiol or its equivalent. Androgen therapy in women is limited by its virilizing properties, and few patients will accept prolonged treatment at more than a few milligrams of methyltestosterone daily.

Intensive physical therapy often produces significant functional and symptomatic improvement. The muscles of the back, hips, and thighs must be strengthened, and a lifelong program of exercise instituted. There is undoubtedly some component of disuse in most osteoporotics, and this must be abolished by a controlled sensible regimen of exercise. Patients must be taught to bend at the hips and knees and not to bend the back in order to pick up objects off the floor, and they must not carry or lift heavy objects. Bed rest is contraindicated except in the acute post-fracture period when it may be necessary for pain relief. Patients should be up and about, and a physical therapy program should be started as soon as possible after an acute vertebral compression. Back braces are usually not indicated, but firm corsets or foundation garments are often very helpful.

Fluoride, given as the sodium salt in doses of 30 to 60 mg daily, also improves calcium balance in many patients, and, in combination with calcium supplements and vitamin D, has apparently increased bone mass in a few patients. Fluoride is known to fit into the apatite crystal lattice in the place of hydroxyl radicals; the resulting fluorapatite is a more stable, less soluble mineral than hydroxyapatite. The bone is thus rendered more resistant to resorptive attack, and the calcium homeostatic system adapts by forcing more effective renal and intestinal calcium conservation.

Prevention. The probable irreversibility of bone atrophy in the aged makes prevention all the more important. There is suggestive evidence that prophylactic estrogen therapy retards postmenopausal bone loss. This effect is in keeping with what is known of estrogen action in bone resorption. Although adequately controlled prospective studies have not yet been performed, it seems likely that prophylactic estrogen therapy may be very useful. It would be particularly desirable to be able to select for such prophylaxis the 25 per cent of the white female population who constitute the high-risk group, but unfortunately this is not yet possible. The best one can suggest is to concentrate on small (less than 140 pounds), very fair-skinned women, with minimal body hair, and usually of Scotch, Irish, or Anglo-Saxon origin. All surveys to date suggest that such women have the highest risk of developing osteoporotic fractures.

Prognosis. There is little information about the natural history of the untreated disease. With adequate treatment, however, most patients can be stabilized and restored to useful functional activity. Hip fractures are probably the principal hazard of the disease; 10 to 15 per cent of patients are dead within three months of such fractures, and the associated enforced bed rest, trauma, and surgery markedly decrease the ultimate functional capacity of those who survive.

881. DISUSE OSTEOPOROSIS

Disuse osteoporosis is a local disorder confined to bones or regions subjected to immobilization or deprived of normal muscle pull. In severe lower motor neuron paralytic disease, such as quadriplegic poliomyelitis or the Guillain-Barré syndrome, virtually the entire skeleton may be involved, but, unlike other osteoporoses, the spine is less severely involved than are the long bones of the extremities. The bone loss develops through a massive increase in bone resorption. This resorption does not appear to be systemically mediated or controllable, and is somehow a consequence of the local withdrawal of mechanical stress. Vascular engorgement within bone occurs during development of the disorder, but it is not known whether this change causes the resorption or is instead caused by it. The pathologic picture is otherwise no different from that of the other osteoporoses. Roentgenographic changes are also nondistinctive except for the localization of disease to the immobilized bones and for a zone of rarefaction in the region of the fused epiphyseal plate, which appears as the first detectable change in involved long bones.

Since immobilized bones are not subjected to mechanical stress, their fragility is of little structural consequence, and the principal significance of the disease lies in the hypercalcemia and hypercalciuria that may be produced by extensive resorption. In poliomyelitis this resorption begins almost immediately and reaches peak values four to five weeks after onset, with urine calcium values sometimes as high as 800 mg per day. If care is not taken to keep these patients hydrated and to maintain a high urine flow, glomerular filtration falls, and hypercalcemia may result. Furthermore, stasis in the urinary tract predisposes to stone formation.

Normal subjects kept at bed rest develop negative calcium balance, with loss predominantly from weight-bearing bones, most particularly the os calcis. A comparable loss occurs as a result of prolonged weightlessness, as in space flight. In flights of up to two months' duration the amount of bone lost is insufficient to pose a risk of fracture. Urine calcium has increased, however, in most astronauts, and in some, up to twice preflight levels.

882. NUTRITIONAL OSTEOPOROSES

Osteoporosis is a frequent manifestation of many nutritional deficiency syndromes in patients of all ages. These include general protein and caloric malnutrition, kwashiorkor, scurvy, chronic alcoholism, and a variety of malabsorption syndromes as well as isolated calcium deficiency. These are specific osteoporoses, due to the malnutrition, and will heal both clinically and roentgenographically, at least in young people, if the underlying cause can be corrected. The osteoporosis is usually a minor part of the over-all syndrome.

Osteoporosis is a common finding in alcoholics of both sexes, and alcoholism should be suspected when osteoporotic fractures are found in men before age 65 and women before age 55. It is not known whether the disorder is due to the generally poor nutrition of alcoholics, to their usually very low calcium intakes, or to large endogenous losses of calcium. Its manifestations and consequences are the same as for ordinary postmenopausal or senile osteoporosis, but because of the coexisting alcoholism it is even harder to treat satisfactorily.

883. ENDOCRINE OSTEOPOROSES

Hyperthyroidism. Bone turnover is accelerated in hyperthyroidism. In some patients bone resorption may exceed formation sufficiently to produce significant osteoporosis. Unlike postmenopausal osteoporosis, this disorder involves all three bony envelopes, including the haversian. Fine-grain roentgenograms will often show significant intracortical tunneling in an otherwise normally thick cortex (cortical striation). The same process, if still more severe, may mimic hyperparathyroidism. The difference seems to be only one of degree. Plasma calcium, phosphorus, and alkaline phosphatase values may all be elevated, and the urine calcium may be normal or high. This too is a specific osteoporosis, treatable by recognizing and treating the hyperthyroidism. Roentgenographic improvement may occur, particularly in younger patients.

Cushing's Syndrome. Osteoporosis occurs in most patients with Cushing's syndrome and may be severe in approximately one third. It is associated with marked depression of osteoblast activity and with defective fracture healing. Similar changes can be produced by administration of glucocorticoids in high doses and are a complication of corticoid therapy, particularly in patients with rheumatoid arthritis. There is marked thinning of the cortex, and except for the accelerated resorption associated with endosteal expansion, bone turnover is generally suppressed. Like postmenopausal osteoporosis, this disorder involves primarily the endosteal envelope. Except for depression of alkaline phosphatase activity, there are no distinctive plasma chemical changes. Urine calcium is usually only moderately elevated, and gastrointestinal calcium absorption is de-

pressed. Improvement is poor, except in young patients, even with satisfactory control of the adrenal secretion.

884. MISCELLANEOUS OSTEOPOROSES

IDIOPATHIC OSTEOPOROSIS

The term "idiopathic osteoporosis" was applied originally to young men or women in whom no demonstrable cause could be found, and who were not postmenopausal or senile (and hence were not considered to have gonadal deficiency as a causal factor). The disease has been described in adolescents and in pregnant women, is commonly more painful than usual postmenopausal osteoporosis, and occurs more often in men than in women. The cause remains unknown. The disease tends to stabilize with time, but does not heal, and except for physical therapy and rehabilitation no treatment has been of much value.

SUDECK'S ATROPHY

After fracture in an extremity, structural turnover in adjacent bones increases markedly. Commonly, osteoporosis develops. Similar changes may also occur without fracture, sometimes following only minor injuries. The term "Sudeck's atrophy" refers to cases with or without fracture in which this osteoporosis comes on very acutely and is associated with severe pain and swelling, tenderness, and sweating in the overlying soft tissue. The disorder is most common in the wrists, hands, and feet, but may involve major portions of the skeleton, or may sometimes be migratory. Abnormal autonomic vasomotor regulation has been implicated as the cause. Sympathetic block may produce profound relief. Although frequently disabling, the disease is usually self-limited and in most instances heals spontaneously over a period of several months to a few years. In particularly severe or protracted cases regional sympathectomy may be indicated.

Bassan, J., Frame, B., and Frost, H.: Osteoporosis: A review of pathogenesis and treatment. Ann. Intern. Med., 58:539, 1963.

Cooke, A. M.: Osteoporosis. Lancet, 1:877, 929, 1955.

deTakats, G.: Sympathetic reflex dystrophy. Med. Clin. North Am., 49:117, 1965.

Heaney, R. P.: A unified concept of osteoporosis. Am. J. Med., 39:877, 1965.

Rich, C., Ensinck, J., and Ivanovich, P.: The effects of sodium fluoride on calcium metabolism of subjects with metabolic bone diseases. J. Clin. Invest., 43:545, 1964.

Rodahl, K., Nicholson, J. T., and Brown, E. M. (eds.): Bone as a Tissue. New York, Blakiston Division, McGraw-Hill Book Company, 1960, Part I: Osteoporosis, pp. 3–102.

Steinbach, H. L.: The roentgen appearance of osteoporosis. Radiol. Clin. North Am., 2:191, 1964.

Urist, M. R.: Osteoporosis. Ann Rev. Med., 13:273, 1962.

THE OSTEOMALACIAS

Robert P. Heaney

885. INTRODUCTION

Definition. The term "osteomalacia," meaning softening of bone, was applied originally to a distinctive clinical syndrome consisting of severe bone pain, skeletal deformity, depressed plasma Ca × P ion product, and wide osteoid borders in bone, all associated with vitamin D deficiency. The term has more recently been extended to include a variety of conditions exhibiting some, but not all, of the features of the full-blown vitamin D deficiency syndrome. This has led to confusion and disagreement concerning the definition of the disorder. Some authorities confine the term to the *clinical syndrome* described above, irrespective of the cause; others choose to base their definition on *morphologic* criteria, i.e., the presence of wide osteoid borders on bone surfaces. For purposes of clarity in exposition, the latter course will be pursued in what follows.

The term "rickets" refers to a series of identical syndromes occurring in childhood, and adds to the picture of adult osteomalacia the features of retarded growth, abnormal proliferation and maturation of the epiphyseal growth plate, and associated periarticular pain.

Morphologic and Roentgenographic Characteristics. Grossly, the skeleton may show little abnormality. In severe cases, bowing of long bones is observed, the pelvic bones are deformed inward, and all bones convey the impression of plastic deformation in response to applied forces. Microscopically, osteoid seams are invariably increased in thickness and in number, both on trabecular surfaces and in newly forming haversian systems. This osteoid fails to show evidence of the normal maturation sequence that must precede mineralization. In some osteomalacias, particularly those with severe vitamin D deficiency, changes of osteitis fibrosa may also be seen.

The principal roentgenographic changes are the deformities described above and, in rickets, widening, fraying, and cupping of all active growth plates. These rachitic changes are most apparent and most severe at sites of rapid growth, particularly the sternal ends of the ribs, the distal end of the radius and ulna, and the proximal ends of the tibia and humerus. In fact, the rachitic lesion is dependent upon growth for its expression. When growth slows or stops for any reason (such as intercurrent illness or increasing malnutrition), calcification of the disordered epiphyseal cartilage slowly occurs, and the roentgenographic lesion appears to heal, even though the basic abnormality remains unchanged. The bone of such persons then shows only osteomalacic lesions. In adults the only characteristic roentgenographic changes are the pseudofractures (Looser's zones, Milkman's lines). These lines are ribbon-like radiolucent zones, perpendicular to free bone surfaces, often bilateral and symmetrical, which give the appearance of incomplete fractures. They are found most commonly along the axillary border of the scapula, in the ischial and pubic rami, in the femoral neck, and in the ribs.

Generalized decrease in bone density is not a feature of osteomalacia per se. However, the disease commonly coexists with osteoporosis and hence may be found in skeletons that show decreased roentgenographic density. This decrease is not due to the osteomalacia per se.

General Pathophysiologic Considerations. The two features most characteristic of the osteomalacias are a low plasma Ca × P ion product and wide osteoid borders in bone. These have usually been considered to be related as cause and effect, and both have been attributed to poor intestinal calcium absorption. However, this simplified relationship is incorrect. As has been stressed before, defective calcium absorption leads to osteoporosis, not to osteomalacia; furthermore, in those osteomalacias caused by vitamin D deficiency small doses of vitamin D sufficient to repair the absorptive defect do not heal the bone lesions; conversely, adequate vitamin D therapy will cure osteomalacia even on a calcium-poor diet.

There are two basic mechanisms that might lead to accumulation of unmineralized osteoid: (1) insufficient concentration of calcium and phosphorus in extracellular fluid to allow crystal nucleation and growth, and (2) abnormalities in the matrix that render it unmineralizable. These mechanisms are not necessarily distinct, for the osteoblasts may well be sensitive to the phosphate concentration of the extracellular fluid, and thus in some cases the matrix abnormality may be due to a metabolic consequence of osteoblast phosphorus deficiency. Probably both defects are involved to varying degrees in the different osteomalacias. Nevertheless, there are undoubted matrix abnormalities in most if not all of the osteomalacias. Both rachitic cartilage and osteomalacic osteoid fail to show staining reactions characteristic of normal premineralization ripening. Some authorities are convinced that absence of a stainable calcification front is a *sine qua non* for the morphologic diagnosis of osteomalacia and is, hence, a more reliable feature than the mere width of osteoid borders. Although rachitic cartilage will mineralize when incubated in normal plasma, osteomalacic osteoid will not, and the first detectable changes in vivo after vitamin D therapy are staining reactions indicative of matrix maturation. These occur prior to measurable changes in plasma calcium or phosphorus concentration.

There can be little doubt that both new matrix production and osteoblast-mediated ripening of osteoid seams are severely depressed. This decrease in individual osteoblast activity is usually compensated for by markedly increased numbers of osteoblasts, which, though working slowly, may succeed in blanketing every available bone surface with a thick layer of poorly mineralizable matrix. The ultimate rate of new bone formation may thus be normal or even high, even though individual osteoblast activity is severely retarded.

886. RICKETS AND OSTEOMALACIA DUE TO VITAMIN D DEFICIENCY

Etiology and Incidence. At the turn of the century approximately 90 per cent of the children of northern European cities had clinical rickets secondary to vitamin D deficiency. For a time vitamin D deficiency became so rare that rickets and osteomalacia of solely nutritional causes were almost unknown in Europe and North America. With the immigration of dark-skinned persons into the industrial cities of northern Europe recently, there has been an increase in vitamin D deficiency disease. In general the disorder is still common in parts of the world where limited exposure to sunlight restricts vitamin D synthesis.

In the United States, vitamin D deficiency osteomalacia is virtually confined to patients with the various malabsorption syndromes, particularly idiopathic sprue, as well as in some patients with the Billroth I type of gastrectomy. Curiously, it is unusual in patients with pancreatic disease, even though the efficiency of vitamin D absorption has been shown to be less in these patients than in those with sprue.

Pathogenesis. Vitamin D deficiency has three main effects: it impairs intestinal calcium absorption, reduces the responsiveness of osteoclasts to parathyroid hormone, and leads to the defects in osteoblast activity mentioned earlier. The decreased sensitivity to parathyroid hormone is compensated for by increased parathyroid gland size and secretion, and this in turn produces markedly enhanced renal tubular responses, i.e., decreased calcium and increased phosphate clearance. Augmented parathyroid hormone levels maximize renal production of the 1,25-derivative from the available 25-HCC, and cause more bone remodeling centers to develop, thus compensating to some degree for the intestinal absorptive defect and the impaired bone resorption. Usually plasma calcium remains normal or nearly so, whereas plasma inorganic phosphate is reduced to low values, often below 2 mg per 100 ml. When skeletal demands for calcium are high, or osteoclast response is sharply reduced, plasma calcium may fall to tetanic levels.

Few patients with pure vitamin D deficiency are in significantly negative calcium balance. Although intestinal absorption is much reduced, it is not zero, and the limited absorption usually allows net recovery of most of the calcium of the digestive juices. Urine calcium is regularly reduced to extremely low values, often unmeasurably low. And thus, with no mechanism for losing calcium, it is not surprising that total bone mass remains at preosteomalacic levels.

Clinical Manifestations. Early in their course, patients with osteomalacia superimposed on gastrointestinal disease may have few symptoms referable to the bone disease; the predominant clinical manifestations are those of the underlying disease. When the osteomalacia becomes more severe, typical symptoms related to the skeleton and the vitamin D deficiency become apparent. These include bone pain, waddling gait, muscle weakness, and anorexia. Aching bone pain is prolonged and is made worse on weight-bearing; the bones may be tender to pressure. Pseudofractures tend to occur in bursts and when present may be associated with severe muscle weakness and bone pain. Experimentally produced hypophosphatemia is itself a cause of weakness; nevertheless the weakness of clinical osteomalacia is better correlated with the appearance of pseudofractures than with fluctuation in phosphate levels. It seems probable therefore that the symptom is due largely to reflex inhibition from bone pain. If the serum calcium falls to low levels, typical hypocalcemic tetany may occur. Occasional patients may have osteomalacia secondary to gluten-sensitive enteropathy, without obvious nutritional or gastrointestinal complaints, and thus may present only with skeletal manifestations.

It should be stressed that the most common bone disease in malabsorption syndromes is osteoporosis, not osteomalacia, and that when osteomalacia occurs it does so not simply because of the malabsorption, but because the patient has become ill enough to lose even casual contact with direct sunlight, thus losing his major source of vitamin D. So long as vitamin D levels remain adequate, however, calcium ion homeostasis works efficiently, and the malabsorption of calcium simply leads to negative calcium balance, which in turn results in osteoporosis. It is for this reason that most of the osteomalacia seen in the United States occurs in patients with pre-existing osteoporosis and represents a combined deficiency state (calcium first, then vitamin D).

Diagnosis. The diagnosis rests securely on a tripod of biopsy, roentgenographic, and biochemical findings. Wide osteoid borders are found on biopsy in all cases. Pseudofractures, when seen in otherwise normal bone, are virtually diagnostic of osteomalacia. The characteristic chemical changes are a normal to low plasma calcium, low plasma phosphate, high alkaline phosphatase, and very low urine calcium. Furthermore, these changes are characteristically found in patients with steatorrhea and with more or less obvious evidence of malabsorption. Occasionally the osteomalacia will be more apparent than the underlying enteropathy, and the observation of the changes described above should lead to a search for an underlying cause. The only differential consideration of consequence relates to other causes of osteomalacia. These include vitamin D resistance, adult hypophosphatasia, and advanced renal disease, all of which will be discussed in succeeding sections.

Treatment. Treatment must be directed at both the vitamin D deficiency and any underlying gastrointestinal disease, which is the usual cause of the deficiency. Uncomplicated vitamin D deficiency responds well to the vitamin in daily doses of as low as 1000 units; the various malabsorption syndromes may require from 10,000 to 50,000 units daily. Requirements in excess of these levels suggest one of the vitamin D resistant forms of osteomalacia (see below). Therapeutic ultraviolet exposure may be particularly helpful in patients with malabsorption syndromes, since skin manufacture of vitamin D bypasses the intestinal absorption block. Healing may be expected to be complete. Any coexisting osteoporosis resulting from calcium malabsorption should be treated by means of a high calcium intake.

887. VITAMIN D RESISTANT RICKETS
(Familial Hypophosphatemia)

Definition and Inheritance. Vitamin D resistant rickets and osteomalacia are distinct syndromes, clinically similar to their vitamin D deficient counterparts, but different in that they fail to respond to usual therapeutic doses of vitamin D. The term "vitamin D resistance" is unfortunate, for there is no evidence of true biochemical refractoriness to the vitamin, or to its metabolites. Instead it is the disease that is resistant, but it is resistant as well to vitamins A, B, C, and E as it is to D, and for the same good reason: it is not caused by deficiency of any one of them. The term "familial hypophosphatemia" is much more apt and describes the essential and invariable expression of the genetic defect that is responsible for the disorder. This defect is most commonly inherited as a sex-linked dominant character with complete penetrance but widely varying expressivity. Other inheritance patterns probably reflect different genetic defects that express themselves as hypophosphatemia. In addition, sporadic cases of resistant rickets, otherwise indistinguishable from the inherited variety, also occur. It is not known whether such patients have offspring who inherit the disease. Furthermore, adults with no sign of childhood rickets or dwarfing can occasionally present with osteomalacia associated with renal tubular hypophosphatemia. These patients give no family history of renal disease. Severe hypophosphatemic osteomalacia, resistant to vitamin D, has been described in association with certain benign tumors, notably sclerosing hemangiomata and neurofibromata. Cure has followed removal of the offending tumor.

Etiology and Pathogenesis. The nature of the genetic defect is unknown. The hypophosphatemia by which it is expressed is probably directly responsible for the osteomalacia. Although the matrix shows the same abnormal staining reactions as in vitamin D deficiency, simple elevation of the plasma phosphate by infusion or phosphate feeding will induce prompt healing and will lead to positive calcium balance. It cannot yet be decided whether the osteoid accumulates simply because there is inadequate mineral to allow crystal nucleation and growth or because the osteoblast suffers from an induced phosphate deficiency. The reason for the hypophosphatemia itself is also obscure. Defective tubular phosphate reabsorption has usually been implicated, and there is no doubt that renal phosphate clearance is greatly increased, but it has been established that tubular phosphate reabsorption in these patients responds normally to parathyroid hormone suppression; i.e., it can be returned to or toward normal by calcium infusion, by immobilization, or by any maneuver that reduces endogenous parathyroid hormone secretion. However, none of these increases the TM_p to normal. It has also been suggested that there is a primary defect in intestinal absorption of calcium leading to secondary parathyroid secretion, which in turn results in phosphaturia. However, it is common to find increased bone density in adults with the untreated disease (even to the extent that the axial skeleton can resemble osteopetrosis); this finding does not suggest lifelong inadequacy of calcium absorption.

Clinical Manifestations. Many affected persons have no demonstrable abnormality except for the hypophosphatemia. The expression of the defect ranges from simple hypophosphatemia without other abnormalities, through histologically demonstrable osteomalacia without clinical symptoms, to mild growth retardation, to typical, severe rickets and osteomalacia. The clinical features of the full-blown syndrome differ from ordinary vitamin D deficiency rickets in several respects. The disease is not common in early infancy and is seen most often after 18 months of age. The plasma calcium is almost always normal, whereas the plasma phosphorus is invariably low. The plasma alkaline phosphatase, although elevated, is rarely as high as in vitamin D deficiency. On biopsy the bone is essentially indistinguishable from that in vitamin D deficiency rickets, and, except for severity, roentgenographic changes do not distinguish between the two types of bone involvement. When the disease presents under the age of three, short stature and bowing of the legs is the characteristic deformity. With onset after three years, knock knee is usually seen. Muscle weakness is not observed in children with resistant rickets; but in adults with either the acquired or the hereditary disease, severe weakness, especially of the lower limbs, is quite common and may even suggest a neurologic disorder. This is believed to be due to hypophosphatemia, but is rarely seen without pseudofractures and pain. Most of these children develop a coxa vara deformity and consequent waddling gait. The limb bones are short and often bowed and there is a tendency to hyperostosis at tendinous insertions which may suggest the diagnosis of achondroplasia. In adolescence the epiphyses close, alkaline phosphatase returns to normal, and the patients become asymptomatic. However,

between 25 and 50 years pseudofractures may occur, especially in the femoral necks or over the convexity of the femoral shafts. These may not be associated with any rise in serum alkaline phosphatase activity.

In children, urinary calcium excretion is of the order of 10 to 20 mg per 24 hours, whereas in adults urinary calcium excretion ranges between 50 and 120 mg per 24 hours. These values are low, especially in children, but should be contrasted to the virtual absence of calcium in vitamin D deficiency rickets and osteomalacia.

Diagnosis. The diagnosis is based primarily on the observation of otherwise typical rickets and osteomalacia in patients without vitamin D deficiency or diseases predisposing thereto and without azotemia or other outspoken renal tubular defects, and on the failure of the bone disease to respond to usual vitamin D therapy. Commonly a positive family history or the familial occurrence of asymptomatic hypophosphatemia can be established. Quite similar bone disorders are seen in patients with multiple renal tubular reabsorptive defects. These defects include reabsorption of amino acids, bicarbonate, and glucose, as well as phosphate. In this group are included the Fanconi syndrome (vide infra) and renal tubular acidosis, as well as renal injury secondary to cystinosis and to lead or cadmium poisoning. Endemic osteomalacia caused by cadmium nephropathy has been described in Japan among persons eating rice irrigated with cadmium-polluted water.

Treatment. Available treatment is not altogether satisfactory, and it is doubtful that asymptomatic patients need any treatment. The disorder does not respond to antirachitic doses of vitamin D or its principal metabolite, 1,25-HCC. The most widely used therapy consists of pharmacologic doses of vitamin D (ergocalciferol, 50,000 to 200,000 units daily). These doses will usually cause roentgenographic changes of the epiphyses to heal. The dose required to do this is always very close to a toxic one. Furthermore, serum levels of phosphorus can never be maintained at normal in these patients without toxicity from vitamin D. Finally, there is little evidence that such therapy improves the growth rate or prevents deformities, despite near toxic levels of vitamin D therapy over a prolonged period of time. The adult syndrome with pseudofractures is best treated by a balanced sodium phosphate mixture containing 1.5 to 2 grams of phosphorus daily. Intake is pushed to levels just short of a cathartic effect. There is a large but transient rise in plasma phosphate after each dose, and divided doses are necessary in order to sustain the effect for a sufficient fraction of each day. A combination of phosphate and vitamin D is commonly employed, and has been reported to increase growth rate better than either agent alone.

888. HYPOPHOSPHATASIA

Hypophosphatasia is a familial skeletal disorder inherited as an autosomal recessive trait. The incidence is about 1 per 100,000 live births. Severe cases present in utero or within six months of birth; less severe cases present in infancy, although occasional cases do not present until late childhood or adult life. The bony disorder consists of severe osteomalacia and rickets which may result in fractures, rickety rosary, soft skull, and bulging fontanelle. The infants fail to thrive, may have fever and convulsions, and frequently die at an early age. Others are stillborn. Milder cases develop during the first year of life with features of rickets. Later, these children may develop craniostenosis. When cases present in adult life, the patients may have pathologic fractures of the pelvis and long bones or compression fractures or biconcavity of the spine indistinguishable from osteoporosis. Stress fractures may occur as in other types of osteomalacia. Histologic features of the disease are characteristic of osteomalacia, with broad osteoid seams lining the bone trabeculae. Serum calcium is normal or slightly elevated, and serum phosphorus is normal, whereas alkaline phosphatase values are always low. Leukocyte alkaline phosphatase is also low. Hypercalciuria is the rule at least in younger persons. All patients excrete phosphoethanolamine in the urine. Urinary pyrophosphate excretion is increased in these patients, and chondrocalcinosis may occur. There is no known effective treatment, although corticosteroid drugs have been used to heal rachitic changes in children, presumably by slowing growth.

889. MISCELLANEOUS OSTEOMALACIAS

Bone changes typical of osteomalacia, but without clinical symptoms, may be observed in many bone diseases, and clinically significant rachitic and osteomalacic skeletal involvement may complicate a variety of disorders. Most important is the bone disease associated with chronic renal insufficiency (see below). Osteomalacic bone changes, with or without symptoms, may occasionally be seen in patients with other bone disorders, such as Paget's disease, hyperparathyroidism, and fluorosis, as well as in patients with neither biochemical changes in the circulating plasma nor predisposing disease. In all such instances osteoid accumulation must be presumed to be due to interference with normal matrix maturation. Only very rarely does such osteomalacia produce clinical symptoms, and it is mentioned here principally because it may present as an incidental finding on bone biopsy.

FANCONI'S SYNDROME

The Fanconi syndrome consists of osteomalacic bone disease associated with renal tubular defect with respect to tubular reabsorption of glucose, amino acids, and phosphate. There may or may not be renal acidosis. The disease is commonly idiopathic, but may also result from renal tubular damage from cystine storage disease, in cadmium or lead poisoning, or from Wilson's disease (hepatolenticular degeneration). When renal acidosis occurs, hypocalcemia is common. Treatment is similar to that of resistant rickets except when acidosis complicates the picture and then it is important to correct acidosis with appropriate alkali therapy as well as to treat the patient with large doses of vitamin D.

Bartter, F. C.: Hypophosphatasia. *In* Stanbury, J. B., Wyngaarden, J. B., and Fredrickson, D. S. (eds.): Metabolic Basis of Inherited Disease. 3rd ed. New York, Blakiston Division, McGraw-Hill Book Company, 1972.

Frame, B., Smith, R. W., Jr., Fleming, J. L., and Manson, G.: Oral phosphates in vitamin-D-refractory rickets and osteomalacia. Am. J. Dis. Child., 106:147, 1963.

Fraser, D.: Hypophosphatasia. Am. J. Med., 22:739, 1957.

Hioco, D.: Osteomalacia. Paris, Editions Masson, 1966.

Stanbury, S. W., and Lumb, G.: Parathyroid function in chronic renal failure. Quart. J. Med., 35:1, 1966.

Williams, T. F., and Winters, R. W.: Familial (hereditary) vitamin D resistant rickets with hypophosphatemia. *In* Stanbury, J. B., Wyngaarden, J. B., and Fredrickson, D. S. (eds.): Metabolic Basis of Inherited Disease. 3rd ed. New York, Blakiston Division, McGraw-Hill Book Company, 1972.

890. RENAL OSTEODYSTROPHY

Definition and Incidence.   The bone disease of persons suffering from chronic uremia presents as a confusing variety of manifestations seemingly different from one part of the world to the next and depending as well on whether the patient is receiving hemodialysis. Typically the bone disease consists of features of osteomalacia, osteitis fibrosa, osteosclerosis, and osteoporosis, the first two being the more important. Although it is not always easy to predict which one of these will predominate in any individual, given time, some form of skeletal disease develops in all uremic patients.

Clinical Manifestations.   Clinical manifestations include bone pain, deformity, fractures, and, in children, growth retardation. Since uremic patients are rarely in very negative calcium balance, total body calcium is usually normal or even high. With the more severe cases of osteitis fibrosa and metastatic calcification there is usually an intrabody shift of mineral from bone to ectopic sites (such as bursae or vascular walls). Frequently the bone marrow is itself a site of metastatic calcification (as in vitamin D intoxication), and this phenomenon may produce or contribute to the roentgenographic appearance of osteosclerosis.

Pathogenesis and Diagnosis.   There is resistance to the action of vitamin D in uremia, which begins to be manifest even at minor degrees of azotemia. At least some of this resistance appears to be due to impaired conversion of 25-HCC to 1,25-HCC, associated either with loss of renal parenchymal tissue or with high plasma phosphate levels, or both. At very high phosphate values, there is apparently some triple hydroxylation to the 1,24,25-derivative. This compound has intestinal but not bone resorptive activity. These defects lead to compensatory parathyroid hyperplasia and hypersecretion. The plasma calcium may be quite low but is more commonly in the low-normal range, and is presumably maintained at even this level only because of sometimes heroic levels of parathyroid hormone secretion.

The parathyroid glands are invariably increased in size, and there appear to be at least a few cases of true autonomous hyperparathyroidism resulting from this long-continued hyperplasia. In general, gland hypertrophy is less severe in those patients with lesions that are predominantly osteomalacic and more severe in patients with predominant osteitis fibrosa and metastatic calcification. The level of phosphatemia depends on a combination of factors, including the degree of renal failure, the level of parathyroid hormone secretion, the phosphate intake, and various therapeutic regimens (principally aluminum hydroxide gels) designed to lower effective phosphate intake. Nevertheless, the plasma phosphate is usually above normal, and the empirical Ca × P product correspondingly elevated. The alkaline phosphatase is usually elevated and roentgenograms demonstrate the features of osteomalacia, osteitis fibrosa, or both. It has been observed that, when the Ca × P product is below 70, the most prominent feature of the bone disease is likely to consist of rickets or osteomalacia, and when above 70, osteitis fibrosa together with varying degrees of metastatic calcification. There is broad overlap between these categories, and the distinction is further complicated by the fact that some degree of osteitis fibrosa, including typical roentgenographic features, is frequent in severe rickets and osteomalacia from any cause, including that seen in the uremic syndrome. The existence of rickets and osteomalacia in the presence of high mineral concentrations presents an interesting and as yet unsolved problem. There has been shown to be a circulating inhibitor of calcification in the plasma of uremic patients. Furthermore, the healing seen with high doses of vitamin D (which produces only trivial changes in Ca × P product in these patients) suggests either systemic removal of this inhibitor or direct vitamin D action on osteoblasts and growth cartilage.

Treatment. If the predominant bony lesion is rachitic (malacic) and if the Ca × P product is lower than 70, then the patient will very likely benefit from vitamin D, which must usually be given in large doses (50,000 to 500,000 units per day) or from dihydrotachysterol. Both the malacic lesions and any associated osteitis fibrosa may heal significantly with these sterols. Recent investigations have shown that as little as 2.5 μg per day of 1,25-HCC (the molar equivalent of 100 I.U. of vitamin D) will return D-dependent functions to normal in uremic subjects. The pure compound is not commercially available, and it is likely that the effect produced by massive doses of the crude D vitamin preparations available is due to the presence of trace quantities of contaminating sterol impurities which act like 1,25-HCC. This, in effect, is the reason why dihydrotachysterol appears to be more effective than calciferol in uremic bone disease. The A-ring of this sterol is sterically similar to 1,25-HCC, and thus the compound circumvents the renal synthetic defect.

If there is little or no malacic component to the bone disease, vitamin D treatment will usually do no good and may, by raising the Ca × P product still further, aggravate an already dangerous propensity to metastatic calcification. It is thus important to evaluate both bone morphology and plasma calcium and phosphate levels before beginning vitamin D treatment. If roentgenographic findings of rickets or osteomalacia are not evident, a bone biopsy should be obtained and an undecalcified section examined for the presence of uncalcified osteoid.

Treatment directed at the uremia itself also has effects on the bone disease and on calcium homeostasis. In general, dialysis does nothing to alter the vitamin D resistance or the tendency to osteomalacia, and by prolonging life may allow osteodystrophy to develop to the point of producing significant disability. Regimens directed at suppressing the plasma phosphate appear to benefit patients with high Ca × P products and with bony lesions predominantly of osteitis fibrosa, whereas slight elevation of dialysis bath calcium has been shown to help the primarily osteomalacic lesion. Successful renal transplantation almost always leads to restoration of normal vitamin D metabolism and corresponding healing of rickets and osteomalacia. Normal vitamin D metabolism returns well before the parathyroid glands can involute, and the sometimes huge residual mass of parathyroid tissue may thus oversecrete parathyroid hormone even when maximally suppressed, producing post-transplantation hypercalcemia. This phenomenon usually becomes apparent as the plasma phosphate falls, but may first make its appearance as much as six months after

transplantation. This situation has been given the unhappy designation "tertiary hyperparathyroidism." It appears to be a true hyperparathyroidism, i.e., hypercalcemia caused by excessive secretion of parathyroid hormone, but in almost all cases is self-limited and subsides as the parathyroid glands complete their involution. In a small minority of cases autonomous parathyroid adenomas exist, and these must be removed surgically. In others the degree of hypercalcemia may be sufficiently severe or prolonged, or the risk of myocardial or pulmonary calcification considered so great, that subtotal parathyroidectomy may be warranted. Several authorities consider that extensive metastatic calcification is an indication for subtotal parathyroidectomy either prior to or soon after renal transplantation.

Kleeman, C. R. (ed.): Divalent ion metabolism and osteodystrophy in chronic renal failure. Arch. Intern. Med., 124:261, 389, 519, 649, 1969.

891. OSTEITIS FIBROSA

Robert P. Heaney

Definition. The term "osteitis fibrosa" is used to designate a pathologic rather than a clinical entity. It refers to the replacement of bone by a highly cellular fibrous tissue, associated with accumulations of osteoclasts, singly and in clumps, together with evidence of increased osteoblastic activity. The terms "osteitis fibrosa cystica" and "von Recklinghausen's bone disease"* have also been used to describe this condition.

Etiology and Incidence. In most cases the morphologic picture comes about because of greatly exaggerated parathyroid hormonal stimulation. It is found in 10 to 25 per cent of patients with primary hyperparathyroidism, is always found as a part of the picture of uremic osteodystrophy, and to variable degrees may be seen in patients with rickets and osteomalacia. In the latter disorders, the presence of osteitis fibrosa depends upon the degree of responsiveness to parathyroid hormone that the bone mesenchyme is able to manifest. However, the identical condition can be produced even without an excess of parathyroid hormone whenever bone turnover is exceedingly rapid, as in certain patients with hyperthyroidism, and locally in rapidly evolving Paget's disease (vide infra).

Pathogenesis and Pathology. In the typical case due to excess parathyroid hormone there is stimulation of all bone cells: osteocytes resorb their perilacunar bone; osteoclasts are found in large numbers and resorb bone on all three bony envelopes; osteoblastic new bone formation is also increased. However, osteoclasts predominate, and as a consequence there is usually a decrease in total skeletal mass. Resorption is particularly prominent in cortical bone immediately beneath the periosteum and is responsible for the typical and characteristic roentgenographic features of the disorder: (1) the presence of a fine lacy pattern of radiolucency at the outer edge of the cortex, particularly in the phalanges and metacarpals; (2) the disappearance of the lamina dura (the equivalent of

---

*The eponym "von Recklinghausen's disease" is also associated with the hereditary disorder neurofibromatosis, which may occasionally exert indirect skeletal effects, chiefly scoliosis and bony erosion by adjacent neurofibromas, and rarely a vitamin D-resistant osteomalacia.

a bone cortex in the tooth socket); and (3) cortical striation seen on fine grain films. When severe, or of long duration, there is virtual loss of detectable bone from the ends of the clavicles and the terminal phalanges ("acro-osteolysis"). Undoubtedly the bony mesenchyme is itself stimulated by parathyroid hormone, and masses of growing fibrous tissue and osteoclasts may expand and destroy the bone cortex, giving rise to what appear, roentgenographically, to be large cystic tumors. Osteoclasts alone may form tumor-like masses that have been designated giant cell tumors. These produce discrete punched-out lesions roentgenographically, particularly in the jaw or facial bones, and in some cases such tumors may be the primary roentgenographic manifestations of osteitis fibrosa. Such tumors are biologically benign and invariably regress if the underlying cause is removed.

Clinical Manifestations.   The principal manifestations of osteitis fibrosa are bone pain and pathologic fractures. Early the pain is not distinctive and is easily mistaken for vague arthritic complaints. There may also be specific arthritides present: both gout and pseudogout have been described in association with osteitis fibrosa. Later the bones become tender to palpation, and in advanced cases the pain may become incapacitating. Pathologic fractures occur through areas weakened by general resorption or giant cell tumor formation, and may involve any bones of the body. Vertebral collapse is common, and compression fractures and acroosteolysis of the terminal phalanges may so shorten those bones as to simulate "clubbing" of the fingers. Since patients may have hypercalcemia, their clinical picture will usually include extraskeletal features described elsewhere in this text (see Ch. 872).

Diagnosis.   The generalized decrease in roentgenographic density must be distinguished from osteoporosis and multiple myeloma, and the cystlike lesions from fibrous dysplasia and true bone tumors. Bone biopsy establishes the true nature of the lesion, and plasma chemical determinations aid in determining its cause, e.g., primary hyperparathyroidism (see Ch. 872), uremia, and osteomalacia.

Treatment.   In primary hyperparathyroidism, removal of the offending adenoma constitutes definitive therapy. Treatment in other conditions producing osteitis fibrosa is less certain or satisfactory. The bone lesions heal with great rapidity when the cause, such as a parathyroid adenoma, can be eradicated. For this reason, giant cell tumors, particularly in the facial bones, should not be treated by mutilating surgical operations until hyperparathyroidism has been excluded as a cause.

Johnson, L. C.: Morphologic analysis in pathology: The kinetics of disease and general biology of bone. *In* Frost, H. M. (ed.): Bone Biodynamics. Boston, Little, Brown & Company, 1964.

Weinmann, J. P., and Sicher, H.: Bone and Bones. St. Louis, C. V. Mosby Company, 1955, pp. 246–251.

BONE INTOXICATIONS

Robert P. Heaney

892. FLUOROSIS

Fluoride is one of the more common constituents of the earth's crust, occurring particularly in association with phosphates, silicates, and calcium. It is abundant in sea water and in many fresh water supplies, and was undoubtedly a component of the environment in which life evolved. It probably functions as an important trace element in human nutrition, though a fluoride deficiency syndrome is not recognized. In optimal concentrations fluoride stabilizes the crystal structure of tooth enamel and probably also that of bone. In high concentrations fluoride acts as a general protoplasmic poison, resulting in death; but between toxic intake levels (> 100 mg) and probably optimal intakes (about 1 mg daily), chronic intake produces changes confined largely to the skeleton. Intoxication occurs because of accidental ingestion of fluoride-containing insecticides, chronic inhalation of industrial dusts (particularly in the aluminum mining and phosphate fertilizer industries), or prolonged drinking of certain fresh waters containing large amounts of fluorides. The skeletal lesions in man vary with the intake but consist of a combination of osteosclerosis and osteomalacia. The malacic lesions are more prominent at higher intake levels and represent interference with matrix maturation or crystal nucleation. Sclerosis consists of coarsening of trabeculae, periosteal new bone deposition, osteophyte formation, and ossification of tendons and ligaments. Severely fluorotic bone is chalky white in appearance and exhibits a crumbly consistency, cutting easily with a knife.

Early there are no specific complaints. As the skeletal disease advances there may be vague pains in the small joints of hands and feet. As osteophyte formation and periosteal bone growth progress, kyphosis, restriction of spine motion, flexion contractures of hips and knees, and ultimately nerve root and spinal cord compression develop. The neurologic involvement produces paresthesias, weakness, and ultimately paralysis. Early the neurologic involvement may simulate peripheral neuropathy, spinal cord tumors, or syringomyelia.

No municipal water supply in the United States contains more than 6 to 8 parts per million of fluoride, and this concentration, although sufficient to produce mottled tooth enamel, almost never produces bone disease. In certain regions of India and Arabia water-related fluoride intake reaches sufficient levels to produce fluoride intoxication. In the Punjab, for example, osteofluorosis is the most common form of bone disease. Deliberate osteofluorosis has sometimes been induced to halt the explosive skeletal demineralization of diseases such as multiple myeloma.

There is no effective treatment for the advanced syndrome except for orthopedic and supportive measures. Effort should be directed at prevention, particularly in the context of industrial exposure. Excess body burdens of fluoride are retained for years after exposure has terminated. Fluoride trapped in bone crystals is released only when bone resorption occurs, and some of the liberated ions are redeposited at sites of new bone formation. If the intake is low, however, urinary excretion will gradually lower the total body content.

893. VITAMIN A INTOXICATION

Although not confined to bone, the effects of chronic excessive vitamin A intake may be most apparent in the skeleton. Such intoxication is rare, and has occurred most frequently in young children who received doses on the order of 100 times the normal daily vitamin requirement and in hunters who ingested large quantities of polar bear liver. The initial bony change is painful periosteal proliferation, particularly of the ulnae, clavicles, and metatarsals. These are readily apparent on roentgenographic examination. Higher doses in small animals produce severe osteoporosis and multiple fractures. The diagnosis is suggested by a history of excessive vitamin intake, and by finding high vitamin A levels in the plasma. Bony healing is usually complete when vitamin exposure ceases.

894. VITAMIN D INTOXICATION

In the past intoxication with vitamin D occurred primarily because of inappropriate and massive vitamin therapy for diseases not caused by vitamin deficiency. The disease is still seen as a complication of more appropriate vitamin D therapy for disorders such as osteomalacia or familial hypophosphatemia, and occasionally occurs in food faddists and in patients with an unusual sensitivity to doses usually considered to lie within the physiologic range. Intoxication results in three principal and closely related effects: hypercalcemia, metastatic calcification, and osteitis fibrosa. The ultimate clinical picture varies, depending upon the relative importance of these effects.

In massive dosage the vitamin (or contaminating trace sterols in the commercial vitamin preparations) directly stimulates both gastrointestinal calcium absorption and osteoclastic bone resorption. Hypercalcemia ensues, and endogenous parathyroid suppression occurs. Plasma inorganic phosphate is therefore normal or high, and thus the Ca × P ion product may rise to extremely high values, probably reaching supersaturated levels in many normally unmineralized tissue regions. In any case large soft-tissue calcium deposits occur, particularly in already damaged regions such as the synovia of arthritic joints, as well as in arterial walls. Urine calcium is initially high, and the renal interstitium is particularly prone to calcification. Such renal calcinosis leads to deterioration of renal function, further phosphate retention, and inability to excrete the excess plasma calcium load. This generates a vicious cycle which may lead to death from hypercalcemia or uremia. Metastatic calcification occurs also in the bone marrow of trabecular bone and may thus lead to the appearance of osteosclerosis. Because of the parathyromimetic effect of vitamin D, osteitis fibrosa is usually seen as well, and the net roentgenographic appearance of bone depends on the balance between these two processes.

Clinical manifestations are caused principally by the hypercalcemia and renal failure, and not by the bone disease itself. These are the same as those of hypercalcemia from any cause, and include anorexia, nausea, vomiting, lassitude, polyuria, dehydration, and ultimately fever, stupor, and death.

The diagnosis of vitamin D intoxication should be considered in the evaluation of patients with hypercalcemia or those found to have extensive soft tissue calcification. It is most readily confirmed by obtaining a history of excessive vitamin D intake and by observing improvement when the vitamin is withdrawn. Treatment consists of management of the hypercalcemia and stopping vitamin D ingestion; this is usually satisfactory unless irreversible kidney damage has occurred.

895. RADIONUCLIDE BONE TOXICITY

Many radioactive isotopes accumulate in the skeleton and, although ingested in doses too small to produce acute systemic effects, may lead years later to severe bone disease. Skeletal damage consists of (1) growth retardation if exposure occurred prior to epiphyseal closure; (2) osteonecrosis, osteomyelitis, and bone abscess; (3) brittleness and tendency to fracture; and (4) osteogenic sarcoma. There are three categories of exposure: (1) strontium-90 and yttrium-91 from radioactive fallout of atom bomb fission products; (2) radium and thorium from industrial and medical exposure; and (3) uranium and the transuranic elements from processing of nuclear reactor fuel and wastes. Strontium and radium, like calcium, are alkaline earth elements and readily form phosphate salts. They are trapped in newly forming bone at the time of its mineralization. The localization of thorium, uranium, and the transuranic elements is less well understood, but appears to be predominantly on bone surfaces adjacent to the innumerable small vessels of bone. Radiation damage in each case is produced by the α and β particles, rather than by the γ radiation. Because of the extremely short range of these particles in bone, the damage is thus confined microscopically to the areas of isotope deposition. Cell death is the usual result, cell sensitivity varying with cell type, as follows: chondroblasts > osteoblasts > osteocytes > osteoclasts. The surrounding bony material, deprived of continuing cellular influence, becomes hard and brittle. Ultimately it is subject to slow resorptive removal. The mechanism of sarcoma production is not known but is presumably the same as for radiation carcinogenesis elsewhere.

Clinical features are variable and not distinctive. Bone pain may be present, and spontaneous fractures may occur through bone that appears roentgenographically normal. Occasionally the long bones may present a punched-out appearance reminiscent of multiple myeloma. Radium dial painters frequently developed necrosis and osteomyelitis of the jaw, related to localization of radium in the periodontal tissues. Radiation damage, once it has occurred, is irrevocable, and no treatment is of any value. Bone localization after acute accidental ingestion of radium and strontium can be minimized by calcium infusion and deliberate production of sustained hypercalciuria.

Barnicot, N. A., and Datta, S. P.: Vitamin A and bone. *In* Bourne, G. H. (ed.): Biochemistry and Physiology of Bone. 2nd ed. Vol. 2. New York, Academic Press, 1971.

Cousins, R. J., and DeLuca, H. T.: Vitamin D and Bone. *In* Bourne, G. H. (ed.): Biochemistry and Physiology of Bone. 2nd ed. Vol. 2. New York, Academic Press, 1971.

Hasterlik, R. J., and Finkel, A. J.: Diseases of bones and joints associated with intoxication by radioactive substances, principally radium. Med. Clin. North Am., 49:285, 1965.

Pugh, D. G.: Roentgenologic Diagnosis of Diseases of Bones. New York, Thomas Nelson & Sons, 1951.

Singh, A., Jolly, S. S., Bansal, B. C., and Mathur, C. C.: Endemic fluorosis; epidemiological, clinical and biochemical study of chronic fluorine intoxication in Punjab (India). Medicine, 42:229, 1963.

Vaughn, J. M.: The effects of radiation on bone. *In* Bourne, G. H. (ed.): Biochemistry and Physiology of Bone. 2nd ed. Vol. 3. New York, Academic Press, 1971.

Weinmann, J. P., and Sicher, H.: Bone and Bones. St. Louis, C. V. Mosby Company, 1955, pp. 246–251.

896.   OSTEOMYELITIS

Paul D. Saville

Definition.   Osteomyelitis is an infection within bone by any bacterial or mycotic organism that infects other tissues.

Pathophysiology.   Before puberty, infection starts in the metaphyseal sinusoidal veins. Because bone tissue is inelastic, local edema accumulates under pressure and leads to necrosis of tissue, breakdown of bone trabeculae, and removal of both matrix and calcium. Infection extends along haversian canals and through the marrow cavity and beneath the periosteum, damaging the vascular channels and causing death of osteocytes. This leads to the formation of a sequestrum. The periosteal new bone formation which takes place on top of already dead bone is known as an involucrum.

Etiology.   Patients can often be shown to have infection elsewhere, particularly in the skin, where *S. aureus* is probably the most common causative organism, but its prevalence has dropped in the United States from 80 per cent in the past to about 50 per cent at present. Gram-negative bacilli occur mainly in adults with vertebral osteomyelitis. *M. tuberculosis* occurs mainly in the spine, especially among economically deprived individuals. Tuberculous and fungal infections of bone can usually be traced back to pulmonary disease. Persons with sickle cell disease have a special susceptibility to Salmonella osteomyelitis. Vertebral osteomyelitis in adults may follow colorectal surgery, or infection of the genital, urinary, or biliary tracts.

Clinical Manifestations.   In the past, over 85 per cent of cases occurred in children under 16. Recently there has been a shift of the disease to older age groups. Infection usually occurs in the metaphyseal region, particularly of the femur and tibia, and multiple bone involvement is not rare. In patients over the age of 50, the most common site of osteomyelitis is the spine.

In children, onset is sudden, with high fever, chills, and pain in a limb. Increasing numbers of patients are seen with atypical features, including low-grade temperatures and even no fever at all. There is usually leukocytosis. Acute local tenderness and swelling may occur because of elevation of the periosteum by pus. In adults, pyogenic spondylitis is seldom heralded by an acute febrile episode. Usually there is simply insidious onset of deep boring pain in the back, aggravated by movement, coughing, sneezing, or straining. Symptoms gradually increase. Patients may complain of abdominal pain when the lumbar vertebrae are involved. Paravertebral or psoas abscesses were once thought to be indicative of tuberculous spondylitis, but today such an abscess in the United States or Western Europe is more likely to be associated with staphylococcal infection than with tuberculosis. In the adult, no changes are visible radiographically, often for many weeks after onset of infection. The first changes are destruction of a disc space and the adjacent vertebral end-plates above and below. Later sclerosis of bone occurs and new bone forms, often with fusion of two vertebrae and obliteration of the intervertebral space. In childhood disease, blood cultures are frequently positive for the causative organism. In adult pyogenic spondylitis, this is rare.

Subacute pyogenic osteomyelitis, known as Brodie's abscess, is usually located in a metaphysis and appears as a lucent lesion sometimes surrounded by slight sclerosis. Its onset is insidious; pain is a prominent symptom, but fever is rare. It is usually due to the presence of *S. aureus,* occasionally *S. albus,* or even more occasionally gram-negative organisms.

Chronic osteitis in the hands or feet is usually due to tuberculosis or syphilis. Asymmetric osteitis in the hands or feet is more likely to be due to group A Streptococcus and *S. aureus.*

Radiographic changes are late in developing in osteomyelitis, but scintigraphy using ^{99m}Tc diphosphonate will point to a lesion early in the disease, either in the spine or in the long bones. This is particularly helpful in the adult in whom there is almost no clinical evidence to indicate spine disease.

Treatment.   It is important to obtain the organism responsible for the infection and to determine the antimicrobial sensitivity. In vertebral osteomyelitis, needle biopsy with aspiration of tissue is necessary. For sensitive organisms, penicillin G is the best antimicrobial and should be used in large doses, preferably 20,000,000 units per day given intravenously. Alternatively, oxacillin, methicillin, or nafcillin may be given in daily doses of 8 to 16 grams intravenously in an adult. Treatment should be maintained for at least four to six weeks. There is no place for oral medication or for bacteriostatic drugs in the initial stages of treatment. Most cases of hematogenous osteomyelitis in children should be surgically drained even when the organism is known and the appropriate antimicrobial is given in large doses.

When osteomyelitis has been clinically cured, it can be assumed that viable organisms remain in haversian and Volkmann canals. It may recur up to four decades later because of the same organisms. These recurrences are often precipitated by trauma.

OSTEOMYELITIS DUE TO CONTIGUOUS INFECTION

Osteomyelitis may be caused by infection gaining entrance to a bone from a compound fracture or through surgical operation, especially with internal fixation. Infection of the phalanges of the hands and feet may occur from soft tissue infections, especially in the hands. Infection of the jaws occurs from dental abscesses and radiation. Infection from the frontal or ethmoid sinuses causes osteomyelitis of the frontal bone by spread from the blood vessels of the mucosal lining of the sinuses. When the frontal bone is infected, pus collects under the periosteum, causing swelling and edema over the forehead known as Pott's puffy tumor. With frontal osteomyelitis, epidural and even subdural abscesses may occur, with severe headache and signs of increased intracranial pressure.

A local infection occurring after a compound fracture or internal fixation is usually associated with pain, pus, and fever. When infection occurs after introduction of a prosthetic device, there is frequently an insidious onset of pain, which may take months or even years after the surgical procedure to become manifest. Extensive bone destruction may occur without clear-cut signs of infection or fever. The existence of infection may be obscured by the use of prophylactic antimicrobials given at the time of surgery. The diagnosis may be helped by needling of the suspected lesion or by open surgery. Where a prosthetic device has been used, it is often necessary to remove this before the infection can be controlled.

Infections of the bones of the feet or toes occur frequently in patients with diabetes mellitus or with severe peripheral vascular disease. The patients frequently have pain and swelling in the affected limb and may have ulcers. More often than not they have no systemic manifestation such as fever. Response to treatment with antimicrobials is usually unsatisfactory, and amputation is often necessary.

Waldvogel, F. A., Medoff, G., and Swartz, M. N.: Osteomyelitis: A review of clinical features, therapeutic considerations and unusual aspects. N. Engl. J. Med., 282:198, 260, 316, 1970.

897. OSTEONECROSIS

Paul D. Saville

Definition. Osteonecrosis denotes the clinical syndrome associated with death of bone cells in a localized volume of bone. The term osteonecrosis is used here for the condition formerly called *aseptic necrosis of bone* or *avascular necrosis of bone.*

Etiology. Osteonecrosis may result from traumatic disruption of the blood supply of bone. Common sites of this include the femoral head after a subcapital fracture of the hip or traumatic dislocation of the hip; the semilunar, navicular, and scaphoid bones in the wrist; the tibial tuberosity; and the epiphysis of the os calcis before closure. Nontraumatic necrosis is believed to be due to obstruction of bony end-arteries by sludged red cells, gas bubbles, lipid droplets, uric acid crystals, or vasculitis. These may arise in Gaucher's disease, in sickle cell anemia, in caisson disease, in systemic lupus erythematosus, in hyperlipemia associated with alcoholism or pancreatitis, and with corticosteroid therapy. *Perthes' disease* is an osteonecrosis of the femoral head occurring for uncertain reasons, largely in males between four and ten years of age. *Osteochondritis dissecans* of the medial femoral condyle of children is a similar condition, as is osteonecrosis of the weight-bearing portion of the medial femoral condyle seen in older adults. The disease also occurs in the talus, the capitellum, and the humeral head.

Incidence. Osteonecrosis of the femoral head occurs in about 50 per cent of cases of subcapital fracture of the hip and in 50 per cent of patients on immunosuppressive therapy for kidney homograft. Perthes' disease of the hip occurs in one of 820 boys and one of 4500 girls.

Clinical Manifestations and Diagnosis. In adults, pain may occur up to three years after the original subcapital fracture. The disease which occurs in alcoholics and immunosuppressed patients, as well as the idiopathic variety, usually manifests itself with sudden bone pain. At first, there are no radiographic changes, but after two months there may be a small radiolucent zone in bone under the articular cartilage. High resolution bone scans with agents such as ^{99m}Tc diphosphonate invariably reveal a focus of intense isotope uptake before radiographic changes become apparent. Later, increased bone density indicates attempted healing of the lesion. Before healing can occur, the resorptive phase leads to weakened bone which may collapse on weight bearing and result in bone deformity. This leads to secondary osteoarthrosis.

Treatment. Treatment consists of stopping weight bearing until healing has occurred. This may take up to three years. Some surgeons use bone grafts inserted through the femoral neck into the head to speed up the healing process in the hip. When osteonecrosis affects bones in the wrist, severe osteoarthrosis of the joint is common and wrist fusion may be required to relieve pain. Prostheses may be used with success when deformity of bone and secondary osteoarthritis occur in weight-bearing joints.

Ahlback, S., Bauer, G. C. H., and Bohne, W. H.: Spontaneous osteonecrosis of the knee. Arthritis Rheum., 11:705, 1968.

CONGENITAL AND/OR HEREDITARY DISORDERS INVOLVING BONE

Paul D. Saville

898. OSTEOGENESIS IMPERFECTA
(Psathyrosis, Fragilitas Ossium, Lobstein's Disease)

Definition. Osteogenesis imperfecta is an inherited disorder of collagen maturation resulting in defects in connective tissue, manifested by increased fragility of the skeleton and blue sclerae.

Inheritance. About half the cases are sporadic, presumably caused by mutations. In the majority of the remaining cases, the disease is inherited as an autosomal dominant trait. There is also a rarer and very severe recessive type. Clinical expression of disease can vary widely; this has been responsible for confusion in classification and terminology. The disease is not uncommon, but precise incidence figures are lacking.

Pathology and Pathogenesis. The basic chemical defect is unknown. Soluble collagens fail to complete the normal sequence of extracellular changes necessary to convert them into a tough fibrous tissue. Total collagen is quantitatively deficient as well. As a result, tendons and ligaments are thin and subject to rupture; the skin is thin; the sclerae of the eyes are also thin and allow the choroidal pigment to show through, giving a blue color. Woven bone may be seen in adult life and may be the only characteristic microscopic abnormality. The rates of new bone formation and resorption are increased. Unlike acquired osteoporosis, there is a defect at the periosteal envelope which results in decreased appositional growth rate. This causes the unduly narrow bones characteristic of this disease.

Clinical Features. The clinical manifestations are extremely variable; 60 per cent of affected individuals have bone disease, but in the same family 5 per cent will have only an otosclerotic type of deafness while an occasional member will manifest only blue sclerae. In severe cases, multiple fractures occur during birth or in utero, or multiple fractures may occur from trivial trauma during childhood. The tendency to fracture decreases as the child approaches adolescence. The children are small and have an increased basal metabolic rate. Serum calcium and phosphorus are normal, but alkaline phosphatase may be elevated when fractures occur. Serum and urine pyrophosphate may be increased. Lax ligaments are a common clinical finding. Radiographs reveal gracile long bones with narrow cortices; the skull is thin and may be deformed. There is radiolucence of the vertebrae which may be uniformly compressed. This gives an appearance of biconcavity or of platyspondylia and can be indistinguishable from severe osteoporosis or osteomalacia. When the diagnosis is uncertain, the finding of wormian bones in the skull x-ray may be of help. Patients with this disease have no difficulty in forming callus; indeed, extremely exuberant callus formation may occur. This may be mistaken for tumor, and biopsy of such tissue can lead to erroneous diagnosis of osteogenic sarcoma.

Treatment. Fractures are treated by conventional methods of fixation. There is no effective treatment for the bone disease itself. Ascorbic acid has been used in massive doses; sodium fluoride, 5 mg per day, has been claimed to reduce the fracture rate, as has magnesium oxide, 10 to 15 mg per kilogram per day, which also has lowered the elevated serum pyrophosphate levels.

899. OSTEOPETROSIS
(Albers-Schönberg's Disease, Marble Bone Disease)

Marble bone disease is a rare familial disorder of the skeleton characterized by an increase in density of all bones owing to failure of bone resorption and bone remodeling.

There are probably dominant as well as recessive types of inheritance. The severe variety presents in infancy with anemia and hepatosplenomegaly. These children have little or no bone marrow and require blood transfusions. Failure to resorb bone results in optic atrophy, deafness, and hydrocephalus. Osteomyelitis of the jaws from dental infection may require antimicrobials. Early death is frequent. Milder cases may come to medical attention later in childhood or in adult life because of retarded growth or increased bone fragility.

Hypersplenism may require splenectomy for improvement of anemia. There is no specific treatment for the bone disease.

900. MELORHEOSTOSIS

This is a rare disorder of bone resulting in massive endosteal thickening, affecting one or more long bones, which begins proximally and proceeds distally like the flow of wax down a candle. The condition is painful. The cause is unknown, and there is no specific treatment.

901. OSTEOPOIKILOSIS

This condition is inherited as an autosomal dominant trait. It consists of multiple dense zones or streaks occurring throughout the skeleton and frequently is associated with local patches of elastic fiber hyperplasia in the skin. It is of little clinical importance.

902. HEREDITARY HYPERPHOSPHATASIA

Hereditary hyperphosphatasia is a rare disease inherited as an autosomal recessive trait. It is characterized by multiple fractures and bone deformity in childhood, presenting radiologically some of the features of Paget's disease of bone. Plasma alkaline phosphatase is extremely high. Bone turnover is rapid and there is increased urinary hydroxyproline. There may be mental retardation. No effective treatment is known.

903. ELLIS–VAN CREVELD SYNDROME
(Chondroectodermal Dysplasia)

This syndrome is characterized by polydactyly of the hands and, rarely, of the feet, dwarfism, and dysplasia of the fingernails. It is inherited as an autosomal recessive trait. In contrast to classic *achondroplasia*, the shortening of the extremities is more marked proximally than distally. Fusion of the capitate and hamate bones of the wrist and a defect in the lateral aspect of the proximal part of the tibia, producing knock knees, are consistent features. Congenital heart disease is frequently present; atrial septal defect is the most common cardiac malformation. An abnormally short upper lip, bound down by multiple frenula, and premature eruption of the teeth are frequent features. The disease is very rare, but it occurs as the main cause of dwarfism in the inbred socioreligious group known as the Old Order Amish, in Lancaster County, Pennsylvania, where it occurs with a frequency of 5 per 1000 births. One third of those afflicted die before two weeks of age. The condition must be distinguished from familial polydactyly and classic achondroplasia.

McKusick, V. A., Egeland, J. A., Eldridge, R., and Krusen, D. E.: Dwarfism in the Amish, I. The Ellis–van Creveld syndrome. Bull. Hopkins Hosp., 115:306, 1964.

904. OSTEOCHONDRO-DYSPLASIAS

ACHONDROPLASIA

Definition. Achondroplasia is a form of inherited dwarfism caused by retardation of endochondral bone formation. This relatively common disorder is inherited as an autosomal dominant trait.

Pathology and Pathogenesis. The abnormality is confined to cartilage and consists of failure or retardation of interstitial cellular proliferation and growth. As a result bones formed in cartilage are shortened. This is most apparent in the long bones of the extremities and in the bones of the base of the skull, and to a much lesser extent in the vertebrae. Membrane bone formation is normal; thus the bones of the cranial vault are able to grow normally and even accommodate themselves to the restricted growth of the base of the skull. Similarly, bone shafts enlarge normally. Microscopically there is a lack of normal cartilage cell columns at the epiphyseal growth plates, so that formation of the primary spongiosa proceeds very slowly and irregularly.

Clinical Manifestations. Clinically there is dwarfism, with disproportionate shortening of the extremities. Final height is usually less than 1.4 meters. The bridge of the nose is flattened and depressed, and the forehead may appear prominent and bulging. The hands and feet are short, and fingers tend to be nearly equal in length. The vertebrae are slightly and symmetrically flatter than normal. There are usually a dorsal kyphosis and compensatory posterior rotation of the sacrum and pelvis. The hip joints may thus be displaced backward and the pelvic inlet narrowed by the sacral promontory. Achondroplastic dwarfs exhibit entirely normal intelligence, endocrine function, and calcium metabolism, and, apart from their characteristic dwarfing and the problems it imposes, are able to live normal, useful lives.

Diagnosis. Achondroplasia presents such a typical picture that it is not usually confused with other causes of dwarfism except hypophosphatemic rickets. Occasionally patients with osteogenesis imperfecta may have very short extremities because of multiple fractures, but the true nature of the disease is immediately apparent roentgenographically. When diagnosis is difficult, measurement of the interpeduncular distance in the lumbar spine may be helpful. In normal people, interpeduncular distance increases (as one goes down) from T-12 to L-5, but in patients with achondroplasia T-11 or 12 are the widest vertebrae, while the lumbar interpeduncular distance either does not increase or actually decreases. Because of this restricted bony canal in the lumbar region, prolapsed intervertebral discs cause extremely severe symptoms, usually with neurologic sequelae. Paraplegia has been described in some cases. In addition, hydrocephalus is not uncommon and is usually of the communicating type, presumably because of bony restriction in the posterior fossa.

Treatment. There is no treatment.

OLLIER'S DYSCHONDROPLASIA; MULTIPLE ENCHONDROMATOSIS

Ollier's dyschondroplasia is a rare disorder in which projections or islands of epiphyseal cartilage proliferate down into the metaphysis. These cartilage remnants fail to undergo the changes required for mineralization but retain the growth potential of the epiphyseal plate, and under continued stimulation by growth hormone may expand slowly until much of the normal metaphyseal architecture is destroyed. There may be gross enlargement of the metaphysis. On the roentgenogram the lesions vary from elongated radiolucent patches to a fragmented, expanded picture that conveys the impression of a violent internal explosion within the metaphysis. Growth may cease and calcification may take place after puberty, but the inclusions may continue to enlarge throughout life, sometimes developing into chondrosarcomas. One side of the body is usually more severely involved than the other, but the lesions are fundamentally bilateral. The long bones and the ilia are most commonly involved, and when severe the disease may result in crippling and invalidism. The only treatment available consists of orthopedic procedures for correction of deformities and pathologic fractures.

HEREDITARY MULTIPLE EXOSTOSES

Probably the most common of the osteodyschondroplasias, the syndrome of hereditary multiple exostoses consists of irregular bony protuberances with a cartilage growth cap that project out from the subepiphyseal metaphyseal cortex and backward along the shaft. Lesions are bilateral, though not truly symmetrical, and represent more an abnormality of development of bony contour than a true exostosis. The metaphyseal cortex extends out around the periphery of the protuberances, and their trabecular structure and marrow spaces are continuous with that of the adjacent metaphysis. The disease occurs in families, but the mode of transmission is not known. Although the lesions begin to develop early in childhood, they rarely become apparent for several years. The basic abnormality is not known, but the disorder behaves as if portions of the zone of proliferating cartilage extended down the side of the metaphysis and in the process of growing split off from the growth plate and migrated back along the shaft, leaving a wake of normal endochondral bone behind them. The lesions are confined to the metaphyses of bones with active growth plates, and when severe may limit joint motion. Growth usually ceases when the epiphyses fuse. Very rarely the cartilaginous cap of an exostosis may develop into a chondrosarcoma.

MORQUIO'S DISEASE
(Morquio-Brailsford Syndrome, Morquio-Ullrich Syndrome)

See Ch. 938.

McKusick, V. A.: Heritable Disorders of Connective Tissue. 4th ed. St. Louis, C. V. Mosby Company, 1972.

Rubin, P.: Dynamic Classification of Bone Dysplasias. Chicago, Year Book Medical Publishers, Inc., 1964.

905. PAGET'S DISEASE OF BONE: OSTEITIS DEFORMANS

Paul D. Saville

Definition. Paget's disease of bone is a chronic, progressive disorder of bone of unknown cause that is characterized grossly by deformity of both external bony contours and internal architecture and microscopically by replacement of normal structure by a morphologically and chemically abnormal bone.

Incidence. The disease is almost unknown before age 30; the incidence increases from 0.5 per cent at 40 to 10 per cent at 90 years of age. Men are affected twice as often as women. It is rare in Scandinavia and in Asia, and more common in Australia and New Zealand.

Schmorl described a 3 per cent prevalence in persons over 40. There appears to be a slight familial tendency, but the mode of genetic transmission (if such exists) is unknown.

Pathology and Pathogenesis. The disease is an essentially local, asymmetrical phenomenon. It may, however, ultimately spread to involve a major fraction of the skeleton. It commonly involves weight-bearing bones. The sacrum and pelvis are most frequently involved, followed closely by the tibia and femur, and then in descending order by the lumbar, thoracic, and cervical vertebrae. Although the bones of the upper extremity are rarely involved, the skull is frequently affected.

The disease is characterized by rapid bone formation and resorption in involved regions. Resorption and the consequent osteoporosis comprise the primary abnormality, and the reparative processes follow along in their wake. When the disease begins in the shaft of a long bone, the first detectable abnormality roentgenographically is indeed a zone of rarefaction, but microscopic examination of the roentgenographically normal bone into which the osteoporotic front is advancing reveals that this bone is already qualitatively abnormal. Furthermore, the repair is achieved by deposition of a primitive and, in some cases, highly abnormal bone that may amount to little more than a kind of metastatic calcification of an areolar, myxoid matrix. This is particularly true of rapid periosteal proliferation.

The replacement bone is thus architecturally and chemically abnormal and is subject to rapid, random remodeling and replacement. It is an unstable structure and may have little mechanical significance.

Microscopically the repeated waves of resorption and repair leave behind a bone with a striking mosaic appearance, created by the pattern of cement lines. There is little or no structural orientation. Some of the repair bone may be osteomalacic, and thus wide osteoid seams are frequently found. Extremely rapid resorption may reproduce locally the picture of osteitis fibrosa.

Clinical Manifestations. Many patients with Paget's disease do not have symptoms. The principal clinical manifestation is bone deformity; much less common is pain. When Paget's disease occurs in the pelvis, osteoarthritis of the hip is a frequent association. The long bones are commonly enlarged, feel hot to the touch, and are bowed. Stress fractures are common along the convex borders of bowed long-bone cortices. Pathologic fractures may occur through these.

Enlargement of the skull, associated with headaches and sometimes cranial nerve palsies, especially nerve deafness, is common. Vertebral enlargement and platyspondyly cause kyphosis and occasionally paraplegia. The course of the disease varies widely, but in most cases it is only very slowly progressive. Massive skeletal involvement is rare. When this occurs, however, serum alkaline phosphatase activity rises to very high levels, and because of the extreme vascularity of the bone, high output cardiac failure may develop. Indeed, when more than 30 per cent of the skeleton is involved, cardiac enlargement is the rule. The disease predisposes to two malignant bone tumors: malignant osteoclastoma and osteogenic sarcoma. Osteogenic sarcoma after age 40 is a rare disorder, and there is no doubt that most cases occurring in older patients do so in pre-existing Paget's disease. The incidence is probably of the order of one per 4000 Paget patients per year.

Roentgenographic Manifestations. The first detectable change may be a sharply circumscribed zone of bone resorption. The lesion in the skull previously called osteoporosis circumscripta is now known to be an early manifestation of Paget's disease. Later the normal bony architecture of the skull is replaced by a greatly thickened, fluffy appearance. A roentgenographic characteristic of Paget's disease is replacement of normal bony architecture by coarse, abnormal-looking trabeculae, enlargement of the external contours of a bone, and flame-shaped lucent zones which start at the ends of the long bones and slowly progress up the shaft. Paget's disease of bone is occasionally the cause of so-called ivory vertebrae, the sclerotic end stage of Paget's disease.

Diagnosis. The plasma calcium and phosphorus are usually normal. Urinary calcium excretion is frequently increased and may lead to stone formation. However, the alkaline phosphatase is invariably high if any significant fraction of the skeleton is involved; indeed, it reaches higher values in this disease than in any other. Acid phosphatase values are also slightly elevated at times. Thus, without specific determination of prostatic acid phosphatase, this test may not be of much help in distinguishing Paget's disease from osteoblastic metastases of prostatic carcinoma. This differential problem arises chiefly when lesions are confined to the pelvis, for there carcinomatous infiltration beneath the periosteum may provoke a periosteal reaction that enlarges the contours of the pubic and ischial rami, thus simulating Paget's disease. In few other bony regions do osteoblastic metastases produce such change in external bony contour, and thus usually there is little diagnostic problem. The ordinary clinical and roentgenographic features are too distinctive to be confused with those of any other disease.

Treatment. Most cases of Paget's disease have no symptoms and require no treatment. Osteoarthrosis of the hip can be treated like any other case of osteoarthrosis with analgesics or by total hip prosthesis. Fractures are treated successfully by internal fixation, although problems may arise because of the unusually large marrow cavity and also because bowing makes passage of metal rods down the cavity difficult.

Three drugs have been shown to control disease activity. *Mithramycin* is believed to have a toxic effect on osteoclasts. One regimen consists of 15 to 25 μg per kilogram per day as an intravenous injection either for five consecutive days each week for four weeks or once or twice weekly for many months. Decrease in pain and other symptoms occurs within two weeks of the onset of treatment. In addition, alkaline phosphatase and increased urinary hydroxyproline decrease. Nausea is a troublesome side effect and begins several hours after the drug has been given. When the platelet count falls below 150,000 per cubic millimeter, the drug should be withheld. Favorable effects have been demonstrated with human, porcine, and salmon *calcitonin*. Variable dose schedules have been tried, including 100 to 200 MRC units subcutaneously once daily or 50 MRC units three times a week. There are infrequent dermal allergic reactions and nausea rarely, but no other important adverse effects. After prolonged treatment, there is a tendency for relapse despite continued medication. Synthetic human calcitonin may not have these disadvantages. Finally, the *diphosphonates* have been shown to be effective in Paget's disease. The drug disodium ethane-1-hydroxy-1,1-diphosphonate (EHDP) has been used in a single oral dose of 20 mg per kilogram per day before breakfast for periods of up to seven months. Treatment results in lowering of both serum alkaline phosphatase and urinary hydroxyproline and in clinical improvement as well. The only known adverse effects are increase in osteoid seams and hyperphosphatemia when the drug is given in large dose. These effects are reversible.

Paraplegia or cauda equina compression can be successfully treated with laminectomy and decompression procedures. Pathologic fractures through pagetoid bone heal well but are technically difficult to deal with. Internal fixation is necessary, but is complicated by large marrow cavities, which often necessitate several rods being packed together, and by bowing which may prevent rods from being thrust down the femoral shaft, as well as by extreme vascularity of bone which causes severe hemorrhage. Sarcomas must be watched for carefully and treated surgically as soon as they become apparent.

De Deuxchaisnes, C. N., and Krane, S. M.: Paget's disease of bone: Clinical and metabolic observations. Medicine, 43:233, 1964.

Frame, B., Parfitt, A. M., and Duncan, H. (eds.): Clinical Aspects of Metabolic Bone Disease. Amsterdam, Excerpta Medica, 1973. (See especially pp. 516–554 for articles by various authors on treatment of Paget's disease.)

Johnson, L. C.: Morphologic analysis in pathology: The kinetics of disease and general biology of bone. In Frost, H. M. (ed.): Bone Biodynamics. Boston, Little, Brown & Company, 1964.

Pugh, D. G.: Roentgenologic Diagnosis of Diseases of Bones. New York, Thomas Nelson & Sons, 1951.

Snapper, I.: Bone Disease in Medical Practice. New York, Grune & Stratton, 1957.

906. FIBROUS DYSPLASIA

Paul D. Saville

Fibrous dysplasia, a developmental disorder of the bone mesenchyme, is characterized by replacement of bone by large masses of cellular fibrous tissue containing immature bone spicules and islands of cartilage. Except for the cartilage component, the histologic features are very similar to those of osteitis fibrosa, as is the roentgenographic appearance, but the two diseases differ in many respects. Fibrous dysplasia is a local disorder, and, although lesions may be widespread, there is always normal, uninvolved bone somewhere; furthermore, the disease is relatively slowly progressive and lacks the rapid bone resorption and formation of osteitis fibrosa. When the disease occurs in young girls, there are sometimes associated precocious puberty and patchy brownish skin pigmentation. This triad is known as "Albright's syndrome." Since large doses of estrogens produce a similar metaphyseal lesion in very young animals, it is not clear whether the precocious puberty of Albright's syndrome is simply a part of the picture or a contributing cause of the bone disease. The disorder may also be associated with hyperparathyroidism, gigantism, or hyperthyroidism.

The cause is unknown. Snapper contends that the disorder is fundamentally a lipoid granuloma, others that it is a disturbance of mesenchymal differentiation.

The age of onset is usually unknown and the disease first becomes apparent between ages 5 and 15, commonly because of deformity or pathologic fractures. Typical roentgenographic changes are cystlike lesions of meta-

physeal or shaft bone, with expansion of the cortex and sometimes severe destruction of bony architecture. Areas of increased density are frequently seen, and as the patient ages the lesions gradually acquire a uniform, ground-glass type of opacity. Plasma calcium and phosphorus are normal; the alkaline phosphatase is usually normal, but may be elevated when the disease is extensive.

Bone involvement is commonly unilateral. The femur and pelvis are frequently involved, as is the skull. Repeated fractures through involved areas of the upper femur lead to the characteristic "shepherd's crook" deformity. In the skull, however, lesions are osteomatoid, rather than fibrous, and roentgenograms reveal dense, featureless opacification and distortion of the facial bones and the base of the skull. Encroachment on cranial nerves may produce neurologic symptoms.

Growth is slow throughout childhood and usually ceases entirely in adolescence. The principal significance of the disorder lies in the production of fractures and deformity, but occasionally osteogenic, fibro-, or chondrosarcoma may occur. Except for indicated orthopedic procedures, no treatment is available.

See references for Ch. 905.

907. HYPERTROPHIC OSTEOARTHROPATHY

Paul D. Saville

Hypertrophic osteoarthropathy is a syndrome consisting of clubbing of the fingers, painful swelling and periosteal new bone deposition in the long bones of the extremities, and sometimes moderate joint swelling and tenderness, particularly at the wrists, ankles, and knees. The disorder is almost always associated with disease elsewhere in the body. It occurs in association with intrathoracic malignancies, usually a lung cancer or mesothelioma, but also with metastatic malignancies and mediastinal tumors, as well as bronchiectasis. Clubbing is common with chronic intestinal diseases; true osteoarthropathy is rare but has been described with ulcerative colitis, portal cirrhosis, and juvenile biliary cirrhosis. Very rarely it exists without apparent predisposing disease, and there is also a distinct hereditary form of the disorder, *pachydermoperiostosis*, associated with thickening of the skin of the scalp, face, and hands. In pachydermoperiostosis onset is usually at puberty. A family history of the disorder can be obtained in about one fourth of the cases.

In the finger tips the predominant changes are edema, hyperemia, and soft-tissue fibrous proliferation; bony changes are variable and usually not prominent. Grossly the fingertips appear bulbous, and there is increased curvature of the nails in all directions. The most typical bony lesions are found in the distal shafts of the bones of the forearm and leg, where there is distinct periosteal new bone deposition. Overlying tissues may be edematous, and the entire region is painful and tender to pressure. More advanced disease may involve the entire forearm and leg bones, and later the femur and humerus are affected.

The cause is unknown. The changes are probably mediated by alterations in periosteal blood flow. There is reason to suspect abnormal visceral reflex patterns, triggered by centrally located disease. Innominate artery aneurysms have been reported in association with osteoarthropathy confined to the involved extremity. In any case, surgical correction of lung lesions responsible for the disorder frequently produces dramatic relief of pain and swelling and prompt healing on roentgenographic examination.

Early in the course of the disorder the arthritic complaints may be misdiagnosed as rheumatoid arthritis. The later periosteal manifestations must be differentiated from disorders such as scurvy, syphilitic periostitis, polyarteritis nodosa, and progressive diaphyseal dysplasia. The skin changes of pachydermoperiostosis may suggest a diagnosis of acromegaly; however, absence of sinus enlargement and presence of periosteal reaction allow differentiation by roentgenography.

The disorder is important for two reasons. It usually serves as an indicator of serious disease elsewhere in the body, and in many cases, particularly of pulmonary neoplasms, may be the first such sign. Second, it is usually painful and may contribute significantly to the over-all disability of the primary disease.

The treatment must obviously be directed at the underlying disease. Analgesics, and sometimes narcotics, are required for symptomatic relief. Vagotomy has also been reported to provide relief.

Fischer, D. S., Singer, D. H., and Feldman, S. M.: Clubbing, a review, with emphasis on hereditary acropachy. Medicine, 43:459, 1964.
Herman, M. A., Massaro, D., Katz, S., and Sachs, M.: Pachydermoperiostosis—clinical spectrum. Arch. Intern. Med., 116:918, 1965.
Pugh, D. G.: Roentgenologic Diagnosis of Diseases of Bones. New York, Thomas Nelson & Sons, 1951.

908.   TUMORS OF BONE

Paul D. Saville

PRIMARY BONE TUMORS

Primary bone tumors present some of the most difficult diagnostic and therapeutic problems in clinical medicine. Adequate treatment for the malignant lesions is almost always mutilating, and the decisions that must be made in order to determine appropriate surgery require the utmost skill and cooperation between surgeon, pathologist, and radiologist. These problems cannot be adequately summarized within the scope of a textbook of medicine. The reader is referred to texts dealing specifically with bone tumors, such as those listed at the end of this chapter.

METASTATIC BONE TUMORS

By far the most common malignant skeletal tumors are metastatic from primary sites elsewhere in the body. Virtually any malignant tumor may metastasize to bone, but there are a few that do so with such regularity that they constitute most skeletal metastatic lesions. In one autopsy series of 1000 cases, two thirds of all patients with breast cancer, one third with lung cancer, and one fourth with renal cancer had skeletal metastases. In addition, approximately one eighth of the patients with cancer of stomach, pancreas, colon, and rectum have bony metastases. More than half of the patients with carcinoma of the prostate have osseous metastases. Thyroid carcinoma frequently and characteristically metastasizes to bone. Thus breast, lung, kidney, thyroid, and prostate account for the bulk of skeletal metastases. In addition leukemias and lymphomas commonly produce significant osseous involvement. Half the patients with Hodgkin's disease at autopsy are found to have osseous lesions.

Clinical Manifestations. Skeletal metastases present because of pain or pathologic fracture, or as an incidental finding on roentgenograms taken for another purpose. When lesions are widespread and related to a known primary site elsewhere, there is usually no diagnostic problem; but when an isolated lesion is discovered, the physician is faced with important differential considerations. He must decide whether the lesion represents a metastatic focus or a primary bone disorder. This may be just as important when the patient has a known primary malignancy as when he does not, for patients with cancer are as prone to unrelated bone disease as anyone else, and it is a serious mistake to assume the presence of metastatic spread if it does not really exist.

Many patients with skeletal metastases, especially from breast, prostate, kidney, and thyroid, live for years, and whether these years are spent productively and comfortably will depend on the therapeutic approach taken by the physician. It is worth stressing that such patients may have more years of useful productive life ahead of them than do many patients with diabetes, valvular heart disease, or emphysema, among others.

Most skeletal metastatic lesions are predominantly osteolytic. As tumors expand, the surrounding bone is destroyed, and the resulting focus appears roentgenographically as a radiolucent zone, sometimes sharply demarcated, sometimes with vague margins. These are referred to as osteolytic lesions. However, almost all tumors, except for multiple myeloma, provoke some degree of bone healing, and on microscopic examination new bone deposition and osteoblastic proliferation are frequently observed in and around metastatic foci. This osteoblastic activity is most pronounced in metastatic spread from cancers of prostate and breast, and to a lesser extent in spread from cancers of the urinary bladder. Breast lesions are fundamentally lytic, but superimposed bone reaction may predominate in many cases, producing patchy areas of increased roentgenographic density. These are referred to as osteoblastic metastases. Prostatic cancer, on the other hand, usually has no detectable lytic component. Metastatic cell clumps provoke such intense bone formation on trabecular surfaces that cancer foci literally have no room to expand peripherally, and instead they are pushed along bone tissue spaces by the evoked closure of those spaces behind them. Leukemic infiltration produces bone pain, lytic lesions, and in some cases pathologic fractures. Involvement with Hodgkin's disease produces a combination of lytic and blastic responses, involves the pelvis, vertebrae, ribs, and femora most commonly, and may sometimes evoke such an overwhelming osteoblastic response as to lead to near total opacification of involved regions.

Biochemical Manifestations. Plasma or urine biochemical changes reflect in general the extent and degree of activity of skeletal metastases. Quiescent or slowly progressive lesions usually produce no detectable change from normal values. Active or extensive osteolytic disease produces a large calcium load, which must be disposed of. This leads to hypercalciuria, hypercalcemia, and secondary suppression of endogenous parathyroid activity; if not arrested, it may produce renal calcinosis, renal failure, and death. Prominent osteoblastic activity or healing of pathologic fractures is usually reflected in an elevated alkaline phosphatase (although this same change can be produced by liver metastases), and in prostatic carcinoma disease activity usually, but not always, produces a rise in acid phosphatase. Cancer not metastatic to bone may sometimes produce changes identical with primary hyperparathyroidism. This syndrome has been observed most often with breast, lung, and kidney tumors, and is in fact a true hyperparathyroidism, for the tumor produces a parathyroid hormone-like agent.

Diagnosis. Multiple lesions in patients with obvious primaries present no diagnostic problem, but isolated lesions, or lesions with uncertain relation to a possible primary, should be subjected to biopsy. This point cannot be stressed too strongly. Open surgical biopsy is preferable in most cases, but needle biopsy may be best for inaccessible lesions, such as involvement of vertebral bodies.

Persistent skeletal pain without obvious roentgenographic changes can frequently be investigated by isotopic techniques, employing bone-seeking isotopes such as fluorine-18, strontium-85, or technetium-99m diphosphonate. Such isotopic scanning methods are four times as likely to reveal bony metastases as routine roentgenograms. Before attempting radical surgical removal of primary tumors of sites, such as breast, known to metastasize to bone, a skeletal scan is advisable. The inevitable reparative reaction to tumor metastases is responsible for a striking increase in local uptake of these isotopes, and the finding of such tracer localization confirms the existence of real bone involvement, even though no changes are present roentgenographically.

Treatment. A significant fraction of patients with breast, prostate, kidney, and thyroid metastases can be helped by appropriate treatment. Hypernephromas exhibit a tendency toward apparently solitary metastases, and in some cases combined removal of the primary plus the metastatic focus may result in several years of symptom-free life before other metastatic lesions become apparent. Breast, prostate, and thyroid carcinomas commonly retain a dependency on their hormonal environment, and their growth can be controlled by manipulation of that environment. Breast cancer in women prior to the menopause, and even for a few years thereafter, responds to oophorectomy and hypophysectomy; prostatic cancer to orchiectomy and estrogen treatment; thyroid cancer to iodine-131 administration and TSH-suppression produced by exogenous thyroid hormone treatment. Estrogen-dependent metastases of breast cancer may also respond to androgens and to certain nonvirilizing experimental androgen analogues. The extreme virilization produced by ordinary androgens severely limits the acceptability and value of these agents. In older women with metastatic breast cancer high dosages of estrogens are frequently of value (see Ch. 877).

Other adjunctive treatment includes the use of radiation therapy to troublesome or isolated lesions, and sometimes regional perfusion with chemotherapeutic agents should be considered. Considerable relief of pain and healing of disabling pathologic fractures can be provided by such means. When pain is not relieved by milder analgesics, adequate doses of narcotics, preferably morphine, should be employed as frequently as necessary.

Dahlin, D. C.: Bone Tumors. Springfield, Ill., Charles C Thomas, 1957.

Lichtenstein, L.: Bone Tumors. 4th ed. St. Louis, C. V. Mosby Company, 1972.

MacDonald, I.: Endocrine ablation in disseminated mammary carcinoma. Surg. Gynecol. Obstet., 115:215, 1962.

Symposium on the Role of Hormones in the Origin and Control of Abnormal and Neoplastic Growth. Cancer Res., 17:421, 1957.

Part XX

CERTAIN CUTANEOUS DISEASES WITH SIGNIFICANT SYSTEMIC MANIFESTATIONS

909. INTRODUCTION

Clayton E. Wheeler, Jr.

The history of medicine contains numerous examples of diseases such as lupus erythematosus and sarcoidosis that were first described on the basis of their dermatologic characteristics but were later recognized as having important manifestations elsewhere in the body. Cutaneous lesions are in fact described in connection with scores of diseases classified in other parts of this textbook. The disorders presented here are often treated by the specialist in dermatology, but they deserve mention in a textbook of medicine because their pathogenesis may provoke lesions in organs other than the skin and because some knowledge of them is needed by the general practitioner or the specialist in internal medicine.

910. CUTANEOUS MANIFESTATIONS OF INTERNAL MALIGNANCY

Clayton E. Wheeler, Jr.

Skin manifestations of internal malignancy are of two types: those in which there is invasion with malignant cells and those in which malignant cells cannot be identified.

Almost any internal malignant process may invade the skin. Lymphomas, melanomas, and metastases from carcinoma of the breast, kidney, prostate, lung, bronchus, stomach, colon, thymus, ovary, and testicle are the most common. Infiltration with malignant cells may produce firm to hard, nontender macules, papules, nodules, tumors, or plaques, which may be skin-colored, pink, red, violet, brown, or black. Lesions may be single or multiple, intact or ulcerated. Alopecia may appear at the infiltrated site. An erysipelas- or scleroderma-like picture may be produced by lymphatic involvement, especially in carcinoma of the breast. Colored, configurate, or ulcerated lesions are more likely to occur in lymphomas, and the skin of generalized exfoliative dermatitis may contain lymphoma cells. All areas should be examined carefully when internal malignancy is suspected; lesions of the scalp, umbilicus, and anogenital region are frequently overlooked.

Tumor cells cannot be identified in the skin in a wide variety of cutaneous manifestations of internal malignancy. In most of these there is no real understanding of pathogenesis; hormonal, immunologic, enzymatic, and toxic mechanisms have been postulated. Although patterns produced in the skin are often highly suggestive of internal malignancy, they may also be caused by benign conditions. The relationship of the skin manifestation to malignancy has been proved in many instances by subsidence of cutaneous changes upon removal of the tumor and recurrence with tumor regrowth at the original or metastatic sites. Cutaneous changes may antedate, coincide with, or follow clinical diagnosis of malignancy. A brief account of these cutaneous manifestations follows.

Pruritus may be localized, generalized, intermittent, migratory, constant, mild, or severe. It may be unassociated with detectable abnormalities of the skin except for punctate and linear excoriations or prurigo-like nodules, or it may accompany lichenoid, eczematous, or bullous eruptions. It is often recalcitrant to the usual symptomatic measures; at times it can be relieved only by successful treatment of the underlying malignant disease. It is more common with lymphomas, especially Hodgkin's disease.

Pallor of anemia or, rarely, *erythema* and *cyanosis* of polycythemia may be present. A tan to dark brown color may result from diffuse *melanosis*. This may be localized to small areas or may be generalized with accentuation of normally hyperpigmented sites. The mechanism of melanosis is obscure in most carcinomas and lymphomas; infrequently, tumors that secrete melanocyte-stimulating hormone may be found. *Altered keratinization* may result in localized or diffuse dryness and scaling that may closely resemble ichthyosis. Hyperkeratosis of the palms and soles, alopecia, and varying degrees of cutaneous atrophy may also be present. This type of acquired ichthyosis is most likely to occur with Hodgkin's disease.

Toxic erythema, urticaria, erythema nodosum, or *erythema multiforme* may be due to any type of internal malignant disease. Chronic forms of erythema multiforme (figurate erythemas) characterized by persistent or migratory rings, arcs, or polycyclic lesions are suggestive of internal carcinoma.

Persistent, circumscribed, or diffuse *eczematous dermatitis* may signify internal malignancy. Pruritus, excoriation, lichenification, and secondary pyoderma may be present, especially if associated with lymphomas.

Generalized exfoliative dermatitis that may be associated with alopecia, loss of nails, lymphadenopathy, defective temperature regulation, and increased peripheral blood flow is more often a manifestation of lymphoma. Skin biopsy may show cells characteristic of the lymphoma or nonspecific inflammation.

Vesicular and *bullous eruptions* that resemble dermatitis herpetiformis, bullous pemphigoid, or pemphigus may be due to internal carcinoma or, less commonly, lymphoma.

Purpura may be due to vasculitis, thrombocytopenia, hypoprothrombinemia, and hypofibrinogenemia. *Migratory, superficial thrombophlebitis*, which is often refractory to treatment with anticoagulants, may affect the extremities or trunk. It may be due to carcinoma of the lung, stomach, ovary, or pancreas. In some instances there is an associated thrombocytosis.

Cold urticaria, acral cyanosis, or *gangrene* may occur in lymphomas or myelomas in association with cryoglobulinemia and macroglobulinemia.

Alopecia mucinosa is characterized by grouped follicular papules or plaques, usually on the scalp, face, or neck. Alopecia is due to mucinous degeneration of the hair follicle. In older patients the condition may be an early manifestation of mycosis fungoides or other lymphomas.

Acanthosis nigricans, as discussed in Ch. 915, is often associated with adenocarcinoma arising in the abdomen or pelvis.

Dermatomyositis in patients over 40 years of age is frequently associated with an internal malignant disease, usually carcinoma. Myopathy without dermatitis, various neuropathies, and myasthenic states may also be associated with an internal malignant condition.

Clubbing of the digits, periostitis, osteoarthropathy, and *gynecomastia* may be associated with carcinoma of the lung or other tumors.

Pachydermoperiostosis is characterized by cutaneous thickening, coarsening of facial features, cutis verticis gyrata, keratosis of the palms, excessive sweating and sebaceous gland secretion, macroglossia, clubbing, osteoarthropathy, and enlargement of the hands. The condition may be confused with acromegaly. It is usually seen in males with carcinoma of the lung.

Reduced resistance to infection is frequently present in persons with internal malignant conditions, especially lymphomas. Pyodermas are likely to be deep and severe and may result in generalized infections, at times with more than one microbial species. There is an increased incidence of herpes zoster, which tends to be accompanied by a chickenpox-like eruption. Herpes simplex infections are more extensive, deeper, and longer in duration. Progressive vaccinia may occur. Complicating tuberculosis, moniliasis, histoplasmosis, cryptococcosis, aspergillosis, mucormycosis, and cytomegalic inclusion disease tend to be progressive and fatal.

Bowen's disease is characterized by one or more circumscribed, scaly, crusted, erythematous plaques that may resemble psoriasis or eczema. Lesions may be found anywhere on the skin and may occur on mucous membranes. Intra-epidermal carcinoma is present microscopically. The long-held idea that a higher than expected percentage of patients with Bowen's disease eventually develop internal malignancies seems untenable from recent studies, except possibly in instances in which the Bowen's disease is related to arsenic exposure.

Paget's disease usually produces eczematoid changes of the nipple as an indication of an underlying ductal carcinoma. Extramammary Paget's disease of the perineum is associated with carcinoma of underlying apocrine glands or carcinoma of the rectum.

Primary amyloidosis associated with multiple myeloma may produce macroglossia, purpura, bullae or acquired epidermolysis bullosa, and waxy, flesh-colored papules, nodules, or plaques on the face, trunk, or extremities.

Gardner's syndrome is characterized by dominant inheritance, multiple cutaneous cysts, osteomas, and polyps in the colon. Carcinoma of the colon develops in over half of these patients by the age of 40.

Anderson, S., Nielsen, A., and Reymann, F.: Relationship between Bowen's disease and internal malignant tumors. Arch. Dermatol., 108:367, 1973.

Brewer, L. M., and Brindley, G. V., Jr.: Unusual manifestations of primary malignant tumors of the thorax. Surg. Clin. North Am., 52:375, 1972.

Kierland, R. R.: Cutaneous signs of internal malignancy. South Med. J., 65:563, 1972.

Rosato, F. E., Shelley, W. B., Fitts, W. T., Jr., and Miller, L. D.: Nonmetastatic cutaneous manifestations of cancer of the colon. Am. J. Surg., 117:277, 1969.

Starke, W. R.: Bowen's disease of the palm associated with Hodgkin's lymphoma. Cancer, 30:1315, 1972.

911. ERYTHEMAS

Clayton E. Wheeler, Jr.

Disorders to be discussed under this heading are toxic erythema, erythema multiforme, and erythema nodosum. Urticaria, a close relative, is described in Ch. 75. Although the erythemas vary in morphology, there are features which group them into a common category. All result from reactions of small blood vessels in the skin or subcutaneous tissue. All are doubtless secondary manifestations of a wide variety of underlying disorders, although in many instances the basic condition cannot be identified. Finally, a given underlying disorder (drug reaction, for example) may cause toxic erythema, erythema multiforme, erythema nodosum, or urticaria in different individuals or simultaneous combinations of these vascular reactions in a single individual.

TOXIC ERYTHEMA

Toxic erythema is an extremely variable eruption that ranges from diffuse faint erythema to a generalized morbilliform exanthem. It is secondary to a wide variety of disorders, the most common of which are drug reactions and microbial diseases. Almost any drug may be incriminated, and infection with almost any organism may be involved. In addition, the eruption may be associated with foods and with noninfectious systemic diseases such as lymphomas, internal malignant processes, and the diseases of connective tissue. In a significant number of patients the underlying condition cannot be determined. When the causative disorder is established, the term toxic erythema is frequently discarded in favor of an etiologic diagnosis. Some examples of this are scarlet fever, infectious mononucleosis, drug reactions, and scarlatiniform eruptions produced by staphylococci.

Cutaneous manifestations result from vascular dilatation and mild inflammation in and about small blood vessels. Pathogenesis is often uncertain and probably varies with the underlying cause. Vascular changes may result from toxins, hypersensitivity reactions, or direct involvement with infectious agents.

Onset is usually abrupt with the appearance of diffuse erythema or erythematous macules. Small areas may be involved initially, but the eruption tends to become generalized and may be universal. In some instances there is a characteristic pattern of distribution and evolution—e.g., measles, scarlet fever, and erythema infectiosum—and in others there is random distribution. There is a tendency for the eruption to begin and to remain more intense at sites of minor irritation. Diffuse eruptions may be faint pink or bright red and are often scarlatiniform. Macular eruptions frequently coalesce to produce a morbilliform pattern. Erythema usually disappears with pressure on the skin, but a purpuric component may be present. Mild eruptions are transient and disappear without sequelae, whereas more severe reactions last for several days, and are followed by scaling or desquamation. The cutaneous changes may induce no symptoms or various degrees of itching, burning, or chilliness. Conjunctivitis is a common accompaniment, and the oral or genital mucous membrane may be involved.

Systemic manifestations depend primarily upon the underlying disorder. Fever is common, and chills may occur. Lymphadenopathy is frequent. Arthralgia or arthritis is occasionally present. Leukocytosis or leukopenia occurs, and the differential count may be abnormal.

The diagnosis depends upon clinical manifestations. Sometimes the eruption is so characteristic as to indicate the nature of the underlying disorder, but more often it is nonspecific. Final diagnosis of the primary condition depends upon careful history, physical examination, and laboratory study.

The primary objective of treatment is elimination of the underlying disease. Treatment of the cutaneous component is unnecessary in mild instances. In more severe cases symptomatic measures such as colloidal baths, topical calamine liniment, and oral antihistaminics may be helpful. Dry, scaly skin may be benefited by application of a bland emollient.

ERYTHEMA MULTIFORME

Definition. Erythema multiforme is an acute inflammatory systemic disease that produces a spectrum of clinical patterns from a few inconsequential lesions on skin or mucous membrane to a severe, sometimes fatal multisystemic disorder. The disorder is a symptom complex secondary to a wide variety of diseases and conditions.

Division of the disease into types such as erythema multiforme minor (Hebra) or erythema multiforme major (*Stevens-Johnson syndrome*) based on the severity or extent of the morbid process seems only to confuse the picture. The disease pattern in many instances falls between these extremes and therefore defies classification into such a scheme. Although of historical importance, synonyms such as *ectodermosis erosiva pluriorificialis, dermatostomatitis, new eruptive fever,* and *mucosal-respiratory syndrome* offer no special advantage. Descriptive titles such as erythema multiforme iris, erythema multiforme bullosum, and erythema multiforme exudativum place too much emphasis upon single morphologic features.

Etiology.   There are two main theories concerning etiology: (1) The disease has a single cause, probably some infectious agent. (2) It is a symptom complex secondary to a variety of underlying disease states. In favor of the single cause theory is a close clinical resemblance to the acute exanthems. Efforts to identify specific bacterial, fungal, or viral agents have been negative or inconclusive, and there is no epidemiologic evidence that the disease is contagious. The symptom complex theory finds support in the large number of conditions with which erythema multiforme has been associated. An incomplete list of these follows: (1) microbial diseases including pneumonia, meningitis, cholera, glanders, typhus, measles, mumps, herpes simplex, vaccinia, orf, mycoplasmal pneumonia, lymphogranuloma venereum, psittacosis, and malaria; (2) drug reactions from antimicrobials, anticonvulsants, codeine, thiouracil, arsenic, barbiturates, antipyrine, belladonna, quinine, mercury, aspirin, butazolidine, chlorpropamide, and antitoxins; (3) vaccination against poliomyelitis, smallpox, or tuberculosis (BCG); (4) internal malignant conditions, including carcinoma and lymphoma; (5) deep x-ray therapy; (6) contact dermatitis, especially poison ivy; and (7) connective tissue disease.

Present consensus is that erythema multiforme is always secondary, but there remains a significant number of cases in which no underlying cause can be identified despite extensive diagnostic effort.

Incidence and Prevalence. Figures are heavily weighted in favor of the unusually severe forms of the disease, e.g., Stevens-Johnson syndrome, which are reported in preference to milder examples. If all degrees of severity are included, erythema multiforme is a common disease. Severe forms are rare in infancy, early childhood, and old age, and males are affected about twice as often as females. The disease is worldwide and there is no racial predilection.

Pathology. Nonspecific inflammatory changes, including vasculitis, are present in skin, mucous membranes, and internal organs. The degree of inflammation correlates with clinical manifestations. The pathogenesis is incompletely understood. A symptom complex secondary to many diseases and drug reactions points to a mechanism of toxicity or hypersensitivity. The relatively common simultaneous occurrence with erythema nodosum and the frequent appearance of urticarial lesions in mild forms of erythema multiforme are further reasons to consider hypersensitivity. The appearance of the disorder a few days to three weeks after herpes simplex, vaccination for smallpox, infection with *Coccidioides immitis,* administration of penicillin, contact dermatitis from poison ivy, or deep x-ray therapy suggests that immunologic mechanisms play a role. The development of erythema multiforme after administration of antipyrine to certain persons, especially blacks, may indicate that genetic enzymatic defects or differences are involved.

Clinical Manifestations.   Perhaps half the patients experience a prodromal period of a day to two weeks, characterized by fever, malaise, cough, coryza, sore throat, chest pain, vomiting, muscular aches, and arthralgia in various combinations and severity. After this, or in patients without prodrome, skin or mucous membrane lesions develop suddenly, together with some systemic reaction and often with evidence of visceral involvement.

Skin lesions are often the first and sometimes the only clinically detectable manifestations of the disorder. They usually develop rapidly, are distributed symmetrically and in crops. There may be few lesions, or almost the entire skin may be involved. There is a predilection for wrists, backs of the hands, ankles, tops of the feet, knees, elbows, face, palms, and soles. No area is exempt, although the scalp is affected infrequently. The polymorphous eruption usually includes red or violet macules, wheals, papules, vesicles, and bullae in various combinations. When vesicles and bullae are present they usually develop in pre-existing macules, papules, or wheals. Hemorrhage into the affected areas is common. Lesions are usually sharply demarcated from normal skin and tend to assume an annular configuration. Merging produces gyrate, serpiginous, or arciform patterns. At times central fluid-containing areas are surrounded by concentric rings of varying shades of erythema or purpura; these are the *target, iris,* or *bull's eye* forms which should bring the consideration of erythema multiforme into focus. As the disease progresses, erosions, superficial ulcerations, crusts which are often hemorrhagic, and scaling areas may occur. Paronychias and shedding of nails occur in severe cases. In mild cases healing takes place in a few days to three weeks without scarring, although hyperpigmentation or depigmentation may persist much longer. In severe cases scarring may result, and healing may take six weeks or more.

Mucous membrane involvement usually accompanies the cutaneous eruption, but in mild forms either may occur separately. One or all mucous membranes may be affected, and few or many lesions may be present. The spectrum includes macular erythema, edema, vesiculation, bleb formation, erosion, ulceration, crusting, fissuring, and bleeding. On mucous membranes vesicles and bullae rupture early, forming erosions or ulcerations. A gray or white pseudomembrane may form at the sites of previous blisters, especially in the mouth. The mouth is the most commonly involved orifice. In severe cases the lips are red, swollen, fissured, eroded, and covered with a bloody crust. The gums are swollen, eroded, and bleed easily. The tongue, buccal mucosa, pharynx, and larynx show any or all of the mucous membrane changes described above. As a result there may be pain, difficulty in eating, drinking, and salivation, fetor oris, and hoarseness. Depending upon severity, the process lasts a few days to several weeks and usually heals without scarring. Lesions in the nose cause bleeding, crust formation, and obstruction. Tenesmus and bleeding may accompany anal disease. Urethral lesions, especially in the male, may cause dysuria, hematuria, pyuria, and even urinary retention in severe instances. Balanitis has led to adherence of glans to prepuce, and in females vulvovaginitis can result in formation of fibrotic bands or in partial stenosis of the vagina.

The eye is the site of attack almost as often as the mouth. The eyelids may be swollen and covered with any of the various skin lesions. Mild cases show transitory conjunctivitis. Purulent or membranous conjunctivitis is present in more severe instances. Subconjunctival hemorrhage occurs, and vesicles and bullae may appear. The cornea is usually spared except in severe cases, when it may be eroded or perforated. Iritis, iridocyclitis, and panophthalmitis have been seen. Inflammation usually subsides in a few days in mild cases but may persist for weeks. Partial or complete loss of vision may result from scarring of the cornea or panophthalmitis. Adhesions of bulbar to palpebral conjunctiva have occurred. Severe ocular damage has been less frequent since the advent of antimicrobial drugs.

Systemic manifestations may occur at any time in relation to skin or mucosal manifestations. Symptoms include fever, malaise, dehydration, muscle and joint pains, toxemia, and prostration. Respiratory manifestations include cough with or without sputum, hemoptysis, dyspnea, cyanosis, bronchitis, pneumonitis, pulmonary consolidation, and pleural effusion. Arthralgia and arthritis, often of multiple joints, have occurred frequently. Possible gastrointestinal symptoms are nausea, vomiting, dysphagia, hematemesis, abdominal pain, diarrhea, and melena. Inflammatory changes of the esophagus or colon account for most of these symptoms. Urinary tract findings have included albuminuria, hematuria, urinary retention, and anuria. Nephritis and uremia may develop, at times when skin and mucous membrane lesions are improving. Nervous system symptoms have been drowsiness, convulsion, confusion, coma, delirium, radiculitis, nystagmus, unequal pupils, and abnormal tendon reflexes. Cardiac arrhythmia, pericarditis, and electrocardiographic changes suggesting myocarditis have occurred. Regional lymphadenopathy has been common but generalized lymphadenopathy infrequent. Splenic and hepatic enlargement are rare. Endoscopic examinations have shown annular, erosive, or ulcerative pseudomembranous lesions of the esophagus, larynx, and colon.

No laboratory test is specific for erythema multiforme. Abnormalities depend upon structures involved and degree of damage. Some degree of leukocytosis is common, although the leukocyte count may be normal or decreased. Eosinophilia occurs occasionally. The platelet count is usually normal but it may be much decreased. Rarely, tourniquet tests are positive. Albuminuria, pyuria, hematuria, and casts are not uncommon. On rare occasions there may be increased cells and protein in the cerebrospinal fluid. Roentgenograms of the chest may show patchy pneumonitis or changes similar to those of mycoplasmal pneumonia. Electrocardiographic abnormalities include conduction defects and alterations suggesting myocarditis. Laboratory studies for infectious agents, tumors, and "collagen diseases" may establish the underlying cause.

Diagnosis. The diagnosis depends upon the presence of skin and mucous membrane lesions. An incomplete symptom complex without involvement of skin or mucous membrane has not been recognized. Polymorphous skin lesions that form annular and configurate patterns and bullous erosive involvement of mucous membranes usually differentiate erythema multiforme from the acute exanthems. *Pemphigus* is more protracted in course, usually exhibits less polymorphism and configuration, and skin biopsy shows acantholysis. *Pemphigoid* and *bullous dermatitis herpetiformis* are more chronic and have less mucous membrane involvement and fewer systemic symptoms; biopsy may be helpful. *Bullous contact dermatitis* can usually be distinguished by location and configuration, suggesting external factors, by lack of mucous membrane or systemic involvement, and by history and patch test. *Lymphomas* at times give rise to polymorphous skin lesions, but the clinical picture and biopsy usually suffice for differentiation. Severe forms of erythema multiforme may be confused with *septicemia* or *systemic lupus erythematosus,* but consideration of the nature of skin and mucous membrane involvement and other clinical and laboratory findings makes differential diagnosis possible.

Treatment. Underlying disease should be sought and eliminated when possible. Mild erythema multiforme requires little treatment: topical application of calamine liniment, oral antihistamines, and colloidal baths. Severe forms of the disorder require prompt active treatment of many types. Fluid and electrolyte imbalance caused by improper intake, vomiting, diarrhea, and renal dysfunction must be corrected. Secondary bacterial infection, especially of the eye, in which staphylococcal infection may be prominent, must be combated with topical or systemic antimicrobials or both. High doses of corticotrophin or adrenal steroids are often helpful in severe erythema multiforme and usually need be given only for short periods of time.

Prognosis. Data concerning duration, complications, recurrences, and mortality are generally based upon studies of patients with severe forms of the disease (Stevens-Johnson syndrome). They are worthless therefore in considering erythema multiforme as a whole. Mild forms, which constitute the majority of cases, subside in a few days to two or three weeks without sequelae. Severe forms last three to six weeks or longer; sequelae include neurologic changes, corneal opacities, blindness, keratoconjunctivitis sicca, conjunctival, vaginal, or preputial synechiae, and esophageal strictures. When all forms of erythema multiforme are included, the mortality rate is low (less than 0.5 per cent). The mortality rate in severe cases has been reported as high as 10 per cent. Treatment appears to decrease the duration and severity of the disease and the mortality rate. Recurrences are likely in some forms of the disease (reports give recurrence rates as high as 25 per cent). The pattern of recurrence is variable. Some attacks are severe and some mild; some patients have only skin or mucous membrane changes, and others have most of the features of the symptom complex. Oral or hidden anogenital herpes simplex infections should be sought in recurrent erythema multiforme.

Ackerman, A. B., Penneys, N. S., and Clark, W. H.: Erythema multiforme exudativum. Distinctive pathological process. Br. J. Dermatol., 84:554, 1971.

Bloom, A., and Lovel, T. W. I.: Erythema multiforme with renal and myocardial injury. Proc. R. Soc. Med., 57:175, 1964.

Brenner, S. M., and Delany, H. M.: Erythema multiforme and Crohn's disease of the large intestine. Gastroenterology, 62:479, 1972.

Gordon, A. M., and Lyell, A.: Mycoplasmas and erythema multiforme. Lancet, 1:1314, 1969.

Shelley, W. B.: Herpes simplex virus as a cause of erythema multiforme. J.A.M.A., 201:153, 1967.

ERYTHEMA NODOSUM

Definition. Erythema nodosum is probably a hypersensitivity reaction characterized by inflammatory nodules in the dermis and subcutaneous tissue. It is regarded as secondary to a variety of underlying disorders, especially bacterial, fungal, and viral infections, and drug reactions.

Etiology. In the light of present knowledge, the cause should be regarded as hypersensitivity vasculitis caused by a multiplicity of diseases and conditions, the most common of which are viral, bacterial, and fungal infections, and drug reactions. Among the associated disorders are tuberculosis, streptococcal pharyngitis, primary atypical pneumonia, leprosy, whooping cough, gonorrhea, lymphogranuloma venereum, measles, cat scratch disease, histoplasmosis, coccidioidomycosis, trichophytosis, chronic ulcerative colitis, syphilis, sarcoidosis, and reactions to iodides, oral contraceptives, sulfonamides, bromides, salicylic acid, arsphenamine, phenacetin, or other drugs. In spite of extensive clinical study, an underlying disorder cannot be diagnosed in one quarter to one half of the patients. This probably reflects

inability to recognize a primary condition and does not mean that erythema nodosum is a disease *sui generis*.

Incidence and Prevalence. The disorder occurs at any age but is rare in early childhood and in the elderly. After puberty it is considerably more common in women. The underlying cause varies from one geographic area to another. Thus, in New England, streptococcal pharyngitis is regarded as the most common cause; in Scandinavia, primary tuberculous infection or sarcoidosis is frequently the underlying disorder; and in the San Joaquin Valley of California, primary infection with *Coccidioides immitis* is the most common cause.

Pathology. The pathologic picture is characteristic irrespective of the underlying cause. Inflammatory changes appear in the interlobular septa of the upper subcutaneous tissue and in the dermis. Vasculitis, especially endothelial reaction in veins, is associated with infiltration with neutrophils, lymphocytes, histiocytes, and, occasionally, eosinophils. In later stages lymphocytes, epithelioid cells, and foreign body giant cells predominate.

Pathogenesis. The extensive epidemiologic and clinical studies of coccidioidomycosis carried out in California have provided useful information on the pathogenesis of one form of erythema nodosum. Typical skin lesions develop in approximately one of twenty persons during primary infection with this fungus. Lesions make their appearance ten to twenty days after the onset of the infection, at about the same time the coccidioidin skin test becomes positive. Erythema nodosum accompanied by a strongly positive skin test indicates an excellent prognosis for complete recovery from the fungal infection. This seems to link the cutaneous nodules with the delayed, or tuberculin, type of sensitivity reaction. Complement-fixing antibodies appear in the serum much later in the course of coccidioidomycosis and, therefore, seem unrelated. In tuberculosis, also, erythema nodosum appears at about the time the skin test becomes positive; in fact, skin tests with tuberculin may precipitate or aggravate the disorder.

Clinical Manifestations. Erythema nodosum is characterized by red, tender nodules which usually develop in skin and subcutaneous tissue over the shins. The anterior thighs and extensor surfaces of the forearms are not uncommonly involved, and more rarely lesions appear on the backs of the upper arms and about the head, face, and eyes. A few to several dozen lesions appear, often in crops. The lesions are usually discrete, and an individual nodule reaches 2 to 5 cm in diameter or larger. As the lesion develops it becomes red, hot, and tender; as it involutes, the bright red color gives way to darker red and finally varying shades of green or yellow which simulate a bruise. During healing a fine cigarette-paper scale may appear on the surface. Individual lesions last a few days to two or three weeks, and usually heal without suppuration, depression, or scar formation.

Many of the symptoms associated with erythema nodosum are doubtless due to the underlying disorder or to the hypersensitivity reaction of which the cutaneous nodules are but one manifestation. There may be no systemic symptoms or varying degrees of malaise, chills, fever, sore throat, and cough. Cervical lymphadenopathy is common. Joint symptoms, present in about 75 per cent of patients, may precede, coincide with, or follow skin lesions, and they range from arthralgia to arthritis. Joint involvement has probably led to the idea that erythema nodosum is a manifestation of rheumatic fever, but follow-up studies indicate that there is only an occasional association.

Transient albuminuria and mild secondary anemia may be present. The total leukocyte count may be normal, decreased, or increased. The sedimentation rate is often elevated, and gamma globulin may be increased. Depending upon the underlying disease, skin tests with tuberculin, coccidioidin, and streptococcal antigens are positive. Chest roentgenograms have shown hilar lymphadenopathy and various types of pulmonary infiltration and pleural reaction. Some of these changes may have been due to underlying sarcoidosis or pulmonary infection. The electrocardiogram is usually normal.

Diagnosis. Clinical manifestations usually suffice for diagnosis. Biopsy is rarely necessary. The inflammatory lesions of adipose tissue that occur in *Weber-Christian disease* usually appear on the thighs, although other areas of subcutaneous or visceral fat may be involved. These lesions tend to break down and discharge an oily liquid, and involution is usually associated with a depressed scar. *Erythema induratum* affects the calves more than pretibial regions, and the lesions are more indolent, often ulcerate, and heal with scarring. The shape of the lesion of *migratory thrombophlebitis* often proclaims its association with a blood vessel. Nodules of *sarcoidosis, polyarteritis nodosa*, pancreatic fat necrosis, and *metastatic neoplasm* occasionally simulate erythema nodosum on the legs or other sites.

Treatment. The most important aspect of management is identification of the underlying cause. Symptomatic treatment for the erythema nodosum, such as bed rest, salicylates, or other analgesics, is usually sufficient. Corticotrophin or adrenal cortical steroids cause involution of the lesions, but these agents are indicated only in the most severe cases and should be used only when the underlying disease will not be worsened by them.

Prognosis. Erythema nodosum usually disappears in three or four weeks, but perhaps 10 per cent of the patients have continuing croplike appearance of new lesions or recurrences after free intervals.

Cronin, E.: Skin changes in sarcoidosis. Postgrad. Med. J., 46:507, 1970.
Kibel, M. A.: Erythema nodosum in children. S. Afr. Med. J., 44:873, 1970.
Kirby, J. F., Jr., and Kraft, G. H.: Oral contraceptives and erythema nodosum. Obstet. Gynecol., 40:409, 1972.
Sams, W. M., Jr., and Winkelmann, R. K.: The association of erythema nodosum with ulcerative colitis. South. Med. J., 61:676, 1968.
Sellers, T. F., Jr., Price, W. N., Jr., and Newberry, W. M., Jr.: An epidemic of erythema multiforme and erythema nodosum caused by histoplasmosis. Ann. Intern. Med., 62:1244, 1965.
Weinstein, L.: Erythema nodosum. D. M., 1–30, June 1969.

912. CONTACT DERMATITIS
(Dermatitis Venenata)

Clayton E. Wheeler, Jr.

Definition. Contact dermatitis is an inflammatory, frequently eczematous dermatitis that results from contact of the skin surface with a variety of substances. It is usually classified as (1) allergic contact dermatitis, (2) primary irritant dermatitis, or (3) contact photodermatitis.

ALLERGIC CONTACT DERMATITIS

Etiology. A specific sensitization process is required for the development of allergic contact dermatitis, which appears to be a form of delayed hypersensitivity.

Although almost anything that touches the skin of man may induce or elicit allergic contact dermatitis, several broad groups of substances are frequently involved. These include cosmetics, clothing, dyes, topical medicaments, industrial chemicals, plants, insecticides, detergents, cleansers, foodstuffs, costume jewelry, paints, varnishes, lacquers, rubber, and plastics.

Incidence and Prevalence. Allergic contact dermatitis, a common disorder, affects both sexes and all races. It is rare in infancy and unusual in early childhood, and the incidence declines in old age. Many occupations provide special exposure that results in contact dermatitis.

Pathology. Allergic contact dermatitis shows spongiosis (intracellular edema) and intraepithelial vesicle formation with many mononuclear cells in the vesicles. Edema and perivascular infiltrate with mononuclear cells appear in the dermis.

Pathogenesis. Four phases are recognized during sensitization: (1) In the *refractory phase* the allergen contacts the skin without initiating sensitization. This phase lasts usually a few days to a few weeks, but substances that have touched the skin for years may finally sensitize. Materials that sensitize a high percentage of contacts (strong sensitizers) tend to initiate the process rapidly; weak sensitizers may contact the skin over prolonged periods before sensitizing. Some patients may never become sensitive even after multiple exposures to strong sensitizers, some become sensitive quickly upon exposure to weak sensitizers, and some show weak reactions to strong agents or vice versa. Both sensitizer and person, as well as the degree and manner of exposure, are important in the net result. In addition, damaged skin appears to become sensitized more easily than normal skin. (2) The *period of incubation* is the time between onset of sensitization and clinical evidence of sensitivity. This interval may be as short as 5 days or as long as several weeks, but it is usually between 7 and 21 days. The refractory phase plus the period of incubation results in an interval of 10 days to several weeks between initial exposure and evidence of sensitivity. If allergic contact dermatitis appears within 5 days after exposure, prior sensitivity existed to the agent or a close chemical relative. (3) The *reaction time* is the interval between exposure to the allergen and development of dermatitis in a sensitized person. The usual interval is 24 to 48 hours, but it may be less than 12 hours or more than 90. An important point is that there is always a latent interval between exposure and clinical evidence of dermatitis. (4) The *period of persisting sensitivity* is usually months or years and may be a lifetime.

The hypersensitivity produced is specific for the allergen involved or for close chemical relatives (cross-sensitivity). There are many examples of cross-sensitization, but only one will be given here: Primary sensitization to benzocaine may result in sensitivity to procaine, paraphenylenediamine, para-aminobenzoic acid, and the sulfonamides. The phenomenon of cross-sensitization introduces a complicating factor in diagnosis and treatment since the patient now reacts to many substances, and removal of the original allergen may not eliminate the dermatitis because of unrecognized continued exposure to chemical relatives.

Allergic contact dermatitis is usually restricted to the point of contact of the allergen with the skin. If the patient is highly sensitive or if large amounts of antigen are used, the reaction may become generalized. In addition, sites of previous dermatitis may become active when minute amounts of allergen are applied to remote areas, a reaction lacking satisfactory explanation. The entire skin is usually sensitive, but there are infrequent instances of localized sensitivity, especially to heavy metals.

Clinical Manifestations.   The first symptom is usually itching, burning, or erythema; in mild cases the dermatitis may subside at this stage. With greater exposure or a higher degree of sensitivity, vesiculation and edema appear in a few hours, and these are followed by weeping and crusting. Provided that there is no further exposure, the skin becomes dry and scaly, loses its erythema, and finally heals, usually without scarring, in one to three weeks. More severe reactions may be associated with hemorrhagic vesicles, bullae, or small areas of denudation, but actual necrosis is unusual. Repeated exposures result in continuing or intermittent dermatitis that is likely to induce lichenification and hyperpigmentation or hypopigmentation. Secondary infection with staphylococci or streptococci, injudicious treatment, and excessive rubbing and scratching may complicate the picture.

Systemic symptoms are usually absent, but extensive dermatitis may result in chilliness, impaired temperature regulation, shocklike symptoms, leukocytosis, eosinophilia, and decreased serum protein.

Diagnosis.   The morphologic diagnosis and specific allergen may be evident at a glance, or the nature and cause of the dermatitis may elude the best efforts. The first requirement for diagnosis is an inflammatory or eczematous dermatitis that exhibits a location and configuration compatible with an external source. Given proper morphology, the diagnosis may be established and the offending allergen identified by history of exposure and proper time relationships. In more difficult cases helpful information may be gained by removal of the patient from the suspected source, which should result in healing, and then re-exposure, which should cause recurrence. Once the list of suspected allergens is cut to a reasonable number, skin tests may be helpful in identifying the specific agent.

Two types of skin test are commonly performed. In each, nonirritating concentrations of test substances are applied to the skin. In one method, useful with liquids or semisolids, the substance is applied to a small area on two or three successive days without covering. The other method involves application of test material and covering with an adhesive, which is usually left in place 48 hours. In both tests, persistent erythema or vesiculation confined to the test site constitutes positive results. False positive results occur with irritating concentrations, sensitivity to agents having nothing to do with the dermatitis, reaction to adhesive, contamination of test substances, and over-reactive skin. False negative results occur with inappropriate concentrations, poor contact with skin, or application of the wrong chemical. The complexity of skin testing makes experienced handling mandatory, and results must be interpreted in conjunction with clinical manifestations.

Disorders to be differentiated from allergic contact dermatitis are primary irritant dermatitis, contact photodermatitis, lichen simplex chronicus, superficial fungal infection, atopic eczema, seborrheic dermatitis, and infectious eczemoid dermatitis.

Treatment.   The most important part of management is elimination of exposure to the allergen. Otherwise, treatment consists of nonirritating symptomatic measures calculated to allow the skin to heal. Mild dermatitis may require no treatment. When erythema, edema, and vesiculation are present, open wet compresses of 1 per cent magnesium sulfate solution for two to three hours twice a day alternated with calamine liniment applied six to eight times a day are helpful. As the reaction subsides and the skin becomes dry, these measures are replaced by bland creams or ointments which may contain adrenal corticosteroids. Generalized eruptions may require colloidal baths. If secondary infection is present, antimicrobials may be incorporated in calamine liniment or bland ointment. Systemic antimicrobials may be utilized in the case of extensive or deep secondary infection. Antihistamines may allay itching and may provide some helpful sedative effect. Systemic adrenal steroids or corticotrophin should be used only for extensive and severe dermatitis and only if there are no contraindications to their use.

Desensitization is of little benefit (poison ivy included); indeed, institution of this procedure during active dermatitis may be harmful. Protective clothing and barrier creams are helpful in some instances.

Prognosis.   Cure can be attained if the allergen is identified and removed. If this cannot be accomplished, the dermatitis is likely to persist or recur, although it may decrease in intensity with time.

Prophylaxis.   Federal regulations guard against release of highly sensitizing food preservatives or colorings, drugs, clothing, cosmetics, and other items. Physicians in industry are continuously on guard against sensitizing agents, recommending the use of materials with low sensitizing capacity whenever possible, protective clothing, proper cleansing and ventilation, and other measures.

CONTACT PHOTODERMATITIS

Contact photodermatitis is an inflammatory reaction in skin from topical application of a photosensitizing compound and exposure to light. The dermatitis is localized to light-exposed sites such as the face, V of the neck, backs of the hands, forearms, and lower legs. Areas which are less involved or spared are the hairy scalp, upper eyelids, undersurface of the chin, and flexor surfaces of the arms. Two types of contact photodermatitis occur. Phototoxic dermatitis usually resembles an exaggerated sunburn and, under proper conditions, it occurs in a large percentage of the population upon first exposure. Photoallergic dermatitis is likely to be eczematous. It occurs in only a small percentage of exposed individuals, and it is a result of specific sensitization. Diagnosis of contact photodermatitis may be aided by photo-patch testing. Treatment is the same as for other forms of contact dermatitis with added avoidance of exposure to light.

PRIMARY IRRITANT DERMATITIS

Primary irritant dermatitis, the most common type of contact dermatitis, is due to exposure of the skin to irritating and cytotoxic chemical and physical agents. Immunologic mechanisms are not involved; sufficient exposure will result in dermatitis in all persons. The eczematous nature of the dermatitis and its location and configuration often provide morphologic resemblance to allergic contact dermatitis. Primary irritant dermatitis is less likely to be intermittent, it is not elicited by nonirritating materials, and the latent period between exposure and dermatitis is short or absent. Primary irritants can, of course, be sensitizers, and some patients present combinations of allergic and primary irritant dermatitis. Treatment is similar to that for allergic contact dermatitis, but it is usually easier to identify and eliminate the cause of primary irritant dermatitis. Complete avoidance of offending agents is often not necessary for cure since the skin may be able to tolerate irritants in small amounts.

Baer, R. L., Ramsey, D. L., and Biondi, E.: The most common contact allergens, 1968–1970. Arch. Dermatol., 108:74, 1973.

Epstein, E.: Shoe contact dermatitis. J.A.M.A., 109:1487, 1969.

Epstein, E., Rees, W. J., and Maibach, H. I.: Recent experience with routine patch test screening. Arch. Dermatol., 98:18, 1968.

Fisher, A. A.: Contact Dermatitis. Philadelphia, Lea & Febiger, 1973.

Ison, A. E., and Tucker, J. B.: Photosensitive dermatitis from soaps. N. Engl. J. Med., 278:81, 1968.

Odom, J. C., and O'Quinn, S. E.: Allergic contact dermatitis. A study of 100 consecutive cases. South. Med. J., 61:1378, 1968.

913. BEHÇET'S DISEASE

Clayton E. Wheeler, Jr.

Definition. Behçet's disease is a multisystemic disease characterized by ulcers (aphthae) of the mouth and genitalia, inflammatory eye disorders, joint manifestations, bowel disease, superficial and deep thrombophlebitis, and nervous system abnormalities.

Etiology. The cause is unknown; viral infection and autoimmune disease have been postulated. Autoantibodies against oral mucosa, esophageal cells, and polymorphonuclear leukocytes have been found. Vasculitis plays a prominent role in pathogenesis and symptomatology.

Incidence and Prevalence. The disease is most prevalent in the Middle East and usually affects young adult males. However, recent studies suggest that the disease is more common, more widely distributed geographically, and more frequent in women than was previously recognized and that many cases are currently missed or misdiagnosed.

Pathology. Biopsies of affected areas of skin, mucous membrane, eyes, and joints usually show perivasculitis and vasculitis of venules and arterioles with frequent thrombosis. A mixed lymphocytic and plasmacytic cellular infiltration is present. Vasculitis of medium-sized and large arteries and veins may lead to aneurysms and thrombosis.

Clinical Manifestations. Behçet's disease is characterized by variability in clinical manifestations, by chronicity, and by frequent recurrences which occur at irregular intervals, vary in duration and intensity, and involve several systems in a changing pattern. There is often a long interval between onset of the disease and manifestations in different organs.

Oral lesions may be the initial manifestation, and they occur in almost all cases at some time during the disease. They may resemble canker sores or may be larger and deeper. Genital changes consist of various pyodermas, herpes-like lesions, and ulcers of the scrotum, vulva, urethra, and vagina. Epididymitis is found occasionally. An outstanding and almost constant feature is pyoderma, which includes pustules, impetigo, folliculitis, furuncles, acne-like lesions, cellulitis, and ulcers. Nodose lesions that resemble erythema nodosum may appear on the legs or elsewhere. Subungual, flame-shaped hemorrhages have been reported. A peculiar feature is the development of papules and pustules after pricking with a sterile needle or injection of sterile saline.

Eye involvement is the most frequent cause of disability; the most common lesions are iridocyclitis and uveitis with hypopyon. Chronic, recurring inflammation often leads to partial or complete loss of vision. This may begin unilaterally, but in time both eyes are affected. Other ocular changes are conjunctivitis, keratitis, retinitis, choroiditis, optic neuritis, optic atrophy, and retinal vessel occlusions.

Most patients experience arthralgias and some develop polyarthritis. Despite years of synovitis, there is usually no joint space narrowing and no osseous erosion. Thrombophlebitis is found in a quarter or more of the cases. This may be migratory, superficial thrombophlebitis or deep vein thrombophlebitis. There have been several reports of superior or inferior (or both) vena caval thrombosis. Aneurysms of large arteries such as the aorta and popliteal may occur. Neurologic complications are being recognized with increasing frequency; they include multiple sclerosis-like disorders, cranial nerve palsies, brainstem syndromes, meningomyelitis, meningoencephalitis, encephalopathies, seizures, and confusional states. Pulmonary and gastrointestinal symptoms develop occasionally. It may be that some patients develop colitis indistinguishable from chronic ulcerative colitis, and acute pancreatitis has been reported.

Fever and malaise often accompany exacerbations and recurrences of the disease, and leukocytosis, elevated sedimentation rate, and nondiagnostic serum protein abnormalities are common (elevation of alpha$_2$ globulin, gamma globulin, IgA, IgG, and IgM). Antinuclear factor has been negative, and complement levels have been normal. Anticytoplasmic antibodies to cadaver esophagus have been demonstrated by indirect immunofluorescent techniques.

Diagnosis. Because of the variability in clinical manifestations, the long delay in appearance of some of the symptoms, and the lack of specific laboratory tests, diagnosis is difficult and often made late. Some insist upon the clinical triad of uveitis, oral aphthae, and genital ulcers, but any two of these with skin lesions, thrombophlebitis, nervous system involvement, ulcerative colitis, or joint disease should bring Behçet's disease into consideration.

Treatment. Topical and systemic corticosteroids may control some of the inflammatory signs and symptoms, but they probably influence the basic course of the disease very little. Systemic antimicrobials are indicated for specific infectious complications. Immunosuppressives (cyclophosphamide, azathioprine, chlorambucil, methotrexate) and fibrinolytics (phenformin, ethyloestrenol) have been used with variable results. Fresh blood transfusions have caused apparent benefit in a few patients.

Prognosis. Prognosis is unpredictable. Spontaneous cures occur, or recurrences may continue relentlessly until blindness results. Central nervous system complications are serious, and most deaths occur in this group. Large vessel disease (thrombosis, emboli, aneurysms) is also of grave significance.

Chajek, T., and Farinaru, M.: Behçet's disease with decreased fibrinolysis and superior vena caval occlusion. Br. Med. J., 1:782, 1973.

Enoch, B. A., et al.: Major vascular complications in Behçet's syndrome. Postgrad. Med. J., 44:453, 1968.

Kansu, E., et al.: Behçet's syndrome with obstruction of the venae cavae. Quart. J. Med., 41:162, 1972.

Mamo, J. G., and Azzam, S. A.: Treatment of Behçet's disease with chlorambucil. Arch. Ophthalmol., 84:446, 1970.

O'Duffy, J. D., and Deodhar, S.: Behçet's disease. Report of 10 cases, 3 with new manifestations. Ann. Intern. Med., 75:561, 1971.

914.   PEMPHIGUS

Clayton E. Wheeler, Jr.

Definition. Pemphigus vulgaris is an uncommon disease characterized by bullae and erosions on the skin and mucous membranes, acantholysis, intercellular antiepithelial antibodies, chemical alterations in the blood, and high mortality rate.

Etiology. The cause remains unknown despite extensive search for toxic, viral, metabolic, immunologic, and enzymatic factors.

Incidence and Prevalence. The disease affects either sex and all races; there is a higher incidence among Jews. It usually begins between the ages of 40 and 60; onset earlier in life is unusual.

Pathogenesis. Although the mechanism of bulla formation is unknown, the characteristic histologic feature of acantholysis indicates that defective intercellular attachment is involved. In acantholysis, the cells of the malpighian layer lose their prickles, become separated from each other, and lie singly or in clumps in blister fluid. On electron microscopy tonofilaments retract from their desmosomal attachments and clump in the cytoplasm of the cell. The role of recently demonstrated intercellular antiepithelial autoantibodies in acantholysis is not clear.

Defective intercellular attachment accounts for the *Nikolsky sign,* characteristic of all forms of pemphigus: Firm pressure with a finger on the top of an intact blister results in extension at the edge, or application of a steady shearing force to the skin with a tongue depressor causes the top layers of the epidermis to slide over underlying cells. Epidermal separation demonstrated by this sign takes place at the site of most prominent acantholysis.

Blister fluid contains water, electrolytes, and protein. The composition resembles serum, although total protein is usually lower and albumin higher. Loss of these substances into bullae and from denuded areas explains most of the changes in the blood, which parallel the duration and severity of the disorder. Total serum protein may fall as low as 3.6 grams and there may be a correspondingly low level of albumin. Alpha$_1$ and alpha$_2$ globulins are increased. Gamma globulin and fibrinogen are usually increased. Sodium, chloride, and calcium are decreased and potassium is normal or increased. Plasma and interstitial fluid volume are increased. Anemia is common and may be due to inanition, serum loss, and in-

fection. Anemia and increased globulin, especially fibrinogen, probably account for the increased sedimentation rate. The leukocyte count is usually elevated with an increase of immature forms. Cutaneous inflammation and infection are important causes of leukocytosis. Eosinophilia may be present.

Pathology. Characteristic changes develop in the skin and orificial mucosa. Intercellular edema in the lower malpighian layer is followed by loss of intercellular bridges, acantholysis, and cleft formation. An intraepithelial bulla is formed just above the basal layer. Healing may result in normal-appearing epidermis or there may be hyperkeratosis, acanthosis, and papillomatosis. Simple or granulomatous inflammation is present in the dermis, and tissue eosinophilia is often prominent.

There are no specific changes in internal organs. Examination of persons dying early in the course of pemphigus may show surprisingly little. Common but variable findings are pulmonary congestion and edema, atelectasis, bronchopneumonia, hydropericardium, focal myocarditis, and brown atrophy. Myeloid hyperplasia of the bone marrow and increased numbers of normoblasts are common. Adrenal changes have included depletion of lipoid, degeneration, and inflammation followed by scar and regeneration, hemorrhage, necrosis, and vein thrombosis. Nonspecific degeneration may involve areas of brain, cord, or ganglia.

Clinical Manifestations. Flaccid or tense bullae are characteristic. These lesions often spread at the edges and show little tendency to heal, and they rupture easily. Localized involvement may be present for months or the disease may begin with a generalized eruption. Skin lesions are randomly distributed, but there is a predilection for areas of friction or pressure. Frequently affected sites are the scalp, axillae, groin, elbows, knees, back, inframammary area, umbilicus, hands, feet, nose, and eyelids. Bullae arise on normal-appearing skin or at previously involved sites. Coalescence and extension often result in large denuded areas. The contents of bullae may be serous, seropurulent, or hemorrhagic, and crusting often develops. Healing takes place with little or no scarring. Secondary infection is a common complication, and hyperpigmentation, hypopigmentation, and milium formation are frequent sequelae. Itching is usually mild or absent. Denudation often causes burning or pain. The Nikolsky sign is positive over intact bullae and sometimes can be elicited over normal-appearing skin.

The oral mucosa is involved in almost all patients with pemphigus vulgaris. In half to two thirds of the cases mouth lesions precede skin lesions by weeks to a year or more. The thin-walled bullae rupture early, leaving erosions which often assume figured patterns. The gums, sides of the tongue, and buccal mucosa along the bite line are preferential sites. The lips frequently become fissured, crusted, or warty. Pain, salivation, and bleeding may make eating and drinking difficult. Bullae, erosions, and inflammation commonly involve the mucosa of the pharynx, larynx, nose, conjunctiva, genitalia, and anus.

Extensive skin and mucous membrane involvement, loss of fluid, electrolytes, and protein, inability to eat and drink, and secondary cutaneous and systemic infection contribute to weakness, weight loss, toxemia, and the severely ill appearance of these patients.

Other Types of Pemphigus. Other types are pemphigus

vegetans, pemphigus foliaceus, pemphigus erythematosus, and fogo selvagem. *Pemphigus vegetans* is less severe than pemphigus vulgaris, of which it is probably a variant, and is characterized by warty, vegetating, pustular, and hyperkeratotic lesions at the axillae, groin, anogenital area, interdigital spaces, and lips. *Pemphigus foliaceus* is characterized by incompletely formed bullae, more crusting and scaling, frequent absence of mucous membrane involvement, milder but longer course, lower mortality rate, more spontaneous cures, and higher position of the bullae in the epidermis. It usually begins on the face or upper trunk and slowly becomes generalized, at which time it resembles exfoliative dermatitis. *Pemphigus erythematosus* may be an abortive form of pemphigus foliaceus or pemphigus vulgaris. Crusting and erythema about the face, mid upper back and chest produce a superficial resemblance to seborrheic dermatitis and lupus erythematosus. *Fogo selvagem* (Brazilian wildfire) resembles pemphigus foliaceus except for its endemicity in central South America and its frequent onset at an early age.

Diagnosis. The clinical diagnosis should be confirmed by biopsy and smears of skin and mucosal lesions. Multiple sampling of lesions may be necessary to show acantholysis. Intercellular antiepithelial autoantibodies can be demonstrated in skin lesions and serum by immunofluorescence. The most difficult differential diagnosis is that of *pemphigoid,* a chronic bullous disease of unknown cause in which the bullae are usually smaller, more tense, rupture less easily, and often show grouping or arise on an inflamed base. Mouth involvement is less severe and less frequent; systemic symptoms are less intense, and the mortality rate is lower. Bullae are subepidermal, acantholysis is absent, and autoantibodies are found in the basal membrane area. Bullous *erythema multiforme* shows more polymorphism and configuration, the onset is acute, fever is often high, the disease is self-limited, and acantholysis is absent. Bullous *drug eruption* follows the pattern of bullous erythema multiforme. Benign *mucous membrane pemphigoid* is characterized by chronic bullous and erosive lesions of the mucous membranes, especially of the eye, in which scarring is prominent. *Contact dermatitis* can usually be differentiated by localization and configuration of lesions, lack of systemic symptoms, infrequent mucosal involvement, and self-limited course. In *familial benign chronic pemphigus,* lesions are usually limited to the neck, axillae, groin, and small areas of the trunk. Mucous membrane involvement and systemic symptoms are absent, and biopsy is usually characteristic. *Pemphigus neonatorum* is a bullous form of impetigo which can be differentiated by age, cultures, and response to appropriate antimicrobials. *Exfoliative dermatitis* lacks bulla formation and mucosal involvement, and biopsy shows chronic dermatitis without acantholysis.

Treatment. Adrenal corticosteroids and corticotrophin were the first medications shown to be truly effective in treatment of pemphigus. These agents control but do not cure the disease. The dose depends upon clinical and serologic response (serum antibody levels to epithelial intercellular substance) and varies from patient to patient. The objective is to bring the disease under control as rapidly as possible and then to decrease the dose gradually until a maintenance level is attained. On some occasions remissions occur and maintenance medication can be stopped, but most patients require continued treatment. An initial dose of 120 to 300 mg per day of prednisone usually suffices to stop new lesions and start healing of old lesions in a week or two. After complete healing of skin and mucous membrane the amount of drug is cautiously reduced until the maintenance level is reached; this is usually between 15 and 30 mg per day of prednisone or its equivalent. The maintenance dose can often be switched to an every-other-day schedule. Some patients require higher doses than outlined above, and a rare patient seems to be unresponsive. Measures must be taken to combat complications of corticosteroid administration such as salt and water retention, potassium depletion, osteoporosis, and peptic ulcer.

Psychotic disturbances caused by pemphigus or corticosteroids may require tranquilizers or sedatives. Transfusions and replacement of serum proteins and electrolytes are often necessary. Cutaneous and internal infections (bacteremia, bronchopneumonia, and urinary tract infections) must be combated with appropriate topical and systemic antimicrobials. Good nursing care, encouragement to eat and drink, soothing mouthwashes, and a cheerful environment are important. Colloidal or potassium permanganate baths and topical calamine liniment add to the patient's comfort.

In addition to corticosteroids, methotrexate, cyclophosphamide, azathioprine and gold sodium thiomalate also influence the course of pemphigus. The exact role of these agents in the treatment of pemphigus has not been established. Moderate and severe cases of pemphigus are best brought under control with corticosteroids. Immunosuppressives may then be used to reduce the dosage of corticosteroids or replace them altogether as the maintenance medication. Mild, early cases of pemphigus may be controlled with the agents listed above without initial administration of corticosteroids. The most recent trend appears to favor azathioprine or gold sodium thiomalate if these agents are to be used.

Prognosis. The mortality rate of untreated pemphigus vulgaris confirmed by biopsy is greater than 90 per cent. Average duration of life after onset is fourteen months, with a range of one month to six or seven years and, rarely, longer. In addition, the uncomfortable state of the patients during much of their course adds greatly to the gloomy picture. Patients die of toxemia, cachexia, shock from protein and electrolyte abnormalities, pulmonary edema, bronchopneumonia, sepsis, or adrenal insufficiency.

Current therapy has cut the mortality rate approximately in half. This is only part of the story, because control of the disease allows most patients to lead comfortable and useful lives. Complications of steroid therapy, such as perforated peptic ulcer, congestive heart failure, suicide, uncontrollable infection, and thromboembolic phenomena, must be added to the list of causes of death, but judicious management keeps these to a minimum.

Ebringer, A., and Mackay, I. R.: Pemphigus vulgaris successfully treated with cyclophosphamide. Ann. Intern. Med., 71:125, 1969.

Lever, W. F.: Pemphigus and Pemphigoid. Springfield, Ill., Charles C Thomas, 1965.

Lever, W. F., and Goldberg, H. S.: Treatment of pemphigus vulgaris with methotrexate. Arch. Dermatol., 100:70, 1969.

Peck, S. M., Osserman, K. E., Weiner, L. B., Lefkovits, A., and Osserman, R. S.: Studies in bullous diseases. Immunofluorescent tests. N. Engl. J. Med., 279:951, 1968.

Penneys, N. S., et al.: Gold sodium thiomalate treatment of pemphigus. Arch. Dermatol., 108:56, 1973.

Roenigk, H. H., Jr., and Deodhar, S.: Pemphigus treatment with azathioprine. Arch. Dermatol., 107:353, 1973.

915. ACANTHOSIS NIGRICANS

Clayton E. Wheeler, Jr.

Definition. Acanthosis nigricans is an uncommon dermatosis characterized by hyperpigmentation and epidermal hypertrophy. Two forms are recognized: (1) malignant or adult, associated with internal cancer, and (2) benign or juvenile, which may be related to developmental, endocrine, or metabolic abnormalities. This terminology is illogical, however, because the dermatosis itself is never malignant and because the adult type may be seen in children and the juvenile form in adults.

Etiology. By definition, malignant acanthosis nigricans is always associated with internal malignancy; adenocarcinoma is the predominant type of cancer, although epidermoid carcinoma, osteogenic sarcoma, and malignant lymphoma have been reported. Almost 70 per cent of the associated malignancies arise in the stomach and more than 90 per cent in the abdomen and pelvis. Sites of origin are the stomach, colon, esophagus, liver, gallbladder, pancreas, ovary, uterus, chorion, kidney, lung, bronchus, mediastinum, breast, and thyroid. Skin changes appear before clinical evidence of carcinoma in 20 per cent; the two appear simultaneously in 60 per cent; and acanthosis follows the diagnosis of malignancy in 20 per cent. Progression of the dermatosis parallels the course of the carcinoma. In a few instances acanthosis has regressed after x-ray or surgical treatment of cancer, only to recur with reactivation of the malignancy.

Benign acanthosis nigricans may be associated with a large number of developmental, metabolic, or endocrine abnormalities that seem to have little in common in the light of present knowledge. These include diabetes mellitus, pituitary tumors, adrenal hyperplasia, hypogonadism, acromegaly, gigantism, congenital total lipodystrophy, hypothyroidism, Addison's disease, Stein-Leventhal syndrome, von Recklinghausen's neurofibromatosis, arachnodactyly, achondroplasia, epilepsy, mental retardation, and degenerative disease of the cord. Familial incidence and occurrence in two and three generations suggest that hereditary factors are important. Lupoid hepatitis and administration of nicotinic acid, stilbestrol, and corticosteroids have been associated with skin lesions resembling acanthosis nigricans.

Incidence and Prevalence. The disorder is worldwide, affects all races, and occurs in either sex. The peak incidence of malignant acanthosis nigricans is between the ages of 40 and 60, but it occurs at all ages. Benign acanthosis nigricans usually appears between the ages of 10 and 20, but the disorder may be present at birth, and it occurs in early childhood and middle age. Intensification and spread commonly occur at puberty if the disorder has existed previously.

Pathology. Characteristic changes are limited to the epidermis, where there are hyperkeratosis, acanthosis (increased thickness of the prickle cell layer), and papillomatosis. Melanin is increased in the basal layer. Benign and malignant forms do not differ histologically, and cancer is not found in the skin in the malignant type.

Pathogenesis. The pathogenesis of acanthosis nigricans is unknown. In the malignant type, theories include humoral or biochemical effects of the cancer, peculiarities of the host triggered by carcinoma, or a common cause for acanthosis and carcinoma. Benign acanthosis nigricans may be related to disturbances of germ plasm or endocrine function.

Clinical Manifestations. Skin changes in malignant acanthosis nigricans are bilateral and symmetrical and exhibit a predilection for flexural and intertriginous areas. The axillae, groin, genital region, and neck are the most common sites of involvement; other areas in approximate order of frequency are face, inner thighs, flexor surfaces of elbows and knees, umbilicus, perianal areas, and eyelids. The palms and soles occasionally become hyperkeratotic, the backs of the fingers are sometimes involved, and in extreme and rare instances the disorder becomes generalized. Involved skin is usually dark brown or black, although light brown and yellow may be seen. The epidermis becomes thickened, and normal skin lines are exaggerated. A soft, velvety, papillomatous appearance develops, and frequently pedunculated growths or warty lesions are scattered over the area. The disorder is distinctly localized, with involved regions blending imperceptibly into normal skin. In some cases there may be loss of scalp or eyebrow hair, and dystrophy of nails may occur. The lips, mouth, tongue, epiglottis, and vagina may be affected. Involved mucous membrane becomes thickened, granular, and warty.

Benign acanthosis nigricans shows the same changes, but the degree and extent are often less, and mucous membrane involvement is unlikely. The cutaneous lesions of both forms are asymptomatic. Systemic symptoms depend upon associated internal disease.

Diagnosis. The diagnosis is based on clinical appearance, histologic findings, and associated internal disease.

Addison's disease and *hemochromatosis* cause more generalized hyperpigmentation, and involved sites lack epidermal hypertrophy, papillomatosis, and warty changes. *Arsenical hyperpigmentation* is generalized, and arsenical keratoses are small and hard and uncommonly affect flexural or intertriginous sites. *Ichthyosis hystrix* shows less predilection for flexural and intertriginous areas, there is more hyperkeratosis, and the palms and soles are more often involved. Obese persons, especially brunets, sometimes develop hyperpigmentation, acanthosis, and papillomatosis of the axillae, groin, and neck. These alterations have been called pseudo-acanthosis nigricans, but they probably represent a form of benign acanthosis nigricans.

Treatment. The most important aspect of management is determination of whether internal malignancy is present. If it is, prompt treatment should be instituted. In the benign type, associated developmental or endocrine disorders may require treatment. There is no effective therapy for the dermatosis, although temporary amelioration of cutaneous changes may occur after irradiation or surgical treatment of carcinoma. Correction of endocrine abnormalities appears to have little or no influence on the skin changes.

Prognosis. The outlook for the patient with acanthosis nigricans and malignancy is gloomy. The associated carcinoma is highly malignant, and average survival after its discovery is one year. Seldom do persons live longer than two years after the skin lesions appear, and progressive skin changes are a bad omen. Few, if any, have been cured, but earlier discovery and improved methods of treatment may alter the picture. The prognosis in benign acanthosis nigricans is good and depends upon associated abnormalities and their amenability to treatment.

The dermatosis tends to progress when associated with malignancy. Skin lesions in the benign form are likely to reach a peak and remain static or regress slowly.

Brown, J., and Winkelmann, R. K.: Acanthosis nigricans: A study of 90 cases. Medicine, 47:33, 1968.

Curth, H. O., Hilberg, A. W., and Machachek, G. F.: The site and histology of the cancer associated with malignant acanthosis nigricans. Cancer, 15:364, 1962.

Garrott, T. C.: Malignant acanthosis nigricans associated with osteogenic sarcoma. Arch. Dermatol., 106:384, 1972.

Hollingsworth, D. R., and Amatruda, T. T., Jr.: Acanthosis nigricans and obesity. Arch. Intern. Med., 124:481, 1969.

Reed, W. B., Dexter, R., Corley, C., and Fish, C.: Congenital lipodystrophic diabetes with acanthosis nigricans. Arch. Dermatol., 91:326, 1965.

916. MAST CELL DISEASE
(Mastocytosis)

Clayton E. Wheeler, Jr.

Mast cell disease will be discussed under two divisions: (1) urticaria pigmentosa of childhood and (2) systemic mastocytosis.

URTICARIA PIGMENTOSA OF CHILDHOOD

Definition. This chronic disease usually begins in early childhood and disappears partially or completely by adolescence. Characteristic skin lesions are single or multiple pigmented macules or nodules that urticate on rubbing and contain large numbers of mast cells.

Incidence. Although uncommon, the disorder is seen yearly in most dermatologic and pediatric practices. Light-skinned persons are affected most often, and it is slightly more common in males. The disorder has been reported in a parent and child in several families and in both members of monozygotic twins. More than 10 per cent of cases are present at birth; over half develop by six months; and the majority appear before puberty. Onset after puberty raises the question of systemic mastocytosis.

Etiology. The probable origin of mast cells from connective tissue cells of histiocytic type suggests that the disorder is one of the reticuloendothelioses. Urticaria pigmentosa may be a systemic disorder, but its benign course appears to separate it from systemic mastocytosis.

Pathogenesis. Human mast cells contain histamine, heparin, and possibly hyaluronic acid. The function of these cells is incompletely understood, but they may be important in connective tissue formation, repair, or maintenance. Local release of histamine on rubbing results in capillary dilatation and edema with erythema and wheal formation, whereas its absorption into the general circulation causes flushing, a shocklike state, and gastrointestinal disturbance. Pigmentation of cutaneous lesions is due to increased melanin production, which presumably results from repeated inflammatory episodes.

Pathology. The characteristic finding is accumulation of mast cells in the dermis. The number of cells determines the macular or nodular nature of the lesion. Mast cells are large and contain round or oval nuclei. The cytoplasm contains large basophilic granules that stain metachromatically and can be demonstrated by fixation with 10 per cent formalin or absolute alcohol followed by staining with Giemsa, methylene blue, or toluidine blue. Lesions that have been rubbed may show edema, eosinophilia, and degranulation of mast cells. Melanin is increased in the basal layer and dermal chromatophores.

Clinical Manifestations. One, few, or innumerable lesions may be present. Frequently they appear in crops for weeks before the final extent of the disease is reached. The trunk is the site of predilection, but the neck, face, scalp, extremities, palms, soles, and oral mucosa may be involved. Although macular eruptions predominate, nodular and plaquelike forms are common. Superimposed bullae or vesicles may occur in young children. Lesions are round, oval, or irregular and vary from a few millimeters to several centimeters. They are discrete except in extensive cases. The color varies from yellow to brown or sepia.

A significant number of patients display symptoms of histamine release into the general circulation. These include episodic bright red flushing, itching, hypotension, weakness, dizziness, headache, dermographism, nausea, vomiting, and diarrhea.

Although the extent of mast cell infiltration has been incompletely studied, the occasional finding of lymphadenopathy, splenomegaly, increased mast cells in bone marrow, and cystic or proliferative bone lesions suggests that urticaria pigmentosa is a systemic disease. Rarely, skin is diffusely infiltrated with mast cells, with or without bulla formation and cobblestoning. This type of patient may develop significant bleeding tendencies, and systemic involvement is likely.

Diagnosis. The diagnosis can usually be made when pigmented lesions exhibit erythema and edema upon rubbing *(Darier's sign)*. This sign is absent in some cases, especially when previous stroking has exhausted the supply of histamine. Biopsy confirms the diagnosis. Increased eosinophil content of the blood is sometimes found, and increased amounts of histamine may be present in the urine.

Pigmented nevi, nevoxanthoendothelioma, xanthoma, myoblastoma, lymphoma, insect bites, and Letterer-Siwe disease can usually be differentiated by histologic findings and the absence of Darier's sign.

Treatment. Treatment is relatively ineffective. Antihistamines, including cyproheptadine, may attenuate some of the symptoms. Trauma should be avoided. Aspirin and codeine degranulate mast cells and may aggravate symptoms. Solitary lesions may be excised. Once systemic mastocytosis is excluded, watchful waiting and reassurance of the parents are essential features of management.

Prognosis. Aside from cosmetic considerations and uncomfortable effects of histamine release, the disease is generally benign. Lesions disappear completely by adolescence in the majority of patients; in the remainder pigmented macules persist without activity. Very rarely, patients develop serious complications such as infected bullae, peptic ulcer, and bleeding tendencies.

SYSTEMIC MASTOCYTOSIS

Systemic mastocytosis, a rare, recently recognized disease, is being reported with increasing frequency. It affects both males and females and usually begins in adult life. The cause is unknown. The clinical manifestations and course may resemble those of lymphoma or leukemia, and it seems likely that the disorder should be classified with the reticuloendothelioses.

Skin or mucous membrane lesions may resemble childhood urticaria pigmentosa, but significant differences that indicate systemic mastocytoses are (1) onset after puberty, (2) multiple, small, confluent macules with persistent telangiectasia, (3) papules and nodules resembling leukemia cutis, (4) chronic lichenified dermatitis, (5) generalized infiltration of skin with a "scotch-grain" appearance, (6) less pigmentation, (7) less tendency to redden and urticate on stroking, (8) extensive involvement of oral, nasal, or rectal mucosa, and (9) progressive cutaneous change.

Histamine release into the general circulation is less likely than in childhood urticaria pigmentosa, yet patients may have flushing, shocklike episodes, and increased histamine in the urine. Diarrhea is often a prominent feature, and peptic ulcer occasionally develops.

Persistent or progressive cutaneous eruption may be the only evidence of the disease, although asymptomatic bone changes can be demonstrated by roentgenographic examination in many cases. These changes consist of solitary or multiple, irregular or round lytic lesions or local or general new bone formation, which causes thickening of the cortex and trabeculae and narrowing of marrow spaces. In more severe instances, lymphadenopathy, splenomegaly, and hepatomegaly are prominent early manifestations, and bone marrow aspiration shows abnormal accumulations of mast cells. The disorder may remain static at this point or may progress with weakness, weight loss, cachexia, nausea, vomiting, diarrhea, and malaise. In these patients anemia, leukopenia, thrombocytopenia, and leukemoid features develop, presumably from the proliferative effect of mast cells in bone marrow. Other blood abnormalities are eosinophilia, lymphocytosis, and monocytosis. Liver function may be impaired by mast cell invasion and associated periportal fibrosis. A malabsorption syndrome may develop. Bleeding tendencies are usually due to combinations of thrombocytopenia and prothrombin deficiency, but there may be a circulating heparin-like substance. Tissue mast cell leukemia, somewhat like other leukemias, is found on rare occasions. Abnormal numbers of mast cells are found at autopsy in almost all tissues. In mild forms, mast cells appear normal, but in severe forms, especially leukemia, anaplasia indicates malignant transformation.

Prognosis varies with the form of the disorder. Disease confined to skin and bone is compatible with long life and little morbidity, but there is always the threat of extension of the morbid process. Extensive reticuloendothelial involvement results in death in a few months to several years. Patients die from pancytopenia, infection, hemorrhage, cachexia, gastroenteritis, perforated peptic ulcer, and leukemia. Therapy is palliative and symptomatic and includes transfusions, antimicrobials, antihistamines, adrenal steroids, corticotrophin, roentgen irradiation, and nitrogen mustard.

Barer, M., Peterson, L. F. A., Dahlin, D. C., Winkelmann, R. K., and Stewart, J. R.: Mastocytosis with osseous lesions resembling metastatic malignant lesions in bone. J. Bone Joint Surg. (Am.), 50:142, 1968.

Burgoon, C. F., Graham, J. H., and McCaffree, D. L.: Mast cell disease. Arch. Dermatol., 98:590, 1968.

Caplan, R. M.: The natural course of urticaria pigmentosa. Arch. Dermatol., 87:146, 1963.

Clement, A. C., Fishbone, G., Levine, R. J., James, A. E., and Janower, M.: Gastrointestinal lesions in mastocytosis. Am. J. Roentgenol. Radium Ther. Nucl. Med., 103:405, 1968.

Sagher, F., and Even-Paz, Z.: Mastocytosis and the Mast Cell. Chicago, Year Book Publishers, Inc., 1967.

Simone, T. J., and Hayes, W. T.: Bullous urticaria pigmentosa with bleeding. J. Pediatr., 78:160, 1971.

917. LETHAL CUTANEOUS AND GASTROINTESTINAL ARTERIOLAR THROMBOSIS (Degos' Disease)

Clayton E. Wheeler, Jr.

Lethal cutaneous and gastrointestinal arteriolar thrombosis is a progressive, often fatal disease in which characteristic cutaneous, gastrointestinal, and central nervous system lesions result from spotty occlusive vascular disease. The cause is unknown. Most cases of this uncommon disorder occur in young adult males. Cutaneous manifestations usually precede gastrointestinal or nervous system symptoms by weeks or months, although the reverse sequence may occur. Indolent, slowly progressive, rose-colored papules 2 to 5 mm in size appear on the trunk or proximal extremities and occasionally elsewhere. In a few days or weeks the papules develop porcelain-like central umbilication covered by white scale and surrounded by a slightly elevated violaceous telangiectatic border. In time the entire lesion becomes white, depressed, and atrophic. There are usually fewer than 100 lesions, and they appear in crops, so that several stages of development are represented at any one time.

Central nervous system symptoms may be mild, localized, evanescent, and migratory in the initial phases, but eventually they become severe, extensive, and permanent. Numbness, weakness, headache, slurred speech, aphasias, seizures, hemiparesis, paraplegia, optic atrophy, and cranial nerve palsies may be found. To date, gastrointestinal involvement has not been reported in patients with prominent central nervous system disease.

Initial gastrointestinal symptoms may be mild and vague and may be associated with asthenia and weight loss, or the onset may be abrupt with signs indicating perforation, ileus, and peritonitis. Laparotomy reveals multiple, oval, white, subserosal patches of atrophy varying from pinpoint to 2 cm in size and irregularly distributed in stomach, ileum, jejunum, and colon. Perforation and peritonitis frequently occur, and there may be localized areas of gangrene.

The basic pathologic abnormality is an obliterative endothelial reaction affecting small arteries and arterioles and corresponding veins. Ischemic infarcts, necrobiosis, or atrophy occurs at involved sites in all layers of the skin and intestinal tract, and similar lesions are found in the central nervous system. The mouth, esophagus, rectum, anus, liver, pancreas, genitalia, bladder, kidney, lung, pleura, heart, retina, choroid, sclera, and conjunctiva have also been involved. Disease of smaller vessels, with emphasis on endothelial reaction, appears to distinguish the disorder from Buerger's disease and periarteritis nodosa.

In 45 reported cases, 23 patients have died (20 with bowel and 3 with cerebral disease), and 7 are alive but have systemic disease. Skin lesions have been present for over three years in 13 of the 15 who have only skin disease. In fatal cases the interval between onset and death has usually been less than one year.

Treatment with antimicrobials, adrenal corticosteroids, anticoagulants, and methotrexate is ineffectual. Surgical intervention in persons with gastrointestinal symptoms is of temporary or no benefit because of the multiplicity and recurrence of lesions. Patients succumb to either gastrointestinal or nervous system involvement.

Howard, R. O., Klaus, S. N., Slavin, R. C., and Fenton, R.: Malignant atrophic papulosis (Degos' syndrome). Arch. Ophthalmol., 79:262, 1968.

Jensen, N. E.: Malignant atrophic papulosis (Degos' syndrome). Br. J. Dermatol., 57:394, 1972.

Lomholt, G., Hjorth, N., and Fischermann, K.: Lethal peritonitis from Degos' disease (malign and atrophic papulosis). Acta Chir. Scand., 134:495, 1968.

Winkelmann, R. K., Howard, F. M., Jr., Perry, H. O., and Miller, R. H.: Malignant papulosis of skin and cerebrum. Arch. Dermatol., 87:54, 1963.

918. ANGIOKERATOMA CORPORIS DIFFUSUM (Fabry's Disease)

Clayton E. Wheeler, Jr.

Definition. Fabry's disease is an inherited disorder of glycolipid metabolism characterized by telangiectatic skin lesions, hypohidrosis, corneal opacities, acral pain and paresthesias, febrile episodes, gastrointestinal symptoms, renal failure, cardiovascular disease, and central nervous system disturbances.

Etiology. An X-linked, incompletely recessive error in glycolipid metabolism is manifested by a deficiency of ceramide trihexosidase with accumulation of ceramide trihexoside and other neutral glycolipids. Trihexosidase activity is essentially absent from intestinal mucosa and leukocytes of hemizygotic males and is less than normal in heterozygotic females.

Prevalence. The disease is uncommon. Males exhibit the full-blown disorder. Females are asymptomatic carriers or develop mild forms of the disease.

Pathology. A glycolipid that is doubly refractile, periodic acid–Schiff positive, and has an affinity for Sudan black B and other histochemical properties is deposited in endothelial cells and smooth muscle of blood vessels, arrectores pilorum muscles, and heart muscles. Similar deposits are found in cells of the renal glomeruli, distal convoluted tubules, loop of Henle, urinary sediment, cornea, sweat glands, central nervous system, spleen, liver, lymph nodes, and bone marrow. On electron microscopy lipid inclusions show a concentrically arranged, lamellar structure. Skin biopsies may show glycolipid in vessels or appendages at sites distant from telangiectases. Telangiectases are dilated vessels in the upper dermis or blood-filled spaces enclosed by epidermis. Cultured skin fibroblasts accumulate ceramide trihexoside and stain metachromatically with toluidine blue.

Clinical Manifestations. Cutaneous lesions usually appear in childhood or around puberty and consist of telangiectatic spots varying in size from barely visible to several millimeters. They are bright red to blue-black, and some are covered with slight scale. They are nonpulsatile lesions that may be partially blanched on diascopy. Telangiectases tend to cluster about the umbilicus, glans penis, scrotum, buttocks, hips, and thighs; but they occur anywhere, including the oral mucosa. A few lesions are found initially, but as the disease progresses they may appear in profusion. Skin lesions may be absent. Sweating is often decreased. Hair may be scanty; many patients shave infrequently. Paresthesias of the hands and feet and episodes of very severe burning pain in the extremities, at times accompanied by fever, may be early symptoms that may be precipitated by exposure to heat or cold or by physical exertion. Attacks of nausea, diarrhea, and abdominal pain are common. A Raynaud-like phenomenon and pain in the muscles and joints may also occur. Patients may complain of dizziness, weakness, and headache. Edema may occur in the absence of renal or cardiac failure.

Dilated, tortuous venules may be found in the palpebral and bulbar conjunctiva and the retina. Corneal opacities are usually, if not always, present and lens opacities may be found. Hypertension develops in older persons, and there may be evidence of myocardial infarction, congestive failure, or cerebrovascular disease.

An early finding, which may be discovered at routine examination, is albuminuria. "Maltese cross" material may be found in the urine on polaroscopy. "Mulberry cells" containing glycolipid may be discerned in the urinary sediment. Later in the disease there are casts, hematuria, and low, fixed specific gravity, azotemia, and anemia.

Diagnosis. Cutaneous telangiectases, albuminuria, glycolipid in cells of skin and renal biopsies, glycolipid in urinary sediment (both ceramide trihexoside and ceramide dihexoside), and a positive family history are diagnostic. In addition, slit-lamp examination of the cornea shows characteristic findings, even in female carriers.

Senile angiomas (de Morgan or ruby spots) are usually brighter red, are more numerous on the upper trunk, and do not cluster together. Angiokeratomas of the scrotum (Fordyce) are common lesions of older men. Lesions of Osler-Weber-Rendu disease are brighter red, less grouped, and occur chiefly in the mouth, nose, and lips and on the fingers. Angiokeratomas identical to those of Fabry's disease have been reported in alpha-1-fucosidase deficiency.

Treatment. In addition to treatment for renal failure, kidney transplants may provide effective enzyme replacement. Administration of purified placental ceramide trihexosidase has temporarily decreased ceramide trihexoside blood levels. These treatments are still in experimental phases but hold promise for the future.

Prognosis. The disease is slowly progressive in males, who usually die in the fourth or fifth decades of renal failure complicated by cardiovascular disease. Longevity is essentially uninfluenced by the mild form that occurs in women.

Brady, R. O., et al.: Replacement therapy for inherited enzyme defect (use of purified ceramidetrihexosidase) in Fabry's disease. N. Engl. J. Med., 289:9, 1973.

Epinette, W. W., et al.: Angiokeratoma corporis diffusum with alpha-L-fucosidase deficiency. Arch. Dermatol., 107:754, 1973.

Ferrons, V. J., Hibbs, R. G., and Burda, C. D.: The heart in Fabry's disease. Am. J. Cardiol., 24:95, 1969.

Matalon, R., Dorfman, A., Dawson, G., and Sweeley, C. C.: Glycolipid and mucopolysaccharide abnormality in fibroblasts in Fabry's disease. Science, 164:1522, 1969.

Philippart, M., Franklin, S. S., and Gordon, A.: Reversal of inborn sphingolipidosis (Fabry's disease) by kidney transplantation. Ann. Intern. Med., 77:195, 1972.

Philippart, M., Sarlieve, L., and Manacorda, A.: Urinary glycolipids in Fabry's disease. Pediatrics, 43:201, 1969.

919.   INCONTINENTIA PIGMENTI
(Bloch-Sulzberger Syndrome)

Clayton E. Wheeler, Jr.

Incontinentia pigmenti is a congenital disorder characterized by bizarre skin lesions and defects in many structures of epidermal and mesodermal origin. The cause is unknown. Maternal viral infection appears unlikely. Evidence suggests that the disorder is inherited as an X-linked trait that is lethal for males. Only 8 of 232 cases have been males.

Cutaneous lesions are usually present at birth but may not appear for a few weeks or a year or two. The process is likely to be localized initially but tends to spread and become generalized. The lesions are papules, vesicles, and bullae that arise in areas of inflammation. At first there is little tendency toward a configurate pattern but, later, groups, patches, and lines are observed. Lesions often come and go in crops, and the pattern shifts from time to time. After weeks or months, the inflammatory phase either passes directly to a pigmented macular stage or blends into a warty or papillomatous stage that subsequently develops into pigmented macules. The most characteristic feature of the skin involvement is the striking and bizarre pattern assumed by pigmented macules and, to a lesser extent, by preceding warty and inflammatory lesions. Streaks, flecks, lines whorls, patches, spidery forms, arborizations, and zebra and marble and fudge ripple patterns are found. The lines and streaks do not correspond to nerve, blood vessel, or dermatome distribution and frequently cross the midline. The macules are usually chocolate-brown, gray-brown, or slate-colored. After a few years pigmented macules often fade gradually, leaving little or no residuum by adult life. The hair may be thin, and a common finding is localized atrophic alopecia of the scalp. Occasionally other cutaneous defects develop such as dystrophic nails, localized atrophy, small keratotic areas, tylosis of palms and soles, and areas simulating localized scleroderma.

Other abnormalities of structures of ectodermal or mesodermal origin occur in approximately two thirds of the patients. *Dental anomalies* include delayed eruption, fewer teeth than normal, and conical crowns of the incisors, canines, and bicuspids. Both deciduous and permanent teeth are affected. Possible *eye changes* are strabismus, corneal opacities, cataracts, optic atrophy,

blue scleras, retinal pigmentary abnormalities, retrobulbar glioma, and ablatio falciformis. *Nervous system involvement* includes spastic paralysis, motor disturbances, epilepsy, microcephaly, mental retardation, nystagmus, decreased hearing, and homonymous hemianopsia. Osseous change, retarded growth and development, patent ductus arteriosus, urachal cyst, supernumerary ears, absence of or supernumerary nipples, and unilateral lack of breast tissue occasionally occur in patients with incontinentia pigmenti.

In the inflammatory, vesicular phase of the disease, blood eosinophilia of 30 to 50 per cent is common, and vesicle fluid eosinophilia may reach 95 per cent. Anemia occasionally occurs at this time.

Diagnosis is difficult in the vesicular or bullous phase. Blood and tissue eosinophilia and roentgenograms of unerupted teeth in infants may be helpful. As the bizarre configuration and the warty and pigmented macular phases develop, diagnosis usually becomes easy. Bullous incontinentia pigmenti must be differentiated from dermatitis herpetiformis, congenital syphilis, epidermolysis bullosa, erythema multiforme, bullous impetigo, virus diseases, and contact dermatitis. Warty and pigmented macular phases resemble systematized epithelial nevi. Hypomelanosis of Ito presents bizarre hypopigmented areas in marble-cake, swirling patterns, but this appears to be a separate disease—not just a hypopigmented phase of incontinentia pigmenti. Roentgenographic dental changes must be distinguished from congenital syphilis and congenital ectodermal defect.

No effective prevention or treatment is known. Adrenal steroid administration has had temporary beneficial effect on the bullous phase but has not been fully evaluated.

Morbidity and longevity depend upon the structures affected and the severity of the process. Cutaneous involvement alone or in association with minor defects of other structures is compatible with a normal life. Involvement of the nervous system or heart may carry a serious prognosis.

Carney, R. G., and Carney, R. G., Jr.: Incontinentia pigmenti. Arch. Dermatol., 102:157, 1970.

Jelenek, J. E., Bart, R. S., and Schiff, G. M.: Hypomelanosis of Ito (incontinentia pigmenti achromians). Arch. Dermatol., 107:596, 1973.

Schmidt, H., Hvidberg-Hansen, J., and Christensen, H. E.: Incontinentia pigmenti with associated lesions in two generations. Acta Derm. Venereol. (Stockh.), 52:281, 1972.

Simonsson, H.: Incontinentia pigmenti, Bloch-Sulzberger syndrome, associated with infantile spasms. Acta Paediatr. Scand., 61:612, 1972.

920.   HEREDITARY ANHIDROTIC ECTODERMAL DEFECT

Clayton E. Wheeler, Jr.

Hereditary anhidrotic ectodermal defect is an uncommon, genetically determined developmental defect of ectodermal, entodermal, and mesodermal structures in which dysgenesis of the epidermis and its appendages is the main feature. Predominance of the disease in males is explained by X-linked inheritance. Dominant and recessive autosomal inheritance have not been excluded in some cases. Defective development probably arises in the second or third month of embryonic life when epidermal appendages are being differentiated.

The *facies* is often so characteristic that unrelated persons appear to be siblings. Wide, high, scanty eyebrows, prominent frontal bones, saddle nose, thick swollen lips with radiating furrows, underdeveloped maxillas and mandibles, and pointed chin are distinctive features. The patient may be small and delicately proportioned, and the skin is likely to be thin, dry, white, and soft, producing a feminine appearance. Petechiae and purpura are occasionally seen, and the tourniquet test may be positive.

Absence of or greatly decreased numbers of sweat glands, which are often rudimentary, account for restricted sweating or none at all. Regulation of bodily temperature in a hot environment is defective because of inadequate sweating; thus, the disorder is one of the causes of fever, especially in the newborn. Lanugo, scalp, eyebrow, eyelash, axillary, and pubic hair are scant or absent. Sebaceous glands are decreased in number and activity. Nails may be normal or exhibit slow growth, ridging, or decreased thickness. Permanent and deciduous teeth may be absent or decreased in number and they are likely to be widely spaced, peg-shaped or conical, pigmented or fragile. Abnormalities of the lens include cataracts, subluxation, and absence. Mucous glands of the mouth, pharynx, larynx, trachea, and bronchi may be essentially absent. This may predispose to frequent respiratory tract infections. Chronic rhinitis contributes to the development of saddle nose. Defective lacrimal glands result in deficient tearing. Body odor is absent because of lack of sweating. Sparse amniotic fluid has been reported at birth. Lack of sweat pores of the palmar dermal ridges and x-ray evidence of defective dentition have diagnostic value.

In accordance with X-linked inheritance, the full-blown syndrome is most often seen in males, but females may show minor abnormalities of teeth, hair, or sweating. Decreased numbers of sweat pores may or may not be found in heterozygous females.

Less common abnormalities include primary hypogonadism, hypospadias, epispadias, absence of nipples, absence of mammary glands, satyr ears, cleft palate, mental deficiency, central nervous system defects, supernumerary fingers and toes, and micro-ophthalmia.

Histologically, the skin shows decreased epidermal and dermal thickness, absence of or rudimentary sweat glands, absence of or small pilosebaceous apparatus, and poorly developed arrectores pilorum muscles.

Treatment is entirely symptomatic and includes protection from heat, use of dentures, and plastic repair of nasal defects. Measures to improve appearance are morale builders. Longevity is usually good. Patients should choose occupations where as little sweating as possible is required for body cooling and where respiratory tract irritants can be avoided.

Beahrs, J. O., et al.: Anhidrotic ectodermal dysplasia: Predisposition to bronchial disease. Ann. Intern. Med., 74:92, 1971.

Crump, I. A., and Danka, D. M.: Hypohidrotic ectodermal dysplasia. J. Pediatr., 78:466, 1971.

Frias, J. L., and Smith, D. W.: Diminished sweat pores in hypohidrotic ectodermal dysplasia. J. Pediatr., 72:606, 1968.

Richards, W., and Kaplan, J. M.: Anhidrotic ectodermal dysplasia. An unusual cause of pyrexia in the newborn. Am. J. Dis. Child., 117:597, 1969.

Verbov, J.: Hypohidrotic (or anhidrotic) ectodermal dysplasia—an appraisal of diagnostic methods. Br. J. Dermatol., 83:341, 1970.

921. NEUROFIBROMATOSIS OF VON RECKLINGHAUSEN

Clayton E. Wheeler, Jr.

Neurofibromatosis is a relatively common disease (one case in about 3000 births) characterized by dominant inheritance, café au lait spots, freckling, and neurofibromas of the skin and internal organs. Cause and pathogenesis are unknown.

Café au lait spots occur in more than 90 per cent of the cases. They are often present at birth, but more may appear up to adult life. In old age the number may decrease. The spots are light brown macules that vary considerably in shape and size. More than five such lesions over 1.5 cm in size are diagnostic (small numbers occur in normal persons). Axillary or generalized freckling, when present, is a characteristic sign. Normal or increased numbers of melanocytes are present in pigmented spots and normal-appearing skin. Giant pigment granules may be found in prickle cells and melanocytes.

Neurofibromas appear at any cutaneous site, including the genitalia, palms, and soles. There may be few or many, and they vary greatly in size and shape. The tumors are of two types: (1) small, dome-shaped, or nipple-like, violaceous dermal lesions that can often be pressed into the skin like small hernias, and (2) subcutaneous nodules along the course of nerves. These may be knotted, plexiform, or pendulous and may attain great size.

The most frequent sites of internal involvement are bone, central nervous system, and pheochrome tissue. Neurofibromas in or near bone produce localized proliferative erosions or cystic lesions. Other frequent bony abnormalities are scoliosis, lordosis, kyphosis, and pseudoarthrosis. Neurofibromas may develop in almost any part of the central nervous system or in the eyes; the symptoms depend upon the size and location of the tumor. Nodules of the iris, hamartomas of the retina, and glaucoma may be found. Of the cranial nerves, the acoustic and optic are most often involved. Mental deficiency is not unusual. There may be an increased number of brain tumors that are not neurofibromas. The incidence of pheochromocytoma in neurofibromatosis is probably less than 1 per cent. On the other hand, 5 to 20 per cent of patients with pheochromocytoma have neurofibromatosis. Other internal involvement includes gastrointestinal bleeding, intestinal obstruction, lung cysts, pulmonary fibrosis, coarctation of the aorta, constricting bands of large vessels, urinary tract obstruction, jaundice, and hypertension caused by abnormalities of renal arteries. Sarcomatous degeneration of neurofibroma is reported in 2 to 16 per cent of cases, depending upon the series studied. Patients are often underdeveloped somatically and sexually, and fertility may be decreased. Precocious sexual development occurs in children. Gigantism and elephantiasis may involve extremities or digits.

Diagnosis is based upon café au lait spots, neurofibromas, bone roentgenograms, the histologic picture, and a positive family history. Treatment is palliative and includes surgical removal of neurofibromas that are large or interfere with function, sarcomas, pheochromocytomas, and various brain tumors. Prognosis is usually good, but it is influenced by malignancy, pheochromocytoma, and skeletal deformities.

Benedict, P. H., Szabo, G., Fitzpatrick, T. B., and Sinesi, S. J.: Melanotic macules in Albright's syndrome and in neurofibromatosis. J.A.M.A., 205:618, 1968.

Crowe, F. W.: Axillary freckling as a diagnostic aid in neurofibromatosis. Ann. Intern. Med., 61:1142, 1964.

Fenoan, N. T., and Yakovac, W. C.: Neurofibromatosis in childhood. J. Pediatr., 76:339, 1970.

Knight, W. A., et al.: Neurofibromatosis associated with malignant neurofibromas. Arch. Dermatol., 107:747, 1973.

Mena, E., et al.: Neurofibromatosis and renovascular hypertension in children. Am. J. Roentgenol. Radium Ther. Nucl. Med., 118:39, 1973.

922. AINHUM
(Dactylolysis Spontanea)

Clayton E. Wheeler, Jr.

Ainhum is characterized by spontaneous amputation of the fifth toe. The disorder is rare in the United States but common in parts of Africa. It affects primarily blacks and other dark-skinned persons, and shows a peak incidence between 30 and 40 years of age. The fifth toe is usually affected, although the fourth toe may be involved. Bilateral cases are common. Hyperkeratotic constriction develops at the undersurface of the toe at or between the plantar creases. This gradually encircles and constricts the toe until bone absorption occurs and the distal portion hangs by a thin pedicle. Inflammation or ulceration is often present. After months or years (average five years) the toe undergoes spontaneous, bloodless amputation. Neurologic and circulatory changes (plethysmographic studies are normal) are absent. Varying degrees of pain are common owing to sepsis, ulceration, and possibly pressure on nerves. There are no constitutional symptoms. Pathologic findings are nonspecific and probably result from chronic inflammation. The cause is unknown, but a plausible theory is that the small toes are predisposed to spontaneous amputation following trauma, chronic infection, and inflammation. The condition may be related to poor protection and care of the feet; most of the patients have gone barefoot. Cure is accomplished by spontaneous or surgical amputation.

Baerg, P. H.: Ainhum (dactylolysis spontanea): A review of the literature and a report of two cases. J. Am. Podiatry Assoc., 61:44, 1971.

Browne, S. G.: True ainhum: Its distinctive and differentiating features. J. Bone Joint Surg. (Br.) 47:52, 1965.

Cole, G. J.: Ainhum. An account of fifty-four patients with special reference to etiology and treatment. J. Bone Joint Surg. (Br.), 47:43, 1965.

Reque, C. J. et al.: Pseudoainhum constricting bands of the extremities. Arch. Dermatol., 105:434, 1972.

923. TOXIC EPIDERMAL NECROLYSIS
(Lyell's Disease, Scalded Skin Syndrome)

Clayton E. Wheeler, Jr.

Definition. Toxic epidermal necrolysis (TEN) is characterized by cutaneous erythema, epidermal loosening and stripping, and a scalded appearance.

Etiology. Two types are recognized: (1) Staphylococcal TEN is due to infection with the group II, usually type 71, staphylococcus and is caused by a toxin elaborated by the organism. (2) Drug-induced TEN may be caused by sulfonamides, butazones, salicylates, aminopyrine, phenacetin, antimicrobials, antihistamines, or anticonvulsants. At times the cause of the TEN cannot be identified.

Incidence. Staphylococcal TEN usually affects infants and young children, whereas drug-induced TEN usually affects adults and sometimes older children.

Pathogenesis and Pathology. Staphylococcal TEN results from infection in the nose, throat, ear, eye, skin, urogenital tract, heart valves, or elsewhere. Staphylococci often cannot be cultured from the erythematous or scalded skin, although sometimes they can. Animal experiments indicate that the Staphylococcus elaborates a toxin called epidermolysin which causes the scalded skin syndrome. Microscopically, the epidermis is damaged at the granular layer with subsequent shedding of this layer along with the horny layer. There is surprisingly little inflammatory or vascular change below the granular layer.

Drug-induced TEN causes necrosis, separation and loss of the entire epidermis, along with upper dermal damage and inflammation.

Clinical Manifestations. In staphylococcal TEN the infant or child is often noted to have a respiratory tract or skin infection. In the course of this infection there develops a diffuse scarlatiniform erythema with accentuation in the body folds and intertriginous sites. The skin is tender and painful to touch. Within a few hours the horny layer loosens and rubs off easily with movement, handling of the child, or friction against the bed, leaving a red, glistening surface resembling a scald. The extent of involvement is variable, true TEN lesions being limited to only a few intertriginous sites or becoming generalized. With proper treatment the process may not progress beyond the stage of erythema (staphylococcal erythema) or may do so only in some areas. With treatment, there is rapid healing, provided the child survives. Healing is accompanied by drying, lessening erythema, and a flaky scaling or peeling over a week or two. Mucous membranes are unlikely to be involved unless directly infected by the Staphylococcus.

In drug-induced TEN the patient is usually ill to begin with and is taking one or several drugs. Patchy or generalized erythema develops over a few hours or days. The entire thickness of the epidermis loosens and is easily stripped away from the dermal bed, leaving a white or pink glistening surface and a scalded appearance. A relatively small amount of the body surface may be affected, or much of the body surface may be involved. The patient suffers great discomfort from the denuded areas in the more extensive cases. Fluid and electrolyte losses are likely to be excessive. The patient may exhibit shock. Epidermal regeneration is slow, taking two to three weeks before significant epidermal barrier function is restored. In this form of TEN the mucous membranes are likely to be involved as well as skin. Secondary bacterial or mycotic infection is likely to be a problem.

Diagnosis. Infection of an infant or child with the group II Staphylococcus followed by erythema, epidermal necrosis, and separation at the granular layer suffices for diagnosis of staphylococcal TEN. History of drug exposure followed by erythema, necrosis, and separation of full-thickness epidermis in an adult or older child suggests drug-induced TEN.

In the adult or drug-induced type, the major differential diagnosis is erythema multiforme of the Stevens-Johnson type. TEN lacks the round, configurate lesions, the tense, well-formed bullae, and the intense dermal inflammation of erythema multiforme. Erythema multiforme lacks the scalded appearance.

Treatment. In staphylococcal TEN, the Staphylococcus is usually penicillin and tetracycline resistant so that cloxacillin, methicillin, erythromycin, or other systemic antimicrobials are used in large doses. The child is kept in a warm room, handled carefully, and subjected to expert nursing care. Pouring calamine liniment on the affected areas and spreading it out gently with gloved fingers may be soothing. Analgesics, antipyretics, and other symptomatic measures may be necessary. Replacement of fluid and electrolytes lost through the skin is most important.

Treatment of the adult, drug-induced TEN is more difficult. The causative agent should be removed if it can be identified. Fluid, electrolytes, and macromolecules should be replaced as they are lost. Secondary bacterial or mycotic infection should be combated with appropriate antimicrobials. Systemic corticosteroids are usually administered as soon as possible, but there is question about their effectiveness, especially after the epidermal damage is done. The patient should be kept in a warm room, handled as little as possible, and kept as comfortable as possible with analgesics, antipyretics, and good nursing care.

Prognosis. In general, the staphylococcal type has a good prognosis. This depends upon the underlying infection, the extent of the TEN, and the promptness of treatment. Unrecognized, untreated cases have a mortality rate of 10 to 25 per cent. Drug-induced TEN has a poor prognosis. Even when recognized and treated early, it has a mortality rate of 25 to 50 per cent, depending largely upon the extent of involvement.

Lillibridge, C. B., Melish, M. E., and Glasgow, L. A.: Site of action of exfoliative toxin in the staphylococcal scalded skin syndrome. Pediatrics, 5:728, 1972.

Lowney, E. D., et al.: The scalded skin syndrome in small children. Arch. Dermatol., 95:359, 1967.

Melish, M. E., and Glasgow, L. A.: The staphylococcal scalded-skin syndrome. N. Engl. J. Med., 282:1114, 1970.

Melish, M. E., Glasgow, L. A., and Turner, M. D.: The staphylococcal scaled-skin syndrome: Isolation and partial characterization of the exfoliative toxin. J. Infect. Dis., 125:129, 1972.

Reid, L. H., Weston, W. L., and Humbert, J. R.: Staphylococcal scalded skin syndrome. Adult onset in a patient with deficient cell-mediated immunity. Arch. Dermatol., 109:239, 1974.

924. DISORDERS OF MELANIN PIGMENTATION

Aaron B. Lerner

Melanin is the brown to black pigment that colors the skin, hair, and eyes. It is formed in the cytoplasm of melanocytes by the oxidation of tyrosine catalyzed by tyrosinase, a copper-containing enzyme. Under normal conditions pigment is transferred from melanocytes to keratinocytes so that the color of skin depends upon the presence of melanin within both the pigment and epidermal cells. Melanocytes are derived embryologically from the neural crest. Before the third month of fetal life these cells migrate to their resting places in the skin at the epidermal-dermal junction, in the eyes along the uveal tract, and in the central nervous system in the leptomeninges. In the conversion of tyrosine to melanin the first compound formed is dopa. After several reactions the melanin polymer is made. The pigment of red hair, and perhaps even that of freckles, results from a side reaction in which dopa is combined with cysteine to form 5-S cysteine dopa. It is the oxidation and polymerization of 5-S cysteine dopa that produces the red pigment.

Pigmented nevi are composed of clusters of melanocytes. Most of them form after birth, although occasionally large pigmented nevi are present at birth as a result of an abnormal proliferation of melanocytes in the skin in utero.

Most disorders of *hypopigmentation,* such as vitiligo, albinism, partial albinism, and phenylketonuria, are under genetic control, whereas the disturbances of *hyperpigmentation* usually occur in patients with endocrine abnormalities.

Hypopigmentation. Albinism and vitiligo are the two most important disturbances of hypopigmentation. In *albinism* there is an absence or decrease of tyrosinase in melanocytes. In *partial albinism* there is a congenital absence of melanocytes in the white patches. The light color of the skin in patients with *phenylketonuria* may result from an inhibition of tyrosinase by the presence of excess phenylalanine. In *vitiligo* and in *graying of hair* pigment cells that were present at birth are destroyed. Vitiligo occurs in about 1 per cent of the population and is transmitted as a dominant trait. Pigment is lost in exposed areas, particularly the face and dorsal aspects of the hands; in the axillae and genitalia; in surrounding body orifices such as the mouth, eyes, nose, nipples, and rectum; at sites of pressure and trauma; about pigmented nevi; and in hair. Patients with vitiligo are usually in good general health. However, the incidence of vitiligo is increased 5- to 15-fold in patients with hyperthyroidism, pernicious anemia, adrenocortical insufficiency, and melanomas. Vitiligo tends to occur in patients who are becoming hyperpigmented, so that there may be lightening in some areas and darkening in others. The loss of melanocytes in these patients probably results from a combination of autocytotoxic and autoimmune processes. Hypopigmentation distinct from vitiligo is seen in patients with scleroderma. Patches of white skin and, less frequently, partial albinism are seen in patients with *tuberous sclerosis.*

Hyperpigmentation. In most clinical states accompanied by hyperpigmentation, endocrine function is abnormal. Specific hormones activate adenyl cyclase on the cell surface to increase the levels of cyclic AMP within melanocytes. When the melanocyte-stimulating hormone, β-MSH, is released in excessive quantities by the pituitary gland, darkening of the skin occurs in patients with adrenocortical insufficiency. Pituitary activity increases as a result of decreased steroid production by the adrenal cortex. However, the same kind of hyperpigmentation can occur in the presence of a pituitary tumor that releases an excess of MSH. Usually pituitary tumors first produce increased amounts of corticotrophin, stimulating the adrenals and leading to the development of Cushing's syndrome. If a pituitary tumor is not suspected and the patient undergoes bilateral adrenalectomy, the tumor will continue to grow, and the skin may become very dark. Initially the tumor produces only large amounts of corticotrophin, but later

MSH peptides are also made. In some patients a pituitary tumor may release excess MSH but not corticotrophin, so that hyperpigmentation without adrenocortical hyperplasia occurs.

A few patients with *metastatic carcinomas* develop similar problems of hyperpigmentation. The carcinomas produce peptides related to or identical with corticotrophin and MSH. Some of these patients develop both Cushing's syndrome and hyperpigmentation, although others show only hyperpigmentation. Assay of some of the tumors has shown the presence of MSH and corticotrophin-like substances. Hyperpigmentation also may be seen in 10 to 15 per cent of women receiving potent synthetic progesterones and estrogens for birth control. Although these substances are not as effective darkeners of melanocytes as are the MSH and MSH-like peptides, they do produce facial pigmentation or *melasma*.

Severe hyperpigmentation is seen occasionally in patients with hyperthyroidism, xanthomatous biliary cirrhosis, sprue, or hemochromatosis. It is likely that in these individuals there are increased amounts of cyclic AMP within melanocytes as a result of either more adenyl cyclase activity or less phosphodiesterase function within the cells. Chronic illness or ingestion of drugs such as busulfan (Myleran) or 4-aminopteroyl glutamic acid (Aminopterin) also produces hyperpigmentation. Again, these substances probably work by increasing cyclic AMP levels within pigment cells.

Melanoma.   All adults have many nevi, and most melanomas arise from nevi. Melanoma accounts for about 1.5 per cent of cancer deaths. Ten to 20 per cent of patients with melanomas develop vitiligo. At times the primary lesion is destroyed even though the tumor is metastasizing at a rapid rate. The relationship between the destruction of normal melanocytes and that of some malignant melanocytes in patients with melanomas is not known. In a few patients with metastatic melanoma moderate amounts of tyrosine oxidation products made in the tumors are carried by the blood to the kidneys and excreted in the urine. In air they become oxidized to melanin, giving the urine a dark color, and the patients are said to have *melanuria*. In exceptional cases of metastatic melanoma, great quantities of tyrosine oxidation products form, reach the skin, and are converted to melanin. The patient first acquires the slate gray color of argyria and later becomes intensely brown or black.

Conference on Pigment Cell Biology. Yale J. Biol. Med., Vol. 46, Dec. 1973.

Lerner, A. B.: On the etiology of vitiligo and gray hair. Am. J. Med., 51:141, 1971.

McGovern, V. J., and Russell, P. (eds.): Mechanisms in Pigmentation. Proceedings of the 8th International Pigment Cell Conference in Sydney, Basel, S. Karger, 1972.

925. ACATALASIA

Alexander G. Bearn

Acatalasia is a rare, autosomal, recessively inherited trait characterized by a deficiency of catalase in many tissues of the body, including the erythrocytes, bone marrow, liver, and skin. The disease is particularly common among Japanese, Koreans, and Chinese, but has also been reported from Germany, Switzerland, and Israel. Manifestations are usually restricted to the oral cavity and are related to the increased susceptibility to tissue damage by normal microbial flora. Oral sepsis may lead to severe gangrenous lesions, including alveolar bone destruction. Approximately 50 per cent of acatalasic subjects are asymptomatic; after puberty gangrenous lesions in the oral cavity are rare. An absence of catalase in individuals homozygous for the trait and intermediate values for the clinically normal heterozygous carriers are characteristic of the families reported from Japan. Homozygotes from Germany, Switzerland, and Israel commonly show residual catalase activity and are symptomatically normal. When hydrogen peroxide is added to acatalasic blood, it turns a brownish black color owing to the formation of methemoglobin; by contrast normal blood bubbles vigorously and remains pink. At least two forms of acatalasia exist in Japan where more than 50 patients with the disease have been reported. Genetic heterogeneity is suggested both from the variations in the clinical expression of the disease and in the level and stability of residual catalase activity in different populations. The estimated frequency in Japan is approximately 1 in 50,000, and the heterozygote frequency is approximately 1 per cent. Variations in the gene frequency within Japan have been reported. Local surgical excision, extraction of teeth, and antimicrobial therapy have been employed. A similar disease occurs in mice, guinea pigs, dogs, and the domestic fowl.

Aebi, H., and Suter, H.: Acatalasemia. *In* Harris, H., and Hirschhorn, K. (eds.): Advances in Human Genetics. Vol. 2. New York, Plenum Press, 1971.

Wyngaarden, J. B., and Howell, R. R.: Acatalasia. *In* Stanbury, J. B., Wyngaarden, J. B., and Fredrickson, D. S. (eds.): The Metabolic Basis of Inherited Disease. 3rd ed. New York, McGraw-Hill Book Company, 1972.

926. ALBINISM
(Oculocutaneous Albinism)

Alexander G. Bearn

The term albinism has come to refer to a genetically heterogeneous group of disorders in which there is an inherited defect in melanin metabolism. It is characterized by a decrease of melanin in the skin, hair, and eyes, and is due to a failure of melanocytes to produce normal melanin. The metabolic defect may involve melanocytes in more than one system (oculocutaneous albinism) or be restricted to one system (ocular albinism). Several independent genetic defects in tyrosine metabolism lead to the same phenotypic effect. Oculocutaneous albinism occurs in two distinct autosomal recessively inherited forms. In one form, the melanocytes lack the enzyme tyrosinase, leading to "tyrosinase-negative" albinism; in the second the enzyme is present and the defect is probably due to a limitation in the availability of tyrosine, the melanogenic substrate for the enzyme.

"Tyrosinase-negative" albinism occurs with a frequency of about 1 in 34,000 and is equally common in whites and blacks. The skin and hair color are strikingly white and do not darken with age. The skin is particularly susceptible to sunlight and often appears wrinkled. Precancerous keratoses in the areas exposed to sunlight are common, and there is a marked increase in frequency of basal cell and squamous cell carcinomas of the skin. Photophobia, astigmatism, and severe defects in visual acuity are common. Horizontal nystagmus is almost invariable. The ocular fundus of albinos is bright orange-red, and the vessels are prominent.

"Tyrosinase-positive" albinism is more frequently found among blacks than among whites. In the black population the phenotypic frequency is 1 in 14,000, whereas in the white population the frequency is approximately 1 in 60,000. In contrast with "tyrosinase-negative" albinism, the pigmentation of the skin and eyes increases with advancing age. Blacks with "tyrosinase-positive" albinism may be darker than many blonde Caucasoids. Freckles and pigmented nevi are common. Photophobia is less pronounced, and not all patients exhibit nystagmus.

Ocular albinism is a very rare variety in which the defect in pigmentation is restricted to the iris and fundus of the eye. Nystagmus, head-nodding, and defective vision also occur. It is inherited as an X-linked recessive trait.

Cutaneous albinism (partial albinism, piebald trait) is limited to the skin and hair. In almost all patients a triangular white forelock is present. The trait is inherited in a dominant fashion.

Fitzpatrick, T. B., and Quevedo, W. C.: Albinism. *In* Stanbury, J. B., Wyngaarden, J. B., and Fredrickson, D. S. (eds.): The Metabolic Basis of Inherited Disease. 3rd ed. New York, McGraw-Hill Book Company, 1972.

Witkop, C. J., Jr.: Albinism. *In* Harris, H., and Hirschhorn, K. (eds.): Advances in Human Genetics. Vol. 2. New York, Plenum Press, 1971.

927. DYSAUTONOMIA (Riley-Day Syndrome)

Alexander G. Bearn

Dysautonomia is a rare recessively inherited disease of childhood, occurring almost exclusively in Ashkenazi Jews. The anatomic basis of the disease is an absence of unmyelinated nerve fibers in the peripheral and autonomic nerves. Features include defective lacrimation, absence of the fungiform papillae of the tongue, vasomotor instability including blotching of the skin, relative indifference to pain, poor motor coordination, and absent deep tendon reflexes. Dysphagia in childhood may be the presenting symptom. Many patients die in childhood from secondary aspiration pneumonia.

The differential diagnosis includes the congenital and hereditary sensory neuropathies which may present with insensitivity to pain.

Brunt, P. W., and McKusick, V. A.: Familial dysautonomia. A report of genetic and clinical studies, with a review of the literature. Medicine, 49:343, 1970.

928. EHLERS-DANLOS SYNDROME

Clayton E. Wheeler, Jr.

Definition. The Ehlers-Danlos syndrome consists of a group of inherited systemic connective tissue disorders in which the major manifestations are fragility and hyperelasticity of skin, easy bruising, atrophic scars and soft pseudotumors, calcified cysts, hyperextensibility of joints with frequent luxations, bleeding tendency, and visceral anomalies.

Etiology. The chief abnormalities of connective tissue are increased fragility and friability and capacity to stretch to an unusual length and return to the original position. Elastic tissue deficiency appears unlikely, because the tissue returns to its original position after stretching. Since toughness and limited extensibility are characteristics of normal collagen, fragility and hyperelasticity seem to indicate a collagen defect. It is conjectural whether the defect is molecular or involves the arrangement of molecules into fibrils or fibrils into bundles, or whether different types of the disease have different defects, because evidence is accumulating that the Ehlers-Danlos syndrome is composed of a heterogeneous group of disorders. Six types have been postulated and more may be expected. Types I to IV are probably inherited as dominant, Type V as X-linked recessive, and Type VI as autosomal recessive traits. Type VI appears to be due to a deficiency in lysyl-protocollagen hydroxylase with defective cross-linking of collagen.

Incidence. The Ehlers-Danlos syndrome is most prevalent among white persons of European ancestry, although dark-skinned people are occasionally affected. Males are involved slightly more often than females. Skin and joint changes usually appear at an early age, but may not be evident until adult life. The disorder, including mild and incomplete forms, is undoubtedly much more common than case reports in the literature indicate.

Pathology. No consistent abnormality of the corium has been demonstrated by microscopic examination. Normal, increased, or decreased amounts of elastic tissue or collagen, fragmentation of elastic tissue, and derangement of architecture of collagen have all been reported. Some of these findings may be late effects of overstretching and fragility rather than primary abnormalities. Limited study with the electron microscope has shown normal-appearing elastic tissue and collagen. No consistent microscopic abnormality has been found in blood vessels. Subcutaneous nodules are composed of encapsulated fat, which is often calcified. Pseudotumors show connective tissue proliferation, increased vascularity, islets of fatty degeneration, and cyst formation.

Pathogenesis. Defective, friable collagen that allows abnormal extensibility and normal elastic tissue that provides return to the original position explain many of the clinical features: hyperelastic skin, scars, pseudotumors, easy bruising, hyperextensibility of joints with luxations, hemarthroses and arthritis, rupture of the lung with emphysema, and fragility and bleeding from the bowel. Defective supporting tissue of vessel walls or surrounding structures accounts for much of the abnormal bleeding, but functional and structural abnormalities of platelets have been reported, and some abnormality in collagen-platelet relationships has been found.

Clinical Manifestations. Clinical features are variable because of mild and incomplete forms and because several genetic or biochemical types may exist. The facies may be normal, or there may be widely spaced eyes, epicanthal folds, broad nasal bridge, and "lop ears." Mentality is usually normal. The patient is likely to be small, short, and poorly developed.

The most striking feature of the soft, velvety skin is its capacity to be pulled abnormally far from underlying structures and to return promptly to its original position. The entire skin is usually hyperelastic, but some regions exhibit this property more than others. With age, elasticity of localized areas, especially about the elbows, may be lost so that the skin hangs in loose folds. Skin of the palms and soles is likely to become lax, furrowed, and redundant, and resembles loose-fitting gloves or moccasins. Despite increased elasticity, the skin is abnormally fragile or brittle, as shown by its tendency to bruise easily and by the development of scars and soft pseudotumors at sites of minor injury. Paper-thin atrophic scars develop over the elbows, knees, shins, and elsewhere. The scars are shiny, brown or red-violet, and often show telangiectasia. Subcutaneous spherules or nodules 2 to 8 mm in size may appear on the legs and forearms. These are easily movable and often calcify. Minor blows result in purpura or hematomas that may organize to form tumors. Retraction of tissues prevents excessive bleeding from skin injury, but minor trauma or surgery produces a gaping, fish-mouth wound that is hard to close and heals slowly.

Hyperextensibility of joints is often striking; the head, extremities, and digits may be placed in abnormal positions ("India rubber men" and "human pretzels"). Because of hyperextensibility of the joints and poor muscular development or tone, infants may show delayed sitting or walking and unsteadiness that occasions frequent falling and subsequent fractures. Other consequences of loose joints and muscle atony or weakness are frequent joint effusions or hemarthroses, arthritis, and habitual dislocations of the hip, shoulders, patella, radius, and clavicle. In addition, flat feet, genu recurvatum, kyphoscoliosis, and loose-end clavicles are seen. Other musculoskeletal abnormalities that have been associated with the Ehlers-Danlos syndrome are spina bifida occulta, arachnodactyly, high arched palate, club foot, spondylolisthesis, pigeon breast, and osteolytic changes of distal phalanges. There may be too few, too many, or poorly formed teeth. Umbilical and inguinal hernias are common. Muscle cramps may involve the legs at night.

Recognition of internal manifestations will undoubtedly increase with further study. Dissecting aortic aneurysm, intracranial aneurysms, spontaneous rupture of large arteries, aneurysm of the sinus of Valsalva and aortic insufficiency, spontaneous rupture of the lung with mediastinal and subcutaneous emphysema, and fragility of the bowel with bleeding or perforation have been reported. Congenital anomalies of the heart, gastrointestinal, respiratory, or genitourinary tracts also occur. Bleeding may occur into the skin or from the lung, vagina, rectum, nose, gums or tooth sockets, or after tonsillectomy, after operation on joints, or post partum.

Beighten classifies the Ehlers-Danlos syndrome into five types and McKusick adds a sixth. (1) Ehlers-Danlos syndrome I, or gravis type, is characterized by striking skin hyperextensibility, fragility and bruisability, and severe joint hypermobility. Friable tissues make operations difficult, and early rupture of fetal membranes may cause prematurity. (2) Ehlers-Danlos syndrome II, or mitis type, is characterized by mild cutaneous and joint manifestations. Tissue friability and prematurity are not problems. (3) Ehlers-Danlos syndrome III, or benign hypermobile type, is characterized by generalized and marked joint hypermobility with frequent complications, but cutaneous manifestations are minimal. (4) Ehlers-Danlos syndrome IV, or ecchymotic type, is characterized by thin, pale skin, prominent venous network, and little cutaneous hyperextensibility. Joint hypermobility is largely limited to the digits. The main feature is severe, easy bruisability. Ruptures of the bowel and great vessels are found predominantly in this type. (5) Ehlers-Danlos syndrome V, or X-linked form, shows striking skin extensibility, and there are moderate fragility, cigarette-paper scarring, and bruising. Joint hypermobility is limited. (6) Ehlers-Danlos syndrome VI, or the hydroxylysine-deficient collagen type, is characterized by autosomal recessive inheritance and paucity of hydroxylysine residues in collagen owing to deficient lysyl hydroxylase activity.

Diagnosis. Two or more of the following clinical features usually suffice for diagnosis: (1) cutaneous hyperelasticity, (2) hyperextensibility of joints, (3) easy bruising, (4) atrophic scars and pseudotumors, (5) calcified subcutaneous cysts, and (6) typical cases in the family.

Cutis laxa is characterized by loose, inelastic skin that hangs in folds. In late stages of the Ehlers-Danlos syndrome, localized areas of skin may become lax, but otherwise there seems to be no relation between the two disorders. Hypermobility of joints occurs as a genetic trait distinct from the Ehlers-Danlos syndrome, and it is part of *Marfan's syndrome, osteogenesis imperfecta, mongolism, cretinism,* and *cachexia.* Blue sclerae are probably essential features of the Ehlers-Danlos syndrome and do not signify a relationship to osteogenesis imperfecta. Besides having hyperelastic joints and skin,

patients with the *Bonnevie-Ullrich-Turner syndrome* show dwarfism, web neck, cubitus valgus, gonadal dysgenesis, and female phenotype with male genotype.

Treatment. There is no treatment for the basic disorder. Trauma to skin and joints should be avoided. Careful suturing, immobilization, and taping may promote wound healing. Hematomas occasionally require drainage. Orthopedic measures, including exercises, braces, reduction of dislocations, and drainage of hemarthroses, may be necessary. Dissecting aneurysm, hemorrhage, intestinal perforation, and various anomalies may require surgical intervention. Surgical procedures should be undertaken with great care because of the friability and hyperelasticity of skin and internal structures. Severed tissues separate abnormally, sutures are difficult to place and often do not hold, and wound dehiscence is a definite threat.

Prognosis. Prognosis for life is usually good, although deaths occur from various internal manifestations. Patients may be comfortable or may suffer considerable inconvenience and morbidity from cutaneous and musculoskeletal abnormalities. The joints tend to become more stable as the patient ages.

Beighton, P., Price, A., Lord, J., and Dickson, E.: Variants of the Ehlers-Danlos syndrome. Ann. Rheum. Dis., 28:228, 1969.

Hines, C., Jr., and Davis, W. D.: Ehlers-Danlos syndrome with megaduodenum and malabsorption syndrome secondary to bacterial overgrowth. Am. J. Med., 54:539, 1973.

Krane, J. M., Pinnell, S. R., and Erbe, R. W.: Lysylprotocollagen hydroxylase deficiency in fibroblasts from siblings with hydroxylysin-deficient collagen. Proc. Natl. Acad. Sci. U.S.A., 69:2899, 1972.

McKusick, V. A.: Heritable Disorders of Connective Tissue. 4th ed. St. Louis, C. V. Mosby Company, 1972.

929. FAMILIAL MEDITERRANEAN FEVER
(Periodic Fever, Periodic Disease, Familial Recurrent Polyserositis, Benign Paroxysmal Peritonitis, Periodic Polyserositis, Recurrent Polyserositis)

Paul B. Beeson

Definition. Familial Mediterranean fever is a familial disease characterized by recurrent short attacks of febrile illness in which there are signs of peritonitis, pleuritis, and arthritis. It is especially common in people of Eastern Mediterranean or Middle East origin, i.e., Jews, Arabs, Turks, and Armenians, but because of their wanderings the disorder is now encountered in all parts of the world. In addition, cases which seem clinically indistinguishable from familial Mediterranean fever are sometimes encountered in persons of quite different ethnic background. The name familial Mediterranean fever will be employed in this edition of the textbook because of current usage, but it has undesirable features. Some of the synonyms, notably recurrent polyserositis, would seem preferable. The most definitive studies of the disorder have been carried out in Israel, and the review by Sohar and colleagues is the best single source of information.

Genetics. Extensive investigation of families in Israel has led to the conclusion that familial Mediterranean fever is inherited as a single recessive autosomal trait, although the somewhat higher incidence in males (3.2) has not been adequately explained.

Pathology. Exudates from the peritoneum, pleura, or joint cavities during acute attacks reveal a preponderance of polymorphonuclear leukocytes and no evidence of microbial invasion. Biopsies of inflamed serosal surfaces usually show mild acute inflammation without underlying vascular disease. The most serious pathologic lesion is amyloidosis, which affects arterioles throughout the body and can seriously injure the kidneys, liver, spleen, lung, and adrenals.

Clinical Manifestations. An affected person shows no evidence of abnormality until the onset of the first attack, usually during the first or second decade of life. Between attacks, until amyloidosis becomes clinically manifest, the patient looks and feels well. Attacks are of short duration, usually one to four days, and consist of fever, which may be moderately high, together with manifestations of acute inflammation of the peritoneum, pleura, or synovial membranes. The peritoneal form is by far the most common, and consequently most sufferers have been subjected to laparotomy. Occasionally the joint manifestations assume more chronic form in which one or two large joints are the sites of painful swelling for weeks or months. In a few instances severe destruction of the hip has necessitated surgical treatment. Sometimes cutaneous lesions resembling erysipelas develop on the legs during an attack.

The serious hazard of this disease lies in the tendency to develop amyloidosis. This process is progressive, and most often causes death in renal failure. The rarity of familial Mediterranean fever in subjects over 40 years of age implies that amyloidosis develops in a high proportion of cases, causing death during adolescence or early adult life.

Differential Diagnosis. Inasmuch as a specific diagnostic test is lacking, the label of familial Mediterranean fever in an individual person must depend largely on ethnic background and the characteristic course of the disease. Obviously the disorder can mimic various infectious and "collagen" diseases, and a diagnosis of appendicitis is almost always considered at some time.

Treatment. No treatment other than symptomatic measures has been found effective in familial Mediterranean fever. Surprisingly, steroids, despite their antipyretic effects, seem to have little value in management of the acute bouts of illness. Recently there has been a report of benefit from regular administration of colchicine, 0.6 mg one to three times a day. There has also been a claim of suppression of attacks by use of indomethacin, 25 mg three times a day. These symptomatic measures deserve further trial. Eliakin and Licht have reported, in a small series of patients, dramatic suppression of attacks by long-term therapy consisting of colchicine, 0.02 mg per kilogram of body weight once a day, and aspirin, 0.5 gram twice a day. This deserves further trial. Nothing can be done to retard the progression of the amyloidosis which is the cause of death in a high proportion of cases.

SYNDROMES RESEMBLING FAMILIAL MEDITERRANEAN FEVER

Periodic Disease. Reimann has directed attention to a collection of syndromes which have the common features of periodic recurrence and intervals of well-being. Among the syndromes he has described are *periodic fever, periodic peritonitis* (familial Mediterranean fever?), *periodic neutropenia, periodic edema, periodic purpura, periodic arthralgia,* and *periodic psychosis.* Bodel and Dillard report that some cases of periodic fever have been ameliorated by administration of conjugated estrogens. The treatment regimens varied between patients, and their report should be studied for details.

Bodel, P., and Dillard, G. M.: Suppression of periodic fever with estrogen. Arch. Intern. Med., 131:189, 1973.
Eliakin, M., and Licht, A.: Colchicine-aspirin for recurrent polyserositis (familial Mediterranean fever). Lancet, 2:1333, 1973.
Goldfinger, S. E.: Colchicine for familial Mediterranean fever. N. Engl. J. Med., 287:1302, 1972.
Özer, F. L., Kaplaman, E., and Zileli, S.: Familial Mediterranean fever in Turkey. Report of twenty cases. Am. J. Med., 50:336, 1971.
Reimann, H. A.: Perplexities of a periodic entity. J.A.M.A., 190:241, 1964.
Siegal, S.: Familial paroxysmal polyserositis: Analysis of fifty cases. Am. J. Med., 36:893, 1964.
Sohar, E., Jafni, J., Pras, M., and Heller, H.: Familial Mediterranean fever. A survey of 470 cases and review of the literature. Am. J. Med., 43: 227, 1967.

930. LAURENCE-MOON SYNDROME

Alexander G. Bearn

The salient features of this recessively inherited syndrome are mental retardation, retinitis pigmentosa, hypogonadism, obesity, and polydactyly. There is a high parental consanguinity rate, and in Switzerland, where the disease appears to be particularly common, consanguinity has been established in more than 50 per cent of the affected sibships. Rigid classification is not possible, and the limits of the syndrome are poorly defined. Although retinitis pigmentosa appears relatively late, it is a common and well-defined feature. Other ocular signs include atypical retinal changes and retinitis without pigmentation. Mental retardation is only moderately severe and is usually noted soon after entering school. Unexplained obesity before the age of ten associated with polydactyly and hypogonadism should arouse suspicion of the disease.

Warkany, J.: Congenital Malformations. Chicago, Year Book Medical Publishers, 1971.

931. LIPOATROPHIC DIABETES

Alexander G. Bearn

The features of this disfiguring and invariably fatal disease include a loss of subcutaneous and body fat, hyperlipemia, hepatomegaly caused by fatty infiltration, phallic enlargement, hyperpigmentation and hypertrichosis with acanthosis nigricans, and insulin-resistant hyperglycemia.

The disease, which is probably due to hypothalamic-pituitary dysfunction, is inherited in a recessive fashion and affects dopamine-β-hydroxylase. Since this enzyme is rate limiting in the conversion of dopamine to norepinephrine, dopamine accumulates in the brain and is accompanied by a relative decrease in the quantity of norepinephrine. It has been suggested that the excess dopamine and decreased norepinephrine may cause an increase in the hypothalamic releasing factors (corticotrophin-releasing hormone, luteinizing-releasing hormone, and melanocyte-stimulating hormone) which can then be detected in the peripheral blood. The possibility that dopamine receptor blockers might influence the course of the disease has been raised and requires further investigation.

Mabry, C. C., Hollingsworth, D. R., Upton, G. V., and Corbin, A.: Pituitary-hypothalamic dysfunction in generalized lipodystrophy. J. Pediatr., 82:625, 1973.

932. LIPOID PROTEINOSIS
(Hyalinosis Cutis et Mucosae)
Alexander G. Bearn

This recently recognized rare autosomal recessively inherited disease, particularly common in South Africa, is characterized by the combination of a husky voice from birth and scarring maculopapular eruptions around the face, arms, and trunk. The mucous membranes of the mouth, tongue, and larynx are diffusely infiltrated with hyaline-like material. Recurrent painful parotitis may occur. Calcification of the hippocampal gyri is an inconstant but pathognomonic sign of the disease. No consistent biochemical abnormalities have been reported. The disease must not be confused with porphyria. Although there is no clear-cut evidence for their effectiveness, corticosteroids have been employed in the treatment of this disorder.

Gordon, H., Gordon, W., and Botha, V.: Lipoid proteinosis in an inbred Namaqualand community. Lancet, 1:1032, 1969.

933. MARFAN'S SYNDROME
(Arachnodactyly, Dolichostenomelia)
Alexander G. Bearn

Marfan's syndrome is a generalized disorder of connective tissue with skeletal, ocular, and cardiovascular manifestations. The molecular nature of the defect is not precisely known, and abnormalities of collagen as well as elastin have been implicated. The condition occurs equally in the sexes, and is inherited as a dominant trait with variable expression. Its prevalence has been estimated to be 1.5 per 100,000 of the population,

and approximately 15 per cent of all cases are due to new mutations. The average age of fathers of those patients with Marfan's syndrome owing to "new mutations" is about seven years in excess of the mean age of fathers generally.

Manifestations. *Skeleton.* The extremities are characteristically long and thin. The arm span is greater than the height, and the lower segment measurement (pubis-to-sole) is in excess of the upper segment (pubis-to-vertex). Excessive longitudinal growth gives rise to arachnodactyly, pectus excavatum or pigeon breast, dolichocephaly, long narrow face, and high arched palate. This last feature, contrary to common opinion, is not specific for Marfan's syndrome, because it may be seen in congenital myopathy and myotonic dystrophy. Weakness and reduplication of ligaments and joint capsules lead to "double-jointedness," backward curvature of the knees, flat feet, and recurrent dislocation of the hips, patella, and other joints. Cutaneous striae may be present, and probably reflect the abnormal elastic fibers. An unexplained sparsity of subcutaneous fat is a feature in many patients. Femoral hernias are not uncommon.

Eyes. The eyes show subluxation of the lens (ectopia lentis). Although this is usually severe and bilateral, minor degrees of subluxation require careful slit-lamp examination for their detection. Diagnosis of Marfan's syndrome in the absence of subluxation or redundancy of the suspensory ligament and without affected family members should be made with extreme caution. Other ocular signs include tremor of the iris and glaucoma. Severe myopia and spontaneous retinal detachment are common and often lead to gross impairment of vision.

Cardiovascular Defects. Disruption and loss of the elastic fibers of the media, associated with an increase in collagen and smooth muscle, is the primary basic defect. The lack of elasticity results in progressive diffuse dilatation of the proximal segment of the ascending aorta and severe aortic regurgitation. The aorta is widest at the sinuses of Valsalva. Aortic regurgitation, owing to dilatation and stretching of the aortic cusps, may occur in the absence of roentgenographic evidence of aortic dilatation. An early systolic click is commonly heard at the apex as well as at the aortic area. *Mitral regurgitation* is being observed with increasing frequency, and appears to be due to stretching of the chordae tendineae. Myxomatous transformation of the mitral ring may occur. Heart failure and rupture of the aorta resulting from *dissecting aneurysm* are the most common causes of death. Prominence of the pulmonary artery is frequently seen, and is due to displacement of the dilated aortic ring as well as to dilatation of the pulmonary artery. Bacterial endocarditis may be superimposed on the cardiac lesion. Cystic disease of the lung may occur as an integral part of Marfan's syndrome.

Differential Diagnosis. Marfan's syndrome must be distinguished from *homocystinuria,* which clinically it may closely resemble. It has been estimated that 5 per cent of patients with nontraumatic ectopia lentis, one of the cardinal signs of classic Marfan's syndrome, have homocystinuria. Ectopia lentis, pectus excavatum, and pigeon breast are common to both syndromes. The lens is more likely to be dislocated upward in Marfan's syndrome but downward in homocystinuria. The presence of a malar flush, generalized osteoporosis, and moderate to severe mental retardation are characteristic of homocystinuria and are not found in Marfan's syndrome; patients with homocystinuria do not develop dissecting aneurysm. Homocystinuria is inherited as a recessive trait. The diagnosis can be made by a positive urinary nitroprusside test or, definitively, by paper electrophoresis of the urine. The primary defect in homocystinuria is a deficiency of cystathionine synthetase in the liver. This deficiency can also be revealed in cultured skin fibroblasts. Rats given β-aminoproprionitrile (or seeds of *Lathyrus odoratus*) develop skeletal changes and dissecting aortic aneurysm reminiscent of some of the features of Marfan's syndrome.

McKusick, V. A.: Heritable Disorders of Connective Tissue. 4th ed. St. Louis, C. V. Mosby Company, 1972, pp. 61–200.

THE MUCOPOLYSACCHARIDOSES
Alexander G. Bearn

934. HURLER'S SYNDROME
(Mucopolysaccharidosis I H, MPS I H)

Definition. Hurler's syndrome is an autosomally inherited abnormality of mucopolysaccharide metabolism characterized by skeletal abnormalities, hepatosplenomegaly, corneal clouding, mental retardation, and increased mucopolysaccharide excretion in the urine.

Etiology. The disease, which has a prevalence of approximately 1 in 40,000, is caused by excessive intracellular accumulation of the mucopolysaccharides dermatan sulfate (chondroitin sulfate B) and heparan sulfate (heparatin sulfate). These substances are preferentially deposited in those tissues and organs in which they normally occur. An increased intracellular deposition of mucopolysaccharides can be demonstrated in cultured fibroblasts derived from patients with Hurler's syndrome and their heterozygous relatives, using metachromatic dyes as well as chemical methods. Recent evidence indicates that the primary inherited defect in Hurler's syndrome is deficiency of the lysosomal enzyme α-L-iduronidase which is responsible for the degradation of the polysaccharide side chains of dermatan sulfate and heparan sulfate. Particularly noteworthy is the discovery that the same enzymatic defect, which can be detected in cultured fibroblasts, occurs in *Scheie's syndrome* (see Ch. 935). This biochemical finding indicates that Hurler's syndrome and Scheie's syndrome, long thought to be closely related, are caused by allelic genes.

Pathology. The most characteristic pathologic feature of the disease is the excessive accumulation of intracellular mucopolysaccharides. Cells of the nervous system, liver, reticuloendothelial system, endocrine glands, cartilage, bone, and heart muscle are involved. Abnormal deposits are also present in the cornea, meninges, epicardium, pericardium, chordae tendineae, heart valves, tracheobronchial cartilages, upper air passages, and coronary and larger peripheral arteries. Distention of fibroblasts with this material causes the appearance of "clear" or "gargoyle" cells.

Clinical Manifestations. Although the patient may appear normal at birth, the disease becomes evident during the first year or two of life and progresses during childhood and adolescence. In the full-blown disorder, the head is large and there is hyperostosis of the sagittal suture that sometimes extends onto the forehead. The facial features are usually coarse and ugly. A broad saddle nose, wide nostrils, thick lips, large tongue, open mouth, and noisy breathing are characteristic. Skeletal abnormalities include short neck, dorsal and lumbar kyphosis with gibbus, short stature, and flaring of the costal margins. The hands are broad with stubby fingers, and there is a tendency for the fifth finger to bend radially. There may be a deformity of joints such as genu valgus, coxa valga, pes planus, or talipes equinovarus. The skin, especially over the upper extremities and thorax, is ridged and grooved, and may present nodular thickenings. Fine lanugo hairs are prominent over much of the cutaneous surface, and the extremities are likely to show profuse growth of large coarse hair. The heart is enlarged, and valvular involvement produces murmurs that may simulate those of rheumatic heart disease. Disease of coronary arteries may give rise to angina or other evidence of occlusive disease. The abdomen is large and protuberant, and the liver and spleen are commonly enlarged. Umbilical and inguinal hernias are frequent. Clouding of the cornea is extremely common; slit-lamp examination of the eyes may be needed to detect the corneal opacification in the early stages of the disease. Mental deterioration is severe and progressive.

Abnormalities demonstrable by roentgenogram include a large skull with frontal and occipital hyperostosis, hypertelorism, long shallow sella turcica with anterior pocketing, and deformities of the facial bones. Gibbus is associated with wedge-shaped deformities and anterior hooklike projections of the vertebral bodies. The ribs are broad, spatulate, and saber shaped. The terminal phalanges of the hands are broad and short, and the long bones, especially of the arms, show swollen shafts from expansion of medullary cavities. The heart is often enlarged, and pulmonary congestion may be present.

Diagnosis. Diagnosis depends upon recognition of the characteristic clinical manifestations, biopsy, blood and bone marrow studies, and examination of the urine for increased mucopolysaccharide content. A simple screening test for this consists of adding acidified bovine serum albumin to the urine. A positive result is indicated by a dense white precipitate owing to the reaction of albumin and acid mucopolysaccharide at low pH. A more specific screening test can be performed by allowing urine to dry on filter paper and adding acetic acid and toluidine blue O. A purple color develops in the urine of patients with Hurler's syndrome. Metachromatic granules in the cytoplasm of circulating lymphocytes (*Reilly bodies*) are usually demonstrable and are useful diagnostic adjuncts. Since the primary inherited defect, a decrease in α-L-iduronidase, occurs in both Hurler's syndrome (MPS I H) and Scheie's syndrome (MPS I S), the distinction between the two syndromes must still be made on clinical grounds (see accompanying table). That Hurler's and Scheie's syndromes should be so different clinically yet have the same enzymatic defect is compatible with genetic allelism. The same gene undergoes mutation in both diseases but at different points on the same codon. An analogous situation exists with hemoglobin SS and hemoglobin CC disease.

Hurler's syndrome has features of cretinism but

The Principal Inherited Mucopolysaccharidoses

Designation	Clinical Features	Primary Inherited Deficiency
Hurler's syndrome (MPS I H)	Early corneal clouding, death before age ten; mental retardation	α-L-Iduronidase deficiency
Scheie's syndrome (MPS I S)	Corneal clouding, stiff joints, aortic incompetence; mental retardation	α-L-Iduronidase deficiency
Hunter's syndrome (MPS II)	No corneal clouding; milder course than Hurler's syndrome	Sulfoiduronate sulfatase deficiency
Sanfilippo's syndrome A (MPS III)	Mild somatic changes, severe mental retardation	Heparan sulfate sulfatase deficiency
Sanfilippo's syndrome B (MPS III)	Identical phenotype	N-acetyl-α-D-glucosaminidase deficiency
Morquio's syndrome (MPS IV)	Severe bone changes, cloudy cornea; normal intelligence	Unknown
Maroteaux-Lamy syndrome (MPS VI)	Severe bone and corneal change; normal intelligence	Unknown.

All are autosomally inherited except Hunter's syndrome, which is X-linked.

differs in that bone age is normal, tests of thyroid function are normal, and the patient is active.

Treatment. Although enzyme replacement with α-L-iduronidase may provide a new therapeutic approach to this disease, further work is needed to establish its clinical usefulness.

935. SCHEIE'S SYNDROME
(Mucopolysaccharidosis I S, MPS I S)

This rare autosomal variant of Hurler's syndrome is characterized by near normal intelligence, marked clouding of the cornea, and excretion of increased quantities of dermatan sulfate and heparan sulfate. The frequency of the disease is approximately 1 in 500,000 births. Aortic regurgitation and the carpal tunnel syndrome are common features of this mucopolysaccharidosis. The primary inherited defect is deficiency of α-L-iduronidase. A deficiency of α-L-iduronidase also occurs in Hurler's syndrome (see Ch. 934).

936. HUNTER'S SYNDROME
(Mucopolysaccharidosis II, MPS II)

This is the only mucopolysaccharidosis known to be inherited in an X-linked recessive fashion. The disease is similar to but clinically less severe than classic Hurler's syndrome. At birth Hunter's syndrome is one and one half times as frequent as Hurler's syndrome without regard to sex. In males, Hunter's syndrome is three times as common. Clouding of the cornea is minimal or absent, and mental deterioration occurs more slowly. Nodular thickening of the skin and deafness are common. Cardiac enlargement and pulmonary hypertension may be features of the disease. Increased urinary excretion of dermatan sulfate and heparan sulfate is the rule. Abnormal accumulations of mucopolysaccharides can be observed in cultured fibroblasts from affected individuals and heterozygous carriers of the abnormal gene. Deficiency of the enzyme *sulfoiduronate sulfatase* is characteristic of Hunter's syndrome. The deficiency can be detected in cultured fibroblasts.

937. SANFILIPPO'S SYNDROME
(Mucopolysaccharidosis III, MPS III)

Sanfilippo's syndrome is rare and is characterized by severe progressive mental retardation with relatively minor somatic changes. Corneal clouding is most uncommon, and dwarfism and hepatosplenomegaly are only moderately severe. The disease is inherited as an autosomal recessive and occurs in approximately 1 in 10,000 to 1 in 200,000 individuals. Many patients languish in mental institutions undiagnosed. As in the other mucopolysaccharidoses, cultured fibroblasts from affected individuals and heterozygous carriers demonstrate increased mucopolysaccharides. An increased urinary excretion of heparan sulfate, but not of dermatan sulfate, is diagnostic. Two clinically indistinguishable forms of Sanfilippo's syndrome have been found to have different enzymatic deficiencies. In one type, Sanfilippo A, the enzyme heparan sulfatase is deficient, whereas in Sanfilippo B, the enzyme N-acetyl-α-D-glucosaminidase is lacking.

938. MORQUIO'S SYNDROME
(Morquio-Brailsford Syndrome, Chondro-osteodystrophy, Mucopolysaccharidosis IV, MPS IV)

Patients with this recessively inherited syndrome are strikingly dwarfed. The characteristic radiologic features of the disease become evident after the age of two and consist of marked osteoporosis, platyspondyly, abnormalities of the femoral heads, and knock knees. Severe skeletal changes may lead to symptoms of spinal cord or medullary compression. Intelligence is unimpaired or trivially decreased. The disease has an estimated frequency of 1 in 40,000 births. Although not invariably present, an increased excretion of keratan sulfate in the urine is diagnostic. The urinary excretion of dermatan sulfate and heparan sulfate is normal. The basic defect is unknown.

939. MAROTEAUX-LAMY SYNDROME
(Mucopolysaccharidosis VI, MPS VI)

Early corneal clouding and normal intelligence are the distinguishing features of this rare autosomal variant of Hurler's syndrome. An increased excretion of dermatan sulfate can be demonstrated. Unlike Scheie's syndrome, the skeletal abnormalities are severe and aortic disease is absent. The enzyme defect in this disease is not yet elucidated.

The comparative clinical and biochemical features of the various mucopolysaccharidoses discussed in Ch. 934 to 939 are summarized in the table.

Dorfman, A.: Heritable diseases of connective tissue: The Hurler syndrome. *In* Stanbury, J. B., Wyngaarden, J. B., and Fredrickson, D. S. (eds.): The Metabolic Basis of Inherited Disease. 3rd ed. New York, McGraw-Hill Book Company, 1972.

McKusick, V. A.: Heritable Disorders of Connective Tissue. 4th ed. St. Louis, C. V. Mosby Company, 1972, pp. 521–686.

Neufeld, E. F.: The biochemical bases for mucopolysaccharidoses and mucolipidoses. *In* Steinberg, A. G., and Bearn, A. G. (eds.): Progress in Medical Genetics. Vol. X. New York, Grune & Stratton, 1974.

PORPHYRIA

Rudi Schmid

940. INTRODUCTION

Porphyrins are tetrapyrrole pigments in which four monopyrroles are linked by four carbon bridges to form a planar ring structure. Each of the pyrroles has two substituent side chains, and the various porphyrins such as uro-, copro-, and protoporphyrin differ only in the nature of these side chains. Their sequential arrangement in specific porphyrins determines the structural isomer type, numbered I to IV. In nature, only porphyrins of the isomer types I and III have been identified. With the exception of protoporphyrin IX (belonging to the isomer type III series), which in the form of ferroprotoporphyrin (heme) serves as the prosthetic group of hemoglobin and other essential heme proteins, porphyrins apparently neither possess physiologic functions nor act as metabolic intermediates. Rather, they are metabolic by-products that have escaped from the biosynthetic path to heme by irreversible oxidation of the corresponding reduced porphyrinogens (see accompanying figure). The latter are intermediates in heme biosynthesis and are formed from the monopyrrole porphobilinogen (PBG), which in turn is synthesized by condensation of 2 moles of δ-aminolevulinic acid (ALA). The overall rate of heme and porphyrin biosynthesis is regulated primarily by the activity of ALA synthetase, which condenses glycine and succinyl-CoA to ALA. This mitochondrial enzyme system is reversibly repressed and inhibited by the final product, heme, and it is likely that this and other regulatory mechanisms are responsible for preventing both overproduction of heme and accumulation of metabolic intermediates. In porphyria, the increased excretion of ALA, PBG, or porphyrins results from an inherited defect or an acquired dysfunction of individual enzyme systems or control mechanisms of heme biosynthesis. Catabolism of hemoglobin and other heme proteins does not lead to formation of porphyrins; instead, the ferroprotoporphyrin ring is cleaved to biliverdin and bilirubin which are linear tetrapyrroles.

Although all aerobic cells can synthesize heme-containing chromoproteins, heme formation is particularly active in the erythroid elements of bone marrow and in liver. The small quantities of porphyrins and porphyrin precursors excreted normally in urine and bile are derived primarily from these sources. Similarly, the metabolic defects in porphyria that result in the accumulation and consequent increased excretion of porphyrins or their precursors usually can be traced to the erythroid cells of the bone marrow or to the liver, or to both. This distinction serves as a convenient basis for the classification of the porphyrias that follows:

A. Congenital erythropoietic porphyria
B. Hepatic porphyrias
   1. Genetic forms
      a. Acute intermittent porphyria
      b. Hereditary coproporphyria
      c. Variegate porphyria
   2. Porphyria cutanea tarda
   3. Acquired and secondary porphyrinuria
C. Erythrohepatic protoporphyria

The classification indicates the major sites of the metabolic disturbance and separates the hereditary forms of porphyria from those with an uncertain genetic basis and from the rare instances in which porphyrinuria appears to be acquired.

It should be noted that increased urinary excretion of porphyrins or precursors, including ALA and PBG, occurs in a variety of conditions other than porphyria. Chronic lead poisoning is commonly associated with increased ALA, and elevated PBG occasionally has been observed in carcinomatosis, Hodgkin's disease, cirrhosis, and affections of the nervous system. Normal urine contains only traces of uroporphyrin, but increased concentrations may be present in heavy metal poisoning and occasionally in parenchymal liver disease; gross uroporphyrinuria has been reported in patients with benign or malignant tumors of the liver. Coproporphyrin frequently is increased in lead poisoning, hemolytic and refractory anemia, hepatitis, cirrhosis, infectious mononucleosis, and alcoholism. In liver disease, coproporphyrinuria may not indicate increased formation of the pigment, but rather its diversion from bile to urine. Protoporphyrin, which has only 2 carboxyl groups and consequently is poorly soluble in water, does not appear in urine, but is excreted exclusively in the bile. The feces regularly contain copro-, proto-, and deuteroporphyrin, but these pigments may be derived in part from food, intestinal hemorrhage, and colonic microflora. Because of the wide range in fecal porphyrin concentration, values up to 200 μg per gram dry weight may not be indicative of porphyria without additional diagnostic evidence.

BIOSYNTHESIS OF HEME

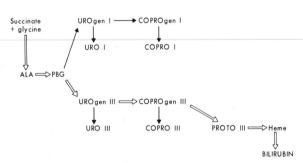

The metabolic pathway from glycine and succinate to heme.

Abbreviations: ALA, δ-aminolevulinic acid; PBG, porphobilinogen; UROgen, uroporphyrinogen; COPROgen, coproporphyrinogen; URO, uroporphyrin; COPRO, coproporphyrin; PROTO, protoporphyrin; I, III, isomer types I and III.

941. CONGENITAL ERYTHROPOIETIC PORPHYRIA
(Congenital Photosensitive Porphyria, Günther's Disease)

This very rare disease is due to a hereditary defect of porphyrin metabolism in the erythroid cells that leads to chronic photosensitivity, hemolytic anemia, and increased urinary excretion of uroporphyrin. Only about 80 cases in both sexes have been reported. Inheritance is by autosomal recessive transmission; heterozygous individuals appear clinically normal.

Excretion of pinkish urine usually begins shortly after birth, whereas cutaneous lesions on exposed parts, increased hemolysis, and splenomegaly may not be detected until later. Hypertrichosis and erythrodontia are virtually always present. Urine contains high concentrations of uroporphyrin I and coproporphyrin I, but excretion of ALA and PBG is normal. Hemoglobin frequently is decreased, and reticulocytes and fecal urobilinogen are increased. Erythrocytes contain much uroporphyrin I, and normoblasts and reticulocytes exhibit intense red fluorescence. The metabolic defect involves faulty conversion of PBG to uroporphyrinogen III in the maturing erythroid cells of the bone marrow. Death may occur in childhood, but if patients live to maturity, they usually exhibit severe scarring and mutilation of hands and face. Successful pregnancy with delivery of phenotypically normal children has been reported. Treatment is symptomatic and prophylactic, consisting essentially of rigorous protection from sunlight. In some instances hemolytic anemia, photosensitivity, and porphyrin excretion have been improved by splenectomy.

942. HEPATIC PORPHYRIAS

ACUTE INTERMITTENT PORPHYRIA

Definition, Incidence, and Genetics. Acute intermittent porphyria (synonyms: *acute porphyria, porphyria hepatica, pyrroloporphyria, Swedish type*) is an abnormality of pyrrole metabolism inherited as a dominant trait. It is associated with recurrent attacks of abdominal pain, gastrointestinal dysfunction, and neurologic manifestations. It is probably the most common form of porphyria, with an over-all incidence of approximately 1 per 100,000 population, but, because of its occurrence in large families, regional incidence may be much higher. The total number of reported cases suggests that people of Scandinavian, Anglo-Saxon, and German ancestry are affected more frequently, whereas the disease is very rare in blacks.

Acute attacks are rarely seen before puberty; they most often begin in the third or fourth decade, and occur more frequently in women. Manifestations may appear only in later life, or recurrent symptoms may be so vague and protean as to escape recognition. Indeed, persons carrying the genetic abnormaltiy may remain free of clinical manifestations throughout life; such latent porphyria tends to be more frequent in men. This probably accounts for the alleged preponderance of porphyria in women of child-bearing age.

Clinical Manifestations. Moderate to severe abdominal pain, often colicky, is frequently the initial or most prominent symptom. The pain may be localized, generalized, or radiating to the back or loins, but the abdomen usually is soft. Abdominal tenderness and distention may exist, but are much less striking than would be expected from the intensity of the pain. Leukocytosis and mild fever may be present. Diarrhea occasionally occurs. Severe vomiting and persistent constipation are frequent and may be accompanied by lack of bowel sounds and dilatation of the stomach. Roentgenograms of the abdomen may reveal distended intestinal loops proximal to areas of spasm; volvulus and gangrene have been reported. Gastrointestinal complications commonly lead to weight loss and occasionally to severe emaciation. Prolonged vomiting may cause dehydration, oliguria, and azotemia.

Neurologic disturbances frequently, though not always, are associated with abdominal manifestations and may involve the peripheral, central, or autonomic nervous system. Peripheral neuropathy usually is predominantly motor, may be asymmetrical, and may vary from mild weakness in one extremity to complete flaccid quadriplegia. These motor disturbances may be preceded or accompanied by severe pain, particularly in the legs. Deep tendon reflexes are usually diminished or absent and, although subjective sensory symptoms are frequent, objective sensory loss is less common. Cranial nerve involvement leads to optic atrophy, ophthalmoplegia, facial palsy, dysphagia, and vocal cord paresis. Weakness of abdominal, intercostal, or diaphragmatic musculature may progress to respiratory paralysis, which has a poor prognosis and ranks as the chief cause of death. Wasting and contracture of affected muscles frequently occur but are reversible to a surprising degree during prolonged remissions.

Many patients have a long history of nervousness, emotional instability, and functional disturbances that may remain unexplained until an acute attack occurs. Striking psychiatric abnormalities include personality changes, hysteria, psychoses, and confusional states. With more severe central nervous system involvement, delirium, coma, and epileptic seizures may occur; on occasion they have followed ingestion of barbiturates or maladvised surgical exploration of the abdomen.

Sinus tachycardia frequently accompanies acute attacks, and the pulse rate has been found to be a good index of the activity of the disease. This is believed to be due to vagal neuropathy, which also may account for nonspecific electrocardiographic abnormalities. Transient hypertension is often present, and on occasion spasm of retinal arteries has been observed. Frank photosensitivity does not occur in acute intermittent porphyria, but mild and apparently reversible pigmentation, particularly of exposed parts of the body, may accompany acute phases of the disease.

Acute episodes vary widely in duration and frequency. Some patients complain merely of occasional and intermittent abdominal pain, whereas in others the initial attack may begin almost explosively and may terminate fatally within days to several weeks. In the majority of cases, distinct attacks recur at irregular intervals over months or years, but tend to decrease in frequency and severity with age. There is strong evidence that attacks may be precipitated by a variety of drugs, including barbiturates, sulfonamides, griseofulvin, estrogens, and contraceptives, all of which are metabolized by microsomal enzyme systems of the liver, that contain hemoproteins. Occasionally, periodic exacerbations are correlated with the menstrual cycle, or latent porphyria may become clinically manifest late in pregnancy or shortly after delivery.

Laboratory Findings and Pathogenesis. The most characteristic laboratory finding is excessive ALA and PBG in the urine. PBG is a colorless chromogen giving a red complex with Ehrlich aldehyde (p-dimethylaminobenzaldehyde in HCl) which after neutralization cannot be extracted with chloroform or butanol (*Watson-Schwartz test*). By contrast the red color produced by Ehrlich aldehyde with urobilinogen or indoles is readily extractable with chloroform or butanol. Ingestion of antipyrine or admixture of methyl red (Zephiran) results in urine that turns red on acidification alone, whereas compounds of the phenolphthalein group show red only in alkaline urine. During acute episodes of porphyria, the Watson-Schwartz test is almost always strongly positive; if the reaction is faintly pink or negative, the diagnosis remains doubtful. In latent porphyria or in patients recovered from an acute attack, urinary excretion of PBG frequently is less pronounced or may be normal so that the Watson-Schwartz test may be negative. In these instances, urinary ALA and PBG should be quantitated by chromatographic methods, which commonly but not invariably reveal increased excretion of these porphyrin precursors. Freshly passed urine may be normal in color and usually contains relatively little preformed uro- and coproporphyrin. It darkens on standing because of conversion of PBG and other precursors to porphyrins and porphobilin, a dark brown pigment of unknown structure. Fecal porphyrins are within normal limits or moderately increased.

Except for a moderate reduction in the circulating red cell volume, hematologic abnormalities usually are absent. Conventional liver function tests frequently yield normal results except for increased BSP retention. The urine may contain increased concentrations of amino acids and indoles; the latter sometimes give an atypical Ehrlich reaction. Elevated protein-bound iodine, cholesterol, and β-lipoprotein levels have been reported. During acute attacks hyponatremia may become an alarming complication; although this often can be ascribed to prolonged vomiting or excessive intravenous fluid replacement, inappropriate secretion of antidiuretic hormone has been demonstrated. The liver is microscopically normal or shows mild focal or centrilobular necrosis and fatty changes. It usually does not exhibit porphyrin fluorescence, but contains much PBG. Inconstant neuropathologic changes include patchy demyelination of the peripheral or central nervous system and chromatolysis of anterior horn cells.

The inherited biochemical defect consists of a partial deficiency of the enzyme *uroporphyrinogen synthetase* which converts PBG to uroporphyrinogen. The ensuing impairment of heme synthesis secondarily leads to derepression of ALA synthetase, which results in increased formation and urinary excretion of ALA and its condensation product, PBG. Although this enzymatic defect is demonstrable in a variety of tissues, including circulating erythrocytes, its functional expression appears to be limited to the liver. Drugs and hormones known to aggravate the disease have been shown to induce the activity of hepatic ALA synthetase. The pathogenesis of the abdominal and nervous manifestations is unknown, but a toxic effect of ALA or PBG has not been ruled out.

Diagnosis and Differential Diagnosis. The diagnosis rests primarily on the determination of increased urinary excretion of ALA and PBG. As a screening procedure, the qualitative Watson-Schwartz test usually is adequate, but for a definitive diagnosis, quantitative determination with chromatographic methods is essential. In prepubertal children and in asymptomatic adults suspected of having latent porphyria, urinary ALA and PBG may be normal; in these instances detection of the inherited defect requires demonstration of reduced uroporphyrinogen synthetase activity in erythrocytes or other tissues. Lead intoxication may produce severe abdominal pain and neuropathy, but the urine rarely contains sufficient PBG to give a positive Watson-Schwartz test, although ALA excretion frequently is increased.

The possibility of porphyria should always be considered in the presence of unexplained abdominal pain, because the disease has been mistaken for cholelithiasis, renal colic, peptic ulcer, appendicitis, bowel obstruction, pancreatitis, and pelvic disorders. Some patients have undergone several surgical procedures before the correct diagnosis was established. Acute attacks seldom last less than 48 hours, and very brief episodes of pain followed by complete remission rarely occur. Obscure neurologic disturbances, especially unexplained peripheral neuropathy, regional muscle weakness, flaccid paralysis, or bulbar palsy, should suggest the possibility of porphyria. Similarly, if hysterical behavior, psychoneurosis, psychosis, or unexplained epilepsy is aggravated by barbiturates, coincides with the menstrual cycle, or is noted in patients under treatment with contraceptives, porphyria should be suspected.

Persistent tachycardia, muscle weakness, and elevated protein-bound iodine may lead to confusion with hyperthyroidism. Occasionally weakness, abdominal pain, pigmentation, and hyponatremia may suggest Addison's disease. During the last trimester of pregnancy, hypertension, vomiting, and oliguria suggestive of eclampsia may in reality be due to porphyria. Provocative diagnostic tests by deliberate administration of barbiturates should be discouraged.

Treatment and Prognosis. There is no specific treatment for acute intermittent porphyria, and therapy remains symptomatic and prophylactic. Acute pain and psychic manifestations usually can be alleviated or controlled with phenothiazines, reserpine, or meperidine. Oral phenothiazines, such as chlorpromazine (25 to 100 mg four times daily), are the preferred treatment for abdominal and muscle pain. Neuropsychiatric manifestations frequently respond to relatively small doses of reserpine. Meperidine (Demerol) by intramuscular injection in doses of 50 to 100 mg may give prompt though transient relief; but, in general, use of opiates should be limited, because the severity and chronicity of the pain render porphyric patients particularly susceptible to addiction. When recurrent manifestations are clearly related to the menstrual cycle, prolonged androgenic suppression has given promising results.

Acute attacks often can be aborted by prompt administration of carbohydrate ("glucose effect"). Intravenous infusion of glucose or fructose at a rate of 10 to 15 grams per hour for 24 hours, or comparable amounts of oral carbohydrates, may result in striking remissions, particularly in patients whose attacks were precipitated or aggravated by anorexia, nausea, and vomiting. In addition, supportive treatment is of great importance. Dehydration and hyponatremia should be prevented. If bulbar signs are present, respiratory paralysis should be anticipated and a mechanical respirator made available. When fever and leukocytosis in excess of 12,000 per cubic millimeter are suggestive of occult infection, most often of the respiratory or urinary tract, sulfonamides should not be used. Drugs in general and barbiturates, griseofulvin, glutethimide, estrogens, and contraceptives in particular should be avoided.

In the earlier literature, the prognosis of acute intermittent porphyria was considered grave, with a mortality of 80 per cent within five years of the first attack. This figure undoubtedly is high; indeed, more recent reports set it around 25 per cent. Death occurs most frequently during the second and third decades, whereas beyond this age manifestations tend to be less severe and the prognosis distinctly improves.

HEREDITARY COPROPORPHYRIA

Hereditary coproporphyria was recognized only recently as a distinct entity. Clinically it resembles variegate porphyria except that a larger percentage of affected individuals remain asymptomatic, or photosensitivity may be the only symptom. As in acute intermittent and variegate porphyria, drugs may precipitate acute attacks which are associated with increased urinary excretion of ALA and PBG. The unique biochemical abnormality is the striking increase in fecal coproporphyrin excretion, whereas fecal protoporphyrin concentration usually is low. During acute attacks, urinary coproporphyrin excretion also may be very high. The disease is inherited as a dominant trait, and the sexes are equally affected. Treatment is the same as for acute intermittent porphyria.

VARIEGATE PORPHYRIA

Definition, Incidence, and Genetics. Variegate porphyria (synonyms: *porphyria cutanea tarda, protocoproporphyria hereditaria, mixed hepatic porphyria, South African genetic porphyria*) is a hereditary abnormality of porphyrin metabolism associated with chronic cutaneous manifestations alone or in conjunction with acute, transient attacks of abdominal pain and neuropathy. The disease is inherited as a dominant trait and the sexes are equally affected. Because of its occurrence in large family groups, the incidence varies widely in different parts of the world. Among white settlers of South Africa it is estimated at 3 per 1000. It undoubtedly is very much less elsewhere, although reliable figures are not available.

Clinical Manifestations. Cutaneous symptoms consist of dermal abrasions, superficial erosions, and blister formation after trivial trauma, and commonly are first noted during the second or third decade. The excessive mechanical fragility is usually limited to exposed parts of the skin. The lesions tend to heal slowly, often leave pigmented or slightly depressed scars, and are subject to secondary infection. Direct sensitivity to sunlight is infrequent, but the distribution of the cutaneous lesions leaves little doubt that light exposure is an important

pathogenic factor. Hyperpigmentation of the face and hands is common, and women often exhibit hypertrichosis, particularly of the temporal margins. The extent of these manifestations varies considerably, but after increased fragility of the skin has developed, it rarely disappears completely. In some instances the abnormality is minimal and remains unnoticed, whereas in others chronicity and secondary infection lead to severe scarring and disfigurement. Cutaneous lesions are uncommon before puberty; they are usually milder in women, but during pregnancy become more pronounced.

Although in many patients manifestations remain limited to the skin, acute episodes of abdominal pain, neuropathy, and encephalopathy, similar in all aspects to those in acute intermittent porphyria, are not uncommon. Barbiturates, sulfonamides, general anesthetics, and excessive amounts of ethanol or estrogens frequently appear to be precipitating or aggravating factors. During acute episodes mortality is approximately 25 per cent, but since many patients never develop acute manifestations, the over-all mortality of variegate porphyria is much lower. Genetic studies from South Africa suggest that before the widespread use of barbiturates and sulfonamides, kinships with porphyria survived and propagated as well as the unaffected population. Unless they terminate fatally, acute attacks commonly resolve completely, although neuropathy and muscle weakness may persist for several months. Evidence of hepatic dysfunction and histologic abnormality, including steatosis, fibrosis, or cirrhosis, is not uncommon, and biopsy material from the liver frequently shows extensive porphyrin fluorescence.

Laboratory Findings and Pathogenesis. The characteristic finding in variegate porphyria is the large amount of copro- and particularly protoporphyrin in the bile and feces. Fecal excretion of these pigments is continuous throughout the course of the disease, and takes place even in those patients with minimal cutaneous manifestations and in asymptomatic children with the genetic trait. PBG and porphyrin levels in the urine are usually slightly elevated, but the qualitative test for PBG is frequently negative. During acute attacks urinary excretion of ALA, PBG, and, at times, uro- and coproporphyrin is greatly increased, and may reach values comparable to those in acute intermittent porphyria in relapse. Azotemia, hypochloremia, hyponatremia, and jaundice may be present, but readily resolve as the acute attack subsides and the disease converts to its cutaneous form.

The exact nature of the inherited biochemical defect is unclear, but it undoubtedly involves increased formation of ALA, PBG, and porphyrins in the liver. Chronic exposure to sunlight is important in the pathogenesis of the cutaneous lesions, but the mechanism underlying the abnormal mechanical fragility of the skin is unclear.

Diagnosis and Differential Diagnosis. The diagnosis can best be established by demonstrating increased porphyrin in the feces. The following qualitative test frequently suffices. A small piece of stool is thoroughly mixed with four parts of ethyl ether and one part of glacial acetic acid, the mixture is filtered, and the filtrate is extracted with 5 per cent hydrochloric acid. Under ultraviolet light with a Wood filter, extracts of porphyric feces exhibit intense red fluorescence, which is faint or absent with normal stool. In quantitative determinations, values in excess of 40 μg of protoporphyrin per gram of dry feces are suggestive of porphyria. During acute attacks the diagnosis can be ascertained by demonstrating increased ALA and PBG excretion in the urine.

Chronic cutaneous lesions limited to exposed parts, abnormal skin fragility, a positive family history, and increased fecal porphyrin excretion usually permit distinction of variegate porphyria from most other skin diseases. Erythrohepatic protoporphyria is the only other light-sensitive dermatosis associated with increased fecal porphyrins, but in this condition erythrocyte or plasma protoporphyrin is usually increased, and the reaction to light is prompt and transient. During acute attacks it may be difficult to distinguish between variegate and acute intermittent porphyria, except that the former diagnosis is suggested by concomitant skin involvement or a positive personal or family history of cutaneous manifestations.

Treatment. Treatment is symptomatic and prophylactic. Management of acute attacks is the same as for acute intermittent porphyria. Exposure to direct sunlight should be minimized and the hands protected from mechanical trauma by gloves. Of paramount importance is avoidance of drugs known to precipitate porphyria.

PORPHYRIA CUTANEA TARDA

Porphyria cutanea tarda (synonyms: *porphyria cutanea tarda symptomatica; constitutional* or *idiosyncratic porphyria; symptomatic porphyria*) is a relatively frequent sporadic form of cutaneous porphyria, characterized by chronic skin lesions, hepatic dysfunction, and uroporphyrinuria. Abdominal and neurologic manifestations are absent. The disease is more common in males and usually begins insidiously, most often in the fourth to sixth decade. It occurs in all parts of the world, but is most frequent in the Bantus of South Africa. Exposed skin shows abnormalities similar to those of variegate porphyria, ranging from slight dermal fragility to severe chronic scarring and disfiguration. The lesions often are more active in summer and tend to heal in winter. Hyperpigmentation and hirsutism are frequent and may be the presenting symptoms. Hepatomegaly with chemical and histologic evidence of liver disease, often caused by chronic alcoholism, is present in the great majority of patients. Disseminated lupus erythematosus appears to occur in porphyria cutanea tarda more frequently than can be accounted for by coincidence. In addition to uroporphyrin, variable degrees of hemosiderosis are frequently found in the liver. Although hepatic hemosiderosis may not differ from that seen in nonporphyric patients with chronic liver disease, recent evidence suggests that cutaneous manifestations and porphyrin excretion may be improved by repeated venesection.

Urinary excretion of uro-type porphyrins and, to a lesser extent, coproporphyrin is greatly increased, and urine may be pink or brownish. Fecal porphyrins are normal or slightly increased, and excretion of ALA or PBG is almost never elevated. The excreted porphyrins undoubtedly are derived from the liver, but the underlying biochemical defect is unknown. Because of the absence of a positive family history, the disturbance is generally assumed to be acquired, usually in association with some other form of liver disease, frequently one caused by alcoholism. However, since only a very small percentage of patients with chronic liver disease develop porphyria, the possibility of a genetically determined but normally undetected defect activated by hepatic injury cannot be ruled out. Treatment is symptomatic and directed toward the primary liver disease. Abstinence in alcoholic patients results in significant improvement or disappearance of the porphyria. Chloroquine and cholestyramine may be useful in reducing the photosensitivity, but both compounds need further clinical evaluation.

In rare instances, intoxications may lead to a form of hepatic porphyria that is *acquired*. Porphyria characterized by cutaneous manifestations, hepatic dysfunction, and uroporphyrinuria has been reported in population groups accidentally exposed to hexachlorobenzene or biphenyls.

943. ERYTHROHEPATIC PROTOPORPHYRIA (Erythropoietic Protoporphyria)

In this recently recognized form of porphyria, high concentrations of protoporphyrin in erythrocytes, plasma, and feces are associated with solar urticaria or solar eczema. Short exposure to sunlight results in intense pruritus, erythema, and edema of exposed skin. These lesions appear during or immediately after exposure, subside in 12 to 24 hours, and usually heal without significant scarring, atrophy, or pigmentation. Occasionally cutaneous manifestations develop only after prolonged exposure to sunlight, or the initial acute skin lesions may progress to a chronic eczematous stage, persisting for weeks and healing with superficial scar formation. Skin manifestations commonly begin during childhood or adolescence, are more severe in summer, and recur throughout life. Affected skin shows neither abnormal mechanical fragility nor blister formation characteristic of the other forms of photosensitive porphyria. Erythrodontia, hirsutism, hyperpigmentation, and neurologic manifestations are lacking. Photosensitivity is mediated by protoporphyrin in plasma or skin and is evoked by near-ultraviolet light in the 400 nm range, in which porphyrins absorb maximally. The excessive protoporphyrin in plasma and feces is derived primarily from the liver, the erythroid cells serving as a minor source. Fasting increases the plasma protoporphyrin level, whereas carbohydrate administration reduces both protoporphyrin formation and photosensitivity. Urinary porphyrin excretion is normal.

The disturbance occurs in both sexes and appears to be inherited as a dominant trait. A significant percentage of persons carrying the genetic abnormality remain clinically asymptomatic, and detection may be possible only by repeated determination of erythrocyte and fecal protoporphyrin concentration. The disease generally has a good prognosis, and neither results in permanent disability nor influences normal life expectancy. However, the incidence of cholelithiasis is distinctly increased, and chronic intrahepatic cholestasis progressing to cirrhosis has been reported. Treatment is prophylactic and consists largely in protection from direct sunlight.

Dean, G.: The Porphyrias. 2nd ed. London, Pitman Medical Publishing Company, 1971.

Goldberg, A.: Porphyrins and porphyrias. *In* Goldberg, A., and Brain, M. C. (eds.): Recent Advances in Haematology. Edinburgh and London, Churchill Livingstone, 1971.

Marver, H. S., and Schmid, R.: The porphyrias. *In* Stanbury, J. B., Wyngaarden, J. B., and Fredrickson, D. C. (eds.): The Metabolic Basis of Inherited Disease. 3rd ed. New York, McGraw-Hill Book Company, 1972.

Meyer, U. A., and Schmid, R.: Hereditary hepatic porphyrias. Fed. Proc., 32:1649, 1973.

Miescher, P. A., and Jaffe, E. R. (eds.): Porphyria and disorders of porphyrin metabolism. Semin. Hematol., 5:293, 1968.

Tschudy, D. P.: Porphyrin metabolism and the porphyrias. *In* Bondy, P. K., and Rosenberg, L. E. (eds.): Duncan's Diseases of Metabolism. 7th ed. Philadelphia, W. B. Saunders Company, 1974.

Waldenström, J., and Haeger-Aronsen, B.: The porphyrias: A genetic problem. Prog. Med. Genet., 5:58, 1967.

Watson, C. J.: The problem of porphyria—some facts and questions. N. Engl. J. Med., 263:1205, 1960.

944. PSEUDOXANTHOMA ELASTICUM

Clayton E. Wheeler, Jr.

Definition. Pseudoxanthoma elasticum is an uncommon, inherited disorder of connective tissue characterized by yellow skin lesions at flexural areas, retinal angioid streaks, chorioretinitis, arterial disease, and visceral bleeding tendencies. The combination of cutaneous lesions and angioid streaks is called the *Grönblad-Strandberg syndrome.*

Etiology. The primary defect appears to be genetically determined premature degeneration and calcification of connective tissue of the skin, eyes, and cardiovascular system. Elastic tissue is probably the abnormal component, although abnormality of collagen has not been excluded. Autosomal recessive inheritance with partial limitation to the female is found most often, but dominant inheritance may occasionally occur.

Incidence. The disorder occurs in all races, in both sexes, and at any age. Skin lesions occur slightly more frequently in females, and angioid streaks more frequently in males. The disease may be present at birth or infancy, but the diagnosis is made most frequently in the third to fifth decades.

Pathology. The histologic picture of cutaneous lesions is diagnostic. The epidermis and upper corium are normal. Characteristic changes consist of granular or rodlike accumulations of basophilic material and calcium deposits in the middle and lower dermis. The basophilic material stains like elastic tissue but shows the periodicity of collagen when examined by the electron microscope. The eye shows basophilia and rents of Bruch's elastic lamina, sclerosis of choroidal vessels, and scleral changes that simulate those of the skin. Elastic tissue degeneration affects the media of vessels of medium and larger size. White plaques histologically resembling those in the skin have been found on the pericardium and endocardium of the ventricles and right atrium, and some investigators suspect specific involvement of the mitral valve.

Clinical Manifestations. The three major areas affected are skin, eyes, and cardiovascular system. Combined skin and eye changes are found in approximately 60 per cent of the cases, skin alone in 10 per cent, and eyes alone in 30 per cent. Cardiovascular abnormalities are present in nearly 80 per cent of the patients if careful search is made. The impression has been gained that the disorder is more severe when skin lesions are well developed, but instances of advanced cardiovascular or eye involvement occur in the absence of clinical cutaneous abnormalities.

Cutaneous lesions are small, soft, chamois-colored papules arranged parallel to skin lines and folds; the result is a crepelike or Moroccan leather appearance. A network of fine telangiectatic vessels sometimes outlines the papules. Coalescence produces circumscribed or diffuse plaques. In mild cases the lesions may be seen only after the skin is stretched. In advanced cases the skin is thickened, hangs in loose, inelastic folds, and resembles the skin of a plucked chicken. Sites of most frequent involvement are the sides of the neck, axillae, groin, cubital and popliteal fossae, and the periumbilical area, but the face, breasts, undersurface of the penis, and the perianal area may be affected as well as the mucosa of the mouth, palate, vagina, and rectum. Papular and arcuate lesions of elastosis perforans serpiginosa may occur in pseudoxanthoma elasticum as well as in Ehlers-Danlos syndrome and other connective tissue diseases.

Angioid streaks of the retina are the most characteristic eye lesions. These lie behind the retinal vessels. They are most numerous around the optic disc, which they may encircle and from which they course like vessels over the fundus. They are flat, serrated streaks varying from narrow lines to three or four times the diameter of retinal veins. They are red, brown, gray, or black, and there may be hemorrhage or white areas of connective tissue proliferation along their course. The streaks are usually bilateral, although not symmetrical, and tend to progress slowly or to become stationary. When the streaks involve the macula, loss of vision occurs. Other eye changes are central chorioretinitis that may also involve the macula, pigmented stippling of the fundus, and hemorrhage from retinal vessels.

Patients often have premature and advanced arterial changes indistinguishable from arteriosclerosis or atherosclerosis with predilection for medium-sized arteries. These changes may result in weak or absent peripheral pulses of the arms or legs, easy fatigability of the legs, intermittent claudication, angina, arrhythmias, cerebrovascular accidents, and mental deterioration. Hypertension occurs in about half the cases. Renal hemangioma and abnormalities of renal arteries may be found. Left ventricular hypertrophy, congestive heart failure, and coronary thrombosis may occur, and mitral valvular disease has been reported. Pulse wave studies of involved extremities show decreased amplitude and velocity, and the dicrotic notch may be lost.

Internal hemorrhage is a special feature of the vascular disease. Bleeding from the gastrointestinal tract occurs in about 10 per cent of the cases, and it may be severe or fatal. Bleeding may arise in peptic ulcer, hiatal hernia, or ulcerative colitis, or its clinical origin may not be demonstrable. Other sites of hemorrhage are skin, subarachnoid space, kidney, uterus, bladder, nasal mucosa, and joints.

The association of thyrotoxicosis, diabetes mellitus, diabetes insipidus, low fertility, amenorrhea, and impotence with pseudoxanthoma elasticum has been suggested but seems doubtful.

Diagnosis. Cutaneous lesions are diagnostic, especially if confirmed by biopsy. Diagnostic histologic changes may be present when clinical findings are minimal or absent. Senile elastosis, a degenerative disease of dermal connective tissue, resembles pseudo-xanthoma elasticum, but it affects only exposed sites. The histologic appearance rules out pseudoxanthoma. Angioid streaks are highly suggestive but not pathognomonic, because they are seen in sickle cell disease and in a small percentage of patients with Paget's disease of bone. Structures resembling angioid streaks occur in rupture of the choroid, choroidal arteriosclerosis, perivascular choroidal pigmentary atrophy, and pigmented streaks of retinal detachment. Cardiovascular changes must be accompanied by typical changes of the eye or skin before their association with pseudoxanthoma elasticum can be ascertained.

Treatment. There is no effective treatment of the basic disease. Symptomatic therapy is indicated for hypertension, congestive failure, subarachnoid or gastrointestinal hemorrhage, cerebrovascular accident, angina, and intermittent claudication. Plastic surgery is sometimes helpful for correction of cosmetic cutaneous defects.

Prognosis. Cutaneous lesions are usually of small consequence. The majority of patients develop angioid streaks, and approximately three quarters of these undergo visual impairment from damage to the macula. Complete blindness, which is unusual, results from glaucoma, vitreous hemorrhage, or retinal detachment. Morbidity and death may result from cerebrovascular accident, heart disease, or internal hemorrhage at any age; however, many patients live a normal span.

Huang, S., Kumar, G., Steele, H. D., and Parker, J. O.: Cardiac involvement in pseudoxanthoma elasticum. Am. Heart J., 74:680, 1967.
McKusick, V. A.: Heritable Disorders of Connective Tissue. 4th ed. St. Louis, C. V. Mosby Company, 1972.
Olinder, I., and Boström, H.: Clinical studies on a Swedish material of pseudoxanthoma elasticum. Acta Med. Scand., 19:273, 1972.
Percival, S. P. B.: Angioid streaks and elastorrhexis. Br. J. Ophthal., 52:297, 1968.
Wilhelm, K., and Paver, K.: Sudden death in pseudoxanthoma elasticum. Med. J. Aust., 2:1363, 1972.

945. WILSON'S DISEASE
(Hepatolenticular Degeneration)

Alexander G. Bearn

Wilson's disease is a rare, autosomal recessively inherited disease characterized by degenerative changes in the brain, particularly in the basal ganglia, and cirrhosis of the liver. A brownish pigmented ring at the corneal margin, the Kayser-Fleischer ring, is pathognomonic of the disease.

Clinical Manifestations. The disease is frequently insidious in onset, manifesting itself as tremor and incoordination in the second or third decade of life. Deteriorating handwriting and difficulty in speech may be common early symptoms. While the patient is at rest, the tremor is often minimal and can be alleviated by resting the hands on a table or placing them in a pocket. Attempts to perform purposive movements are less successful, and a wild ataxia frequently develops. Rarely, symptoms occur as early as four years of age or may be delayed until the fourth decade of life. In late childhood and early adolescence, the disease is more likely to be rapidly progressive; rigidity, dysarthria, and dysphagia occur more frequently than tremor. Uncontrollable choreoathetotic movements and staggering may be particularly distressing. The sensory system is unaffected, and pyramidal signs are usually absent. In the terminal stages of the disease the patient is frequently febrile and emaciated. Muscular rigidity, contractures, and mental deterioration dominate the clinical picture, and the patient becomes completely bedridden.

In adults, clinical signs of severe hepatic insufficiency are uncommon, although slight abnormalities in liver function can be detected, and cirrhosis can be recognized by liver biopsy. In childhood, however, the disease commonly presents as atypical or prolonged hepatitis, which may be indistinguishable from juvenile cirrhosis. Signs of central nervous system dysfunction are minimal or absent. Portal hypertension can frequently be demonstrated, and ascites and hepatic coma may supervene. Rarely, massive bleeding from esophageal varices may be the first manifestation of the disease. Jaundice may be an early symptom, and is frequently followed by several years of normal health.

Behavioral and personality changes, acute schizophrenic episodes, transient hemiparesis, and unexplained Coombs-negative hemolytic anemia may also herald the onset of the disease. Unusual pigmentation of the lower extremities, azure lunulae of the nails, and bone lesions may be found.

Genetics. The disease is ubiquitous and occurs in approximately 1 in 200,000 persons. It is particularly common in populations with a high inbreeding coefficient. As anticipated in a rare autosomal recessive disease, an increased consanguinity in the parents of affected persons is extremely common; in one series the frequency of marriages among first cousins was 36 per cent. Clinically normal heterozygous carriers of the gene have been estimated to occur with a frequency of approximately 1 in 500.

Pathogenesis. A decrease in the biliary excretion of copper is the primary disturbance in Wilson's disease; this results in an accumulation of copper in the brain, liver, kidney, and other tissues, including Descemet's membrane of the cornea, where it gives rise to the characteristic *Kayser-Fleischer ring*. The copper first accumulates in the liver and is stored initially in the hepatocytes, and later in the lysosomes. As the disease progresses, the accumulation of copper causes hepatocellular damage with release of copper from within the hepatocyte. The copper released from the liver is distributed and deposited in various tissues of the body, giving rise to cellular and organ damage.

In normal persons, approximately 95 per cent of the copper in serum is bound to ceruloplasmin whereas the remaining 5 per cent is loosely bound to serum albumin. In patients with Wilson's disease, there is a decrease in the concentration of serum ceruloplasmin and total serum copper and an increase in the easily dissociable albumin-bound copper. The excretion of copper in the urine is usually considerably increased. Exceptionally, and particularly in girls with chronic active hepatitis or cirrhosis, the serum copper and ceruloplasmin levels may be normal. Accumulation of copper in the kidneys selectively damages the proximal renal tubules. Aminoaciduria, glycosuria, phosphaturia, uricosuria, and calciuria may be present. The serum phosphate and serum uric acid also may be decreased.

Pathology. Although it is assumed that accumulation of copper in the tissues is responsible for the symptoms, the brain may appear surprisingly normal at autopsy. Slight generalized atrophy is common, particularly of the basal ganglia. An accumulation of large astrocytes is found throughout the central nervous system and is more marked in the basal ganglia and cerebral cortex. In the rare acute form of the disease, cavitation of the putamen, globus pallidus, caudate nucleus, and cerebral cortex may be evident. In the asymptomatic stage of the disease, the liver is grossly and histologically normal despite an increase in the hepatic concentration of copper. As the disease progresses, liver damage occurs and the characteristic pathologic changes of chronic active hepatitis or postnecrotic cirrhosis become evident. Glycogen degeneration of hepatic cell nuclei, with the accumulation of cytoplasmic fat droplets, is frequently observed.

Diagnosis. The disease should be suspected in all cases of unexplained tremor and rigidity, particularly in early adult life. The differential diagnosis includes Parkinson's syndrome, cerebellar ataxia, chorea, and choreoathetosis. In children and young adults, the disease frequently presents with symptoms resulting from chronic active hepatitis, and the disease should be suspected in all cases of juvenile cirrhosis. The presence of *Kayser-Fleischer rings* is pathognomonic of the disease, but these may be absent in children under the age of ten. They are golden brown or green-brown, and are located at the limbus and may encircle the entire cornea. In the early stages of the disease, a careful slit-lamp examination may be needed to demonstrate their presence with certainty. Needle biopsy of the liver and determination of the hepatic copper concentration should be undertaken in all patients in whom the diagnosis is suspected. In most patients with Wilson's disease the copper content of the liver is usually greater than 200 μg per gram dry weight (normal, less than 50 μg per gram dry weight); in some patients it may reach a level of 2000 μg per gram. A decrease in serum ceruloplasmin (less than 20 mg per 100 ml) can nearly always be observed and, in the absence of malnutrition, sprue, or the nephrotic syndrome, is virtually diagnostic. The disease is difficult to diagnose unequivocally in the first six months of life, because decreased ceruloplasmin and increased hepatic copper are common in normal children.

Treatment. The aim is to decrease the total body copper and prevent its reaccumulation. A high-protein, low-copper diet with the addition of sulfurated potash, technical (20 mg three times daily, with meals), is often recommended, although it is not as important as intensive and continued drug therapy. The administration of D-penicillamine (β, β-dimethylcysteine), 1 to 2 grams a day, depending on body weight, is the treatment of choice and should be continued indefinitely. A "sensitivity" reaction associated with fever, arthralgia, and leukopenia may occur. Desensitization with steroids should be undertaken and penicillamine therapy cautiously reinstituted. Except for the occasional occurrence of skin reactions, toxic reactions are seldom seen. The nephrotic syndrome has been reported in a few patients, and the urine should be monitored regularly for proteinuria. Pyridoxine deficiency, as a result of treatment with penicillamine, may give rise to optic neuritis but can be prevented by administration of pyridoxine, 50 mg daily.

Persistent decrease in serum ceruloplasmin accompanied by elevated hepatic copper in an asymptomatic sib of a patient with Wilson's disease is an indication to begin therapy. In newborn infants treatment should be delayed until it is apparent that the decreased serum ceruloplasmin and increased hepatic copper have persisted beyond the normal physiologic period of three to six months. When penicillamine treatment is started early and continued indefinitely, symptomatic improvement is usually dramatic and long continued. In the absence of treatment the disease is invariably fatal.

Bearn, A. G.: Wilson's Disease. *In* Stanbury, J. B., Wyngaarden, J. B., and Fredrickson, D. S. (eds.): The Metabolic Basis of Inherited Disease. 3rd ed. New York, McGraw-Hill Book Company, 1972.

Sass-Kortsak, A.: Hepatolenticular degeneration (Kinnear-Wilson's disease). *In* von Schwiegk, H. (ed.): Handbuch der Inneren Medizin. 5th ed. Berlin, Springer-Verlag, 1974.

Sternlieb, I.: Evolution of the hepatic lesion in Wilson's disease (hepatolenticular degeneration). *In* Popper, H., and Schaffner, F. (eds.): Progress in Liver Diseases, Vol. IV. New York, Grune & Stratton, 1972.

946. WERNER'S SYNDROME

Alexander G. Bearn

This rare, recessively inherited syndrome is characterized by scleroderma-like changes in the skin, especially in the extremities, symmetrical growth retardation with absence of the adolescent growth spurt, a senile appearance, and premature graying of the hair. Cataract, soft tissue and vascular calcifications, and premature arteriosclerosis are common. Diabetes mellitus occurs in 50 per cent of the patients and is of the insulin-resistant type. Certain features of Werner's syndrome resemble scleroderma, progeria, and myotonic dystrophy.

Epstein, C. J., Martin, G. M., Schultz, A. L., and Motulsky, A. G.: Werner's syndrome. A review of its symptomatology, natural history, pathologic features, genetics and relationship to the natural aging process. Medicine, 45:177, 1966.

Part XXII
NORMAL LABORATORY VALUES OF CLINICAL IMPORTANCE

947. THE USE AND INTERPRETATION OF LABORATORY-DERIVED DATA

James B. Wyngaarden

When you can measure what you are speaking about, and express it in numbers, you know something about it. Lord Kelvin, 1889.

The basic workup of a patient begins with the acquisition of data. The experienced clinician will insist upon a discerning and sensitive history, a thorough physical examination, and such laboratory tests as are necessary to evaluate the general health of his patient, to arrive at a specific diagnosis, to assess the functional status of involved organs, and to provide a basis for monitoring effectiveness of therapy.

The inclusion of a panel of chemical tests or enzyme assays of blood (or urine) as a part of a basic medical evaluation is in a state of evolution. A decade ago many physicians would have ordered a fasting blood sugar and blood urea nitrogen determination as a part of the general workup, and other tests only if suggested by a differential diagnosis constructed from the clinical evaluation.

In 1966 Thiers published a provocative study comparing the results of a screening battery of eleven tests run by an automated multichannel analyzer with those of tests specifically ordered on the same patients by physicians as part of the admission workup. The screening battery detected twice as many abnormal test results of significance to the patient as were uncovered by selective ordering. The most common findings were elevated glucose or uric acid concentration values. Ensuing developments were rapid. Ingenious automated analyzers have brought an increasing number and variety of tests of diagnostic utility within the reach of all practitioners. In the larger hospitals and teaching centers it is now common practice to include a "Chem 12," or "Chem 18," as a standard component of the initial workup. The cost of such a screening battery is now no greater than that of three or four selected tests run manually a decade ago.

This new practice has profound implications in the teaching of medical students and house officers. One can no longer evaluate the reasoning process which led the house officer to order a serum calcium determination. Some of the intellectual discipline of the construction of a logical differential diagnosis is now gone. The information comes automatically by a computer print-out. Attention has shifted from the selective acquisition of data to the interpretation and use of it, including the evaluation of significance of test results and (perhaps) the selection of a second round of tests and studies. The gains surely outweigh the losses. Since many diseases present initially with rather nonspecific constitutional symptoms, the clinical approach may not suggest the most appropriate laboratory tests, and the initial laboratory screen may disclose unexpected hypercalcemia, acidosis, azotemia, or evidence of liver disease.

In order to utilize the results of laboratory tests intelligently (and economically), the physician must be able to evaluate the validity of the test result, he must understand principles of variation and distribution of values, and he must be able to integrate the data received from the laboratory with the information he has acquired from the patient. If the test result deviates from values found in a healthy control population, is the difference trivial, or is it indicative of important dysfunction? Should the test be repeated? How often need a particular measurement be followed? What additional tests or studies are indicated on the basis of these leads?

The more information the physician has about his patient, the more effective the physician should be in caring for him. To ensure that this is the result requires a sophisticated knowledge of medical science, excellent clinical judgment, and a profound respect for the limitations of the laboratory. One of the best ways of acquiring the constructively critical attitude so essential to the proper evaluation of laboratory test results is for the student or house officer to work in a laboratory for a while. There is an irony in the present pattern of medical education: at a time of unparalleled reliance upon an ever-expanding universe of laboratory tests in the practice of medicine, first-hand learning experiences in the laboratory are being progressively eliminated from the medical curriculum.

SOME LIMITATIONS OF THE LABORATORY

Criteria for Evaluation of Laboratory Methods. A trustworthy laboratory test must pass critical evaluations of specificity, sensitivity, accuracy, and precision.

Specificity refers to the detection of the substance in question and no other. It is doubtful that any test is absolutely specific for the substance being measured. There is always some other substance around that is capable of reacting. In biochemical analyses this limitation is most serious in tests dependent upon color development, less in the case of assays dependent upon degradation by purified enzymes, and perhaps least in such procedures as atomic absorption spectroscopy.

Sensitivity refers to the ability of the test to detect the substance in question at the required concentrations, namely, those at which the compound exists in body fluids.

Accuracy refers to the quantitative detection of the

correct amount of the substance being measured. This property rests upon both specificity and sensitivity. A test may be accurate in the absence of certain interfering drugs, and only in a certain range of values. It may fail this criterion under other conditions.

Precision embodies *repeatability,* the obtaining of the same result on samples analyzed in replicate fashion, and *reproducibility,* representing quality control over time. Precision rests upon the specificity, sensitivity, and accuracy of the method, and characterizes the procedure under conditions of actual use in the diagnostic laboratory.

The "Law of Errors." Early in the nineteenth century, the German mathematician and physicist, Johann C. F. Gauss, introduced the "law of errors." This law states that in repeated measurements of the *same* object or substance, the random component on the errors will be distributed about the mean as a frequency function. This distribution, which is bell shaped, is often called "normal" or "gaussian." Note that the law applies to repeated measurements of the same item. Its extension to a population of those items is justifiable only under certain circumstances, for not all distributions are bell shaped, and not all bell-shaped distributions are gaussian. The matter of distributions will be discussed further below, when we consider the topic of the "normal range" of a biological variable. First, however, it may be pertinent to emphasize the topic of error, for every laboratory measurement is subject to it.

SOURCES OF ERROR

These are legion, and include some factors under the control of the clinician, such as the dietary preparation of the patient, and the techniques of collection and handling of samples. Reduction of the error factor to an acceptable minimum requires continuous compulsive attention to every detail of the process.

Laboratory Errors. There is imprecision in every measurement. In tests run by hand, pipetting, timing, reading, and recording errors occur. They are more frequent when technicians are overworked or fatigued. It is common to find greater scatter of results of replicate tests at the end of the day than at the beginning. Technician fatigue can be largely eliminated by automation, but there will always remain the technical limitations of machines and the human error in the preparation of reagents, in the standardization of instruments, and in the copying of test results. The last is not totally avoided by the computer print-out, as even typewriters make mistakes. Quality control of laboratory performance is both a science and an art. Control criteria vary widely from laboratory to laboratory. Split samples submitted to different laboratories may show surprising disparities in results.

Drug Interference. According to Osler, man is distinguished from all other members of the Animal Kingdom by his desire to take drugs. Since many patients do not regard proprietary pain remedies or vitamins as drugs, the physician may obtain a negative drug history unless questions are appropriately phrased. Drugs have great potential for interference with laboratory tests. High resolution chromatography of urine yields about 300 peaks of ultraviolet absorbing materials. Two hundred and fifty of these disappear if the "normal sub-

ject" abstains from salicylates and vitamins for a few days. Salicylates and vitamins also produce chromogens which interfere with certain analytic methods employed in automated tests, particularly of the urine.

DISTRIBUTIONS OF VALUES

There is widespread belief among medical students and graduate physicians that if the sample of test results from a healthy population is large enough, the distribution will be "normal" (gaussian); that on this assumption one may justifiably determine a mean value ($\bar{x}$) and its standard deviation (δ); that the value, $\bar{x} \pm 2\delta$, will include the central 95 per cent of all measurements; that this segment of the distribution is the "normal range;" and that values which fall outside this range are by definition "abnormal." All these beliefs are erroneous in most instances. The experimental fact is that for most physiological variables the distribution is smooth, unimodal, and skewed, and that $\bar{x} \pm 2\delta$ does not cut off the desired central 95 per cent. Among the distributions of serum calcium, inorganic phosphorus, magnesium, alkaline phosphatase, total proteins, albumin, uric acid, and blood urea, only that of albumin is gaussian. All others are skewed, leptokurtic, or both. The value $\bar{x} \pm 2\delta$ will cut off many more measurements in one tail of the distribution than the other. The uncritical application of principles of normal distributions in situations in which variables are not normally distributed leads occasionally to values of $\bar{x} - 2\delta$ which are negative, surely a biological absurdity.

Once we discard the notion that the distribution of values in healthy persons is gaussian, the question of estimating the mean and standard deviation does not arise. One is then spared the awkward exercise of fitting skewed distributions to bell-shaped curves by constructing histograms of logarithms of the data (a technique which has the effect of compressing the skewed tail to create a "log-gaussian distribution"), or by constructing plots of cumulative frequencies of values (or log-values) on probability paper in search of the linear relationship indicative of a normal distribution (see accompanying figure).

These pitfalls can be circumvented by use of *nonparametric* methods for estimating the normal range, that is, methods which do not involve any a priori assumption regarding the parental distribution shape except that it is continuous. Two nonparametric methods of normal range estimation are the method of *percentile estimates* with associated nonparametric confidence intervals, and the method of nonparametric *tolerance intervals* which include a specified proportion of the population with a specified probability. The required sample sizes of healthy persons for the normal value studies are large, just as they are with parametric methods.

The percentile method of expressing interindividual variation in many kinds of data has been in use for a long time. Physicians are familiar with its use in pediatric growth charts of height and weight. The method avoids the arbitrary distinction of normal and abnormal. It also removes the aura of precision of the standard deviation, expressed to two or more decimal places. The percentile method appropriately fits the real world of nongaussian distributions.

From every laboratory test for which a good normal-

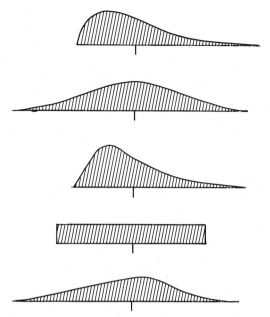

Five distributions with the same mean and standard deviation ($\bar{x} = 4$, $\delta = 2.83$). From top to bottom: χ_r^2 normal, lognormal, rectangular, and mixture of two normals. (From Elveback, L. R.: Mayo Clinic Proc. 47:93, 1972; with permission.)

value study has been done, the laboratory can report not only the result but also the percentile corresponding to that result and appropriate to the age and sex of the patient under study. With this information the clinician can know how common or how unusual the test result is. This information obviates the necessity of remembering a large number of complicated relationships. The percentile method is superior to an arbitrary definition of a normal range, such as $\bar{x} \pm 2\delta$, even in those few cases in which a distribution is gaussian, for it indicates for each test result the relationship of that result to the healthy population. The percentile method is also superior to the definition of the normal range as the range of all observed values in a healthy sample population, for this method seriously underestimates any selected segment, e.g., the central 95 per cent, in small samples, and overestimates it in large samples.

The percentile method does not systematically over- or underestimate any selected range, regardless of sample size. If one wishes to cut off the lowest and highest 2.5 per cent, or 5 per cent, one simply orders all values and finds the value that cuts off the desired percentage of observations at either tail of the distribution. The complete percentile range is readily defined. No assumptions are required about distribution shape except that it is continuous. From the size of the healthy population represented in the distribution, the confidence limits of a given percentile may be ascertained, with known probability, by reference to standard tables. The method should particularly appeal to clinicians who utilize local norms, which are often based on small samples.

The "Normal Range." From this discussion, it is clear that "normal range" is an arbitrary and potentially misleading term. By whatever method it is defined, the normal range will exclude observations of the parental distribution of healthy subjects and will very likely include some values of other distributions. What

is desired by the clinician is an expression of cut-off points at either end of a distribution, such that by far the largest number of values of healthy individuals is included in the central segment, and as few values as possible are included that are part of another distribution, i.e., that the number of false positives and false negatives are both minimized. Ingrained habits, perhaps now indelible, will probably lead us to continue to select the central 95 per cent of the parental distribution as "clinical limits," even though there is no magic in this number. Some clinical investigators have advocated use of the central 90 per cent.

Influence of Age. The distributions of values of many plasma constituents vary with age in the healthy population. For example, plasma cholesterol concentrations, mean and 90 per cent limits, are 180 (120 to 240) mg per 100 ml in the "normal" 20- to 29-year age group, and 245 (160 to 330) mg per 100 ml in the "normal" 50- to 59-year age group. Whether values of 325 mg per 100 ml in the older age group are biologically "normal" simply because they fall in the 90 to 95 percentile range could be debated.

Influence of Sex. Distributions in men may differ from those in women. For example, plasma urate concentration values, mean and 90 per cent limits, are 4.9 (2.7 to 7.2) mg per 100 ml in men, and 4.0 (2.5 to 6.3) mg per 100 ml in premenopausal women. Mean serum calcium values in normal men decline 0.0068 mg per 100 ml per year from age 20 to age 80. Those of women show no regression against age. This is an important point in the diagnosis of hyperparathyroidism which is chiefly a disease of the older age group.

Biological Rather Than Statistical Norms. This concept has been alluded to above, in the suggestion that the clinical norms of serum cholesterol concentrations should perhaps be defined in terms of age-related values that are noninjurious, rather than as a 90 percentile range. Perhaps the 5 to 50 percentile range should be selected as the "clinical limits" or "normal" range in the older population. Such an approach requires a biological rather than statistical definition, but data are not yet available to set reliable limits in this manner.

A more secure example concerns urate concentration values. An electrolyte solution with the sodium concentration of plasma is saturated with urate at 6.4 to 6.8 mg per 100 ml. In addition, proteins of plasma bind urate equivalent to about 5 per cent of the amount in solution. Values above 7.0 (perhaps 7.2) mg per 100 ml represent supersaturation and are "abnormal" in that they are associated with increased risk of renal stone and clinical gout. The risk factors increase as urate concentration values increase above 7.0 mg per 100 ml. The 95 per cent limits of serum urate values in "healthy" male New Zealand Maoris are 4 to 10 mg per 100 ml, and 10 per cent of adult males develop gout. Surely the central 95 per cent of the distribution of the general male population cannot be considered "normal," even though the reference sample is appropriately selected by the usual criteria.

Discontinuous Distributions. Some traits may be distributed bimodally, or trimodally. Such relationships are most likely to emerge from studies of families in which there is a monogenetic disease characterized by a chemical abnormality. For example, measurements of galactose-1-phosphate uridyltransferase activity in the families of patients with transferase deficiency galactosemia are distributed trimodally. The effects of two and of one mutant allele are clearly distinguishable from the normal and from each other. Assay values in the three modes are zero, 7.5 to 13.5 units, and 19.5 to 32 units. The intermediate enzyme assay values are found in subjects who are presumed heterozygotes by pedigree analysis. It is common to hear the term "heterozygote value" applied to an enzyme activity value approximately one half of normal. This practice is justifiable only when assay data are combined with pedigree data, for there may be other reasons for a reduced enzyme assay value that have nothing to do with genetics.

An apparent continuous distribution with marked skewing may at times be dissected into two or even three distribution modes by appropriate clinical and pedigree studies. For example, the distribution of plasma cholesterol concentrations in familial hypercholesterolemia displays marked overlap between subjects who are clinically normal and those who are heterozygotes by pedigree analysis. Similarly, there is considerable overlap between heterozygotes and abnormal homozygotes. Only a complete family pedigree permits adequate definition of the range of values in each distribution mode.

THE PHYSICIAN AND THE LABORATORY TEST RESULT

The tables that follow contain values which define the limits of the clinical norms. They represent the best data currently available, but are subject to all the un-certainties discussed above. In some instances more selective data of an age- and sex-matched control population will need to be consulted by the physician.

Clinical judgment rather than exclusive reliance on published normal ranges will always be required. For example, a serum BUN concentration of 22 mg per 100 ml is not a normal value for a patient on a rice diet. Also, electrolyte test results of sodium 145 mEq per liter, potassium 3.5 mEq per liter, chloride 96 mEq per liter, and CO_2 30 mEq per liter may indicate metabolic alkalosis even though all individual values fall within published normal ranges.

Laboratory tests are critical to the diagnosis of disease and management of patients. They have both great value and inherent imprecision. The doctor must know the limits of reliability and usefulness of each test result in the clinical setting of the individual patient. This is particularly true when all deviant test results have returned to normal but the patient is not improving. It is especially when laboratory data provide little or no help that the patient needs a doctor.

Bryan, D. J., Wearne, J. L., Viau, A., Musser, A. W., Schoonmaker, F. W., and Thiers, R. E.: Profile of admission chemical data by multichannel automation: An evaluative experiment. Clin. Chem., 12:137, 1966.

Elveback, L. R., Guillier, C. L., and Keating, F. R.: Health, normality, and the ghost of Gauss. J.A.M.A., 211:69, 1970.

Keating, F. R., Jones, J. D., Elveback, L. R., and Randall, R. V.: The relation of age and sex to distribution of values in healthy adults of serum calcium, inorganic phosphorus, magnesium, alkaline phosphatase, total proteins, albumin, and blood urea. J. Lab. Clin. Med., 73:825, 1969.

Mainland, D.: Remarks on clinical "norms." Clin. Chem., 17:267, 1971.

948. NORMAL LABORATORY VALUES OF CLINICAL IMPORTANCE

Rex B. Conn

NORMAL HEMATOLOGIC VALUES

For some procedures the normal values may vary, depending upon the methods used.

Acid hemolysis test (Ham)		No hemolysis
Alkaline phosphatase, leukocyte		Total score 14–100
Bleeding time		
Ivy		Less than 7 min
Duke		1–7 min
Carboxyhemoglobin		Up to 5% of total
Cell counts		
Erythrocytes: Males		4.6–6.2 million/cu mm
Females		4.2–5.4 million/cu mm
Children (varies with age)		4.5–5.1 million/cu mm
Leukocytes		
Total		5000–10,000/cu mm

Differential	Percentage	Absolute
Myelocytes	0	0/cu mm
Juvenile neutrophils	3– 5	150– 400/cu mm
Segmented neutrophils	54–62	3000–5800/cu mm
Lymphocytes	25–33	1500–3000/cu mm
Monocytes	3– 7	285– 500/cu mm
Eosinophils	1– 3	50– 250/cu mm
Basophils	0– 0.75	15– 50/cu mm

(Infants and children have greater relative numbers of lymphocytes and monocytes)

Platelets	150,000–350,000/cu mm
Reticulocytes: Adults	25,000–75,000/cu mm
	0.5–1.5% of erythrocytes
Newborns	4–6% of erythrocytes
Clot retraction, qualitative	Begins in 30–60 mm
	Complete in 24 hours
Coagulation factors:	
Factor activity	
Factors II, V, VII, IX, X, XI	70–120%
Factor VIII	60–120%
Coagulation time (Lee-White) (room temp.)	5–15 min (glass tubes)
	19–60 min (siliconized tubes)
Cold hemolysin test (Donath-Landsteiner)	No hemolysis
Corpuscular values of erythrocytes	
(Values are for adults; in children, values vary with age)	
M.C.H. (mean corpuscular hemoglobin)	27–31 picogm
M.C.V. (mean corpuscular volume)	80–105 cu micra
M.C.H.C. (mean corpuscular hemoglobin concentration)	32–36%
Fibrinogen	200–400 mg/100 ml
Hematocrit	
Males	40–54 ml/100 ml
Females	37–47 ml/100 ml
Newborn	49–54 ml/100 ml
Children (varies with age)	35–49 ml/100 ml
Hemoglobin	
Males	14.0–18.0 grams/100 ml
Females	12.0–16.0 grams/100 ml
Newborn	16.5–19.5 grams/100 ml
Children (varies with age)	11.2–16.5 grams/100 ml
Hemoglobin, fetal	Less than 1% of total
Hemoglobin A_2	1.5–3.0% of total
Hemoglobin heat stability	No precipitation
Hemoglobin oxygen affinity (p50)	26–28 mm Hg

NORMAL HEMATOLOGIC VALUES (*Continued*)

Hemoglobin, plasma	0–5.0 mg/100 ml
Methemoglobin	0.03–0.13 gram/100 ml
Osmotic fragility of erythrocytes	
Immediate	10% lysis in 0.45–0.50% NaCl
	50% lysis in 0.40–0.45% NaCl
	90% lysis in 0.35–0.42% NaCl
After 24 hours incubation	10% lysis in 0.57–0.66% NaCl
	50% lysis in 0.47–0.60% NaCl
	90% lysis in 0.28–0.50% NaCl
Partial thromboplastin time	35–45 sec
Prothrombin consumption	Over 80% consumed in 1 hr
Prothrombin content	100% (calculated from prothrombin time)
Prothrombin time (one stage)	12.0–14.0 sec
Sedimentation rate	
Wintrobe: Males	0–5 mm in 1 hr
Females	0–15 mm in 1 hr
Westergren: Males	0–15 mm in 1 hr
Females	0–20 mm in 1 hr
(May be slightly higher in children and during pregnancy)	
Thromboplastin generation test	Compared to normal control
Tourniquet test	Ten or fewer petechiae in a 2.5 cm circle after 5 min with cuff at 100 mm Hg

Bone marrow, differential cell count	Range	Average
Myeloblasts	0.3– 5.0%	2.0%
Promyelocytes	1.0– 8.0%	5.0%
Myelocytes: Neutrophilic	5.0–19.0%	12.0%
Eosinophilic	0.5– 3.0%	1.5%
Basophilic	0.0– 0.5%	0.3%
Metamyelocytes ("juvenile" forms)	13.0–32.0%	22.0%
Polymorphonuclear neutrophils	7.0–30.0%	20.0%
Polymorphonuclear eosinophils	0.5– 4.0%	2.0%
Polymorphonuclear basophils	0.0– 0.7%	0.2%
Lymphocytes	3.0–17.0%	10.0%
Plasma cells	0.0– 2.0%	0.4%
Monocytes	0.5– 5.0%	2.0%
Reticulum cells	0.1– 2.0%	0.2%
Megakaryocytes	0.03– 3.0%	0.4%
Pronormoblasts	1.0– 8.0%	4.0%
Normoblasts	7.0–32.0%	18.0%

NORMAL BLOOD, PLASMA, AND SERUM VALUES

For some procedures the normal values may vary depending upon the methods used.

Acetone, serum	
Qualitative	Negative
Quantitative	0.3–2.0 mg/100 ml
Aldolase, serum	0.8–3.0 milliunits/ml (IU) (30°) (Sibley-Lehninger)
Alpha amino nitrogen	4–6 mg/100 ml
Ammonia nitrogen, blood	75–196 μg/100 ml
plasma	56–122 μg/100 ml
Amylase, serum	80–160 Somogyi units/100 ml
Ascorbic acid	See Vitamin C
Base, total, serum	145–160 mEq/liter
Bilirubin, serum	
Direct	0.1–0.4 mg/100 ml
Indirect	0.2–0.7 mg/100 ml
	(Total minus direct)
Total	0.3–1.1 mg/100 ml
Calcium, serum	4.5–5.5 mEq/liter
	(9.0–11.0 mg/100 ml)
	(Slightly higher in children)
	(Varies with protein concentration)

NORMAL BLOOD, PLASMA, AND SERUM VALUES (*Continued*)

Calcium, serum, ionized	2.1–2.6 mEq/liter
	(4.25–5.25 mg/100 ml)
Carbon dioxide content, serum	24–30 mEq/liter
	Infants: 20–28 mEq/liter
Carbon dioxide tension (Pco_2), blood	35–45 mm Hg
Carotene, serum	50–300 μg/100 ml
Ceruloplasmin, serum	23–44 mg/100 ml
Chloride, serum	96–106 mEq/liter
Cholesterol, serum	
Total	150–250 mg/100 ml
Esters	68–76% of total cholesterol
Cholinesterase, serum	0.5–1.3 pH units
RBC	0.5–1.0 pH units
Copper, serum	
Male	70–140 μg/100 ml
Female	85–155 μg/100 ml
Cortisol, plasma	6–16 μg/100 ml
Creatine, serum	0.2–0.8 mg/100 ml
Creatine phosphokinase, serum	
Male	0–50 milliunits/ml (IU) (30°)
Female	0–30 milliunits/ml (IU) (30°) (Oliver-Rosalki)
Creatinine, serum	0.7–1.5 mg/100 ml
Cryoglobulins, serum	0
Fatty acids, total, serum	190–420 mg/100 ml
Fibrinogen, plasma	200–400 mg/100 ml
Folic acid, serum	7–16 nanogm/ml
Glucose (fasting)	
blood, true	60–100 mg/100 ml
Folin	80–120 mg/100 ml
plasma or serum, true	70–115 mg/100 ml
Haptoglobin, serum	40–170 mg/100 ml
Hydroxybutyric dehydrogenase, serum	0–180 milliunits/ml (IU) (30°) (Rosalki-Wilkinson)
	114–290 units/ml (Wroblewski)
17-Hydroxycorticosteroids, plasma	8–18 μg/100 ml
Immunoglobulins, serum	
IgG	800–1500 mg/100 ml
IgA	50–200 mg/100 ml
IgM	40–120 mg/100 ml
Iodine, butanol extractable, serum	3.2–6.4 μg/100 ml
Iodine, protein bound, serum	3.5–8.0 μg/100 ml
	(May be slightly higher in infants)
Iron, serum	75–175 μg/100 ml
Iron binding capacity, total serum	250–410 μg/100 ml
% saturation	20–55%
17-Ketosteroids, plasma	25–125 μg/100 ml
Lactic acid, blood	6–16 mg/100 ml
Lactic dehydrogenase, serum	0–300 milliunits/ml (IU) (30°) (Wroblewski modified)
	150–450 units/ml (Wroblewski)
	80–120 units/ml (Wacker)
Lipase, serum	0–1.5 units (Cherry-Crandall)
Lipids, total, serum	450–850 mg/100 ml
Magnesium, serum	1.5–2.5 mEq/liter
	(1.8–3.0 mg/100 ml)
Nitrogen, nonprotein, serum	15–35 mg/100 ml
Osmolality, serum	285–295 mOsm/kg serum water
Oxygen, blood	
Capacity	16–24 vol % (varies with Hb)
Content Arterial	15–23 vol %
Venous	10–16 vol %
Saturation Arterial	94–100% of capacity
Venous	60–85% of capacity
Tension, Po_2 Arterial	75–100 mm Hg

NORMAL BLOOD, PLASMA, AND SERUM VALUES (*Continued*)

pH, arterial, blood	7.35–7.45
Phenylalanine, serum	Less than 3 mg/100 ml
Phosphatase, acid, serum	1.0–5.0 units (King-Armstrong)
	0.5–2.0 units (Bodansky)
	0.5–2.0 units (Gutman)
	0.0–1.1 units (Shinowara)
	0.1–0.63 unit (Bessey-Lowry)
Phosphatase, alkaline, serum	5.0–13.0 units (King-Armstrong)
	2.0–4.5 units (Bodansky)
	3.0–10.0 units (Gutman)
	2.2–8.6 units (Shinowara)
	0.8–2.3 units (Bessey-Lowry)
	30–85 milliunits/ml (IU)
	(Values are higher in children)
Phosphorus, inorganic, serum	3.0–4.5 mg/100 ml
	(Children: 4.0–7.0 mg/100 ml)
Phospholipids, serum	6–12 mg/100 ml as lipid phosphorus
Potassium, serum	3.5–5.0 mEq/liter
Proteins, serum	
Total	6.0–8.0 grams/100 ml
Albumin	3.5–5.5 grams/100 ml
Globulin	2.5–3.5 grams/100 ml
Electrophoresis	
Albumin	3.5–5.5 grams/100 ml
	52–68% of total
Globulin	
Alpha$_1$	0.2–0.4 gram/100 ml
	2–5% of total
Alpha$_2$	0.5–0.9 gram/100 ml
	7–14% of total
Beta	0.6–1.1 grams/100 ml
	9–15% of total
Gamma	0.7–1.7 grams/100 ml
	11–21% of total
Pyruvic acid, plasma	1.0–2.0 mg/100 ml
Serotonin, platelet suspension	0.1–0.3 μg/ml blood
serum	0.10–0.32 μg/ml
Sodium, serum	136–145 mEq/liter
Sulfates, inorganic, serum	0.8–1.2 mg/100 ml (as S)
Thyroxine, serum	4.4–9.9 μg/100 ml
Thyroxine, free, serum	1.0–2.1 nanogm/100 ml
Thyroxine binding globulin (TBG), serum	10–26 μg/100 ml
Thyroxine iodine (T$_4$), serum	2.9–6.4 μg/100 ml
Transaminase, serum	
SGOT	0–19 milliunits/ml (IU) (30°) (Karmen modified)
	15–40 units/ml (Karmen)
	18–40 units/ml (Reitman-Frankel)
SGPT	0–17 milliunits/ml (IU) (30°) (Karmen modified)
	6–35 units/ml (Karmen)
	5–35 units/ml (Reitman-Frankel)
Triglycerides, serum	0–150 mg/100 ml
Urea, blood	21–43 mg/100 ml
plasma or serum	24–49 mg/100 ml
Urea nitrogen, blood (BUN)	10–20 mg/100 ml
plasma or serum	11–23 mg/100 ml
Uric acid, serum	
Male	2.5–8.0 mg/100 ml
Female	1.5–6.0 mg/100 ml
Vitamin A, serum	20–80 μg/100 ml
Vitamin B$_{12}$, serum	200–800 picogm/ml
Vitamin C, blood	0.4–1.5 mg/100 ml

NORMAL URINE VALUES

Acetone and acetoacetate	0
Alcapton bodies	Negative
Aldosterone	3–20 μg/24 hrs.
Alpha amino nitrogen	50–200 mg/24 hrs
	(Not over 1.5% of total nitrogen)
Ammonia nitrogen	20–70 mEq/24 hrs
Amylase	35–260 Somogyi units/hr
Bence Jones protein	Negative
Bilirubin (bile)	Negative
Calcium	
Low Ca diet (Bauer-Aub)	Less than 150 mg/24 hrs
Usual diet	Less than 250 mg/24 hrs
Catecholamines	
Epinephrine	Less than 10 μg/24 hrs
Norepinephrine	Less than 100 μg/24 hrs
Chloride	110–250 mEq/24 hrs
	(Varies with intake)
Chorionic gonadotrophin	0
Copper	0–30 μg/24 hrs
Creatine	
Male	0–40 mg/24 hrs
Female	0–100 mg/24 hrs
	(Higher in children and during pregnancy)
Creatinine	15–25 mg/kg of body weight/24 hrs
Cystine or cysteine, qualitative	Negative
Delta aminolevulinic acid	1.3–7.0 mg/24 hrs

Estrogens	Male	Female
Estrone	3–8	4–31
Estradiol	0–6	0–14
Estriol	1–11	0–72
Total	4–25	5–100

(Units above are μg/24 hrs)
(Markedly increased during pregnancy)

Glucose (reducing substances)	Less than 250 mg/24 hrs
Gonadotrophins, pituitary	5–10 rat units/24 hrs
	10–50 mouse units/24 hrs
	(Increased after menopause)
Hemoglobin and myoglobin	Negative
Homogentisic acid, qualitative	Negative
17-Hydroxycorticosteroids	
Male	3–9 mg/24 hrs
Female	2–8 mg/24 hrs
	(Varies with method used)
5-Hydroxyindole-acetic acid (5-HIAA)	
Qualitative	Negative
Quantitative	Less than 16 mg/24 hrs
17-Ketosteroids	
Male	6–18 mg/24 hrs
Female	4–13 mg/24 hrs
Osmolality	38–1400 mOsm/kg water
pH	4.6–8.0, average 6.0
	(Depends on diet)
Phenylpyruvic acid, qualitative	Negative
Phosphorus	0.9–1.3 gm/24 hrs
	(Varies with intake)
Porphobilinogen	
Qualitative	Negative
Quantitative	0–0.2 mg/100 ml
	Less than 2.0 mg/24 hrs
Porphyrins	
Coproporphyrin	50–250 μg/24 hrs
Uroporphyrin	10–30 μg/24 hrs

NORMAL URINE VALUES (*Continued*)

Potassium	25–100 mEq/24 hrs (Varies with intake)
Pregnanetriol	Less than 2.5 mg/24 hrs in adults
Protein	
Qualitative	0
Quantitative	10–150 mg/24 hrs
Sodium	130–260 mEq/24 hrs (Varies with intake)

Solids, total	30–70 grams/liter, average 50 grams/liter
	(To estimate total solids per liter, multiply
	    last two figures of specific gravity by 2.66,
	    Long's coefficient)

Specific gravity	1.003–1.030
Sugar	0
Titratable acidity	20–40 mEq/24 hrs
Urobilinogen	Up to 1.0 Ehrlich unit/2 hrs (1–3 P.M.) 0–4.0 mg/24 hrs
Vanillylmandelic acid (VMA)	1–8 mg/24 hrs

NORMAL VALUES FOR GASTRIC ANALYSIS

Basal gastric secretion (one hour)

	Concentration Mean ± 1 S.D.	Output Mean ± 1 S.D.
Male	25.8 ± 1.8 mEq/liter	2.57 ± 0.16 mEq/hr
Female	20.3 ± 3.0 mEq/liter	1.61 ± 0.18 mEq/hr

After histamine stimulation

Normal	Mean output = 11.8 mEq/hr
Duodenal ulcer	Mean output = 15.2 mEq/hr

After maximal histamine stimulation

Normal	Mean output 22.6 mEq/hr
Duodenal ulcer	Mean output 44.6 mEq/hr

Diagnex blue (Squibb):	Anacidity	0–0.3 mg in 2 hrs
	Doubtful	0.3–0.6 mg in 2 hrs
	Normal	Greater than 0.6 mg in 2 hrs

Volume, fasting stomach content	50–100 ml
Emptying time	3–6 hrs
Color	Opalescent or colorless
Specific gravity	1.006–1.009
pH (adults)	0.9–1.5

NORMAL VALUES FOR CEREBROSPINAL FLUID

Cells	Fewer than 5 cu mm, all mononuclear
Chloride	120–130 mEq/liter (20 mEq/liter higher than serum)
Colloidal gold test	Not more than 1 in any tube
Glucose	50–75 mg/100 ml (20 mg/100 ml less than blood)
Pressure	70–180 mm water
Protein, total	15–45 mg/100 ml
Albumin	52%
Alpha$_1$ globulin	5%
Alpha$_2$ globulin	14%
Beta globulin	10%
Gamma globulin	19%

NORMAL VALUES FOR SEMEN

Volume	2–5 ml, usually 3–4 ml
Liquefaction	Complete in 15 min
pH	7.2–8.0; average 7.8
Leukocytes	Occasional or absent
Count	60–150 million/ml
	Below 60 million/ml is abnormal
Motility	80% or more motile
Morphology	80–90% normal forms

NORMAL VALUES FOR FECES

Bulk	100–200 grams/24 hrs
Dry matter	23–32 grams/24 hrs
Fat, total	Less than 6.0 grams/24 hrs
Nitrogen, total	Less than 2.0 grams/24 hrs
Urobilinogen	40–280 mg/24 hrs
Water	Approximately 65%

TOXICOLOGY

Arsenic, blood	3.5–7.2 μg/100 ml
Arsenic, urine	Less than 100 μg/24 hrs
Barbiturates, serum	0
	Coma level: Phenobarbital approximately 11 mg/100 ml; most other barbiturates 1.5 mg/100 ml
Bromides, serum	0
	Toxic levels above 17 mEq/liter
Carbon monoxide, blood	Up to 5% saturation
	Symptoms occur with 20% saturation
Dilantin, blood or serum	Therapeutic levels 1–11 μg/ml
Ethanol, blood	Less than 0.005%
Marked intoxication	0.3–0.4%
Alcoholic stupor	0.4–0.5%
Coma	Above 0.5%
Lead, blood	0–40 μg/100 ml
Lead, urine	Less than 100 μg/24 hrs
Lithium, serum	0
	Therapeutic levels 0.5–1.5 mEq/liter
	Toxic levels above 2 mEq/liter
Mercury, urine	Less than 10 μg/24 hrs
Salicylate, plasma	0
Therapeutic range	20–25 mg/100 ml
Toxic	Over 30 mg/100 ml
Death	45–75 mg/100 ml

LIVER FUNCTION TESTS

Bromsulphalein (B.S.P.)	Less than 5% remaining in serum 45 minutes after injection of 5 mg/kg of body weight
Cephalin cholesterol flocculation	0–1 in 24 hours
Galactose tolerance	Excretion of not more than 3.0 grams galactose in the urine 5 hours after ingestion of 40 grams of galactose
Glycogen storage	Increase of blood glucose 45 mg/100 ml over fasting level 45 minutes after subcutaneous injection of 0.01 mg/kg body weight of epinephrine
Hippuric acid	Excretion of 3.0–3.5 grams hippuric acid in urine within 4 hours after ingestion of 6.0 grams sodium benzoate

or

Excretion of 0.7 gram hippuric acid in urine within 1 hour after intravenous injection of 1.77 grams sodium benzoate

Thymol turbidity	0–5 units
Zinc turbidity	2–12 units

PANCREATIC (ISLET) FUNCTION TESTS

Glucose tolerance tests	Patient should be on a diet containing 300 grams of carbohydrate per day for 3 days prior to test.
Oral	After ingestion of 100 grams of glucose or 1.75 grams glucose/kg body weight, blood glucose is not more than 160 mg/100 ml after 60 minutes, 140 mg/100 ml after 90 minutes, and 120 mg/100 ml after 120 minutes. Values are for blood; serum measurements are approximately 15% higher.
Intravenous	Blood glucose does not exceed 200 mg/100 ml after infusion of 0.5 gram of glucose/kg body weight over 30 minutes. Glucose concentration falls below initial level at 2 hours and returns to preinfusion levels in 3 or 4 hours. Values are for blood; serum measurements are approximately 15% higher.
Cortisone-glucose tolerance test	The patient should be on a diet containing 300 grams of carbohydrate per day for 3 days prior to test. At 8½ and again 2 hours prior to glucose load patient is given cortisone acetate by mouth (50 mg if patient's ideal weight is less than 160 lb, 62.5 mg if ideal weight is greater than 160 lb). An oral dose of glucose, 1.75 grams/kg body weight, is given and blood samples are taken at 0, 30, 60, 90, and 120 minutes. Test is considered positive if true blood glucose exceeds 160 mg/100 ml at 60 minutes, 140 mg/100 ml at 90 minutes, and 120 mg/100 ml at 120 minutes. Values are for blood; serum measurements are approximately 15% higher.

RENAL FUNCTION TESTS

Clearance tests (corrected to 1.73 sq meters body surface area)

Glomerular filtration rate (G.F.R.)

Inulin clearance, Mannitol clearance, or Endogenous creatinine clearance
- Males 110–150 ml/min
- Females 105–132 ml/min

Renal plasma flow (R.P.F.)

p-Aminohippurate (P.A.H.), or Diodrast
- Males 560–830 ml/min
- Females 490–700 ml/min

Filtration fraction (F.F.)

$$FF = \frac{G.F.R.}{R.P.F.}$$
- Males 17–21%
- Females 17–23%

Urea clearance (C_u)
- Standard 40–65 ml/min
- Maximal 60–100 ml/min

Concentration and dilution
- Specific gravity >1.025 on dry day
- Specific gravity <1.003 on water day

Maximal Diodrast excretory capacity T_{M_D}
- Males 43–59 mg/min
- Females 33–51 mg/min

Maximal glucose reabsorptive capacity T_{M_G}
- Males 300–450 mg/min
- Females 250–350 mg/min

Maximal PAH excretory capacity $T_{M_{PAH}}$
- 80–90 mg/min

Phenolsulfonphthalein excretion (P.S.P.)
- 25% or more in 15 min
- 40% or more in 30 min
- 55% or more in 2 hrs
- After injection of 1 ml P.S.P. intravenously

THYROID FUNCTION TESTS

Protein bound iodine, serum (P.B.I.)	3.5–8.0 μg/100 ml
Butanol extractable iodine, serum (B.E.I.)	3.2–6.4 μg/100 ml
Thyroxine iodine, serum (T_4)	2.9–6.4 μg/100 ml
Free thyroxine, serum	1.4–2.5 nanogm/100 ml
T_3 (index of unsaturated T.B.G.)	10.0–14.6%
Thyroxine-binding globulin, serum (T.B.G.)	10–26 μg T_4/100 ml
Thyroid-stimulating hormone, serum (T.S.H.)	0 up to 0.2 milliunit/ml
Radioactive iodine (I^{131}) uptake (R.A.I.)	20–50% of administered dose in 24 hrs
Radioactive iodine (I^{131}) excretion	30–70% of administered dose in 24 hrs
Radioactive iodine (I^{131}), protein bound	Less than 0.3% of administered dose per liter of plasma at 72 hrs
Basal metabolic rate	Minus 10% to plus 10% of mean standard

GASTROINTESTINAL ABSORPTION TESTS

d-Xylose absorption test	After an 8 hour fast 10 ml/kg body weight of a 5% solution of d-xylose is given by mouth. Nothing further by mouth is given until the test has been completed. All urine voided during the following 5 hours is pooled, and blood samples are taken at 0, 60, and 120 minutes. Normally 26% (range 16–33%) of ingested xylose is excreted within 5 hours, and the serum xylose reaches a level between 25 and 40 mg/100 ml after 1 hour and is maintained at this level for another 60 minutes.
Vitamin A absorption test	A fasting blood specimen is obtained and 200,000 units of vitamin A in oil is given by mouth. Serum vitamin A level should rise to twice fasting level in 3 to 5 hours.

NORMAL VALUES FOR SEROLOGIC PROCEDURES

Anti-hyaluronidase	Less than 1:200. Significant if rising titer can be demonstrated at weekly intervals.	
Anti-streptolysin O titer	Normal up to 1:128. Single test usually has little significance. Rise in titer or persistently elevated titer is significant.	
Bacterial agglutinins	Significant only if rise in titer is demonstrated or if antibodies are absent.	
Complement fixation tests	Titers of 1:8 or less are usually not significant. Paired sera showing rise in titer of more than two tubes are usually considered significant.	
C reactive protein (C.R.P.)	Negative	
Heterophile titer	Low titers may be present normally, but these antibodies are absorbed by Forssman antigen (guinea pig kidney). In infectious mononucleosis an elevated heterophile titer is present. The titer is only minimally reduced after incubation with guinea pig kidney but is significantly reduced after incubation with beef red cell stroma.	
Proteus OX-19 agglutinins	1:80	Negative
	1:160	Doubtful
	1:320	Positive
R.A. test (latex)	1:40	Negative
	1:80–1:160	Doubtful
	1:320	Positive
Rose test	1:10	Negative
	1:20–1:40	Doubtful
	1:80	Positive
Tularemia agglutinins	1:80	Negative
	1:160	Doubtful
	1:320	Positive

Castleman, B., and McNeely, B. U.: N. Engl. J. Med., 290:39, 1974.
Davidsohn, I., and Henry, J. B.: Clinical Diagnosis by Laboratory Methods. 15th ed. Philadelphia, W. B. Saunders Company, 1974.
Department of Laboratory Medicine, The Johns Hopkins Hospital: Clinical Laboratory Handbook, Baltimore, July 1, 1974.
Henry, R. J.: Clinical Chemistry–Principles and Techniques. New York, Harper & Row, 1964.
Long, C.: Biochemists' Handbook. Princeton, D. Van Nostrand Company, 1961.
Miale, J. B.: Laboratory Medicine–Hematology. 4th ed. St. Louis, C. V. Mosby Company, 1972.
Miller, S. E., and Weller, J. M.: Textbook of Clinical Pathology. 8th ed. Baltimore, Williams and Wilkins Company, 1971.
Stewart, C. P., and Stolman, A.: Toxicology, Mechanisms and Analytic Methods. New York, Academic Press, 1960.
Sunderman, F. W., and Boerner, F.: Normal Values in Clinical Medicine. Philadelphia, W. B. Saunders Company, 1949.
Tietz, N. W.: Fundamentals of Clinical Chemistry. 2nd ed. Philadelphia, W. B. Saunders Company, 1975.
Wintrobe, M. M.: Clinical Hematology. 6th ed. Philadelphia, Lea & Febiger, 1967.

Index

Note: In this index the expression "vs." has been used to denote "differential diagnosis." Thus "Addison's disease, vs. acanthosis nigricans" is the equivalent of "Addison's disease, differential diagnosis from acanthosis nigricans." **Boldface entries and folios** in the index indicate main discussions in the text. *Italic folios* indicate illustrations and tables.

Abdomen
actinomycosis of, 387
acute, 1274–1277
distention of, in pneumococcal pneumonia, 282, 285
pain in, in acute appendicitis, 1274
in hepatic disease, 1332
in irritable colon, 1189
in Zollinger-Ellison syndrome, 1209
pyogenic infections of, enteric bacteria in, 369
surgery of, air travel after, 74
symptoms in, in dissecting aneurysm, 1062
Abdominal angina, 1284
Abdominal lymphoma, Mediterranean-type, 1548
Abducens nerve, disorders of, 782
Abetalipoproteinemia, *24,* **765,** 1233, **1635**
Abortion, septic, hypofibrinogenemia in, 1575
Abscess(es)
anorectal, 1307
appendiceal, vs. regional enteritis, 1261
at sites of subcutaneous injections, 369
brain, 672–674
amebic, 498
cerebrospinal fluid in, *670*
enteric bacteria causing, 369
epilepsy associated with, 724
in head injury, 755
presenting as "acute meningitis," 674
vs. cerebral infarction, 659
vs. herpes simplex encephalitis, 693
vs. intracranial tumor, 740
vs. subdural empyema, 675
vs. viral encephalitis, 690
vs. viral meningitis, 690
Brodie's, 1838
Candida, 454
cerebellar, 674
cerebral, 672–674. See also *Abscess(es), brain.*
cerebral epidural, 675
cerebrospinal fluid in, *670*
frontal lobe, 674
gas, 348
in staphylococcal infection, 318
injection, "atypical" mycobacteria causing, 412
ischiorectal fossa, 1307
liver, acute, 1342–1343
amebic, 497, 498, 499
lung, 845–847
air travel and, 74
cavitary, vs. pulmonary tuberculosis, 399
metastatic, 845
vs. pulmonary paragonimiasis, 521
myocardial, in acute infective endocarditis, 312
paravertebral, in staphylococcal osteomyelitis, 322

Abscess(es) (*Continued*)
parietal lobe, 674
pelvic, tuberculous, 404
pelvirectal, 1307
perianal, 1307
perinephric, 1145
perirectal, enteric bacteria causing, 369
tuberculous, 404
peritonsillar, in streptococcal pharyngitis, 296
skin, in heroin addiction, 589
spinal epidural, 677, 678
cerebrospinal fluid in, *670*
primary, 324
vs. transverse myelitis, 679
splenic, 1553
subdiaphragmatic, pleural involvement in, 877
submucous, 1307
subphrenic, 1288
temporal lobe, 673
"Welch," 348
Absense attack, 726
Absorption, gastrointestinal
normal mechanisms of, 1217–1220
tests of, 1892
Absorption atelectasis, 843
Abstinence syndrome
in alcohol abuse, 566, 600, 601
in central nervous system depressant abuse, 591
in opiate abuse, 588
in sedative abuse, 604
Acalculia, 556
Acalculous cholecystitis, 1313
Acanthamoeba castellani, 502
Acanthocytosis, 765, 1233
Acanthosis nigricans, 1856–1857
in internal malignancy, *1803,* 1847
Acarina, infections carried by, 94
Acatalasia, *25,* **1865**
Accelerated idioventricular rhythms, 1032–1033, *1033*
Accidental poisoning, common, 52–57
Acervuli, 1702
Acetaminophen
as analgesic, 608, *609*
as aspirin substitute in classic hemophilia, 1568
liver injury caused by, 1344
Acetazolamide
in acute mountain sickness, 79
in chronic airway obstruction, 834
in epilepsy, *731,* 732
in familial periodic paralysis, 799
in heart failure, *899,* 900
in renal cysts, 1170
metabolic acidosis after, 1592
Acetohexamide, in diabetes mellitus, 1615, *1615*

Acetophenetidin, as analgesic, *609*
Acetylcholine, in regulation of gastric secretion, 1201
Acetylsalicylic acid. See *Aspirin.*
Acetylstrophanthidin, as diagnostic test for adequacy of digitalization, 894
Achalasia, *1180,* **1181–1182,** *1181*
esophageal carcinoma and, 1182, 1291, 1292
Achondroplasia, 1840–1841
genetic counseling in, 37
Acid(s). See names of specific acids.
Acid-base balance, disturbances of, 1579, 1589–1599
Acidemia, isovaleric, *23*
Acidophilic adenoma, acromegaly and, 1689, 1696
Acidosis
hyperchloremic, in chronic renal failure, 1095
in total parenteral nutrition, 1393
lactic, in gram-negative bacteremia, 370
in septic shock, 905
metabolic acidosis from, 1591, 1593
metabolic, 1590–1594
causes of, *1590*
in delirium, *549*
in hyperparathyroidism, 1811
in respiratory failure, 837
vs. asthma, 828
renal, 1591, 1594
in chronic renal failure, 1098
renal tubular, *25,* **1152–1153**
in chronic renal failure, 1099
respiratory, 1590, 1596–1598
in delirium, *549*
in respiratory failure, 837
Aciduria
argininosuccinic, *23, 1641,* 1644
dietary restriction in, 36
beta-aminoisobutyric, *1642, 1645,* 1661
beta-hydroxyisovaleric, *23*
L-glyceric, 1629
glycolic, 1628
methylmalonic, *23*
orotic, *24,* 1661
prevention and management of, 37
xanthurenic, *24*
Acinar cells, dysfunction of, in chronic pancreatitis, 1250
Acinar emphysema, focal proximal, 857
Acne vulgaris, pustular, 320
Acoustic neuroma, 739
Acoustic trauma, hearing loss in, 621
Acro-asphyxia, 1077
Acrocyanosis, 1077–1078
in internal malignancy, 1847
vs. ergotism and methysergide toxicity, 1078
Acrodynia, 61, 1161

i